Orthognathic Surgery

Orthognathic Surgery

Principles, Planning and Practice

Edited by

Farhad B. Naini

BDS (Lond.), MSc (Lond.), PhD (KCL), FDS.RCS (Eng.), M.Orth.RCS (Eng.),

FDS.Orth.RCS (Eng.), GCAP (KCL), FHEA

Consultant Orthodontist
Kingston Hospital and St George's Hospital and Medical School
London, UK

Daljit S. Gill

BDS (Hons), BSc (Hons), MSc (Lond.), FDS.RCS (Eng.),

M.Orth.RCS (Eng.), FDS (Orth) RCS (Eng.), FHEA

Consultant Orthodontist
Great Ormond Street Hospital NHS Foundation Trust and UCLH Eastman Dental Hospital
London, UK

WILEY Blackwell

Registered office:
John Wiley & Sons, Ltd, The Atrium, Southern Gate, Chichester, West Sussex, PO19 8SQ, UK

Editorial offices:
9600 Garsington Road, Oxford, OX4 2DQ, UK
The Atrium, Southern Gate, Chichester, West Sussex, PO19 8SQ, UK
1606 Golden Aspen Drive, Suites 103 and 104, Ames, Iowa 50010, USA

For details of our global editorial offices, for customer services and for information about how to apply for permission to reuse the copyright material in this book please see our website at www.wiley.com/wiley-blackwell

Library of Congress Cataloging-in-Publication Data applied for.

9781118649978 (Hardback)

A catalogue record for this book is available from the British Library.

Wiley also publishes its books in a variety of electronic formats. Some content that appears in print may not be available in electronic books.

Set in 9.5/12pt PalatinoLTStd by Aptara Inc., New Delhi, India

1 2017

Dedication

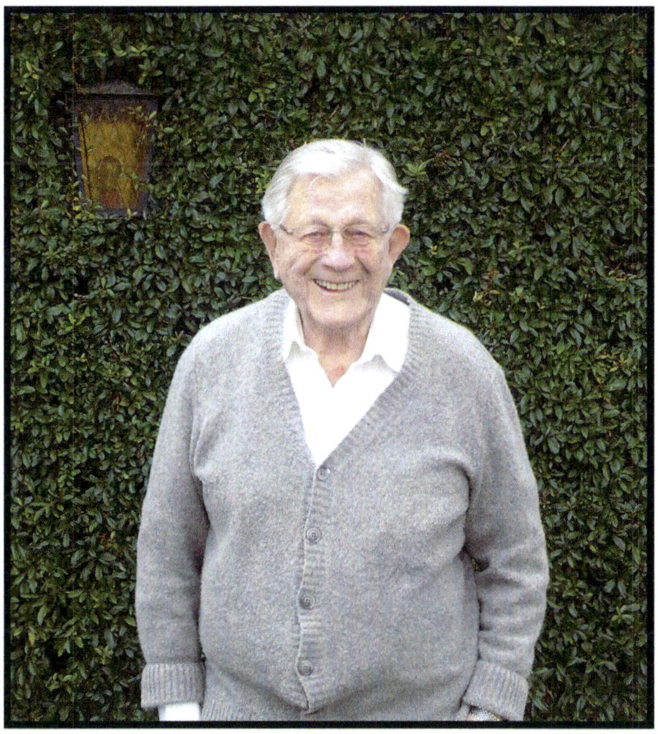

Hugo L. Obwegeser

MD, DMD, FDS.RCS (Eng.), Hon. FRCS (Eng.), Hon. FDS.RCPS (Glas.), Hon. FFD.RCS (Ire.)
Emeritus Professor of Oral Diagnosis and Oral Surgery, Dental School, and Director of the Department of Cranio-Maxillofacial Surgery, University Hospital, Zürich, Switzerland
Pioneer of Maxillofacial and Reconstructive Surgery of the Facial Skeleton and father of modern Orthognathic Surgery

Contents

Foreword

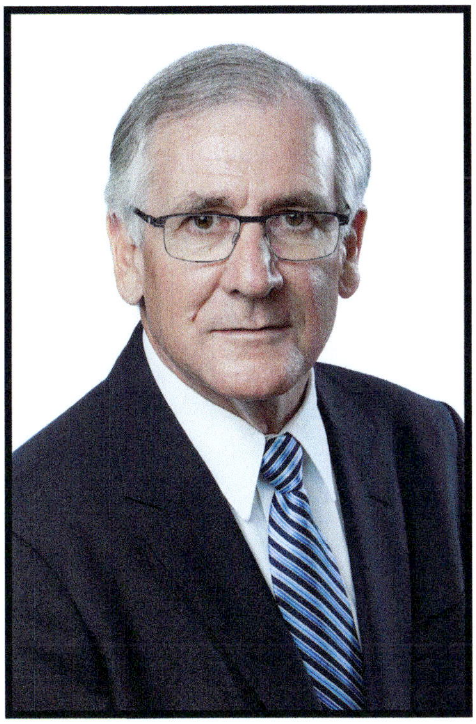

Auguste Comte (1798–1857) said: *'One does not know a science completely without knowing its history.'* It is, therefore, appropriate that this book is dedicated to Professor Hugo Obwegeser and introduced by him in a most informative and delightful contribution – 'A Life's Work.'

History has provided us with several great clinicians, 'giants' in their own right, on whose shoulders we could stand. This comprehensive book on modern orthognathic surgery edited (and authored) by Farhad B. Naini and Daljit S. Gill, is proof of the sound foundation laid by 'giants' and the subsequent development of the science by succeeding generations of clinicians.

Several factors distinguish surgical orthodontic correction of dentofacial deformities from most clinical treatment approaches:

Firstly, the diagnosis, treatment planning and correction of dentofacial deformities requires the expertise of several specialized clinicians. In this respect, the key players are the Orthodontist and the Maxillofacial surgeon, while the expertise of the Periodontist, Prosthodontist, general dental practitioner, and medical practitioner may be required in some cases.

Secondly, the treatment goals in orthognathic surgery are multifactorial. The major factors that should be considered when planning treatment are: improving facial aesthetics, the establishment of a functional occlusion, maintaining or increasing the airway space, the establishment and/or maintenance of periodontal health, healthy temporomandibular joints and, certainly, resolving the patient's main complaints.

Thirdly, there are very few treatments in the medical and dental fields that can provide such accuracy in planning and predictability of treatment outcomes before commencement of treatment.

Finally, according to a well-known proverb, 'a sorrow shared is halved while a pleasure shared is doubled.' Successful orthognathic treatment outcomes can be shared and enjoyed equally by the surgeon, the orthodontist and, most importantly, the patient. The fact that the functional and aesthetic changes that follow orthognathic surgery are in most cases life changing allows the patient to appreciate the aesthetic and functional changes and share the pleasure with their families and friends, which is unique in respect of the correction of dentofacial deformities.

In the text, the editors have assembled an extremely talented and knowledgeable group of authors from a variety of specialties and have addressed a wide range of topics from basic diagnosis and treatment planning to the treatment of complex cases. The book is clearly a culmination of passion and exceptional hard work and offers current and scientific orthognathic treatment approaches.

A sound scientific approach, experience, and effective and efficient technical craft will all come together to make the treatment of patients occur smoothly and successfully. Orthognathic surgery, however, also demands an artistic approach as well as an imagination. Armand Trousseau (1801–1867), a French surgeon, told his students:

'Medicine consists of science and art in a certain relationship to each other, yet wholly distinct. Science can be learned by anyone, even the mediocre. Art, however, is a gift from heaven. So you cannot count yourselves amongst the great doctors by simply acquiring knowledge. Knowledge ... gives the artist fresh inspiration. Therefore, learn as much as you can ... but your learning must be the basis for your art, not an end to itself. A little less science and a little more art, Messieurs!'

Albert Einstein's (1879–1955) view of the importance of an imagination is equally interesting:

> *'Imagination is more important than knowledge. For knowledge is limited to all we know now and understand, while imagination embraces the entire world, and all there ever will be to know and understand.'*

Orthognathic surgery is a science and an art. This landmark publication will not only serve as an important scientific reference and guide to many clinicians, but also as an inspiration to develop the art and imagination required to treat patients with dentofacial deformities successfully. I believe that this reference text will find its way onto the bookshelf of every clinician interested in the management of patients with dentofacial deformities.

Johan P. Reyneke
BChD, MChD, FCOMFS(SA), PhD
July, 2016

Preface

'Aesthetics and Function in Harmony'

Orthognathic surgery holds a unique position within medicine and surgery. Firstly, it is a subspecialty of two distinct surgical specialties: Oral and Maxillofacial Surgery and Orthodontics. Secondly, orthognathic surgical treatment, from the intricate details of diagnosis and treatment planning through to the finesse of surgical technique, requires the perfect blend of art and science. Finally, unlike many other parts of medicine and surgery, patients do not just 'need' such treatment; they also 'desire' the treatment, and the combined functional and aesthetic improvements may be, quite literally, life-changing for the orthognathic patient.

> 'It is astonishing with how little reading a doctor can practice medicine, but it is not astonishing how badly he may do it.'
>
> Sir William Osler (1849–1919)

The fundamental purpose of this book is to provide clinicians with comprehensive information regarding diagnosis and treatment planning, and detailed, up-to-date, step-by-step descriptions of the specific operative techniques in orthognathic surgery and relevant procedures from allied specialties.

There is some 'method' in the arrangement of the book. Considerable thought was given to the order of the chapters, which have been grouped into themed sections. This format should provide a logical sequence to the reader. Attempts have been made to reduce repetition, other than where a similar procedure has been described with certain nuances of technique, which readers may find useful. Any clinician faced with a difficult situation will always benefit from knowledge of several methods to deal with the problem at hand.

The first chapter is a special introduction by Professor Hugo Obwegeser, the leading pioneer of orthognathic surgery. It is a pleasure to dedicate this textbook to Professor Obwegeser. Countless patients owe him the possibility to lead a normal life, and many surgeons owe him success and satisfaction in their profession. The photograph of Professor Obwegeser at the beginning of the book was taken by Hengameh Naini, in the Obwegesers' garden in Schwerzenbach, Switzerland. Professor Obwegeser asked if we didn't mind if he didn't wear a suit and tie. He wanted to be shown as himself, 'not all dressed up.' 'I was raised on a farm, and that is still where my heart lies.' Professor Obwegeser expressed his enthusiasm for this book, and his desire 'to hold the book in his hands.' The editors hope that he is pleased with the result.

The rest of the book is separated into two parts. A house cannot be built on sand – a firm foundation is required. Therefore the chapters in Part I (Principles and Planning) cover the fundamental principles, background considerations and essential information that should be firmly grasped by the orthognathic clinician. Part II (Clinical Practice and Techniques) is separated into four sections. Section 1 covers Orthognathic surgical planning and techniques; Section 2 covers Adjunctive surgery; Section 3 covers Orthognathic surgery in the cleft patient and orthognathic aspects of craniofacial surgery; and finally Section 4 has two chapters that will provide useful 'food for thought' for the orthognathic clinician.

Many of the authors invited to contribute chapters to this book are *the* internationally renowned leaders in their field, and all have established reputations in their respective sphere of interest. The list of contributing authors reads like a veritable *Who's Who* of the masters of Orthognathic Surgery and allied specialties. The contributing authors remit was to provide chapters that were comprehensive and practical, to analyse the scientific literature for their chosen subjects, and, more importantly, to augment their chapters with technical knowledge and wisdom gathered from long-term clinical experience and careful scrutiny of their techniques and clinical results, which legitimately deserves to be considered as a vital part of our 'evidence base'. Referencing has been thorough, but selective rather than exhaustive.

The most important part of learning orthognathic surgery remains the apprenticeship – when basic knowledge has been learned, and the higher trainee spends time with an experienced surgeon and orthodontist team. Observing an experienced clinical team with a patient and their family on the clinic or on the ward is invaluable, and teaching surgical technique in the operating theatre is almost invariably a one-to-one experience. To paraphrase a famous Oslerian maxim: *to study [orthognathic surgery] without books it to sail an uncharted sea, while to study books without patients is not to go to sea at all*. To compile and write a comprehensive book chapter on a specialist topic must be a labour of love because the intellectual and emotional effort put into such an endeavour is incalculable. The editors' desire is that the chapters in this book will be used by higher trainees to enhance higher surgical training on diagnostic and treatment planning clinics, on the ward and in the operating theatre.

Throughout the book there is an emphasis on accurate diagnosis and logical treatment planning, as well as the step-by-step description of technical procedures, and the intricacies of surgical technique, detailed in such a way that both the experienced clinician and the higher surgical trainee may understand the technical subtleties.

It may be reasoned that undertaking research educates the researcher more thoroughly than anyone else; by the same token, having had the opportunity to edit manuscripts from the most accomplished individuals in the field of orthognathic surgery, has been of enormous value to us. We sincerely hope that our readers derive as much pleasure and benefit from reading this book as we have from compiling and editing it.

Farhad B. Naini and Daljit S. Gill
March 2016

Acknowledgements

No project of this magnitude is complete without acknowledgements. Individual credits to the museums, libraries, archives and medical journals for permission to reproduce and redraw some of the figures are provided in the respective figure legends throughout the book.

I am very grateful to the following museums, libraries and foundations for their kind help: The Librarians and staff of the Royal Library for their kindness in allowing me to select a number of illustrations from the Leonardo da Vinci drawings in The Royal Collection at Windsor Castle, by Gracious Permission of Her Majesty Queen Elizabeth II. Thank you also to the Freud Museum London (especially Bryony Davies, Assistant Curator), London, UK; Charles Dickens Museum, London, UK; Countway Library of Medicine, Harvard Medical School, Boston, USA; Historical Collections and Archives, Oregon Health and Science University, USA; Casa Buonarroti, Florence, Italy; US National Library of Medicine; and the Blond McIndoe Research Foundation (especially Mrs Jacqui Pinney and Mr Anthony Metcalfe), Queen Victoria Hospital, East Grinstead, Kent, UK.

A number of individuals require special mention. First and foremost, my sincere thanks are due to Professor Johan Reyneke for his enthusiasm for this project from the outset, for providing the Foreword and two superb chapters.

My sincere thanks are due to the late and much missed Mr Raymond Edler (Consultant Orthodontist) and Mr Peter Blenkinsopp (Consultant Oral and Maxillofacial Surgeon - retired). At the age of 23, as a young House Surgeon, it was on their orthognathic clinics at the Norman Rowe Maxillofacial Unit that I first experienced the life-changing results of orthognathic surgery, undertaken at the highest level of expertise.

My thanks to my friend Professor Aron D. Wahrman, Professor of Plastic and Reconstructive Surgery, Temple University, Pennsylvania, whose knowledge of the history of medicine and surgery appears inexhaustible, and to the Robert H. Ivy Society of Plastic Surgeons, for a number of the figures in Chapter 2.

My thanks also to Dr Friedrich Peter Carls, Dr Elif Keser, Professor Paul Thomas, Professor Daniel Hrušák, and Professor Darko Macan for their generous help and kindness, and to Dr Anna Gibilaro and Professor William Proffit for their help in organizing Chapter 18.

Thank you to Lisa Randazzo of Dolphin Imaging for providing a number of figures for Chapter 10, and to Mr Paul Robinson, Consultant Oral and Maxillofacial surgeon (retired) at Guy's Hospital, for helpful advice. Thanks also to my orthodontic colleagues Allan Jones and Lucy Davenport-Jones. My thanks also extend to a number of my former and current trainees, particularly Drs Priti Acharya, Sarah Akram, Georgina Cartwright, Christopher Clayton, Joanne Collins, Leila Khamashta-Ledezma, Paul Mooney, Rachel O'Brien, Sapna Radia, Thushala Ubaya and Sophia Wahla.

My sincere and heartfelt appreciation goes to my Consultant Maxillofacial surgical colleagues, Mehmet Manisali, Helen Witherow, Andrew Stewart and Ashraf Messiha. They are all dear friends, a pleasure to work with, and incredibly talented surgeons. The quality of postoperative results in my chapters is thanks to their dedication and efforts. Special thanks are due to all my patients for the privilege of treating them, and for their permission to use their photographs in this book.

Though impossible to fully express in words, my enduring love and deepest appreciation goes to my parents and brother. I have had the honour to proof read a number of my father's books over the years, and his exploration of the greatest minds of past ages. However, one sentence always remains in my mind - the opening words of wisdom from his book *The Genuine Face of Omar Khayyam* – and that is 'You are what you read.' Finally, to my wife Hengameh - my heart and soul – whose kindness and wisdom are simply wonderful. Hengameh is an animal behaviourist, and her chosen profession is also her deep passion. Yet she made time in her already packed schedule to create the illustrations for my chapters. This book would simply not have been possible without her dedication.

Farhad B. Naini
March 2016

I would like to thank my grandparents and parents for their unfailing help, and thank my wife, Balpreet, and my children, Aran and Anika, for their love and patience.

Daljit S. Gill
March 2016

Our thanks to the staff at Wiley-Blackwell, particularly Jessica Evans, for their enthusiasm for this project; our thanks also to Carolyn Holleyman, and particularly to Shiela Salcedo, Gayle Mak and Shalini Sharma for their invaluable assistance in preparing the final proofs.

We are donating part of the royalties for this book to *Changing Faces*, the leading UK charity that supports and represents people who have disfigurements to the face, hand or body from any cause, thereby complementing medical and surgical interventions by addressing the psychological and social challenges posed by such disfigurements. We are donating the rest of the royalties to animal welfare charities chosen by Hengameh Naini, and support her hope that the human species will eventually look beyond considerations of narrow self-interest and learn to include animals within our sphere of morality.

Farhad B. Naini and Daljit S. Gill
March 2016

Contributors

Keith Altman, MBBS, BDS, FDS.RCS, FRCS (Maxfac)
Consultant Oral and Maxillofacial Surgeon
Department of Oral and Maxillofacial Surgery
Brighton and Sussex University Hospitals NHS Trust
Brighton, UK

Daniel Archer, MBBS, FDS.RCS, FRCS
Consultant Oral and Maxillofacial Surgeon
Head and Neck Unit, Royal Marsden Hospital
Northwick Park/St George's Hospitals
London, UK

Farhad Ardeshirpour, MD
Assistant Professor and Director
Division of Facial Plastic and Reconstructive Surgery
Department of Head and Neck Surgery
Loma Linda University Medical Center
Loma Linda, CA, USA

Mehran Armand, PhD
Senior Scientist/Adjunct Professor
Applied Physics Laboratory/Department of Mechanical Engineering
Faculty of Orthopaedic Surgery, School of Medicine
The Johns Hopkins University
Baltimore, MD, USA

Scott P. Bartlett, MD
Professor of Surgery
Chief of the Division of Plastic Surgery
The Perelman School of Medicine at the University of Pennsylvania
The Children's Hospital of Philadelphia
Philadelphia, PA, USA

Dale S. Bloomquist, DDS, MS
Professor Emeritus of Oral and Maxillofacial Surgery
Department of Oral and Maxillofacial Surgery
School of Dentistry
University of Washington
Seattle, WA, USA

Anne S. Blyth, MBChB, FFARCSI
Consultant Anaesthetist
Department of Anaesthesia
St George's Hospital
London, UK

Vinicius Boen, BSc
Software Engineer
Department of Orthodontics and Pediatric Dentistry
University of Michigan
MI, USA

Jonathan Britto, BSc, MBBS, MD, FRCS, FRCS (Plast.)
Consultant Plastic and Craniofacial Surgeon
Craniofacial Unit
Great Ormond Street Hospital
London, UK

Alexander C. Cash, BDS (Lond.), MSc (Lond.), FDS.RCS (Edin.), M.Orth.RCS (Edin.), M.Orth.RCS (Eng.), FDS.Orth.RCS (Edin.)
Head of Service / Clinical Director / Consultant Orthodontist
South Thames Cleft Service
St. Thomas' Hospital
London, UK

Lucia Cevidanes, DDS, MS, PhD
Assistant Professor
Department of Orthodontics and Pediatric Dentistry
University of Michigan
MI, USA

Robert A.C. Chate, BDS, D.Orth.RCS (Eng.), D.Orth.RCPS (Glasg.), M.Orth.RCS (Eng.), M.Surg Dent.RCS (Ed.), FDS.RCS (Ed.)
Consultant Orthodontist
Essex County Hospital/Colchester University Hospital
Colchester, UK

Alistair R.M. Cobb, MBBS, BDS, FRCS (OMFS), FDS.RCS (Eng), MFSEM (UK)
Consultant Oral and Maxillofacial Surgeon/Honorary Senior Clinical Lecturer
South West UK Cleft Service
Bristol Dental Hospital/University of Bristol
Bristol, UK

Richard Cobb, BDS, MBBS, DHMSA, MFDS (Eng.), MRCS (Eng.)
Specialist Registrar
Department of Oral and Maxillofacial Surgery
Whipps Cross/The Royal London Hospital
Barts Health NHS Trust
London, UK

Martyn T. Cobourne, BDS (Hons), MSc, PhD, FDS.RCS, M.Orth.RCS, FDS.Orth.RCS, FHEA
Professor and Honorary Consultant in Orthodontics
Head of Department of Orthodontics and Craniofacial Development
King's College London
Guy's and St Thomas NHS Foundation Trust
London, UK

Gisela I. Contasti-Bocco, DDS
Assistant Professor
Department of Orthodontics
Nova University
Fort Lauderdale, Florida, USA;
Formerly, Director of the Santa Rosa Orthodontics Center
Orthodontics Department
Dental School
Central University of Venezuela
Caracas, Venezuela

Canice E. Crerand, PhD
Principal Investigator, Center for Biobehavioral Health
The Research Institute at Nationwide Children's Hospital;
Assitant Professor, Department of Pediatrics
The Ohio State University College of Medicine
Columbus, OH, USA

David J. David, AC, MD, MBBS, FRCS, FRACS
Professor of Cranio-Maxillofacial Surgery
University of Adelaide
Head of Australian Craniofacial Unit
Adelaide, Australia

Jelena Devic, MBChB, FRCA
Consultant Anaesthetist
Department of Anaesthesia
St George's Hospital
London, UK

Stephen Dover, BDS, FDSRCS (Eng.), MBChB, FRCS (Eng.)
Consultant Oral, Maxillofacial and Craniofacial Surgeon
University Hospitals Birmingham NHS Trust;
Honorary Senior Lecturer, Faculty of Medicine and Surgery, University of Birmingham;
Consultant Maxillofacial Surgeon, West Midlands Craniofacial Unit, Birmingham Children's Hospital
Birmingham, UK

Peter Doyle, FDS.RCS, FRCS (OMFS)
Consultant Oral and Maxillofacial Surgeon
Department of Oral and Maxillofacial Surgery
Chesterfield Royal Hospital
Chesterfield, UK

Tirbod Fattahi, MD, DDS, FACS
Associate Professor and Chair
Department of Oral and Maxillofacial Surgery
University of Florida College of Medicine
Jacksonville, FL, USA

Carlo Ferretti, BDS, MDent (MFOS), FCD (SA), MFOS
Professor of Oral and Maxillofacial Surgery
Department of Maxillofacial and Oral Surgery
University of Witwatersrand
Johannesburg, South Africa

Joel Ferri, MD, PhD, HDR
Professor, Head and Chairman
Department of Oral and Maxillofacial Surgery
University Hospital of Lille
Lille, France

Umberto Garagiola, DDS, PhD
Professor of Orthodontics
Biomedical Surgical and Dental Department
Maxillo-Facial and Odontostomatology Unit
Fondazione Cà Granda IRCCS Ospedale Maggiore Policlinico
School of Dentistry
University of Milan
Milan, Italy

Daljit S. Gill, BDS (Hons), BSc (Hons), MSc (Lond.), FDS.RCS (Eng.), M.Orth.RCS (Eng.), FDS (Orth.) RCS (Eng.), FHEA
Consultant Orthodontist
Great Ormond Street Hospital NHS Foundation Trust and UCLH Eastman Dental Hospital
London, UK

Brent Golden, MD
Oral and Maxillofacial Surgeon
Department of Oral and Maxillofacial Surgery
University of North Carolina
Chapel Hill, NC, USA

Chad R. Gordon, DO, FACS
Co-Director, Face Transplant Program
Assistant Professor of Plastic and Reconstructive Surgery
Department of Plastic and Reconstructive Surgery
The Johns Hopkins Hospital
Johns Hopkins University School of Medicine
Baltimore, MD, USA

Gerald Grant, DMD
3D Medical Applications Center
Department of Radiology
Walter Reed National Military Medical Center
Bethesda, MD, USA

Cesar A. Guerrero, DDS
Assistant Professor
Division of Oral and Maxillofacial Surgery
Department of Surgery
University of Texas Medical Branch
Galveston, Texas, USA;
Formerly Professor and Director
Santa Rosa Maxillofacial Surgery Center
Oral and Maxillofacial Surgery Department
Dental School
Central University of Venezuela
Caracas, Venezuela

Raquel Guijarro-Martínez, MD, DDS, PhD
Maxillofacial Surgeon
Maxillofacial Institute
Barcelona, Spain

Ben Gurney, MBChB, BDS, FRCS (OMFS)
Senior Registrar in Oral and Maxillofacial Surgery
Maxillofacial Unit
Royal Surrey County Hospital
Guildford, UK

Bahman Guyuron, MD, FACS
Emeritus Professor of Plastic Surgery
Department of Plastic and Reconstructive Surgery
Case Western Reserve University
Cleveland, OH, USA.

Piet Haers, MD, DMD, FDS.RCS, PhD
Professor of Oral and Maxillofacial Surgery
Head of South Thames Cleft Service, Guy's Hospital;
Consultant Oral, Maxillofacial and Cleft Surgeon
Royal Surrey Hospital
Guildford, UK

Andrew Heggie, MBBS (Melb), BDSc (Melb), MDSc (Melb), LDS (Vic), FRACDS, FFD.RCS, FRACDS (OMS), FRCS (Edin.), FICD, FADI, FPFA
Professor and Head of Maxillofacial Surgery
Melbourne Craniofacial Unit
Department of Plastic and Maxillofacial Surgery
Melbourne, VIC, Australia

Manolis Heliotis, BDS, MBChB, MSc, FDS.RCS, FRCS
Consultant Oral and Maxillofacial Surgeon
North West London Regional Maxillofacial Unit
Clinical Director of the Head and Neck Directorate
Northwick Park Hospital
London, UK

Federico Hernández Alfaro, MD, DDS, PhD, FEBOMS
Professor of Maxillofacial Surgery
Head of the Oral Surgery and Maxillofacial Department of the International University of Catalonia;
Maxillofacial Institute
Barcelona, Spain

Christoph Huppa, MD
Consultant Oral and Maxillofacial Surgeon
Department of Oral and Maxillofacial Surgery
King's College Hospital London
London, UK

Shamique Ismail, BDS, FDS.RCS, MSc, M.Orth.RCS, FDS.Orth.RCS
Consultant Orthodontist
Department of Orthodontics
North West London Hospitals NHS Trust
London, UK

Tate Jackson, DDS, MS
Assistant Professor
Department of Orthodontics
University of North Carolina
Chapel Hill, NC, USA

Ronald Jacobson, DDS, MS
Associate Professor (Adjunct)
University of Detroit Mercy School of Dentistry
Attending Orthodontist
Ann and Robert Lurie Children's Hospital
Chicago, IL, USA

Rahul Jayaram, MBBS, BDS (Hons), MDS (OMFS), MFDS.RCS (Edin.), MRCS (Eng.), FRCS (OMFS)
Senior Registrar in Oral and Maxillofacial Surgery
Maxillofacial Unit
St George's Hospital
London, UK

Paul Johnson, BSc, MA, BchD (Hons), MB.Bchir, FDS.RCS, FRCS
Consultant Oral and Maxillofacial Surgeon
Maxillofacial Unit
Royal Surrey Hospital
Guildford, UK

Donald R. Joondeph, DDS, MS
Professor Emeritus of Orthodontics
Department of Orthodontics
School of Dentistry
University of Washington
Seattle, WA, USA

Leonard B. Kaban, DMD, MD, FACS
Chief of Oral and Maxillofacial Surgery
Massachusetts General Hospital
Walter C. Guralnick Distinguished Professor and Head (Retired)
Department of Oral and Maxillofacial Surgery
Harvard School of Dental Medicine
Boston, MA, USA

Leila Khamashta-Ledezma, BDS (Lond), MJDF.RCS (Eng.), MSc (KCL), M.Orth.RCS (Edin.), FDS.Orth.RCS (Edin.), GCAP (KCL), FHEA
Consultant Orthodontist
Department of Orthodontics
Guy's and St Thomas's NHS Foundation Trust
London, UK

Katherine P. Klein, DMD, MS
Specialist Orthodontist and Co-Director of the Orthognathic Surgical Team
Department of Oral and Maxillofacial Surgery
Massachusetts General Hospital and Harvard School of Dental Medicine
Boston, MA, USA

Maarten J. Koudstaal, MD, DMD, PhD
Consultant Maxillofacial Surgeon
Department of Oral and Maxillofacial Surgery
Erasmus University Medical Center, Sophia Children's Hospital
Rotterdam, The Netherlands;
Honorary Consultant
Craniofacial Department
Great Ormond Street Hospital
London, UK;
Research Associate
Boston's Children's Hospital
Boston, MA, USA

Wayne F. Larrabee, MD, MPH
Professor and Head
Department of Otolaryngology – Head and Neck Surgery
University of Washington
Seattle, WA, USA

Gavin Mack, BDS, MSc, MFDS, M.Orth, FDS.Orth.RCS
Consultant Orthodontist
Department of Orthodontics
King's College Hospital London
London, UK

Caitlin Magraw, DDS
Resident, Department of Oral and Maxillofacial Surgery
University of North Carolina
Chapel Hill, NC, USA

Mehmet Manisali, MSc, FFD.RCSI, FRCS (Edin.), FRCS (OMFS)
Consultant Maxillofacial Surgeon
Maxillofacial Unit
St George's Hospital
London, UK

N. Shaun Matthews, BDS, MBBS, FDS.RCS, FRCS (Edin.), FRCS (OMS)
Consultant Oral and Maxillofacial Surgeon
Department of Oral and Maxillofacial Surgery
King's College Hospital London
London, UK

James McInnes, BSc (Hons), MIMPT
Chief Maxillofacial Technologist
Maxillofacial Laboratory Manager
Wexham Park Hospital NHS Foundation Trust
Berkshire, UK

Ashraf Messiha, BDS, MBBCh, BAO, MFDS, MRCS, FRCS, FRCS (OMFS)
Consultant Oral and Maxillofacial Surgeon
Maxillofacial Unit
St George's Hospital
London, UK

Pushkar Mehra, DMD, MS
Professor and Chairman
Department of Oral and Maxillofacial Surgery
Associate Dean for Hospital Affairs
Boston University Henry M. Goldman School of Dental Medicine
Boston, MA, USA

Declan Millett, BDSc, DDS, FDS.RCPS (Glasg.), D.Orth.RCS (Eng.), M.Orth.RCS (Eng.)
Professor and Head
Department of Orthodontics
Cork University Dental School and Hospital
University of Cork
Cork, Ireland

Sima Molavi, MD
Research Fellow
Department of Plastic and Reconstructive Surgery
University Hospitals Case Medical Center
Cleveland, OH, USA

Craig Murakami, MD, FACS
Clinical Professor
Department of Otolaryngology – Head and Neck Surgery
University of Washington
Virginia Mason Medical Center
Seattle, WA, USA

Tania Murphy, BDS, MMedSci (Oral Surg), MFDS.RCS (Edin.), MMedSci (Orth), MOrth, FDS.Orth.RCS (Edin.)
Consultant Orthodontist
Department of Orthodontics
Montagu Hospital
Mexborough, UK

Alison Murray, BDS, MSc, FDS.RCPS, M.Orth.RCS
Consultant Orthodontist
Department of Orthodontics
Royal Derby Hospital
Derby, UK

Foad Nahai, MD, FACS
Professor of Surgery
Division of Plastic and Reconstructive Surgery
Department of Surgery
Emory University School of Medicine
Atlanta, GA, USA

Farhad B. Naini, BDS (Lond.), MSc (Lond.), PhD (KCL), FDS.RCS (Eng.), M.Orth.RCS (Eng.), FDS.Orth.RCS (Eng.), GCAP (KCL), FHEA
Consultant Orthodontist
Maxillofacial Unit
Kingston Hospital and St George's Hospital and Medical School
London, UK

Tung Nguyen, DDS, MS
Associate Professor
Department of Orthodontics
University of North Carolina
NC, USA

Joe Niamtu III, DMD, FAACS
Oral and Maxillofacial Surgeon
Private Practice, Cosmetic Facial Surgery
Richmond, Virginia, USA

Romain Nicot, MD
Fellow of the Department of Oral and Maxillofacial Surgery
University Hospital of Lille
Lille, France

Hugo L. Obwegeser, MD, DMD, FDS.RCS (Eng.), hon. FRCS (Eng.), Hon. FDS.RCPS (Glas.), Hon. FFD.RCS (Ire.)
Emeritus Professor of Oral Diagnosis and Oral Surgery, Dental School;
Director of the Department of Cranio-Maxillofacial Surgery (Retired)
University Hospital
Zürich, Switzerland

Jonas Osher, MFDS, MRCS, FRCS
Consultant Maxillofacial Surgeon
Department of Maxillofacial Surgery
King's College Hospital London
London, UK

Beatriz Paniagua, PhD
Computer Scientist
Department of Psychiatry
University of North Carolina,
NC, USA

Pravin K. Patel, MD, FACS
Professor and Chief of Craniofacial Surgery
The Craniofacial Center
Chicago, IL, USA;
Chief of Pediatric Plastic and Craniofacial Surgery
University of Illinois, Chicago, IL, USA;
Chief of Plastic and Maxillofacial Surgery
Shriners Hospitals for Children, Chicago, IL, USA

Ceib Phillips, MPH, PhD
Professor, Department of Orthodontics
University of North Carolina
Chapel Hill, NC, USA

Katharine A. Phillips, MD
Professor of Psychiatry and Human Behavior
Department of Psychiatry and Human Behavior
Warren Alpert Medical School of Brown University;
Director of Research for Adult Psychiatry
Director, Body Dysmorphic Disorder Program
Rhode Island Hospital
Providence, RI, USA

David S. Precious, DDS, MSc FRCDC, FRCS
Dean Emeritus
Professor of Oral and Maxillofacial Surgery
Dalhousie University
Halifax, Nova Scotia, Canada

Johan P. Reyneke, BChD, MChD, FCMFOS (SA), PhD
Director of the Centre for Orthognathic Surgery
Sunninghill Hospital
Johannesburg, South Africa;
Clinical Professor
Department of Oral and Maxillofacial Surgery
University of Florida College of Dentistry
Gainesville, FL, USA;
Honorary Professor
Department of Maxillofacial and Oral Surgery
University of Witwatersrand
Johannesburg, South Africa

David Rice, BDS, MSc, PhD, FDS, M.Orth, FDS.Orth.RCS
Professor and Head of Orthodontics
Faculty of Medicine
University of Helsinki
Helsinki, Finland

Aura Marina Rodriguez, DDS
Director
La Cascada Orthodontics Center, Los Teques
Orthodontics Department
Dental School
Central University of Venezuela
Caracas, Venezuela

Harvey Rosen, MD, DMD
Chief of the Division of Plastic Surgery
Pennsylvania Hospital;
Clinical Associate Professor of Surgery
University of Pennsylvania School of Medicine
Philadelphia, PA, USA

Jonathan Sandler, BDS (Hons), MSc, PhD, FDS.RCPS, M.Orth.RCS
Consultant Orthodontist
Chesterfield Royal Hospital, UK
Professor of Orthodontics
Sheffield University
Sheffield, UK

Jocelyn M. Shand, MBBS (Melb), MDSc (Melb), BDS (Otago), FDS.RCS (Eng.), FRACDS (OMS)
Consultant Oral and Maxillofacial Surgeon
Melbourne Craniofacial Unit
Melbourne, VIC, Australia

Henrietta Spalding, BA (Hons)
Head of Policy and Practice
Changing Faces Charity
London, UK

Simon Stapleton, MD, FRCS
Consultant Neurosurgeon
Department of Neurosurgery
St George's Hospital
London, UK

Andrew Stewart, MBBS (Hons) (Lond.), BDS (Hons) (Lond.), FDS.RCS (Eng.), FRCS (Glasg.)
Consultant Oral and Maxillofacial Surgeon
Maxillofacial Unit
St Helier, Kingston and St George's Hospitals
London, UK

Martin Styner, PhD
Computer Scientist
Department of Psychiatry
University of North Carolina
NC, USA

Harlyn K. Susarla, DMD, MPH
Department of Plastic and Reconstructive Surgery
The Johns Hopkins Hospital, Johns Hopkins University School of Medicine;
Department of Oral and Maxillofacial Surgery
Massachusetts General Hospital
Harvard Medical School
Boston, MA, USA

Seenu Susarla, MD, DMD, MPH
Department of Plastic and Reconstructive Surgery
The Johns Hopkins Hospital, Johns Hopkins University School of Medicine;
Department of Oral and Maxillofacial Surgery
Massachusetts General Hospital
Harvard Medical School
Boston, MA, USA

Edward W. Swanson, MD
Department of Plastic and Reconstructive Surgery
The Johns Hopkins Hospital, Johns Hopkins University School of Medicine
Baltimore, MD, USA

Jesse A. Taylor, MD
Associate Professor of Surgery
Mary Downs Endowed Chair of Craniofacial Surgery
Division of Plastic Surgery
The Perelman School of Medicine at the University of Pennsylvania
The Children's Hospital of Philadelphia
Philadelphia, PA, USA

Nigel Taylor, MDSc, BDS, FDS.RCS (Ed.), M.Orth.RCS (Ed.)
Consultant Orthodontist
Department of Orthodontics
Royal Surrey County Hospital
Guildford, UK

Ali Totonchi, MD
Professor of Plastic Surgery
Medical Director of Craniofacial Deformity Clinic
Director of Plastic Surgery Residency, MH Hospital
Plastic Surgery Division
MetroHealth Medical Center
Cleveland, OH, USA

Maria J. Troulis, DDS, MSc
Chief of Oral and Maxillofacial Surgery
Massachusetts General Hospital;
Walter C. Guralnick Professor of Oral and Maxillofacial Surgery
Chair of the Department of Oral and Maxillofacial Surgery
Harvard School of Dental Medicine
Boston, MA, USA

Natalie N. Tung, DDS, MD
Assistant Professor of Oral and Maxillofacial Surgery
Director of Predoctoral OMFS and Oral Surgery Clinic
Division of Oral and Maxillofacial Surgery
Herman Ostrow School of Dentistry
University of Southern California
Los Angeles, CA, USA

Kelly Wade-McBane, BSc (Hons), PGDip (Human Nutrition and Dietetics)
Senior Head and Neck Specialist Dietician
Department of Nutrition and Dietetics
St George's Hospital
London, UK

Helen Witherow, BDS (Birm.), FDS.RCS (Eng.), MBChB (Bristol), FRCS (Eng.), FRCS (OMFS)
Consultant Oral and Maxillofacial Surgeon
Maxillofacial Unit
St George's Hospital
London, UK

Larry M. Wolford, DMD
Clinical Professor of Oral and Maxillofacial Surgery
Baylor College of Dentistry and Baylor University Medical Center
Dallas, TX, USA

Michael Yaremchuk, MD
Chief of Craniofacial Surgery
Massachusetts General Hospital
Clinical Professor of Surgery
Harvard Medical School
Boston, MA, USA

Linping Zhao, PhD
Assistant Professor of Surgery (Research)
Department of Plastic and Cranio-Maxillofacial Surgery
University of Illinois, Chicago, USA

Chapter 1

Introduction: Orthognathic Surgery – A Life's Work

Hugo L. Obwegeser

Introduction

Dr Farhad B. Naini has asked me to write an introduction to this definitive textbook on Orthognathic Surgery. I am very grateful for the honour. My intention is to compose a commentary on the development of orthognathic surgery. Firstly, however, I must express my gratitude to my teachers. It is due to them that I developed the ability to produce new ideas (Figure 1-1). I initially received general surgical training for six months in the military services and an equivalent period in a country hospital in my native town. Following this I had the privilege to train for two years with Hermann von Chiari at his Viennese Institute for Pathology and Microbiology. I then spent six years training in dentistry and maxillofacial surgery with my teacher Richard Trauner at the Maxillofacial Unit of the Dental School of the University of Graz. I spent another five months training in plastic and reconstructive surgery with Sir Harold Gillies in Basingstoke, London, and later six months with Eduard Schmid in Stuttgart. Norman Rowe and Paul Tessier were very good friends and colleagues of mine, and we learned from each other. All I know I owe to my teachers.

Historical remarks

The wish to correct deformities of the maxillo-mandibular complex is an old desire. It was mainly mandibular anomalies that led to a desire for the development of corrective surgery. V.P. Blair (1907),[1] F. Kostečka (1934),[2] and others developed ideas and techniques to cut the body or the ramus of the mandible for repositioning into a planned new occlusion. Their procedures did not satisfy my teacher Richard Trauner, as the results had too many problems. He suggested that we needed to develop another osteotomy that would produce broad contacting bone surfaces and as such have better prerequisites for early bony union and reduce the likelihood for relapse.

How did the sagittal splitting procedure come into being?

Due to my teacher's request it was my obligation to develop an idea for a procedure that would fulfil his intentions. As I very much disliked skin incisions in the visible regions of the face for surgery on the facial

Orthognathic Surgery: Principles, Planning and Practice. Edited by Farhad B. Naini and Daljit S. Gill.

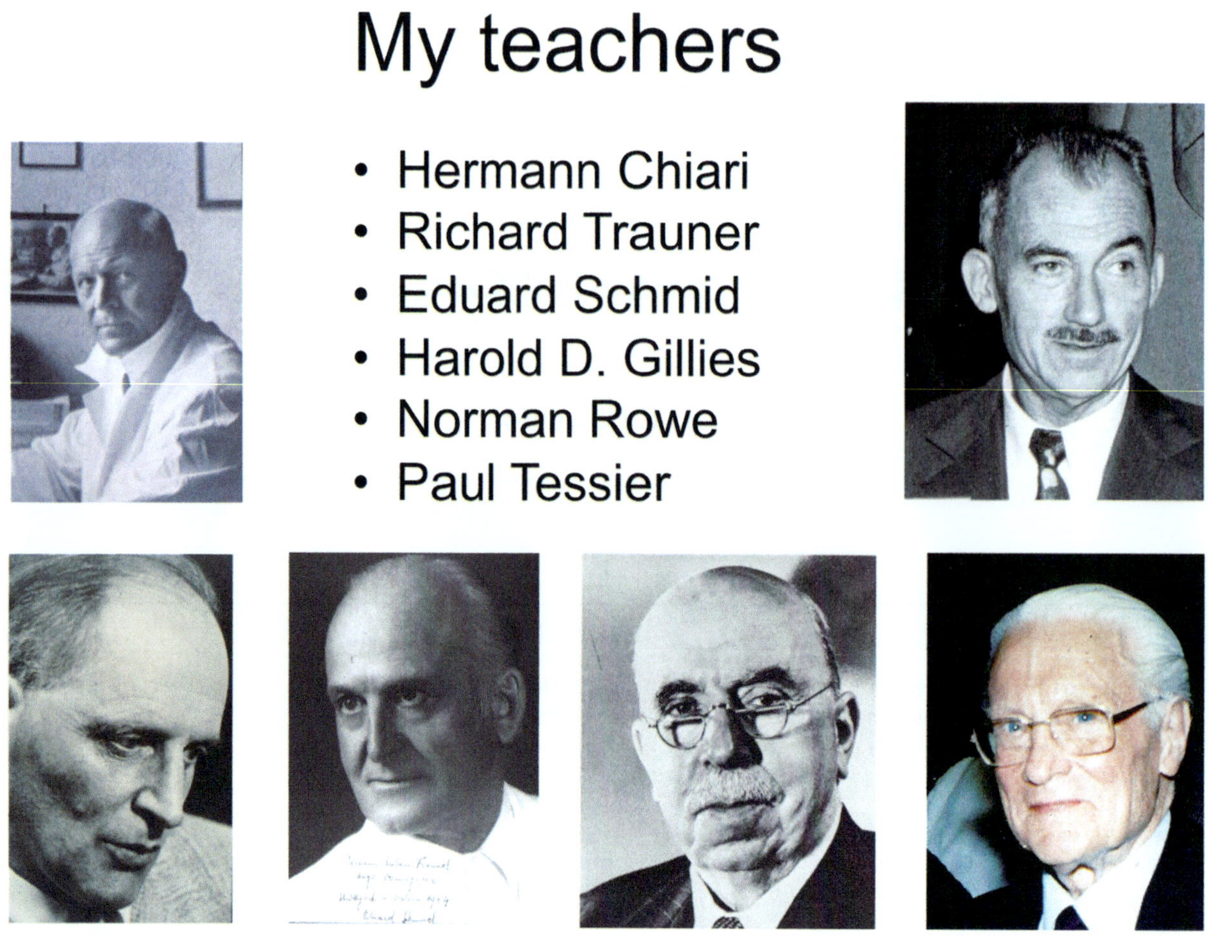

Fig. 1-1 My teachers (anticlockwise): Professor Hermann von Chiari, Chief of the Institute of Pathology and Microbiology of the University of Vienna. Professor Richard Trauner, Chief of Dentistry and Maxillofacial Surgery, University of Graz, Austria. Professor Eduard Schmid, Chief of the Klinik für Gesichtschirurgie, Marienhospital, Stuttgart. Sir Harold Gillies, International founder of Plastic and Reconstructive Surgery, Basingstoke, England. Mr Norman Rowe, Chief of Department of Oral Surgery, Basingstoke, England. Dr Paul Tessier, Chief of the Department of Plastic Surgery, Military Hospital, Paris.

skeleton, I had to find a transoral procedure. I took a cadaveric mandible and turned it around in my hands in order to view it from every direction. By doing so I realised that the vertical splitting of the ramus would produce the ideal situation in relation to the desired goal. However, how could it be split without damaging the mandibular nerve in its canal? In order to find that out I decided to make horizontal cuts about every five millimetres in the ramus. The resultant findings proved very promising. No instrument should touch the area of the mandibular canal. It became obvious that I had to cut the lingual cortical plate of the mandible just above the entrance of the mandibular nerve into the mandible. Another cut of the lateral cortical plate had to be placed somewhere close to the angle, either above or in front of it, but towards the angle in order to correct an unpleasant angle anomaly. That would provide enough raw bone surface contact for fast bony union, independently of whether the mandible would be repositioned in a posterior or an anterior position, or even when a rotation of the mandible was necessary (Figure 1-2).

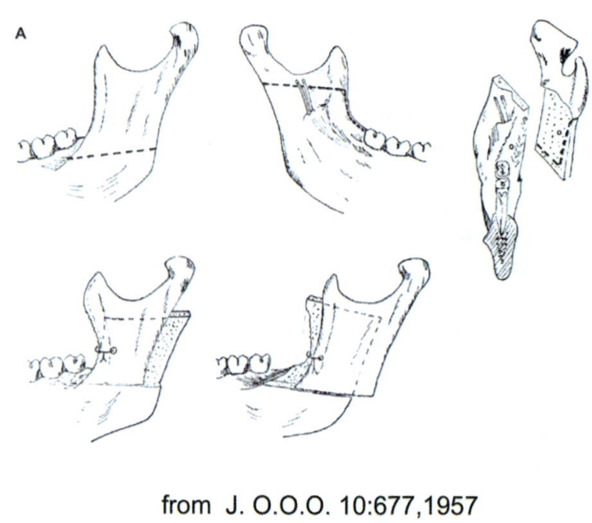

Fig. 1-2 Drawings of my sagittal splitting technique (from: Obwegeser, 1957).[3]

Trauner's inverted L-shaped osteotomy of the ramus

My chief, Richard Trauner, liked my idea. He himself had the intention to perform his idea, an inverted L-shaped osteotomy of the ramus. Trauner's technique required both a transoral and a transfacial approach. The first patient in whom we attempted to produce our ideas was an edentulous young lady, on 17 February 1953. Due to the use of the acrylic splints fixed to the jaws for intermaxillary fixation, the surgery became rather chaotic and somewhat of a mess.

My first successful sagittal splitting of the mandibular ramus

The next case was a 24-year-old female with an intact dentition, but with a protruding position of the mandible. We operated on her on 22 April 1953. This time the procedure went very well (Figure 1-3). The patient's right side was operated using Trauner's technique of the inverted L-shaped osteotomy; it was satisfactory.

I now had the opportunity to perform my first sagittal splitting procedure of the mandibular ramus on the patient's left side. My operation proceeded without any problems. The segments of the split ramus fitted together nicely after the mandible was fixed in the new occlusal position by intermaxillary fixation. It did not require any further fixation. So I proceeded to close the soft tissues tidily over the anterior ramal rim. The result was very pleasing and remained stable over 33 years (Figure 1-4).

My final technique for many years (Figure 1-5)

In the early days, when I was forming my ideas into practical procedures, we operated under sedation and local anaesthesia. General intubation anaesthesia was, in those days, only available for the radical surgery required in cancer cases. Nowadays, the orthognathic patient almost invariably receives general anaesthesia, usually with nasal intubation. A rubber prop is placed between the upper and lower teeth on one side, which keeps the mouth open while operating on the contralateral side. The vestibular mucosa is infiltrated with a 1% local anaesthetic solution plus vasoconstrictor, from the premolar region up to the coronoid process. The incision goes through the mucosa and the periosteum, almost in the depth of the vestibulum, and follows cranially along the anterior crest. The periosteum is elevated in the areas of the bone cuts to be performed, inferiorly above the angle and cranially above the lingula back to the posterior border. Next, the cortical cuts are undertaken. For that I cut on the lingual side the anterior rim with a carbonate burr in order to allow good vision further posteriorly. I use a 3 mm fissure burr to cut the lingual cortical bone above the lingula, to the depth that blood points appear, as far back as the posterior border. The lateral cut is normally performed in the angle area; however, in cases of severe retromandibulism I may go forward to the extent that I will be close to the mental foramen. To connect both osteotomies I produce a vertical cut. For that I use, for safety reasons, a rose burr, making one perforation after the other on the lingual side of the crest, just through the cortical plate. Finally, they are

(a) (b) (c)

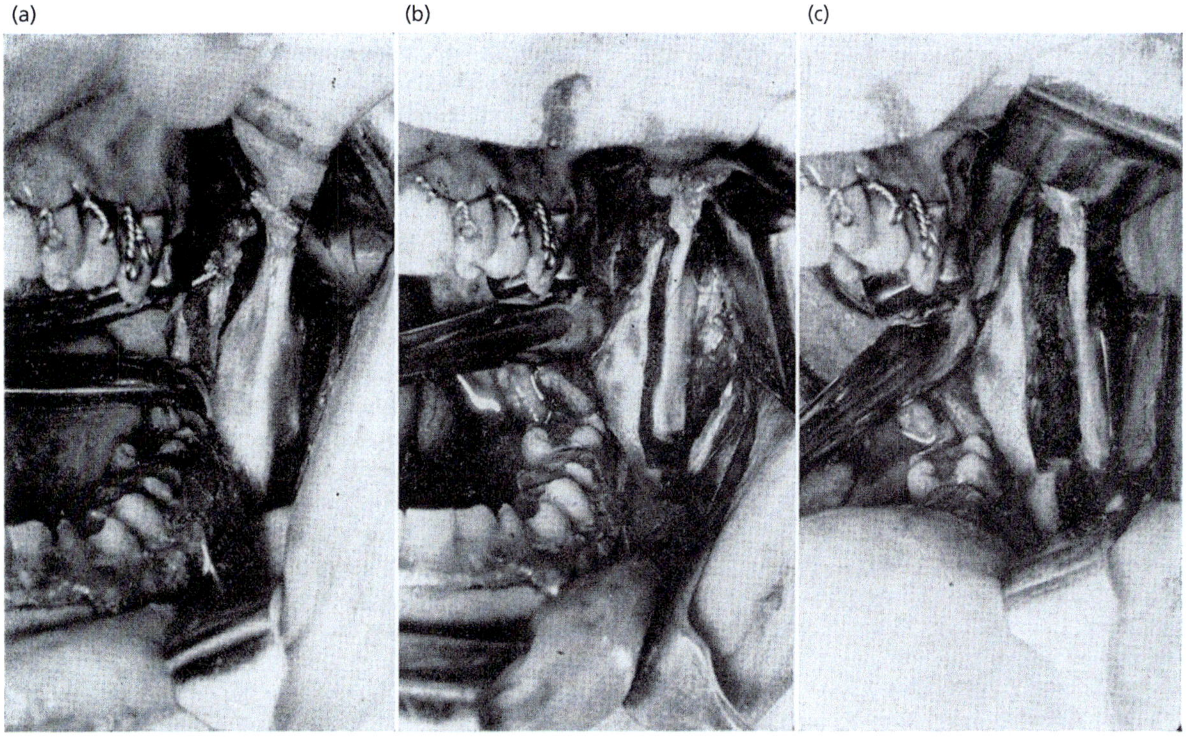

Fig. 1-3 Intraoperative photographs (from: Obwegeser, 1957).[3]

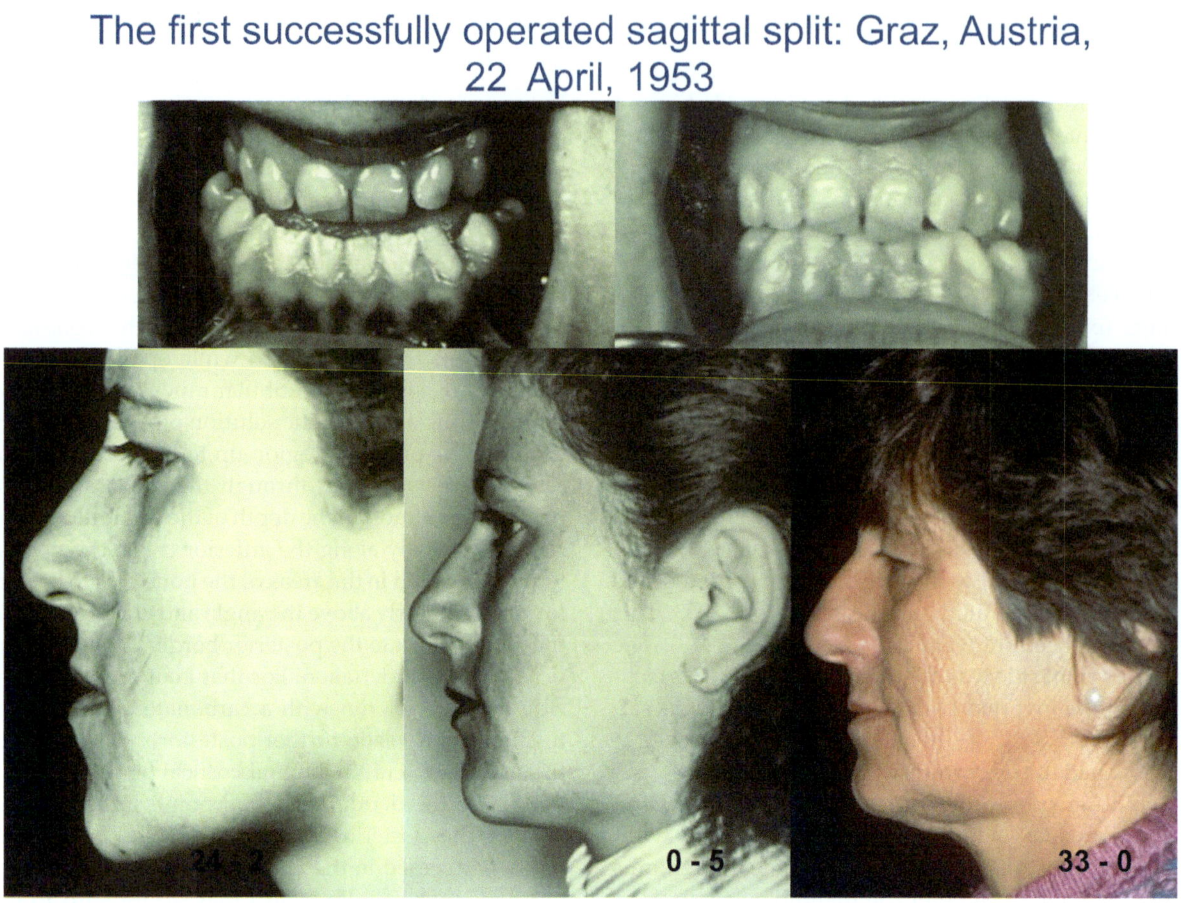

Fig. 1-4 My first successful sagittal splitting case (from: Obwegeser HL. Mandibular Growth Anomalies. Springer, 2001).[31]

connected with a bone cutting burr. I want to be certain that I will not be too deep in the ramus, thereby reducing the risk of damage to the mandibular nerve. My nephew, Joachim Obwegeser, prefers to make this connecting cut by the use of a saw. Using the wedge osteotome, I open the cut gently and not too deeply. Next I use my bone spreader forceps, inserted into the vertical cut, in order to open the cortical plates (see Figure 1-5). Normally, the split opens the cortical plates right through to the posterior border; if not, the posterior border is cut under direct vision with a broad splitting osteotome. By employing this technique I was able to avoid damage to the nerve. Fixation screws will have to be carefully placed.

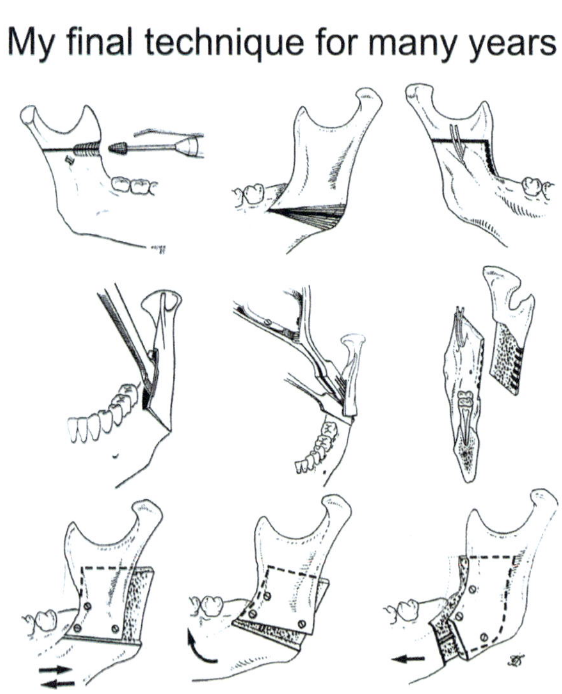

Fig. 1-5 My final technique for the sagittal splitting procedure for many years (from: Obwegeser HL. Mandibular Growth Anomalies. Springer, 2001).[31]

International reaction

After publication of the sagittal splitting osteotomy procedure in *Oral Surgery, Oral Medicine, Oral Pathology and Oral Radiology* (1957),[3] I was invited to lecture on the subject in various countries. The transoral sagittal splitting procedure went around the world after I had published it in detail and had finally lectured on it in a postgraduate course to the American Association of Oral Surgeons, in 1966, at the Walter Reed Hospital. This procedure conquered the professional world all around the globe. It is now in daily use, probably in every country in the world. It is the procedure of choice for every specialist dealing with maxillomandibular anomalies.

Transoral chin correction

The same is true with the transoral sliding chin correction, a procedure that I published together with the

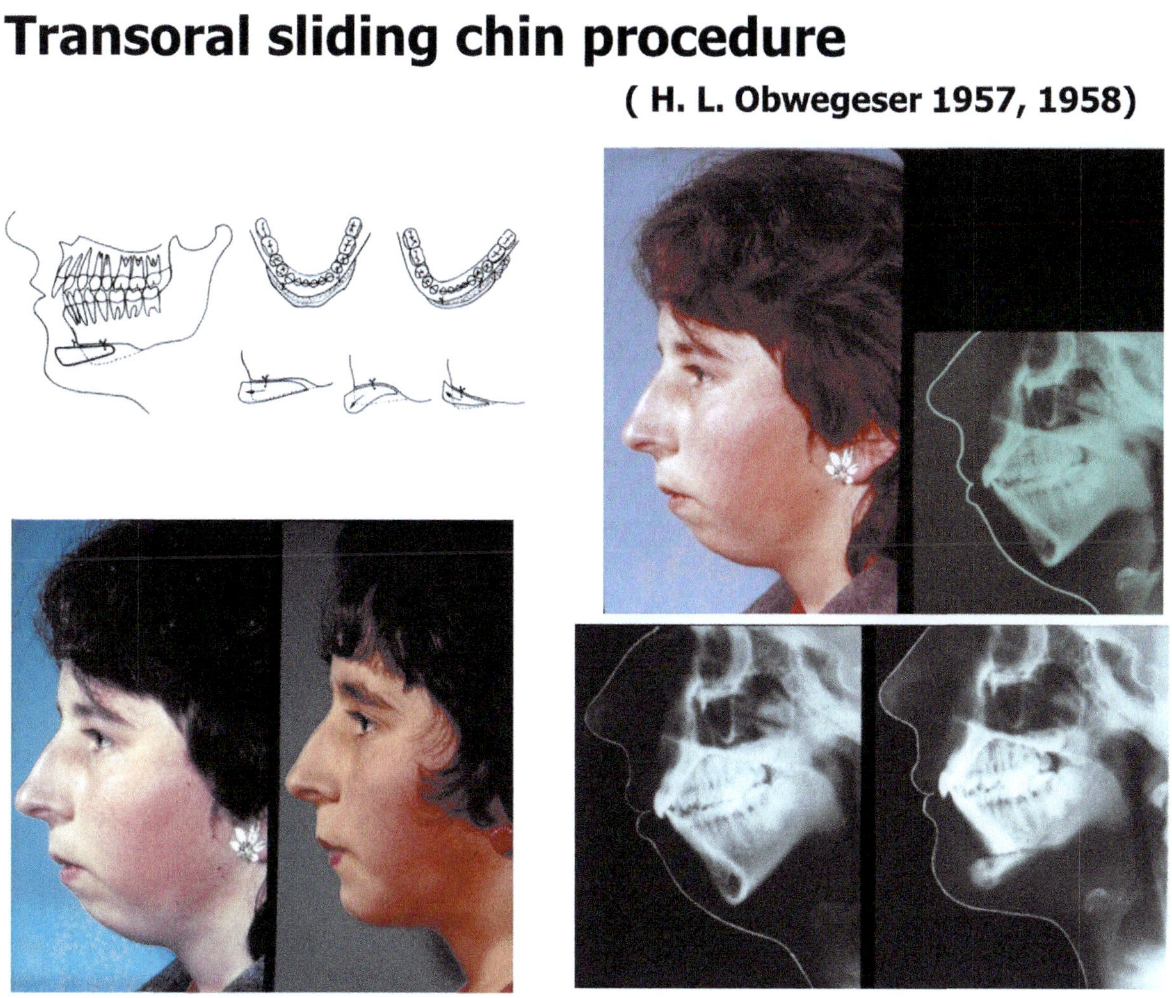

Fig. 1-6 My technique and first case of transoral sliding chin procedure (from: Obwegeser HL. Mandibular Growth Anomalies. Springer, 2001).[31]

sagittal splitting procedure (1957).[3] It does not require a detailed description here (see Chapters 3 and 33). Otto Hofer (1942)[4] was obviously the first to have the idea to increase the prominence of the chin by cutting its inferior rim off the mandibular body. However, he demonstrated the procedure on a cadaver via an extraoral approach. I got the idea when I investigated the lateral cephalometric radiograph of a patient with a very retruded chin. It was so obvious that there was the material I needed. I performed it right away on the patient. The technique was simple and the result very convincing (Figure 1-6). My personal friend and colleague, Otto Neuner (1965),[5] developed the idea of using a double step, in order to obtain greater increase in chin prominence. I, eventually, also performed a triple step procedure (1970a).[6]

The mobilization of the maxilla – its history

The mobilization of the maxilla had been the intention of many surgeons who desired to correct maxillomandibular anomalies. Georg Axhausen from Kiel, Germany, published three articles describing osteotomies of the maxilla, for the correction of its position after trauma (1934),[7] and in cases due to other aetiological factors resulting in anomalies of the maxilla (1936 and 1939).[8,9] However, his publications did not describe the technique in a way that would permit other surgeons to carry out the procedure. In 1942, Karl Schuchardt,[10] from Hamburg, published the mobilization of the dislodged upper jaw of a war injury and its repositioning using traction weight. He wrote that the procedure would be hardly used for the correction of maxillary deformities in secondary cleft cases.

Sir Harold Gillies worked hard on this subject, as did Norman Rowe. During my training with Sir Harold, in 1951–52, I had on several occasions the privilege to watch or even assist him. He was definitely the pioneer for the final mobilization procedure of the maxilla, because he opened the cleft and rotated the palatally dislocated alveolar segments laterally so far that they could fit with the mandibular teeth. However, he did not dislocate them anteriorly. He filled the very large steps in the canine fossae with cancellous bone grafts from the iliac crest. To the great surprise of his observing visitors the grafts healed, without infection, despite the fact that the region was not completely covered with a vestibular flap or any other mucous membrane on its raw surface on the sides of the maxillary and nasal cavities. That pioneering

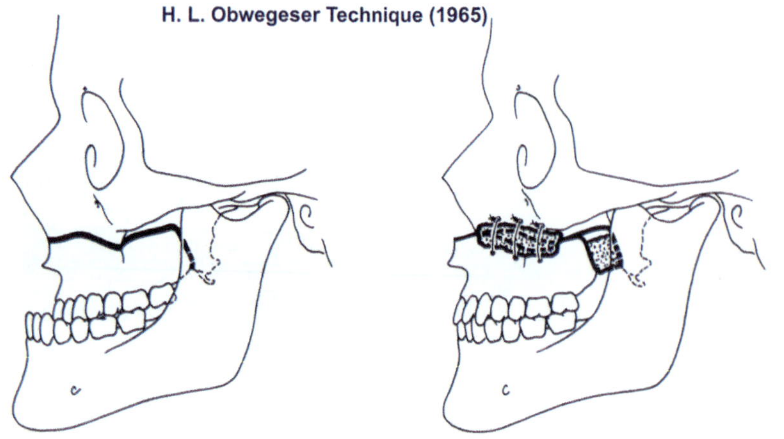

Fig. 1-7 Drawings of my technique of Le Fort I anterior repositioning (from: Obwegeser, 1969).[28]

step allowed me to advance the mobilized maxilla up to 20 millimetres and more. These bone grafts, together with the graft that I always place behind the tuberosity and the pterygoid processes, have become to me a conditio sine qua non (Figure 1-7). In 1986, R. Drommer published a very interesting article on 'The History of the Le Fort I Osteotomy'.[11] He stated very clearly that 'Hugo Obwegeser' was the first to publish a procedure that every experienced surgeon should be able to perform. It was in 1962 at the South American International Conference on Oral Surgery in Buenos Aires, Argentina, when I first reported on my successful mobilization of the maxilla (Obwegeser, 1962).[12] The procedure could be performed together with the transoral splitting of the rami. However, the first patient in whom I operated on both jaws was on 5 September 1969; that is, 16 years after the first publication of the sagittal splitting of the mandibular ramus and 7 years after the publication of the Le Fort I-type osteotomy and mobilization of the maxilla.

Operative technique for mobilization of the maxilla

The patient normally receives nasal intubation anaesthesia. In addition, I infiltrate the vestibulum with 1% local anaesthetic solution plus a vasoconstrictor. The incision goes all the way round in the vestibulum, however, only when the palatal mucosa is free of scars. Next, the periosteum is raised cranially. In the piriform aperture, the mucosa is raised from the floor of the nose and from the septum for at least 15 mm. The septum osteotome separates it from the palate. I use an oscillating saw for the circular osteotomy. Just prior to this, I separate the tuberosity from the pterygoid process with an elastic special tuber osteotome. This prevents the saw cutting further posteriorly and avoids damage to the regional blood vessels.

For many years I used the anterior down fracture technique to get the maxilla loose. My nephew, Joachim Obwegeser (1997),[13] suggested to me to start in the posterior region with down fracturing, by the use of my bone separating forceps. Only after that, with the same instrument, the anterior down fracture is performed. The maxilla must be mobilized to the extent that it can easily be overcorrected with a pair of tweezers. The fixation of the maxilla in the new position has to follow the plan. In cases when the mandible also has to be repositioned a preoperatively prepared occlusal splint guarantees the position in which the maxilla has to be fixed. Next the mandibular osteotomy is completed and then fixed in the new occlusion. Whether the jaws are fixed with wires, or plates and screws, you always have to keep in mind that the tendency of the pull of the musculature is to bring the jaws back to their initial position. This means that some use of intermaxillary elastics may be useful to maintain the new dental occlusion.

With these three procedures, orthognathic surgery experienced an explosion throughout the world.

Modifications of the procedures

I received visiting observers from all over the world. Some had the idea to alter the position or the direction of the cortical cuts in the sagittal splitting of the mandibular rami, and went on to name the modified procedure according to their own name (K. Schuchardt, 1954;[14] Dal Pont, 1959 and 1961;[15,16] E.E. Hunsuck, 1968;[17] B.V. Epker, 1977;[18] etc.). However, I still believe that my original technique for the mandible as well as for the maxilla remains the best solution to the clinical problems.

New procedures

In September 1967 Paul Tessier published for the first time his techniques for the mobilization of the middle third of the facial skeleton (Le Fort III-type osteotomy) and for dislocating the orbital coni including their contents (hypertelorism operation).[19]

Between 1953 and 1967 several ideas were published for repositioning the whole mandible.[20,21] I myself published a technique that I named the transoral angle

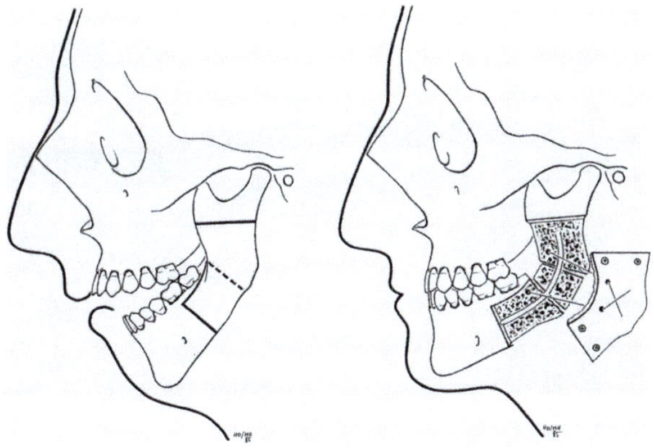

Fig. 1-8 Drawings of my transoral angle osteotomy (from: Obwegeser HL. Mandibular Growth Anomalies. Springer, 2001).[31]

osteotomy (1964) (Figure 1-8).[22] In cases of posterior vertical maxillary excess, Karl Schuchardt (1954)[14] had the idea of cranially repositioning the lateral maxillary segments, thereby allowing the mandible to autorotate anteriorly and close the occlusion (Figure 1-9 a–d). In my experience, in a very high percentage of cases, that procedure led to relapse of the anterior open bite.

For the correction of an edentulous antemandibulism I wanted to get rid of the internal fixation with the help of acrylic splints, fixed to both jaws. For that reason I produced a bilateral sagittal splitting as far anterior and close to the mental foramen as possible. By doing so I was able to fix the large segments of the

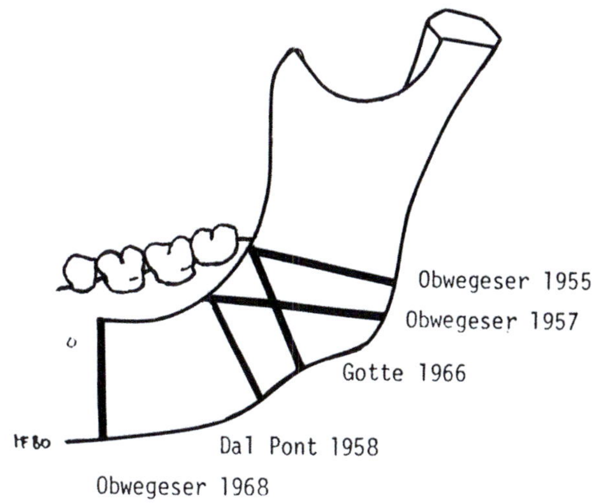

Fig. 1-10 Some variations of lateral cortical cut for the sagittal splitting procedure by different authors (from: Obwegeser, 1968).[23]

mandible in the desired position using a circumferential wire in the ramus region as well as in the body of the mandible (1968).[23] There are many minor alterations of the original sagittal split osteotomy, and it is not possible to mention them all in detail (Figure 1-10).

Segmental alveolar osteotomies

Heinz Köle deserves the honour of various segmental osteotomies of the alveolar processes in the maxilla as

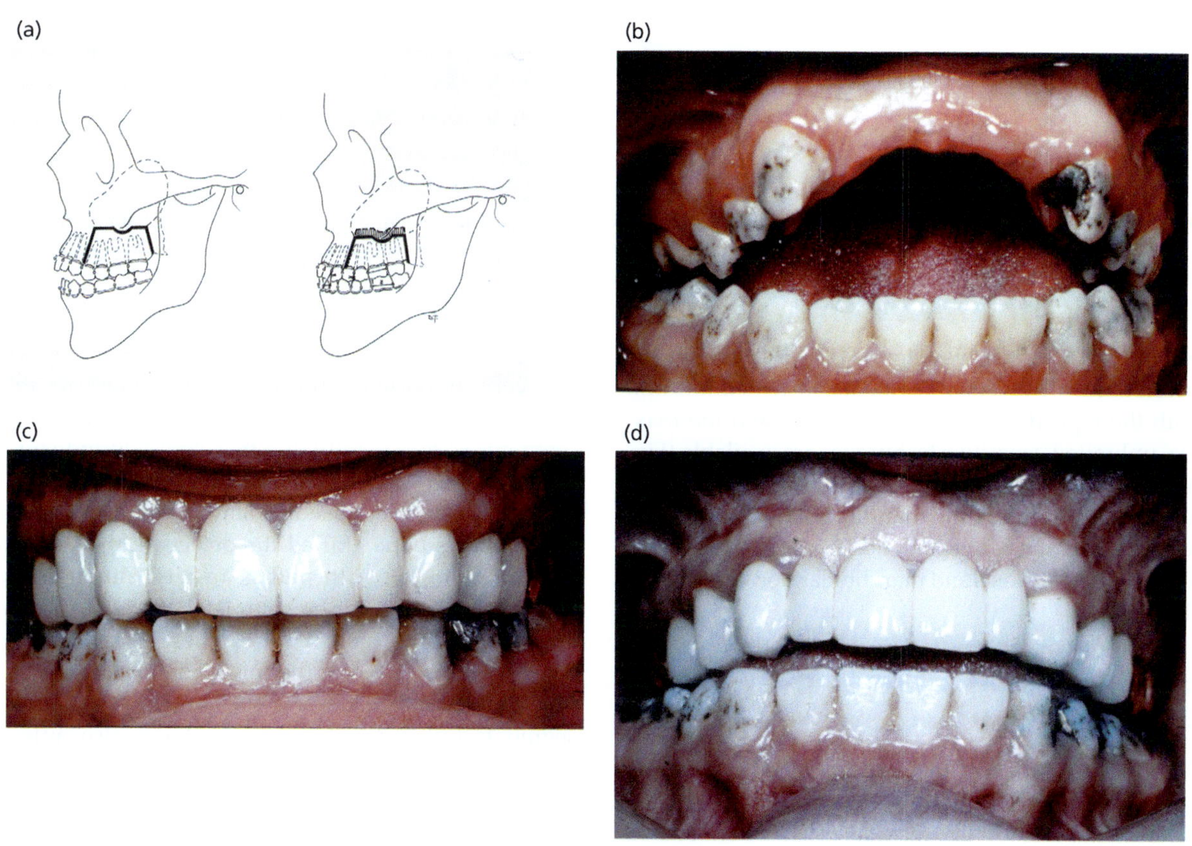

Fig. 1-9 Schuchardt's procedure for correcting a maxillary open bite: (a) technique; (b) case before surgery; (c) occlusion after additional bridge work; (d) amount of relapse after one year.

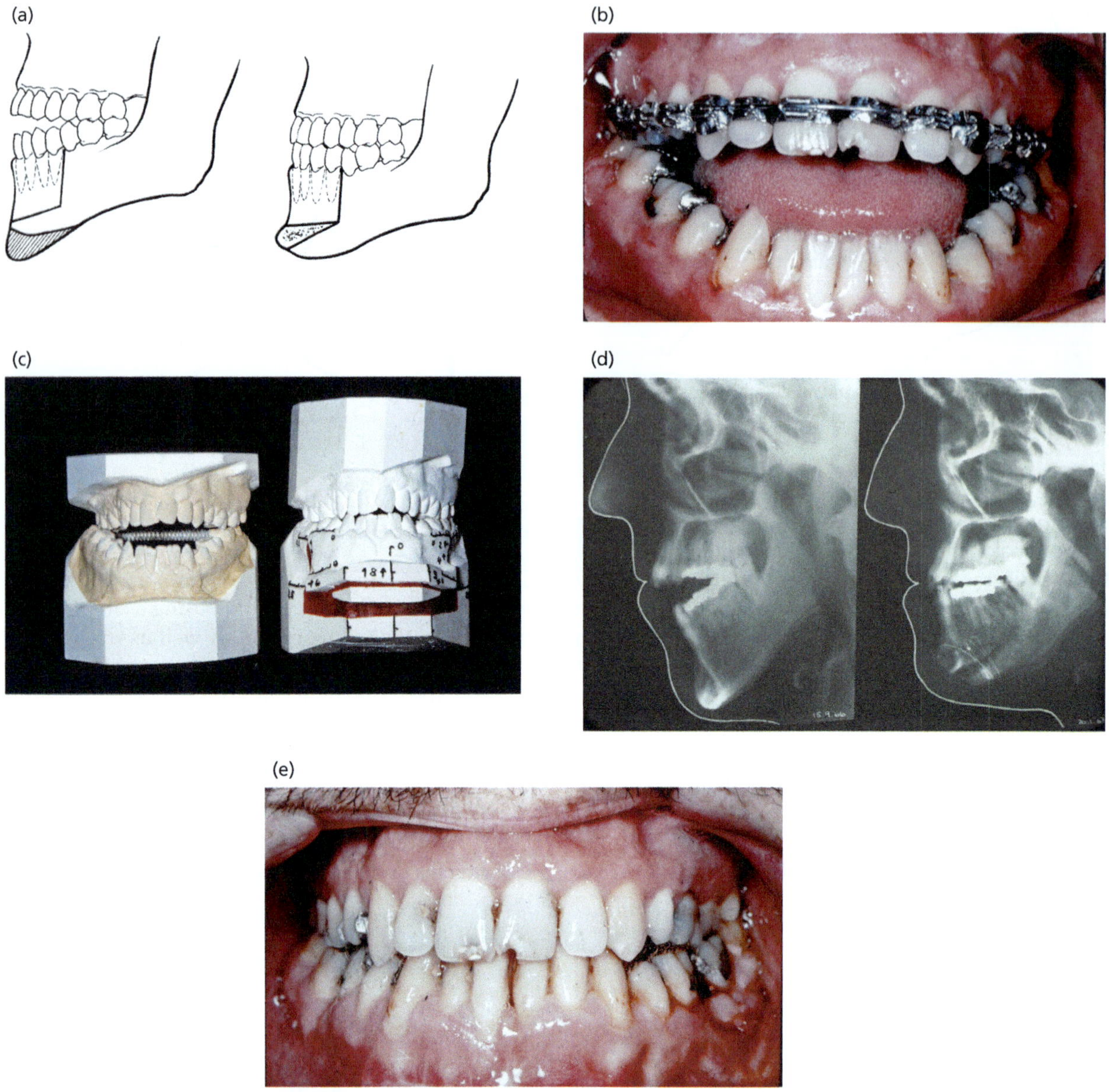

Fig. 1-11 H. Köle's technique for closing an anterior mandibular open bite: (a) The technique in a drawing; (b) Case before surgery; (c) Model operation; (d) Lateral skull radiographs before and after surgery; (e) Occlusion after one year. (From: Obwegeser HL. Mandibular Growth Anomalies. Springer, 2001.)[31]

well as in the mandible (Figure 1-11 a–e).[24] With the possibilities of alveolar segmental osteotomies, and with the repositioning of the mandible and the maxilla, unlimited corrective techniques are available (Figure 1-12 a–c). Joachim Obwegeser (1987)[25] described a circular splitting of the mandible, which is a useful technique for the correction of certain types of cases of independent occlusal and mandibular body anomalies (Figure 1-13).

Problems of maxillary anomalies in secondary cleft deformity cases

Severe deformities of the maxilla tend to occur in secondary cleft deformity cases. Nevertheless, the dislocated parts of the maxilla must be mobilized and repositioned. Accurate model surgery defines the amount and the direction of the required repositioning of the alveolar segments. Sir Harold Gillies undertook the very important and pioneering work in this subject. He, together with Norman Rowe, rotated the segments so far laterally that they could occlude with the mandible (Gillies and Rowe).[26] For that the cleft had to be widely reopened and in a later session closed again. Gillies bone grafted the defects in the steps of the canine fossae with perfect results, although the bone grafts could not be completely covered on the side to the antral and nasal cavities. That step was the pioneering work for the correction of severely collapsed maxillary arches. He only rotated the alveolar segments but did not reposition them also anteriorly; that was my contribution to the Le Fort I repositioning.

The secondary cleft deformity cases are the most challenging to correct properly. However, it is a fascinating subject and very pleasing for both the surgeon

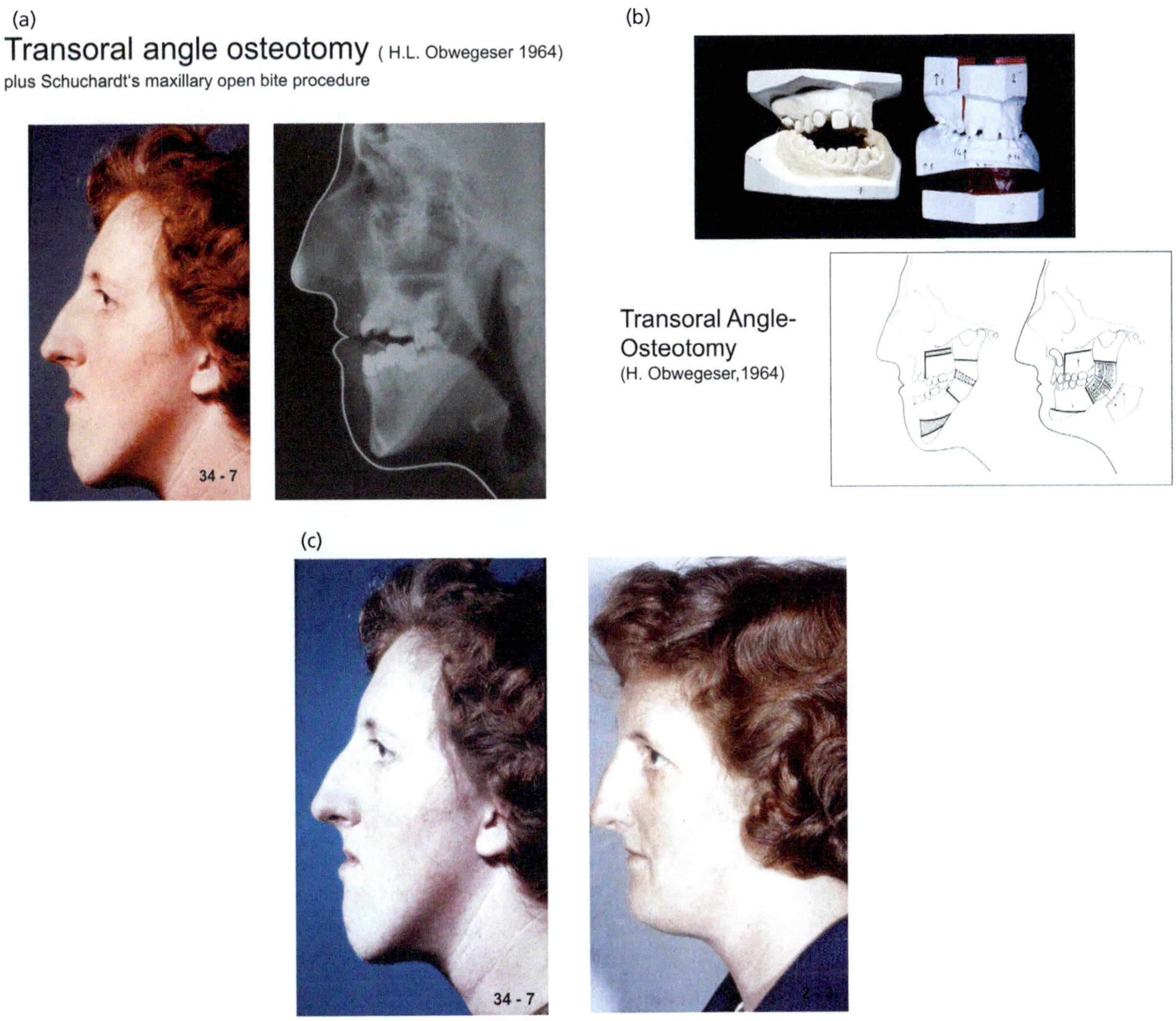

Fig. 1-12 Case of maxillomandibular long face plus open bite: (a) Before surgery; (b) Model operation plus drawings of planned surgery; (c) Result of surgery.

and even more so for the patient. The planning is undertaken as for any orthognathic surgery case: first, on a tracing of the lateral cephalometric radiograph, the ideal profile line is drawn. The model surgery shows all the details of the required osteotomies. The surgeon will have to decide the technical feasibility of reproducing in the patient what the model surgery demonstrates is required (Figure 1-14 a–d).

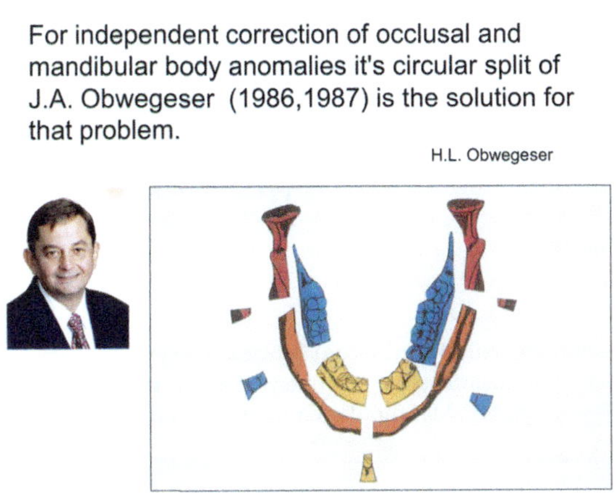

Fig. 1-13 Joachim Obwegeser's circular splitting of the mandible (from: Obwegeser HL. Mandibular Growth Anomalies. Springer, 2001).[31]

The Le Fort III + I osteotomy

After I had the privilege to observe Dr Paul Tessier perform a Le Fort III-type osteotomy, I then performed it. However, soon I had a case to correct presenting with severe micro- and retromaxillism. It was obvious that the forward repositioning of the middle third would not produce a satisfactory result. There would still remain some lack of vertical height. For that reason, in addition to the Le Fort III osteotomy, I separated the maxillary complex with an additional Le Fort I mobilization. That allowed me (Obwegeser, 1969)[27,28] to reposition the maxilla in a good occlusal relationship with the inferior dentition (Figure 1-15). The gap that remained then between the cranial half of the middle third and the maxilla I filled with cancellous bone grafts from the iliac crest. The final result was very pleasing and with it a new

(a)

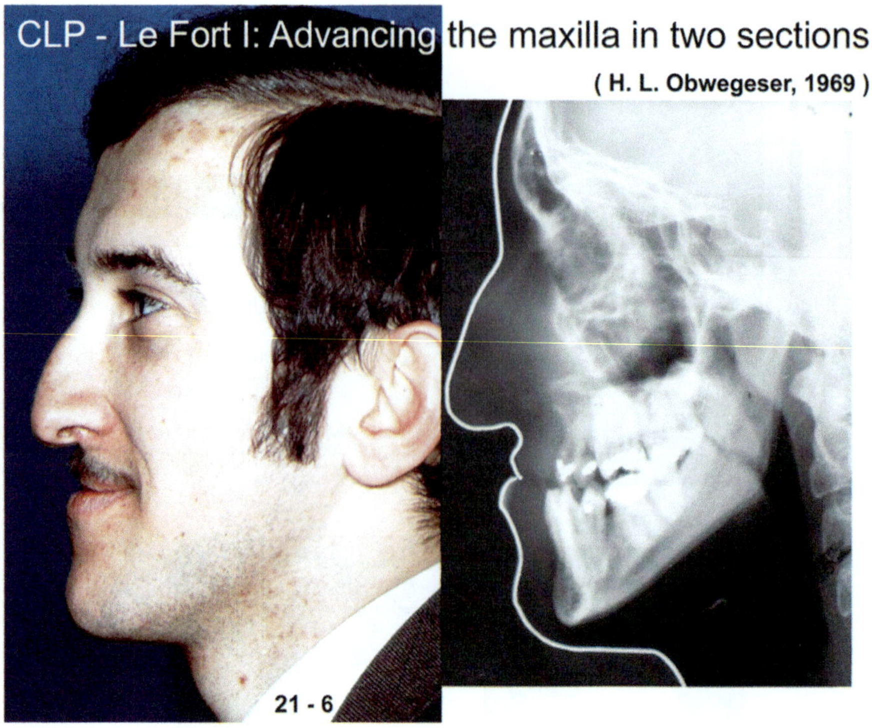

(b)

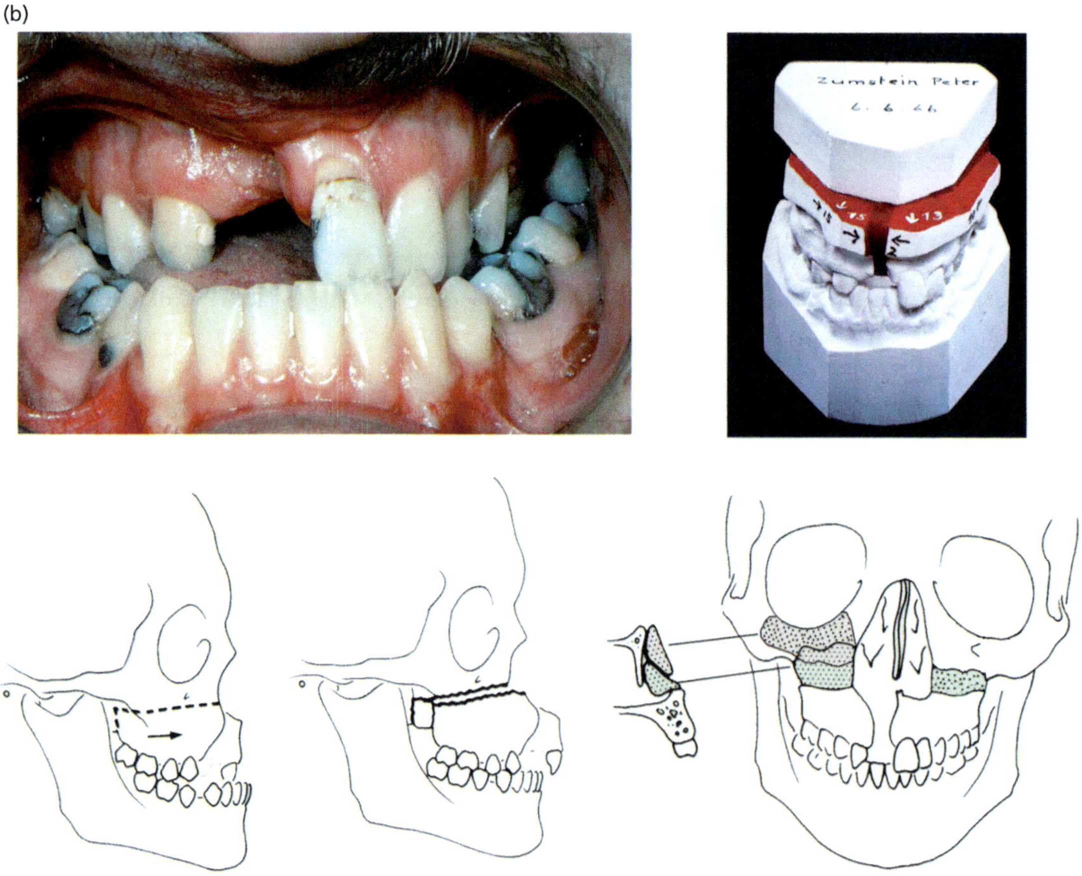

Fig. 1-14 Case of secondary cleft deformity: Retromaxillism plus collapse of the maxillary arches: (a) Before surgery; (b) Model operation and drawings of planned surgery; (c) Lateral skull radiographs and occlusion before and one year and three months after surgery; (d) Profile view before and three months after surgery. (From: Obwegeser HL. Mandibular Growth Anomalies. Springer, 2001.)[31]

(c)

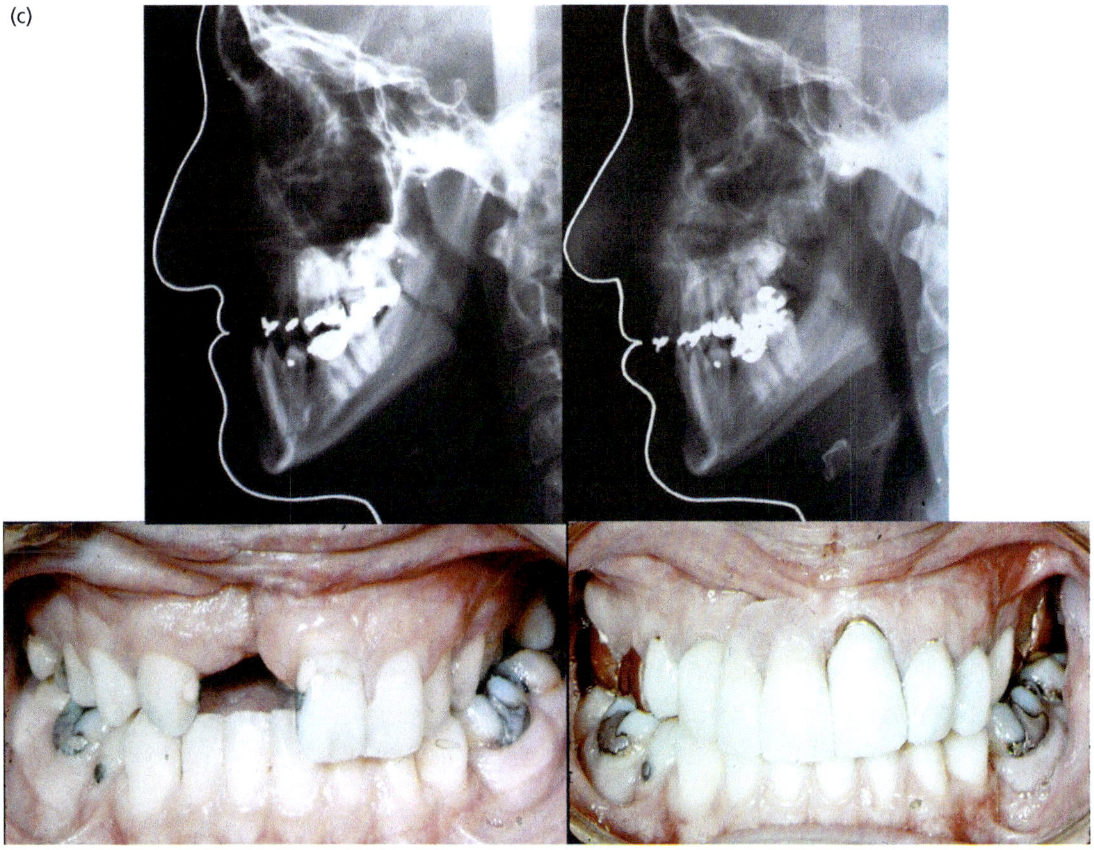

(d)

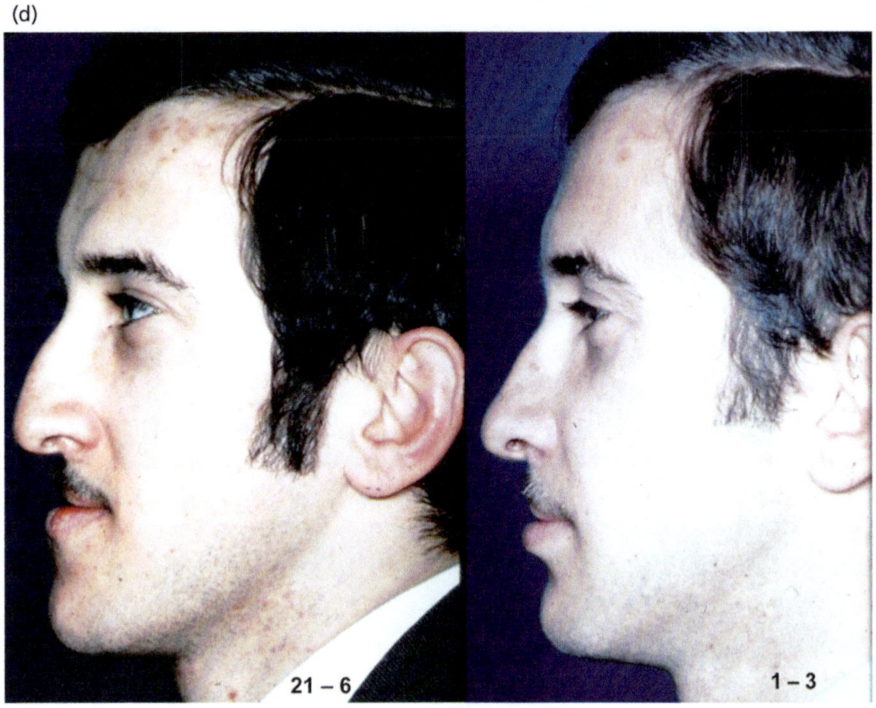

Fig. 1-14 *(Continued)*

variation of the middle third advancement was born (Figure 1-16 a,b).

The correction of hypertelorism

Dr Paul Tessier described the principal technique of rotating dislocated orbital coni together with their contents. His transcranial approach is the key to the problem. A subcranial approach was also published, but is more complicated than the approach described above.

The correction of a unilateral dislocation of the orbit is a straightforward procedure, producing a good result. A symmetrical bilateral dislocation is not much more difficult to correct (Figure 1-17 a–d). There is no question that we have to operate on these patients in

LF III + LF I, H. L. Obwegeser, 1969

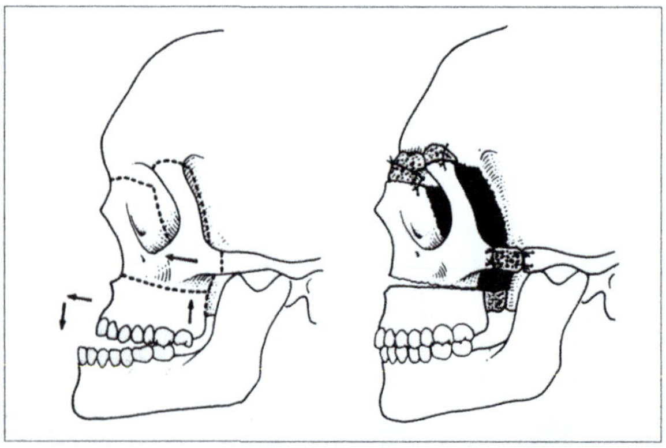

Fig. 1-15 H.L. Obwegeser's technique for a combined Le Fort III+I operation. (From: Obwegeser, 1969.)[28]

childhood because of their eyes, although we are fully aware that such early correction may interfere with the subsequent growth of the maxilla. That means we have to inform the patient that after the age of 18 years a second operation will be required to obtain the final result. I learned this by treating a very convincing case – Antonio – which I describe as the case of my life (H. Obwegeser, G. Weber, H.P Freihofer, H.F. Sailer, 1978) 'Facial duplication – the unique case of Antonio'. J Maxillofacial Surgery 6: 179–198).[29]

Antonio was referred to me at the age of 10 years (Figure 1-18). He was born with a median facial cleft, two complete noses and two fully developed premaxillae and altogether seven incisor teeth. My treatment plan was formulated based on Tessier's procedure for the correction of hypertelorism (Figure 1-19).

(a)

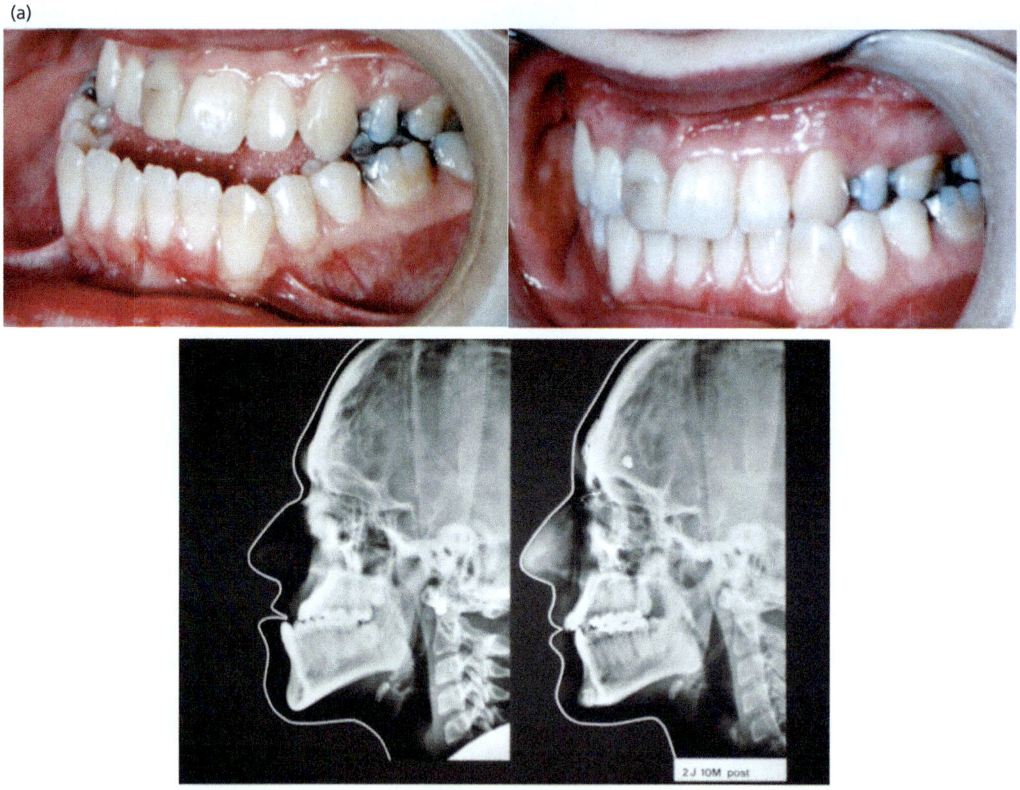

(b)

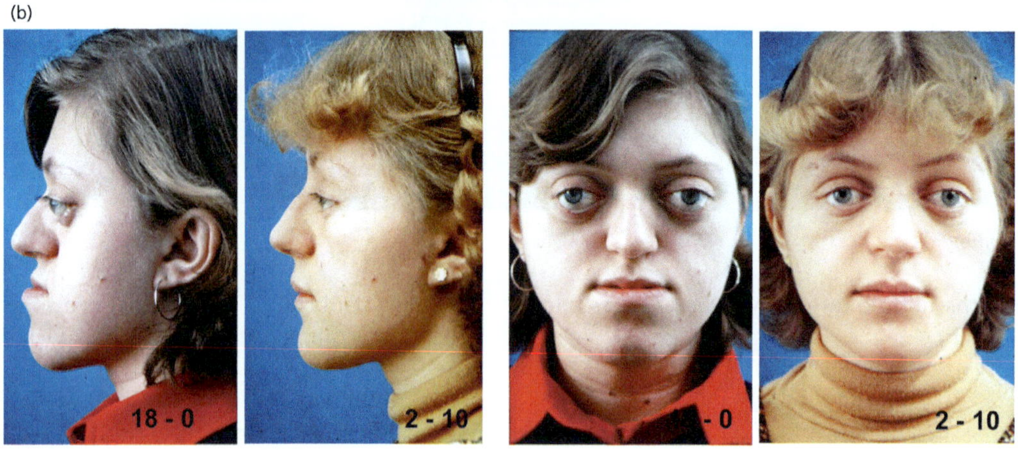

Fig. 1-16 Case of micro-retromaxillism: (a) Occlusion and lateral skull radiographs before and after surgery; (b) Profile and front views of case before and 2 years and 10 months after surgery. (From: Obwegeser HL. Mandibular Growth Anomalies. Springer, 2001.)[31]

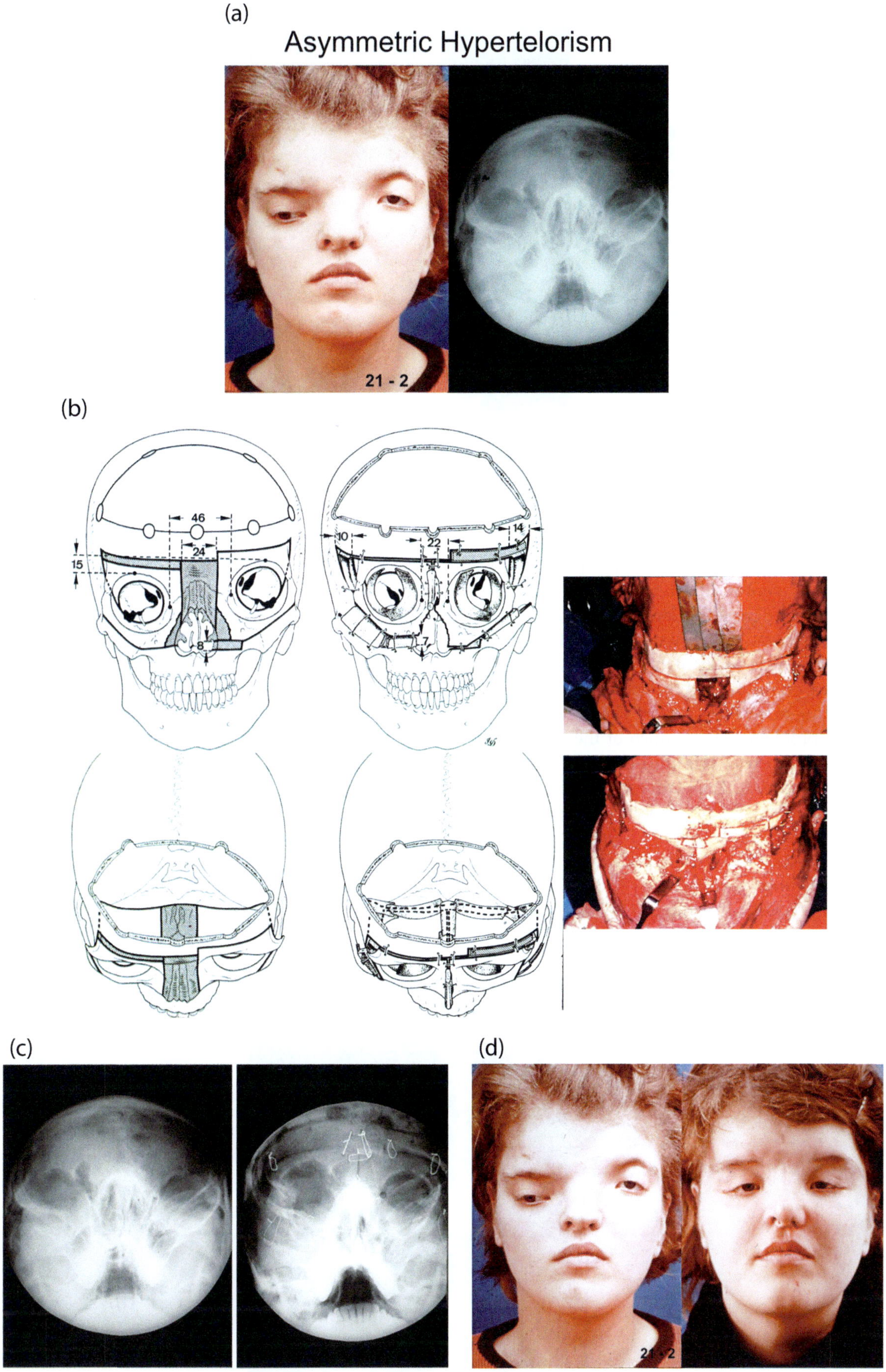

Fig. 1-17 Case of asymmetric hypertelorism. (a) Front view and semi-axial skull radiograph before surgery; (b) Planned operation and operation pictures; (c) Semi-axial radiographs of the skull before and after the correction; (d) Patients front views before and after the correction.

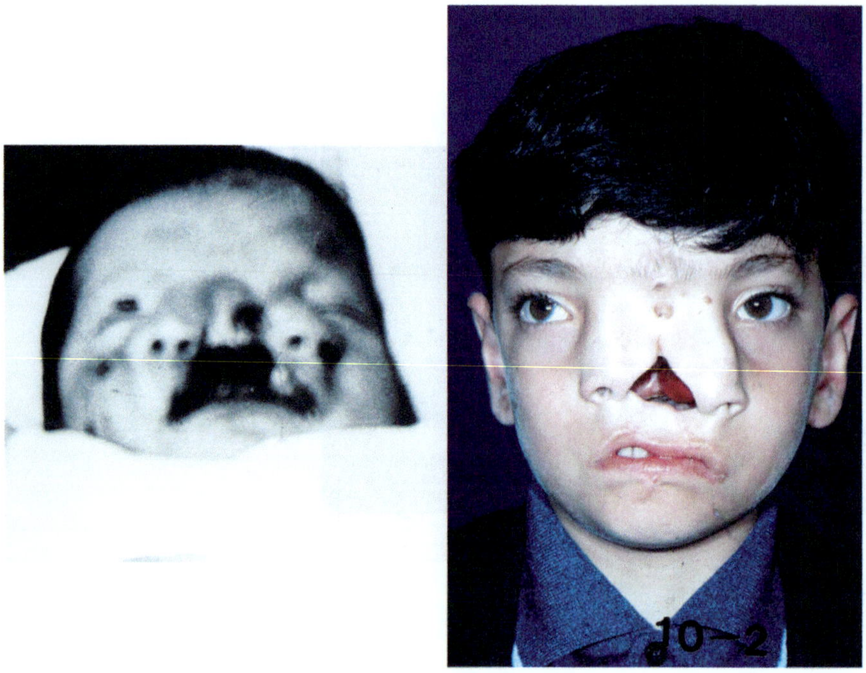

Fig. 1-18 Antonio – the case of my life. (From Obwegeser et al., 1978.)[29] Patient presented with midfacial duplication and medial facial cleft. Left: situation after birth; Right: at age of 10.

The operation was performed on the 4 July 1969. The first operation went well. After the neurosurgeon (G. Weber) had raised the skull flap he found, to our great surprise, two cristae galli. In those days neither tomography nor MRI was yet available. That meant I had to plan the case on the basis of conventional radiographs and according to my imagination. The two cristae galli solved the problem of how much of the cranial base I would have to excise (Figure 1-20) – they provided the answer (Figure 1-21). I planned the operation with military precision, step by step, including the necessary time that would be required for each step. This was typed and handed to every person working on the case. The operation was started at 8.00 in the morning and ended precisely according to my written plan at 3.00 o'clock the following morning. I had to resect both premaxillae with the seven incisor teeth.

Eventually, we achieved a result that allowed a good functional occlusion for mastication and acceptable anterior dental aesthetics, so that nobody would miss his front teeth! However, at this stage there was still a long way to go. The primary result was very pleasing, but a purulent infection compelled the neurosurgeon to remove the large bone flap of the skull and I removed the bone grafts for the reconstruction of the lateral orbital defects. The Children's Hospital managed to treat the meningitis. In due course, the patient was discharged home with a helmet. Ten months later he returned with a severe discrepancy of the middle third of the face and the mandible. The latter was far

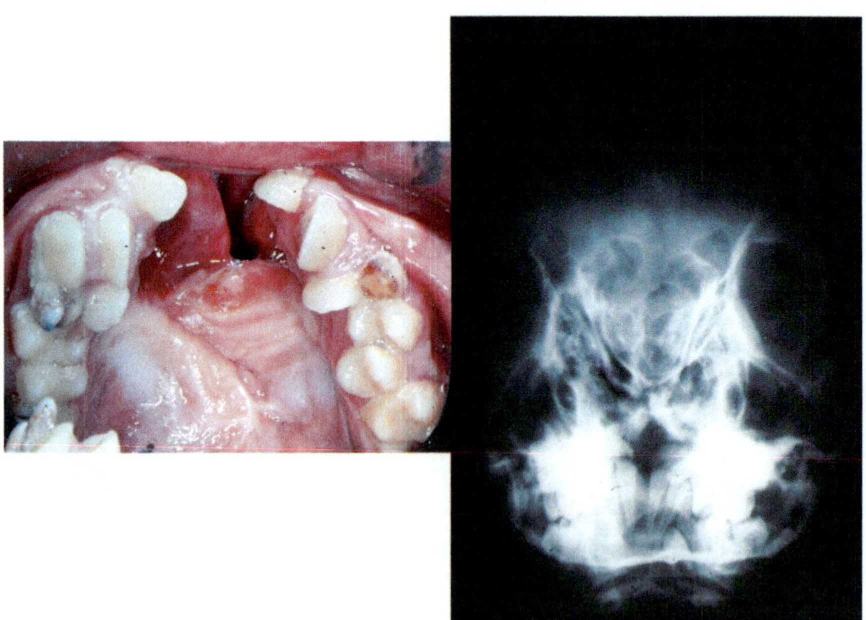

Fig. 1-19 Patients maxilla with two premaxillae plus skull semi-axial radiograph.

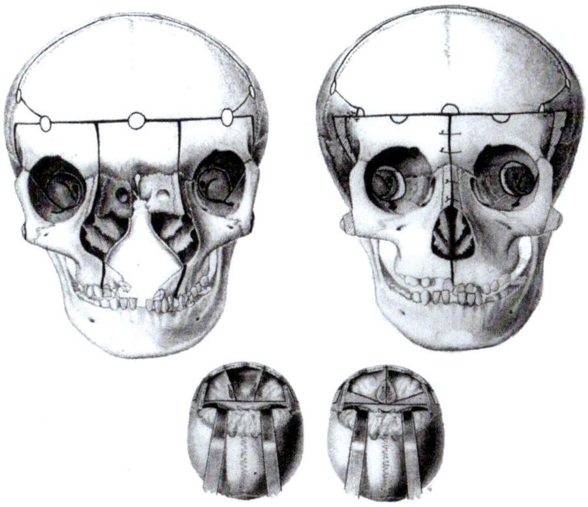

Fig. 1-20 Drawings of planned operation.

in front of the maxilla, as the mandible had grown forward but the maxilla had not. I corrected the condition with a Le Fort I advancement in two sections and a repositioning of the anterior mandibular alveolus. The primary result was quite pleasing (Figure 1-22).

Thirteen months later the neurosurgeon reimplanted the skull flap again after he had autoclaved it. The same immediate infection caused him to remove it again. I said to him do not worry; I will make him a new skull covering. So I did, 10 months later. I took from the right side of the chest four ribs, and from the left three ribs. As they had been taken already during the first intervention the regeneration was somehow sclerosed bone. Despite this I managed to split the ribs. So I had 14 half-ribs for the reconstruction of the large skull defect. There were no postoperative problems. The patient could now leave without a helmet. Finally, the whole defect was covered with bone made from his own ribs (Figure 1-23). However, the face changed very much in the following years (Figure 1-24). I decided to wait until he was at least 18 years of age. When he returned the presentation was that of a severe midface retrusion and mandibular prominence, due to lack of forward growth of the maxilla and zygomatic bones and lower half of the nose, and overgrowth of the mandible – the patient described his own appearance as 'monstrous' (Figure 1-25). After evaluation of the situation it was obvious that I had to posteriorly reposition the mandible in addition to its anterior alveolar segment, and the maxilla and the inferior periorbital region had to advance (Figure 1-26). The result was very convincing (Figure 1-27). In addition, the missing columella had to be reconstructed. For that I planned a caterpillar flap with an L-shaped cartilage taken from the ribs (Figure 1-28). There were no complications but a nice result of the nose and the profile was produced. The patient was discharged home as a man with a normal face, albeit with some scars. He could eat everything. The missing incisors were not obvious. The quality of his speech

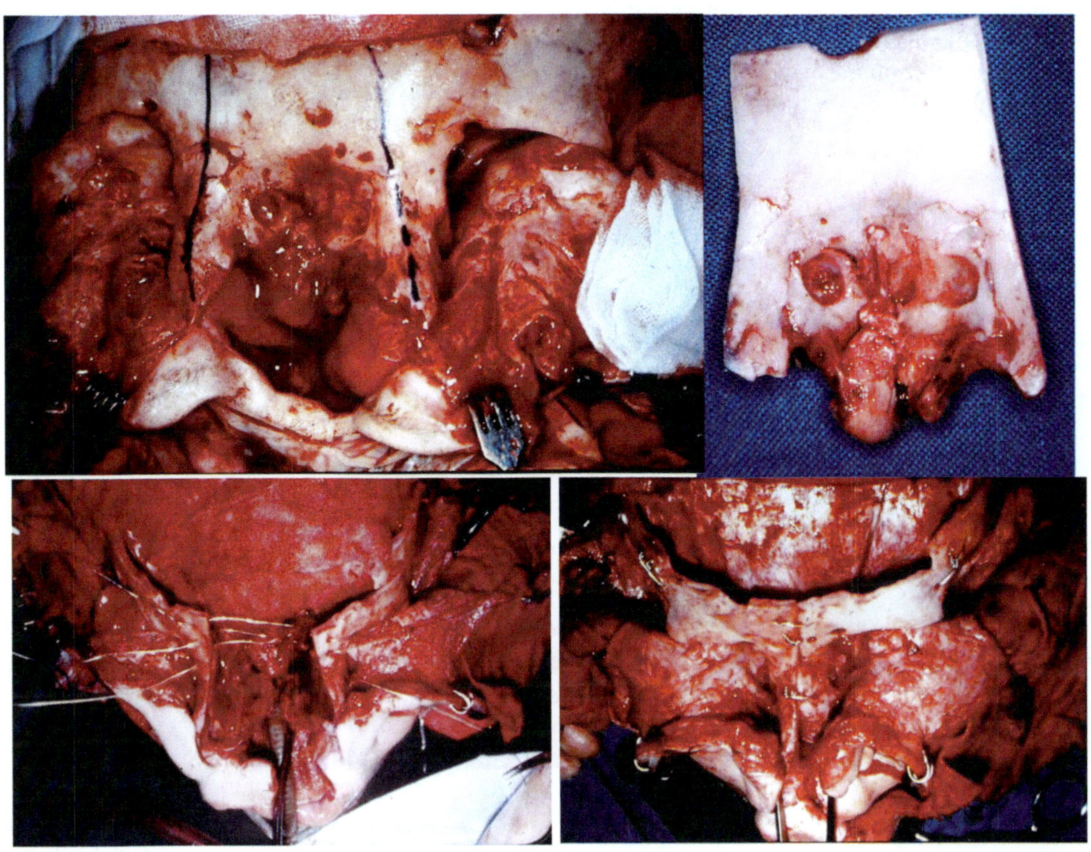

Fig. 1-21 Skeletal situation during and after correction plus excised part of forehead area.

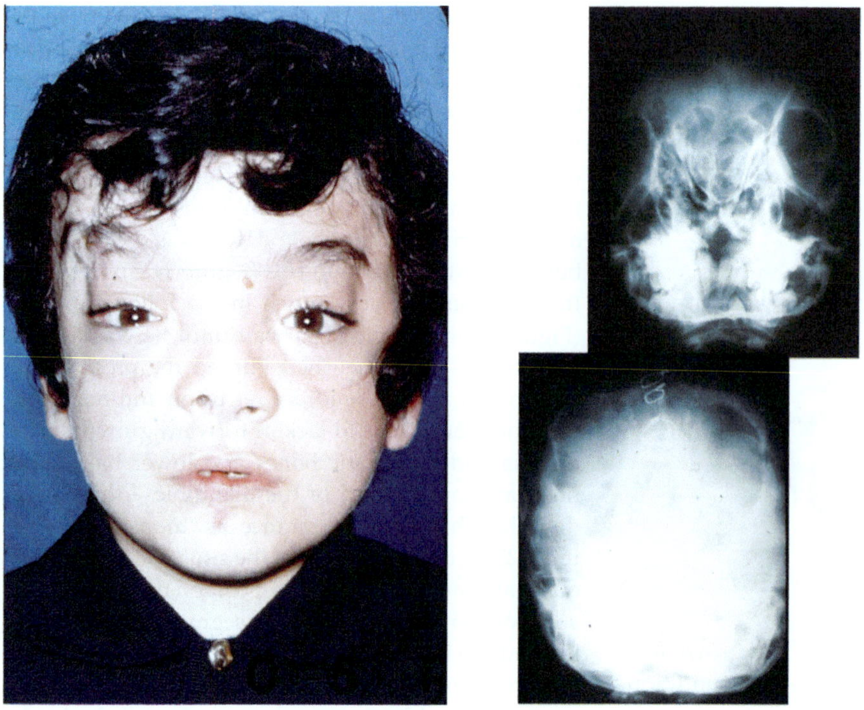

Fig. 1-22 Patient after surgery plus radiograph.

was good enough for his native town to employ him in the city's telephone business (Figures 1-29 and 1-30). His nasal airway was excellent and so was the view of the nose from below (Figure 1-31). Twenty-five years later I visited him in his home town in southern Italy. We met on the road like father and son, with much enthusiasm on both sides (Figure 1-32).

In summary, I must confess that I learnt a great deal by treating Antonio. First, to never give up, and second, to avoid operating on the maxilla until its growth has ceased. That is what I now advise every young colleague.

Recurrence

There are many possibilities for relapse and recurrence of a deformity. While a patient's skeletal growth has not ceased, there will always remain the possibility that further growth will alter the result of surgery. The mandible will continue to grow normally as long as the condyles have not been involved. On the contrary, the maxilla will almost cease to grow after it has been surgically exposed. A further cause for a postoperative change may be due to hyperactivity in the condyles growth regulators. We believe that there are two; one for growth in length and the other for growth of mass

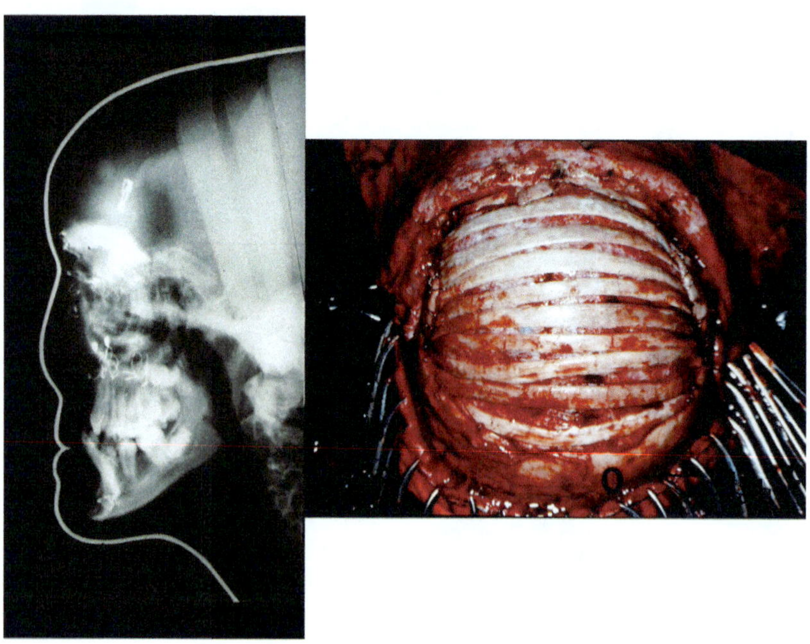

Fig. 1-23 Patients lateral skull radiograph after removal of cranial plate due to infection plus view of reconstruction of skull defect with 14 half ribs.

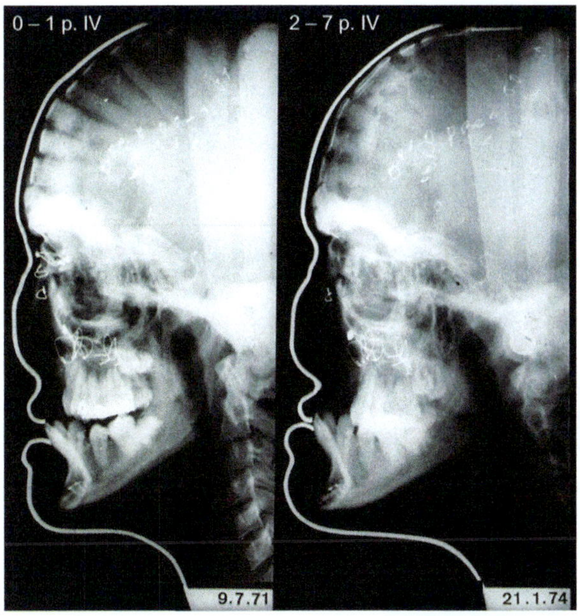

Fig. 1-24 Lateral scull view with slight retromaxillism on the left side and 2.5 years later with severe facial deformity.

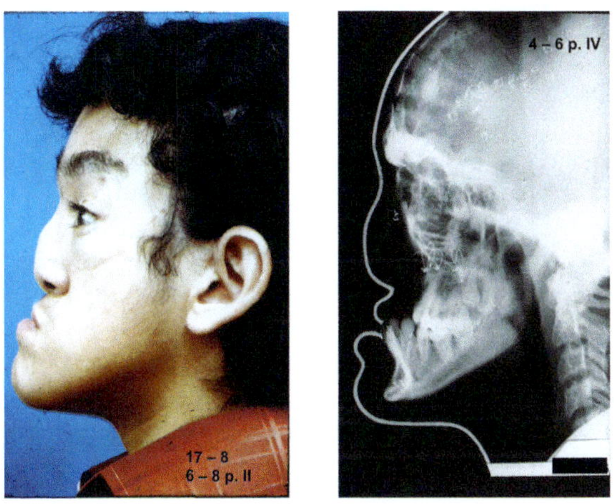

Fig. 1-25 Patients profile at age 17 years and 8 months and his lateral radiograph at age 18.

(Obwegeser and Makek, 1986).[30] The relapse following Schuchardt's procedure for correction of an anterior open bite due to the inferior position of the lateral maxillary alveolar segments is probably due to the fact that the maxillary sinuses are reduced in their size, without an additional connection to the nasal cavity. That was John Hovell's explanation when I discussed the problem with him; I think he was right. Muscular force may be another cause for relapse, certainly in cases with greater neuromuscular aetiology.

Special instruments

For all the procedures that I have developed, I also developed special instruments in order to make the surgery less difficult. These instruments facilitate the surgery to a great extent. For me, it was mandatory for these instruments to be available when I was operating. These surgical instruments are sold all over the world by various companies as 'Obwegeser Instruments'. Most of them are of no use in my hands as they have been altered from my original designs. Only the Medicon Company (in Tuttlingen, Germany) and KLS-Martin-Company (also in Tuttlingen, and in Jacksonville, PO Box 50249, Florida 32250-0244 USA) have asked me to check their instruments from time to time to guarantee permanent best quality according to my original designs.

The same is true with the surgical hand piece for the drill burr. The usual hand pieces are too short for our work in the depth of our operating fields. I asked W & H Dentalwerk Bürmoos (GmbH. Austria, 5111 Bürmoos), a famous Austrian hand piece producer for drill burrs, to make a longer hand piece, which can hold any burr with a shaft of 2.35 mm diameter. They were able to make it to my great satisfaction. I recommend it very much for working on the skull, in particular for the sagittal splitting technique. The same company also produces a special electro motor for use in surgery in the operating room.

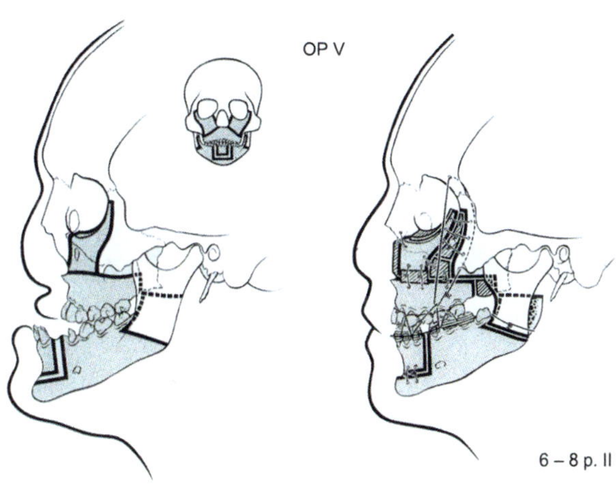

Fig. 1-26 Drawings of the skeletal situation and the planned correction.

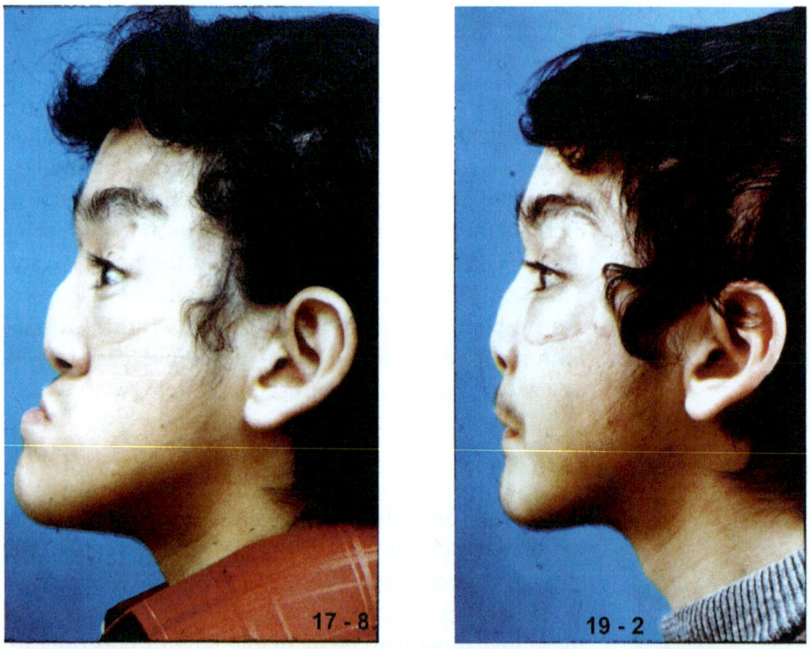

Fig. 1-27 Profile before and after surgical correction.

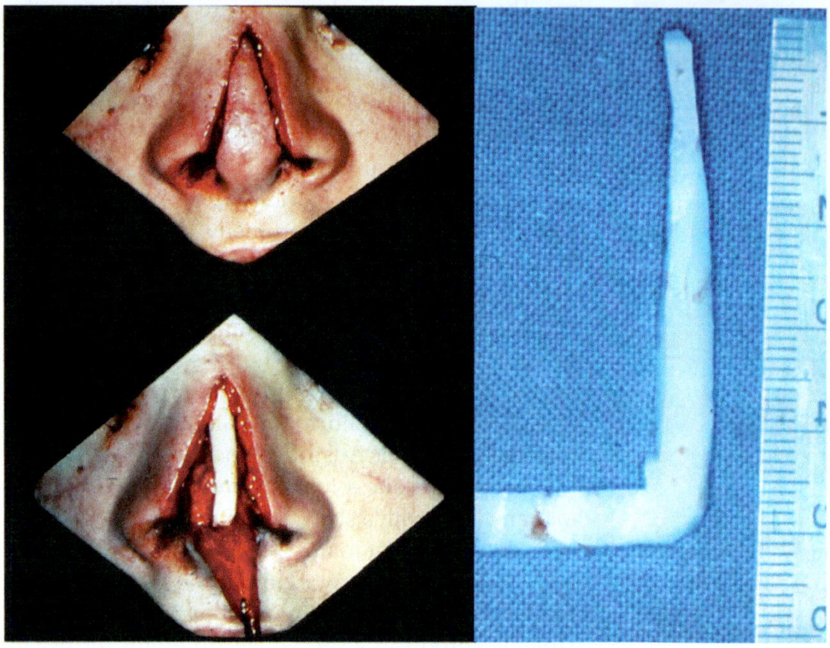

Fig. 1-28 Reconstruction of the missing columella by a caterpillar flap and reconstruction of the framework of the septum by an L-shaped cartilage graft from the ribs.

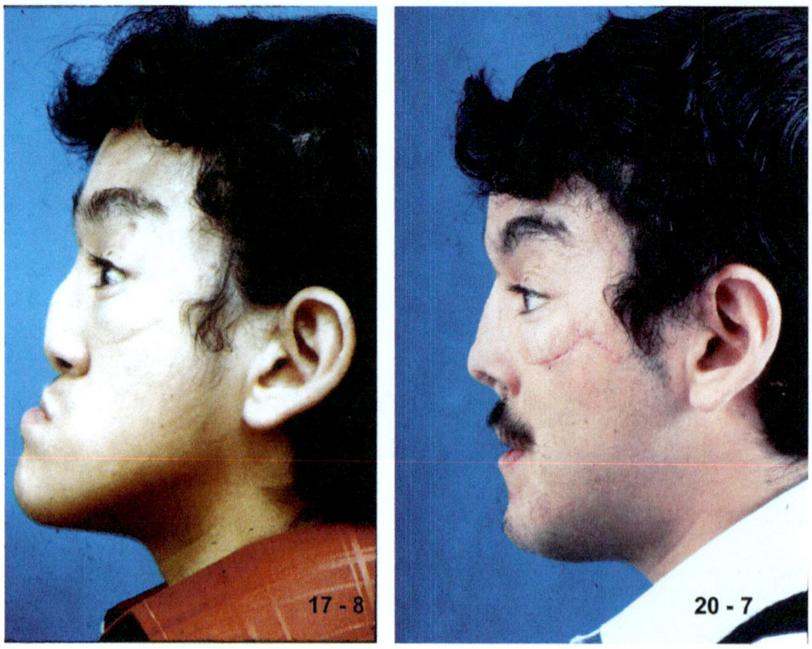

Fig. 1-29 Profile view of patient at age 17 years and 8 months, and 20 years and 7 months.

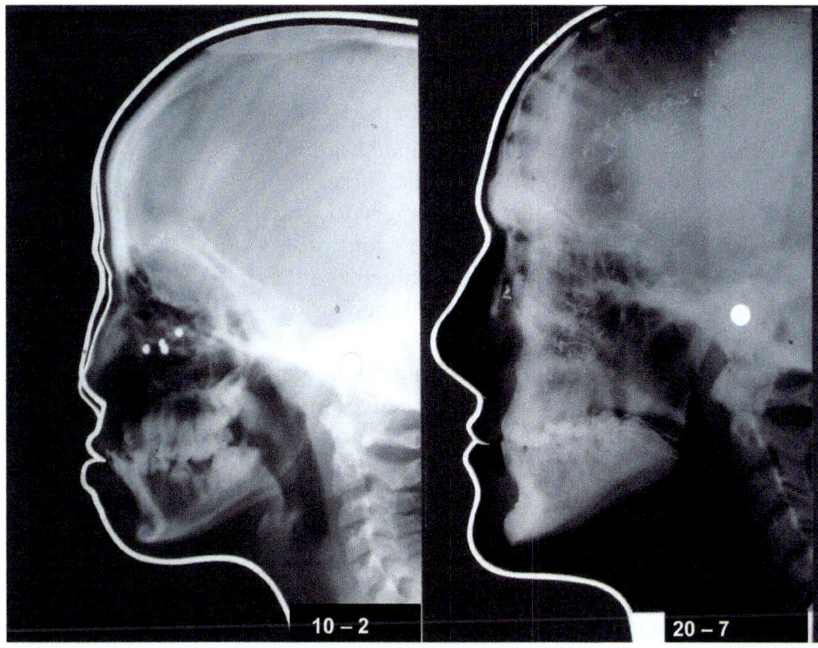

Fig. 1-30 Presurgical and final lateral cephalometric radiograph of the skull.

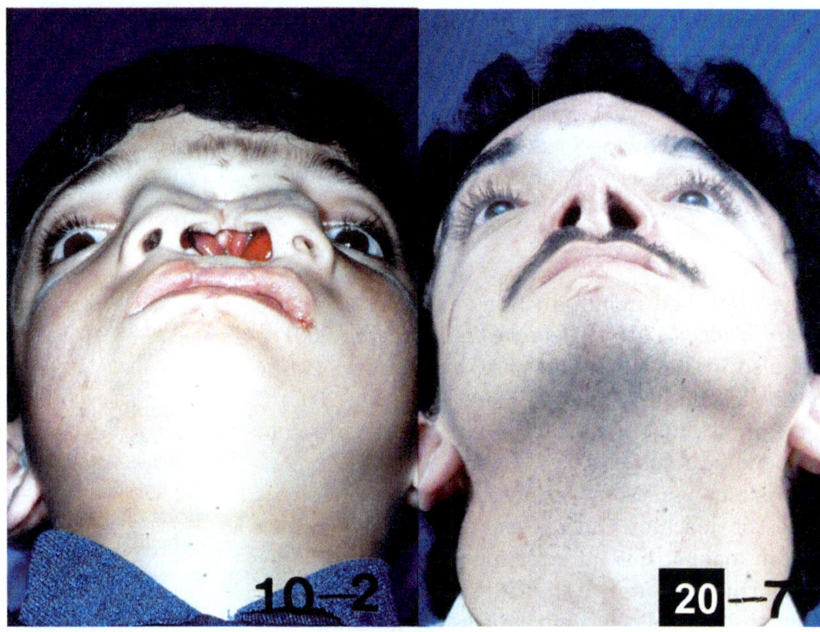

Fig. 1-31 View of the nose before surgery and the final result.

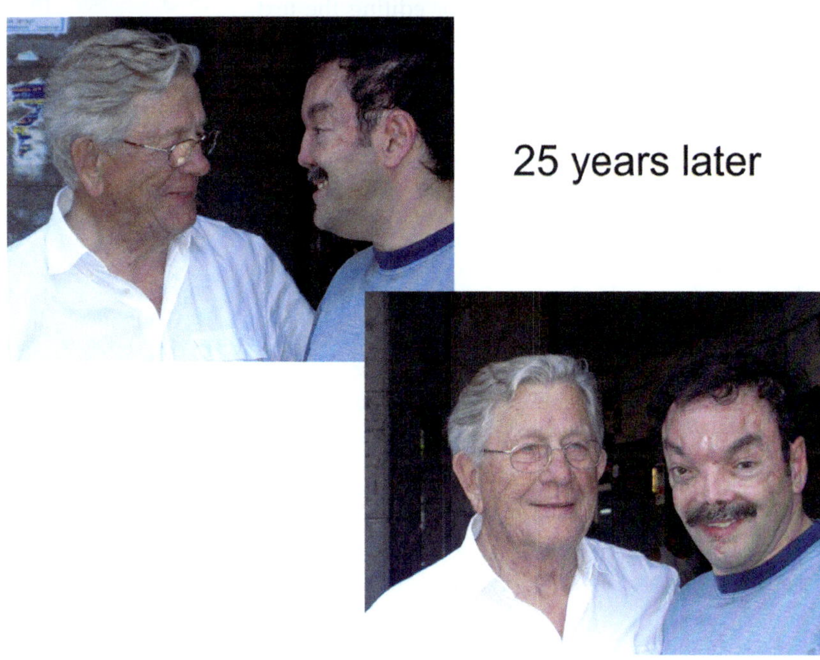

Fig. 1-32 The patient and his surgeon again 25 years after surgery.

Concluding remarks

I am delighted to be honoured with the dedication of this reference textbook on orthognathic surgery, the subspecialty of cranio-maxillofacial surgery to which I have devoted most of my working life and professional career. Dr Naini has gathered together many of the most famous names from around the world, in all the fields relevant to the treatment of the orthognathic patient – from cranio-maxillofacial surgery, orthodontics, facial plastic and reconstructive surgery, otorhinolaryngological surgery, psychiatry and other related specialties. As I write this introduction, at the age of 92, I am well aware that many of the distinguished contributing authors in this book have been my students, or students of my students. As such, many internationally-renowned centres devoted to cranio-maxillofacial and orthognathic surgery, around the world, are training second- and third-generation 'Obwegeser' students. It fills me with immense pride to know that the procedures I pioneered for the correction of dentofacial and craniofacial deformities are helping to improve the quality of life of countless patients, and allowing great professional satisfaction for the clinicians serving these patients.

Acknowledgements

I have published an introduction on this subject in my book *Mandibular Growth Anomalies* (Springer, 2001)[31] and also in an article published in *Clinics in Plastic Surgery* (Edited by Pravin K. Patel, Elsevier, 2007)[32]. Some of the illustrations used in this chapter are from these publications.

I wish to express my sincere thanks to my nephew, Professor Joachim Obwegeser, for his tremendous help in making this introduction possible for me by transferring my original slide illustrations onto a computer system. I also wish to express my gratitude and compliments to Dr Farhad Naini for editing the text and transferring it into proper English.

References

1 Blair VP. Operations on the jaw-bone and face. Surg Gynecol Obstet. 1907;4:67–78.
2 Kostečka F. Die chirurgische Therapie der Progenie. Zahnärztliche Rundschau. 1931;16:670–88.
3 Obwegeser HL. Surgical procedures to correct mandibular prognathism and reshaping of the chin. In: Trauner R, Obwegeser HL (Eds). The surgical correction of mandibular prognathism and retrognathia with consideration of genioplasty. Oral Surg Oral Med Oral Pathol. 1957;10:677–89.
4 Hofer O. Operation der Prognathie und Microgenie. Dtsch Zahn Mund Kieferheilk. 1942;9:121–32.
5 Neuner O. Chirurgische Orthodontie. Schweiz Monatschr Zahnheilkunde. 1965;75:940–4.
6 Obwegeser HL. Die einzeitige Vorbewegung des Oberkiefers und Rückbewegung des Unterkiefers zur Korrektur der extremen 'Progenie'. Schweiz Monatschr Zahnheilk. 1970;80:547–55.
7 Axhausen G. Zur Behandlung veralteter disloziert verheilter Oberkieferbruche. Dtsch Zahn Mund Kieferheilk. 1934;1:334–42.
8 Axhausen G. Ueber die korrigierende Osteotomie am Oberkiefer. Dtsch Z Chir. 1936;248:515–22.
9 Axhausen G. Die operative Orthopädie bei den Fehlbildungen der Kiefer. Dtsch Zahn Mund Kieferheilk. 1939;6:582–600.
10 Schuchardt K. Ein Betrag zur chirurgischen Kieferorthopädie unter Berucksichtigung ihrer Bedeutung fur die Behandlung angeborener und erworbener Kieferdeformitaten bei Soldaten. Dtsch Zahn Mund Kieferheilkd Zentralbl. 1942;9:73–89.
11 Drommer RB. The history of the 'Le Fort I osteotomy'. J Maxillofac Surg. 1986;14:119–22.
12 Obwegeser HL. Cirugia del 'mordex apertus'. Rev Asoc Odont Argent. 1962;50:430–41.
13 Obwegeser JA. Personal communication (1997).
14 Schuchardt K. Die chirurgie als helferin der kieferorthopädie. Fortschr Kieferorthop. 1954;15:1–25.
15 Dal Pont G. L'osteotomia retromolare per la correzione della progenia. Minerva Chir. 1959;14:1138–41.
16 Dal Pont G. Retromolar osteotomy for the correction of prognathism. J Oral Surg Anaesth Hosp D Serv. 1961;19:42–47.
17 Hunsuck EE. A modified intraoral sagittal splitting technique for correction of mandibular prognathism. J Oral Maxillofac Surg. 1968;26:250–3.
18 Epker BV. Modifications in the sagittal osteotomy of the mandible. J Oral Surg Anaesth. 1977;35:157–9.
19 Tessier P, Guiot G, Rougerie J, Delbet JP, Pastoriza J. Ostéotomies cranio-naso-orbito-faciales, hypertelorisme. Chir Plast. 1967;12:103.
20 Obwegeser HL. In: Trauner R, Obwegeser HL (Eds). Zur Operationstechnik bei der Progenie und anderen Unterkieferanomalien. Dtsch Zahn Mund Kieferheilkunde. 1955;23:11–26.
21 Obwegeser HL. Die Kinnvergrösserung. Oesterr Zschr Stomatol 1958;55:535–41.
22 Obwegeser HL. Der offene Biss in chirurgischer Sicht. Schweiz Monatschr Zahnheilk. 1964;74:668–87.
23 Obwegeser HL. Operative Behandlung der zahnlosen Progenie ohne intermaxilläre Fixation. Schweiz Monatschr Zahnheilk. 1968; 78:416–25.
24 Köle H. Kinnostektomie nach Köle. In: Reichenbach E, Köle H. (Eds). Chirurgische Kieferorthopädie, 2. Leipzi: Aufl Joh Ambros Barth, 1970.
25 Obwegeser JA. Eine neue Operationsmethode zur Osteotomie des gesamten Unterkiefer-Alveolarfortsatzed – vorläufiger Bericht. Dtsch Zahn Kiefer Gesichtschir. 1987;11:276–7.
26 Gillies HD, Rowe NL. L'ostéotomie du maxillaire supérieur enoisagée essentiellement dans le cas de bec-de-lièvre total. Rev Stomatol. 1954;55:545–52.
27 Obwegeser HL. Paper read at the First International Conference on Cleft Lip and Palate (1969).
28 Obwegeser HL. Surgical corrections of small or retrodisplaced maxillae. Plast Reconstr Surg. 1969;43:352–65.
29 Obwegeser HL, Weber G, Freihofer HP, Sailer HF. Facial duplication – the unique case of Antonio. J Maxillofac Surg. 1978;6:179–98.
30 Obwegeser HL, Makek MS. Hemimandibular hyperplasia – hemimandibular elongation. J Maxillofac Surg. 1986;14:183–208.
31 Obwegeser HL. Mandibular Growth Anomalies. Berlin Heidelberg: Springer, 2001.
32 Obwegeser HL. Orthognathic surgery and a tale of how three procedures came to be: A letter to the next generation of surgeons. In: Patel PK (Ed.). Orthognathic Surgery. Clin Plast Surg. 2007;34:331–55.

Part I: Principles and Planning

Chapter 2

Historical Evolution of Orthognathic Surgery

Farhad B. Naini

Introduction

'If you would understand anything, observe its beginning and its development.'

Aristotle (384–322 BC)[1]

A description of the historical evolution of orthognathic surgery will focus, inevitably, on which surgeon introduced which surgical procedure. However, despite the obvious importance of this information, orthognathic surgery is far more than just a series of surgical procedures used to move the jaws, or segments thereof. Diagnosis, including a four-dimensional analysis of a growing and ageing craniofacial complex, covered by a manifestly variable soft tissue envelope, and treatment planning with its intricacies and complexities, are the cornerstones of successful treatment. The developments in modern orthodontics permit accurate three-dimensional repositioning of the teeth with respect to their own jaw, making orthognathic surgery easier and more predictable (see Chapter 12); and developments in craniofacial imaging, particularly cephalometrics, has advanced diagnosis, planning and the analysis of treatment outcomes. Following on from all the technical procedures, the individual patient's psychosocial well-being determines the ultimate success of treatment. Therefore, all the individuals that have contributed to the understanding of the craniofacial complex, in terms of growth and development, ageing changes, diagnosis and treatment planning, the technical developments in surgery and orthodontics, and the psychological understanding of dentofacial and craniofacial deformities, have been significant in the development of this unique subspecialty of cranio-maxillofacial surgery and orthodontics.

The development of any specialty is almost always due to a universal, step-by-step progress. It is the culmination of the creativity of and improvements made by individuals that leads to the progress of medicine and science as an entity. The purpose of this chapter is to describe some of the milestones and pioneers in the historical evolution of orthognathic surgery.

A perfect chronological history of the evolution of orthognathic surgery is impossible. Various surgical procedures to reposition the maxilla, mandible and chin were being developed by different surgeons in different countries, sometimes simultaneously. The description that follows attempts to describe the evolution of the different surgical procedures based on each jaw, and the type of surgical procedure

Orthognathic Surgery: Principles, Planning and Practice. Edited by Farhad B. Naini and Daljit S. Gill.

undertaken, following chronological history as far as possible.

Mandibular osteotomies

'Study the past, if you would divine the future.'
Confucius (c. 551–479 BC)[2]

Mandibular body ostectomies and osteotomies

The first known surgical procedure that may be described as 'orthognathic' appears to have been by the American surgeon **Simon P. Hullihen** (1810–57) in 1849 (Figure 2-1).[3] Hullihen was born in Pennsylvania, and obtained his medical degree from Washington Medical College in Baltimore at the age of 22. He eventually settled in Wheeling, Virginia, where he decided to devote his practice to dentistry, oral surgery and surgery of the head and neck. The medical community treated him with disdain, and two medical students were put up to taking a chicken with a broken leg to Hullihen as a 'patient'. Instead of accepting this as an obvious practical joke, Hullihen accepted the 'patient', splinted its leg, and kept, fed and looked after it for 10 days, until its leg had healed. When the two popinjays predictably refused to pay, Hullihen took them to court and thereby obtained his fee.[4]

For his leadership in oral surgery, the Baltimore College of Dentistry (now the University of Maryland Dental School) awarded Hullihen an Honorary Doctor of Dental Surgery in 1842. Providing his Valedictory Address to the School's graduating class of 1850, He said: 'An efficacious union of medical and mechanical skill is the only course, the only plan to make an accomplished dental surgeon'.[4–6]

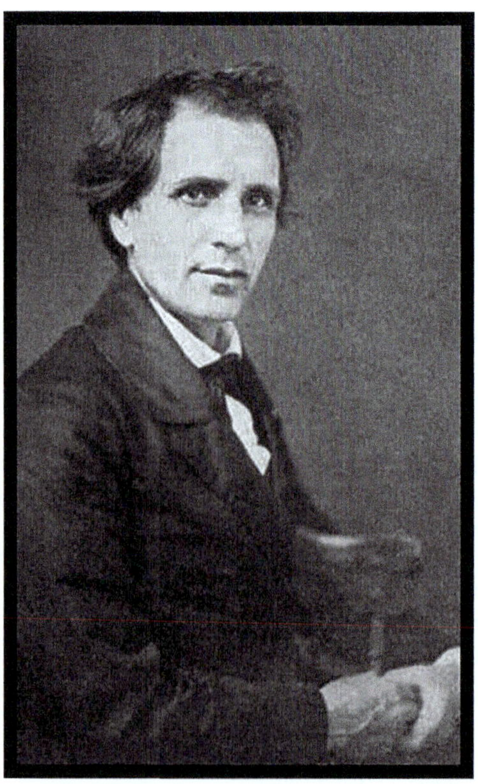

Fig. 2-1 Simon P. Hullihen (1810–1857).

Hullihen reported a case of surgical correction of a prognathic mandibular open bite deformity, which had developed in a female patient, 'Mary S' aged 20, secondary to severe burns of her neck and chest at the age of 5, with subsequent scar contractures. At the age of 7, two distinguished surgeons in New York had attempted a correction by dissecting underneath the scar, elevating her head, and leaving the exposed areas to heal by secondary intention. The patient presented to Hullihen with prominent mandibular incisors and anterior mandible, anterior open bite and an inferiorly positioned and everted lower lip (Figure 2-2a). Hullihen wrote:[3]

> 'Miss Mary S, aged 20, daughter of the Hon. Wm S., of Ohio, came to Wheeling in the Spring of 1848, to obtain relief from the effects of a very severe burn, which she received fifteen years before. The burn was primarily confined to the neck and lower part of the face, and its cicatrix produced a deformity of the most dreadful character. Her head was drawn forward and downward – the chin was confined within an inch of the sternum – the underlip was so pulled down that the mucous membrane of the left side came far below the chin – the under

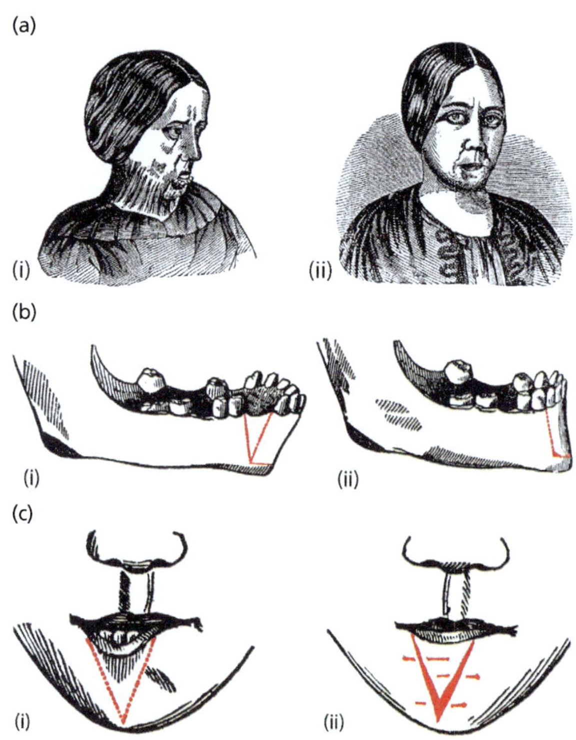

Fig. 2-2 (a)(i): Preoperative view of female patient, aged 20 years, following severe burns to the neck and chest 15 years earlier, and subsequent scar contractures and deformity of the anterior mandible. Hullihen undertook a wedge ostectomy and set-back of the anterior mandible via an intraoral approach, followed by two further surgical procedures for scar revision and lower lip revision. (a)(ii) 3 weeks postoperative result, following the final surgical procedure. (b)(i): Anterior subapical osteotomy and ostectomy; (b)(ii) Rotational set-back of the anterior mandibular dentoalveolar segment. (c): Diagram of the lip revision surgery. (After Hullihen,[3]).

jaw was bowed slightly downward, and elongated, particularly in its upper portion, which made it project about one inch and three eighths beyond the upper jaw… She was barely able to turn her head to either side… she could not close her jaws but for an instant, and then only by bowing her head forward; she could not retain her saliva for a single instant, and as might be expected, her articulation was very indistinct.'

On 12 June 1848, Hullihen removed a V-shaped wedge section bilaterally from the anterior mandible via a subapical osteotomy, and the anterior segment was repositioned, being posteriorly inclined and set-back, and fixed with wire ligatures (Figure 2-2b). On the right side an edentulous space between the canine and first premolar was utilized for the wedge resection and in the left quadrant by removing the first premolar. Impressions were taken to create dental stone models, on which he constructed a silver plate occlusal splint, which was cemented and left in situ for 6 weeks, allowing bony union. Hullihen specified that correcting her dental occlusion was important to help restore function. The patient was said to have complained of very little discomfort. On the 31 July, Hullihen mobilized a flap from her left shoulder and, having freed the contractures, secured the pedicled flap to her neck and chin. A month later, Hullihen revised the lower lip with a V-type incision and V-Y closure (Figure 2-2c). This pioneering procedure by Hullihen is all the more remarkable as it was performed intraorally, used the concept of immobilization of the osteotomized segments by means of an intraoral occlusal splint, and all without general anaesthesia or antibiotics.

Tragically, Hullihen's career was cut short at the age of 47, when he contracted typhoid pneumonia. His obituary in Wheeling read: 'amongst American surgeons he had no superior, probably no equal. In dentistry he was not equaled in America'.

Another operation to reduce mandibular prognathism was not undertaken again for almost 50 years. James Whipple (1898)[7] reported a patient, 'Mr K', whom he had followed up for a number of years noting, 'the lower maxilla was found to be significantly prognathic, with a space appearing between the first and second bicuspids.'

Note:

The etymology of the term 'maxilla' requires explanation (*Latin* 'maxilla': a jawbone, either upper or lower).[8] In early anatomical texts the term 'maxilla' literally meant 'jaw', i.e. 'upper maxilla' referred to the maxilla, and the 'lower maxilla' referred to the mandible. This is the etymology of the term **bimaxillary**, which means pertaining to the maxilla and mandible, e.g. bimaxillary prognathism, bimaxillary surgery etc. The alternative term for 'bimaxillary' is 'maxillomandibular.' Early texts and published articles often referred to the mandible as the 'lower maxilla' or 'inferior maxilla'.

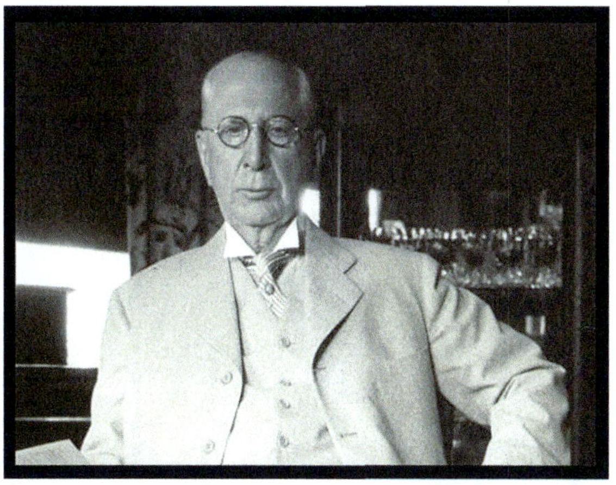

Fig. 2-3 Edward Hartley Angle (1855–1930) (Courtesy of The University of Arizona).

Whipple referred the patient to **Edward H. Angle** (1855–1930) in 1896 (Figure 2-3), recognized as one of the pioneers of modern orthodontics, who suggested 'a double resection of the lower maxilla to correct a severe protrusion'.[9] The patient decided against having the surgery. In 1897, **Vilray Papin Blair** (Figure 2-4) (1871–1955) performed the first 'double resection of the mandible' on the same patient, which was essentially a bilateral ostectomy of the mandibular body via an extraoral approach, with parallel cuts in the premolar regions and removal of the osteotomized blocks. Copper wire interosseous ligatures secured the bony segments (Figure 2-5). Four months later Whipple constructed gold crowns for the posterior dentition to 'improve the occlusion'. Following Whipple's publication of Blair's procedure,[7] which was written without Blair who was out of the country

(a)

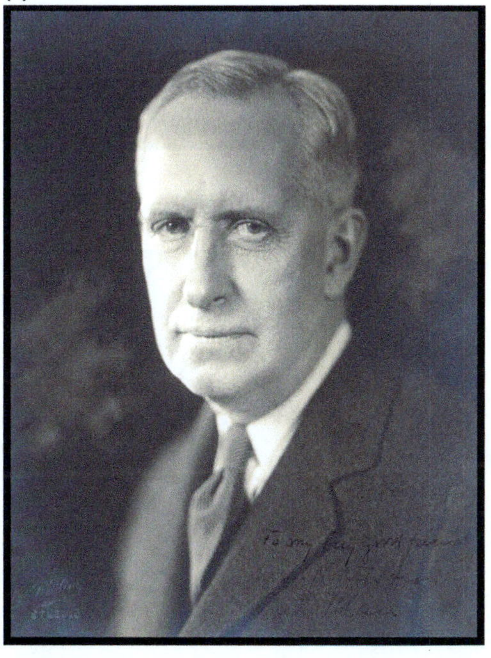

Fig. 2-4 Vilray Papin Blair (1871–1955), through the ages.

(b)

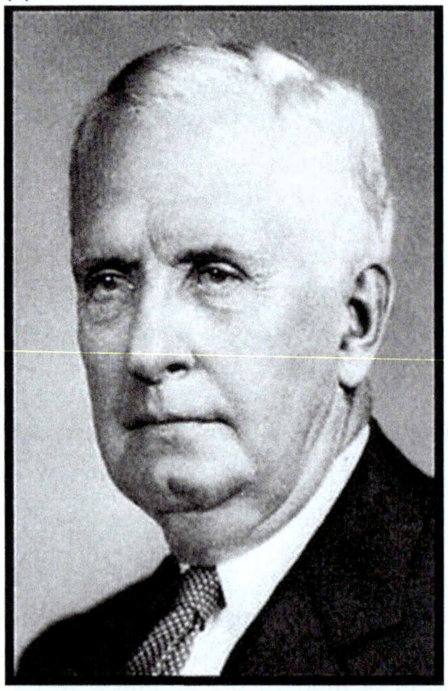

(c)

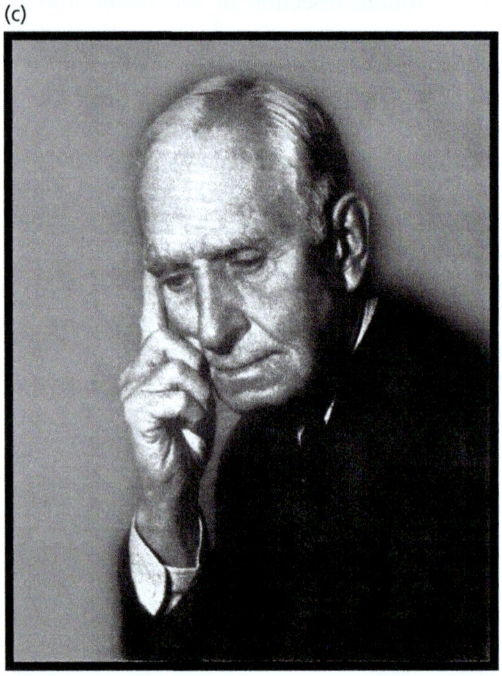

Fig. 2-4 (*Continued*).

(a)

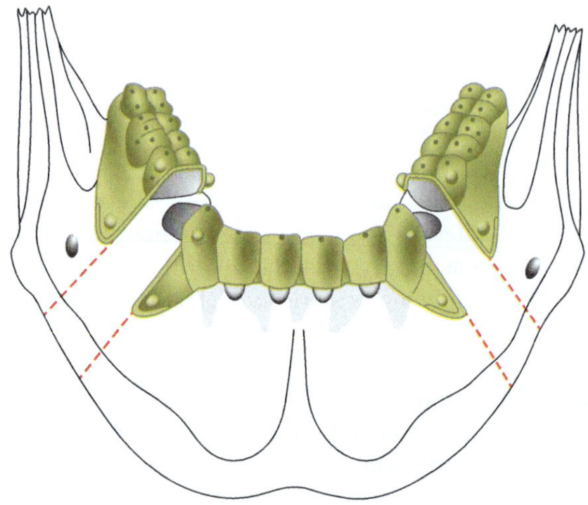

(b)

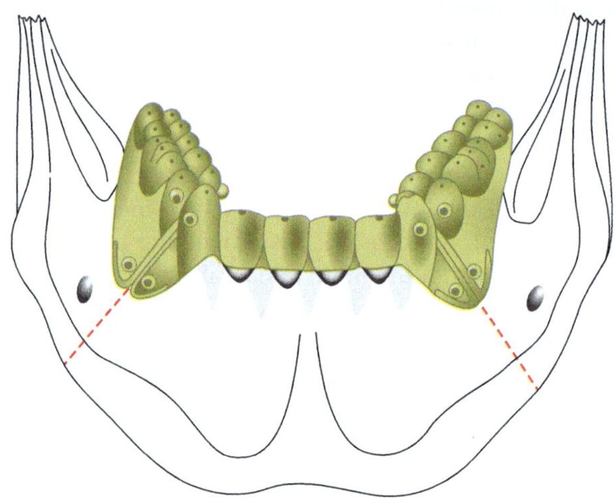

Fig. 2-6 Cast gold splints for postoperative fixation, suggested by Edward Angle, (a): pre-mandibular body ostectomy, (b): postoperative.

at the time, Angle commented that a V-section should have been used, as well as cast gold splints for postoperative fixation (Figure 2-6). **Rodrigues Ottolengui** (1861–1937) (Figure 2-7),[10] a leading American dentist and orthodontist, criticized Angle's splint, and suggested that a single template splint should have been

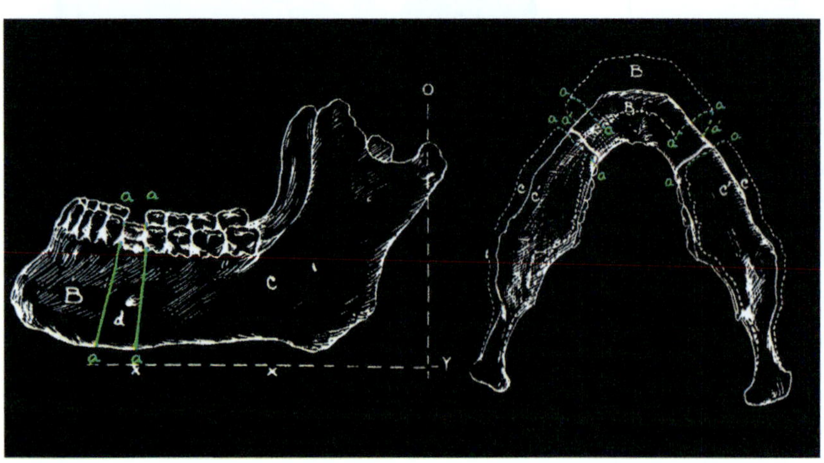

Fig. 2-5 Blair's mandibular body ostectomy, undertaken in 1897.

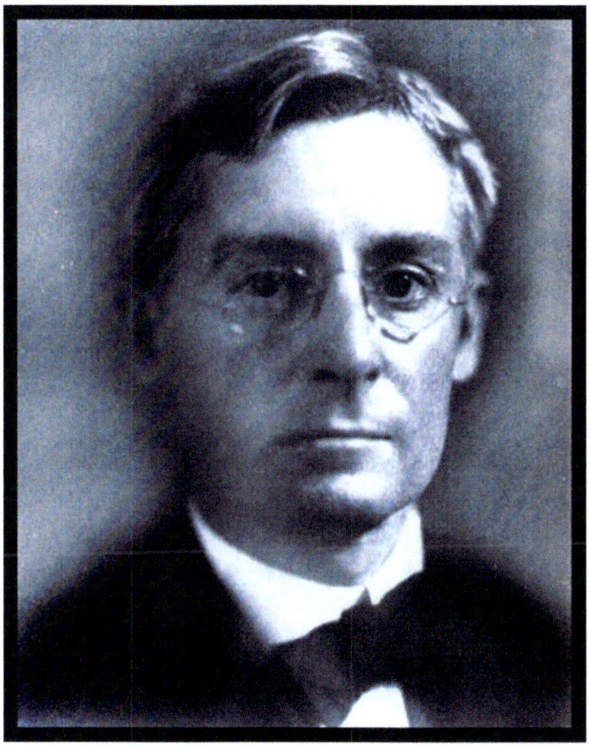

Fig. 2-7 Rodrigues Ottolengui (1861–1937).

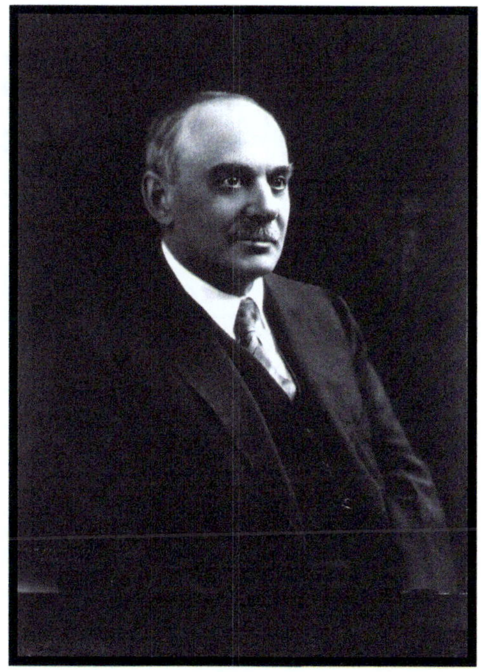

Fig. 2-9 Max Ballin (1869–1934).

used, representing the predetermined postoperative dental occlusion, with the teeth being cemented to the splint following the ostectomy (Figure 2-8). In this respect, Ottolengui appears to have been ahead of his time, as modern surgical wafer splints are a modification of this advice. Nevertheless, Ottolengui did state the following: 'I have no doubt that in advancing the proposed procedure, Dr Angle aims to aid surgeons of the future who might undertake this operation in collaboration with dentists, or, better still, with orthodontists.' Blair, who had performed the operation in 1897, only gave his account in 1906.[11,12] Although Hullihen's procedure had been performed without anaesthesia, Blair had used chloroform, though antibiotics were still not available. In 1908, **Max Ballin** (1869–1934) (Figure 2-9), a surgeon from Detroit (Michigan),[13] suggested removing the teeth at the site of the proposed mandibular body ostectomy a few months prior to the surgery. He wrote:

> 'I would recommend ... to extract the teeth, necessary to remove for the resection, first, and then wait some months until the extraction wound is completely healed and atrophy of the alveolar process on the place of extraction has taken place. Then the surgeon can proceed, as in our case; that is, excise a piece of the jaw without entering the oral cavity ... '

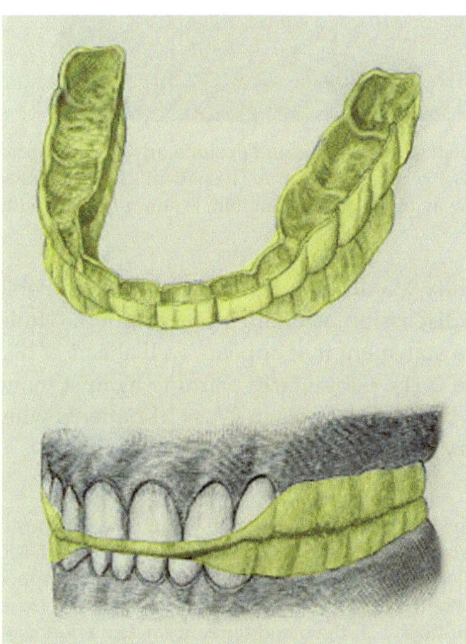

Fig. 2-8 Ottolengui surgical splint.

Therefore, as the mandibular body ostectomies were being undertaken via an extraoral approach, this would potentially reduce the contamination of the external surgical site from intraoral pathogens. Ballin's paper was presented before the American Society of Orthodontists at Detroit, and the paper published in the journal edited by Ottolengui (Figure 2-10a–c). The discussion following Ballin's presentation is noteworthy. The chairman, Dr Pullen, said:[13]

> 'I assure you it has been a great treat to me to hear a clinical talk of this kind by so eminent a surgeon as Dr Ballin has proclaimed himself to be by the results attained in treatment. *It is the first time in the history of the American Society of Orthodontists that such a clinic has been given*, and we are glad to have such a record as the work which has been done so successfully for its kind as shown this morning... .Now we, as orthodontists, do not pretend to tell the surgeon anything that is new to him, but there is no doubt that the medical profession can profit by suggestions from the dental profession, and vice

(a) (b) (c)

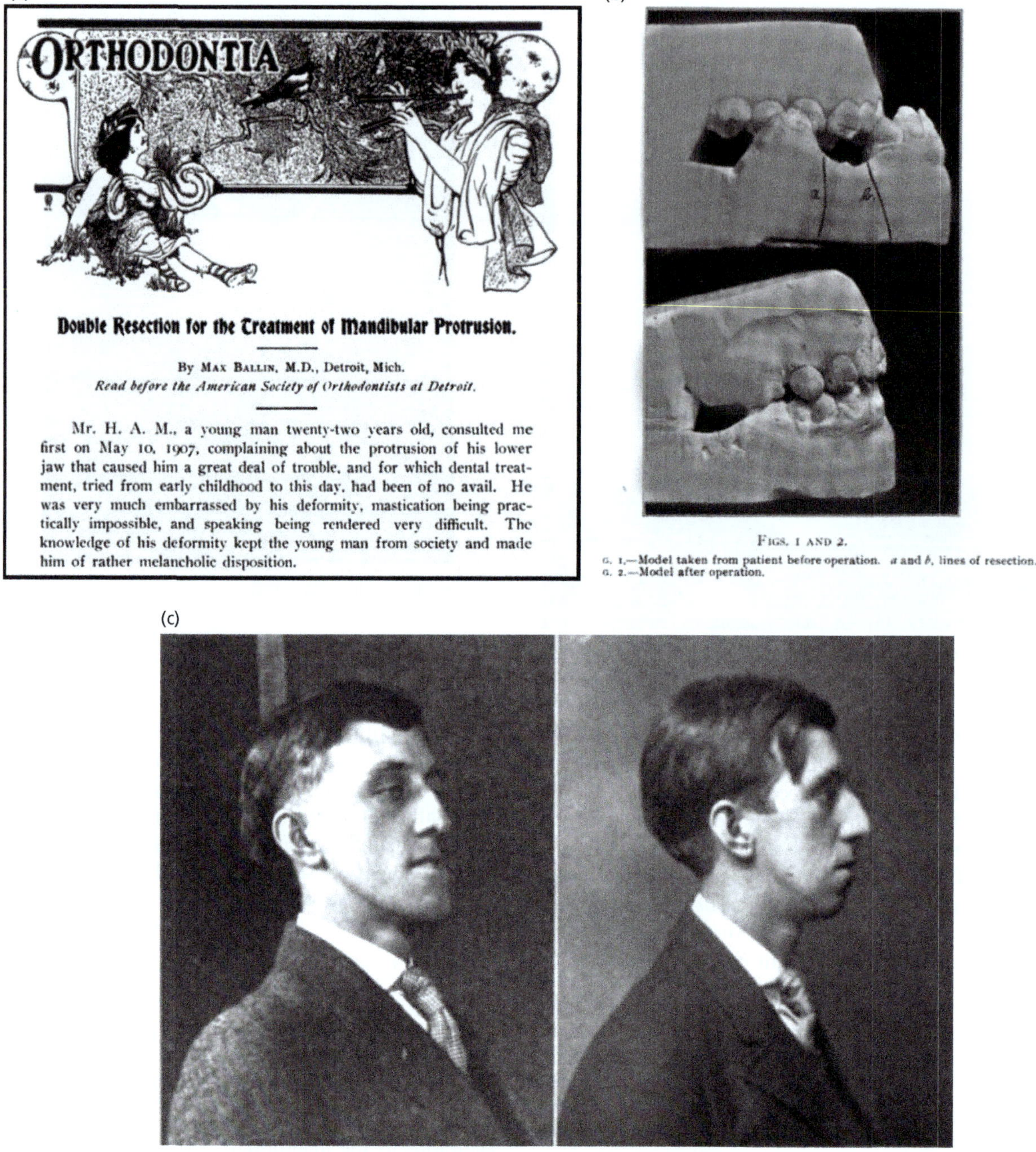

ORTHODONTIA

Double Resection for the Treatment of Mandibular Protrusion.

By Max Ballin, M.D., Detroit, Mich.
Read before the American Society of Orthodontists at Detroit.

Mr. H. A. M., a young man twenty-two years old, consulted me first on May 10, 1907, complaining about the protrusion of his lower jaw that caused him a great deal of trouble, and for which dental treatment, tried from early childhood to this day, had been of no avail. He was very much embarrassed by his deformity, mastication being practically impossible, and speaking being rendered very difficult. The knowledge of his deformity kept the young man from society and made him of rather melancholic disposition.

a
b
Figs. 1 and 2.
G. 1.—Model taken from patient before operation. *a* and *b*, lines of resection.
G. 2.—Model after operation.

Fig. 2-10 (a): Ballin's paper from 1908;[13] (b): Patient's dental models; (c): Patient's preoperative and postoperative facial appearance. Towards the end of his presentation, Ballin said: 'The result, as you can see, is a very favorable one. The patient's facial expression is very much improved, and the young man, who formerly was shy and kept away from society, I am told, is now a favorite with young ladies.'

> versa, and by this cooperation we will further and better our practices and benefit humanity thereby.' [Emphasis added]
>
> The chairman went on to say, 'We want to know more about it [jaw surgery] so as to be able to speak with absolute authority with reference to these operations. We want to see more of them.'

The patient presented by Ballin would today probably benefit from bimaxillary surgery, with a maxillary advancement and mandibular set-back. Historically, the ability to reposition the mandible in a stable manner long preceded the ability to reposition the maxilla. As a consequence, many patients underwent only mandibular surgery to correct a primarily maxillary deformity. Maxillary surgery was not yet available, but in the discussion of Ballin's presentation, Ottolengui made a statement that appears well ahead of his time (Figure 2-11), particularly warning against mandibular set-back procedures in Class III patients when the primary aetiology was maxillary retrusion:[13]

> '... the resection of a portion of a mandible which is of normal size in order to make it fit an upper arch which is underdeveloped, is analogous to the extraction of two upper teeth to make the upper arch harmonize with a lower arch which is too small... .If the mandible is normal an effort should be made to put the abnormal part (in this case the maxilla) right, *thus making the abnormal fit the normal.*' [Emphasis added]

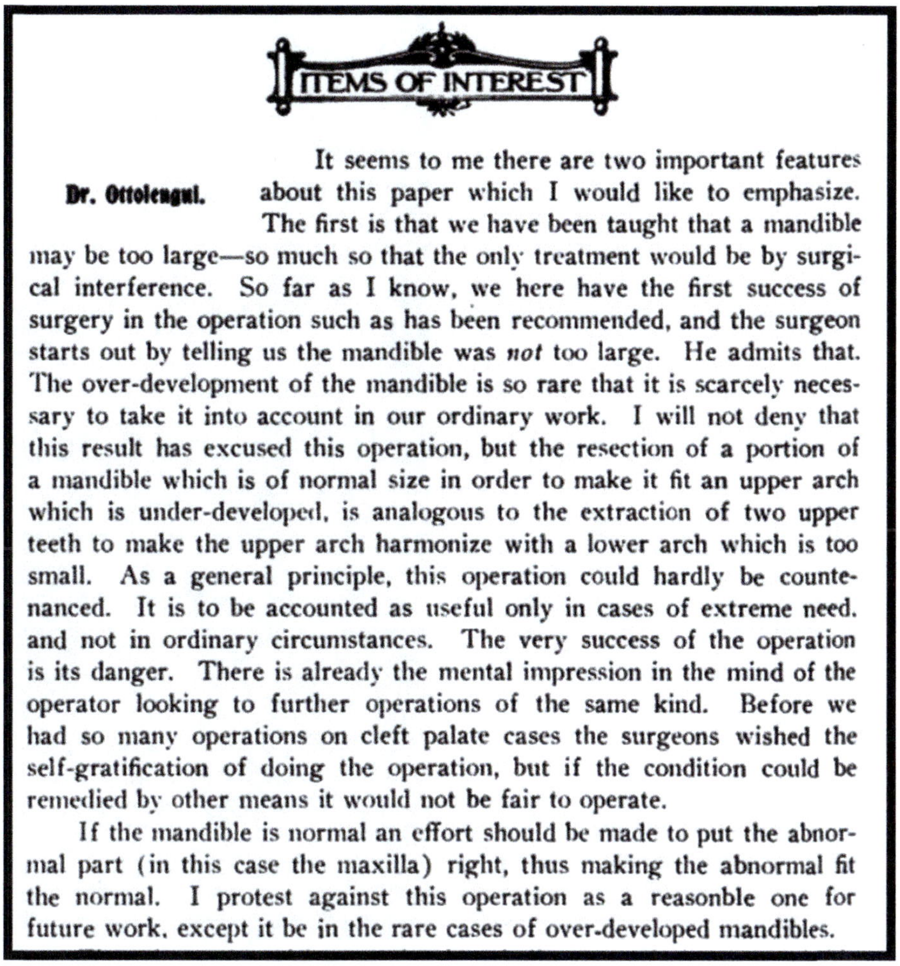

ITEMS OF INTEREST

Dr. Ottolengui. It seems to me there are two important features about this paper which I would like to emphasize. The first is that we have been taught that a mandible may be too large—so much so that the only treatment would be by surgical interference. So far as I know, we here have the first success of surgery in the operation such as has been recommended, and the surgeon starts out by telling us the mandible was *not* too large. He admits that. The over-development of the mandible is so rare that it is scarcely necessary to take it into account in our ordinary work. I will not deny that this result has excused this operation, but the resection of a portion of a mandible which is of normal size in order to make it fit an upper arch which is under-developed, is analogous to the extraction of two upper teeth to make the upper arch harmonize with a lower arch which is too small. As a general principle, this operation could hardly be countenanced. It is to be accounted as useful only in cases of extreme need, and not in ordinary circumstances. The very success of the operation is its danger. There is already the mental impression in the mind of the operator looking to further operations of the same kind. Before we had so many operations on cleft palate cases the surgeons wished the self-gratification of doing the operation, but if the condition could be remedied by other means it would not be fair to operate.

If the mandible is normal an effort should be made to put the abnormal part (in this case the maxilla) right, thus making the abnormal fit the normal. I protest against this operation as a reasonble one for future work, except it be in the rare cases of over-developed mandibles.

Fig. 2-11 Ottolengui's response to Ballin's paper. (From Ballin,[13]).

Matthew Henry Cryer (1840–1921) (Figure 2-12),[14] the English-born American Professor of Oral Surgery at the University of Pennsylvania (and uncle to Robert H. Ivy) founded the first hospital dental service in America, at the Philadelphia General Hospital, developed an electrically operated surgical engine for cutting bone in jaw surgery, and gave his name to the 'Cryer's elevators' used in surgical dentistry. Cryer suggested a semi-circular osteotomy near the angle of the mandible, which permitted vertical rotation of the mandibular body (Figure 2-13). However, the technique resulted in a posterior open bite and did not win favour. Interestingly, Cryer pointed out:[14]

> 'It may be possible in some cases to make the incision high enough in the ramus to avoid cutting the inferior dental nerve and vessels, or, if the incision were made so that the center of the curve could come above the inferior dental foramen, the severing of the nerve might be avoided. The parts could be held together by wire sutures, assisted by a maxillo-mandibular splint, which should be made before the operation. There would be no danger of septic conditions if the operation were performed with surgical care, but when a section is removed from the body of the bone it is impossible to avoid infection.'

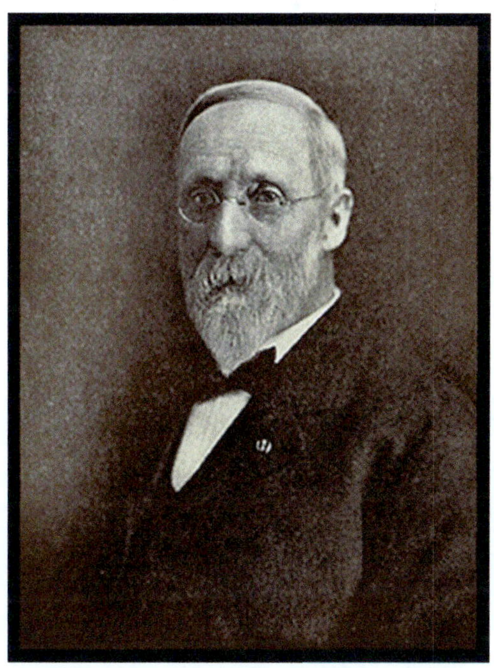

Fig. 2-12 Matthew Henry Cryer (1840–1921). (Courtesy of Historical Collections & Archives, Oregon Health & Science University).

A number of surgeons continued body ostectomies of the mandible from an extraoral approach, but

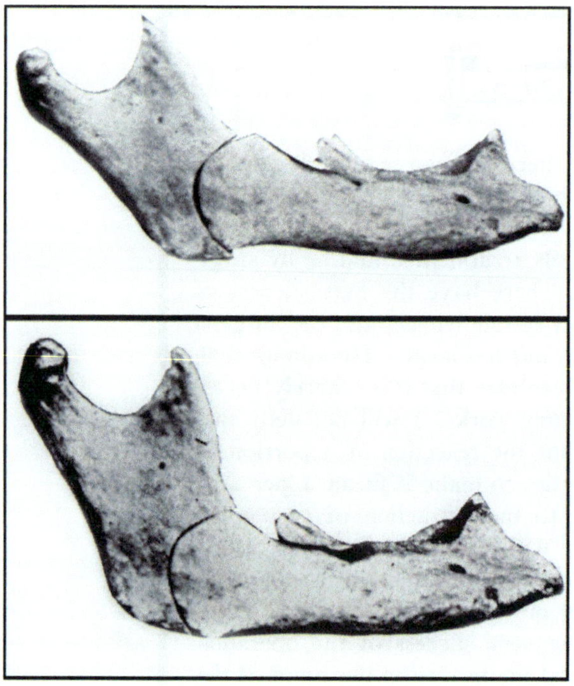

Fig. 2-13 Cryer's semi-circular osteotomy (1913). (From Cryer,[14]).

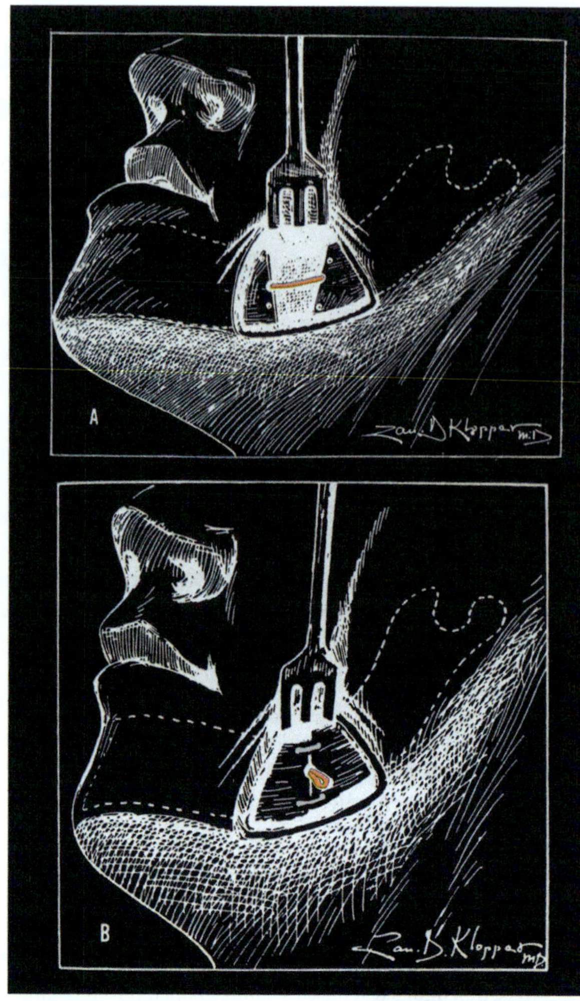

Fig. 2-15 Harsha's extraoral mandibular body resection, maintaining the integrity of the neurovascular bundle (1912). (After Harsha,[16]).

contamination of the extraoral wound created postoperative complications. In 1917, **Thomas G. Aller**[15] described removal of the bony wedge via an intraoral approach (Figure 2-14). At the end of his paper, Aller noted, 'We consider the banding of several teeth on each side the best fixation for occlusion… A competent dentist, preferably an orthodontist, should be associated with all such cases, as the upper jaw may need to be widened before the operation on the mandible is undertaken. Likewise the services of the orthodontist may be needed for some time after the operation.' However, all these techniques compromised the neurovascular bundle. Nevertheless, 5 years earlier, **William M. Harsha** (1912)[16,17] performed an extraoral mandibular body resection, but managed to maintain the integrity of the neurovascular bundle (Figure 2-15). In 1931, at the Second International Orthodontic Congress held in London, Kazanjian (see later) presented five cases of mandibular prognathism that he had treated with body ostectomies using an extraoral approach, both using a Gigli saw and a surgical bur, with postoperative immobilization using an intraoral orthodontic appliance. These cases were subsequently published in 1932 (Figure 2-16a–f).[18]

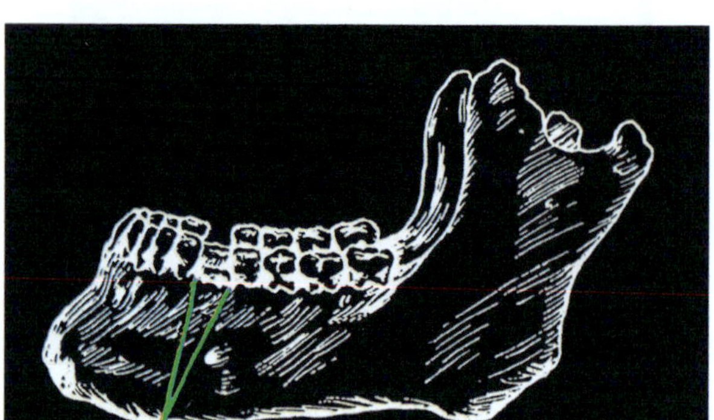

Fig. 2-14 Aller's description of removal of a bony wedge via an intraoral approach (1917). (After Aller,[15]).

The importance of postoperative immobilization to prevent non-union of the segments was gaining recognition. In 1906, **Anton Freiherr von Eiselsberg** (1860–1939) (Figure 2-17a), Professor of Surgery in Vienna and previously a student of Theodor Billroth,[19] suggested a step-ostectomy to increase the surface area for contact (Figure 2-17b), and his technique was advocated by Hans Pichler and Richard Trauner in 1948.[20] The respected British oral surgeons **Ben Fickling** and **Gordon Fordyce** (1955) (Figure 2-18),[21] and **John Herbert Hovell** (1910–88) (1956) (Figure 2-19),[22] an oral surgeon and orthodontist at the Royal Dental and St Thomas' Hospitals in London, suggested the use of cancellous bone chips from the iliac crest to promote bony union, and Edward C. Armbrecht et al. (1957)[23] suggested using cancellous bone from the resected bone of the mandible. Hovell[22] also warned against

(a) (b)

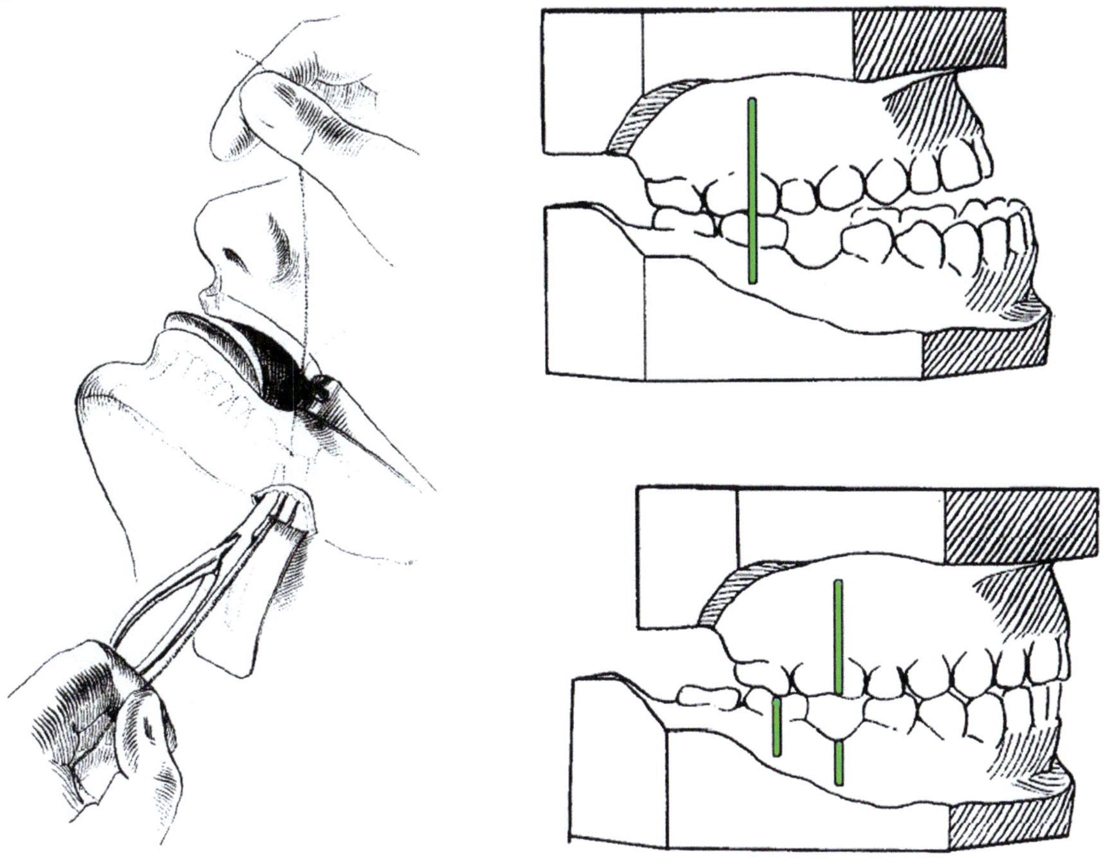

(c) (d)

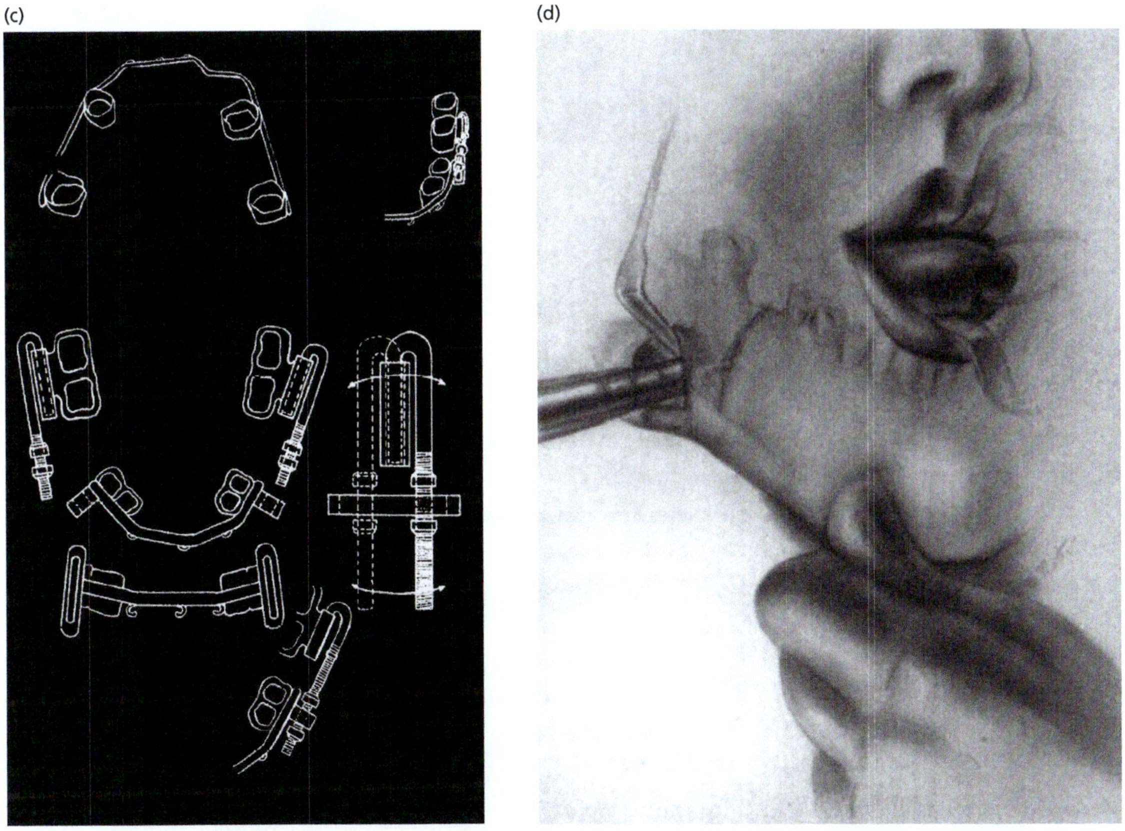

Fig. 2-16 (a): Kazanjian's use of a Gigli saw for a mandibular body ostectomy and set-back (1932). (b): measuring the amount of bone removal required using study models; (c): Orthodontic splint, cemented preoperatively; (d): Use of a surgical bur for an ostectomy (on a different patient), for mandibular set-back and closure of an anterior open bite. (e): Preoperative anterior open bite; (f): Postoperative result. Kazanjian achieved this by (a): 'cut through the mandible at the molar region on each side and elevate the anterior segment to meet the maxillary teeth.' This is an early description of closure of an anterior open bite with an isolated mandibular procedure. (After Kazanjian,[18]).

(e)

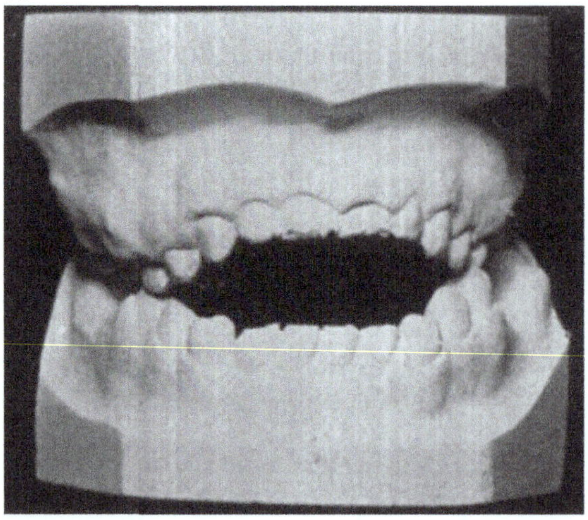

(f)

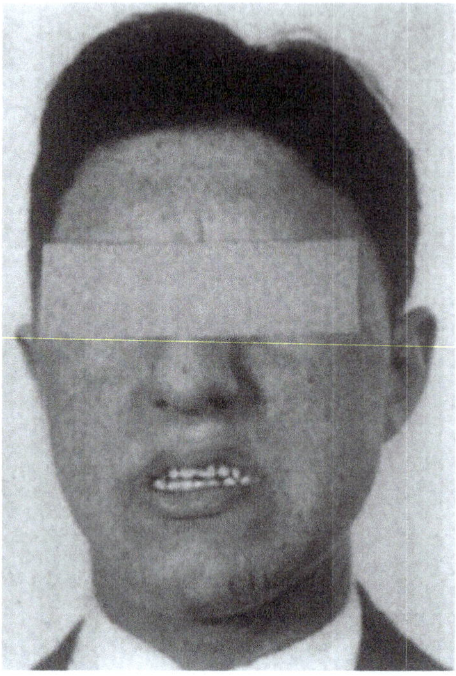

Fig. 2-16 (*Continued*)

(a)

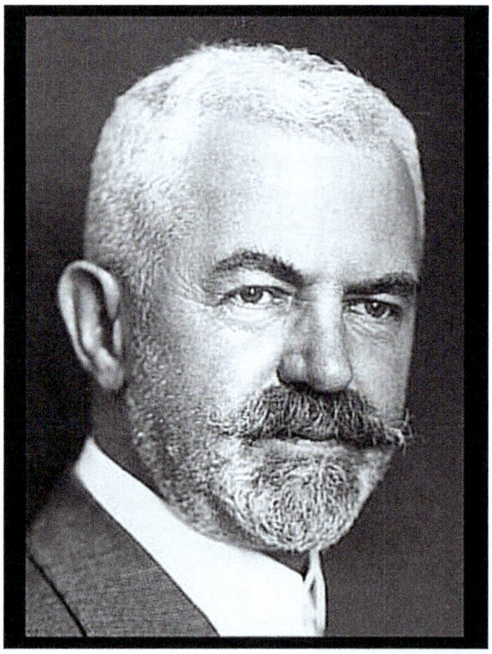

(b)

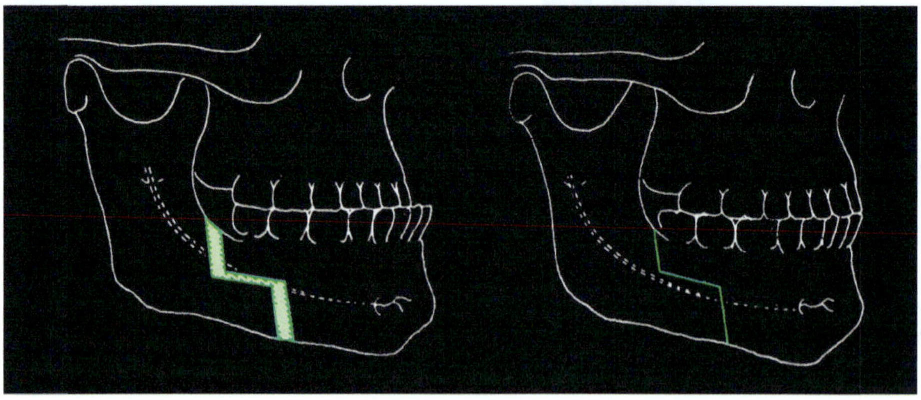

Fig. 2-17 (a): Anton Freiherr von Eiselsberg (1860–1939). (b): step-ostectomy. (After von Eiselsberg,[19]).

31 *Section of Odontology* 989

anæsthesia. 12.3.55: Cavity has completely healed. Almost completely recovered from mental anæsthesia. Radiograph shows bone cavity filling with great rapidity. 2.4.55: No mental anæsthesia.

Pathological report (Professor R. B. Lucas).—(1) Fragments of normal bone and blood clot. There is no epithelium or connective tissue present and no evidence of odontogenic cyst formation or of neoplasia. The appearances are in keeping with the diagnosis of hæmorrhagic bone cyst. (2) The |5 shows an occlusal cavity but is not otherwise grossly abnormal.

Mandibular Osteotomy for Facial Asymmetry.—B. W. Fickling, F.R.C.S., F.D.S., and G. L. Fordyce, F.D.S.

S. F., female, aged 19.

History.—Congenital facial asymmetry. No familial history. No evidence of condylar hyperplasia. Marked deviation of the mandible to the right side with slight prognathism.

Preparation.—13.12.54: 8|8 removed. Models of teeth mounted on plaster mandible. New articulation devised and cosmetic result assessed. Site and amount of sections determined. Splints fitted to the teeth and pre-arranged locking bars prepared.

Operation.—9.2.55: Bilateral mandibular osteotomy with chip bone graft from right iliac crest. The inferior dental bundles were exposed prior to section and were not divided. On the left side 7 mm. of bone were removed in |8 region and on the right side the mandible was merely sectioned. The posterior fragments were immobilized by interosseus wiring to the main body fragment, which was held by cap splints to the upper jaw.

Follow-up.—Ninth day: Patient discharged home. No mental anæsthesia. Fifth week: *All fixation discarded;* firm clinical union. Seventh week: Case demonstrated.

Fig. 2-18 Fickling and Fordyce technical note describing iliac crest bone graft (1955,[21]).

the stretching of the muscles attached to the mandibular ramus and the potential for relapse:

> 'The relapse to an anterior open bite which may occur if union is delayed or fixation is removed too soon is due to a different cause. It is, I think, muscular imbalance and due to the pull of the internal pterygoid upon the backwardly displaced ascending ramus. This question of muscular imbalance is, I think, a most important one. The words of a well known orthopaedic surgeon with whom I discussed this question were, "If you're fighting muscle, you must look out for trouble". I do not think it possible permanently to stretch muscles, and if an elevator, for example the internal pterygoid, is stretched as must be the case in many ascending ramus slides either it will produce a relapse or retention must be maintained until there is actual shift of the muscle attachment. We know that this type of shift occurs during growth and I think that it happens after ascending ramus slides. But it takes time, and is another reason why prolonged retention may be necessary in these cases. Using the open approach, I find no difficulty in stripping the attachment of the internal pterygoid, and thus facilitating its reattachment in a new position.'

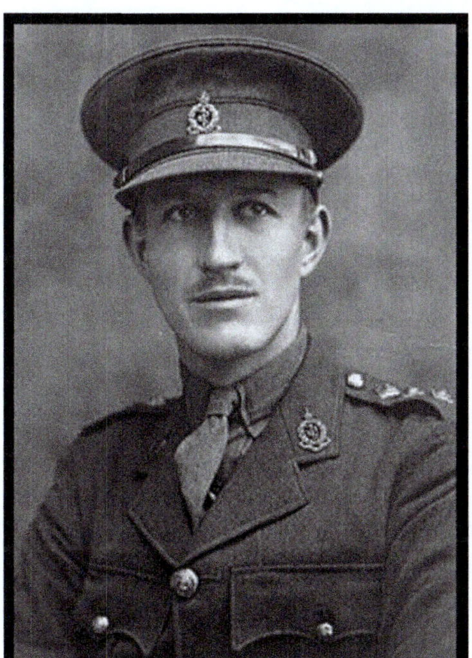

Fig. 2-19 John Herbert Hovell (1910–1988). (Courtesy of Journal of Medical Biography, Sage Publications).

Hovell[22] also described another potential problem that may follow a mandibular set-back procedure, that of excessive submental fullness:

> 'There is one more point to be mentioned. That is the question of the excessive bag of soft tissue which often remains below the mandible. In performing body resections I have recently joined my two incisions and excised a wedge of skin and subcutaneous tissue. The result is excellent, the bag is obliterated and the scar line tucks up into an invisible position under the jaw (Figure 2-20).'

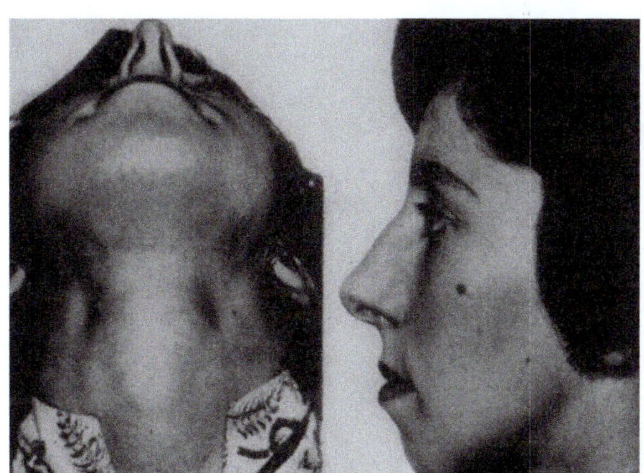

Fig. 2-20 Hovell described the potential detrimental effects on the submental-cervical region from a significant mandibular set-back, and its surgical management by removal of a wedge of submental skin. (From Hovell,[22]).

Note:

In an excellent biography of Hovell, Gelbier[24] has pointed out that in 1960, albeit with the support of the orthodontist Clifford Ballard, Hovell proposed the formation of the Consultant Orthodontist Group (COG) and chaired the first meeting. The COG later became part of the British Orthodontic Society when the various British orthodontic organizations merged. Before going overseas to serve in World War II, Hovell went to Rooksdown House, Basingstoke (London), where members of six Army Maxillofacial Units were trained by **Sir Harold Gillies** (1882–1960) and **Martin Amsler Rushton** (1903–1970), an oral surgeon and later Professor of Oral Pathology at Guy's Dental School. Hovell was instrumental in pushing for surgeons and orthodontists to work together in the correction of jaw deformities, and appears to have been the first surgeon in the UK to carry out an Obwegeser bilateral sagittal split osteotomy of the ascending rami of the mandible in December 1958 (Figure 2-21).

The **mandibular subapical alveolar osteotomy**, originally described by Hullihen in 1849 was not described further until 1936, when Hofer described an anterior mandibular subapical osteotomy to advance the mandibular labial dentoalveolar segment,[25] (Figure 2-22). Hofer's incision severed the mental nerves. **Heinrich Köle** (1959) (Figure 2-23) suggested a modification of this procedure, using a vestibular incision, preservation of the mental nerves, and creating the horizontal osteotomy 10 mm below the mandibular incisor apices, which avoided damage to the incisor roots, allowed advancement of the segment up to 20 mm, and provided greater bone contact for healing.[26–28] The osteotomized segment was stabilized with an intraoral splint and by a circumferential wire passing through a previously prepared hole in the segment and twisted over the splint (Figure 2-24). If

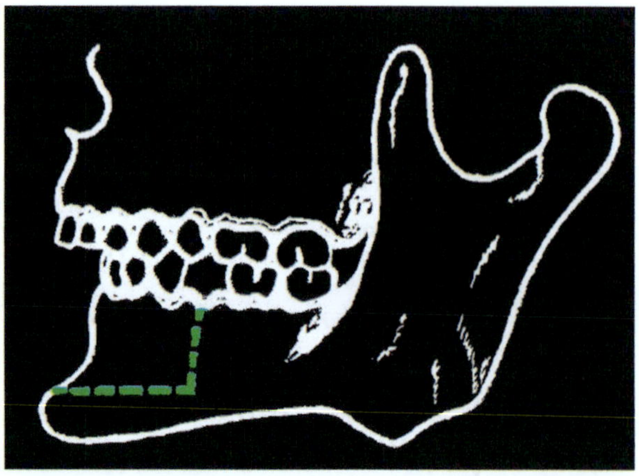

Fig. 2-22 Hofer's anterior mandibular subapical osteotomy to advance the mandibular labial dentoalveolar segment (1936) (After Köle,[26–28]).

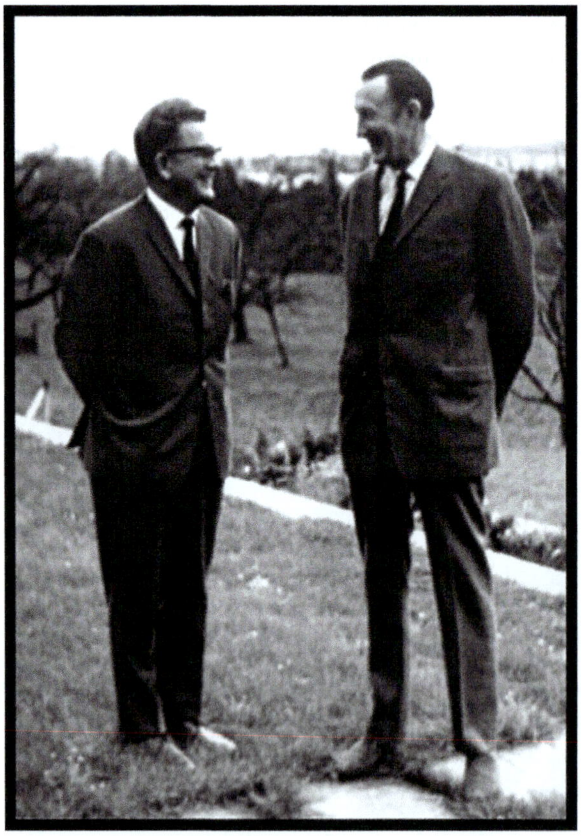

Fig. 2-21 Hovell with his friend Hugo Obwegeser in Zurich. (Courtesy of Journal of Medical Biography, Sage Publications).

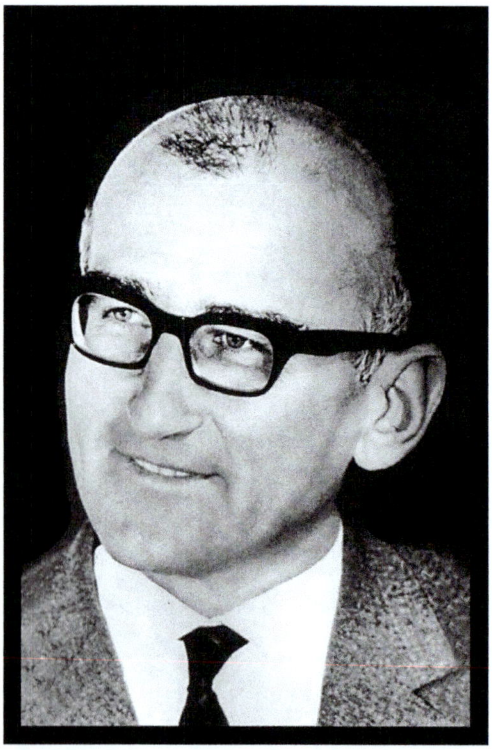

Fig. 2-23 Heinrich Köle. (Courtesy of the Journal of Cranio-Maxillofacial Surgery).

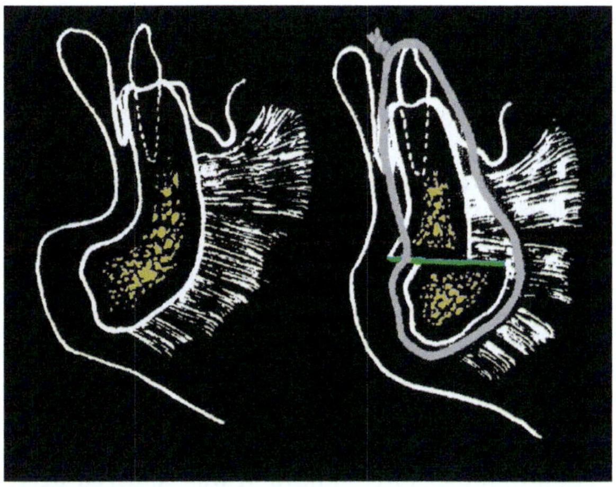

Fig. 2-24 Köle subapical anterior mandibular advancement osteotomy (After Köle,[26–28]).

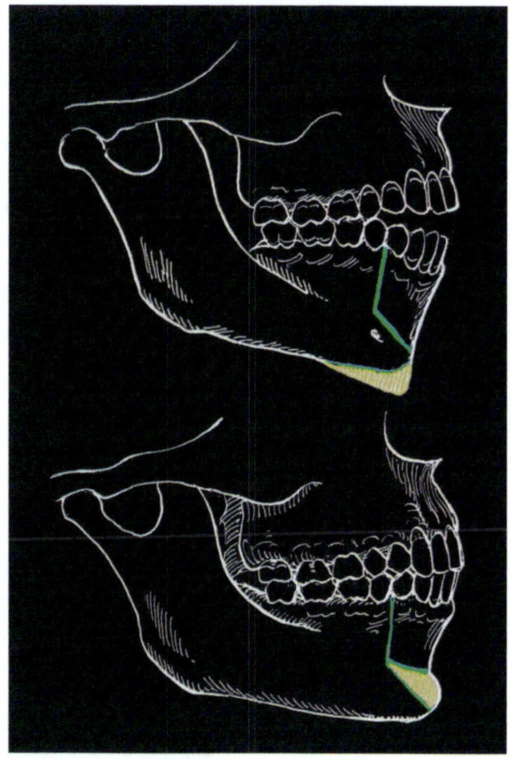

Fig. 2-25 Köle subapical anterior mandibular advancement osteotomy and closure of an anterior open bite, with bone graft taken from the inferior border of the chin, concomitantly reducing vertical chin height (After Köle,[26–28]).

the osteotomized anterior mandibular alveolar segment needed to be elevated to help close an anterior open bite, bone could be taken from the chin and used as a bone graft in the vertical step created inferior to the dentoalveolar segment (Figure 2-25).

Useful variations of anterior mandibular subapical alveolar osteotomies have been described. **John Sowray** and **Richard Haskell** (1968)[29,30] described the reduction in length of the mandibular body by the bilateral ostectomy of a first premolar and associated socket with concomitant ostectomy of a vertical segment from the midline of the mandibular symphysis to reduce the chin width and feminize the appearance. The three ostectomy sites were connected by a horizontal cut inferior to the apices of the anterior teeth (Figure 2-26). Obwegeser (1969)[31] described a similar procedure, but with elevation of the osteotomized anterior dentoalveolus to close an anterior open bite, with a bone graft taken from the inferior border of the chin and wedged into the space inferior to the dentoalveolar segment.

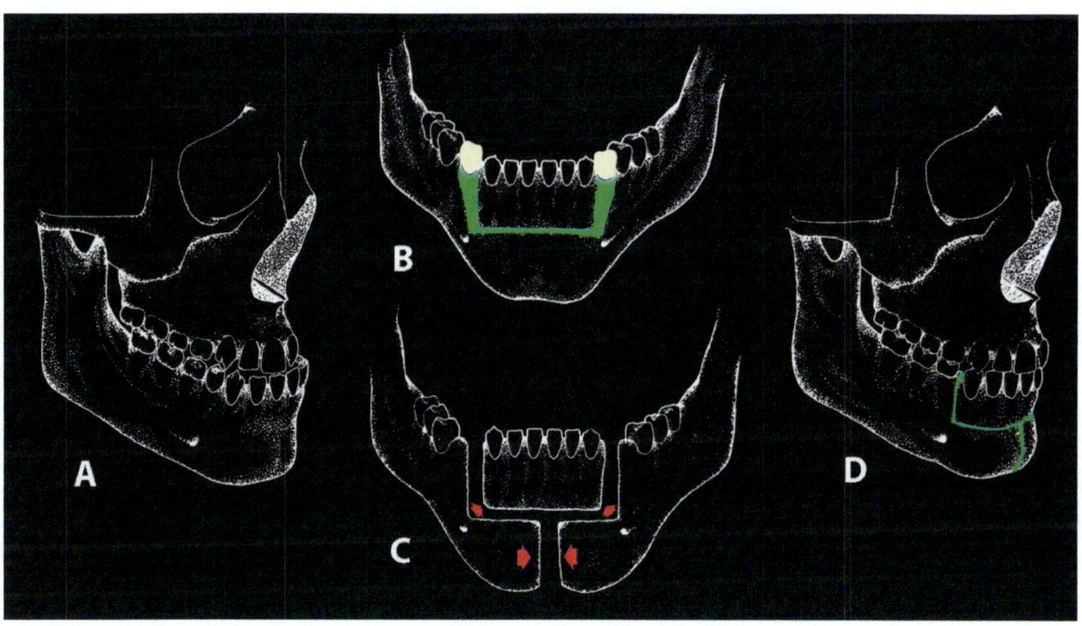

Fig. 2-26 Sowray and Haskell Y-body ostectomy (1968) (After Henry,[30]): (a): Preoperative skeletal Class III with mandibular prognathism; (b): Extraction of mandibular first premolars and localized anterior alveolar osteotomy, permitting segmental set-back; (c): Midline symphyseal ostectomy, permitting anterior constriction; (d): Postoperative result.

> **Note:**
>
> Richard 'Dick' Haskell (1936–2000) was consultant oral and maxillofacial surgeon at Guy's Hospital in London. He had worked under Professor John Sowray at King's College Hospital before moving to Guy's. As an undergraduate student I had the great pleasure of sitting in on his consultant clinics. He was undoubtedly one of the most respected consultants at Guy's and had a contagious enthusiasm for this specialty. He was a true intellectual, and is remembered fondly for his unique teaching style, which was often interspersed with lines from Shakespeare.

A further development to the anterior subapical mandibular osteotomies was the total mandibular subapical (alveolar) osteotomy, permitting mobilization and subsequent repositioning of the entire mandibular dentoalveolar process, described by the American oral surgeon **Robert Bruce MacIntosh** in 1974,[32] (Figure 2-27). MacIntosh described three potential indications for this osteotomy:[32–34]

- Infantile apertognathia, i.e. open bite from the molars forward that develops early in childhood. Ramus height and masticatory muscle relationship in such cases disallow many of the conventional ramus osteotomies, and anterior alveolar osteotomies do not improve the molar occlusion.
- Cases in which prior ramus osteotomies have been carried out but have led to relapse during the postoperative period.
- A third, rather rare, indication was condylar agenesis/hypoplasia in which the functional condylar-ramus masticatory muscle relationships should be left as undisturbed as possible.

The historical development and indications for this procedure are discussed further in Chapter 39.

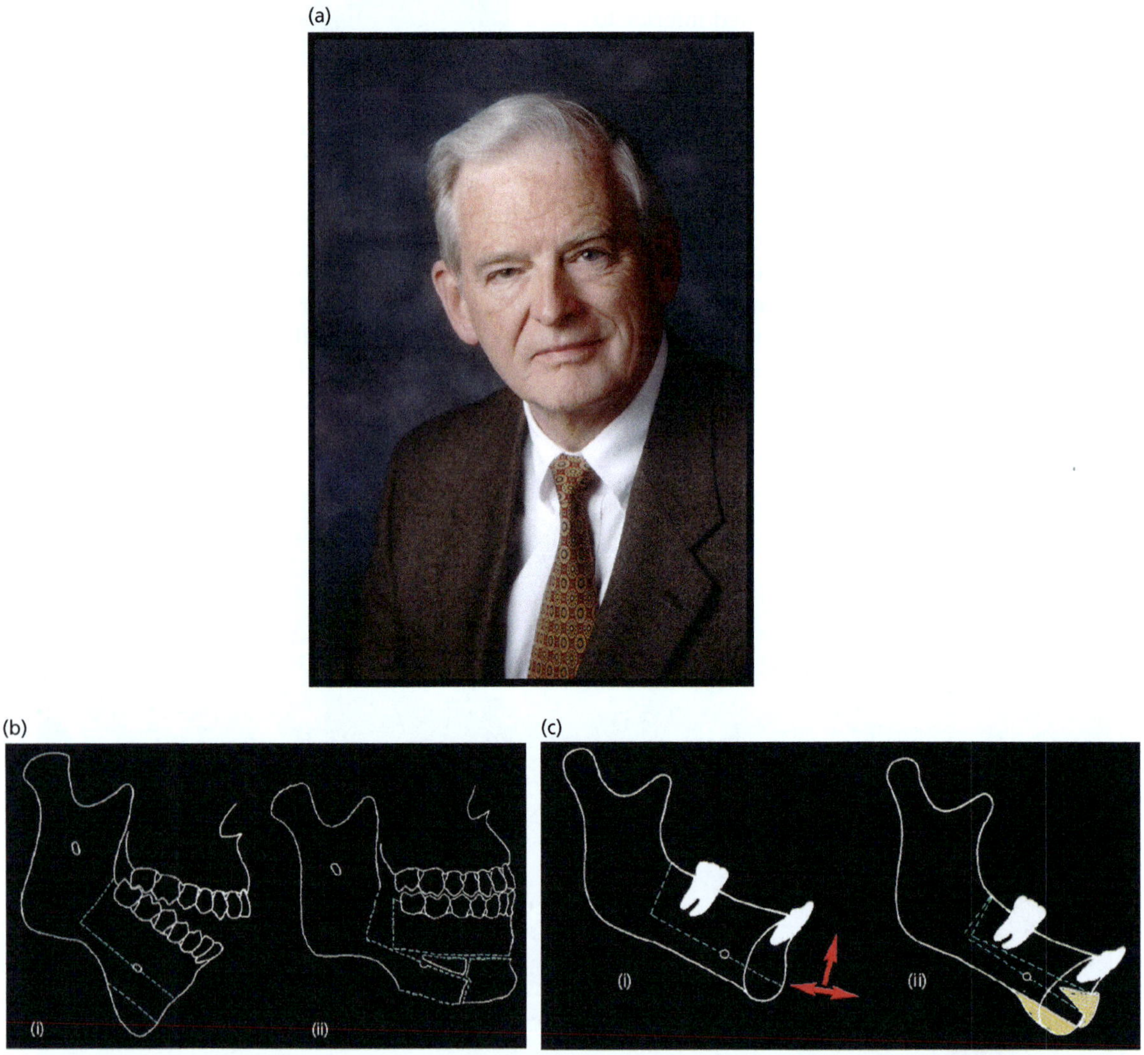

Fig. 2-27 (a): Robert Bruce MacIntosh (Courtesy of Dr R. Bruce MacIntosh). (b): Total mandibular subapical (alveolar) osteotomy - original description by MacIntosh (1974,[32]); (i) Position of the osteotomy at the base of the alveolus, and another horizontal osteotomy of the osseous chin. (ii) The repositioned alveolar process supported by the transposed chin fragment and an augmenting iliac bone graft (After MacIntosh, 1974,[32]). (c): Subsequent description by MacIntosh (1985,[34]); (i) Describing the potential repositioning of the entire mandibular dentoalveolar segment in the direction of the desired correction, (ii) Diagram of the surgical procedure used to reduce lower face height and augment the chin, modified from Köle (After MacIntosh, 1985,[34]).

Surgery to the condyle and condylar neck

The first condylar resection appears to have been undertaken by the British surgeon **Sir George Murray Humphry** (Figure 2-28) (1820–96) at Addenbrooke's Hospital in Cambridge in 1856, to treat a case of temporomandibular joint 'chronic rheumatic arthritis' in a female patient aged 21.[35] Interestingly, Humphry's description of the patient appears to be that of a right-sided condylar hyperplasia leading to a progressive mandibular asymmetry. Resection of the right condyle from an extraoral approach was reported to be successful in correcting the mandibular asymmetry, dental occlusion and improved the patient's chewing ability. The patient was stable at a 9-month review. However, the first bilateral condylectomy (resection of the condyles) to correct mandibular prognathism was undertaken by **Paul Berger** (Figure 2-29) (1845–1908) in 1897 in Paris.[36] Berger was Clinical Professor of Surgery and Pathology at the Faculté de Médecine in Paris, and is credited with being the first surgeon to wear a surgical mask whilst operating in 1897, in order to reduce the possibility of postoperative infection. In 1898, two renowned French surgeons from Lyon, **Mathieu Jaboulay** (Figure 2-30) (1860–1913) and **Léon Bérard** (Figure 2-31) (1870–1956), reported the results of their cases, by removing the condyles 'piece by piece' using 'tooth-forceps' via a preauricular incision.[37] The condylectomy was predominantly advocated for the correction of mandibular asymmetry or prognathism resulting from condylar pathology. **Robert Henry Ivy**[38] (1881–1974) (Figure 2-32), the double-qualified British-born American surgeon influential in the development of plastic surgery in the United States, pointed out that bilateral condylectomy used to set-back a prognathic mandible usually resulted in a less than ideal dental occlusion.

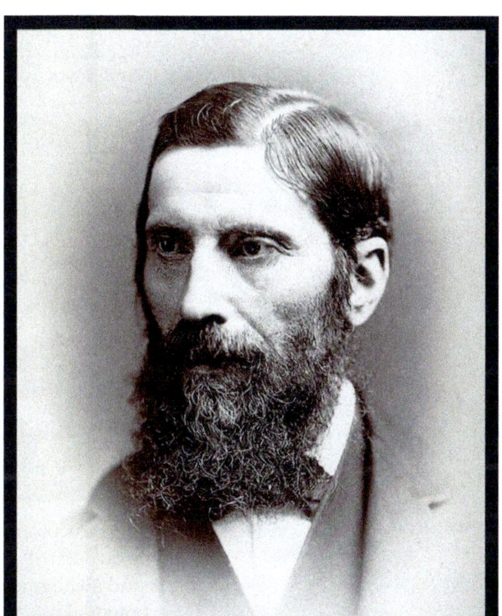

Fig. 2-28 Sir George Murray Humphry (1820–1896).

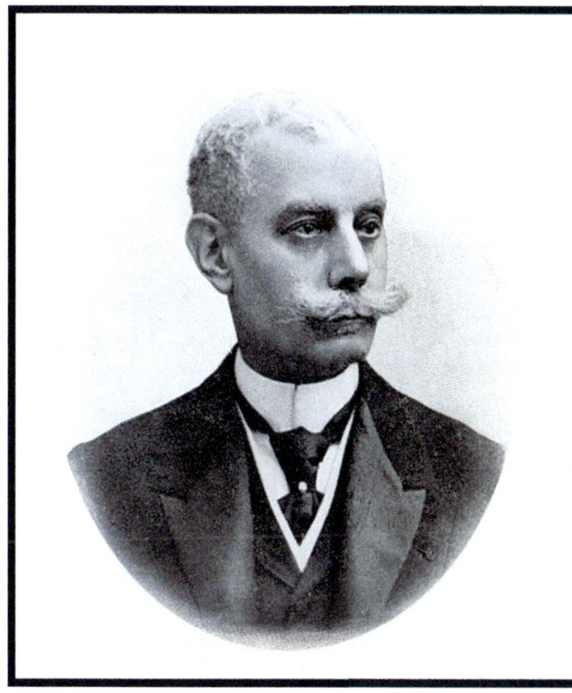

Fig. 2-29 Paul Berger (1845–1908).

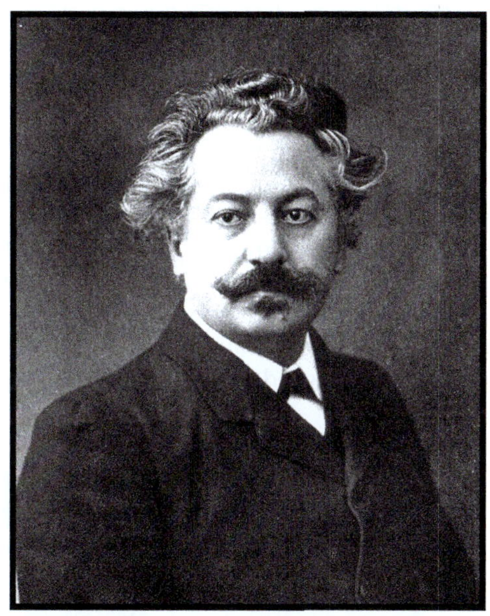

Fig. 2-30 Mathieu Jaboulay (1860–1913).

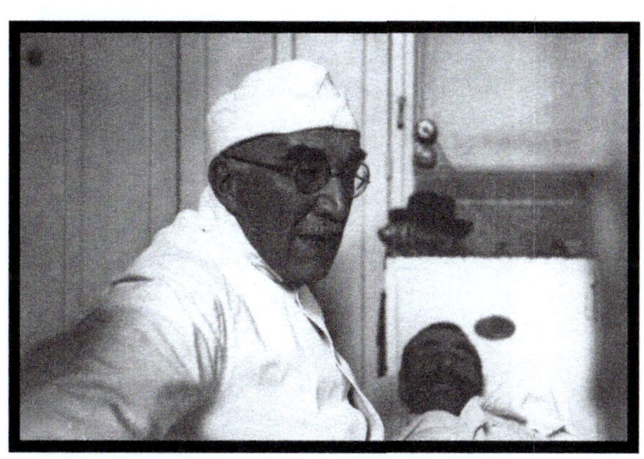

Fig. 2-31 Léon Bérard (1870–1956).

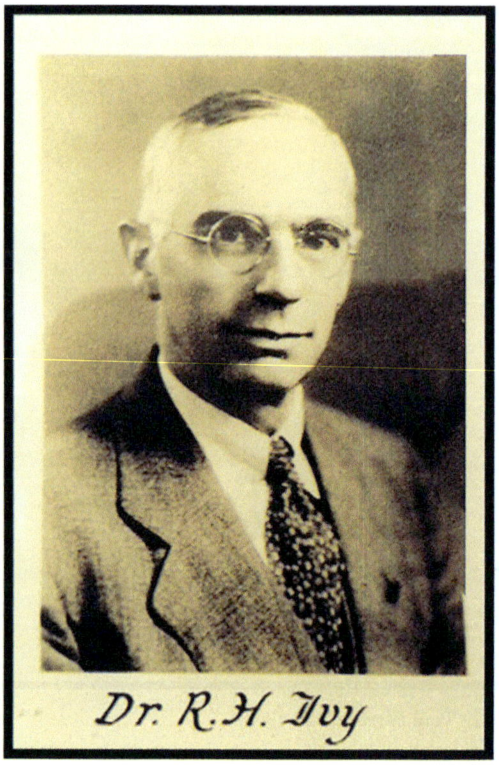

Fig. 2-32 Robert Henry Ivy (1881–1974) (Courtesy of Professor Aron Wahrman and the Robert H. Ivy Society of Plastic Surgeons).

An alternative surgical technique was to osteotomize the condylar neck. In 1921 **Léon Dufourmentel** (Figure 2-33) (1884–1957) described such a technique in Paris.[39] However, in 1928 **František Kostečka** (1893–1951) (Figure 2-34a) from Prague,[40,41] described and popularized the technique using an extraoral approach (with minimal incisions) and Gigli saw, previously designed by the Florentine surgeon

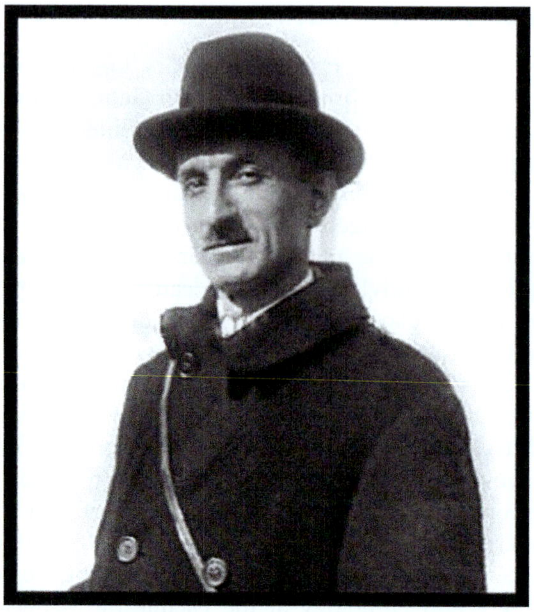

Fig. 2-33 Léon Dufourmentel (1884–1957).

Leonardo Gigli (1863–1908) (Figure 2-34b) (Figure 2-35).[42] Kostečka wrote:[41]

'The advantage of this operation is its easy technic. It can be performed in a few minutes under local anesthesia. No incisions are made in the skin, and the needle punctures heal without leaving any traces. Any injury to the large vessels, nerves or musculature is quite impossible. The general appearance of the patient is thereby vastly improved. I am, however, convinced that it is impossible to recommend only one method for the operation for open-bite, because the varieties of this anomaly are numerous. It is necessary to know the results obtained from all the methods which have been used up to now, in order that a method may be chosen which will have the best result for each individual case. It happens sometimes that the operator must modify one method or combine several methods during the operation.'

(a) (b)

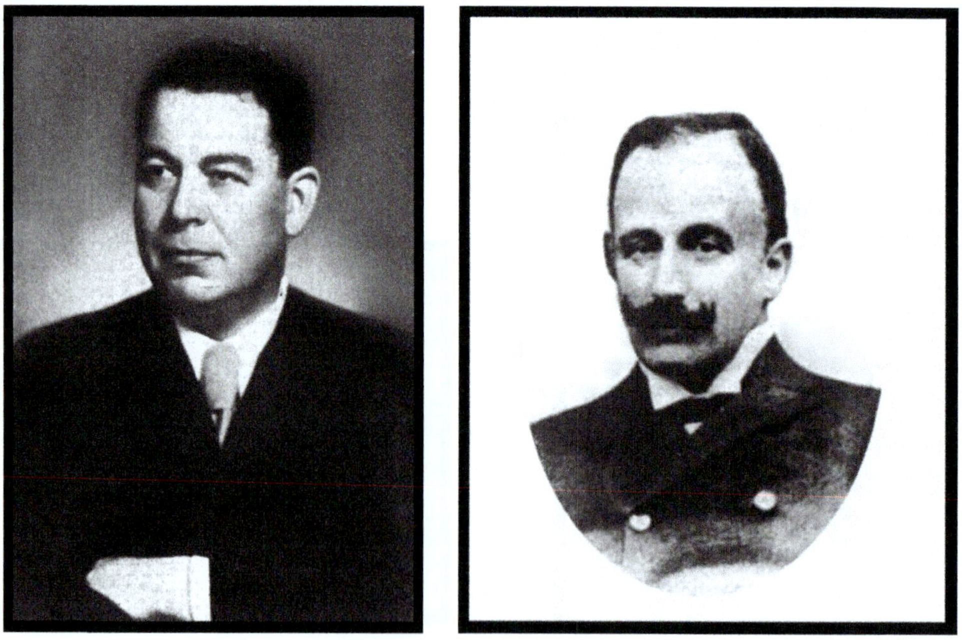

Fig. 2-34 (a): František Kostečka (1893–1951) (Courtesy of Professor Daniel Hrušák). (b): Leonardo Gigli (1863–1908).

(a)

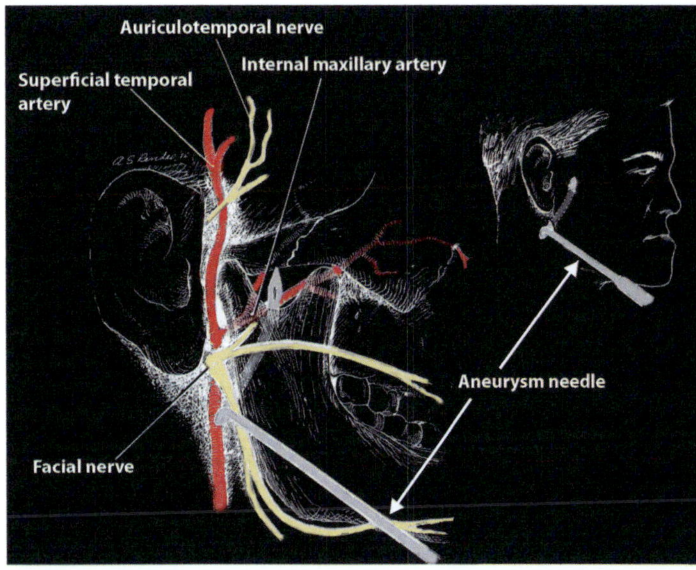

(b)

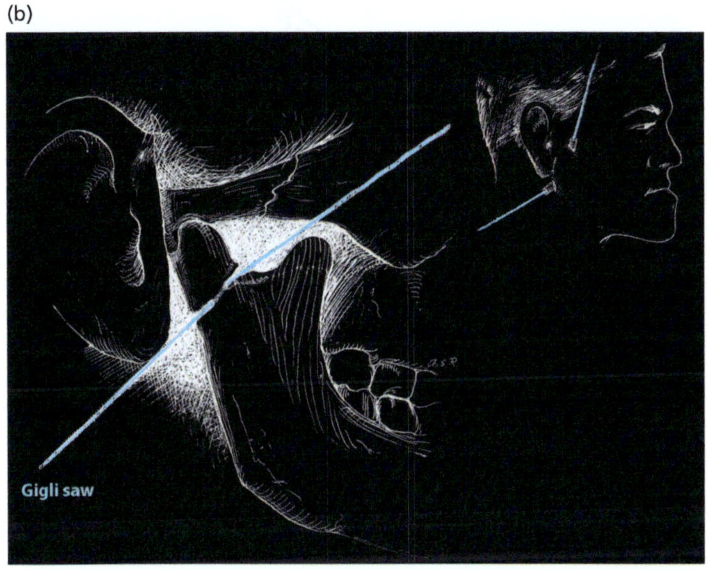

(c)

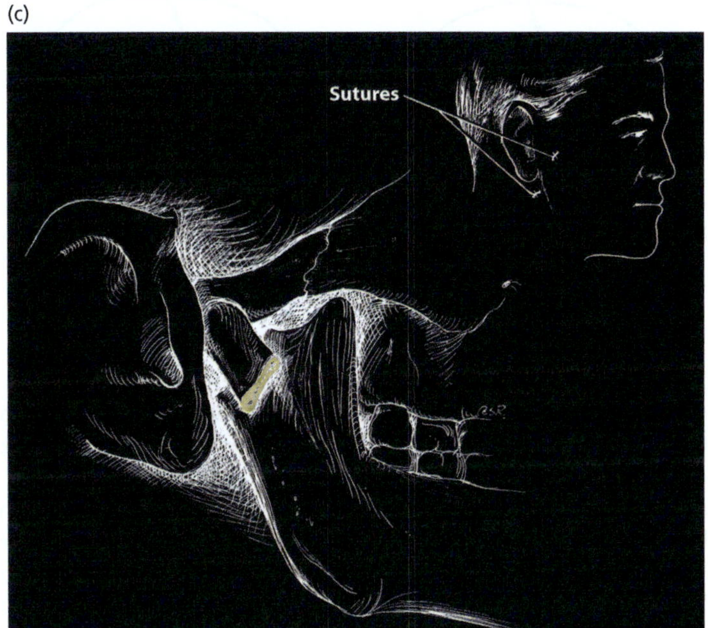

Fig. 2-35 (a): Kostečka's condylar neck osteotomy using an extraoral approach and Gigli saw (1928) (After Spilka,[42]), demonstrating insertion of aneurysm needle and the structures to be avoided; (b) Gigli saw in position; (c) Position of mandibular condyle and ramus after condylar neck osteotomy and set-back of the mandible. (d): Various approaches to closing an anterior open bite with mandibular surgery (From Kostečka, 1934,[41]). (e): Kostečka's technique, demonstrating insertion of the curved needle and the Gigli saw (From Kostečka, 1934,[41]). (f): Kostečka's technique, demonstrating the osteotomy of the mandibular ramus between the posterior ramal border and the centre of the sigmoid notch, and pushing the mandible up into occlusion after the osteotomy (From Kostečka, 1934,[41]).

(d)

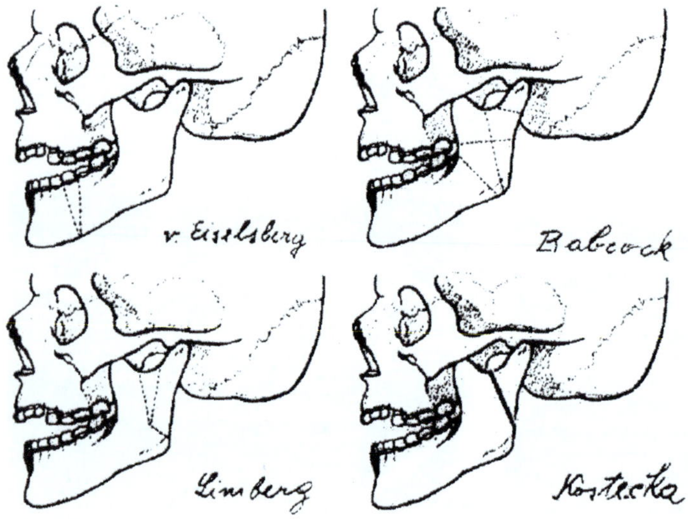

(e)

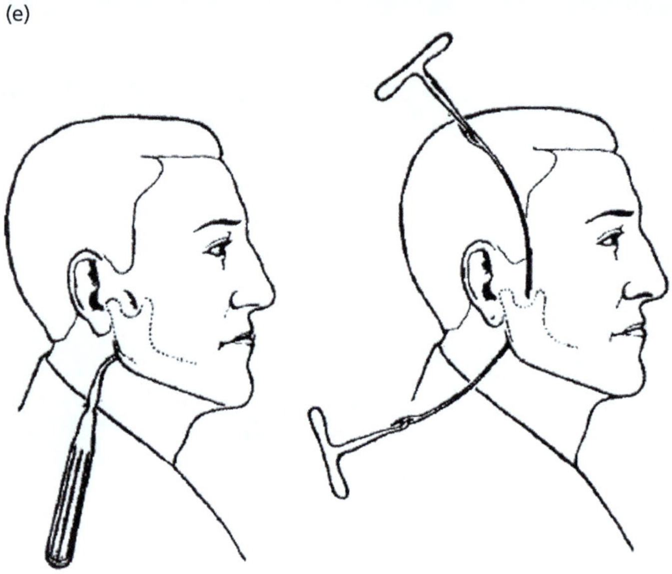

(f)

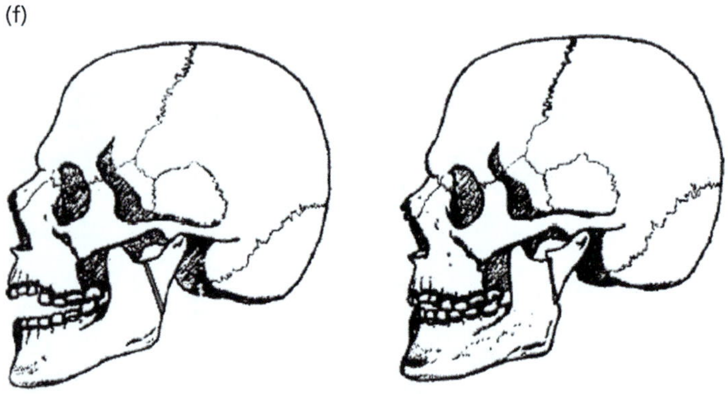

Fig. 2-35 *(Continued)*

Kostečka's procedure found its way to the UK via Major C. Konig, Chief Dental Surgeon of the Czechoslovak Armed Forces. Cast metal interdental cap splints were constructed for each jaw separately and a rod and tube device for locking the two members together was arranged on each side so that the splint could only be locked up when the jaw had been pushed backwards to the precise predetermined position of the upper and lower teeth. On the day before operation, the upper and lower members of the splint were separated and cemented respectively on the teeth. Both sides having been anaesthetized by mandibular block and subcutaneous infiltration, Kostečka's needle was passed behind the posterior border of the left ramus and was made to emerge through the cheek close to the angle made by the anterior border of the ramus and the inferior edge of the zygomatic arch. The Gigli wire saw was attached and drawn back through the wound. With very few strokes the condylar neck of the ramus was bisected. The right side was similarly sectioned (Figure 2-36).[43] There was no difficulty in pushing the jaw back and

(a)

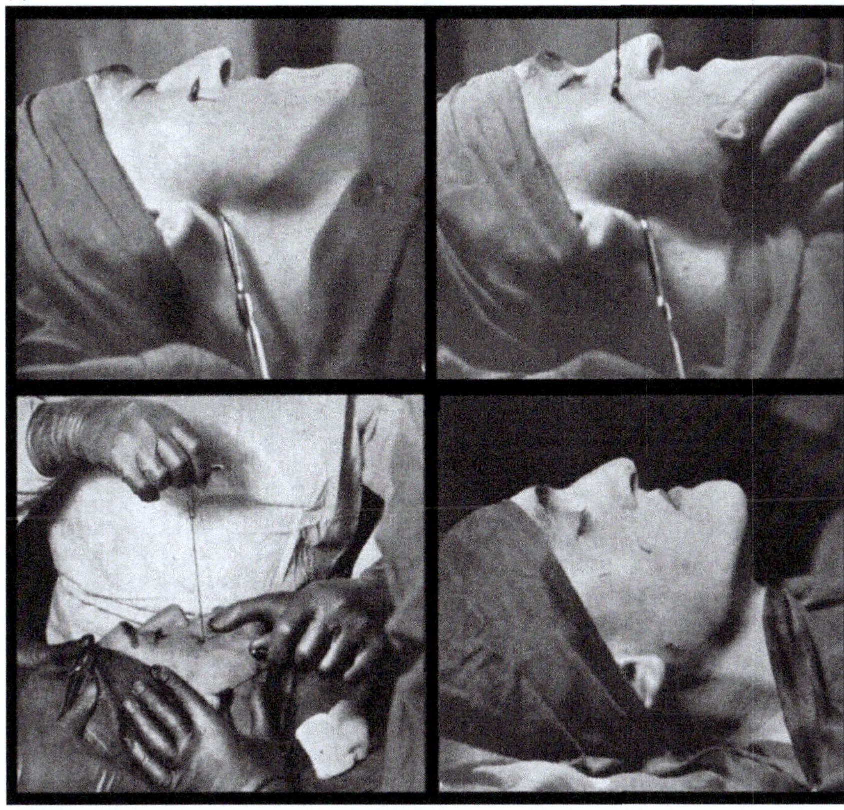

(b)

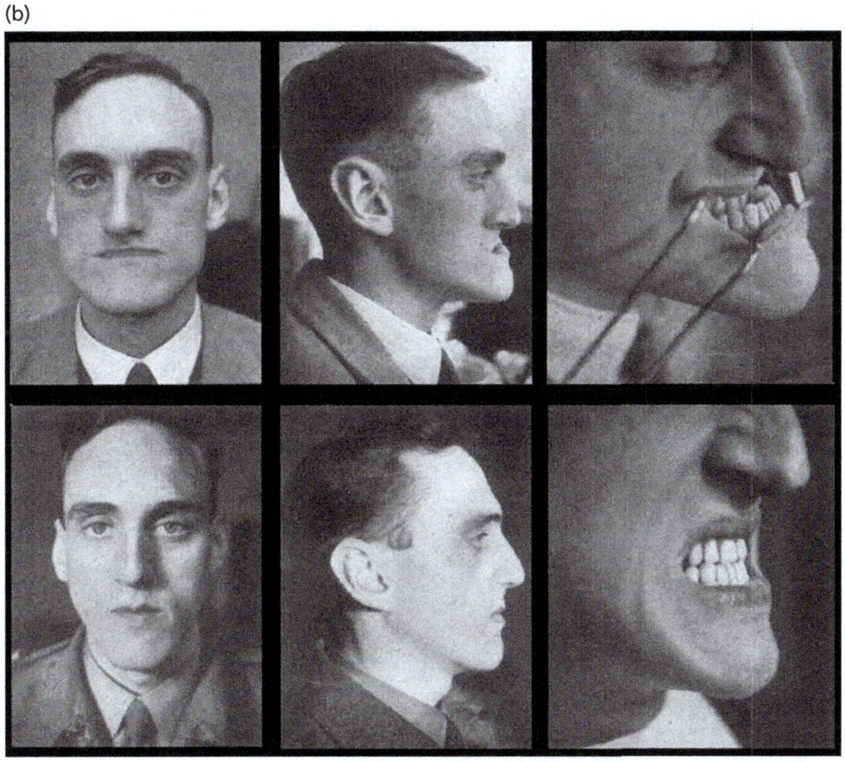

Fig. 2-36 (a): An example of Kostečka's condylar neck osteotomy using an extraoral approach and Gigli saw. (b): Patient treated using Kostečka's technique (preoperative images above, postoperative images below). (From Bowdler Henry,[43]).

immediately locking the splints in the predetermined position by passing the rods through the interdigitating tubes. Kostečka advocated splinting for 12 weeks.

In 1940, **Arthur E. Smith** from Los Angeles (and Johnson),[44] suggested the removal of a small rectangle of bone from the sigmoid notch, followed by a horizontal osteotomy of the condylar neck, to set-back the mandible (Figure 2-37). It seems that few regions of the mandible escaped the attention of surgeons attempting to find ways to set-back the mandible.

Mandibular ramus osteotomies

The first description of an ascending ramus osteotomy appears to be from **Sir William Arbuthnot Lane** (1856–1943) (Figure 2-38), a pioneering British

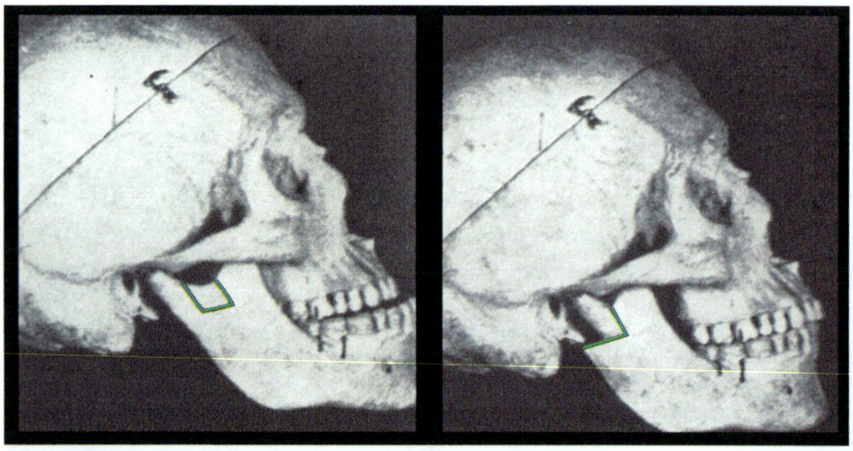

Fig. 2-37 Smith and Johnson's sigmoid notch ostectomy and condylar neck osteotomy to set-back the mandible (1940). (From Smith and Johnson,[44]).

surgeon and physician trained at Guy's Hospital in London, in a Monograph published in 1905. Lane divided the ramus transversely just above the level of the mandibular foramen and lingula, allowing the body of the mandible to slide back. He then joined the fragments of the rami in this position with plates.[15] In 1907, Blair performed a similar procedure via an extraoral approach using a Gigli saw, with the horizontal osteotomy made between the sigmoid notch and the lingula. He successfully advanced the mandible just over 9 mm (Figure 2-39).[45,46] In this classic paper, Blair wrote:[45]

> 'While surgeons for centuries have expended early talent and energy upon the correction of deformities of almost all kinds, from clubfoot to malrelation of the teeth, both for cosmetic and utilitarian reasons, yet little study or work seems to have been done to alleviate those distressing conditions that arise from excessive asymmetry of the dental arches. Where this deformity was too great to be corrected by orthodontic appliances, the victims have, so far as I can determine, with the exception of a few isolated cases, been compelled to go through life without relief.'

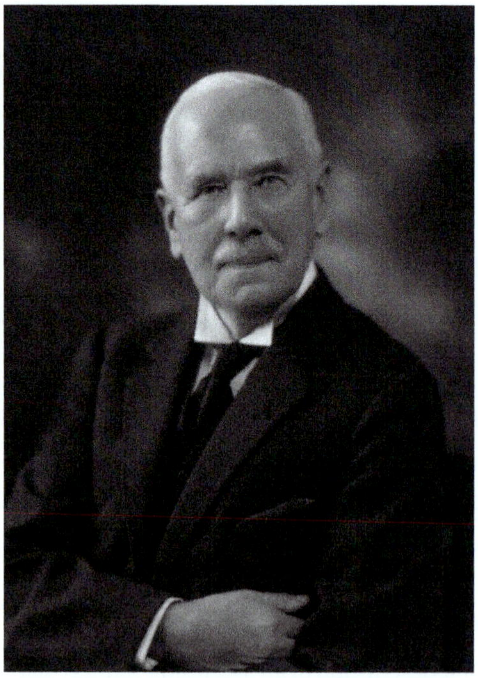

Fig. 2-38 Sir William Arbuthnot Lane (1856–1943).

He also recognized that there were three distinct problems in jaw surgery:

'(1) the cutting of the bone, (2) the placing of the jaw in its new position, and (3) holding it there.'

A year later, **William Wayne Babcock** (1872–1963) (Figure 2-40), Professor of Surgery in Temple University and of Oral Surgery in the Philadelphia Dental College, applied the same technique for the correction of mandibular prognathism and anterior open bite. Babcock also described other techniques in which mandibular prognathism with anterior open bite could be treated.

The German dentist **Christian Bruhn** (Figure 2-41) (1868–1942) established the Oral and Maxillofacial Surgery services in Düsseldorf during and following the First World War. In both 1920 and 1927, Bruhn described an extraoral approach to the mandibular ramus, from a lateral direction.[48] In 1927, Bruhn stated in an English language journal: 'Gradually a new sphere of medical and dental science arose, and soon a new system became possible. Thus a new way was found to remove the deformation of the lower jaw, especially the so-called macrognathy and micrognathy.' This was one of the few significant exchanges of ideas or concepts prior to 1960 between American and European surgeons. Interestingly, it was under the direction of Professor Bruhn that Herbert Hofrath (1889–1952) developed the cephalostat and cephalometric radiography in 1931 (a more sophisticated version was developed independently by the American orthodontist B. Holly Broadbent in the same year).[49] Following the retirement of Bruhn in 1934, **August Lindemann** (Figure 2-42) (1880–1970) was appointed Professor of Oral and Maxillofacial Surgery in Düsseldorf. Lindemann also described an extraoral approach to the mandibular ramus, similar to Bruhn.[50,51] Lindemann also pioneered the use of iliac bone grafts and reconstructive surgery of the mandible following World War I. Lindemann

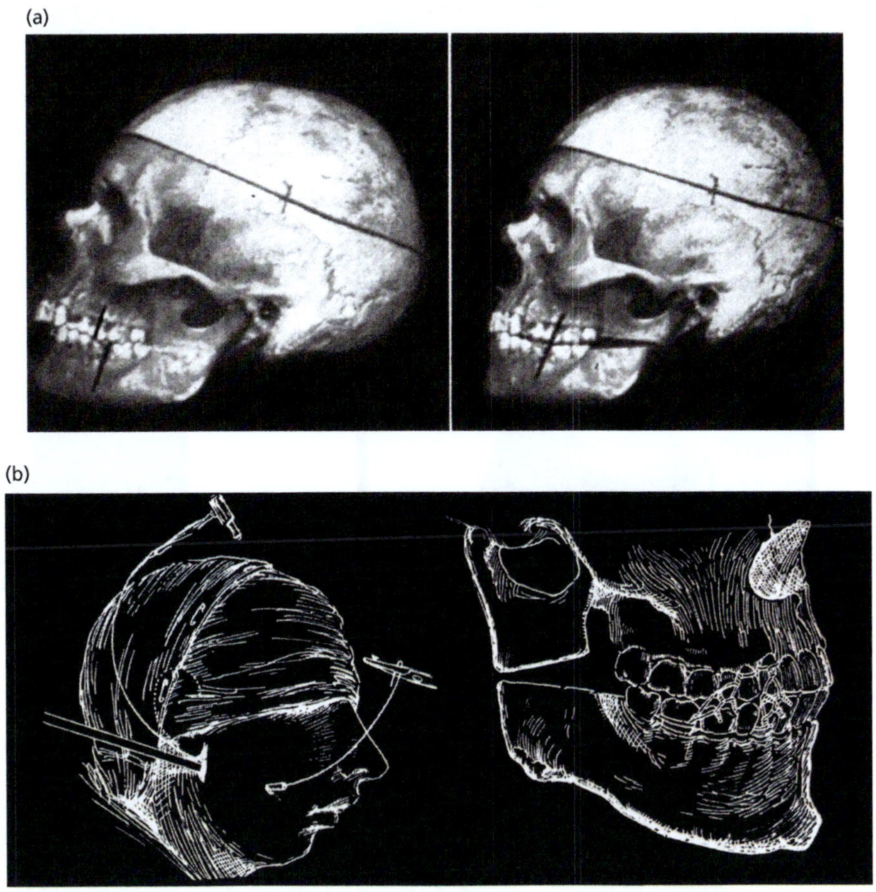

Fig. 2-39 (a): Blair's horizontal ramus osteotomy to advance the mandible (From Blair, 1907,[45]). (b): Blair's use of the Gigli saw for his horizontal ramus osteotomy (After Blair,[12]).

retired in 1950 and was succeeded by Karl Häupl (1893–1960).

The pioneering Armenian-born American surgeon **Varaztad Hovhannes Kazanjian** (Figure 2-43) (1879–1974) suggested tapering the horizontal ramus osteotomy obliquely from the medial to the lateral aspect of the ramus in order to obtain a wider area of bone contact, undertaking the procedure via an extraoral approach (Figure 2-44).[52–54]

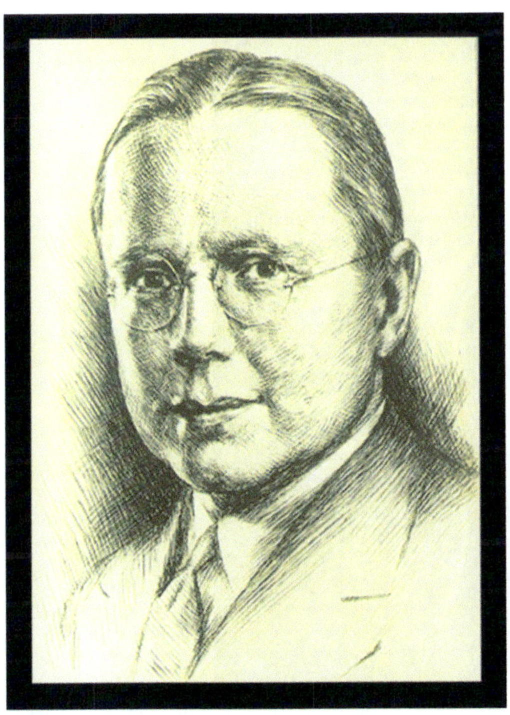

Fig. 2-40 William Wayne Babcock (1872–1963).

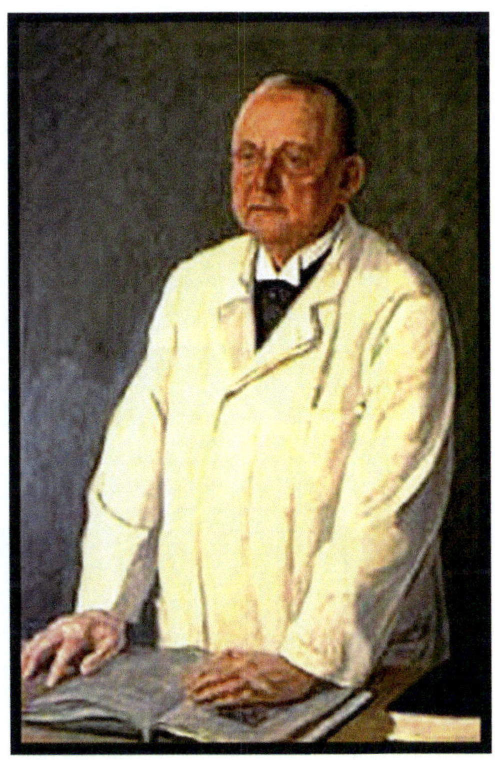

Fig. 2-41 Christian Bruhn (1868–1942).

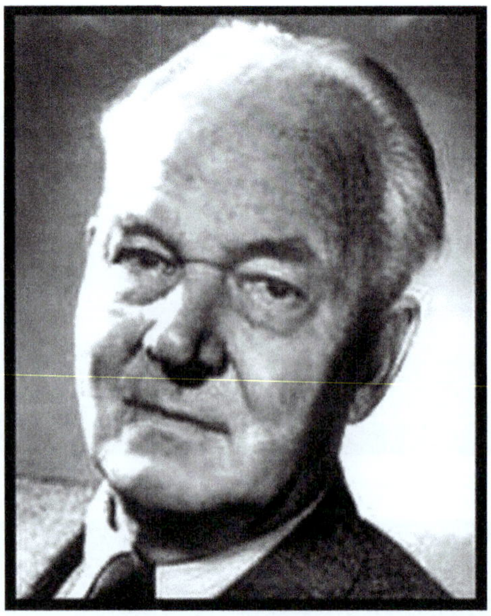

Fig. 2-42 August Lindemann (1880–1970).

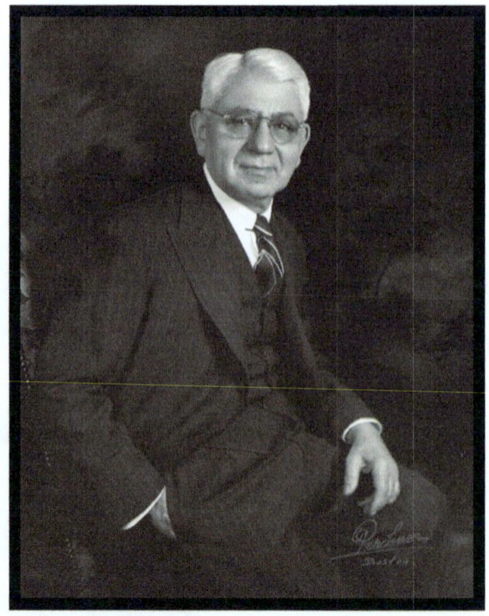

Fig. 2-43 Varaztad Hovhannes Kazanjian (1879–1974).

(a)

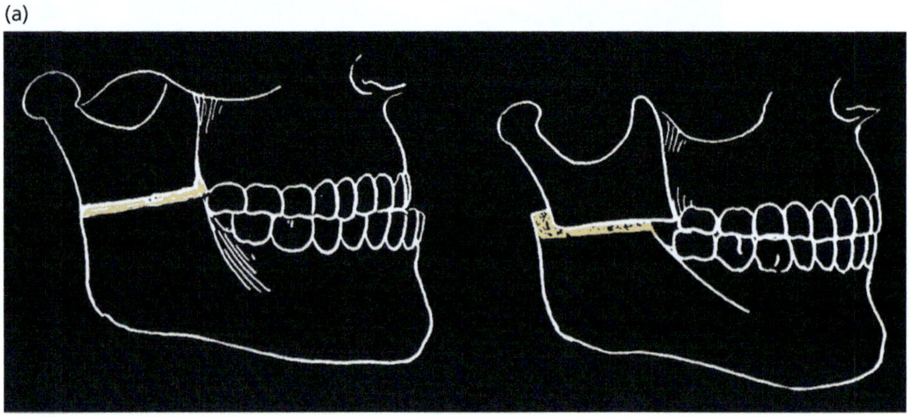

(b)

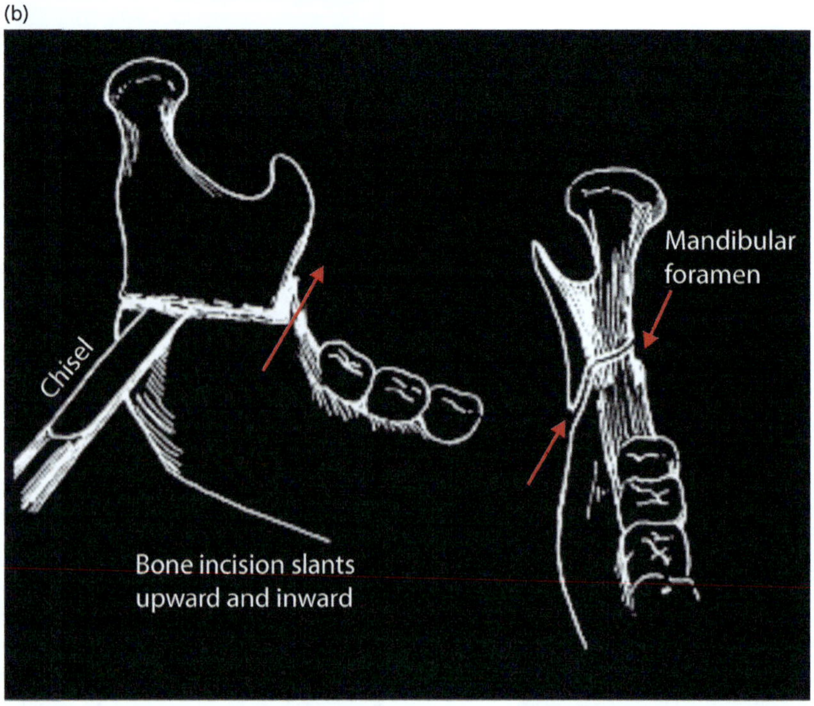

Fig. 2-44 (a,b): Kazanjian's horizontal osteotomy tapering obliquely from the medial to the lateral aspect of the ramus in order to obtain a wider area of bone contact (1951). (After Kazanjian,[53]).

Note:

Varaztad Kazanjian is rightly regarded as one of the founding fathers of facial plastic, maxillofacial and reconstructive surgery. He was born in the city of Erzincan in Western Armenia on the 18 March 1879, and was smuggled out of the country to escape the Ottoman genocide in his country. In Worcester, Massachusetts, he took evening classes while working in a wire mill, eventually entering Harvard Dental School, graduating in 1905. He obtained his MD from Harvard in 1921, and went on to become Professor of Clinical Oral Surgery and in 1941 Harvard's first Professor of Plastic Surgery.[55]

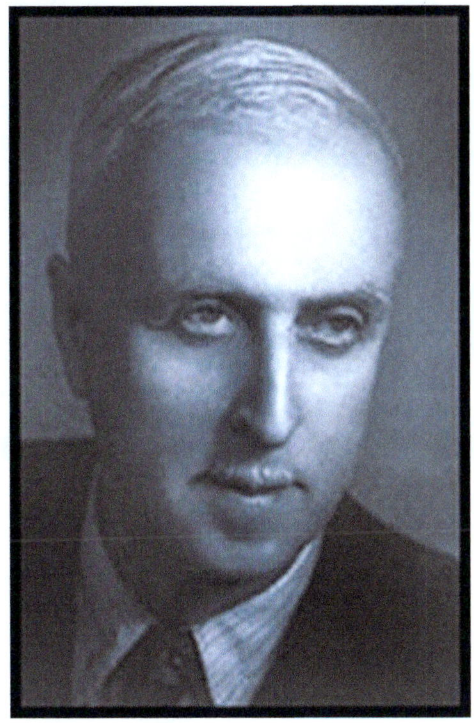

Fig. 2-45 Alexander Limberg (1894–1974).

In 1922, the double-qualified Russian oral surgeon **Alexander Limberg** (1894–1974) (Figure 2-45), Professor of 'Odontologia' and Head of the Stomatological Department and Dental Clinic of the Medical Institute in what was then Leningrad, carried out an oblique vertical osteotomy of the ascending rami via an extraoral approach to close an anterior open bite in a female patient aged 20. He presented his result before the Russian Odontological Congress in Moscow in 1923, and subsequently published the case in 1925 (Figure 2-46).[56] Limberg emphasized the use of classical canons of proportion in facial analysis, and emphasized the importance of orthodontic preparation for jaw surgery, stating, 'The orthodontic treatment must precede the surgical interference, as its aim consists in obtaining conformity of the upper and lower dental arches… Before an operation on the mandible for the correction of the occlusion is performed, it is often necessary to treat the patient first by orthodontic means.'

Skaloud (1951)[57] advocated a combined extraoral and intraoral approach to the horizontal ramus osteotomy by passing a Gigli saw from the skin behind the jaw into the mouth. He undertook transosseous wiring of the bone segments together by passing a wire over the sigmoid notch to a hole drilled through the lower segment of the ramus (Figure 2-47). As with previous osteotomy techniques, osseous fixation remained a stumbling block.

The pioneering German surgeon **Martin Wassmund** (1892–1956) (Figure 2-48) described a smoothly transitioning inverted 'L' type osteotomy of the mandibular

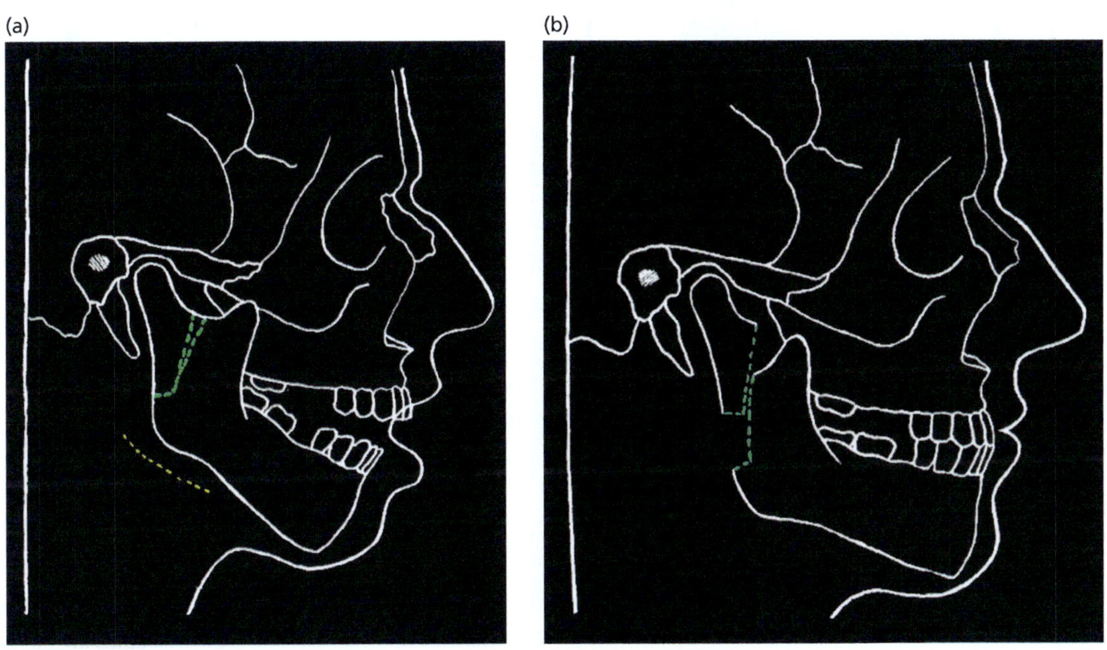

Fig. 2-46 (a): Limberg's ramus osteotomy to close an anterior open bite. (After Limberg,[56]). (b): Following ramus osteotomy. (After Limberg,[56]). (c): Patient before and after Limberg osteotomy (1925). (From Limberg,[56]).

(c)

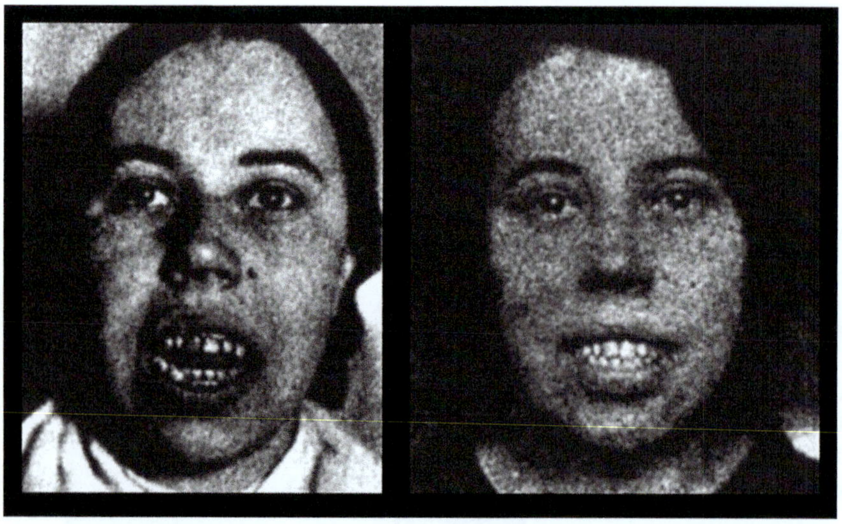

Fig. 2-46 (*Continued*).

(a) (b)

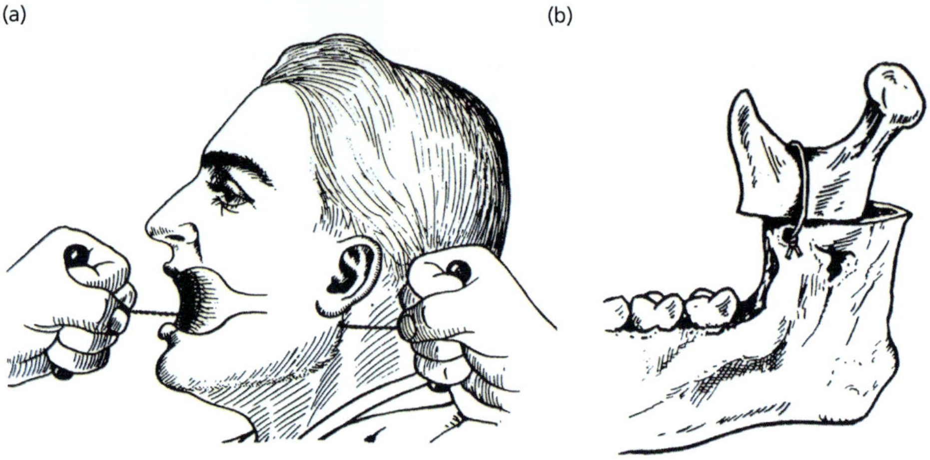

Fig. 2-47 (a): Skaloud (1951) advocated a combined extraoral and intraoral approach to the horizontal ramus osteotomy using a Gigli saw and, (b): undertaking transosseous wiring of the bone segments. (From Skaloud,[57]).

(a) (b)

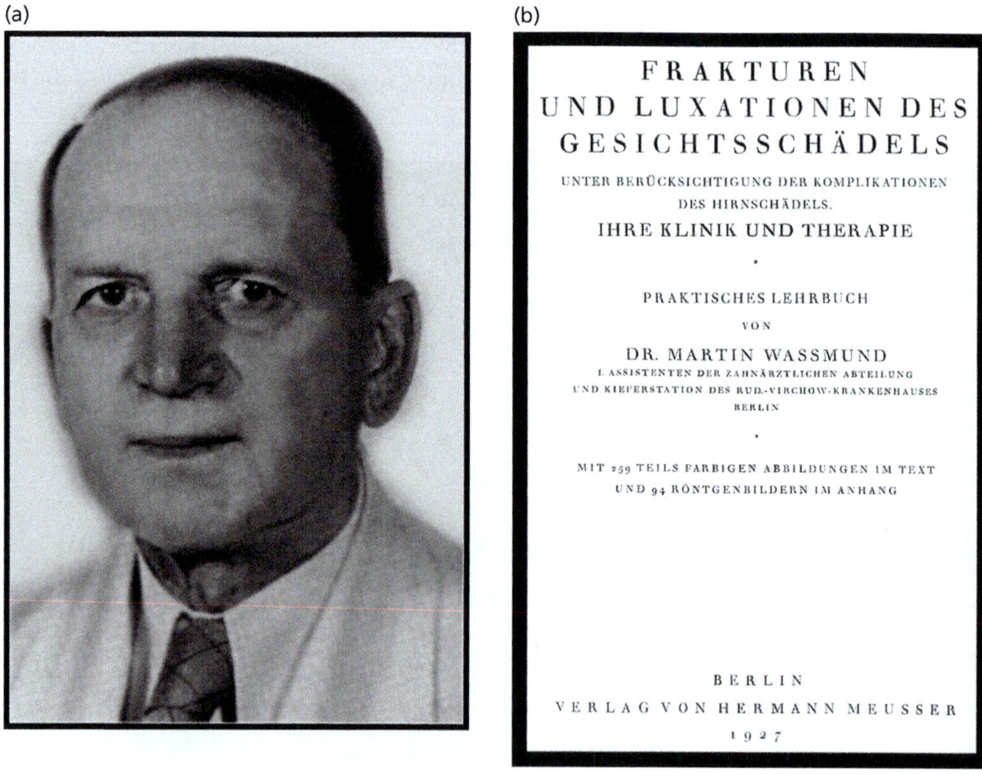

FRAKTUREN
UND LUXATIONEN DES
GESICHTSSCHÄDELS
UNTER BERÜCKSICHTIGUNG DER KOMPLIKATIONEN
DES HIRNSCHÄDELS.
IHRE KLINIK UND THERAPIE

PRAKTISCHES LEHRBUCH
VON
DR. MARTIN WASSMUND
I. ASSISTENTEN DER ZAHNÄRZTLICHEN ABTEILUNG
UND KIEFERSTATION DES RUD.-VIRCHOW-KRANKENHAUSES
BERLIN

MIT 259 TEILS FARBIGEN ABBILDUNGEN IM TEXT
UND 94 RÖNTGENBILDERN IM ANHANG

BERLIN
VERLAG VON HERMANN MEUSSER
1927

Fig. 2-48 (a): Martin Wassmund (1892–1956). (b): Wassmund's textbook (1927).

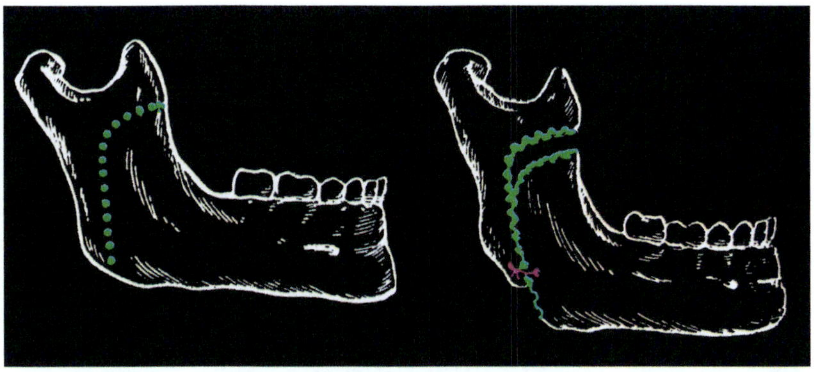

Fig. 2-49 Wassmund's smoothly transitioning inverted 'L' type osteotomy of the mandibular rami via an extraoral approach, used to advance the mandible and potentially close an anterior open bite (1927). (After Wassmund,[58]).

rami via an extraoral approach in 1927, which could be used to advance the mandible and potentially close an anterior open bite (Figure 2-49).[58]

The earliest description of an attempt at a sagittal-type osteotomy of the mandibular rami, albeit undertaken via an extraoral approach, appears to be by the German surgeon **Georg Clemens Perthes** (1869–1927) in 1922 (Figure 2-50), a pioneer of diagnostic radiography.[59] However, Perthes appears to have been describing a procedure undertaken by another surgeon, **A. Schlössmann**. Moreover, the Schlössmann-Perthes technique was an oblique horizontal osteotomy, not a true sagittal split (Figure 2-51). Kazanjian published a very similar technique via an extraoral approach in 1951 (see Figure 2-44).[53]

The move from an extraoral to a completely intraoral approach to the mandibular ramus took place in the 1940s and 50s, but interestingly the first horizontal ramus osteotomy via an intraoral approach was undertaken in Berlin by the double-qualified surgeon **Franz Ernst** (1887–1947) in 1938.[60] The approach did not catch on, and ramus surgery via an extraoral approach continued. In 1942 **Karl Schuchardt** (1901–85) (Figure 2-52), who had trained under Wassmund, developed a stepped horizontal osteotomy of the mandibular ramus from an intraoral approach (Figure 2-53).[61] However, it was in 1953 that a talented surgeon named **Hugo Lorenz Obwegeser**, then aged 33 and working with the renowned surgeon **Richard Trauner** (Figure 2-54) (1900–80) in the Maxillofacial Unit of the Dental School of the University of Graz in Austria, decided to solve the problem of mandibular surgery once and for all.[62]

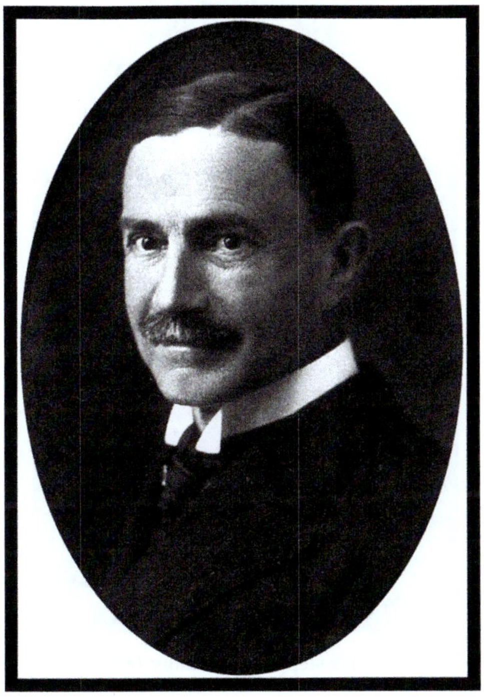

Fig. 2-50 Georg Clemens Perthes (1869–1927).

Note:

Obwegeser's sagittal split osteotomy

'Fortis imaginatio generat casum'
(A powerful imagination generates the event)
Philosophical axiom

My wife, Hengameh, and I visited Professor Obwegeser at his home in Schwerzenbach, Switzerland, on a beautiful afternoon on the 23 March 2012 (Figure 2-55). Professor Obwegeser described with characteristic clarity how he had devised the sagittal split osteotomy. He explained that he had held a cadaveric mandible in his hands, turning it around and observing it from different angles, determined not to put it down until the solution to the problem of mandibular surgery had presented itself. He decided that if the mandibular ramus could be split along its sagittal plane, there would be a wide bony surface contact, required for healing. He had seen mandibles fractured along this plane twice previously. He then proceeded to create multiple cross-sections of a dry cadaveric mandible, and thereby became certain that the mandibular canal and its contents could be protected. The term **'sagittal splitting'** of the mandibular ramus was coined by Professor Obwegeser. One of the distinct advantages of this technique is that no bone grafting is required for mandibular advancement surgery. Professor Obwegeser's second wish was that the procedure would be undertaken intraorally, with no external facial scars, which he also accomplished. Further description of the first procedure in 1953 together with the images may be found in Professor Obwegeser's account in Chapter 1.

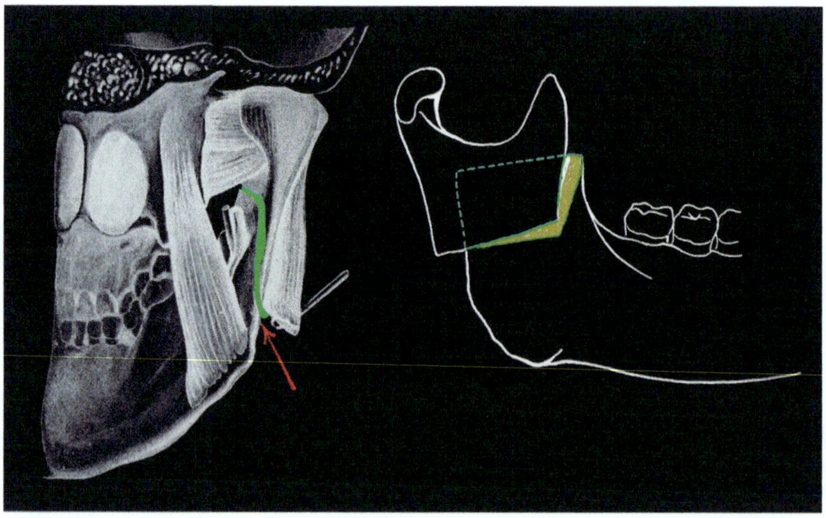

Fig. 2-51 Schlössmann–Perthes oblique horizontal ramus osteotomy (1922). (After Perthes,[59]).

The first sagittal split osteotomy of the mandibular ramus was performed by Obwegeser on the 17 February, 1953 (see Chapter 1) (Figure 2-56a). It was undertaken unilaterally via an intraoral approach, and the contralateral side was operated on by Trauner using his inverted L osteotomy, via a combined intraoral and extraoral approach (Figure 2-57).

In 1957, an Italian surgical trainee named **Giorgio Dal Pont** visited Zurich and assisted Professor Obwegeser in the operating theatre. Through observation and discussion, Dal Pont suggested that the lateral corticotomy could be moved anteriorly, and vertically directed along the body of the mandible. Obwegeser undertook the procedure with Dal Pont assisting, and it was successful (Figure 2-56b, and see Figure 1-10). Unfortunately, upon his return to Italy, Dal Pont made the unconventional decision of publishing this technique, failing to add as co-authors or even to mention that the case being published was operated on by Hugo Obwegeser.[63,64] Dal Pont never performed the operation himself after his return to Italy. Obwegeser continued to make minor modifications to his sagittal split technique.[65] Further modifications were later suggested by the American military oral surgeon Colonel **Ervin Eugene Hunsuck** (1927–97) (1968),[66] who advocated an incomplete horizontal osteotomy of the medial side of the ramus, ending behind the lingula rather than progressing to the posterior border of the ramus, and relying on vertical cleavage lines within the mandible to complete the split (Figure 2-56c). This reduced the possibility of inadvertently cutting vessels posterior

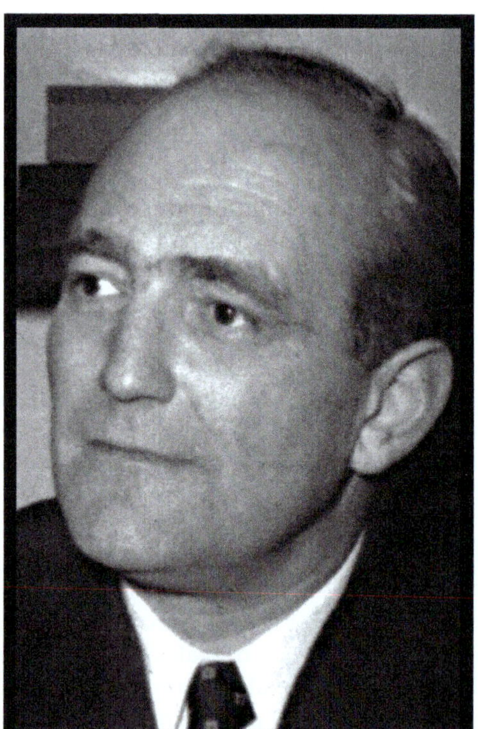

Fig. 2-52 Karl Schuchardt (1901–1985).

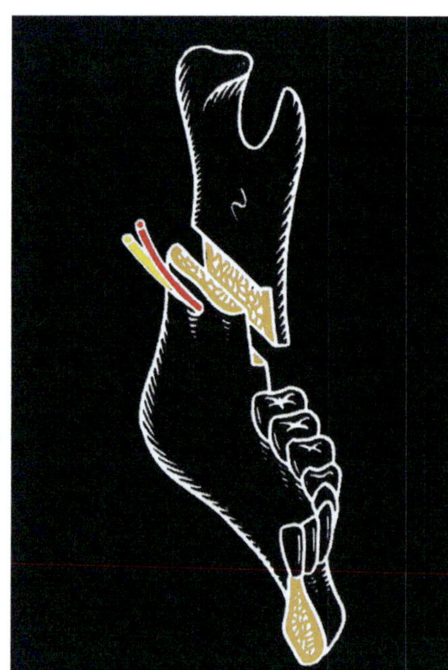

Fig. 2-53 Schuchardt's stepped osteotomy. (After Schuchardt,[61]).

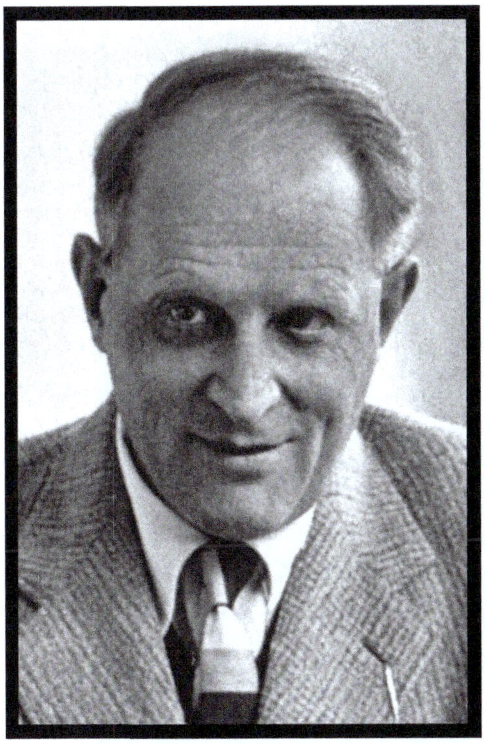

Fig. 2-54 Richard Trauner (1900–1980).

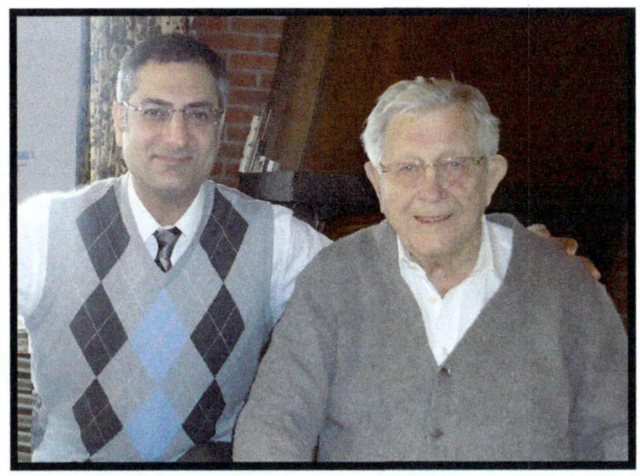

Fig. 2-55 The author with Professor Hugo Obwegeser, Schwerzenbach, Switzerland, 23 March, 2012.

to the ramus, and thereby reduced the potential for bleeding. Later **Bruce Epker** (1977)[67] advocated further modification to the Hunsuck approach. He advised minimal soft tissue dissection (reducing postoperative oedema), suggesting that the periosteum and masseter muscles should not be reflected from the mandibular ramus laterally, and that stripping of the pterygomasseteric sling at the inferior-posterior border of the mandible was unnecessary, as the proximal segment was not being repositioned.

Vertical osteotomies of the mandibular ramus are also sometimes undertaken to set-back the mandible. Following on from the Kostečka condylar neck osteotomy (1928),[40] Robinson (1958),[68] Thoma (1961)[69] (Figure 2-58), and Hinds et al. (1962)[70] described very similar procedures via an extraoral approach. However, in 1954, the American military oral

(a)

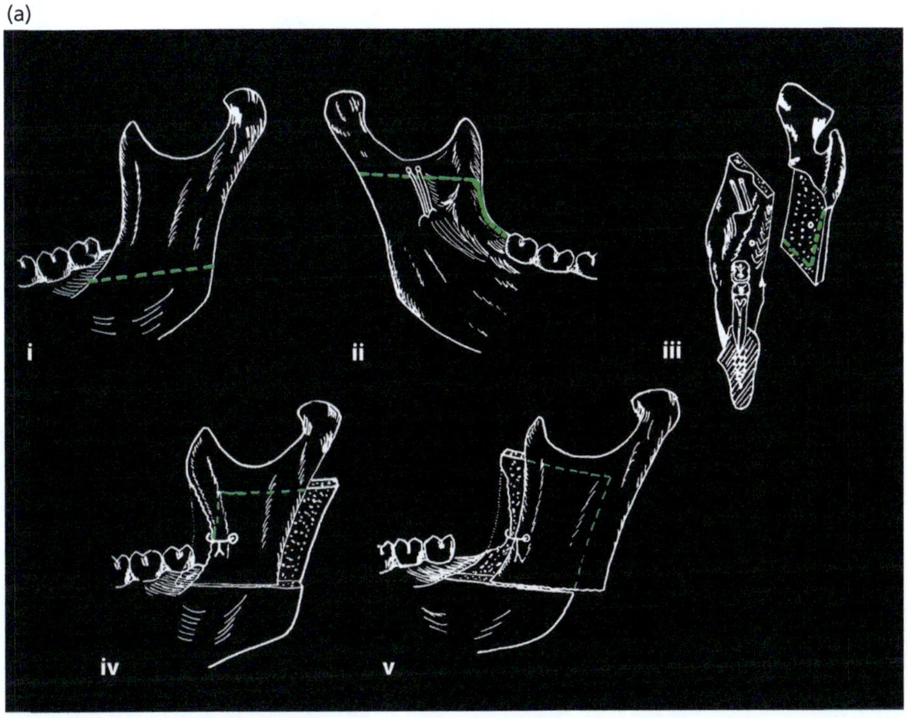

Fig. 2-56 (a): Obwegeser's original sagittal split osteotomy (1957); (i) Buccal osteotomy; (ii): Lingual osteotomy; (iii): Proximal and distal segment after split osteotomy; (iv) and (v): Mandibular set-back and advancement, respectively, with wire fixation in situ (After Obwegeser, 1957,[62]). (b): Obwegeser's modification (with Dal Pont) (After Obwegeser, 1964,[65]); (i) and (ii) buccal and lingual cuts; (iii) separation of the segments in the sagittal plane; (iv) set-back to correct mandibular prognathism; (v) advancement to correct mandibular retrognathia; (vi) correction of anterior open bite by rotation of the distal segment. (c): Hunsuck modification, (i) Buccal view; (ii) Lingual view.

(b)

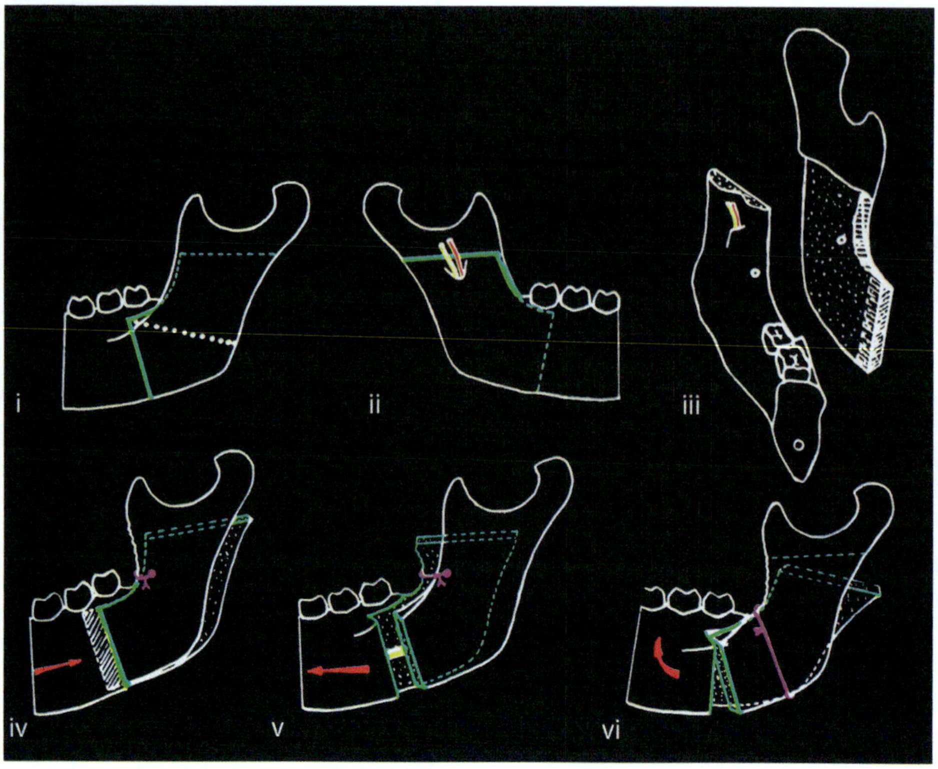

(c)i

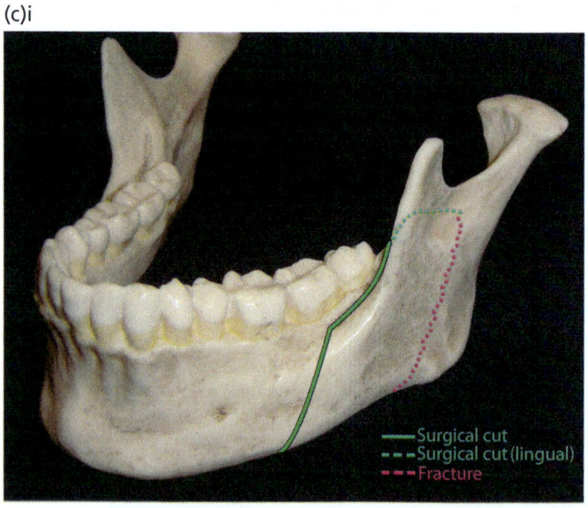

(c)ii

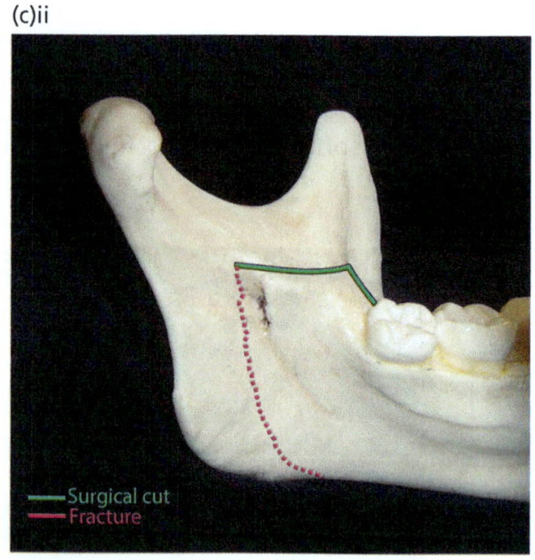

Fig. 2-56 (*Continued*)

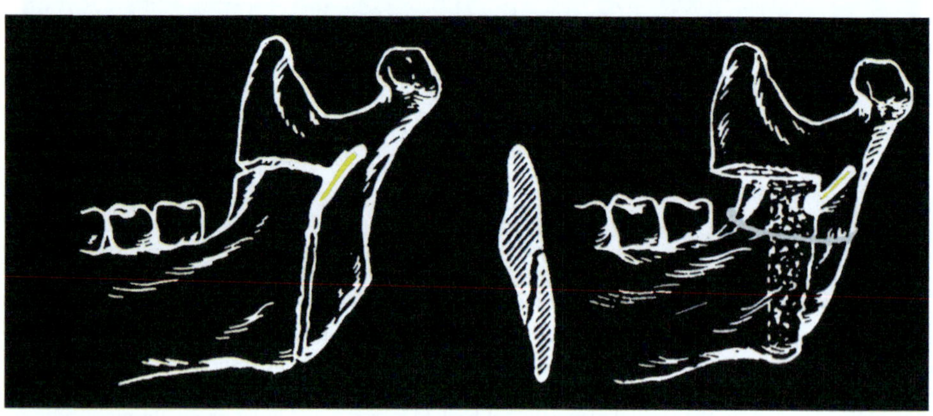

Fig. 2-57 Trauner and Obwegeser's inverted 'L' osteotomy. (After Trauner and Obwegeser,[62]).

surgeons Colonel **Jack B. Caldwell** (Figure 2-59) (1914–86) and **Gordon S. Letterman** (1954)[71] described a true vertical osteotomy of the mandibular ramus via an extraoral approach, the so-called **vertical subsigmoid osteotomy (VSSO)**, used to set-back the mandible in cases of severe mandibular prognathism. This was differentiated from the previous oblique vertical osteotomies in that the inferior aspect of the surgical cut extended to a point anterior to the gonial angle (Figure 2-60). Caldwell et al. (1968)[72] later described a mandibular osteotomy to advance the mandible, which was essentially a modification of the inverted L osteotomy, with an extended anterior curvature undertaken inferiorly leading to a short vertical cut of the inferior mandibular border. They referred to the procedure as a 'vertical L' osteotomy, but it is now commonly referred to as a 'C' osteotomy (Figure 2-61). In 1970, Hebert, Kent and Hinds[73] described the vertical subsigmoid osteotomy via an intraoral approach, using a Stryker saw with a short right angle blade. However, they stated that lack of visibility was a

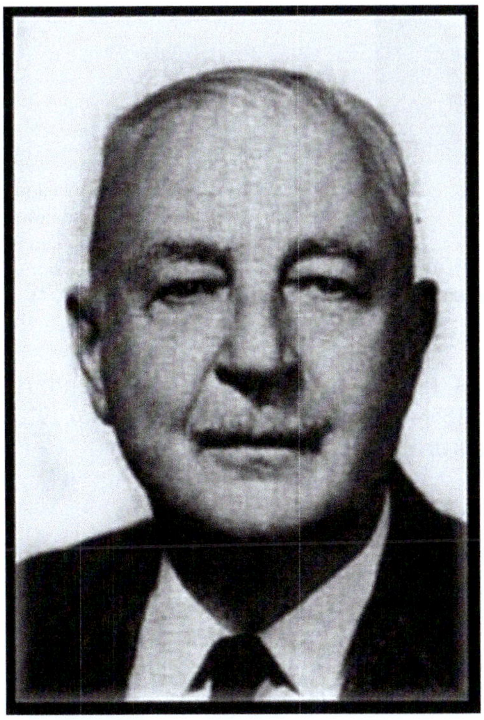

Fig. 2-58 Kurt H. Thoma (1883–1972) – Swiss-born American oral surgeon.

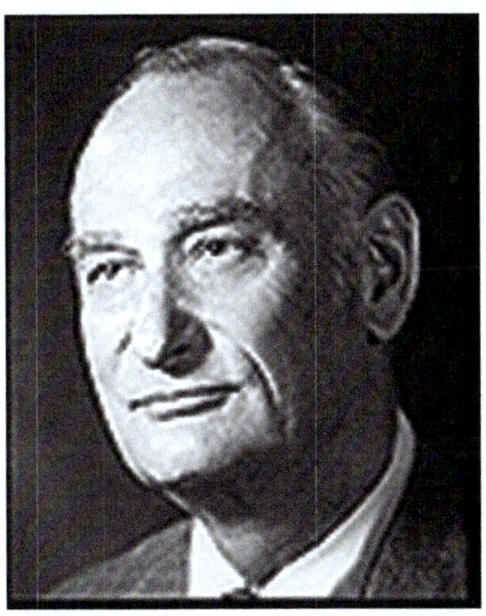

Fig. 2-59 Jack B. Caldwell (1914–1986).

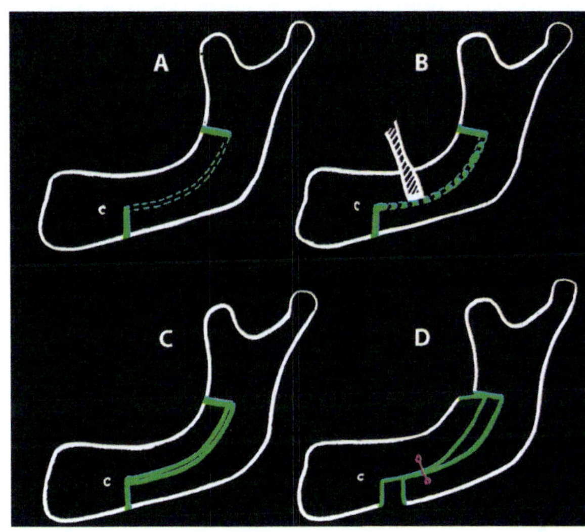

Fig. 2-61 Caldwell's C osteotomy. (After Caldwell et al.[72]).

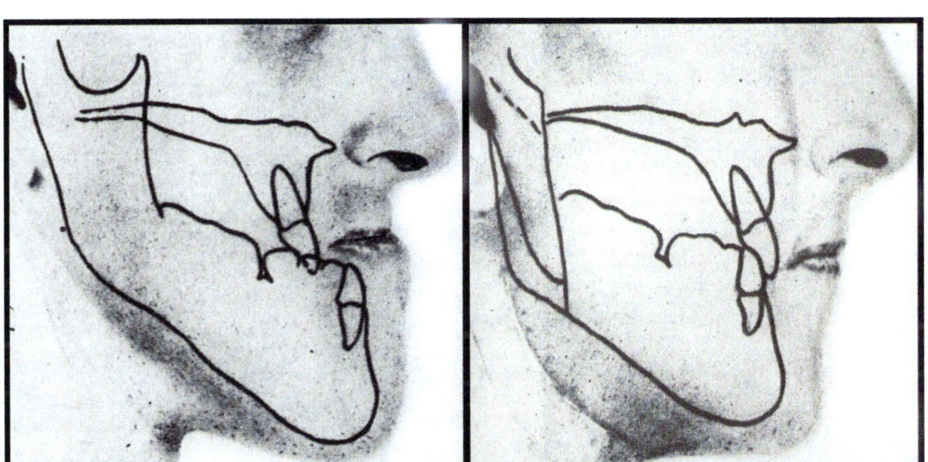

Fig. 2-60 Caldwell and Letterman's vertical subsigmoid osteotomy (via an extraoral approach) for mandibular set-back (1954). (From Caldwell and Letterman,[71]). Hebert, Kent and Hinds later described the procedure via an intraoral approach (1970).[73]

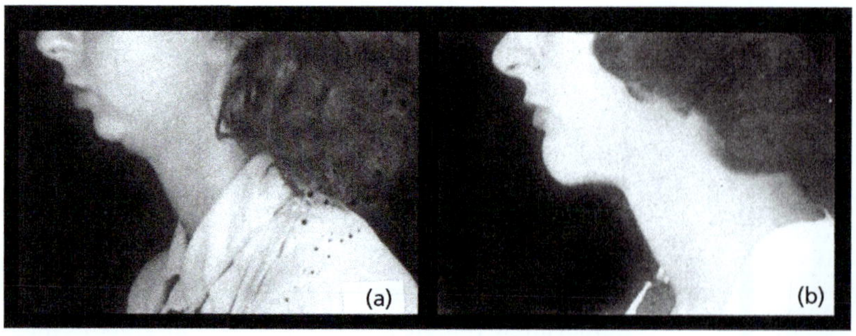

Fig. 2-62 Iliac bone graft to the osseous chin placed via a submental incision and resection of submental adipose tissue (patient had orthodontic treatment to improve the dental occlusion prior to surgery) (From Kazanjian, 1952,[74]).

disadvantage of the intraoral approach, as direct vision of the bone cut was not always possible, and suggested reserving the approach for patients prone to keloid scar formation and those who object to extraoral incisions.

Osseous genioplasty

Grafts and implants have been used for many years in the attempt to increase the prominence of a receding chin. Until the 1950s, onlays placed via a submental skin incision, both autogenous grafts, such as bone,[74] (Figure 2-62), or alloplastic implants, were the methods of choice. Problems were inevitable, such as eventual resorption of the bone grafts, infection, displacement and bony erosion by alloplastic materials. The osseous genioplasty, which is essentially *an osteotomy of the inferior border of the anterior part of the mandible*, was the solution to these problems.

The first recorded report of an osseous surgical procedure to advance a recessive chin is from 1942, undertaken by the surgeon **Otto Hofer**.[75] Hofer had been trained by **Hans Pichler** (1887–1949) (Figure 2-63) in Vienna,[76] the distinguished oral surgeon famous for operating on Sigmund Freud (Figure 2-64) (1856–1939) more than 30 times from 1923 until Freud's death in 1939.

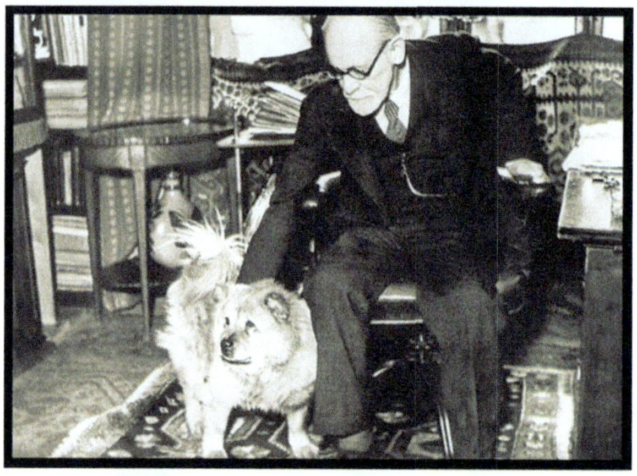

Fig. 2-64 Sigmund Freud (1856–1939), the 'father of psychoanalysis', in his study with his beloved Chow Chow, named Jo-fi (c.1936). Jo-fi was his constant companion. Freud admired the lack of pretension in the behaviour of dogs, which he felt was sadly lacking in humans.

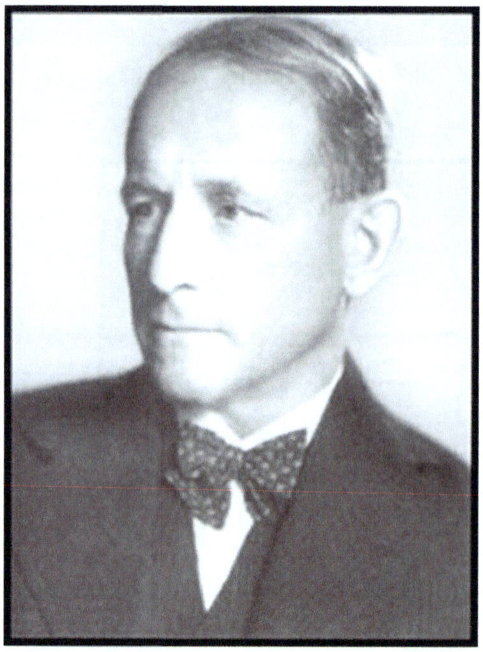

Fig. 2-63 Hans Pichler (1887–1949).

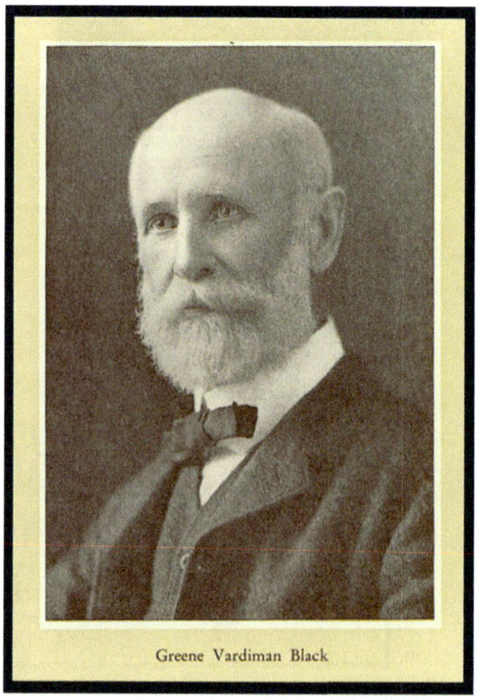

Fig. 2-65 Greene Vardiman (GV) Black (1836–1915).

Note:

Pichler trained in dentistry after his medical education, and spent a year with GV Black (1836–1915) (Figure 2-65), regarded as the pioneer of dentistry in the United States.[76] Therefore, he was able to operate on Freud's maxillary carcinoma by removing much of the right side of his maxilla, part of his mandible and cheek, and to create the maxillofacial prosthesis following surgical reconstruction (Figure 2-66). Freud found the prosthesis, which he dubbed 'the monster', difficult to wear, as it was sore but could not be left out due to the risk of soft tissue shrinkage. He also found it difficult to speak, and refused to eat in public due to embarrassment. In 1931, Dr Brunswick, a friend of Freud, invited Varaztad Kazanjian, then travelling through London and Paris for congresses, to visit Vienna and see Freud. Kazanjian initially refused, but was persuaded by Princess Maria of Greece. Kazanjian worked with Pichler, and made Freud a new prosthesis, which was more tolerable, and which he managed to wear for 3 years (Figure 2-67). Kazanjian and Pichler remained life-long friends.[77]

Hofer advanced the osseous chin via an extraoral approach (Figure 2-68), though the procedure was undertaken on a cadaver, which Hofer failed to mention in his paper. Sir Harold Gillies mentions some form of advancement osteotomy of the chin from an external approach, which was reported in 1957.[78] However, the osseous genioplasty from an intraoral

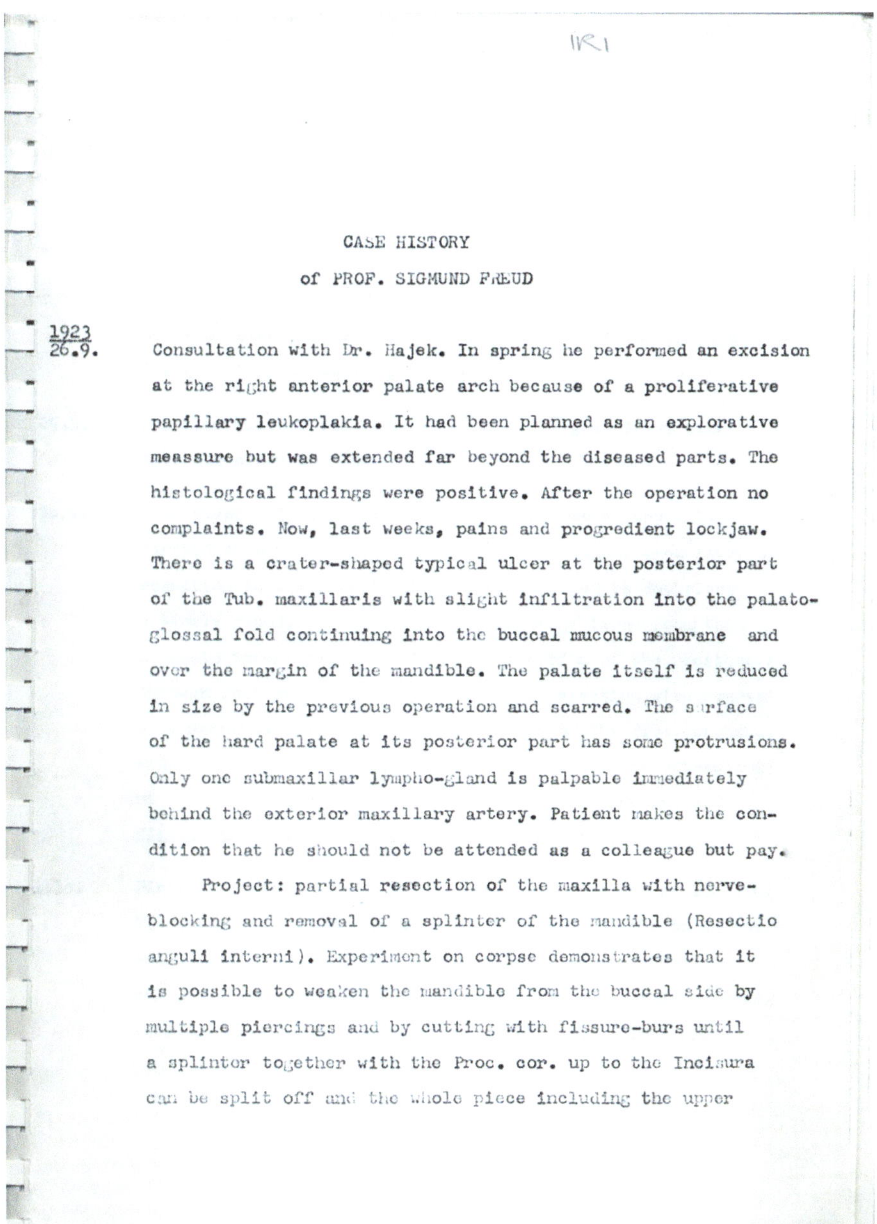

1181

CASE HISTORY

of PROF. SIGMUND FREUD

1923
26.9. Consultation with Dr. Hajek. In spring he performed an excision at the right anterior palate arch because of a proliferative papillary leukoplakia. It had been planned as an explorative meassure but was extended far beyond the diseased parts. The histological findings were positive. After the operation no complaints. Now, last weeks, pains and progredient lockjaw. There is a crater-shaped typical ulcer at the posterior part of the Tub. maxillaris with slight infiltration into the palato-glossal fold continuing into the buccal mucous membrane and over the margin of the mandible. The palate itself is reduced in size by the previous operation and scarred. The surface of the hard palate at its posterior part has some protrusions. Only one submaxillar lympho-gland is palpable immediately behind the exterior maxillary artery. Patient makes the condition that he should not be attended as a colleague but pay.

Project: partial resection of the maxilla with nerve-blocking and removal of a splinter of the mandible (Resectio anguli interni). Experiment on corpse demonstrates that it is possible to weaken the mandible from the buccal side by multiple piercings and by cutting with fissure-burs until a splintor together with the Proc. cor. up to the Incisura can be split off and the whole piece including the upper

Fig. 2-66 First page of case history notes of Professor Sigmund Freud by Professor Hans Pichler (Courtesy of Freud Museum London).

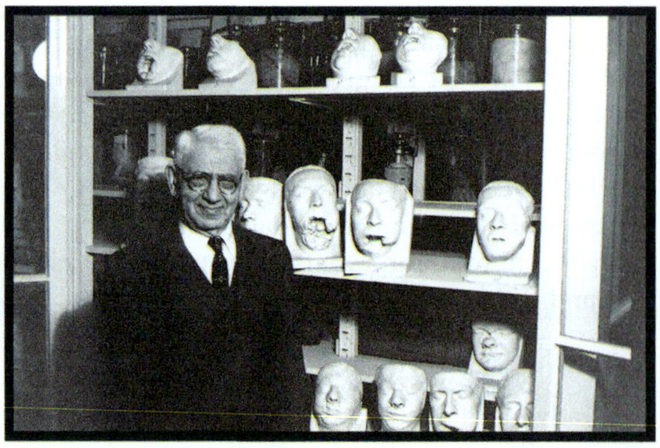

Fig. 2-67 Varaztad Kazanjian in his laboratory.

approach, and in fact the term 'genioplasty', were introduced by Obwegeser in 1957 (see Chapter 1 and Figure 1.6).[62] In 1964, John Marquis Converse and Donald Wood-Smith published an article presenting various modifications of the osseous genioplasty to advance the chin while simultaneously reducing or increasing osseous chin height, as well as correcting osseous chin asymmetry (Figure 2-69a–d).[79] Various modifications have been introduced to this incredibly versatile procedure, including double-step advancement, suggested by **Otto Neuner** (1965) (Figure 2-70),[80] and triple-step advancement as described by Obwegeser in 1970.[81]

Maxillary osteotomies

'One does not know a science completely without knowing its history.'

Auguste Comte (1798–1857)[82]
French philosopher and mathematician

The Le Fort I-type maxillary osteotomy

The fund of knowledge drawn upon in the development of modern maxillary orthognathic surgical procedures had diverse historical origins and contributions. The removal of nasal and nasopharyngeal polyps via hemimaxillary osteotomy was being undertaken in Europe in the mid-19th century, notably by the German surgeon **Bernhard Rudolf Konrad von Langenbeck** (1810–87) (Figure 2-71) in Berlin (von Langenbeck had succeeded Johann Friedrich Dieffenbach as director of the Clinical Institute of Surgery at Charité Hospital in Berlin).[83] The first maxillary procedure that would today be described as a total Le Fort I-type osteotomy appears to have been undertaken

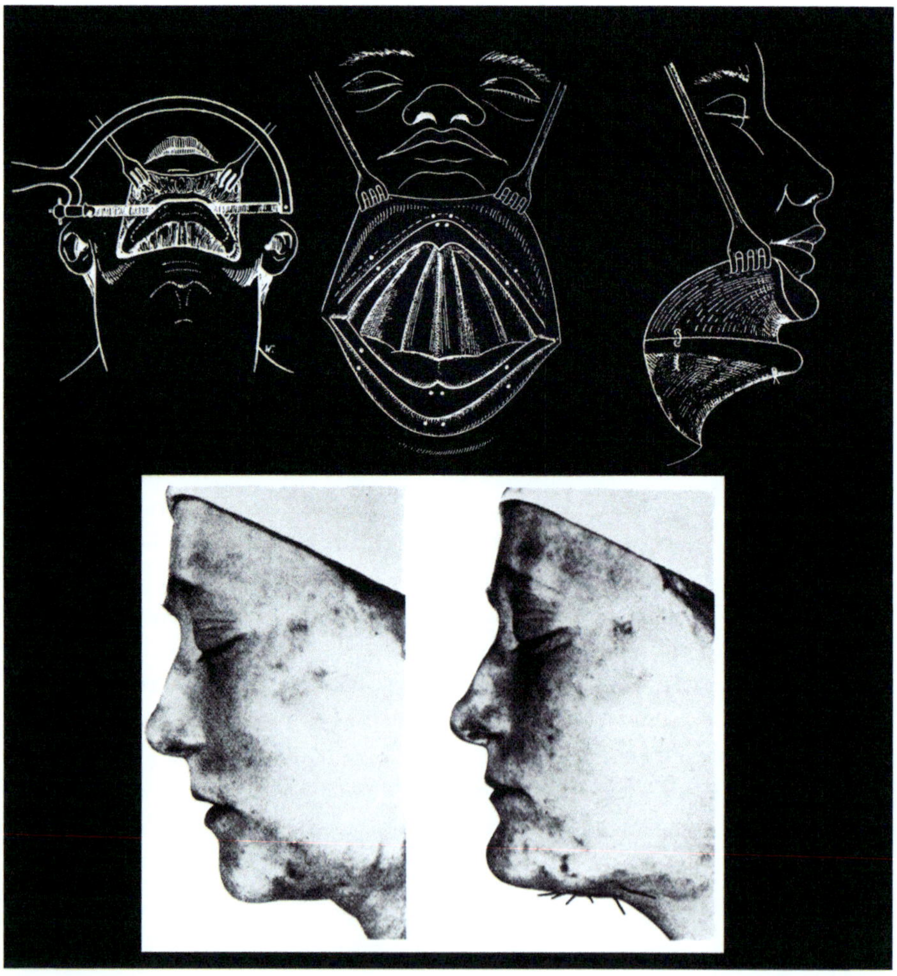

Fig. 2-68 Hofer's advancement genioplasty of the osseous chin, undertaken via an extraoral approach on a cadaver (After Hofer, 1942,[75]) (Courtesy of Professor Hugo Obwegeser).

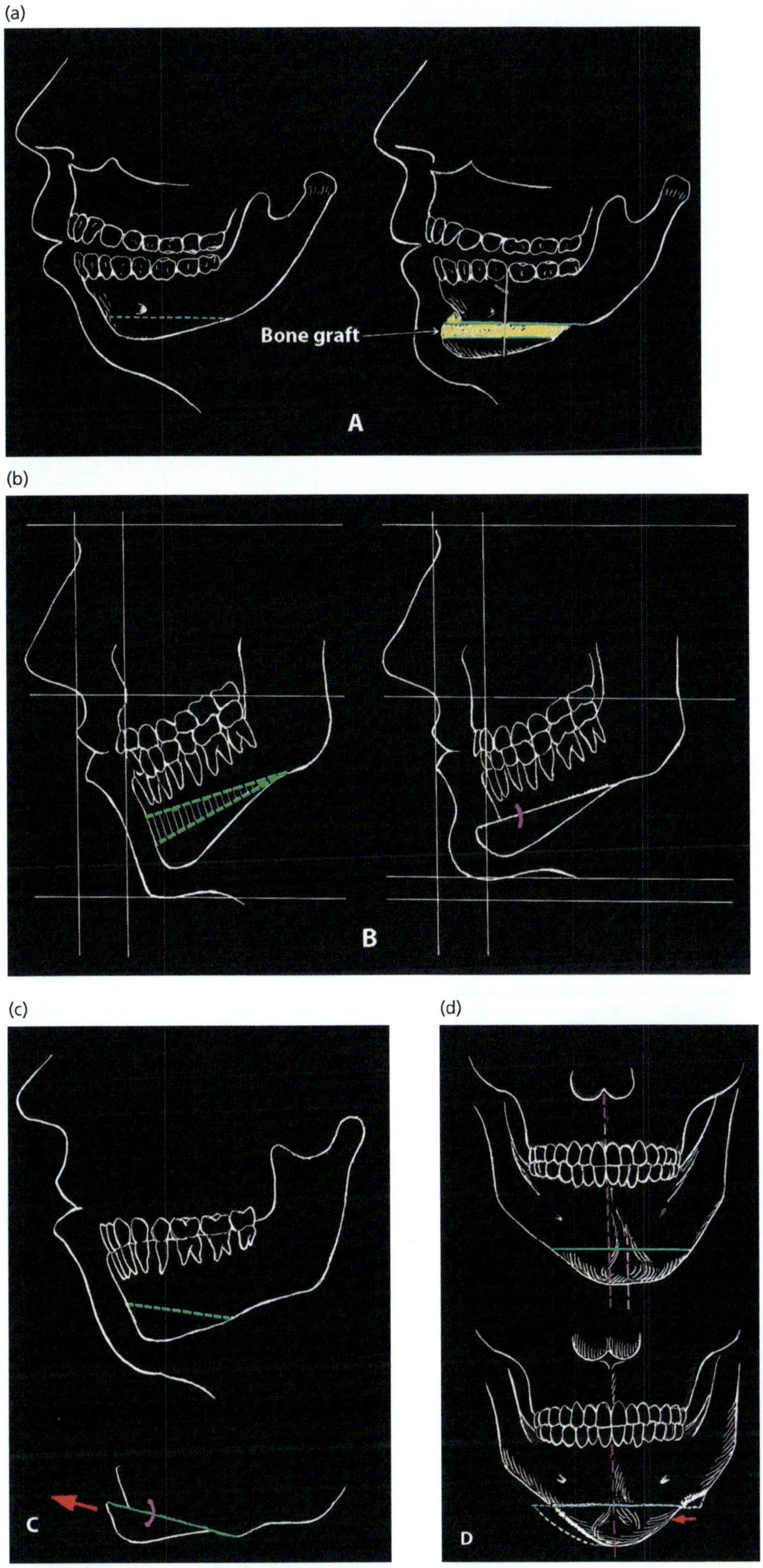

Fig. 2-69 (a): The 'sandwich' procedure, used to advance and increase the height of the chin; (b): Advancement genioplasty with resection of a bony segment to reduce chin height; (c): Oblique osteotomy to advance and reduce height of chin; (d): Correction of osseous chin asymmetry – the broken line outlines bone to be resected to obtain a smooth contour (After Converse and Wood-Smith, 1964,[79]).

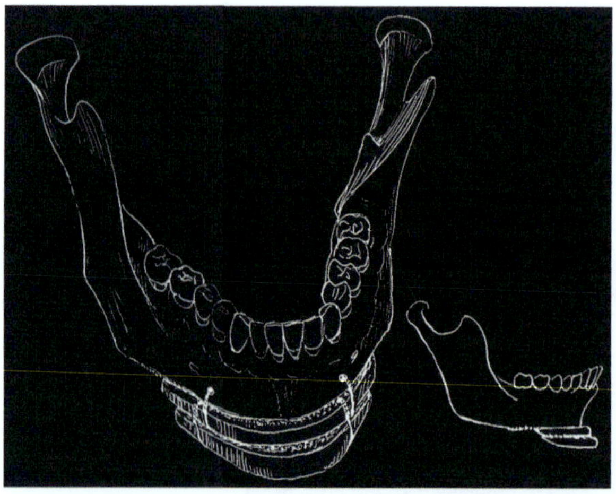

Fig. 2-70 Neuner's double-step advancement genioplasty (1965). (After Neuner,[80]).

in 1868 by the American surgeon **David Williams Cheever** (Figure 2-72) (1831–1915) in Boston City Hospital, to provide surgical access for removal of a large nasopharyngeal polyp.[84] One year prior to this, in 1867, Cheever had undertaken a downfracture of the right hemimaxilla for similar surgical access in another patient, who had made a complete recovery.[85] The total downfracture of the maxilla at the Le Fort I level performed in 1868, described as Cheever's 'double operation', though technically successful, had an unfortunate postoperative outcome in that the patient subsequently died 5 days later, though probably not as a direct result of the maxillary procedure.[86,87] A friend of Cheever, John Collins Warren from Harvard wrote to von Langenbeck in Germany to ask whether a 'double operation' had been undertaken in Europe, and

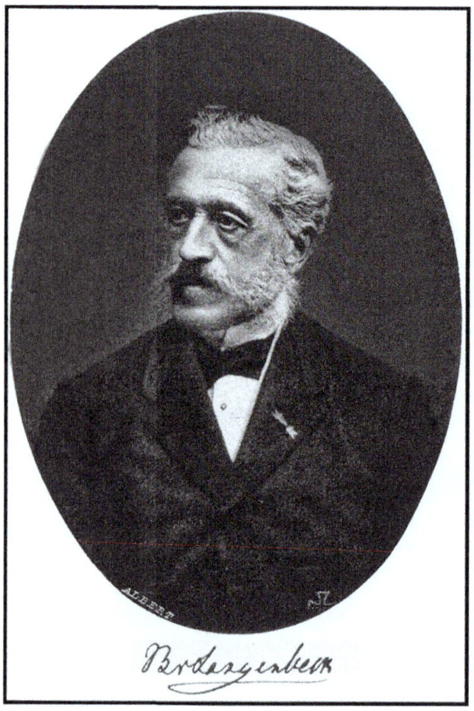

Fig. 2-71 Bernhard von Langenbeck (1810–1887).

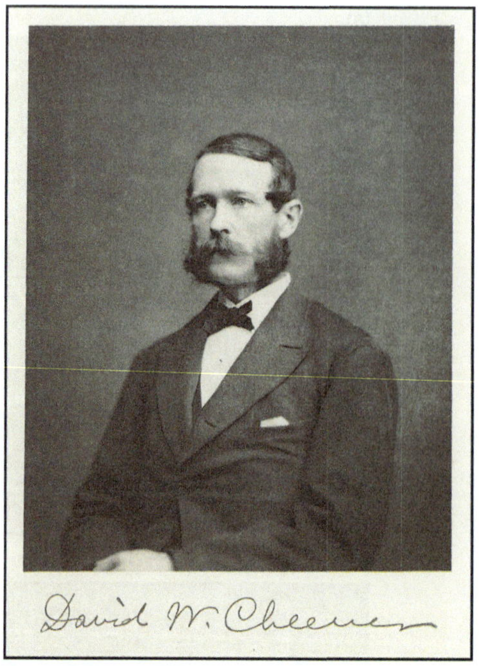

Fig. 2-72 David W. Cheever (1831–1915) (c.1875, Courtesy of Harvard Medical School).

von Langenbeck apparently replied that to the best of his knowledge such a procedure had not been undertaken anywhere else.[87]

In 1901, a French surgeon from Lille named **René Le Fort** (1869–1951) (Figure 2-73) conducted experiments using blunt trauma to intact cadaveric faces, from different directions and varying magnitudes, and thereby described the natural planes of maxillary and facial fractures,[88,89] now known as the Le Fort classification of facial fractures. The names of the Le Fort I, II and III-type osteotomies are due to their similarity

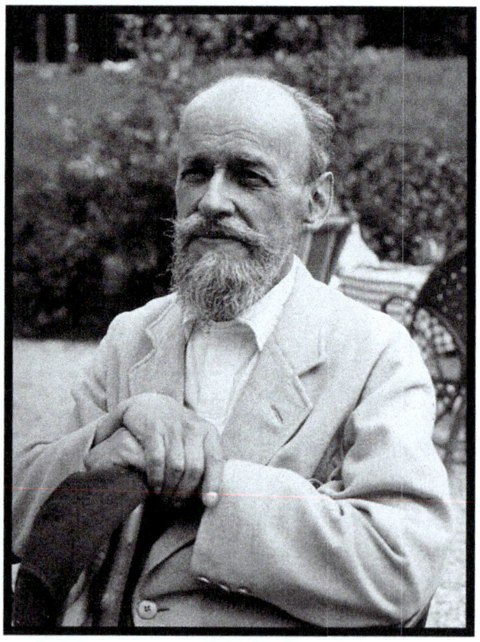

Fig. 2-73 René Le Fort (1869–1951).

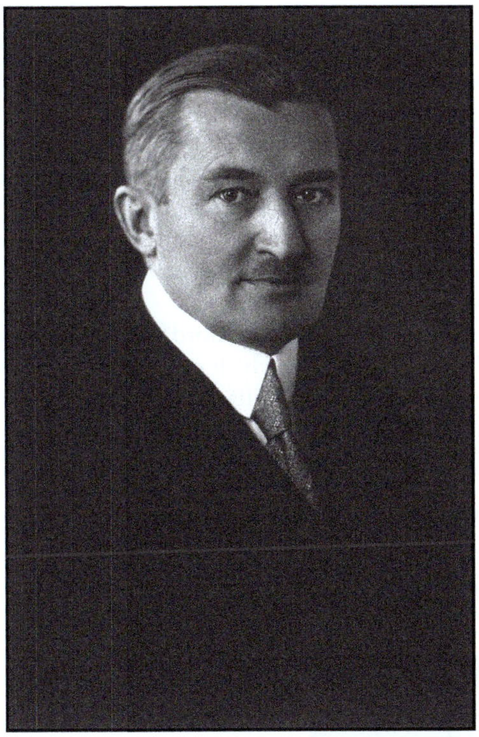

Fig. 2-74 Georg Axhausen (1877–1960) (Courtesy of the National Library of Medicine).

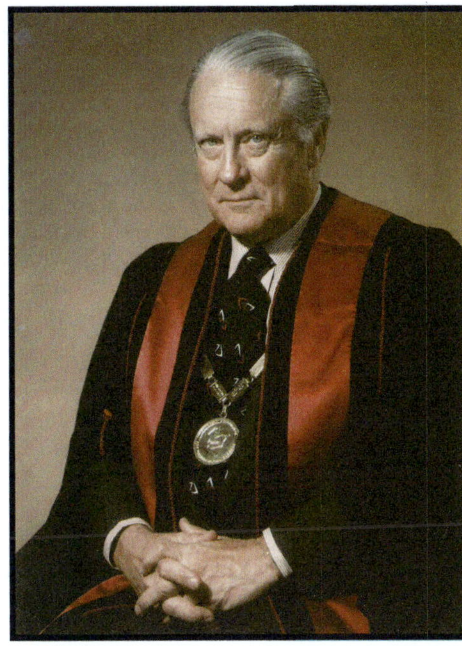

Fig. 2-75 Norman Lester Rowe (1915–1980). Professor Rowe was appointed consultant in oral surgery at Rooksdown House in Basingstoke (1949-59) and worked there with Sir Harold Gillies. Norman Rowe's stature as a clinician and statesman grew after Rooksdown House was transferred to Queen Mary's University Hospital, Roehampton, in 1959. Roehampton became *the* centre for oral and maxillofacial surgeons throughout the world as a result of his reputation as a surgeon and his extensive writing, particularly the textbook *Fractures of the Facial Skeleton*. He made friends wherever he went and was affectionately known as 'Uncle' to both senior and junior colleagues, which reflected his perceived wisdom and his willingness to give help whenever it was asked of him. He became a lifelong friend to Professor Hugo Obwegeser. (Courtesy of Mr Peter Blenkinsopp, Consultant Oral and Maxillofacial Surgeon, and head of the former Norman Rowe Maxillofacial Unit at Queen Mary's University Hospital, Roehampton, UK).

to the Le Fort fractures. The Le Fort I fracture is sometimes referred to as a Guérin fracture, after its original description by the French surgeon **Alphonse François Marie Guérin** (1816–1895) in 1866.

In 1927, Wassmund carried out a maxillary osteotomy at the Le Fort I level, without pterygoid plate disjunction or mobilization at the time of surgery.[90] He used elastics to close an anterior open bite, without placing a bone graft, which subsequently relapsed. In 1934, Axhausen (Figure 2-74) in Berlin described advancement of the maxilla at the Le Fort I level, which was incompletely mobilized, again with postoperative elastic traction.[91] In 1942, in order not to impair the vascular supply to the maxilla, Schuchardt described a two-stage Le Fort I osteotomy, the second stage involving pterygomaxillary separation, and use of external postoperative traction using weights hung from an overhead pulley system to advance the maxilla.[92] In 1949, Moore and Ward recommended horizontal transection of the pterygoid plates for maxillary advancement.[93] In 1954, Gillies and Rowe (Figure 2-75) described a maxillary osteotomy in a cleft patient with advancement and use of autogenous bone grafts, though the mandible also had to be set-back and the profile was 'flattened', suggesting that the required maxillary advancement was not achieved.[94] Gillies and Rowe demonstrated further cases in cleft patients.

Most of the techniques described partial mobilization the maxilla, followed by placement of some form of external orthopaedic force for repositioning. Inevitably, relapse rates were considerable.

Modern Le Fort I-type osteotomy was developed by Obwegeser,[95,96] in that he fully mobilized the maxilla, and performed pterygomaxillary disjunction between the maxillary tuberosities and the pterygoid plates. This proved to be a major advance (see Chapter 1 for further description of the development of this technique). Obwegeser also suggested the use of a bone graft between the pterygoid plate and maxillary tuberosity bilaterally.

Note:

Hugo Obwegeser – the father of modern orthognathic surgery

Professor Hugo Obwegeser was the invited speaker for a series of lectures at the Walter Reed Army Medical Center in Washington D.C., in mid-June of 1966. This appearance is widely regarded as the inspiration hailing the beginning of many subsequent contributions to orthognathic surgery, particularly in the United States. As such, it is also widely regarded as the beginning of modern orthognathic surgery. Time magazine (1 July 1966) commented:

> '... last week, 500 of the most eminent U.S. oral surgeons sat on the edges of their chairs at Washington's Walter Reed Army Medical Center as a respected Swiss practitioner described his radical jaw-splitting procedures... American oral surgeons have never been so impressed... '

His subsequent publications, including the first description of a simultaneous bimaxillary procedure (Le Fort I-type maxillary advancement and inferior repositioning osteotomy and bilateral sagittal split set-back osteotomy of the mandible) undertaken on 5 September 1969 (Figure 2-76), paved the way for the development of modern orthognathic surgery as a distinct field.

A useful modification to the Le Fort I-type maxillary advancement was suggested by **Josef Kufner** (1924–1995) (Figure 2-77a) from Prague (1971),[97] which was to undertake a 'high' Le Fort I-type osteotomy including a part of the inferior orbital rim and zygoma (also described as the Kufner modification of the Le Fort III-type osteotomy), in order to improve a flat facial contour higher up in the face rather than just at the lower part of the maxilla, i.e. malar-maxillary advancement (Figure 2-77b).

In 1985, Bennett and Wolford[98] described the Le Fort I 'step' osteotomy, which prevented the potential ramping effect with maxillary advancements (Figure 2-78).

Segmental maxillary osteotomies

The first maxillary osteotomy undertaken to correct a malocclusion, which may thereby be referred to as

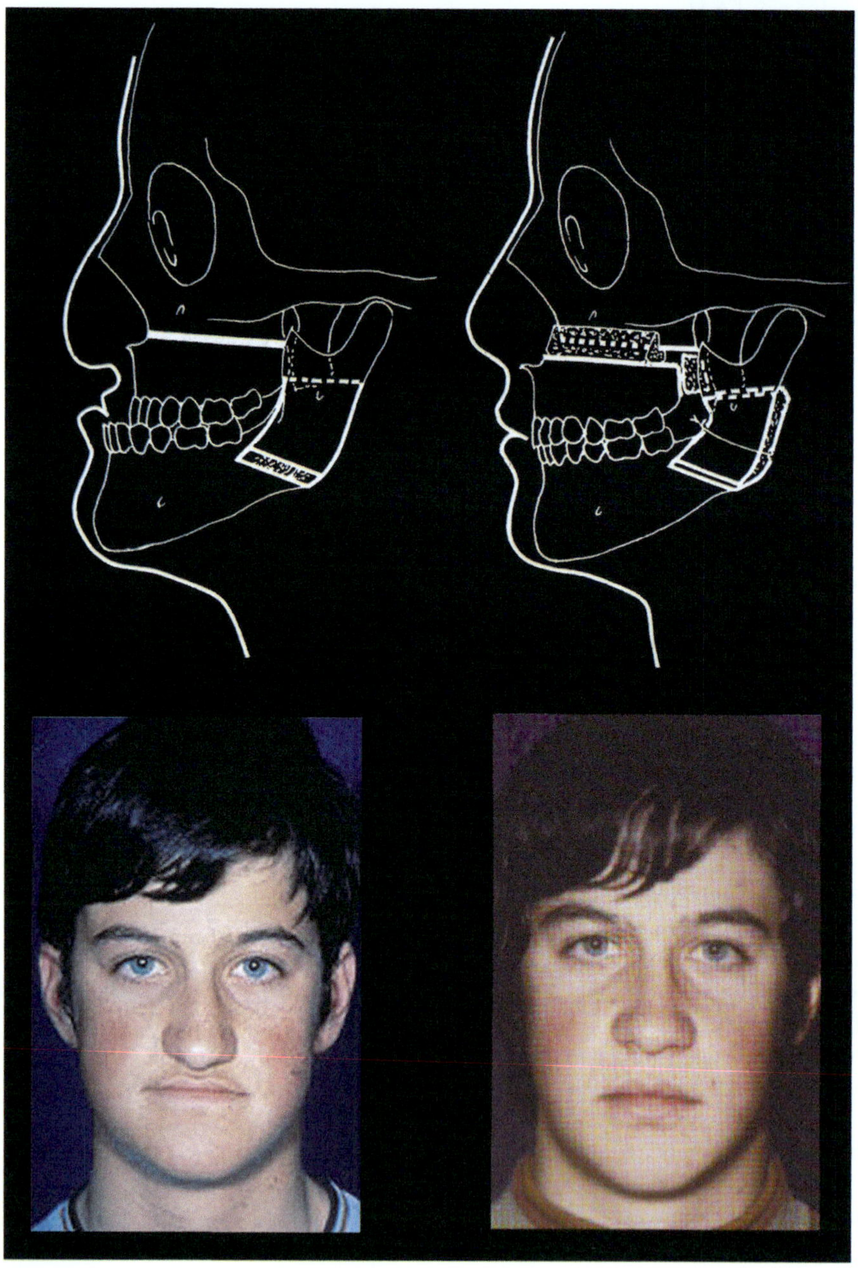

Fig. 2-76 Obwegeser's first description of a simultaneous bimaxillary osteotomy (undertaken in 1969, published in 1970,[81]).

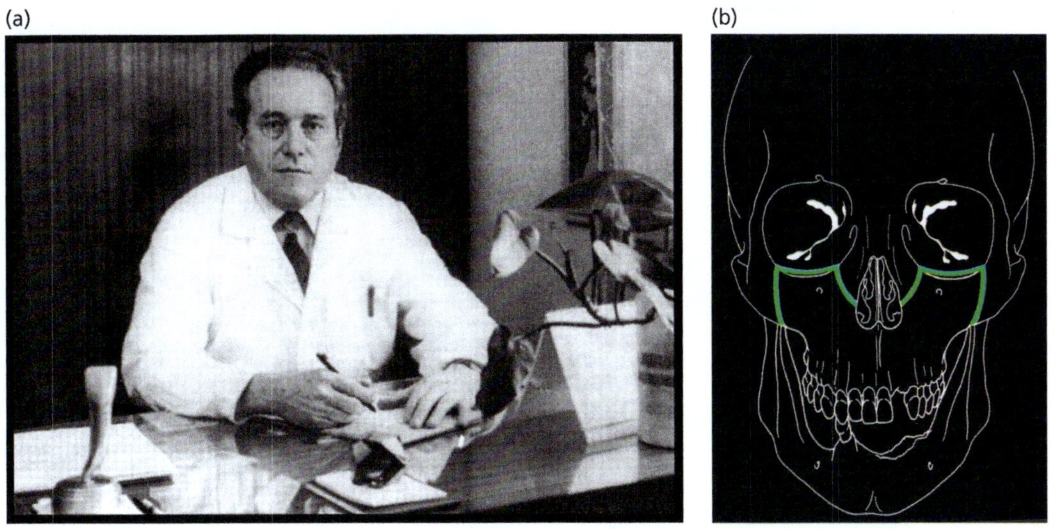

Fig. 2-77 (a): Josef Kufner (1924–1995) (Courtesy of Professor Daniel Hrušák). (b): Kufner's extended osteotomy of the maxilla, i.e. Kufner modification of the Le Fort III-type osteotomy (After Obwegeser).

the first maxillary orthognathic procedure, was undertaken by the German surgeon **Günther Cohn-Stock** (1889–1983) (Figure 2-79) in 1920, and published in 1921.[99,100] His technique involved the extraction of a maxillary premolar bilaterally, a palatal approach to the anterior maxillary dentoalveolus, the removal of a wedge-shaped segment of bone, and retroclination of the dentoalveolus. The technique was thereby useful for retroclination of a proclined anterior maxillary dentoalveolus, but not for bodily retrusion of a prominent dentoalveolus, as the maxillary incisors would inevitably retrocline (Figure 2-80). Cohn-Stock was Jewish, and thereby left Germany in 1939 through the help of Prince Bernhard of Holland, and immigrated to London. In 1965 he retired to Northern California.[100]

In 1935, Wassmund described his now famous segmental set-back of the anterior maxillary dentoalveolus (Figure 2-81).[101] Wassmund's procedure was in two stages; first, removal of palatal bone via the palate; and second, a month later, removal of bone from a buccal approach and set-back of the anterior maxilla. In 1954 **Ivo Čupar** (1901–1981) (Figure 2-82) from Zagreb described an osteotomy of the maxillary labial segment (canine-to-canine region), based on palatal blood supply.[102] The Čupar osteotomy involved a maxillary vestibular incision from first premolar to premolar. The mucoperiosteum was elevated through this

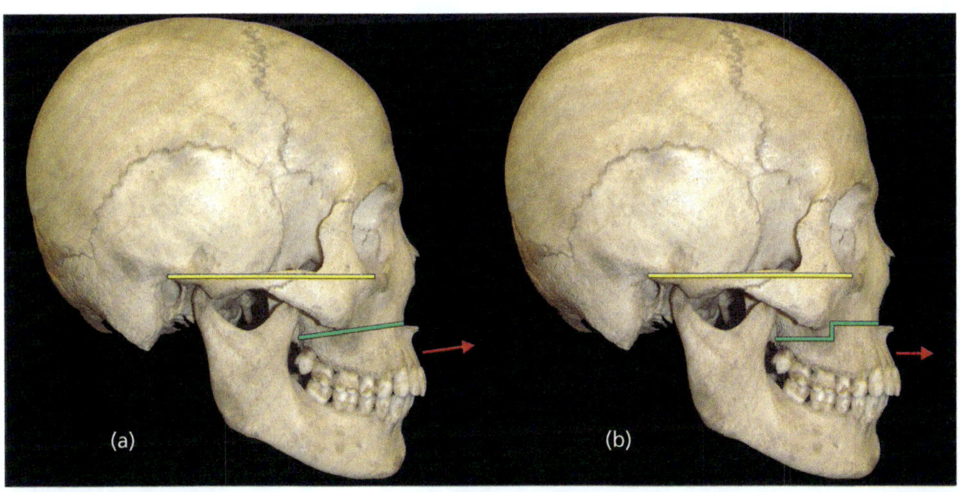

Fig. 2-78 (a): Traditional Le Fort I-type osteotomy, from the piriform rim region, approximately 5 mm above the roots apices, to the pterygoid plate region. The osteotomy is designed to avoid the root of the canine and the maxillary buttress, and thereby tends to have an anterior-superior inclination. Advancement of the maxilla creates a ramping effect and inadvertent vertical movement. (b): Bennett and Wolford's Le Fort I 'step' osteotomy (1985), which prevents the potential ramping effect by keeping the horizontal cuts parallel to the true horizontal plane (or Frankfort plane if it is horizontal). The anterior cut is made from the piriform rim, approximately 4–5 mm above the root of the maxillary canine, to the zygomatic buttress. In the buttress region, a vertical step is created (approximately 5–8 mm), following which a further horizontal cut is continued at an inferior level towards the pterygoid plates. The osteotomy design eliminates the ramping effect. Significant maxillary advancement may require grafting of the step region.

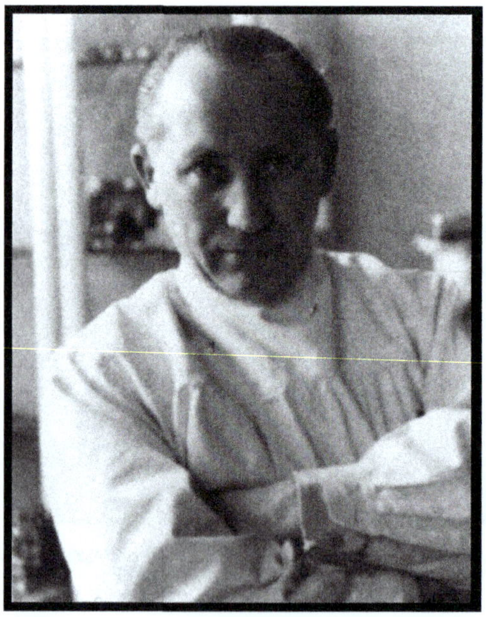

Fig. 2-79 Günther Cohn-Stock (1889–1983) (Courtesy of Journal of Cranio-Maxillofacial Surgery – Elsevier).

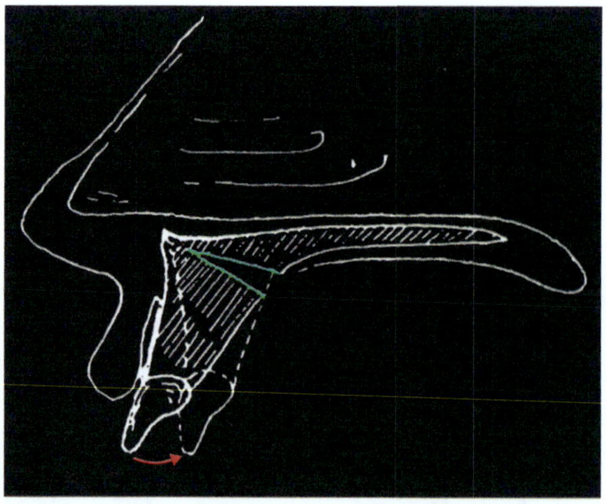

Fig. 2-80 The first recorded maxillary anterior segmental osteotomy (Cohn-Stock, 1921). The greenstick type osteotomy of the anterior maxillary segment relapsed within a month of the procedure. (After Cohn-Stock,[99]).

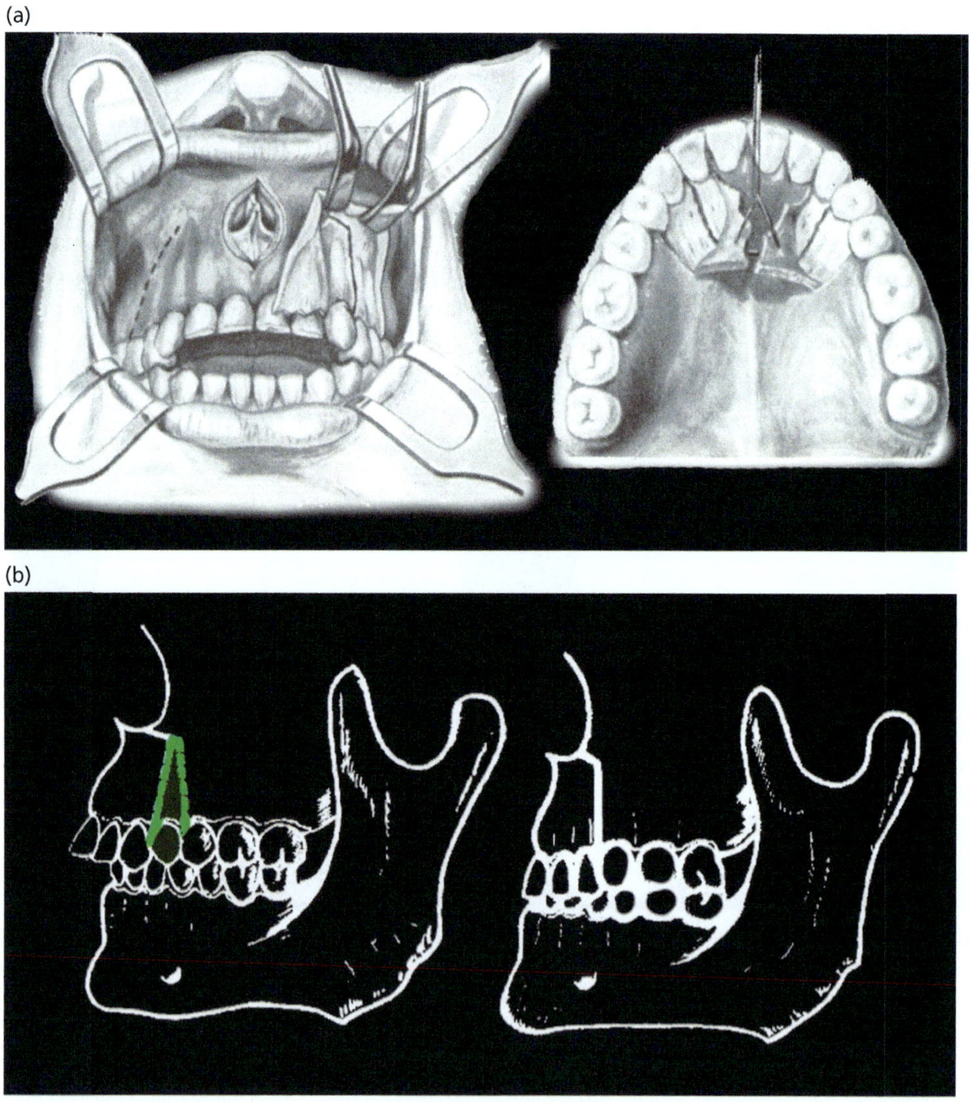

Fig. 2-81 (a): Wassmund's two-stage segmental set-back of the anterior maxillary dentoalveolus (1935). (From Wassmund,[101]). (b): Wassmund's procedure increases the incisor overbite (After Köle, 1959,[26–28]).

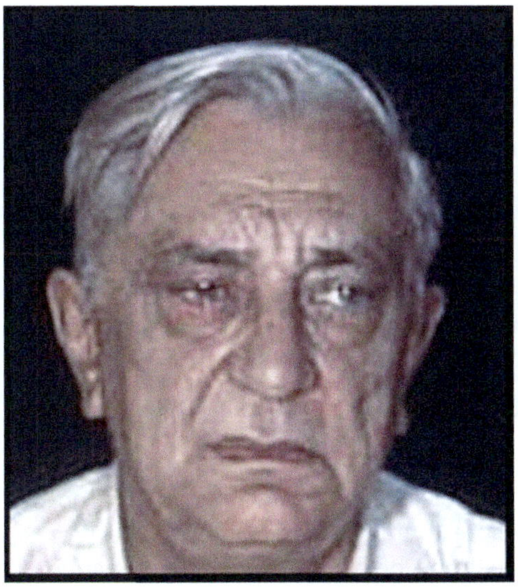

Fig. 2-82 Ivo Čupar (1901–1981) (Courtesy of Professor Darko Macan).

incision to expose the piriform aperture and anterior wall of the maxilla up to the canine fossa. Maxillary first premolars were extracted bilaterally. Palatal tunnelling was undertaken via the extraction sockets converging at the midline. Keeping the gingivoperiosteal flap intact and well retracted a maxillary osteotomy was carried out from the socket of the extracted premolars to the piriform aperture bilaterally followed by the palatal osteotomy. After completing the osteotomy, the anterior maxillary segment was downfractured and superiorly and posteriorly repositioned.

In 1959, Köle[26–28] described a number of variations of segmental maxillary osteotomies (Figure 2-83). In 1962, **Siegfried Wunderer** in Vienna described a modification to Wassmund's procedure, as a single procedure from a palatal approach that preserved a broad labial mucoperiosteal pedicle; the technique also bears his name (Figure 2-84).[103]

(a)

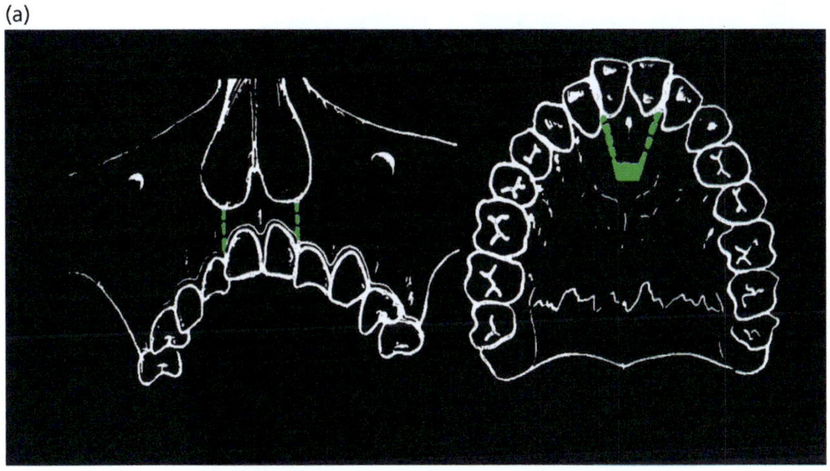

(b)

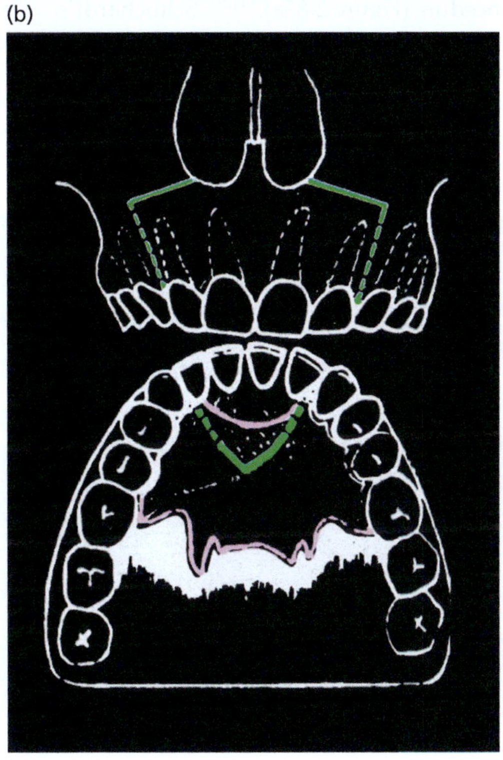

Fig. 2-83 (a, b): Köle described variations of segmental maxillary osteotomies (After Köle, 1959,[26–28]).

(c)

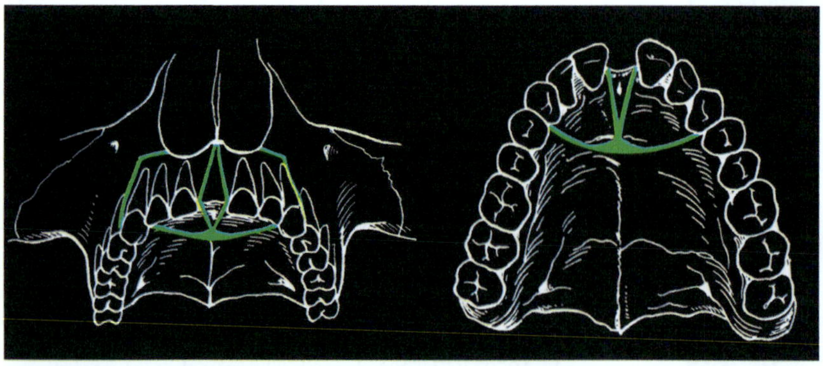

Fig. 2-83 (*Continued*).

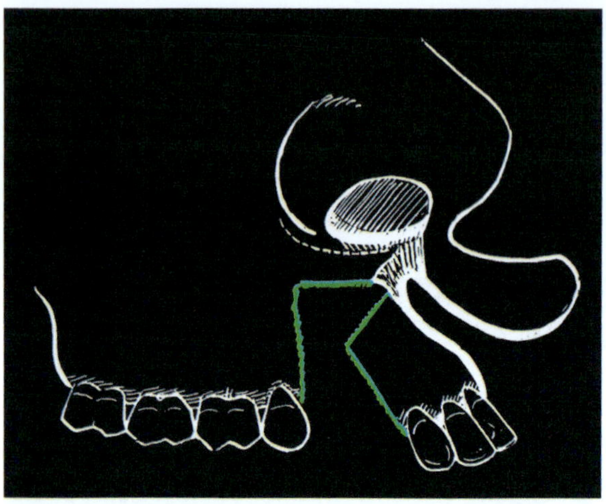

Fig. 2-84 Wunderer's osteotomy is a single-stage procedure from a palatal approach that preserves a broad labial mucoperiosteal pedicle (After Converse).

Posterior segmental impaction of the maxillary dentoalveolus was described by Schuchardt as a two-stage procedure (Figure 2-85a).[104,105] Schuchardt's procedure involved bilateral impaction of the posterior dentoalveolar processes of the maxilla, allowing forward mandibular autorotation and closure of an anterior open bite. The first stage of the procedure involved release of the mucoperiosteum on the hard palate, preserving the greater palatine artery. A sagittal osteotomy of the hard palate was undertaken on both sides of the alveolar process starting behind the maxillary canine on the palate and extending along the palatal roots as far as the maxillary tuberosity. The mucoperiosteum was then sutured back in position. After 3 to 6 weeks, the second stage of the procedure was undertaken, with a horizontal incision in the buccal vestibule, and a horizontal strip of bone removed from the lateral wall of the maxilla above the roots of the premolar and molar teeth. The ostectomy terminated vertically behind the terminal molar. With either finger pressure or a stroke with a mallet, the alveolar process was mobilized and superiorly repositioned, and dental splints and intermaxillary wiring used for fixation. One of the main drawbacks to the procedure was that by the second stage, the initial palatal osteotomy sites had already begun to fuse. In addition, the maxillary tuberosity region required further trauma to move the osteotomized segment. Kufner[106,107] (Figure 2-85b) later described a one-stage modification of the Schuchardt osteotomy. A vestibular incision was made from the apex of the first premolar as far as the apices of the maxillary molars. Horizontal bony strips were removed from the lateral wall of the maxilla above the roots of the posterior teeth,

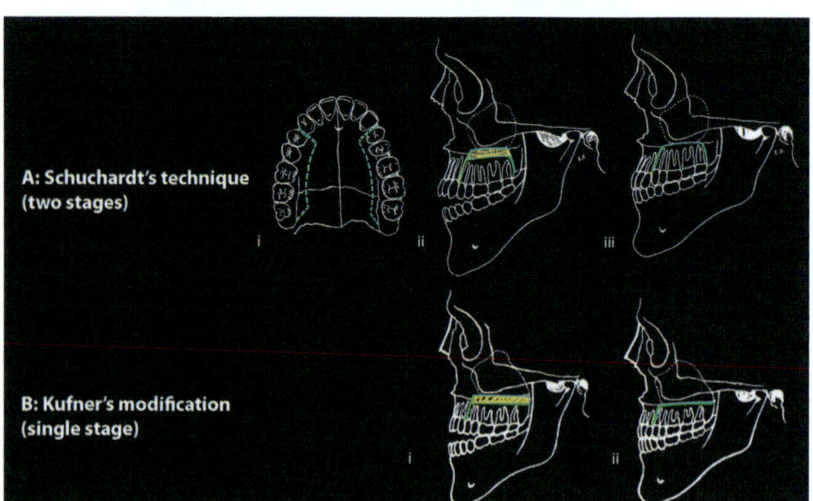

Fig. 2-85 (a): Schuchardt's posterior segmental osteotomy was developed in the mid-1950s. Initially described as a two-stage procedure, (i) with bilateral palatal alveolar osteotomies performed, followed by reapplication of the palatal flap, and (ii and iii) buccal osteotomies undertaken as a second procedure after 3–6 weeks to elevate the posterior maxillary dentoalveolar segments. The posterior segment could also be inferiorly repositioned, and the residual space bone grafted, in the presence of a lateral open bite. (b): Kufner's one-stage modification of the Schuchardt posterior segmental osteotomy. (After Kufner,[97]).

from the first premolar region to the pterygopalatine fissure. Kufner noted:[107]

> 'Following removal of this strip of bone, a horizontal incision is made in the mucous membrane of the maxillary sinus making the posterior wall of the maxillary tuberosity and the palatal side accessible. In these locations a cut is enough, and an ostectomy is not necessary because the upward positioning of the alveolus is not blocked. The mucous membrane of the palatal wall of the maxillary sinus is not cut to the whole extent of the wound. Bridges of the mucous membrane are saved to improve the nutrition of the floor of the sinus. Nutrition is also received through the interdental gingiva which is nourished from the untouched palatal mucous membrane. After total mobilization, the alveolar process is hinged upon only a small bony bridge between the canine and the first premolar. There is no difficulty in removing this bridge with a narrow, flat chisel. The movable alveolar processes on both sides are then simultaneously shifted into the maxillary sinus. The best way to achieve this shift is through a slow biting by the patient.'

Note:

The advances in orthodontic techniques and mechanics in repositioning the teeth prior to surgical repositioning of the jaws have reduced the need for segmental surgery.

Blood supply to the osteotomized maxilla

From the late 1960s, revascularization studies undertaken by the American oral and maxillofacial surgeon **William H. Bell** helped to advance the understanding of the biological basis of maxillary (and mandibular) surgery and thereby its techniques.[108–119] It was demonstrated that the maxilla could be sectioned at the Le Fort I level and furthermore segmented and repositioned with only transient ischaemic effects and minimal discernible effects on revascularization and bone healing. Microangiography and histological methods demonstrated that the vascular circulation to the anterior maxillary segment was maintained when a soft tissue pedicle remained intact. The biological importance of maintaining a viable labial/buccal or palatal pedicle and thereby a blood supply to an osteotomized segment, which had been known clinically, was confirmed (Figure 2-86). Non-pedicled segments were shown to undergo necrosis within one week. As long as vascularity was not compromised following an osteotomy, bony union occurred within six weeks and dental pulp vascularity was maintained so long as the osteotomies were undertaken at some distance from the root apices.

Rigid fixation

Another advance in the evolution of orthognathic surgery occurred with the introduction and application of rigid and semi-rigid fixation between osteotomized segments with plates and screws, as opposed to wire osteosynthesis. The advantages were improved postoperative stabilization of the bony segments and considerable reduction in the need for

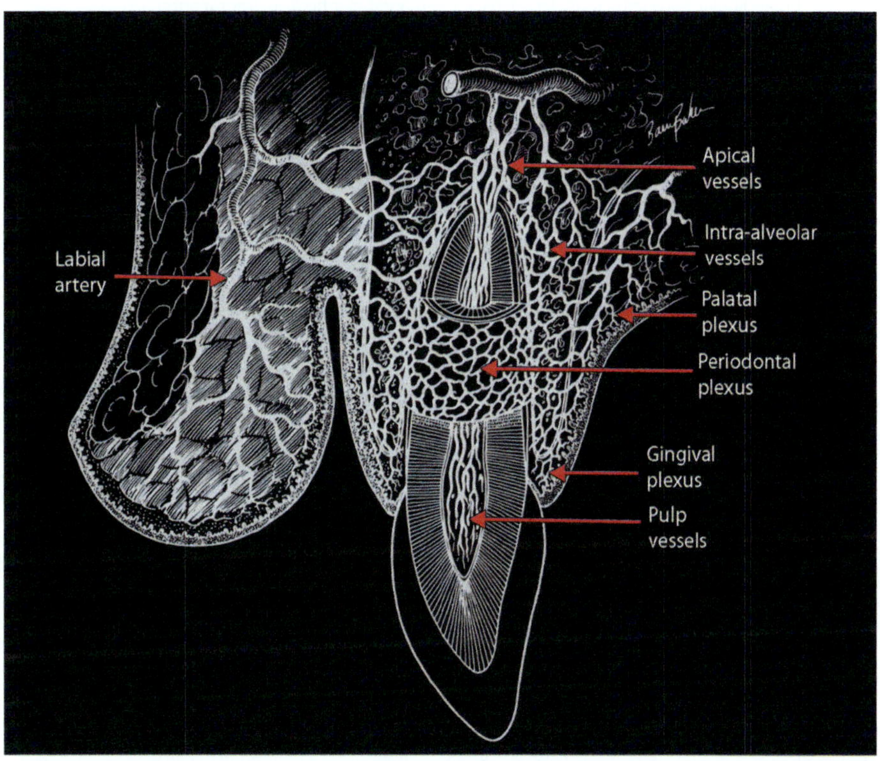

Fig. 2-86 Schematic diagram of the blood supply to the anterior maxillary dentoalveolus from various anastomosing vessels, which permits maxillary osteotomies to be undertaken without compromising vascularity (After Bell, 1972,[112]).

intermaxillary fixation. The origin of the technique stems from orthopaedic trauma surgery. The first bone plating in the maxillofacial region was carried out by the German general surgeon **Johannes Soerensen** in 1917,[120] using a gold wedding ring transformed into a small gold plate for the fixation of a mandibular fracture.[121] The application of rigid fixation in orthognathic surgery begins with **Bernd Spiessl** (1921–2002) (Figure 2-87), from Nittenau in Germany, who was appointed as Chair of Maxillofacial Surgery at Basel University in Switzerland in 1965. In 1974, Spiessl described rigid fixation of the mandible following a sagittal split osteotomy using compression lag screws, and explained its importance in relation to significant reduction in postoperative skeletal relapse.[122] Another German maxillofacial surgeon, **Hans Luhr** (1932–date), currently Emeritus Professor of Maxillofacial Surgery at the University of Göttingen, helped advance the understanding of rigid fixation techniques for maxillofacial trauma and eventually orthognathic surgery. Luhr trained and worked in Schuchardt's unit in Hamburg in the 1960s, and

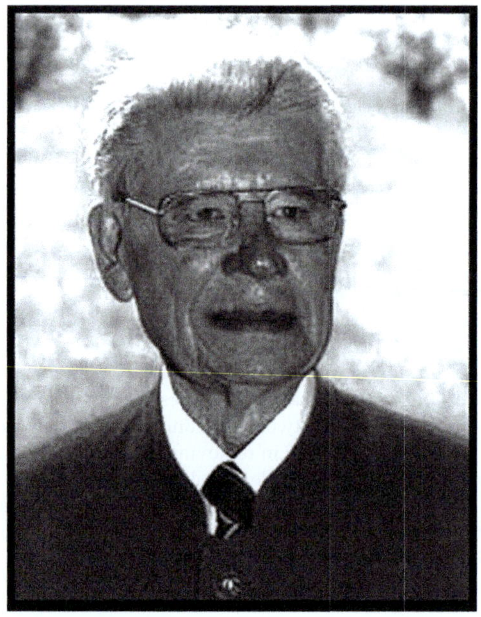

Fig. 2-87 Bernd Spiessl (1921–2002).

Table 2-1 Some landmark dates in the development of orthognathic surgery. Colour code: Maxillary procedures (purple); Mandibular procedures (green); chin procedures (yellow); other (blue)

Date	Clinician(s)	Description
1849	Hullihen[3]	Anterior mandibular subapical osteotomy and set-back, intraoral approach.
1859	von Langenbeck[83]	Hemimaxillary osteotomy for access to nasopharyngeal polyp.
1868	Cheever[84]	Maxillary osteotomy and downfracture at what is now termed the Le Fort I level for access to a nasopharyngeal polyp.
1905	Lane	Horizontal ramus osteotomy to set-back the mandible, extraoral approach.
1906	Blair[11]	Mandibular body ostectomy to set-back the mandibular body, extraoral approach; (procedure undertaken in 1897, but published in 1906).
1907	Blair[12]	Horizontal ramus osteotomy to advance the mandible, extraoral approach.
1909	Babcock[47]	Horizontal ramus osteotomy to set-back the mandible, extraoral approach; (procedure undertaken in 1908, but published in 1909).
1912	Harsha[17]	Performed a mandibular body ostectomy, extraoral approach;maintained the integrity of the neurovascular bundle.
1913	Cryer[14]	Described a semi-circular osteotomy near the angle of the mandible, extraoral approach.
1917	Aller[15]	Described removal of the bony wedge from the mandibular body, via an intraoral approach.
1921	Cohn-Stock[99]	Segmental retroclination of the anterior maxillary dentoalveolus (procedure undertaken in 1920).
1925	Limberg[56]	Posterior oblique vertical ramus osteotomy, extraoral approach.
1927	Wassmund[58]	Inverted 'L' type ramus osteotomy, extraoral approach.
1927	Wassmund[58]	Le Fort I osteotomy with the pterygomaxillary junction left intact; elastic forces were used to advance the maxilla.
1928	Kostečka[40]	Condylar neck osteotomy using Gigli saw to set-back the mandible, extraoral approach (but with minimal incisions).
1934	Axhausen[91]	Le Fort I osteotomy with postoperative advancement using elastic traction.
1935	Wassmund[101]	Segmental set-back of the anterior maxilla (2-stage procedure: first palatal approach; 4 weeks later buccal approach).
1936	Hofer[25]	Described an anterior mandibular subapical osteotomy to advance the mandibular labial dentoalveolar segment; extraoral approach; severed the mental nerves.
1936	Kazanjian[52]	Oblique horizontal osteotomy of the ramus, extraoral approach.
1938	Ernst[60]	The first horizontal ramus osteotomy via an intraoral approach.
1942	Hofer[75]	Osseous genioplasty - horizontal forward sliding osteotomy of a receding chin, extraoral approach (on a cadaver).
1942	Schuchardt[92]	Stepped horizontal osteotomy of the ramus, intraoral approach.
1942	Schuchardt[92]	Staged Le Fort I osteotomy, followed by pterygomaxillary separation; external postoperative traction using a pulley and weights was used to advance the maxilla.
1949	Moore and Ward[93]	Recommended horizontal transection of the pterygoid plates for maxillary advancement.

Table 2-1 (*Continued*)

Date	Clinician(s)	Description
1953	Obwegeser,[62]	Sagittal split osteotomy of the ramus, intraoral approach, (published in 1957).
1954	Gillies and Rowe[94]	Described a maxillary osteotomy in a cleft patient with advancement and use of autogenous bone grafts.
1954	Čupar[102]	Described a single-stage anterior segmental maxillary osteotomy (intraoral approach).
1954	Caldwell and Letterman[71]	Vertical subsigmoid osteotomy of the ramus, extraoral approach.
1957	Trauner and Obwegeser[62]	Osseous genioplasty, intraoral approach.
1959	Obwegeser (and Dal Pont)[64]	Modification of the original Obwegeser sagittal split osteotomy, moving the lateral corticotomy anteriorly, and vertically directed along the body of the mandible (published by Dal Pont, see text).
1959	Köle[26–28]	Described an anterior mandibular subapical osteotomy to advance the mandibular labial dentoalveolar segment; intraoral approach; preserved the mental nerves.
1959	Schuchardt[105]	Described a two-stage segmental impaction of the posterior maxillary dentoalveolus (Developed in mid-1950s).
1960	Kufner[106]	Modified the Schuchardt two-stage posterior segmental maxillary impaction as a one-stage procedure.
1965	Neuner[80]	Described the double-step advancement osseous genioplasty.
1965	Obwegeser[95]	Fully mobilized the maxilla; in a single step brought it into the predicted position.
1966	Obwegeser	Walter Reed Army Medical Center – series of lectures – described as the beginning of modern orthognathic surgery.
1966	Wunderer[103]	Segmental set-back of the anterior maxilla (1-stage procedure, palatal approach).
1968	Caldwell et al.[72]	'C' type ramus osteotomy.
1968	Hunsuck[66]	Advocated a modified Obwegeser sagittal split osteotomy, suggesting an incomplete horizontal osteotomy of the medial side of the ramus, ending behind the lingula and relying on vertical cleavage lines within the mandible to complete the split.
1969 to mid-1990s	Bell[108–119]	Investigations on the blood supply and revascularization following orthognathic procedures, particularly in the maxilla.
1970	Hebert, Kent, and Hinds[73]	Vertical subsigmoid osteotomy of the ramus, intraoral approach.
1970	Obwegeser	Report of first bimaxillary orthognathic procedure, performed in 1969, published in 1970 (see Chapter 1).
1974	Spiessl[122]	Described rigid fixation of the mandible following a sagittal split osteotomy using compression lag screws;Luhr's maxillofacial fixation system was in development from the 1960s, including plates and screws.
1974	MacIntosh[32]	Described the total subapical mandibular osteotomy.
1977	Epker[67]	Advocated further modification to the Hunsuck approach to the Obwegeser sagittal split osteotomy, suggesting minimal soft tissue dissection.
1985	Bennett and Wolford[98]	Described the Le Fort I 'step' osteotomy, which prevented the potential ramping effect with maxillary advancement.

while training developed an interest in finding better methods to unite maxillofacial fractures. He eventually developed his own maxillofacial fixation system in the late 1960s, which included plates and screws.[123] Luhr continued developing his system over the next few decades, and other clinicians also began using rigid fixation in orthognathic surgery. In the early 1970s, the French surgeon **Francois Michelet**, from Bordeaux, described cases using miniplate fixation of sagittal split osteotomies.[124,125] Another French surgeon, **Maxime Champy**, from Strasbourg, described the use of miniplates for Le Fort I osteotomies.[126] The problems with compression lag screws and rigid fixation leading to condylar displacement and resultant dental occlusal aberrations led to a move by surgeons, such as **Helmut Lindorf**, from Nürnberg, to advocate the use of non-lag 'position' screws.[127] Other advances continue to be made in this field, including the use of resorbable fixation.

Some of the landmark dates and major surgical contributions to orthognathic surgery are provided in Table 2-1.

Influence of craniofacial surgery

'… a true creator is necessity, which is the mother of our invention.'

Plato (c. 429–347 BC)[128]

The teeth and jaws are an integral part of the craniofacial complex. As such, some of the greatest advances in orthognathic surgery were inextricably linked to pioneering efforts to improve reconstructive surgery of the entire facial skeleton. For facial reconstructive surgery, the 'necessity' for surgical inventiveness came with the horrific facial injuries suffered by soldiers in the First World War and, particularly, Air Force pilots in the Second World War. Some injuries were predominantly to the soft tissues, particularly involving burns, which required radical new techniques for reconstruction. Other injuries involved the facial skeleton and overlying soft tissues, which necessitated the reconstructive correction of the supporting skeletal framework of the face in order to permit reconstruction of the overlying soft tissue envelope. At the forefront of these advances was the pioneering work of the British surgeon and father of modern plastic surgery, **Sir Harold Gillies** (Figure 2-88) (see Box 2.1).[129–134]

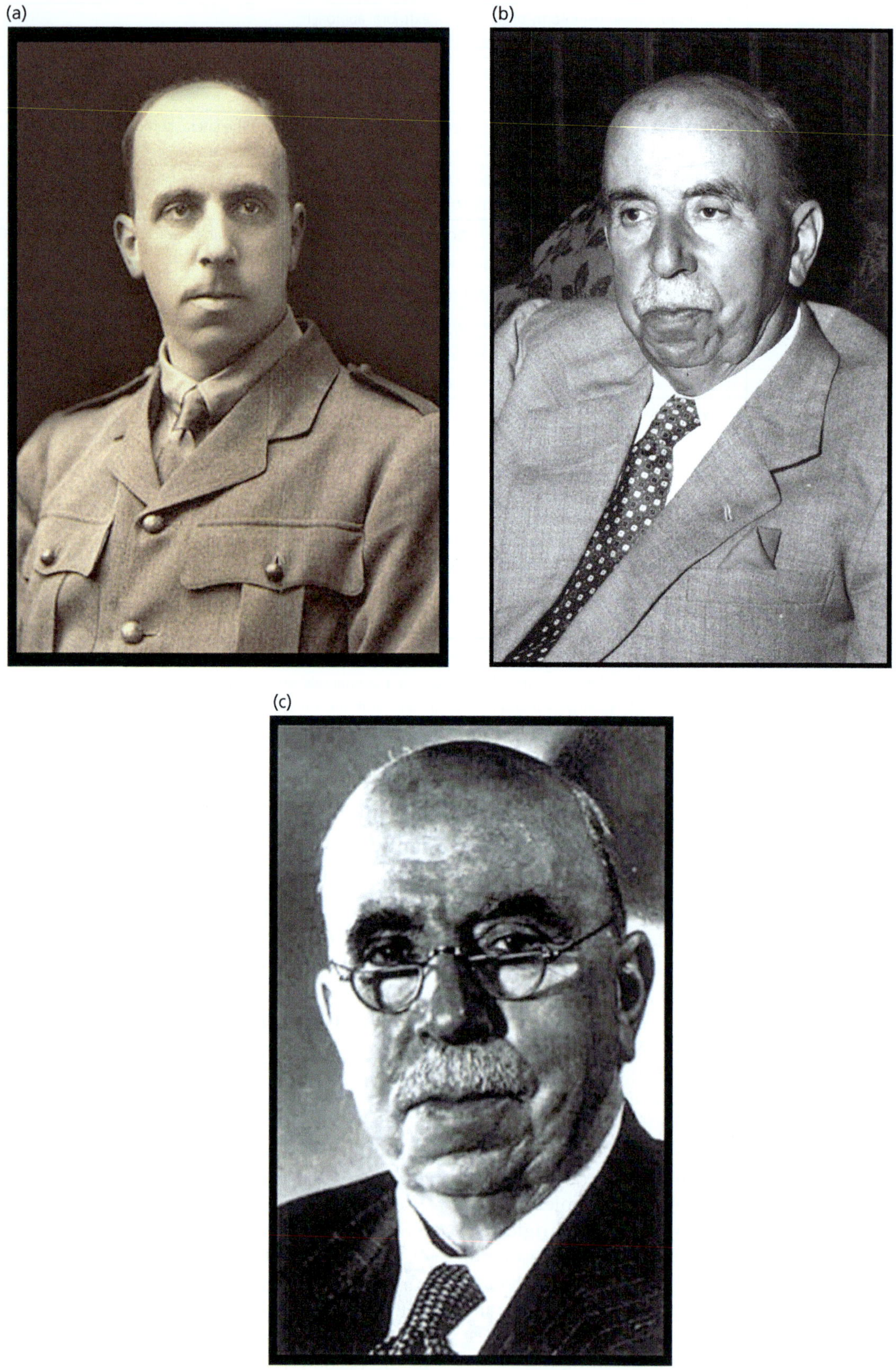

Fig. 2-88 Sir Harold Gillies (1882–1960), through the ages.

Box 2-1 Sir Harold Gillies – the father of modern plastic surgery

'We [Paul Tessier and I] had primarily different routes to the fascinating field of reconstructive surgery of the facial skeleton. However, both of us had for some period the same teacher – Sir Harold Gillies of London, Basingstoke – the most important pioneer of modern plastic surgery. He was the first to try to bring the middle third of the facial skeleton forward.'

Professor Hugo Obwegeser
Speech at bestowal of Chevalier de la Légion d'Honneur to Dr Paul Tessier (2005).[135]

Harold Delf Gillies was born in Dunedin, New Zealand, on the 17 June 1882, the youngest of eight children. His father died when he was just 4. He was sent to boarding school in England at the age of 8, and returned to school in New Zealand when he was 12. In 1901 he returned to England to attend Gonville and Caius College, Cambridge. He was awarded a scholarship in his first year and qualified from St Bartholomew's Hospital in 1906, becoming a Fellow of the Royal College of Surgeons of England four years later. He overcame the obstacle of a stiff elbow sustained sliding down the banisters at home in childhood and managed to row for Cambridge in the 1904 Boat Race and also to play golf for England against Scotland, and win the Royal St George Grand Challenge Cup at Sandwich in 1913 (Figure 2-89). Noted as the best house surgeon at St Bartholomew's Hospital in his time, he became an ear, nose and throat surgeon under the tutelage of Sir John Milsom Rees (1866–1952).

Following the outbreak of World War I he joined the Royal Army Medical Corps and the British Red Cross. Initially posted to Wimereux, near Boulogne, he acted as medical minder to a French-American dentist, **Auguste Charles Valadier** (1873–1931), who was not allowed to operate unsupervised but was attempting to develop maxillofacial repair work (Valadier went on to become a pioneer in the treatment of jaw injuries, later becoming a naturalized British citizen and receiving a Knighthood).[136] Gillies, eager after observing Valadier, decided that facial reconstructive surgery was for him. He left for Paris to visit the renowned surgeon **Hippolyte Morestin** (1869–1918) (Figure 2-90), originally from the French colony of Martinique, at the Val-de-Grâce Military Hospital. He saw him remove a tumour from a patient's face, and repair the area with skin taken from the patient. After observing Morestin operate, Gillies wrote: 'this was the one job in the world I wanted to do.' Gillies became enthusiastic about the work and on his return to England persuaded the army's chief surgeon, Sir William Arbuthnot Lane, that a facial injury ward should be established at the Cambridge Military Hospital in Aldershot. Following the number of injured soldiers from the first day of the Battle of the Somme (1 July 1916), it became clear that larger facilities would be needed. With the help of Arbuthnot Lane, a new hospital devoted to facial repairs was developed at Sidcup in Kent. The Queen's Hospital opened in June 1917 and with its convalescent units provided over 1000 beds. There Gillies and his colleagues developed many techniques of plastic surgery; more than 11,000 operations were performed on over 5000 men, mostly soldiers with facial injuries, usually from gunshot wounds. The hospital, later to become

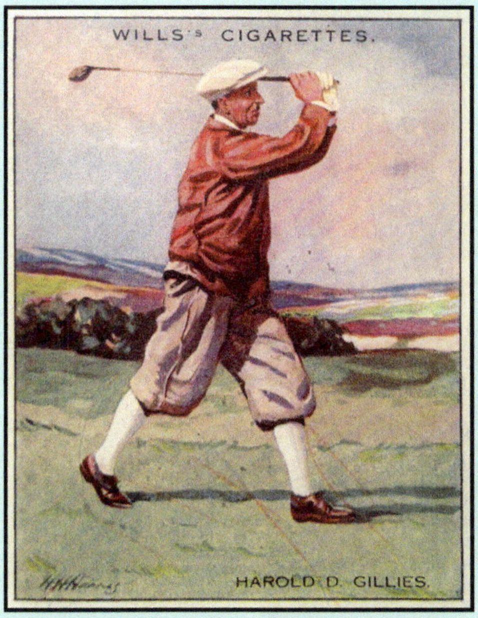

Fig. 2-89 Gillies playing golf (Courtesy of Dr Aron D. Wahrman, Professor of Plastic Surgery, Temple University School of Medicine, Philadelphia, USA).

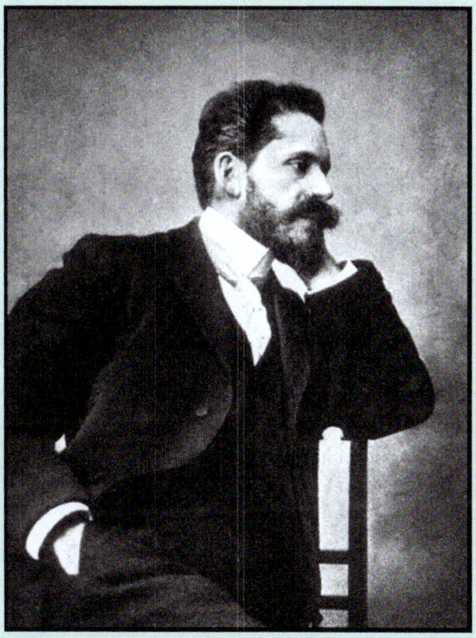

Fig. 2-90 Hippolyte Morestin (1869–1918).

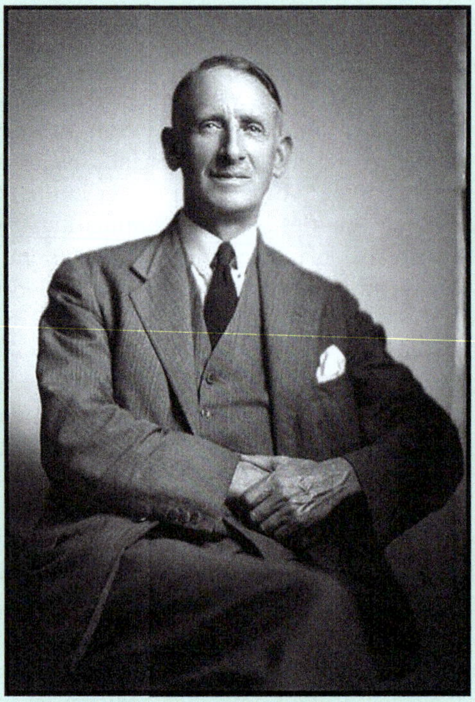

Fig. 2-91 Henry Percy Pickerill (1879–1956).

Queen Mary's Hospital, was at Frognal House (the birthplace and property of Thomas Townsend, Lord Sydney, after whom Sydney, Australia was named). In 1917, the British dental surgeon **Henry Percy Pickerill** (1879–1956) (Figure 2-91), who had become the first Dean of the University of Otago's Dental School in Dunedin, New Zealand, took leave from the University of Otago and returned to England to fulfill his wartime duties with the New Zealand Medical Corps. In 1918, Pickerill's unit was transferred to Queen's Hospital Sidcup, where he also established a reputation in facial reconstructive and plastic surgery. Gillies led the British section and Pickerill the New Zealand section at Queen's Hospital, and there was a 'healthy' rivalry between the two men. Following the First World War, Pickerill returned to New Zealand. Pickerill made substantial contributions to the development of facial plastic, reconstructive and jaw surgery.

Gillies' reputation continued to grow. American surgeons in France such as Ivy and Kazanjian did pioneering work (Figure 2-92), but would send difficult cases to Sidcup, as indeed would Valadier in due course. At his unit in Sidcup, Gillies worked with a team, including dentists, physicians, radiologists, dental technicians, artists, sculptors and photographers. He had a keen interest in art, which is often a mainstay for facial aesthetic and reconstructive surgery (Figure 2-93).

Gillies and his consultant plastic surgeon colleague from Sidcup, **Thomas Pomfret (Tommy or TP) Kilner** (1890–1964), who held the only chair in plastic surgery in the UK, remained the only two dedicated plastic surgery specialists in England until the 1930s (in Kilner's obituary, Robert Ivy wrote: 'Kilner was greatly respected and beloved by all American plastic surgeons who knew him, and was looked upon as their chief ambassador of good-will with their British colleagues').[137] However, they were eventually joined by **Arthur Rainsford Mowlem** (1902–86)[138] and **Archibald McIndoe**

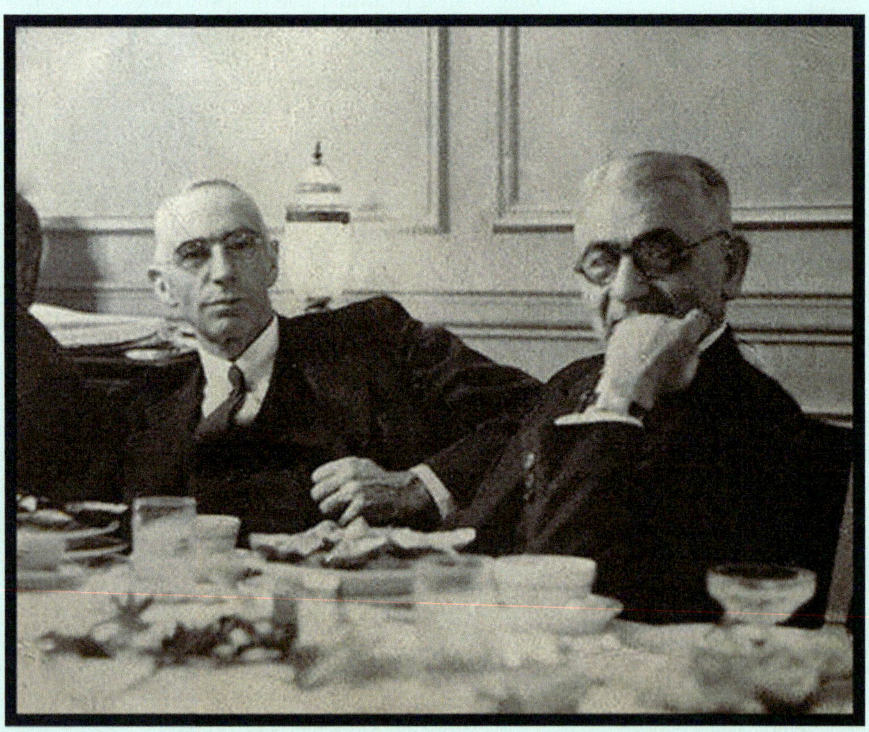

Fig. 2-92 Robert Ivy and Varaztad Kazanjian (c.1950) (Courtesy of Countway Library of Medicine, Boston, USA).

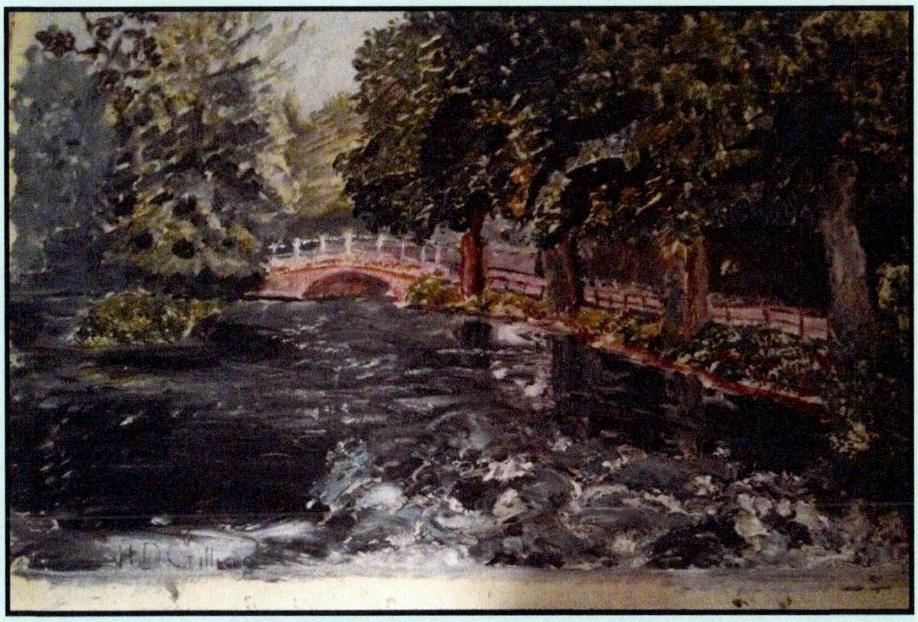

Fig. 2-93 'Bossington on the Test' – painting by Sir Harold Gillies (Courtesy of Dr Aron D. Wahrman, Professor of Plastic Surgery, Temple University School of Medicine, Philadelphia, USA).

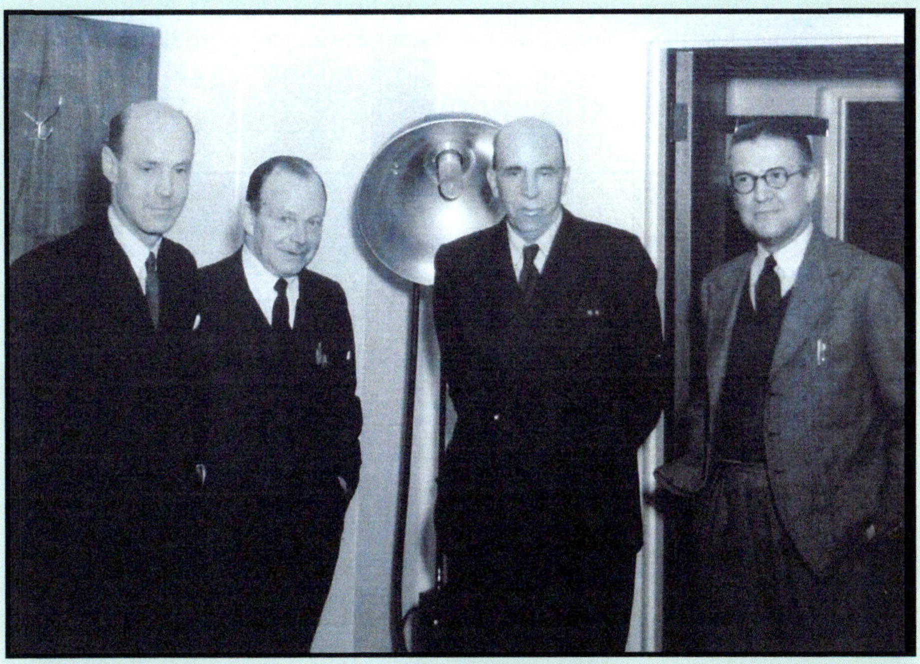

Fig. 2-94 The 'Big Four' – Mowlem, Kilner, Gillies and McIndoe (from left to right).

(1900–60). These four were the only plastic surgeons in the UK at the outbreak of the Second World War (Figure 2-94). Retained as an advisor to the armed forces and with **Sir William Kelsey Fry** (1889–1963), the dental and oral surgeon with whom he had worked at Sidcup, Gillies was instrumental in the organization of plastic surgery services. This time the idea of a single hospital was abandoned; Sidcup was well within range of enemy aircraft (indeed it was bombed twice) and it was decided to split the service. Gillies had already found a base at Rooksdown House, at Park Prewett Hospital near Basingstoke and it was here that the main centre for the army was established. Mowlem went to St Albans, Kilner to Roehampton and McIndoe was appointed to the RAF designated hospital at East Grinstead. Gillies made innumerable contributions to the development of facial reconstructive surgery. For his war services Gillies was knighted in the King's Birthday Honours list of June 1930.

Note:

Sir Archibald McIndoe and 'the town that didn't stare'

Archibald Hector McIndoe was born in Dunedin, New Zealand on the 4 May 1900. He was the cousin of Sir Harold Gillies. Whilst studying medicine at the University of Otago he met the visiting William Mayo, one of the founders of the Mayo Clinic. Mayo offered McIndoe a fellowship, which he accepted, eventually spending five years at the Mayo Clinic. His wife, Adonia, eventually joined him, and found work playing piano in the hotel opposite the clinic, earning a higher wage than Archibald. Whilst at the Mayo, McIndoe (unknowingly) operated on Al Capone's younger brother, for which he received 1000 dollars from a member of the entourage, who said 'Al told me to say thank you for all you did for his kid brother.'[139]

In 1931, the McIndoe family came to England. Archibald began work on his Royal College of Surgeons Fellowship, and his cousin, Sir Harold Gillies, found him work at St Bartholomew's Hospital and in his own private practice. From 1932 to 1939, McIndoe assisted Gillies, refining his surgical skills, and recognizing the importance of Gillies' approach of treating the 'whole' patient, not just their injuries, and rebuilding their confidence and self-esteem. With the outbreak of World War II, McIndoe set up the plastic and maxillofacial unit (called the Centre for Plastic and Jaw Surgery) at the Queen Victoria Hospital in East Grinstead, where he pioneered the treatment of servicemen with an array of facial injuries sustained in conflict (Figure 2-95). The 'airman's burn' was an unfortunately typical injury, referring to severe burns of the face and hands when aircraft fuel tanks ignited before the pilots could parachute to safety. Pilots often removed their gloves and goggles to have better control of the aircraft, thereby sustaining more severe injuries.

McIndoe was a very skilled and innovative surgeon, and what he didn't know, he invented. However, as well as making enormous technical surgical advances, McIndoe deserves special recognition for understanding and leading the rehabilitation and reintegration of burns survivors into society. In 1941, the **Guinea Pig Club** (so-called as so many of the pioneering surgical procedures being undertaken on the injured servicemen were experimental) was founded at the Queen Victoria Hospital, with Sir Archibald (affectionately known as 'the boss' or 'the maestro') as its first president. McIndoe's wonderful sense of humour was part of the Guinea Pig rehabilitation. This is evident in the Club's constitution, which

(a)

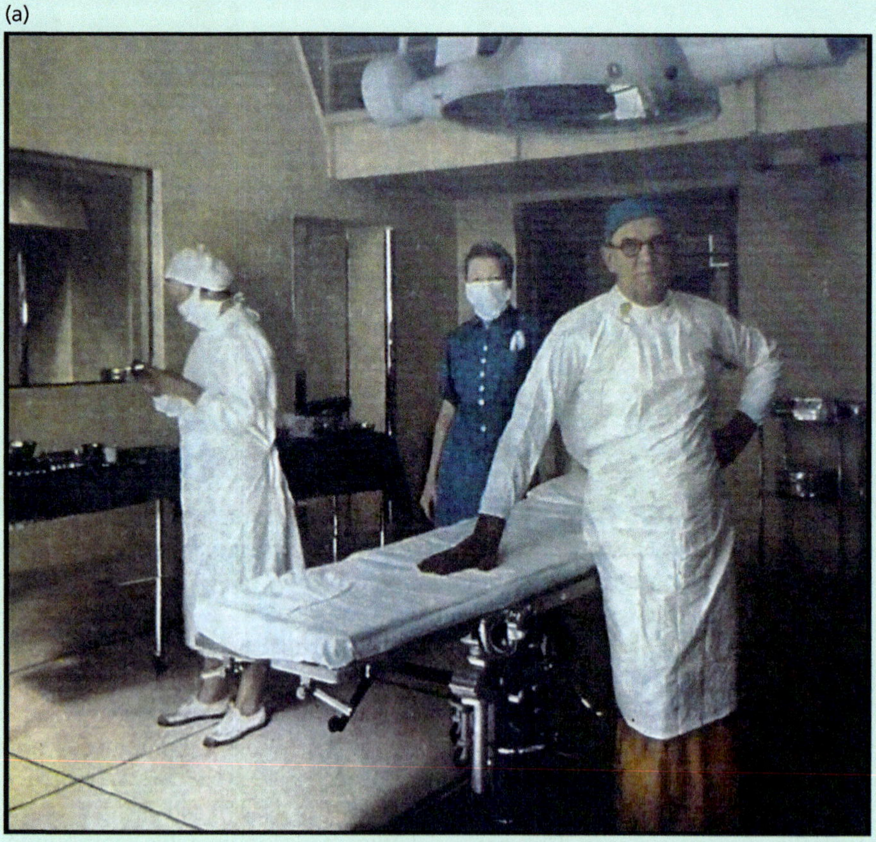

Fig. 2-95 (a): McIndoe in the main operating theatre, with theatre Sister, Miss Mullens, behind. (b): McIndoe in the operating theatre (Courtesy of Mrs Jacquie Pinney, CEO, Blond McIndoe Research Foundation, Queen Victoria Hospital, East Grinstead, UK).

(b)

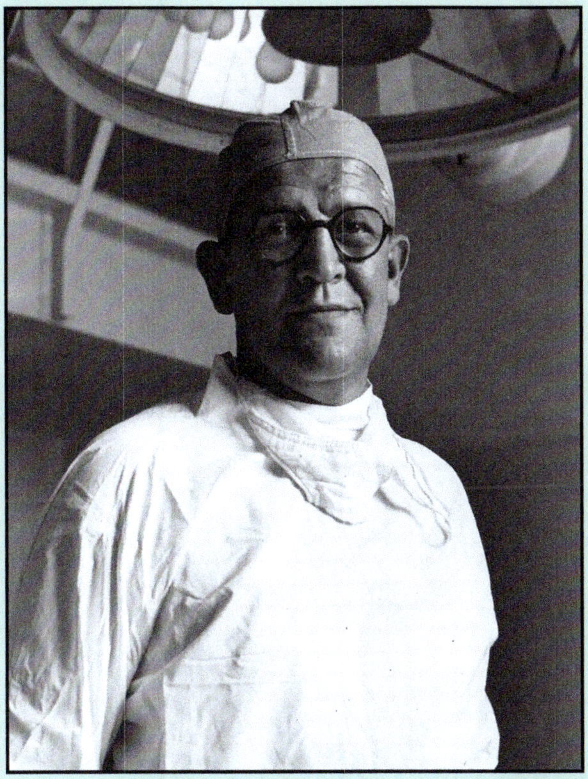

Fig. 2-95 (*Continued*).

included a first secretary with severely damaged fingers 'to discourage excessive minute taking', and a treasurer with severely injured legs to reduce the risk of his 'walking off' with the Club funds! Members were servicemen who had undergone at least two operations by McIndoe. One of McIndoe's unique qualities was to be unconventional. He disposed of the 'convalescent uniforms' provided for patients by the hospital and his 'boys' were allowed to wear their own service uniforms whilst recovering. A beer keg was always kept for them on the recovery ward, with McIndoe saying: 'After what these boys have been through, nothing is too good for them.' The facial injuries of many of the servicemen were found to be too much to bear by their wives or girlfriends, who ended their relationships at the worst time possible for a patient's morale. However, many of the men eventually married nurses from the hospital, who saw past their injuries, realising that once you get to know the real person, a facial disfigurement just fades in your vision.

Outside the safety of the hospital, members of the public, who owed their lives to these brave men, would stare at them and sometimes shout abuse at them, simply because of their facial appearance. One of the servicemen remembers a visit to London by train, and hearing a member of the public looking at him and remarking offensively: 'They shouldn't let them out.' It is heartbreaking to remember that these were the same RAF servicemen of whom Sir Winston Churchill (1874–1965) said:

> 'The gratitude of every home in our Island... goes out to the British airmen who, undaunted by odds, unwearied in their constant challenge and mortal danger, are turning the tide of the World War by their prowess and their devotion. Never in the field of human conflict was so much owed by so many to so few' (Figure 2-96).[140]

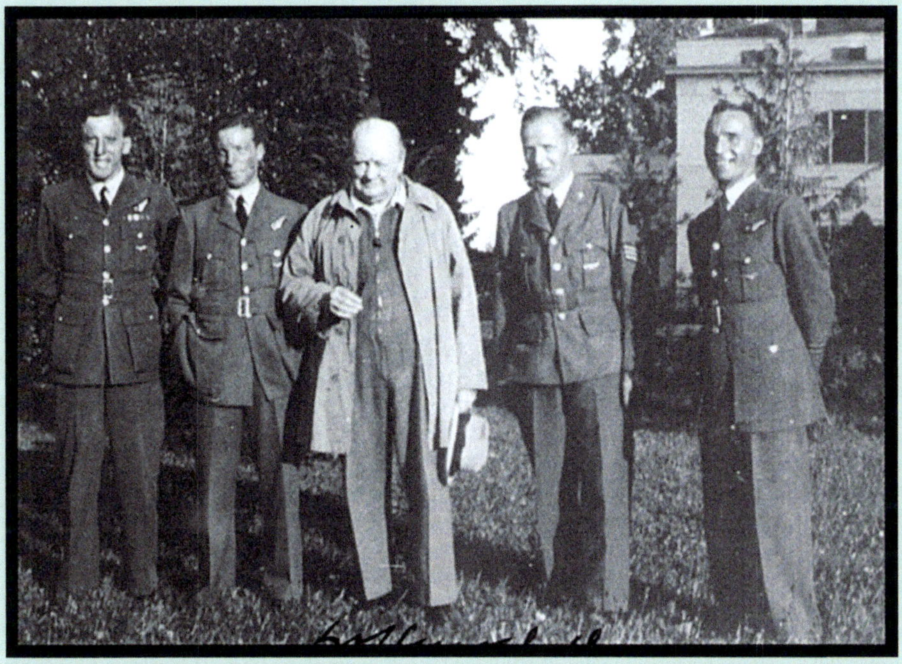

Fig. 2-96 Sir Winston Churchill with 'the few' (Courtesy of Mrs Jacquie Pinney, CEO, Blond McIndoe Research Foundation, Queen Victoria Hospital, East Grinstead, UK).

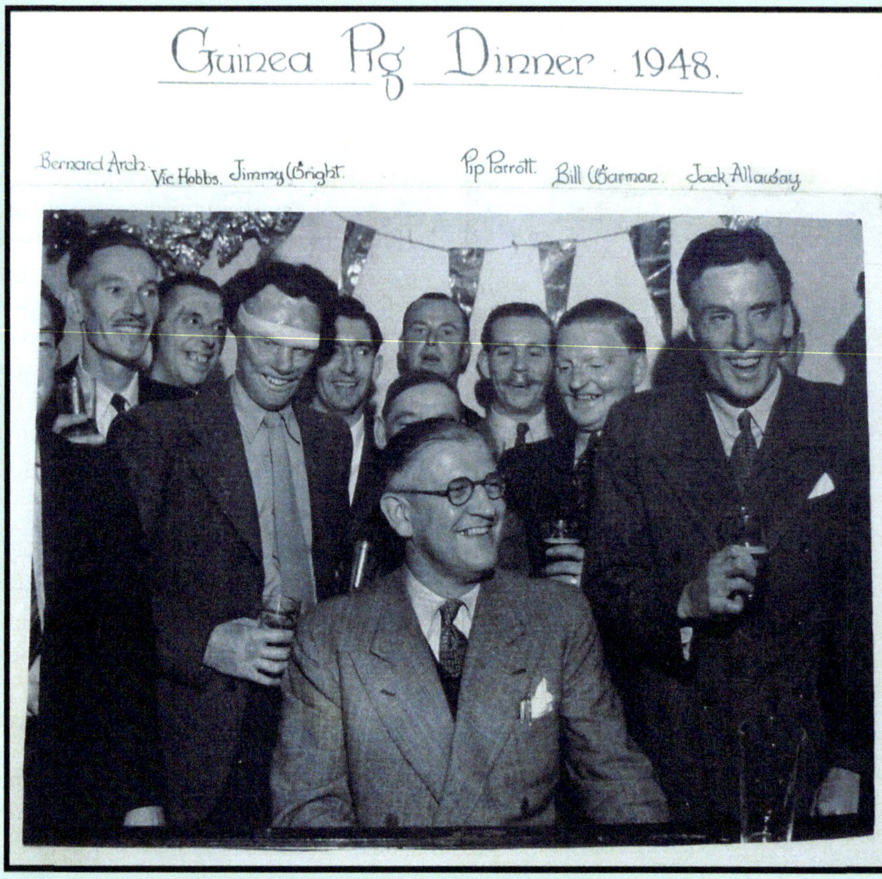

Fig. 2-97 Sir Archibald McIndoe playing the piano at a Guinea Pig Club dinner (Courtesy of Mrs Jacquie Pinney, CEO, Blond McIndoe Research Foundation, Queen Victoria Hospital, East Grinstead, UK).

(a)

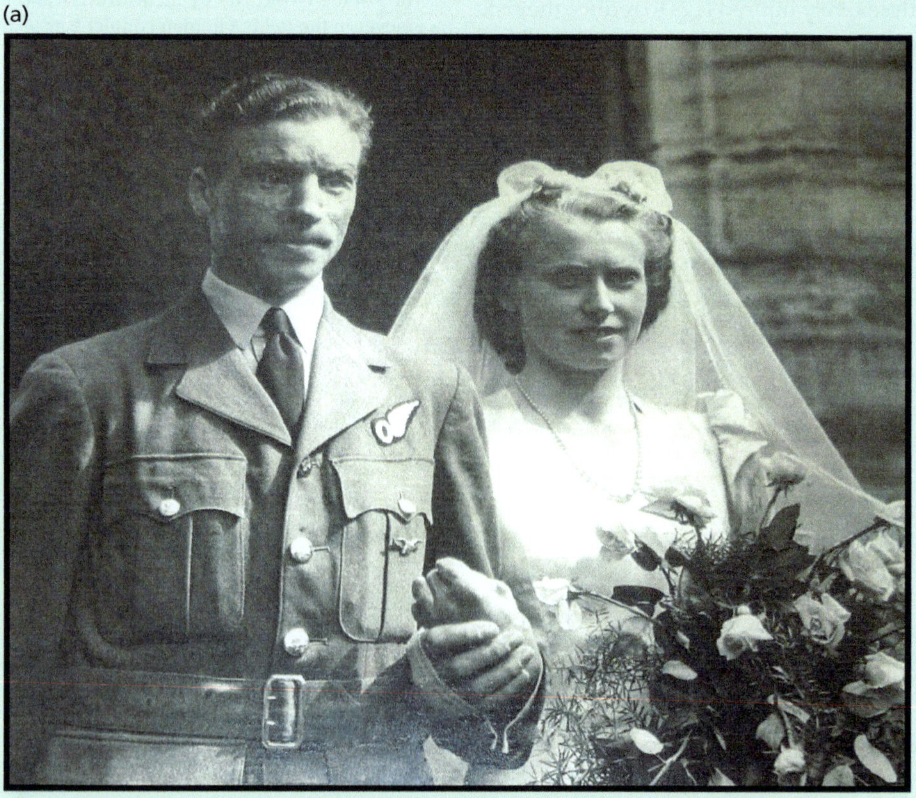

Fig. 2-98 (a): Airman Bill Foxley on his wedding day. (b): Bill Foxley (photograph by Lucinda Marland, Courtesy of Mrs Jacquie Pinney, CEO, Blond McIndoe Research Foundation, Queen Victoria Hospital, East Grinstead, UK).

(b)

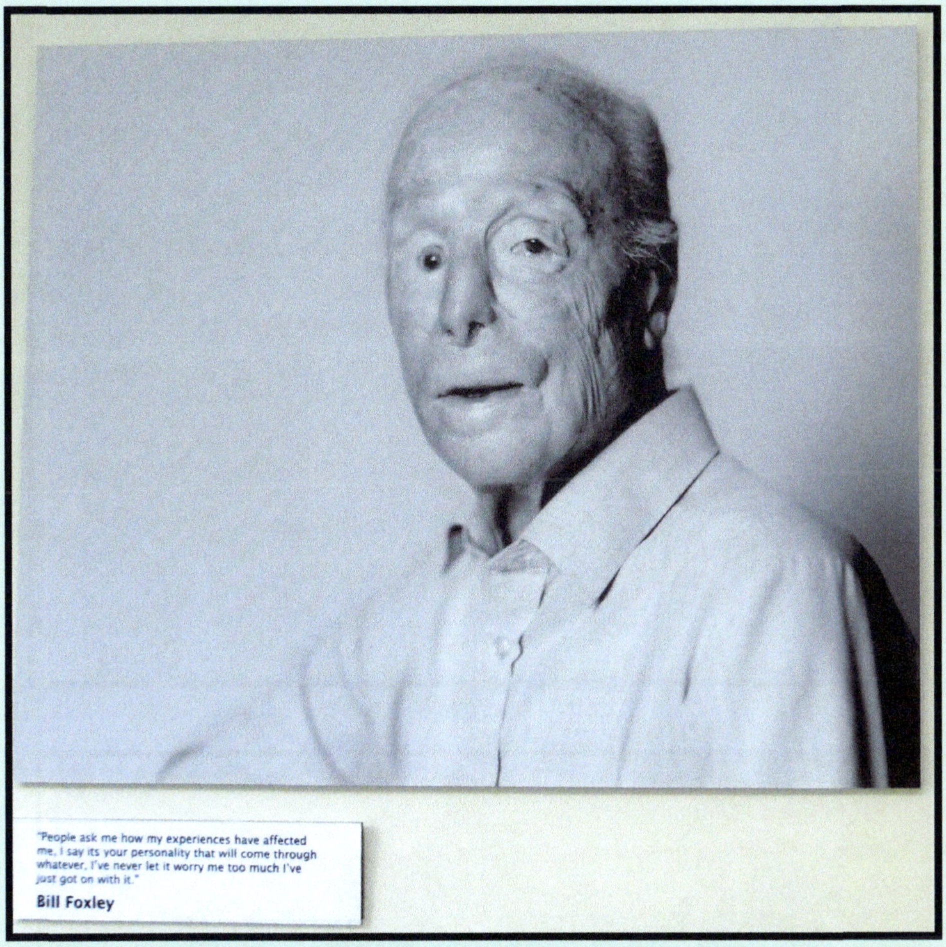
"People ask me how my experiences have affected me, I say its your personality that will come through whatever, I've never let it worry me too much I've just got on with it."
Bill Foxley

Fig. 2-98 (*Continued*).

These men were 'the few' to who people owed their freedom. Becoming aware of this mire of ignorance, McIndoe realised that the public had to be educated. *McIndoe's next move was simply inspired and demonstrates his understanding of the importance of psychosocial functioning on patients with facial deformities.* McIndoe requested that hospital staff spread the word in East Grinstead that injured servicemen in town should be made to feel part of the community, and be regarded as 'normal young men who happen to be in temporary difficulty.' He went on to say: 'Think of these boys as human beings – think how you would treat them if they were your own sons – and remember that you're not doing them a favour by visiting them; they're doing you a favour by speaking to you' (Figure 2-97). The warmth of the people of East Grinstead and their understanding of the importance of Sir Archibald's request earned the town the accolade of 'the town that didn't stare'. Many of the Guinea Pigs eventually reintegrated back into society (Figure 2-98).

In the late 1940s, Sir Archibald visited East Africa and began farming in the foothills of Mount Kilimanjaro. Being a consummate philanthropist, he co-founded the African Medical and Research Foundation (AMREF) in 1957, together with two of his former trainees, **Thomas Rees** (who went on to become an internationally respected plastic surgeon) and Michael Wood, to help treat the rural population of the region.

Sir Archibald's legacy and indomitable spirit lives on. The Guinea Pig Club, now with HRH Prince Phillip, Duke of Edinburgh, as its president, continues to look after members or their widows, in the UK and abroad. In 1944, Archibald McIndoe said:[139] 'We are the trustees of each other … it is one thing to die for your country, but it's a great deal more important to live for it' (Figure 2-99).

(a)

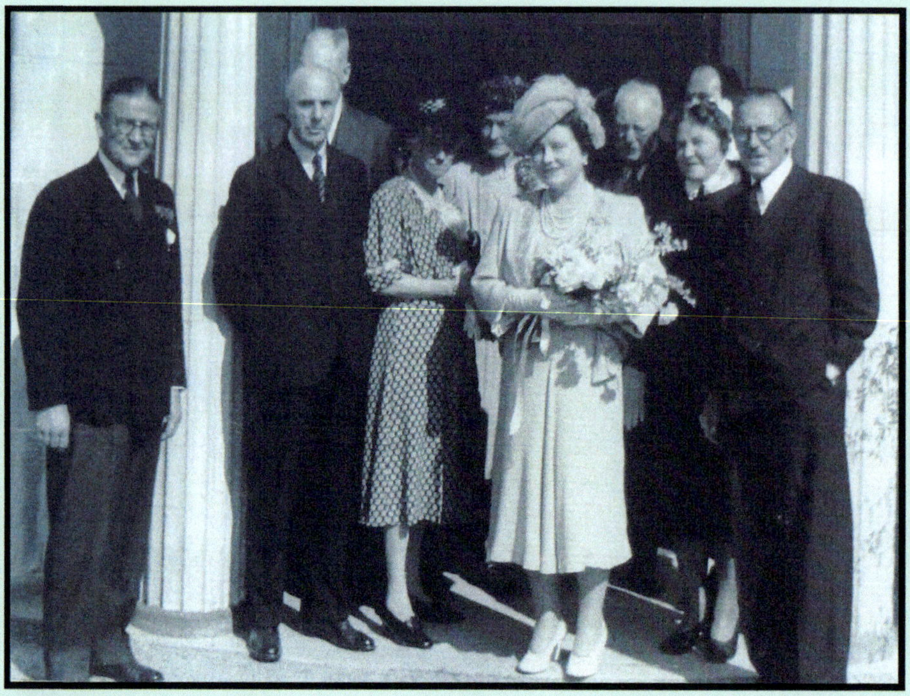

(b)

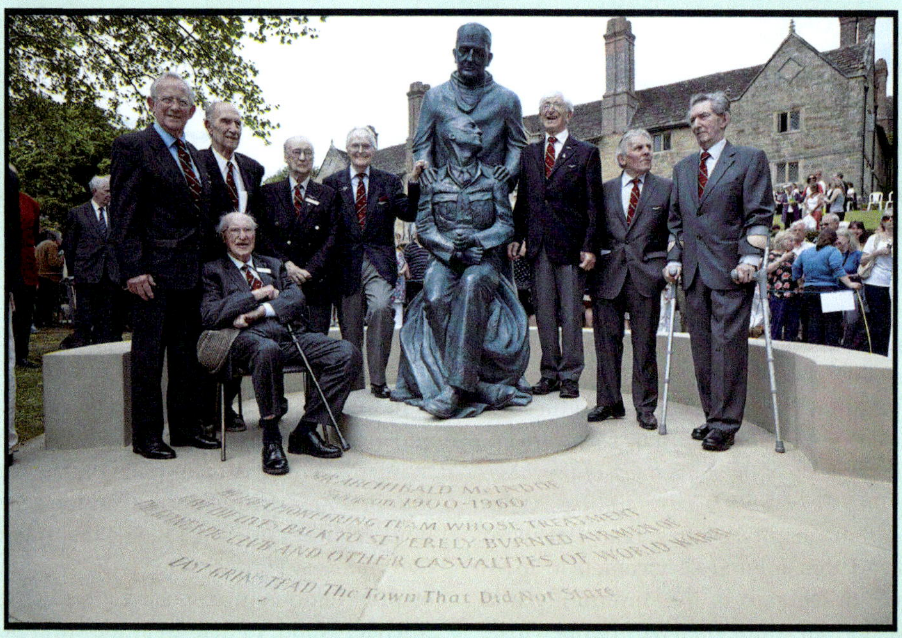

Fig. 2-99 (a): The Queen (later The Queen Mother) visiting Queen Victoria Hospital, with Sir Archibald McIndoe (left) and Sir William Kelsey Fry (right). (b): The larger than life bronze McIndoe Memorial Statue, unveiled on the 9 June 2014, by HRH The Princess Royal, is situated in a prominent location in front of Sackville College in East Grinstead on the route Sir Archibald took daily to the Queen Victoria Hospital. It is the work of the renowned British sculptor, Martin Jennings, who has created such masterpieces as 'John Betjeman' (Sir John Betjeman – 1906–84 – former Poet Laureate) now standing in all its glory in St Pancras railway station, London, and 'Charles Dickens' in Portsmouth. Martin's desire was to create a statue which visually captured not only McIndoe's physical appearance but also projected the content of his character. In order to achieve this Martin carried out extensive research. McIndoe is displayed wearing his surgeon's gown, and his hands are on the RAF soldier's shoulders – he was not just their surgeon, but acted as their guardian. The soldier is looking up both at Sir Archibald, and to the sky where he flew to defend freedom. This statue is particularly personal to Martin, as Sir Archibald had operated on Martin's father, Michael Jennings, who had sustained severe injuries when his tank caught fire after being hit by a shell towards the end of World War II. The RAF soldier's hands are based on Martin's memory of his father's hands. The statue is placed on an inscribed stone plinth with a semi-circular stone seat to enable visitors to interact and 'be with' the statue. (Courtesy of Mrs Jacquie Pinney, CEO, Blond McIndoe Research Foundation, Queen Victoria Hospital, East Grinstead, UK).

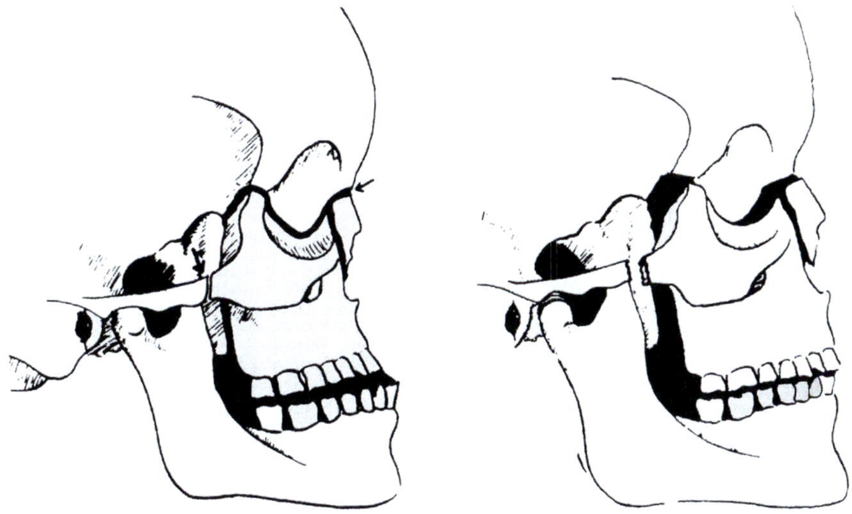

Fig. 2-100 Gillies performed the first elective Le Fort III-type advancement osteotomy on a patient with a severe developmental midfacial retrusion (From Gillies and Harrison, 1950,[141]).

In 1940, a Royal Air Force pilot suffered a Le Fort III fracture. A year later, Gillies reopened the fractures and placed traction to the entire facial segment using weighted pulleys.[78] In 1942, Gillies attempted a similar procedure on a patient with a congenital midfacial retrusion. The case was published in 1950 (Figure 2-100).[141] There was considerable relapse and Gillies was not fond of the procedure, but he was already aware that had bone grafts been used, the procedure may have been more stable. However, a young French surgeon named **Paul Tessier** (Figure 2-101), who had spent a great deal of time training under Gillies and McIndoe in England, revived the interest in this procedure, and went on to become the leader in the field of craniofacial surgery.

Paul Tessier and high level facial osteotomies

'Monsieur… my dear friends,
I excuse myself for being seated before you, broken and quavering.

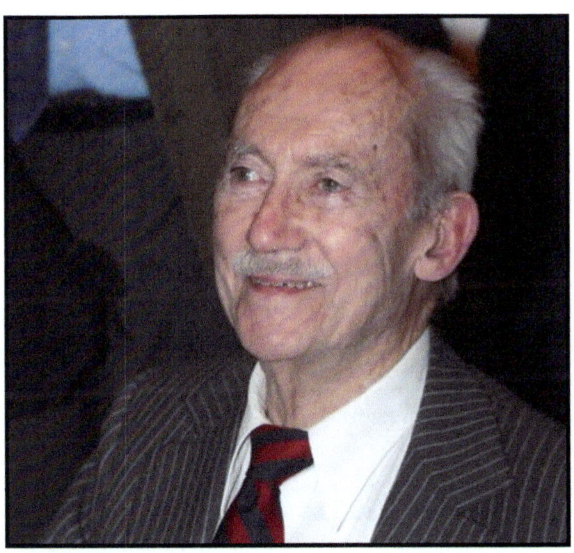

Fig. 2-101 Paul Tessier (1917–2008).

My thanks first of all to M. Pouliquen, one of our 40 Immortals of the Academia Francaise… like the 10,000 Persian 'Immortals' of Cyrus the Great.'

Paul Tessier (1917–2008)
First lines of acceptance speech on the bestowal of Chevalier de la Légion d'Honneur (2005)[142]

The **Le Fort III-type osteotomy** is a true craniofacial disjunction, with the entire maxilla, the zygomas and nose being advanced as a unit. Importantly, orbital cavity volume increases, reducing exorbitism. The facial changes are marked, and often significantly improved. Tessier worked on and improved his procedures systematically from the late 1950s, though his work became internationally recognized in the late 1960s and early 70s.[143–145]

Note:

Paul Tessier – the father of craniofacial surgery

'This world is but a school of inquiry.'
Michel de Montaigne (1533–1592)[146]

Paul Louis Ernest Tessier was a great surgical innovator. He devised and described original techniques for craniofacial reconstruction, which had an immense impact on facial plastic and maxillofacial surgery, and revolutionized the treatment of craniofacial birth defects and developmental deformities. He essentially created the new subspecialty of craniofacial surgery, thereby giving hope to many with severe facial deformities that were previously thought to be untreatable. His trainees recall that he was never content that a patient should look 'better than they did before we started' but he declared 'if it is not normal, it is not enough'.[147]

Tessier was born in Héric, near Nantes, in 1917. He entered Nantes medical school in 1936. In 1940 he became a prisoner of war, and was only released as he contracted typhoid. During his surgical residency in 1943, he narrowly escaped death again when his on-call room was destroyed by a bomb during an attack on Nantes – Tessier was at a celebratory picnic arranged by students he was mentoring.

Tessier developed an interest in the treatment of facial deformities from observing cleft lip and palate repair during his surgical residency in Nantes. After the destruction of Nantes, he eventually moved to Hôpital Foch in Paris, joining the paediatric department.[142]

After the war he began spending a few months in England twice each year with the 'big four' of plastic surgery – Gillies, McIndoe, Mowlem, and Kilner – but particularly with McIndoe and Gillies, from whom he learnt a great deal, describing his time with them as 'a revelation'. He developed a fondness for England which remained with him.

In 1957 Dr Tessier was consulted by a young man with Crouzon syndrome, which results in a facial deformity with severe maxillary hypoplasia, exorbitism and respiratory obstruction. Tessier sought to clarify the difficulties by planning various approaches on dry skulls at home and then on cadavers. Since he had not been to medical school in Paris the medical establishment denied him access to an anatomy room. Characteristically he did not give up but travelled regularly to Nantes at the end of his working day to carry out dissections, returning on the 2.30am train to be back at work in Paris by morning. This painstaking preparatory work typified his thoroughness and dedication. Finally, when he was ready, Tessier operated on his patient, completely separating the facial skeleton from the cranium, advancing it by 25 mm, and securing it by the novel use of bone grafts.[147] The procedure was successful, despite Tessier being denied access to the dental laboratory for the creation of surgical splints, hitherto always used to stabilise facial fractures, because of a historic and decidedly infantile dispute between the plastic and maxillofacial services at Foch.

An excellent 2-volume biography of Tessier, called *A Man from Héric*, has been written by the American craniofacial surgeon S. Anthony Wolfe.[142] Wolfe recounts that having undertaken Le Fort III-type osteotomies, Tessier was presented with a number of patients with orbital hypertelorism. He discussed the possibility of a transcranial approach with his neurosurgical colleague at Hôpital Foch in Paris, Gerard Guiot, and Guiot's reply was, 'Pourquoi pas?' Interestingly, *Pourquoi Pas* was also the name of the boat used by the polar explorer Jean-Baptiste Charcot, the grandson of the great Victor Hugo, and became the motto of the International Society of Craniofacial Surgery, which was founded in 1983, with Tessier as honorary president.[142]

Over the ensuing years Dr Tessier not only pursued and developed his ideas but trained the first generation of craniofacial surgeons worldwide. In 1972 he carried out the first of his craniofacial procedures in the United Kingdom at Great Ormond Street Hospital for Children, where he continued to visit, teaching in the operating theatre and clinics, for 25 years.[147]

Note:

In 1969, Professor Obwegeser performed simultaneously combined Le Fort III and I osteotomies (see Chapter 1). Obwegeser and Tessier became lifelong friends (Figure 2-102).

Tessier continued to make improvements to his techniques throughout his career, and the specialty of craniofacial surgery which he was instrumental in forming went from strength to strength. In 1971, Kufner described a modification of the Le Fort III-type osteotomy for malar-maxillary advancement in patients with a normal nose (see Figure 2-77b),[97] though a high Le Fort I-type maxillary advancement and malar implants has a potentially lower morbidity and thereby is more likely to be undertaken for such a skeletal discrepancy today. In 1978, the Mexican plastic surgeon **Fernando Ortiz-Monasterio** (1923–2012) (Figure 2-103) described the monobloc fronto-facial osteotomy, permitting advancement of the entire orbital framework and midface in one 'monobloc' piece in adolescent children.[148]

One of the least commonly undertaken midfacial procedures is the **Le Fort II-type osteotomy**. It is usually indicated in patients presenting with severe nasomaxillary retrusion. It is not known who performed the first Le Fort II-type advancement osteotomy, though both Tessier and Obwegeser were involved in its development. Henderson and Jackson described

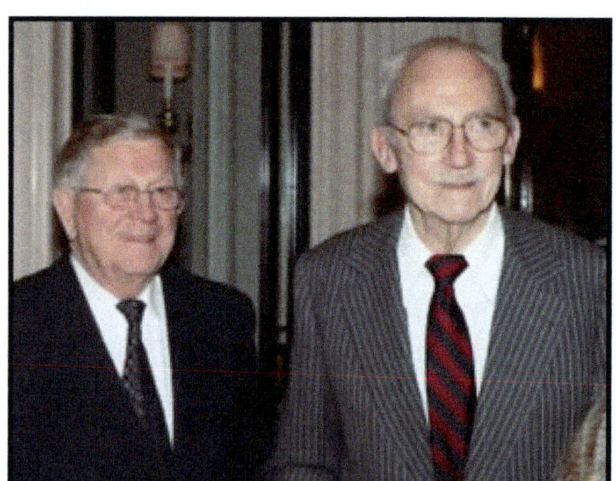

Fig. 2-102 Professor Hugo Obwegeser and Dr Paul Tessier (in 2005).

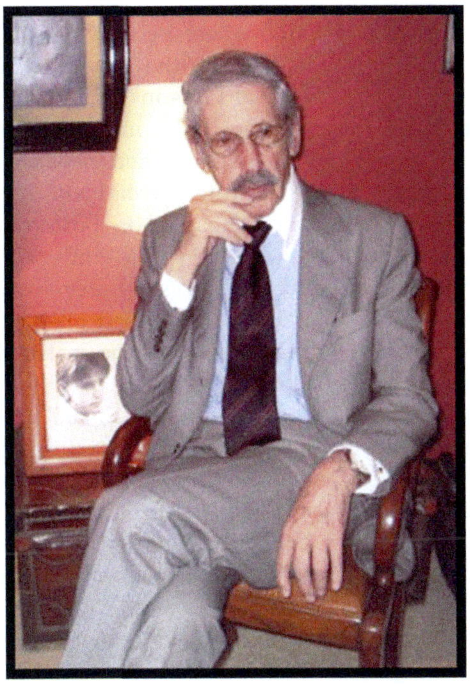

Fig. 2-103 Fernando Ortiz-Monasterio (1923–2012).

the procedure in 1973;[149] **Derek Henderson** was one of the leading oral and maxillofacial surgeons in the UK, with a specific interest in orthognathic surgery.

Distraction osteogenesis

Another advance in craniofacial surgery came with the introduction of **distraction osteogenesis** of the maxillofacial skeletal structures. The technique, designed to lengthen and create new bone by stretching the callus of an osteotomy site, was introduced by **Gavril Abramovich Ilizarov** (1921–92) (Figure 2-104) in the 1960s. Ilizarov was born in the Caucasus, but worked in the Kurgan region of Siberia.[150,151] However, two decades passed before the concept reached the West, and another decade before it was adopted for cranio-maxillofacial procedures (see Chapters 45, 46, 57 and 58).

Psychosocial implications of facial deformities

'We need more psychology. We need more understanding of human nature, because the only real danger that exists is man himself.'

Carl Gustav Jung (1875–1961)
Swiss psychologist
(BBC interview, 1959)

Social conditions and prevailing societal attitudes have produced unnecessary human misery and suffering throughout the ages. For an individual with a noticeable dentofacial deformity, the stigma, discrimination and despair they suffer often results from the public's lack of the human elements of compassion, understanding and empathy – all of which result from a lack of public education. The impact of Sir Archibald McIndoe and 'the town that didn't stare', described above, demonstrates the vital role that psychosocial issues play in the treatment of patients with facial deformities, and the importance of public education. McIndoe understood that there was a psychosocial rehabilitation that was part and parcel of having a facial deformity, and he became a forerunner for what should today be a routine part of any facial surgical treatment – psychosocial therapy.

A number of other individuals have been instrumental in improving our understanding of the importance of psychosocial functioning in the treatment of facial deformities, but the work of two individuals deserves special mention.

Frances Cooke Macgregor

Professor Frances Cooke Macgregor (1906–2001) was a renowned social scientist and the first scholar whose research and writing on the psychosocial significance of visible facial differences led directly to the first acknowledgement of disfigurement as a disability (Figure 2-105). Her publications document 40 years of research.[152]

Her work on facial disfigurement began during World War II while photographing patients at the

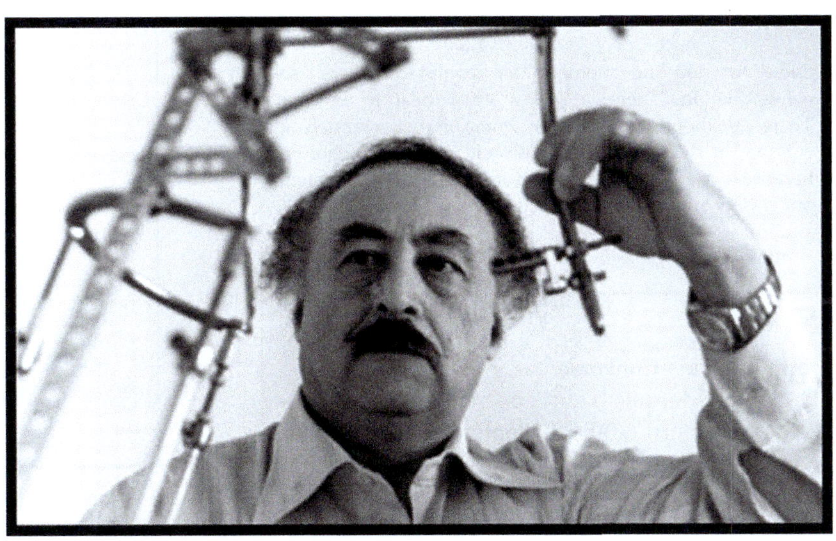

Fig. 2-104 Gavril Abramovich Ilizarov (1921–1992).

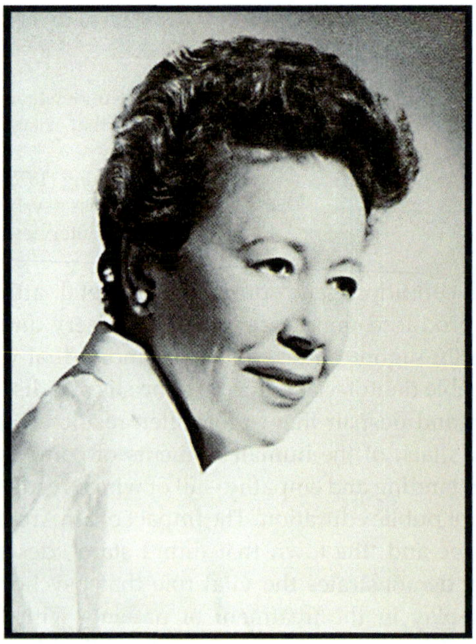

Fig. 2-105 Frances Cooke Macgregor (1906–2001). (From: Naini FB. Facial Aesthetics: Concepts and Clinical Diagnosis. Oxford: Wiley-Blackwell, 2011; reprinted with permission).

Ellis Fischel Cancer State Hospital in Columbia, Missouri. Shortly after the war, she met plastic surgeon Dr **John Marquis Converse**, who helped repair the shattered and burned faces of English and French pilots. His specialty coincided with her interest in the social and psychological ramifications of facial disfigurement. Converse supported her suggestion to conduct an exploratory study of his patients at a time when the existing literature on physical disabilities was limited almost entirely to functional impairments. Her work eventually led to the World Health Organization adding facial disfigurement to its list of disabilities. In 1951 the Society for the Rehabilitation of the Facially Disfigured was established, now known as the National Foundation for Facial Reconstruction (NFFR).

When she was honoured with a Special Citation for Distinguished Service from the Society for the Facially Disfigured (now the NFFR), Frances Cooke Macgregor said:[152]

> 'Now is not the moment for complacency or self-congratulation. There is still a great deal to be done. There are thousands and thousands of men, women and children in this world like those you see today who, only because of the way they look, are among the least accepted in our society and the most neglected.'

Note:

John Marquis Converse

Dr John Marquis Converse (1909-81) (Figure 2-106) was born on the 29 September 1909 in San Francisco, USA.[153] His father was Chief Physician of the American Hospital in Paris, and Converse moved early to Paris, where he was raised. He graduated in medicine from the American Hospital in the University of Paris in 1935 and again from Massachusetts General Hospital in Boston in 1938. His early training in plastic and maxillofacial surgery was under the tutelage of Kazanjian in Massachusetts General Hospital in Boston, and subsequently from Sir Harold Gillies while serving with the American armed forces in Europe during World War II. In 1952 he established his base in New York, becoming Director of the Institute of Reconstructive Plastic Surgery in 1957. He published a seminal work on traumatic maxillofacial surgery with his mentor Kazanjian, and founded the annual Kazanjian lectures in 1962. Converse conceived and established the Society for the Facially Disfigured (now NFFR), and his flair for fundraising promoted both his clinical, academic and philanthropic work. He was editor of the monumental multivolume textbook *Reconstructive Plastic Surgery*. He contributed to tissue transplantation research and was instrumental in founding the Transplantation Society. He had a particular interest in maxillofacial surgery, emanating from his earlier training with Kazanjian and Gillies. His name is associated with the orbital floor 'blow out' fracture and with the preservation of olfactory sensation in the surgical correction of orbital hypertelorism. He was married from 1964 until his death to Veronica B. Cooper, widow of legendary film actor Gary Cooper.

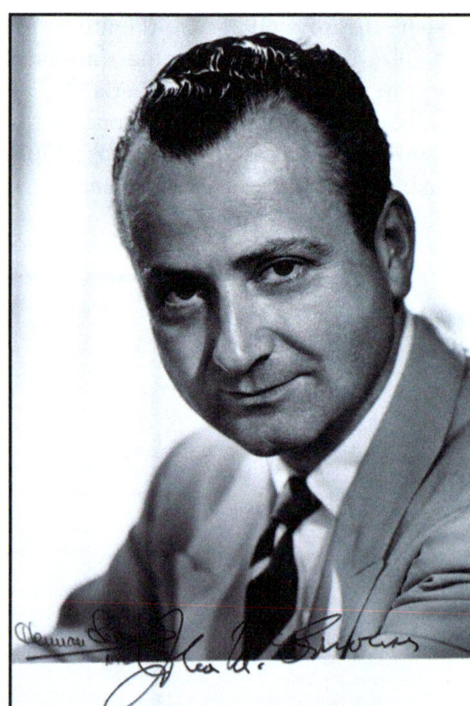

Fig. 2-106 John Marquis Converse (1909–1981) (Courtesy of the National Library of Medicine).

Katharine Phillips

The Italian professor of psychiatry Enrico Morselli (1852–1929) described a condition termed 'dysmorphophobia' in 1891. Now named **body dysmorphic disorder (BDD)**, this seriously debilitating condition can take hold of an affected patient's life, and if undiagnosed, will have potentially disastrous consequences for treating surgeons. The internationally recognized authority and researcher on BDD is Katharine A. Phillips, MD, Professor of Psychiatry and Human Behavior and Director of Research Training for the General Psychiatry Residency Training Program at the Alpert Medical School of Brown University (Figure 2-107). Dr Phillips is also Senior Research Scientist, Director of Research for Adult Psychiatry, and Director of the Body Dysmorphic Disorder Programme at Rhode Island Hospital.

Dr Phillips' research on BDD has been continuously funded by the National Institute of Mental Health since 1995. She has received numerous honours and awards for her research, clinical work, and other academic contributions, including a Special Presidential Commendation from the American Psychiatric Association for her research accomplishments. For more than 20 years, her research has focused primarily on BDD, a disorder that causes marked impairment in social, occupational and academic functioning and is associated with high rates of suicidality.

When she began her research on BDD, virtually no systematic scientific research had been done on the disorder, and thus very little was known about it. One major focus of her work has been to develop and test effective treatments for BDD, both psychotherapeutic and pharmacological. Her other major focus has been psychopathology research to elucidate BDD's clinical features, including symptoms, suicidality, insight, comorbidity, and impairment in psychosocial functioning, as well as BDD's relationship to other disorders, such as obsessive-compulsive disorder and social anxiety disorder. She has also conducted studies of BDD's prevalence and course of illness over time, developed widely used BDD and insight measures, and collaborated on neuroimaging, molecular genetics, and neuropsychological studies of BDD. More than 180 of her 275 publications focus primarily on BDD. She has authored and co-authored a number of books, including the acclaimed *The Broken Mirror: Understanding and Treating Body Dysmorphic Disorder*.[154]

Dr Phillips has stated: 'The overall goal of my past and ongoing work is to better understand and develop effective treatments for BDD, an under-recognized and often debilitating disorder. I hope that this work, in turn, will alleviate the profound suffering and impairment that this disorder so often causes' (see Chapter 9).

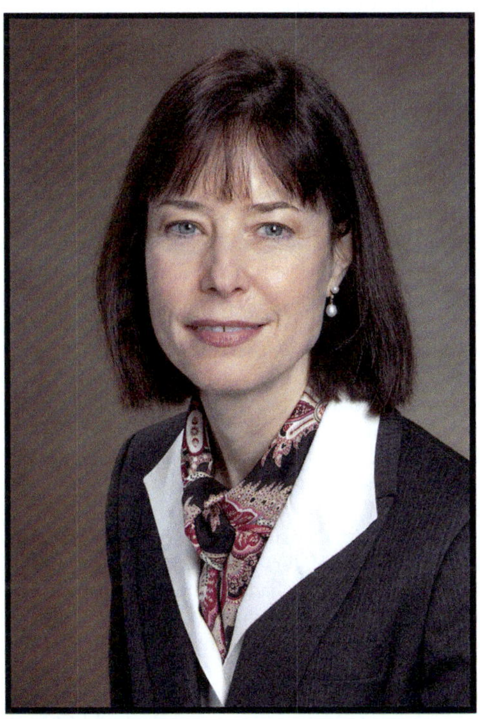

Fig. 2-107 Katharine Phillips (Courtesy of Professor Katharine Phillips).

Conclusion

> 'Progress, far from consisting in change, depends on retentiveness. When change is absolute there remains no being to improve and no direction is set for possible improvement: and when experience is not retained, as among savages, infancy is perpetual. *Those who cannot remember the past are condemned to repeat it*.' [Emphasis added]
>
> George Santayana (1863–1952)[155]
> Spanish-born American philosopher

The accumulated knowledge, achievements and experiences of the pioneers of orthognathic surgery, which have been committed to literature and thereby transmitted to the modern day, are the connective tissue of the specialty and remain a guide for future progress. A specialty that fails to remember, misapprehends or misinterprets its historical development loses that guidance, and those who cannot learn from history or who fail to learn from the mistakes of their predecessors are destined to repeat them. Moreover, those who stand on the shoulders of these giants will inevitably lead the future of the specialty.

References

1 Aristotle. The Works of Aristotle. Ross WD (Ed.). 12 vols. Oxford: Clarendon, 1908.
2 Confucius. The Analects or The Conversations of Confucius With his Disciples and Certain Others. Trans. Soothill WE. Oxford: Oxford University Press, 1945.
3 Hullihen SP. Case of elongation of the under-jaw and distortion of the face and neck, caused by a burn, successfully treated. Am J Dent Sci. 1849;9:157–65.
4 Armbrecht EC. Hullihen, the oral surgeon. Int J Orthod Oral Surg. 1937;23:377, 511, 598, 711.
5 Goldwyn R. Simon P. Hullihen: pioneer oral and plastic surgeon. Plast Reconstr Surg. 1973;52:250–7.

6 Aziz SR. Simon P. Hullihen and the origin of orthognathic surgery. J Oral Maxillofac Surg. 2004;62:1303–7.
7 Whipple JW. Double resection of inferior maxilla for protruding lower jaw. Dental Cosmos. 1898;40:552–7.
8 Naini FB. Regional aesthetic analysis: The maxilla and midface. In: Naini FB. Facial Aesthetics: Concepts and Clinical Diagnosis. Oxford: Wiley-Blackwell, 2011.
9 Angle EH. Double resection of lower maxilla. Dental Cosmos 1898;40:635–8.
10 Ottolengui RD. A friendly criticism of Dr Angle's proposed technique in surgical correction of mandibular protrusion. Dental Cosmos 1903;45:454–7.
11 Blair VP. Report of case of double resection for correction of protrusion of mandible. Dental Cosmos. 1906;48:817–20.
12 Blair VP. Surgery and Diseases of the Mouth and Jaws (Ed. 3). St. Louis: The C.V. Mosby Company, 1918.
13 Ballin M. Double resection for treatment of mandibular protrusion. Dent Items. 1908;30:422–7. Discussion 427–31.
14 Cryer MH. Studies of the anterior and posterior occlusion of the teeth, with suggestions as to treatment. Dental Cosmos. 1913;55:673–91.
15 Aller TG. Operative treatment of prognathism. Dental Cosmos. 1917;59:394–9.
16 Harsha WM. Prognathism with operative treatment. J Am Med Ass. 1912;59:2035.
17 Harsha WM. Bilateral resection of the jaw for prognathism. Surg Gynecol. Obstet. 1912;15:51–3.
18 Kazanjian VH. Surgical treatment of mandibular prognathism. Internat J Orthodont Oral Surg Radiogr. 1932;18:1224–39.
19 Von Eiselsberg A. Uber plastic bei ektropium des unterskiefers (progenie). Wiener Klinische Wechenschrift. 1906;19:1505.
20 Pichler H, Trauner R. Mund. Und Kieferchirurgie, Part I, Vol. 1 and 2. Vienna: Urban Schwarzenberg, 1948.
21 Fickling BW, Fordyce GI. Mandibular osteotomy for facial asymmetry. Proc R Soc Med. 1955;48:989.
22 Hovell JH. The surgical construction of variations in the facial skeletal pattern. Proc R Soc Med. 1956;49:546–56.
23 Armbrecht EC, Clarke G, Kline KK. Bilateral ostectomy for correction of prognathism – report of a case. J Oral Surg. 1957;15:63–6.
24 Gelbier S. John Herbert Hovell (1910-1988), TD, MRCS, LRCP, FRCS, FDSRCS (Eng), FFD (Ire), DOrth. J Med Biogr. 2014 May 15.
25 Hofer O. Die vertikale osteotomie zur verlangerung des einseitig verkurxten aufsteigenden unterkieferastes. Atschr Stomatol. 1936;34:826.
26 Köle H. Surgical operations on the alveolar ridge to correct occlusal abnormalities. Oral Surg Oral Med Oral Pathol. 1959;12(3):277–88.
27 Köle H. Surgical operations on the alveolar ridge to correct occlusal abnormalities. Oral Surg Oral Med Oral Pathol. 1959;12(4):413–20.
28 Köle H. Surgical operations on the alveolar ridge to correct occlusal abnormalities. Oral Surg Oral Med Oral Pathol. 1959;12(5):515–29.
29 Sowray JH, Haskell R. Ostectomy at the mandibular symphysis. Br J Oral Surg. 1968;5:97–102.
30 Henry TC. Localized osteotomy in cases of mild inferior protrusion. Pp.80–92. In: Walker RV (Ed.): Oral Surgery: Transactions of the Third International Conference on Oral Surgery, 1968. Edinburgh and London: E & S Livingstone, 1970.
31 Obwegeser H. Die bewegung des unteren alveolarfortsatzes zur korrektur von kieferstellungsanomalien. Dtsch Z Zeitschrift. 1969;24:5–15.
32 MacIntosh RB. Total mandibular alveolar osteotomy: encouraging experiences with an infrequently indicated procedure. J Maxillofac Surg. 1974;2:210–8.
33 Macintosh RB, Carlotti AE. Total mandibular alveolar osteotomy in the management of skeletal (infantile) apertognathia. J Oral Surg. 1975;33:921–8.
34 Pangrazio-Kulbersh V, MacIntosh RB. Total mandibular alveolar osteotomy: an alternate choice to other surgical procedures. Am J Orthod. 1985;87:319–37.
35 Humphry GM. Excision of the condyle of the lower jaw. Br Assoc Med J. 1856;4:61–2.
36 Berger P. Du traitement chirurgical du prognathisme. Theèse (Thesis): Meédecine. Lyon: A. Rey, 1897.
37 Jaboulay M, Bérard L. Traitement chirurgical du prognathisme inférieur. Presse Med Paris. 1898;6:173–6.
38 Ivy RH. Surgery in relation to orthodontia and facial harmony. Internat J Orthodont Dent Child. 1933;19:888–98.
39 Dufourmentel L. Le traitement chirurgical du prognathisme. Presse Medicale 1921;29:235.
40 Kostečka F. Surgical correction of protrusion of the lower and upper jaws. J Am Dent Ass. 1928;15:362.
41 Kostečka F. A contribution to the surgical treatment of openbite. Am J Orthodont Oral Surg. 1934;20:1082–92.
42 Spilka CJ. Surgical correction of mandibular prognathism. Oral Surg Oral Med Oral Pathol. 1956;9:1255–66.
43 Bowdler Henry C. A case of Kostecka's operation for the correction of the prognathous mandible. Proc R Soc Med. 1946;39:646–8.
44 Smith AE, Johnson JB. Surgical treatment of mandibular deformations. JADA. 1940;27:689–700.
45 Blair VP. Operations on the jaw bone and face. Surg Gynecol Obstet. 1907;4:67–8.
46 Ivy RH. Vilray Papin Blair, A.M., M.D., F.A.C.S.: Honorary Member, British Association of Plastic Surgeons. Br J Plast Surg. 1953;5:224–7.
47 Babcock WW. The surgical treatment of certain deformities of the jaw associated with malocclusion of the teeth. JAMA. 1909;53:833–9.
48 Bruhn C. The surgical-orthopedical removal of the deformations of the jaws. Internat J Orthodont Oral Surg Radiogr. 1927;13:65–79.
49 Naini FB. Cephalometry and cephalometric analysis. In: Naini FB. Facial Aesthetics: Concepts and Clinical Diagnosis. Oxford: Wiley-Blackwell, 2011.
50 Lindemann A. Die Wehrchirurgie des Gesichtsschädels – Nachbehandlung und Nachoperation. Dtsch Z Zahn Mund Kieferheilk. 1936;3:105.
51 Lindemann A, Hofrath H. Die Kieferosteotomie. Chirurg. 1938;10:745–70.
52 Kazanjian VH. Surgical correction of deformities of the jaws and its relation to orthodontia. Internat J Orthodont Oral Surg. 1936;22:259–82.
53 Kazanjian VH. The treatment of mandibular prognathism with special reference to edentulous patients. Oral Surg Oral Med Oral Pathol. 1951;4:680–88.
54 Kazanjian VH. The surgical treatment of prognathism; an analysis of sixty-five cases. Am J Surg. 1954;87:691–700.
55 Deranian HM. Miracle Man of the Western Front: Dr Varaztad H. Kazanjian, Pioneer Plastic Surgeon. Worcester, Massachusetts: Chandler House Press, 2007.
56 Limberg A. Treatment of open-bite by means of plastic oblique osteotomy of the ascending rami of the mandible. Dental Cosmos. 1925;67:1191–1200.
57 Skaloud F. A new surgical method for correction of prognathism of the mandible. Oral Surg Oral Med Oral Pathol. 1951;4:689–94.
58 Wassmund M. Frakturen und Luxationen des Geishtschädels. Unter Berücksichtigung der Komplikationen des Hirnschädels. Ihre Klinik und Therapie. Praktisches Lehrbuch. Berlin: H. Meusser, 1927.
59 Perthes G. Operative Korrektur der Progenie. Zbl Chir. 1922;49:1540–1.
60 Ernst F. Uber die chirurgische beseitigung der prognathie des unterkiefers (Progenie). Zentralbl Chir. 1938;65: 179.

61 Schuchardt K. Ein Betrag zur chirurgischen Kieferorthopädie unter Berucksichtigung ihrer Bedeutung fur die Behandlung angeborener und erworbener Kieferdeformitaten bei Soldaten. Dtsch Zahn Mund Kieferheilkd Zentralbl. 1942;9:73–89.
62 Obwegeser HL. Surgical procedures to correct mandibular prognathism and reshaping of the chin. In: Trauner, R and Obwegeser, HL (Editors). The surgical correction of mandibular prognathism and retrognathia with consideration of genioplasty. Part I. Surgical procedures to correct mandibular prognathism and reshaping of chin. Oral Surg Oral Med Oral Pathol. 1957;10:677–89.
63 Dal Pont G. L'osteotomia retromolare per la correzione della progenia. Minerva Chir. 1959;14:1138–41.
64 Dal Pont G. Retromolar osteotomy for correction of prognathism. J Oral Surg Anesth Hosp D Serv. 1961;19:42–7.
65 Obwegeser H. The indications for surgical correction of mandibular deformity by the sagittal splitting technique. Br J Oral Surg. 1964;1:157–71.
66 Hunsuck EE. A modified intraoral sagittal splitting technique for correction of mandibular prognathism. J Oral Maxillofac Surg. 1968;26:250–3.
67 Epker BN. Modifications in the sagittal osteotomy of the mandible. J Oral Surg. 1977;35:157–9.
68 Robinson M. Prognathism corrected by open vertical subcondylotomy. J Oral Surg (Chic). 1958;16:215–9.
69 Thoma KH. Oblique osteotomy of mandibular ramus: special technique for correction of various types of facial defects and malocclusion. Oral Surg. 1961;14 Suppl 1:23–46.
70 Hinds EC, Galbreath JC, SillsAH. Selection of procedure in the management of jaw deformities. Plast Reconstr Surg Transplant Bull. 1962;29:176–85.
71 Caldwell JB, Letterman GS. Vertical osteotomy in the mandibular rami for correction of prognathism. J Oral Surg (Chic). 1954;12:185–202.
72 Caldwell JB, Hayward JR, Lister RL. Correction of mandibular retrognathia by vertical L osteotomy: a new technic. J Oral Surg. 1968;26:259–64.
73 Hebert JM, Kent JN, Hinds EC. Correction of prognathism by an intraoral vertical subcondylar osteotomy. J Oral Surg. 1970;28:651–3.
74 Kazanjian VH. Bone transplanting of the mandible. Am J Surg. 1952;83:633–9.
75 Hofer O. Operation der prognathie und mikrogenie. Dtsch Zahn Mund Kieferheilkd. 1942;9:121–32.
76 Trauner R. In memory of Professor Otto Hofer, D.D.S. Osterr Z Stomatol. 1972;69:112–3.
77 Personal communication, Freud Museum London.
78 Gillies HD, Millard Jr. DR. The Principles and Art of Plastic Surgery. London: Butterworth and Co. Ltd., 1957.
79 Converse JM, Wood-Smith D. Horizontal osteotomy of the mandible. Plast Reconstr Surg. 1964;34:464–71.
80 Neuner O. Chirurgische Orthodontie. Schweiz Monatschr Zahnhlkd. 1965;75:940–4.
81 Obwegeser HL. Die einzeitige Vorbewegung des Oberkiefers und Rückbewegung des Unterkiefers zur Korrektur der extremen "Progenie". Schweiz Monatschr Zahnheilk. 1970;80:547–55.
82 Comte A. The positive philosophy of Auguste Comte. Freely translated and condensed by Harriet Martineau (1855). London: George Bell & Sons, 1896.
83 Von Langenbeck B. Beitrange zur osteoplastik. In: Goschen A (Ed.). Die osteoplastiche resektion des oberkierers. Deutsche Klinik. Berlin: Reimer, 1859.
84 Cheever D. Displacement of the upper jaw. Med Surg Rep Boston City Hosp. 1870;1:156.
85 Cheever D. Naso-pharyngeal polpus, attached to the basilar process of occipital and body of the sphenoid bone successfully removed by a section, displacement, and subsequent replacement and reunion of the superior maxillary bone. Boston Med Surg. 1867;8:162.
86 Moloney F, Worthington P. The origin of the Le Fort I maxillary osteotomy: Cheever's operation. J Oral Surg. 1981;39:731–4.
87 Halvorson EG, Mulliken JB. Cheever's double operation: the first Le Fort I osteotomy. Plast Reconstr Surg. 2008;121:1375–81.
88 Le Fort R. Étude expérimentale sur les fractures de la mâchoire supérieure. Rev Chir. 1901;1:208, 260, 479.
89 Le Fort R. Experimental study of fractures of the upper jaw (paper of 1901 translated by Paul Tessier). Plast Reconstr Surg. 1972;50:497–506.
90 Wassmund M. Frakturen und luxationen des gesichtsschädels. Leipzig: Meusser, 1927.
91 Axhausen G. Zur behandlung veralteter disloziert geheilter oberkieferbruche. Dtsch Zahn Mund Kieferheilk. 1934;1: 334–9.
92 Schuchardt K. Ein Betrag zur chirurgischen Kieferorthopädie unter Berucksichtigung ihrer Bedeutung fur die Behandlung angeborener und erworbener Kieferdeformitaten bei Soldaten. Dtsch Zahn Mund Kieferheilkd Zentralbl. 1942;9:73–89.
93 Moore FT, Ward TG. Complications and sequelae of untreated fractures of the facial bones and their treatment. Br J Plast Surg. 1949;1:257–67.
94 Gillies H, Rowe N. L'ostéotomie du maxillaire supérieur enoisagée essentiellement dans le cas de bec-de-lièvre total. Rev Stomatol. 1954;55:545–52.
95 Obwegeser H. Surgery of the maxilla for the correction of prognathism. SSO Schweiz Monatsschr Zahnheilkd. 1965;75:365–74.
96 Obwegeser HL. Surgical correction of small or retrodisplaced maxillae. The 'dish-face' deformity. Plast Reconstr Surg. 1969;43:351–65.
97 Kufner J. Four-year experience with major maxillary osteotomy for retrusion. J Oral Surg. 1971;29:549–53.
98 Bennett MA, Wolford LM. The maxillary step osteotomy and Steinmann pin stabilization. J Oral Maxillofac Surg. 1985;43:307–11.
99 Cohn-Stock G. Die chirurgische immediatregulierung der kiefer, speciell die chirurgische behandlung der prognathie. Vierteljahrsschr Zahnheilk. 1921;3:320.
100 Wolfe SA. Günther Cohn-Stock, M.S., D.D.S., father of maxillary orthognathic surgery. J Cranio-Maxillofacial Surg. 1989;17:331–4.
101 Wassmund M. Lehrbuch der praktischen chirurgie des mundes und der kiefer. Leipzig: Meusser, 1935.
102 Cupar I. Die chirurgische behandlung der form und stellungsveränderungen des oberkiefers. Ost Z Stomatol. 1954;51:565–77.
103 Wunderer S. Die prognathie-operation mittels frontal gestielten maxillafragment. Osterr Z Stomatol. 1962;59:98–102.
104 Schuchardt K. Formen des offenen bisses und ihre operativen behandlungmöglichkeiten. Stuttgart: Fortschr Kiefer Gesichts-Chir., 1955.
105 Schuchardt K. Experiences with the surgical treatment of some deformities of the jaws: prognathia, micrognathia, and open bite. In: Wallace AB (Ed.). Transactions of Second Congress, International Society of Plastic Surgeons. London, 1959. Edinburgh: E & S Livingstone Ltd., 1961.
106 Kufner J. Nove notedy chirurgickeho leceni otereneho skusu. Čslka Stomat. 1960;60:5.
107 Kufner J. Experience with a modified procedure for correction of open bite. pp 18-23. In: Walker RV (Ed.). Oral Surgery: Transactions of the Third International Conference on Oral Surgery, 1968. Edinburgh and London: E & S Livingstone, 1970.
108 Bell WH. Revascularization and bone healing after anterior maxillary osteotomy: a study using adult rhesus monkeys. J Oral Surg. 1969;27:249–55.

109 Bell WH, Levy BM. Revascularization and bone healing after anterior mandibular osteotomy. J Oral Surg. 1970; 28:196–203.
110 Bell WH, Levy BM. Healing after anterior maxillary osteotomy. J Oral Surg. 1970;28:728–34.
111 Bell WH, Levy BM. Revascularization and bone healing after posterior maxillary osteotomy. J Oral Surg. 1971; 29:313–20.
112 Bell WH, Levy BM. Revascularization and bone healing after maxillary corticotomies. J Oral Surg. 1972;30:640–8.
113 Bell WH. Biologic basis for maxillary osteotomies. Am J Phys Anthropol. 1973;38:279–89.
114 Bell WH, Fonseca RJ, Kenneky JW, Levy BM. Bone healing and revascularization after total maxillary osteotomy. J Oral Surg. 1975;33:253–60.
115 Bell WH, Schendel SA, Finn RA. Revascularization after surgical repositioning of one-tooth dento-osseous segments. J Oral Surg. 1978;36:757–65.
116 Scheideman GB, Kawamura H, Finn RA, Bell WH. Wound healing after anterior and posterior subapical osteotomy. J Oral Maxillofac Surg. 1985;43:408–16.
117 Quejada JG, Kawamura H, Finn RA, Bell WH. Wound healing associated with segmental total maxillary osteotomy. J Oral Maxillofac Surg. 1986;44:366–77.
118 Storum KA, Bell WH, Nagura H. Microangiographic and histologic evaluation of revascularization and healing after genioplasty by osteotomy of the inferior border of the mandible. J Oral Maxillofac Surg. 1988;46:210–6.
119 Bell WH, You ZH, Finn RA, Fields RT. Wound healing after multisegmental Le Fort I osteotomy and transection of the descending palatine vessels. J Oral Maxillofac Surg. 1995;53:1425-33; discussion 1433–4.
120 Soerensen J, Warnekros L. Chirug und Zahnarzt. Berlin: Springer Verlag, 1917.
121 Steinhäuser EW. Historical development of orthognathic surgery. J Craniomaxillofac Surg. 1996;24:195–204.
122 Spiessl B. Osteosynthese bei sagittaler osteotomie nach Obwegeser-Dal Pont. Fortschr Kiefer Gesichtschir. 1974;18: 145–8.
123 Luhr HG. Indications for use of a microsystem for internal fixation in craniofacial surgery. J Craniofac Surg. 1990;1: 35–52.
124 Michelet FX, Benoit JP, Festal F, Despujols P, Bruchet P, Arvor A. Fixation without blocking of sagittal osteotomies of the rami by means of endo-buccal screwed plates in the treatment of antero-posterior abnormalities. Rev Stomatol Chir Maxillofac. 1971;72:531–7.
125 Michelet FX, Deymes J, Dessus B. Osteosynthesis with miniaturized screwed plates in maxillo-facial surgery. J Maxillofac Surg. 1973;1:79–84.
126 Champy M. Surgical treatment of midface deformities. Head Neck Surg. 1980;2:451–65.
127 Lindorf HH. Sagittal ramus osteotomy with tandem screw fixation. Technique and results. J Maxillofac Surg. 1986;14:311–6.
128 Plato. The Republic (Book II). In: Hamilton E, Cairns H (Eds). The Collected Dialogues of Plato. Princeton, NJ: Princeton University Press, 1961.
129 Bamji AN. The Macalister archive: records from the Queen's Hospital, Sidcup, 1917-1921. J Audiov Media Med. 1993;16:76–84.
130 Bamji A. Sir Harold Gillies: surgical pioneer. Trauma 2006; 8: 143–156.
131 Holdsworth WG. Sir Harold Gillies. Ann Plast Surg. 1979;3:464–68.
132 Matthews DN. Gillies: mastermind of modern plastic surgery. Br J Plast Surg. 1979;32:68–77.
133 Millard DR. Sir Harold Gillies. Ann Plast Surg. 1979;3: 454–63.
134 Negus V. Sir Harold Gillies. Arch Otolaryngol. 1966;83: 372–8.
135 Personal communication, Professor Hugo Obwegeser.
136 McAuley JE. Charles Valadier: a forgotten pioneer in the treatment of jaw injuries. Proc R Soc Med. Aug 1974;67: 785–9.
137 Ivy RH. T. Pomfret Kilner, C.B.E., F.R.C.S. Emeritus Professor of Plastic Surgery, University of Oxford. Plast Reconstr Surg. 1964;34:313–4.
138 Griffiths RW. Arthur Rainsford Mowlem (1902–1986), plastic surgeon. J Med Biogr. 2013;21:180–92.
139 Pinney J, Metcalfe AD. Sir Archibald McIndoe and the Guinea Pig Club. PMFA News 2014;1:21–4.
140 Sir Winston Churchill. 20th August 1940, Speech delivered in The House of Commons. 'The Few'. The Churchill Centre and Museum. Retrieved 7th October, 2014.
141 Gillies HD, Harrison SH. Operative correction by osteotomy of recessed malar maxillary compound in a case of oxycephaly. Br J Plast Surg. 1950;3:123–7.
142 Wolfe SA. A Man from Héric: The Life and Work of Paul Tessier, MD, father of Craniofacial Surgery: Volumes I and II. Raleigh, NC: Lulu.com, 2012.
143 Tessier P. Surgical treatment of rare orbito-facial malformations. J Genet Hum. 1966;15:Suppl:322–55.
144 Tessier P. Total facial osteotomy. Crouzon's syndrome, Apert's syndrome: oxycephaly, scaphocephaly, turricephaly. Ann Chir Plast. 1967;12:273–86.
145 Tessier P. The definitive plastic surgical treatment of the severe facial deformities of craniofacial dysostosis. Crouzon's and Apert's diseases. Plast Reconstr Surg. 1971; 48:419–42.
146 Montaigne. The Complete Essays of Montaigne. Trans. Frame DL. Stanford, CA : Stanford University Press, 1958.
147 Jones B. Paul Louis Tessier. BMJ. 12, 2008; 337(7661): 118.
148 Ortiz-Monasterio F, del Campo AF, Carrillo A. Advancement of the orbits and the midface in one piece, combined with frontal repositioning, for the correction of Crouzon's deformities. Plast Reconstr Surg. 1978;61:507–16.
149 Henderson D, Jackson IT. Nasomaxillary hypoplasia – the Le Fort II osteotomy. Br J Oral Surg. 1973;11:77–93.
150 Ilizarov GA. The principles of the Ilizarov method. Bull Hosp Jt Dis Orthop Inst. 1988;48:1–11.
151 Golyakhovsky V. Gavriel A. Ilizarov: 'The magician from Kurgan'. Bull Hosp Jt Dis Orthop Inst. 1988;48:12–16.
152 Naini FB. Psychological ramifications of facial deformities. In: Naini FB. Facial Aesthetics: Concepts and Clinical Diagnosis. Oxford: Wiley-Blackwell, 2011.
153 Thompson N. John Marquis Converse 1909–1981. Chirurgia Plast. 1981;6:149–51.
154 Phillips KA. The Broken Mirror: Understanding and Treating Body Dysmorphic Disorder. Oxford: Oxford University Press, 2005.
155 Santayana G. Reason in Common Sense (1905). In: Santayana G. The Life of Reason or the Phases of Human Progress (1905-1906). New York: Charles Scribner's Sons, 1920.

Chapter 3

Orthognathic Surgery: Preliminary Considerations

Farhad B. Naini and Daljit S. Gill

Inter Artem et Scientiam Concordia
'Art and Science in Harmony'
Motto of the British Orthodontic Society
(Registered with the College of Arms)

Definition of orthognathic surgery

Orthognathic surgery may be defined as the surgical repositioning of the maxilla and/or mandible, and/or their segments thereof, with or without orthodontic repositioning of the teeth, in order to improve dentofacial function and aesthetics (in a stable manner) and health-related quality of life. The term 'orthognathic' is derived from the Greek *orthos*: correct or straight, and *gnathos*: jaw.[1]

Orthognathic surgery is also sometimes defined as the combined orthodontic-surgical correction of dentoskeletal deformities. Though this is almost always the case, the inaccuracy of the definition lies in the fact that, occasionally, surgical camouflage only is undertaken, e.g. genioplasty, or very rarely in patients where the postoperative dental occlusion will be satisfactory without orthodontics. These cases do not involve orthodontics, but are still classified as orthognathic surgery. Additionally, bimaxillary advancement to open the airway for sleep apnoea does not always require orthodontic treatment, but again is orthognathic surgery. However, it remains that for the vast majority of patients, orthodontic treatment is part and parcel of modern orthognathic surgery.

> **Note:**
>
> In clinical practice, the terms *orthognathic surgery* and *orthognathic clinic* are preferable to any terms that mention the word 'deformity'. It is insensitive and tactless to use terms such as 'dentofacial deformity' or 'facial deformity clinic' in any environment where a patient or their family may be confronted with it.

Orthognathic Surgery: Principles, Planning and Practice. Edited by Farhad B. Naini and Daljit S. Gill.

Aetiology of dentofacial deformities

> '... and now remains that we find out the cause of this effect,
> Or rather say, the cause of this defect,
> For this effect defective comes by cause.'
> William Shakespeare (1564–1616)
> *Hamlet* (c.1600)[2]

The term 'aetiology' (derived from Old Latin: *aetiologia*; from Greek *aitia*: cause, and *logia*: -logy, used to denote the study of something) refers to the investigation and assignment of the cause of any disorder.

Nature vs. nurture

The aetiology of any dentofacial or craniofacial deformity may be genetic, environmental or multifactorial, i.e. a combination of the two. The question of the influence of genetics vs. environment is often labelled with the 'nature vs. nurture?' cliché derived from Shakespeare's final solo-authored play *The Tempest* (1611):[3]

> 'A devil, a born devil, on whose nature
> Nurture can never stick... '

Many craniofacial syndromes have a known genetic determination (see Chapter 55). The presenting **craniofacial phenotype**, i.e. the characteristic craniofacial appearance of many syndromic patients is usually consistent enough to provide a visual impression of the diagnosis at any age and for any ethnic background. However, the craniofacial phenotype of some craniofacial syndromes evolves with age.

The fact that genetic factors play a predominant role in the aetiology of many malocclusions has been established,[4] and each facial bone is likely to have a genetically predetermined size and growth potential.[5] However, it has also been suggested that the facial bones are influenced by functional muscle attachments and oronasopharyngeal function, collectively known as the **functional matrix**.[6,7] *There is an interaction of genetic and environmental factors in the aetiology of dentofacial disproportion and malocclusion.* We need to find out which genes are involved, how much influence they really exert and how strong or weak is the genetic influence for different facial features.[8,9]

For any malocclusion or dentofacial deformity, e.g. mandibular prognathism, the question is whether the trait is primarily genetically or environmentally determined. Orthodontics as a rule works by *altering the environment* of the teeth, and dentofacial orthopaedics works by altering the environment of the developing dentition and growing jaws. This is important as the greater the genetic determination of a malocclusion, the worse the prognosis for a successful outcome by means of orthodontic or dentofacial orthopaedic intervention,[9] and, as such, the greater the likelihood of a requirement for orthognathic surgical correction.

It is only our genes that we inherit from our parents, referred to as the **genotype**. How these genes are expressed, referred to as the **phenotype** (e.g. our facial features) depends on the manner in which the genes interact with our environment during growth and development. The separate contributions of heredity and environment are not always equivalent for each facial characteristic. For example, iris pigmentation is relatively independent of environmental factors. Conversely, an anterior open bite due to only a digit-sucking habit is environmentally determined. However, other facial features, e.g. the length of mandible, *may* be more affected by the environment. The dilemma that exists is that only the combined, final result of the nature–nurture interaction can be directly observed. In the case of a single individual, there is no accurate way to gauge the separate contributions of genetics or environment to any one dentofacial characteristic. However, to overcome this problem, it is possible to obtain an idea of the relative contribution of each using two methods: **family studies**, and the **twin method**.

The Hapsburgs were a royal European family, and over 23 generations portrait painters captured images of the Hapsburgs, and they all exhibited the same mandibular prognathism and protrusive lower lip. The 'Hapsburg jaw' is a good example of a genetically inherited characteristic in a family. However, there are very few long-term family studies available. The alternative method used to investigate genetic determination is the twin method, first described by Sir Francis Galton in *Fraser's Magazine* (1875). Monozygotic (identical) twins result from one sperm fertilizing one egg, and the resultant zygote splitting into two. Therefore, monozygotic twins are genetically identical and any differences between them may be attributed, with some confidence, to the environment. Monozygotic twins may be compared with same-sex dizygotic (non-identical) twins, who share only 50% of their genes. Differences between such twin pairs may be compared and contrasted.

The heritability of the various dentofacial phenotypes (i.e. malocclusions and associated dentofacial features) has been studied.[9] Harris[10] undertook extensive familial cephalometric studies in **Class 2 division 1** malocclusions, and found the mandible to be significantly more retruded than in Class I patients, the body of the mandible to be smaller, and the overall mandibular length reduced. Kloeppel[11] found a strong familial occurrence for **Class II division 2** malocclusion, and in a clinical and cephalometric study of 48 twin pairs Marcovic[4] found identical twins 100% concordant for Class II division 2 malocclusion and non-identical twins 90% discordant, concluding that genetics is the main aetiological factor in Class II division 2 malocclusion. For the **Class III** malocclusion, Schulze and Weise[12] studied mandibular prognathism in twins and found that concordance in identical twins was 6 times higher than in non-identical twins, and an extensive literature review and family study undertaken by Litton et al.[13] found strong familial occurrence for Class III malocclusion, no association

Table 3-1 Degree of concordance of malocclusions in twins (Based on data from Lundstrom, 1984)[14] *Note*: Class II division 1 and Class II division 2 malocclusions were not separated.

Malocclusion	Identical twins (%)	Non-identical twins (%)
Class I	87.3	84.6
Class II	67.7	23.8
Class III	83.3	10.0

with gender, and different modes of transmission in different families or populations. In a famous study of twins, Lundstrom[14] found the strongest genetic predisposition for Class III malocclusions, but that different types of malocclusion did occur in identical pairs of twins (Table 3-1). Unfortunately, the problem with this study was that he did not separate Class II division 1 and Class II division 2 cases.

Bearing in mind the results of Marcovic's study,[4] it appears that the Class II division 2 malocclusion has a higher genetic determination than the Class II division 1. Lundstrom[14] concluded that 'the type of malocclusion and jaw relationship is strongly influenced by heredity, but is affected likewise by the environment.'

The genetic determination of the facial **vertical dimension** has also been investigated.

Hunter[15] found that vertical skeletal dimensions have a stronger genetic determination than sagittal dimensions. This was verified in a three-dimensional study of twins by Naini and Moss,[16] which also found that vertical facial dimensions have a stronger genetic determination than sagittal dimensions.

The **clinical implications** of such research are that facial dimensions with a lower genetic determination are more open to influence by dentofacial orthopaedic correction than are facial proportions with a high genetic determination. The evidence cited above from twin studies and family studies on the genetic determination of the various malocclusions and associated dentofacial deformities appears to indicate that the strongest genetic determination is for Class III and Class II division 2 malocclusions, and vertical skeletal discrepancies. As such, these malocclusions are less likely to be amenable to orthodontic and dentofacial orthopaedic correction, and more likely eventually to require orthognathic surgical correction.

Note:

Although the extent of further growth cannot be accurately predicted, the pattern of growth is unlikely to change. Therefore, the mild to moderate Class III skeletal pattern of a growing patient will either stay mild to moderate, or may become severe, and a patient with a severe Class III skeletal pattern presenting at a young age is likely to remain a severe Class III.

Classification of dentofacial deformities

Classification may be defined as the process by which the complexity of a series of associated or disparate parameters is organized into a list of discrete and well-defined categories according to predetermined clinical signs. For the patient with a dentofacial deformity these parameters are the dentoskeletal and soft tissue units and subunits of the craniofacial complex.

Devising an accurate and all-encompassing classification of dentofacial deformities is fraught with difficulties due to the interrelationships of the many dentofacial parameters. There are different dental and dentoalveolar relationships, different soft tissue parameters (e.g. size, morphology and activity of the tongue and circumoral musculature), and the skeletal (basal bone) variations in the different planes of space, all of which may co-exist, with various parameters cross-cutting one another, e.g. an anterior open bite may be skeletal, soft tissue or dentoalveolar, or any combination of these aetiological elements. However, it is still worthwhile attempting to bring some form of order by classifying these morphological relationships, despite the limitations.

A number of classification systems have been suggested, though some are far too simple and leave out too many relevant parameters, whereas others are too complex to be of practical benefit. A potentially useful and practical approach to the classification of dentofacial deformities is based on the recognition and description of the *primary morphological parameter of the deformity*, referred to as the **primary descriptor**, followed by any highly relevant additional morphological relationships (**secondary descriptors**), and an attempt at identifying the aetiological factors.

Morphological–aetiological classification of dentofacial deformities

The description of a dentofacial deformity often involves a number of dentoskeletal parameters and their structural interrelationships, e.g. the sagittal, vertical and transverse skeletal relationships, the sagittal, vertical and transverse dentoalveolar relationships, and any relevant soft tissue parameters. The **aetiology** is usually also described, as far as possible, in order to explain *why* the morphological and structural relationships are as they are, which is relevant for diagnosis, treatment planning and the prognosis for postoperative stability.

The primary descriptor of a dentofacial deformity may be one parameter, e.g. sagittal mandibular excess, or a commonly recognized combination of parameters, e.g. posterior vertical maxillary excess and posterior rotation of the mandible. Though other skeletal discrepancies may be present as well, the primary descriptor is the most obvious and severe. The primary descriptors may be described separately for the maxilla, mandible and chin, followed by their commonly recognized combinations (Table 3-2).

Table 3-2 Classification of dentofacial deformities based on primary and secondary descriptors (Primary descriptors are *predominantly* skeletal in aetiology; Secondary descriptors may have a multifactorial aetiology)

<table>
<tr><th>Maxillary deformities</th><th>Primary descriptor</th><th>Potential secondary descriptors</th></tr>
<tr><td rowspan="7"></td><td>Sagittal maxillary excess
Prominence of the maxilla due to an excessive size (macrognathia), excessive forward position (prognathism), or both</td><td rowspan="18">Dentoalveolar parameters:
• Sagittal dentoalveolar relationships
∘ Incisor relationships (Class I, II/1, II/2, III)
∘ Canine relationships
∘ Molar and premolar relationships
• Vertical dentoalveolar relationships
∘ Incisor overbite
▪ Average
▪ Deep
▪ Reduced
▪ Anterior open bite (AOB)
∘ Buccal segment overbite
▪ Average
▪ Scissors bite
▪ Lateral open bite
▪ Posterior open bite
• Transverse dentoalveolar relationships
∘ Dental crossbites/scissors bites

Aesthetic parameters:
• Maxillary incisor exposure in repose and animation
• Gingival exposure in repose and animation
• Incisor inclinations

Soft tissue parameters:
• Lip seals
∘ Complete (lip competence)
∘ Incomplete (lip incompetence)
∘ Potential lip competence – due to interposed maxillary incisors
• Lip heights – increased or reduced lip heights may have functional considerations (see lip seals) as well as aesthetic considerations in relation to incisor exposure
• Lower lip trap – lower lip caught behind maxillary incisors in a Class II patient, causing their proclination.
• Soft tissue thicknesses
∘ Upper lip
∘ Lower lip
∘ Chin pad
• Tongue
∘ Position – e.g. forward resting position between the incisors thereby impeding their full eruption
∘ Activity – e.g. endogenous tongue thrust leading to a soft tissue anterior open bite and excessive incisor proclination</td></tr>
<tr><td>Sagittal maxillary deficiency
Reduced size of the maxilla (micrognathia) in the sagittal dimension, posterior positioning of the maxilla in relation to the craniofacial complex (retrognathia), or both</td></tr>
<tr><td>Vertical maxillary excess (VME)
Excessive vertical growth of the maxilla and associated dentoalveolus in an inferior direction
• Total
• Posterior
• Anterior – usually due to overeruption of the maxillary incisors</td></tr>
<tr><td>Vertical maxillary deficiency (VMD)
Reduced vertical growth of the maxilla and associated dentoalveolus in an inferior direction
• Total
• Anterior – due to impeded eruption of the maxillary incisors (by the tongue or a prolonged digit sucking habit)</td></tr>
<tr><td>Transverse maxillary excess
Excessive transverse width of the maxilla, potentially leading to bilateral scissors bite</td></tr>
<tr><td>Transverse maxillary deficiency
Severely narrow maxillary width, leading to dental crossbites, biting of the tongue and possibly food accumulation in the palate (if high and narrow palatal vault)</td></tr>
<tr><td>Maxillary asymmetry
• Bodily translation to left or right (uncommon)
• Transverse canting of the maxillary occlusal plane (usually secondary to a mandibular asymmetry)</td></tr>
<tr><td>Mandibular deformities</td><td>Primary descriptor</td></tr>
<tr><td rowspan="5"></td><td>Sagittal mandibular excess
Prominence of the mandible due to an excessive size (macrognathia), excessive forward position (prognathism), or both</td></tr>
<tr><td>Sagittal mandibular deficiency
Reduced size of the mandible (micrognathia) in the sagittal dimension, posterior positioning of the mandible in relation to the craniofacial complex (retrognathia), or both</td></tr>
<tr><td>Anterior (forward or clockwise) mandibular growth rotation</td></tr>
<tr><td>Posterior (backward or anticlockwise) mandibular growth rotation</td></tr>
<tr><td>Mandibular asymmetry
• Hemimandibular elongation
• Hemimandibular hyperplasia
• Unilateral condylar hyperplasia
• Unilateral lack of growth</td></tr>
<tr><td>Chin deformities</td><td>Primary descriptor</td></tr>
<tr><td rowspan="2"></td><td>Chin excess (osseous)
• Sagittal
• Vertical
• Combined</td></tr>
<tr><td>Chin deficiency (osseous)
• Sagittal
• Vertical
• Combined</td></tr>
</table>

Table 3-2 (*Continued*)

Combined bimaxillary deformities	**Primary descriptor**	**Functional parameters:** • Mandibular displacements ◦ Anterior – in Class III patients ◦ Lateral – leading to a pseudo-asymmetry • Mandibular postural resting position, freeway space and overclosure
	Class III skeletal pattern Sagittal maxillary deficiency and sagittal mandibular excess	
	Tall face deformity Increased face height, particularly lower anterior face height, due to VME (total or posterior), backward rotation of the mandible, an increased mandibular plane angle ± vertical chin excess	
	Short face deformity Reduced lower anterior face height due to VMD and mandibular overclosure, forward rotation of the mandible, a reduced mandibular plane angle, usually associated with relative chin prominence due to mandibular overclosure	
	High angle deformity A 'high angle' deformity refers to patients with an increased mandibular plane angle and an increased, obtuse gonial angle, usually associated with an increased lower anterior face height and either an anterior open bite or VME; the sagittal skeletal pattern may be Class I, II or III.	
	Low angle deformity A 'low angle' deformity refers to patients with a reduced mandibular plane angle and reduced gonial angle, usually associated with a reduced lower anterior face height and a deep incisor overbite; the sagittal skeletal pattern may be Class I, II or III.	

Note:

A useful descriptive test is to imagine that one is describing a patient's dentofacial relationships to a colleague *verbally only*, e.g. over the telephone. Within a few short statements, one's colleague should be able to form a relatively accurate mental image of the patient's dentofacial relationships. For example, 'the patient has a Class II division 1 incisor relationship on a severe Class II skeletal pattern due to mandibular retrognathia, with a reduced lower anterior face height and low mandibular plane angle'.

Terminology for orthognathic surgical procedures

The orthognathic surgical procedures most routinely undertaken involve the repositioning of the tooth-bearing segments of the maxilla or mandible in a variety of directions in relation to the craniofacial complex.

The following terminology is commonly used:

Maxillary surgery (Le Fort I level osteotomy)

- Repositioning in the sagittal plane
  - Anterior repositioning or advancement
  - Posterior repositioning or set-back (pushback)
- Repositioning in the vertical plane
  - Superior repositioning or impaction
  - Inferior repositioning or setdown (downgraft)
- Repositioning in the transverse plane
  - Bodily translation/transverse repositioning to the left or right
  - Transverse expansion
- Repositioning in relation to the sagittal axis
  - Differential impaction/setdown of the right side of the maxillary occlusal plane in relation to the left side (to correct a transverse occlusal plane cant)
- Repositioning in relation to the vertical axis
  - Maxillary rotation to the left or right
- Repositioning in relation to the transverse axis
  - Differential impaction/setdown of the posterior aspect of the maxillary occlusal plane in relation to the anterior aspect.

Mandibular surgery

- Repositioning in the sagittal plane
  - Advancement
  - Set-back (or pushback)

Additionally, dentoalveolar segments of the maxilla and mandible may be surgically repositioned in relation to the three planes of space and three axes of rotation (see Chapter 5).

Mandibular autorotation

This term describes the rotation of the mandible round the transverse axis (in this case the hinge axis), which usually follows vertical repositioning of the maxilla. There are two types of mandibular autorotation:

- Forward (anticlockwise or counterclockwise) – i.e. in the direction of mouth closing, usually in response to a superior repositioning of the posterior aspect of the maxilla.
- Backward (clockwise) – i.e. in the direction of mouth opening, usually in response to an inferior repositioning of the posterior aspect of the maxilla.

> **Note:**
>
> The terms 'clockwise' or 'anticlockwise' rotation of the mandible relate to the observer assessing the patient's *right profile* view. Some authorities commonly use the patient's left profile view (usually anatomists and plastic surgeons), in which case the terms clockwise or anticlockwise rotation become obsolete. It is generally good practice to add the phrase 'in the direction of mouth opening' or 'in the direction of mouth closing' after clockwise or anticlockwise rotation, respectively, to avoid any confusion.

Chin surgery (osseous genioplasty)

The osseous genioplasty is a very versatile procedure, which may be used for the following movements of the bony chin:

- Advancement
- Set-back
- Vertical augmentation
- Vertical reduction
- Transverse (lateral) expansion
- Transverse (lateral) reduction
- Asymmetrical

Prevalence of dentofacial deformities

It is very difficult to find accurate data on the prevalence of dentofacial deformities potentially requiring orthognathic surgery within different populations. Based on the results of a study undertaken in the UK in the mid-1980s,[17] between 5–19% of children referred to an orthodontist for potential treatment were diagnosed as having a malocclusion too severe for orthodontic treatment alone.

The British Association of Oral and Maxillofacial Surgeons (BAOMS) Commissioning Guide (2013) published by the Royal College of Surgeons of England and endorsed by the British Orthodontic society (BOS) stated that there were over 2718 orthognathic surgical procedures undertaken in England in 2012, though there was a wide variation in numbers treated across England.[18]

In the USA, based on an analysis of the third National Health and Nutrition Estimation Survey (NHANES-III) undertaken between 1989 to 1994, which included estimates of malocclusions from 14,000 individuals aged 8 to 50 years, Proffit et al.[19] estimated that approximately 2% of the US population had malocclusions severe enough to be 'disfiguring' and at the limit for orthodontic correction; i.e. dentofacial deformities severe enough that they would potentially require orthognathic surgery.

Objectives of orthognathic surgery

The following are the objectives of orthognathic surgery, which will be discussed in greater detail in the following chapters:

1. Aesthetics

Improved dentofacial appearance, away from deformity and towards normality, is usually the primary motivation of patient's seeking orthognathic surgical treatment. Although this is an anecdotal observation, clinicians involved in the treatment of orthognathic patients are aware that for many patients the aesthetic considerations are often more important than the functional problems.[20]

2. Function

In most patients improved function is an important motivator, and in some patients, it is the primary motivator for treatment.[21,22] The following are some of the functional problems with which patient's may present:

Incising food

Difficulty in incising food; is a particular problem in patient's with anterior open bites, as they are unable to bite through food with their anterior teeth, or in cases of severe anterior open bite extending to the molars, with any teeth.

Mastication

Difficulty in mastication may potentially lead to digestive problems, but one of the major concerns for patients is the embarrassment of eating in public, particularly with significant anterior or lateral open bites, and severe Class III malocclusions.

> **Note:**
>
> An additional concern, which is becoming more common with the increase in the popularity of snorkelling and diving, is the inability to undertake these activities for an individual with an anterior open bite.

Deglutition

The difficulty in forming a lip seal may make swallowing difficult and again is a source of embarrassment for some patients in public.

Trauma

Trauma may be a factor in different situations:

- **Biting the tongue** – tends to occur if the maxillary width is very constricted;
- **Traumatic occlusion** – traumatizing the anterior palatal mucosa or labial gingivae in the mandibular

incisor region due to a traumatic anterior dental occlusion, leading to potentially significant discomfort and stripping of the mucosa.

Attrition

Tooth wear due to repetitive occlusal contact between the teeth, which may be a particular problem in edge-to-edge incisor relationships.

Respiration and sleep apnoea

Obstructive sleep apnoea/hypopnoea syndrome is now understood to be a debilitating condition (see Chapter 44). The opening of the airway with maxillary and/or mandibular and/or osseous chin advancement surgery may provide life-changing benefits.

Temporomandibular joint dysfunction

Temporomandibular joint dysfunction (TMD) related to dental occlusal problems may be a significant problem for some patients, though it should be borne in mind that the link between the two is by no means proven. The aetiology of TMD is usually multifactorial, and orthognathic surgery should not be undertaken as a cure for TMD. Patients with pre-existing TMD-type symptoms should be warned that there is no evidence that orthognathic treatment will relieve such symptoms.

Speech

Speech problems may be due to the inability to place the teeth and oral soft tissues in relation to each other in order to produce speech sounds.

Drooling

Drooling, also referred to as ptyalism or sialorrhoea, is defined as the unintentional flow of saliva outside the mouth, which may be due to excess saliva production or problems with swallowing, but may also be due to weak or underdeveloped circumoral musculature or an anterior open bite associated with excessive lower anterior face height and an incomplete lip seal (lip incompetence), leading to an inability to retain saliva in the mouth (salivary incontinence).

3. Stability

A stable skeletal and dental-occlusal end result is of paramount importance.

It is important to strike a pragmatic balance between these three objectives. Aesthetic improvement is of primary significance, as the vast majority of patients' desire an improvement in their dentofacial appearance. However, clinical facial evaluation must always be critical of dentofacial morphology and aesthetic relationships as it relates to dentofacial function. As in architecture, *form and function are intimately related.* Orthognathic treatment should avoid, as far as possible, altering one to the detriment of the other.

Effectiveness of orthognathic surgery

Clinical effectiveness (from Latin *efficere*: to accomplish) refers to whether a treatment modality is successful in producing a desired or intended result. The objectives of orthognathic surgery are improved dentofacial function and aesthetics in a stable manner, leading to an improved **health-related quality of life**. The quality of life benefits of orthognathic surgery have been demonstrated.[23–27] Additionally, most patients undergo orthognathic treatment in their formative years, either late teenage years or early twenties; as such, the enduring benefits of such treatment are potentially lifelong.

A number of studies have demonstrated significant improvements in oral function following orthognathic surgery using **oral health-related quality of life** measures.[24,25,27–29] Systematic reviews of the literature have demonstrated that patients undergoing orthognathic treatment have improved self-confidence, body image, psychological health and social adjustment,[30] and improved well-being.[22]

In a decisive study, Cunningham et al.[31] demonstrated the monetary **cost-effectiveness** of orthognathic treatment, based on cost per quality-adjusted life-year (QALY), a measure that takes into account both the quantity and quality of life generated by healthcare interventions, i.e. in crude terms, the value for money of orthognathic surgery. They demonstrated that orthognathic treatment provides good outcomes for a relatively low cost, compared with other surgical or medical procedures in the UK.

Every surgical procedure carries an element of risk. The risk-benefit considerations of orthognathic treatment are discussed in more detail in Chapter 5. However, the risks and potential morbidity of orthognathic treatment are relatively low, and usually short-term. The low prevalence of postoperative complications was confirmed by Sousa and Turrini's[32] review of the literature, which found approximately 12% altered sensation, 3.4% infection, 2.5% fixation problems, 1.8% unfavourable fracture during the osteotomy (1.8%). Iannetti et al.[33] reviewed 3236 patients and found irreversible sensory deficits in only 2% of patients.

Orthognathic surgery has a vitally important role in improving the airway in patients with **obstructive sleep apnoea/hypopnoea syndrome** (OSAHS), which has otherwise serious long-term consequences for a patient's physiological health and their quality of life (see Chapter 44). Although orthognathic surgery is not a treatment modality for patients presenting with **temporomandibular joint dysfunction** (TMD), a meta-analysis found that 'patients having orthognathic treatment for dentofacial deformities and who are also suffering from TMD, appear more likely to see improvement in their signs and symptoms than deterioration'.[34] Hassan et al.[35] reviewed **the effects of orthognathic surgery on speech**, though no clear evidence directly relating malocclusions to speech discrepancies was found. Furthermore, it was difficult to draw any firm conclusions with respect to the effect of orthognathic surgery on speech. It may be logically posited that a better dental/incisor relationships may allow certain speech sounds to be more easily generated. However, this area requires further investigation.

Treatment need – who will benefit from orthognathic surgery?

Skeletal discrepancies associated with dental malocclusions are often graded as mild, moderate or severe, though the distinction between these categories is not absolutely clear. A pragmatic distinction is that malocclusions associated with **mild** skeletal discrepancies may be treated by orthodontic treatment alone, whereas malocclusions associated with **moderate** skeletal discrepancies will require an element of growth modification/dentofacial orthopaedics in the growing patient and/or camouflage orthodontic treatment. However, a skeletal discrepancy associated with a malocclusion is deemed **severe** if it is obvious that *neither growth modification nor orthodontic camouflage treatment can significantly improve the facial aesthetic and dental-occlusal relationships.*

Therefore, to answer the question 'who will benefit from orthognathic surgery?' – The potential patient must fulfil two important criteria:

1. A skeletal discrepancy severe enough that neither orthodontic camouflage, growth modification or even orthodontic treatment combined with surgical camouflage treatment (e.g. genioplasty) will be able to provide the ideal facial aesthetic and dental-occlusal relationship; and
2. A desire to have orthognathic surgery – This may appear obvious, but there are patients who will certainly benefit from orthognathic treatment, but, having been given the information required to make an informed decision, will simply not wish to go ahead with such treatment.

Measurable criteria

Certain **measurable criteria** have been provided in order to help the decision-making process as to when a patient is beyond orthodontic correction and likely to require orthognathic surgery, though these should be viewed only as *rough guidelines* and, as always, each treatment plan must be tailored to the specific needs of the patient. For the Class II adolescent patient, Proffit et al.[36] suggested the following criteria as indications for orthognathic surgery:

- Incisor overjet: >10 mm
- Pogonion–nasion-perpendicular distance: >18 mm
- Mandibular body length (gonion–menton): <70 mm
- Skeletal face height (nasion–menton): >125 mm

For the Class III patient Kerr et al.[37] found that the threshold values for the ANB angle and mandibular incisor inclination below which orthognathic surgery was almost always carried out were –4 and 83 degrees, respectively.

Index of Orthodontic Treatment Need (IOTN)

It is also possible to take an inferential approach to orthognathic treatment need, i.e. to presume the presence of a skeletal discrepancy likely to require orthognathic surgical correction based on the dental-occlusal relationship. The **Index of Orthodontic Treatment Need (IOTN)** was developed in the UK in the mid-1980s,[17] and is now used to assess the need for orthodontic treatment in the National Health Service (NHS).[38] The IOTN is a rather general method of determining the level of treatment need for an individual patient by reference to an index that incorporates dental health/functional and aesthetic components. The dental health component of the IOTN is divided into five grades, each subdivided into a number of distinct categories. The IOTN grades a malocclusion based on the worst characteristic. Grade 1 signifies no treatment need, and grade 5 a 'very great' need for treatment. Patients falling into grades 4 and 5 are eligible to receive orthodontic treatment under the English NHS. The specific categories under grades 4 and 5, which are potentially relevant to the orthognathic patient, are described in Table 3-3.

In relation to orthognathic surgical treatment need, the problem with the IOTN is that there are certain dentofacial deformities with little impact on the dental occlusion, i.e. a facial deformity due to a jaw malrelationship, but essentially normal dental occlusion. For example, a severe tall face patient with excess incisor and gingival exposure at rest and in animation, but a Class I dental occlusion, will score low on the IOTN, but will have a potentially high orthognathic surgical treatment need.

Table 3-3 IOTN dental health component grades 4 and 5 with subcategories potentially relevant to the orthognathic patient (Adapted from Brook and Shaw[17] and Fox[38])

Grade 5	• Increased overjet >9 mm • Reverse overjet >3.5 mm with reported masticatory or speech difficulties • Defects of cleft lip and palate and/or other craniofacial abnormalities
Grade 4	• Increased overjet >6 mm but ≤9 mm • Reverse overjet >3.5 mm with no masticatory or speech difficulties • Reverse overjet >1 mm but <3.5 mm with recorded masticatory and speech difficulties • Anterior or posterior crossbites with >2 mm discrepancy between the retruded contact position and intercuspal position • Extreme lateral or anterior open bites >4 mm • Increased and complete overbite with gingival or palatal trauma

Index of Orthognathic Functional Treatment Need (IOFTN)

The use of IOTN has limitations as a measure of functional and health need in orthognathic treatment provision. As discussed above, certain severe malocclusions and their associated dentofacial deformities would not be eligible for UK National Health Service funding for orthognathic treatment using IOTN. For example, excessive maxillary incisor and gingival exposure with evidence of gingival and/or periodontal effects, complete scissor bites, or facial asymmetries with marked effects on the occlusal plane. In addition, IOTN makes no mention of orthognathic treatment for sleep apnoea.

With these limitations in mind, a new index has been developed in the UK to help in the prioritization of severe malocclusions not amenable to orthodontic treatment alone.[39] In a joint venture, the School of Oral and Dental Sciences at the University of Bristol and the Orthodontic Department at the Eastman Dental Hospital in London, with the aid of the Consultant Orthodontist Group of the British Orthodontic Society, created a new **Index of Orthognathic Functional Treatment Need (IOFTN)**, based on and where possible using the same traits as used in the IOTN dental health component, but with modifications and additions to reflect the functional indications of treatment need for orthognathic patients. The index has been found to feel familiar to those already using the IOTN, and to be valid, reliable and quick and easy to use.[39]

As with the IOTN, the single-most severe trait is used for scoring the patient (Table 3-4). It is important, particularly when scoring from study models alone, that additional clinical and facial aesthetic information is provided, e.g. the degree of maxillary incisor exposure, as well as potential psychological issues. It is important to bear in mind that the IOFTN concerns the *functional indicators* for orthognathic treatment. As such, other clinical, aesthetic and psychological indicators must also be considered in the evaluation of treatment need for potential orthognathic patients. Nevertheless, it is certainly a step in the right direction.

Table 3-4 Index of Orthognathic Functional Treatment Need

This index applies to those malocclusions that are **not amenable to orthodontic treatment alone, due to skeletal deformity**,and will ordinarily apply to those patients who will have completed facial growth prior to surgery (commonly 18 years of age and older). It relates only to the **functional** need for treatment and should be used in combination with appropriate psychological and other clinical indicators.

5. Very Great Need for Treatment
- 5.1 Defects of cleft lip and palate and other craniofacial anomalies
- 5.2 Increased overjet greater than 9 mm
- 5.3 Reverse overjet ≥ 3 mm
- 5.4 Open bite ≥ 4 mm
- 5.5 Complete scissors bite affecting whole buccal segment(s) with signs of functional disturbance and or occlusal trauma
- 5.6 Sleep apnoea not amenable to other treatments such as MAD or CPAP (as determined by sleep studies)
- 5.7 Skeletal anomalies with occlusal disturbance as a result of trauma or pathology

4. Great Need for Treatment
- 4.2 Increased overjet ≥ 6 mm and ≤ 9 mm
- 4.3 Reverse overjet ≥ 0 mm and < 3 mm with functional difficulties
- 4.4 Open bite < 4 mm with functional difficulties
- 4.8 Increased overbite with evidence of dental or soft tissue trauma
- 4.9 Upper labial segment gingival exposure ≥ 3 mm at rest
- 4.10 Facial asymmetry associated with occlusal disturbance

3. Moderate Need for Treatment
- 3.3 Reverse overjet ≥ 0 mm and < 3 mm with no functional difficulties
- 3.4 Open bite < 4 mm with no functional difficulties
- 3.9 Upper labial segment gingival exposure < 3 mm at rest, but with evidence of gingival/periodontal effects
- 3.10 Facial asymmetry with no occlusal disturbance

2. Mild Need for Treatment
- 2.8 Increased overbite but no evidence of dental or soft tissue trauma
- 2.9 Upper labial segment gingival exposure < 3 mm at rest with no evidence of gingival/periodontal effects
- 2.11 Marked occlusal cant with no effect on the occlusion

1. No Need for treatment
- 1.12 Speech difficulties
- 1.13 Treatment purely for TMD
- 1.14 Occlusal features not classified above

Note:

A noteworthy point is that there is a potential distinction in the functional indication of treatment for an anterior open bite (AOB). Anterior open bites vary both in their **degree of vertical separation** of the maxillary and mandibular incisors (i.e. the size of the open bite in millimetres), and in their **lateral extent**, e.g. canine-to-canine or molar-to-molar (Figure 3-1). The canine-to-canine open bite essentially leads to a problem with incising food, whereas the molar-to-molar may also lead to problems of mastication. Both will have aesthetic and social implications, such as embarrassment in eating in public.

Facial attractiveness research studies

Finally, **data from facial attractiveness research studies** may provide an insight into the degree of deviation of any facial parameter from the average at which observers begin to find the deviation to be unattractive, as well as the threshold values of desire for surgical correction. The use of observers of different age groups, both genders, and different ethnic backgrounds are important due to inter-observer variability. Additionally, the use of preoperative orthognathic patients, as well as lay people and clinicians as observers may be particularly useful.[40–49] Such data will be presented in the relevant chapters of this book.

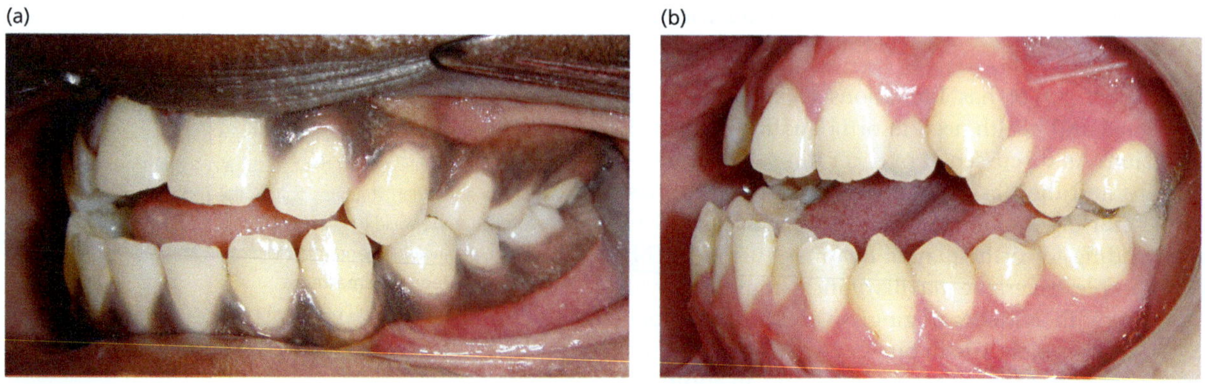

Fig. 3-1 (a): Anterior open bites predominantly in the incisor or canine-to-canine region are a problem for incising food. (b): Anterior open bites that extend further posteriorly will also be a problem for mastication.

Scope of orthodontic treatment and growth guidance

This book focuses on orthognathic surgery. However, as well as the orthodontist, it is incumbent upon every clinician involved in orthognathic treatment to have an understanding of the scope and limitations of orthodontic treatment, particularly for younger patients presenting with a skeletal element to their malocclusions. Where dental development and dentofacial growth are concerned, appropriate referral to the orthodontist at the appropriate time is paramount.

Dentofacial orthopaedics/growth guidance

'Medicine is not only a science; it is also an art... it deals with the very processes of life, which must be understood before they can be guided.'

Paracelsus (1493–1541)[50]
Swiss–German physician

The terms **growth guidance**, **growth modification** and **dentofacial orthopaedics** essentially refer to the same treatment phenomenon, though different authorities often have their own preferential term. The concept of dentofacial orthopaedics, as opposed to orthodontics, refers to the use of appliances utilizing greater **orthopaedic forces** applied to the dentition and/or jaws *of an actively growing patient* in order to either restrict, enhance or potentially alter the direction of growth, as opposed to light orthodontic forces required to move the teeth.

Note:

The term 'orthopaedic' is derived from the title of a book by the French physician **Nicolas Andry de Bois-Regard** (1658–1742), a professor at the University of Paris, who invented the term in the first book written on the subject in the West. The book, entitled *L'Orthopédie, ou, L'art de prevenir et corriger dans les enfants les difformitez du corps*, was published in Paris in 1741. The title of the English translation from 1743 reads *Orthopaedia: or the art of correcting and preventing deformities in children.*[51]

Andry explains that he formed the title from the Greek words: '*Orthos*, which signifies straight, free from deformity, and *Pais*, a child. Out of these two words I have compounded that of Orthopaedia, to express in one term the design I propose, which is to teach the different methods of preventing and correction of deformities of children.'[51] However, the work is particularly famous for an engraving on the frontispiece that shows a crooked young tree that has been tied to a straight stake (Figure 3-2). This depicts the deformed child as analogous to the sapling and therefore suggests that bone is a structure that responds to carefully applied stimuli. It is an excellent visual metaphor for dentofacial orthopaedics used as a form of dentoskeletal growth guidance.

For over 100 years, orthodontists have been intrigued by the concept of dentofacial orthopaedics, and the possibility of altering dentofacial form *without surgery*. In an average growing individual, the average displacement of the maxilla and mandible is in a forward and downward direction away from the cranium (Figure 3-3). A number of types of growth modifying appliances are available if such growth is aberrant:

Functional appliances

The use of **functional** or **myofunctional appliances**, also termed **functional jaw orthopaedics**, describes the use of appliances that work primarily by anterior posturing of the retrusive mandible. The action of this family of appliances depends upon the activity of the orofacial musculature and soft tissues, as the forward posturing of the mandible alters the activity of the orofacial musculature, leading to changes in the dentoskeletal relationships. The mode of action of these appliances is still not fully understood, but perhaps up to 3/4 of the Class II correction is thought to be due to dentoalveolar changes and 1/4 due to enhancement or acceleration of mandibular growth by allowing the full expression of the mandible's genetic potential to

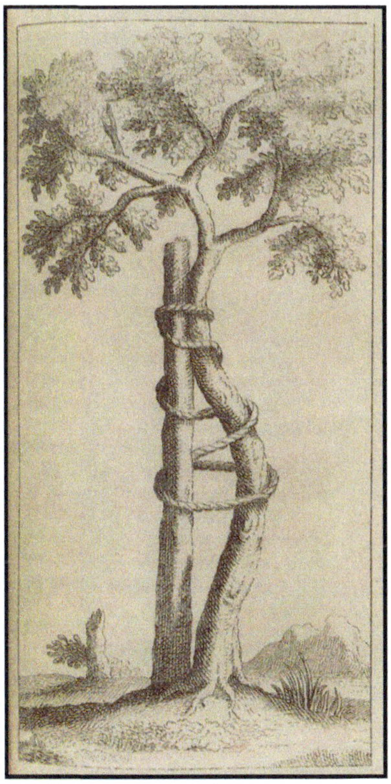

Fig. 3-2 Andry's tree (1741).

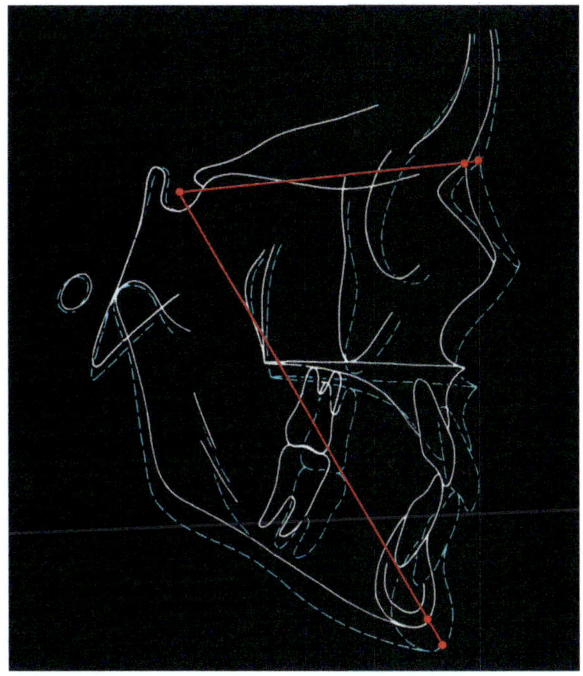

Fig. 3-3 In an average growing individual, the average displacement of the maxilla and mandible is in a forward and downward direction away from the cranium.

express. Functional appliances also remove abnormal or restrictive muscular activity that may be preventing normal development. Ideally, these appliances should be worn close to full time during the pubertal growth period (Figure 3-4).

There is another family of functional appliances termed **Class III functional appliances**, which may be used to help correct a *mild* Class III malocclusion, e.g. a Class III Twin Block or function regulator type-III (FRIII). These appliances posture the mandible posteriorly and rotate it open. Their mode of action is predominantly dental, with proclination of the maxillary incisors and retroclination of the mandibular incisors, whilst effective mandibular prominence is somewhat reduced by downward and backward rotation of the mandible. The appliances are contraindicated in patients with increased lower face height.

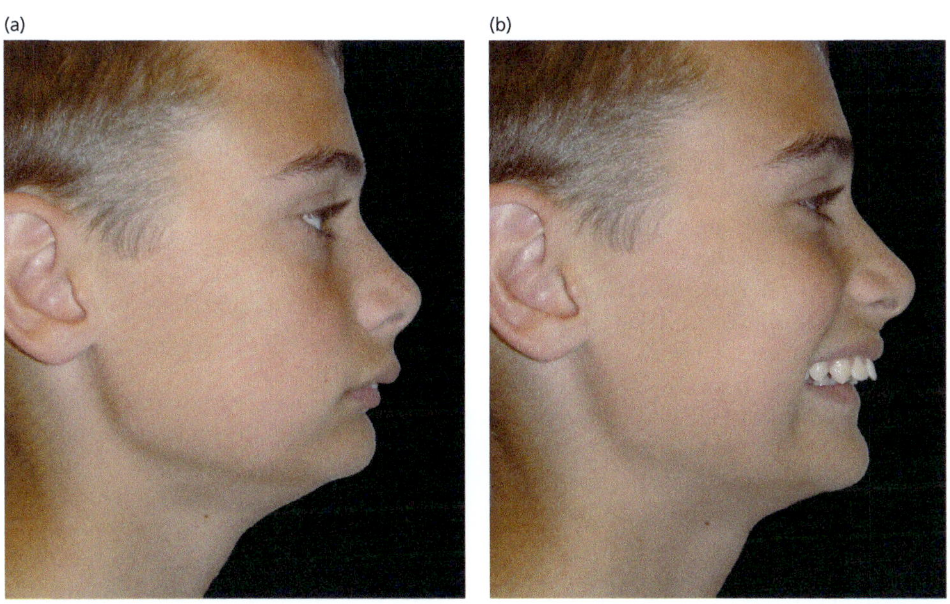

Fig. 3-4 (a)–(c): Pretreatment photographs of a patient with Class II division 1 incisor relationship on a moderate Class II skeletal pattern. (d), (e): After 12-months of functional appliance treatment, demonstrating incisor overjet correction. The lateral open bites are to be expected with a Twin Block functional appliance, and will reduce with a period of part-time wear of the appliance. (f), (g): Following removal of fixed orthodontic appliances.

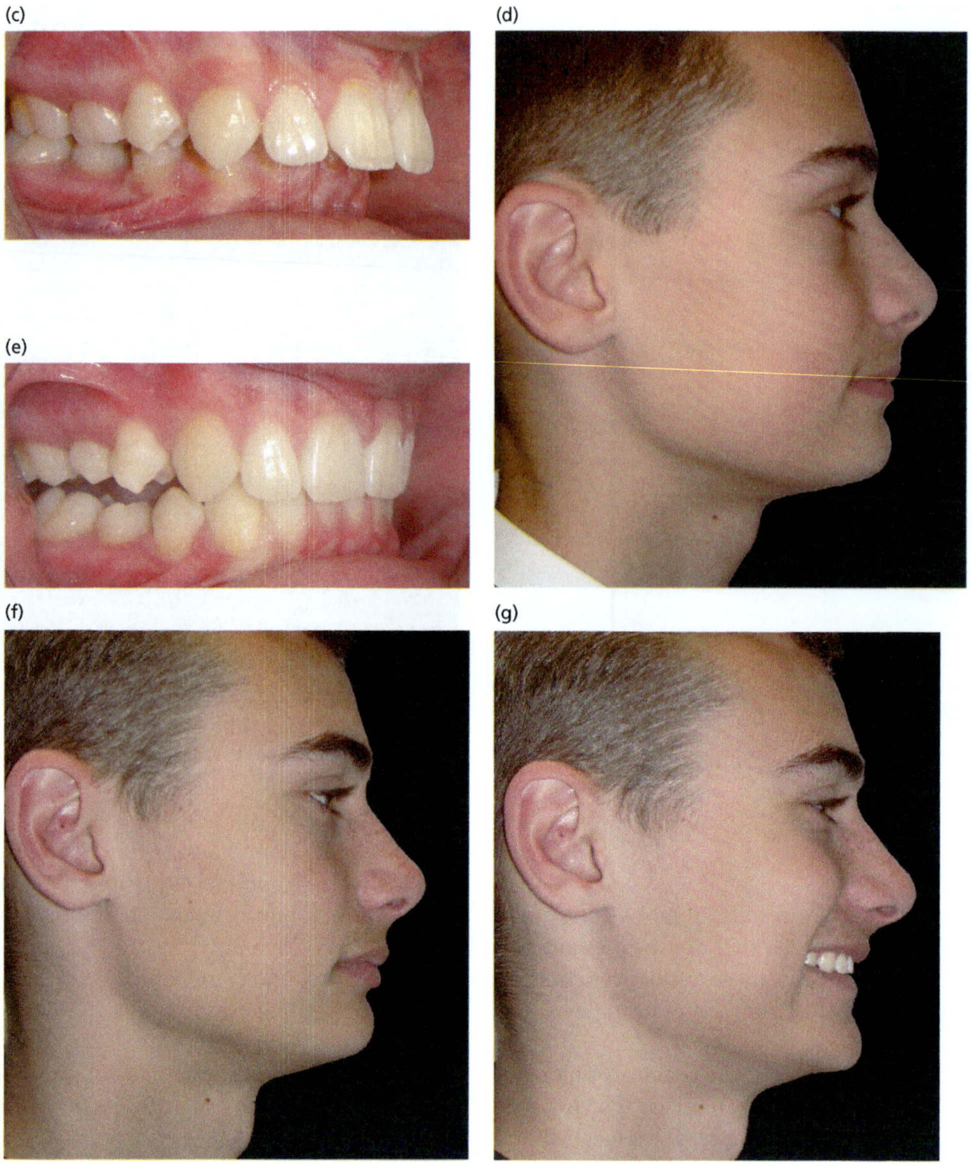

Fig. 3-4 (*Continued*).

In growing patients with asymmetrical growth of the jaws, a **hybrid functional appliance** may be considered.[52] The purpose of these appliances is potentially to enhance growth of the condyle on the growth deficient side, as well as permitting vertical eruption of the posterior teeth on the vertically deficient side while impeding eruption on the contralateral side. The wax construction bite should be taken with the patient symmetrically postured forward in the best sagittal position, as well as the best vertical and transverse positions. Unilateral posterior bite blocks help impede eruption, whereas lingual and buccal shields keep the tongue and cheek away from the posterior dentition allowing unimpeded eruption on the contralateral side, where vertical development is desired. These appliances only work if the patient is actively growing. It is important to bear in mind that there is no evidence that such appliances can enhance condylar growth and/or improve significant mandibular asymmetry.

Orthopaedic headgear

The term **headgear** is used to describe an extraoral appliance that makes use of the cranium to apply forces to the maxilla and/or teeth, for the purposes of growth modification or tooth movement, respectively (Figure 3-5). The headgear elastics are applied to the dentition via a facebow attached to the dentition or appliance. The magnitude and direction of force depend on the intended treatment objectives. Headgear may be used for **extraoral anchorage** (~250 g of force per side), to prevent the posterior maxillary dentition from moving forward during orthodontic treatment, or for **extraoral traction** (~500 g of force per side), to distalize the posterior maxillary dentition. However, **orthopaedic headgear** applies heavier orthopaedic forces (~800 g per side for at least 12 hours per day) to the maxilla via the maxillary first molars, a maxillary splint or a functional appliance, in order to impede maxillary growth. The direction of pull of

(a) (b) (c)

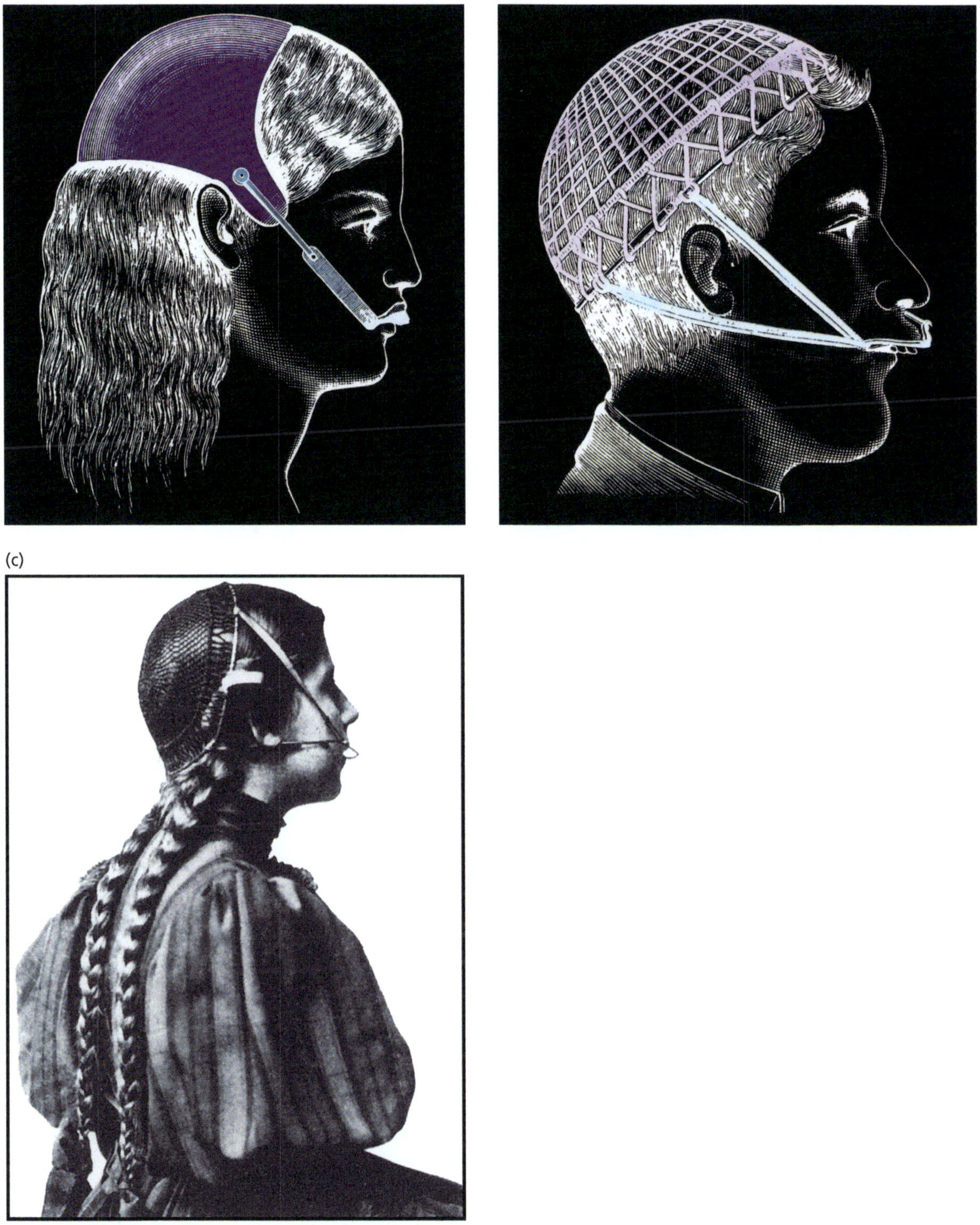

Fig. 3-5 (a): Norman Kingsley's headgear (1861) (After Goddard, 1897). (b): Edward Angle's headgear (After Goddard, 1897). (c): Edward Angle's headgear (1907).

the headgear varies depending on the facial growth pattern; the more vertical the growth pattern, the higher the direction of pull (Figure 3-6).

Protraction headgear (facemask or reverse-pull headgear)

Extraoral force may be used to protract the entire maxillary dentoalveolus and influence the growth direction of the maxillary basal bone, at least in the short term. The protraction facemask may be used in the treatment of a Class III malocclusion due to *mild to moderate maxillary retrusion* in the growing patient, ideally with a low mandibular plane angle and reduced lower anterior face height. The presence of an anterior crossbite and reverse incisor overjet should lead the diagnosing clinician to assess for an anterior mandibular displacement. Such patients can

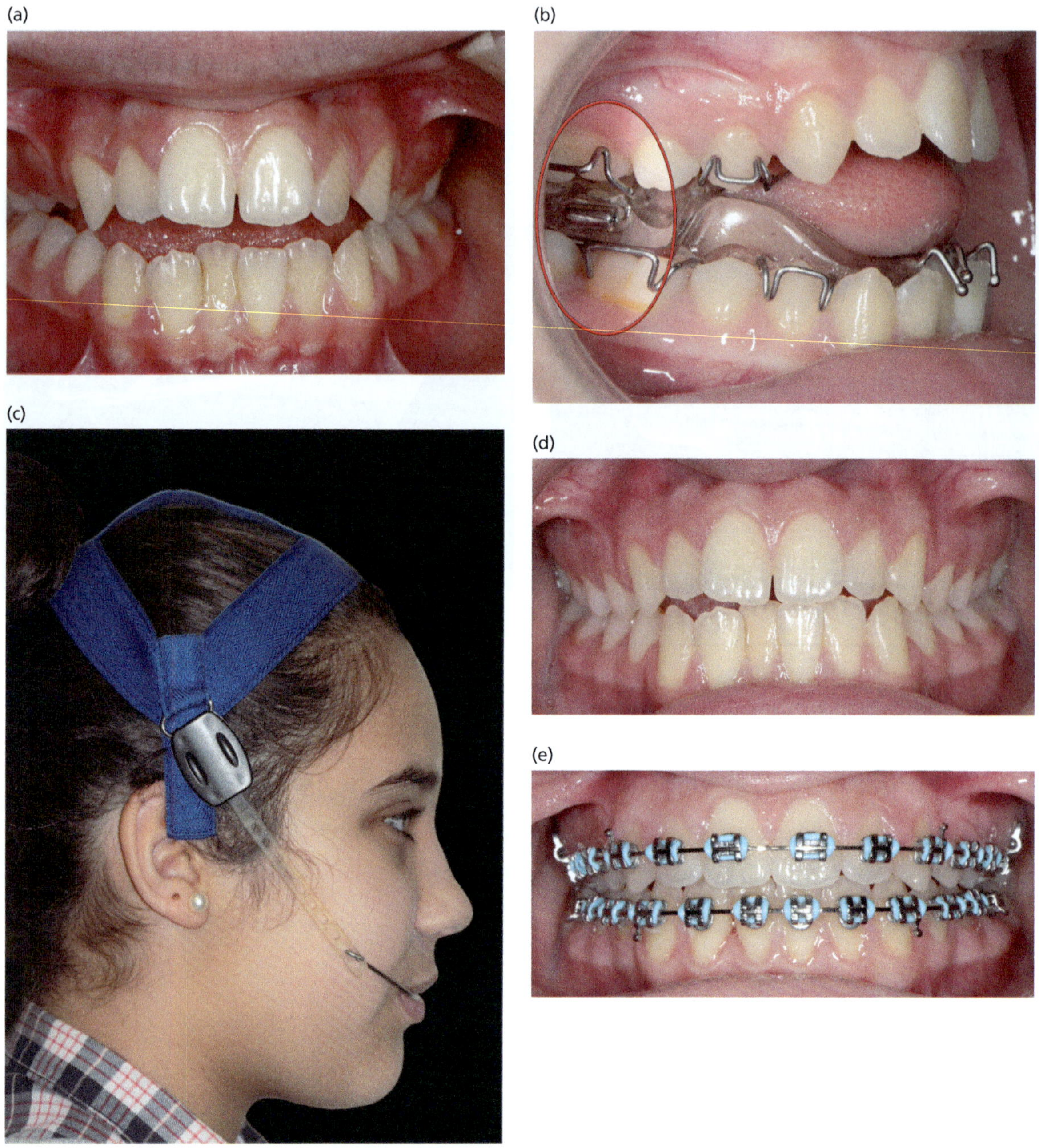

Fig. 3-6 (a): Pretreatment photograph demonstrating an anterior open bite in a growing Class II patient. (b): Twin Block functional appliance for sagittal dental occlusal correction, with flying extraoral traction (EOT) tubes for attachment of the headgear facebow to the upper component of the appliance. (c): High pull headgear in situ. (d): End of functional appliance phase of treatment. (e): Patient in fixed appliances, and continuing with headgear to the maxillary first molars, with correction of the anterior open bite.

often achieve an almost edge-to-edge incisor relationship and posture their mandible anteriorly in order to achieve maximum intercuspation of their posterior dentition. As such, the degree of required anterior movement of the maxilla and maxillary incisors is not excessive, and the overall opening of the bite and downward and backward rotation of the mandible is beneficial. The original facemask was developed by Jean Delaire in France in the early 1970s,[53] though the design has been somewhat modified. It is comprised of two resting pads that contact the forehead and chin in the midline. The pads are connected by an adjustable vertical midline framework, to which is connected an adjustable horizontal bar. Elastic traction is applied from an intraoral appliance on the maxillary dentition to the horizontal bar, in order to protract the maxilla, using ~500 g of force pre side for 12 hours per day.[54] The force is applied relatively anteriorly, usually in the canine or first premolar regions, and the force vector is downward and forward in order to reduce any undesirable tilting of the maxillary occlusal plane (round the transverse axis of rotation) and opening of the bite (Figure 3-7). The facemask is used in conjunction with a removable or fixed appliance attached to the maxillary dentition, but lateral expansion is almost always used concomitantly, in order to 'loosen' the

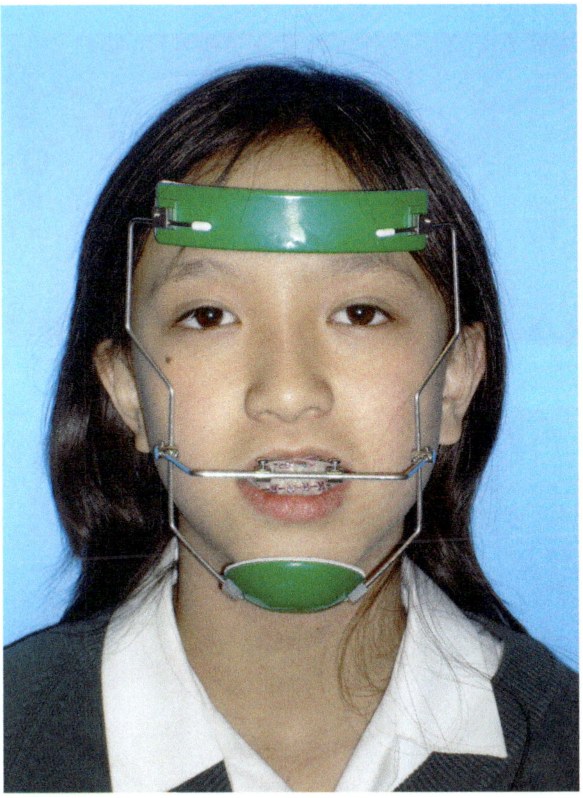

Fig. 3-7 Facemask.

circum-maxillary sutural system, which have not yet fused in the young growing child (the effectiveness of simultaneous lateral expansion requires further investigation). Therefore, the optimal age for such treatment is considered to be between 7 to 8 years, permitting up to 5 mm of maxillary skeletal protraction.[54] The treatment is effective in older growing patients, but with diminishing skeletal response and greater dentoalveolar change. Patients will often require a few millimetres of overcorrection of the incisor overjet, and a Class III functional appliance as a retainer. Patients reverting back to a reverse overjet with continued growth are likely to require orthognathic correction.

Chin cup

The chin cup, or chin cap, is an extraoral appliance consisting of a cup that fits on the patient's chin, which is attached to a headstrap with an elastic force vector in a posterosuperior direction. The concept is to direct forces through the mandibular condyles in order to impede and/or redirect mandibular growth. It is used in growing patients with Class III malocclusions due to mild to moderate mandibular prognathism. The force vector may be more vertically directed in patients with a vertical jaw growth pattern. Orthopaedic forces of ~800 g per side for 12 hours per day may be used. When used, the treatment may be through the pubertal growth period and thereby prolonged. Discontinuation of the treatment invariably leads to a continuation of a Class III growth pattern. Though still used in the Far East, the use of chin cups has diminished in the UK.

Rapid maxillary expansion (RME)

Rapid maxillary expansion (RME) will be described in detail in Chapter 13, but is essentially a technique to increase the maxillary palatal width in the growing patient by opening and expanding apart the midpalatal suture before it has fully fused (Figure 3-8).

Orthodontic camouflage

Camouflage (from *Italian* camuffare: to disguise) orthodontic treatment refers to the treatment of a malocclusion where the skeletal discrepancy is not corrected, but the teeth are repositioned through their supporting alveolar bone in order to improve the dental occlusion. Such treatment usually requires the extraction of teeth to provide space to retrocline and retract the incisor and canine teeth (usually maxillary first premolars in a Class II malocclusion, and mandibular first premolars in a Class III malocclusion). Camouflage treatment may help to improve facial aesthetics, e.g. retroclination and retraction of proclined and protruded maxillary incisors in a Class II patient will improve smile aesthetics and reduce excessive upper lip prominence. However, camouflage treatment undertaken incorrectly may worsen facial appearance, e.g. in a Class II malocclusion predominantly due to mandibular retrognathia, with the maxillary incisor sagittal position essentially normal, any retraction of the maxillary incisors to reduce the incisor overjet may have significant detrimental effects on the nasolabial and facial profile aesthetics. In such patients, it may be better to align the teeth and maintain the incisor overjet.

The important parameters to bear in mind when considering orthodontic camouflage treatment are:

- Complete (total) or partial camouflage?
  Where there is a moderate to severe skeletal discrepancy, complete camouflage and dental-occlusal correction may be difficult to achieve, with potential detrimental effects on facial aesthetics. In such situations, consideration may be given to **partial occlusal correction**. For example, in a patient with a Class II skeletal discrepancy, consideration may be given to alignment with partial overjet correction; i.e. an attempt to improve the maxillary incisor inclination and position in relation to the upper lip, otherwise alignment of the teeth only and accepting a degree of increase in the incisor overjet (Figure 3-9), rather than excessively retracting the maxillary incisors, with potential detrimental effects on nasolabial and facial aesthetics, just in order to achieve a Class I incisor relationship.

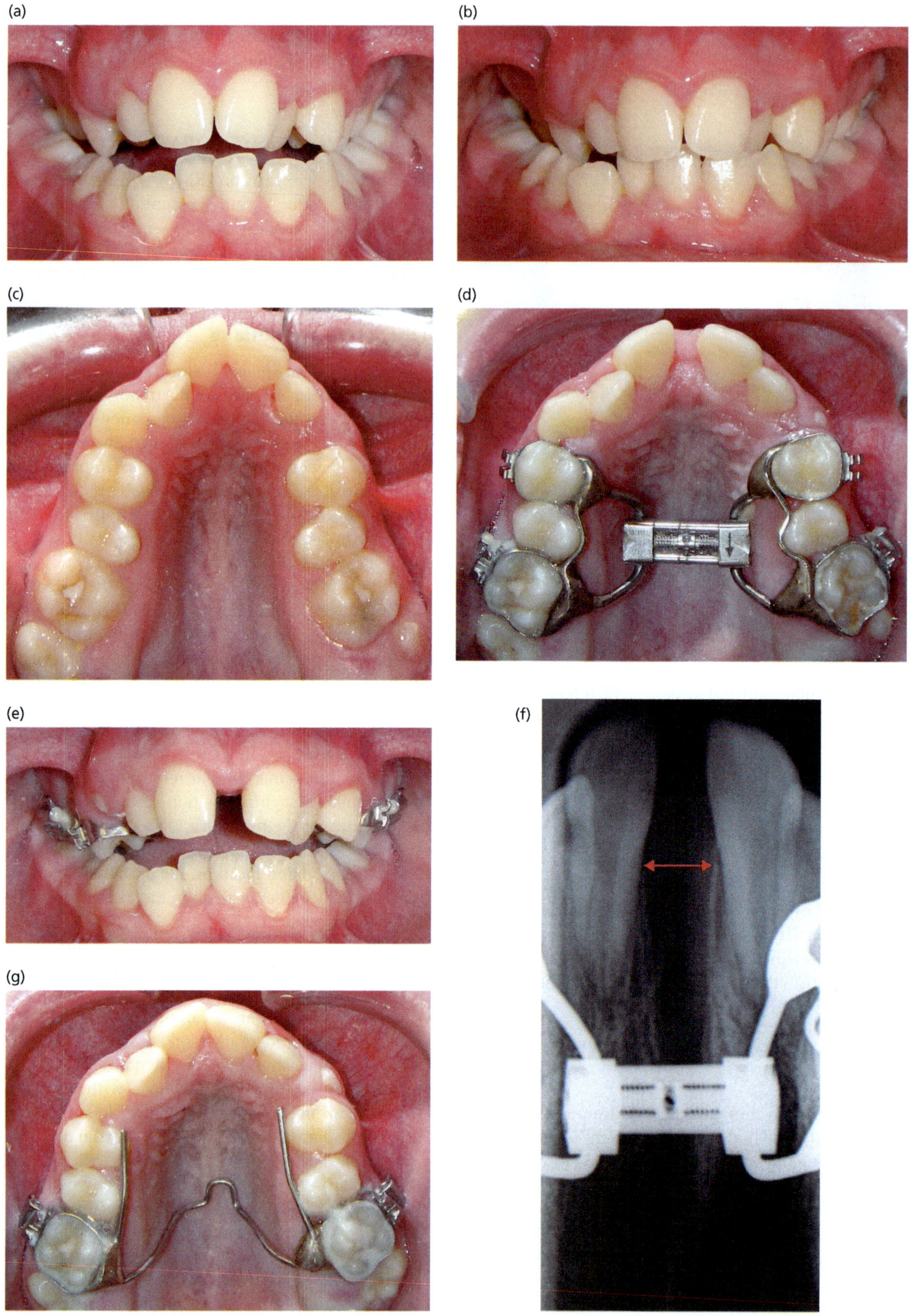

Fig. 3-8 (a): Narrow maxilla, patient is displacing her mandible to her right to obtain maximum intercuspation of her teeth. (b): Undisplaced occlusion, demonstrating bilateral posterior crossbites. (c): Maxillary occlusal view. (d): (e): Rapid maxillary expansion (RME) appliance in situ at 3 weeks, demonstrating the diastema that will form. (f): Maxillary occlusal radiograph at 3 weeks demonstrating separation of the midpalatal suture. (g): At 3 months, RME appliance is removed and a transpalatal arch is placed. The diastema has closed spontaneously, due to the action of the transseptal fibres.

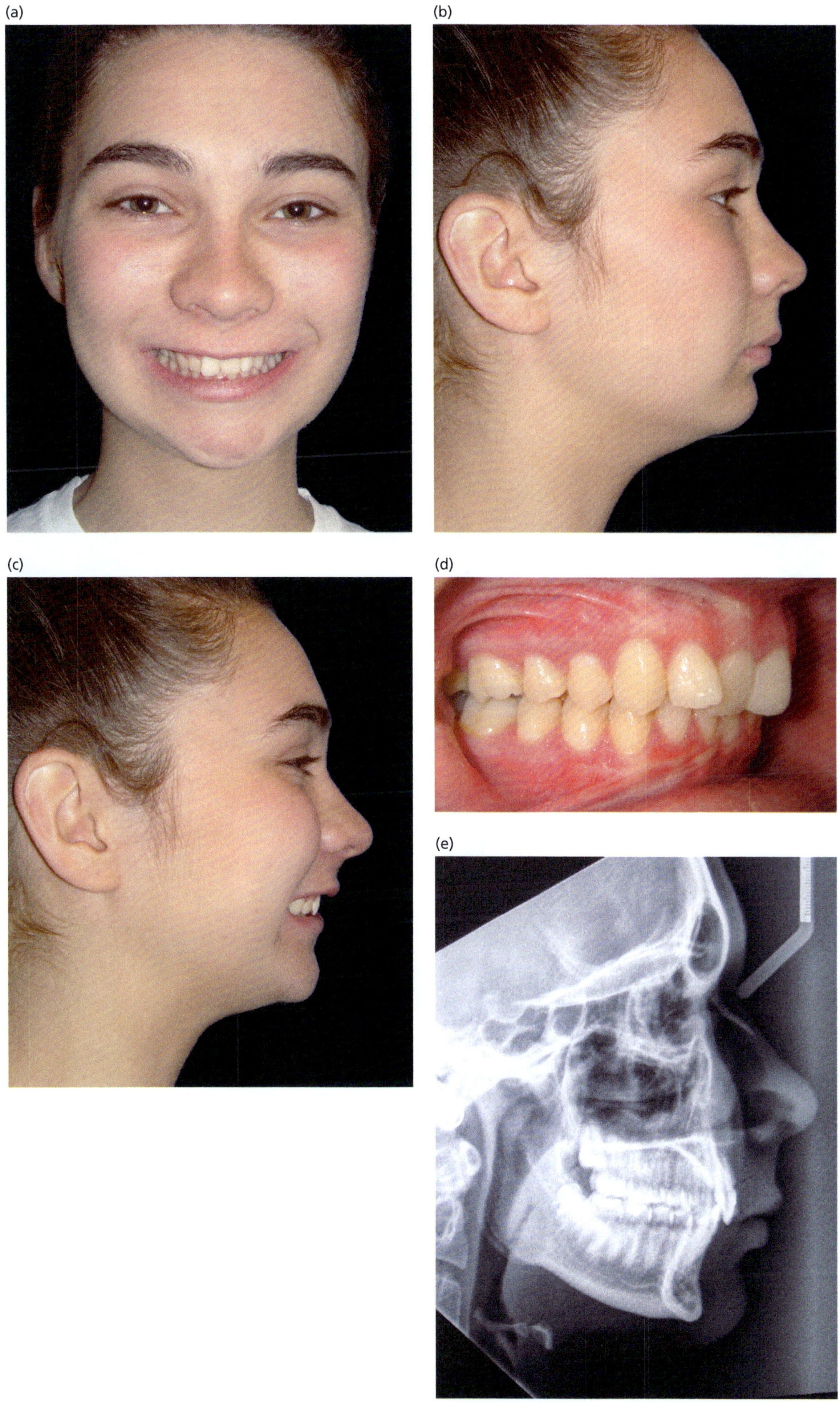

Fig. 3-9 Orthodontic camouflage treatment with partial occlusal correction in a patient with a Class II division 2 incisor relationship with mild to moderate mandibular retrognathia. The patient did not desire orthognathic surgery. The maxillary arch was aligned and the maxillary incisor inclination corrected to achieve an acceptable lip-incisor relationship. The increased incisor overjet and Class II buccal occlusion was accepted. (a)–(e): Pretreatment images. (f)–(j): End of treatment.

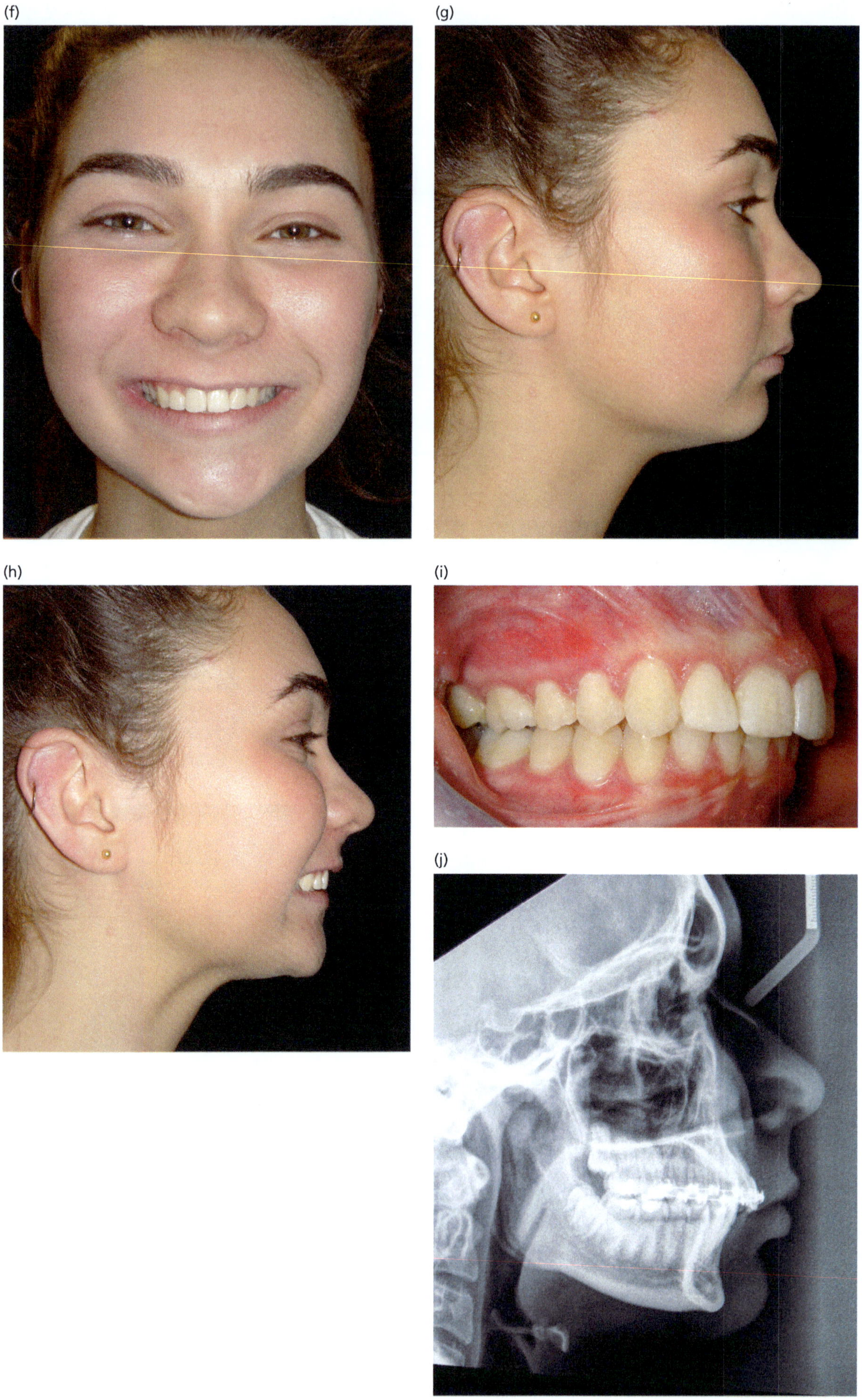

Fig. 3-9 (*Continued*)

- **Is there space or does space need to be created?** One of the most important factors to consider is that *there has to be scope to alter the incisor inclination(s)* for successful orthodontic camouflage treatment. Incisor inclination alteration may be achievable on a non-extraction basis if there are spaced dental arches, or space creation without dental extractions is possible, e.g. distal movement of teeth, or interdental enamel reduction. Alternatively, dental extractions may be undertaken, providing space to alter incisor inclinations in one or both dental arches (Figure 3-10).
- **Subsequent growth must be taken into account** It is important to bear in mind that *the pattern of jaw growth is unlikely to alter*. This is particularly relevant for Class III patients. If orthodontic camouflage treatment is undertaken early in a growing Class III patient with mandibular premolar extractions and retroclination and retraction of the mandibular incisors, it is possible that subsequent skeletal growth may turn a moderate Class III into a severe Class III pattern, with the patient desiring surgical correction. Subsequent orthodontic decompensation and proclination of the mandibular incisors will thereby reopen the premolar extraction spaces. As such, where the degree of further potential growth is difficult to determine, treatment is better delayed.

It is important not to underestimate what orthodontics can achieve, but this is dependent on accurate diagnosis and appropriate treatment planning, and referral at an appropriate age where growth modification is achievable. It is also important for the orthodontist to realise that much of the changes achieved with dentofacial orthopaedics tend to be dentoalveolar, and severe skeletal discrepancies will usually require surgical correction.

A specific problem – the young severe Class III patient

One of the difficult issues facing the orthognathic team is the patient presenting with a severe Class III skeletal discrepancy that obviously will require orthognathic surgical correction in the future, but who is simply too young to begin treatment.

If the patient is too young to be aware of a problem, it is important for the clinician not to draw any unnecessary attention to the dental occlusion or facial appearance. The parent's should be informed in the most discreet and considerate way possible that there is treatment available to improve the malocclusion and jaw discrepancy when the patient is older. For example, the young patient may be taken by the nurse to a nearby consultation room, e.g. 'to be given a sticker because you are such a great patient', while the clinician discusses potential future treatment with the parents. The parents, and other family members/older siblings, should also be advised not to draw unnecessary attention to such issues in the home environment. In somewhat older or adolescent patients who understand the issues, which usually begins when they have been subjected to teasing or bullying on account of their dentofacial appearance, the future treatment should be discussed in a thoughtful way, and the patient should be reassured that the treatment is not uncommon or unique in any way, and is not essential but an option the patient can consider for the future. Showing the patient images of previously treated patients may be very helpful (see Chapter 10). If there is severe narrowing of the maxilla or obvious crowding and/or rotations of the maxillary dentition, patients may request an initial course of orthodontic treatment in the maxillary arch only. This may be provided so long as the patient is aware that future treatment will still be prolonged.

If the patient is too young for orthognathic surgery, but is also borderline Class III in terms of potential future orthognathic treatment need, the treatment decision can be rather complicated as future growth is difficult to predict. Growth patterns are unlikely to change and Class III patterns tend to become worse, but the extent is difficult to predict with any degree of accuracy. Ideally, it is better to wait until the end of adolescence to assess any further unfavourable growth, or only to treat the maxillary arch until the patient s older. However, some patients may appear adamant that they will not desire orthognathic surgery in the future, and would like orthodontic camouflage treatment while they are still growing. In such situations, the clinician must be confident that the patient and parents fully appreciate that further unfavourable growth will make the dentofacial appearance worse, and informed consent is vitally important.

Surgical camouflage

Surgical camouflage refers to surgical procedures that partially mask the facial soft tissue appearance due to an underlying skeletal discrepancy, and thereby improve the facial aesthetic appearance to some extent, whilst avoiding repositioning of the jaws with full blown orthognathic surgery. Examples include:

- Genioplasty (Figure 3-11)
- Rhinoplasty
- Soft tissue augmentation or other soft tissue camouflage surgery

Note:

Single jaw surgery in a patient ideally requiring bimaxillary surgery may be considered, in certain situations, as surgical camouflage.

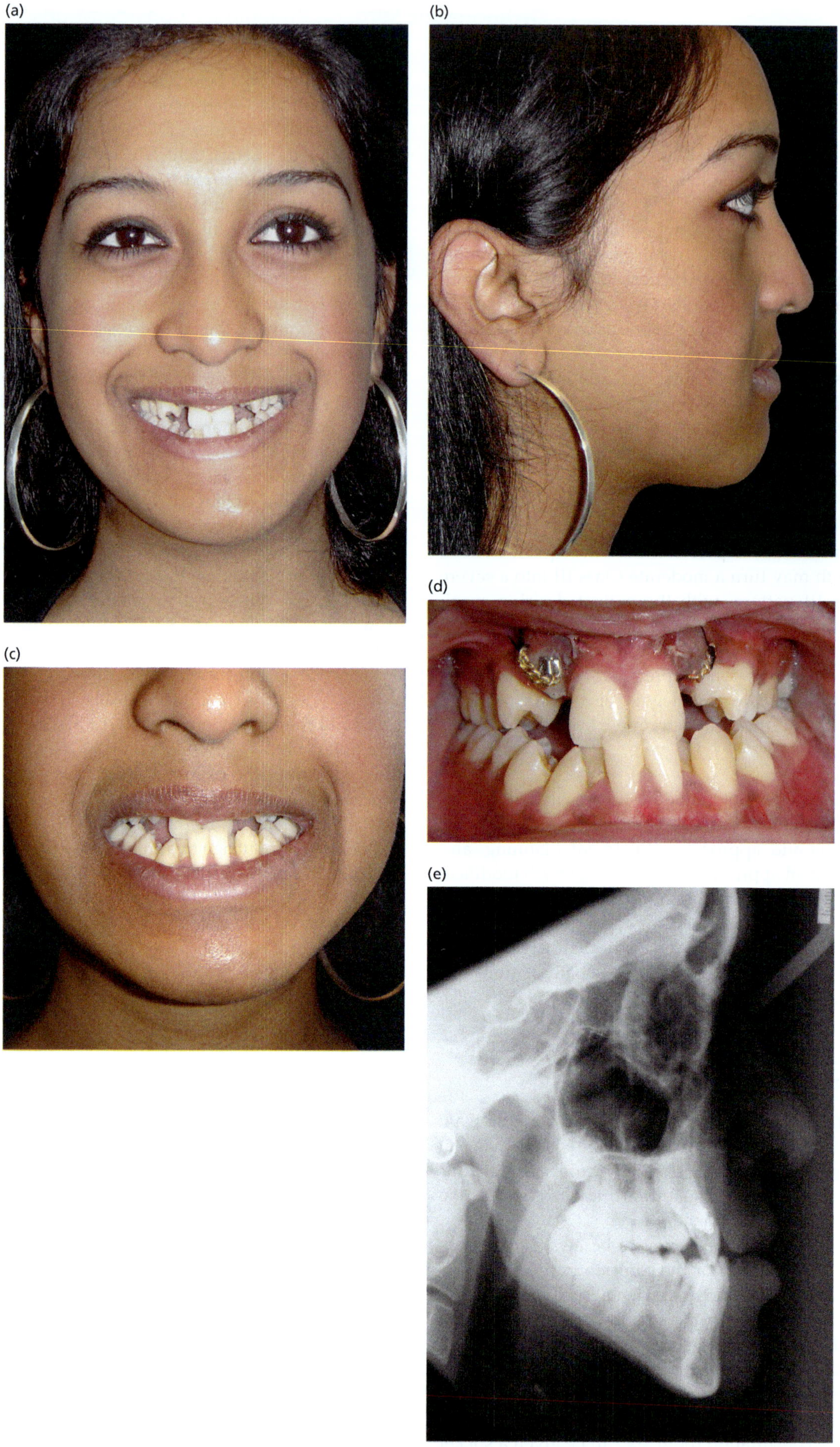

Fig. 3-10 Orthodontic camouflage treatment of a Class III patient, with missing maxillary lateral incisors. (a)–(e): Pretreatment photographs. Mandibular first premolars were extracted to permit alignment and retroclination of the mandibular incisors with fixed orthodontic appliances; the maxillary canines were aligned next to the central incisors, and reshaped. (f)–(j): End of treatment.

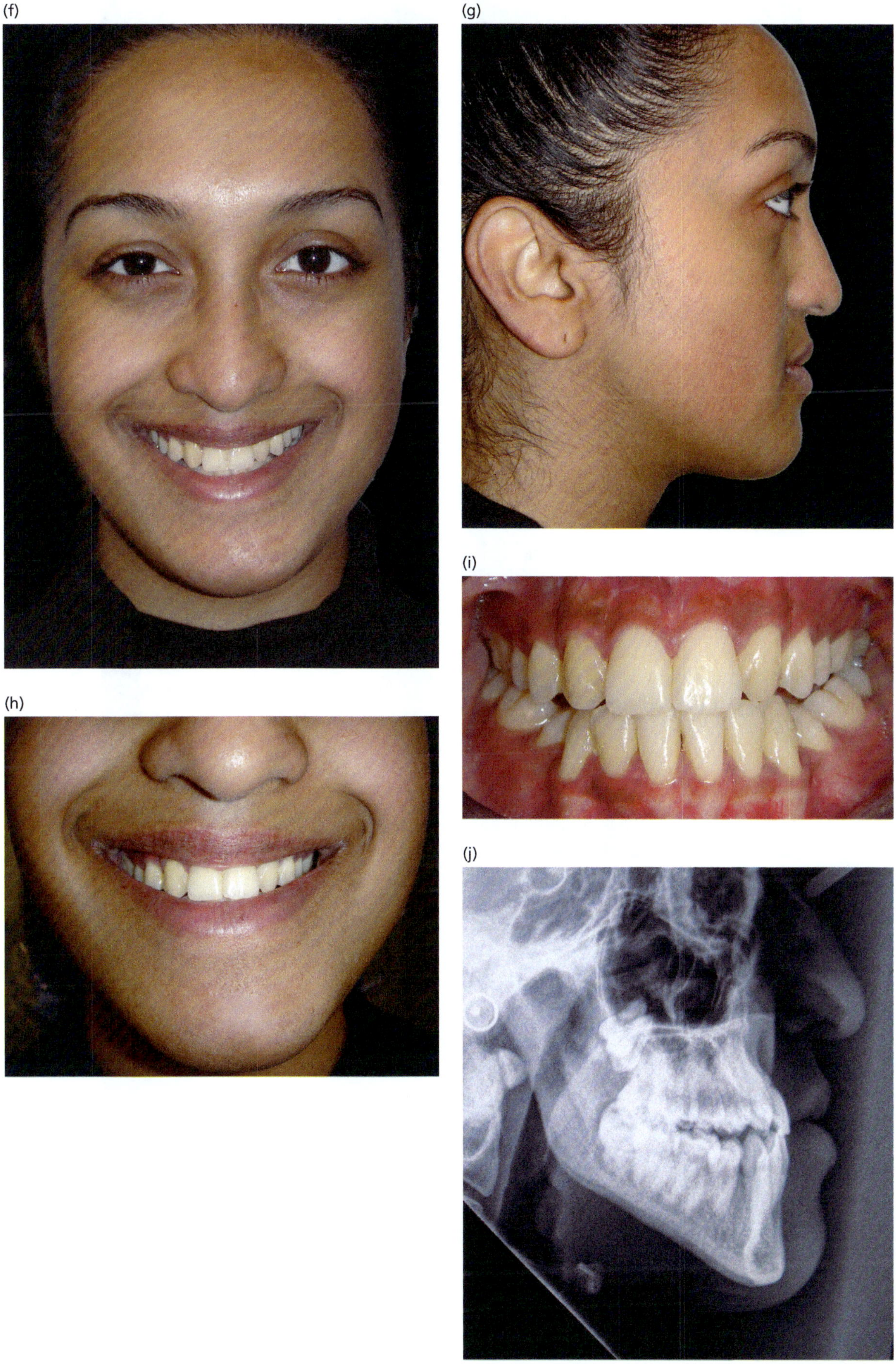

Fig. 3-10 (*Continued*)

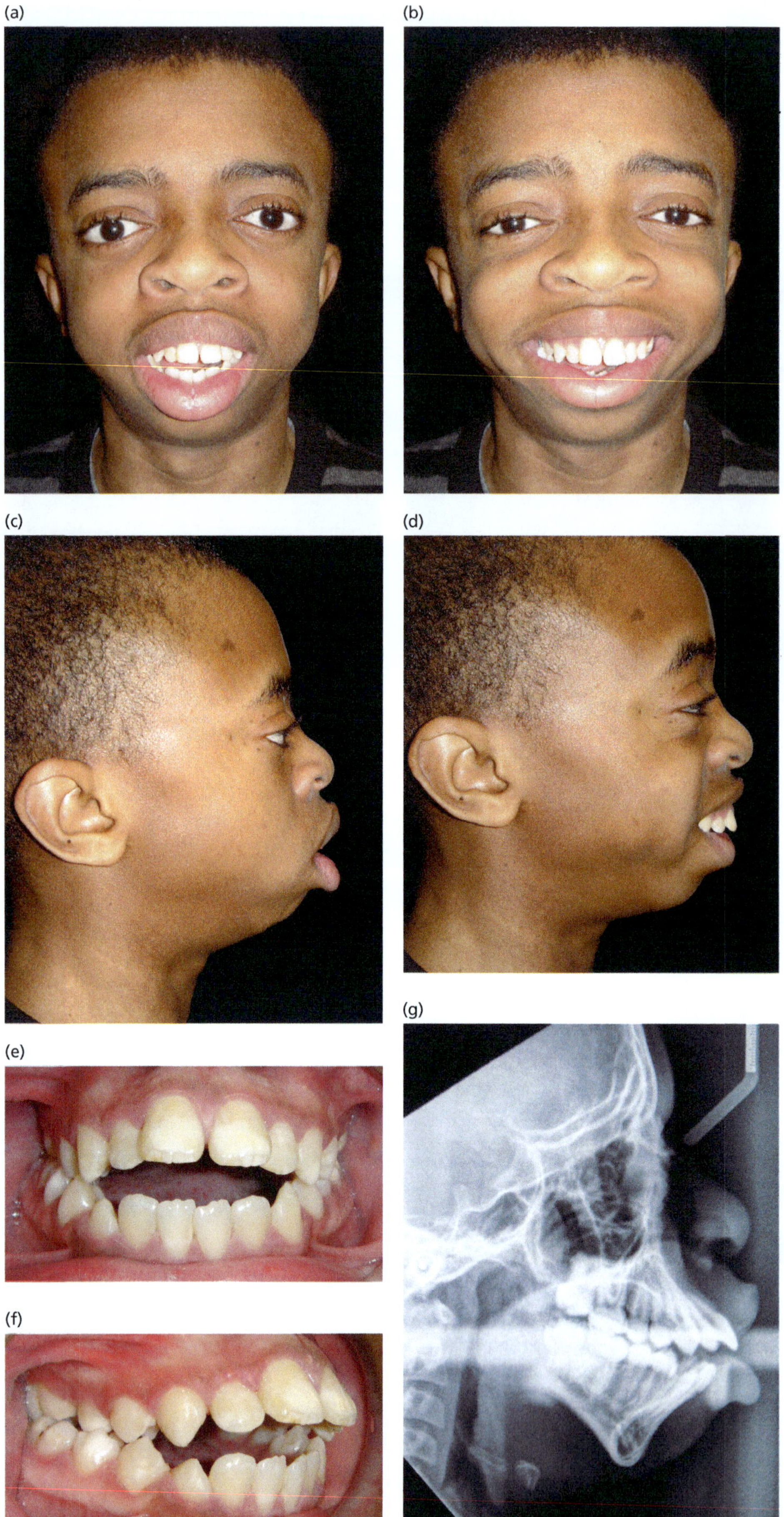

Fig. 3-11 Patient with Noonan syndrome, with severe bimaxillary dental proclination, anterior open bite, severe mandibular retrognathia and retrogenia, and reduced mandibular ramus height. The patient did not desire bimaxillary orthognathic surgery, but following camouflage orthodontic treatment to retrocline the incisor teeth and reduce the anterior open bite, decided on an advancement genioplasty, which in this case is a form of surgical camouflage. (a)–(g): Pretreatment. (h)–(n): Following orthodontic camouflage treatment, with extraction of first premolar teeth and retroclination of the anterior teeth. (o)–(r): 8-days following double-step advancement genioplasty. (s): Before and after genioplasty.

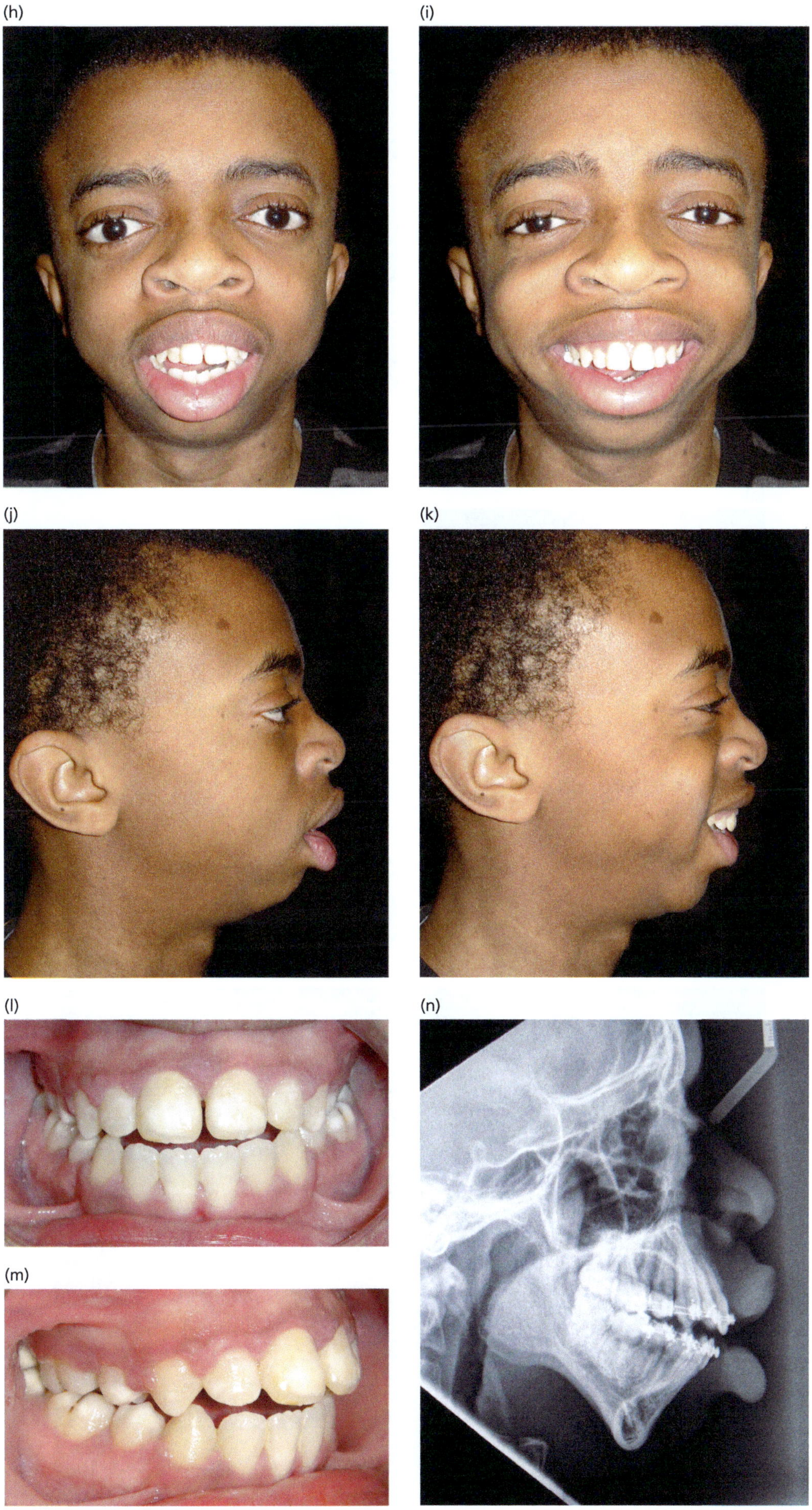

Fig. 3-11 (*Continued*)

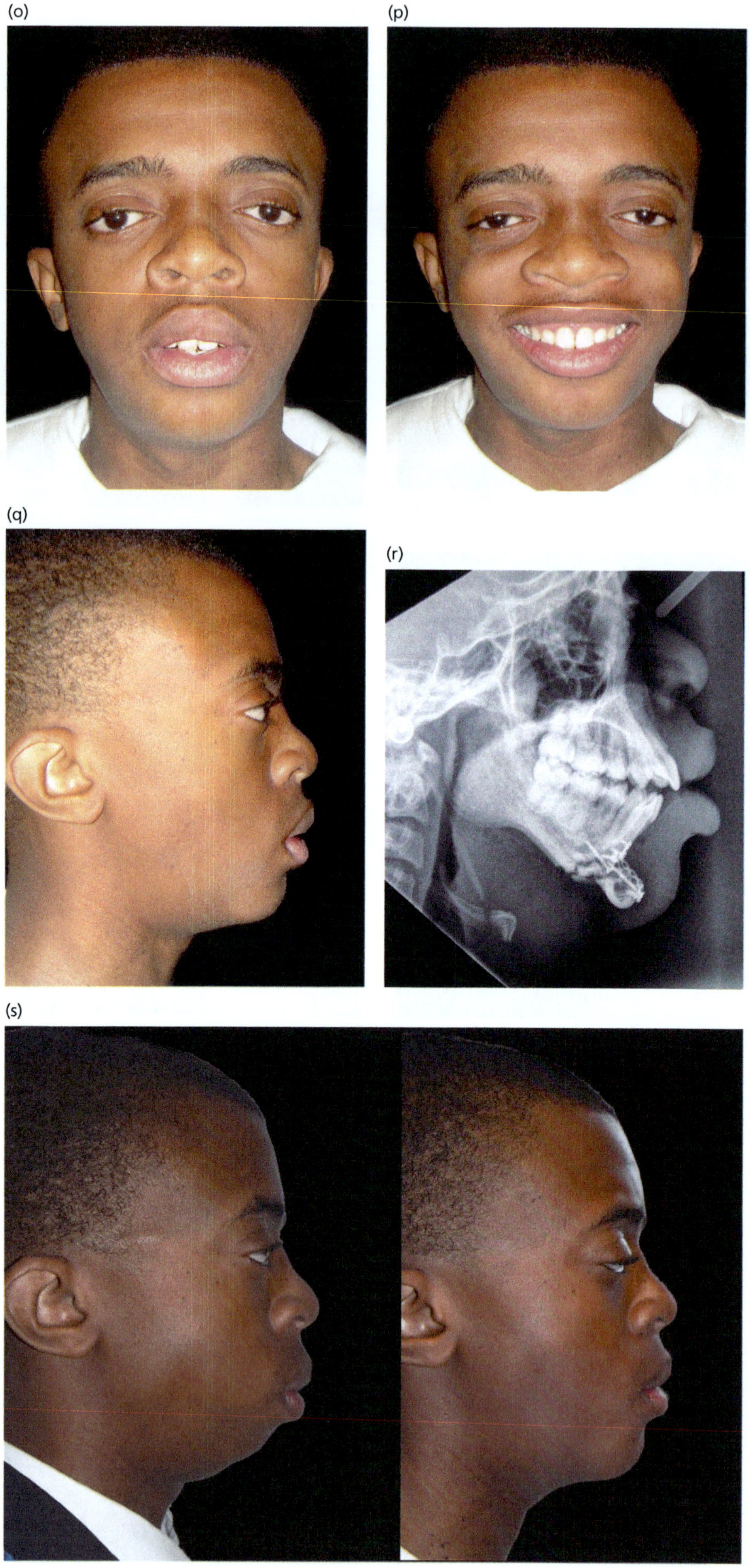

Fig. 3-11 *(Continued)*

References

1 Naini FB. Facial Aesthetics: Concepts and Clinical Diagnosis. Oxford: Wiley-Blackwell, 2011.
2 Shakespeare W. The Tragedy of Hamlet, Prince of Denmark (c.1600). London: New Penguin Shakespeare, 1972.
3 Shakespeare W. The Tempest (1611). London: New Penguin Shakespeare, 1971.
4 Marcovic MD. At the cross-roads of orofacial genetics. Eur J Orthod. 1992;14:469–81.
5 van der Linden FP. Genetic and environmental factors in dentofacial morphology. Am J Orthod. 1966;52:576–83.
6 Moss ML, Salentijn L. The capsular matrix. Am J Orthod. 1969;56:474–90.
7 Moss ML, Salentijn L. The primary role of functional matrices in facial growth. Am J Orthod. 1969;55:566–77.
8 Mossey PA. The heritability of malocclusion: Part 1 Genetics, principles and terminology. Br J Orthod. 1999;26:103–13.
9 Mossey PA. The heritability of malocclusion: Part 2. The influence of genetics in malocclusion. Br J Orthod. 1999;26:195–203.
10 Harris JE. Genetic factors in the growth of the head: Inheritance of the craniofacial complex and malocclusion. Dent Clin North Am. 1975;19:151–60.
11 Kloeppel W. Deckbiss bei Zwillingen. Fortschr Kieferorthop 1953;14:130–5.
12 Schulze C, Weise W. Zur vererburg der progenie. Fortschr fte Kieferorthop. 1965;26:213–29.
13 Litton SF, Ackermann LV, Isaacson RJ, Shapiro BL. A genetic study of Class 3 malocclusion. Am J Orthod. 1970;58:565–77.
14 Lundström A. Nature versus nurture in dento-facial variation. Eur J Orthod. 1984;6:77–91.
15 Hunter WS. A study of the inheritance of craniofacial characteristics as seen in lateral cephalograms of 72 like-sexed twins. Rep Congr Eur Orthod Soc. 1965;41:59–70.
16 Naini FB, Moss JP. Three-dimensional assessment of the relative contribution of genetics and environment to various facial parameters with the twin method. Am J Orthod Dentofacial Orthop. 2004;126:655–65.
17 Brook PH, Shaw WC. The development of an index of orthodontic treatment priority. Eur J Orthod. 1989;11: 309–20.
18 British Association of Oral and Maxillofacial Surgeons (BAOMS) Commissioning Guide (2013): Royal College of Surgeons of England, UK.
19 Proffit WR, Fields HW Jr, Moray LJ. Prevalence of malocclusion and orthodontic treatment need in the United States: estimates from the NHANES III survey. Int J Adult Orthodon Orthognath Surg. 1998;13:97–106.
20 Obwegeser HL. Surgical correction of small or retrodisplaced maxillae. The 'dish-face' deformity. Plast Reconstr Surg. 1969;43:351–65.
21 Proothi M, Drew SJ, Sachs SA. Motivating factors for patients undergoing orthognathic surgery evaluation. J Oral Maxillofac Surg. 2010;68:1555–9.
22 Alanko OM, Svedström-Oristo AL, Tuomisto MT. Patients' perceptions of orthognathic treatment, well-being, and psychological or psychiatric status: a systematic review. Acta Odontol Scand. 2010;68:249–60.
23 Cunningham SJ, Garratt AM, Hunt NP. Development of a condition-specific quality of life measure for patients with dentofacial deformity: I. Reliability of the instrument. Community Dent Oral Epidemiol. 2000;28:195–201.
24 Cunningham SJ, Garratt AM, Hunt NP. Development of a condition-specific quality of life measure for patients with dentofacial deformity: II. Validity and responsiveness testing. Community Dent Oral Epidemiol. 2002;30:81–90.
25 Lee S, McGrath C, Samman N. Impact of orthognathic surgery on quality of life. J Oral Maxillofac Surg. 2008;66:1194–9.
26 Motegi E, Hatch JP, Rugh JD, Yamaguchi H. Health-related quality of life and psychosocial function 5 years after orthognathic surgery. Am J Orthod Dentofacial Orthop. 2003;124:138–43.
27 Esperão PT, de Oliveira BH, de Oliveira Almeida MA, Kiyak HA, Miguel JA. Oral health-related quality of life in orthognathic surgery patients. Am J Orthod Dentofacial Orthop. 2010;137:790–5.
28 Øland J, Jensen J, Melsen B. Factors of importance for the functional outcome in orthognathic surgery patients: a prospective study of 118 patients. J Oral Maxillofac Surg. 2010;68:2221–31.
29 Murphy C, Kearns G, Sleeman D, Cronin M, Allen PF. The clinical relevance of orthognathic surgery on quality of life. Int J Oral Maxillofac Surg. 2011;40:926–30.
30 Hunt OT, Johnston CD, Hepper PG, Burden DJ. The psychosocial impact of orthognathic surgery: a systematic review. Am J Orthod Dentofacial Orthop. 2001;120:490–7.
31 Cunningham SJ, Sculpher M, Sassi F, Manca A. A cost-utility analysis of patients undergoing orthognathic treatment for the management of dentofacial disharmony. Br J Oral Maxillofac Surg. 2003;41:32–5.
32 Sousa CS, Turrini RN. Complications in orthognathic surgery: A comprehensive review. J Oral Maxillofac Surg Med Pathol. 2012;24:67–74.
33 Iannetti G, Fadda TM, Riccardi E, Mitro V, Filiaci F. Our experience in complications of orthognathic surgery: a retrospective study on 3236 patients. Eur Rev Med Pharmacol Sci. 2013;17:379–84.
34 Al-Riyami S, Cunningham SJ, Moles DR. Orthognathic treatment and temporomandibular disorders: a systematic review. Part 2.Signs and symptoms and meta-analyses. Am J Orthod Dentofacial Orthop. 2009;136:626.e1–16.
35 Hassan T, Naini FB, Gill DS. The effects of orthognathic surgery on speech: a review. J Oral Maxillofac Surg. 2007;65:2536–43.
36 Proffit WR, Phillips C, Tulloch JF, Medland PH. Surgical versus orthodontic correction of skeletal Class II malocclusion in adolescents: effects and indications. Int J Adult Orthodon Orthognath Surg. 1992;7:209–20.
37 Kerr WJ, Miller S, Dawber JE. Class III malocclusion: surgery or orthodontics? Br J Orthod. 1992;19:21–4.
38 Fox N. The Index of Orthodontic Treatment Need. In: Gill DS, Naini FB (Eds). Orthodontics: Principles and Practice. Oxford: Wiley-Blackwell, 2011.
39 Ireland AJ, Cunningham SJ, Petrie A, Cobourne MT, Acharya P, Sandy JR, Hunt NP. An Index of Orthognathic Functional Treatment Need (IOFTN). J Orthod. 2014;41:77–83.
40 Naini FB, Cobourne MT, McDonald F, Donaldson AN. The influence of craniofacial to standing height proportion on perceived attractiveness. Internat J Oral Maxillofac Surg. 2008;37:877–85.
41 Naini FB, Donaldson ANA, McDonald F, Cobourne MT. Assessing the influence of asymmetry affecting the mandible and chin point on perceived attractiveness in the orthognathic patient, clinician and layperson. J Oral Maxillofac Surg. 2012;70:192–206.
42 Naini FB, Donaldson ANA, McDonald F, Cobourne MT. Influence of chin height on perceived attractiveness in the orthognathic patient, clinician and layperson. Angle Orthod. 2012;82:88–95.
43 Naini FB, Donaldson AN, Cobourne MT, McDonald F. Assessing the influence of mandibular prominence on perceived attractiveness in the orthognathic patient, clinician and layperson. Eur J Orthod. 2012;34:738–46.
44 Naini FB, Donaldson ANA, McDonald F, Cobourne MT. Assessing the influence of lower facial profile convexity on perceived attractiveness in the orthognathic patient, clinician and layperson. Oral Surg Oral Med Oral Pathol Oral Radiol. 2012;114:303–11.
45 Naini FB, Donaldson ANA, McDonald F, Cobourne MT. Assessing the influence of chin prominence on perceived attractiveness in the orthognathic patient, clinician and layperson. Internat J Oral Maxillofac Surg. 2012;41:839–46.

46 Naini FB, Donaldson ANA, McDonald F, Cobourne MT. The influence of combined orthodontic-orthognathic surgical treatment on perceptions of attractiveness: A longitudinal study. Eur J Orthod. 2013;35:590–8.
47 Naini FB, Donaldson ANA, McDonald F, Cobourne MT. How does variation in lower anterior face height influence perceived attractiveness? A quantitative investigation. J Orthod. 2013;40:206–17.
48 Naini FB, Cobourne MT, McDonald F, Wertheim D. The aesthetic impact of upper lip inclination on orthodontics and orthognathic surgery. Eur J Orthod. 2015;37:81–6.
49 Naini FB, Cobourne MT, McDonald F, Wertheim D. Aesthetic impact of the upper component of the nasolabial angle: a quantitative investigation. J Oral Maxillofac Surg Med Pathol. 2015;27:470–6.
50 Paracelsus. Die Grosse Wundarznei (1536). Berlin: Verlag, 1963.
51 Andry N. Orthopaedia: or, the art of correcting and preventing deformities in children: by such means, as may easily be put in practice by parents themselves, and all such as are employed in educating children (1741). Translated from the French. London: A. Millar, 1743.
52 Vig PS, Vig KW. Hybrid appliances: a component approach to dentofacial orthopedics. Am J Orthod Dentofacial Orthop. 1986;90:273–85.
53 Delaire J. Manufacture of the 'orthopedic mask'. Rev Stomatol Chir Maxillofac. 1971;72:579–82.
54 Ngan P. Biomechanics of maxillary expansion and protraction in Class III patients. Am J Orthod Dentofacial Orthop. 2002;121:582–3.

Chapter 4

Orthognathic Surgery: The Patient Pathway

Farhad B. Naini and Daljit S. Gill

'The physician requires ordered thinking, and treatment requires a logical progression... founded upon evidence from close observation of patients and empirical investigation.'

Pür Sina (Latinized: Avicenna, or Ibn Sina) (AD 980–1037)
Persian physician-polymath, *Canon Medicinae (The Canon of Medicine)*[I]

Introduction

The purpose of this Chapter is to describe the members of the orthognathic team and define their responsibilities, to discuss the clinician's role throughout orthognathic treatment, and to detail the sequencing of treatment and the coordination of care throughout the orthognathic patient pathway.

The orthognathic team

'Great advances in science are almost always due to individuals... but, to be effective and efficient, the practice of medicine requires the physician-surgeon to work with and lead a highly-trained team.'

Zakariya Razi (Latinized: Rhazes) (AD 865–925)
Persian physician-polymath, *Outcomes of the Science of Medicine*[II]

Orthognathic surgery carries a rather unique position within medicine and surgery as it requires the working together of two distinct surgical specialties throughout the treatment process, over a relatively prolonged period for each patient.

[I] Avicenna's *Canon of Medicine* has been described as the first book on evidence-based medicine in history.[1] This vast tome, consisting of more than a million words, surveyed the entire field of medical knowledge from ancient times to the most up-to-date techniques. Its comprehensive and systematic approach meant that when it was translated into Latin in the 12th century, it became the standard medical textbook for seven centuries throughout Europe.[2] Sir William Osler (1849–1919) (Figure 4-1) described Avicenna as the 'author of the most famous medical textbook ever written,' noting that Avicenna's *Canon of Medicine* remained 'a medical bible for a longer time than any other work'.[3] Avicenna's name has been used internationally in a number of universities, and his portrait hangs in the hall of the Avicenna Faculty of Medicine, the oldest medical school in the University of Paris. His Mausoleum is in the city of Hamedan, Iran.

[II] The English historian Edward G. Browne (1862–1926) considered Razi as 'probably the greatest and most original of all the physicians and one of the most prolific as an author'.[4] He is best known for discovering alcohol and its medical application, and is regarded as 'the father of paediatric medicine' as he authored the first book on the subject, entitled *The Diseases of Children*.

Orthognathic Surgery: Principles, Planning and Practice. Edited by Farhad B. Naini and Daljit S. Gill.

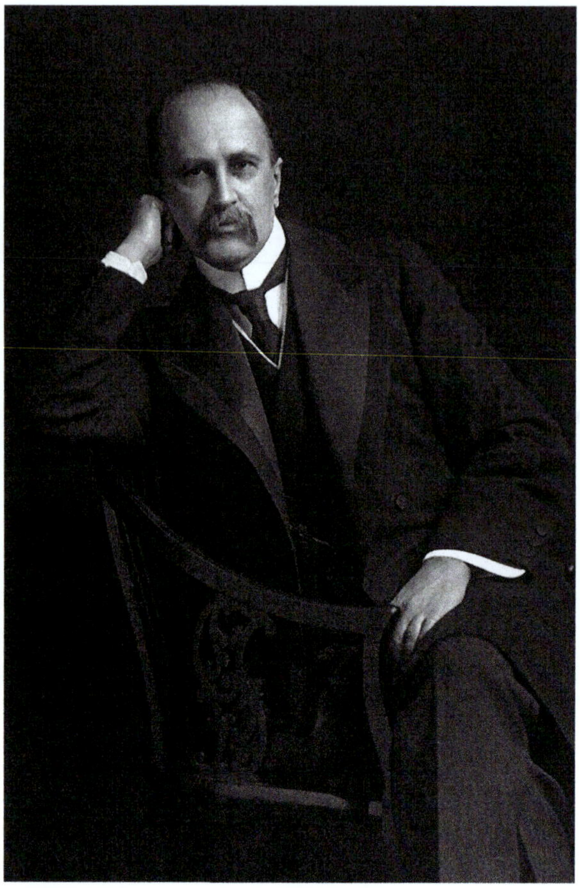

Fig. 4-1 Sir William Osler (1849–1919).

The principal players in the orthognathic team are the consultant surgeon and consultant orthodontist (in the UK, the 'consultant' is the clinician with ultimate responsibility for the care of a patient in the hospital service). The relationship between the surgeon and orthodontist is almost symbiotic. Orthognathic treatment is the perfect blend of art and science, and the potentially life-changing nature of the treatment for patients makes it incredibly rewarding for both surgeon and orthodontist.

Consultant maxillofacial surgeon

Oral and maxillofacial surgery, also referred to as cranio-maxillofacial surgery (Professor Hugo Obwegeser's preferred term) is a surgical specialty requiring a long and arduous training. In the UK, and many other countries, this requires a dual qualification in medicine and dentistry, as well as general surgical training and a firm background in other specialties dealing with the head and neck. Upon being appointed a hospital consultant, a maxillofacial surgeon in the UK usually chooses a subspecialty interest: orthognathic surgery, head and neck oncology or trauma surgery. It may be argued that a special interest in orthognathic and/or craniofacial surgery should be deemed mandatory, permitting high volume surgery, appropriately monitored with accurate clinical audit.

Note:

Clinical audit is a process of quality improvement, seeking to improve patient care and treatment outcomes through systematic review of care against explicit predetermined criteria, and an ideal known as the gold standard, and the implementation of changes and improvements until the gold standard is achieved. The importance of clinical audit for each orthognathic team should not be underestimated. The key component of clinical audit is that performance is reviewed (or audited) to ensure that what *should* be done is *being* done, and if not it provides a framework to enable improvements to be made. Without it, it is difficult to know if one is doing the right thing.

Consultant orthodontist

The term 'consultant' is used on purpose – orthognathic surgery is a distinct subspecialty of both maxillofacial surgery and orthodontics that requires higher training. In the UK, at least 2 years of training *following* orthodontic specialization is required to become a hospital consultant. Orthognathic surgery is not easy and misguided attempts to provide such treatment without adequate understanding and training will inevitably result in problems for the patient and considerable confusion and distress for the orthodontist.

Clinical psychologist/liaison psychiatrist

The psychologist or psychiatrist on the orthognathic team should have a special interest in body image disorders, particularly body dysmorphic disorder (BDD) (see Chapter 9). The importance of such a clinician on the team cannot be overemphasized.

Maxillofacial technologist

The role of the maxillofacial technologist is to undertake the model surgery and to construct the splint wafers (see Chapter 13).

Orthodontic technologist

The orthodontic technician is required to construct various aspects of fixed appliances, e.g. transpalatal arches, and removable appliances during treatment, and to construct the retainers following debond of the appliances.

Specialist orthognathic nurse

There is perhaps no greater calling in life than nursing. Where possible, it is extremely useful for every orthognathic team to have an experienced specialist orthognathic nurse, who attends all the joint clinics and has a good understanding of the various stages of the treatment process.

Note:

Patients often find it very useful to have contact with such a nurse, both as a source of information and advice, and as a stable and empathetic base of support for the patient and their parents/family members to rely upon as and when required.

Specialist maxillofacial/head and neck dietician
The dietician is required to provide preoperative and postoperative advice to the orthognathic patient (see Chapter 15).

Speech and language therapist
A speech therapist is usually not required for the routine orthognathic patient, but commonly required and vitally important in the clinical treatment of cleft orthognathic patients (see Chapter 56).

General medical and dental practitioners
The general medical and dental practitioner should be considered part of the team and the patient's care should be coordinated with them.

Consultant anaesthetist
Ideally, the anaesthetist should have a special interest in head and neck surgery (see Chapter 14).

Orthognathic treatment pathway – the clinician's role

The clinician's step-by-step role in the management of the orthognathic surgical patient may be described using the acronym 'DAATTARS' (Table 4-1).

Sequencing of treatment and coordination of care

The sequence of treatment in the orthognathic patient pathway is demonstrated in Figure 4-2. Comprehensive details of each stage of treatment are described in the appropriate Chapters. The purpose of this section

Table 4-1 The clinician's role in the orthognathic treatment pathway

Stage	Description
Diagnosis	An accurate diagnosis is followed by the formation of a **problem list**, ideally ordered from the most to the least severe.
Aetiology	The aetiology of a dentofacial deformity is always relevant in diagnosis and treatment planning, as well as in the prognosis for stability, e.g. a significant tongue thrust will make the prognosis for long-term stability questionable.
Aims of treatment	The objectives of treatment should be decided before any treatment begins, and include the desired facial soft tissue appearance and contours, the skeletal moves required to achieve the ideal soft tissue outcome, and the orthodontic treatment required to achieve the most ideal static and dynamic functional dental-occlusal outcome.
Treatment plan	The treatment plan ultimately chosen by the clinicians in conjunction with the patient should form the gold standard plan for the correction of the presenting dentofacial deformity for the individual patient. Explanation of the risks and benefits of treatment and informed consent are mandatory.
Treatment mechanics	A step-by-step road map is required for the successive stages of treatment: • preoperative orthodontic preparation, • the surgical procedure(s), • the required postoperative orthodontics, • retention, • any potential secondary or adjunctive procedures.
Alternative treatment plan(s)	Other than the gold standard approach, are there any other alternative treatment approaches: • simpler surgical solutions – e.g. single-jaw rather than bimaxillary surgery, or • surgical camouflage (if orthodontics not desired), or • orthodontic camouflage (if surgery not desired).
Retention regime	The purpose of retainers is to maintain the new position of the teeth until the surrounding bony and soft tissues have stabilized and to prevent unwanted changes due to long-term growth. Active retainers may occasionally be required for the application of Class II or III elastics following orthognathic surgery (see Chapter 12). The retention regime depends to a great extent on the original skeletal discrepancy and associated malocclusion, and any soft tissue parameters, and is often unique for each patient depending on a variety of other factors, such as the degree of interdigitation of the final dental occlusion. In the absence of major concerns regarding stability, a retention regime of 3–4 months close to full-time wear, followed by 9 months evenings and nights, a year of nights only, gradually reducing to part-time wear for an indefinite period is advised. The patient should be advised before the start of treatment that they will be 'married to their retainers' on a long-term basis.
Stability	The prognosis for both surgical/jaw bone repositioning and dental/orthodontic stability is an indicator of treatment success (see Chapter 18).

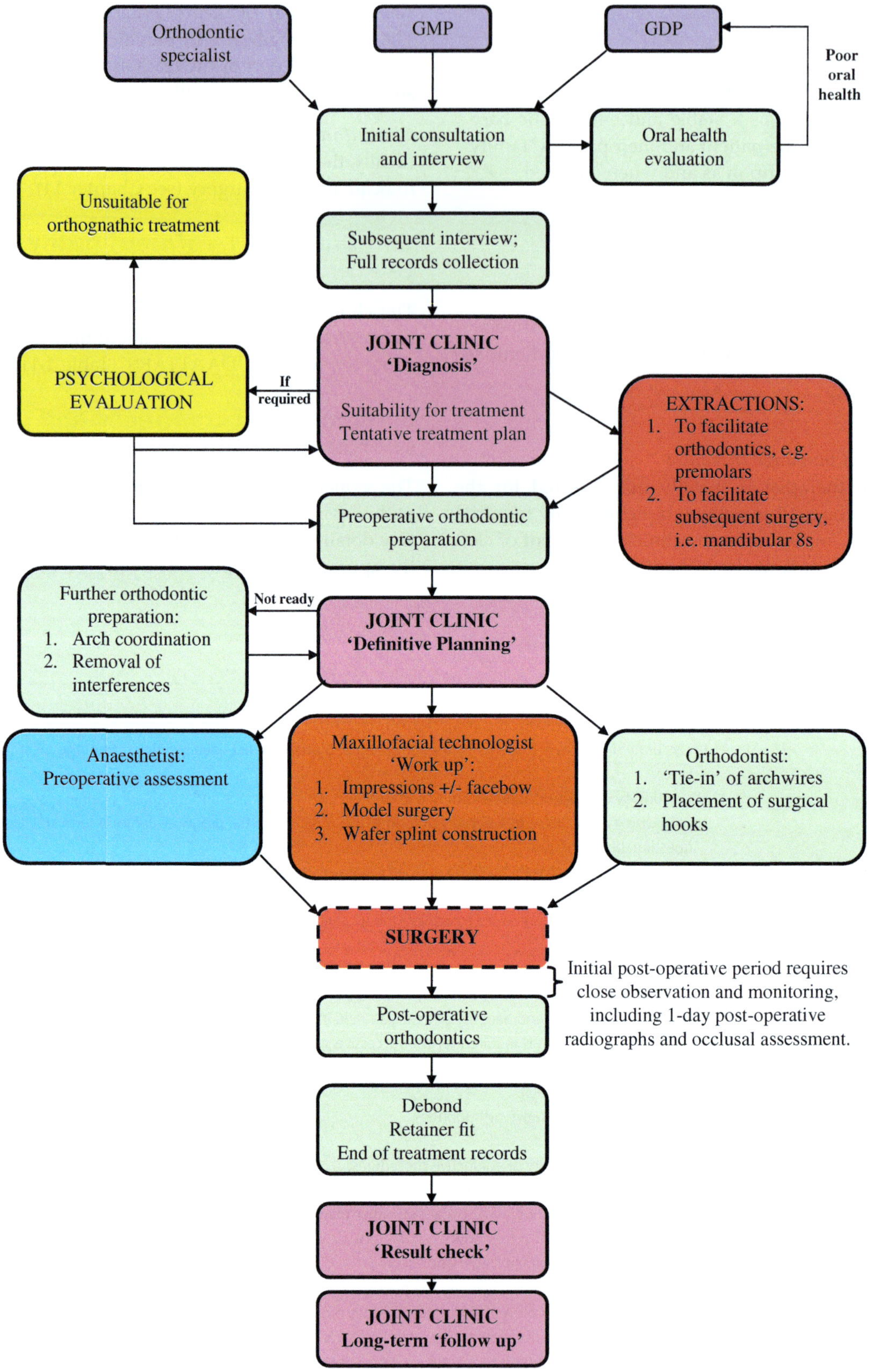

Fig. 4-2 The orthognathic patient pathway. GDP, General Dental Practitioner; GMP, General Medical Practitioner.

is to provide a brief overview of the orthognathic treatment pathway.

Initial referral

The initial referral to the orthognathic surgery unit in a hospital department may be from a variety of sources, including the general medical practitioner (GMP), but more commonly from either the general dental practitioner (GDP) or an orthodontist in specialist practice. Although the initial appointment may be with the consultant surgeon, more often than not it is with the consultant orthodontist.

Initial consultation and interview

The purpose of the initial consultation and interview is mainly to undertake an introductory discussion with the patient and to make a preliminary evaluation of the suitability of the patient for orthognathic surgical treatment. A comprehensive clinical and radiographic **oral health evaluation** is undertaken and the patient referred back to the general dental practitioner (GDP) if any dental or periodontal treatment or an improvement in oral hygiene is deemed to be required. The patient should be provided with preliminary information about orthognathic treatment, including potential downsides and complications (see Chapter 10) and provided with information leaflets to read, and potentially an information DVD to watch, in the comfort of their own home. An appointment may be made for a subsequent consultation after a few months, providing the patient with a period of time for contemplation. The patient should also be asked to write down and bring any further questions they have to the following consultation. If parents/spouses have not accompanied the patient to the initial consultation, it is important to ask for them to be present at the subsequent consultation.

Subsequent consultation and interview

In the subsequent consultation and interview it is always useful to ask the patient some questions about the information provided at the previous consultation and contained in the information leaflets. Questioning is simply to evaluate the patient's attitude towards treatment, and the clinician's manner and tone should be congenial and not appear like an interrogation. The clinician may begin by asking the patient: 'Did you have time to read the information leaflet?' This may be followed by asking whether they remember how long the treatment would take, and what the potential complications could be? The inability to answer these questions should be a red flag signal. If all appears well and the patient seems to be suitable for treatment, any additional records may be taken (e.g. impressions for dental study models) and an appointment made to see the patient on the joint clinic with the surgeon. At this point, the patient and their family must be informed that the ultimate decision as to whether they will be accepted for treatment will be a joint decision by the surgeon and orthodontist at the joint clinic.

Note:

What is the 'joint clinic'?
The term 'joint clinic' or 'joint orthognathic clinic' refers to a specific set of appointments during the orthognathic treatment pathway where the patient is seen jointly by the consultant surgeon and orthodontist. These are of the utmost importance, as defining decisions regarding the patient's treatment are often made at these clinics. Although they may be required at various stages of the treatment pathway, the set joint clinics are the following:

- Initial joint 'diagnosis' clinic
- Preoperative joint 'definitive planning' clinic
- Immediate postoperative period – In the immediate postoperative period, patients may also be seen on a formal joint clinic, though often the requirement for very close observation and monitoring requires weekly reviews, which are arranged between the surgeon and orthodontist, and require excellent communication between the two.
- Joint 'result check' clinic
- Joint 'follow up' clinics.

Note:

It is useful for the specialist orthognathic nurse to speak with the patient before they enter the consultation room for a joint clinic. The presence of the surgeon and orthodontist and a number of senior trainees, particularly in a teaching unit, may be rather intimidating for patients if they are not prepared. The patient should be informed beforehand if trainees will be present, and every member of the team should politely introduce themselves and help to put the patient and their parents/family members at their ease. Patients rarely mind this situation so long as the importance of teaching is explained to them, and they are made to feel as part of the process, and not as a looker-on.

Joint 'diagnosis' clinic

This is the initial clinic where the patient is seen by both the consultant surgeon and consultant orthodontist, together with all the necessary initial patient records. The primary objective is to agree on the patient's **suitability for orthognathic treatment** and to confirm a **definitive diagnosis** (see Chapter 5). An open and honest discussion of the **risks/costs and benefits** of treatment is covered, usually by the surgeon, though at this stage the patient should be well aware of these issues from previous discussions with the orthodontist (see Chapters 5 and 11). Additionally, a **tentative surgical treatment plan** is provided, though this is rather general (e.g. single-jaw surgery or bimaxillary surgery, and possible requirement for a genioplasty) and the patient should be informed that the plan may be subject to modification depending on preparatory orthodontic treatment. Arrangements may be made for a further appointment should the clinicians feel that the patient still requires more time to think of the options for treatment. Alternatively, arrangements may be made for the patient to see a clinical psychologist or liaison psychiatrist if this is deemed necessary.

A logically ordered, practical **orthodontic treatment plan** is also determined, which is akin to a road map; it points out the final destination based on realistic objectives and often the best way to achieve those objectives.

If the patient is suitable for orthognathic surgery, arrangements may also be made for any necessary **dental extractions**:

- **To facilitate preparatory orthodontics**, e.g. premolar extractions.
- **To facilitate subsequent mandibular surgery**, i.e. surgical removal of impacted mandibular third molar teeth. This is usually undertaken carefully by the consultant surgeon or an experienced member of their team, in order to preserve as much bone as possible. Ideally, this should be undertaken as soon as possible, preferably at least 1 year before mandibular surgery. The orthodontist should not place bonded tubes or bands on the mandibular second molars until the third molars have been removed, which allows better surgical access and prevents potential intraoperative dislodgement of the orthodontic attachments.

Preoperative orthodontics

The length of preparatory orthodontic treatment is variable and may take anything from 12 to 24 months, depending on the degree of tooth movement required and associated patient factors (see Chapter 12). When the preparatory orthodontics is deemed to be complete, **full records** (preoperative radiographs, photographs, 'snap' study models, and any necessary measurements) are taken and the patient booked onto the joint 'definitive planning' clinic.

Joint 'definitive planning' clinic

This is the joint clinic after the preparatory orthodontic treatment has been completed and the patient is essentially ready for surgery. The patient is seen by the consultant surgeon in conjunction with the consultant orthodontist, together with all the necessary preoperative patient records. The treating orthodontist will have undertaken a full 'work-up', including a potential provisional plan. The surgeon will undertake a comprehensive evaluation of the patient and their records (see Chapter 6). It is always useful for the surgeon to undertake this procedure before the orthodontist has discussed the provisional plan, as this in itself is a method of checking the plan and that nothing has been missed. At this stage, an experienced surgeon and orthodontist team will almost always have an obvious treatment plan on which they agree, though there is sometimes an element of mild bartering over the number of millimetres of movements required. The definitive, final decision must be made jointly by the surgeon and orthodontist, and it is unusual for experienced teams not to agree at this stage.

Advice regarding postoperative oral hygiene and nutrition should be provided at this appointment, and re-iterated at subsequent appointments as required.

If for any reason the patient is not ready for surgery, for example, if arch coordination in the canine-to-canine region is not well-prepared or a dental-occlusal interference is found requiring further orthodontic preparation, then this must be undertaken. *Delaying surgery is preferable to error.*

Once a definitive treatment plan has been decided and a date agreed for the surgery, three almost simultaneous preparatory stages are required:

- **Orthodontist** – For tying-in of the archwires with stainless steel ligatures and placement of surgical hooks (see Chapter 12).
- **Maxillofacial technologist** – A surgical planning form is completed and used by the maxillofacial technologist for the surgical 'work up', which includes the model surgery and construction of the wafer splints (see Chapter 13). The model surgery is checked by both surgeon and orthodontist, and the splint wafers tried in by the surgeon, usually one week prior to the surgery.
- **Anaesthetist** – For anaesthetic preoperative assessment (see Chapter 14).

Surgery

On the day of the operation the patient attends starved as per previously provided instructions. The length of surgery is variable and depends on the type of operation, but a useful guideline to provide parents/spouses of the patient is *approximately* 2 hours for a single-jaw procedure and under 4 hours for a bimaxillary procedure. After a short recovery, the patient returns to the ward.

Initial postoperative period

In the first few postoperative days and weeks the patient requires close observation and monitoring. Initially, the surgeon will see the patient both in recovery and the ward, in particular assessing the dental occlusion in relation to the planned position. Light intermaxillary elastics may be applied as required. The orthodontist will usually see the patient on the following morning, ideally together with the surgeon. Having assessed the dental occlusion, **postoperative radiographs** are taken and assessed at this stage (see Chapter 12). The postoperative hospital stay is usually short, perhaps one or two nights, but the recovery at home is relatively prolonged. The patient and their family are also seen by the **specialist dietician** prior to discharge, in addition to being provided with further instructions regarding the importance of maintaining a good level of oral hygiene (see Chapter 15). The patient is seen weekly for the first four weeks by the orthodontist and by the surgeon as required during this time.

Postoperative orthodontics

Active orthodontic treatment usually begins after the first few postoperative weeks, and will take approximately 6 ± 3 months. When the final dental occlusion is deemed satisfactory and the patient is happy, arrangements are made for removal of the orthodontic appliances, fitting of retainers and final treatment records.

Joint 'result check' clinic

The results of treatment are assessed by the surgeon and orthodontist and compared with the pretreatment and preoperative treatment plans. Any regions of paraesthesia are noted carefully in the patient's records for comparative purposes at subsequent follow-up appointments. This is often a very useful teaching clinic for senior trainees. The orthodontist will make arrangements for review of retainer wear as required.

Joint 'follow up' clinics

Orthognathic patient should be followed up on a long-term basis in order to monitor the stability of the post-operative result and improvements in any regions of paraesthesia, particularly the lower lip, chin and gingivae. It is recommended that records are taken at 1, 2, 5 and 10 years for comparative purposes and clinical audit.

References

1 Sharma V, Minhas R. Explanatory models are needed to integrate RCT and observational data with the patient's unique biology. J R Soc Med. 2012;105:11–24.
2 Naini FB. Avicenna and the Canon Medicinae. J R Soc Med. 2012;105:142.
3 Osler W. The Evolution of Modern Medicine. New Haven: Yale University Press, 1913.
4 Browne EG. Literary History of Persia. Vol. 2. London: T. Fisher Unwin, 1901.

Chapter 5

Patient Evaluation and Clinical Diagnosis

Farhad B. Naini and Daljit S. Gill

'Many look, but few see.'
Leonardo da Vinci (1452–1519)[1]

Introduction

Diagnosis remains the single most important step in the clinical management of any patient. It is often said that 'a journey of a thousand miles begins with a single step.' In terms of clinical treatment, it thereby follows that if this step is in the wrong direction, then no matter the speed of treatment or expertise in technique, one is nevertheless travelling in the wrong direction. Comprehensive clinical diagnosis of the craniofacial complex and the analysis of diagnostic records have been described elsewhere (presented in detail in *Facial Aesthetics: Concepts and Clinical Diagnosis*).[2] The purpose of this chapter is to provide a step-by-step guide to clinical diagnosis specifically for the orthognathic surgical patient.

Patient interview

The initial step in reaching a clinical diagnosis is the information obtained from the patient interview.[3] Any breakdown in communication at this stage may be irreparable. As such, it is important for the clinician's approach to be courteous and professional, while avoiding being over-familiar.

'I've learned that people will forget what you said, people will forget what you did, but people will never forget how you made them feel.'
Maya Angelou (1928–2014) (attributed)
African-American author and poet

One of the principles of clinical diagnosis is that *the observation of the patient begins from the moment they enter the consultation room*. The clinician should look for any signs of physical illness or potential psychosocial disturbances, which may be evident in the patient's posture, demeanour or their general manner, and

Orthognathic Surgery: Principles, Planning and Practice. Edited by Farhad B. Naini and Daljit S. Gill.

particularly in the relationship between younger patients and their parents.

The format of the patient interview should be a well-organized, **structured conversation**, in which the clinician directs the interview but the patient is allowed to ask questions as required. The patient should be sitting comfortably at the clinician's eye level and the interview should be free from interruption. Sufficient time should be allowed for an unhurried first consultation, both to gain the trust of the patient and to avoid errors of omission on the part of the clinician. The patient interview should never appear rushed; patients will sense this, leading to an unsuccessful consultation. The clinician also should avoid appearing to be an automaton, with a set of questions to go through, and simply writing notes without looking at the patient. Such obvious lack of empathy demonstrates poor practice.

The main purpose of the interview in the potential orthognathic surgical patient is to answer two questions:

- What are the patient's **concerns**? I.e. are they aesthetic or functional, or both?
- What is the patient's **attitude** towards their concern?

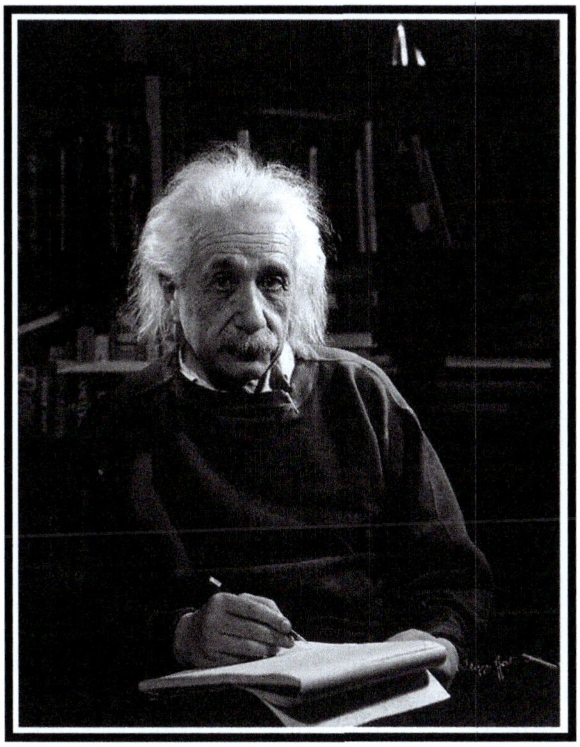

Fig. 5-1 Albert Einstein (1879–1955).

Note:

Avoid preconceptions

'It is easier to split an atom than a preconception.'
Albert Einstein (1879–1955) (attributed)

Einstein recognized human fallibility and the ease with which our preconceptions may effect our decisions (Figure 5-1). It should always be recognized that human beings are complex, and that the clinical environment is not a natural environment for a patient. In practice, the clinician should avoid forming opinions of the patient's motivation for seeking treatment too early in the consultation process. Ryan et al.[4] proposed that the everyday problems of living with a dentofacial deformity and the motivation for seeking treatment could be classified either as exclusively practical (including functional and structural), exclusively psychological (including psychosocial and aesthetic), or a combination. In some patients, the motivation for seeking treatment may not relate to the impact of their condition but to a complex array of other factors such as personality, upbringing, and interpersonal relationships. They concluded that clinicians should take care not to make assumptions but explore these factors 'on an individual basis without preconceived ideas'.

Presenting complaint

As in all of medicine and surgery, the patient's presenting complaint is very important. However, the clinician should be aware that patient's often attend their first consultation with mixed emotions and may find it difficult to convey their reasons for seeking advice or treatment.

The patient should be encouraged to speak honestly, and the clinician should take notes using the patient's own words. **Leading questions**, which suggest an answer (e.g. are you concerned about the prominence of your chin?), should be avoided. Instead, **open questions**, which do not suggest an answer (e.g. do you have any specific concerns?), should be used, although **closed questions**, which usually have a 'yes or no' answer may be asked *during* the interview process to extract specific information.

Note:

Avoid medical jargon

'You must learn to talk clearly.'
Martin H. Fischer (1879–1962)[5]
German-born American physician

Medical and surgical jargon is indecipherable to the layperson. A clinician must avoid obscure language and learn to translate the cryptography of surgical jargon into plain language that the patient can understand.

As well as avoiding medical jargon the clinician should demonstrate empathy throughout the consultation. Clinicians must never be, or appear to be, indifferent, unsympathetic or judgemental to a patient's concerns.[3]

> **Note:**
>
> **Demonstrate empathy**
>
> 'You never really understand a person until you consider things from his point of view ... until you climb into his skin and walk around in it.'
>
> '... you never really know a man until you stand in his shoes and walk around in them.'
>
> Harper Lee
> To Kill a Mockingbird (1960)[6]
>
> It is important for the clinician to have genuine empathy for their patients, but also to be able to demonstrate their empathy without appearing condescending. Sir William Osler wrote:[7]
>
> 'The motto of each of you as you undertake the examination and treatment of a case should be "put yourself in his place." Realize, so far as you can, the mental state of the patient, enter into his feelings ... '

A kind word and sympathetic look will put the patient at their ease. The medical maxim stands true: 'The patient will know if you care, well before they care if you know.'

History of presenting complaint

The main question for the potential orthognathic patient is, 'Why did the patient decide to have the problem corrected *now*?' The duration of a patient's concern is an important indicator of their primary motivation for treatment. Decisions resulting from recent life alterations, e.g. unemployment or divorce, with a desire that surgery will improve such issues in life, are likely to result in an unhappy patient in the long-term.

> **Note:**
>
> Patients rarely present the history of their complaint in a logical order. Some patients may be verbose, whereas others are reticent or possibly unclear and ambiguous. The art of 'taking a patient history' lies in eliciting all potentially relevant information from a thorough interview, censoring inessential or irrelevant information and arranging the facts in a logical order. It is often better to write notes after the patient has given their preliminary information, at which time the facts may be rechecked by the clinician whilst making a concise yet accurate written record of the patient's history in a logical order. Patients also prefer talking to a clinician who is looking at them, rather than constantly writing notes.

Psychosocial history

Dissatisfaction with the results of orthognathic surgery is uncommon, but when they do occur is often due to an underlying psychological or emotional disturbance in the patient, *unidentified* at the patient interview stage. More than one consultation appointment may well be required for the clinician to comprehensively evaluate the patient's:

- Perception
- Motivation
- Expectation(s)
- Cooperation
- Support network

Perception

The **patient's perception** of their dentofacial appearance is of primary importance. The clinician's first objective is to determine whether a dentofacial deformity exists and if so, *whether the patient's perception of the deformity ties in with the clinician's evaluation*.[3] Excessive concerns about a minor or imperceptible deformity, a history of 'doctor shopping', particularly if treatment was refused by previous clinicians, or vague concerns are usually a danger signal of a potential problem, and may require referral to a clinical psychologist or liaison psychiatrist, as these may be evidence of an underlying psychiatric disorder, such as **body dysmorphic disorder** (BDD) (see Chapter 9). Phillips et al.[8] found that up to a quarter of patients requiring orthognathic surgery have some forms of underlying psychiatric disorder.

> **Note:**
>
> **Considerations of priming effects**
>
> In this context, the term 'priming' refers to some cue from the patient provided in their history, such as a specific admission or information that induces the clinician to become potentially susceptible to misunderstanding or misapprehending further information from the patient, i.e. something the patient says is misinterpreted and affects the clinician's judgment for the rest of the interview. Psychologists refer to this as **associative activation**, e.g. if you have recently seen the word 'eat' or 'food', you are more likely to complete the word fragment SO_P as SOUP, whereas the word 'wash' would more likely lead you to complete the word fragment as SOAP.[9] The relevance to the patient interview is that the clinician should beware of incorrectly linking something the patient has said, relating it to the clinician's previous experience with other patients, and allowing that to colour their judgement throughout the rest of the interview. For example, a patient seeking orthognathic surgery informs the clinician that they are recently divorced. This is important information, but the clinician should not immediately think that the recent divorce is the only reason for the patient seeking treatment. The clinician should be careful not to become self-convinced of any issue until all the relevant information has been gathered and contemplated.

Motivation

> 'What you think of yourself is more important than what people think of you.'
>
> Persian proverb

Patients who demonstrate **external (extrinsic) motivation** for seeking orthognathic treatment, e.g. the desire to obtain a promotion or find a partner, are less likely to be happy with the results of treatment than those who have **internal (intrinsic) motivation**, i.e. they desire an improved facial appearance or function for themselves. The clinician should listen carefully for clues and cues from the patient during the interview. Sir William Kelsey Fry (1889–1963) (see Figure 2.99A), the pioneering dental and oral surgeon who, with Sir Harold Gillies, was one of the founders of British maxillofacial and plastic surgery, always stressed the importance of listening intently to patients during a consultation:[10]

> 'God gave you ears, eyes and hands; use them on the patient in that order.'

Expectation(s)

Socially well-adjusted patients with relatively stable lives and realistic expectations are likely to benefit from treatment. However, patients with **unrealistic expectations**, both in terms of the potential aesthetic result of treatment *and* the potential effects of treatment on their life (e.g. assuming better job prospects), will inevitably be unhappy with the results of treatment. It is important for the clinician not to downplay issues such as the prolonged length of treatment and potential complications. Skirting around or soft-pedalling these issues is not in the patient's best interests in the long-term. It is also vitally important not to over-promise a result, but to inform the patient of the likely result that may be realistically achieved, e.g. patients with facial asymmetries must comprehend that their postoperative result will never be perfectly symmetrical.

Cooperation

The likely level of cooperation must be gauged by the clinician during the interview process.[11] Orthognathic surgery is prolonged and requires a considerable commitment from the patient, and often their family. The **risk/cost benefit considerations** of proposed orthognathic treatment compared to alternatives such as orthodontic camouflage, surgical camouflage or no treatment must be considered and discussed until the clinician is comfortable that the patient understands the pros and cons of each approach.

> **Note:**
>
> **Risk/cost vs. benefit considerations**
> An open and honest discussion regarding the risk/cost vs. benefit considerations of orthognathic treatment is mandatory (see Chapter 11).

> Clinicians should remember that *what you tell a patient before treatment is sound professional advice; what you tell them after treatment is viewed as an excuse.* Both the orthodontist and surgeon should be absolutely candid and unambiguous about the details and potential risks of treatment, even if such information causes the patient to decline treatment. The orthognathic surgical pathway is a lot to go through for any patient, though patient satisfaction with the results of treatment tends to be high (see Chapter 20). The patient should be fully aware of the potential **risks** associated with both the orthodontic treatment, e.g. decalcification, root resorption etc., and the surgery (see Chapter 10). The surgical risks involve those that are short term and very likely to occur, e.g. postoperative discomfort, oedema, trismus, difficulty eating etc., and those that may be long-term, e.g. altered sensation or loss of sensation to the lower lip and chin. The **cost** of treatment does not equate to monetary cost in the UK National Health Service, but to the imposition of treatment on a patient's daily life, i.e. the **inconveniences** and **sacrifices** required of the patient in undergoing treatment, both in terms of **social costs**, e.g. time off school, university or work, the potential social impact of having fixed orthodontic appliances on a long-term basis, extra effort required in maintaining a very high standard of oral hygiene, avoidance of certain dietary products due to having an orthodontic appliance, and **emotional costs**, such as acceptance of the initial worsening of the dentofacial appearance following orthodontic decompensation. Only when the balance between risks/costs and benefits has been discussed unequivocally with the patient and the proposed treatment has a high likelihood of success should treatment proceed.

Support network

The importance of a patient's **social support network**, particularly **family support**, should never be underestimated. The clinician should meet and gauge the support and feelings of the immediate family. Ideally, parents and spouses should be collaborators in the treatment, providing much needed emotional support for patients. This is particularly important during the high-stress chapters of the treatment process, e.g. the week before and the first few weeks after surgery. However, parents or spouses may not want the patient to undergo treatment for a variety of reasons. If full family support is not obvious, it is important for the reasons to be explored until some form of consensus is reached before instigating treatment.

Medical history

A thorough medical history is mandatory (see Chapter 14). Standardized, self-administered questionnaires may be helpful in encouraging more truthful responses to sensitive questions. Patients may complete such a questionnaire prior to the consultation, though the responses must be double-checked by the clinician, ideally at the end of the consultation when rapport has been built.[3]

For the orthognathic patient, particularly relevant aspects of the medical history are past or present **psychological or psychiatric illness**, **anxiety** and **depression** or any **body image disturbances**, such as anorexia or bulimia nervosa.[3] In addition, any medical condition that may affect subsequent surgical treatment should be noted, and where required, confirmation sought from the general medical practitioner.

Suitability for orthognathic treatment

At the end of the consultation the patient should always be given an opportunity to ask any questions. *It is useful to actively ask the patient if they have any questions*, as the patient may be anxious or perhaps even somewhat intimidated by the clinical environment, particularly when trainees are present on a teaching clinic.

At the end of the initial consultation and interview the patient should be given information leaflets about potential treatment options and any other sources of information that the clinician feels may be useful (see Chapter 10). So long as no major 'red flag' signs are noted, a **second consultation interview** may be arranged. The patient should also be asked to write down any further questions they may think of and bring these to the second consultation. *A reasonable time between the initial and second interview should be provided, permitting a period of contemplation for the patient and their family.*

At the second interview, it is always useful to ask the patient to briefly summarise the information provided at the first interview by the clinician. Although a patient should not be expected to remember everything discussed at the initial interview, if they demonstrate an overly confused recollection of the information previously provided, demonstrate a preference to gloss over the potential downsides of orthognathic treatment (such as the prolonged length of treatment or possible complications), appear somewhat bewildered, or provide vague or odd answers, this in itself may be a cause for concern. If it is decided that the patient will benefit both functionally and aesthetically from orthognathic surgical treatment, *the bottom line for the clinician is whether the patient is psychologically and emotionally suitable for treatment*. If having completed the consultation interviews the clinician has any doubt regarding whether to accept a patient for treatment, any feeling of bravery on the part of the clinician is best tempered by caution.

If an underlying psychological issue is suspected, the patient should be informed in a straightforward and polite way that the clinician is acting in their best interest, and referral to a clinical psychologist or liaison psychiatrist may be arranged (see Chapter 9).

If the patient is suitable for treatment, any further records may be taken at this appointment, and arrangements made to see the patient on the 'joint clinic'.

Clinical diagnostic records

> 'It is not difficult to find a solution to a problem; it is only difficult to identify the problem.'
>
> Hugo Obwegeser[12]

Accurate diagnostic records are an important supplemental tool to clinical patient evaluation in orthognathic surgery.[13]

Purpose of clinical records

Clinical records are required for:

- **Diagnosis** – provide additional data to the clinical evaluation.
- **Treatment planning** – preliminary records are required to help form a tentative plan prior to orthodontic preparation. The preoperative records are vital for accurate preoperative planning.
- **Treatment analysis** – analysis of treatment results by comparing pretreatment, preoperative and postoperative records is important in evaluating the effects of treatment, whether the objectives were met, and to help improve future treatment strategies for similar patients.
- **Patient communication.**
- **Teaching, audit and research.**
- **Medicolegal documentation.**

Mandatory records for orthognathic surgery

A number of records are mandatory for the orthognathic surgical patient.

Orthopantomograph (OPT)

The **rotational tomograph** is alternatively termed the **dental panoramic tomograph (DPT)**. As the name suggests it is very useful for an overall assessment of dental development, but also particularly useful for analysing mandibular asymmetry (see Chapter 34).

Lateral cephalometric radiograph

This vitally important **diagnostic and planning tool** is a specific lateral skull radiograph, which provides standardized and reproducible images due to the use of a head-holding device termed a cephalostat (Figure 5-2). **Serial cephalometric radiographs** are useful for **monitoring craniofacial growth changes**, in particular the direction of jaw growth, and for **monitoring treatment changes**.

(a) (b)

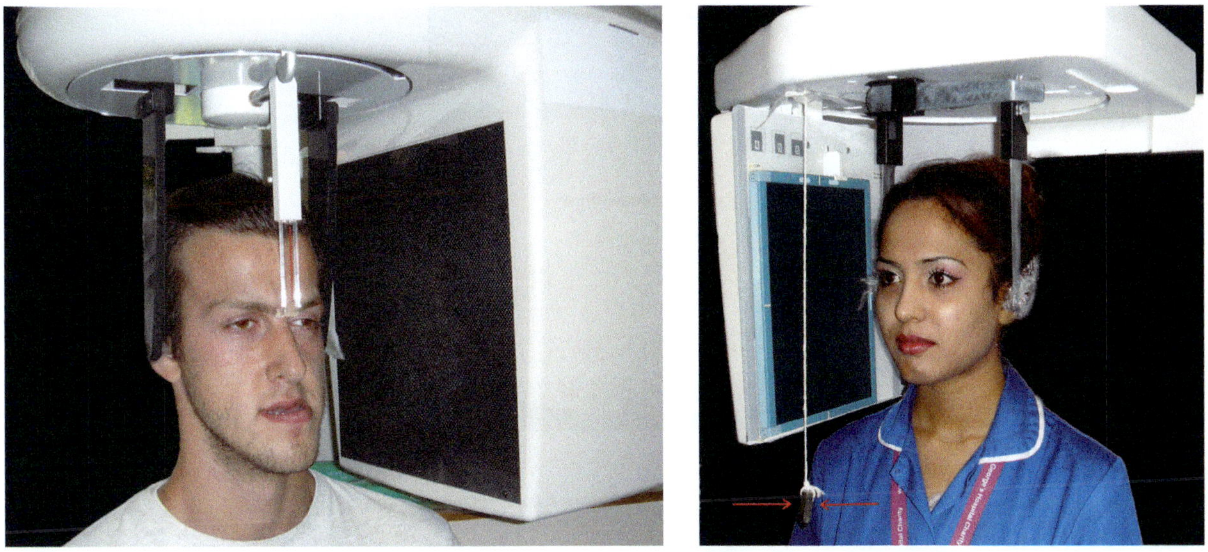

Fig. 5-2 (a) Head-holding device known as the cephalostat. (b) Modified technique for taking the lateral cephalometric radiograph, with the patient in natural head position (NHP), and using a plumb (shown with red arrow) and plumb line, which will appear on the cephalometric radiograph and act as the true vertical (see Figure 5-14).

Clinical photographs

Extraoral and intraoral colour photographs are required at the start of treatment, at the preoperative stage and at the end of treatment. Intraoperative photographs are also useful. Photographs are used for both diagnosis and planning, monitoring treatment progress and changes, and as a form of medicolegal documentation.

Study models

Dental study casts, or study models, are required in any patient undergoing orthognathic surgery involving planned alteration of the dental occlusion, or craniofacial surgery involving movement of the jaws. The impressions should be fully extended into the labial and buccal sulci and record all the erupted teeth. The models are trimmed in a special way, referred to as **Angle's trimmed**, so that the bases are symmetrical, enabling the occlusion to be evaluated at varying angles with the models placed on a flat surface and making it easier to analyse arch form and symmetry (Figure 5-3). Preoperative **'snap' study models** may be hand articulated into the proposed postoperative dental occlusion, in order to assess arch coordination and potential occlusal interferences (Figure 5-4).

In patients requiring *maxillary* orthognathic surgery, the preoperative models may be mounted onto an **adjustable articulator** (a mechanical device that represents the temporomandibular joints, to which the maxillary and mandibular casts are attached, with the intention of reproducing mandibular movements), using a **facebow transfer** (a facebow is a device used to record the relationship of the maxillary dental arch to the condylar hinge axis of the temporomandibular joints), in order to permit model surgery and splint wafer fabrication (see Chapter 13).

Anthropometric measurements

> 'If you cannot measure it, you cannot improve it.'
>
> William Thomson, Lord Kelvin (1824–1907)[14]

Many craniofacial measurements may be obtained from the cephalometric radiographs and study models. However, a number of initial baseline anthropometric measurements, as well as preoperative and postoperative measurements may be very helpful in

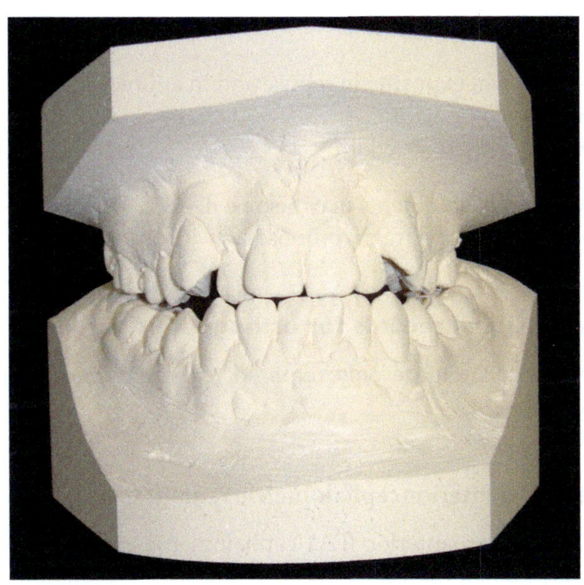

Fig. 5-3 Angle's trimmed pretreatment study models.

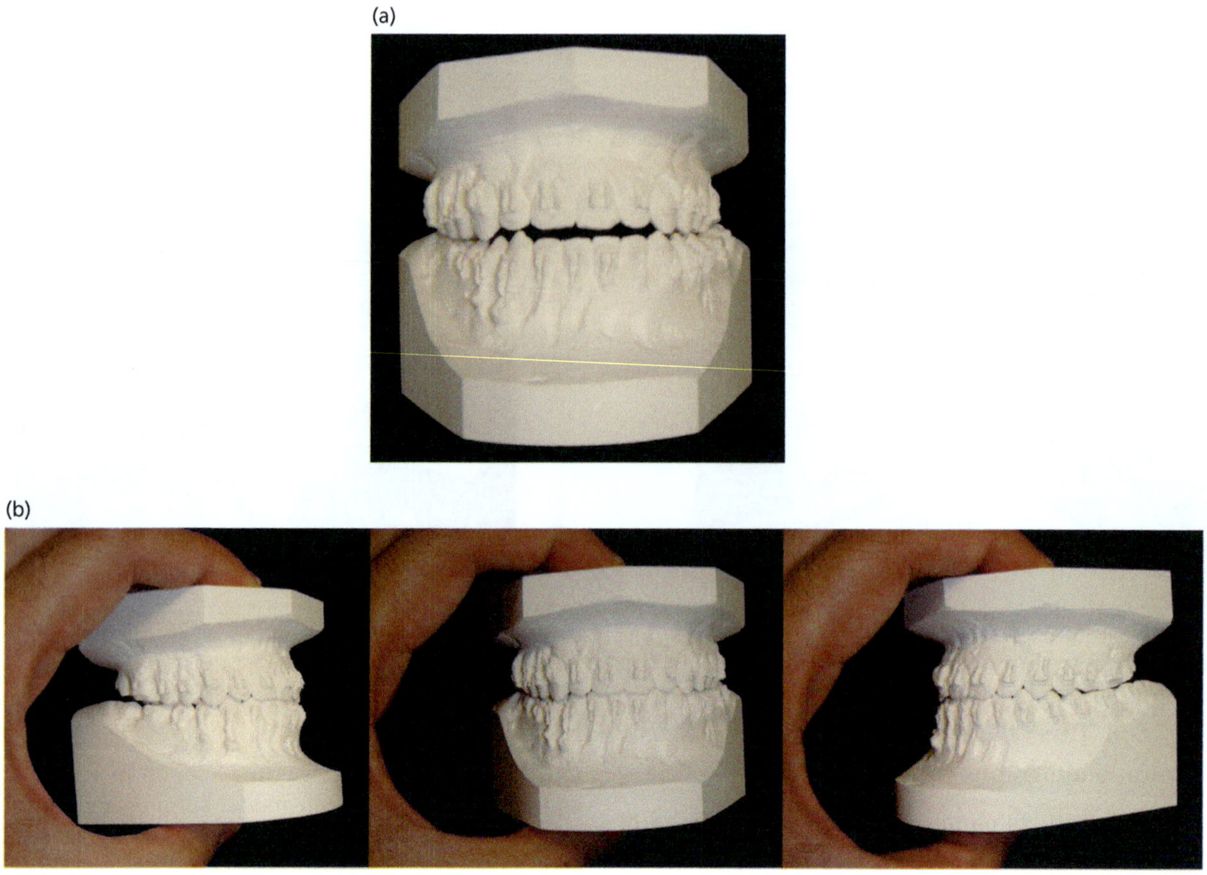

Fig. 5-4 (a) Preoperative 'snap' study models of a Class III patient with an anterior open bite. (b) Hand articulating the 'snap' models to assess proposed postoperative arch coordination and potential occlusal interferences.

analysing treatment effects and results. Anthropometric measurements may be taken with anthropometric precision instruments, such as the **spreading caliper** and **sliding caliper**, or alternatively with a **ruler** and a **compass divider caliper** (Figure 5-5). The following anthropometric measurements are particularly useful when maxillary surgery is proposed:

- Upper lip height
- Maxillary incisor exposure in repose and in animation
- Gingival exposure in repose and in animation
- Nasal base width
- Nasal interalar width

Other measurements may also be desired, depending on the type of surgery proposed.[13]

Additional records for orthognathic surgery

Some records are only required for specific orthognathic cases.

Posteroanterior cephalometric radiograph

The posteroanterior (PA) cephalometric radiograph may be helpful as an adjunct to clinical evaluation in patients with skeletal facial asymmetry.

Computed tomography (CT)

CT is a technique that may be used to generate a detailed three-dimensional (3D) image of both the dentoskeletal complex and enveloping facial soft tissues. The skeletal images may be used to create 3D stereolithographic models, which are particularly useful in planning complex craniofacial surgery. Cone beam CT is a useful technological adjunct and is described in detail in Chapter 8.

3D facial soft tissue scans

The potential for combining 3D soft tissue scans with a dentoskeletal CT is attractive for planning purposes. Systems are currently under development (see Chapter 6).

Serial height measurements

For the younger patient contemplating potential orthognathic surgery, serial height measurements may provide an indication of **growth cessation**, as growth in standing height is well correlated with jaw growth.

Weight and height measurements

The **body mass index (BMI)** is a measure of *relative weight* based on an individual's mass and height. It

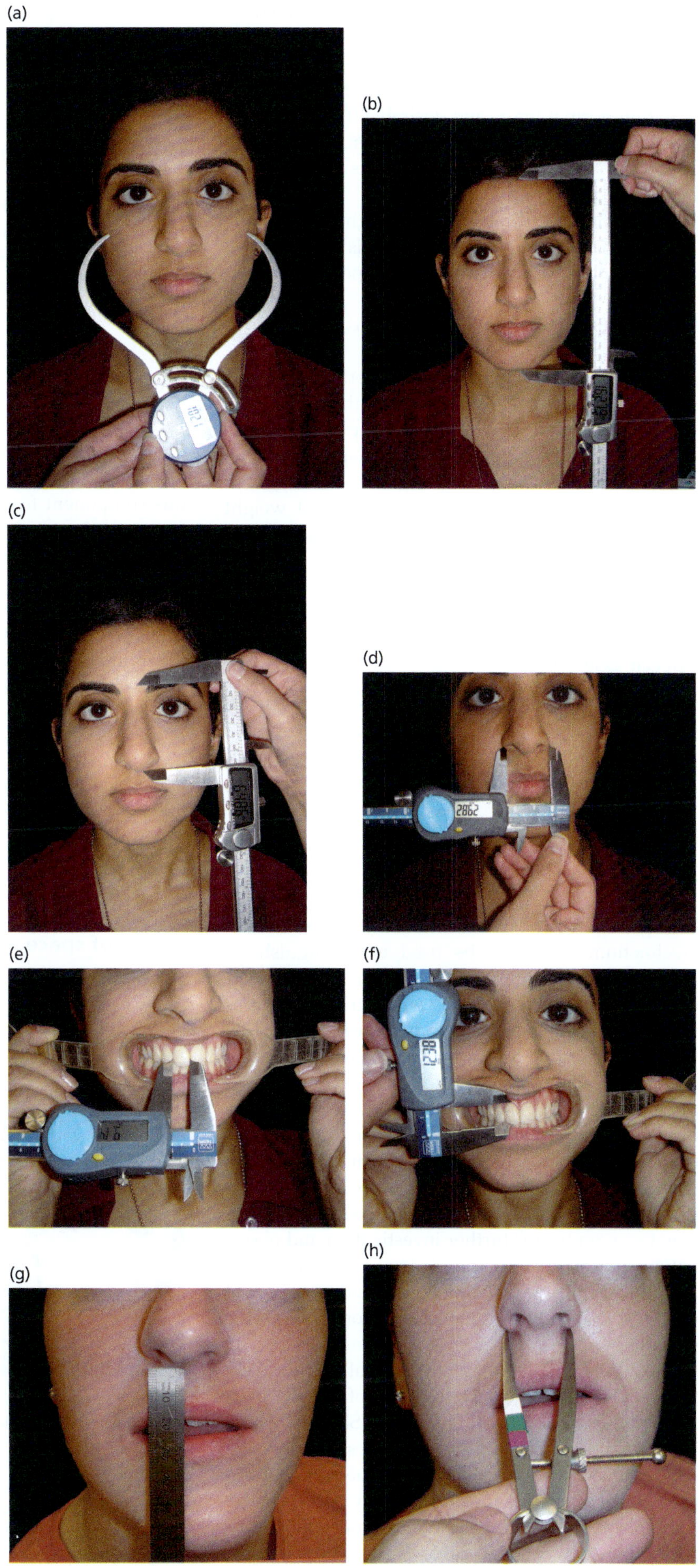

Fig. 5-5 Examples of anthropometric measurements: (a) The arms of spreading calipers are curved, allowing the instrument to fit round larger curved regions of the face. (b) The sliding caliper to measure total face height. (c) Measuring midfacial height with a sliding caliper. (d) Measuring nasal base width with a sliding caliper. (e) Measuring maxillary incisor crown width; the tips of the caliper have been thinned with a stone to improve the accuracy of measurements. (f) Measuring maxillary incisor crown height with a sliding caliper. (g) Measuring upper lip height and maxillary incisor exposure in repose with a ruler. (h) Measuring nasal base width with a divider caliper.

is defined as the individual's body mass divided by the square of their height. The BMI is used in a wide variety of contexts as a simple method to assess how much an individual's body weight departs from what is within normal limits and desirable (from a clinical point of view) for a person of his or her height.

The current BMI value settings are as follows:

- 18.5 to 25 may indicate optimal weight.
- Lower than 18.5 suggests the person is underweight.
- Greater than 25 may indicate the person is overweight.
- Greater than 30 suggests the person is obese.

However, these are only guidelines. Perhaps the most useful aspect of the BMI is to allow the clinician to discuss overweight and underweight problems more objectively with their patients (see Chapter 10). *Baseline measurements of height and weight* should be undertaken pretreatment and preoperatively, and weight measurements should be monitored postoperatively (usually by the patient, unless there is a specific concern).

Speech assessment

Preoperative speech assessment by a speech and language therapist is rarely required in orthognathic surgery, except in cleft patients, particularly where large maxillary advancements are planned (see Chapter 56).

Nuclear medicine (scintigraphy)

The gamma-emitting, bone seeking isotope ^{99m}Tc (Technetium-99m) may be used to distinguish an active rapidly growing condyle from the contralateral condyle in patients with asymmetrical mandibular growth due to unilateral condylar overgrowth. This short-lived isotope becomes concentrated in areas of active bone deposition, such as the alveolar ridges during the eruption of the teeth. The condyles are not normally areas of intense imaging and a 'hot' condyle is evidence of active condylar growth. This technique cannot by itself rule out excessive unilateral condylar growth as false negatives do occur. A negative scan means further investigation and observation of growth is required. However, false positive images are rare. Therefore, a positive unilateral condylar 'hot spot' is a good indication of excessive growth.

More recent and potentially useful advances in nuclear imaging include the use of single photon emission computed tomography (SPECT), which increases image contrast and improves lesion detection and localization.[15] The technique has demonstrated enhanced diagnostic accuracy for condylar hyperplasia and hemimandibular hyperplasia compared with conventional planar ^{99m}Tc scanning.[16]

Patient evaluation – the basics

'The eye sees only what the mind is prepared to comprehend.'
Robertson Davies (1913–1995)[17]
Canadian author and man or letters

Prior to instigating the clinical patient evaluation, it is important to discuss two important principles in facial aesthetic analysis. The first is an understanding of the **modified subunit principle**, and the second is how each craniofacial unit and subunit is positioned relative to the **three planes of space** and the **three axes of rotation**.[2]

Modified subunit principle

Facial beauty has been defined as 'the assemblage of graceful features that pleases the eye and mind of an observer'.[18] The **assemblage** describes how the various component features fit together, *like a mosaic*, to form each face. As such, the craniofacial complex may be thought of as being comprised of a number of **units** and each unit as being comprised of a number of **subunits**. It is useful to think of the units and subunits as cranio-dento-skeletal elements, which form the framework for their overlying soft tissue units and subunits.[2] *Each subunit is essentially a part of the craniofacial complex that may be independently altered with treatment* (Figure 5-6).[2] For example, the smallest subunit of the maxillary complex is the maxillary central incisor, which may be moved in relation to the three planes of space and in relation to the three axes of rotation, independently of the rest of the craniofacial complex.

Planes of space and axes of rotation

The entire craniofacial complex and the relative position of each facial unit and its constituent subunits

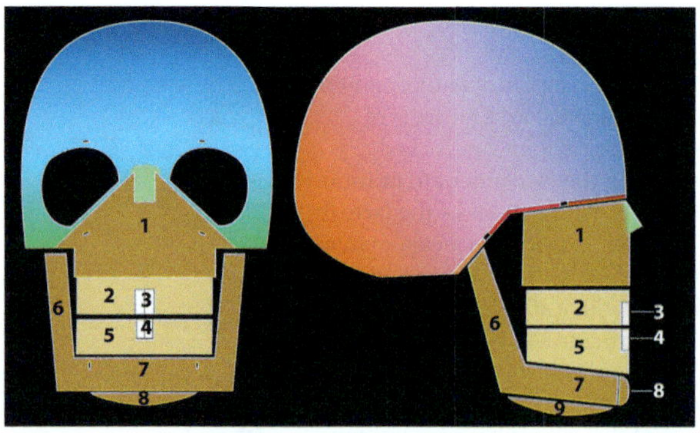

Fig. 5-6 Dentoskeletal subunits of the bimaxillary complex. 1. Nasomaxillary complex. 2. Maxillary dentoalveolus. 3. Maxillary incisors. 4. Mandibular incisors. 5. Mandibular dentoalveolus. 6. Mandibular ramus. 7. Mandibular body (corpus). 8. Mandibular symphysis (osseous chin). 9. Inferior border of the mandible. (From: Naini FB. Facial Aesthetics: Concepts and Clinical Diagnosis. Oxford: Wiley-Blackwell, 2011; modified and reprinted with permission.)

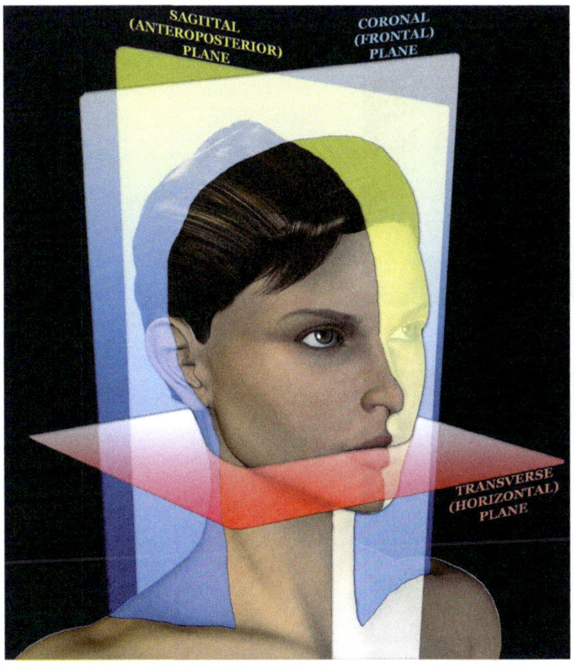

Fig. 5-7 The facial planes. (From: Naini FB. Facial Aesthetics: Concepts and Clinical Diagnosis. Oxford: Wiley-Blackwell, 2011; reprinted with permission.)

may be evaluated in relation to the **three planes of space** (Figure 5-7):

- Sagittal (anteroposterior) plane
- Coronal (frontal) plane
- Transverse (horizontal) plane

In addition, the structural relationships and potential surgical and/or orthodontic movements of the component parts of the craniofacial complex may be described in relation to the **three axes of rotation** (Figure 5-8a–c):

- Sagittal (anteroposterior) axis
- Vertical (longitudinal) axis
- Transverse axis

A useful illustrative example may be described in relation to the maxilla. If the maxillary dental arch is level, the maxillary occlusal plane may be thought of as an imaginary table top on which the maxillary dentition sits. Therefore, in relation to the three planes of space, the maxilla and maxillary occlusal plane may be too far forward (prognathic) or back (retrognathic), too far up (vertical maxillary deficiency) or down (vertical maxillary excess), too far to the left or right (an asymmetry due to bodily translation to the left or right). In relation to the three axes of rotation, the maxilla and maxillary occlusal plane may be rotated round the sagittal axis (i.e. leading to a transverse cant of the maxillary occlusal plane), rotated round the vertical axis (leading to a midline deviation due to rotation of the jaw), or rotated round the transverse axis, (i.e. posterior aspect at a different vertical level to the anterior) (Figure 5-9).

Every craniofacial unit and subunit may be thought of in the same way.

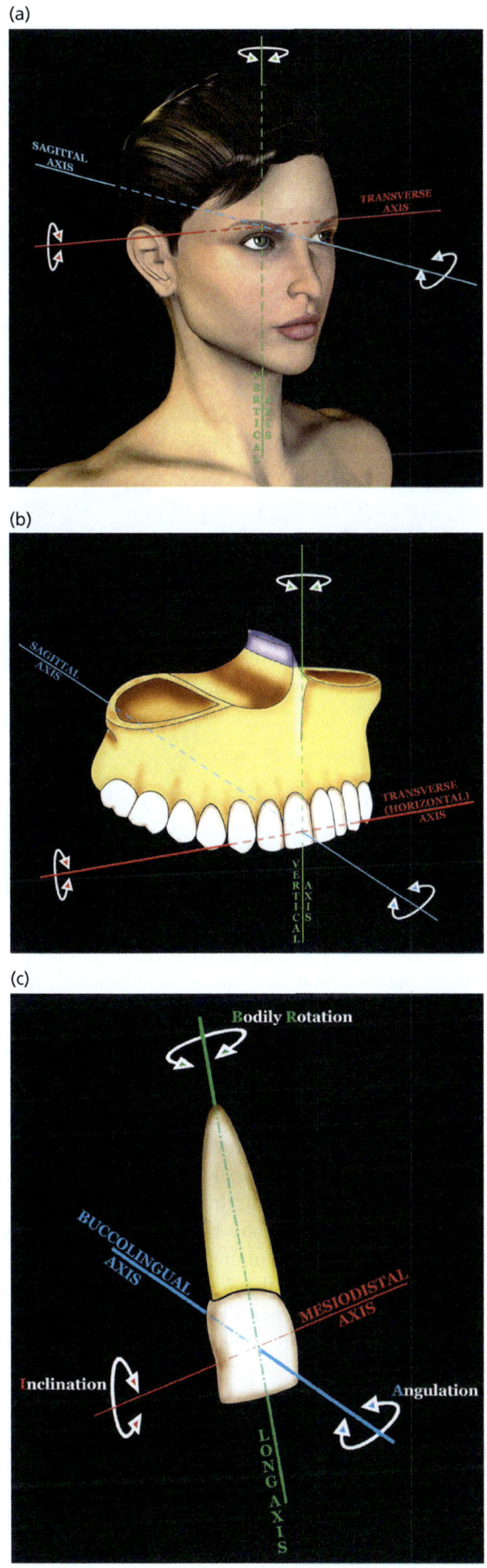

Fig. 5-8 (a) The axes of rotation. (b) Maxillary rotation around the three axes of rotation. (c) Maxillary incisor rotation around the three axes of rotation. (From: Naini FB. Facial Aesthetics: Concepts and Clinical Diagnosis. Oxford: Wiley-Blackwell, 2011; reprinted with permission.)

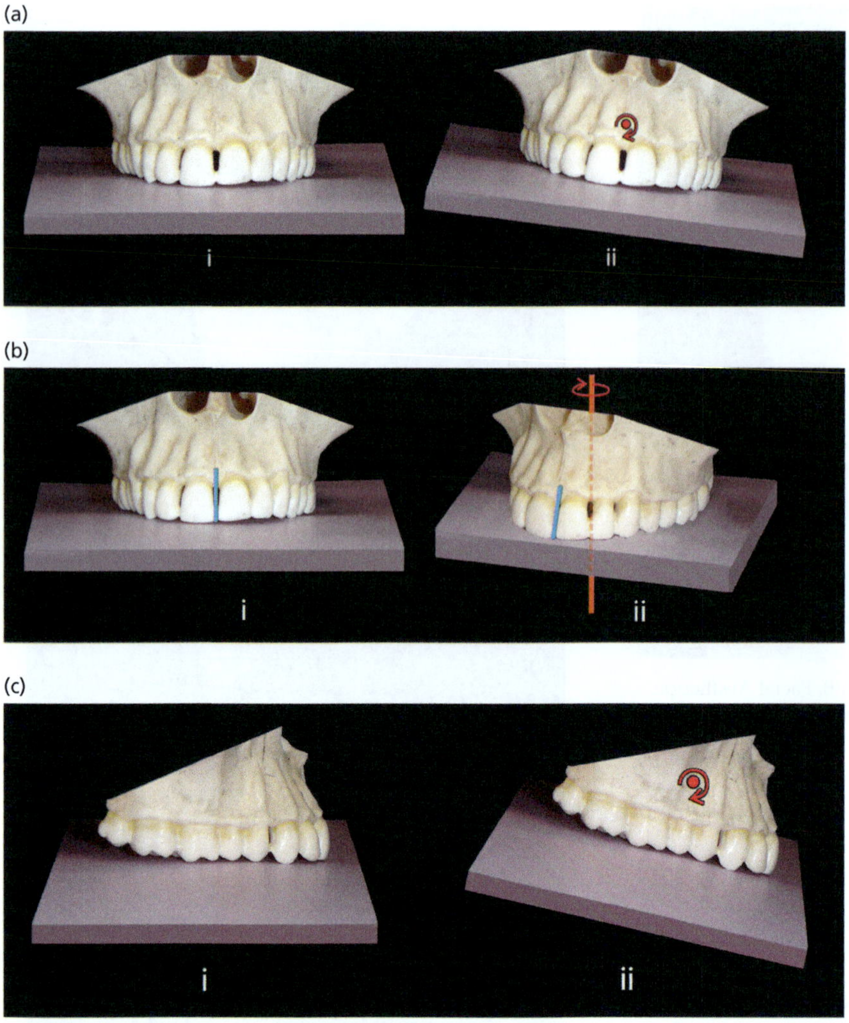

Fig. 5-9 Rotation of the maxilla and maxillary occlusal plane round the axes of rotation: (a) Rotation round the sagittal axis, leading to a transverse cant of the maxillary occlusal plane. (b) Rotation round the vertical axis, leading to a maxillary dental midline deviation. (c) Rotation round the transverse axis, leading to a difference in the vertical level of the anterior and posterior regions of the maxillary occlusal plane.

Evaluation in repose and animation

> 'What sunshine is to flowers, smiles are to humanity. These are but trifles, to be sure; but scattered along life's pathways, the good they do is inconceivable.'
>
> Joseph Addison (1672–1719) (attributed)

Patients should be evaluated with their facial soft tissues in repose, but also in the animated states of speech and smiling. Mandibular incisor exposure tends to be greater in speech, and this increases with age; the degree of exposure may be observed in normal speech. A number of parameters should be evaluated in smiling, in particular the degree of elevation of the upper lip and resultant maxillary incisor and gingival exposure, and the width of the smile (see below and Chapter 7).

Cephalometric landmarks and definitions

Facial aesthetic analysis and both two-dimensional and three-dimensional cephalometric analysis require a thorough familiarity with anthropometric and cephalometric landmark locations and their definitions. A thorough description of anthropometric and cephalometric landmarks, lines, planes and volumes has been provided elsewhere.[19] Relevant anthropometric landmarks are defined throughout the rest of this chapter as they arise, but in terms of orthognathic surgery the most relevant skeletal and soft tissue landmarks are presented in Figures 5-10 (definitions in Table 5-1) and 5-11 (definitions in Table 5-2).

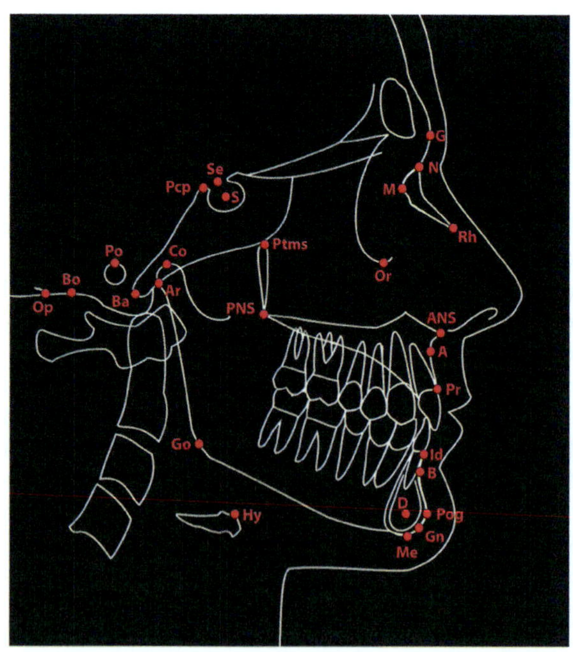

Fig. 5-10 Hard tissue (skeletal) lateral cephalometric landmarks (see Table 5-1 for definitions).

Table 5-1 Hard tissue lateral cephalometric (skeletal) landmarks (Figure 5-10).

Landmark (abbreviation)	Definition
Anterior facial landmarks (from superior to inferior)	
Glabella (G)	The most prominent point of the anterior contour of the frontal bone in the midsagittal plane, in the supraorbital and frontal sinus region
Nasion (N or Na)	The intersection of the internasal and frontonasal sutures, in the midsagittal plane
Frontonasomaxillary point (FNM or M-point)	The point at the junction of the nasofrontal and nasomaxillary sutures, designated as M-point by the craniofacial surgeon Jean Delaire; it is used to construct the 'superior cranial base line' by joining M-point with the apex of the posterior clinoid process (Pcp) in the Delaire craniofacial analysis.
Orbitale (Or)	The lowest point on the inferior orbital rim (bilateral)
Anterior nasal spine (ANS)	The tip of the bony anterior nasal spine; this point corresponds to the anthropological point 'acanthion'
A-point (Point A; subspinale)	The point at the deepest midline concavity on the maxillary *alveolus* between anterior nasal spine and prosthion
Prosthion (Pr; Supradentale, Sd)	The most inferior anterior point on the maxillary alveolar process, between the maxillary central incisors, in the midsagittal plane
Infradentale (Id)	The most superior anterior point on the mandibular alveolar process, between the mandibular central incisors, in the midsagittal plane
B-point (Point B; supramentale)	The point at the deepest midline concavity on the mandibular *alveolus* between infradentale and pogonion
D-point (point D)	This is the centre of the body of the mandibular symphysis (bony chin) in the midsagittal plane and is estimated visually. The angle SND was described by the orthodontist Cecil Steiner to provide an assessment of the sagittal position of the **mandibular skeletal base** in relation to the anterior cranial base.
Pogonion (Pog)	The most anterior point on the contour of the mandibular symphysis, in the midsagittal plane
Gnathion (Gn)	The most anterior inferior point on the mandibular symphysis (bony chin), in the midsagittal plane. It may be determined by inspection, or constructed as the point of intersection of a vertical tangent to pogonion and a horizontal tangent to menton, extending the bisector through the anterior inferior curvature of the mandibular symphysis
Menton (Me)	The most inferior point of the mandibular symphysis, in the midsagittal plane
Posterior facial landmarks (approximately from superior to inferior)	
Sella entrance point (Se)	The midpoint of the entrance to the sella turcica
Sella (S)	The point representing the geometric centre of the pituitary fossa (sella turcica), in the midsagittal plane
Porion (Po)	The 'anatomical' porion is the most superior point of the outline of the external auditory meatus (bilateral). The use of ear rods in the cephalostat often makes anatomic porion difficult to locate, in which case the superior margin of the glenoid fossa of the temporomandibular joint that lies at the same level may be substituted for constructing the Frankfort plane. The term 'machine' porion refers to the most superior point of the image of the ear rods, which some authorities use as an alterative
Condylion (Co)	The most posterior superior point on the head of the mandibular condyle (bilateral)
Condylar midpoint (Con)	This is the arbitrary centre of the mandibular condyle in lateral view; it is estimated visually (alternative term is **capitulare**). An imaginary line through point Con of both mandibular condyles forms the **condylar hinge axis** around which the mandible may rotate during the initial part of the opening movement.
Articulare (Ar)	The point of intersection of the images of the posterior border of the mandibular ramus and the inferior border of the basilar part of the occipital bone (bilateral). It may be used as a substitute for condylion if the latter is not readily discernible; articulare is often the most superior point on the mandibular ramus that can be consistently identified. It was defined by the orthodontist Arne Björk. Any opening or closing movements of the mandible will alter its position.
Basion (Ba)	The most inferior point on the anterior margin of the foramen magnum, in the midsagittal plane
Opisthion (Op)	The most inferior point on the posterior margin of the foramen magnum, in the midsagittal plane
Bolton point (Bo)	The highest point on the upward curvature of the outlines of the retrocondylar fossae of the occipital bone, approximating the centre of the foramen magnum; named by the orthodontist Birdsall Holly Broadbent in honour of the philanthropist Charles B. Bolton
Pterygomaxillare superius (Ptms)	The pterygomaxillary fissure is a bilateral teardrop-shaped area of radiolucency, the anterior surface of which represents the posterior surfaces of the maxillary tuberosities. The landmark is the most superior point of the pterygomaxillary fissure (bilateral)
Pterygomaxillare (Ptm)	The most inferior point at the junction of the anterior and posterior borders of the pterygomaxillary fissure (bilateral); this point is in very close proximity to PNS
Posterior nasal spine (PNS)	The most posterior point on the bony hard palate, in the midsagittal plane. It may be located by extending the anterior wall of the pterygomaxillary fissure inferiorly to intersect the hard palate
Gonion (Go)	The most inferior posterior point on the contour of the angle of the mandible (gonial angle). It may be determined by inspection, or constructed as the point of intersection of the posterior ramal plane and mandibular plane, extending the bisector through the curvature of the gonial region of the mandible (bilateral)
Hyoid point (Hy)	The most anterior superior point on the body of the hyoid bone, also termed hyoidale

Used with permission from *Facial Aesthetics: Concepts and Clinical Diagnosis*.[2]

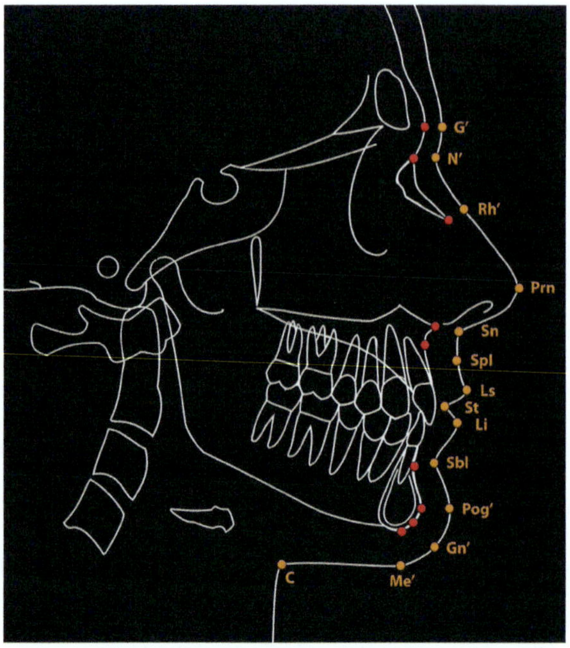

Fig. 5-11 Soft tissue lateral cephalometric landmarks (see Table 5-2 for definitions).

Table 5-2 Soft tissue lateral cephalometric landmarks (Figure 5-11).

Landmark (abbreviation)	Definition
Glabella (G′)	The most prominent point of the soft tissue anterior contour of the forehead in the midsagittal plane, in the supraorbital brow ridge region, in the midsagittal plane
Nasion (N′ or Na′)	Cephalometric soft tissue nasion is *usually* the point of deepest concavity of the soft tissue contour of the root of the nose, in the midsagittal plane. Soft tissue nasion (N′) and skeletal nasion (N) should be at the same vertical level. In some individuals there is an anterior curvature of the superior portion of the nasal bones; in such patients the deepest point of the nasal radix is termed 'sellion' (or 'subnasion'), which is inferior and usually posterior to soft tissue nasion
Rhinion (Rh′)	The soft tissue point overlying the caudal end of the nasal bones in lateral view, marking the osseocartilaginous nasal junction
Pronasale (Prn)	The most prominent point of the nasal tip, in the midsagittal plane
Subnasale (Sn)	The point where the base of the nasal columella meets the upper lip, in the midsagittal plane
Soft tissue A-point (supralabiale, Spl)	The point of greatest concavity of the facial contour of the upper lip between subnasale and labrale superius, in the midsagittal plane
Labrale superius (Ls)	The point representing the mucocutaneous vermilion border of the upper lip, in the midsagittal plane
Stomion superius (Sts)	The most inferior point of the upper lip, in the midsagittal plane
Stomion (St)	The most anterior point of contact between the upper and lower lip, in the midsagittal plane. If the lips are held apart in repose, a superior and inferior stomion point may be distinguished
Stomion inferius (Sti)	The most superior point of the lower lip, in the midsagittal plane
Labrale inferius (Li)	The point representing the mucocutaneous vermilion border of the lower lip, in the midsagittal plane
Soft tissue B-point (sublabiale, Sbl)	The point of greatest concavity of the facial contour of the lower lip between labrale inferius and soft tissue menton. It is the deepest point of the mentolabial fold.
Pogonion (Pog′)	The most anterior point on the contour of the soft tissue chin, in the midsagittal plane
Gnathion (Gn′)	The most anterior inferior point on the soft tissue chin contour, in the midsagittal plane. It may be determined by inspection, or constructed as the point of intersection of a vertical tangent to soft tissue pogonion and a horizontal tangent to soft tissue menton, extending the bisector through the anterior inferior curvature of the soft tissue chin pad
Menton (Me′)	The most inferior point of the soft tissue chin, in the midsagittal plane
Cervical point (C)	The innermost point between the submental region and the anterior surface of the neck, in the midsagittal plane. It is located at the intersection of a horizontal tangent to the submental plane and a vertical tangent to the anterior neck plane

Used with permission from *Facial Aesthetics: Concepts and Clinical Diagnosis.*[2]

Systematic clinical evaluation

As already stated, comprehensive clinical facial aesthetic analysis and the wide array of cephalometric analyses have been described in detail elsewhere (presented in *Facial Aesthetics: Concepts and Clinical Diagnosis*).[2] Such information is extremely valuable in the understanding of craniofacial relationships, and for research purposes. However, the purpose of this section is not to reproduce all this information, but to provide a pragmatic approach to the initial patient evaluation. A logically ordered and step-by-step approach to clinical evaluation is more practical, effective and user-friendly. The emphasis is not so much on numerical measurements but on grasping the overall structural and proportional relationships that lead to an understanding of the morphology of the orthognathic patient.

> 'State first what you see; cultivate your powers of observation.'
>
> Sir William Osler (1849–1919)[20]

Diagnosis requires a *disciplined collection of objective information*. However, such factual information does not automatically lead to a diagnosis, just as a collection of specific words does not automatically form a rational sentence. It is the logical arrangement of these facts that allows the clinician to form a coherent picture, and the relative interrelationships of these objective facts forms the basis of accurate clinical diagnosis. In orthognathic surgery, *diagnosis is founded upon observation*. Therefore, it is incumbent upon the clinician to cultivate the habit of keen observation, always based on accurate scientific and artistic knowledge and background considerations.[2]

The diagnostic process

> 'Thoroughness is the most difficult habit to acquire.'
>
> Sir William Osler (1849–1919)[21]

It is only by the *systematic, accurate and thorough evaluation* of the craniofacial complex that factual information may be collected, which may then be logically ordered to form a diagnosis. *A methodical approach to diagnosis helps to avoid errors of omission on the part of the clinician.*

The clinical evaluation of the prospective orthognathic patient essentially consists of three consecutive stages:[2]

1. **Initial qualitative evaluation** (i.e. observe) – observation of the patient required to acquire preliminary data, albeit somewhat subjective.

> **Note:**
>
> The initial qualitative evaluation is based primarily on the **visual impression** formed from observation of the patient. At this stage, actual linear and angular measurements are not as important as the overall visual impression, and *notes made by the clinician should be qualitative*. For example, angular parameters may be visually separated into upper and lower components, and a qualitative decision made as to whether they are obtuse, average or acute (Figure 5-12). The initial, qualitative visual impression may subsequently be checked, using actual measurements, by clinical, photographic and cephalometric analysis.

2. **Quantitative analysis** (i.e. measure and analyse) – this stage requires anthropometric and cephalometric measurement and analysis.
3. **Subsequent qualitative evaluation** (i.e. re-observe) – assiduous and reflective re-observation of the patient in light of the previous findings.

The clinician must synthesize the data from the initial qualitative evaluation and the quantitative analysis. The question is 'does the subsequent qualitative evaluation corroborate the combined quantitative analysis and initial qualitative evaluation?' If it does, the descriptive clinical diagnosis may be made; if not, the process must be started again in order to find out where the discrepancy has arisen.

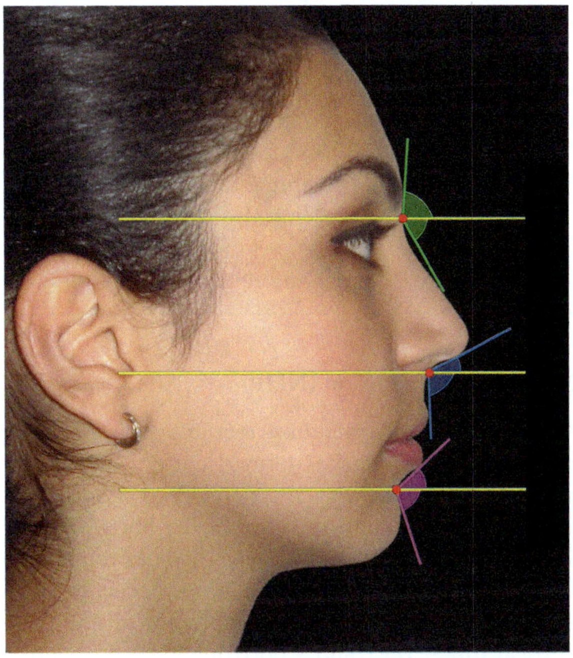

Fig. 5-12 Angular profile parameters may be visually separated into upper and lower components and a *qualitative* decision made as to whether they are obtuse, average or acute. The patient should be in natural head position. The nasofrontal, nasolabial and mentolabial angles are demonstrated separated into upper and lower components by a true horizontal line.

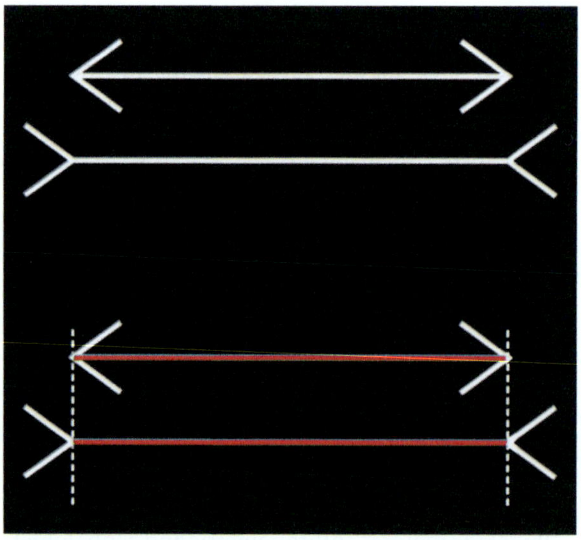

Fig. 5-13 Two sets of arrows that exhibit the Müller–Lyer optical illusion. The set on the bottom demonstrates that all the shafts of the arrows are of the same length.

Note:
It is important to measure and analyse, then re-observe

Despite the supreme importance of observation in clinical diagnosis, the consequence of not just accepting the results of the initial qualitative observation may be demonstrated by an optical illusion termed the **Müller–Lyer illusion**, devised by the German sociologist Franz Carl Müller-Lyer in 1889 (Figure 5-13). When viewing the two horizontal lines of apparently different lengths with appended fins pointing in opposite directions, it is clear that the bottom line is longer – that is the result of observation alone. However, measuring the lines clearly confirms that they are identical in length. This illusion illustrates the potential for misinterpreted perception that may occur from observation alone. In clinical diagnosis, potential illusional visual impressions may be mitigated by measurement, analysis and re-observation.

Natural head position (NHP)

Accurate clinical evaluation requires the patient to be positioned in what is termed natural head position (NHP).[22] NHP may be defined as a standardized and reproducible position of the head in space when the subject is focusing on a distant point at eye level. In NHP, the visual axis is thought to be horizontal. This allows an extracranial vertical line (**true vertical line – TrV**), and a horizontal line perpendicular to that vertical (**true horizontal line – TrH**), to be used as reference lines for facial aesthetic analysis (Figure 5-14).[13] This is important as the inclination or sagittal cant of all anatomical reference lines and planes, such as the Frankfort plane, is subject to biological variation.[13,23] This is particularly important

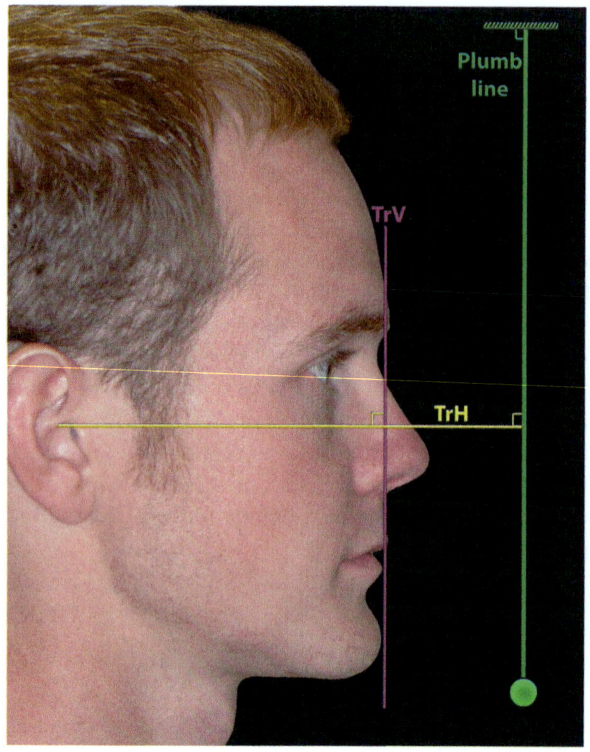

Fig. 5-14 A patient in natural head position (NHP), demonstrating the true facial vertical (TrV) and true horizontal (TrH) lines used to evaluate facial aesthetics. The true vertical may be taken as a line parallel to a plumb line hanging from the ceiling. The true horizontal will be at right angles to this. In some patients the Frankfort plane may be parallel to the true horizontal; however the inclination of the Frankfort plane is subject to individual variability. (From: Naini FB. Facial Aesthetics: Concepts and Clinical Diagnosis. Oxford: Wiley-Blackwell, 2011; reprinted with permission.)

in the orthognathic and craniofacial surgical patient, as the greater the aberration in craniofacial morphology from the average, the more likely that anatomical reference planes will not be horizontal (Figure 5-15).[24] The logical progression to the use of anatomical reference planes is to take facial photographs and cephalometric radiographs with the patient in physiological NHP (with the subject standing upright and looking straight ahead into the image of his/her own eyes in a small mirror located at a distance, at the level of the eyes) and to derive a true horizontal plane and a true vertical plane to which all the craniofacial structures may be related.[13]

For the clinical evaluation, the patient should be asked to stand relaxed, with their head in the most natural position for them, while looking straight ahead.

Viewing (observational) position and distance

A practical viewing position is required for the initial qualitative facial evaluation. The patient should be examined in natural head position (NHP), and their head should be level with that of the clinician. Ideally, the patient and clinician may stand facing one another, unless there is a significant height difference, in which case one or both may be seated on adjustable seats, whilst maintaining the patient's head in NHP. An

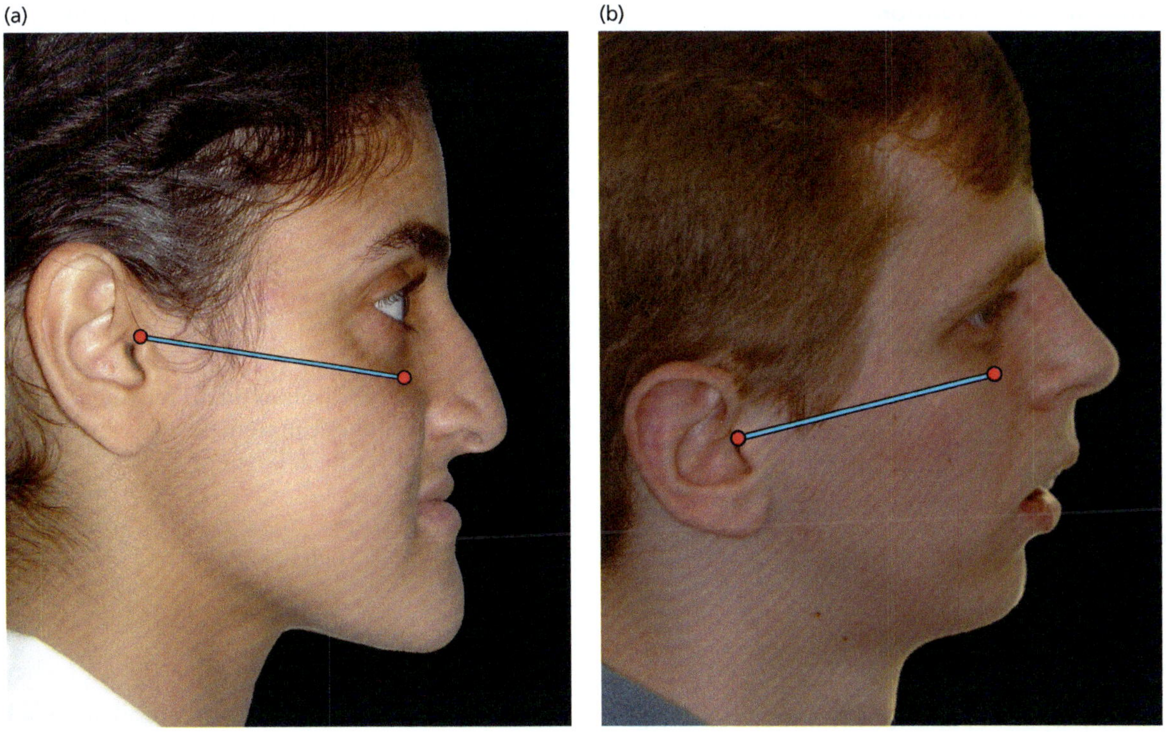

Fig. 5-15 (a) Facial profile of a patient with a significant Class III jaw relationship in natural head position (NHP), demonstrating a marked downward inclination of the Frankfort plane in relation to the true horizontal. (b) Facial profile of a patient with a significant Class II jaw relationship in natural head position (NHP), demonstrating a marked upward inclination of the Frankfort plane in relation to the true horizontal.

initial viewing distance of approximately 1 metre is recommended.

Note:

Anamorphosis – a word of caution

The importance of a correct viewing position of the clinician in relation to the patient may be illustrated by describing an optical illusion. In art, **anamorphosis** refers to a distorted projection or perspective requiring the viewer to occupy a specific vantage point to reconstitute the image. One of the earliest known definitive examples of perspective anamorphosis was drawn by Leonardo da Vinci, and is known as *Leonardo's eye* (c. 1485), which only appears as an eye when viewed from a specific position (Figure 5-16). The point is simple; *if you view the object from an incorrect position, the image will appear distorted*. The relevance of this point to clinical evaluation is clear, in that any aspect of the craniofacial complex may appear distorted if viewed from an odd angle, e.g. the patient lying flat and the clinician looking obliquely from above and behind.

For example, dental midline deviations should be evaluated from the frontal view. Clinicians will be aware that a dental midline deviation often appears somewhat different when viewed from above and behind the patient compared to being viewed from the frontal aspect.

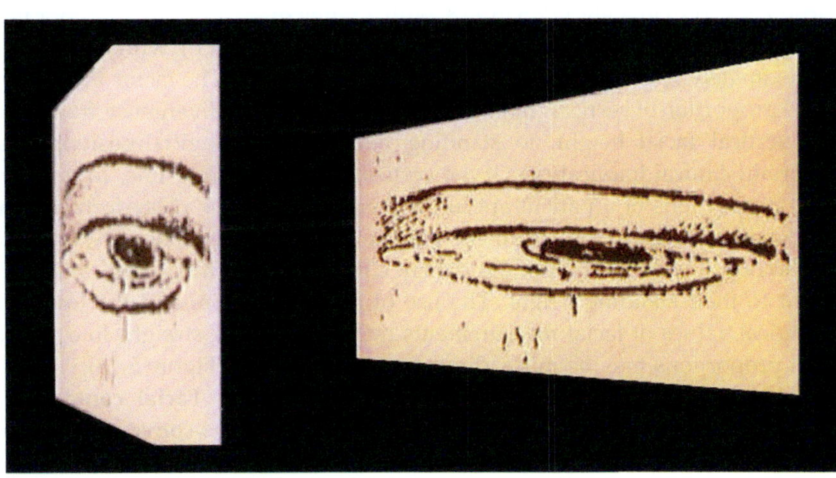

Fig. 5-16 Leonardo's eye (c.1485) is the earliest example of a drawing using anamorphic perspective, and only appears as an eye when viewed from a specific position and angle.

Clinical facial evaluation

There is variation in the classical, Renaissance and neoclassical proportional canons, variability in modern anthropometric and cephalometric normative population values and in the results of attractiveness research studies. Additionally, the diagnosing clinician must bear in mind that facial aesthetic considerations are influenced by ethnic and gender variation, cultural influences and variation in any specific patient's desires.[2] This demonstrates that the aesthetic 'ideals' described below, and the numerous others described in *Facial Aesthetics: Concepts and Clinical Diagnosis*,[2] are a useful first step in the clinical evaluation of dentofacial relationships, but only as *guidelines*. It is important to remember that each patient must be evaluated as an individual, and treatment planning decisions must be tailored to the individual patient.[2]

> **Note:**
>
> For the purposes of descriptive clarity, the next section will be divided broadly into frontal evaluation followed by profile evaluation. However, there is no strict demarcation between the two and it should be borne in mind that in clinical practice, the clinician will often need to evaluate various facial parameters from both frontal, oblique lateral and profile views, and some parameters need to be evaluated from a number of other directions.

Relationship of head height and size to standing height and stature

The clinician should begin analysing the patient from the moment they walk in through the door. The proportional relationship of the patient's standing height to their craniofacial height is an important starting point, as is the overall size of the head in relation to overall body stature.

Based on classical, Renaissance and neoclassical 'ideal' proportions,[25] normative anthropometric data,[26,27] and the results of attractiveness research,[28] the ideal craniofacial height to standing height proportion is approximately 1/7.5 to 1/8, with a range of 1/7 to 1/8.5. This equates to vertical face height being approximately 1/10 of standing height.

The proportion of vertical craniofacial (head) height, and vertical facial height, to standing height has important clinical implications. If the vertical craniofacial proportions of a patient are to be altered with orthognathic surgery, the treatment plan must take into account the proportion of the patient's total face height to their standing height. The use of absolute numerical values of facial measurements rather than facial proportions may be misleading, as the vertical facial height of a patient who is 1.8 m (6 ft) tall will be different to that of a patient 1.5 m (5 ft) tall.[29]

In terms of stature and physical build, it is likely that a larger head and broader face type may appear in better proportion in relation to a stocky physical build, whereas a smaller, leaner head and face is likely to appear more proportionate with a thinner physique. This issue was discussed by the Renaissance artist Albrecht Dürer and is logical, but not scientifically proven.[25,27]

Facial type

There is great variation in **facial shape**. However, a simple assessment will allow an overall categorization of the basic facial shape in frontal view, which may be any combination of the following:[30]

- Overall facial shape: Round, square or triangular
- Vertical facial height: Reduced, normal or increased
- Transverse facial width: Broad (wide), normal or narrow

Variations in facial height and width result in an innumerable variety of the three basic facial shapes (round, square and triangular).

The **facial height to width ratio** helps to describe the overall facial type, such as 'tall', 'thin', 'short' or 'square' face (Figure 5-17). Bizygomatic facial width, measured from the most lateral point of the soft tissue overlying each zygomatic arch (zygion), is approximately 70–75% of vertical facial height. In addition, bitemporal width, measured from the most lateral point on each side of the forehead, is 80-85% of bizygomatic width. Bigonial width, measured from the soft tissue overlying the most lateral point of each mandibular angle (soft tissue gonion), is usually 70–75% of bizygomatic width.

Two parameters for facial type should be evaluated in profile view:

- Facial divergence
- Facial contour

Facial divergence describes *the slope or inclination of the face in profile view*.[30] It is determined by the sagittal position of soft tissue pogonion (Pog′) and subnasale (Sn) relative to a vertical line dropped from glabella (G′), with the subject's head in natural head position. The factor that discriminates and distinguishes facial divergence from profile convexity or concavity is the sagittal position of subnasale (Sn) relative to the G′-Pog′ line. In order for the face to diverge anteriorly or posteriorly, yet not to exhibit signs of convexity or concavity, subnasale (Sn) must be on or nearly on the G′-Pog′ line; i.e. the **upper facial plane** (UFP, G′-Sn) and the **lower facial plane** (LFP, Sn-Pog′) are in a straight line, but diverge anteriorly or posteriorly (Figure 5-18).

Facial contour in profile view may be described as **convex**, **straight** or **concave**.[30] With the patient in

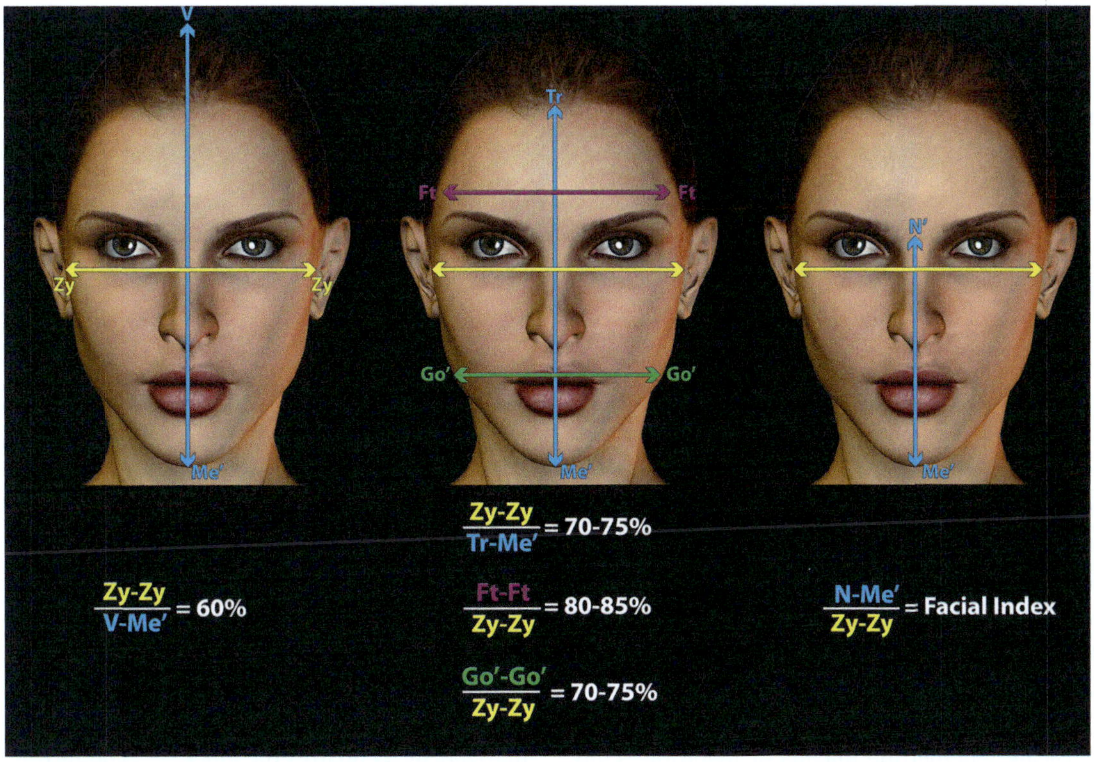

Fig. 5-17 Facial height-to-width ratios. (From: Naini FB. Facial Aesthetics: Concepts and Clinical Diagnosis. Oxford: Wiley-Blackwell, 2011; reprinted with permission.)

natural head position, the overall contour of the facial profile may be described by the relationship between two lines: the **upper facial plane** (UFP), connecting glabella (G′) to subnasale (Sn), and the **lower facial plane** (LFP), connecting subnasale to soft tissue pogonion (Pog′). In a **straight profile**, these two lines form a nearly straight line. Such a facial profile is termed **orthognathic** (Greek *orthos*: correct or straight; *gnathos*: jaw). An angle between these two lines indicates **facial profile convexity** (pogonion behind relative to subnasale in the sagittal plane), or **facial profile concavity** (pogonion ahead relative to subnasale in the sagittal plane). A convex profile indicates a skeletal Class II jaw relationship (and/or sagittal chin deficiency) and a concave profile indicates a skeletal Class III jaw relationship (and/or sagittal chin excess).

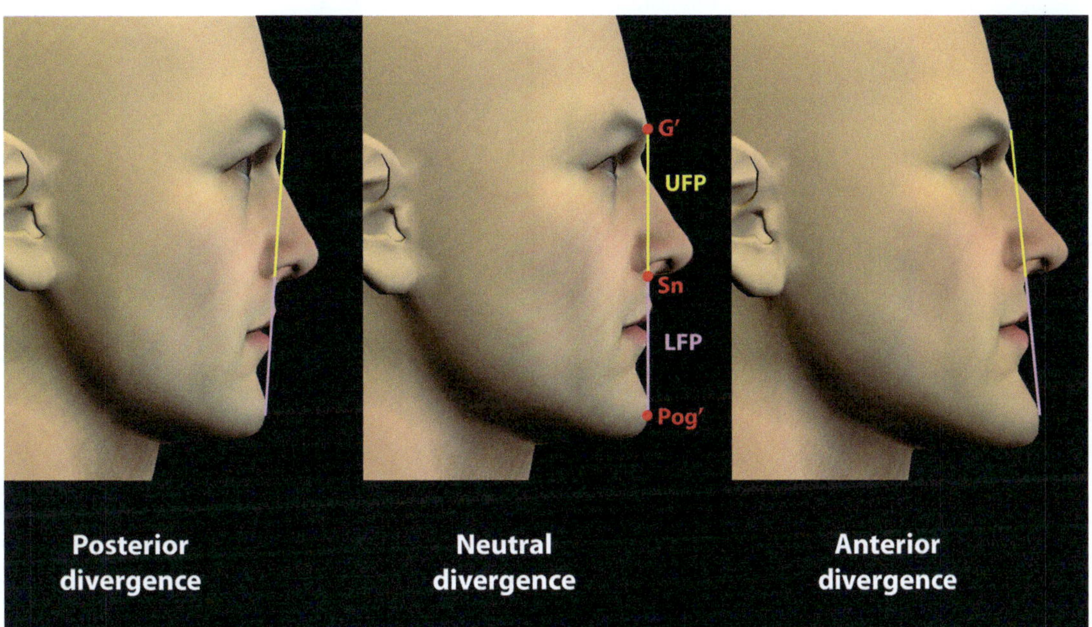

Fig. 5-18 Facial divergence. (From: Naini FB. Facial Aesthetics: Concepts and Clinical Diagnosis. Oxford: Wiley-Blackwell, 2011; reprinted with permission.)

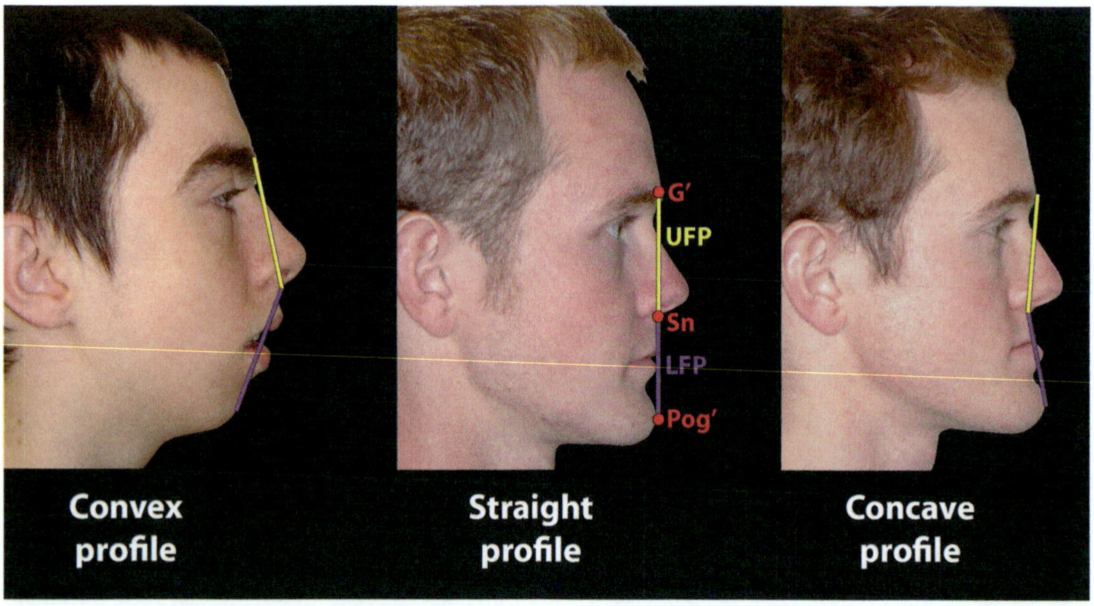

Fig. 5-19 Facial profile contours. (From: Naini FB. Facial Aesthetics: Concepts and Clinical Diagnosis. Oxford: Wiley-Blackwell, 2011; reprinted with permission.)

However, profile convexity or concavity does not of itself indicate whether the maxilla or mandible/chin is at fault (Figures 5-19–5-21).

Vertical facial evaluation

A useful starting point is the evaluation of the vertical facial thirds. This proportional canon, known as the **vertical facial trisection (Vitruvian trisection)**, was described by the Roman architect Vitruvius and popularized by Leonardo da Vinci.[25,27] The face may be vertically divided into thirds:

- Upper facial third: trichion (hairline) to glabella;
- Middle facial third: glabella to subnasale;
- Lower facial third: subnasale to soft tissue menton. The lower facial third may be slightly greater than the middle third in males.

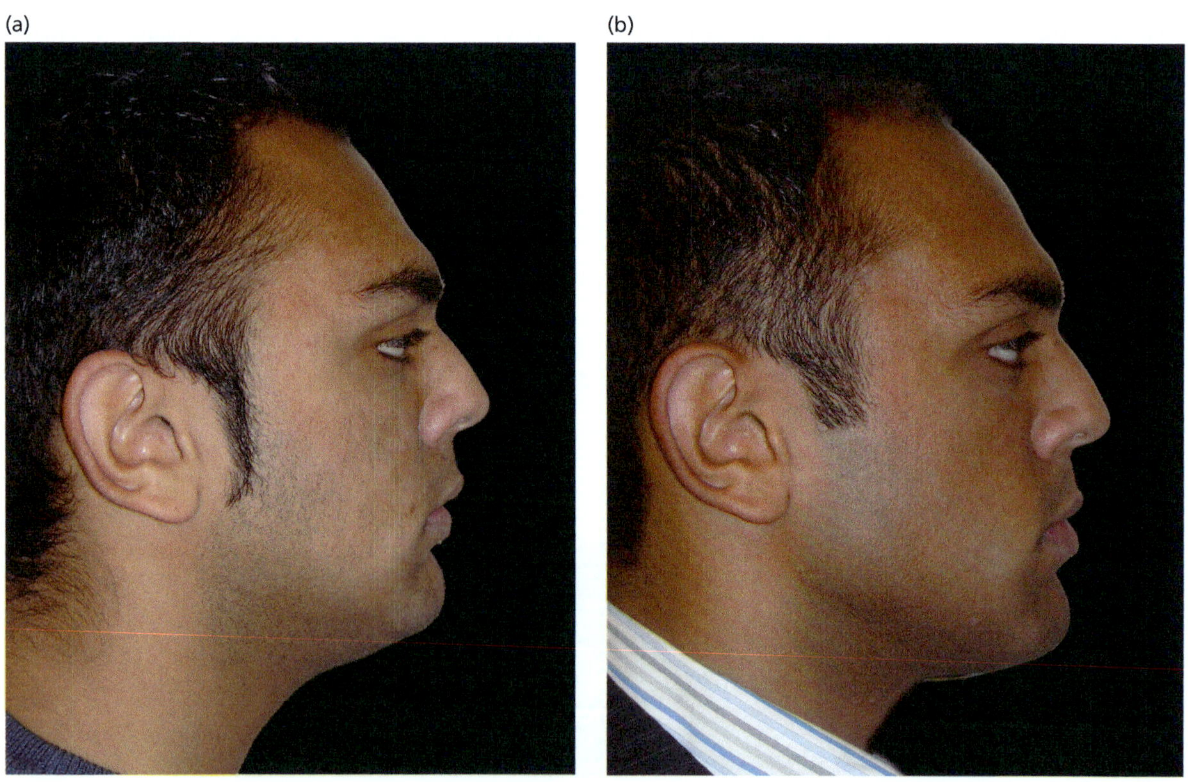

Fig. 5-20 (a) Pretreatment Class II patient with mandibular retrognathia, demonstrating a convex facial profile contour. (b) Following mandibular advancement osteotomy, demonstrating a relatively straight or orthognathic facial profile contour.

(a) (b)

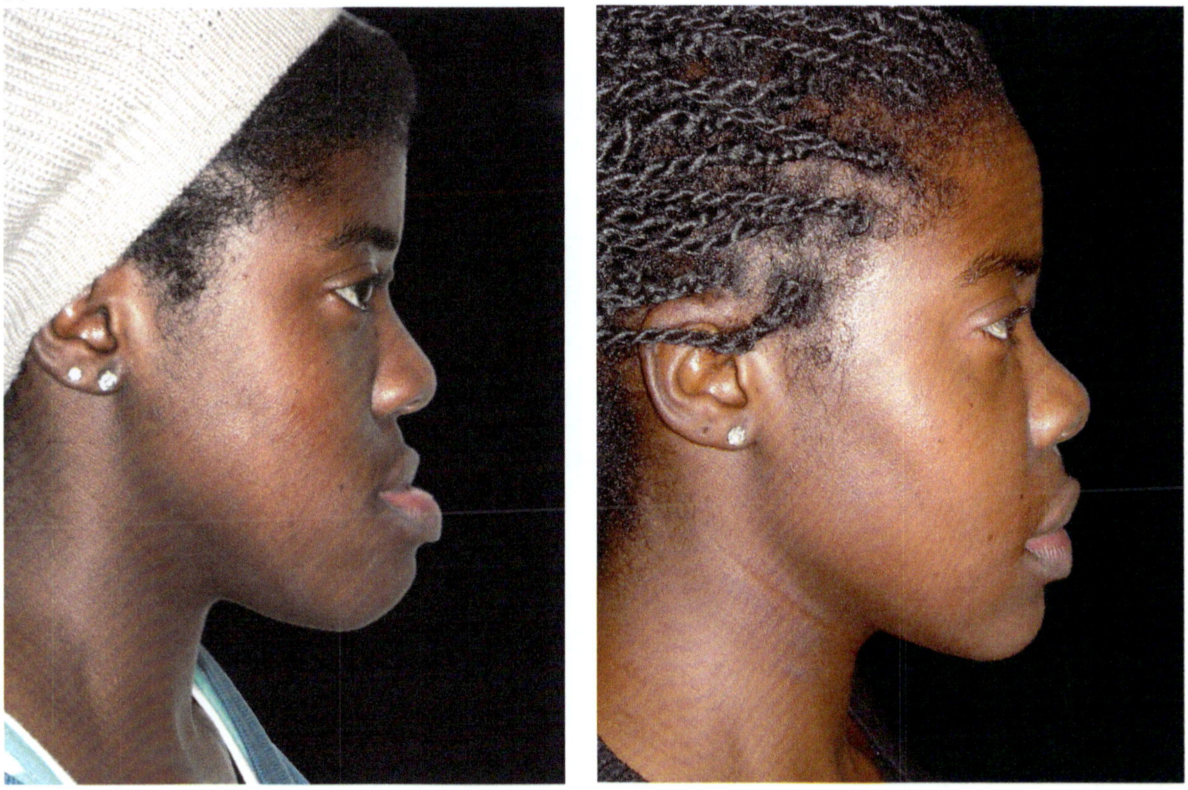

Fig. 5-21 (a) Preoperative Class III patient with maxillary retrognathism and mandibular prognathism, demonstrating a concave facial profile contour. (b) Following maxillary advancement at the Le Fort I level and mandibular set-back, demonstrating a relatively straight facial profile contour, within the norm for the ethnic background.

The **lower facial third** may be further subdivided. Leonardo da Vinci described the upper lip as forming the upper third and the lower lip and chin forming the lower two-thirds. Albrecht Dürer subdivided the lower anterior face height into quarters, with the upper lip height $^1/_4$ of lower facial height.[27] Subsequent attractiveness research has found that Leonardo's proportion appears to be the ideal, though a range of variability exists from the upper lip being anything from $^1/_2$ to $^1/_4$ of LAFH.[31,32]

The **lower anterior face height (LAFH)** and its proportional relationships have important clinical implications in the orthognathic patient. An increase or reduction in LAFH may be due to two parameters:

- **Vertical maxillary position** – **Total vertical maxillary excess (total VME)** results from excessive inferior development of the maxilla (Figure 5-22). This is often accompanied by excessive maxillary incisor exposure in repose and excessive gingival display at rest and on smiling, sometimes referred to in lay terminology as a 'gummy smile'. Treatment, therefore, centres on superior repositioning of the maxilla. In certain cases **anterior VME** may be due to excessively over-erupted maxillary incisors and canines (for example, Class II division 1 or 2 malocclusion) (Figure 5-23), in which case the treatment of choice will either be an anterior segmental impaction of the maxilla, or orthodontic intrusion of the maxillary incisors and associated gingivae. Alternatively, a reduction in LAFH may be due to **vertical maxillary deficiency (VMD)**, due to lack of inferior development of the maxilla, which is often accompanied by reduced maxillary incisor exposure. Treatment usually centres on inferior repositioning of the maxilla (Figure 5-24). **Anterior VMD** may occur as a result of an impediment to the eruption of the maxillary incisors, usually from a forward resting tongue position (Figure 5-25). VME and VMD are described further in Chapters 26 and 27 respectively.
- **Vertical chin height** – An excessively increased chin height, leading to a lower facial disproportion (Figure 5-26), may require a vertical reduction genioplasty. Alternatively, a reduced chin height may require vertical augmentation (Figure 5-27). However, sagittal correction of mandibular position often alters the appearance of the mentolabial fold region and lower facial height proportions, potentially improving the chin height to face height proportion. Therefore, in such cases, vertical reduction or augmentation genioplasty may be undertaken as a secondary procedure if required.

Finally, the **mandibular plane angle**, formed between the mandibular plane (tangent to the inferior border of the mandible) and the true horizontal plane (or Frankfort plane if it is horizontal) in profile view, should be assessed. The advantage of this variable is that it

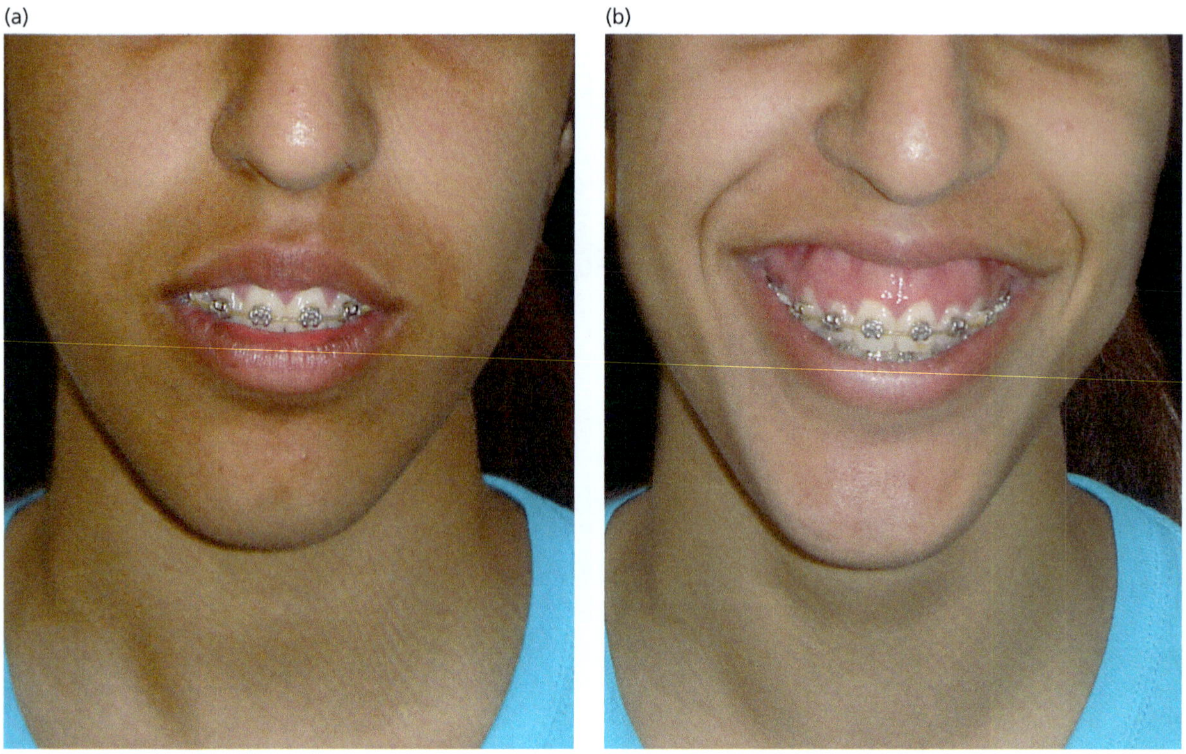

Fig. 5-22 Total vertical maxillary excess (total VME): (a) Excessive maxillary incisor exposure in repose (b) Excessive maxillary gingival exposure on smiling.

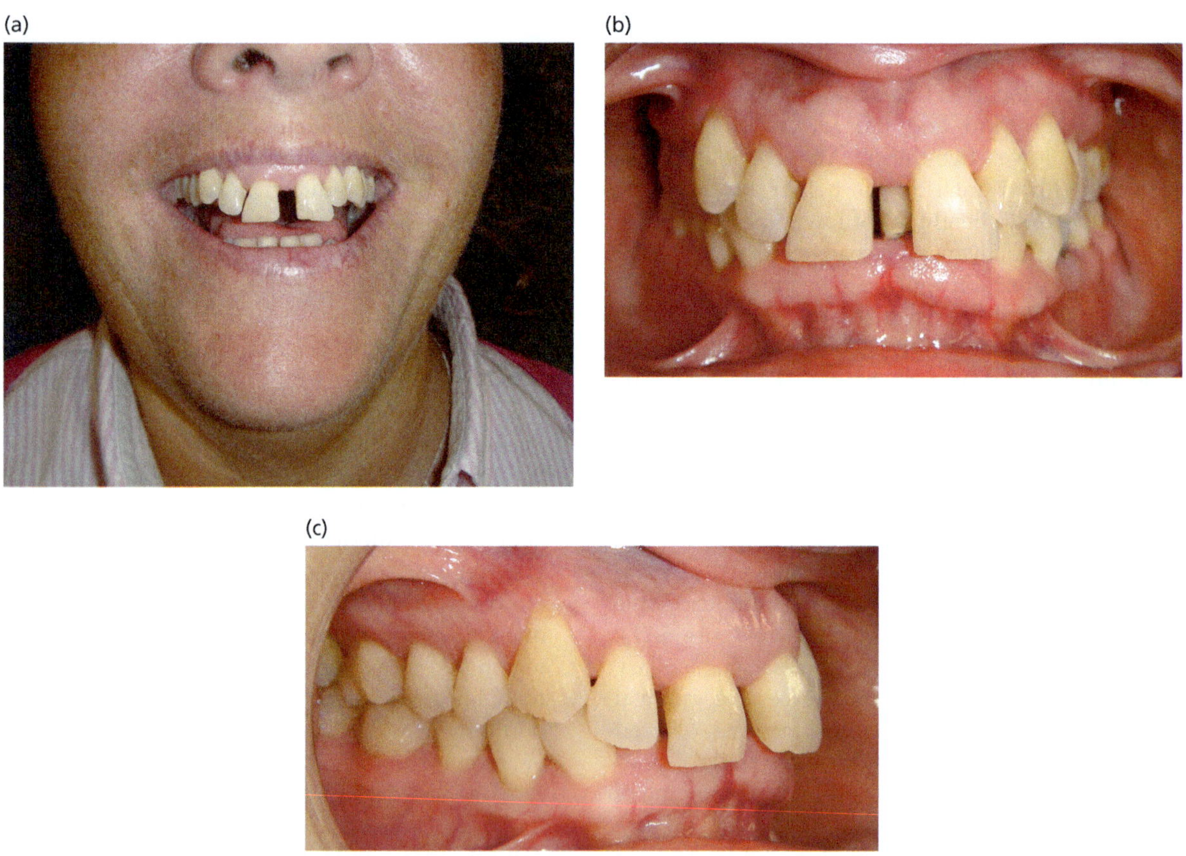

Fig. 5-23 (a–c) Anterior vertical maxillary excess (anterior VME) – this is due to excessive eruption of the maxillary incisor teeth and associated gingivae, i.e. the ‘gummy smile’ is only evident anteriorly.

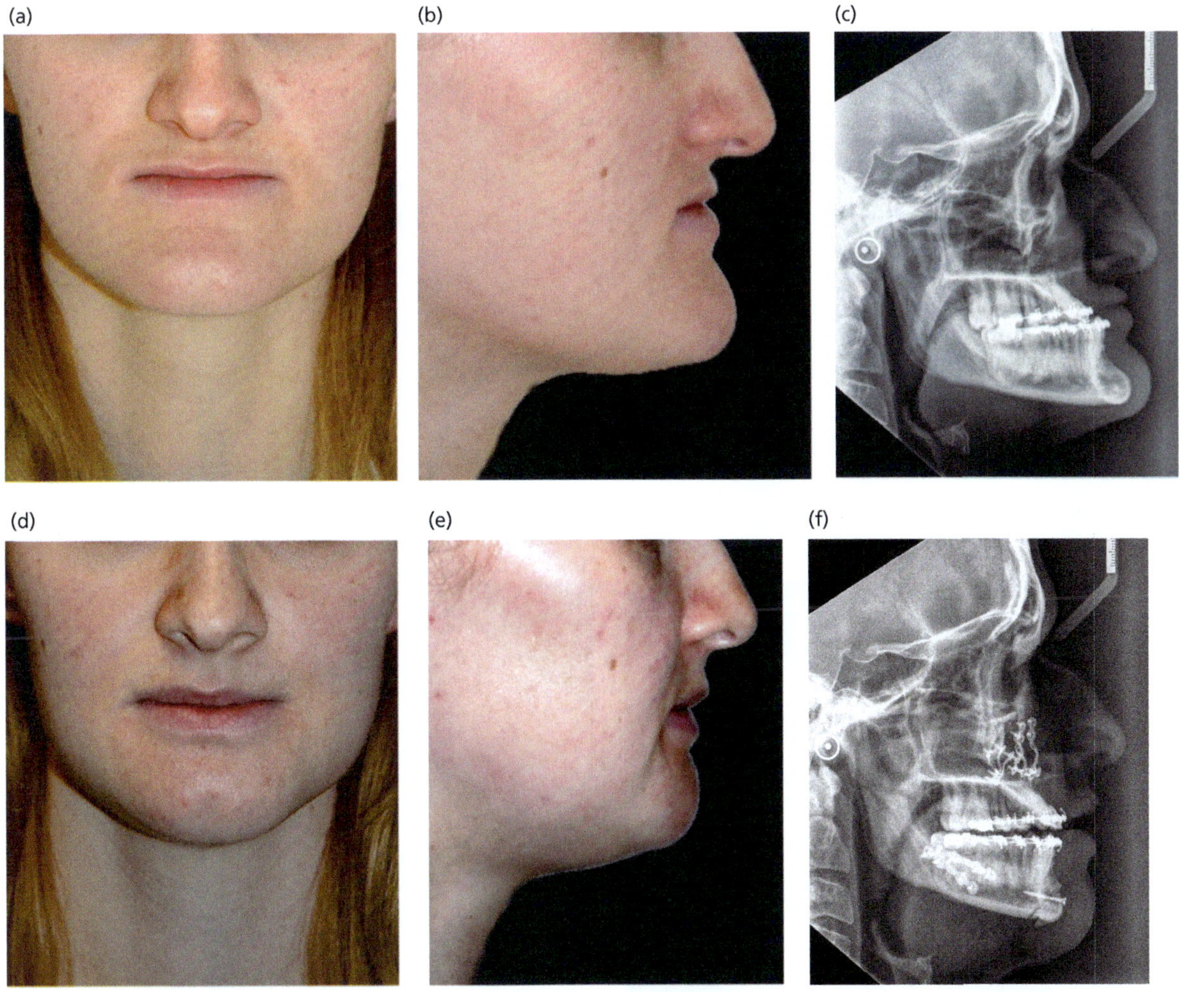

Fig. 5-24 Total vertical maxillary deficiency (total VMD): (a–c) Preoperative photographs and lateral cephalometric radiograph demonstrating VMD and mandibular overclosure and reduced lower anterior face height (LAFH). (d–f) Following maxillary advancement and inferior repositioning, mandibular set-back and set-back genioplasty, with improved LAFH to total face height proportion.

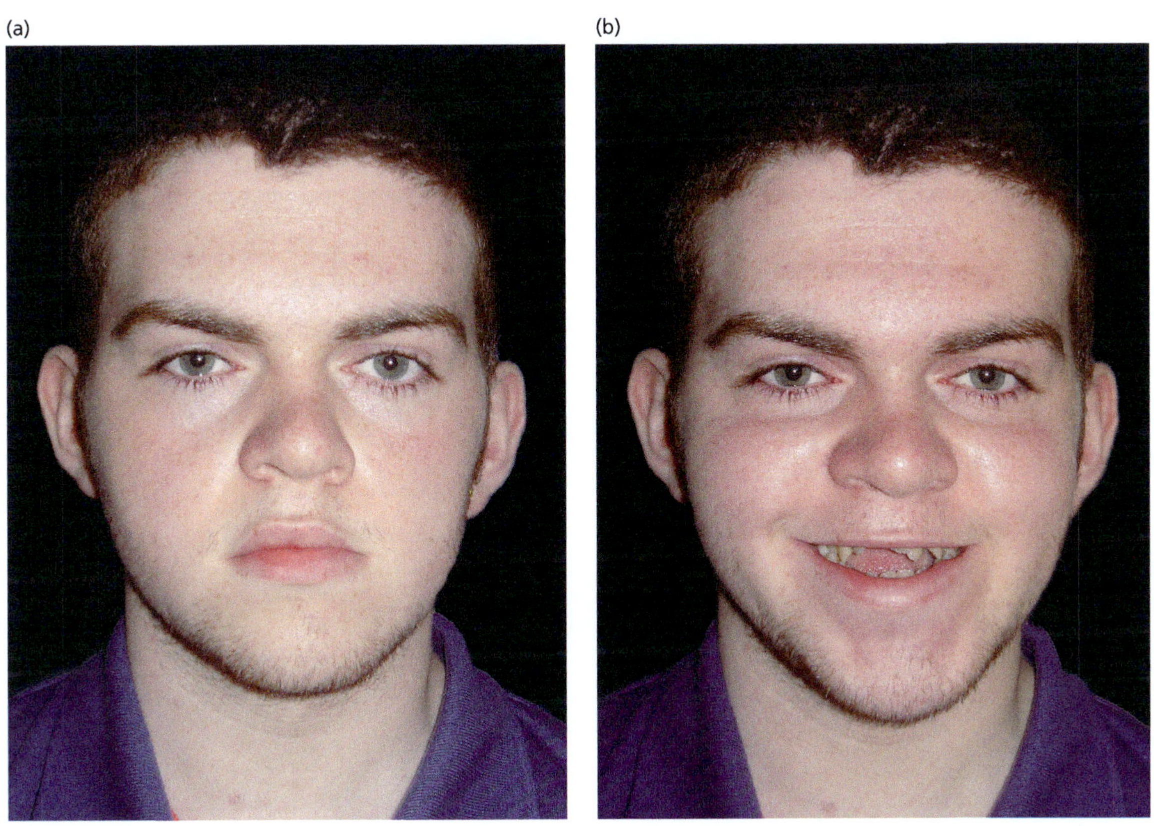

Fig. 5-25 (a–d) Anterior vertical maxillary deficiency (anterior VMD), due to impeded eruption of the maxillary incisors and associated alveolus, with an adaptive tongue to lower lip swallow pattern secondary to a long-standing digit sucking habit. The lower anterior face height is normal.

(c) (d)

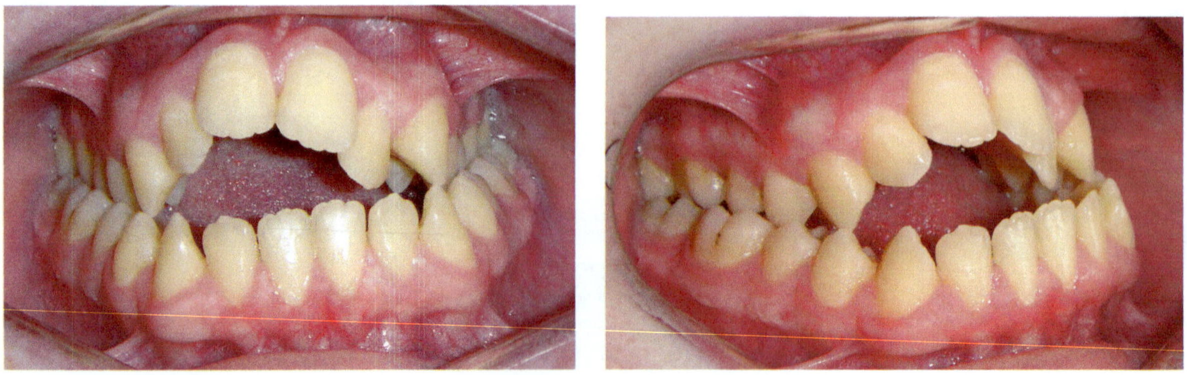

Fig. 5-25 (*Continued*).

(a) (b)

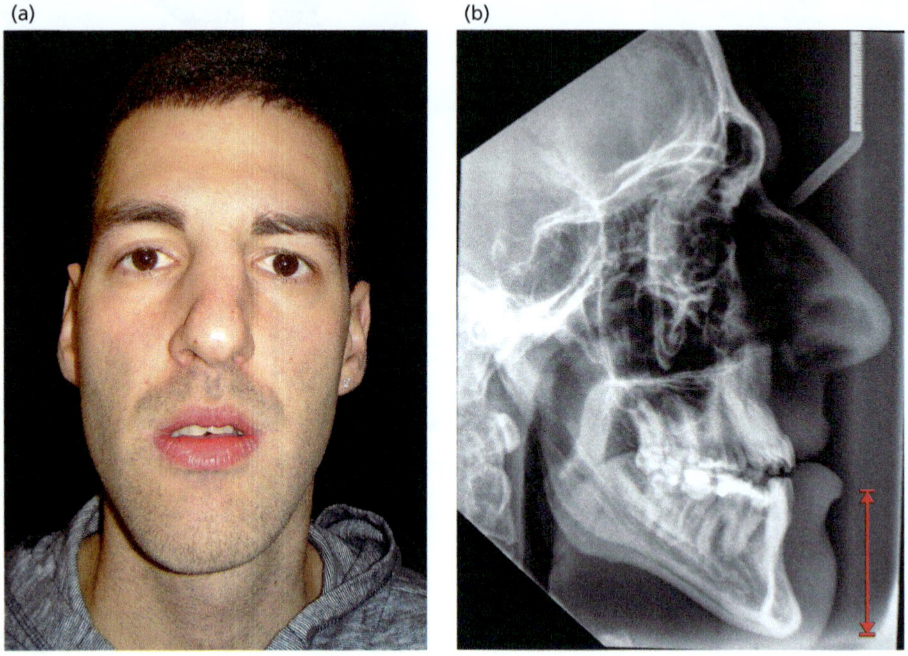

Fig. 5-26 (a, b) Increased chin height, albeit on a tall face.

(a) (b)

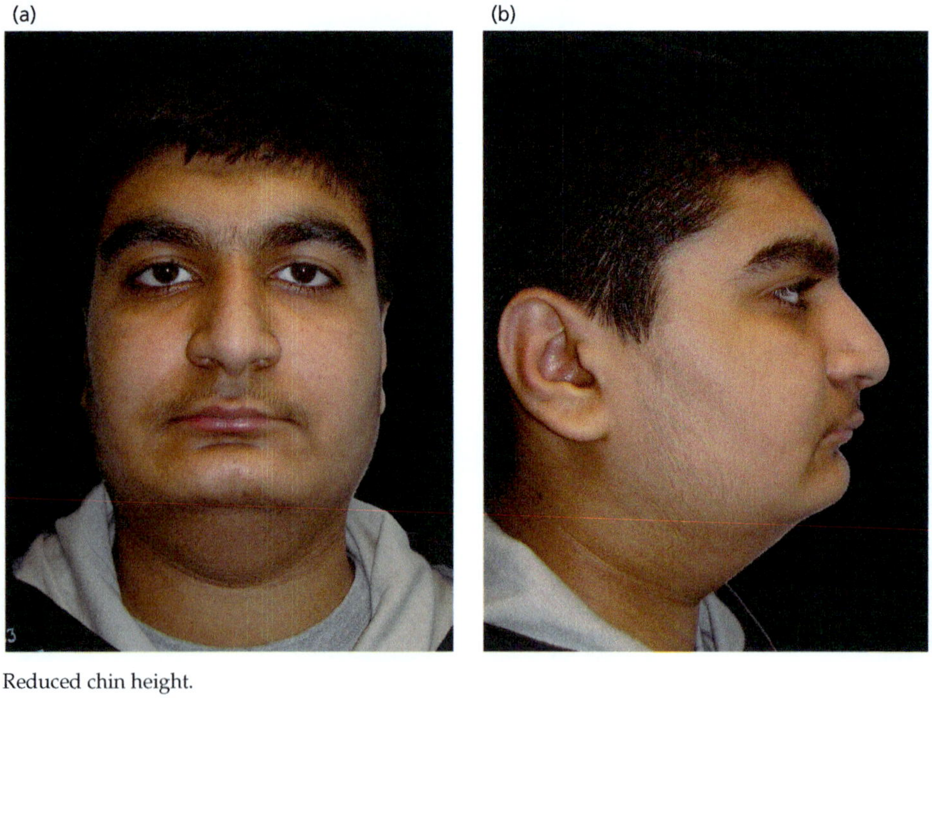

Fig. 5-27 (a–c) Reduced chin height.

(c)

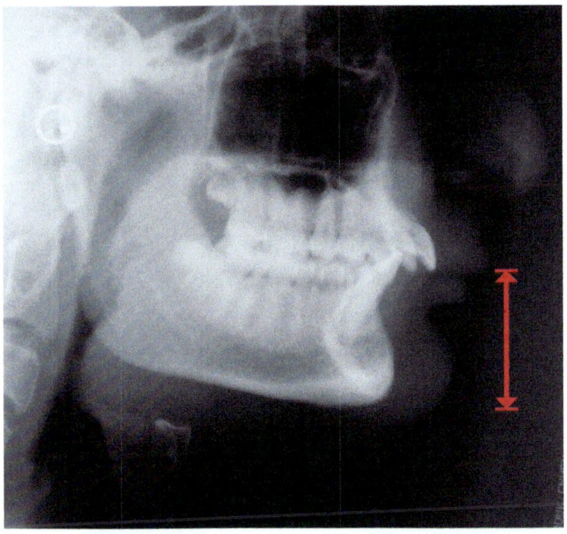

Fig. 5-27 (*Continued*).

may be assessed clinically by placing a finger or dental mirror handle along the inferior lateral border of the mandible (Figure 5-28).

Transverse facial evaluation

The **rule of fifths** describes the ideal transverse proportions of the face to comprise of equal fifths, each roughly equal to one eye width. It is a practical and convenient guideline to use in clinical practice. The alar base width should be approximately equal to the intercanthal width. This is important clinically as anterior and/or superior repositioning of the maxilla tends to increase the alar base width. This may be partially counteracted by the placement of an 'alar cinch suture' at the time of surgery to maintain the alar base width, thought his may have a tendency to elevate the nasal tip (see Chapter 22). Alternatively, some clinicians prefer rhinoplastic alar wedge resection as a secondary procedure (see Chapter 48).

The inherent ethnic variation in alar base width must be taken into account in diagnosis and treatment planning. The following anthropometric values for **alar base width** are useful guidelines:

- White male: 33 ± 2 mm
- White female: 31 ± 2 mm
- African-American male: 40 ± 5 mm
- African-American female: 38 ± 4 mm

The medial fifths of the face are measured from the lateral to the medial canthi of the eyes. **Mouth width** at rest is approximately equal to the distance between the medial iris margins (Figure 5-29). **Bigonial width** is slightly greater than biocular width (distance from the left to the right lateral canthus), i.e. the line from the lateral canthi of the eyes (outer border of the medial fifth of the face) should be approximately coincident with the antegonial region. Bigonial width should be approximately 70–75% of bizygomatic width. Increased bigonial width may occur in patients with increased skeletal bigonial width, or in patients with masseter muscle hypertrophy; the gonial angles will be lateral to the outer border of the medial fifth of the face (Figure 5-30). Conversely, patients with reduced bigonial width may require gonial angle implants to correct this proportion.

(a)

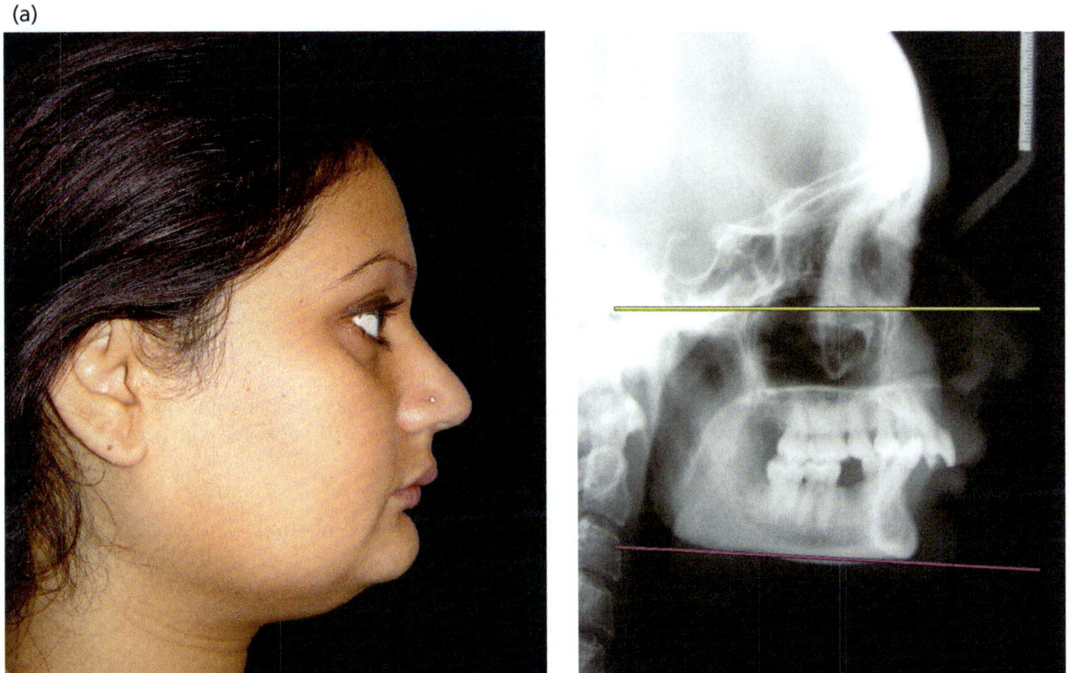

Fig. 5-28 (a) Reduced mandibular plane angle. (b) Increased mandibular plane angle.

(b)

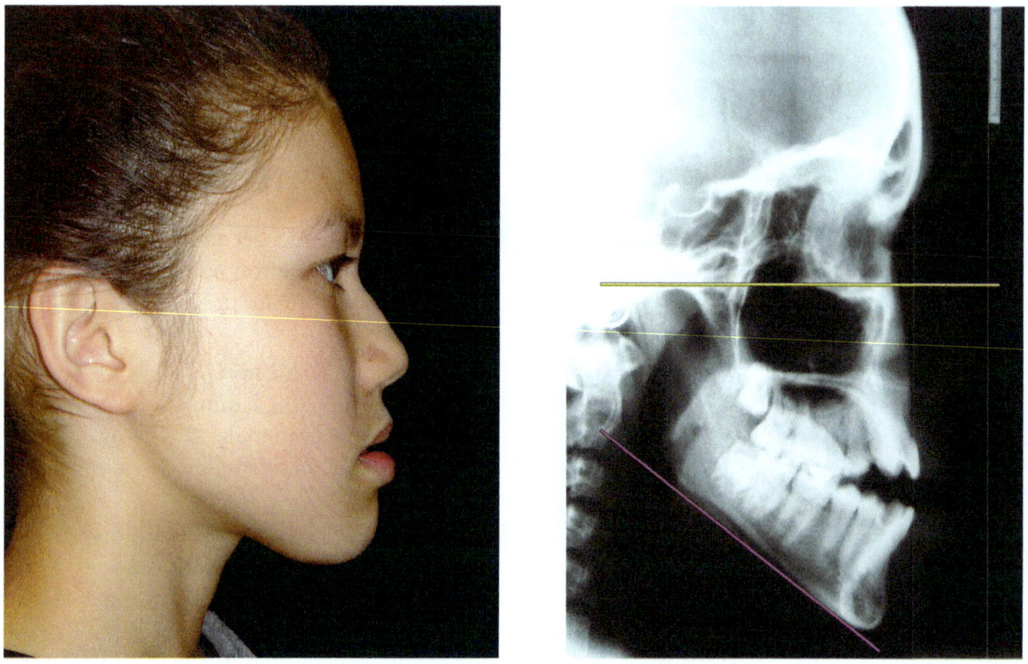

Fig. 5-28 (*Continued*).

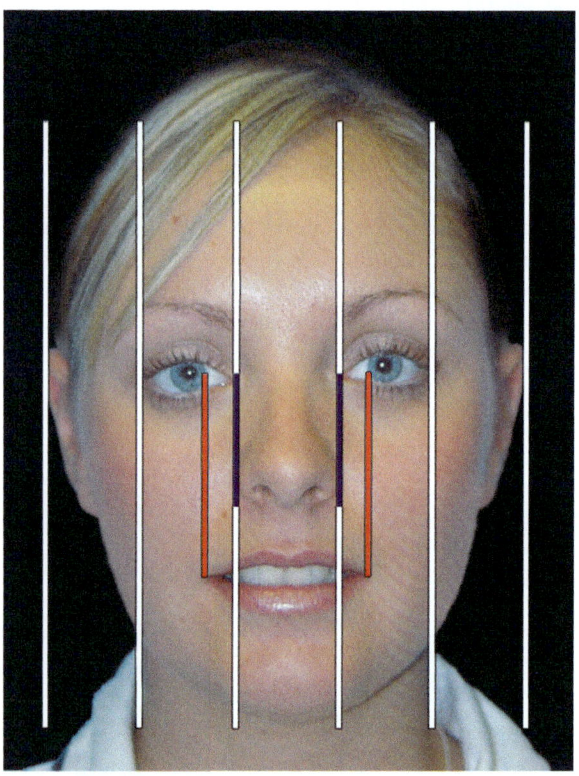

Fig. 5-29 Transverse facial proportions. The 'rule of fifths' states that transverse facial dimensions may be divided into equal fifths, each the width of an eye. The nasal alar base width should be equal to the intercanthal distance. The mouth width is equal to the distance between the medial iris margins. (From: Naini FB. Facial Aesthetics: Concepts and Clinical Diagnosis. Oxford: Wiley-Blackwell, 2011; reprinted with permission.)

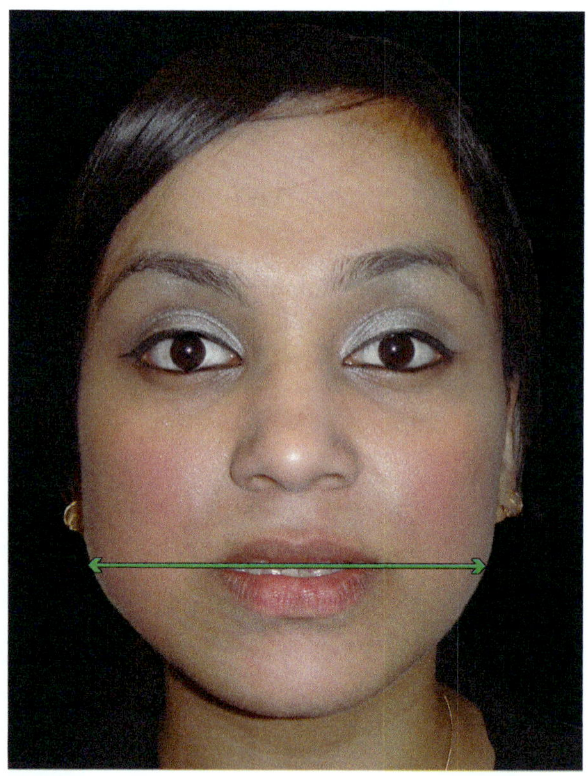

Fig. 5-30 Increased bigonial width. (From: Naini FB. Facial Aesthetics: Concepts and Clinical Diagnosis. Oxford: Wiley-Blackwell, 2011; reprinted with permission.)

Facial symmetry

The face must also be examined for **bilateral symmetry** in frontal view, bearing in mind that a small degree of asymmetry is present in most individuals and essentially normal. The **facial midline** can be constructed using two main landmarks. The mid-philtrum of the upper lip (Cupid's bow) will be in the midline of the face except in exceptional circumstances, e.g. an operated cleft lip or severe nasal asymmetry leading to a lateral deviation of the upper lip. A line joining this point to the mid-glabellar region

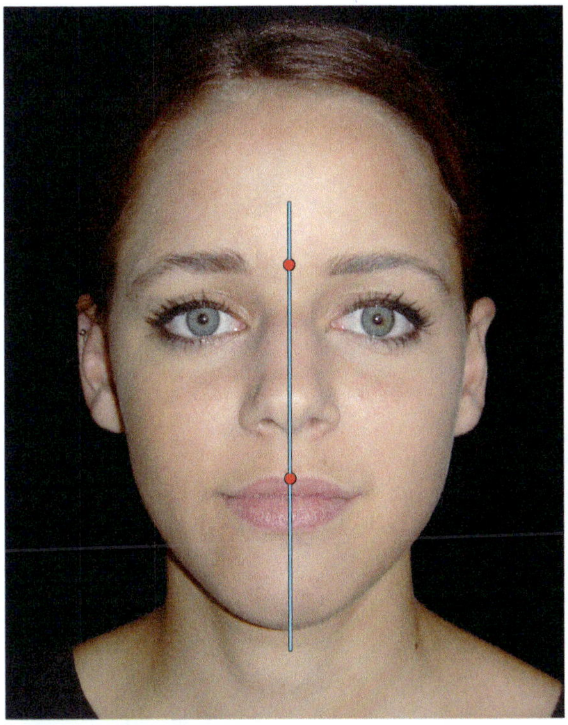

Fig. 5-31 Facial midline, connecting glabella and the mid-philtrum of the upper lip (midpoint of Cupid's bow).

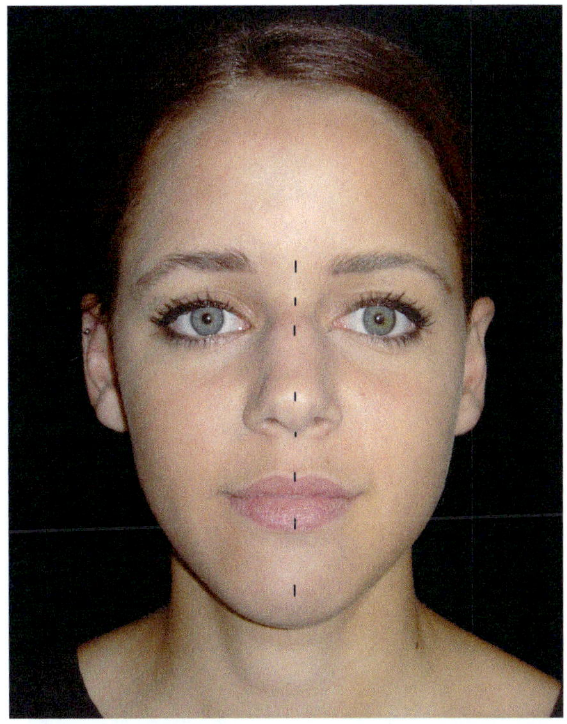

Fig. 5-32 The midpoints of different structures may be marked on the patient's face with a skin pencil to demonstrate any deviations from the facial midline.

(glabella), midway between the eyebrows, forms the facial midline (Figure 5-31). In the symmetrical face, this line will extend to the midpoint of the chin. Midline points should lie approximately on the facial midline, and bilateral facial structures should be approximately equidistant from this line. The midpoints of various facial structures may be marked with a skin pencil to permit more accurate clinical assessment (Figure 5-32).[33]

Palpation of the skeletal and soft tissue structures is also useful, and wherever possible both sides of the face should be examined simultaneously.

The presence of a **cant in the transverse maxillary occlusal plane** (i.e. rotation round the sagittal axis) may be assessed in relation to the interpupillary line (or a true horizontal plane) with the patient biting on a wooden spatula, or by the clinician holding a dental mirror handle against the maxillary dental occlusal surfaces, both in the incisor/canine region and the premolar/molar region (Figure 5-33). In the absence of a maxillary cant and/or vertical orbital dystopia, the transverse maxillary occlusal plane should be parallel to the interpupillary line. Further information may be found in Chapter 34.

Dental midlines

The relationship of the dental midlines to their respective jaws and to the facial midline must be assessed. The **maxillary dental midline** can be assessed in relation to the midpoint of the upper lip (Cupid's bow). In addition to the relationship of the maxillary incisors to the facial midline, their **transverse angulation** must also be assessed, as increased transverse angulation in frontal view reduces dentofacial aesthetics (Figure 5-34). The **mandibular dental midline** is assessed in relation to the maxillary dental midline and to the midpoint of the chin. Angulation as well as bodily deviation should be noted.

Smile width and buccal corridors

The **buccal corridor** or 'negative space' is the space revealed between the buccal surface of the posterior teeth and the commissures of the lips when a patient smiles. The presence of dark buccal corridors (excessive lateral negative space) may be due to:[34]

- **Transverse narrowing of the maxilla, especially in the premolar region:** When excessively narrow, expansion of the maxillary arch may be required in order to improve the arch form and dental occlusion; an additional advantage is that such expansion helps to fill the corners of the smile.
- **Palatal inclination of the maxillary posterior dentition:** The terminal tooth exposed in smiling is often the first or second premolar. As such, *it is important that maxillary premolar crowns are not palatally inclined.* Where this is the case, increased buccal crown inclination and/or expansion of the posterior maxillary dentition, primarily in the premolar region, are required. In aesthetic dentistry, an increase in the thickness of the buccal aspect of ceramic restorations on the premolar teeth may help to fill out the smile.
- **Retropositioned maxilla:** Maxillary advancement is the treatment of choice, as moving the maxilla anteriorly permits a wider part of the dental arch to move forward and reduce the lateral negative space (Figure 5-35).

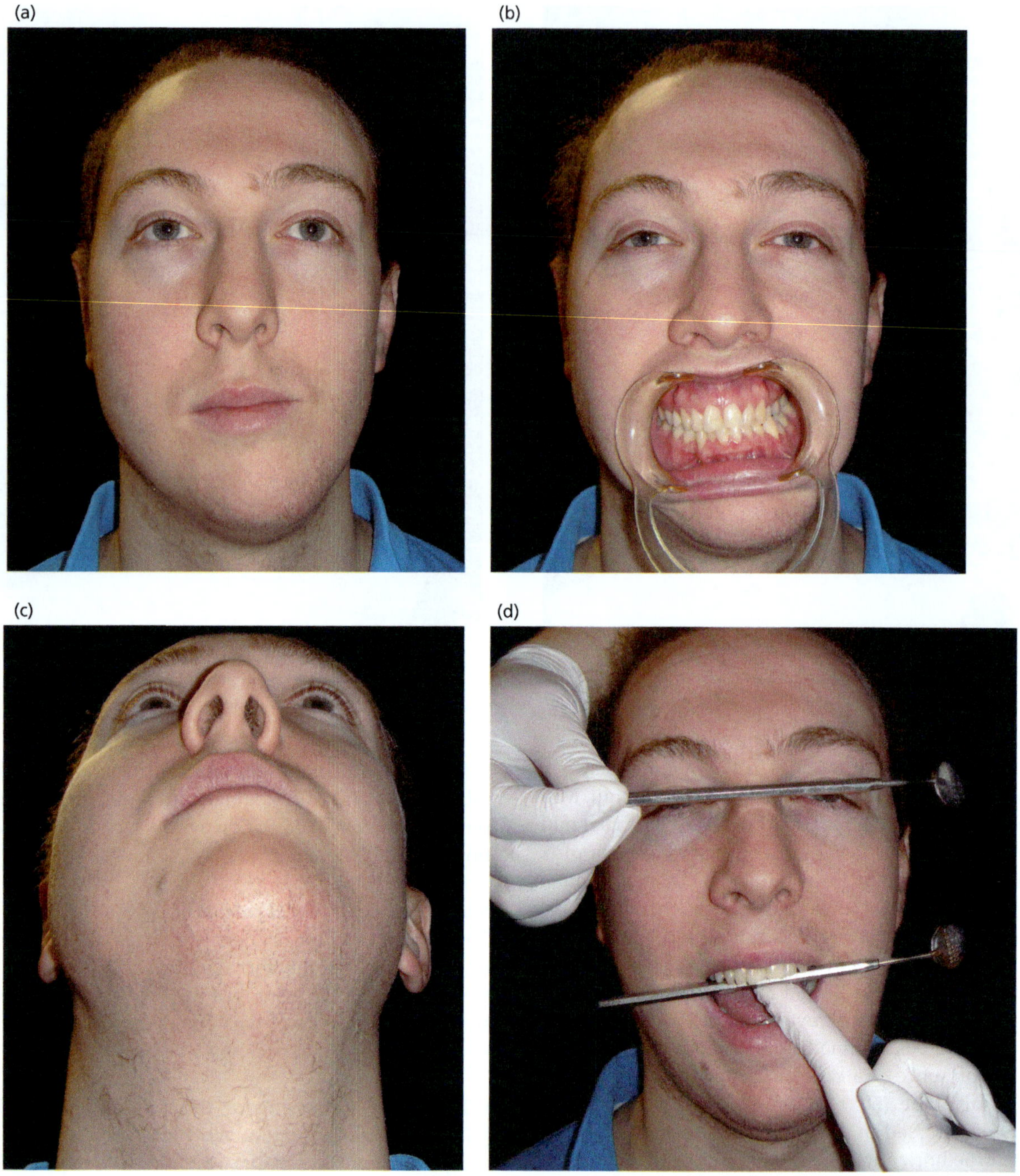

Fig. 5-33 (a) Significant asymmetry of the lower face, with the mandible and chin point to the patients left, and transverse cant of the rima oris (left and right commissures at different vertical levels) and the inferior chin plane. (b) Transverse cant of the maxillary occlusal plane evident, canted down on the patient's right. (c) Inferior view highlights asymmetry of the chin and lower lip in relation to the upper lip. (d) Dental mirror handle held against the maxillary dentition demonstrates a transverse cant in relation to the interpupillary plane.

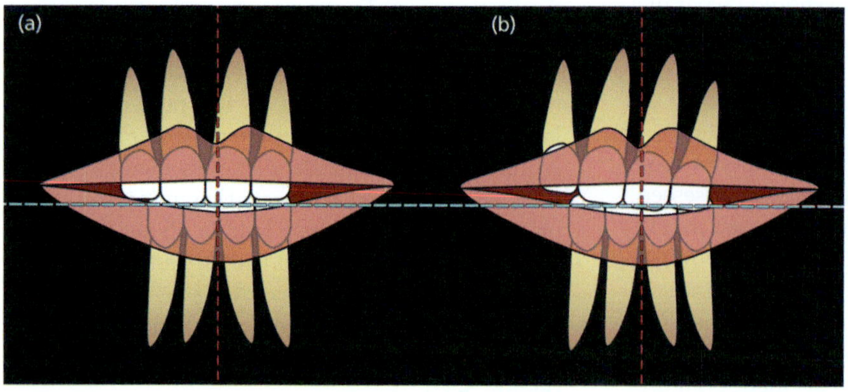

Fig. 5-34 Maxillary dental midline shift of 2 mm to the right of the patient's facial midline: (a) Maxillary incisors are correctly angulated, with the mesial and distal contact areas of their crowns parallel to the facial midline. (b) Excessive maxillary incisor angulation to the patient's right and thereby a transverse cant of the incisal edge plane. (From: Naini FB. Facial Aesthetics: Concepts and Clinical Diagnosis. Oxford: Wiley-Blackwell, 2011; reprinted with permission.)

(a)

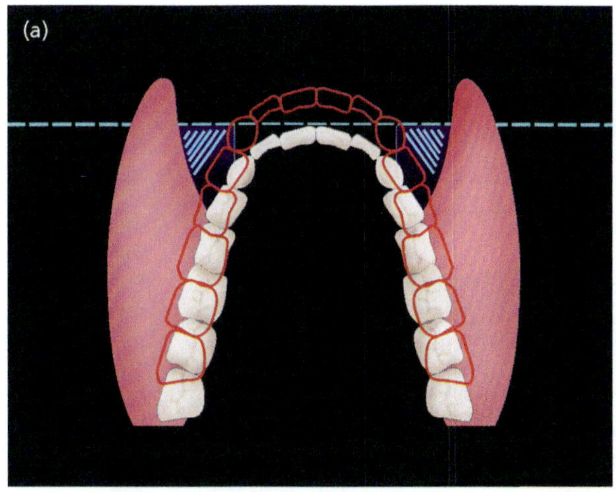

(b) (c)

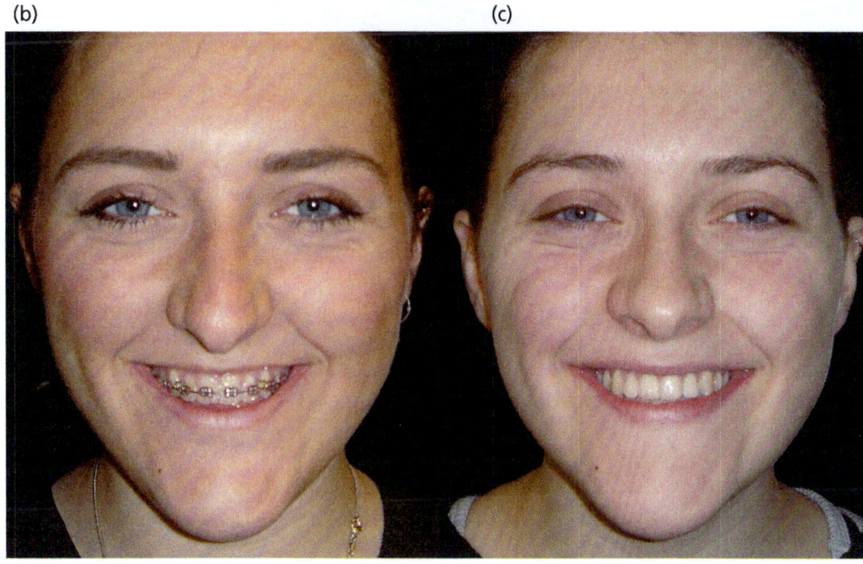

Fig. 5-35 (a) Maxillary advancement permits a wider part of the dental arch to move forward and reduce the lateral negative space. (From: Naini FB. Facial Aesthetics: Concepts and Clinical Diagnosis. Oxford: Wiley-Blackwell, 2011; reprinted with permission.) (b, c) Maxillary advancement reduces the buccal corridors, 'filling' the corners of the smile.

- **Dynamic inter-commissure distance:** Normal values for inter-commissure distance (i.e. mouth width) in repose have been provided:[26]
  - Male: 55 ± 3 mm
  - Female: 50 ± 3 mm

  Data on changes in mouth width in the dynamic state of smiling is limited. However, Rigsbee et al.[35] demonstrated that, in an 'attractive' smile, the mouth increased to 130% of its original width. There is likely to be considerable individual variation in the degree of increase in inter-commissure distance in smiling. The greater this increase, the greater the potential for lateral negative space in smiling.
- **The vertical dimension:** It has been demonstrated that an increased lower anterior face height (measured from subnasale to soft tissue menton) and, in particular, the lower lip-chin height (measured from stomion to soft tissue menton), are negatively correlated with the **buccal corridor area**, i.e. the two-dimensional area visible in frontal view. This is thought to be due to increased stretch of the lower facial soft tissues in patients with increased lower face height, and thereby reduced buccal corridors in smiling.[36]

Note:

The concealed premolar smile

A great deal of attractiveness research has been carried out on the influence of buccal corridors on the perceptions of smile attractiveness. Orthodontists do not like buccal corridors, yet the results of research indicate that laypeople do not share the orthodontists' dislike. In denture prosthetics a degree of lateral 'negative space' (buccal corridors) is planned, and thought to give a more natural appearance. Overall, it is likely that the parameter leading to the perception of smile attractiveness is not the presence or absence of buccal corridors, but the ***visibility of the posterior dentition distal to the maxillary canine teeth.*** In patients with adequate visibility of the premolar teeth when observed in frontal view, the presence of buccal corridors is unlikely to be perceived as unattractive; conversely, in patients with a narrow 'canine to canine' smile with the premolars *concealed* behind the canine teeth ('concealed premolar smile'), the smile attractiveness is likely to be unsatisfactory (Figure 5-36).[34]

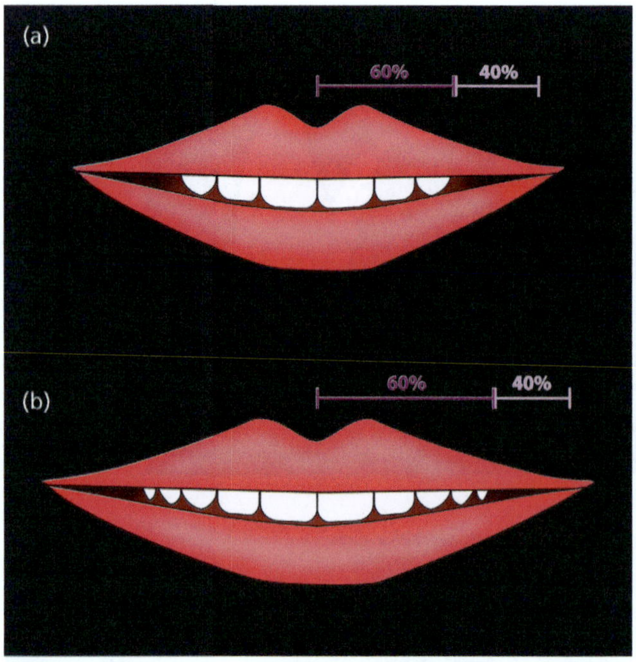

Fig. 5-36 The 'concealed premolar' smile: it is likely that the parameter leading to the perception of smile attractiveness is not the presence or absence of buccal corridors, but the visibility of the posterior dentition distal to the maxillary canine teeth. (a) Narrow 'canine to canine' smile with the premolars 'concealed' behind the canine teeth. (b) Adequate visibility of the premolar teeth when observed in frontal view. In both situations, the percentage of visible dentition to buccal corridor is identical, but the visibility of the premolar teeth distal to the canines in (b) improves the smile aesthetics. (From: Naini FB. Facial Aesthetics: Concepts and Clinical Diagnosis. Oxford: Wiley-Blackwell, 2011; reprinted with permission.)

A summary of the frontal facial evaluation is provided in Table 5-3.

Aesthetic evaluation of the lips

The lips are a significant aesthetic parameter and form an important part of the lower face in both frontal and profile view. As such, aesthetic evaluation of the lips forms an essential part of clinical assessment of the orthognathic patient. Systematic clinical evaluation of the lips requires analysis of a number of parameters, which may be conveniently remembered with the acronym LAMPP: lip lines, activity (function), morphology (form), posture and prominence (Table 5-4).[37]

Table 5-3 Frontal facial evaluation.

Vertical proportions	• Facial trisection: hairline (trichion) to glabella, glabella to subnasale, subnasale to soft tissue menton should be *approximately* equal.
	• Anterior lower facial third is often slightly greater than middle third, especially in males.
	• Anterior lower facial third is further subdivided into:
	  ○ Upper lip (subnasale to stomion): 1/3
	  ○ Lower lip and chin (stomion to soft tissue menton): 2/3
	• Vertical face height is ~1/10 of standing height.

Transverse proportions	• Rule of fifths – Each fifth is approximately the width of an eye. • Mouth width approximately equal to the distance between the medial iris margins. • Alar base width approximately equal to the intercanthal distance. • Bitemporal width is ~80–85% of bizygomatic width. • Bigonial width is ~70–75% of bizygomatic width.
Facial height to width ratios	• Helps to describe the overall facial type, e.g. 'tall', 'thin', 'short' or 'square' face. • Bizygomatic facial width is ~70–75% of vertical facial height.
Sagittal parameter assessment in frontal view	• Increased sclera exposure above the lower eyelid and below the iris is a sign of midface deficiency. • Paranasal hollowing/flatness is a sign of maxillary retrusion. This may be observed in frontal and profile examination of the face.
Bilateral facial symmetry	• Mid-philtrum of upper lip (Cupid's bow) and glabella used to construct facial midline. • Minor asymmetry is essentially normal. • Transverse occlusal plane parallel to interpupillary line in absence of transverse maxillary occlusal plane cant or vertical orbital dystopia.
Maxillary dental midline	• Assessed in relation to middle of philtrum of upper lip (Cupid's bow) and to facial midline. • Mesiodistal incisor angulation should be correct in relation to the maxillary occlusal plane (in the absence of a transverse cant).
Mandibular dental midline	• Assessed in relation to midpoint of chin, maxillary dental midline and to the facial midline. • Mesiodistal angulation should be assessed as well as lateral midline deviation.
Excessive dark 'buccal corridors' on smiling	May be due to (major considerations): • Transverse maxillary deficiency • Palatally inclined maxillary posterior teeth • Sagittal maxillary deficiency

Summarized from *Facial Aesthetics: Concepts and Clinical Diagnosis*, with permission.[2]

Table 5-4 Aesthetic evaluation of the lips.

Lip lines	Defined as the vertical position of the upper and lower lips in relation to the anterior dentition. • Maxillary incisor exposure at rest: 2–5 mm (usually greater in females than males). • Depends on upper lip height and vertical maxillary incisor position (see Table 5-5). • Lower lip should cover incisal third of maxillary incisors. • Upper and lower **lip lines** may be **high** or **low** in relation to maxillary incisors.
Lip activity (function)	**Lip tonicity** refers to the muscular tone of the lips, related to the production of normal muscular contraction and function. The lips may be **hypertonic** (overactive) or **hypotonic** and possibly flaccid: • A strap-like lower lip often retroclines the incisors (commonly occurs in Class II division 2 malocclusions). • Flaccid lips are less likely to significantly alter position with anteroposterior dental and even skeletal movement. Patients with an increased incisor overjet or a significant anterior open bite may develop an **adaptive anterior oral seal** for swallowing, and the *soft tissue resting position and function* often worsens the malocclusion, e.g. a lower lip trapped behind the maxillary incisors will tend to procline the incisors.
Lip morphology (form)	**Lip heights** may be evaluated in terms of linear measurements compared to population norms, as well as proportional relationships. **Lip thickness** is an important aesthetic parameter, and correlated with lip prominence. • Full, thick lips are less likely to significantly alter position with anteroposterior dental or skeletal movement. • Thin lips are more likely to 'flatten' with incisor retraction or set-back osteotomies. • There is significant ethnic variation. **Lip curvature** (frontal view) – the contour of the upper lip at rest in frontal view depends mainly on the differential height of the mid-philtrum and the bilateral oral commissures. • If the mid-philtrum height is excessively short in relation to the oral commissures, surgical 'lengthening' of the philtrum region may be required (see Chapter 53). **Lip curl (profile view)** – a mild sagittal anterior curvature or 'curl' of the upper lip in profile view is an important aesthetic parameter. • Reduced curl – may result from reduced dentoalveolar support and poorly planned orthodontic treatment or orthognathic surgery. • Excessive curl – may occur as a result of a reduced LAFH or mandibular overclosure, compressing the lips together. **Lip inclination** – the inclination of the upper and lower lips in profile view is important. • **Upper lip inclination** (in relation to the true horizontal line through subnasale) forms the lower component of the nasolabial angle (ideal value ~80–85°).[38] • **Lower lip inclination** – forms the upper component of the mentolabial angle. • Everted lips may be due to interposed proclined maxillary incisor teeth. • Flat or backward sloping lips give an 'aged' appearance to the facial profile. **Vermilion exposure** • Very thin vermilion and reduced vermilion exposure may be rather unattractive. • Vermilion height of upper lip should be ~1/3 of upper lip height. • Vermilion exposure of lower lip is usually slightly greater than upper lip (by 2–3 mm) • There is significant ethnic variability.
Lip posture	**Lip posture** may be defined as the characteristic way in which an individual, in natural head position, maintains their normal lip position in repose, i.e. with normal muscular tone and without excessive muscular contraction.[37] • **Complete lip seal** – Lips held together at rest without excessive muscular effort, also referred to as lip competence. • **Incomplete lip seal** – Lips habitually held apart at rest by more than 3–4 mm, also referred to as lip incompetence (Figure 5-37). • **Potential lip competence** – lips are unable to be held together due to interposed maxillary incisor teeth (Figure 5-38).
Lip prominence	**Lip prominence** is visually evaluated *relative* to the prominence of the nose and chin in profile view. Wide arrays of analyses have been described to evaluate lip prominence.[37] Two useful methods, combining three analyses, may be used together: • **Subnasale vertical (SnV)** – This is a true vertical line through subnasale; labrale superius of the upper lip should be just anterior to SnV, and labrale inferius should be on or just behind (Figure 5-39). • **Combined Burstone–Ricketts 'triangle'** – The Burstone line (Sn-Pog**'**)[39] and Ricketts E-line (Pr-Pog**'**)[40,41] are drawn, and the lips should fall within the triangle formed between the two lines, with the upper lip slightly ahead of the lower lip (Figure 5-40). Additional analyses that may be employed are (values based on North American white individuals): • 'Esthetic' line (Ricketts E-line)[40,41] – Joins the nasal tip to soft tissue pogonion. The upper lip should be 4 mm and the lower lip 2mm behind this line in adults. This is very dependent on nasal and chin projection. • Steiner line (S-line)[42,43] – Joins soft tissue pogonion to the midpoint between subnasale and nasal tip. The lips should touch this line. • Harmony line (H-line)[44,45] – A line from soft tissue pogonion touching the upper lip should bisect the nose. • Profile line (Z-line of Merrifield)[46] – A tangent to the chin and vermilion border of the most prominent lip should ideally bisect the nose. • Riedel plane[47] – The chin (soft tissue pogonion) should be on a line drawn tangent to both lips.

Summarized from *Facial Aesthetics: Concepts and Clinical Diagnosis*, with permission.[2]

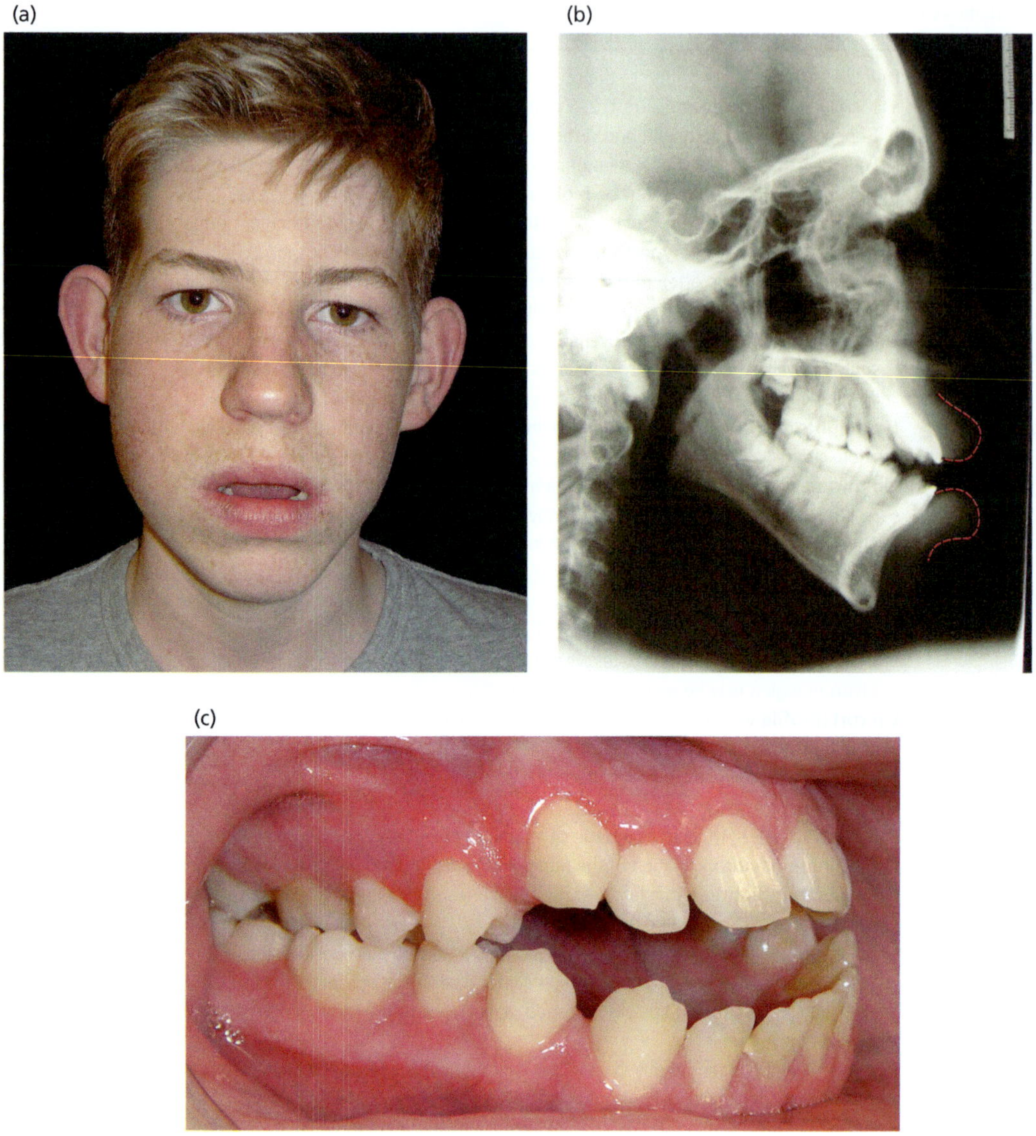

Fig. 5-37 (a–c) Incomplete lip seal (incompetent lip posture) – the posterior teeth are in occlusion, but there is an increased lower anterior face height, significant anterior open bite and bimaxillary incisor proclination, all of which have led to the observed lip posture in repose.

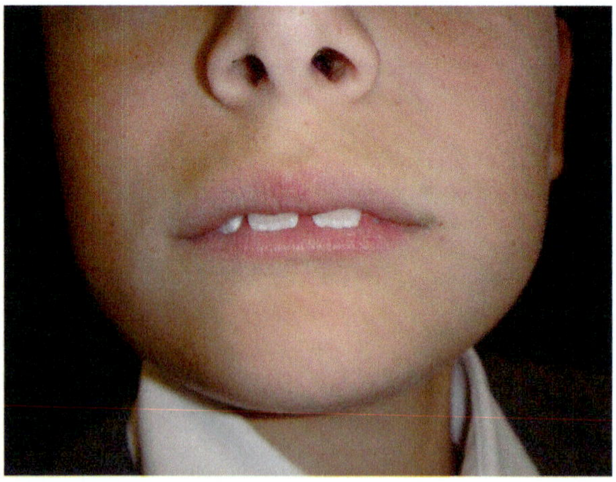

Fig. 5-38 Potentially competent lips, with maxillary incisors interposed between the upper and lower lips.

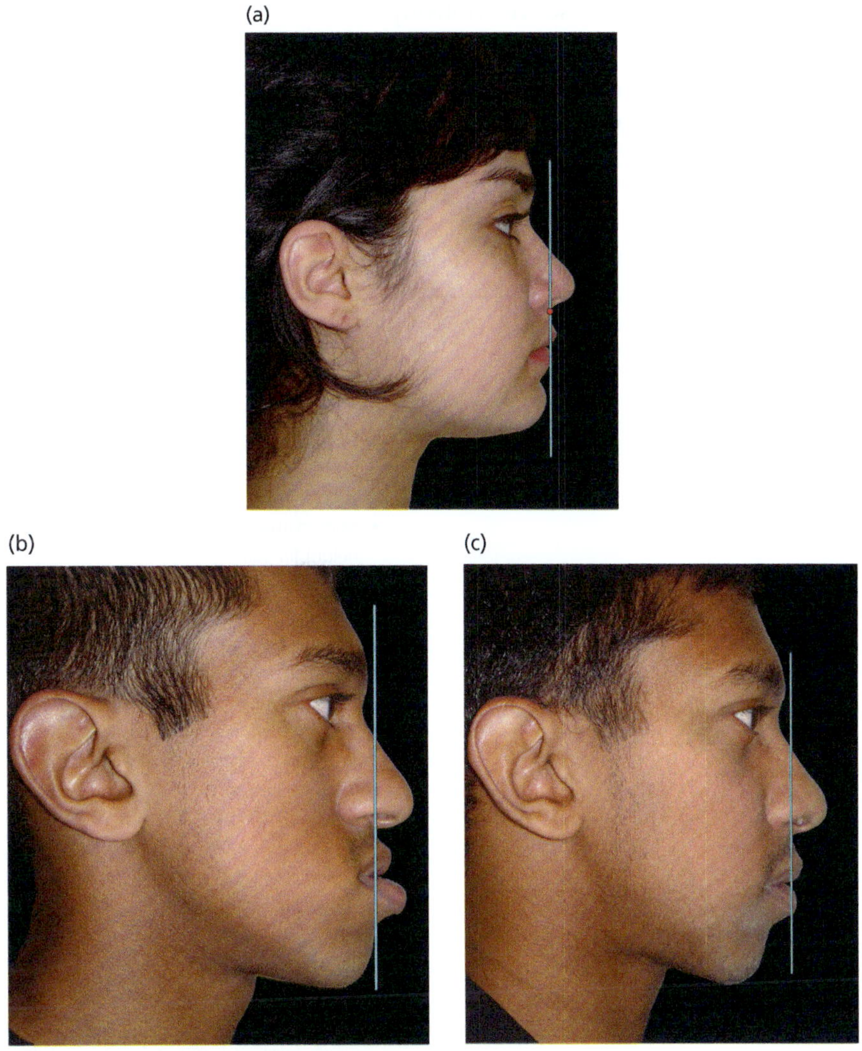

Fig. 5-39 (a) The subnasale vertical (SnV) line is a true vertical line through subnasale; labrale superius of the upper lip should be just anterior to SnV, and labrale inferius should be on or just behind. (b) A Class III patient with maxillary retrognathism and mandibular prognathism. Subnasale is retruded, therefore the SnV line will be posteriorly positioned, but it demonstrates the relative sagittal discrepancy between the prominence of the upper and lower lips. (c) Following maxillary advancement and mandibular set-back, the sagittal relationship of the upper and lower lips is improved. (The patient may have benefited from, but did not desire, an advancement genioplasty as a secondary procedure).

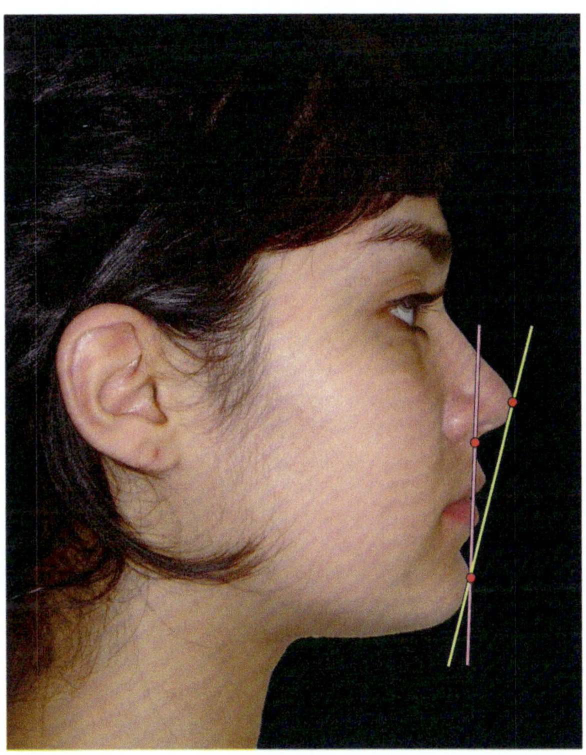

Fig. 5-40 The combined Burstone–Ricketts 'triangle' is formed between the Burstone line (Sn-Pog′) and Ricketts E-line (Pr-Pog′); the lips should fall within the triangle formed between the two lines, with the upper lip slightly ahead of the lower lip.

Upper lip–maxillary incisor relationship

The relationship of the maxillary incisors to the upper lip forms the foundation stone of treatment planning in orthognathic surgery (see Chapter 6). Aesthetic evaluation of this 'lip–incisor' relationship should take seven specific parameters into consideration (Table 5-5) (Figure 5-41).[34]

Table 5-5 Upper lip to maxillary incisor relationship

Upper lip height	Increased upper lip height will tend to reduce maxillary incisor exposure and vice versa. • Normal upper lip height: ∘ Adult males 22 ± 2 mm ∘ Adult females 20 ± 2 mm • Upper lip height comprises roughly one-third of lower anterior face height. • Upper lip height increases by approximately 3 mm between the ages of 10 and 20 years in male and female individuals. • Mid-philtrum height is approximately equal to, or 1–2 mm less than commissure height (in adults). • Reduced mid-philtrum height results in an unattractive inverted arc appearance of the upper lip, which may require surgical procedures to increase upper lip height.
Smile curtain	Defined as the muscular capacity to elevate the upper lip. • The elevation of the upper lip from repose to full smile exhibits considerable individual variability, averaging 7–8 mm (range 2–12 mm).[48] • An increased muscular capacity to raise the upper lip higher than average on smiling may lead to excessive gingival exposure ('gummy smile'). • If the lip–incisor relationship at rest is correct, a 'gummy smile' may have to be accepted, or botulinum toxin type A injections may be used to the levator muscles of the upper lip (see Chapter 26); alternatively surgery to reduce the elevation of the upper lip may be required (see Figure 53-31). • The Le Fort I incision tends to slightly reduce the smile curtain, at least temporarily.
Vertical position of the anterior maxilla and incisor teeth	The more inferior the position of the anterior maxilla, the greater the exposure of the maxillary incisors, and vice versa. • **Vertical Maxillary Excess (VME)** leading to a 'gummy smile' may result from *excessive inferior development of the maxilla;* often accompanied by excessive gingival display at rest and on smiling. Treatment centres on superior repositioning of the maxilla. • In certain cases **anterior VME** may be due to *excessively over-erupted maxillary incisors* (e.g. Class II division 2 malocclusion); the treatment of choice will either be an anterior segmental impaction of the maxilla, or orthodontic intrusion of the maxillary incisors and associated gingivae. • **Vertical Maxillary Deficiency (VMD)** may lead to reduced incisor exposure. • **Anterior dentoalveolar VMD** may be due to a digit sucking habit or forward resting tongue position preventing normal incisor eruption.
Sagittal position of the anterior maxilla and incisor teeth	The more anterior the position of the maxillary incisors, the greater the exposure of the maxillary incisors, and vice versa. • Incisor exposure increases with maxillary advancement, and reduces with maxillary set-back surgery – this must be taken into consideration, and concomitant maxillary impaction or inferior repositioning may be required in order to obtain an adequate upper lip–incisor relationship.
Maxillary incisor inclination	Should always be evaluated in relation to the facial profile and a true vertical line (Figure 5-42). • Increased proclination reduces incisor exposure. • Retroclination of proclined incisors towards the correct inclination increases incisor exposure, as the teeth rotate round their centre of resistance (Figure 5-43).
Maxillary incisor crown height	• Maxillary central incisor crown height is approximately 10 mm (range: 9–12 mm). • Incisal wear reduces incisor exposure.
Labial gingival margins of maxillary incisors	• A vertically more incisal gingival attachment, or any gingival hypertrophy will reduce incisor exposure, and may require gingivectomy (in the absence of gingival inflammation). • Incisor gingival margins may migrate gingivally until late adolescence when normal crown height is achieved (delayed apical migration)

Summarized from *Facial Aesthetics: Concepts and Clinical Diagnosis*, with permission.[2] (see Figure 5-41)

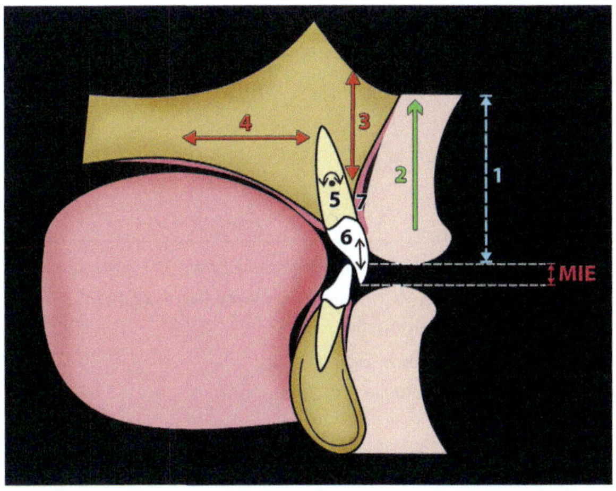

Fig. 5-41 The 'lip–incisor relationship' and maxillary incisor exposure (MIE) depends on the following factors: 1. Upper lip height. 2. Smile curtain – the muscular capacity to elevate the upper lip. 3. Vertical position of the anterior maxilla and incisor teeth. 4. Sagittal position of the anterior maxilla and incisor teeth. 5. Inclination of the maxillary incisor teeth. 6. Maxillary incisor crown height. 7. Vertical level of the labial maxillary incisor gingival margins. (From: Naini FB. Facial Aesthetics: Concepts and Clinical Diagnosis. Oxford: Wiley-Blackwell, 2011; reprinted with permission.)

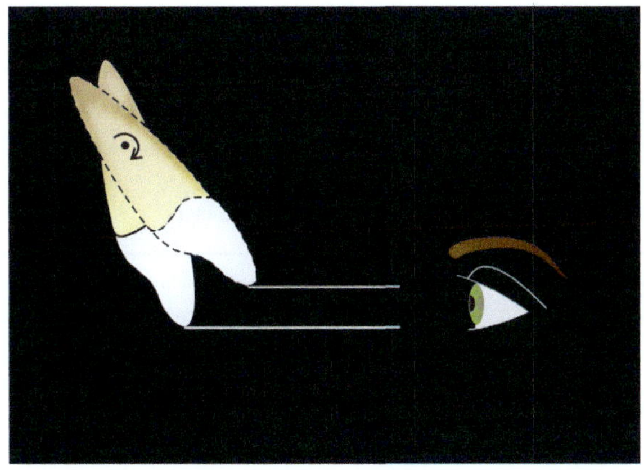

Fig. 5-43 Retroclination of proclined maxillary incisors towards the correct inclination increases the incisor exposure, as the teeth rotate around their centre of resistance.
(From: Naini FB. Facial Aesthetics: Concepts and Clinical Diagnosis. Oxford: Wiley-Blackwell, 2011; reprinted with permission.)

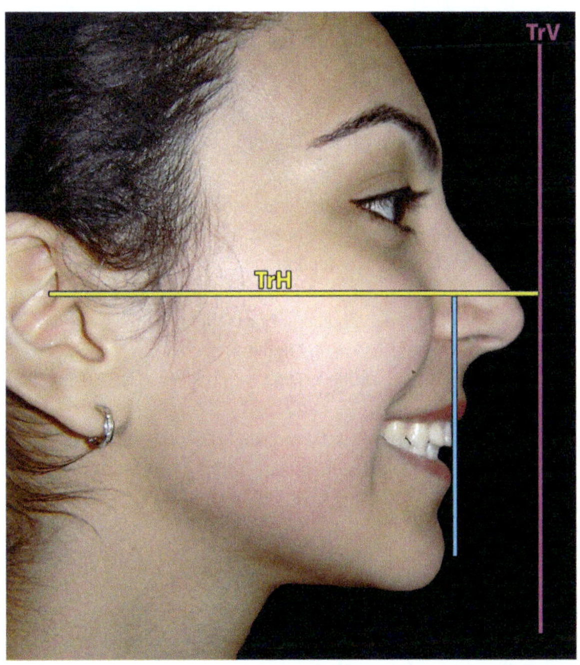

Fig. 5-42 The most accurate measurement of maxillary incisor crown inclination is that of a tangent to the labial face of the maxillary central incisor in relation to the true horizontal plane (TrH), with the patient in natural head position. TrV, true vertical. (From: Naini FB. Facial Aesthetics: Concepts and Clinical Diagnosis. Oxford: Wiley-Blackwell, 2011; reprinted with permission.)

Specific profile parameters

A number of profile parameters that require thorough aesthetic evaluation have been described above. However, there are a further number of *specific* profile parameters that also require assessment (Table 5-6).

Table 5-6 Evaluation of specific profile parameters.

Sagittal position of maxilla	• True vertical line (TrV or facial vertical) from soft tissue nasion, soft tissue glabella or a point midway between the two (perpendicular to the true horizontal line), with patient in natural head position (NHP) (see Figure 5-14). Subnasale and soft tissue A-point are ~ on this line. • Paranasal hollowing/flatness is a sign of maxillary retrognathism (Figure 5-44).

Relationship of upper lip to nasal columella (**nasolabial region**)	The **nasolabial angle (NLA)** is formed between the nasal columella and the upper lip slope.
	• Significant ethnic and gender variability:
	  ○ White males: 100° ± 12°
	  ○ White females: 105° ± 10°
	  ○ African-American males: 72° ± 15°
	  ○ African-American females: 74° ± 15°
	• Varies depending on sagittal position of maxillary incisors and anterior maxilla, the morphology of the upper lip, as well as the vertical position of the nasal tip
	• NLA should be separated into upper and lower component parts using a TrH line through subnasale (with patient in NHP) (see Figure 5-12), as *component angles vary independently*:
	  ○ Upper component of NLA (columella tangent to TrH): ideal value ~12–24° (range 8–30°).[49]
	  ○ Lower component of NLA (upper lip inclination to TrH): ideal value ~80–85°.[38]

Maxillary incisor inclination in profile smiling view	• The inclination of the labial face of the maxillary incisor should be evaluated in a smiling profile view of the patient in NHP. • A tangent to the labial face of the maxillary central incisor should be approximately parallel to a true facial vertical line (TrV) (Figure 5-45).[34]
Maxillary incisor position in sagittal plane	• Clinically, the maxillary incisors should be approximately level with a true vertical line dropped from soft tissue nasion, glabella or a point between the two, depending on the morphology of the glabellar-nasal region (Figure 5-46). • Cephalometrically, the maxillary incisors should be approximately 4 mm anterior to the nasion-perpendicular (which is very similar to their proposed position in relation to the true vertical dropped from soft tissue nasion).
Sagittal lip prominence	See 'lip prominence' section of Table 5-4

Relationship of lower lip to chin (**mentolabial fold region**)	• Mentolabial (labiomental) angle is formed between the lower lip and soft tissue chin; average value ~130°.
	• Significant individual variability:
	  ○ White males: 115° – 145°
	  ○ White females: 120° – 130°
	• Varies depending on the mandibular incisor inclination, skeletal and soft tissue chin morphology, lower lip posture, and lower anterior face height.
	• Mentolabial angle should be separated into upper and lower component parts using a TrH line through soft tissue B-point (with patient in NHP) (see Figure 5-12), as *component angles vary independently*.
	• Excessively proclined mandibular incisor teeth, a prominent chin and a reduced lower anterior face height may lead to an acute labiomental angle.

Sagittal chin position	• True vertical line (TrV or facial vertical) with patient in NHP – Soft tissue pogonion should be ~0 ± 2 mm to this line • If the patient has normal sagittal projection of the midface, subnasale (rather than soft tissue nasion) may be used to drop a TrV line, perpendicular to the true horizontal line (TrH) with the patient in NHP. This analysis is useful for planning treatment in mandibular retrognathia or retrogenia, where the maxillary position is correct. • The sagittal prominence of the soft tissue chin ideally should not be further ahead than the lower lip (Figure 5-47). • It is vital to assess the soft tissue thickness anterior to the bony chin (observe on lateral cephalograph, and palpate), as an over-projection of the chin may be entirely due to the soft tissue thickness.

Relationship of submental–cervical region	• **Lower lip–chin–submental plane angle**: average 110° ± 8°. This is obtuse if mandibular retrognathia, retrogenia, excessive lower lip projection or increased submental fat are present.
	• **Submental–cervical angle** describes the contour of the transition from the submental plane to the anterior aspect of the neck: average 110° (range 100–135°).
	• **Submental length** (soft tissue menton to C-point, which is the junction of submental plane and vertical plane of the anterior aspect of the neck).
	  ○ Linear value ~50 mm
	  ○ Proportional value: ~80% of LAFH (Figure 5-48).
	• An excessively reduced submental length is a relative contraindication to significant mandibular set-back, which could result in the formation of submental fullness or a 'double chin' appearance (Figure 5-49).[50]

Summarised from *Facial Aesthetics: Concepts and Clinical Diagnosis*, with permission.[2]

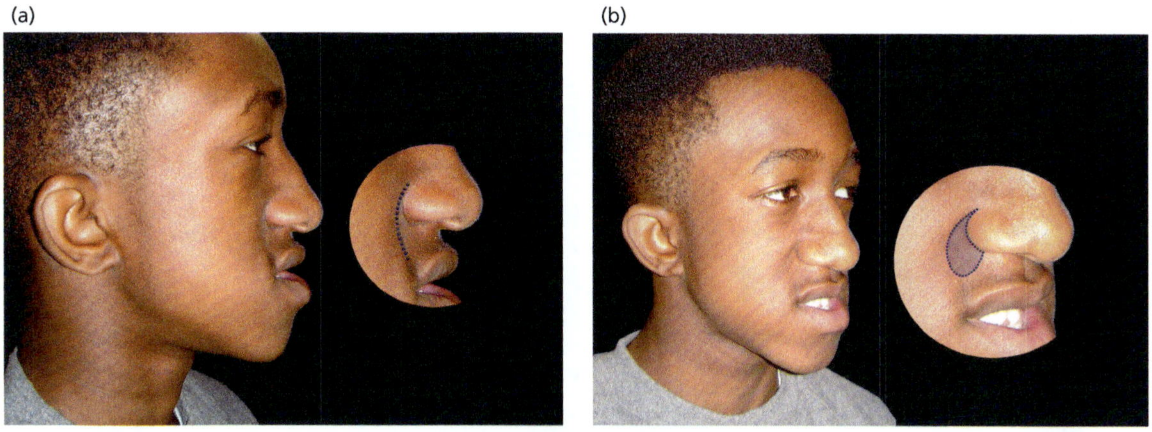

Fig. 5-44 (a, b) Paranasal hollowing is a sign of maxillary retrognathism.

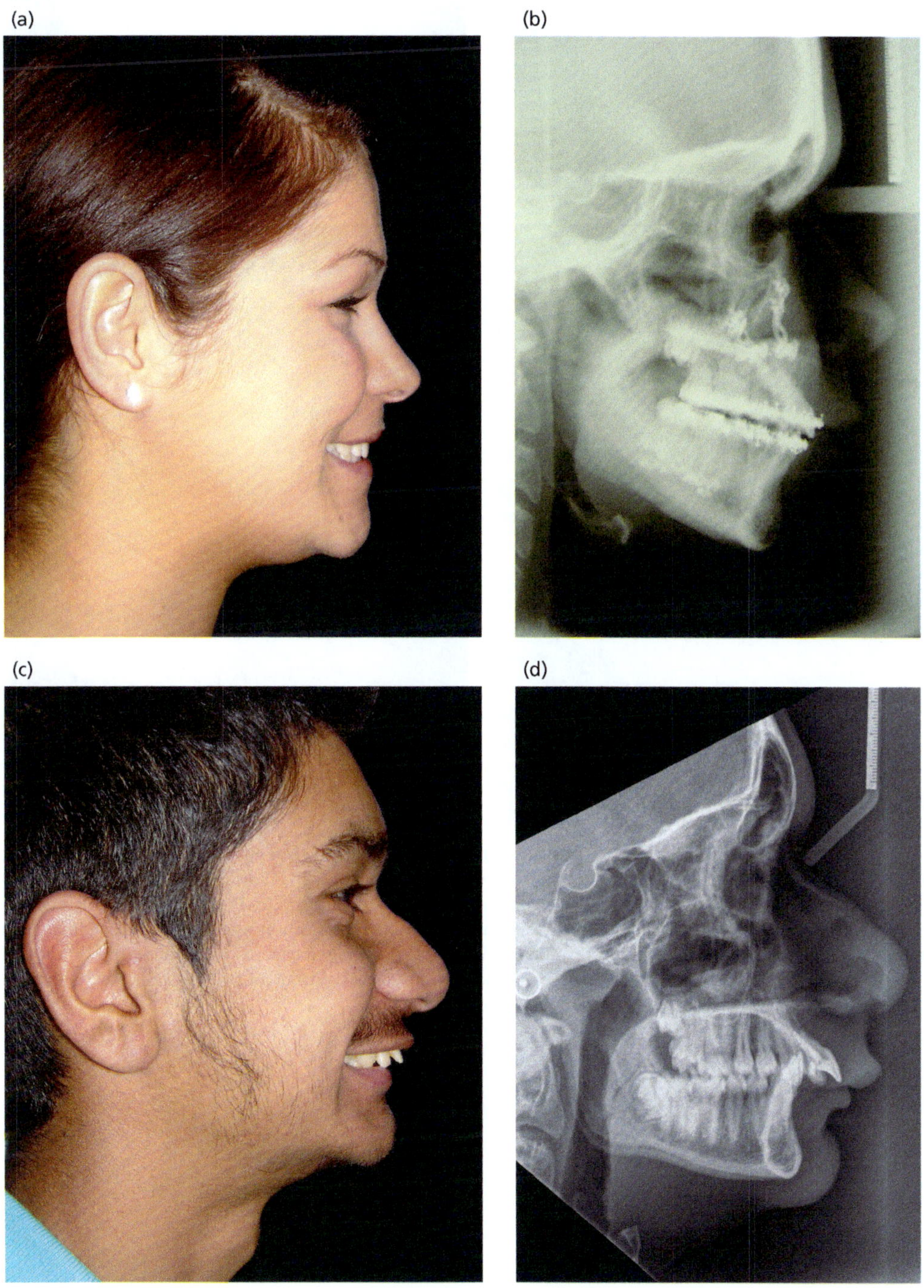

Fig. 5-45 (a, b) Post-treatment profile smiling view. A tangent to the labial face of the maxillary central incisor is approximately parallel to a true facial vertical line, which is the ideal inclination of the maxillary incisor crown. (c, d) Pretreatment profile smiling view. A tangent to the labial face of the maxillary central incisor is proclined relative to a true facial vertical line.

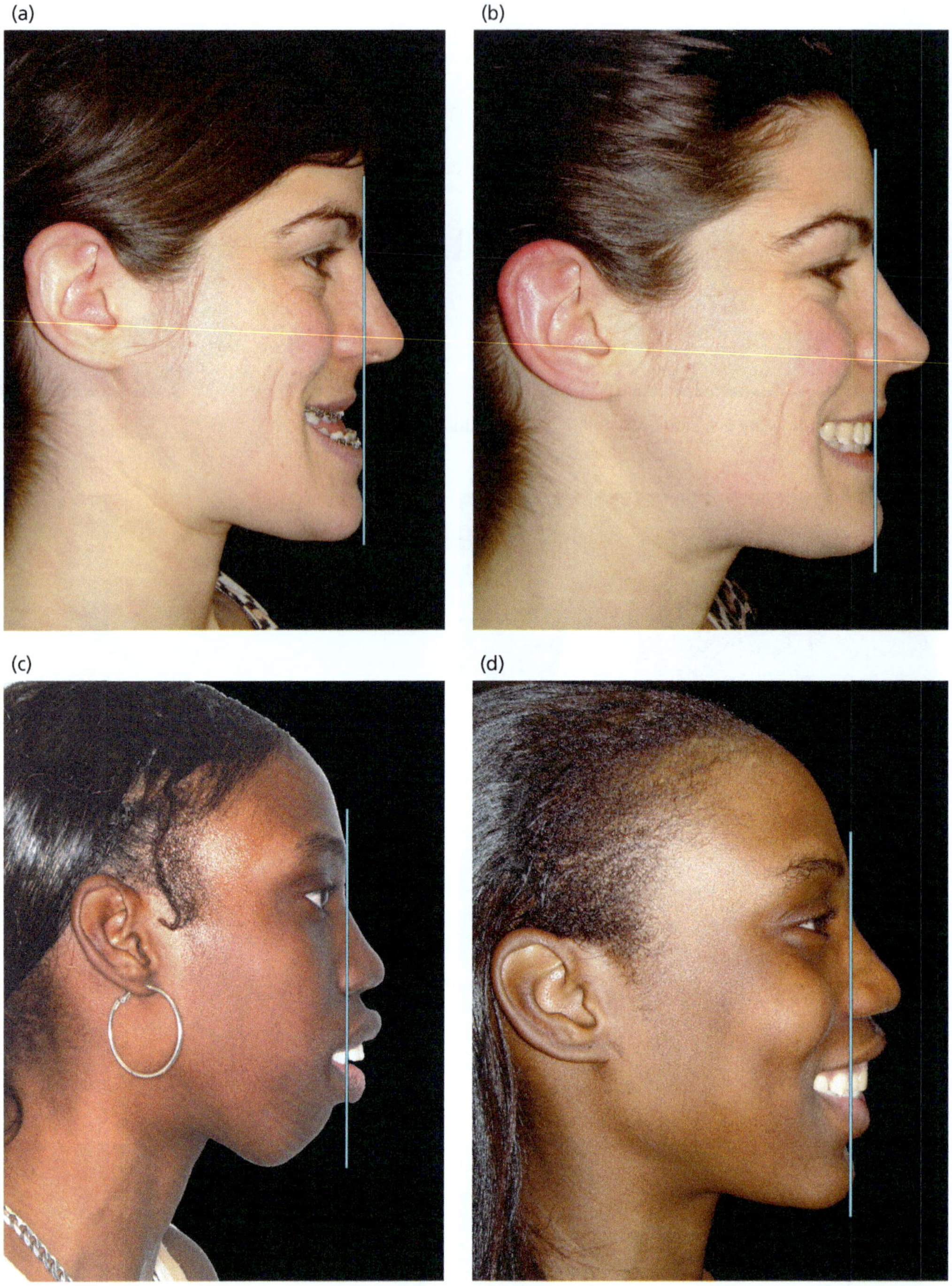

Fig. 5-46 (a) Preoperative profile smiling view of a Class III patient. The maxillary incisor crowns are significantly behind a true vertical line (TrV) dropped from glabella. (b) Following maxillary advancement at the Le Fort I level and mandibular set-back osteotomy. The sagittal position of the maxillary incisor crowns are very close to the TrV. (c) Pretreatment profile view of a Class II patient with maxillary dentoalveolar protrusion, vertical maxillary excess, mandibular retrognathia and retrogenia. The maxillary incisor crowns are significantly in front of a true vertical line (TrV) dropped from glabella. (d) Following orthodontic maxillary incisor retraction, maxillary incisor impaction and small set-back, mandibular advancement and advancement genioplasty. The sagittal position of the maxillary incisor crowns are very close to the TrV.

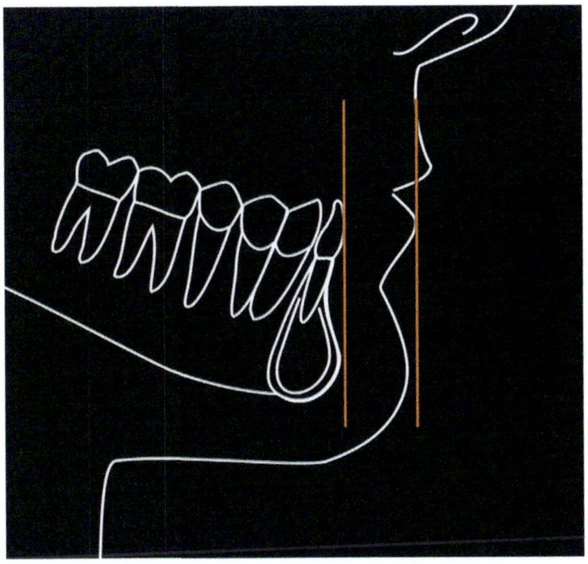

Fig. 5-47 The sagittal prominence of the soft tissue chin ideally should not be further ahead than the lower lip. The innermost point in the depth of the mentolabial fold (soft tissue B-point, also termed sublabiale) should be behind both the lower lip and chin, creating a smooth S-shape in the transition between the lower lip and chin. This shape also occurs in the dentoskeletal support, with the labial surface of the mandibular incisor on a vertical line with osseous pogonion, and skeletal B-point behind this line.

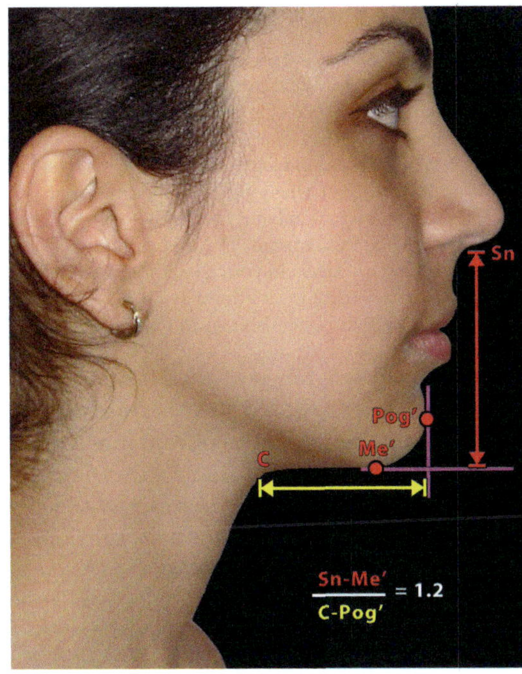

Fig. 5-48 Lower vertical height–depth ratio. (From: Naini FB. Facial Aesthetics: Concepts and Clinical Diagnosis. Oxford: Wiley-Blackwell, 2011; reprinted with permission.)

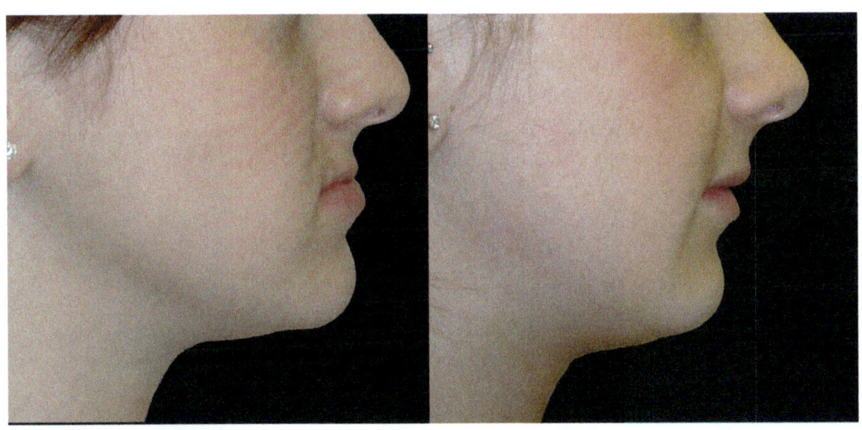

Fig. 5-49 Following a mandibular set-back osteotomy, submental fullness has increased and the submental–cervical angle become obtuse.

Examination of the temporomandibular joints (TMJ)

The condyles should be palpated and any deviation in the path of opening and closure of the mandible observed both from frontal view and by standing behind the patient and looking from above. The joints are examined for tenderness and noises, including clicking (from movement of the articular disc) and crepitus (potentially from arthritic problems). The range of mouth opening and lateral excursions should be assessed and the muscles of mastication gently palpated for any signs of tenderness.

Note:

Range of mouth opening

The lower limit of the range of normal (unstrained) mouth opening is approximately 35 mm in women and 40 mm in men; less than this is considered reduced mouth opening. The lower limit of normal excursive movements is approximately 8 mm, best evaluated by measuring the deviation of the dental midlines on excursion.[51] *Pretreatment and preoperative baseline measurements should be recorded for postoperative comparative purposes.*

Cephalometric analysis

> 'In physical science the first essential step in the direction of learning any subject is to find principles of numerical reckoning and practicable methods for measuring some quality connected with it. I often say that when you can measure what you are speaking about, and express it in numbers, you know something about it; but when you cannot measure it, when you cannot express it in numbers, your knowledge is of a meagre and unsatisfactory kind; it may be the beginning of knowledge, but you have scarcely in your thoughts advanced to the state of *Science*, whatever the matter may be.'
>
> William Thomson, Lord Kelvin (1824–1907)[14]

An incredibly diverse range of cephalometric analyses have been described, and their normative values are based on varying sample sizes from different populations. Each analysis has advantages and shortcomings, and *no claim can be made for the universal application of any specific analysis*.[19] Comprehensive cephalometric analysis has been described elsewhere.[19] *The purpose of this section is to describe only the specific cephalometric relationships directly relevant to the orthognathic patient.*

Note:

Interpreting cephalometric analysis

> 'Take nothing for granted if you can check it.'
>
> Rudyard Kipling (1865–1936)[52]

For an in-depth understanding of the structural and morphological relationships of the craniofacial complex, it is important to have a detailed understanding of the application of the various cephalometric analyses to each dentoskeletal and soft tissue parameter. *Cephalometric analysis is essentially applied geometry*.[19] Occasionally, the interpretations of different cephalometric analyses exploring the same parameter may disagree. For this reason, *the results of each cephalometric analysis should be re-checked with another, and always in relation to the clinical findings*.

In addition, comparison of a patient's craniofacial measurements to population normative values, though useful, should be undertaken with care. There is significant **individual variability**, even within a relatively homogenous population from a similar ethnic background, and variations due to age and gender. This is reflected in wide ranges of normative values and their standard deviations.

The vitally important purpose of cephalometric analysis is that with practice, it teaches the clinician's eye to see, in the same way that a professional architect will view a building differently to a layperson. Linear and angular normative values become less important, compared with the observation and evaluation of the inter-relationships between the various dentofacial parameters that create each individual face.

Sagittal skeletal relationships

Two useful methods of analysing sagittal skeletal relationships are the nasion perpendicular, which provides linear measurements, and a group of angular measurements which relate the maxilla (SNA angle), mandible (SNB angle) and chin (SND angle; SN-Pog angle) to the anterior cranial base (sella-nasion or SN plane). An extension of the latter is the ANB angle, which relates the maxilla to the mandible.

Nasion perpendicular (McNamara) (Figure 5-50): With the patient's head oriented in NHP, the most direct method to determine the sagittal position of the maxilla and mandible is to measure the horizontal linear distance to the nasion perpendicular (N-perpendicular), a vertical line perpendicular to the true horizontal, dropped from bony nasion. McNamara's original data was based on the Frankfort plane rather than the true horizontal plane. Points anterior to N-perpendicular are assigned a positive value, and posterior a negative value. In white Caucasian patients:[53]

- Maxillary point A is on or slightly ahead of nasion perpendicular (0 to +1 mm)
- Mandibular point B is 2–3 mm behind nasion perpendicular
- A–B difference (horizontal distance between points A and B when both are projected onto the true horizontal) is approximately 4 mm

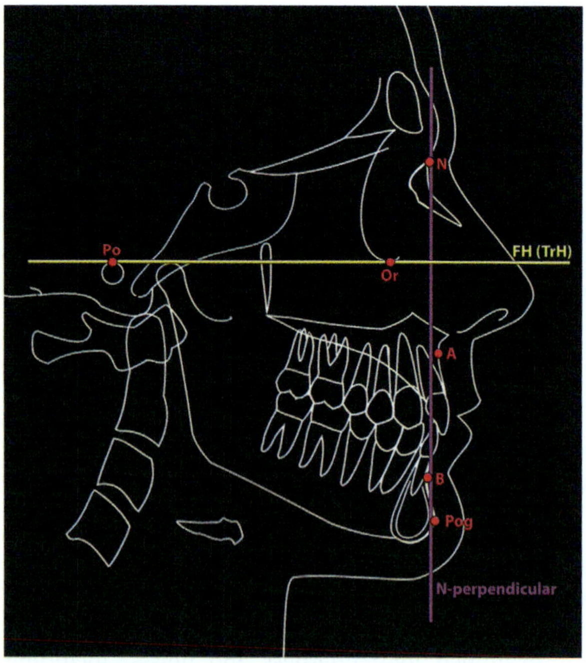

Fig. 5-50 The nasion perpendicular is a vertical line perpendicular to the Frankfort Horizontal (FH) plane, or ideally the true horizontal plane (TrH), dropped from bony nasion. (From: Naini FB. Facial Aesthetics: Concepts and Clinical Diagnosis. Oxford: Wiley-Blackwell, 2011; reprinted with permission.)

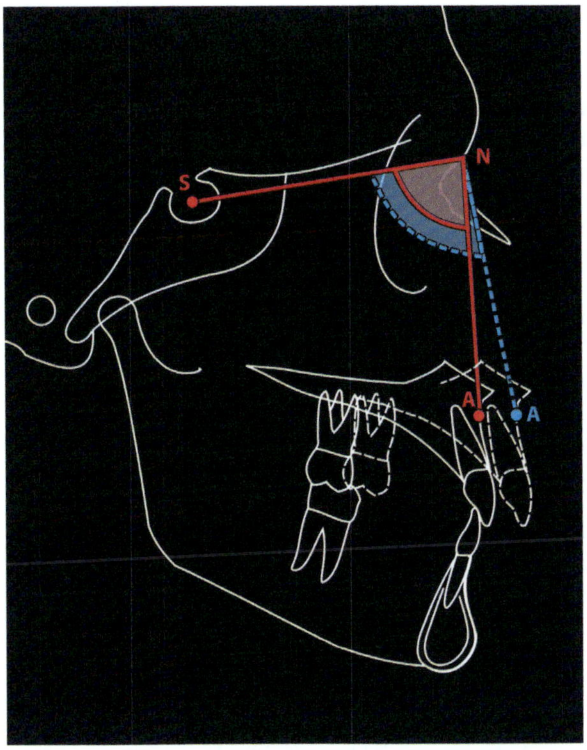

Fig. 5-51 An increase in the SNA angle *may* indicate protrusion of the maxillary dentoalveolus, assuming the SN plane has a normal inclination, and sella and nasion are in normal sagittal and vertical positions. (From: Naini FB. Facial Aesthetics: Concepts and Clinical Diagnosis. Oxford: Wiley-Blackwell, 2011; reprinted with permission.)

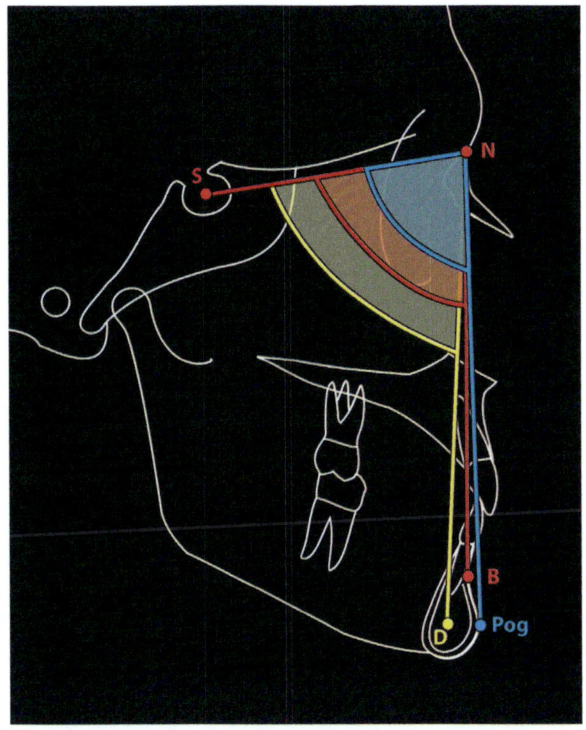

Fig. 5-52 The SNB, SND and SN-Pog angles provide an indication of the sagittal position of the mandibular apical base, mandible, and chin, respectively, in relation to the anterior cranial base and in relation to each other. (From: Naini FB. Facial Aesthetics: Concepts and Clinical Diagnosis. Oxford: Wiley-Blackwell, 2011; reprinted with permission.)

- Hard tissue pogonion (the most anterior point on the bony chin) is:
  - –4 to 0 mm behind N-perpendicular (in adult women)
  - –2 to +5 mm to N-perpendicular (in adult men).

SNA angle (82 ± 3°): relates the sagittal position of the maxillary apical base (A-point) to the anterior cranial base (SN). The SNA angle provides an *indication* of the sagittal position of the maxilla relative to the anterior cranial base (Figure 5-51).

SNB angle (79 ± 3°): relates the sagittal position of the mandibular apical base (B-point) to the anterior cranial base (SN). The SNB angle provides an *indication* of the sagittal position of the mandible relative to the anterior cranial base (Figure 5-52).

It should be noted that A-point and B-point are alveolar points and do not necessarily represent the true position of the skeletal bases, though they tend to provide a useful indication of the relative sagittal position of the maxilla and mandible. Additionally, the inclination of the SN plane is variable, therefore these analyses may only be employed if the SN plane has a normal inclination of 6–7° relative to the true horizontal, and sella and nasion are in normal sagittal and vertical positions.

SND angle (76–77°): Point 'D' is the centre of the body of the symphysis (bony chin) and is estimated visually. The SND angle provides an assessment of the *sagittal position of the mandibular skeletal base* in relation to the anterior cranial base (see Figure 5-52).

SN-Pog angle (80 ± 3°): This angle is formed between the most anterior point on the bony chin (pogonion) and the SN plane. It is important to compare the value of SNB to SN-Pog. In patients with a prominent chin but mandibular dentoalveolar (apical base) retrusion, the facial profile may be acceptable even though the dentoalveolar relationship is unfavourable. This relationship is common in Class II division 2 type malocclusions. If SN-Pog is smaller than SNB, the patient is likely to have an excessively recessive bony chin in the sagittal plane (see Figure 5-52).

ANB angle (3 ± 1°): The ANB angle represents the difference between the SNA and SNB angles, providing an indication of the sagittal discrepancy between the maxillary and mandibular apical bases (Figure 5-53). The ANB angle is positive if point A lies anterior to NB. If NA and NB coincide, the ANB angle is zero. If point A lies posterior to NB, ANB will be negative. The skeletal pattern is described as:

- Class I: the ANB angle is in the range 2–4°;
- Class II: if ANB angle greater than 4°;
- Class III: if ANB angle less than 2°.

When assessing sagittal skeletal pattern using the angle ANB, it should be borne in mind that variations

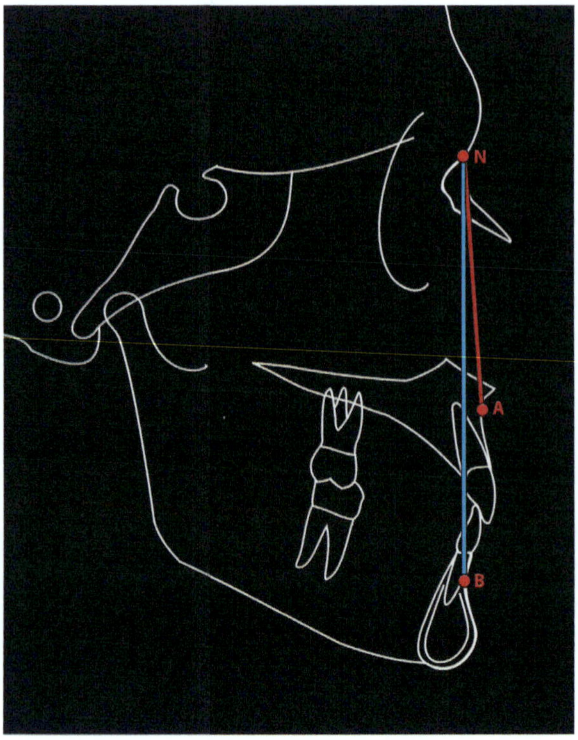

Fig. 5-53 The ANB angle represents the difference between the SNA and SNB angles, providing an indication of the sagittal discrepancy between the maxillary and mandibular apical bases. (From: Naini FB. Facial Aesthetics: Concepts and Clinical Diagnosis. Oxford: Wiley-Blackwell, 2011; reprinted with permission.)

in the position of nasion will affect the ANB angle. Additionally, the sagittal skeletal and dental-occlusal relationships do not always match due to dentoalveolar compensation, e.g. a significant sagittal skeletal Class II may have a relatively small incisor overjet if the mandibular incisors are excessively proclined.

Vertical skeletal relationships

There is no single cephalometric variable that reliably distinguishes normal from vertically abnormal individuals.[19] Therefore, it is necessary to analyze both **linear** anterior and posterior vertical dimensions, both as absolute measurements and proportional relationships, and **angular** measurements comparing posterior and anterior vertical dimensions.

Relative inclination of horizontal facial planes: The orthodontist Viken Sassouni described the importance of analysing the relative inclination of the horizontal planes of the dentoskeletal complex.[54] A slightly modified version of this analysis may be employed, utilizing the following five horizontal facial planes (Figure 5-54):[19]

- Anterior cranial base (S-N) plane;
- True horizontal plane (or Frankfort plane if it is horizontal);
- Maxillary (palatal) plane;
- Occlusal plane;
- Mandibular plane.

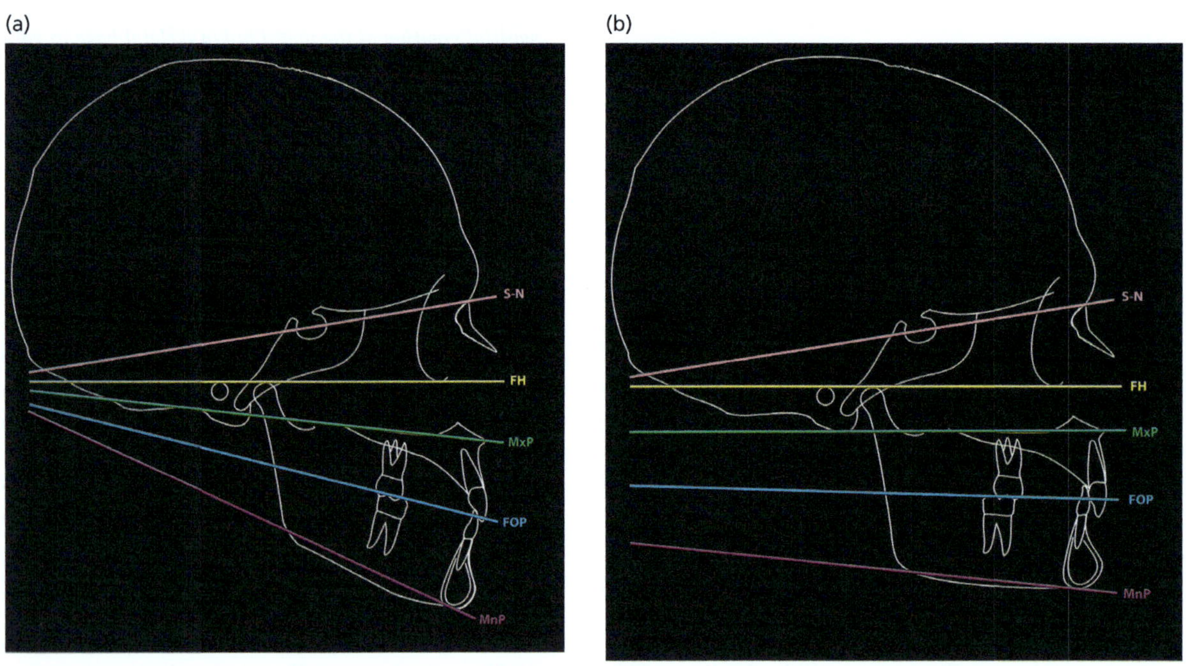

Fig. 5-54 (a) According to the Sassouni analysis, in a well-proportioned face, the horizontal facial planes should *converge* symmetrically toward an approximate *area of intersection located near the occiput*. If any part of the face is vertically disproportionate, its associated plane will not converge with the others. (b) If the area of convergence of the horizontal facial planes is positioned well behind the occiput, the planes will be nearly parallel; this skeletal pattern is associated with similar anterior and posterior facial heights, and correlates with a deep overbite tendency, termed a 'skeletal deep bite'. (c) If the area of convergence of the horizontal facial planes is positioned in front of the occiput, towards the face, the planes will diverge anteriorly; this skeletal pattern is associated with markedly different anterior and posterior facial heights, and correlates with an anterior open bite tendency, termed a 'skeletal open bite'. MxP, maxillary plane; MnP, mandibular plane; FOP, functional occlusal plane; FH, Frankfort Horizontal plane; SN, sella–nasion plane. (From: Naini FB. Facial Aesthetics: Concepts and Clinical Diagnosis. Oxford: Wiley-Blackwell, 2011; reprinted with permission.)

(c)

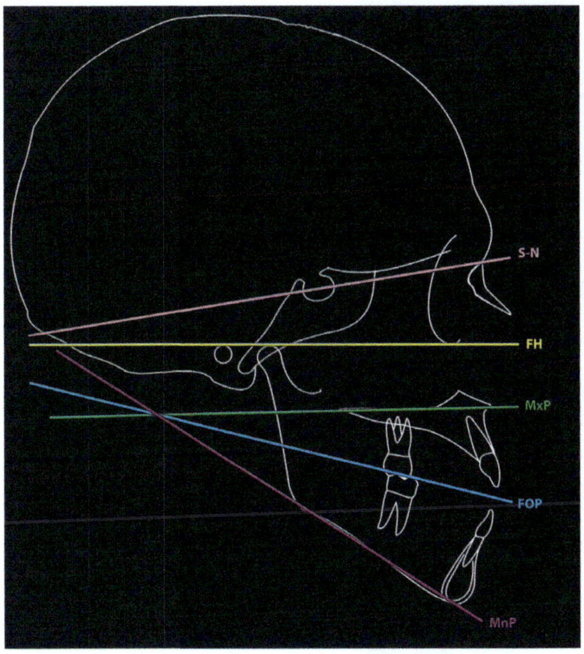

Fig. 5-54 (*Continued*).

In a well-proportioned face, these horizontal facial planes should *converge* symmetrically toward an approximate *area of intersection located near the occiput* (back of the skull). If any part of the face is vertically disproportionate, its associated plane will diverge from the others.

Anterior face height ratio (Figure 5-55): Horizontal lines are projected from G, N, ANS and Me onto the true vertical. The middle anterior face height (MAFH) may be measured from the projection of either G or N to that of ANS. The lower anterior face height (LAFH) is measured from the projection of ANS to that of Me. The proportional relationship of MAFH:LAFH is approximately 50:50% or 45:55%, depending on which uppermost point is used. This proportional relationship is more important than any absolute measurements.

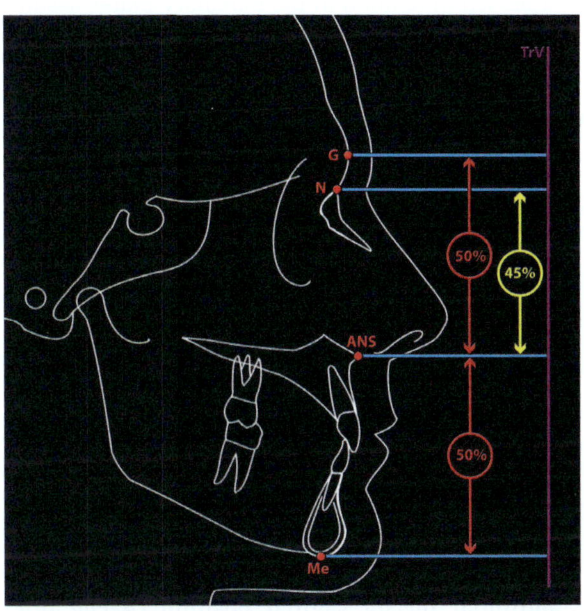

Fig. 5-55 Anterior face height ratios (proportional relationship of lower to middle anterior face height). (TrV: true vertical plane). (From: Naini FB. Facial Aesthetics: Concepts and Clinical Diagnosis. Oxford: Wiley-Blackwell, 2011; reprinted with permission.)

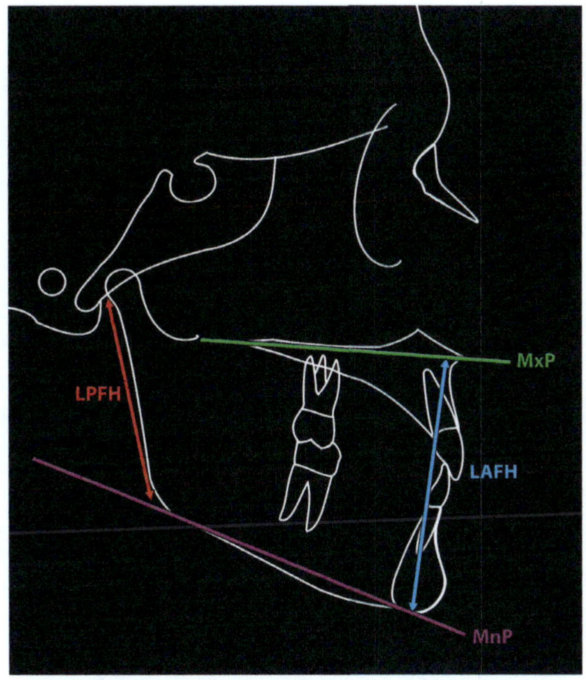

Fig. 5-56 Facial Height Index (FHI: Proportional relationship of anterior to posterior lower face height) is the ratio of LAFH to LPFH, and should be from 0.65 to 0.75. If the LPFH is less than 65% or more than 75% of the lower anterior face height, there is likely to be a vertical skeletal discrepancy. MxP, maxillary plane; MnP, mandibular plane. (From: Naini FB. Facial Aesthetics: Concepts and Clinical Diagnosis. Oxford: Wiley-Blackwell, 2011; reprinted with permission.)

Anterior to posterior face height ratio (Facial Height Index, FHI) (Figure 5-56): This is the ratio of the LAFH to the lower posterior face height (LPFH), and should be approximately between 0.65 to 0.75.[55] Hence, if the LPFH is less than 65% or more than 75% of the LAFH, there is likely to be a vertical skeletal discrepancy. The FHI must be analysed in conjunction with the anterior face height ratio, in order to assess whether the discrepancy lies in the anterior or posterior face height, or both.

Maxillary–mandibular planes angle (MMPA) (Figure 5-57): This is largely determined by the ratio of anterior and posterior intermaxillary heights. It should be assessed in conjunction with the anterior face height ratio. The average value is 27° ± 5°.

Gonial angle (Figure 5-58): The angle Ar-Go-Me (average value between 120°–130°) is formed between the inclination of the posterior border of the mandibular ramus and the mandibular plane. It helps to describe the morphology of the mandible, in particular the relationship between the ramus and the body. It is highly correlated with the

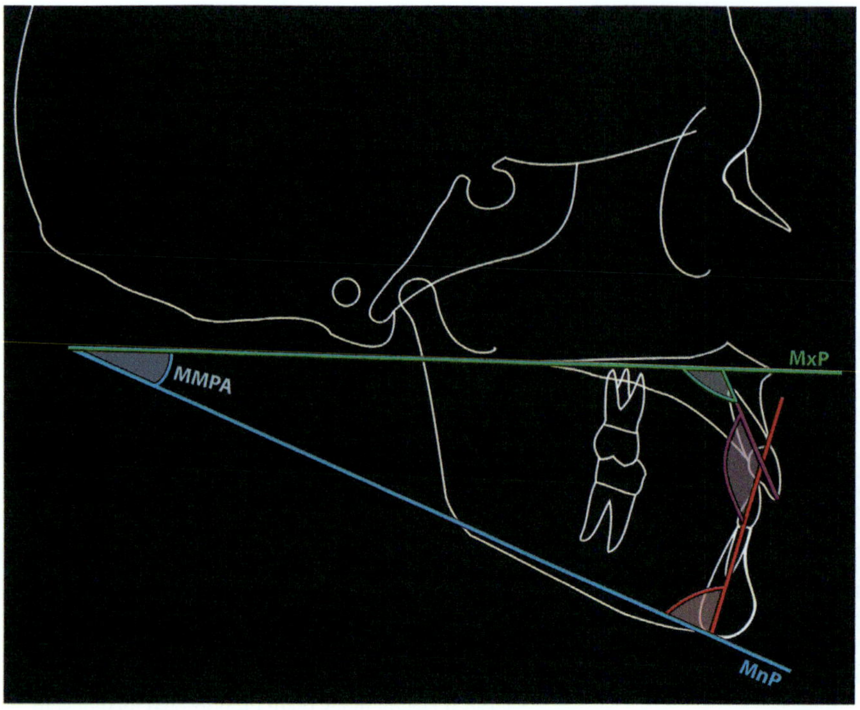

Fig. 5-57 The maxillary–mandibular planes angle (MMPA) is the anterior angle formed by the intersection of the maxillary plane and the mandibular plane. The interincisal angle is the posterior angle formed by the intersection of the long axes of the maxillary and mandibular central incisors; the sum of the MMPA, maxillary incisor to maxillary plane inclination, mandibular incisor to mandibular plane inclination and interincisal angle should be 360°. (From: Naini FB. Facial Aesthetics: Concepts and Clinical Diagnosis. Oxford: Wiley-Blackwell, 2011; reprinted with permission.)

mandibular plane angle. The gonial angle may be divided into upper and lower component parts, by drawing a **facial depth line** (nasion–gonion). The **upper component** of the gonial angle (50 ± 2°) identifies the inclination of the ramus and the **lower component** identifies the inclination of the body of the mandible.

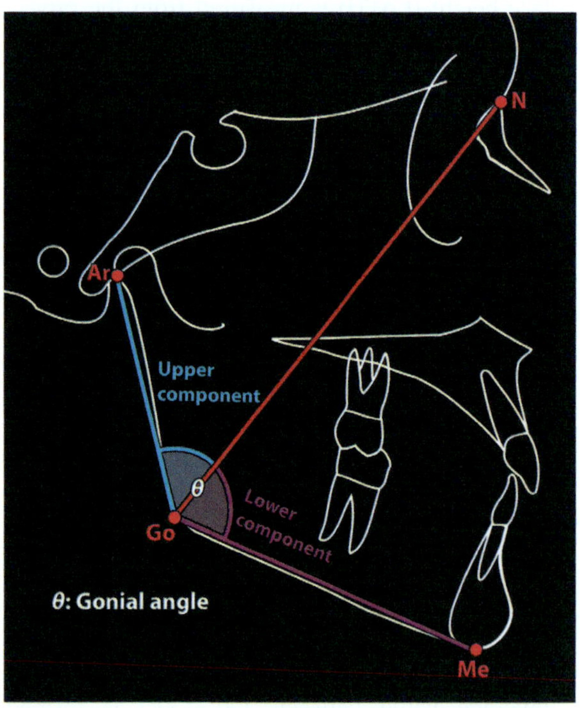

Fig. 5-58 The gonial angle may be divided into an upper and lower component in order to determine the relative contribution of the ramus and body inclination to mandibular morphology. (From: Naini FB. Facial Aesthetics: Concepts and Clinical Diagnosis. Oxford: Wiley-Blackwell, 2011; reprinted with permission.)

Dentoalveolar relationships

Maxillary incisor inclination: As already described above, the inclination of the labial face of the maxillary incisors is of paramount importance in both diagnosis and treatment planning. It is assessed clinically in relation to the smiling profile view of the patient, which demonstrates the aesthetic impact of the maxillary incisor inclination in relation to the face and smile. However, it may also be assessed cephalometrically (Figure 5-59).

Maxillary incisor inclination may also be assessed in relation to the maxillary plane, assuming an average maxillary plane inclination and a normal crown-root angle for the maxillary central incisor. Average value is: 109–112° ± 6°.

Mandibular incisors inclination: This may be assessed in relation to the mandibular plane (see Figure 5-57). Average value is: 92° ± 5°. There is an important inverse geometrical relationship between this value and the MMPA, *which is important for treatment planning of mandibular autorotation in orthognathic surgery*. If the MMPA is increased, there tends to be a compensatory retroclination of the mandibular incisors. Conversely, in 'low angle' patients, the mandibular incisors may be proclined. The combined mandibular incisor inclination and MMPA should be approximately 120°. Hence, for every degree the MMPA exceeds its average value, the expected value of the mandibular incisor inclination should be reduced by 1°, and vice versa.

Mandibular incisor sagittal position (A-Pog line) (Figure 5-60): This is the perpendicular distance of the mandibular central incisor edge to the A-Pog line.[56] It represents the degree of mandibular incisor protrusion in relation to the lower face. In

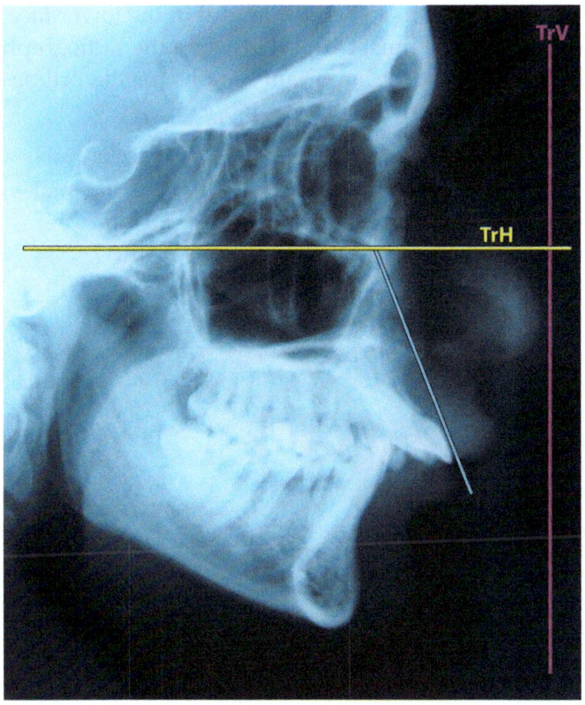

Fig. 5-59 Excessive maxillary incisor proclination may be evaluated on a profile smiling photograph and a lateral cephalometric radiograph taken with the patient in natural head position. TrH, true horizontal; TrV, true vertical. (From: Naini FB. Facial Aesthetics: Concepts and Clinical Diagnosis. Oxford: Wiley-Blackwell, 2011; reprinted with permission.)

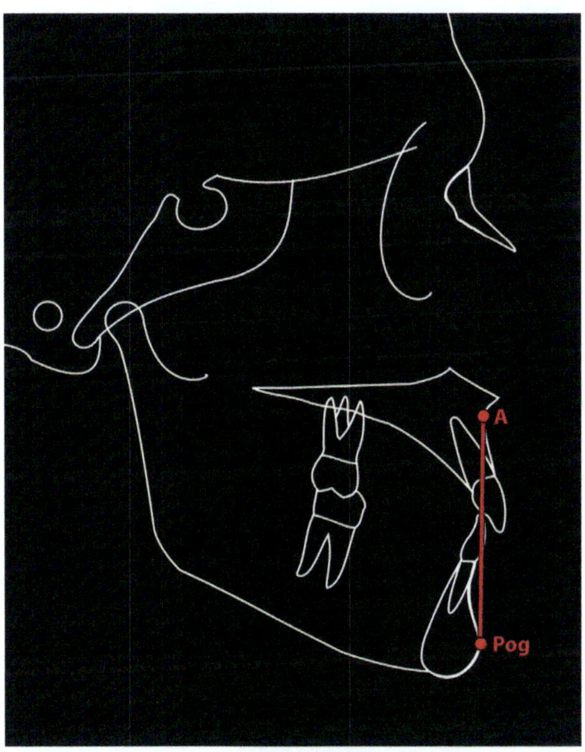

Fig. 5-60 In individuals with good dentofacial aesthetics and good dental occlusions, the mandibular incisor edge lies on or close to the A-Pog line. (From: Naini FB. Facial Aesthetics: Concepts and Clinical Diagnosis. Oxford: Wiley-Blackwell, 2011; reprinted with permission.)

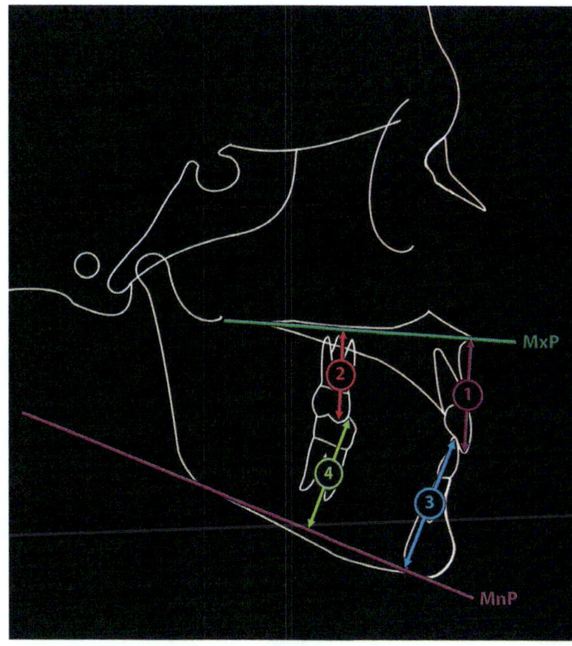

Fig. 5-61 1: Anterior maxillary dental height; 2: Posterior maxillary dental height; 3: Anterior mandibular dental height; 4: Posterior mandibular dental height. (From: Naini FB. Facial Aesthetics: Concepts and Clinical Diagnosis. Oxford: Wiley-Blackwell, 2011; reprinted with permission.)

individuals with good dentofacial aesthetics and good dental occlusions, the *mandibular incisor edge lies on or close to the A-Pog line*. It is important to bear in mind that the orientation of the A-Pog is influenced by the sagittal position of maxillary A-point and the prominence of the chin.

Vertical dentoalveolar heights (Figure 5-61): The anterior and posterior maxillary and mandibular dental heights should be evaluated. The **anterior maxillary dental height** (average ~28 ± 3 mm) should be evaluated bearing in mind the upper lip height and maxillary incisor inclination. An increase in this dimension may indicate over-eruption of the maxillary incisors or anterior vertical maxillary excess. A decrease may occur if the anterior vertical incisor eruption has been impeded, e.g. patients with an anterior open bite of soft tissue aetiology or those with prolonged digit sucking habits. **Posterior maxillary dental height** is on average only a few millimetres less than the anterior. An increase in this dimension may be due to posterior vertical maxillary excess. The roots of the maxillary molars should be at, or no more than 3 mm inferior to the height of the palatal vault.

Anterior mandibular dental height is on average between 40 to 45 ± 3 mm. An increase may indicate excessive eruption of the mandibular incisor teeth and/or increased vertical chin height. A decrease in this dimension may be due to impeded eruption of the mandibular incisor teeth or reduced vertical chin height. **Posterior mandibular dental height** is usually approximately 5–6 mm less than anterior mandibular dental height.

Soft tissue thickness

The thickness of the facial soft tissues, particularly in the lower face, is an important diagnostic and treatment planning parameter. Thick soft tissues may effectively mask a significant underlying dentoskeletal discrepancy (Figure 5-62 and 5-63). In addition to clinical palpation, the thickness of the soft tissues may be gleaned from the lateral cephalometric radiograph. However, for this to be meaningful in the lower face, the lip posture must be relaxed when the radiograph is taken. The most important regions for the orthognathic patient are (Figure 5-64):

- Upper lip thickness: 15 mm
- Lower lip thickness: 15 mm (slightly less in females)
- Mentolabial fold region thickness: ~10 mm
- Soft tissue chin pad thickness: 10 ± 2 mm

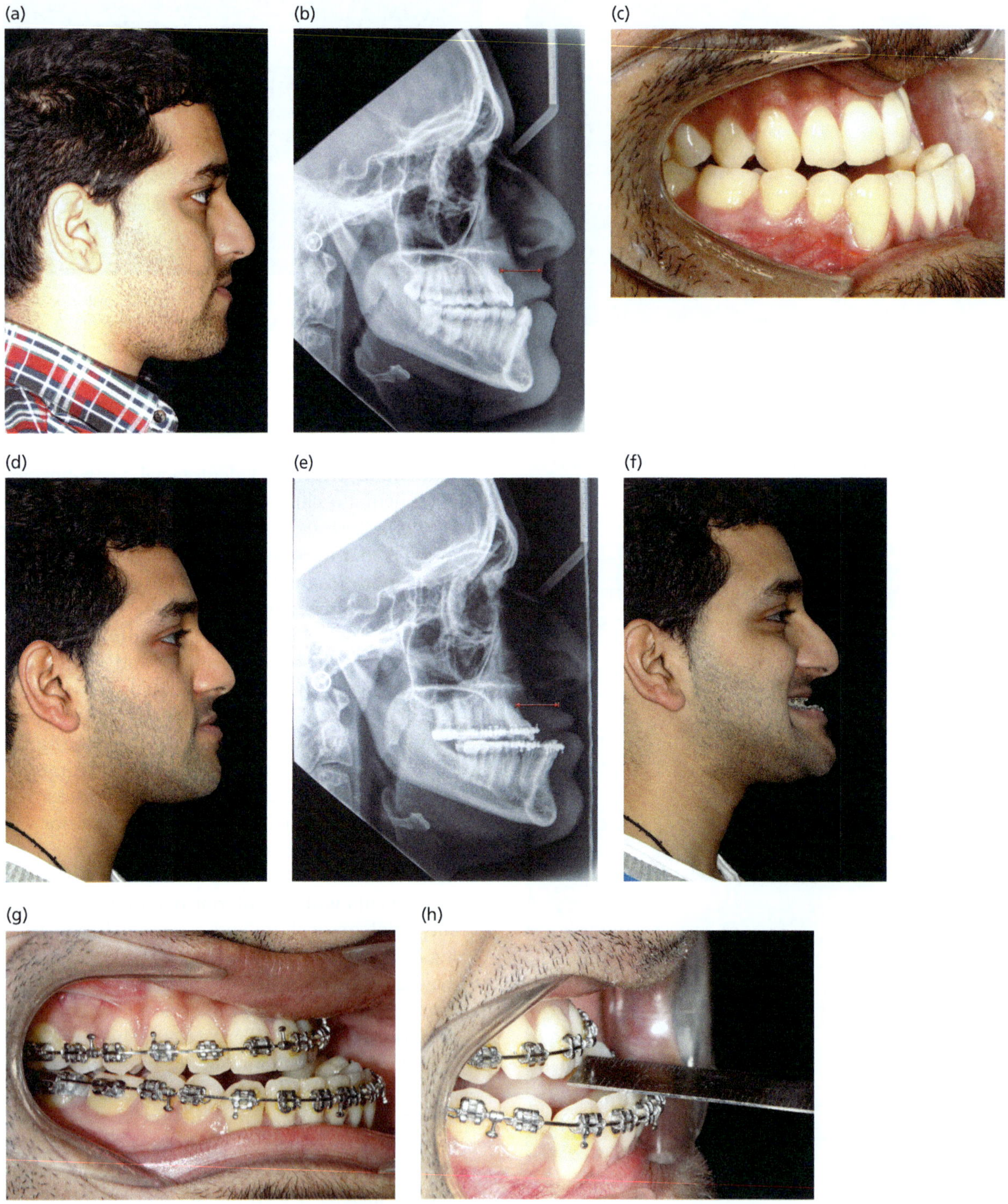

Fig. 5-62 Thick soft tissues may effectively mask a significant underlying dentoskeletal discrepancy. (a–c) Pretreatment images for a patient with a severe Class III skeletal discrepancy, but the increased thickness of the upper lip masks much of the underlying skeletal discrepancy. (d–h) Preoperative views after orthodontic decompensation, demonstrating a 10 mm reverse incisor overjet, requiring approximately 12–13 mm of bimaxillary sagittal repositioning to obtain a Class I incisor relationship. The profile smiling view provides a better indication of the extent of the sagittal discrepancy. However, despite decompensation, the thickness of the upper lip still masks much of the extent of the skeletal discrepancy. (i–k) End of treatment views, following maxillary advancement at the Le Fort I level and mandibular set-back.

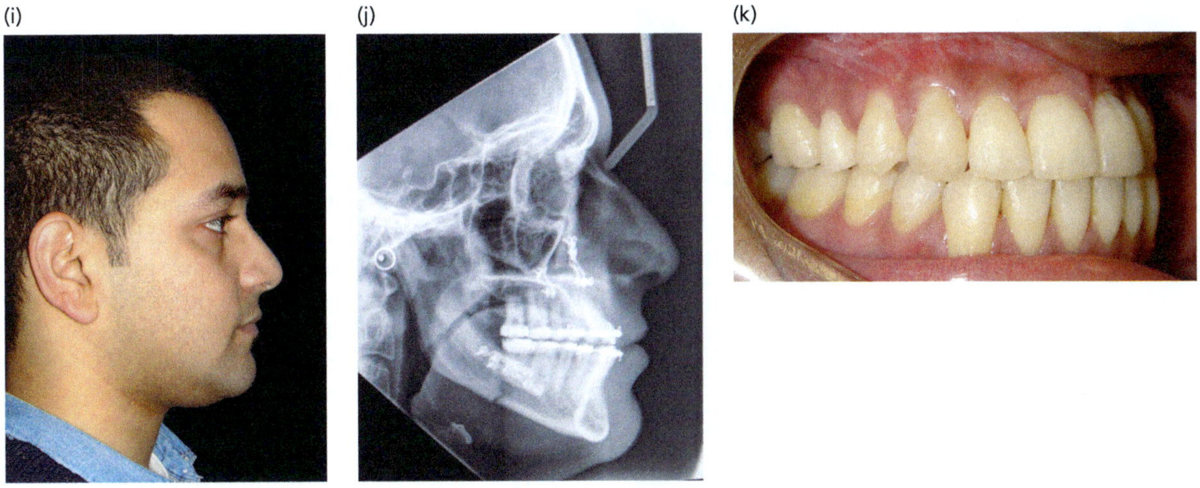

Fig. 5-62 (*Continued*).

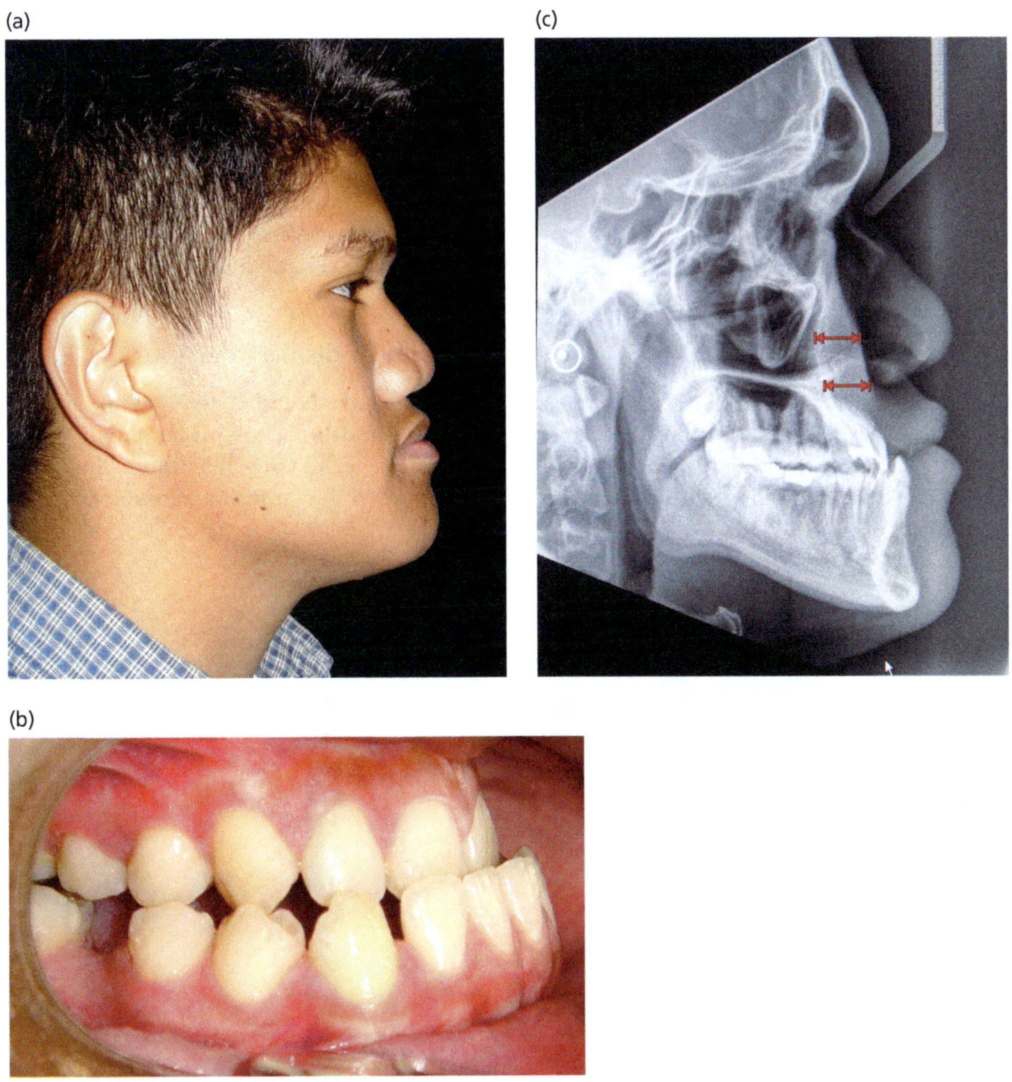

Fig. 5-63 (a–c) Patient with a significant Class III skeletal discrepancy, where the maxillary retrognathism is partially masked by the thickness of the soft tissues of the cheek.

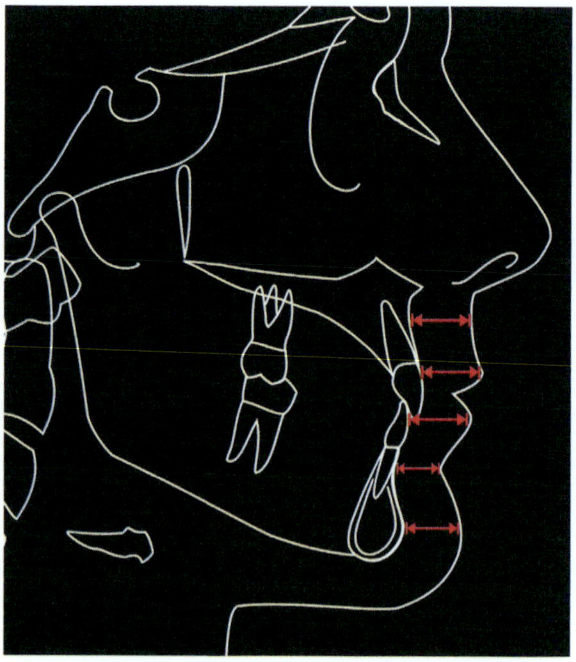

Fig. 5-64 Soft tissue thicknesses of the upper lip, lower lip, mentolabial (labiomental) fold region and the chin pad.

Dental-occlusal relationship evaluation

Oral health

The initial **intraoral evaluation** should routinely check for defective restorations and any signs of dental, periodontal or soft tissue disease, which must be controlled and treated prior to embarking on orthognathic surgical treatment. **Teeth of poor prognosis** should be noted, as they will form part of the treatment plan, and may need to be extracted in place of other routinely extracted teeth, should dental extractions be required. Areas exhibiting a **thin gingival biotype** or **gingival recession** should be noted and photographed. Where alveolar bone and enveloping gingival tissues are thin, preparatory dental movements may exacerbate the recession. This may be particularly relevant to mandibular incisor proclination in the orthodontic decompensation of skeletal Class III patients. In such situations, consideration may need to be given to partial decompensation of the teeth. It is also vitally important to use the lightest possible forces with which to move the teeth, in order to reduce the possibility of exacerbating the gingival recession (Figure 5-65). Excellent preoperative records and informed consent is such situations are paramount.

Freeway space and mandibular overclosure

The **freeway space**, which is the distance between the occlusal surfaces of the maxillary and mandibular dentitions when the mandible is in the rest position, should be evaluated. It is usually in the order of 2–3 mm. An excessively deep incisor overbite may be related to **overclosure** of the mandible. In such cases, which may be associated with a Class II division 1, Class II division 2 or Class III malocclusion, the posterior dentition may be in infraocclusion, or there is relative posterior **vertical maxillary deficiency** (relative VMD). As such, the *freeway space may be increased, leading to excessive forward mandibular rotation on closure, i.e. overclosure* (Figure 5-66).

Mandibular displacements

The clinician should actively look for **anterior** or **lateral mandibular displacements**, which may be present in achieving maximum intercuspation of the teeth. If an **anterior crossbite** is present, the

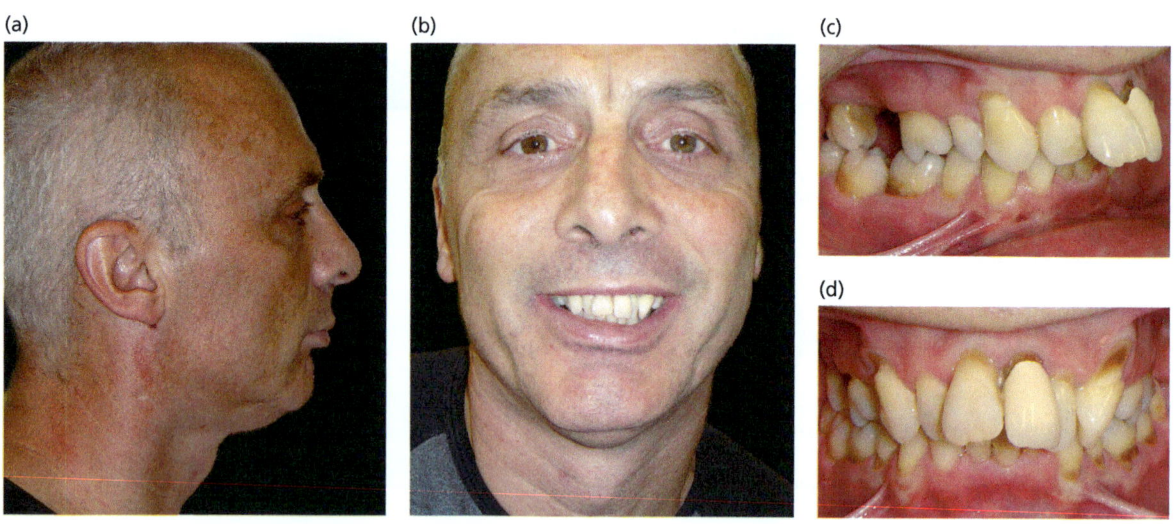

Fig. 5-65 (a–e) Pretreatment photographs of a patient with a Class II division 1 incisor relationship with proclined maxillary incisors, on a Class II skeletal pattern due to mandibular retrognathia. There is extensive gingival recession and both generalized and further localized alveolar bone loss. Orthodontic treatment was carried out with very light forces, and patience, with light round nickel–titanium archwires and round stainless steel archwires, prior to a mandibular advancement osteotomy. (f–j) End of treatment photographs, following orthodontic treatment, mandibular advancement osteotomy and restorative dentistry to restore the buccal abrasion cavities and old restorations.

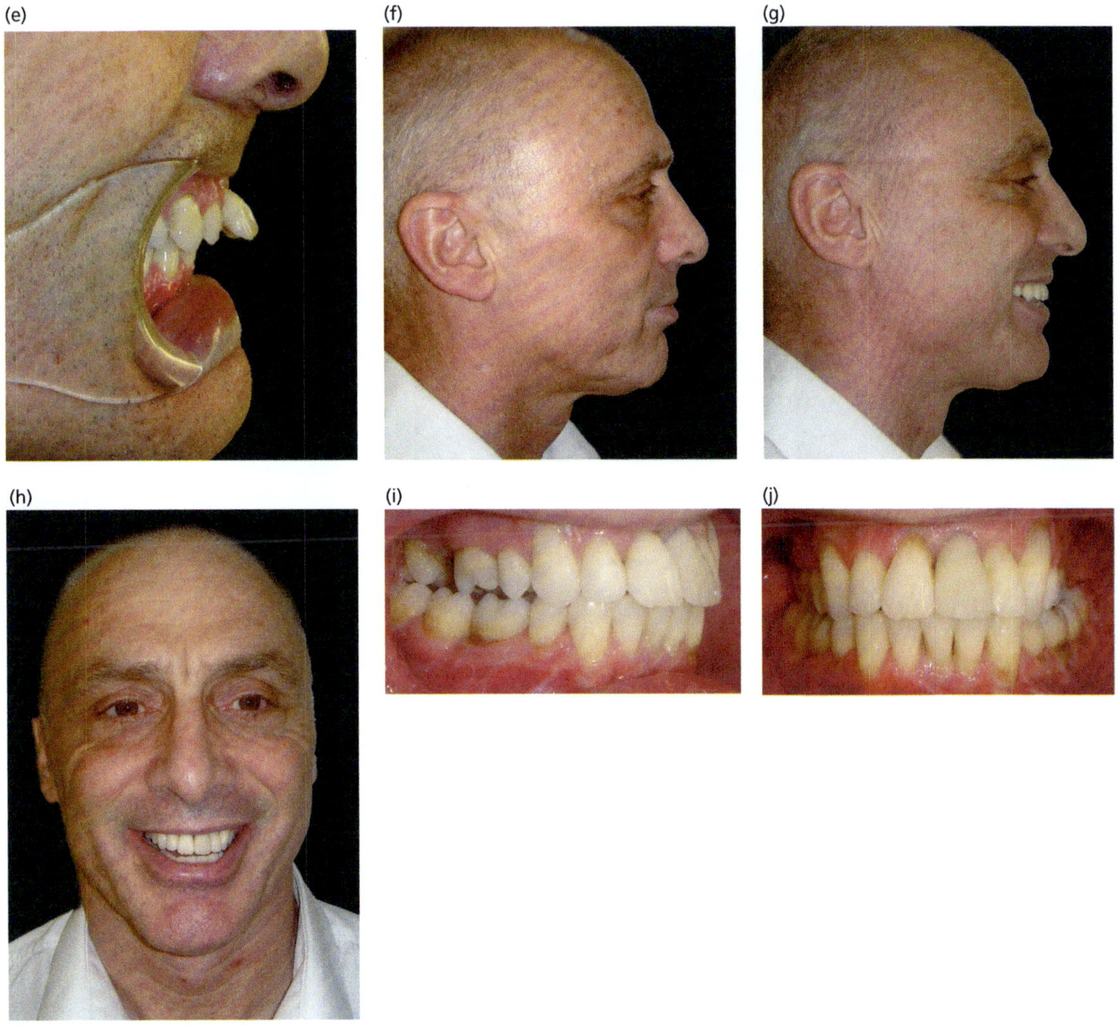

Fig. 5-65 (*Continued*).

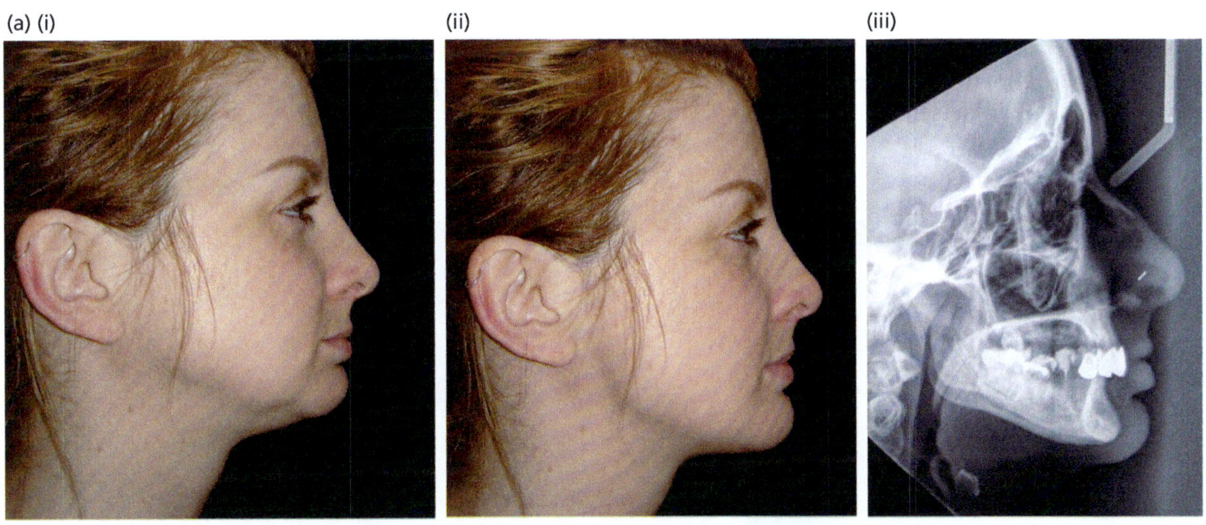

Fig. 5-66 Mandibular overclosure and excessive freeway space. (a)(i) In a Class II patient, in overclosed position. (a)(ii) Patient posturing mandible forward and downward, demonstrating change in lower facial profile aesthetics. (a)(iii) Lateral cephalometric radiograph in the overclosed position, demonstrating vertical maxillary deficiency. (b)(i) A Class III patient in overclosed position. (b)(ii) Patient with the mandible in a relaxed, open position (intraorally there would be an increased freeway space), demonstrating the change in profile aesthetics as the mandible has rotated downward and backward, reducing the Class III appearance. (b)(iii) Intraoral view showing overclosure. (b)(iv) Lateral cephalometric radiograph demonstrating vertical (and sagittal) maxillary deficiency.

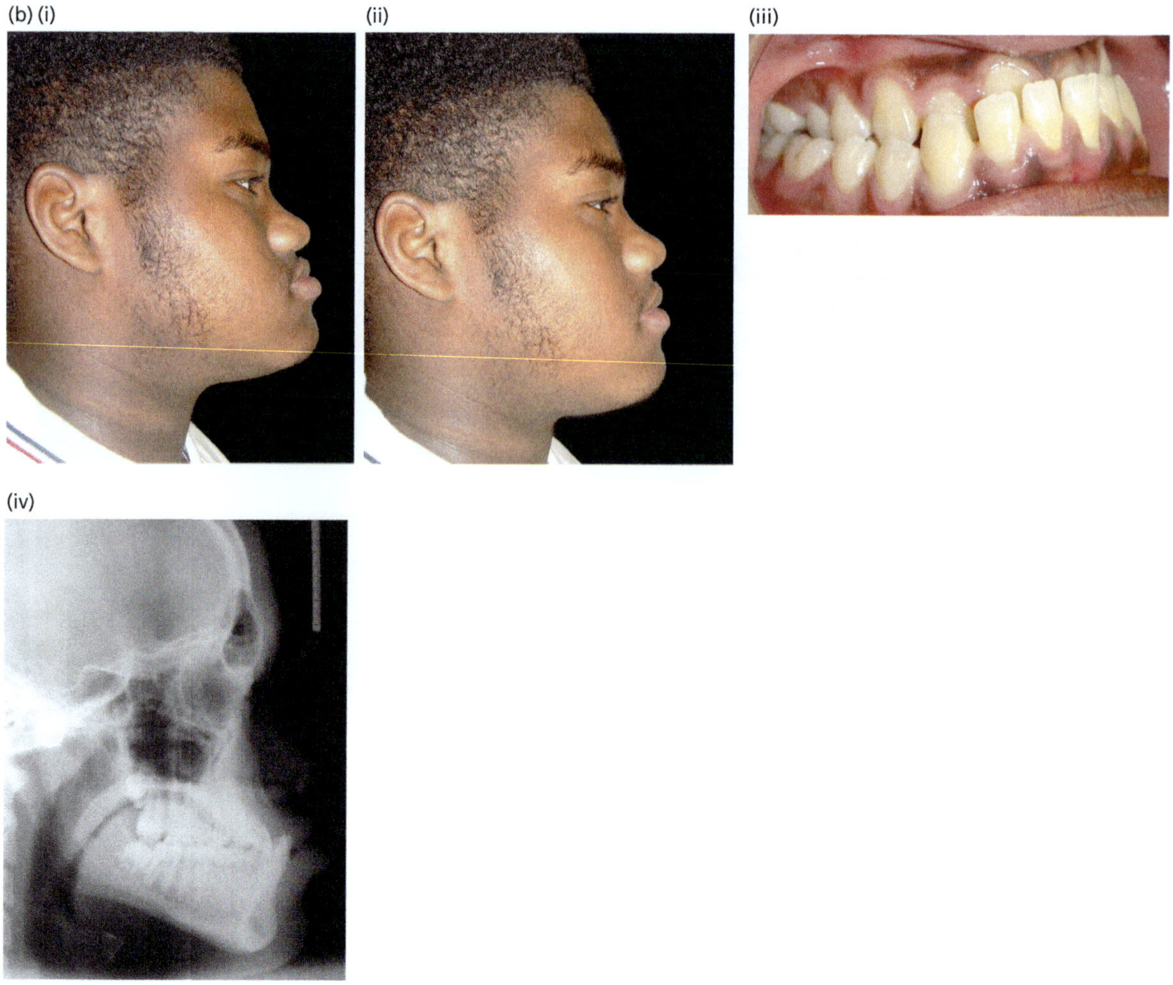

Fig. 5-66 (*Continued*).

clinician should assess whether the patient can achieve, or almost achieve, an edge-to-edge incisor relationship, from which position they displace the mandible anteriorly to achieve maximum intercuspation of their posterior teeth (Figure 5-67). If a **unilateral posterior crossbite** is present, it is vitally important to search for an associated **lateral mandibular displacement** (Figure 5-68).[33] Such displacements are usually due to a **premature contact** between the maxillary and mandibular dentitions and, as such, will often resolve following preparatory orthodontic decompensation of the teeth.

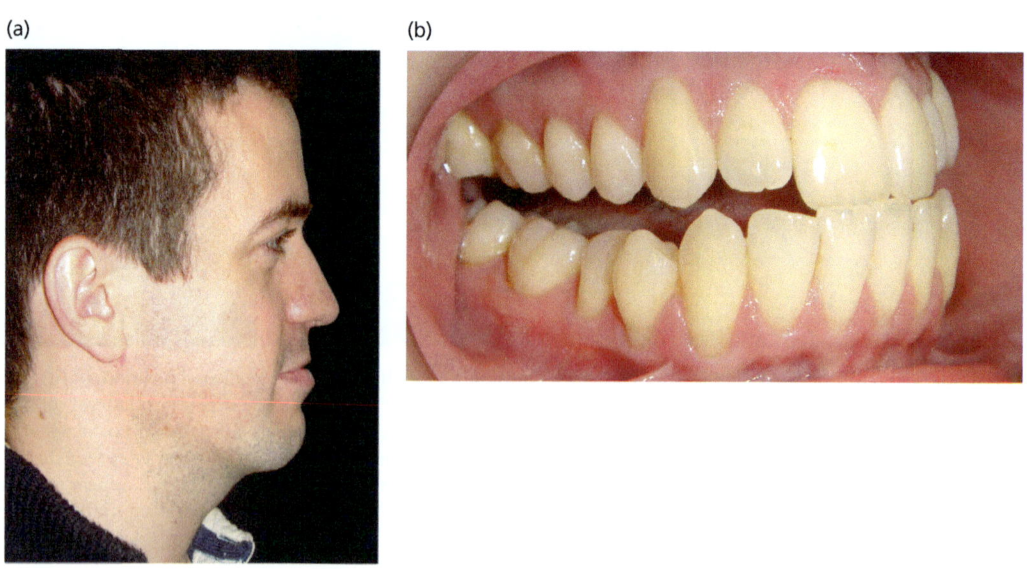

Fig. 5-67 (a, b) Patient profile and intraoral views in the mandibular rest position.

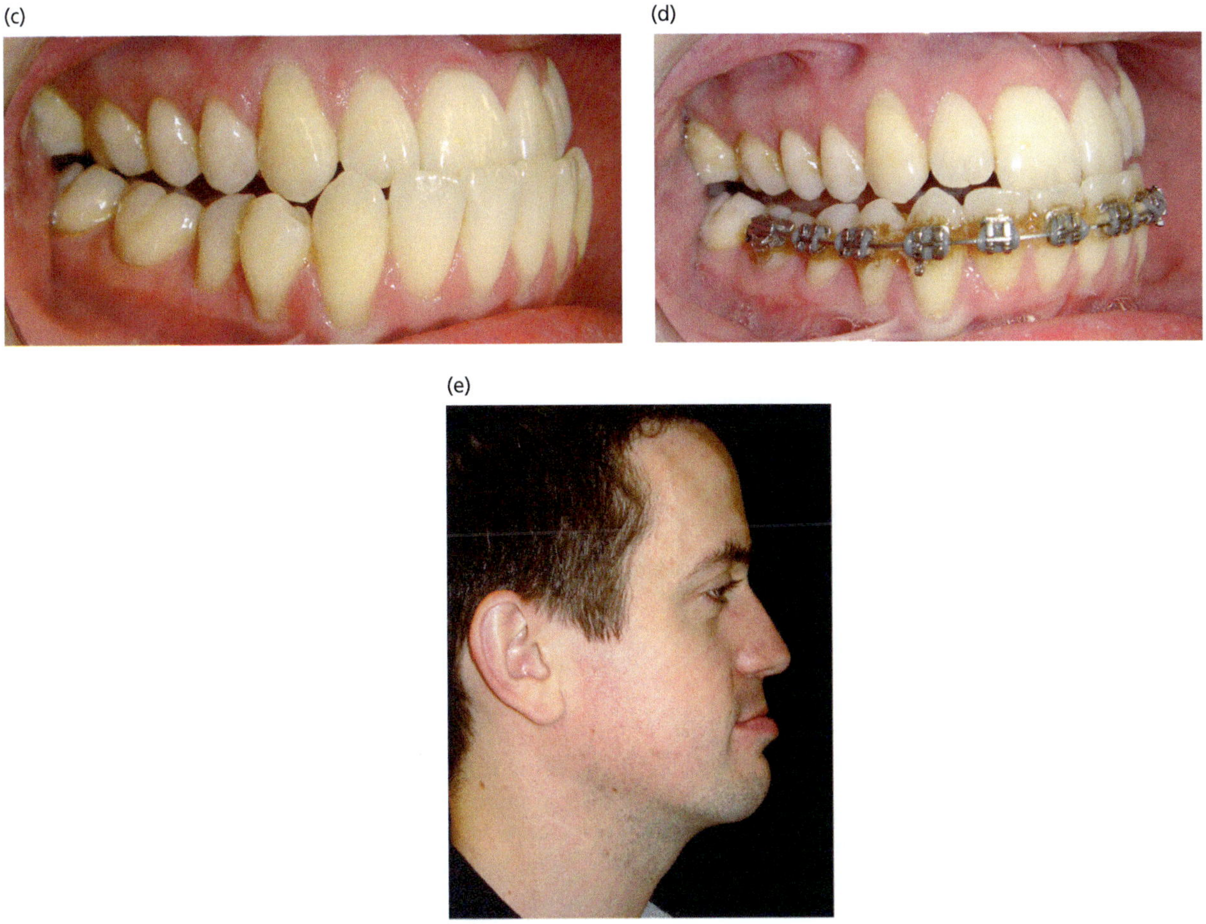

Fig. 5-67 (*Continued*) (c) Patient posturing his mandible forward to achieve maximum intercuspation of the posterior dentition. In this particular patient, this displaced position was uncomfortable and the patient had to strain to maintain the occlusion. (d) After two visits of orthodontic alignment and decompensation (proclination of the mandibular incisors), this was the dental occlusion achieved without any strain. (e) The change in facial profile is evident even in this early phase of mandibular incisor decompensation.

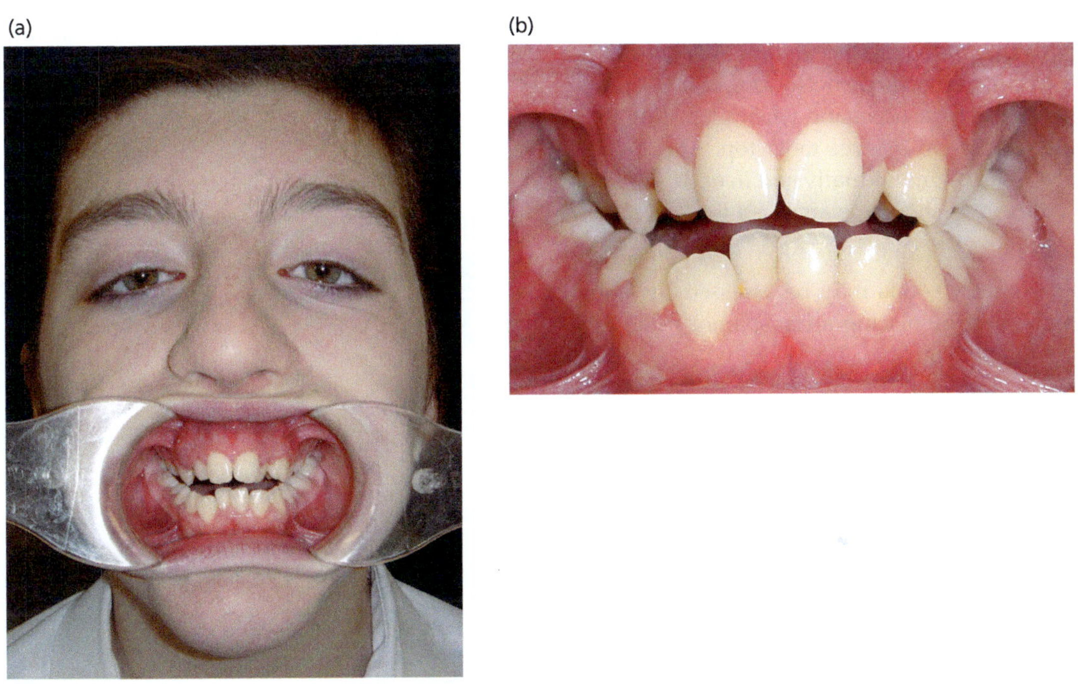

Fig. 5-68 (a, b) Undisplaced position, with mandibular dental midline almost coincident with the maxillary dental midline. (c, d) Lateral mandibular displacement to the patient's right in order to achieve maximum intercuspation of the teeth, with the mandibular dental midline significantly to the patient's right.

(c)

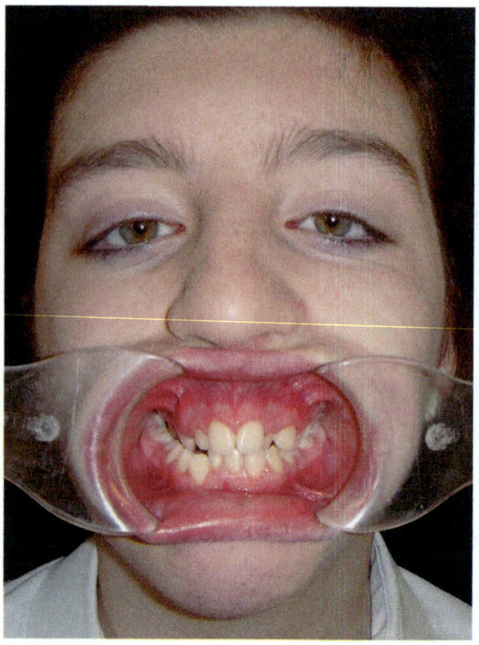

(d)

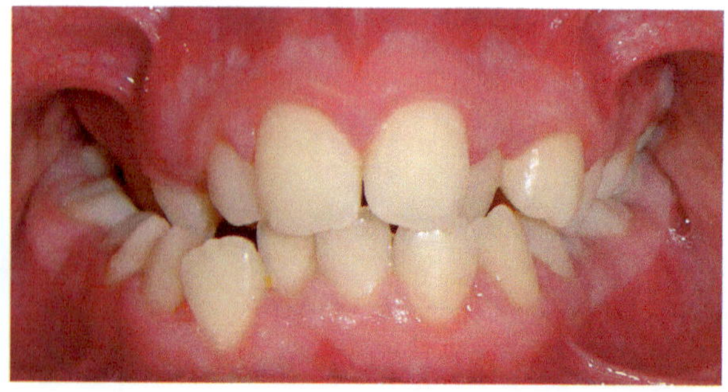

Fig. 5-68 (*Continued*).

Tongue evaluation

The size, activity and resting position of the tongue should be evaluated, particularly in the presence of an anterior open bite or excessive bimaxillary dental proclination (Figure 5-69).

Dental study models

Dental study models (study casts) are an indispensible three-dimensional record of the orthognathic patient for initial and preoperative diagnosis, as well the analysis of treatment results. The models should be **Angle's trimmed** in centric occlusion, such that they will remain in centric occlusion when placed on their posterior surface on a level table top. The models should be assessed individually and in occlusion. The individual models should be analysed for:

- **Arch symmetry** – this may be assessed by visual inspection and by placing a transparent ruled grid over each dental arch.

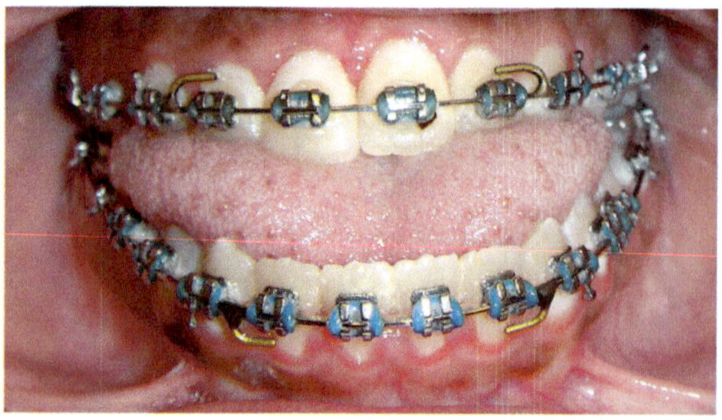

Fig. 5-69 Large tongue in a patient with a Class III anterior open bite.

- **Crowding/spacing/rotations** – the degree of these parameters should be assessed.
- **Curve of Spee** (in the mandible) and the associated sagittal curve in the maxillary dental arch may be evaluated by holding each dental arch against the flat under surface of the opposing model (Figure 5-70).

The models should be assessed in occlusion for:

- **Incisor, canine and molar relationships** – should be assessed in the sagittal, vertical and transverse planes (Figure 5-71).

(a)

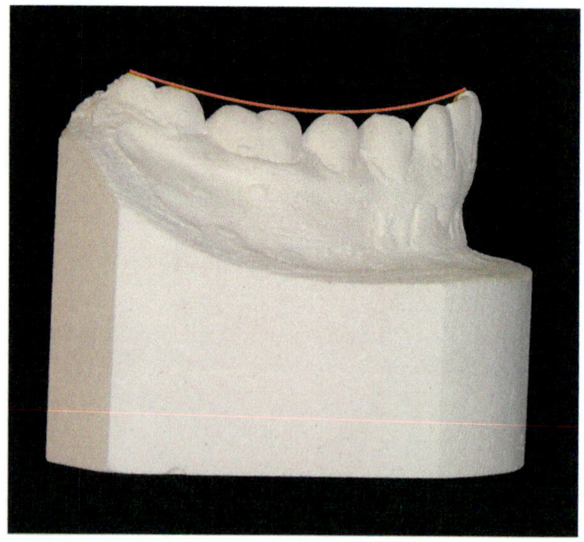

Fig. 5-70 (a) Excessive curve of Spee evident in the mandibular dental arch.

(b) (c)

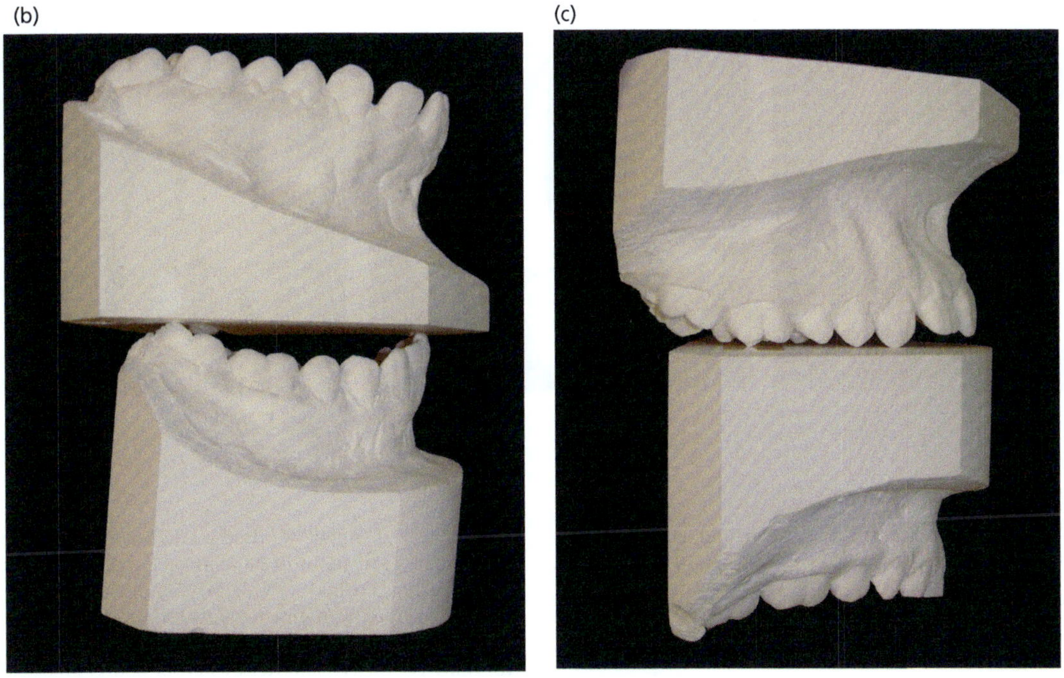

Fig. 5-70 (*Continued*) (b) The curve of Spee in the mandibular arch and (c) the sagittal occlusal curve in the maxillary dental arch may be evaluated by holding each dental arch against the flat under surface of the opposing model.

(a) (b)

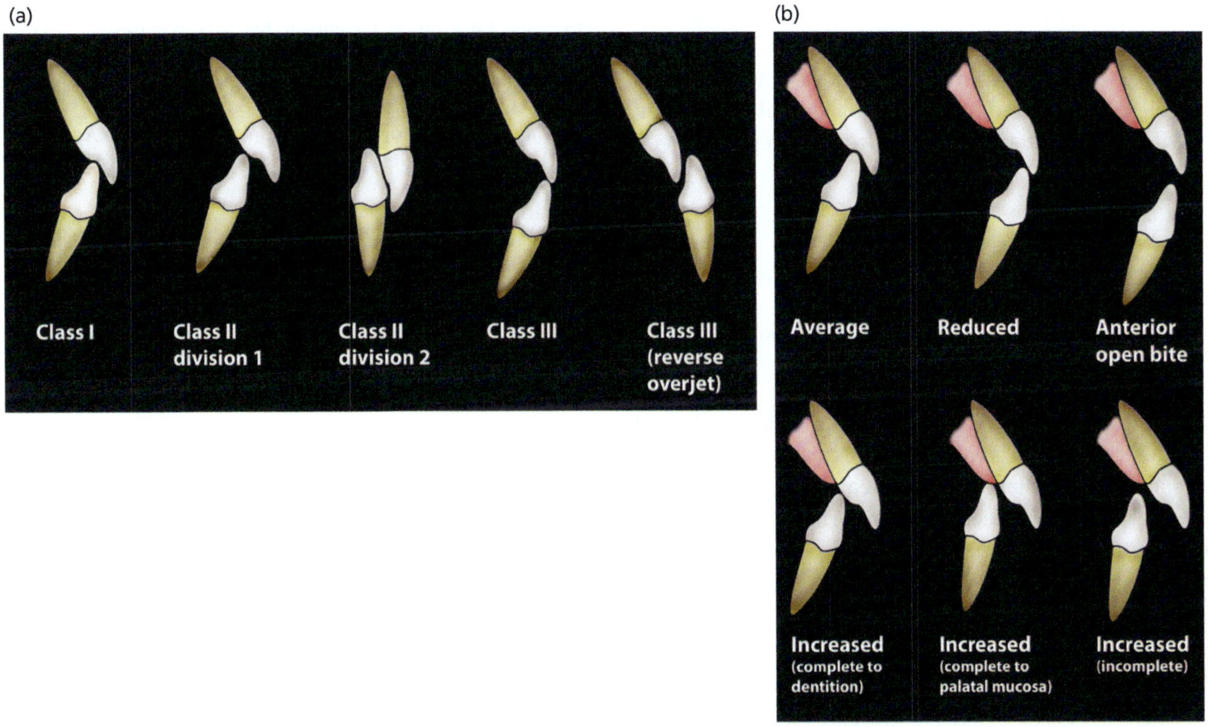

Fig. 5-71 (a) Sagittal incisor relationships.
Class I: The mandibular incisor edges occlude with or lie immediately below the cingulum plateau of the maxillary central incisors.
Class II: The mandibular incisor edges lie posterior to the cingulum plateau of the maxillary central incisors. There are two divisions:
division 1: the overjet is increased; the maxillary central incisors are proclined or of average inclination.
division 2: the maxillary central incisors are retroclined; the overjet is usually minimal but may be increased.
Class III: The mandibular incisor edges lie anterior to the cingulum plateau of the maxillary central incisors. The overjet is reduced or reversed. (b) Classification of incisor overbite. (c) Class I buccal segment relationship: in a Class I molar relationship, the distobuccal cusp of the maxillary first molar occludes between the distobuccal cusp of the mandibular first molar and the mesiobuccal cusp of the mandibular second molar (Andrews Class I). The mesiobuccal cusp of the maxillary first permanent molar falls within the buccal groove between the mesial and middle cusps of the mandibular first permanent molar (Angle's Class I). Sagittal discrepancies may be distinguished as $^1/_4$, $^1/_2$, $^3/_4$ or full unit discrepancies, with a 'unit' being the mesiodistal width of one premolar. The canines and premolars exhibit a cusp-to-embrasure relationship buccally and a cusp-to-fossa relationship lingually. (d) Class II (full unit) buccal segment relationship. (e) Class III (full unit) buccal segment relationship. (From: Naini FB. Facial Aesthetics: Concepts and Clinical Diagnosis. Oxford: Wiley-Blackwell, 2011; reprinted with permission.)

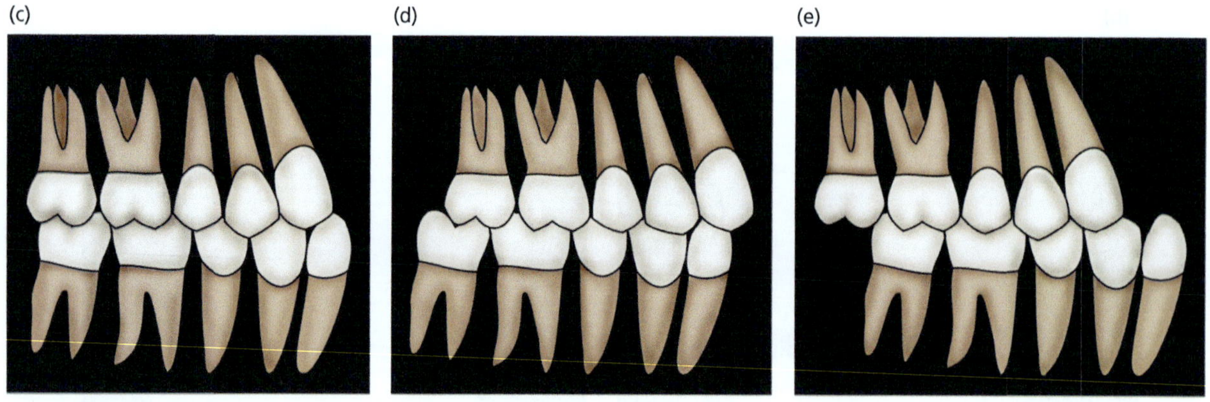

Fig. 5-71 (*Continued*).

- **Arch widths** – potential requirements for arch coordination should be evaluated, particularly the intercanine width coordination between the opposing dental arches.
- **Potential interferences** – assess for any potential dental interference, such as hanging palatal cusps of maxillary second molars or other overerupted teeth.
- **Hand articulating the study models** – holding the models in the *approximate postoperative relationship of the skeletal bases* permits the clinician to see what dental movements may be required to permit a well-interdigitated, functional dental occlusion when the skeletal bases are surgically repositioned.

Concluding remarks

'I suppose it is tempting, if the only tool you have is a hammer, to treat everything as if it were a nail.'

Abraham Maslow (1908–70)[57]
US psychologist

The importance of an accurate diagnosis should not be underestimated. Without it, the treatment plan and all subsequent steps in the treatment process will inevitably be incorrect. It is important to remember that *the diagnosis dictates the surgical procedure(s) required, not vice versa.*

References

1 Richter JP. Literary Works of Leonardo da Vinci (2nd Ed). Oxford: Oxford University Press, 1939.
2 Naini FB. Facial Aesthetics: Concepts and Clinical Diagnosis. Oxford: Wiley-Blackwell, 2011.
3 Naini FB. Patient Interview and Consultation. In: Naini FB. Facial Aesthetics: Concepts and Clinical Diagnosis. Oxford: Wiley-Blackwell, 2011.
4 Ryan FS, Barnard M, Cunningham SJ. Impact of dentofacial deformity and motivation for treatment: a qualitative study. Am J Orthod Dentofacial Orthop. 2012;141:734–42.
5 Fabing H, Marr R (Eds). Fischerisms. Springfield, IL: Charles C. Thomas, 1944.
6 Lee H. To Kill a Mockingbird. Philadelphia, PA: J. B. Lippincott & Co., 1960.
7 Penfield W. Neurology in Canada and the Osler centennial. Can Med Assoc J. 1949;61:69–73.
8 Phillips C, Bennett ME, Broder HL. Dentofacial disharmony: psychological status of patients seeking treatment consultation. Angle Orthod. 1998;68:547–56.
9 Morewedge CK, Kahneman D. Associative processes in intuitive judgment. Trends Cog Sci. 2010;14:435–40.
10 Ward TG. Sir William Kelsey Fry. Br J Surg. 1966;53:317.
11 Macgregor FC. Uncooperative patients: some cultural interpretations. Am J Nurs. 1967;67:88–91.
12 Obwegeser HL. Mandibular Growth Anomalies. Berlin Heidelberg: Springer, 2001.
13 Naini FB. Clinical Diagnostic Records, Natural Head Position and Craniofacial Anthropometry. In: Naini FB. Facial Aesthetics: Concepts and Clinical Diagnosis. Oxford: Wiley-Blackwell, 2011.
14 Thomson W (Baron Kelvin). Popular Lectures and Addresses (Vol. 1) (1891–1894). Cambridge: Cambridge University Press, 1894.
15 Sarikaya I, Sarikaya A, Holder LE. The role of single photon emission computed tomography in bone imaging. Semin Nucl Med. 2001;31(1):3–16.
16 Pripatnanont P, Vittayakittipong P, Markmanee U, Thongmak S, Yipintsoi T. The use of SPECT to evaluate growth cessation of the mandible in unilateral condylar hyperplasia. Int J Oral Maxillofac Surg. 2005;34(4):364–8.
17 Davies R. Tempest-Tost. Toronto, ON: Clarke Irwin & Co., 1951.
18 Naini FB. Facial Beauty. In: Naini FB. Facial Aesthetics: Concepts and Clinical Diagnosis. Oxford: Wiley-Blackwell, 2011.
19 Naini FB. Cephalometry and Cephalometric Analysis. In: Naini FB. Facial Aesthetics: Concepts and Clinical Diagnosis. Oxford: Wiley-Blackwell, 2011.
20 Bean RB, Bean WB (Eds.). Sir William Osler: Aphorisms from his bedside teachings and writings. New York: Henry Schuman, 1950.
21 Osler W. The Student Life (1892). In: Osler W. Aequanimitas, with other addresses to Medical Students, Nurses, and Practitioners of Medicine. (3rd Ed.). Philadelphia: Blakiston, 1932.
22 Moorrees CFA, Kean MR. Natural head position: a basic consideration in the interpretation of cephalometric radiographs. Am J Phys Anthropol. 1958;16:213–34.
23 Naini FB. The Frankfort plane and head positioning in facial aesthetic analysis: The perpetuation of a myth. JAMA Facial Plast Surg. 2013;15:333–4.
24 Zebeib A, Naini FB. Variability of the inclination of anatomical horizontal reference planes of the craniofacial complex in relation to the true horizontal line in orthognathic patients. Am J Orthod Dentofacial Orthop. 2014;146: 740-7.
25 Naini FB. Facial Proportions: Classical Canons to Modern Craniofacial Anthropometry. In: Naini FB. Facial Aesthetics:

Concepts and Clinical Diagnosis. Oxford: Wiley-Blackwell, 2011.

26 Farkas LG. Anthropometry of the Head and Face (Ed. 2). New York: Raven Press, 1994.

27 Naini FB. Facial Proportions. In: Naini FB. Facial Aesthetics: Concepts and Clinical Diagnosis. Oxford: Wiley-Blackwell, 2011.

28 Naini FB, Cobourne MT, McDonald F, Donaldson AN. The influence of craniofacial to standing height proportion on perceived attractiveness. Int J Oral Maxillofac Surg. 2008;37:877–85.

29 Naini FB, Moss JP, Gill DS. The enigma of facial beauty: esthetics, proportions, deformity, and controversy. Am J Orthod Dentofacial Orthop. 2006;130:277–82.

30 Naini FB. Facial Type. In: Naini FB. Facial Aesthetics: Concepts and Clinical Diagnosis. Oxford: Wiley-Blackwell, 2011.

31 Naini FB, Donaldson ANA, McDonald F, Cobourne MT. Influence of chin height on perceived attractiveness in the orthognathic patient, clinician and layperson. Angle Orthod. 2012;82:88–95.

32 Naini FB, Donaldson ANA, McDonald F, Cobourne MT. How does variation in lower anterior face height influence perceived attractiveness? A quantitative investigation. J Orthodont. 2013;40:206–17.

33 Naini FB. Facial Symmetry and Asymmetry. In: Naini FB. Facial Aesthetics: Concepts and Clinical Diagnosis. Oxford: Wiley-Blackwell, 2011.

34 Naini FB, Gill DS. Smile Aesthetics. In: Naini FB. Facial Aesthetics: Concepts and Clinical Diagnosis. Oxford: Wiley-Blackwell, 2011.

35 Rigsbee OH 3rd, Sperry TP, BeGole EA. The influence of facial animation on smile characteristics. Int J Adult Orthodon Orthognath Surg. 1988;3:233–9.

36 Yang IH, Nahm DS, Baek SH. Which hard and soft tissue factors relate with the amount of buccal corridor space during smiling? Angle Orthod. 2008;78:5–11.

37 Naini FB. Regional Aesthetic Analysis: The Lips. In: Naini FB. Facial Aesthetics: Concepts and Clinical Diagnosis. Oxford: Wiley-Blackwell, 2011.

38 Naini FB, Cobourne MT, McDonald F, Wertheim D. The aesthetic impact of upper lip inclination in orthodontics and orthognathic surgery. Eur J Orthod. 2015;37:81–6.

39 Burstone CJ, James RB, Legan H, Murphy GA, Norton LA. Cephalometrics for orthognathic surgery. J Oral Surg. 1978;36:269–77.

40 Ricketts RM. A foundation for cephalometric communication. Am J Orthod. 1960;46:330–57.

41 Ricketts RM. The value of cephalometrics and computerized technology. Am J Orthod. 1972;42:179–99.

42 Steiner CC. Cephalometrics for you and me. Am J Orthod. 1953;39:729–55.

43 Steiner CC. Cephalometrics in clinical practice. Angle Orthod. 1959;29:8–29.

44 Holdaway RA. A soft tissue cephalometric analysis and its use in orthodontic treatment planning. Part I. Am J Orthod. 1983;84:1–28.

45 Holdaway RA. A soft tissue cephalometric analysis and its use in orthodontic treatment planning. Part II. Am J Orthod. 1984;85:279–93.

46 Merrifield LL. The profile line as an aid in critically evaluating facial esthetics. Am J Orthod. 1966;52:804–22.

47 Riedel RR. An analysis of dentofacial relationships. Am J Orthod. 1957;43:103–19.

48 Rubin LR. The anatomy of a smile: its importance in the treatment of facial paralysis. Plast Reconstr Surg. 1974;53:384–87.

49 Naini FB, Cobourne MT, McDonald F, Wertheim D. Aesthetic impact of the upper component of the nasolabial angle: a quantitative investigation. J Oral Maxillofac Surg Med Pathol. 2015;27:470–6.

50 Naini FB. Regional Aesthetic Analysis: Submental–cervical Region. In: Naini FB. Facial Aesthetics: Concepts and Clinical Diagnosis. Oxford: Wiley-Blackwell, 2011.

51 Naini FB. Dental-Occlusal Relationships: Terminology, Description and Classification. In: Naini FB. Facial Aesthetics: Concepts and Clinical Diagnosis. Oxford: Wiley-Blackwell, 2011.

52 Kipling R. Something of myself: For my friends known and unknown. London: Macmillan & Co. Ltd., 1937.

53 McNamara JA Jr. A method of cephalometric evaluation. Am J Orthod. 1984;86:449–69.

54 Sassouni V. A roentgenographic cephalometric analysis of cephalo-facio-dental relationships. Am J Orthod. 1955;41:735–64.

55 Horn A. (1992) Facial height index. Am J Orthod Dentofacial Orthop. 1992;102:180–6.

56 Downs WB. Analysis of the dentofacial profile. Angle Orthod. 1956;26:191–212.

57 Maslow AH. The Psychology of Science: A Reconnaissance. New York: Harper and Row, 1966.

Chapter 6

Principles of Orthognathic Treatment Planning

Farhad B. Naini and Daljit S. Gill

Introduction

> 'Everything should be made as simple as possible, but not simpler.'
>
> Albert Einstein (1879–1955) (attributed)

It is very easy to *overcomplicate* the treatment planning process. Though the accurate analysis of soft tissue and dentoskeletal relationships is vitally important, the use of the numerical values obtained from such analyses is to *enhance* the clinician's observation, not to take the place of observation. *Trained observation and quantitative analysis are both required.* Excessive reliance just on numbers from linear and angular measurements of the facial soft and hard tissues without an understanding of proportional relationships and the interrelationship of adjacent facial units and subunits to the whole, may lead to missing the big picture, i.e. missing the wood for the trees. Knowledge of cephalometric analysis (2D and 3D) is vital for the understanding of the growth and development of the craniofacial complex and for diagnosis, treatment planning and the analysis of treatment results. However, the *essence of treatment planning* in orthognathic surgery still involves the *educated eye* of the clinician.

There are two key stages within the orthognathic treatment pathway in which treatment planning is required. At the initial 'diagnostic' joint clinic, a **provisional treatment plan** is provided to the patient. This is often not much more than a discussion of the potential type of surgery that will be required, e.g. single jaw or bimaxillary, with or without genioplasty, and the preoperative orthodontic treatment required. However, the **definitive preoperative treatment plan** is reached after the completion of the preoperative orthodontic preparation, at the preoperative 'planning' joint clinic. The remainder of this chapter will focus mainly on the definitive, final preoperative treatment planning process.

The **preoperative treatment planning process** (numbered 1 to 4 below) essentially follows the 4-stage sequence below:

1. **Preoperative diagnosis** (qualitative and quantitative) – this is the most important stage, and is based predominantly on clinical observation of the patient (and palpation), as well as analysis of craniofacial measurements, proportional relationships and symmetry, in order to evaluate which part(s) of

Orthognathic Surgery: Principles, Planning and Practice. Edited by Farhad B. Naini and Daljit S. Gill.

the craniofacial complex (jaws, teeth, soft tissues) is at fault?

2. **Vectorial analysis** (qualitative) – based predominantly on clinical observation of the patient and preoperative records, the purpose of this stage is to determine the **essential movements** of each jaw, or segments thereof, required to obtain the best facial aesthetic and dental-occlusal relationship, the **direction** each jaw or jaw segment should be moved, and the **approximate magnitude** (i.e. amount) of movement required?
3. **Prediction planning** (quantitative) – Cephalometric and photographic (2D or 3D) planning to obtain the accurate linear movements of the teeth and jaws (number of mm), and angular changes (number of degrees) required to achieve the said result, and to assess whether it is realistically achievable?
4. **Model surgery** (quantitative) – using dental models (usually on an articulator) and/or 3D models to check the feasibility of the planned surgery.

> **Note:**
>
> Stages 3 and 4 are always undertaken bearing in mind, and consistently referring to, the results of stages 1 and 2.

1. Preoperative diagnosis

'I would like to see the day when somebody would be appointed surgeon somewhere who had no hands, for the operative part is the least part of the work.'

Harvey Cushing (1869–1939)[1] (Figure 6-1)
Pioneer of modern neurosurgery and man of letters

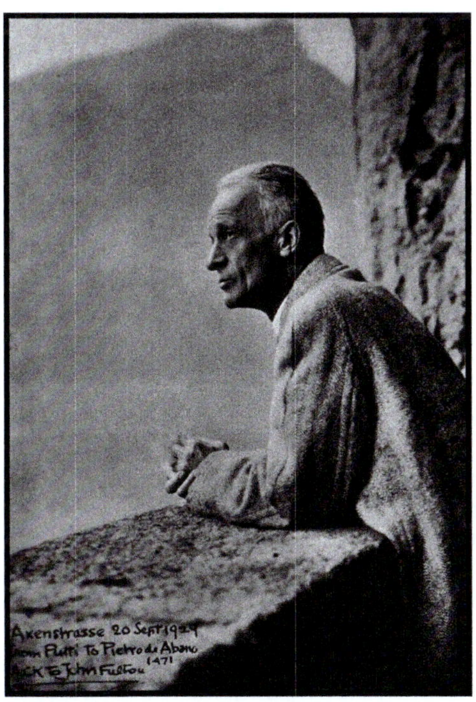

Fig. 6-1 Harvey Cushing (1869–1939).

Evaluation of principle diagnostic parameters

Clinical diagnosis has been described in detail in Chapter 5.[2] The purpose of this section is to describe the **principle aesthetic diagnostic parameters** that *need to be reassessed preoperatively* at the definitive treatment planning clinic, when the preoperative orthodontic treatment has been completed (Table 6-1). Rather than the traditional method of assessing the frontal view followed by the profile view, and assessing soft tissue clinical parameters followed by cephalometric analysis, it is proposed that an approximate top–down approach to analysis of the craniofacial complex be employed,[2] with the patient, cephalometric and other radiographs and preoperative 'snap' dental models all at hand.

> **Note:**
>
> In both diagnosis and treatment planning, always plan the relative position of every craniofacial unit and subunit by considering it relative to its next larger context – the maxillary incisors in relation to the upper lip, the maxillary incisor-upper lip complex in relation to the nose and lower lip, the nasolabial complex in relation to the forehead and chin etc.

Every craniofacial complex should be metaphorically 'taken to pieces', and every parameter or feature (unit and subunit) analysed in terms of its morphology, and in relation to its neighbouring features and the whole. Thorough and accurate **analysis** permits the next stage – **synthesis** of the separate parameters, i.e. 'putting the pieces back together', only in a new and improved configuration. In the process of synthesis, the clinician should always bear in mind the three cardinal aims of treatment – improving dentofacial aesthetics, improving function and attaining a stable final result.

Chair side techniques to aid clinical diagnosis

Nothing is as useful as the actual result of an orthognathic surgical procedure in demonstrating the appropriateness of the original treatment plan – hence the importance of analysing and auditing clinical results. However, any diagnostic modality that permits simulation of a potential final operated result is extremely useful in the treatment planning stages of orthognathic surgery. A number of simple techniques may be used at the chair side to aid **prognostic visualization** in treatment planning.

Masking

Masking any of the facial regions, particularly in profile view, reduces the visual influence of the masked

Table 6-1 Preoperative diagnostic parameters and their relevance to treatment planning

Diagnostic parameter		Relevance to treatment planning
Scleral exposure above lower eyelid and below the iris		Increased scleral exposure is usually a sign of high level maxillary retrusion, and may suggest the requirement for a higher level Le Fort I maxillary advancement. If severe, may indicate need for a Le Fort III advancement.
Paranasal hollowing		A sign of maxillary retrusion and hypoplasia, thereby may suggest requirement for maxillary advancement (Figure 6-2).
Nasolabial angle (NLA):	Columella inclination (upper component of NL angle)[2,3]	This is likely to increase with maxillary advancement (Figure 6-3). If there is drooping of the nasal tip and a reduced columella inclination, maxillary advancement will elevate the nasal tip and improve nasolabial aesthetics. If the columella inclination is already increased (up-turned nasal tip), maxillary advancement will exacerbate this, which may be an aesthetic problem.
	Upper lip inclination (lower component of NL angle)[2,4]	If the upper lip is inclined backwards, which is evident in profile view, this may be a sign of maxillary dentoalveolar retrusion, and an indication for maxillary advancement or dentoalveolar protrusion. If the upper lip is excessively inclined forward, this may suggest requirement for a maxillary set-back or perhaps if due to proclined maxillary incisors, it may be improved either by their orthodontic retroclination (Figure 6-4) or their relative retroclination following differential posterior maxillary impaction.
Nasal alar base width (in relation to intercanthal width)		Is it narrow, average or broad? If contemplating maxillary advancement or impaction, this will broaden – can it aesthetically accommodate being broader (Figure 6-5)? Will an alar cinch suture be required, or potentially post-orthognathic wedge resection rhinoplasty?
Vertical face height ratios:	UFH : MFH : LAFH	The upper (UFH), middle (MFH) and lower anterior face heights (LAFH) should be approximately equal, bearing in mind some variation.[5]
	Upper lip height : lower lip height : chin height	ULH ~1/3 : LLH ~1/3 : CH ~1/3 is a useful starting point, though there is a range of normal variability, from a relationship of ULH ~1/2 : LLH and CH ~1/2, particularly in females with slightly reduced LAFH, to ULH $\frac{1}{4}$ of LAFH in males.
	Lower posterior face height (LPFH) to LAFH	LPFH (measured cephalometrically) should be approximately between 65 to 75% of LAFH, otherwise there is likely to be a vertical skeletal discrepancy.[5]
Mandibular plane inclination and gonial angle		The inclination of the mandibular plane may be judged relative to the true horizontal line, and may be measured clinically by placing a finger or dental mirror handle along the inferior lateral border of the mandible (Figure 6-6a).[6] The gonial angle is a measure of the angle formed between the slope of the posterior border of the mandibular ramus and the mandibular plane. It helps to describe the morphology of the mandible, and is highly correlated with the mandibular plane angle (Figure 6-6b).[6]
Upper lip height (short, average or increased?)		Relevant to maxillary incisor exposure – an excessively short upper lip may be surgically 'lengthened'. Excessive upper lip height may have to be accepted (particularly in men), though surgical procedures to reduce upper lip height are available (see Chapter 53).
Maxillary incisor exposure in relation to upper lip	In repose	Anything from 2–5 mm in men, and perhaps a little greater in women, is deemed attractive. This relationship forms the foundation stone of treatment planning (see section below). If reduced, it will improve with maxillary advancement, but may also require downgrafting (inferior repositioning) of the anterior maxilla. If excessive, may require maxillary impaction if primarily skeletal, or attempts to reduce elevation of the upper lip on smiling, if predominantly a problem of hyperelevation of the upper lip on smiling (excessive smile curtain) (Figure 6-7).
	On smiling	Ideally no more then 1–3 mm of gingival exposure should be displayed on full smiling. Assess the smile arc, particularly if planning differential posterior maxillary impaction (Figure 6-8).
Transverse cant of the maxillary occlusal plane (at incisors, canines, premolars and molars)		This should be assessed visually in frontal view with the aid of orthodontic cheek retractors (Figure 6-9a) and/or photographic retractors (Figure 6-9b), and with placement of a dental mirror handle or tongue spatula on the occlusal plane (Figure 6-9c). The maxillary occlusal plane should be level with a true horizontal (or the interpupillary plane in the absence of vertical orbital dystopia), unless a cant correction is being planned, in which case the decision is which side to impact and/or which side to set-down, or combinations thereof, depending on the degree of cant correction required to level the occlusal plane, obtain the ideal maxillary incisor exposure, lower face height and stability (impactions are more stable than set-downs).

Table 6-1 (*Continued*)

Maxillary incisor inclination – correct to face, proclined or retroclined?	This is ideally evaluated in the profile smiling view, with the patient in natural head position (NHP). A tangent to the labial face of the maxillary central incisor crown should be approximately parallel to a true facial vertical line preoperatively (Figure 6-10), unless a differential posterior impaction of the maxilla is planned, in which case the incisor inclination is prepared by proclining the teeth preoperatively, allowing automatic correction with the surgery.
Maxillary incisor sagittal position – prominent, average or retrusive?	With the patient in natural head position (NHP), the sagittal position of the maxillary central incisors should be approximately in line with a true vertical line dropped from soft tissue nasion, soft tissue glabella or somewhere between the two, depending on the morphology of the glabellar-nasal region (Figure 6-10).
Incisor overjet (or reverse overjet)	This is relevant to the degree of relative jaw movement possible, e.g. 6 mm reverse overjet, means ~8–9 mm overall sagittal jaw movement to achieve a Class I incisor relationship.
Sagittal relationship of upper lip, lower lip, mentolabial fold and chin relative to one another	The aesthetic relationship of these neighbouring soft tissue parameters is usually closely related to the underlying dentoskeletal discrepancy (Figure 6-11).
Maxillary dental midline in relation to mid-philtrum of upper lip and facial midline	Midline landmarks may be drawn on the patient's face with a skin pencil, in order to assess the deviation of the dental midlines (Figure 6-12). If there is bodily deviation of the dental midline (i.e. not an angulation problem), this may be corrected by rotation of the maxilla round the vertical axis, but no more than 3–4 mm, otherwise it may lead to posterior occlusal disturbances. If very mild bodily deviation of 1–2 mm, may decide to accept if maxillary surgery is otherwise not required. If greater deviation than 3–4 mm, may require partial or complete correction by further orthodontic treatment (with dental extractions). If there is an angulation problem, then if due to a transverse maxillary cant, it will be corrected automatically with the surgical cant correction. If the angulation problem is purely dental (usually due to incorrect bracket positioning on anterior teeth), then it will require further orthodontic alignment to correct. Maxillary dental midline deviations may be due to a combination of the above factors (Figure 6-13).
Mandibular dental midline in relation to maxillary dental midline and facial midline	Are they coincident? Will the mandibular dental midline be corrected with the proposed surgery, or is further orthodontic treatment required? Is there a lateral mandibular displacement?
Mandibular incisor inclination	Is autorotation of the mandible being planned? If yes, the mandibular incisor inclination will alter relative to the mandibular plane following surgery; therefore the incisor inclination should be orthodontically prepared preoperatively, such that the inclination will be correct following autorotation (Figure 6-14). If no autorotation is planned, mandibular incisor inclination should be corrected preoperatively.
Transverse cant of the mandibular occlusal plane	This should be assessed visually in frontal view with the aid of orthodontic cheek retractors and/or photographic retractors, and with placement of a dental mirror handle or tongue spatula on the occlusal plane (Figure 6-15). If related to rotation of the mandible round the sagittal axis (e.g. hemimandibular hyperplasia), then this will be improved with the surgery to correct the overall bimaxillary cant (Figure 6-16). Otherwise it should be levelled preoperatively.
Mandibular dental midline in relation to midpoint of chin	Should be coincident with the midpoint of the chin if there is a mandibular/chin asymmetry that is planned for surgical correction.
Chin position in transverse plane	If a significant transverse bodily displacement of the chin is observed, assess if this is secondary to a mandibular asymmetry, in which case it will be corrected with the mandibular surgery, or whether it is an isolated chin asymmetry, which may require corrective genioplasty.[7]
Transverse inclination (cant) of the inferior chin plane	If due to mandibular asymmetry (usually hemimandibular hyperplasia), then will be improved with the mandibular surgery; otherwise, may require symmetry-correcting genioplasty (Figure 6-17).
Sagittal chin prominence	This should be assessed in repose and in animation – in some patients, particularly Class III patients with dentoalveolar compensation (Figure 6-18a–c), and Class II patients with osseous chin prominence (Figure 6-18d–f), the chin is effaced and appears prominent only on smiling.
Mentolabial fold morphology, angle and depth	This is very relevant to whether a genioplasty is required – the presence of a gentle S-shape from the lower lip, through the mentolabial fold and to the chin is arguably more important than the sagittal position of the chin.[8,9]

(*continued*)

Table 6-1 (*Continued*)

Vertical position of bilateral inferior mandibular borders	Assess the vertical height of the inferior borders for symmetry – if significant asymmetry, then consider inferior border augmentation or reduction to improve symmetry, or accept.
Submental-cervical angle (acute, average or obtuse)	This will alter with sagittal movement of the mandibular body (advancement improves this region by stretching the submental soft tissues, and set-back usually leads to a more obtuse angle and potentially poor aesthetics), and autorotation of the mandible (improves with forward rotation of the mandible stretching the submental soft tissues, and vice versa).
Submental-cervical length (reduced, average or increased)	Mandibular or chin advancement lengthens this region and stretches the submental soft tissues, usually improving aesthetics (Figure 6-19). Mandibular or chin set-back reduces submental length and usually increases submental fullness, potentially deteriorating submental-cervical aesthetics.

Note: For the purposes of this stage of patient evaluation, *normative values are not as important as proportional relationships*. It is important to visually assess whether specific linear or angular measurements are essentially greater or less than average (e.g. it is more important to assess whether a specific angular relationship, such as the nasolabial angle, is acute, average or obtuse, rather than its exact numerical value).

(a) (b)

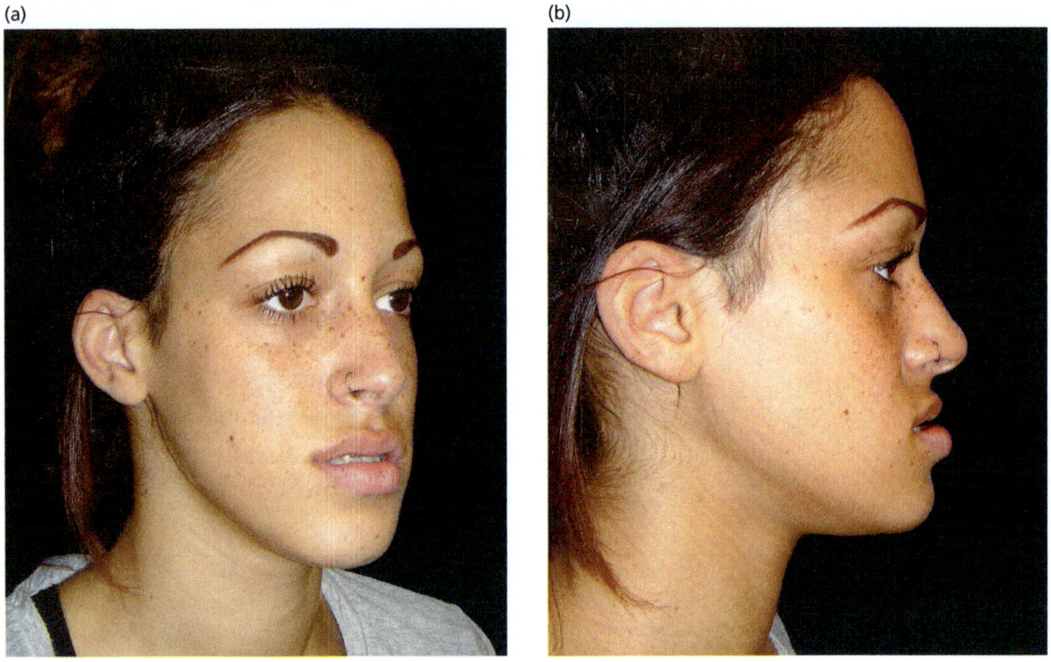

Fig. 6-2 Paranasal hollowing. (a): Oblique lateral view. (b): Profile view.

(a) (b)

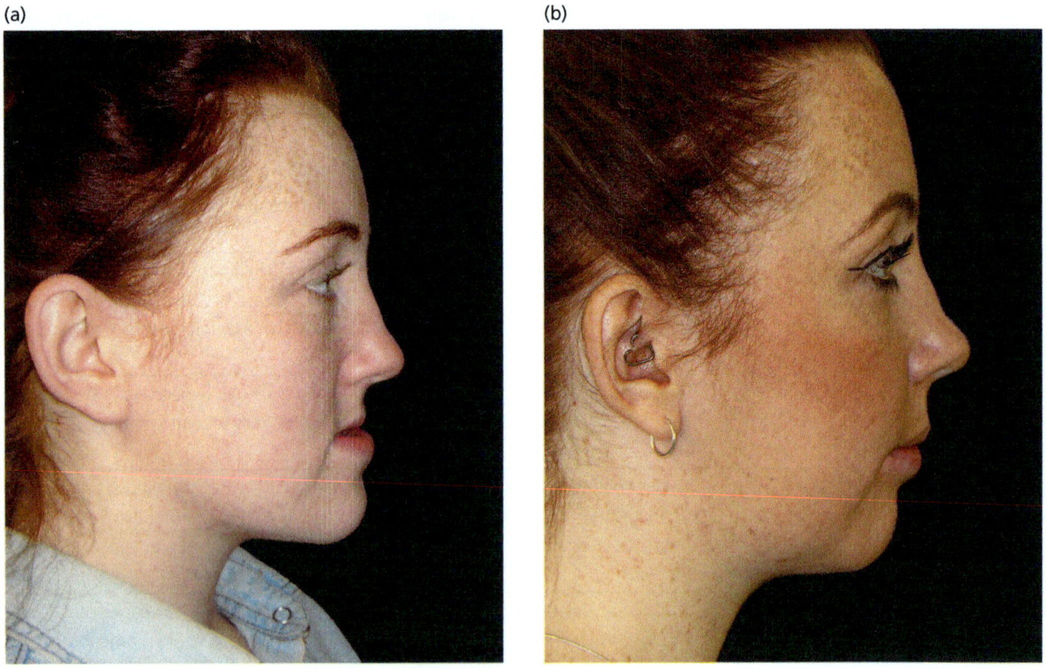

Fig. 6-3 Nasal columella inclination (upper component of the nasolabial angle) tends to increase with maxillary advancement. (a): preoperative profile view. (b): Following maxillary advancement.

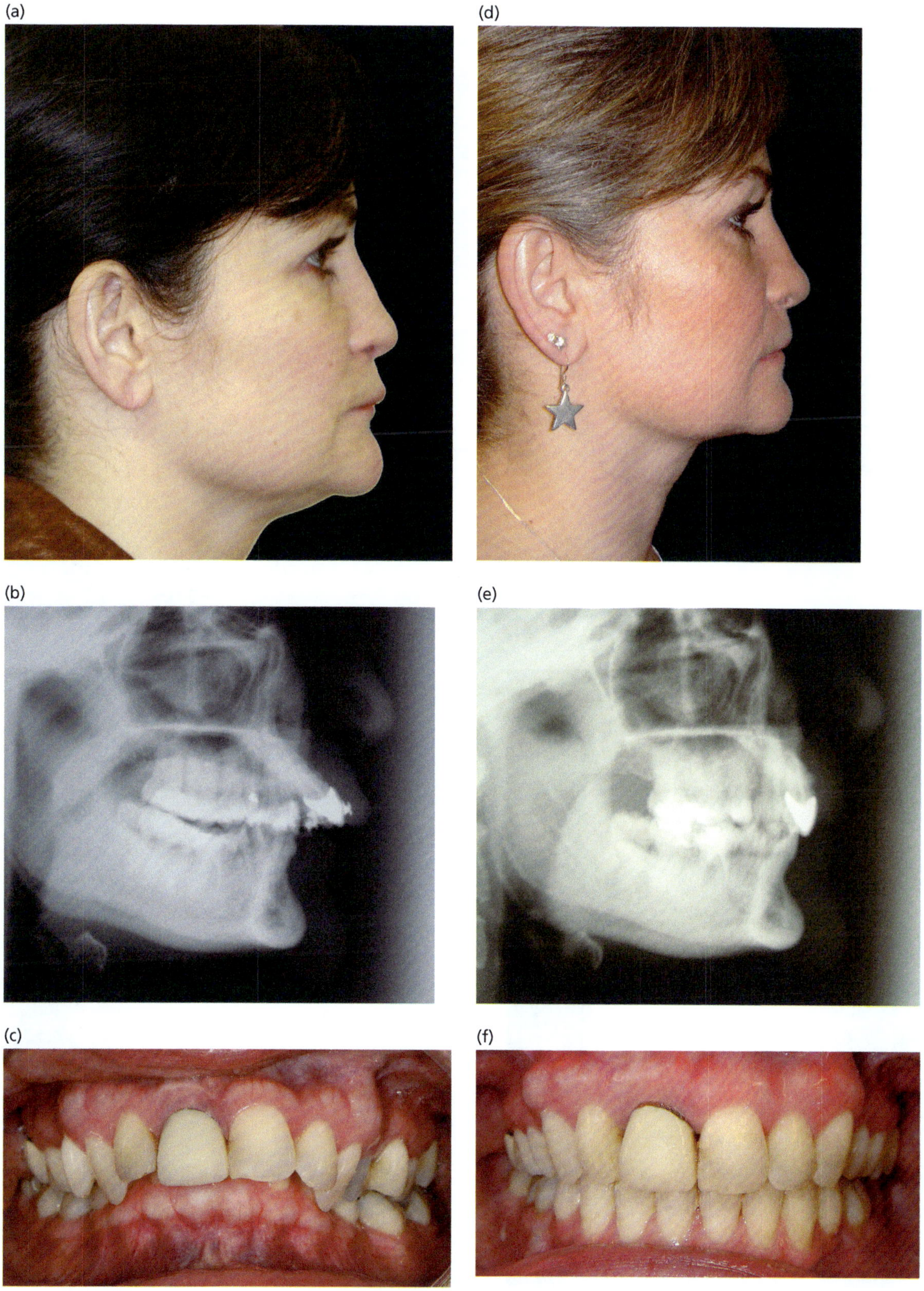

Fig. 6-4 Upper lip inclination (lower component of nasolabial angle) will alter with orthodontic or surgical changes to the inclination of the maxillary incisors. (a–c): Pretreatment views of a patient with proclined maxillary incisors, proclined upper lip and deep incisor overbite. (d–f): Following orthodontic retroclination of the maxillary incisors by 30°, the nasolabial angle increased by 20°, though all the increase was in the upper lip inclination (from 60° to 80°). (Figures 7.4b and e from Naini et al.[4]; reprinted with permission).

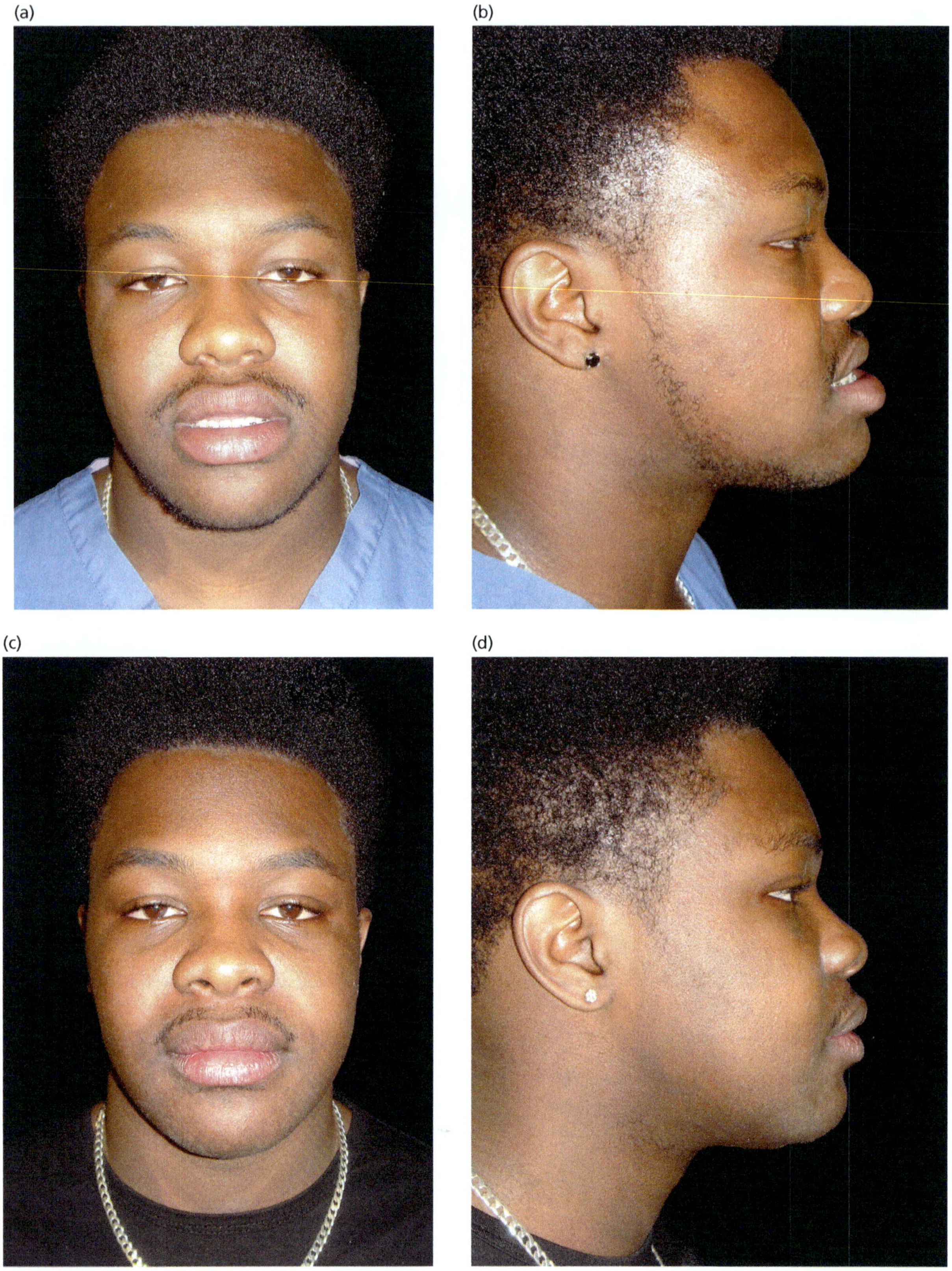

Fig. 6-5 Class III patient (a, b) preoperative views, (c, d): following maxillary advancement and mandibular set-back osteotomies. The nasal alar base width (an alar cinch suture was employed intraoperatively) and nasal columella inclination have increased, despite an overall improvement in the facial aesthetics.

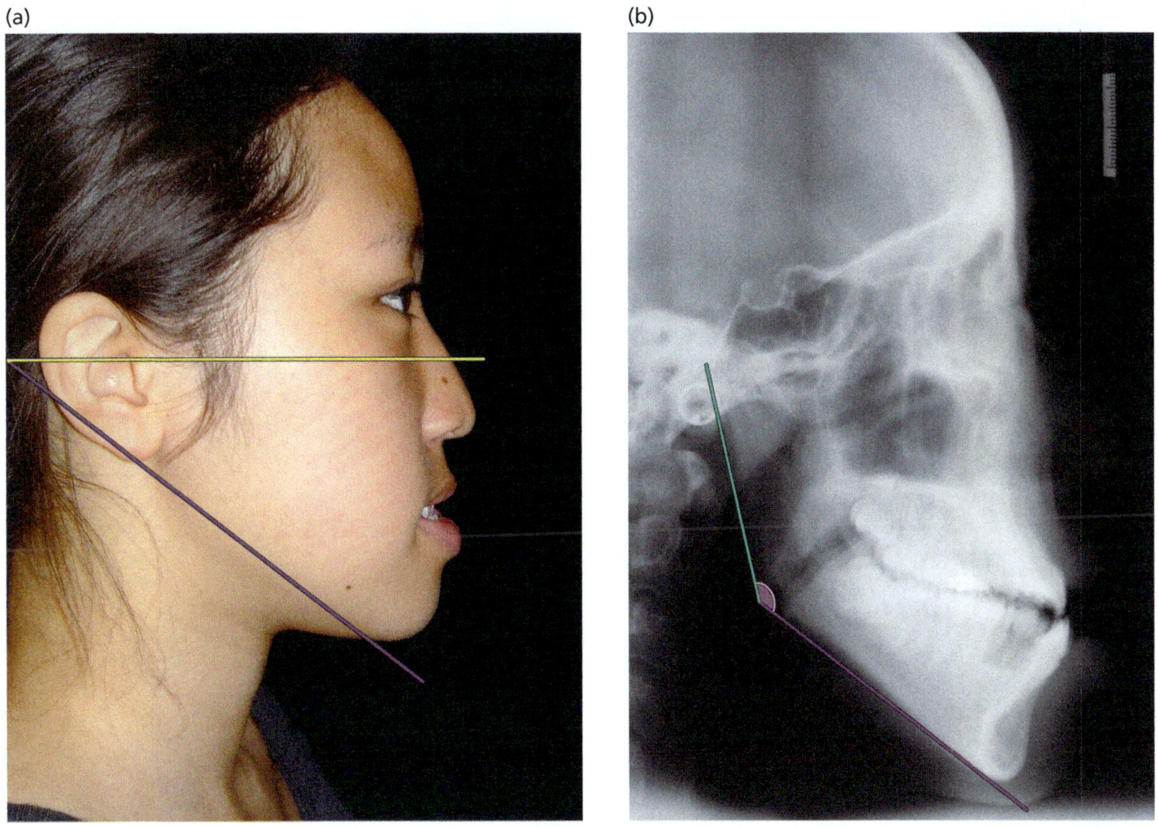

Fig. 6-6 (a): Increased mandibular plane angle. (b): Increased gonial angle.

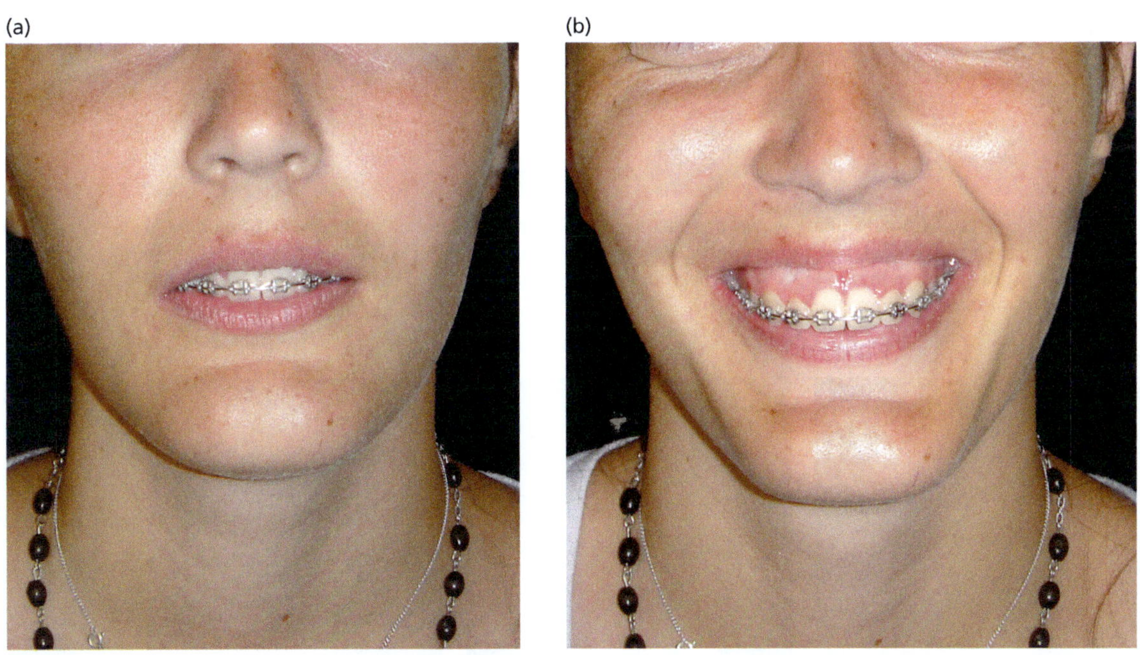

Fig. 6-7 Maxillary incisor exposure at rest (a) is very slightly increased, and on smiling (b) there is excessive gingival exposure due to hyperelevation of the upper lip. The maxilla should not be impacted more than a few millimetres, if at all, bearing in mind that maxillary incisor exposure will reduce with ageing.

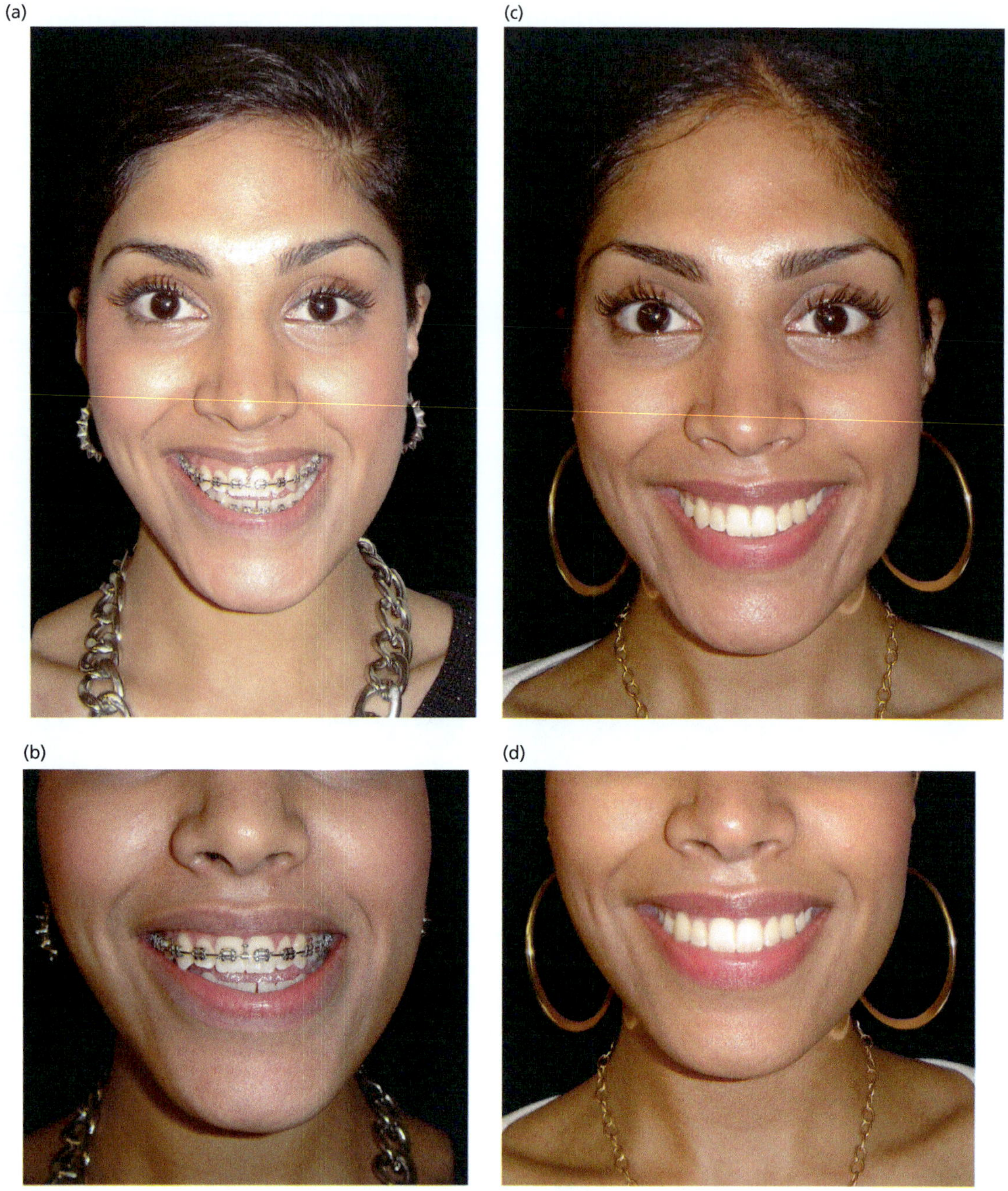

Fig. 6-8 (a, b) Preoperative frontal smiling views, demonstrating a flat smile arc. Patient underwent differential posterior maxillary impaction and slight advancement, forward mandibular autorotation and asymmetrical set-back. (c, d) End of treatment views, demonstrating improvement in the smile arc relationship following effective surgical retroclination of the maxillary incisors with differential posterior maxillary impaction.

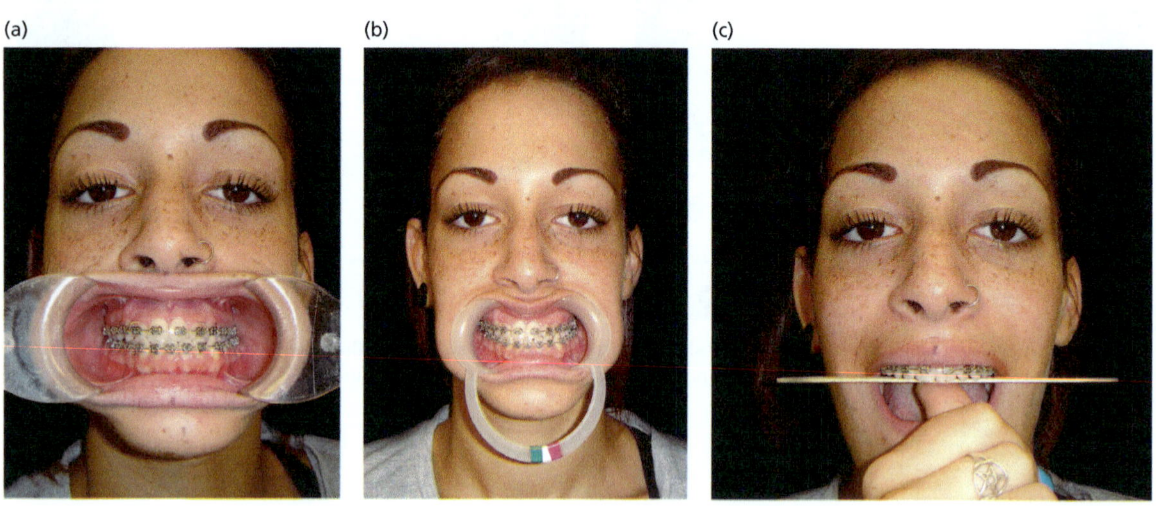

Fig. 6-9 Transverse canting of the maxillary occlusal plane should be assessed visually in frontal view with the aid of (a) photographic retractors and/or (b) orthodontic cheek retractors, and (c) with placement of a wooden tongue spatula (or dental mirror handle) on the occlusal plane.

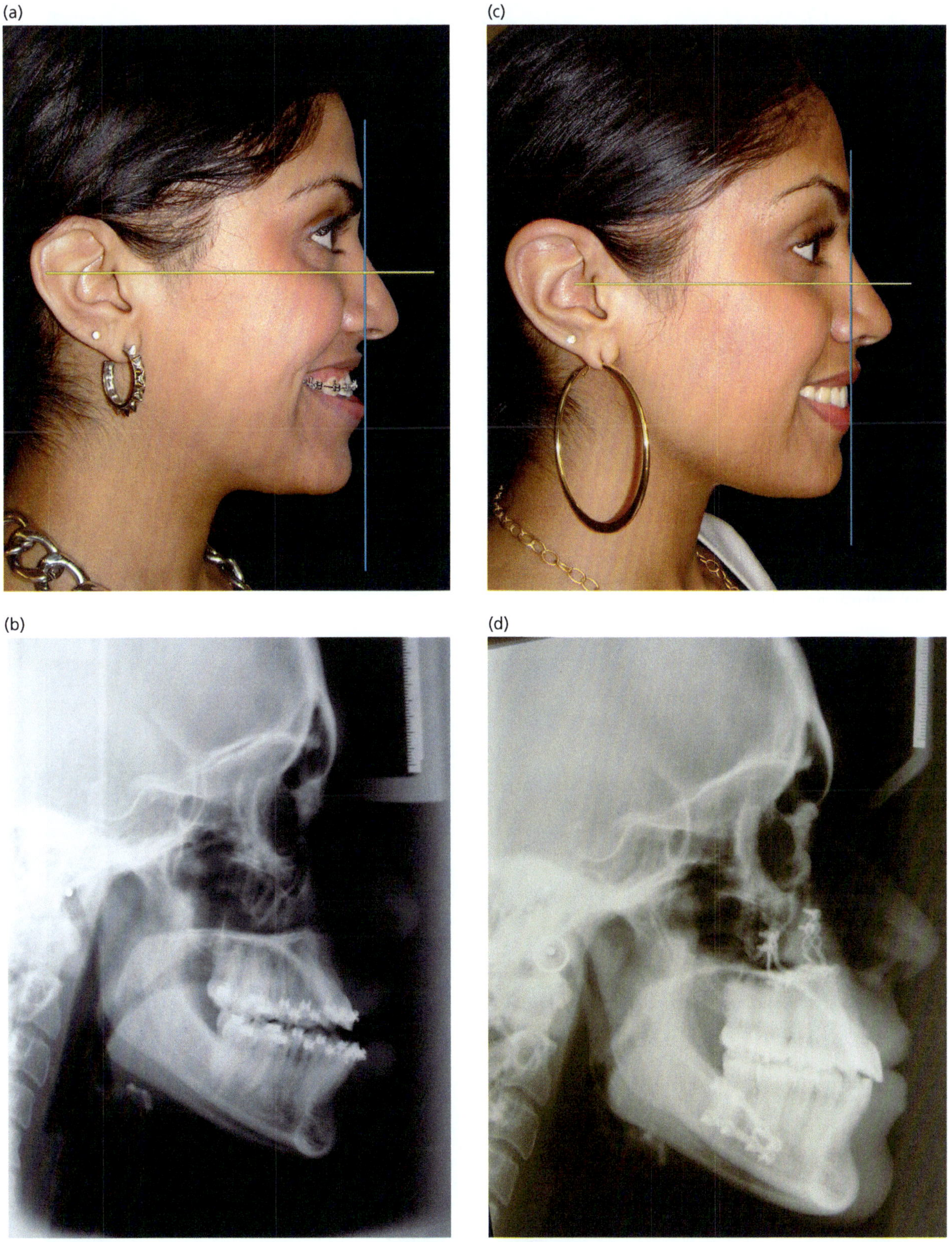

Fig. 6-10 Maxillary incisor inclination and sagittal position: (a, b): Preoperative profile smiling view and lateral cephalometric radiograph of patient shown in Figure 6-8. The maxillary incisors are slightly proclined and the maxilla retrognathic, with the incisors behind the true vertical line from soft tissue glabella. (c, d): Following differential posterior maxillary impaction and advancement, the inclination and sagittal position of the maxillary incisors has improved.

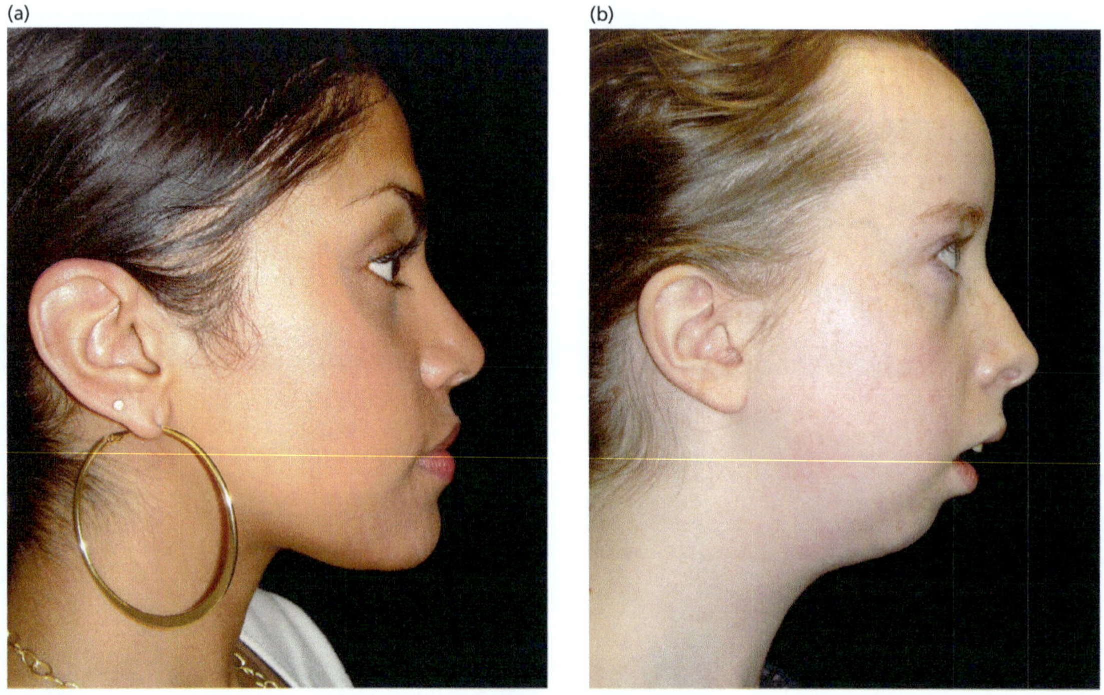

Fig. 6-11 The relationship of the upper lip, lower lip, mentolabial fold and chin is of paramount importance in facial aesthetics. (a): The upper lip is usually just slightly ahead of the lower lip, which is almost in line or just ahead of soft tissue pogonion. However, perhaps more important than the sagittal position is the transition between these neighbouring structures, which should be smooth and S-shaped. (b): This patient has mandibular retrognathia, retrogenia and posterior rotation of the mandible, but the retrogenia is more of an aesthetic problem as there is no depth to the mentolabial fold and thereby no S-shape in the transition between the mentolabial region and the chin.

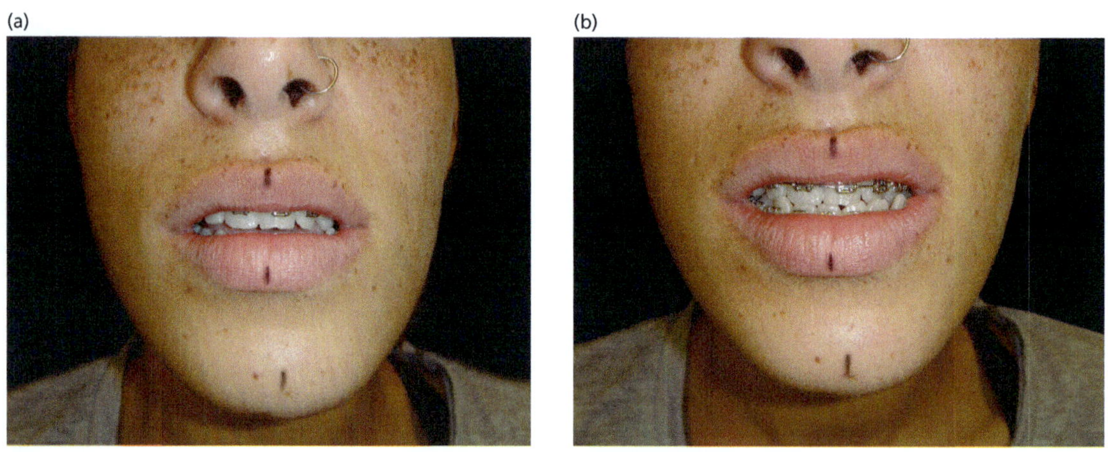

Fig. 6-12 Midline markings made at the chair side to assess dental midline deviations in relation to the upper lip, lower chin and chin. (a): In repose. (b): In occlusion.

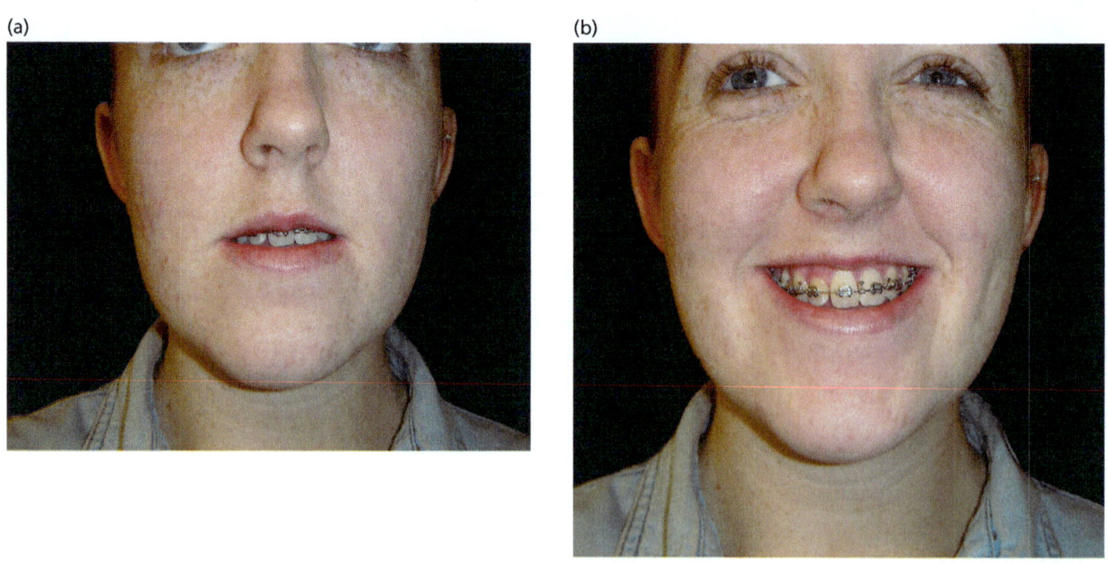

Fig. 6-13 (a–c): Preoperative views of a Class III patient with maxillary dental midline deviation to her left, and with the incisors angulated to her left due to the maxillary occlusal plane being canted down on her right.

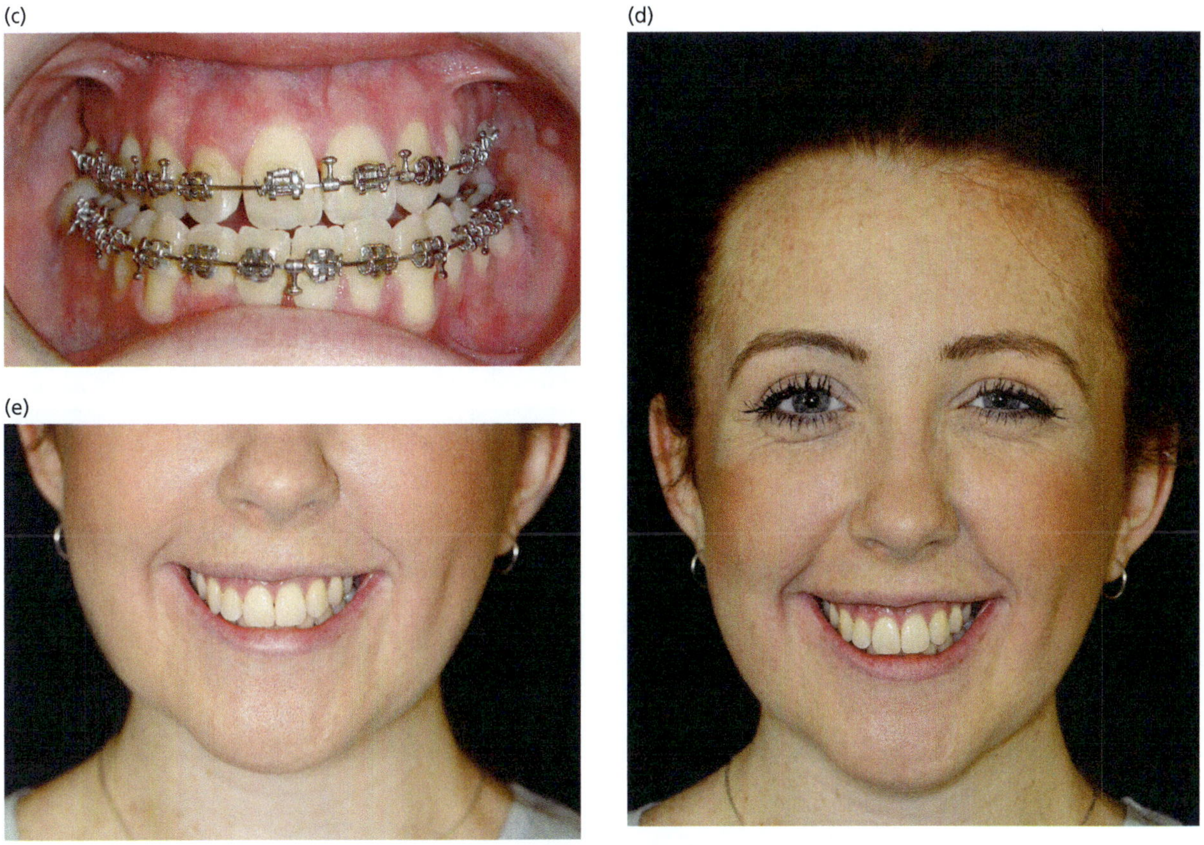

Fig. 6-13 (d,e): Postoperative smiling views, following maxillary impaction on the patient's right side to level the transverse cant, and maxillary rotation to her right to correct the midline discrepancy. The maxilla was also advanced and mandible set-back. The maxillary left lateral incisor was missing, and the canine has been masked in the lateral incisor position.

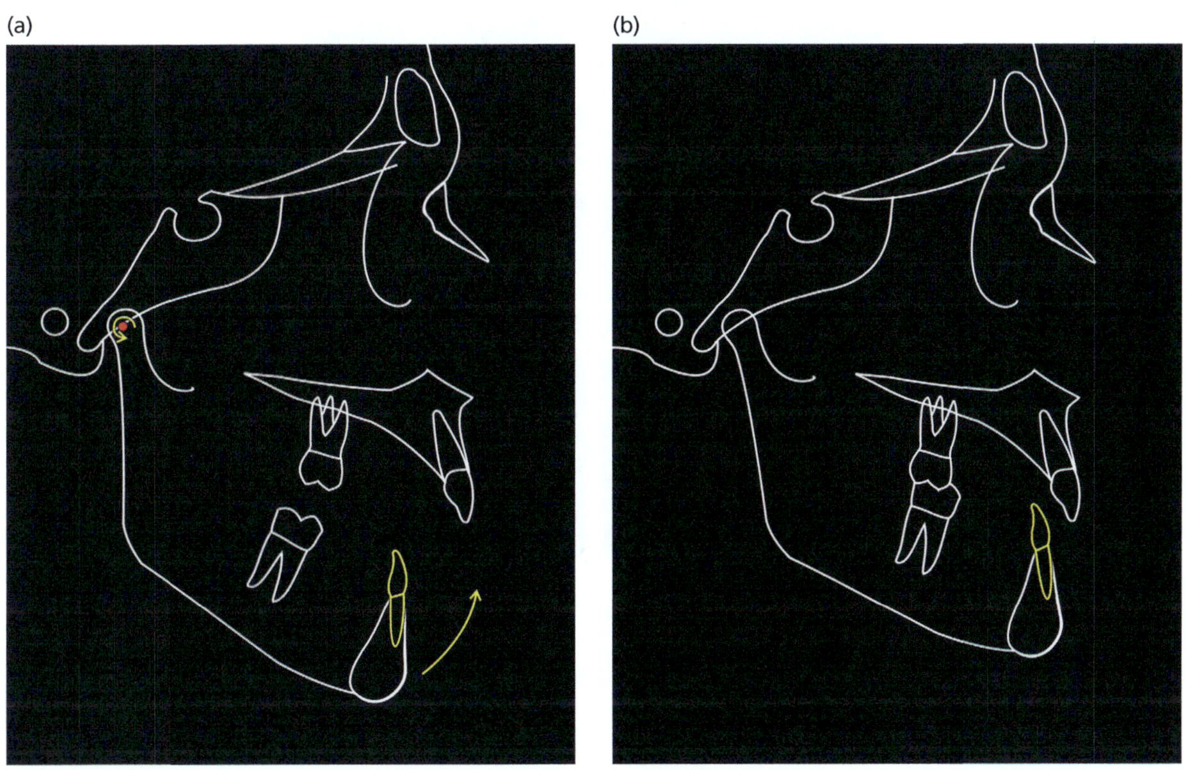

Fig. 6-14 Mandibular incisor inclination preparation for mandibular autorotation. (a) If the mandibular incisor inclination is not orthodontically prepared prior to forward mandibular autorotation, then (b) the incisor inclination will be incorrect following autorotation. (c) The mandibular incisor inclination has been orthodontically prepared (in this case by proclination). In this situation, the mandibular incisors may appear excessively proclined, but clinicians should be aware that this is their *planned* position. (d) With forward autorotation of the mandible; (e) the mandibular incisor inclination will be correct.

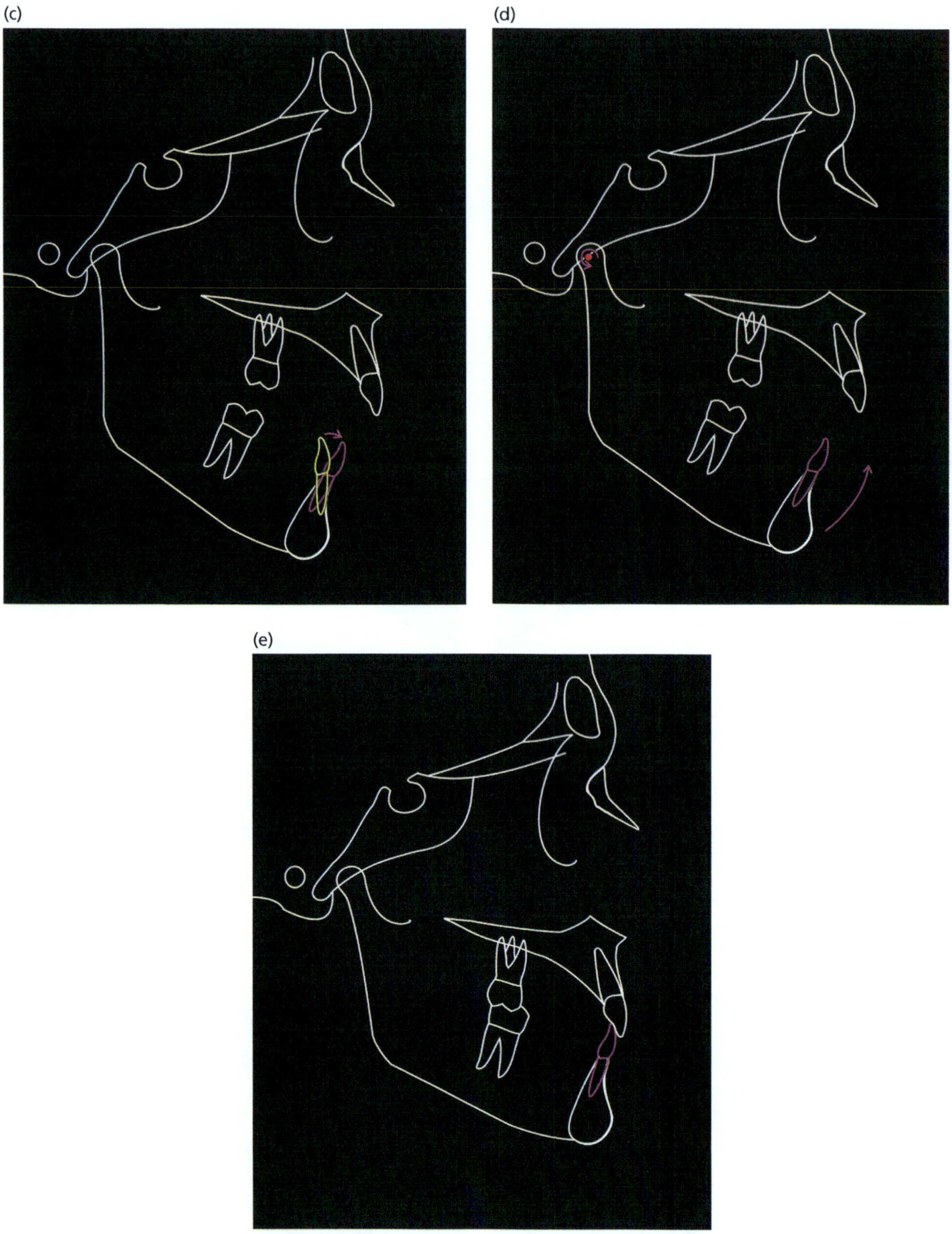

Fig. 6-14 (*Continued*)

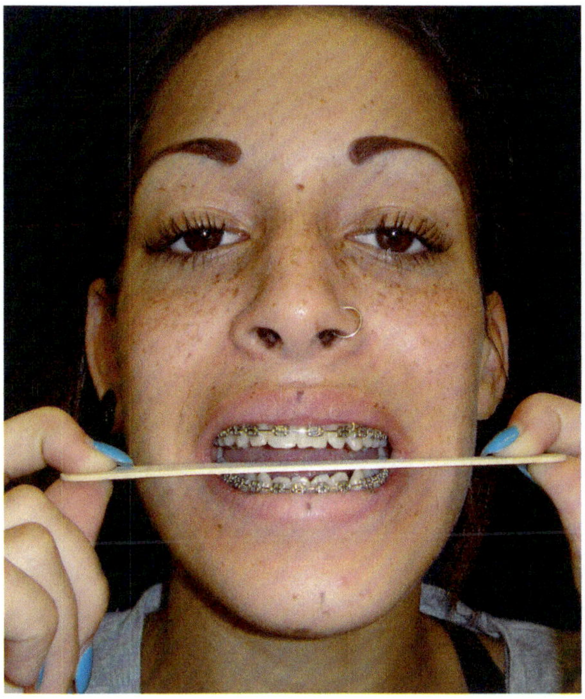

Fig. 6-15 Transverse canting of the mandibular occlusal plane may be assessed using a wooden tongue spatula.

region on the adjacent structures. The relationship of the forehead, nose, midface, upper lip, lower lip, chin and submental-cervical region may be evaluated by **masking** any of these regions whilst evaluating the relationships of the other structures (Figure 6-20).[10] This may be undertaken clinically by holding a piece of card over a region, e.g. the lower face. Alternatively, this technique may be undertaken on a clinical profile photograph. One of the most important uses of this technique is to reduce or eliminate the **illusional effects** of relative structures on the perception of one another, where what is visually perceived differs from objective reality (Figure 6-21).

Cotton wool roll technique

If a treatment plan is not clear cut, the degree of relative movement of the maxilla, mandible, and chin required to provide ideal facial soft tissue profile aesthetics may be rather difficult to ascertain. For example, in some Class III patients, the relative degree of maxillary advancement compared with mandibular set-back may be difficult to determine.

A simple and relatively quick chair side technique for evaluating the potential facial profile change with

(a)

(b)

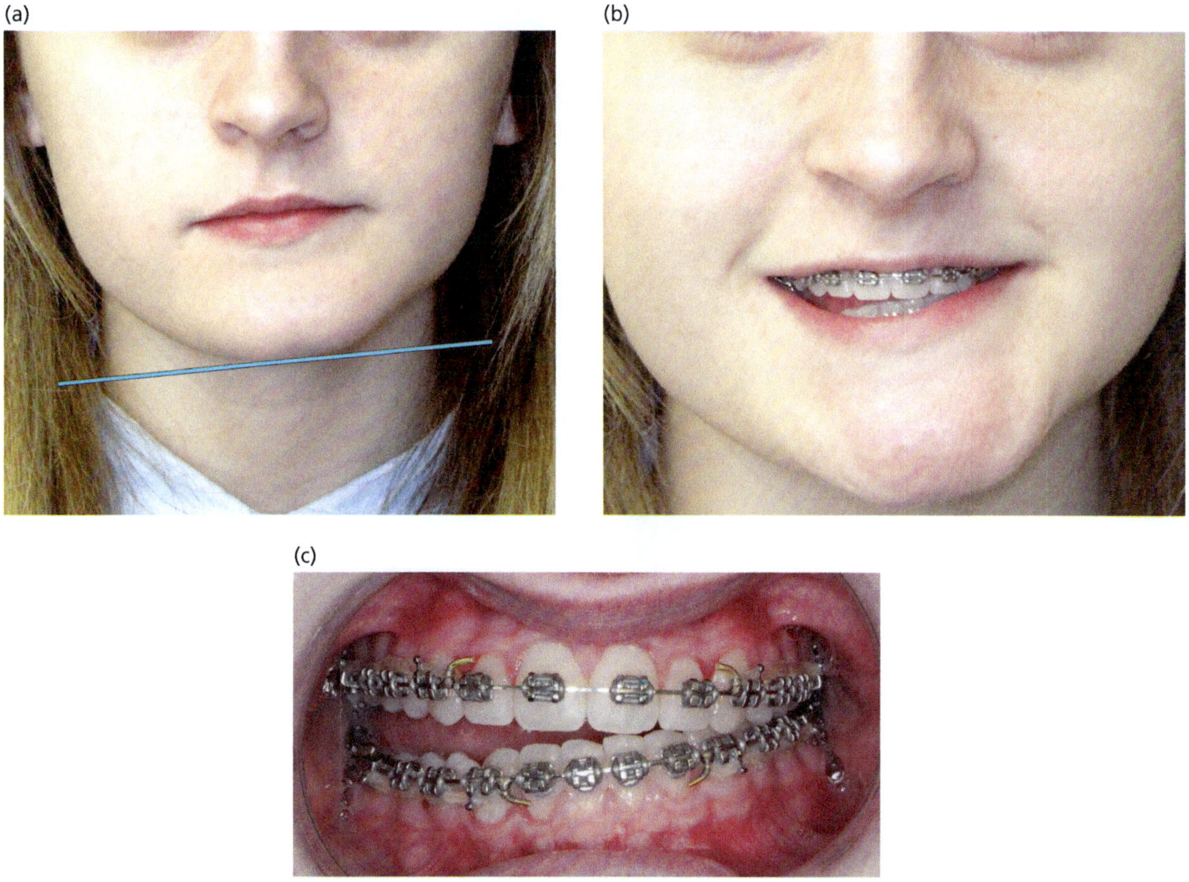

(c)

Fig. 6-16 (a–c): Patient with right-sided hemimandibular hyperplasia, where the tongue has prevented overeruption of the maxillary posterior dentition on her right side. There is a transverse cant of the mandibular occlusal plane and the inferior chin plane, which will both correct with rotation of the mandibular body around the sagittal axis.

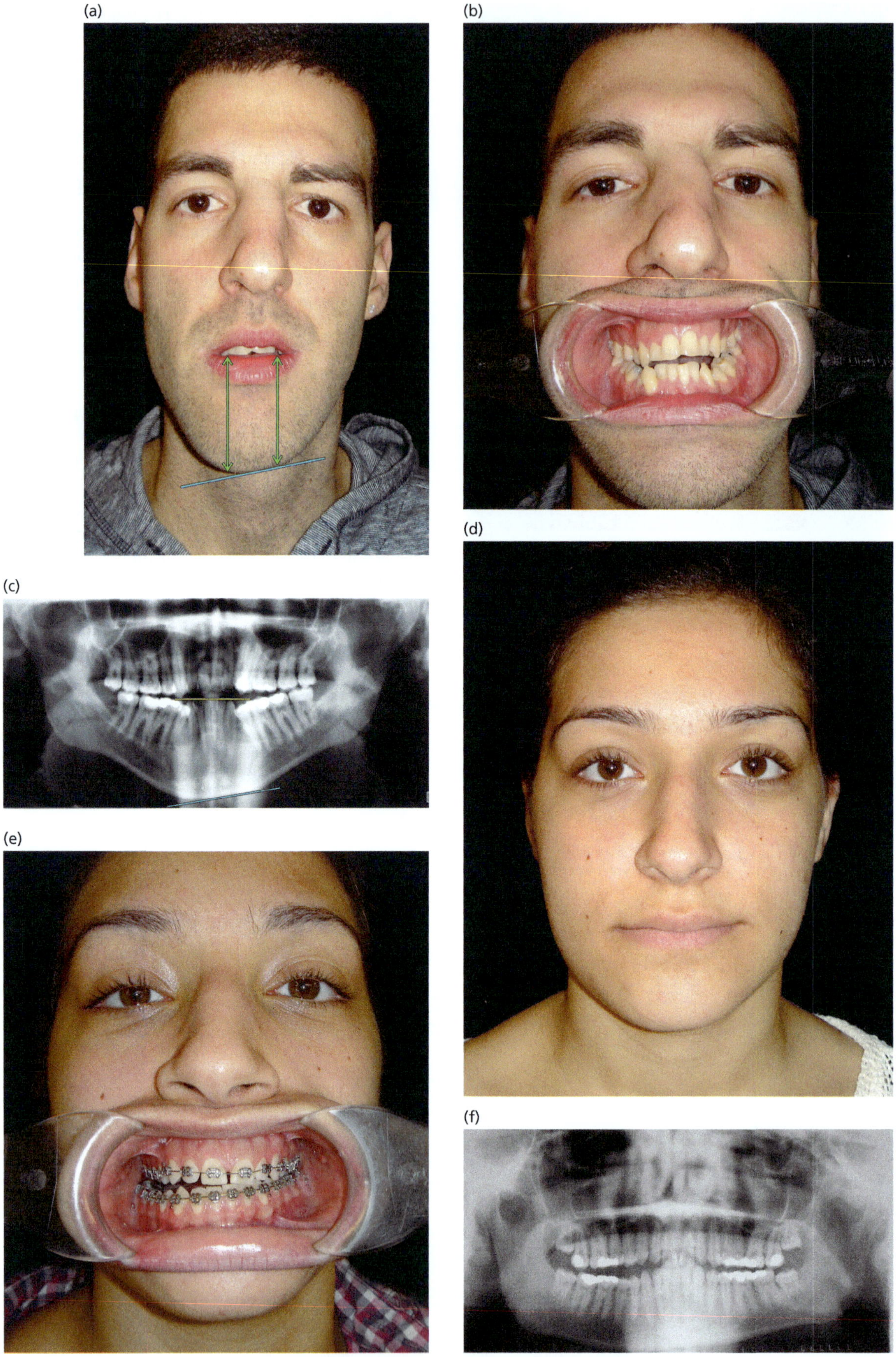

Fig. 6-17 (a–c): Transverse cant of the inferior chin plane due to asymmetry of the bony chin, i.e. greater bony chin height on the patient's right compared with his left. There is minimal transverse cant in the mandibular occlusal plane. The asymmetry of the chin will require a genioplasty. (d–f): Transverse cant of the inferior chin plane due to right-sided hemimandibular hyperplasia, with concomitant transverse cant of the mandibular occlusal plane. The cant of the inferior border of the chin will correct with the surgical repositioning of the mandibular body.

(a) (b) (c) (d) (e) (f)

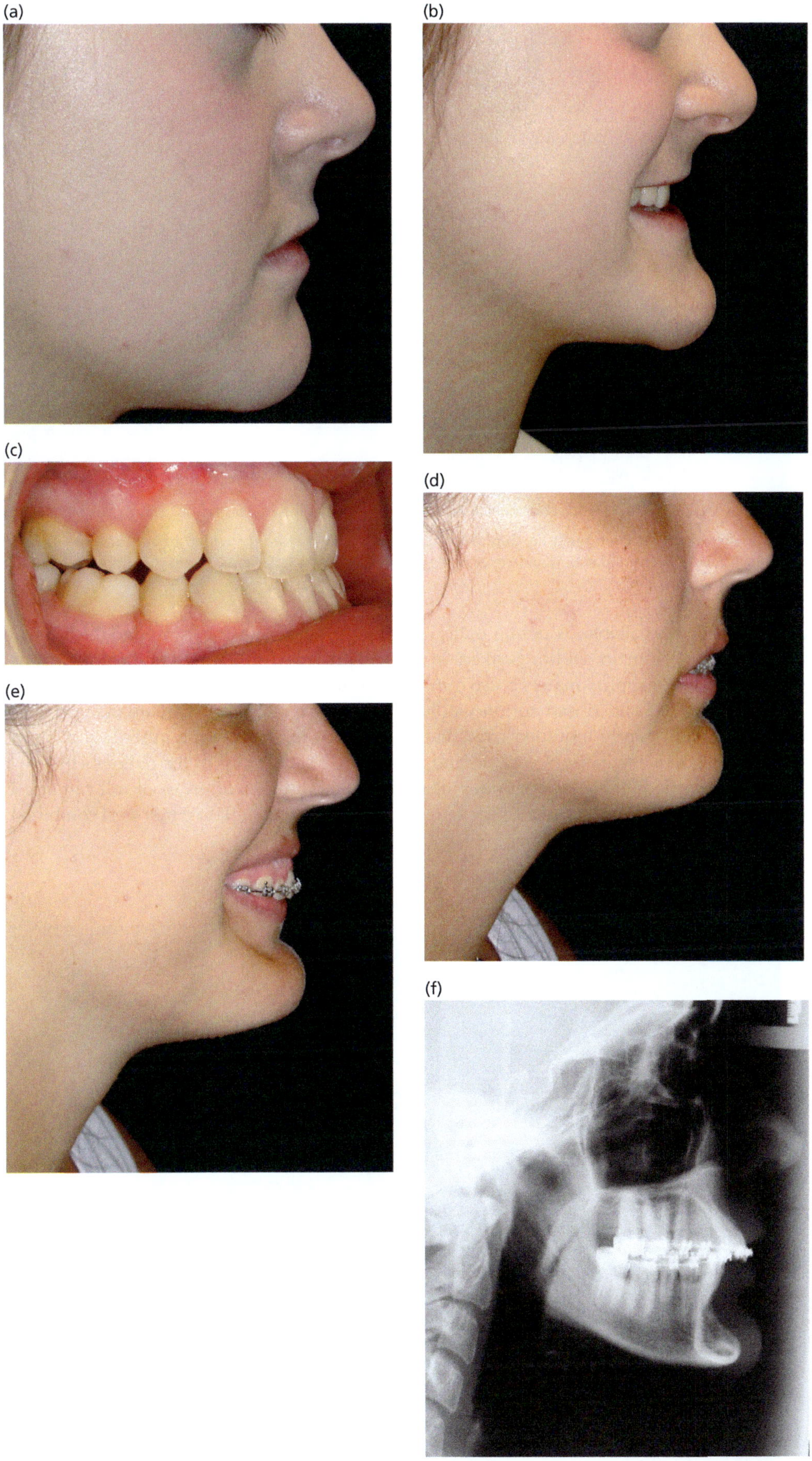

Fig. 6-18 (a–c): Class III patient who has undergone dentoalveolar compensation, with retroclination of the mandibular incisors. The chin is effaced and appears prominent only on smiling. (d–f): Class II patient, preoperative views, showing smile effacing the chin. Lateral cephalometric radiograph demonstrates retrusion of the mandibular dentoalveolus and relative prominence of the bony chin.

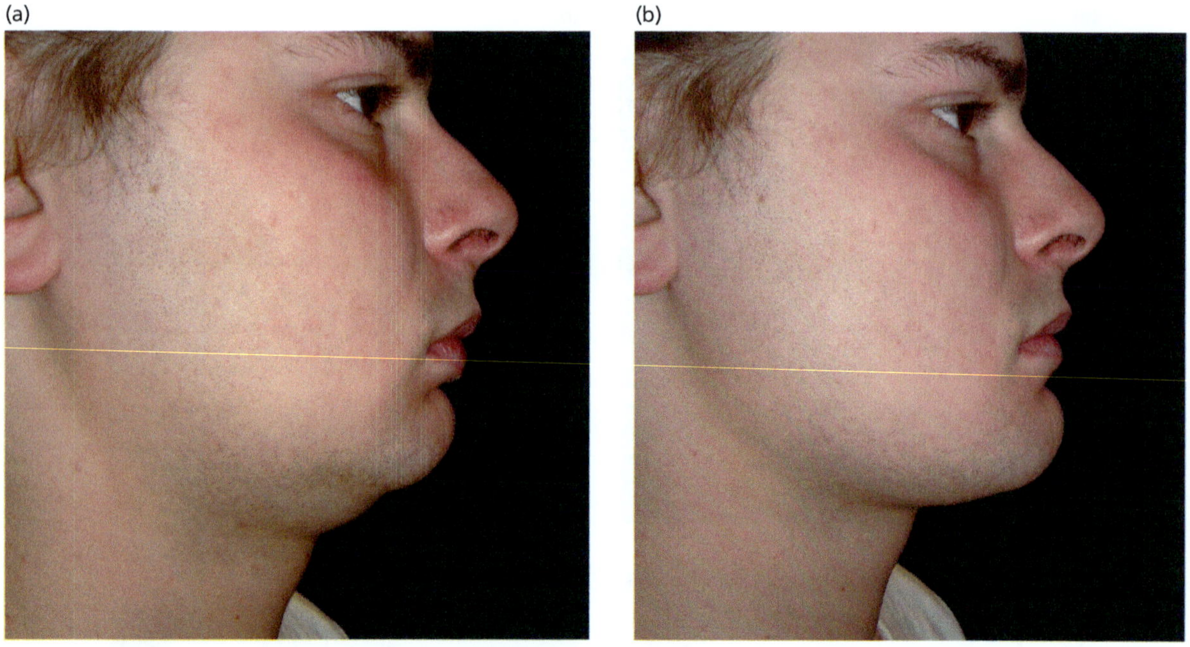

Fig. 6-19 (a) Patient with mandibular retrognathia. (b) Posturing the mandible forward provides an indication of the potential changes in lower facial relationships and submental-cervical region with mandibular advancement osteotomy.

maxillary advancement is available. A dental cotton wool roll is normally 10 mm in width. Soaked in water and gently rinsed, it is approximately 5 to 6 mm in width. As such, a soaked and rinsed cotton wool roll can be positioned and gently moulded over the anterior aspect of the maxillary incisors, just on and slightly superior to the orthodontic brackets, under the upper lip. With the patient in natural head position, the teeth gently in occlusion, and the lips in repose, this will provide a simulation of the potential result of a 5- to 6-mm maxillary advancement on the upper lip and allow the clinician to evaluate the potential change in the facial appearance (Figure 6-22 and Figure 6-23).[10,11] Digital photographs of the patient's profile taken with and without the cotton wool roll can also be used to demonstrate the relative merits of combined maxillary

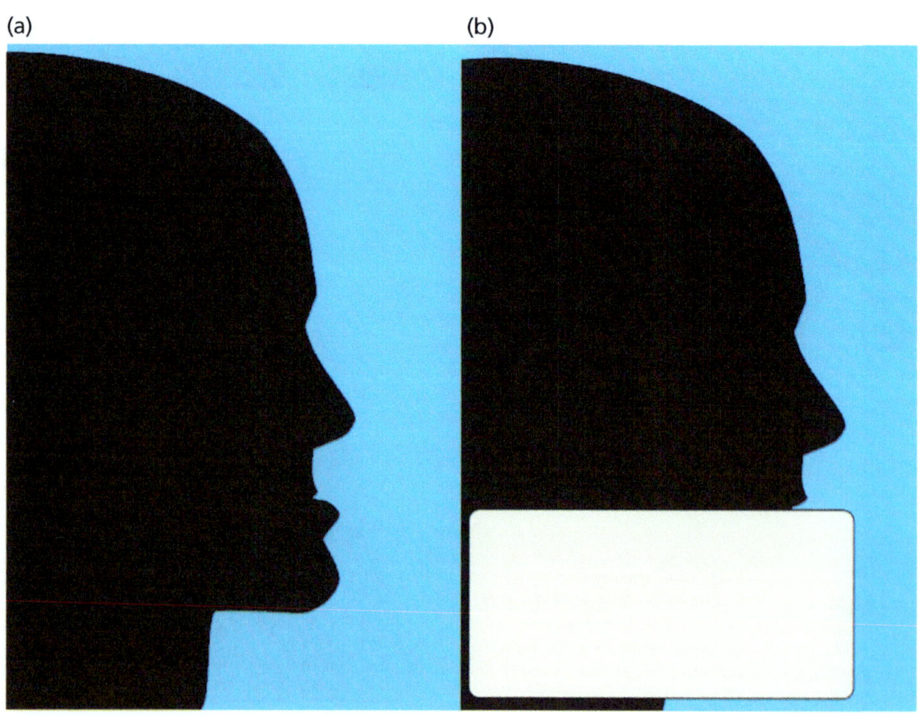

Fig. 6-20 (a): Mandibular excess may create the illusion of upper lip and/or maxillary deficiency. (b): Masking the lower lip and chin demonstrates a normal upper lip prominence. (From: Naini FB. Facial Aesthetics: Concepts and Clinical Diagnosis. Oxford: Wiley-Blackwell, 2011; modified and reprinted with permission.)

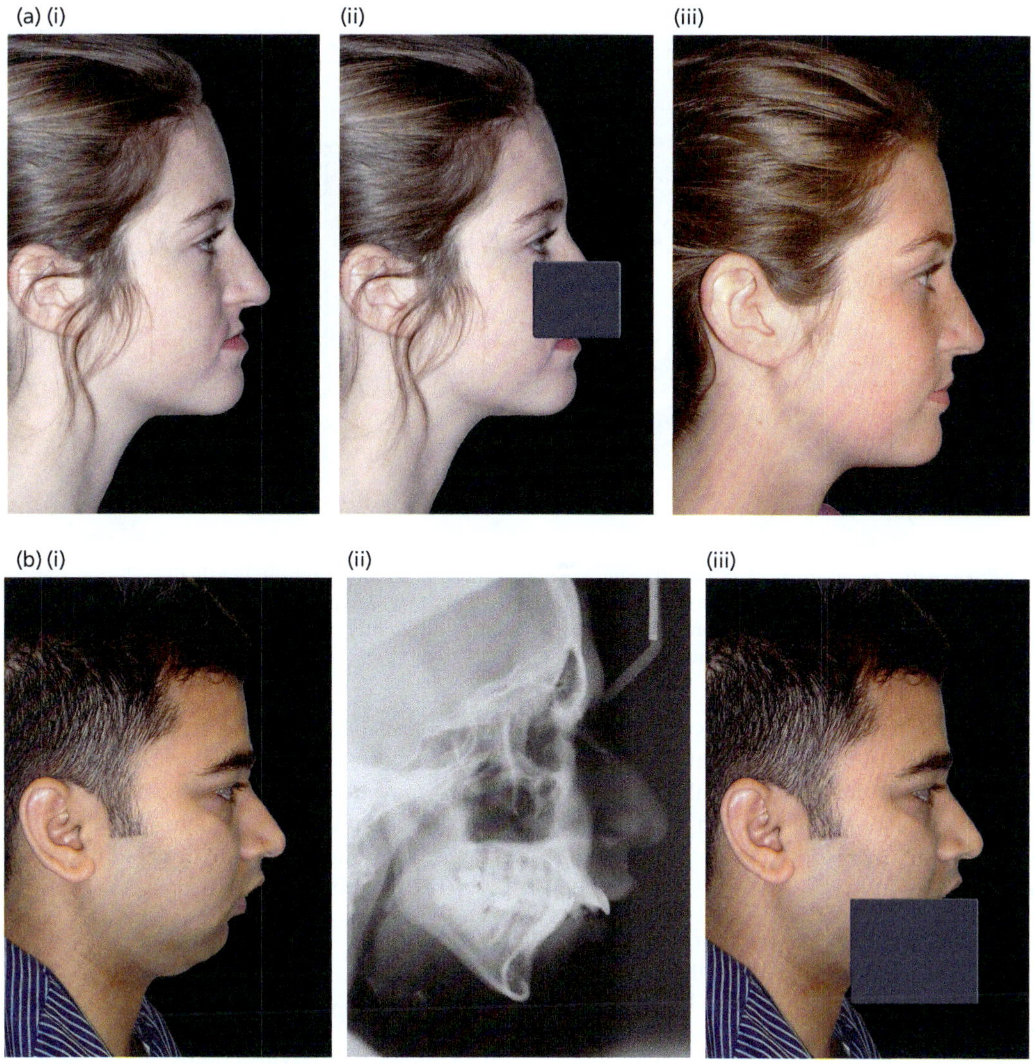

Fig. 6-21 (ai): Class III patient with predominantly maxillary retrognathia. (aii): Masking the midface helps to demonstrate that the sagittal position of the mandible is only mildly prominent. (aiii): Postoperative result following maxillary advancement and very slight mandibular set-back. (bi and ii): Class II patient with mandibular retrognathia. Lateral cephalometric radiograph confirms mandibular retrognathia and demonstrates proclination of maxillary incisors, but (biii) masking the lower lip and chin demonstrates acceptable midface position, with mild proclination of the upper lip.

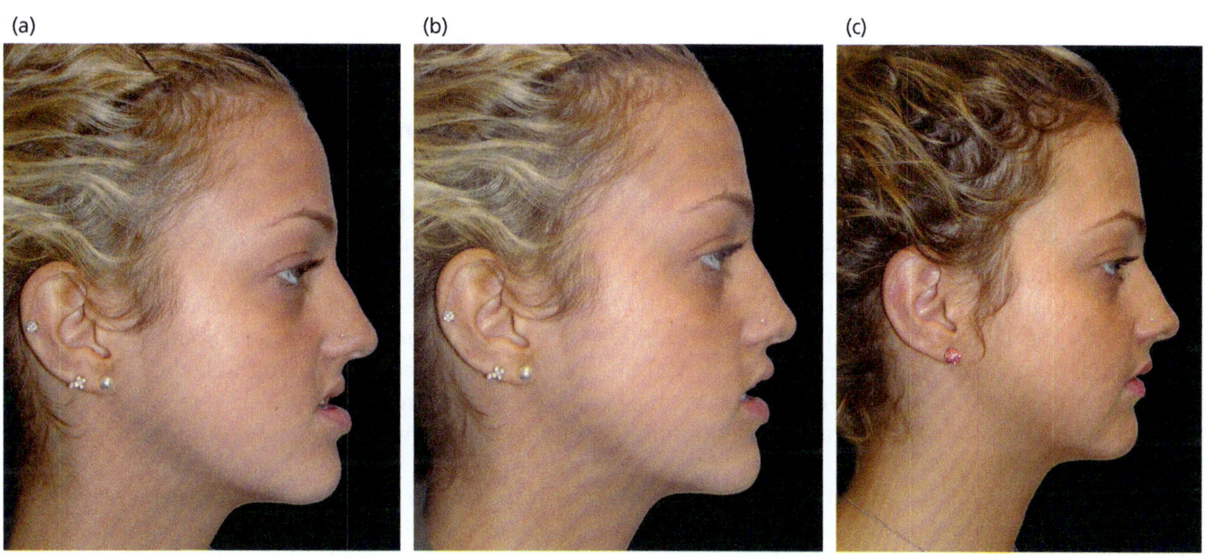

Fig. 6-22 (a): Preoperative profile view of a Class III patient in natural head position, with teeth lightly in occlusion and soft tissues in repose. (b): Soaked and rinsed cotton wool roll positioned under the upper lip simulating the potential effects of a 5–6 mm maxillary advancement. Result demonstrates that mandibular position is essentially normal. (c): Postoperative result following maxillary advancement and very small mandibular set-back to correct the dental occlusion.

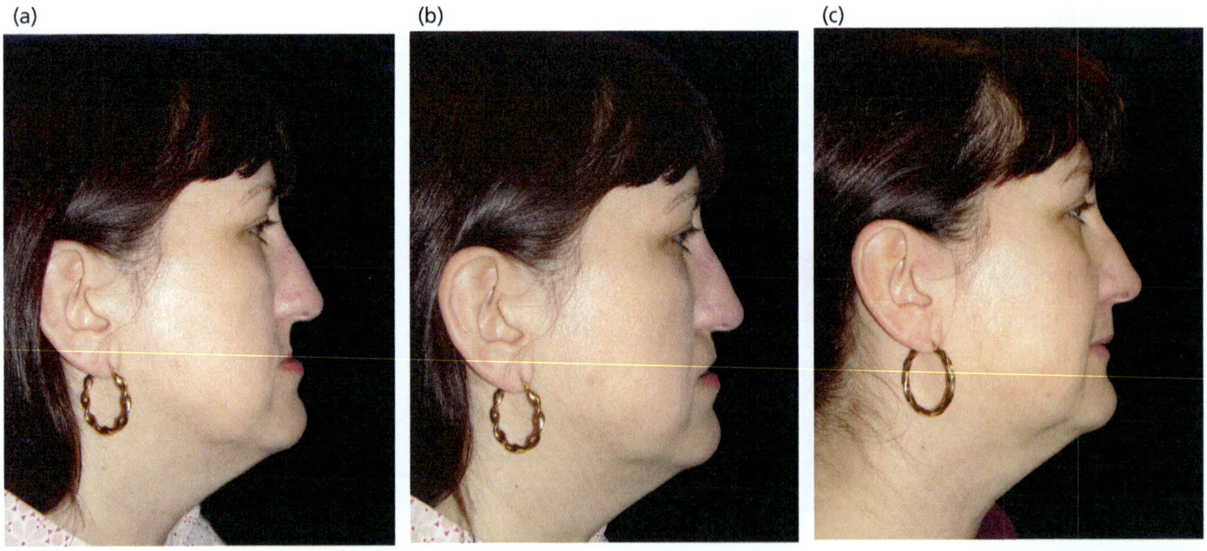

Fig. 6-23 (a): Preoperative profile view of a Class III patient in natural head position, with teeth lightly in occlusion and soft tissues in repose. (b): Soaked and rinsed cotton wool roll positioned under the upper lip simulating the potential effects of a 5–6 mm maxillary advancement. Result demonstrates that mandibular position is still slightly prominent. (c): Postoperative result following maxillary advancement and mandibular set-back.

advancement and mandibular set-back in relation to isolated mandibular set-back to the patient, particularly in situations in which a patient only regards the mandibular prominence as the problem.

Posturing the mandible

In patients presenting with mandibular retrognathia, a general idea of the potential postoperative soft tissue result of mandibular advancement may be gleaned by asking the patient to posture their mandible forward to the desired postoperative incisor relationship. Though not absolutely accurate, this technique provides the clinician with an idea of the change in the facial outline, both in frontal and profile views, which may be achieved with such a procedure (see Figure 6-19). There are two specific parameters that may be checked:

- The change in lower anterior face height (LAFH) and unfurling of the mentolabial fold will aid the decision as to whether further mandibular arch levelling is required to prevent excessive increase in lower face height following a 3-point landing. If the LAFH is to be maintained, the mandibular arch should be orthodontically levelled in the preparatory orthodontic phase of treatment. Alternatively, the greater the desired increase in the LAFH with mandibular advancement, the greater the curve of Spee that must be maintained or created in the mandibular arch with the preparatory orthodontics (Figure 6-24).
- The degree of advancement of the soft tissue chin in relation to the lower lip will aid the decision as to whether an advancement or set-back genioplasty, or vertical augmentation or reduction genioplasty may be required following a proposed mandibular advancement osteotomy.

Very occasionally, if a patient finds it difficult to maintain the postured position, an acrylic wafer splint may be made to the postured position. Digital photographs of the patient in the initial and postured positions may also be shown to the patient, which may help in the information provision required (Figure 6-25).

Genioplasty prediction

If a potential advancement genioplasty is being planned, the clinician may gently squeeze the soft tissue chin pad between the thumb and index finger, in order to simulate the potential soft tissue change that would result following an advancement genioplasty. Though relatively crude, this simple technique can be surprisingly useful at the chair side (Figure 6-26).

Skeletal expansion vs. contraction and effects on the overlying soft tissues

Rosen[12] has eloquently described an important principle in orthognathic surgery – that *the expansion of the dentoskeletal structures in all planes of space provides a more reliable and predictable alteration in the overlying soft tissue contour compared with relative dentoskeletal contraction*. For example, mandibular advancement or advancement and/or set-down osseous genioplasty provide a relatively predictable soft tissue outcome, within reason. However, mandibular set-back, or set-back and/or vertical reduction genioplasty lead to a reduction in the dentoskeletal support for the soft tissues, and may lead to a less predictable and potentially unfavourable soft tissue outcome. The potentially detrimental soft tissue response to skeletal contraction has been described for reduction

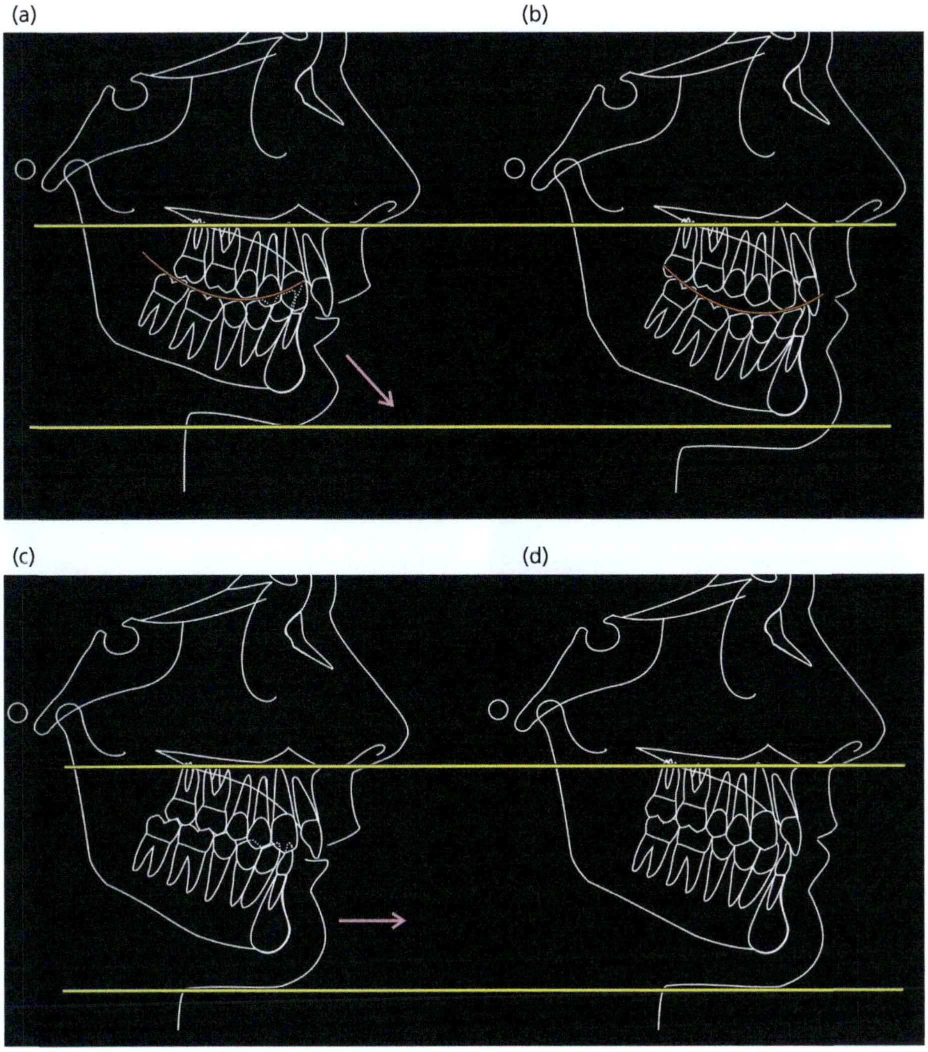

Fig. 6-24 (a) Maintaining or creating an increased curve of Spee prior to mandibular advancement. (b) Mandibular advancement to a 3-point landing (incisors and terminal molars) occurs by a downward and forward vector of movement of the mandibular incisors. This will increase the lower anterior face height (LAFH) and unfurl the mentolabial fold, improving the soft tissue contour of the lower face. The lateral open bites are closed orthodontically by extrusion of the mid-arch mandibular dentition, i.e. *postoperative levelling of the curve of Spee*. (c) If the LAFH does not need to be increased, the mandibular dental arch is levelled in the preoperative orthodontic preparatory phase, i.e. *preoperative levelling of the curve of Spee*. (d) As such, mandibular advancement does *not* lead to any significant change in the LAFH.

genioplasty,[13] and mandibular set-back surgery,[12] as well as for maxillary set-back.[14] Posterior repositioning of the anterior maxilla has even been linked with a prematurely aged appearance.[14,15]

This principle has important treatment planning implications, *as if there is a choice between expanding or contracting the skeletal volume, skeletal expansion is likely to be the better option*. For example, in a Class III patient with combined retrognathic maxilla and prognathic mandible, all things being equal, the ratio of maxillary advancement to mandibular set-back should be increased, i.e. it may be better to advance the maxilla to a greater extent than setting back the mandible. Alternatively, unilateral bowing of the inferior mandibular border may require an inferior border shave, but a more predictable outcome may be achieved by expanding the skeletal volume by placing an implant on the contralateral inferior mandibular border.

2. Vectorial analysis

'In the correction of facial skeletal anomalies the surgeon's eyes, experience and intuition are more important than tracings and computer-planning.' (see Box 6-1)

Hugo L. Obwegeser[16]

A vector may be defined as a quantity having **direction** as well as **magnitude**. It is usually denoted by a line drawn from its original to its final position.

In treatment planning, once the region(s) at fault have been identified (by clinical observation and possibly palpation), the next step may be termed *vectorial analysis*, in which the **direction** of movement of each jaw/subunit is determined, following which the **approximate magnitude** of the movement required is determined.

This process is based predominantly on observation of the patient, and is thereby **qualitative** in nature. It is not, however, entirely subjective; the reason is that

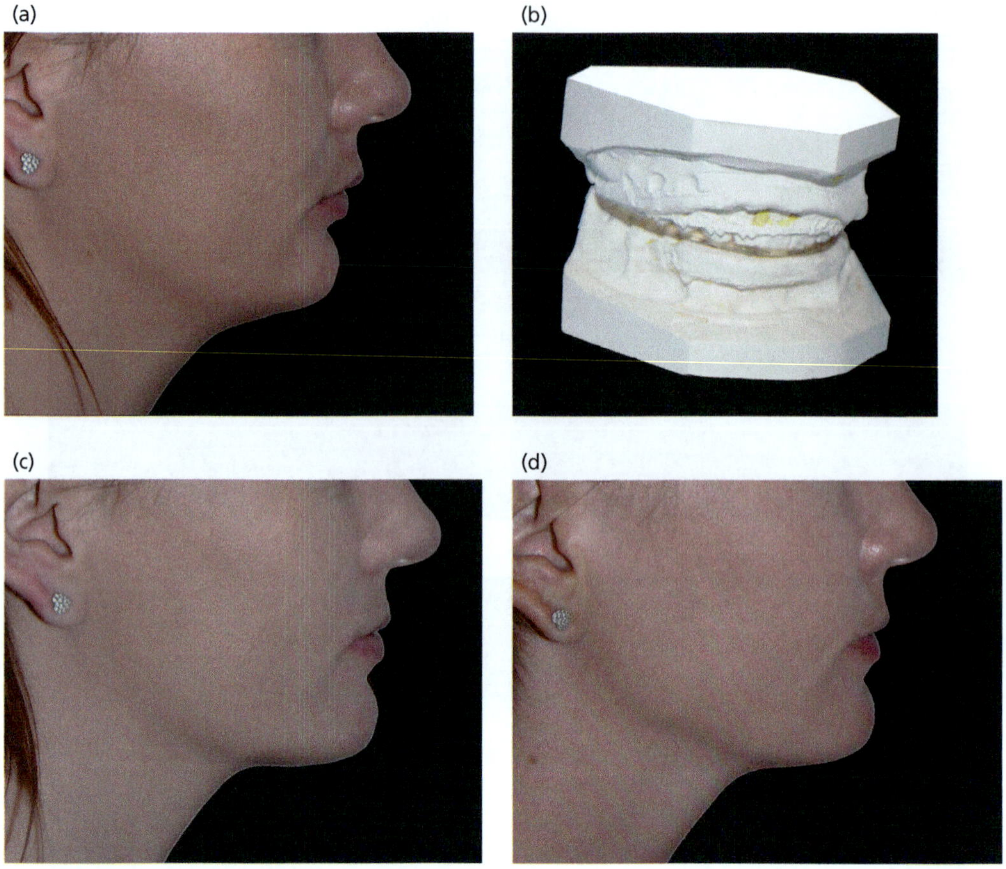

Fig. 6-25 (a): Preoperative profile view of a Class II patient with mandibular retrognathia. (b): Thin acrylic wafer made to the proposed postoperative position with a planned mandibular advancement osteotomy. (c): Postured position using prepared wafer to simulate proposed postoperative position. (d): Postoperative result following mandibular advancement osteotomy.

most trained clinicians are likely to obtain similar findings. After accurate preoperative diagnosis, *vectorial analysis is the most important stage of the treatment planning process.*

Case example

A Class III patient with mandibular asymmetry being assessed preoperatively (Figure 6-27). *Stage 1* – The **preoperative clinical evaluation and diagnosis** demonstrates the following:

In *frontal view,* sequential masking in a top-down approach demonstrates that the upper face is relatively symmetrical. Marking midline structures demonstrates that the nose is asymmetrical, but the facial asymmetry is predominantly affecting the lower face. There is a transverse cant to the maxillary occlusal plane, down on the patient's right. Maxillary incisor exposure is somewhat reduced (1–2 mm), but the midline is essentially coincident with the midphiltrum of the upper lip. Upper lip height is average. The lower lip and chin are to the left of the facial midline, and there is a transverse cant of the inferior

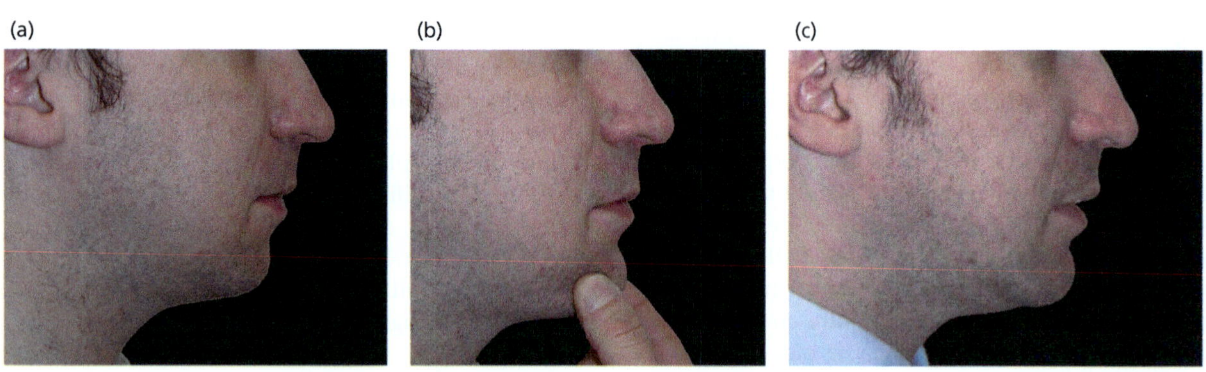

Fig. 6-26 (a): Preoperative profile view of a patient with retrogenia. (b): Gently squeezing the soft tissue chin pad between the thumb and index finger simulates the potential soft tissue change that would result with an advancement genioplasty. (c): Postoperative profile view following advancement osseous genioplasty.

Box 6-1 Treatment planning: intuitive judgement vs. methodical analysis

> 'The value of experience is not in seeing much, but in seeing wisely.'
>
> Sir William Osler (1849–1919)[17]

The role of 'intuition' in treatment planning requires elaboration. The impact of intuition has been extensively investigated and eloquently described by the renowned American psychologist Daniel Kahneman.[18–20] The word intuition refers to the ability to understand something instinctively and immediately, without the intervention of or need for conscious reasoning. It infers a sense of knowing or perceiving something without the evidence or logic of knowing how we know.

In 1985, the Getty Museum paid a staggering sum to buy a kouros, a statue of a youth thought to be from the archaic period of Greek sculpture.[21] A number of the experts viewing the sculpture had an intuitive 'gut' feeling that the statue was a fake. These experts all appeared to agree that the statue was a fake 'without knowing how they knew', which epitomises the concept of intuition. The statue is now labelled 'Greek, about 530 BC, or modern forgery.' This story is often recounted as a triumph of intuition, the implication being that a systematic investigation designed to find the cues that guided these experts would simply have failed. However, Kahneman rejects this conclusion, stating that not only was such an inquiry needed, but that if it had been conducted properly, it would probably have succeeded.[19]

In any field or endeavour, whether scientific or not, some 'experts' are **analytical**, i.e. they undertake calculations and work things out to decide which way to proceed, whereas other 'experts' are more **intuitive**, i.e. appear to 'go with their gut instincts'. In orthognathic surgical treatment planning, the differences between these two approaches to intuition and expertise are often viewed as conflicting.

Intuition as pattern recognition

The intuitive ability of firefighters has been investigated.[19] These individuals work in high risk situations where split second decisions may mean the difference between life and death. When faced with a difficult situation, experienced firefighters would:

> 'draw on a repertoire of patterns that they had compiled during more than a *decade of both real and virtual experience* to identify a plausible option, which they considered first. They evaluated this option by mentally simulating it to see if it would work in the situation they were facing… If the course of action they were considering seemed appropriate, they would implement it. If it had shortcomings, they would modify it. If they could not easily modify it, they would turn to the next most plausible option and run through the same procedure until an acceptable course of action was found.'

This theory of decision making has been called the recognition-primed decision (RPD) model,[19] and applies to a clinician undertaking orthognathic treatment planning as much as it does to firefighters. The process involves two phases:[18]

- Phase 1 – A tentative plan comes to mind by an automatic function of **associative memory** (i.e. you've seen something work before, so the answer is just there for you; you don't have to work it out) – this phase is intuitive, but *requires a solid base of previous experience*;
- Phase 2 – A deliberate process in which the plan is mentally simulated to check if it will work – this phase is analytical, and requires active checking of the plan from phase 1.

This model of intuitive decision making as pattern recognition is developed from ideas initially presented by the American scholar Herbert Simon (1916–2001), the founding father of the study of decision making. Simon's definition of intuition was as follows:[18]

> 'The situation has provided a cue; this cue has given the expert access to information stored in memory, and the information provides the answer. *Intuition is nothing more and nothing less than recognition.*'

Kahneman confirms that the importance of this statement is that 'it reduces the apparent magic of intuition to the everyday experience of memory'.[18] It helps to demystify intuitive expertise, as it becomes clear that such associative memory can only be gained from long years of training, practice, and sound experience.

Acquiring skill in treatment planning

Kahneman[18,20] has also discussed how the information that supports intuition becomes 'stored in memory'? Although certain types of intuition may be acquired very quickly, the intuition associated with 'expertise' in a task or subject takes a long time to develop. Kahneman has pointed out that acquiring expertise in complex tasks is intricate and slow because expertise is not reliant on a single skill but rather on a large collection of skills. The example of a chess master is provided:[18,20]

> 'An expert player can understand a complex position at a glance, but it takes years to develop that level of ability. Studies of chess masters have shown that at least 10,000 hours of dedicated practice (about 6 years of playing chess 5 hours a day) are required to attain the highest levels of performance. During those hours of intense concentration, a serious chess player becomes familiar with thousands of configurations, each consisting of an arrangement of related pieces… '

In the same way, after thousands of hours of good practice and intricate analysis, the experienced orthognathic clinician may appear to be able to diagnose and plan a case almost 'at a glance.'

Environmental requirements for obtaining skill

In order for 'expert' intuitive skills to be valid, the expertise has to be real and based on conditions that are predictable. For example, a clinician who has diagnosed, treatment planned, treated and analysed the final results of many patients with a Class II skeletal pattern and vertical maxillary excess, will have developed real expertise in managing such patients. Such clinicians will also know the limits of their knowledge, and when to seek further advice or the corroboration and critique of colleagues on more complex cases. This is very different from pseudo-experts who have limited understanding of the subject, but often are under the illusion that they are experts. There is a boundary between real expertise, and those who *think* they have such expertise, but don't, and most of what they do comes down to chance.

Kahneman[18] poses the question: 'when do judgements reflect true expertise?' The answer is based on two basic conditions for acquiring a skill:

- An environment that is sufficiently regular to be predictable – The predictability of a task, such as orthognathic surgical treatment planning, is very important in relation to whether your expertise is relevant. For example, specific types of dentofacial deformities with which a patient may present often follow specific patterns of growth and development, and their clinical management may follow a relatively regular pathway; and
- An opportunity to learn these regularities through prolonged practice – i.e. specific training, analysis of cases and hard graft.

It is only under these circumstances that over time, a clinician will develop 'expert intuition'. Kahneman has also described how the opportunity for professionals to develop intuitive expertise depends to a great extent on the quality of feedback received (in orthognathic surgery this 'feedback' relates to the quality of results obtained, and their analysis), as well as on sufficient opportunity to practice. Obtaining such feedback in orthognathic surgery is important, but does not occur quickly, as each orthognathic patient may be under treatment for anything from 18 months to 3 years. Long-term follow up is also essential, in order for the clinician to be aware of the stability of their results.

Conclusions

One of the problems with intuitive thinking is that people usually do not stop to check their answers, because they are sure they are right, and they therefore leave themselves open to making errors. It is important to understand the potential fallibility of our decision making. If there is a possibility that we could be making a mistake, the answer is to slow down, go back to first principles, think logically and **methodically analyse**, or sometimes to just ask a professional colleague for their opinion.

We should be somewhat more humble in what we know. We should look for consistency - are our treatment planning decisions really consistent? Consistent thinking and learning is imperative. One does not want to develop 'paralysis through over-analysis',[18] but one must be aware that *intuition is only useful when it is based on real expertise*, i.e. 'expert intuition.'

The point is that intuition in a specialized field, such as orthognathic surgery, is not something one just develops by a process of osmosis while going through a training programme. So, 'intuitive judgement', in the sense of the 'expert' trainer being asked to explain an orthognathic treatment planning decision replying with an all-knowing glance and wave in the vague direction of the window, 'well, it's an art, not a science!', and thereby dodging the question, is unacceptable. Not attempting to analyse and to find answers, but just relying on 'intuition' in treatment planning is intellectually lazy.

However, there is no doubt that with many hours of training, reading, thinking and methodically analysing patients before, during and after treatment etc., a clinician will develop a level of expertise (just like a professional architect), which will allow the clinician to 'see' dentofacial parameters and their relationships far more acutely than someone with an untrained eye. This may be called 'expert intuitive judgement' - and such expertise takes many years of hard graft to acquire.

chin plane. The mandibular dental midline is coincident with the chin.

In *profile view*, the maxilla is retrusive and the mandibular sagittal position is essentially correct. The 'cotton wool roll' technique helps to provide confirmation of this observation. The submental-cervical angle is increased, which also contraindicates mandibular set-back, to avoid detrimental effects to submental-cervical aesthetics.

Stage 2 – The **vectorial analysis** (direction and approximate magnitude of jaw movements required) provides the following provisional plan: the maxilla needs to be advanced, which will increase the prominence and support to the upper lip, and increase

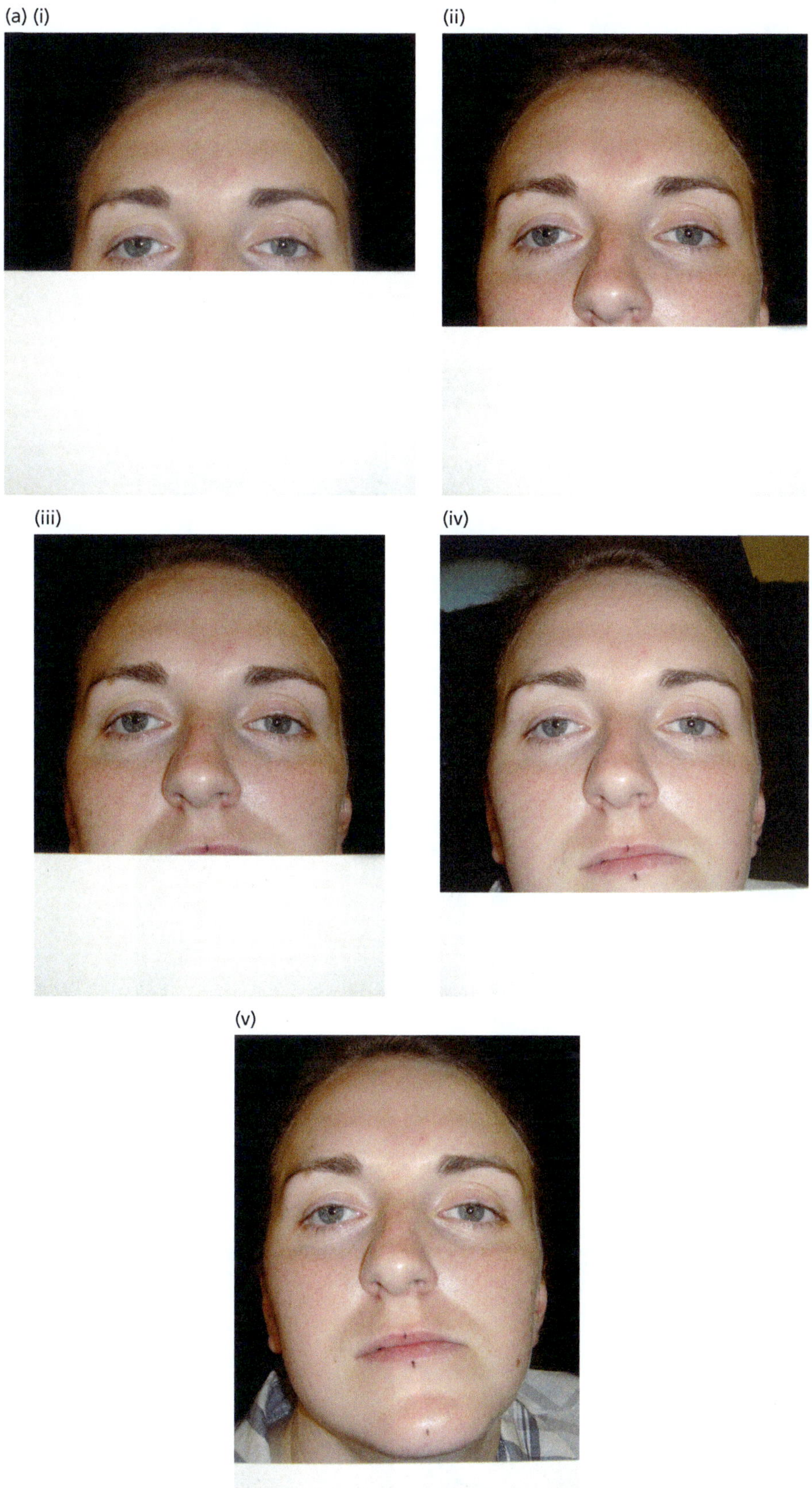

Fig. 6-27 (ai–v): Sequential masking of the face in frontal view, with marking of midline landmarks. (bi–iii): Assessing maxillary incisor exposure, maxillary midline position in relation to mid-philtrum of upper lip, and transverse canting of the maxillary occlusal plane. (c): Upper lip height and maxillary incisor exposure in repose. (d): Assessing the dental-occlusal relationship in relation to the facial morphology. (ei–iv): Sequential masking of the face in profile view. (f): (i) Placement of soaked and rinsed cotton wool roll under the upper lip, in order to (ii) simulate a 5–6 mm maxillary advancement, compared with (iii) preoperative profile. (gi–iii): Preoperative 'snap' models in occlusion. Maxillary dental midline marked in red. Various vertical lines are drawn between the maxillary and mandibular dental models in the preoperative position. (hi–iii): Preoperative 'snap' models hand articulated in the proposed postoperative occlusion. The horizontal distance between the previously drawn vertical lines demonstrates the distance the mandibular body needs to be rotated to the patient's right in order to achieve symmetry and an acceptable dental occlusion.

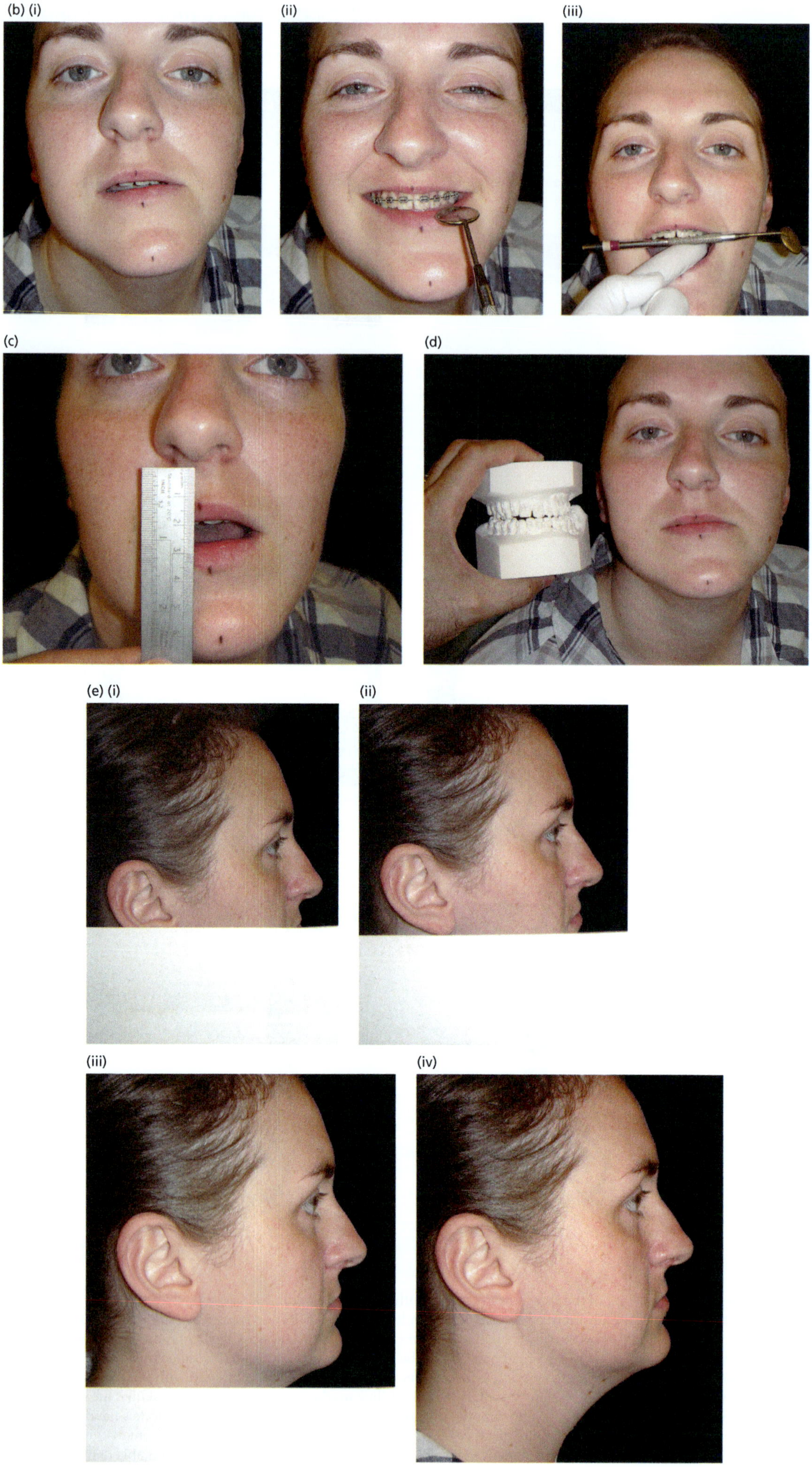

Fig. 6-27 *(Continued)*

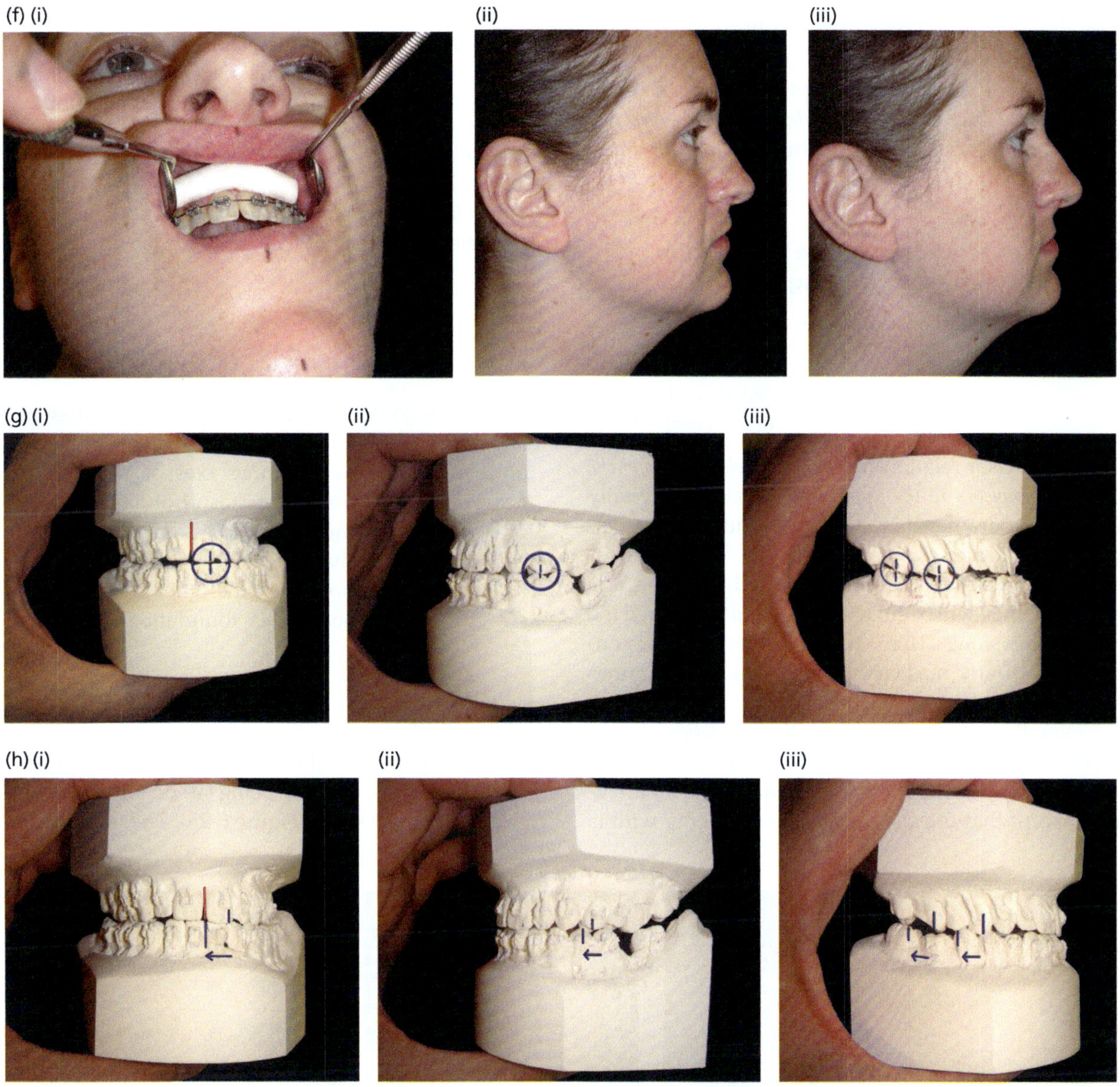

Fig. 6-27 (*Continued*)

maxillary incisor exposure in relation to the upper lip. The mandibular sagittal position is essentially correct. In frontal view, the maxillary occlusal plane cant may be corrected by impaction on the patient's right and set-down on her left, to level the maxillary occlusal plane whilst not reducing incisor exposure. A mandibular osteotomy to correct the asymmetry of the lower lip and chin will provide an acceptable dental occlusion and provide coincidence of the dental midlines to each other and the facial midline. The *direction* and *approximate magnitude* of the surgical moves is now decided.

Following the provisional plan, the next two stages (i.e. *Stage 3* – prediction planning, and *Stage 4* – feasibility model surgery) are **quantitative**, and involve the systematic analysis of diagnostic records, e.g. cephalometric planning, and taking accurate measurements, and model surgery, in order to determine the exact movements required (in millimetres and degrees) and whether the plan from the vectorial analysis is viable (see below).

Note:

Prediction planning may be carried out in preparation for the 'joint planning clinic', for example by a senior trainee with the responsibility of undertaking the patient's treatment. However, *it is advisable for the senior clinicians responsible for the final surgical plan not to look at the prediction planning until they have completed the vectorial analysis. Only then should the prediction planning be viewed, to assess whether it corroborates the clinician's overall treatment plan. If it does, the information passes to the next stage of feasibility model surgery. If it does not, then the process needs to be checked to find out where the discrepancy has arisen.*[2] It is important for the clinicians not to be led by the prediction tracings or results of prediction planning simulation software, i.e. not to be swayed by the results of a computer programme. *The primary objectives should be decided based on clinical observation of the patient*, and the prediction plans are used as a check.

Lip–incisor relationship: The foundation stone of treatment planning

> 'No person who is not a great sculptor or painter can be an architect. If he is not a sculptor or painter, he can only be a *builder*.'
>
> John Ruskin (1819–1900)[22]
> English art and social critic, and man of letters

The 'lip–incisor relationship', i.e. the *relationship of the maxillary incisors to the upper lip in repose*, is a vitally important parameter in clinical diagnosis and treatment planning.

When an architect is designing and planning any structure, they will begin with what is often termed the 'foundation stone'. This is the first stone set in the construction of any masonry project, which determines the position of every other stone and the design of the overall structure. Therefore, *the foundation stone is important since all other stones will be set in reference to it.*

In clinical practice we are very much like an architect, except that the structure we are working with is the craniofacial complex. As such, we can use what is termed the **foundation stone concept**. In orthognathic surgery, the foundation stone of treatment planning is the 'lip–incisor relationship', which describes both:

- the relationship of the maxillary incisors to the upper lip; *and*
- the relationship of the maxillary incisor-upper lip complex to the rest of the craniofacial complex.

Note:

The key is to decide where the maxillary incisors should be positioned in the three planes of space and in relation to the three axes of rotation to achieve the best *postoperative* result, and the vectors of dentoskeletal movement required (orthodontically and surgically) to achieve this position, then to build the position of all the other surrounding structures in relation to this 'foundation stone'.

Case example

A Class III patient with maxillary retrognathism and mandibular prognathism being assessed at the initial, pretreatment stage (Figure 6-28). The 'lip–incisor'

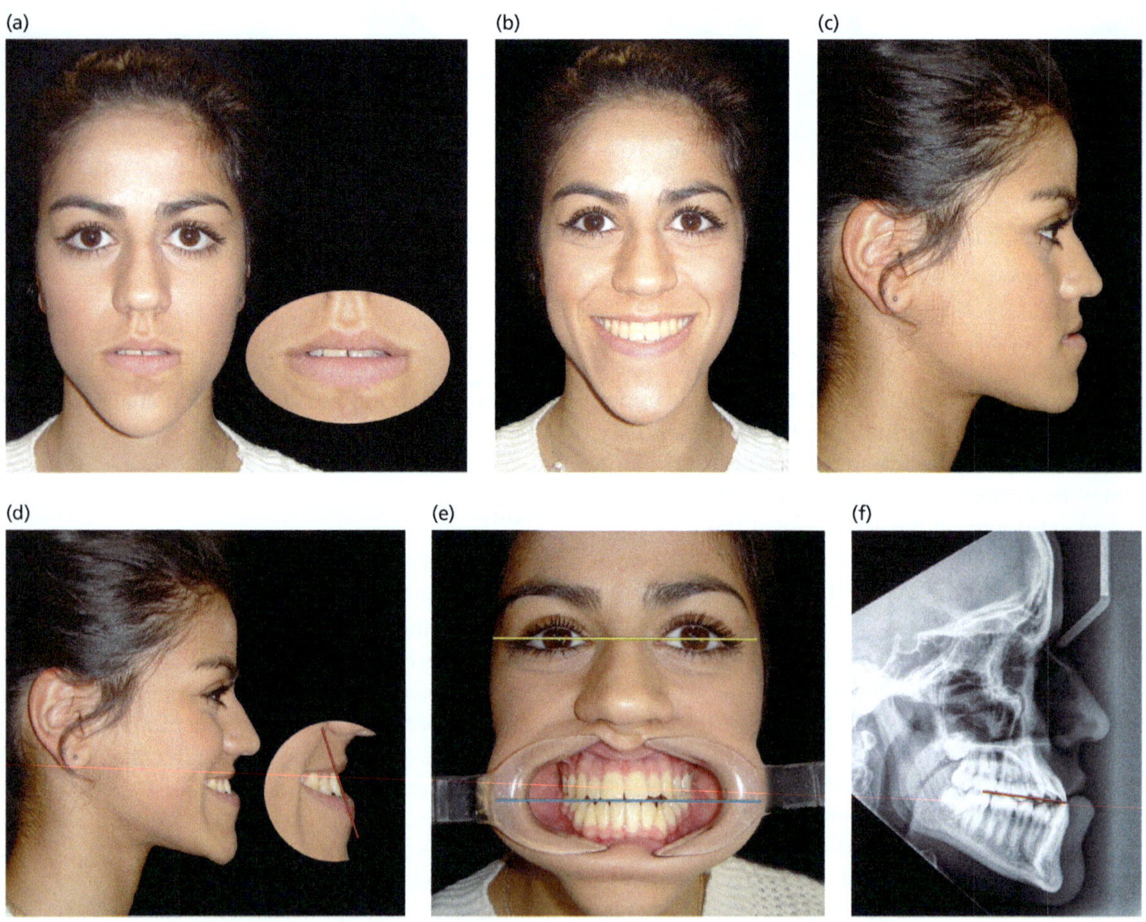

Fig. 6-28 Case example demonstrating the evaluation of the relationship of the maxillary incisors to the upper lip, and the 'lip–incisor' complex to the face (see in conjunction with Table 6-2).

Table 6-2 Case example demonstrating the evaluation of the relationship of the maxillary incisors to the upper lip, and the 'lip–incisor' complex to the face (see in conjunction with Figure 6-28)

Planes of space	Maxillary incisor relationship
Vertical	Maxillary incisor exposure in relation to the upper lip in repose: • ~2 mm in repose, therefore slightly reduced for a young female (Figure 6-28a). Maxillary incisor exposure in animation: • Upper lip elevates to almost the gingival margins, with good incisor exposure on smiling. A few more millimetres of gingival exposure would be acceptable (Figure 6-28b).
Sagittal	There is maxillary retrognathism, with paranasal hollowing (Figure 6-28c). The maxillary incisor crowns are retruded in relation to the face, which is to be expected due to the maxillary retrognathism, but the incisors are proclined (Figure 6-28d).
Transverse	Maxillary dental midline is coincident with the mid-philtrum of the upper lip and the facial midline. The bodily position of the maxilla is not to the patient's left or right, but symmetrically positioned in relation to her face.
Axes of rotation	
Sagittal	There is no transverse cant to the maxillary occlusal plane at the incisors (incisal plane), or at the canines, premolars or molars (Figure 6-28e).
Vertical	There is no dental midline deviation, and the maxilla is not rotated around the vertical axis.
Transverse	There is no sagittal cant to the maxillary occlusal plane, and the incisors and posterior dentition are level in profile view (best assessed on a lateral cephalometric radiograph taken with the patient in natural head position) (Figure 6-28f).
Diagnostic considerations	The maxillary incisors need to be retroclined (decompensated) to their ideal inclination, with a tangent to their labial face parallel to the true vertical. The maxilla will be advanced, and maxillary incisor exposure will increase by a few millimetres, which is aesthetically desirable. The maxilla does not require rotation to the left or right (around the vertical axis), and does not require relative impaction or setdown anteriorly in relation to posteriorly (rotation around the transverse axis). The mandibular incisors will be proclined (decompensated) to their correct inclination for the mandible, and the mandible set-back. Final surgical moves will be decided following the preparatory orthodontic phase of treatment.

relationship may be evaluated systematically in relation to the three planes of space and the three axes of rotation (Table 6-2 and Figure 6-28).

Sequencing the planning process

The essence of treatment planning is to build a coherent picture of *where you are* (based on the diagnosis), *where you want to get to* (the ideal postoperative result, based on the aims of treatment), and *how you are going to get there* (the treatment plan and treatment mechanics). The treatment mechanics are planned according to a **step-by-step navigation protocol**, i.e. each treatment step and the mechanics required in order to achieve it are planned in a step-by-step sequence.

The steps in the planning sequence are essentially as follows, with the patient in natural head position, their teeth lightly in occlusion and the soft tissues in repose (this discussion is relevant to the initial tentative pre-treatment plan, but is mainly for the definitive preoperative plan). *The steps below are described as a series of questions, which the clinician will ask themselves while systematically analysing the patient and their preoperative records*:

1. **Begin with the maxilla and maxillary incisors in the sagittal and vertical planes, and in relation to the transverse axis of rotation:**

Is the anterior maxilla and maxillary incisors too far forward (dentoalveolar protrusion) or too far back (dentoalveolar retrusion)? Is the anterior maxilla too far up (anterior VMD) or down (anterior VME)? Is the posterior maxilla too far up (uncommon) or down (posterior VME)? Are the maxillary incisors proclined, average inclination or retroclined? Is the maxillary occlusal plane inclined too far up or down in the sagittal plane? *The answer to these questions will determine the three-dimensional position of the maxillary complex in relation to the craniofacial complex.*

What is the exposure of the maxillary incisors in relation to the upper lip at rest (i.e. normal, excessive or reduced)? Is the upper lip height normal, reduced or excessive? Can the upper lip height be accepted, or will it require surgical correction? *The answer to these questions will determine whether the anterior maxilla needs to be superiorly or inferiorly repositioned.*

Are the maxillary incisors proclined, at the correct inclination or retroclined? Is the inclination of the maxillary incisors a purely dental issue or is it related to a sagittal cant of the maxillary occlusal plane (i.e. rotation of the maxillary plane round the transverse axis, as in high angle, AOB cases)? *These determine whether the incisor inclination should be corrected in the preparatory orthodontics, or if a degree of proclination needs to be maintained or even created,*

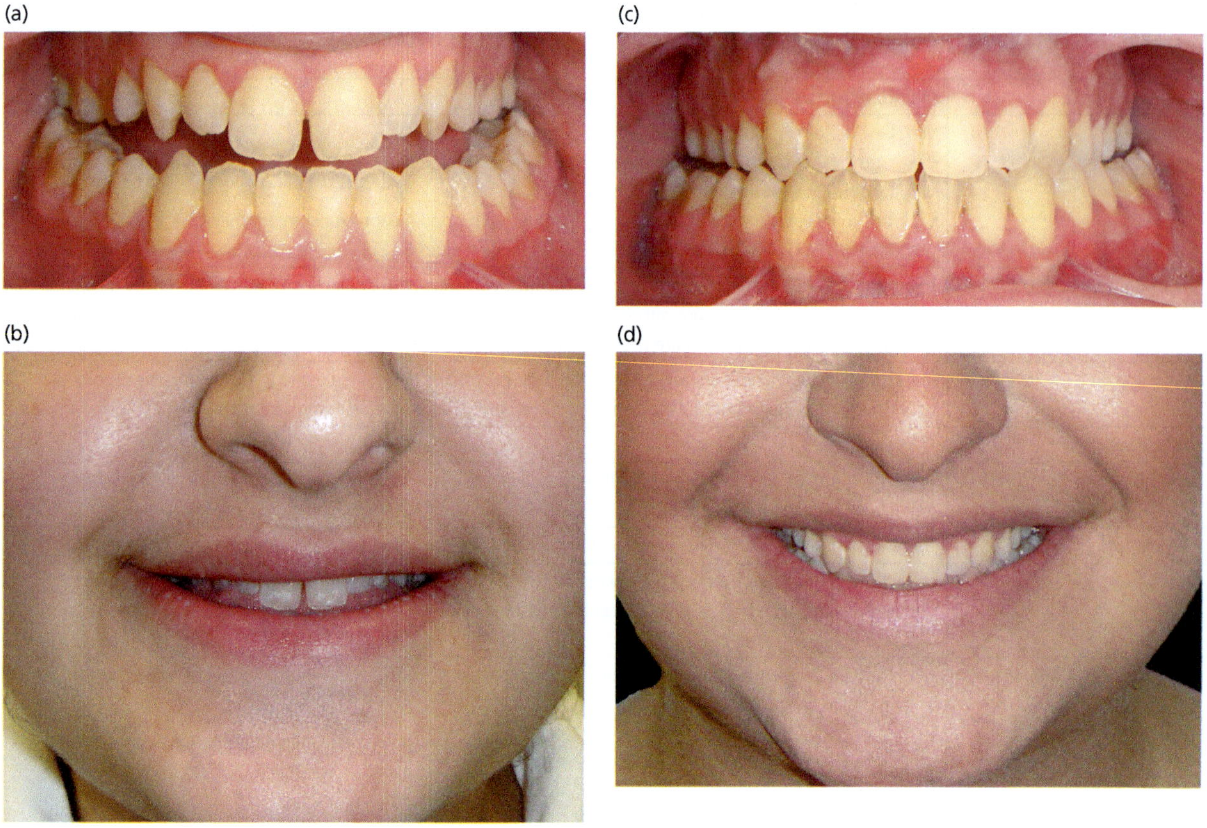

Fig. 6-29 (a, b) Pretreatment Class III patient with broad mandibular dental arch. (c, d) Following maxillary advancement, accepting a planned bilateral posterior crossbite is not a functional or aesthetic problem as long as the maxillary arch is well-aligned and of average width.

in preparation for differential posterior impaction of the maxilla?

Is the anterior maxillary dentoalveolus deficient or excessive in the sagittal or vertical plane? Is the maxilla deficient or excessive in the sagittal or vertical plane? *The degree of tooth exposure, both anteriorly and posteriorly, at rest and on smiling, together with the lower anterior face height proportion in relation to the total face height, will help determine whether the entire maxilla needs to be superiorly repositioned, or just the anterior maxillary dentoalveolus, or whether a differential posterior impaction of the maxilla is required.*

Is the upper lip inclination normal, proclined or retroclined, and is its position related to the maxillary incisors, e.g. proclined upper lip due to proclined maxillary incisors? The inclination of the upper lip is relevant to both maxillary incisor inclination and sagittal position, and to the sagittal position of the maxilla itself.

2. **Next, assess the maxilla and maxillary incisors in the transverse plane, and in relation to the sagittal and vertical axes of rotation:**
   Is there a transverse cant of the maxillary occlusal plane? If so, is there vertical deficiency on one side, vertical excess on the other side, or a combination of both? *This determines whether to impact on one side, set-down the other side, or a combination of both, to level the cant, whilst maintaining or improving the lip–incisor relationship.*

   If there is a cant, are the maxillary incisors angulated in the direction of the cant, and will their angulation self-correct when the maxilla is repositioned, or do the maxillary incisor angulations require further orthodontic correction?

   Is there a maxillary dental midline deviation to the patient's left or right? Can it be corrected with orthodontics (and are dental extractions required in order to create space), or should it be corrected by rotation of the maxilla round the vertical axis?

   Is the maxilla narrow, and if so, is it in the canine, premolar, and/or molar regions? Are there posterior crossbites? If so, can they be accepted (Figure 6-29)? If there is unilateral posterior crossbite, is there an associated lateral displacement of the mandible? Does the maxilla require transverse expansion and if so, how much, and how will it be achieved (orthodontics, surgery or both)?
3. When the postoperative position of the maxilla and maxillary incisors has been planned, **the next stage is to plan the mandibular movements required in the sagittal and vertical planes of space to achieve the best facial aesthetic result, incisor relationship and dental occlusion:**
   If a vertical movement of the maxilla has been planned, how much will the mandible autorotate? On autorotation, will the lower lip and chin become too prominent (following forward rotation) or retrusive (following backward rotation)? Will the

incisor relationship be correct following autorotation, or will it be Class II or Class III?

Will the mandibular body need to be repositioned in the sagittal plane (advanced or set-back)?

Does the mandibular occlusal plane need to be levelled preoperatively (if no increase in lower anterior face height is desired), or does an increased curve of Spee need to be maintained in order to increase the lower anterior face height while advancing the mandible to a 3-point landing?

Depending on autorotation and/or the requirement for sagittal repositioning of the mandible, do the mandibular incisors need to be proclined or retroclined (are dental extraction required to create space if retroclination is required)?

4. **Next, assess the requirement for mandibular repositioning to correct mandibular asymmetry:**
   Is there a mandibular asymmetry? If so, is it unilateral or bilateral, and is it primarily vertical (e.g. hemimandibular hyperplasia) or horizontal (e.g. hemimandibular elongation)?

   Where is the midpoint of the chin in relation to the mandible (i.e. is an asymmetry of the chin due to the asymmetry of the mandible, or is there an additional asymmetry of the chin itself)?

   Where is the mandibular dental midline in relation to the midpoint of the chin? Does the mandibular dental midline need to be made coincident to the midpoint of the chin, which will subsequently be corrected with surgery?
5. **Next, assess the position of the chin in the 3 planes of space and in relation to the 3 axes of rotation:**
   Taking into account the potential sagittal and vertical movements of the maxilla and mandible, will the chin need to be advanced or set-back to correct the sagittal chin position in relation to the rest of the profile?

   Will the potential alterations in the lower anterior face height affect the mentolabial fold depth and contour for the better or worse? Will the sagittal vector of chin movement also require a vertical vector, e.g. antero-inferior advancement of the chin?

   Will any transverse deviations of the chin be corrected with corrective rotation of the mandibular body or will additional genioplasty be required?

   Will there be a requirement for a corrective genioplasty at the same time as the principal orthognathic procedure, or may it be required as a secondary procedure?
6. **Finally, is there or will there be a requirement for adjunctive procedures**?
   If the maxilla is superiorly repositioned or advanced, the nasal alar base will widen, so is there a need for a cinch suture intraoperatively? Will the nasal tip elevate excessively following maxillary advancement? Could there be a need for a rhinoplasty as a secondary procedure?

   Will the submental-cervical region become 'fuller' following mandibular set-back? Could a secondary procedure be required to limit or improve this (neck lift, submental liposuction or platysma plication etc.)?

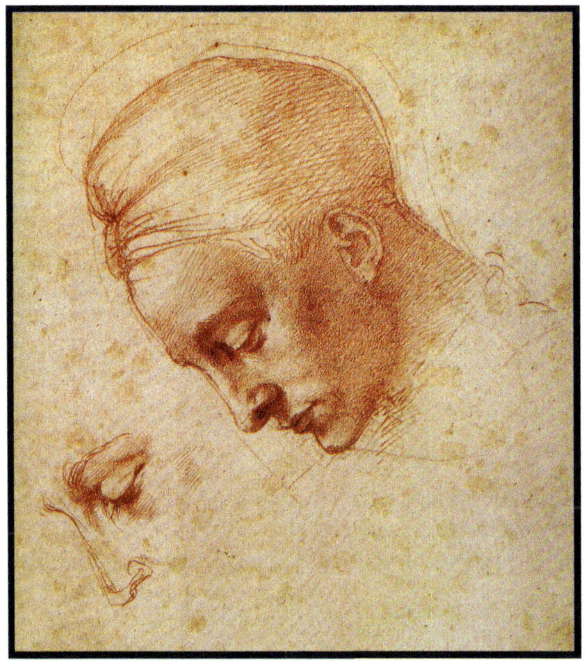

Fig. 6-30 Prior to embarking on a major painting or sculpture, Michelangelo made careful analytical studies, as may be seen in the various profile lines depicted here, and the faint lines demonstrating prominence of the lips and chin in this study (*Study for the Face of Leda*, Michelangelo, c. 1530, Casa Buonarroti, Florence).

3. Prediction planning

> 'In every block of marble I see a statue as plain as though it stood before me, shaped and perfect in attitude and action. I have only to hew away the rough walls that imprison the lovely apparition to reveal it to the other eyes as mine see it.'
>
> Michelangelo Buonarroti (1475–1564) (Figure 6-30) (attributed)

Note:

Michelangelo's views on sculpture has certain parallels to treatment planning in orthognathic surgery, i.e. the experienced clinician will see in their mind's eye the change that is likely to occur to a patient's dentofacial appearance with orthognathic treatment. The clinician should look at a patient's face and 'see' what needs to be achieved, and what will be the resulting end point. However, prediction planning tools may also be valuable.

The purpose of surgical prediction planning is to obtain the *linear movements* of the various components of the dentoskeletal complex (number of mm), and *angular changes* (number of degrees) required to achieve the desired final result, and to assess whether these are realistically achievable. A number of methods are available, some historical and others more modern (essentially refinements based mostly on technological improvements of the said historical methods), though senior trainees should familiarise themselves with all these techniques, as all help to 'educate the eye.'

Cephalometric prediction planning

'And as imagination bodies forth
The form of things unknown, and the poet's pen
Turns them to shapes . . . '

William Shakespeare (1565–1616)
A Midsummer Night's Dream (c.1595–6)[23]

Hand-tracing method

Cephalometric prediction planning for orthognathic surgery has been used for many years (Figure 6-31),[24] and despite its limitations, is a tried and tested method of planning. The principle of the method is to simulate the desired surgical movements by overlaying separate cut-outs of tracing paper of the dentoskeletal segments that will be moved, and pasting them in the desired position. The technique permits visualization of a relatively accurate proposed postoperative dentoskeletal outcome and an estimation of the proposed postoperative soft tissue profile.

The technique involves manually tracing the salient features of the craniofacial complex on transparent acetate tracing paper with a sharp pencil. Following this, separate tracings are made of the dentoskeletal segments that are planned to be moved on separate sheets of tracing paper, which are overlaid on the original in the desired postoperative positions. The overlying soft tissue outlines are drawn based on the type of soft tissue change that is predicted in view of the dentoskeletal movements undertaken.

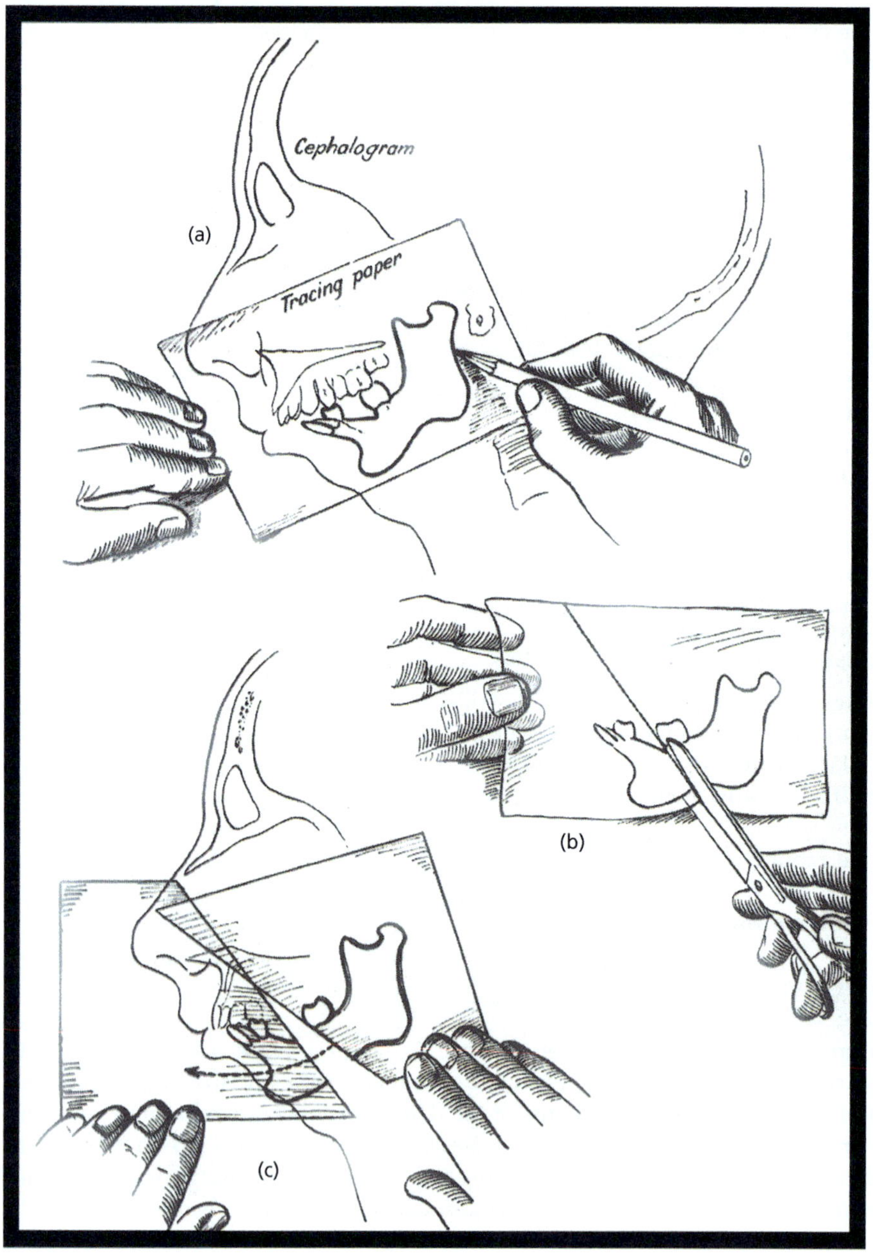

Fig. 6-31 Kazanjian and Converse demonstrating the utilization of cephalometric prediction tracings in planning orthognathic surgery. (a) Tracing the outline of the mandible on tracing paper placed over the lateral cephalometric radiograph. (b) Cutting the mandibular tracing to allow repositioning of the anterior segment. (c) Repositioning the cut segment to permit visualization of the proposed surgical procedure. (From: Kazanjian VH, Converse JM. The Surgical Treatment of Facial Injuries. Second edition. Baltimore: The Williams and Wilkins Company, 1959.)

The starting point in the hand-tracing technique is an accurate preoperative lateral cephalometric radiograph on which the prediction tracing may be undertaken. The cephalometric radiograph should be taken with *the patient in natural head position* and *the soft tissues in repose*. It is particularly important for the lip posture to be relaxed, as many patients develop a habitual closed lip posture by elevating their lower lip and contracting the circumoral musculature. Prior to taking the cephalometric radiograph, the patient should be given a face mirror, and the clinician should clearly explain the lip posture required. Slight digital pressure in the depth of the mentolabial fold will help to relax the mentalis muscle and lower lip.[8]

The lateral cephalometric radiograph is traced on transparent acetate tracing paper, including the relevant hard tissues (cranial base, maxilla and maxillary dentition, mandible and mandibular dentition, including the condyle and chin regions) and overlying soft tissues. It is important to trace the occlusal surfaces of the dentition as accurately as possible (Figure 6-32).

The next step is to trace every segment that is planned to be repositioned on separate pieces of tracing paper, each in a different colour, which makes the eventual interpretation of the superimposed tracing segments easier. For example, in a patient being planned for bimaxillary surgery, a separate tracing of the maxilla and maxillary dentition, and one of the mandible and associated dentition is required.

The maxillary tracing is placed onto the original tracing, and then it is moved the required amount into the planned postoperative position, and secured with transparent adhesive tape. The mandibular tracing is then placed onto this combined tracing. If the maxilla has been superiorly repositioned, the mandibular tracing will autorotate (usually round the centre of the condyle, referred to as the condylar midpoint), until the occlusal surfaces of the mandibular teeth meet those of the maxillary teeth in the proposed postoperative position. Any sagittal movement of the mandible and associated dentition is then carried out by moving the mandibular tracing forward or backward until the desired incisor and occlusal relationships are achieved. This third tracing is also secured with transparent adhesive tape.

The final step is to draw the estimated predicted postoperative soft tissue outline. A new sheet of tracing paper is placed over the composite created dentoskeletal prediction. The unmoved parts of the original tracing are drawn onto the new sheet, as are the new planned postoperative positions of the maxilla and mandible. The soft tissue profile of the forehead and upper half of the nose, which is unlikely to change with orthognathic procedures, is drawn. In cases where maxillary surgery is not being undertaken, the rest of the nose and upper lip may also be drawn. If maxillary surgery has been planned, the soft tissue outline of the lower part of the nose, upper lip, lower lip, mentolabial fold, chin and submental-cervical region is drawn based on the potential alteration from the original, estimated from the hard tissue movements undertaken.

This technique has a number of limitations:

- **Variable soft tissue response** – The postoperative representation of the soft tissues is rather crude and essentially an estimate. *It is impossible with this, or any other technique for that matter, to reproduce with a significant degree of accuracy the anticipated change in the soft tissue contour* of the lips, mentolabial region, chin and submental-cervical region. With the best will in the world, a degree of 'artistic license' will be required. In some patients, certain regions of the overlying soft tissues move almost 1:1 in relation to the underlying dentoskeleton, whereas in others the range of soft tissue to hard tissue movement will be different (see Tables 16-1–16-3). The variability in soft tissue response depends on three parameters:

  1. **Soft tissue morphology and tonicity** – The *initial* morphology, particularly the thickness, and tonicity of the soft tissues are variable. The greater the thickness and the more flaccid the tone, the greater the **compressibility** of the soft tissues and the less the potential movement of the lips in relation to the underlying dentoskeletal framework (Figure 6-33).
  2. **'Dead space'** – The potential 'dead space' between the labial surfaces of the dentoskeletal regions and the inner surface of the lips is variable (Figure 6-34). The greater the dead space, the less the movement of the soft tissues in relation to the underlying dentoskeleton.
  3. **Change in soft tissue morphology** – The morphology of the soft tissues may alter quite considerably depending on the underlying dentoskeletal movements. For example, anterior-inferior repositioning of the mandible and/or bony chin will tend to unfurl the mentolabial region (Figure 6-35).

Note:

Predicting soft tissue to hard tissue movement ratios

Though difficult to predict with any degree of exceptional accuracy due to the factors described above, the potential soft tissue prediction remains a vitally important part of the treatment planning process. The predicted soft tissue to hard tissue movement ratios are derived from data based on the results of previous research investigating the average soft tissue to hard tissue movements resulting from different types of orthognathic surgical procedures (see Tables 16-1–16-3). These are termed **baseline predictions**, i.e. they are based on algorithms derived from average ratios, which are likely to be relatively accurate for the 'average' patient. Computerised planning

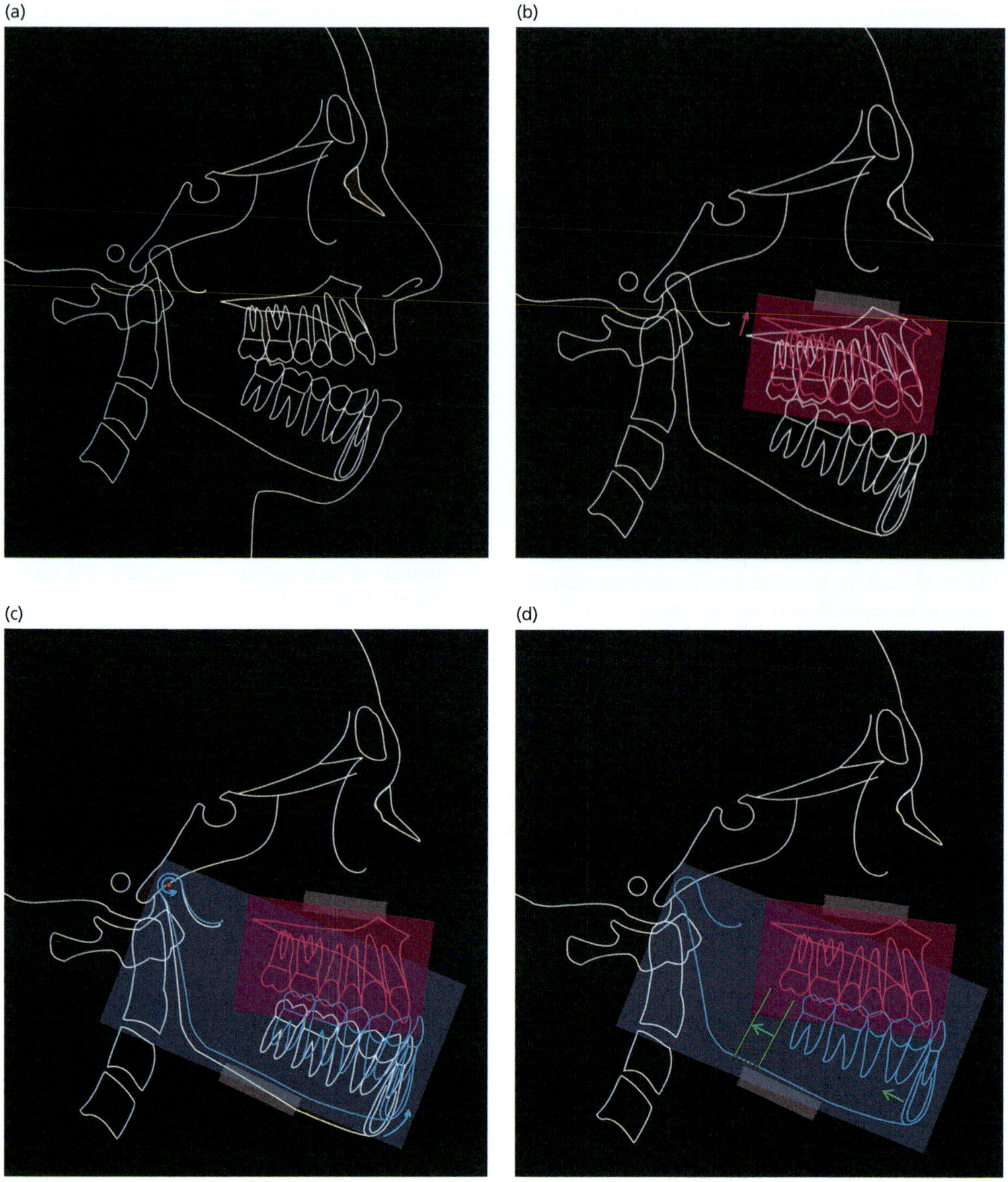

Fig. 6-32 Hand tracing technique for cephalometric prediction tracing. The example is for a Class III, anterior open bite patient with posterior vertical maxillary excess, mandibular prognathism, increased lower anterior face height, and a flat pogonion. (a): The preoperative lateral cephalometric radiograph is traced on transparent acetate tracing paper, including the relevant hard tissues, including the occlusal surfaces of the dentition, and overlying soft tissues. (b): The maxilla and maxillary dentition are traced on a separate piece of tracing paper (shown in red). The maxillary tracing is placed onto the original tracing, and then it is moved the required amount into the planned postoperative position (in this case with a posterior differential impaction and advancement), and secured with transparent adhesive tape. (c): A separate mandibular tracing is made and placed onto the combined tracing (shown in blue). As the maxilla has been superiorly repositioned, the mandibular tracing will autorotate (usually round the centre of the condyle, referred to as the condylar midpoint), until the occlusal surfaces of the mandibular teeth meet those of the maxillary teeth. As there is mandibular sagittal excess, this places the mandibular incisors into a reverse overjet. (d): Sagittal set-back of the mandibular body and associated dentition is then carried out by moving the mandibular tracing backward until the desired incisor and occlusal relationships are achieved. This tracing is also secured with transparent adhesive tape (e). (f): A separate tracing is made of the osseous chin (shown in orange) and placed onto the combined tracing. This is advanced the required amount and secured with transparent adhesive tape. (g): The final step is to draw the estimated predicted postoperative soft tissue outline. A new sheet of tracing paper is placed over the composite created dentoskeletal prediction. The unmoved parts of the original tracing are drawn onto the new sheet, as are the new planned postoperative positions of the maxilla and mandible. The soft tissue profile of the forehead and upper half of the nose, which is unlikely to change with orthognathic procedures, is drawn. As maxillary surgery has been planned, the soft tissue outline of the lower part of the nose, upper lip, lower lip, mentolabial fold, chin and submental-cervical region is drawn based on the potential alteration from the original, estimated from the hard tissue movements undertaken.

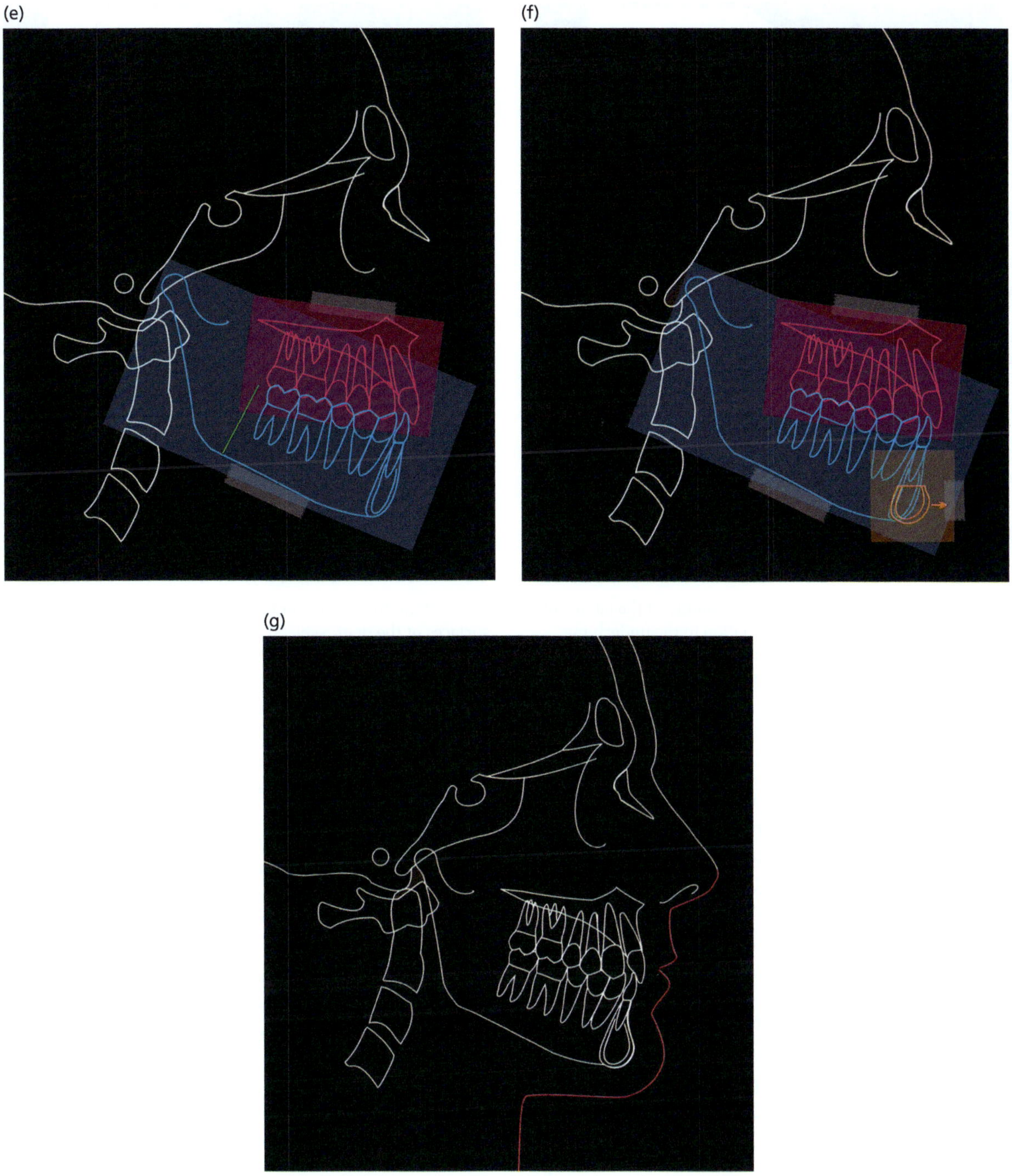

Fig. 6-32 (*Continued*)

software, which will be described later in this chapter, essentially utilises such baseline predictions to create the potential postoperative soft tissue profile. Such ratios are a reasonable basis for a baseline prediction if the planner knows nothing about a patient except the category of surgery that is planned. However, this prediction planning technique may be made rather more accurate by utilising **case-specific information** regarding individual patients, such as their soft tissue tonicity, soft tissue thickness, potential soft tissue compressibility etc., which permit *adjustment of the estimate in the appropriate direction away from the average baseline prediction*. For example, in relation to a maxillary advancement the baseline prediction for soft tissue advancement at labrale superius of the upper lip may be 60%, but case specific-information may be a thick and flaccid upper lip, which means a substantial likelihood for reduced soft tissue movement. Such information may be incorporated into the soft tissue prediction planning process.

- **Accuracy of numbers** – Each lateral cephalometric radiograph has a millimetre rule superimposed on the image in the midline. Therefore, despite the magnification of the image, the

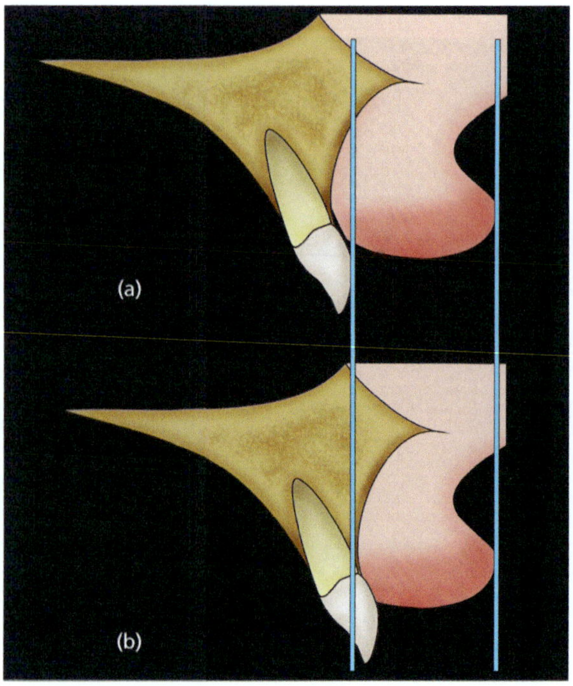

Fig. 6-33 (a, b) The greater the compressibility of the labial soft tissues, the less they will move in relation to the underlying dentoskeletal complex. Compressibility is related to the thickness and tonicity of the soft tissues – thick, flaccid lips move less.

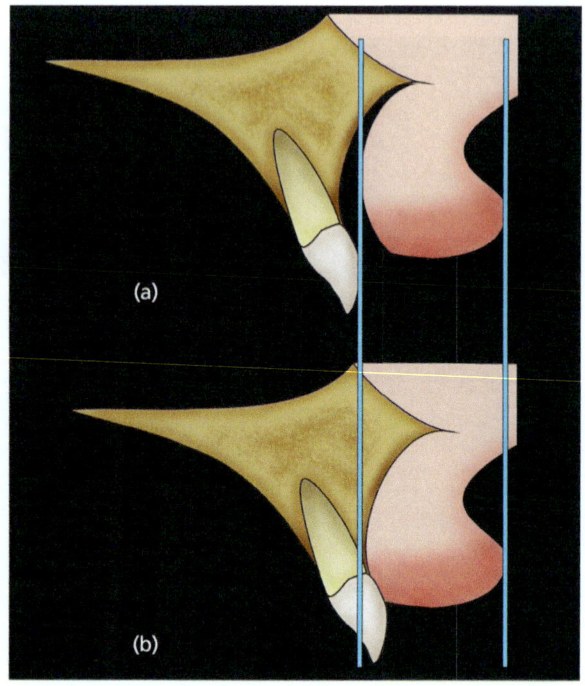

Fig. 6-34 (a, b) The greater the 'dead space' between the labial surfaces of the dentoskeletal regions and the inner surface of the lips, the less the potential movement of the lips in relation to the dentoskeleton.

millimetre rule may be used to measure distances or movements. However, there is a potential for error when measurements are made from structures that are not in the midline, e.g. measuring the degree of posterior impaction from the mesiobuccal cusp of the maxillary first molar, which is not a midline structure. This is the reason that the feasibility of all potential planned surgical moves is also assessed with model surgery and in relation to the clinical diagnosis.

- **Autorotation and the centre of mandibular rotation** – There is some uncertainty and therefore debate as to the location of the point(s) round which the mandible will autorotate following superior or inferior repositioning of the maxilla. Some authorities have suggested that the centre of rotation is located within the mastoid air cells, i.e. posteroinferior to the condyle.[25–27] Others suggest using condylion, which is the most posterior superior point on the head of the mandibular condyle. An investigation comparing the use of different centres for autorotation found little difference between them.[28] Nadjmi et al.[29] suggested that the mandible rotates around the same point following maxillary impaction surgery as during

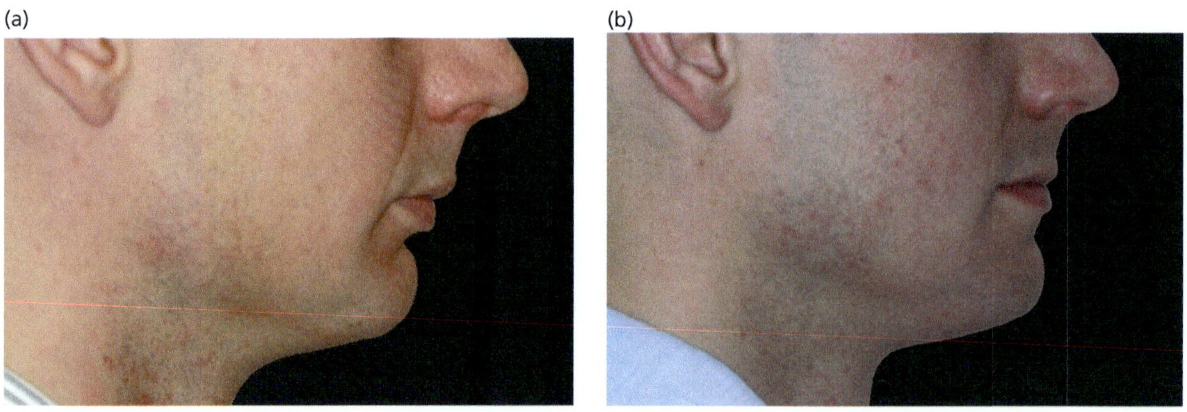

Fig. 6-35 Antero-inferior movement of the mandible, as occurs with mandibular advancement to a 3-point landing, will tend to unfurl the mentolabial fold. (a) Preoperative profile with reduced lower anterior face height (LAFH) and deep mentolabial fold. (b) Following mandibular advancement to a 3-point landing, chin projection is improved, LAFH is increased and the aesthetics of the mentolabial transition improved.

initial jaw opening, and suggested that the centre of mandibular autorotation should be determined on an individual basis. *There is no definitive evidence as to the true centre of rotation of the mandible, due to the potential methodological errors in previous research. Therefore, the condylar midpoint, which is estimated visually, is acceptable.*

Surgical Visual Treatment Objectives (VTO)

A similar, but rather more elaborate method of cephalometric prediction planning is termed the 'surgical VTO'. The purpose is to develop realistic treatment objectives from the lateral cephalometric radiograph tracing and data obtained from clinical evaluation of the patient. The technique is described in detail by Reyneke in Chapter 31.

Photographic 'montage' prediction planning

This historical, but still potentially useful technique involves the creation of a predicted postoperative profile 'montage' using the preoperative photograph. The purpose of the technique was to look at just the soft tissue changes required to achieve the best possible soft tissue profile outcome. The preoperative profile photograph is taken with either a millimetre measuring ruler held near the midline or alternatively a one centimetre square piece of paper on the patient's profile, which allows enlargement of the image and the creation of a 1:1 image. The proposed sections of the facial profile are cut up and reassembled into the proposed postoperative positions. Though rather crude, the results may still be useful, and the technique is a precursor to the photo-cephalometric prediction planning techniques (see below) (Figure 6-36).

Photo-cephalometric prediction planning techniques

Superimposition of the profile photograph with the lateral cephalometric radiograph is a useful technique, permitting cutting of the various dentoskeletal units and subunits together with their overlying soft tissue envelope, and pasting them into the desired postoperative position. This permits the clinicians to check the potential facial aesthetic result in profile view, and to get an idea of whether the planned dentoskeletal movements will permit correction of the dental-occlusal relationships.

Profile line 'transfer' technique (after Obwegeser)

> 'In the treatment planning of facial anomalies, first the profile, then the occlusion.'
>
> Hugo L. Obwegeser[16]

Obwegeser described a planning technique based on drawing an 'ideal' profile line on a patient's preoperative profile photograph, then transferring the said line onto the preoperative lateral cephalometric radiograph.[30] The skeletal movements required to achieve the change in soft tissue profile were then predicted on the radiograph.

The basic steps in the technique are as follows:

The desired profile and facial contours are decided following the clinical evaluation of the patient. Then, a profile photograph is magnified until it is made 1:1 in size in relation to the tracing of the lateral cephalometric radiograph. The surgeon then draws the proposed idealized profile line on the profile photograph. Although this is primarily an artistic endeavour, the surgeon bases the proposed profile line on the results

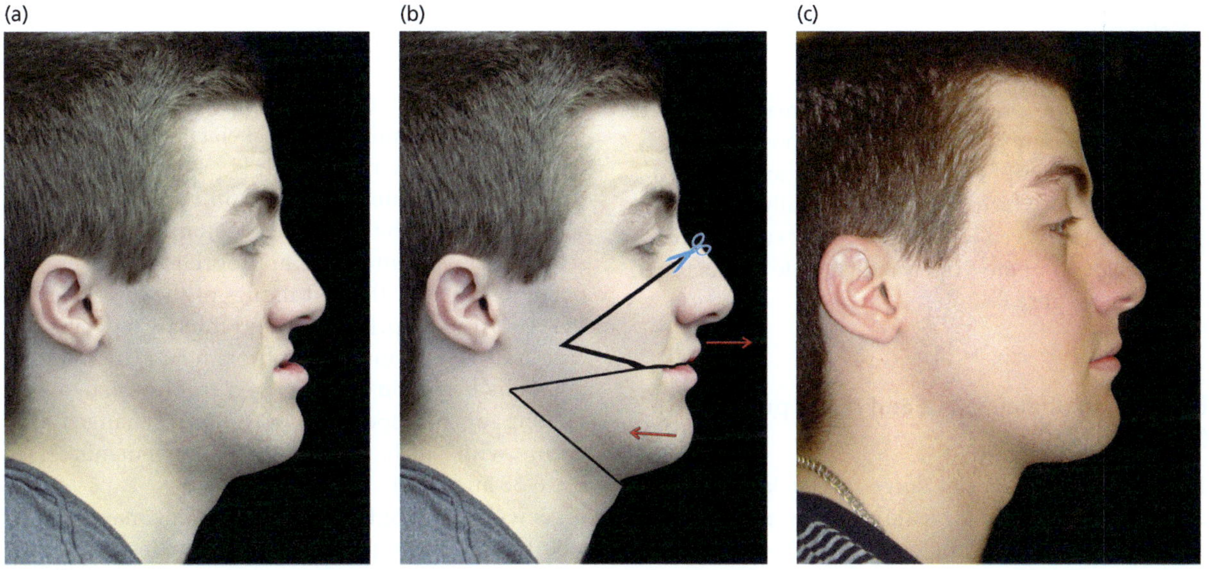

Fig. 6-36 Photographic 'montage' prediction planning. (a) Preoperative profile of a Class III patient with Saerthre–Chotzen syndrome. (b) Predicted soft tissue result with maxillary advancement and slight mandibular set-back. (c) Final postoperative profile view.

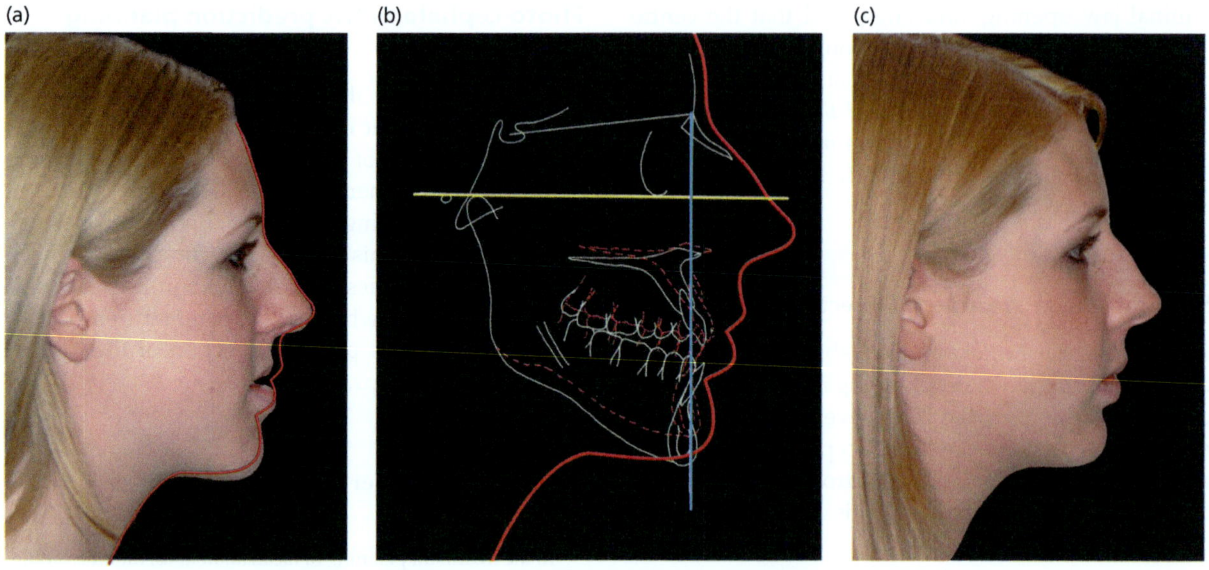

Fig. 6-37 Profile line 'transfer' technique (After Obwegeser). (a) Preoperative profile photograph, with idealized, planned postoperative soft tissue profile line (solid red line) drawn on the preoperative profile. (b) Idealized, planned postoperative profile line (solid red line) transferred onto the preoperative lateral cephalometric radiograph (or a tracing thereof). The dentoskeletal regions are repositioned such that the overlying soft tissue outline will match the planned soft tissue outline. In this case, the patient had a differential posterior impaction and advancement of the maxilla, forward autorotation and set-back of the mandible (in broken red lines). (c) Final, postoperative profile photograph.

of the clinical evaluation as well as proportional guidelines relevant to the said patient's age, stature, gender, ethnic background and even character. The surgeon also has to consider how much soft tissue movement is likely in relation to the proposed skeletal movements. The new planned profile is then transferred and superimposed onto the tracing of the lateral cephalometric radiograph. The maxilla, mandible and chin may then be moved on the tracing into the desired position that will provide the ideal planned profile (Figure 6-37). *The essence of this approach is that the teeth and jaws should be made to fit the idealized planned soft tissue facial contour, not the other way around.*

Note:

It is a useful training exercise to take the preoperative profile photograph of an already treated patient and, without looking at the postoperative profile photograph, attempt to draw an idealized profile on it, which you would ideally desire to have been achieved with orthognathic surgery. You may then compare your prediction to the actual result of surgery.

Photo-cephalometric 'cut and paste' prediction (2D, historical)

The British maxillofacial surgeon Derek Henderson described a technique to create a superimposed profile photograph-lateral cephalometric radiograph composite for profile prediction planning.[31] Henderson defined profile planning as 'reasoned prediction of the probable effects of alternative facial osteotomies (or other hard tissue corrections) on facial profile, and the use of the resulting predictions to formulate a treatment plan.'

The basic steps in the technique are as follows:

Firstly, a lateral cephalometric radiograph is taken with the patient in natural head position, the teeth in light occlusion and the soft tissues in repose. A profile photograph is taken under the same circumstances and positional relationships, as far as possible at approximately the same time. If there is marked overclosure of the mandible, the photograph and radiograph may be taken in the mandibular rest position, by placing a wax wafer of appropriate thickness between the maxillary and mandibular dentition. A facial profile transparency is produced, i.e. a profile photograph printed on a transparent base, which is enlarged to permit accurate superimposition on the soft tissue profile outline of the cephalometric radiograph. A tracing of the required dentoskeletal structures from the cephalometric radiograph is made onto the photograph. The **photo-cephalograph composite** is then sectioned along the planned osteotomy lines, and the sections moved into their appropriate postoperative positions. Finally, the soft tissues of the lower half of the nose, upper lip, lower lip and chin are repositioned (cut and pasted) into the approximate postoperative positions based on data derived from investigations looking at postoperative soft tissue changes that occur with such dentoskeletal movements (Figure 6-38 and 6-39).

As well as being time-consuming, the major downside to this technique is that the changes to the soft tissue contours cannot be made unless significant cutting and pasting is undertaken. Although the technique is still useful to clinicians, patients may find the

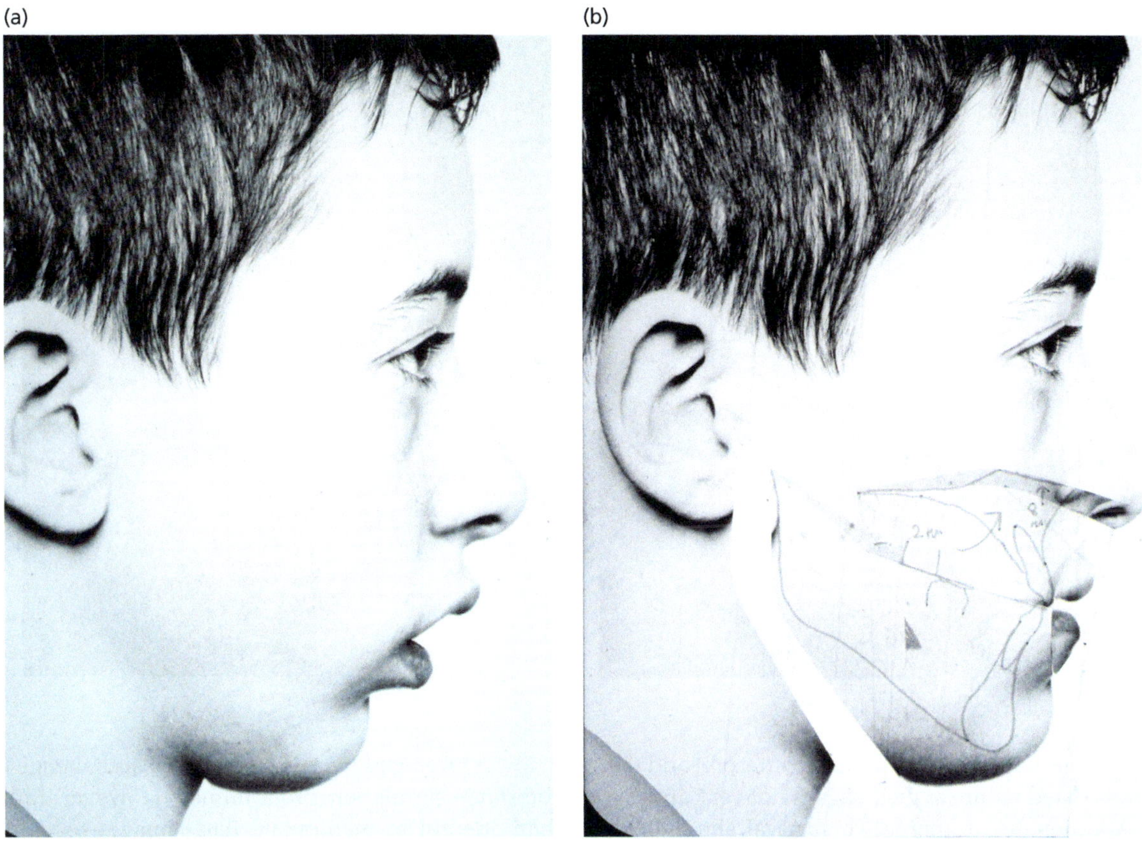

Fig. 6-38 Photo-cephalometric 'cut and paste' prediction planning. (a) Preoperative profile photograph. (b) Preoperative photo-cephalometric profile composite photograph, with segments 'cut and pasted' by hand into proposed postoperative positions. (Courtesy of Mr Raymond Edler.)

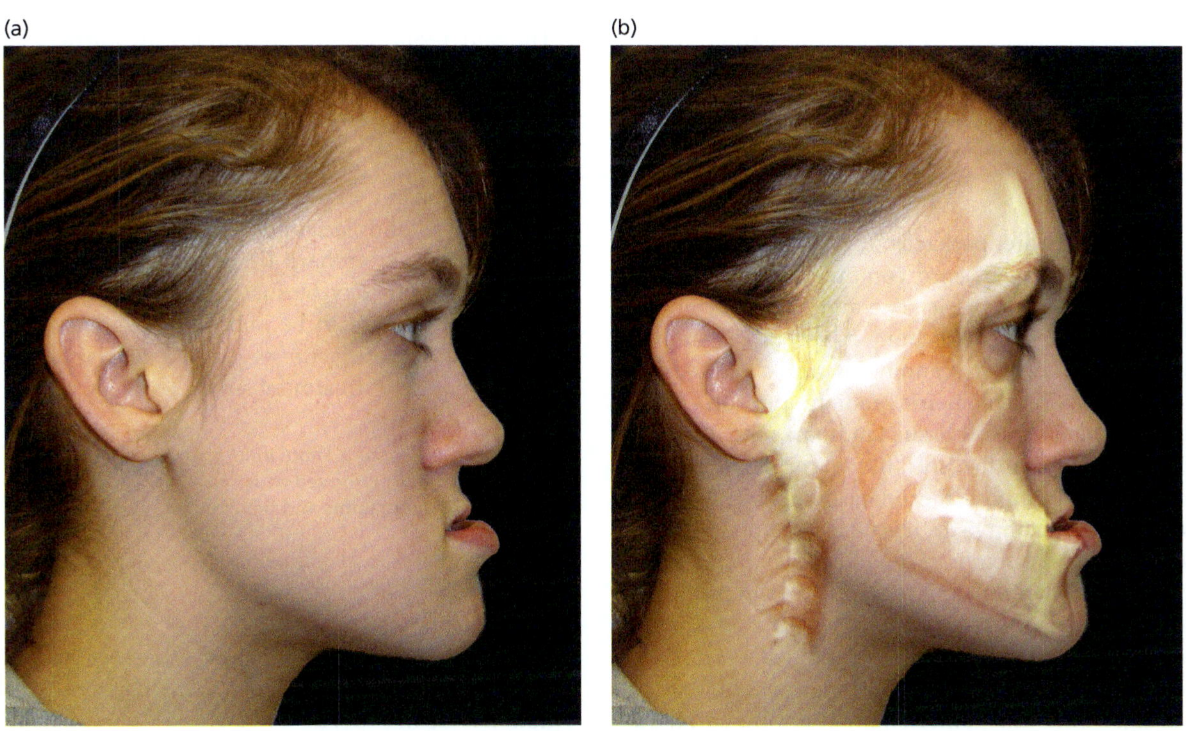

Fig. 6-39 Photo-cephalometric 'cut and paste' prediction planning. (a) Preoperative profile photograph. (b) Preoperative photo-cephalometric profile composite photograph. (c) Prediction planning using 'cut and paste' technique. (d) Final postoperative result.

(c) (d)

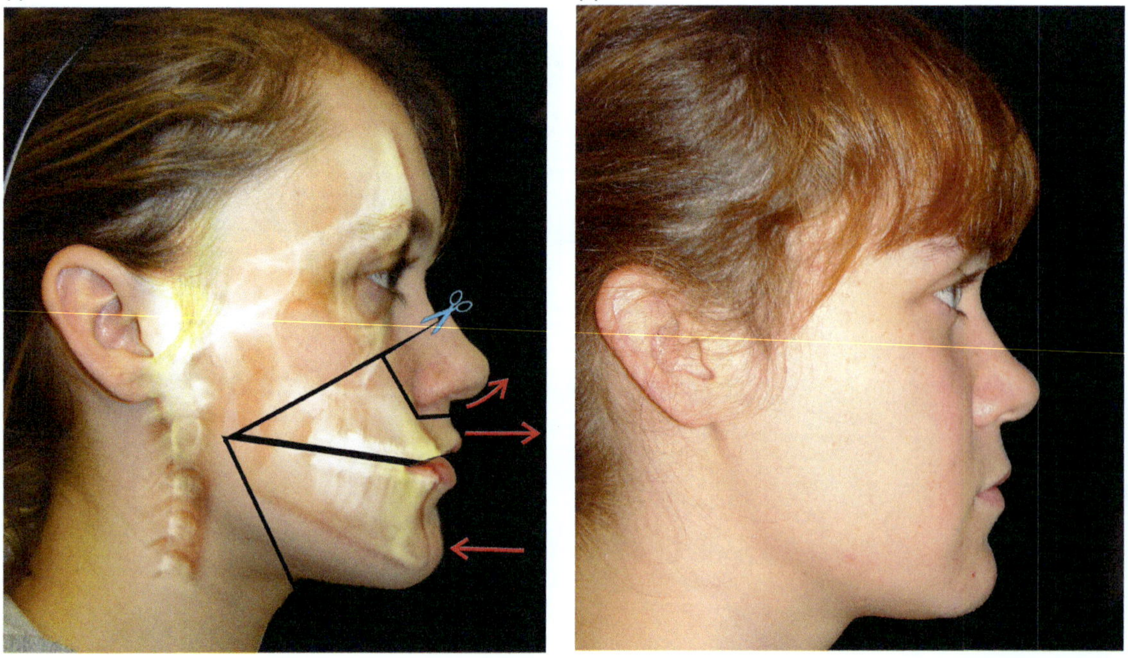

Fig. 6-39 (*Continued*)

potential predicted results difficult to interpret and the cut and pasted nature of the image is not very appealing. Additionally, if alternative surgical simulations are to be compared, the procedure has to be repeated on new photo-cephalograph templates, which makes the procedure even more time-consuming. In order to surmount these shortcomings, computer simulation software packages have been developed (see below).

Computer simulation software prediction (2D, modern)

> 'The computer can show you what you (may) achieve with your planning but cannot plan for you.'
>
> Hugo L. Obwegeser[16]

Modern software packages for surgical-simulation prediction are in essence computerised versions of the photo-cephalometric 'cut and paste' technique described above. The techniques essentially employ digitally entering or scanning a profile photograph and lateral cephalometric radiograph, on which dentoskeletal and soft tissue landmarks are digitised, following which the soft tissue profile outline is used to superimpose the images, creating a photo-cephalometric composite. It is vitally important for the soft tissue image on both the photograph and radiograph to be identical, and for landmark identification to be as accurate as possible, otherwise the superimposition will be inaccurate. Desired dentoskeletal movements are then entered by the clinician, and mathematical algorithms automatically undertake the soft tissue changes relative to the hard tissue movements. The soft tissue contours may also be manipulated, to provide a better outline, though this potentially increases the subjectivity of the method. Vertical soft tissue alterations, e.g. improving lip seal after vertical reduction of lower face height, provide the greatest challenge for computer simulation programmes. However, rather than attempt to manipulate these images too much using image refinement 'touch-up' tools, it may be better to present them to patients so that the 'this is a simulation only' issue becomes obvious (Figure 6-40).

Computerized prediction programmes have a number of advantages:

- The soft tissue profile predictions are carried out automatically, though the predictions still suffer from the same problem as the hand-tracing method, in that the soft tissue to hard tissue changes are difficult to predict with any degree of accuracy, due to variations in muscle tonicity, soft tissue thickness, 'dead space' and variability in soft tissue compression resulting from hard tissue movements. Therefore, the result may be just as misleading. If prediction results are to be shown to patients, most programme manufacturers carry a **disclaimer** on printed copies of treatment simulations, e.g.:

  > 'These images are a simulation of the likely outcome of surgery. This is performed with the assistance of a computer prediction programme and therefore is only an impression of the type of facial change that might be expected. The outcome with the actual operation normally differs from these images to a variable degree.'

  Nevertheless, patients find these images much easier to understand and, as such, patient communication may be improved.
- Though the data entry is still time-consuming, once the photo-cephalometric image has been created it is easier and quicker to undertake several alternative predictions where the treatment plan is not straightforward, in order to compare the results.

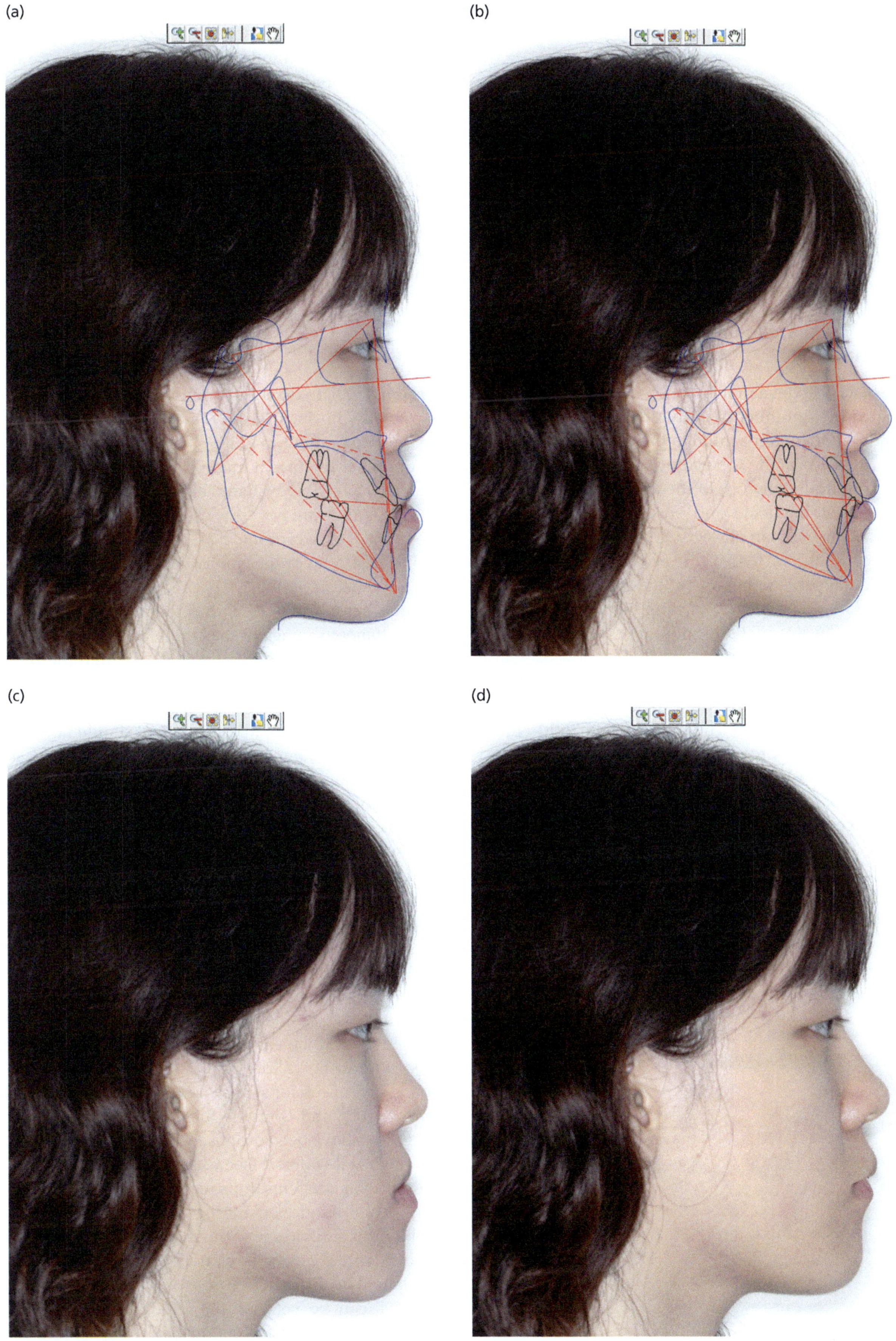

Fig. 6-40 Computer simulation prediction planning (2D). (a) Photo-cephalometric profile as viewed on the computer monitor. (b) Surgical simulation, planning for a 2 mm posterior impaction of the maxilla and 3 mm advancement, with mandibular forward autorotation and set-back of 3 mm to a Class I incisor relationship. (c) Preoperative profile as in image (a), but with cephalometric analysis lines removed. (d) Surgical prediction as in image (b), but with cephalometric analysis lines removed. (Dolphin Imaging software prediction planning used.)

- Storage and subsequent retrieval of image predictions is easy.

Note:

It is worthwhile remembering that a computer and associated software programmes are useful aids, but they do not replace the human eye, ear or brain, and the decision-making process should always proceed with the wise judgement of the treating clinicians.

Computer simulation software prediction (3D, modern)

The historical development of science and medicine is defined by a number of individuals, who made substantial contributions through their inventiveness and dedicated research. The evolution of X-ray radiography is undoubtedly one of the defining achievements throughout medicine and surgery. The pioneering work of the German physicist Wilhelm Conrad Roentgen (or Röntgen, 1845–1923) produced and detected electromagnetic radiation in the wavelength range today known as X-rays, earning him the first Nobel Prize in Physics in 1901. Soon after, the Polish-born French physicist–chemist Marie Sklodowska-Curie (1867–1934) undertook her pioneering work on radioactivity, receiving the Nobel Prize in Physics in 1903. The works of Thomas Wingate Todd (1885–1938), B. Holly Broadbent (1894–1977) and Herbert Hofrath (1889-1952) were instrumental in the development of cephalometric radiography.[32] However, the move from 2D to 3D radiography occurred as a result of work by the English electrical engineer Sir Godfrey Hounsfield (1919–2004), together with the South African-American physicist Allan Cormack (1924-1998), for the development of X-ray computed tomography (CT), earning the Nobel Prize for Physiology or Medicine in 1979. CT is now an internationally utilized diagnostic modality (Figure 6-41), as are its newer generation advances with reduced radiation, such as cone beam CT (CBCT).

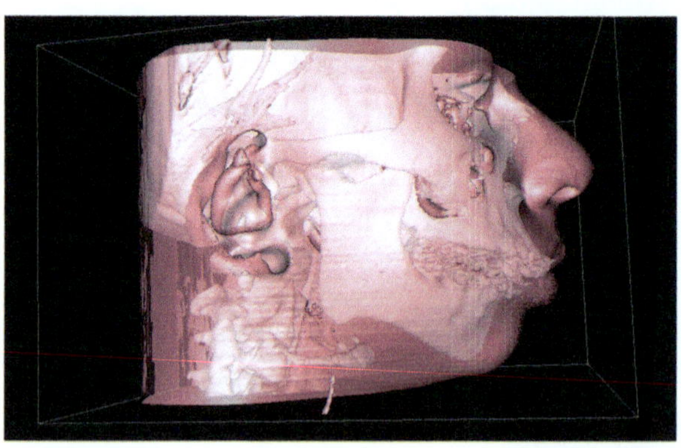

Fig. 6-41 Three-dimensional preoperative computed tomograph (CT) of a patient as viewed on a computer monitor. The image demonstrates the dentoskeleton and overlying soft tissues, and it may be rotated and viewed on the monitor in any direction.

It is with the orthodontic-orthognathic reliance on 2D cephalometric radiography as an aid in both diagnosis and treatment planning that a move towards 3D systems has been inevitable. The ideal 3D orthognathic surgical planning system should have the following requirements:

- Low radiation.
- Accurate, simultaneous capture of the craniodentoskeletal complex and overlying soft tissues, with a life-like appearance.
- Ability to undertake virtual surgical planning and splint-wafer construction in preparation for surgery.

It is important to dispel any myths at the outset – there is currently no such ideal 3D system for orthognathic treatment planning.

A number of current manufacturers advertise commercially available systems able to produce pretty '3D' images, which are nevertheless of little or no use, e.g. the concept of 'wrapping' a 2D facial photograph over a 3D CBCT scan of the cranioskeletal complex is simply nonsensical.

Cone beam CT (CBCT) has the ability to provide a simultaneous image of the craniofacial skeleton and overlying soft tissues (Figure 6-42). Though the radiation exposure is reduced compared with traditional CT, it is still considerably higher than one or two plain radiographs. Additionally, the patient should not have any head positioning pads placed onto the face, as these will cause soft tissue distortion, and the patient should not be supine, but ideally in natural head position, though this may be difficult to achieve with current systems. The soft tissue image is bland and does not resemble the patient's skin tone.

A current technique involves using some form of **3D stereophotogrammetry** or **laser scanning** to capture the facial soft tissue image (Figure 6-43), which may then be superimposed onto the 3D CBCT of the cranioskeletal complex. This superimposition requires the two images to be identical, and the superimposition process itself to be easy and reliable, in order for the procedure to be valid. Techniques to scan the dentition,[33] or impressions/models of the dental-occlusal complex,[34,35] and combine these with the rest of the image also have been proposed, as have techniques to create virtual wafers[33] (see Chapter 42).

Even when systems improve to the extent that accurate virtual surgical planning becomes possible, the problem of individual variability with the alteration of soft tissue changes in relation to hard tissue movements will be difficult to surpass.

CBCT can be very useful for diagnosis, particularly in preparation for craniofacial surgery, and the development of craniofacial implants to improve soft tissue contour defects. However, the use of such systems in orthognathic surgery still requires further development.

(a)

(b)

(c)

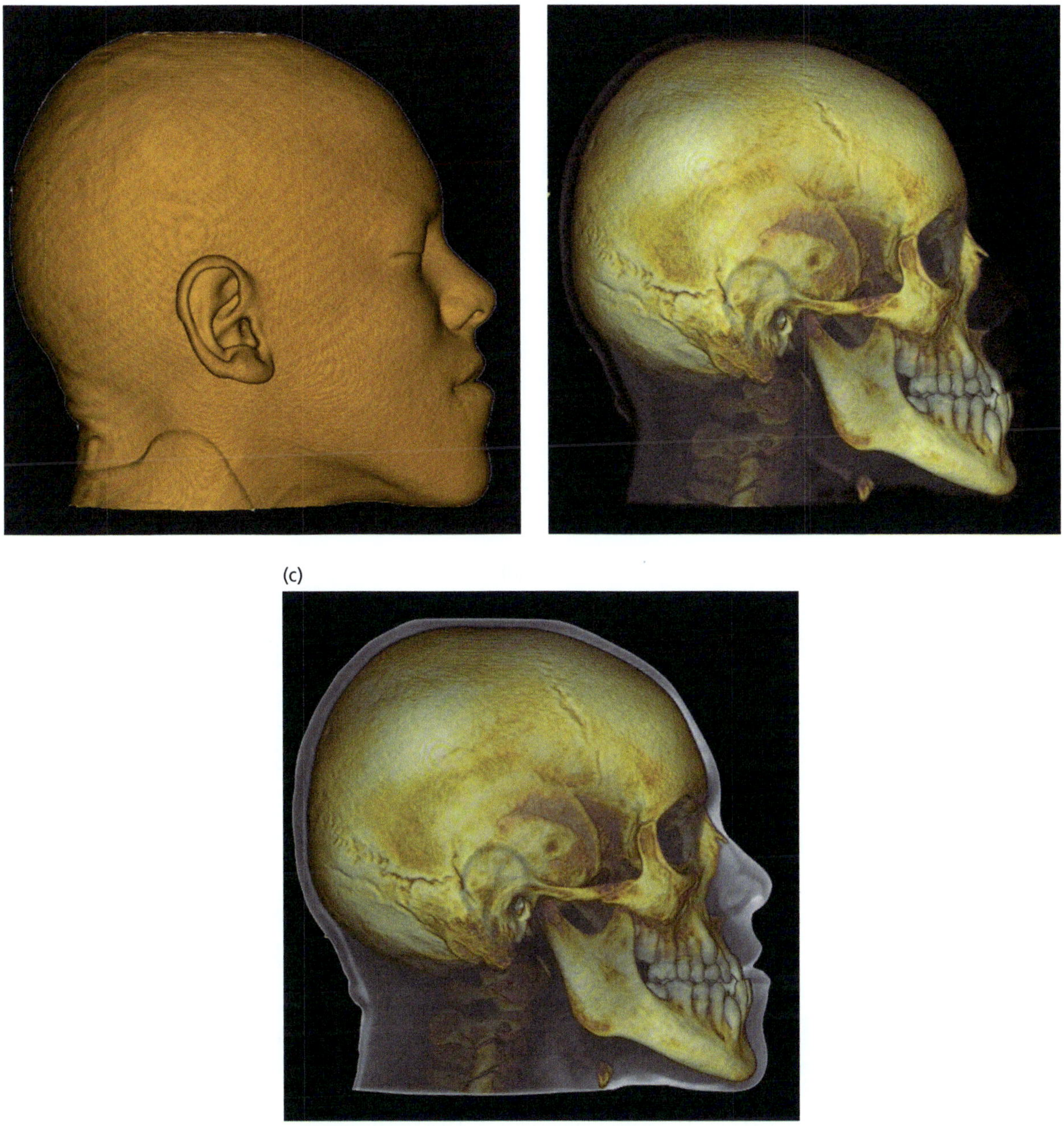

Fig. 6-42 Views obtained from a 3D CT scan of a Class III patient, which simultaneously provides images of the dentoskeleton and overlying soft tissues of the cranio-maxillofacial complex. (Courtesy of Dr Jacques Treil.)

Note:

The final point to remember is that diagnosis and treatment planning have always been based on a 3D model – the patient. While many clinicians today are attempting to use more and more complex 3D imaging and computerized planning systems to try to make treatment planning more accurate and predictable, they would do well remembering to employ the most simple yet complex tool at their disposal – their eyes.

4. Model surgery

Model surgery describes the simulation of the planned surgical procedures on the patient's preoperative articulator-mounted dental models, i.e. it is a trial-run of the planned surgery on the study models. The objectives of model surgery are two-fold:

- To verify that the planned surgical procedures, based on data from the clinical evaluation of the patient and the prediction planning, are realistic; and
- Fabrication of the surgical wafer splints. If bimaxillary surgery is planned, the maxillary cast is repositioned in relation to an unmoved mandibular cast to construct the intermediate wafer; then the mandibular cast is repositioned to create the final wafer.

For a comprehensive description of model surgery technique see Chapter 13.

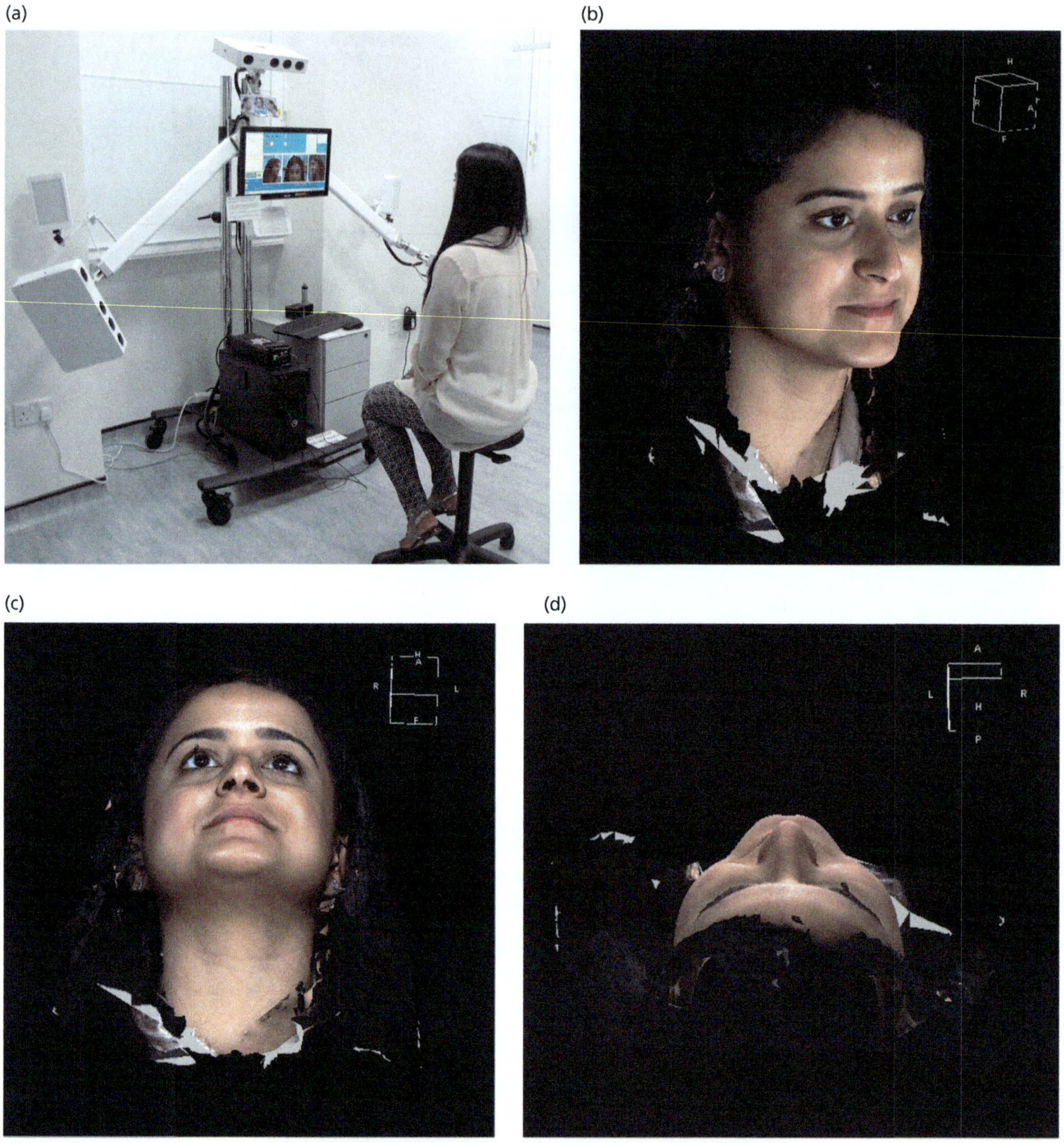

Fig. 6-43 3D stereophotogrammetry. (a) Multiple cameras capture images of the face simultaneously. (b) An example of an image as viewed on a computer monitor, which may be rotated and viewed from different angles, such as (c) a worm's eye view or (d) bird's eye view.

Concluding remarks

> 'I have always thought that one man of tolerable abilities may work great changes, and accomplish great affairs among mankind, if he first forms a good plan, and ... make(s) the execution of that same plan his sole study and business.'
>
> Benjamin Franklin (1706–1790)[36]

An accurate diagnosis invariably directs the clinician to the appropriate treatment plan. However, the gold standard treatment plan may not be appropriate for every patient. For example, a patient may simply not desire orthognathic surgery. Therefore, alternative treatment plans may also be discussed. The clinician's role is to provide each patient with enough information, such that the patient can make the correct decision for themselves.

The essence of treatment planning is to build a coherent picture of where you are, where you want to get to, and how you are going to get there, albeit allowing for contingencies. So long as basic principles are followed, there is no need for treatment planning to be over-complicated.

References

1 Cushing H. Letter to Dr Henry Christian, 20th Nov., 1911. In: Harvey Cushing's Seventieth Birthday Party: April 8, 1939 – Speeches, letters and tributes. Park Ridge, IL: The Harvey Cushing Society, 1939.
2 Naini FB. Facial Aesthetics: Concepts and Clinical Diagnosis. Oxford: Wiley-Blackwell, 2011.
3 Naini FB, Cobourne MT, McDonald F, Wertheim D. Aesthetic impact of the upper component of the nasolabial angle:

a quantitative investigation. J Oral Maxillofac Surg Med. Pathol. 2015;27:470–6.
4 Naini FB, Cobourne MT, McDonald F, Wertheim D. The aesthetic impact of upper lip inclination in orthodontics and orthognathic surgery. Eur J Orthod. 2015;37:81-6.
5 Naini FB. Facial Proportions. In: Naini FB. Facial Aesthetics: Concepts and Clinical Diagnosis. Oxford: Wiley-Blackwell, 2011.
6 Naini FB. Facial Type. In: Naini FB. Facial Aesthetics: Concepts and Clinical Diagnosis. Oxford: Wiley-Blackwell, 2011.
7 Naini FB, Donaldson ANA, McDonald F, Cobourne MT. Assessing the influence of asymmetry affecting the mandible and chin point on perceived attractiveness in the orthognathic patient, clinician and layperson. J Oral Maxillofac Surg. 2012;70:192–206.
8 Naini FB. Regional Aesthetic Analysis: Mentolabial (Labiomental) Fold. In: Naini FB. Facial Aesthetics: Concepts and Clinical Diagnosis. Oxford: Wiley-Blackwell, 2011.
9 Naini FB, Donaldson ANA, McDonald F, Cobourne MT. Assessing the influence of chin prominence on perceived attractiveness in the orthognathic patient, clinician and layperson. Internat J Oral Maxillofac Surg. 2012;41:839–46.
10 Naini FB. Regional Aesthetic Analysis: The Maxilla and Midface. In: Naini FB. Facial Aesthetics: Concepts and Clinical Diagnosis. Oxford: Wiley-Blackwell, 2011.
11 Naini FB. "Cotton wool roll" technique in orthognathic planning. J Oral Maxillofac Surg. 2012;70:e369–e370.
12 Rosen HM. Maxillary advancement for mandibular prognathism: indications and rationale. Plast Reconstr Surg. 1991;87:823–32.
13 Kawamoto HK. Reduction mentoplasty (Discussion). Plast Reconstr Surg. 1982;70:151.
14 van der Dussen FN, Egyedi P. Premature aging of the face after orthognathic surgery. J Craniomaxillofac Surg. 1990;18:335–8.
15 Freihofer HP. Reversing segmental osteotomies of the upper jaw. Plast Reconstr Surg. 1995;96:86–92.
16 Obwegeser HL. Mandibular Growth Anomalies. Berlin Heidelberg: Springer, 2001.
17 Osler W. The Army Surgeon (1894). In: Osler W. Aequanimitas, with other addresses to Medical Students, Nurses, and Practitioners of Medicine. (3rd Ed.). Philadelphia: Blakiston, 1932.
18 Kahneman D. Expert intuition: when can we trust it? In: Kahneman D. Thinking, fast and slow. London: Penguin Books, 2011:234–44.
19 Kahneman D1, Klein G. Conditions for intuitive expertise: a failure to disagree. Am Psychol. 2009;64:515–26.
20 Tversky A, Kahneman D. Judgment under uncertainty: heuristics and biases. Science. 1974;185:1124–31.
21 Gladwell M. Blink. New York: Little, Brown and Company, 2005.
22 Ruskin J. Lectures on Architecture and Painting, delivered at Edinburgh in November, 1853, with illustrations drawn by the author. London: Smith, Elder, and Co., 1855.
23 Shakespeare W. A Midsummer Night's Dream (c.1595–6). Oxford: Oxford World's Classics, 1992.
24 Kazanjian VH, Converse JM. The Surgical Treatment of Facial Injuries. Second edition. Baltimore: The Williams and Wilkins Company, 1959.
25 Brewka RE. Pantographic evaluation of cephalometric hinge axis. Am J Orthod. 1981;79:1–19.
26 Sperry TP, Steinberg MJ, Gans BJ. Mandibular movement during autorotation as a result of maxillary impaction surgery. Am J Orthod. 1982;81:116–23.
27 Nattestad A, Vedtofte P. Mandibular autorotation in orthognathic surgery: a new method of locating the centre of mandibular rotation and determining its consequence in orthognathic surgery. J Craniomaxillofac Surg. 1992;20:163–70.
28 Bryan DC. An investigation into the accuracy and validity of three points used in the assessment of autorotation in orthognathic surgery. Br J Oral Maxillofac Surg. 1994;32:363–72.
29 Nadjmi N, Mommaerts MY, Abeloos JV, De Clercq CA. Prediction of mandibular autorotation. J Oral Maxillofac Surg. 1998;56:1241–7; discussion 1247–8.
30 Obwegeser H. Grundsätzliches zur Korrekturplanung von Kiefer- und Gesichtsanomalien aus chirurgischer Sicht. In: Schuchardt K, Schwenzer N (Eds). Fortschr Kiefer Gesichtchir. Stuttgart: Thieme, 1981;26:9–12.
31 Henderson D. The assessment and management of bony deformities of the middle and lower face. Br J Plast Surg. 1974;27:287–96.
32 Naini FB. Cephalometry and Cephalometric Analysis. In: Naini FB. Facial Aesthetics: Concepts and Clinical Diagnosis. Oxford: Wiley-Blackwell, 2011.
33 Hernández-Alfaro F, Guijarro-Martínez R. New protocol for three-dimensional surgical planning and CAD/CAM splint generation in orthognathic surgery: an in vitro and in vivo study. Int J Oral Maxillofac Surg. 2013;42:1547–56.
34 Swennen GR, Mollemans W, Schutyser F. Three-dimensional treatment planning of orthognathic surgery in the era of virtual imaging. J Oral Maxillofac Surg. 2009;67:2080–92.
35 Swennen GR, Mollemans W, De Clercq C, Abeloos J, Lamoral P, Lippens F, Neyt N, Casselman J, Schutyser F. A cone-beam computed tomography triple scan procedure to obtain a three-dimensional augmented virtual skull model appropriate for orthognathic surgery planning. J Craniofac Surg. 2009;20:297–307.
36 Franklin B. Autobiography (1868). Oxford: Oxford University Press, 1998.

Chapter 7

Smile Aesthetics: Specific Considerations in the Orthognathic Patient

Daljit S. Gill and Farhad B. Naini

Introduction

The face may be subdivided into a number of aesthetic unit and subunit subunits (see Chapter 5), of which the smile must be considered an important component or subunit (Figure 7-1). It is important for the orthognathic team to understand the contributing factors to an aesthetic smile and how orthodontics in combination with orthognathic surgery may influence the smile subunit. As orthognathic surgery may have both positive and negative influences upon the smile, it is essential to discuss these with the patient as a part of informed consent. The important components of the smile can be considered as:

1. The alignment of the teeth – primarily determined by orthodontic treatment.
2. Sagittal position and inclination of the maxillary incisors.
3. The visibility of the dentition and gingivae (dentogingival complex) both in the vertical and transverse dimensions.
4. Symmetry.

This chapter will focus primarily on those parameters of the smile that can be influenced by orthognathic treatment, and should be read in conjunction with Chapters 5 and 6. Readers are referred elsewhere for information regarding the influence of tooth size and shape upon smile aesthetics.[1]

The alignment of the teeth

Tooth alignment is a major factor contributing to a pleasing smile, and orthodontic treatment, particularly with modern fixed appliances, can produce accurate three-dimensional tooth positioning. Andrews (1972)[2] studied the common features contributing to the ideal non-treated dentition and defined six keys producing the ideal natural dental occlusion:

- Correct crown angulation (mesio-distal tip) of the teeth with respect to the occlusal plane.
- Correct crown inclination (labio-lingual angle) of the teeth with respect to the occlusal plane.
- No space between the teeth.
- No rotations of the teeth.
- Class I molars (Andrews Classification cf Angle's Classification) and therefore a correct canine and incisor occlusion.
- A flat to minimal curve of Spee.

Orthognathic Surgery: Principles, Planning and Practice. Edited by Farhad B. Naini and Daljit S. Gill.

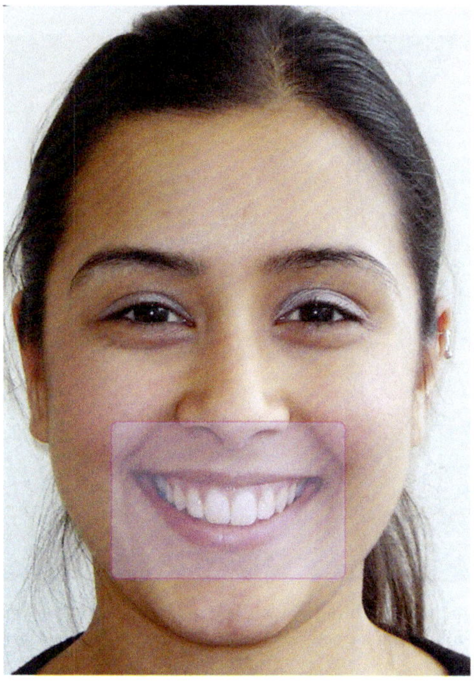

Fig. 7-1 The smile should be considered as an important aesthetic subunit of the face which can be influenced by orthodontics in combination with orthognathic surgery.

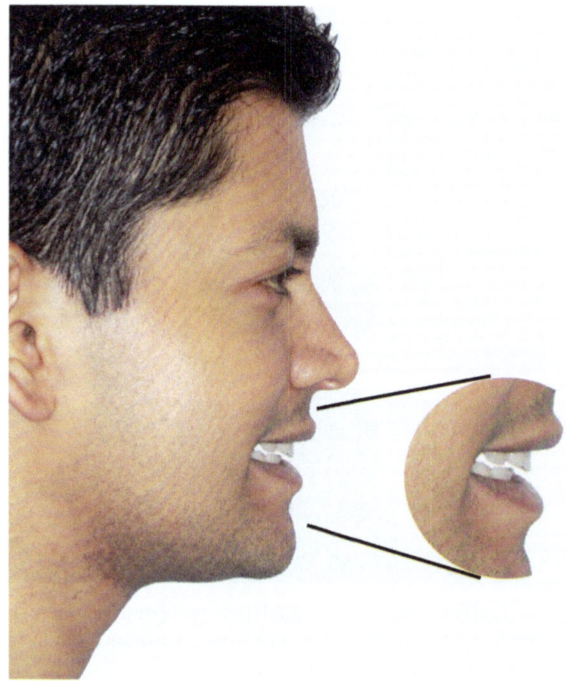

Fig. 7-2 For ideal smile aesthetics the labial face of the maxillary incisors should be vertical or very slightly anteriorly inclined. Cephalometric norms do not necessarily provide the best aesthetic outcomes and a clinical examination of maxillary incisor inclination should be compulsory.

The preadjusted edgewise appliance has attempted to standardize tooth positioning to the ideal. In terms of orthognathic surgery, it is important to plan to achieve the ideal occlusion and incisor inclinations following repositioning of the skeletal bases. Although Andrews judged the maxillary incisor inclination in relation to the occlusal plane, it is far more important to consider the sagittal position and inclination of the maxillary incisors in relation to the face, in order to establish ideal facial and smile aesthetics. The sagittal position and inclination of the maxillary incisors is best considered and judged in profile view.

Sagittal position and inclination of the maxillary incisors

In the profile smiling view, with the patient in natural head position, the sagittal position of the maxillary incisors may be evaluated in relation to a true vertical line dropped from either soft tissue glabella, soft tissue nasion or a point between the two, depending on the aesthetic contour of the glabellar–nasal region.[3] The rationale for using this upper facial reference structure is that there appears to be a correlation between profile smile aesthetics and the incisor–glabellar region relationship.[3,4]

The inclination of the maxillary incisors in profile view also has an impact upon the aesthetics of the smile. Ideally, the inclination of the labial face of the maxillary incisors should be approximately parallel to the true vertical line.[3] Relying solely on the cephalometric evaluation of maxillary incisor inclination can be misleading, as the value is also affected by the inclination of the maxillary plane and not just the maxillary incisor inclination. It is possible for cephalometric analysis to indicate that the maxillary incisor inclination is out of the normal range when clinically the incisor is in a normal aesthetically pleasing relationship. Bearing in mind that it is important to assess this relationship clinically, evidence would suggest that in the profile view the most pleasing smile is achieved when the labial face of the maxillary central incisor is within 3 degrees to the true vertical with the patient in natural head position (Figure 7-2).[5] From the point of view of orthognathic planning it is important that the correct maxillary incisor inclination is achieved following repositioning of the maxilla. So when a posterior maxillary impaction is planned, for example to close an open bite, the preoperative orthodontics should maintain or create an element of maxillary incisor proclination, to enable the surgical move to establish the correct incisor inclination (Figure 7-3). The effect differential movement of the maxilla has on maxillary incisor inclination is proportional to the size of the differential move and the length of the maxilla (Figure 7-4).[6] As a general rule, for an average maxillary length, for every 1 mm of posterior impaction there will be 1.5 degrees of maxillary incisor retroclination (see Chapter 29).

The visibility of the dentition in the vertical dimension

The smile line

The smile line is the vertical relationship between the upper lip and the maxillary dentition during smiling. A high smile line is one where an excessive band

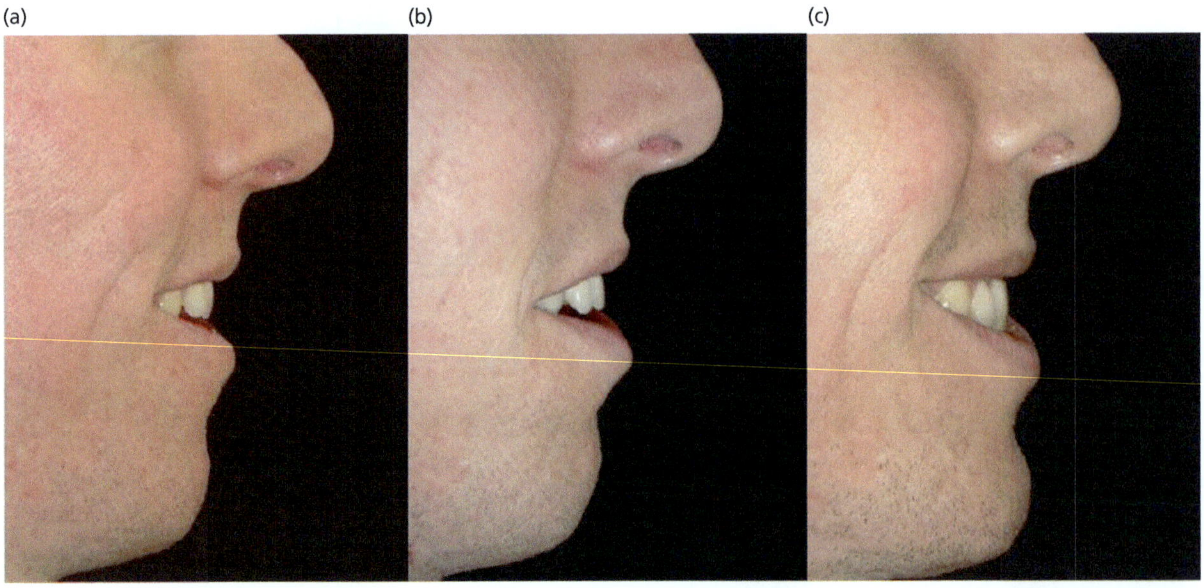

Fig. 7-3 (a) Pretreatment (b) immediately preoperative and (c) post-operative profile smiling views. The maxillary incisors were proclined preoperatively so that a pleasing incisor inclination was achieved following a posterior maxillary impaction. The patient was treated with lingual appliances.

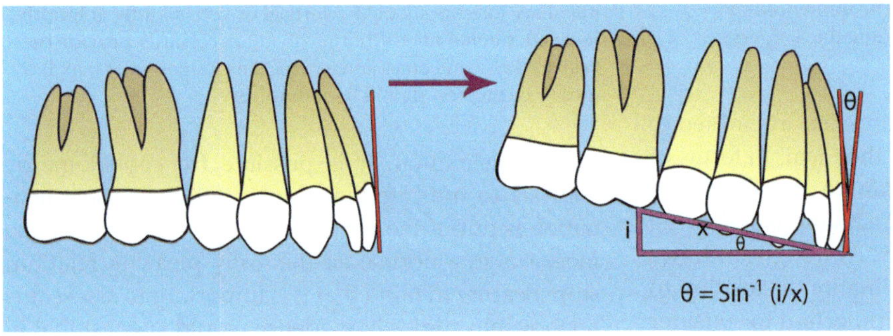

Fig. 7-4 Posterior maxillary impaction has a retroclining effect on the maxillary incisors. The effect is proportional to the amount of impaction (i) and the effective length of the maxilla (x). A formula has been described to calculate the amount of proclination that should be incorporated during preoperative orthodontic treatment.[6]

(typically >2 mm) of gingival tissue is visible during smiling and a low smile line is when less than the ideal amount (<75%) of the vertical crown height of the maxillary central incisor is displayed. One can consider there to be two smile lines; an anterior smile line that determines vertical incisor display and a posterior smile line that determine vertical premolar/molar display. The evidence would suggest that patients generally prefer smiles with 0–2 mm of gingival exposure for both the female and the male smile.[7] Females tend to have a higher smile line than males and there is evidence that the amount of incisor display decreases with ageing.[8,9] A 'gummy' smile may be better tolerated in females than males, and in those with a short facial height than an increased facial height. There appears to be individual variability in what is perceived to be attractive, i.e. no single figure for degree of tooth or gingival exposure will fit everyone, and dentists are more critical of the smile than lay people; therefore it is important to carefully discuss the wishes of the individual patient during treatment planning.

There is limited research on what patients prefer to be an attractive posterior smile line. One study demonstrated that 0–2 mm of gingival exposure in the second premolar region was considered to be most attractive.[10] This figure may be of use when planning the degree of differential movement of the maxilla when planning for the correction of a transverse maxillary cant.

Tables 7-1 and 7-2 list the factors that must be considered in the differential diagnosis of a high and low smile line, some diagnostic features and treatment strategies. Maxillary inferior movement and advancement will increase the incisor exposure (Figure 7-5) and maxillary impaction will reduce it. The anterior vertical position of the maxilla should be planned to achieve the ideal amount of maxillary incisor display at rest (usually 2–5 mm).

The smile arc

Frush and Fisher (1958)[11] first introduced the concept that for a pleasing smile there should be harmony between the curvature of the maxillary incisal edges and canines to the curvature of the lower lip (Figure 7-1). There are many factors that may determine the normal smile arc relationship, including the maxillary occlusal plane angle and the vertical positioning of the incisors.

Table 7-1 Causes, diagnosis and management of excess maxillary gingival exposure

Causes of excess gingival exposure	Diagnosis	Management
Vertical maxillary excess (VME)	Excess maxillary incisor/gingival show at rest and during smiling in the presence of normal upper lip height	Maxillary impaction (moderate- severe cases) Incisor intrusion with orthodontics and temporary anchorage devices (mild cases)
Hypermobility of the upper lip	Normal maxillary incisor exposure at rest 2–5 mm	Botulinum toxin to the elevator muscles of the upper lip
Short upper lip	Decreased lip height: Normal for males = 22 ± 2 mm and females = 20 ± 2 mm.	Surgical lip 'lengthening'
Tooth wear of the maxillary incisors leading to compensatory eruption and migration of the gingival margins	Evidence of tooth wear, central incisor gingival margin apical to lateral incisor, asymmetry in the gingival margins	Orthodontic intrusion to reposition the gingival margin followed by restorative build-up
Delayed migration of the gingival margins	Increased sulcus depth in absence of periodontal disease.	Gingivectomy, Apically repositioned flap

Table 7-2 Causes, diagnosis and management of reduced maxillary gingival exposure

Causes of deficient tooth exposure	Diagnosis	Management
Vertical maxillary deficiency (VMD)	Deficient maxillary incisor/gingival show at rest and during smiling in the presence of normal upper lip height	Inferior maxillary repositioning ± bone graft and maxillary advancement
Microdontia or incisor edge attrition	Reduced incisor dimensions (Normal maxillary incisor height: Males = 10.5 mm and Females = 10 mm)	Restorative dentistry ± orthodontic repositioning
Proclined maxillary incisors	Clinical and cephalometric diagnosis	Orthodontic treatment
Tall upper lip	Increased lip height. Normal for males = 22 ± 2 mm and females = 20 ± 2 mm.	Surgical lip lift
Hypomobile upper lip	Normal maxillary incisor show at rest and reduced amount on smiling.	Facial reanimation surgery for facial nerve palsy

Figure 7-6 illustrates the effect of the maxillary occlusal plane angle on the appearance of the incisal edge curvature. One can appreciate that an optimal occlusal plane angle would help to establish an ideal smile arc relationship. In the orthognathic patient, the occlusal plane angle can be altered with differential vertical repositioning of the maxilla. Patients with a flat occlusal plane angle may be more likely to benefit from such a change to improve the smile arc relationship (Figure 7-7). This may be observed with clockwise rotation of the bimaxillary complex (see Chapter 31).

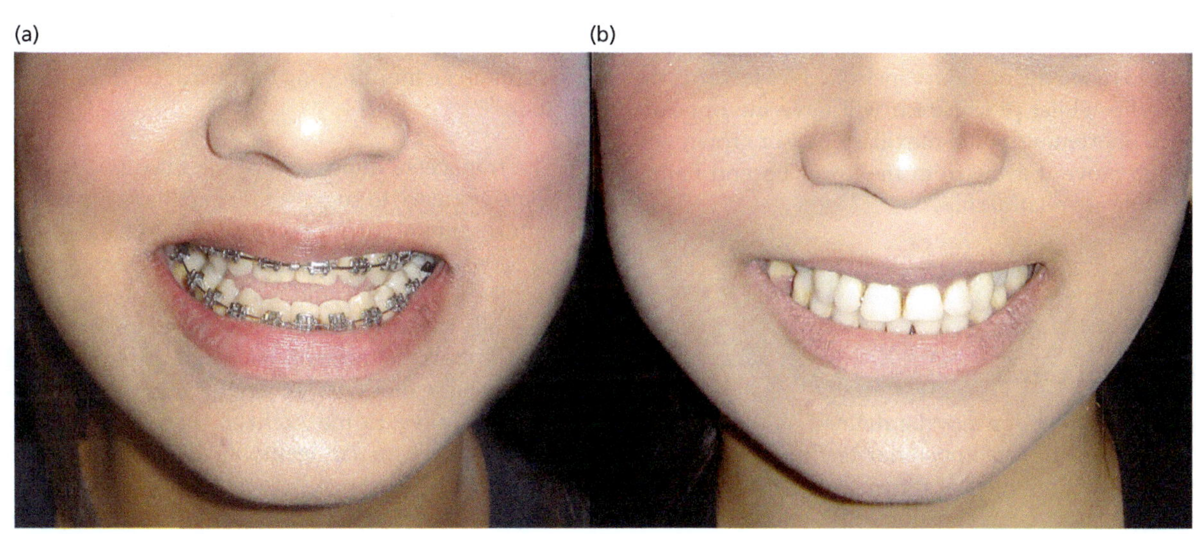

Fig. 7-5 Maxillary advancement and inferior repositioning increases maxillary incisor exposure during smiling. (a) Before and (b) after maxillary surgery.

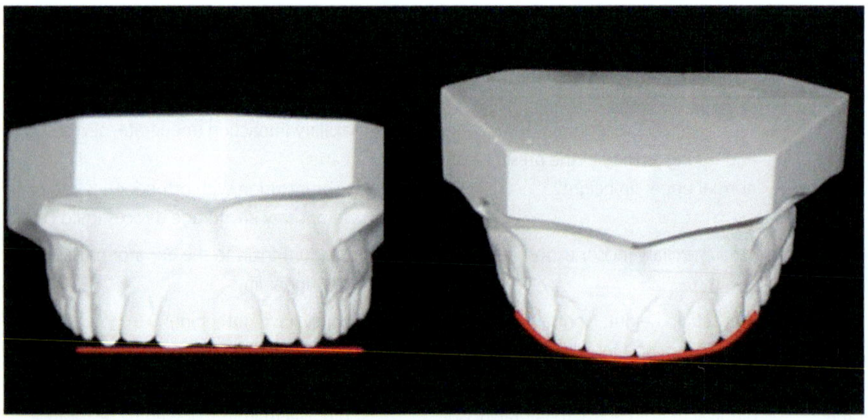

Fig. 7-6 A progressive increase in the occlusal plane inclination increases the effective curvature of the incisor and canine tip edges, which helps to contribute to an improved smile arc relationship.

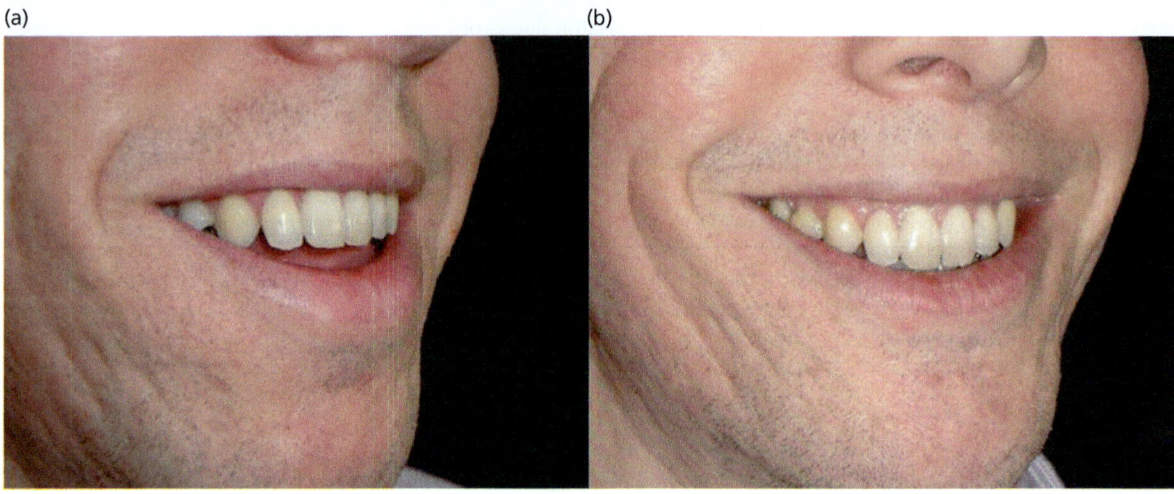

Fig. 7-7 (a) Preoperative and (b) postoperative oblique lateral smile views demonstrating an improvement of the smile arc following posterior maxillary impaction, which increased the maxillary occlusal plane inclination, for the management of an anterior open bite. The patient was treated with lingual appliances.

The vertical height of the maxillary incisors will also influence the relationship of the incisal edges to the lower lip. The height of the incisors can be affected by the anterior vertical maxillary height, the upper incisor inclination and the height of the maxillary incisor crowns. The anterior vertical maxillary height is largely determined by the position of the underlying skeletal base, which can be modified with surgical repositioning. Retroclination of the maxillary incisors tends to move the maxillary incisor edges towards the lower lip whilst proclination will have the opposite effect. Shortening of the maxillary incisor crown will tend to move it away from the lower lip and flatten the smile arc relationship.

The visibility of the dentition in the transverse dimension

The buccal corridors

The buccal corridor may be defined as the distance from the most visible posterior teeth in the smile to the inner commissures of the lips.[11] One study found that the mean buccal corridor width within one sample was 11%.[12] Clinical experience would suggest that some patients do prefer smiles with minimal buccal corridors. The scientific literature is a little more equivocal with some studies supporting better smile aesthetics with narrower buccal corridors,[13,14] and others suggesting that the buccal corridors make little difference to the smile.[15,16] From a clinical viewpoint it is the presenting concerns of the individual patient that are important and it is necessary for the clinician to appreciate what factors contribute to the size of the buccal corridors.

The main factors affecting the buccal corridor width include:[3]

1. The transverse dimension of the maxilla. There is some evidence to suggest that maxillary expansion reduces buccal corridor width.[12] Such changes may be seen with both rapid maxillary expansion and surgically assisted rapid maxillary expansion.
2. Palatally inclined premolars and molars. Andrews found that the normal maxillary premolar and molar inclination was –7 and –9 degrees, respectively, relative to the occlusal plane.[17] The inclination of the molar teeth can be modified with orthodontic treatment.
3. Sagittal maxillary position. As the maxilla is advanced, a wider portion comes to lie within the inter-commissure line resulting in a reduction

in buccal corridor width. Therefore, a Le Fort I advancement is likely to reduce the buccal corridor width.

4. The inter-commissure width. One study suggests that the mean increase in inter-commissure width during smiling is approximately 130% of the resting width.[18] The greater this increase, the greater the likelihood of increased buccal corridor space. The inter-commissure width may increase with age, leading to an age related increase in buccal corridor width.[12]
5. The vertical dimension of the face. There is some evidence for a correlation between increased lower anterior facial height and reduced buccal corridor width.[19] One explanation is that as the facial height increases, the cheek soft tissues become progressively stretched and come to lie closer to the underlying dentition. Therefore, both maxillary and mandibular advancement, which increase the lower facial height, and inferior repositioning of the maxilla may result in a reduction in the buccal corridor width.

Symmetry

A symmetrical dental arrangement is important for good smile aesthetics. As with facial aesthetics, there is a certain degree of tolerance to the existence of asymmetry within the smile and no smile is perfectly symmetrical.

Dental midlines

Ideally, the maxillary dental midline should be both coincident and parallel to the facial midline. In the majority of patients, the facial midline can be constructed by connecting glabella and the mid-philtrum of the upper lip. Evidence would suggest that it is more important for the maxillary incisors to be correctly angulated, and for the dental midline to be parallel to the facial midline than it is for it to be coincident with this line. For example, it has been shown that dental midline discrepancies of less than 2 mm are largely unnoticeable.[20] Whereas, angulation discrepancies of the midline of greater than 6 degrees and 10 degrees to the vertical were found to be unacceptable when judged by orthodontists and laypeople, respectively.[21] An angulated dental midline may be encountered in those with a transverse maxillary occlusal plane cant. In such cases, cant correction will help to improve the dental midline relationship.

Maxillary cants

A transverse cant of the maxillary occlusal plane is most commonly found in those that have a vertical asymmetry of the mandible (e.g. hemimandibular hyperplasia, hemifacial microsomia). Where there is either vertical mandibular over- or under-growth, the maxillary buccal segments will erupt to contact and mirror the position of the lower molars in the majority of patients. A maxillary cant may result in an asymmetry of canine/premolar/molar tooth show and gingival display, and a cant of the maxillary dental midline. When there is a significant underlying soft tissue asymmetry, there may also be a cant of the inter-commissure line which complicates management further. Research would suggest that laypeople may find cants of the maxillary occlusal plane greater than 2–4 degrees less attractive.[22–25]

Conclusions

A number of factors that contribute to the smile that can be influenced by orthognathic surgery have been reviewed. The smile should be evaluated in all three planes of space during routine diagnosis and treatment planning. Orthognathic surgical procedures should be planned in order to maximise smile aesthetics. Optimal smile aesthetics can be achieved within a range of normal values and it is important that aims are patient led as the views of professionals can differ from those of lay people. Liaison with other dental specialities (e.g. Prosthodontics) may be important during the planning stages in order to address issues such as tooth size, shape and colour which are also important for a pleasing smile.

References

1 Naini FB, Gill DS. Dentogingival Aesthetics. In: Naini FB. Facial Aesthetics: Concepts and Clinical Diagnosis. Oxford: Wiley-Blackwell, 2011.

2 Andrews LF. The six keys to normal occlusion. Am J Orthod. 1972;62:296–309.

3 Naini FB, Gill DS. Smile Aesthetics. In: Naini FB. Facial Aesthetics: Concepts and Clinical Diagnosis. Oxford: Wiley-Blackwell, 2011.

4 Schlosser JB, Preston CB, Lampasso J. The effects of computer-aided anteroposterior maxillary incisor movement on rating of facial attractiveness. Am J Orthod Dentofacial Orthop. 2005;127:17–24.

5 Ghaleb N, Bouserhal J, Bassil-Nassif N. Aesthetic evaluation of profile incisor inclination. Eur J Orthod. 2011;33:228–35.

6 Naini FB, Hunt NP, Moles DR. The relationship between maxillary length, differential maxillary impaction, and change in maxillary incisor inclination. Am J Orthod Dentofacial Orthop. 2003;124:526–9.

7 Hunt O, Johnston C, Hepper P, Burden D, Stevenson M. The influence of maxillary gingival exposure on dental attractiveness ratings. Eur J Orthod. 2002;24:199–204.

8 Vig RG, Brundel GC. Kinetics of anterior tooth display. J Prosthet Dent. 1978;39:502–4.

9 Desai S, Upadhyay M and Nanda R. Dynamic smile analysis: Changes with age. Am J Orthod Dentofacial Orthop. 2009;136:310.e1–10.

10 Crawford RWI, Tredwin C, Moles D, Gill D. Smile esthetics: The influence of posterior maxillary gingival margin position. J Prosthodont. 2012;21:270–8.

11 Frush JO, Fisher RD. The dysesthetic interpretation of the dentogenic concept. J Prosthet Dent. 1958;8:55–58.

12 Maulik C, Nanda R. Dynamic smile analysis in young adults. Am J Orthod Dentofacial Orthop. 2007;132:307–15.

13 Moore T, Southard KA, Casko JS, Qian F, Southard TE. Buccal corridors and smile esthetics. Am J Orthod Dentofacial Orthop. 2005;127:208–13.

14 Martin AJ, Buschang PH, Boley JC, Taylor RW, Mckinney TW. The impact of buccal corridors on smile attractiveness. Eur J Orthod. 2007;29:530–7.
15 Kim E, Gianelly AA. Extraction vs nonextraction: arch widths and smile esthetics. Angle Orthod. 2003;73:354–8.
16 Roden-Johnson D, Gallerano R, English J. The effects of buccal corridor spaces and arch form on smile esthetics. Am J Orthod Dentofacial Orthop. 2005;127:343–50.
17 Andrews LF. Straight Wire – The Concept and Appliance. LA Wells Co San Diego, CA 92107. 1989. Chapter 4, p. 32.
18 Rigsbee OH 3rd, Sperry TP, BeGole EA. The influence of facial animation on smile characteristics. Int J Adult Orthodon Orthognath Surg. 1988;3:233–9.
19 Yang IH, Nahm DS, Baek SH. Which hard and soft tissue factors relate with the amount of buccal corridor space during smiling? Angle Orthod. 2008;78:5–11.
20 Johnston CD, Burden DJ, Stevenson MR. The influence of dental to facial midline discrepancies on dental attractiveness ratings. Eur J Orthod. 1999;21:517–22.
21 Thomas JL, Hayes C, Zawaideh S. The effect of axial midline angulation on dental aesthetics. Angle Orthod. 2003;73:359–64.
22 Ker AJ, Chan R, Fields HW, Beck M, Rosenstiel S. Esthetics and smile characteristics from the layperson's perspective: a computer-based survey study. J Am Dent Assoc. 2008;139:1318–27.
23 Geron S, Atalia W. Influence of sex on the perception of oral and smile esthetics with different gingival display and incisal plane inclination. Angle Orthod. 2005;75:778–84.
24 Peck S, Peck L. Selected aspects of the art and science of facial esthetics. Semin Orthod. 1995;1:105–26.
25 McLeod C, Fields HW, Hechter F, Wiltshire W, Rody W, Christensen J. Esthetics and smile characteristics evaluated by laypersons. Angle Orthod. 2011;81:198–205.

Chapter 8

Orthodontic and Orthognathic Surgery Planning Using CBCT

Lucia H.S. Cevidanes, Vinicius Boen, Beatriz Paniagua, Martin Styner and Tung Nguyen

Introduction

Three-dimensional (3D) diagnostic assessment of facial morphology at baseline and overtime now allows more effective and rational clinical decision making for orthodontic and orthognathic surgery patients. Assessments over time and often diagnostic assessment of left and right differences in asymmetry cases now require careful 3D superimposition techniques. With the availability of cone beam CT (CBCT), the preparation of the surgical plan has shifted from using 2D radiographic images to 3D images and models. In the past ten years, a number of research centres and commercial companies have strived to provide software environments that allow preparation of the operative plan on 3D models of the skeletal structures extracted from the CBCT.

Studies on the 3D bone remodelling and displacements with surgery have now helped elucidate clinical questions on variability of outcomes of surgery.[1–3] Accuracy and reliability of this tools, increased costs and radiation exposure are some of the aspects to be discussed in this transition. It is important to validate the clinical application of these methods, and critically assess the difficulty of transferring virtual plans into the operating room and assess long-term treatment outcomes of surgery. The image analysis tools for 3D images, specifically colour maps and 3D *Closest Point* quantification, have been adapted by us for use with cone beam CTs of the craniofacial complex and have brought significant contribution to clinical needs as they broaden the diagnosis and narrow the treatment targets. However, the *Closest Point* method measures displacement that occurs with orthognathic surgery as the smallest separation between the boundaries of the same structure, which may or may not be the appropriate directional distance between equivalent boundaries or landmarks on pre- and post-surgery images. The *Closest Point* method cannot be used to quantify longitudinal changes and fails to quantify rotational and large translational movements. Other 3D morphometric approaches under development will also be discussed in this chapter.

Orthognathic Surgery: Principles, Planning and Practice. Edited by Farhad B. Naini and Daljit S. Gill.

3D CBCT diagnosis and treatment planning

While many clinicians have made routine clinical use of CBCT imaging, 3D CBCT imaging in orthodontics and orthognathic surgery offers diagnostic information for the following complex conditions:

Tooth morphology and relative position within the alveolar bone

Small or medium field of view high resolution images that include an arch quadrant or both upper and lower arches are needed to evaluate buccal and lingual plates of the alveolar bone, bone loss or formation, bone depth and height, presence or absence of unerupted teeth, tooth development, tooth morphology and position, amount of bone covering the tooth, proximity or resorption of adjacent teeth. CBCT findings may lead to modifications in the treatment planning (such as avoid extraction, change plan of which tooth to extract, or placement of bone plates and mini-screws), reduced treatment duration and improved control of additional root resorption and in the ortho-surgical planning.[4–15]

Temporomandibular joint health and disease

The spectrum of the clinical and pathologic presentation of TMJ OA ranges from structural and functional failure of the joint with disc displacement and degeneration to subchondral bone alterations (erosions), bone overgrowth (osteophytes), loss of articular fibrocartilage, and synovitis. For detecting TMJ bony changes, panoramic radiography and MRI have only poor to marginal sensitivity.[16] For this reason, CBCT has recently replaced other imaging modalities as the modality of choice to study TMJ bony changes.[17–19] The Research Diagnostic Criteria for Temporomandibular Disorders (RDC/TMD)[20] was revised recently to include image analysis criteria for various imaging modalities.[16] The RDC/TMD validation project[21–23] concluded that revised clinical criteria alone, without recourse to imaging, are inadequate for valid diagnosis of TMD and had previously underestimated the prevalence of bony changes in the TMJ. TMJ pathologies that result in alterations in the size, form, quality and spatial relationships of the osseous joint components lead to skeletal and dental discrepancies in the three planes of space. In affected condyles, the perturbed growth and/or bone remodelling, resorption, apposition can lead to progressive bite changes that are accompanied by compensations in the maxilla, 'non-affected' side of the mandible, tooth position, occlusion and articular fossa, and unpredictable orthodontic outcomes (Figure 8-1).[24,25]

The temporomandibular joint (TMJ) is prone to a myriad of pathologies that could be didactically divided as 'degenerative pathologies' and 'proliferative pathologies'. Such pathologies can dramatically affect other craniofacial structures and be easily recognized, or the TMJ pathology can be challenging to diagnose even to experts when its progression is subtle and limited even though still clinically relevant (Figure 8-2). In any situation, longitudinal quantification of condylar changes has the potential to improve clinical decision making, by identifying the most appropriate and beneficial therapy.

The TMJ is unique in relation to the other joints in our body. Adult joint bone surfaces are composed by hyaline cartilage but the TMJ. The TMJ has its bone surfaces composed by fibro cartilage that allows a tremendous ability to morphological adaptation due to function. The threshold between functional physiologic stimulus with its positive biochemical effects on the TMJ and joint overloading that lead to degenerative changes is beyond current knowledge.[26–31] Such threshold is influenced by a multitude of factors, including but not limited to the joint loading vectors and their magnitude,[32] patient inherited or acquired (genetic and mostly epigenetic) factors including hormonal and autoimmune imbalances. Current methods to detect pathological conditions in a cross-sectional diagnostic assessment (bone scintigraphy and positron emission tomography) are highly sensitive; however, they do not have enough specificity, as there are no standard normal values for baseline assessments. Longitudinal 3D quantification using CBCTs offer a relative low cost/low radiation technology (compared to PET-CT and bone scintigraphy) and can make a significant difference on treatment planning as an additional biomarker or risk factor tool. The use of biomarkers to aid diagnosis in temporomandibular joint disorders is very promising but it is not novel. Several biomarkers, including C-reactive protein, have previously been identified in blood and in synovial fluid biopsies of patients with TMJ condylar bone resorption and related to the pathological progress.[33–35] Such techniques, still currently restricted to academic environments and research centres, are certainly very promising and will complement CBCT three-dimensional techniques that is already a clinical tool protocol.

Airway assessment

Airway morphology and changes overtime with surgery, growth and its relationship to obstructive sleep apnoea have been recently assessed in CBCTs.[36–42] However, the boundaries of the nasopharynx superiorly with the maxillary and paranasal sinuses, and the boundaries of the oropharynx with the oral cavity anteriorly and inferiorly with the larynx boundary are not consistent among subjects. Additionally, image acquisitions and airway shape and volume will vary markedly with functional stage of the dynamic process of breathing and head posture. If head posture is not correctly reproduced in longitudinal studies, differences in head posture will lead to

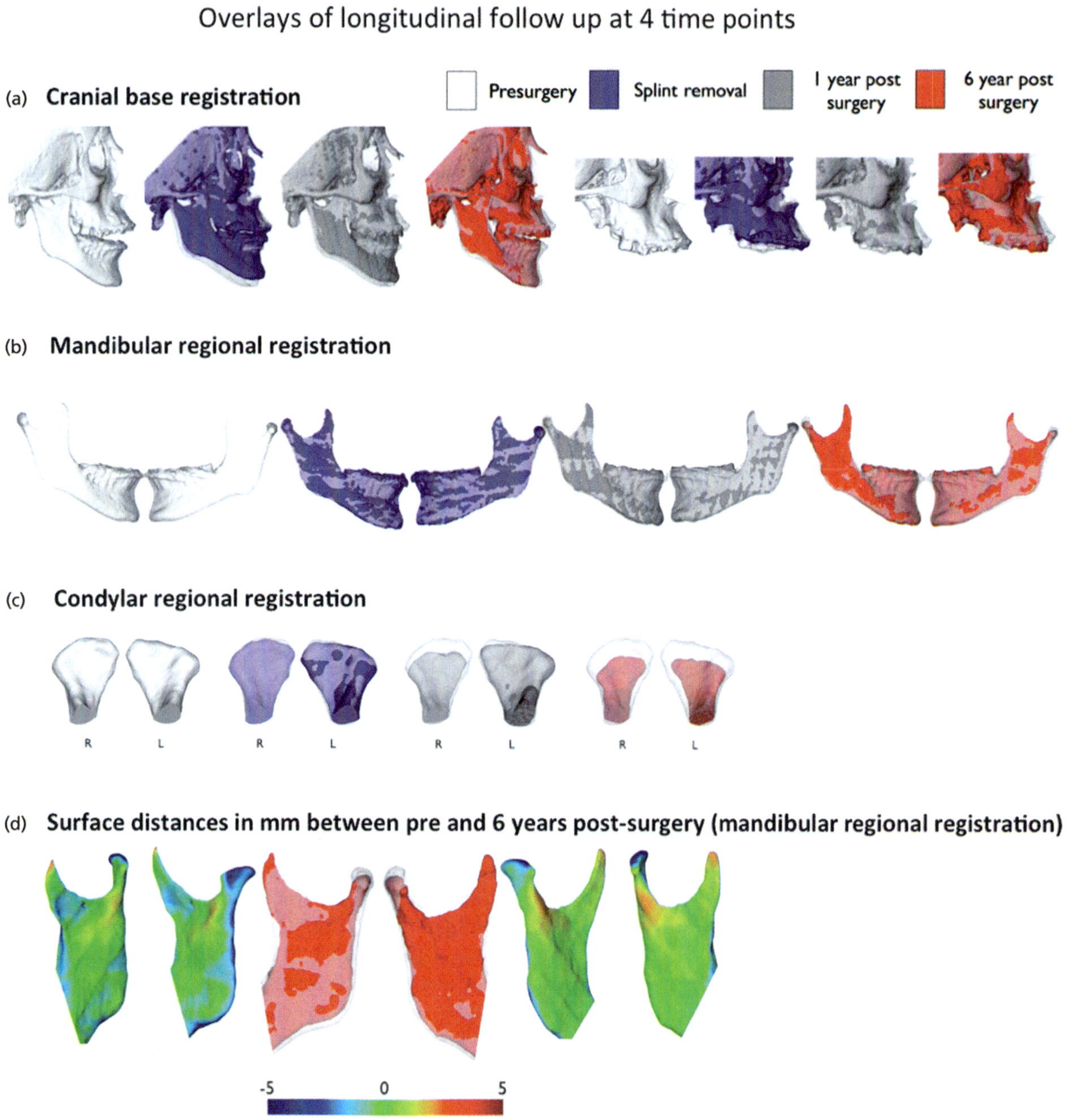

Fig. 8-1 Longitudinal assessment of outcomes of a maxillary impaction surgery for open bite correction. The pre-surgery model is shown in white, splint removal in blue, 1 year post-surgery in grey and 6 years post-surgery in red. The different time points were superimposed using a voxel-based automated registration at different anatomical structures of interest for reference to assess in detail the bone remodelling and displacements over time. (a) Cranial base superimposition shows that at the overall relative rotational displacement of the mandible at splint removable, relapsed 6 years post-surgery as the maxillary impaction relapsed. (b) Mandibular overall changes shown in a mandibular regional superimposition. Note that condylar changes and overall ramus adaptive changes that had began between pre surgery and 1 year post-surgery and progressed further 6 years post-surgery. (c) Condylar regional superimposition showing the progression of condylar resorptive changes in more detail, and that some flattening was already present pre-surgery. (d) Close-up views of the left and right ramus changes between pre surgery and 6 years post-surgery in a mandibular regional superimposition. The colour maps show about 5 mm of condylar changes and in some regions in the ramus surface.

variability in airway dimensions. Longitudinal assessments of mandibular setback have not shown consistent reduction of airway space nor have mandibular propulsion devices shown enlargement of the airway space that might be helpful for obstructive breathing conditions (Figure 8-3). Retroglossal airway changes after four bicuspids extraction and lower anterior teeth retraction or significant surgical mandibular advancement or setback are prone to great variability and still being under scrutiny studies.

Dentofacial deformities and craniofacial anomalies

CBCT imaging offers the ability to analyze facial asymmetry and antero-posterior, vertical and

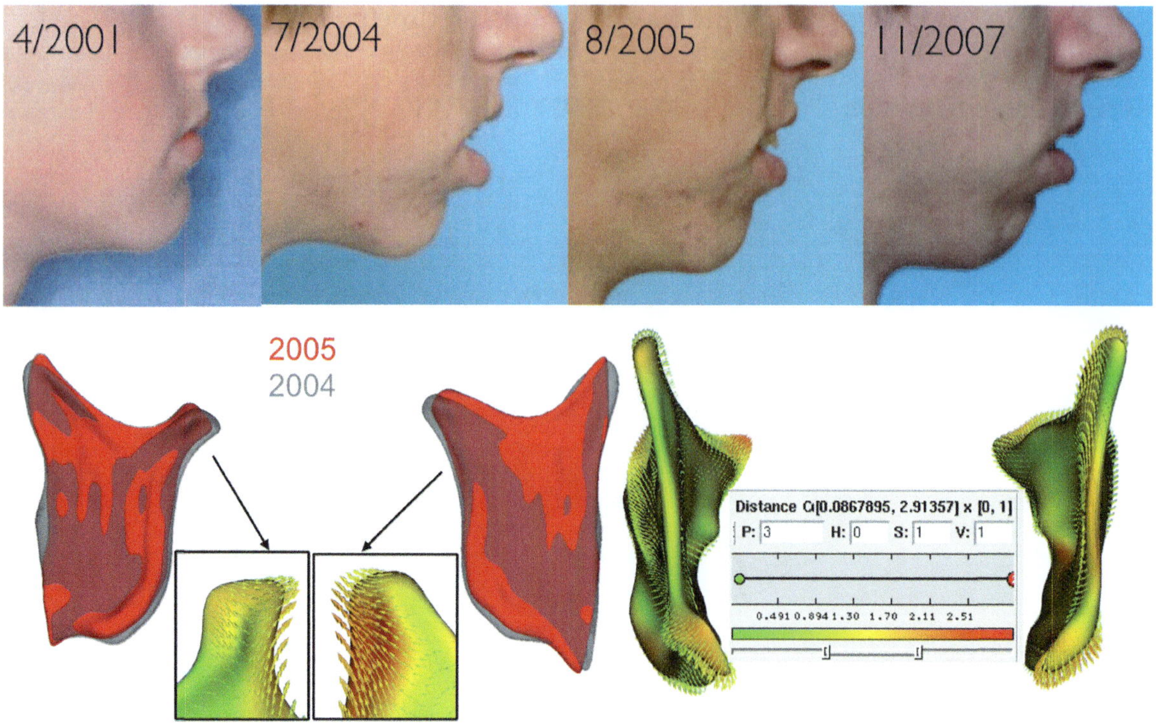

Fig. 8-2 Marked facial changes as a result of idiopathic asymptomatic progressive condylar resorption. Skeletal anteroposterior, vertical and transverse discrepancies shown in surface models.

transverse discrepancies (Figure 8-4). The virtual treatment simulations can be used for treatment planning in orthopaedic corrections and orthognathic surgery and for printing surgical splints. Computer-aided jaw surgery (CAS) is increasingly in use clinically due to the possibility to incorporate a high level of precision for accurately transferring virtual plans into the operating room. In complex cases, follow-up CBCT acquisitions, for growth observation, treatment progress and post-treatment observations, may be helpful to assess stability of the correction overtime.[43–58]

The methods for CAS systems in jaw surgery follow procedures from the image scanners to the operating room and have included commercially a number of systems: Medical Modeling (Texas) and Maxilim (Medicim, Mechelen, Belgium). The advantages of those systems are that they do not require time or computer expertise form the surgeon, and for a service fee, the commercial companies construct surface models from CBCTs and impressions/or digital dental casts registered to the CBCT, perform the virtual surgery and print surgical splints. The CAS steps include: (1) data acquisition: collection of diagnostic data; (2) image segmentation that consists in identification of anatomic structures of interest in the image data sets and visualization of 3D display of the anatomic structures; (3) diagnosis: extraction of clinical information from the 3D representations of the anatomy, for example by using mirroring planes; (4) planning and simulation: preparation of n operative plan by using the virtual anatomy, simulation of the outcome (5) 3D printed surgical guides or individually fabricated synthetic grafts or prosthetic repair; and (6) intraoperative guidance: assistance for intraoperative realization of the virtual plan.

1. Collection of diagnostic records

Diagnosis of skeletal discrepancies is based on visual data coming from different sources: clinical examination, 3D photographic examination, cone beam CT (CBCT), CT, MRI and digital dental models. Computer assisted systems must integrate different records in order to characterize the orthodontic diagnosis and formulate the treatment plan. Multimodality registration is available for a number of commercial software programs, such as 3DMDvultus (3DMD, Atlanta, GA), Maxilim (Medicim, Mechelen, Belgium), Dolphin Imaging (Dolphin Imaging & Management Solutions, Chatsworth, CA), InVivoDental (Anatomage, San Jose, CA), and SimPlant OMS (Materialise, Leuven, Belgium). The CMFApp software (developed under the funding of the Co-Me network[59]) and 3DSlicer[60] (National Alliance for Medical Image Computing, NIH Roadmap) provide uniform medical data handling preoperative grey level image (CBCT, CT,MRI), skeletal models, acquired dental occlusion, operative plans, diagnostic data (3D cephalometry, mirrored structures), planning data (osteotomy lines, repositioning plans), guidance data (registration points and transformations), postoperative image, etc.

2. Segmentation and visualization of anatomical structures of interest

The acquired DICOM files can be imported into diverse 3D image analysis software and exported

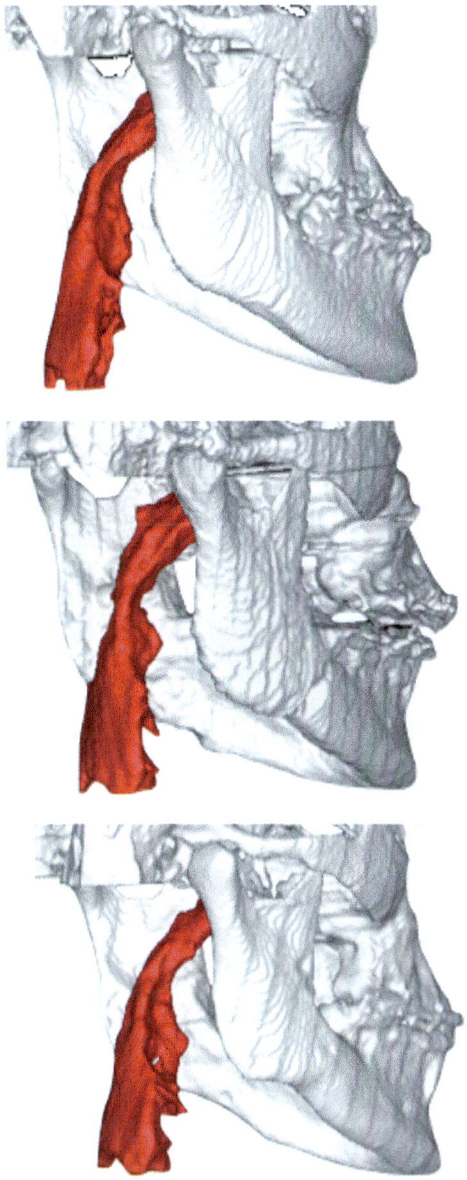

Fig. 8-3 Follow up of mandibular set-back surgery shows that the airway space is reduced at the lower portion of the pharynx at splint removal. Note that the airway space reduction is no longer observed at 1 year post-surgery.

as different formats while keeping the resolution. Next, in a process known as image segmentation, we identify and delineate the anatomical structures of interest in the image. In orthodontics and orthognathic surgery, the goal of segmentation is to obtain a 3D representation of the hard and soft tissues that is usable for virtual planning. Even though image segmentation has been a field of active research for many decades, it remains to be one of the hardest, most time consuming and frequently required steps in image processing systems. There does not and cannot exist a standard segmentation method that can be expected to work equally well for all tasks. The morphology and position of the condyles, internal surface of the ramus and maxilla are critical for careful virtual surgery planning. In order to best capture these and other areas, our method of choice for the segmentation procedures utilizes ITK-SNAP[61] software that has received continuous NIH support for further open-source software development. ITK-SNAP was developed, based on the NIH Visualization Tool Kit (VTK) and Image Tool Kit (ITK), as part of the NIH Roadmap Initiative for National Centers of Biomedical Computing. The automatic segmentation procedures in ITK-SNAP utilize two active contour methods to compute feature images based on the CBCT image gray level intensity and boundaries (Figure 8-5). The first method causes the active contour to slow down near edges, or discontinuities, of intensity. The second causes the active contour to attract to boundaries of regions of uniform intensity. After obtaining the segmentation result, manual post-processing is normally necessary. Artefacts resulting from metallic elements need to be removed. Lower and upper jaws are usually connected due to insufficient longitudinal image resolution and must be separated in the temporomandibular joint and on occlusal surface in particular. For this reason, it has been recommended that the CBCT be taken in centric occlusion with a stable and thin bite registration material.[62] On a laptop computer equipped with 1GB of RAM, the initial mesh generation step typically takes about 15 minutes. Manual post-processing usually takes longer, up to a couple of hours (separation of the jaws can be particularly tedious).

Two technological options are available to visualize these structures three dimensionally. The first are surface-based methods, which require the generation of an intermediate surface representation (triangular mesh) of the object to be displayed, provide very detailed shading of the facial surfaces at any zoom factor. Also, any other three-dimensional structure that can be represented by a triangular mesh can be easily included in the anatomical view (e.g., implants imported from CAD implant databases). The second are volume-based methods, which create a 3D view directly from the volume data.[63] The advantages of surface-based methods are the very detailed shading of the facial surfaces at any zoom factor. The majority of existing CMF surgery planning software programs use surface-based visualization. An obvious disadvantage of surface-based methods is the need for an intermediate surface representation. The advantages of volumetric methods are that not only you have direct visualization of volumetric operations in 3D, but also on cross-sectional image views. Virtual osteotomies are applied on the original image dataset. However, it is difficult to establish the boundaries between tissues and assign the proper colour/transparency values to obtain the desired display. Moreover, the image intensity for a given tissue can vary between patients and scanners (e.g., bone density varies with age and metabolic status; there are variations in scanner calibrations). Virtual cutting operations are much more difficult to simulate in voxel-wise representations. Further evolutions in software and graphics hardware that combine both surface- and volume-based visualization technologies

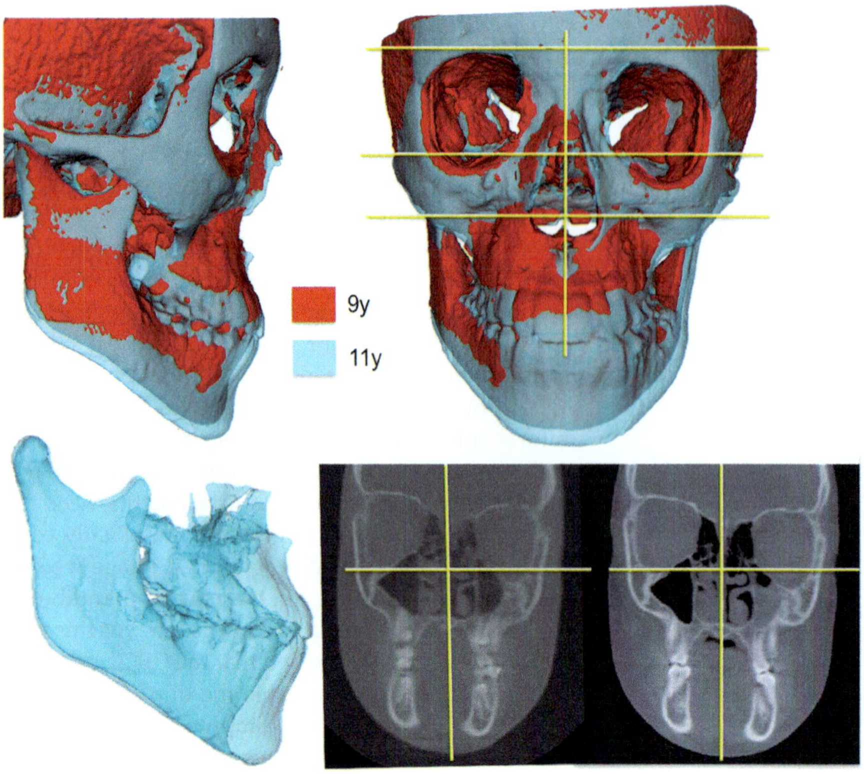

Fig. 8-4 Diagnosis of a patient with facial asymmetry. While the mandibular growth appears asymmetric relative to the cranial base, careful diagnosis using semi-transparent overlays show that the right and left mandibular ramus and corpus are very symmetrical and the multiplanar cross-sections clarify that left orbit and maxillary sinuses are vertically longer than the right side and that the aetiology of the facial asymmetry is located in the midface and not in the mandibular growth.

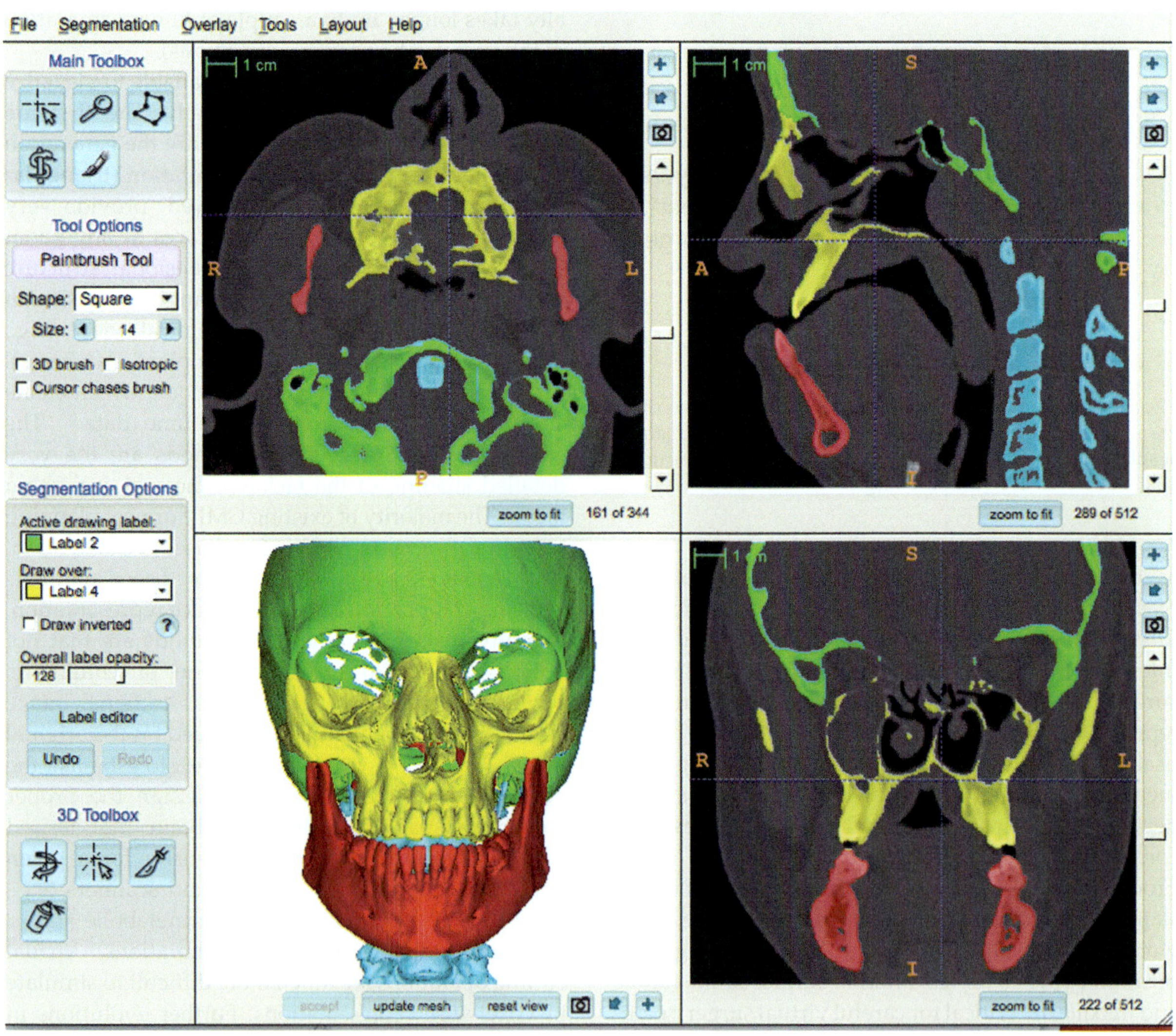

Fig. 8-5 Construction of surface models using ITK-SNAP.

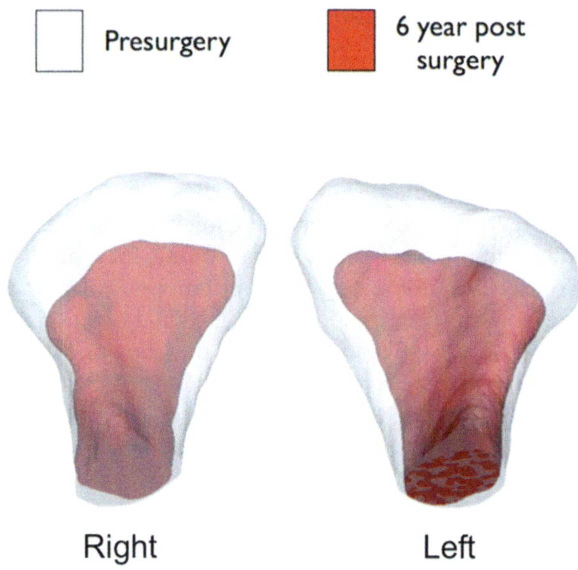

Fig. 8-6 Semi-transparent overlays of pre-surgery (white) and 6 year post-surgery (red) surface models of the mandibular condyles in close-up view of patient shown in Figure 8-1. The condylion landmarks in the pre-surgery and 1 year post-surgery would not be homologous points in the condyles, when marked bone changes have occurred.

have great potential as they offer complementary information and might expedite the whole process.

3. Diagnosis using 3D cephalometry and mirroring techniques

Morphometrics is the branch of mathematics studying shapes and shape changes of geometric objects. Cephalometrics is a subset of morphometrics. Clinical cephalometric analyses have been based on a set of points, either of anatomical meaning or from an abstract definition (such as middle point between two other points) and understanding of facial morphology is described by angles and linear measurements (Figure 8-6). Surface and shape data available in 3D imaging provide new characterization schemes, based on higher order mathematical entities (e.g., spline curves and surfaces). For example, Cutting et al.[64] and Subsol et al.[65] introduced the concept of *ridge curves* for automatic cephalometric characterization. Ridge curves (also known as *crest lines*) of a surface are the loci of the maximal curvature, in the associated principal curvature directions. The ridge lines of a surface convey very rich and compact information, which tend to correspond to natural anatomic features. Lines of high curvature are typical reference features in the craniofacial skeleton. Future studies will establish new standards for three dimensional measurements in the craniofacial skeleton. New developments in this area might lead to comprehensive 3D morphometric systems including surface-based and volume-based computed shape measurements (Figure 8-7). They could also lead to 4D shape information which integrates evolution over time in the analysis, an application of great relevance once allow early diagnosis of post-intervention unexpected positional changes and clinical decision making before further complications.

4. Surgical planning and simulation

After establishment of the diagnosis, the next step is to use the 3D representations of the anatomy to plan and simulate the surgical intervention. In orthognathic surgery, corrective interventions designate procedures that do not require an extrinsic graft and reconstructive interventions are designated for situations in which a graft is used. In corrective procedures, it is important to determine the location of the surgical

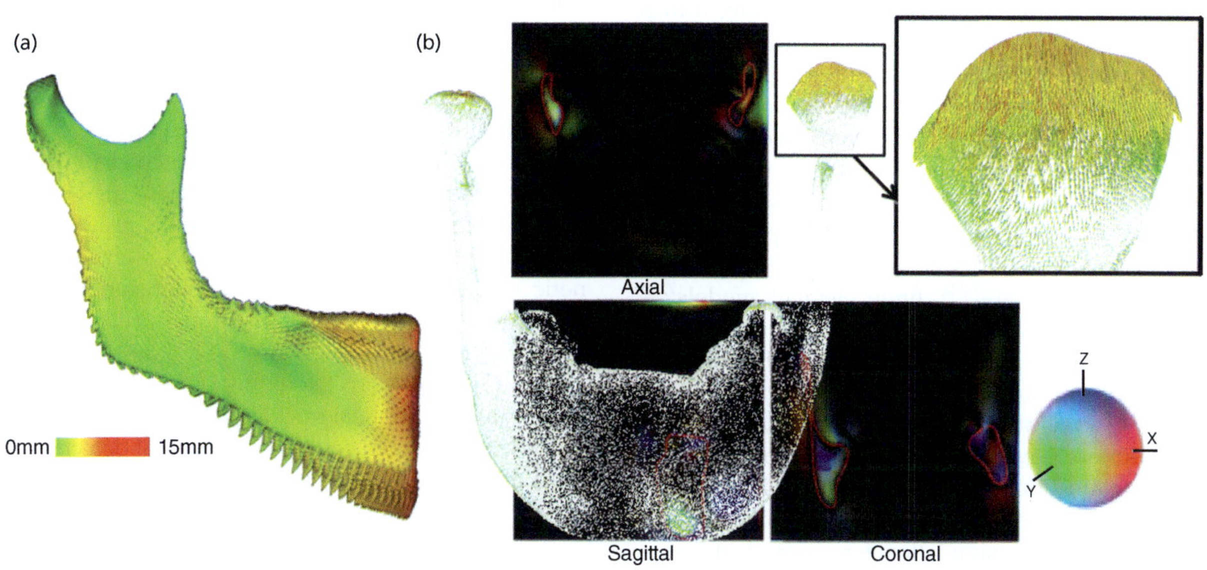

Fig. 8-7 Methods for corresponding surface points for shape analysis. (a) Vectors between correspondent surface points before and after mandibular set-back surgery. The absolute value in mm of the vectors length is displayed in colour-coded maps. (b) Colour-coded maps using tensor based morphometry.

cuts, to plan the movements of the bony segments relative to one another, and to achieve the desired realignment intraoperatively. In reconstructive procedures, problems consist in determining the desired implant or graft shape. In the case of implants and prosthesis, the problems are to select the proper device and shape it, or to fabricate an individual device from a suitable bio-compatible material. With a graft, the difficulties lie in choosing the harvesting site, shaping the graft, and placing the implant or graft in the appropriate location.[66]

Virtual osteotomies allow for planning of cuts, position and size of fixation screws and plates, taking into account the intrinsically complex cranial anatomy; regions of thin (or absent) bone, such as the maxillary sinus anterior wall, create sudden discontinuities in the mesh; and inner structures (e.g., mandibular nerve canal) often included in the surface model. After the virtual osteotomy, the virtual surgery with relocation of the bony segments can be performed with quantification of the planned surgical movements.[67–71] Relocation of the anatomical segments with six degrees of freedom (DOF) is tracked for each of the bone fragments. This allows for the correction of the skeletal discrepancy for a given patient and simultaneous tracking of measurements of X, Y and Z translation and rotation around each of these axes. The segment repositioning produced can be used as an initial suggestion to the surgeon, for discussions of the 3D orthodontic and surgical treatment goals for each patient, and/or for printing surgical splints if high resolution scans of the dental structure are registered to the CT or CBCT and if the software tool presents an occlusion detection functionality to detect occlusal contacts, conflicts and the precise occlusion in the virtual simulations.

Simulation of soft tissue changes

Methods that attempt to predict facial soft tissue changes resulting from skeletal reshaping utilize approximation models, since direct formulation and analytical resolution of the equations of continuum mechanics is not possible with such geometrical complexity. Different types of models have been proposed: displacements of soft tissue voxels are estimated with the movements of neighbouring hard tissue voxels,[72] bone displacement vectors are simply applied on the vertices of the soft tissue mesh,[73] and multi-layer mass-spring models,[74–76] finite element models[77–79] and mass tensor models[80] that assume biological properties of soft tissue response. In any case, thorough validation reports for all these methods are still lacking. Comparisons of the simulation with the postoperative facial surface have not yet been performed. Surgical planning functions generally do not fulfill the requirements enumerated above for preparation of quantitative facial tissue simulation for surgical planning. Other functionalities that have been incorporated into different software systems include: simulation of muscular function,[81] distraction osteogenesis planning[82] and 4D surgery planning.[83]

5. Intraoperative guidance

Surgical navigation

In surgical procedures, achieving the desired bone segment realignment freehand is difficult. Also, segments must often be moved with very limited visibility, e.g., under the (swollen) skin. Approaches used currently in surgery rely largely on the clinician's experience and intuition. In maxillary repositioning, for example, a combination of dental splints, compass, ruler, and intuition are used to determine the final position. It has been shown that in the vertical direction (in which the splint exerts no constraint), only limited control is achieved.[84] While the surgical splint guides the position of the maxilla relative to the mandible, in two-jaw surgeries the spatial position of the two jaws relative to the face is influenced by the splint precision and the trans-surgical vertical assessment. As the splints are made over teeth and guide bone changes away from those teeth, small splint inaccuracies may reflect in significant bone position inaccuracies. The predictability of precise osteotomies in the wide variety patient morphologies and consequent controlled fractures such as in the pterygoid plates, sagittal split osteotomies or interdental cuts are still a concern. In reconstructive procedures, the problems of shaping and placing a graft or implant in the planned location also arises. Surgical navigation systems have been developed to help accurately transfer treatment plans to the operating room.

Tracking technology

Different tracking technologies[85,86] for the tracking of the displacement of a mobilized fragment in the course of an osteotomy can be used with respective advantages and disadvantages: (1) ultrasound where an array of three ultrasound emitters is mounted on the object to be tracked, but the speed of sound value can vary with temperature changes and the calibration procedure is very delicate; (2) electromagnetic tracking where a homogeneous magnetic field is created by a generator coil. Ferromagnetic items such as implants, instruments or the operation table can interfere strongly with these systems, distorting the measurements in an unpredictable way. Newer systems claim reduction of these effects and feature receivers the size of a needle head possibly announcing a renewal of interest for electromagnetic tracking in surgical navigation (examples are the 3D guidance trackstar, Ascension, Burlington, VT, StealthStation® AXIEM, Medtronic, Louisville, CO, and Aurora, Northern Digital Inc., Ontario, Canada); (3) infrared (IR) optical tracking devices rely on pairs or triplets of charged coupled devices that detect positions of IR markers and in these device between the cameras and markers, a free line-of-sight is required.

Longitudinal assessments using CBCT

Over the last dedace we have utilized longitudinal CBCT images for assessment of treatment outcomes.

Even with the availability of 3D images, there are critical barriers that have to be overcome before longitudinal quantitative assessment of the craniofacial complex can be routinely performed:

Radiation from CBCT acquisition

The use of 3D images for treatment planning and follow-up raises concerns regarding radiation dose, that require guidelines for specific applications rather than indiscriminate use. Although the radiation doses from dental CBCT exams are generally lower than CT exams, dental CBCT exams increased radiation doses are of concern because they still deliver more radiation that conventional 2D X-ray exams. Furthermore, the radiation dose concerns are even greater for younger patients since they are more sensitive to radiation.

Construction of 3D surface models

Longitudinal quantitative assessment of growth, surgical correction and stability of results requires construction of 3D surface models. Segmentation, the process of constructing 3D models by examining cross-sections of a volumetric data set to outline the shape of structures, remains a challenge.[87–90] Many standard automatic segmentation methods fail when applied to the complex anatomy of patients with facial deformity. The methods described by Gerig et al.[91] address these technical difficulties, and have been adapted by Cevidanes et al. in our laboratory to construct 3D craniofacial models. The constructed 3D surface models labelled with different colours are used to mask and select specific anatomic structures of interest to be used as reference for the registration/superimposition processes.

Image registration

This is a core technology for many imaging tasks. The two obstacles to widespread clinical use of non-rigid (elastic and deformable) registration are computational cost and quantification difficulties as the 3D models are deformed.[93–95] Non-rigid registration can be used to register images of the same patient for example, a child during growth or to create composite/average of jaw morphologies from different patients.[96] Non-rigid registration means that the registration takes into consideration more than just 6 DOF (three rotational and three translational) changes between two image acquisitions, and also includes changes regarding the scale (size) and/or shape of the face. However, for longitudinal assessments,[97] even if non-rigid (scale and shape) changes are taken into account to compute rotation and translation (rigid registration) between two acquired images, only rotation and translation should be applied, so that the registration process does not distort/morph the images.

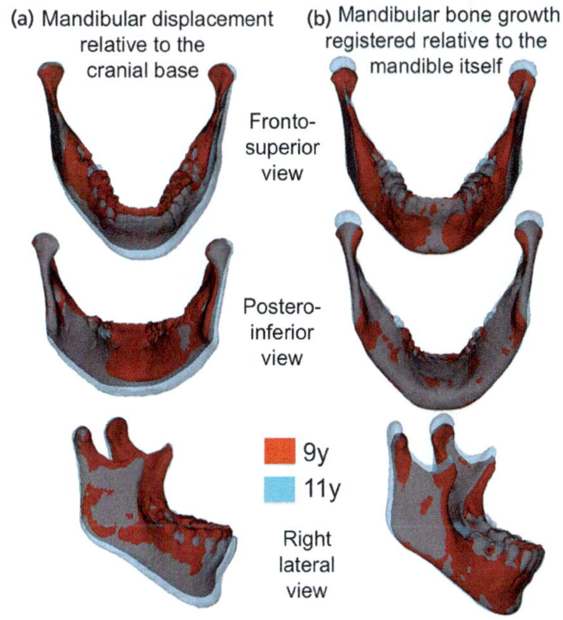

Fig. 8-8 Longitudinal follow-up of growth of the patient with facial asymmetry shown in Figure 8-4. Semi-transparent overlay of surface models of baseline (red), and 2-year growth observation follow-up (cyan), superimposed on the cranial base and in the mandible. (a) Growth displacement to the left relative to the cranial base. (b) Symmetrical growth by bone remodelling of the mandible is noted when the mandibular regional superimposition is used.

The registration procedures can be based on landmarks, surface models or voxel grey intensity and both commercial and open source tools now allow these different options for craniomaxillofacial registration (https://sites.google.com/a/umich.edu/dentistry-image-computing/). We have developed[98–100] a novel sequence of fully automated voxel-wise rigid registration at the cranial base (for overall facial assessments) and regionally (to assess maxillary and mandibular bone remodelling) and superimposition (overlay) methods (Figure 8-8). The major strength of the voxel based registration method is that registration does not depend on the precision of the 3D surface models. In fact, surface models that extend beyond the bone boundaries in the multiplanar images aid the automatic detection of the bone boundaries during the voxel based registration. However, the use of clearly defined anatomical structures of reference for the registration does require prior construction of surface models for all time point grey-level images. The surface models are only used as references to mask anatomic structures that change with growth and treatment. The registration procedures actually compare voxel by voxel of grey-level CBCT images, containing only the cranial base for example, to calculate rotation and translation parameters between the two images.

Registration/superimposition in the cranial base does not completely define the movement of the mandible relative to the maxilla. Future studies are needed to investigate the use of different 3D regional superimposition areas. Currently, superimposition of

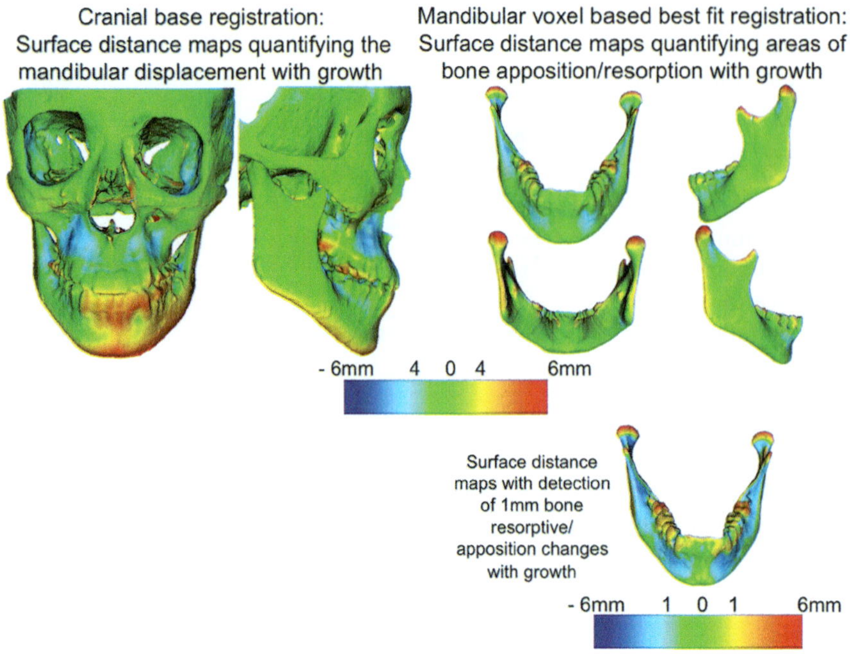

Fig. 8-9 Quantification of surface differences and linear distances between baseline (red), and 2-year growth observation follow-up (cyan), superimposed on the cranial base and in the mandible for patient shown in Figures 8-4 and 8-8. (a) Approximately overall 4 mm of mandibular growth displacement to the left relative to the cranial base. (b) Symmetrical growth by bone remodelling of the mandible is noted with about 6 mm of bone apposition in the condyles. More stringent colour-coded maps detecting changes greater than 1 mm show areas of bone remodelling through out the mandible.

3D surface models is still too time-consuming and computing-intensive to apply these methods in routine clinical use. Our current focus is on developing a simplified analysis so that soon these methods can be used clinically (https://sites.google.com/a/umich.edu/dentistry-image-computing/).

Quantitative measurements

Precise quantitative measurement is required to assess the placement of bones in the desired position, the bone remodelling, the position of surgical cuts and fixation screws and/or plates relative to risk structures. Current quantification methods include:

a) *Volume changes*[96] reflect increase or decrease in size, but structural changes at specific locations are not sufficiently reflected in volume measurements; volume assessment does not reveal location and direction of proliferative or resorptive changes, which would be relevant for assessment clinical results.
b) *Landmark-based*[101] measurements present errors related to landmark identification. Locating 3D landmarks on complex curving structures is not a trivial problem for representation of components of the craniofacial form.[102] As Bookstein[103] noted, there is a lack of literature about suitable operational definitions for the landmarks in the three planes of space (coronal, sagittal, and axial). Gunz et al.[104] and Andresen et al.[105] proposed the use of semi-landmarks, i.e., landmarks plus vectors and tangent planes that define their location, but information from the whole curves and surfaces must also be included. The studies of Subsol et al.[65] and Andresen et al.[105] provided clear advances toward studies of curves or surfaces in 3D, referring to tens of thousands of 3D points to define geometry.
c) *Closest Point measurements* between the surfaces can display changes with colour maps as proposed by Gerig et al.[106] However, the *Closest Point* method measures closest distances, not corresponding distances between anatomical points on two or more longitudinally obtained images (Figure 8-9). For this reason, the *Closest Point* measurements completely fails to quantify rotational and large translational movements, and this method cannot be used for longitudinal assessments of growth or treatment changes, nor the physiologic adaptations, such as bone remodelling that follows surgery.
d) *Shape correspondence:* The SPHARM-PDM framework[107,108] was developed as part of the National Alliance of Medical Image Computing, (NA-MIC, NIH Roadmap for Medical Research), and has been adapted for use with CBCTs of the craniofacial complex.[109,110] SPHARM-PDM is a tool that computes point-based models using a parametric boundary description for the computing of Shape analysis. The 3D virtual surface models are converted into a corresponding spherical harmonic description (SPHARM), which is then sampled into a triangulated surfaces (SPHARM-PDM). This work presents an improvement in outcome measurement as compared to closest point correspondence (CP) based analysis. This standard analysis is currently used by most commercial and academic softwares, but does not map corresponding surfaces based in anatomical geometry and usually underestimates rotational and large translational movements. CP colour maps measure surgical jaw displacement as the smallest separation between boundaries of the same structure which may not be the right anatomical corresponding boundaries on pre- and post-surgery anatomical structures (Figure 8-10).

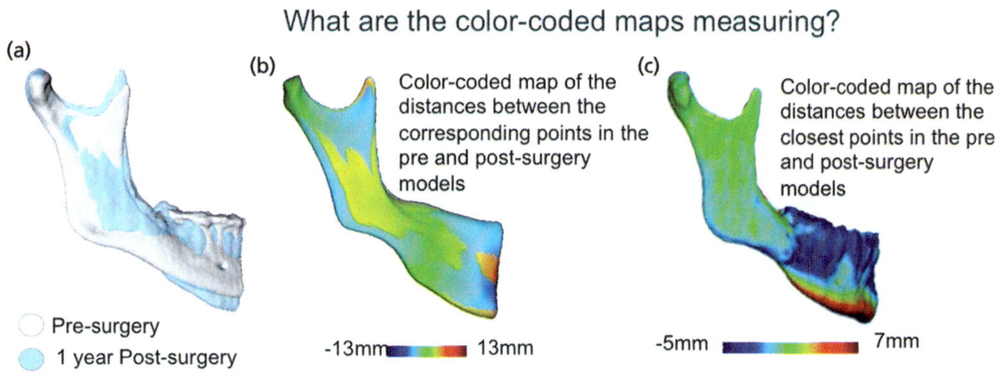

Fig. 8-10 Do you know how to interpret a colour-coded map? The superimposition was performed relative to the cranial base. (a) Overlay of pre-surgery (white) and one year post-surgery (blue) surface models. (b and c) Two different types of colour maps displayed in the 1-year post-surgery model. (b) Correspondent point based colour maps that reflect the pattern of bone changes shown in (a). (c) Closest point surface distance colour maps. Note that because the remodelling of the ramus was marked, the pattern of the closest point colour map does not reflect the actual remodelling/displacement changes and minimizes the measured surface changes.

Conclusions

The clinical use of CBCT imaging in orthodontics and orthognathic surgery now has guidelines proposed by European and American associations,[111,112] and the hardware for image acquisition as well as software for image analysis have continued to develop and evolve dramatically over the recent years. Careful image analysis requires combined multidisciplinary efforts among oral maxillofacial surgeons, orthodontists, radiologists and image analysis experts to properly interpret the wealth of information now available for clinicians.

References

1 Cevidanes LHS, Bailey LTJ, Tucker Jr. GR, Styner MA, Mol A, Phillips CL, Proffit WR. et al. Superimposition of 3D Cone-beam CT models of orthognathic surgery patients. Dentomaxillofacial Radiol. 2005;34:1–9.
2 Carvalho FdeA, Cevidanes LH, da Motta AT, Almeida MA, Phillips C. Three-dimensional assessment of mandibular advancement 1 year after surgery. Am J Orthod Dentofac Orthop. 2010;137(4Suppl): S53.e1–S53.e12.
3 Tucker S, Cevidanes LHS, Styner M, Kim H, Reyes M, Proffit W, Turvey T. Comparison of actual surgical outcomes and 3-dimensional surgical simulations. J Oral Maxillofac Surg. 2010;68(10):2412–21.
4 Molen AD. Considerations in the use of cone-beam computed tomography for buccal bone measurements. Am J Orthod Dentofac Orthop. 2010;137(4 Suppl):S130–5.
5 Leung CC, Palomo L, Griffith R. Hans MG. Accuracy and reliability of cone-beam computed tomography for measuring alveolar bone height and detecting bony dehiscences and fenestrations. Am J Orthod Dentofac Orthop. 2010;137(4 Suppl):S109–119.
6 Tai K, Hotokezak H, Park JH, Tai H, Miyajima K, Choi M, Kai LM, Mishimah K. Preliminary cone-beam computed tomography study evaluating dental and skeletal changes after treatment with a mandibular Schwarz appliance. Am J Orthod Dentofac Orthop. 2010;138(3):262.e1–262.e11.
7 Becker A, Chaushu C, Casap-Caspi N. Cone-beam computed tomography and the orthosurgical management of impacted teeth. J Am Dent Assoc. 2010;141;14S–18S.
8 Botticelli S, Verna C, Cattaneo PM, Heidmann J, Melsen B. Two- versus three-dimensional imaging in subjects with unerupted maxillary canines. Eur J Orthod. 2011;33: 344–9.
9 Katheria BC, Kau CH, Tate R, Chen J-W, English J, Bouquot J. Effectiveness of impacted and supernumerary tooth diagnosis from traditional radiography versus cone beam computed tomography. Ped Dent. 2010;32(4):304–309.
10 Leuzinger M, Dudic A, Giannopoulou C, Killaridis S. Root-contact evaluation by panoramic radiography and cone-beam computed tomography of super-high resolution. Am J Orthod Dentofac Orthop. 2010;137(3):389–92.
11 Tamimi D, ElSaid K. Cone beam computed tomography in the assessment of dental impactions. Semin Orthod. 2009;15:57–62.
12 Van Elslande D, Heo G, Flores-Mir C, Carey J, Major PW. Accuracy of mesiodistal root angulation projected by cone-beam computed tomographic panoramic-like images. Am J Orthod Dentofac Orthop. 2010;137(4 Suppl):S94–S99.
13 Shemesh H, Cristescu RC, Wesslink PR, Wu M-K. The use of cone-beam computed tomography and digital periapical radiographs to diagnose root perforations. JOE. 2011;37(4):513–6.
14 Sherrard JF, Rossouw PE, Benson BW, Carrillo R, Buschang PH. Accuracy and reliability of tooth and root lengths measured on cone-beam computed tomographs. Am J Orthod Dentofac Orthop. 2010;137(4 Suppl):S100–S108.
15 Treil J, Braga J, Loubes J-M, Maza E, Inglese J-M, Casteigt J, Waysenson B. 3D tooth modeling for orthodontic assessment. Semin Orthod. 2009;15:42–47.
16 Ahmad M, Hollender L, Anderson Q, Kartha K, Ohrbach RK, Truelove EL, John MT, Schiffman EL. Research diagnostic criteria for temporomandibular disorders (RDC/TMD): development of image analysis criteria and examiner reliability for image analysis. Oral Surg Oral Med Oral Pathol Oral Radiol Endod. 2009;107(6):844–60.
17 Alexiou K, Stamatakis H, Tsiklakis K. Evaluation of the severity of temporomandibular joint osteoarthritic changes related to age using cone beam computed tomography. Dentomaxillofac Radiol. 2009;38(3):141–7.
18 Helenius LM, Hallikainen D, Helenius I, Meurman JH, Könönen M, Leirisalo-Repo M, Lindqvist C. Clinical and radiographic findings of the temporomandibular joint in patients with various rheumatic diseases: A case control study. Oral Surg Oral Med Oral Pathol Oral Radiol Endod. 2005;99:455–63.
19 Koyama J, Nishiyama H, Hayashi T. Follow-up study of condylar bony changes using helical computed tomography in patients with temporomandibular disorder. Dentomaxillofac Radiol. 2007;36:472–7.

20 S.F. Dworkin and L. LeResche, Research diagnostic criteria for temporomandibular disorders: review, criteria, examinations, and specifications, critique. J Craniomandib Disord. 1992;6:301–55.
21 Schiffman EL, Ohrbach R, Truelove EL, Tai F, Anderson GC, Pan W, Gonzalez YM, John MT, Sommers E, List T, Velly AM, Kang W, Look JO. The Research Diagnostic Criteria for Temporomandibular Disorders. V: methods used to establish and validate revised Axis I diagnostic algorithms. J Orofac Pain. 2010;24(1):63–78.
22 Truelove E, Pan W, Look JO, Mancl LA, Ohrbach RK, Velly AM, Huggins KH, Lenton P, Shiffman EL. The Research Diagnostic Criteria for Temporomandibular Disorders. III: validity of Axis I diagnoses. J Orofac Pain. 2010;24(1):35–47.
23 Schiffman EL, Truelove EL, Ohrbach R, Anderson GC, John MT, List T, Look JO. The Research Diagnostic Criteria for Temporomandibular Disorders. I: overview and methodology for assessment of validity. J Orofac Pain. 2010;24(1):7–24.
24 Kapila S, Conley RS, Harrell Jr WE. The current status of cone beam computed tomography imaging in orthodontics. Dentomaxillofac Radiol. 2011;40:24–34.
25 Bryndahl F, Eriksson L, Legrell PE, Isberg A. Bilateral TMJ disk displacement induces mandibular retrognathia. J Dent Res. 2006;85:1118–23.
26 Ishida T, Yabushita T Soma K. Effects of a liquid diet on temporomandibular joint mechano-receptors. J Dent Res. 2009;88(2):187–91.
27 Blumberg TJ, Natoli RM, Athanasiou KA. Effects of doxycycline on articular cartilage GAG release and mechanical properties following impact. Biotechnol Bioeng. 2008; 100(3):506–15.
28 Burgin LV, Aspden RM. Impact testing to determine the mechanical properties of articular cartilage in isolation and on bone. J Mater Sci Mater Med. 2008;19(2):703–11.
29 Roemhildt ML, Coughlin KM, Peura GD, Badger GJ, Churchill D, Fleming BC Beynnon BD. Effects of increased chronic loading on articular cartilage material properties in the lapine tibio-femoral joint. J Biomech. 2010;43(12): 2301–8.
30 Scott CC, Athanasiou KA. Mechanical impact and articular cartilage. Crit Rev Biomed Eng. 2006;34(5), 347–78.
31 Verteramo A, Seedhom BB. Effect of a single impact loading on the structure and mechanical properties of articular cartilage. J Biomech. 2007;40(16):3580–9.
32 Gallo LM, Gössi DB, Colombo V, Palla S. Relationship between kinematic center and TMJ anatomy and function. J Dent Res. 2008;87(8):726–30.
33 Fredriksson L, Alstergren P. Kopp S. Tumor necrosis factor-alpha in temporomandibular joint synovial fluid predicts treatment effects on pain by intra-articular glucocorticoid treatment. Mediators Inflamm. 2006(6):594.
34 Nordahl S, Alstergren P, Eliasson S, Kopp S. Radiographic signs of bone destruction in the arthritic temporomandibular joint with special reference to markers of disease activity. A longitudinal study. Rheumatol (Oxford). 2001;40(6): 691–4.
35 Alstergren P and Kopp S. Prostaglandin E2 in temporomandibular joint synovial fluid and its relation to pain and inflammatory disorders. J Oral Maxillofac Surg. 2000;58(2):180–88.
36 Abramson Z, Susarla SM, Lawler M, Bouchard C, Troulis M, Kaban LB. Three-dimensional computed tomographic airway analysis of patients with obstructive sleep apnea treated by maxillomandibular advancement. J Oral Maxillofac Surg. 2011;69(3):677–86.
37 Schendel S, Powell N, Jacobson R. Maxillary, mandibular, and chin advancement: treatment planning based on airway anatomy in obstructive sleep apnea. J Oral Maxillofac Surg. 2011;69(3):663–76.
38 Iwasaki T, Saitoh I, Takemoto Y, Inada E, Kanomi R, Hayasaki H, Yamasaki Y. Evaluation of upper airway obstruction in Class II children with fluid-mechanical simulation. Am J Orthod Dentofacial Orthop. 2011;139(2): e135–45.
39 Schendel SA, Hatcher D. Automated 3-dimensional airway analysis from cone-beam computed tomography data. J Oral Maxillofac Surg. 2010;68(3):696–701.
40 Conley RS. Evidence for dental and dental specialty treatment of obstructive sleep apnoea. Part 1: the adult OSA patient and Part 2: the paediatric and adolescent patient. J Oral Rehabil. 2011;38(2):136–56.
41 Lenza MG, Lenza MM, Dalstra M, Melsen B, Cattaneo PM. An analysis of different approaches to the assessment of upper airway morphology: a CBCT study. Orthod Craniofac Res. 2010;13(2):96–105.
42 El H, Palomo JM. Measuring the airway in 3 dimensions: a reliability and accuracy study. Am J Orthod Dentofacial Orthop. 2010;137(4 Suppl):S50.e1–9; discussion S50–2.
43 Agarwal R. Anthropometric evaluation of complete unilateral cleft lip nose with cone beam CT in early childhood. J Plast Reconstr Aesthet Surg. 2011 March 24.
44 Behnia H, Khojasteh A, Soleimani M, Tehranchi A, Atashi A. Repair of alveolar cleft defect with mesenchymal stem cells and platelet derived growth factors: a preliminary report. J Craniomaxillofac Surg. 2011 March 17.
45 Dalessandri D, Laffranchi L, Tonni I, Zoti F, Piancino MG, Paganelli C, Bracco P. Advantages of cone beam computed tomography (CBCT) in the orthodontic treatment planning of cleidocranial dysplasia patients: a case report. Head Face Med. 2011;27:7–6.
46 Ebner FH, Kürschner V, Dietz K, Bültmann E, Nägele T, Honegger J. Craniometric changes in patients with acromegaly from a surgical perspective. Neurosurg Focus. 2010;29(4):E3.
47 Edwards SP. Computer-assisted craniomaxillofacial surgery. Oral Maxillofac Surg Clin North Am. 2010;22(1): 117–34.
48 Jayaratne YSN, Zwahllen RA, Lo J, Cheung LK. Three-dimensional color maps: A novel tool for assessing craniofacial changes. Surg Innov. 2010;17:198 originally published online 11 June 2010.
49 Kim Y-I, Park S-B, Son W-S, Hwang D-S. Midfacial soft-tissue changes after advancement of maxilla with Le Fort I osteotomy and mandibular setback surgery: comparison of conventional and high Le Fort osteotomies by superimposition of cone-beam computed tomography volumes. J Oral Maxillofac Surg. 2011 April 14.
50 Abou-Elfetouh A, Barakat A, Abdel-Ghany K. Computed-guided rapid-prototyped templates for segmental mandibular osteotomies: a preliminary report. Int J Med Robot. 2011 March 16.
51 Lloyd TE, Drage NA, Cronin AJ. The role of cone beam computed tomography in the management of unfavourable fractures following sagittal split mandibular osteotomy. J Orthod. 2011;38(1):48–54.
52 Gateno J, Xia JJ, Teichgraeber JF. New 3-dimensional cephalometric analysis for orthognathic surgery. J Oral Maxillofac Surg. 2011;69(3):606–22.
53 Almeida RC, Cevidanes LH, Carvalho FA, Motta AT, Almeida MA, Styner M, Turvey T, Proffit WR, Phillips C. Soft tissue response to mandibular advancement using 3D CBCT scanning. Int. J Oral Maxillofac Surg. 2011;40(4): 353–9.
54 Cevidanes LHC, Tucker S, Styner M, Kim H, Chapuis J, Reyes M. Proffit W, Turvey T, Jaskolka M. Three-dimensional surgical simulation. Am J Orthod Dentofac Orthop. 2010;138(3):361–71.
55 Orentlicher G, Goldsmith D, Horowitz A. Applications of 3-dimensional virtual computerized tomography technology in oral and maxillofacial surgery: current therapy. J Oral Maxillofac Surg. 2010;68(8):1993–59.
56 Jayaratne YS, Zwahlen RA, Lo J, Tam SC, Cheung LK. Computer-aided maxillofacial surgery: an update. Surg Innov. 2010;17(3):217–25.

57 Popat H, Richmond S. New developments in: three-dimensional planning for orthognathic surgery. J Orthod. 2010;37(1):62–71.
58 Schendel SA, Lane C. 3D orthognathic surgery simulation using image fusion. Semin Orthod. 2009;15:48–56.
59 CMFApp software (http://co-me.ch/) accessed as of March 16, 2016.
60 3DSlicer software (http://www.slicer.org/) accessed March 16, 2016.
61 Yushkevich PA, Piven J, Hazlett HC, Smith RG, Ho S, Gee JC, et al. User-guided 3D active contour segmentation of anatomical structures: significantly improved efficiency and reliability. Neuroimage. 2006;31(3):1116–28.
62 Swennen GR, Mollemans W, De Clercq C, Abeloos J, Lamoral P, Lippens F, et al. A Cone-Beam Computed Tomography Triple Scan Procedure to Obtain a Three-Dimensional Augmented Virtual Skull Model Appropriate for Orthognathic Surgery Planning. J Craniofac Surg. 2009;20(2):297–307.
63 Pommert A, Riemer M, Schiemann T, Schubert R, Tiede U, Hohne KH. Three-Dimensional Imaging in Medicine: Methods and Applications. R Taylor, S Lavallee, G Burdea, and R Mosges, Eds. Computer Integrated Surgery MIT Press Cambridge, MA. 1996:155–74.
64 Cutting CB, Bookstein FL, Taylor RH. Applications of Simulation, Morphometrics, and Robotics in Craniofacial Surgery. R Taylor, S Lavallee, G Burdea, and R Mosges, editors, Computer Integrated Surgery MIT press Cambridge, MA, 1996:641–62.
65 Subsol G, Thirion JP, Ayache N. A scheme for automatically building three-dimensional morphometric anatomical atlases: application to a skull atlas. Med Image Anal. 1998;2(1):37–60.
66 Chapuis J. Computer-Aided Cranio-Maxillofacial Surgery. PhD thesis, University of Bern. 2006.
67 Chapuis J, Schramm A, Pappas I, Hallermann W, Schwenzer-Zimmerer K, Langlotz F, et al. A new system for computer-aided preoperative planning and intraoperative navigation during corrective jaw surgery. IEEE Trans Inf Technol Biomed. 2007;11(3):274–87.
68 De Momi E, Chapuis J, Pappas I, Ferrigno G, Hallermann W, Schramm A, et al. Automatic extraction of the mid-facial plane for cranio-maxillofacial surgery planning. Int J Oral Maxillofac Surg. 2006;35(7):636–42.
69 Krol Z, Chapuis J, Schwenzer-Zimmerer K, Langlotz F, Zeilhofer HF. Preoperative planning and intraoperative navigation in the reconstructive craniofacial surgery. J Med Inform Tech. 2005;9:83–9.
70 Chapuis J, Langlotz F, Blaeuer M, Hallermann W, Schramm A, Caversaccio M. A Novel Approach for Computer-Aided Corrective Jaw Surgery. 3rd International Conference on Computer-Aided Surgery around the Head, Berlin, Germany, 2005 August.
71 Chapuis J, Ryan P, Blaeuer M, Langlotz F, Hallermann W, Schramm A, et al. A new approach for 3D computer-assisted orthognathic surgery – first clinical case. Computer Assisted Radiology and Surgery, Berlin, Germany. 2005 June.
72 Schutyser F, Van Cleynenbreugel J, Ferrant M, Schoenaers J, Suetens P. Image-based 3D planning of maxillofacial distraction procedures including soft tissue implications. Med Image Comput Comput-Assist Intervent. 2000;1935:999–1007.
73 Xia J, Samman N, Yeung RW, Shen SG, Wang D, Ip HH, et al. Three-dimensional virtual reality surgical planning and simulation workbench for orthognathic surgery. Int J Adult Orthod Orthognath Surg. 2000;15(4):265–82.
74 Teschner M, Girod S, Girod B. 3-D simulation of craniofacial surgical procedures. Stud Health Technol Inform. 2001;81:502–8.
75 Keeve E, Girod B, Girod S. Computer-Aided Craniofacial Surgery. HU Lemke (Ed.) Computer Assisted Radiology. Paris, France, 1996.
76 Mollemans W, Schutyser F, Nadjmi N, Maes F, Suetens P. Predicting soft tissue deformations for a maxillofacial surgery planning system: from computational strategies to a complete clinical validation. Med Image Anal. 2007;11(3):282–301.
77 Westermark A, Zachow S, Eppley BL. Three-dimensional osteotomy planning in maxillofacial surgery including soft tissue prediction. J Craniofac Surg. 2005;16(1):100–4.
78 Chabanas M, Luboz V, Payan Y. Patient specific finite element model of the face soft tissues for computer-assisted maxillofacial surgery. Med Image Anal. 2003;7(2):131–51.
79 Schendel SA, Montgomery K. A web-based, integrated simulation system for craniofacial surgical planning. Plast Reconstr Surg. 2009;123(3):1009–1106.
80 Keeve E, Girod S, Kikinis R, Girod B. Deformable modeling of facial tissue for craniofacial surgery simulation. Comput Aided Surg. 1998;3(5):228–38.
81 Zachow S, Gladilin E, Zeilhofer HF, Sader R. Improved 3D Osteotomy Planning in Craniomaxillofacial Surgery. Medical Image Computing and Computer-Assisted Intervention: 4th International Conference Ultrecht, The Netherlands, 2001 October.
82 Gladilin E, Zachow S, Deuflhard P, Hege HC. Anatomy- and physics-based facial animation for craniofacial surgery simulations. Med Biol Eng Comput. 2004;42(2):167–70.
83 Gateno J, Teichgraeber JF, Xia JJ. Three-dimensional surgical planning for maxillary and midface distraction osteogenesis. J Craniofac Surg. 2003;14(6):833–9.
84 Vandewalle P, Schutyser F, Van Cleynenbreugel J, Suetens P. Modeling of Facial Soft Tissue Growth for Maxillofacial Surgery Planning Environments. IS4TH. 2003:27–37.
85 Langlotz F. Localizers and trackers for computer assisted freehand navigation. In: F. Picard, L-P Nolte, A.M. Digiola, B. Jamaraz, editors, Hip and Knee Surgery – Navigation, Robotics, and Computer Assisted Surgical Tools, pp. 51–53. Oxford University Press, 2004.
86 Kim H, Jurgen P, Krol Z, Caversaccio M, Nolte LP, Zeilhofer HF, Gonzales MA. Clinical applications of computer-aided planning and navigation system for cranio-maxillofacial surgery. CAS-H 2009. Leipzig, Germany, Book of Abstracts.
87 Adams R, Bischof L. 'Seeded Region Growing,' IEEE Trans Pattern Anal Machine Intellig. 1994;16:641–7.
88 Ma WY, Manjunath BS. 'Edge Flow: A Technique for Boundary Detection and Image Segmentation,' IEEE Trans. Image Process. 2000;9:1375–88.
89 Lie WN. 'Automatic Target Segmentation by Locally Adaptive Image Thresholding, IEEE Trans. Image Process. 1995;4:1036–41.
90 Moon N, Bullitt E, Leemput K, Gerig G. Model-Based Brain and Tumor Segmentation, Proc. 16th Int Conf on Pattern Recognition ICPR 2002, editors: R. Kasturi, D. Laurendeau, C. Suen, IEEE Computer Society, Aug. 2002, pp. 528–31.
91 Gerig G, Prastawa M, Lin W, Gilmore J. 'Assessing Early Brain Development in Neonates by Segmentation of High-Resolution 3T MRI', SHORT PAPER, Lecture Notes in Computer Science LNCS #2879, pp. 979–80, Nov. 2003.
92 Crum WR, Hartkens T, Hill DL. Non-rigid image registration: theory and practice. Br J Radiol. 2004;77 Spec No 2:S140–53.
93 Christensen GE, Rabbitt RD, Miller MI. Deformable templates using large deformation kinematics. IEEE Trans Image Process. 1996;5:1435–47.
94 Rueckert D, Sonoda LI, Hayes C, Hill DLG, Leach MO, Hawkes DJ. Nonrigid registration using free-form deformations: application to breast MR images. IEEE Trans Med Imag. 1999;18:712–21.
95 Hajnal JV, Hill DLG, Hawkes DJ, editors. In: Medical image registration. CRC Press Boca Raton, 2001.
96 Thompson PM, MacDonald D, Mega MS, Holmes CJ, Evans AC, Toga AW. Detection and mapping of abnormal brain structure with a probabilistic atlas of cortical surfaces. J Comput Assist Tomogr. 1997; 21:567–81.

97 Maes F, Collignon A, Vandermeulen D, Marchal G, Suetens P. Multimodality image registration by maximization of mutual information. IEEE Trans Med Imag. 1997;16:187–98.
98 Cevidanes LHS, Bailey LTJ, Tucker Jr. GR, Styner MA, Mol A, Phillips CL, Proffit WR, et al. Superimposition of 3D Cone-beam CT models of orthognathic surgery patients. Dentomaxillofacial Radiol. 2005;34:1–9.
99 Cevidanes LHS, Phillips CL, Tulloch, JFC, Proffit WR. Superimposition of 3D Cone-beam CT Models of Orthognathic Surgery Patients. In: McNamara JA (Ed.) 3D Imaging. Moyers Symposium Series, 2005.
100 Cevidanes LHS, Styner MA, Proffit WR. Image analysis and superimposition of 3D cone-beam CT models. Am J Orthod Dentofacial Orthop. 2006;129(5):611–8.
101 Rohr K. Landmark-based image analysis: using geometric and intensity models. Volume 21 of Computational Imaging and Vision Series. Dordrecht, Boston, London: Kluwer Academic Publishers, 2001.
102 Dean D, Hans MG, Bookstein FL and Subramanyan K. Three-dimensional Bolton-Brush Growth Study landmark data: ontogeny and sexual dimorphism of the Bolton Standards cohort, Cleft Palate Craniofac J. 2000;37:145–55.
103 Bookstein FL. Morphometric tools for landmark data (1st edn.) Cambridge University Press, Cambridge (1991), p. 435.
104 Gunz P, Mitteroecker P, Bookstein FL. Semi-landmarks in three dimensions. In: Slice DL, editor. Modern morphometrics in physical anthropology. New York: Kluwer Academic Publishers, 2004.
105 Andresen R, Bookstein FL, Conradsen K, Ersboll BK, Marsh JL, Kreiborg S. Surface-bounded growth modeling applied to human mandibles. IEEE Trans Med Imag. 2000;19:1053–63.
106 Gerig G, Jomier M, Chakos M. Valmet: a new validation tool for assessing and improving 3D object segmentation. In: Niessen W, Viergever M (Eds). MICCAI 2001: Proceedings of the International Society and Conference Series on Medical Image Computing and Computer-Assisted Intervention; 2001 Oct 14–17; Utrecht, Netherlands. Berlin: Springer; 2001. pp.516–528.
107 Styner M, Oguz I, Xu S, Brechbuhler C, Pantazis D, Levitt J, Shenton ME, Gerig G. Framework for the statistical shape analysis of brain structures using Spharm-PDM. Special edition open science workshop at MICCAI. Insight J 2006;1–7. Available at: http://hdl.handle.net/1926/215.
108 Gerig G, Styner M, Jones D, Weinberger D, Lieberman J. Shape analysis of brain ventricles using Spharm. MMBIA Proceedings. IEEE 2001; 171–8.
109 Paniagua B, Cevidanes L, Walker D, Zhu H, Guo R, Styner M. Clinical application of SPHARM-PDM to quantify temporomandibular joint arthritis. Comput Med Imaging Graph. 2011;35(5):345–52.
110 Paniagua B, Cevidanes L, Zhu H, Styner M. Outcome quantification using SPHARM-PDM toolbox in orthognathic surgery. Int J Comput Assist Radiol Surg. 2011;6(5):617–26.
111 European Commission. Item 4.2 the Developing Dentition in Protection Radiation No. 172. Cone Beam CT for Dental and Maxillofacial Radiology (Evidence-based Guidelines). (2011), pp. 45–56 Available at: http://ec.europa.eu/energy/nuclear/radiation_protection/doc/publication/172.pdf Accessed Jan 4, 2014.
112 American Academy of Oral and Maxillofacial Radiology: Evans CA, Scarfe WC, Ahmad M, Cevidanes LHS, Ludlow JB, Palomo JM, Simmons KE, White, SC. Clinical recommendations regarding use of cone beam computed tomography in orthodontic treatment. Position statement by the American Academy of Oral and Maxillofacial Radiology. Oral Surg Oral Med Oral Pathol Oral Radiol. 2013;116:238–57.

Chapter 9

Psychological Evaluation and Body Dysmorphic Disorder

Katharine A. Phillips and Canice E. Crerand

Introduction

Surgeons who perform orthognathic procedures need to be familiar with a common and usually severe body image disorder known as body dysmorphic disorder (BDD). Patients with BDD have a distorted view of their appearance, believing that they look abnormal or deformed in some way when they actually do not. A majority of these patients seek and receive cosmetic procedures, including orthognathic surgery, for their perceived appearance defects. This is problematic, because available data indicate that cosmetic treatment usually does not improve BDD symptoms, and individuals with this disorder are typically disappointed with the results. In fact, some patients are so dissatisfied with an objectively acceptable surgical outcome that they sue or are even violent toward the surgeon.

This chapter describes BDD's prevalence, its key clinical features, a patient with BDD, and both ineffective and effective treatment approaches. We also discuss how surgeons can approach these patients so as to improve outcomes for both patient and surgeon.

Prevalence of BDD

Findings from three nationwide epidemiological studies suggest that BDD affects 1.7–2.4% of the general population.[1–3] Among college student samples, BDD's prevalence ranges from 1.3–13%.[4–9] Higher rates have been reported among cosmetic surgery and dermatology patients, due in part to the fact that persons with BDD frequently seek and receive cosmetic treatments to try to correct their perceived appearance 'defects.'[10–13] In dermatology samples, BDD's prevalence ranges from 6.7–14%.[14–17] In cosmetic surgery samples in the U.S., a prevalence of 7–8% has been reported,[18,19] whereas a prevalence of 2.9–53% has been found in international cosmetic surgery populations.[20–33] This broad range is likely accounted for, at least in part, by methodological differences (e.g.,

Orthognathic Surgery: Principles, Planning and Practice. Edited by Farhad B. Naini and Daljit S. Gill.

use of clinical interviews vs. self-report questionnaires vs. validated measures to assess BDD symptoms) and limitations (e.g., small sample size, selection biases). Nonetheless, these studies suggest that BDD is relatively common among individuals presenting for cosmetic procedures.

Case reports have described patients with BDD in dental practices[33,34] and maxillofacial surgery populations.[35,36] One study found that 7.5% of 40 adults seeking orthodontic treatment had BDD.[37] In a study of cosmetic dentistry patients, 9.5% of 91 patients were diagnosed with BDD.[38] Although a small prospective study of 30 patients seeking orthognathic surgery found that none met diagnostic criteria for BDD,[39] a larger study of 160 patients presenting for maxillofacial procedures reported that 10% had BDD.[27] Such findings underscore the importance of understanding BDD and its presentation in these settings, especially since patients with the disorder typically report dissatisfaction with treatment outcomes.

Definition and clinical features of BDD

Definition of BDD

Individuals with BDD (formerly known as 'dysmorphophobia') are preoccupied with one or more perceived defects or flaws in their appearance that to other people are not observable or appear only slight.[40] Patients may use terms such as ugly, unattractive, not right, hideous, or monstrous to describe the disliked body areas. To qualify for a diagnosis of BDD, the preoccupation must cause clinically significant distress or impairment in psychosocial functioning (e.g., social, academic, occupational). In addition, patients must perform one or more excessive repetitive behaviours in response to the appearance concerns, such as excessive mirror checking, excessive grooming, seeking reassurance about how they look, or frequently comparing their appearance to that of other people.[40]

Body areas of concern

BDD preoccupations most often involve the face or head. However, any body area can be the focus of concern, and concern with multiple areas is the norm.[41] The most common areas of concern are the skin (e.g., perceived scarring, acne, colour, wrinkles, marks), hair (e.g., perceived thinning; 'ugly' texture or colour), and nose (e.g., size or shape).[41] In two studies (N = 200 and N = 188), 17% of patients were preoccupied with the appearance of their chin or jaw.[41,42] Twenty percent were preoccupied with the appearance of their teeth and 6% with their mouth. An additional 14% were preoccupied with the appearance of their overall face and an additional 12% with the size or shape of their face, which in some cases involved the structure of the chin/jaw area. More than 25% of individuals with BDD have at least one concern that involves asymmetry (e.g., asymmetric eyes or jaw line).[43]

Core BDD symptoms

Preoccupations and distress

Thoughts about the disliked body areas are intrusive, unwanted, and distressing. They occur, on average, for 3–8 hours a day and sometimes occur for most of a person's waking hours; thus, they are sometimes referred to as 'obsessions.'[44] The preoccupations are usually difficult to resist and control.[44,45] They trigger anxiety, distress, shame, depressed mood, or other painful emotions.[44,45]

Insight

Of particular relevance to surgeons, most individuals with BDD – prior to effective treatment – have poor or absent insight. That is, a majority of patients are completely or mostly convinced that their view of their 'defect' is accurate (complete conviction is also referred to as 'delusional thinking').[41,42] Even if other people tell them that the defect is not visible and that the patient looks normal, the patient typically does not believe this. As a result, many patients do not accept that they have a psychiatric disorder, and they seek cosmetic treatment rather than psychiatric treatment.

Excessive repetitive behaviours

The appearance preoccupations and distressing emotions drive patients to perform excessive, repetitive (sometimes referred to as 'compulsive') behaviours.[44,45] All individuals with BDD, at some time during the course of the disorder, perform these behaviours, which are difficult to control and time-consuming, occurring, on average, for 3 to 8 hours a day.[44,45] Although patients perform these behaviours in order to alleviate their emotional distress, the behaviours often exacerbate their distress.[45]

The repetitive behaviours are usually behavioural (observable) but may also be mental.[41,42] The most common mental compulsion is comparing the disliked body parts with same body parts of other people (including those of the surgeon and his/her office staff). Common excessive behaviours include checking the disliked body parts by looking at them (often at very close range) in mirrors or other reflecting surfaces, or directly; excessively grooming (e.g., cutting, styling, or shaving hair); seeking reassurance or questioning others about how the disliked body areas look; and compulsively seeking and/or receiving cosmetic procedures.[41,42] Additional behaviours include compulsive skin picking (to remove perceived acne) and hair plucking, excessively touching the disliked areas to check them, excessively changing clothes (e.g., to more effectively camouflage disliked areas), compulsively shopping (e.g., for make-up, skin or hair products, or clothes to minimize the 'flaws'), dieting, and excessively exercising or lifting weights to build muscle.[41,42] About one quarter of patients compulsively tan (e.g., to darken 'pale' skin), which can cause burns and increase the risk of skin cancer.[45] Camouflaging one's perceived flaws (e.g., with a hat, makeup, sunglasses, hair, clothes, body position), which more than 90% of patients with BDD do, can be done repeatedly (e.g., reapplying make-up 20 times a day).[45]

Psychosocial functioning and quality of life

Patients with BDD typically have very poor psychosocial functioning and quality of life.[46] On standardized measures of these constructs, individuals with BDD typically score several standard deviation units below normative scores.[46] More severe BDD symptoms are associated with poorer functioning and quality of life.[46] Impairment in functioning can range from moderate (e.g., avoiding dating and some social events but able to attend some social events and school) to extreme and incapacitating (e.g., unable to work, attend school, or have any relationships).[45] Nearly one-third of those with BDD have been completely housebound for at least one week because of BDD;[41] some are housebound for years because they feel too ugly to be seen.[45] Nearly 40% of individuals with BDD have been psychiatrically hospitalized, and more than one quarter attributes at least one psychiatric hospitalization primarily to BDD.[42]

Associated features of BDD

Referential thinking

A majority of individuals with BDD have ideas or delusions of reference (also referred to as 'referential thinking').[41,42] This consists of the false belief that other people take special notice of the patient in a negative way because of how they look (e.g., mock, talk about, or stare at them).[41]

Associated symptoms

Patients with BDD typically have symptoms such as low self-esteem and high levels of social anxiety and avoidance, anxiety, and depressed mood.[45,47] Many individuals are ashamed of their appearance concerns because they worry that other people will consider them vain.[45]

Suicidality

In both clinical and epidemiologic samples, rates of suicidal ideation and suicide attempts appear very high.[3,41,48] Patients often attribute their suicidality to the suffering that BDD causes. Although data on the rate of completed suicide in BDD is minimal, it appears markedly elevated and perhaps even higher than that in depression, bipolar disorder, and other serious mental disorders.[49]

Co-occurring disorders

The most common co-occurring disorders are major depressive disorder, substance use disorders (which often appears to consist of self-medication, secondary to the distress that BDD causes), social anxiety disorder, and obsessive-compulsive disorder.[41,50]

Age at onset and course of illness

BDD usually onsets in early adolescence; two-thirds of individuals have onset before age 18.[51] The disorder appears to usually be chronic, with a high relapse rate among those who remit.[52] However, a majority of patients improve when they receive evidence-based psychiatric treatment (see below).

A patient with BDD

J, a 35-year-old single white male, had been obsessed with his 'funny-looking jaw and chin' since early adolescence. He believed that they 'stuck out' and made the overall shape of his face and head appear abnormal. Even though other people reassured J that he looked normal, J was convinced that he looked 'like a freak.' He thought about these perceived defects for 6–7 hours a day, and he spent 4–5 hours a day performing excessive compulsive behaviours such as comparing his jaw and chin with that of other people, asking his friends if he looked okay, and repeatedly checking his jaw and chin in the mirror and other reflecting surfaces while moving them into various positions to try to make them look better. As a result of these preoccupations, J became anxious and depressed to the point that he had thoughts that life wasn't worth living. He found it difficult to concentrate on his job and was often late for work because it was difficult to leave the mirror. His job performance declined, and he avoided many social situations because he didn't want other people to see him and thought people laughed at his jaw. J consulted five surgeons, none of whom agreed to perform the procedure he requested.

Treatment of BDD

Cosmetic treatment

Because individuals with BDD are typically so distressed and impaired by their perceived appearance defects, and because their insight is usually poor or absent, it is not surprising that many seek cosmetic treatment. Cosmetic surgical procedures and dermatologic treatments[10–13] are most often sought and received by persons with BDD. A study of 250 adults with BDD found that 76% sought cosmetic treatment to fix their perceived 'defects,' and 66% actually received cosmetic treatments.[12] In a study of 200 individuals with BDD, 71% sought and 64% received such treatment.[10] In both studies, dermatologic procedures such as topical acne agents and cosmetic surgical procedures, including rhinoplasty and jaw surgery, were among the most commonly sought and received treatments; dental procedures such as teeth whitening, oral surgery, and braces were also requested and received. Consistent with clinical reports of 'polysurgical addicts'[53] and 'surgiholics,'[54] individuals with BDD often undergo multiple cosmetic treatments, sometimes even on the same feature.[56] Some patients are so desperate to correct perceived defects that they engage in 'do-it-yourself' procedures or injure themselves (e.g., using a hammer to break one's nose) so surgery would then be necessary.[12,45,56]

There is little evidence that cosmetic treatments improve BDD, and patients frequently express dissatisfaction with treatment outcomes.[10,12,13,45,55,56] Although persons with BDD may report temporary improvements in the appearance of the treated body part,[55] over time cosmetic treatments typically produce no change or, even worse, an exacerbation of BDD symptoms.[10,53,55,56] For example, in a study of cosmetic treatment among persons with BDD, only 3.6% of 528 procedures resulted in improvement in overall BDD symptoms.[10] Similarly, another study found that although 43% of procedures led to temporary improvements in appearance and/or preoccupation with the treated body part, these gains were not sustained, and only 2.3% of 87 procedures improved overall BDD symptoms over the longer-term.[55] It is possible that the differences in ratings of temporary vs. longer-term improvement, and different findings for improvement in appearance of the treated body part specifically vs. overall BDD severity, are due to the fact that persons with BDD are typically preoccupied with multiple body parts,[41] and preoccupation with other, untreated 'defects' persists after cosmetic treatment. In addition, persons with BDD frequently report that their appearance concerns shift from one body part to another following cosmetic procedures, which might also contribute to a lack of change in overall BDD severity.[56,57]

Similar results were found in a small prospective study of 24 cosmetic surgery patients who had requested treatment of minimal defects, ten of whom had been diagnosed with BDD prior to surgery. At a 5-year follow-up evaluation, seven of the ten patients with BDD had received cosmetic surgery;[57] only one of the patients who underwent cosmetic surgery experienced a remission from BDD symptoms. The remaining six patients continued to meet criteria for BDD, and five of them developed new appearance concerns. A recent prospective study of 166 persons seeking rhinoplasty found that greater preoperative BDD-like symptoms were predictive of lower satisfaction with treatment outcome and quality of life postoperatively.[58] Although only three patients in this study met criteria for BDD, these findings demonstrate that even subclinical BDD symptoms can have a negative impact on patient satisfaction postoperatively. Additionally, another prospective study of 161 persons with BDD found that receipt of cosmetic treatments did not predict remission from BDD symptoms at 1-year follow-up.[59]

Taken together,[60] these findings suggest that surgeons and other providers of cosmetic treatment should be aware that temporary improvements following cosmetic treatment appear unlikely to be maintained and that longer-term outcomes appear to typically be poor. Indeed, in a survey of 265 cosmetic surgeons, 178 reported having operated on a patient with BDD, with only 1% of cases resulting in BDD improvement.[60]

Of interest, the most common reason for non-receipt of desired cosmetic procedures is physician refusal,[10,12] which suggests that physicians may know or suspect that a patient has BDD or is not a good candidate for cosmetic treatment. However, regarding surgical and minimally invasive treatment specifically, cost is the most common reason such treatment is not received by persons with BDD.[55] And compared to other treatment providers (e.g., dermatologists), surgeons appear to be *less* likely to refuse to perform procedures on persons with BDD.[55] This finding suggests that some surgeons may be missing signs of BDD preoperatively. It could also reflect that some surgeons do not believe that it is inappropriate to operate on patients with BDD. According to a survey of 265 surgeons, only 30% reported that operating on a patient with BDD was always contraindicated.[60,61]

Performing cosmetic procedures on persons with BDD can present risks for treatment providers. Patients with BDD can be demanding and difficult for surgeons and office staff to manage. Even more concerning, case reports describe patients with BDD who have threatened or sued their treatment providers.[60,62,63] A survey of 265 cosmetic surgeons found that 40% had been threatened by a patient with BDD: 29% had been threatened legally, 2% had been threatened physically, and 10% had been threatened both legally and physically.[60] Some patients with BDD fantasize about harming their surgeon, and some individuals with apparent BDD have even murdered their treatment providers.[64–66] Given these safety concerns, coupled with the evidence that cosmetic treatments rarely improve BDD, BDD should be considered a contraindication for cosmetic treatments.[61,67–69]

Psychiatric treatment

Two types of treatment are efficacious for BDD: serotonin-reuptake inhibitors (SRIs, SSRIs) and cognitive-behavioural therapy that is tailored specifically to BDD. Some patients do well with either medication or CBT, whereas others (especially more severely ill patients) benefit from combining the two treatments.[45] There is no evidence that general counselling or supportive therapy are effective treatments for BDD.

Pharmacotherapy

Two blinded controlled trials (with fluoxetine and clomipramine) and four open-label trials (with fluvoxamine, escitalopram, and citalopram) have shown that SRIs often improve core BDD symptoms and associated features such as depression, anxiety, anger–hostility, psychosocial functioning, and quality of life.[45,70] SRIs may also protect against worsening of suicidality and decrease suicidal ideation in patients with BDD.[70] Although data are limited, SRIs appear more efficacious than non-SRI antidepressants or other types of medication.[45,70] SRI monotherapy also appears efficacious for patients with delusional BDD beliefs;[70–72] thus these patients should receive an SRI rather than antipsychotic monotherapy.

It is important to note that although data are limited, mean SRI doses that are often effective for treating BDD appear to be higher than those typically needed to treat many other disorders, such as depression.[45,70] Patients not uncommonly improve, or further improve, when the maximum SRI dose recommended by the manufacturer is reached or exceeded (although the latter should generally not be done with clomipramine and citalopram).[45,71] To determine whether a particular SRI will work, patients should be treated for 12 to 16 weeks while reaching a high dose (if needed and tolerated) for at least 2–4 of those weeks.[45,70]

Small open-label trials suggest that the serotonin-norepinephrine reuptake inhibitor venlafaxine and the antiepileptic medication levetiracetam may be helpful for BDD; however, because data are preliminary these medications are not currently recommended as first-line treatments.[70]

Cognitive-behavioural therapy

CBT is the best-studied psychosocial treatment for BDD; it has been shown to be efficacious in studies that used a waiting-list control group and in case series, although studies with better control groups are needed.[73–75] Effective CBT diminishes core BDD symptoms and associated symptoms such as depression. CBT must address BDD's unique symptoms; using CBT designed for obsessive-compulsive disorder, depression, or another disorder is unlikely to be successful. Because BDD can be difficult to treat and many therapists are not trained to provide the treatment, we recommend use of a treatment manual for BDD[76] by a therapist who has CBT training and experience.

CBT's core elements consist of cognitive restructuring to help patients develop more accurate and helpful beliefs and thoughts; exposure combined with behavioural experiments to decrease avoidance (e.g., of social situations); and ritual (response) prevention to decrease excessive repetitive behaviours.[76] Other recommended elements include perceptual retraining with mirrors, cognitive approaches that target core beliefs (e.g., 'I am worthless'), habit reversal for BDD-related skin picking or hair picking/plucking, and treatment of more severe depressive symptoms if needed.[76] If relevant to a particular patient, treatment should also address a desire for cosmetic treatment.[76] Motivational interviewing techniques are often needed to enhance motivation for treatment both initially and during the course of therapy.[76]

The number and frequency of sessions varies substantially in published reports,[45] but in the authors' clinical experience, most patients need at least six months of weekly hour-long treatment, combined with daily structured homework assignments. Patients should continue to practice CBT skills after treatment has ended, and additional (booster) sessions should be considered.

Assessment of patients with BDD

An estimated 10% of patients presenting for orthognathic surgery have BDD. This statistic, coupled with cosmetic surgery's increasing popularity, means that oral and maxillofacial surgeons are likely to encounter patients with BDD. It is therefore critically important for oral and maxillofacial surgeons to assess patients for BDD symptoms, particularly given the safety concerns associated with treating such patients.

Preoperative screening interview

A screening interview during the initial consultation can be an effective way of identifying patients with BDD. This interview can help safeguard providers against patients who could become litigious or violent; it also provides an opportunity to direct patients with BDD to more effective and appropriate psychiatric treatment. Patients should be informed that these questions are part of the practice's standard initial consultation procedures and are asked of all prospective patients. Such a statement can help reassure patients that they are not being 'singled out' and may encourage an honest disclosure of information.

This interview should include an assessment of (1) appearance concerns and BDD symptoms; (2) patient motivations and expectations for the desired procedure; (3) psychiatric status and history; and (4) observations of the patient's behaviour in the office.[61,67,69] Surgeons can also incorporate questions that focus on the first three items into their standard pre-visit assessment forms, which could be completed by patients before the initial consultation and reviewed together during the appointment.

1. Appearance concerns and BDD symptoms

Surgeons should query patients about their appearance concerns and ask diagnostic questions for BDD. These questions should focus on the following:

1. Is the patient preoccupied with the perceived flaw(s); do they think about it, in total, for at least an hour a day?
2. Does this preoccupation cause clinically significant distress – for example, anxiety, depression, sadness, hopelessness, or feelings that life isn't worth living? The surgeon can ask how upset the patient becomes when they think about their appearance, the emotions they experience, and how severe and prolonged the negative emotions are.

3. Does the preoccupation with perceived appearance flaws cause clinically significant impairment in functioning – for example, decrease in focus or concentration, or difficulty with or avoidance of social, family, school, or work activities?
4. Does the patient perform at least one excessive repetitive behaviour in response to the appearance concerns? As discussed above, these behaviours are either mental (such as comparing their appearance with that of other people) or behavioural, such as scrutinizing the feature of concern in the mirror or other reflecting surfaces; excessive grooming; skin picking; excessive use of make-up or other products; camouflaging the feature of concern with clothing, hats, hairstyles, body positioning; or over-emphasizing other features (e.g., dramatic hairstyle) to distract attention from the feature of concern.[41,42]

Patients with non-existent or minimal flaws who spend at least an hour a day preoccupied with perceived flaws, who experience resulting clinically significant distress or impairment in functioning, and who perform at least one associated repetitive behaviour have BDD.

Patients who present with concerns about minimal or slight defects in appearance (e.g., asymmetry that would typically only be noticeable to a trained professional) should be carefully assessed.[67,68] Although it is not uncommon for patients to present for correction of minimal or slight defects in appearance or for improvement of otherwise normal-appearing features, patients who present with these types of concerns should be asked the above questions. In cases where patients present with minimal or slight defects in appearance, the degree of distress they are reporting and the amount of functional impairment they are experiencing can help differentiate those with and without BDD.[67] For example, a patient who is so concerned about a minimal or slight defect that she refuses to attend school or leave her home likely meets criteria for BDD. In contrast, a patient with a minimal defect who reports feeling self-conscious in some situations but is otherwise functioning well most likely does not have BDD.

Patients with BDD are often secretive about and ashamed of their concerns and the extent of their preoccupation and distress. In our experience, some patients purposely minimize their symptoms in the hope that the surgeon will not discover that they have BDD and refuse to operate. Thus, it is not uncommon for BDD to go undetected preoperatively by surgeons.[60] We recommend that surgeons additionally assess the following 'red flags,' which can suggest that a patient has BDD:

- In general, patients should be able to discuss specific appearance concerns that are readily observable.[69] Patients who present with vague, nonspecific complaints (e.g., comments about being ugly or deformed, 'my jaw just doesn't look right') may have BDD.[67,68]
- Patients who express beliefs that other people are talking about them, laughing at them, or taking special notice of them because of their appearance 'defect' may have BDD.
- Repeated requests for reassurance about the perceived flaw, or insistence that the surgeon agree that the patient looks deformed, suggest that BDD may be present.
- Some patients with BDD bring drawings to the consultation that detail how they would like to change their appearance or photos of celebrities to illustrate their idea of perfection; such behaviours may indicate the extensive amount of time they spend obsessing about their appearance.
- Patients who request unusual procedures, especially when they seem unwarranted to the surgeon, may have BDD.
- Patients who have had multiple procedures on the same body part yet still express dissatisfaction with treatment outcomes may have BDD. Those who have had many previous cosmetic procedures should be carefully queried about their satisfaction with the prior procedures, the nature of their appearance concerns, BDD symptoms, and expectations for treatment outcomes.[77]
- When family members believe the patient should not have surgery, the surgeon should ask them about their concerns (if this is acceptable to the patient). Family members may be aware of signs such as the above, which the patient may be reluctant to reveal to the surgeon.

2. Motivation and expectations

Inquiring about a patient's motivations and expectations for surgery can yield important clues about BDD. Questions may include 'What made you decide to seek treatment at this time?' and 'What do you hope to accomplish by having surgery?' In general, patients should be able to clearly articulate their goals for surgery and express reasonable expectations for how surgery will affect their life. Patients with unrealistic expectations (e.g., believing that surgery will improve a troubled marriage or vastly increase popularity) or who make dramatic statements about how surgery will transform their lives may be suffering from BDD.[61,67,68]

3. Psychiatric history

Another key component of preoperative screening for BDD is information about the patient's psychiatric history.[61,67,69] BDD frequently co-occurs with other psychiatric disorders such as depression and anxiety disorders, and a patient who presents with current symptoms or has a history of being treated for these or other psychiatric disorders should be carefully assessed. Surgeons should directly ask about the patient's history of psychiatric and psychological treatment, including psychiatric hospitalization.

For patients with current symptoms of BDD or a history of psychiatric disorders or psychiatric hospitalization, a preoperative mental health evaluation is recommended before proceeding with surgery.[61,67,69] If a patient discloses that they are currently receiving psychiatric or psychological treatment, the surgeon or staff should request permission to contact the patient's mental health care provider in order to discuss the appropriateness of surgery. (However, surgeons should keep in mind that many patients with BDD do not divulge their BDD symptoms to their mental health clinician, and many clinicians are not familiar with BDD.) Surgeons should be cautious about proceeding with surgery if the patient refuses to allow contact with their mental health care provider.[61,67,69]

4. Office behaviour observations

Surgeons and their staff should pay attention to patients' behaviour in the office. Deviations from expected, typical behaviour may reveal clues about BDD or other psychopathology.[61,67,69] Demands for unusual appointment times (e.g., in the evening or early morning), repeated cancelling and rescheduling of appointments, excessive phone calls, angry or threatening demands to speak with the surgeon, or repeated reassurance seeking from staff about their appearance may be indicative of BDD.[67,68,76] Surgeons may be unaware of these behaviours, particularly if patients are 'on their best behaviour' during their consultation in hopes of convincing the surgeon to perform the desired procedure. Surgeons can consider asking patients to return for a follow-up consultation if the office staff raise concerns. A mental health evaluation is recommended if concerns persist about the patient's behaviour.

Screening questionnaires

In addition to conducting a clinical interview, brief screening instruments for BDD can be used. One such measure is the Body Dysmorphic Disorder Questionnaire-Dermatology Version (BDDQ-DV),[77] a reliable and valid self-report measure that maps onto DSM-IV diagnostic criteria. The Cosmetic Procedure Screening Questionnaire (COPS) is a 9-item instrument that is available to screen for BDD.[78] Both measures are free and available online. Patients who endorse symptoms consistent with BDD can be further screened during the initial consultation and referred to a mental health professional for additional evaluation and treatment.

How surgeons can approach patients with BDD

If the surgeon suspects that a patient has BDD, he/she is encouraged to inform the patient of their impressions and to provide some brief education about the disorder (e.g., 'It sounds like you have a body image problem known as body dysmorphic disorder, a known and treatable condition').[68,77] The surgeon can encourage the patient to learn about BDD by offering educational resources (e.g., www.BDDprogram.com).[45]

We recommend that surgeons inform patients with suspected BDD that they are concerned that the patient will be dissatisfied with the outcome of the surgery and that cosmetic procedures rarely help BDD symptoms, and can in fact make them worse. Then, patients should be briefly made aware that there are effective treatments for BDD, including psychiatric/psychological treatments, and referrals to a psychiatrist and/or psychologist can be made. It can be helpful to provide patients a list of local mental health providers with expertise in BDD or other body image problems and to convey to the patient that effective mental health treatments are available.

A major challenge in making such referrals is the poor or absent insight that is typical of BDD. Patients may resist the diagnosis because they believe that they truly are ugly. It can be helpful for surgeons to note that there is a mismatch between how people with BDD see themselves compared to how others see them, for reasons that are not well understood – that individuals with BDD see themselves as ugly or deformed, whereas other people do not see them this way. It is not helpful, however, to argue with the patient about how they look or to try to convince the patient that you are right and they are wrong, as this is likely to be ineffective. It is more helpful to empathize with and underscore the patient's distress and the impact of their appearance concerns on their daily lives (e.g., 'I can see how worried you are about your jaw and how much it's upsetting you and interfering with your life'); this approach can be helpful in encouraging patients to accept a mental health evaluation and treatment.[77]

In general, it is best to be clear about why a referral to a mental health provider is being made (to get effective treatment for BDD) and to not promise that surgery will be performed after the psychiatric evaluation. It is best to not minimize the patient's concern (e.g., 'it's all in your head'), provide reassurance that they look okay (unless the patient recognizes this to some degree themselves), or say something like 'Well, I see a little something, but it's not that bad'; these strategies are unlikely to be helpful and may even exacerbate the patient's distress. Surgeons are also discouraged from giving in to requests to perform minor procedures or to offer less invasive treatment options to appease the patient,[77] as in our experience patients may have a poor outcome following even minor interventions. Referrals to other surgeons are also discouraged, as this gives patients the implicit message that surgery may be helpful when in fact it appears unlikely to be.

Conclusions

BDD is seen more commonly among persons interested in appearance-altering procedures such as orthognathic surgery than in the general population. Cosmetic surgery and other appearance-altering procedures appear to offer little benefit for most persons with BDD and may do more harm than good, not only for the patients themselves, but potentially for providers. Patients with BDD appear to rarely be satisfied with the outcome of appearance-altering procedures and may threaten lawsuits or even become violent towards the treating physician. Because of these concerns, BDD should be considered a contraindication for orthognathic surgery and other appearance-altering procedures.

A careful preoperative evaluation and/or use of screening instruments for BDD can help to identify patients with BDD. Patients identified as having BDD symptoms should be referred for mental health evaluation and treatment, as psychiatric/psychological treatments (i.e., SRI antidepressants and cognitive-behavioural therapy) are appropriate and effective treatments for this often chronic and debilitating disorder.

References

1 Koran LM, Abujaoude E, Large MD, Serpe RT. The prevalence of body dysmorphic disorder in the United States adult population. CNS Spectr. 2008;13(4):316–22.
2 Rief W, Buhlmann U, Wilhelm S, Borkenhagen A, Brahler E. The prevalence of body dysmorphic disorder: A population-based survey. Psychol Med. 2006;36(6):877–85.
3 Buhlmann U, Glaesmer H, Mewes R, Fama JM, Wilhelm S, Brahler E, et al. Updates on the prevalence of body dysmorphic disorder: A population-based survey. J Psychiatr Res. 2010;178(1):171–5.
4 Liao Y, Knoesen N, Deng Y, Tang J, Castle D, Bookun R, et al. Body dysmorphic disorder, social anxiety and depressive symptoms in Chinese medical students. Soc Psychiatry Psychiatr Epidemiol. 2010;45(10):963–71.
5 Biby EL. The relationship between body dysmorphic disorder and depression, self-esteem, somatization, and obsessive-compulsive disorder. J Clin Psychol. 1998;54(4):489–99.
6 Cansever A, Uzun O, Donmez E, Ozsahin A. The prevalence and clinical features of body dysmorphic disorder in college students: A study in a Turkish sample. Compr Psychiatry. 2003;44(1):60–4.
7 Mayville S, Katz RC, Gipson MT, Cabral K. Assessing the prevalence of body dysmorphic disorder in an ethnically diverse group of adolescents. J Child Fam Stud. 1999;8(3): 357–62.
8 Taqui A, Shaikh M, Gowani S, Shahid F, Khan A, Tayyeb S, et al. Body dysmorphic disorder: Gender differences and prevalence in a Pakistani medical student population. BMC Psychiatry. 2008;8(1):1–10.
9 Callaghan GM, Lopez A, Wong L, Northcross J, Anderson KR. Predicting consideration of cosmetic surgery in a college population: A continuum of body image disturbance and the importance of coping strategies. Body Image. 2011;8(3):267–74.
10 Crerand C, Phillips KA, Menard W, Fay C. Nonpsychiatric medical treatment of body dysmorphic disorder. Psychosomatics. 2005;46:549–55.
11 Hollander E, Cohen LJ, Simeon D. Body dysmorphic disorder. Psychiatr Ann. 1993;23(7):359–64.
12 Phillips KA, Grant J, Siniscalchi J, Albertini RS. Surgical and non-psychiatric medical treatment of patients with body dysmorphic disorder. Psychosomatics. 2001;42:504–10.
13 Veale D, Boocock A, Gournay K, Dryden W, Shah F, Willson R, et al. Body dysmorphic disorder. A survey of fifty cases. Br J Psychiatry. 1996;169(2):196–201.
14 Calderón P, Zemelman V, Sanhueza P, Castrillón MA, Matamala JM, Szot J. Prevalence of body dysmorphic disorder in Chilean dermatological patients. J Eur Acad Dermatol Venereol. 2009;23(11):1328.
15 Uzun O, Basoglu C, Akar A, Cansever A, Ozsahin A, Cetin M, et al. Body dysmorphic disorder in patients with acne. Compr Psychiatry. 2003;44(5):415–9.
16 Phillips KA, Dufresne RG Jr, Wilkel C, Vittorio C. Rate of body dysmorphic disorder in dermatology patients. J Am Acad Dermatol. 2000;42:436–41.
17 Conrado LA, Hounie AG, Diniz JB, Fossaluza V, Torres AR, Miguel EC, et al. Body dysmorphic disorder among dermatologic patients: Prevalence and clinical features. J Am Acad Dermatol. 2010;63(2):235–43.
18 Crerand CE. Rate of body dysmorphic disorder among patients seeking facial cosmetic procedures [Phd Thesis]. Philadelphia, PA: Drexel University; 2004.
19 Sarwer DB, Wadden TA, Pertschuk MJ, Whitaker LA. Body image dissatisfaction and body dysmorphic disorder in 100 cosmetic surgery patients. Plast Reconstr Surg. 1998;101(6):1644–9.
20 Aouizerate B, Pujol H, Grabot D, Faytout M, Suire K, Braud C, et al. Body dysmorphic disorder in a sample of cosmetic surgery applicants. Eur Psychiatry. 2003;18:365–8.
21 Bellino S, Zizza M, Paradiso E, Rivarossa A, Fulcheri M, Bogetto F. Dysmorphic concern symptoms and personality disorders: A clinical investigation in patients seeking cosmetic surgery. Psychiatry Res. 2006;144(1):73–8.
22 Castle DJ, Molton M, Hoffman K, Preston NJ, Phillips KA. Correlates of dysmorphic concern in people seeking cosmetic enhancement. Aust N Z J Psychiatry. 2004;38(6):439–44.
23 Harth W, Linse R. Botulinophilia: Contraindication for therapy with botulinum toxin. Int J Clin Pharmacol Ther. 2001;39:460–3.
24 Ishigooka J, Iwao M, Suzuki M, Fukuyama Y, Murasaki M, Miura S. Demographic features of patients seeking cosmetic surgery. Psychiatry Clin Neurosci. 1998;52(3):283–7.
25 Vargel S, Ulusahin A. Psychopathology and body image in cosmetic surgery patients. Aesthetic Plast Surg. 2001;25(6):474–8.
26 Vindigni V, Pavan C, Semenzin M, Grana S, Gambaro F, Marini M, et al. The importance of recognizing body dysmorphic disorder in cosmetic surgery patients: Do our patients need a preoperative psychiatric evaluation? Eur J Plast Surg. 2002;25:305–8.
27 Vulink NC, Rosenberg A, Plooij JM, Koole R, Berge SJ, Denys D. Body dysmorphic disorder screening in maxillofacial outpatients presenting for orthognathic surgery. Int J Oral Maxillofac Surg. 2008;37(11):985–91.
28 Lai C-S, Lee S-S, Yeh Y-C, Chen C-S. Body dysmorphic disorder in patients with cosmetic surgery. Kaohsiung J Med Sci. 2010;26(9):478–82.
29 Alavi M, Kalafi Y, Dehbozorgi GR, Javadpour A. Body dysmorphic disorder and other psychiatric morbidity in aesthetic rhinoplasty candidates. J Plast Reconstr Aesthet Sur. 2011;64(6):738–41.
30 Picavet VA, Prokopakis EP, Gabriëls L, Jorissen M, Hellings P. High prevalence of body dysmorphic disorder symptoms in patients seeking rhinoplasty. Plast Reconstr Surg. 2011;128:509–17.
31 Mulkens S, Bos AER, Uleman R, Muris P, Mayer B, Velthuis P. Psychopathology symptoms in a sample of female cosmetic surgery patients. J Plast Reconstr Aesthet Surg. 2012;65(3):321–7.
32 Veale D, Eshkevari E, Ellison N, Costa A, Robinson D, Kavouni A, et al. Psychological characteristics and motivation of women seeking labiaplasty. Psychol Med. 2014;44(03):555–66.

33 De Jongh A, Adair P. Mental disorders in dental practice: A case report of body dysmorphic disorder. Spec Care Dentistry. 2004;24(2):61–4.
34 Herren C, Armentrout T, Higgins M. Body dysmorphic disorder: Diagnosis and treatment. Gen Dent. 2003;51: 164–6.
35 Cunningham SJ, Bryant CJ, Manisali M, Hunt NP, Feinmann C. Dysmorphophobia: recent developments of interest to the maxillofacial surgeon. Br J Oral Maxillofac Surg. 1996;34(5):368–74.
36 Cunningham SJ, Harrison SD, Feinman C, Hopper C. Body dysmorphic disorder involving the facial region: a report of 6 cases. J Oral Maxillofac Surg. 2000;58:1180–3.
37 Hepburn S, Cunningham S. Body dysmorphic disorder in adult orthodontic patients. Am J Orthod Dentofacial Orthop. 2006;130(5):569–74.
38 De Jongh A, Aartman IHA, Parvaneh H, Ilik M. Symptoms of body dysmorphic disorder among people presenting for cosmetic dental treatment: a comparative study of cosmetic dental patients and a general population sample. Community Dent Oral Epidemiol. 2009;37(4):350–6.
39 Rispoli A, Acocella A, Pavone I, A. Tedesco, Giacomelli E, Ortiz L, et al. Psychoemotional assessment changes in patients treated with orthognathic surgery: Pre and post-surgery report. World J Orthod. 2004;5:48–53.
40 American Psychiatric Association. Diagnostic and Statistical Manual of Mental Disorders, Fifth Edition. 5th ed. Washington, DC: American Psychiatric Association; 2013.
41 Phillips KA, Menard W, Fay C, Weisberg R. Demographic characteristics, phenomenology, comorbidity, and family history in 200 individuals with body dysmorphic disorder. Psychosomatics. 2005;46(4):317–25.
42 Phillips KA, Diaz S. Gender differences in body dysmorphic disorder. J Nerv Ment Dis. 1997;185(9):570–7.
43 Hart AS, Phillips KA. Symmetry concerns as a symptom of body dysmorphic disorder. J Obsessive Compuls Relat Disord. 2013;2(3):292–8.
44 Phillips KA, Wilhelm S, Koran LM, Didie ER, Fallon BA, Feusner J, et al. Body dysmorphic disorder: Some key issues for DSM-V. Depress Anxiety. 2010;27(6):573–91.
45 Phillips KA. Understanding Body Dysmorphic Disorder: An Essential Guide. New York, NY: Oxford University Press; 2009.
46 Phillips KA, Menard W, Fay C, Pagano M. Psychosocial functioning and quality of life in body dysmorphic disorder. Comprehen Psychiatry. 2005;46:254–60.
47 Phillips KA, Stein DJ, Rauch SL, Hollander E, Fallon BA, Barsky A, et al. Should an obsessive-compulsive spectrum grouping of disorders be included in DSM-V? Depress Anxiety. 2010;27(6):528–55.
48 Phillips KA, Didie ER, Menard W, Pagano ME, Fay C, Weisberg RB. Clinical features of body dysmorphic disorder in adolescents and adults. Psychiatry Res. 2006;141(3):305–14.
49 Phillips KA, Menard W. Suicidality in body dysmorphic disorder: A prospective study. Am J Psychiatry. 2006;163(7): 1280–2.
50 Gunstad J, Phillips KA. Axis I comorbidity in body dysmorphic disorder. Compr Psychiatry. 2003;44:270–6.
51 Bjornsson AS, Didie ER, Grant JE, Menard W, Stalker E, Phillips KA. Age at onset and clinical correlates in body dysmorphic disorder. Compr Psychiatry. 2013;54(7):893–903.
52 Phillips KA, Menard W, Quinn E. A four-year prospective observational follow-up study of course adn predictors of course in body dysmorphic disorder. Psychol Med. 2013;43:1109–17.
53 Fukuda O. Statistical analysis of dysmorphophobia in outpatient clinic. Jap J Plast Reconstruct Surg. 1977;20(6):569–77.
54 Gorney M. Recognition and management of the patient unsuitable for aesthetic surgery. Plastic and Reconstructive Surgery. Plast Reconstruct Surg. 2010;126:2268–71.
55 Crerand CE, Menard W, Phillips KA. Surgical and minimally invasive cosmetic procedures among persons with body dysmorphic disorder. Ann Plast Surg. 2010;65(1):11-6.
56 Veale D. Outcome of cosmetic surgery and 'DIY' surgery in patients with body dysmorphic disorder. Psych Bull. 2000;24(6):218–21.
57 Tignol J, Biraben-Gotzamanis L, Martin-Guehl C, Grabot D, Aouizerate B. Body dysmorphic disorder and cosmetic surgery: Evolution of 24 subjects with a minimal defect in appearance 5 years after their request for cosmetic surgery. Eur Psychiatry. 2007;22(8):520–4.
58 Picavet VA, Gabriels L, Grietens J, Jorissen M, Prokopakis EP, Hellings PW. Preoperative symptoms of body dysmorphic disorder determine postoperative satisfaction and quality of life in aesthetic rhinoplasty. Plast Reconstr Surg. 2013;131(4):861–8.
59 Phillips KA, Pagano ME, Menard W, Fay C, Stout RL. Predictors of remission from body dysmorphic disorder: A prospective study. J Nerv Ment Dis. 2005;193(8):564–7.
60 Sarwer DB. Awareness and identification of body dysmorphic disorder by aesthetic surgeons: Results of a survey of american society for aesthetic plastic surgery members. Aesthet Surg J. 2002;22(6):531–5.
61 Sarwer DB, Crerand CE, Magee L. Body dysmorphic disorder in patients who seek appearance-enhancing medical treatments. Oral Maxillofacial Surg Clin North Am. 2010;22(4):445–53.
62 Leonardo J. New York's highest court dismisses BDD case. Plast Surg News. 2001 July: 1–9.
63 Kaplan R. What should plastic surgeons do when crazy patients demand work? The New York Observer, 2000 March: 1.
64 Phillips KA, McElroy SL, Lion JR. Body dysmorphic disorder in cosmetic surgery patients (letter). Plast Reconstruct Surg. 1992;90:333–4.
65 Yazel L. The serial-surgery murder. Glamour. 1999 May:108–14.
66 Cotterill JA. Body dysmorphic disorder. Dermatol Clin. 1996;14(3):457–63.
67 Crerand CE, Franklin ME, Sarwer DB. Patient safety: Body dysmorphic disorder and cosmetic surgery. Plast Reconstr Surg. 2008;122(4S):1–15.
68 Naini FB, Gill DS. Body dysmorphic disorder: A growing problem? Prim Dent Care. 2008;15(2):62–4.
69 Sarwer DB. Psychological assessment of cosmetic surgery patients. In: Sarwer DB, Pruzinsky T, Cash TF, Goldwyn RM, Persing JA, Whitaker LA, editors. Psychological Aspects of Reconstructive and Cosmetic Plastic Surgery: Clinical, Empirical and Ethical Perspectives. Philadelphia: Lippincott Williams & Wilkins; 2006, pp. 267–83.
70 Phillips KA, Hollander E. Treating body dysmorphic disorder with medication: Evidence, misconceptions, and a suggested approach. Body Image. 2008;5(1):13–27.
71 Hollander E, Allen A, Kwon J, Aronowitz B, Schmeidler J, Wong C, et al. Clomipramine vs desipramine crossover trial in body dysmorphic disorder: Selective efficacy of a serotonin reuptake inhibitor in imagined ugliness. Arch Gen Psychiatry. 1999;56(11):1033–9.
72 Phillips KA, Albertini RS, Rasmussen SA. A randomized placebo-controlled trial of fluoxetine in body dysmorphic disorder. Arch Gen Psychiatry. 2002;59(4):381–8.
73 Veale D, Gournay K, Dryden W, Boocock A, Shah F, Willson R, et al. Body dysmorphic disorder: A cognitive behavioural model and pilot randomised controlled trial. Behav Res Ther. 1996;34(9):717–29.
74 Rosen JC, Reiter J, Orosan P. Cognitive-behavioral body image therapy for body dysmorphic disorder. J Consult Clin Psychol. 1995;63(2):263–9.

75 Wilhelm S, Phillips KA, Didie E, Buhlmann U, Greenberg JL, Fama JM, Keshaviah A, Steketee G. Modular cognitive-behavioral therapy for body dysmorphic disorder: a randomized controlled trial. Behav Ther. 2014;45:314–27.
76 Wilhelm S, Phillips K, Steketee G. Cognitive-behavioral therapy for body dysmorphic disorder: A modular treatment manual: Guilford Publications, Inc.; 2013.
77 Phillips KA, Dufresne RG, Jr. Body dysmorphic disorder: a guide for dermatologists and cosmetic surgeons. Am J Clin Dermatol. 2000;1:235–43.
78 Veale D, Ellison N, Werner TG, Dodhia R, Serfaty MA, Clarke A. Development of a Cosmetic Procedure Screening Questionnaire (COPS) for body dysmorphic disorder. J Plast Reconstr Aesthet Surg. 2011;65(4):530–2.

Chapter 10

Patient Information Provision

Farhad B. Naini, Daljit S. Gill and Umberto Garagiola

Introduction

> 'Time spent in communication (with patients) is never wasted.'
>
> Frances Cooke Macgregor (1906–2001)[1]

The purpose of this chapter is to describe *what information to provide to patients, and how to provide it*. A fully comprehensible account of the orthognathic surgical process, potential outcomes, risks/costs and benefits can be difficult to provide to a prospective patient. Different types of information and information provision techniques may be suitable depending on the patient and the various stages of the orthognathic treatment pathway.

Effective communication

Effective communication is required to increase patient satisfaction and involvement in the consent and decision making process, as well as optimizing the information given to prospective patients regarding all aspects of what is potentially a long and complex treatment pathway.

After interviewing and examining the patient, and thereby having reached a diagnosis, the clinician needs to communicate three things to the patient:

1. Explain the diagnosis and how it has occurred in words the patient can understand.
2. Explain what will happen if no treatment is provided, e.g. will the dentofacial appearance and malocclusion become worse with further growth and development.
3. Explain the treatment options that are available, including their benefits and risks.

Imparting all of this information requires effective communication.

In the clinic and on the ward

The experienced clinician should be a master of the art of making complex issues clear. Patients yearn for a clinician able to communicate in understandable, **jargon-free language**.

The concept of the 'ward round' was introduced into medicine by the Persian physician Avicenna in the 11th century, and introduced into modern medical schools by the pioneering physician Sir William Osler (1849–1919), who always stressed the importance of teaching medical students in the presence of patients on the wards. However, whether at the bedside, in the ward, or on the teaching clinic, patients want their surgeon

Orthognathic Surgery: Principles, Planning and Practice. Edited by Farhad B. Naini and Daljit S. Gill.

to talk to them, not about them. It is prudent to always inform the patient beforehand if their case is going to be discussed with trainees or colleagues on a consultation clinic or on the ward, so that the patient feels part of the process. The patient should never be made to feel like a bystander.

Clinicians routinely discuss a patient's dentofacial appearance and possible surgical solutions in their presence. Although important for teaching purposes, if the patient is not prepared and made to feel part of the process, this may become a frightening, embarrassing and even potentially psychologically traumatic experience for the patient. Although the patient may be sitting quietly in the dental chair and appear outwardly composed, they will be highly sensitive to the remarks, language and behaviour of the clinicians. Terms such as 'deformity', which should never be used in the presence of patients, will be insulting, and terms such as 'incompetent lips' may be misunderstood as referring to an incompetent individual.[2,3] Technical language used between the clinicians and discussion of the proposed surgical procedures, particularly using words such as 'cut', 'surgical fracture', 'split', 'reattach', 'bone removal' etc. will heighten the patient's anxiety. Any signs of indecision or conflicting opinions between clinicians regarding alternative treatment plans or strategies in the presence of a patient are likely to be misinterpreted and thereby may undermine the patient's confidence. The implications for a patient in not fully understanding all the technical dialogue surrounding them is potentially an irretrievable loss of confidence in the process.

To avoid such misapprehensions, it is far better for the clinicians and trainees to discuss a patient's case using the records immediately prior to seeing the patient on the clinic, to avoid undesirable language with negative connotations (e.g. words such as 'deformities') in the patient's presence, to be honest yet reassuring, to involve the patient in any necessary discussions using jargon-free language and to always make the patient feel involved in the treatment process.

Time management

Within most healthcare systems, the clinician's time is a valuable commodity. Unfortunately, this often means that bureaucratic systems reduce the length of appointments and overbook clinics. Despite such problems, the clinician must always bear in mind that without adequate time, it is impossible for the patient to communicate their desires and apprehensions adequately, and difficult for the clinician to convey all required information to the patient. Patients expect and clinicians need time in a consultation. Patients want to feel that the clinician interviewing and examining them is thinking of nothing else. As such, the clinician should never appear to be indifferent to the patient's concerns or in a hurry. Patient dissatisfaction often stems from poor communication or lack of information, leading to a potential surprise at some point during the treatment process. For example, the last thing a surgeon will want to hear from a patient the day before surgery is 'I didn't realise my lower lip could become *permanently* numb after surgery'.

Retention of information

There is some evidence that orthognathic patients may not be well-informed about the reasons, risks and benefits of their treatment.[4] Although clinicians provide patients with information at various stages of the treatment process and obtain a signed 'informed consent' form before proceeding, short-term recall of information has been found to be poor. In one investigation, the preoperative meeting between 16 orthognathic patients (and in some cases their parents) and their orthodontist was audio taped, and the patients were interviewed in person immediately afterwards. Both patients and parents recalled fewer than half the risks given by orthodontists, only 60% of the patient and parent responsibilities, and 70% of the procedures they would undergo. Over 25% of patients recalled no risks. Even when patients and parents recalled some risks, responsibilities, and procedures, these often differed from the specifics given by orthodontists.[4] Another investigation found that the overall recall of the possible risks of orthognathic treatment following the initial information-giving appointment was only 40%.[5] These findings highlight the need for improved communication in preparing patients for orthognathic surgery. Interestingly, there is also evidence that the amount of information that a patient forgets is not usually related to age or intelligence but to the type of information presented, the order of presentation of information and the patient's anxiety level.[6]

Selective recall

Patients may also demonstrate selective recall of information provided to them, with a tendency to recall information about potentially positive outcomes more frequently compared to information about the surgical risks,[7] and to recall information in favour of their decision to undergo orthognathic surgery while suppressing information which may cause them anxiety.[8]

Dissatisfaction with treatment

Satisfaction with orthognathic surgery has been found to be over 90%, though this favourable attitude to orthognathic surgery does not translate to 'cosmetic' surgical procedures.[9,10]

Macgregor[11] presented three major categories for the reasons for dissatisfaction with aesthetic facial surgery, many of which, either directly or indirectly, are a reflection of poor communication:

1. Patient-dependent factors: multiple or serious psychological problems, unrealistic expectations, external motivations for surgery.

2. Surgeon-dependent factors: lack of empathy for postoperative problems, hurried evaluations, and lack of preoperative preparation.
3. Surgeon–patient interaction: poor communication or personality conflict.

Information-seeking behaviour in patients

Health information-seeking behaviour may be defined as 'the purposive search for health-related information to satisfy a query'.[12] Such information forms a significant part of patient education, permitting the patient's informed participation in decisions relating to their health and potential treatment.

Patients may be broadly divided regarding their approach towards health information-seeking behaviour into 'monitors' and 'blunters'.[13] Monitors actively seek information about their medical condition, and the information helps to reduce anxiety and offers reassurance. Conversely, blunters actively avoid information and prefer less information, coping by distracting themselves from the situation. It is worthwhile attempting to find out in which category a prospective patient belongs. Information-seeking behaviour in orthognathic patients has not been investigated. However, there is some evidence relating to orthodontic patients. Stephens et al.[14] found that the preferred method of obtaining information for orthodontic patients was verbal, followed by audiovisual and written. Audiovisual information could be beneficial for those who find reading difficult or who struggle to retain verbal information. Few patients were found to access information via the Internet, and this was attributed to concerns about the reliability of the information.

Methods of information provision

Information may be provided to patients in a number of ways:

Verbal information

Verbal information provision remains the mainstay of medical practice. The **setting for information provision** is important. Ideally, verbal information should be provided in a quiet and relaxed environment, free from interruption and not surrounded by too many people. The descriptions provided by the consultant surgeon or orthodontist, albeit often using information provision aids/tools is vitally important. The avoidance of medical jargon remains paramount. The skill in communication is to ascertain the most important facts that a prospective patient must understand then arrange them in a logical order and provide a condensed version, which will not overwhelm the patient. Part of a transcript from an initial patient consultation is provided (Box 10.1 and Figure 10-1).

Note:

Describing paraesthesia to patients

Postoperative paraesthesia of the lips, chin, tongue, palate and gingivae is very common immediately following orthognathic surgical procedures. Attempting to describe the sensation of paraesthesia was relatively straightforward in the past. For example, the patient would be told that their lip would feel 'like a dental injection wearing off.' However, many younger patients today may have never had an intraoral local anaesthetic injection as they may never have had any dental restorations. An alternative comparative description would be to say to the patient: 'Have you ever slept on your arm for an extended period of time, or sat down for too long in one position? Paraesthesia is the pins and needles feeling you get in your arm or leg after such incidents.'

Note:

Overweight patients

Patients who are overweight may be struggling with emotional issues, and the subject should be approached delicately and with empathy, but it cannot be avoided. Undertaking an elective surgical procedure, such as orthognathic surgery, on a patient who is excessively overweight increases the risks of postoperative complications, such as deep vein thrombosis (DVT). The patient should be informed that the request for them to reduce their body weight is to reduce the risks of surgery. It should be explained that treatment cannot begin until the patient's Body Mass Index (BMI) has been shown to be improving. The patient may be set a reasonable target for weight reduction, and reviewed after 3–4 months. Preparatory orthodontic treatment may be instigated if the patient demonstrates that they are heading in the right direction.

It has been suggested that verbal information should be supplemented by written (see below) and/or visual information, in view of the fact that the method of information provision affects information retention.[15] Examples of **visual information provision tools** that may enhance verbal information provision for the potential orthognathic surgical patient at the chair side include:

Radiographs

The orthopantomograph (OPT) and particularly the lateral cephalometric radiograph may be used at the chair side to demonstrate approximately where the proposed osteotomies are to be made and which

Box 10-1 Patient information provision at the chair side

The following is part of a transcript from an initial patient consultation with a patient presenting with a severe Class III skeletal discrepancy with an anterior open bite. The consultant orthodontist is describing orthognathic treatment to the patient, in the presence of their parents:

'The type of treatment you are contemplating is called orthognathic surgery. "Orthognathic" just means correcting the jaws. The treatment is a combination of orthodontic treatment with fixed braces on your teeth, combined with an operation to reposition your jaws.

The treatment time is prolonged. From the day the braces go on your teeth, to the day the braces are removed, can take up to 3 years. The surgery to reposition the jaws is carried out about two-thirds of the way through the treatment. The braces stay on your teeth all the way through treatment, including during your surgery.

The purpose of the orthodontic braces is to reposition your teeth into the correct position for *their own jaw*, that is, to reposition your upper teeth into the correct position for your upper jaw, and your lower teeth for your lower jaw. This process usually makes your bite worse. If you imagine my hands are your front teeth, and in the average person they normally bite in this sort of relationship to one another (Figure 10-1a). As your jaws have grown away from one another, nature's way of compensating for that is to try to get your teeth to meet. So your lower lip has tilted your lower teeth backwards, and your tongue has pushed your upper teeth forward (Figure 10-1b), reducing your reverse bite. The role of the initial orthodontic treatment is to reposition the teeth into the correct position for their own jaw, by tilting the lower teeth forward and the upper teeth backward, which increases the horizontal gap between them (Figure 10-1c) and worsening your bite. The surgeon can then move your top jaw forward and your lower jaw back the required amount, which reduces the prominence of your lower jaw, improves the relationship between the upper, middle and lower parts of your face, and improves your bite. After the surgery, you will have anything from 3 months to 1 year of further orthodontic brace work to get your bite into the best possible relationship.

I must emphasize that it doesn't matter how long you take to decide whether you would like to pursue jaw surgery. You can take as long as you wish, and my role is to give you enough information so that you can make the right decision for you. But, it's very important that before orthodontic braces go onto your teeth, you are sure, because the tooth movements required to prepare you for surgery are exactly the opposite of those if you want to have brace treatment without surgery. Either way, changing your mind during treatment can be disastrous.

In terms of the surgery itself – it is usually carried out after anything from 1 to 2 years after the brace work begins, but this is an estimate and the time is variable depending on how much tooth movement is required for any one patient, as well as how quickly the teeth move. The surgery is carried out under a general anaesthetic, so you will be fully asleep throughout. The surgery takes about $1^1/_2$ hours if it's just for a single jaw, and about $3^1/_2$ to 4 hours if both jaws are being repositioned; so it is a moderate sized operation. You will need a number of appointments with the surgical team in preparation for the surgery for impressions of your teeth and some measurements. The models made of your teeth are then placed on something called an articulator, which simulates how your teeth bite together, and open and close. The operation is carried out as a trial-run on these models. You will also need to see the anaesthetist for an anaesthetic check. You will normally be admitted to hospital quite early on the morning of your operation, on an empty stomach, and your operation will be some time during that day. Bring a book or some music to keep yourself occupied in case you are waiting some time, but don't eat or drink anything even if one of the nurses offers you something. Blood transfusion is rarely required for this operation nowadays, but it may be required.

The operation itself is carried out mostly from inside the mouth, so you won't have any scars on your face. A breathing tube has to be used to keep you breathing during the operation, and it is usually placed through one of your nostrils. But some surgeons prefer to place the breathing tube in from under your chin, particularly if they are undertaking surgery to the upper jaw. In that case you will have a small scar under your chin, although after about a year it is barely visible.

When you wake up from the operation you will initially be in recovery, (though most patients can't remember this part), and you will then be returned to the ward. You will feel tired and lethargic, swollen and will be in some discomfort. Many of the nerves around your upper and lower lips, chin, tongue, roof of your mouth and gums will have been bruised during the operation as they have to be protected. So, most of these areas will feel quite numb, and this can make you feel even more swollen than you are. Most of the sensation comes back to normal with time, although it can take anything from a few days up to $1^1/_2$ years from the date of the operation for all the feeling to return. Having said that, in some patients, not all the feeling returns and you may be left with an area that feels numb or just different. This happens in about 10% of patients, so if you absolutely do not want to risk this happening, then you shouldn't have the treatment. Having said that, when numbness does occur, most patients just adapt to it and it doesn't appear to be a long-term issue for most patients who have already had this treatment. Remember that we are talking about sensory nerves, which give these areas feeling. This will not affect the movement of your lips.

You may still have an acrylic wafer splint wired to your top brace when you wake up from the operation, although most surgeons now remove this at the end of the operation. You are also likely to have some small orthodontic elastic bands placed between your upper and lower braces, to guide your teeth into position, as you initially may not know exactly where to bite.

After upper jaw surgery, it is quite normal to have a little blood oozing from your nose for a day or so. This is because some blood will have accumulated in the sinuses of the upper jaw. Some gauze will be placed to soak this up if required, and make you more comfortable.

For the first week or so after the operation, you won't be able to open your mouth very much more than 1 to 2 centimetres, and may have small elastic bands between your upper and lower teeth to guide them together. Most patients tend to go home the following day after the operation, but some patients need an extra night in hospital. Overall, the hospital stay is relatively short, but your recovery period at home is quite long. It will take about 6 weeks for the bones to heal in their new position, though the bones are held together with metal plates and screws. The plates and screws are quite small and placed under the skin and muscles, so often you can't feel them. They are made of biocompatible metal called titanium, which is also used for dental implants and false knees and hips, so they don't cause any harm. Once the bones are healed in the new position, the plates and screws become superfluous, and are not really needed any more. But they are usually left in place to avoid another operation to remove them. They are too small to set off alarms in airports. Occasionally, the plates may become infected, or the screws may become loose, in which case there is a small operation to remove them. You will be on a liquidized diet for the first week, and it is common to lose a little weight after this operation, usually about 3 to 4 kilograms, though you will often put the weight back on quite quickly when you begin to eat properly again. The second week after the operation you will be on a soft, fork-mashable diet, and from week 3 you will gradually move onto chewing normally, though nothing hard or sticky. You should be back on normal food consistency after 6 weeks, when the bones will have healed. The first week after the operation is always the worst. You have to remember that you will have been starved before the operation, had a 3 to 4 hour general anaesthetic, lost a little blood, gone through the stress of having an operation, and will be sore, swollen, bruised, and will feel tired and 'beaten up'. It is quite normal for most patients to even feel somewhat down, low in mood and even a little depressed. The thing to remember is that this will only last for the first 5 to 7 days, and most patients feel much better after this time. Nevertheless, you will essentially be resting at home for the first week, though you will need to walk around at home and avoid just lying down. You will probably need about 2 weeks off school or work, though some patients need a little more time. There should be no contact sports for 3 months following the operation, though you can start light training if you like after the first 3 to 4 weeks.

You will have weekly appointments for the first month after your operation, but after that you will return to routine intervals between your appointments. When your braces are removed, which can be anything from 3 months to 1 year after your operation, you will be fitted with removable retainers, which are required to keep your teeth straight. You will wear these almost full time for the first 3 months (except eating and cleaning your teeth), then go onto evenings and nights wear, then nights only, which you will need to continue indefinitely. Some patients gradually reduce their retainer wear, at about 2 years after brace removal, to a few nights per week. We will recommend that you carry on wearing your retainers on a part time basis in the long-term.

We also need to discuss the stability of this form of treatment, in other words, whether the result that we can achieve with orthodontics and surgery will last in the long-term. The retainers are required to keep the teeth straight. The stability of the result of the orthodontic brace treatment will require retainer wear on some kind of part-time basis in the long-term, as the teeth will have a tendency to move throughout life. In the long-term, you may only need to wear removable retainers a few nights per week.

The new position of the bones is usually relatively stable, but some movement can occur over time, which may be in the wrong direction. So, sometimes the bite may slip somewhat over time. We tend to follow up our patients long-term to keep an eye on the stability of the result. In terms of the surgery to reposition the jaw bones, reducing the prominence of your lower jaw should be relatively stable, but there is a possibility of your bite opening somewhat after treatment. It is unlikely to ever return to where it is now, but occasionally the result achieved at the end of treatment may not be perfectly stable.

Sometimes additional surgery may be required at some stage after the main operation to reposition the jaws. Chin surgery may be required as a second procedure. Also, upward and forward movement of the upper jaw tends to slightly flare the nostrils and slightly elevates the tip of the nose. Measures may be taken during the operation to limit these changes, but additional surgery is sometimes required as a second procedure.

We will go through all this information again in more detail during your treatment, and here is an information leaflet which has most of the information we just discussed, so you can read it at home in your own time. There is some space at the back of the leaflet, so if you have any other questions, write them down and we can go over them next time.

Do you have any questions?'

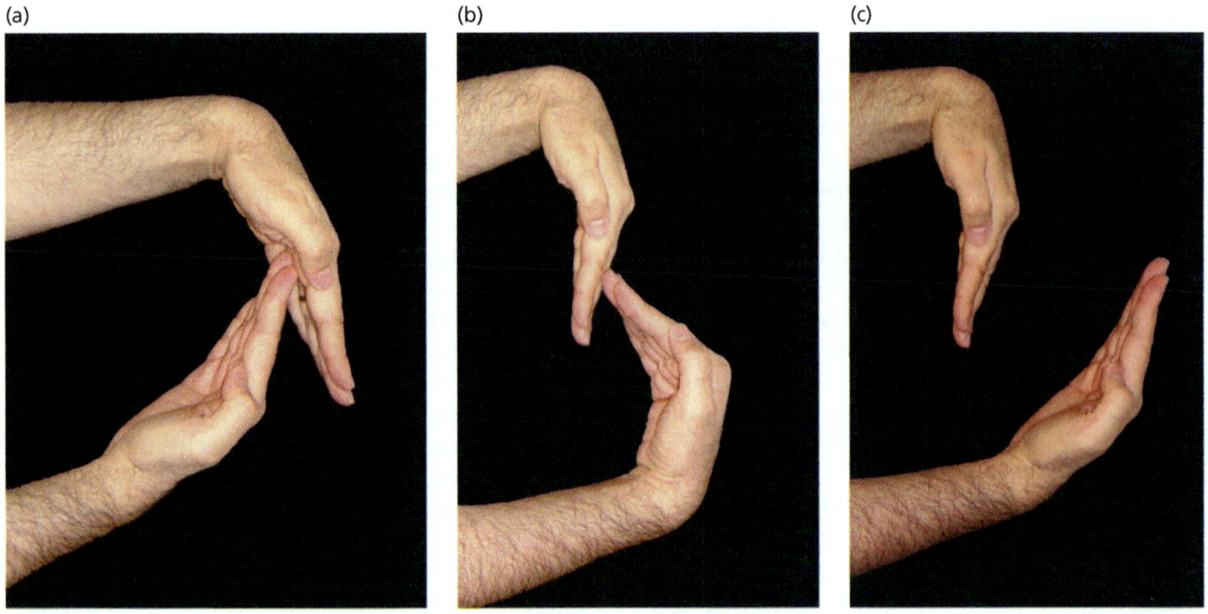

Fig. 10-1 As a very basic descriptive tool, orthodontists often use their hands to mimic the position and relationship of the maxillary and mandibular incisors to each other. (a) An average, Class I incisor relationship, with the incisors at an average inclination. (b) Demonstrating dentoalveolar compensation for a Class III skeletal pattern. (c) Demonstrating the effect of orthodontic decompensation on the incisor inclinations and the 'worsening' of the bite prior to surgical correction.

dentoalveolar or bony segments are to be repositioned. Mandibular third molars and their potentially intimate relationship to the mandibular nerve may be described on the OPT when consenting for their surgical removal. Plates and screws on radiographs of previously operated patients may be useful to demonstrate their positions and size. A particular advantage of the lateral cephalometric radiograph is that it will help to correlate the skeletal relationships to the patient's aesthetic concern with their soft tissue appearance, and usually clarifies why such correction is not achievable with orthodontics only.

Study models

The patient's own dental study models are a useful three-dimensional tool to demonstrate the dental parameters, such as the degree of crowding or rotations, and the dental-occlusal relationships. When dental extractions are required, the teeth to be removed may be pointed out to the patient. Hand articulation of *pretreatment* study models in the approximate postoperative position for the basal bones will demonstrate to the patient why preparatory orthodontics is required. Additionally, hand articulation of *preoperative* study models will demonstrate the potential postoperative dental occlusion.

Photographs

The patient's own photographs may be used to demonstrate areas of soft tissue deficiency or excess, and photographic manipulation software may be used to demonstrate the possible treatment changes with orthognathic surgery (see Chapter 6).

3D imaging

As 3D imaging and manipulation software packages improve, it will be possible to demonstrate potential treatment results of a patient's own proposed surgery to them, though accurate systems demonstrating life-like images are not yet available.

Plastic skull

It is possible to obtain plastic skulls with magnetized segments which may be repositioned at the Le Fort I level in the maxilla, and simulating a mandibular sagittal split osteotomy and osseous genioplasty. This may be a useful adjunct to the verbal description of the procedures.

Images of previously treated patients with similar condition

The potential advantage of using 'before and after' images of previously treated patients, as long as their consent has been provided, is that it avoids the difficulties encountered with patients' expectations when using photographic manipulation software of their own images. The images shown to a prospective patient should be of a patient with as similar a dentofacial discrepancy and malocclusion as possible, and ideally of the same gender and similar ethnic background (Figures 10-2 to 10-6). It is better to have images of patients with a realistic result rather than of patients where the most 'ideal' result was achieved, to avoid the risk of unrealistic expectations. This is particularly true of the dental-occlusal relationships.

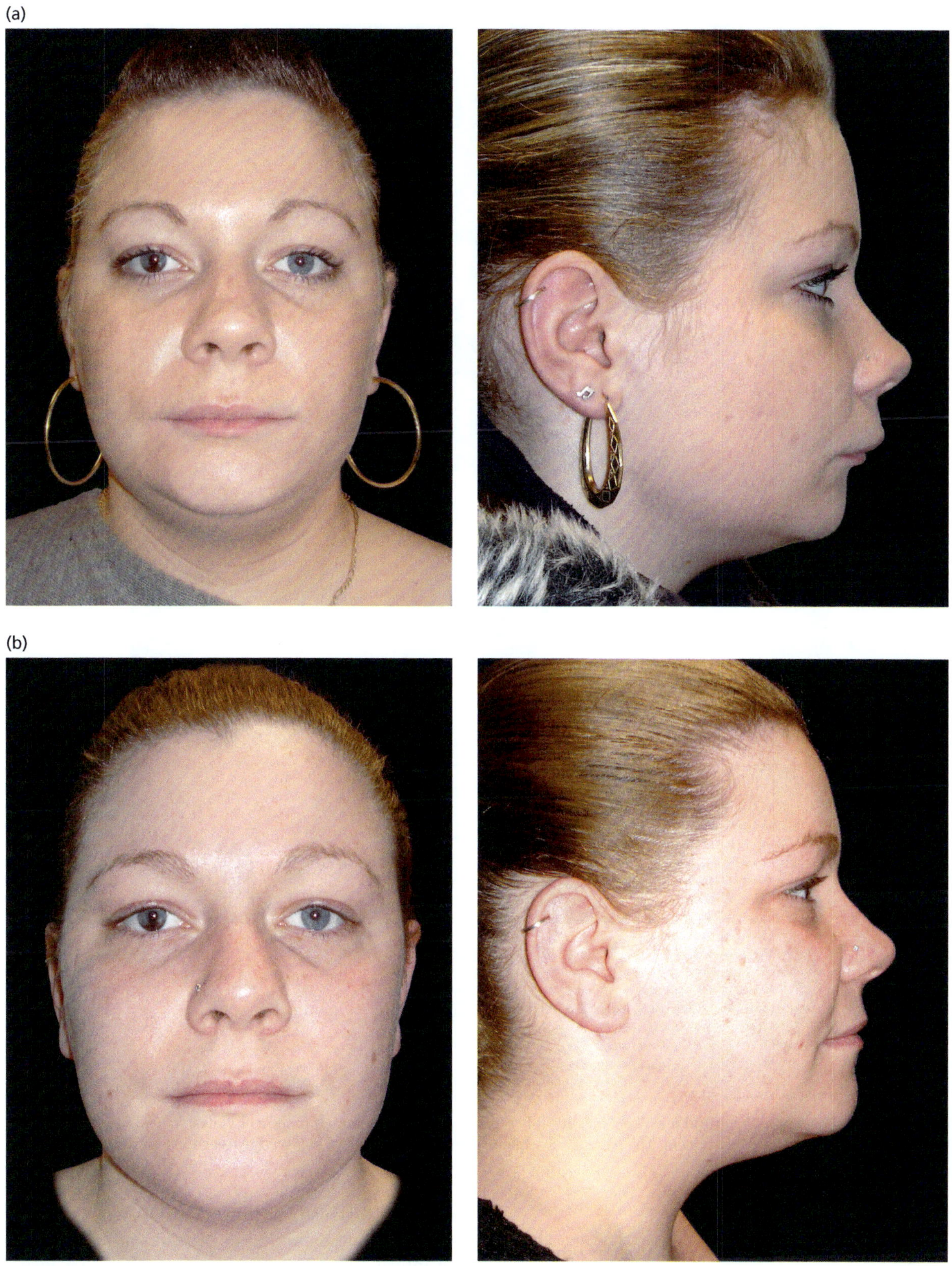

Fig. 10-2 Class II patient with mandibular retrognathism. (a) Pretreatment views. (b) End of treatment views, following mandibular advancement.

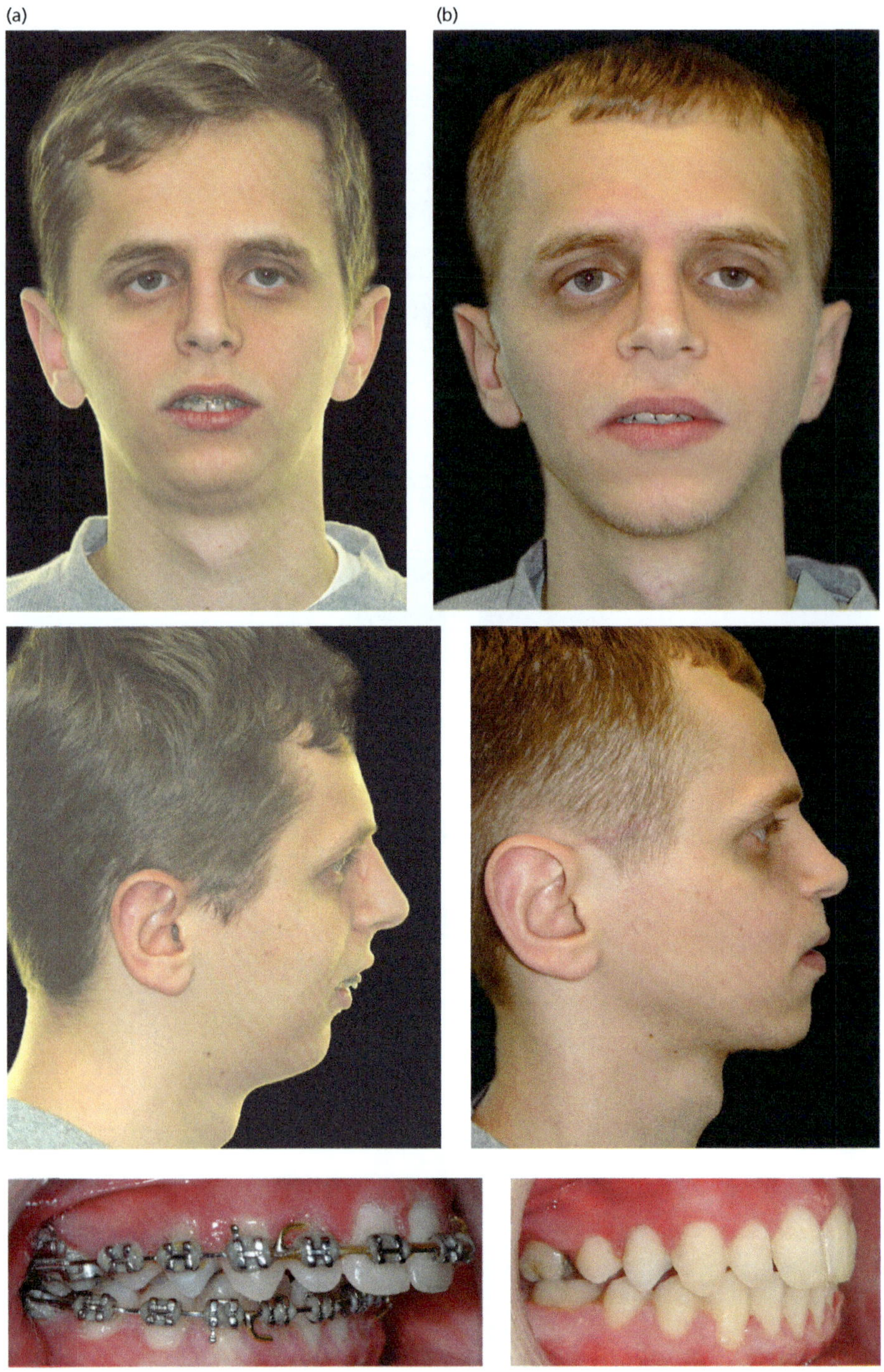

Fig. 10-3 Class II patient with vertical maxillary excess. (a) Preoperative views. (b) End of treatment views, following maxillary impaction and mandibular advancement. The patient subsequently underwent bilateral alar wedge resection to reduce the interalar width.

Schematic images

It is possible to use artist's representation schematic images of various dentofacial deformities and the stages of orthognathic treatment, as well as explaining the location of osteotomies and the relative size and position of plates and screws (Figure 10-7).

Schematic video/computerized demonstrations

Similar to the schematic images, short multimedia videos may be used to demonstrate the various procedures, which may be viewed on a computer monitor while the clinician provides additional verbal information. There is some evidence that visual computer-based information leads to improved retention of information compared to written media in adolescent orthodontic patients.[16]

Speaking with a previously treated patient

There is evidence that orthognathic patients like the opportunity of meeting patients who have undergone a similar procedure in order to ask questions that

(a)

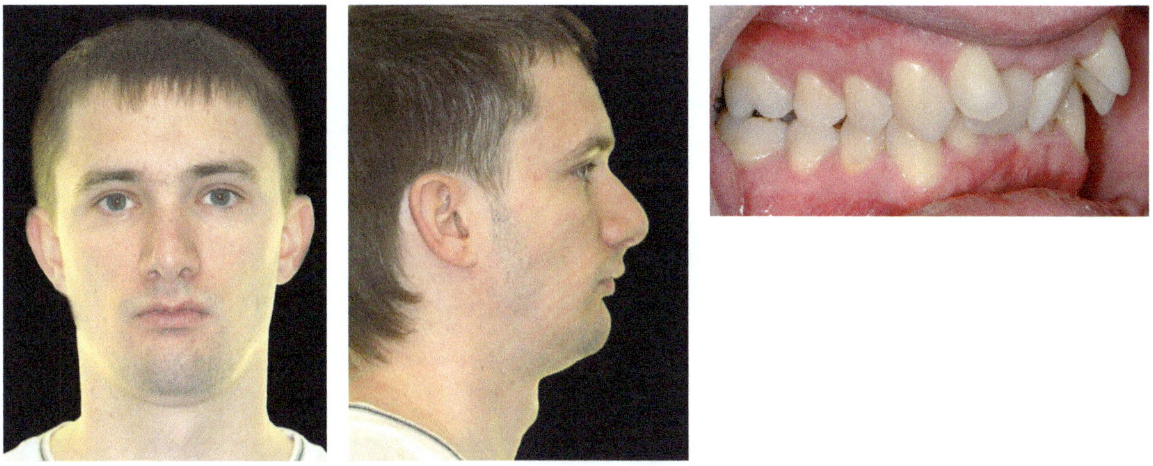

(b)

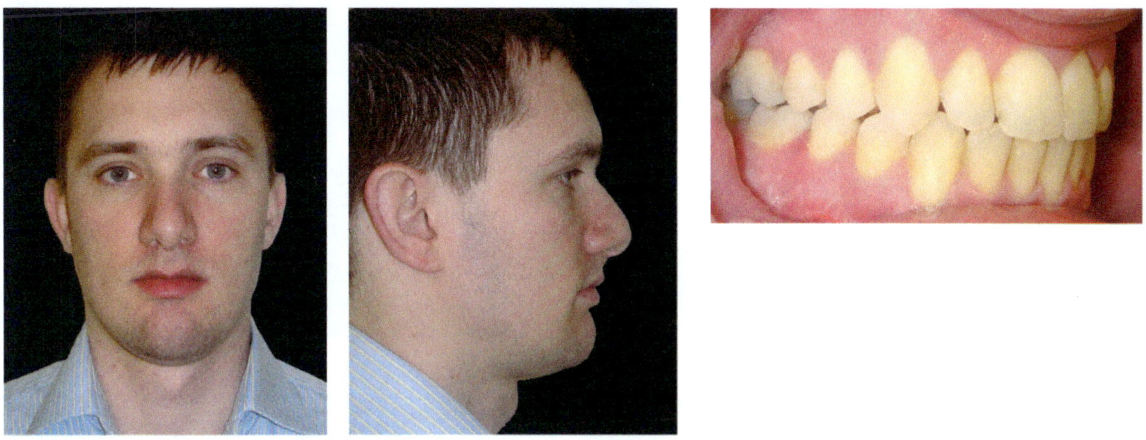

Fig. 10-4 Class II patient with Class II division 2 malocclusion and mandibular retrognathism. (a) Pretreatment views. (b) End of treatment views. The maxillary incisor inclination was corrected, creating an increased incisor overjet, and the mandible advanced.

(a)

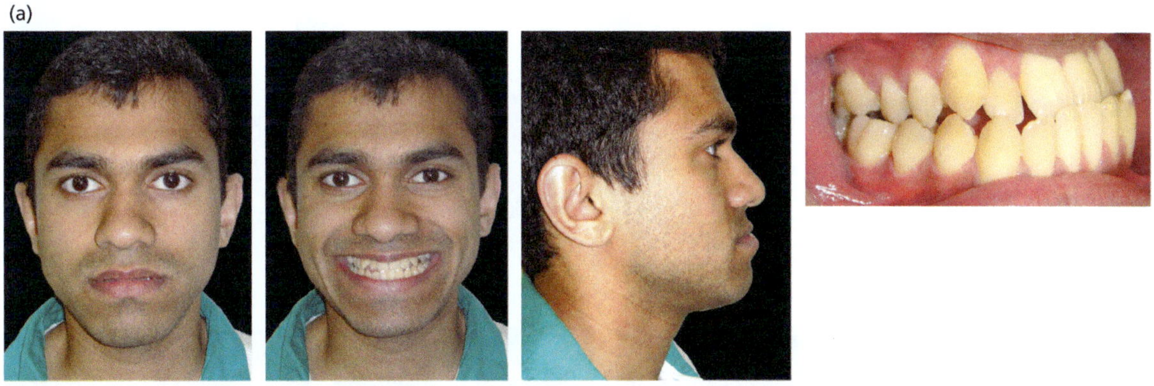

(b)

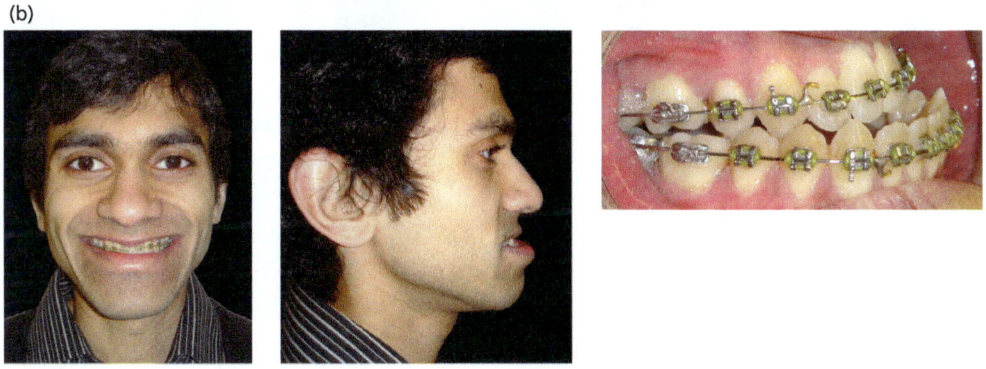

Fig. 10-5 Class III patient with maxillary retrognathism and mandibular prognathism, and average vertical proportions. (a) Pretreatment views. (b) Preoperative views. Maxillary first premolars were extracted to create space for incisor decompensation and alignment. 'Worsening' of the profile and dental occlusion due to decompensation is evident. (c) End of treatment views, following maxillary advancement and mandibular set-back.

(c)

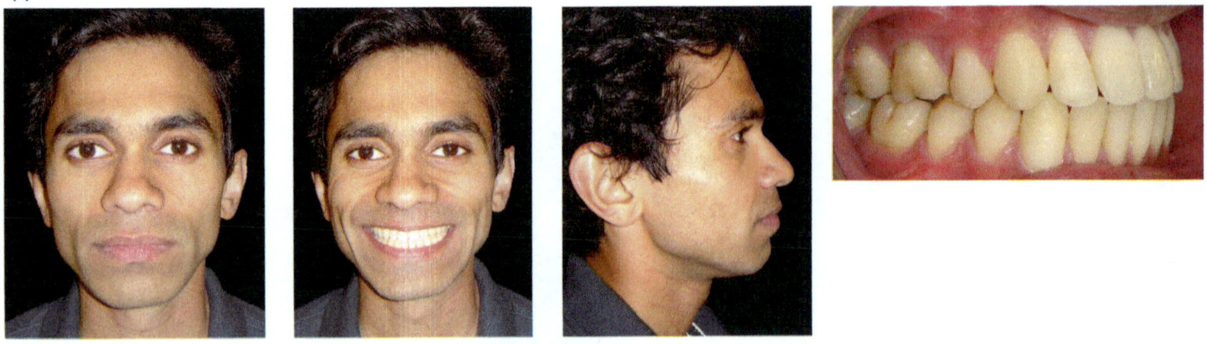

Fig. 10-5 (*Continued*).

(a)

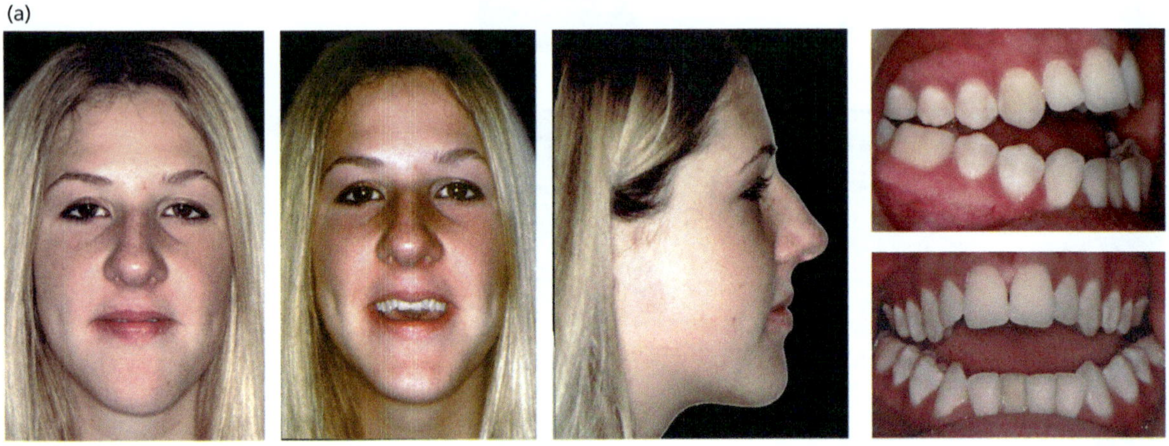

(b)

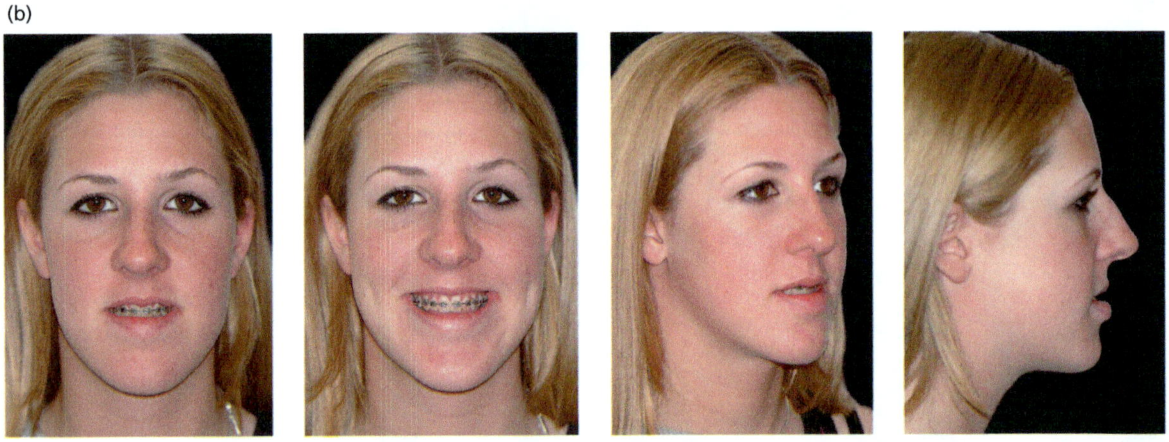

(c)

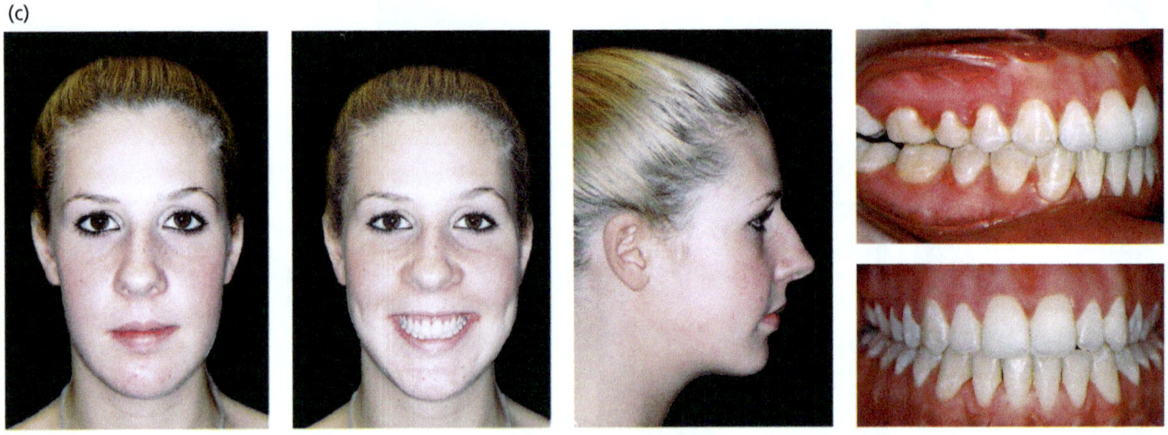

Fig. 10-6 Class III patient with maxillary retrognathism, mandibular prognathism, increased lower anterior face height and skeletal anterior open bite. (a) Pretreatment views. (b) Preoperative view, demonstrating 'worsening' of profile and increased lower lip prominence. (c) End of treatment views, following maxillary differential posterior impaction and advancement, forward mandibular autorotation and set-back.

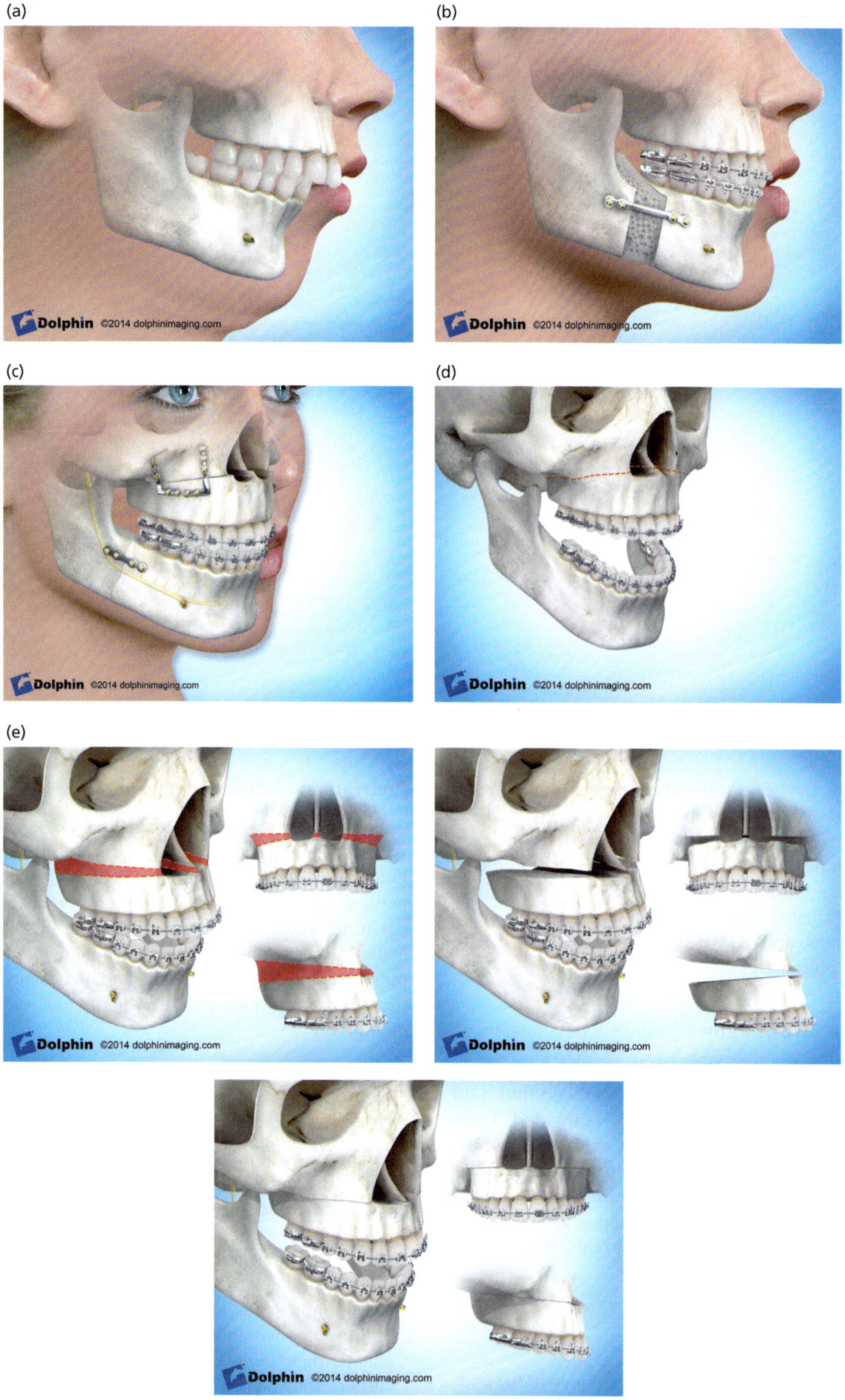

Fig. 10-7 Examples of 3D images showing orthognathic surgery and its effects: (a) Mandibular retrusion; (b) Mandibular advancement; (c) Location of the mandibular nerve; (d) Le Fort I-type osteotomy; (ei–iii) Differential posterior maxillary impaction; (f) Segmental maxillary surgery; (g) Le Fort I-type advancement osteotomy, mandibular advancement osteotomy and advancement genioplasty, showing positions of plates and screws; (h) Airway opening with bimaxillary advancement surgery (Courtesy of Dolphin Imaging; © 2014 www.dolphinimaging.com).

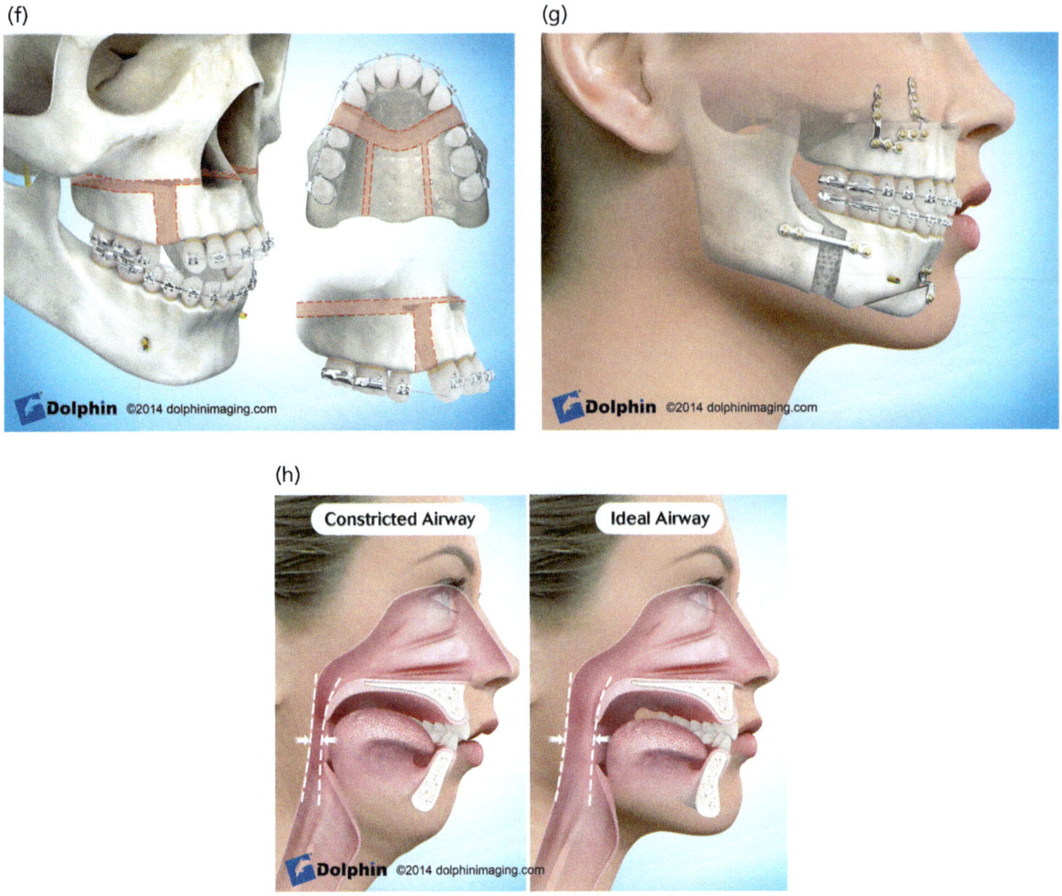

Fig. 10-7 (*Continued*).

clinicians may find difficult to answer due to lack of personal experience of the treatment itself.[10,17] There are issues of confidentiality that must not be breached, but so long as a previously treated patient agrees to this beforehand, prospective patients often find this a very valuable method of obtaining information (see Chapters 60 and 61).[18] This should be arranged without the presence of the clinicians.

Written information

Clear verbal information is paramount, but patients may experience information overload and find it difficult absorbing all the information provided. Therefore, **information leaflets** may be extremely useful at various stages of treatment. Their principal advantage is that patients may read them in their own time, and re-read them as required. Information leaflets should be available in different formats as required, including Braille.

Note:

When an information leaflet is provided at the end of any consultation, patients should be invited to make a list of any questions they may have after reading them, and to bring their list to the next consultation so their questions may be answered.

Pretreatment information leaflet (Box 10.2)

A general pretreatment information leaflet may be valuable for a prospective patient, and should be provided at the end of the initial consultation. The information contained in the leaflet should corroborate verbal information already provided by the clinician. The leaflet also contains useful information for the preoperative phase of treatment, and it is worthwhile providing another copy to the patient a few weeks preoperatively.

Note:

Changing your mind during treatment
The patient should be advised to take their time in coming to a decision as to whether to proceed with orthognathic surgical treatment. However, they should be informed in no uncertain terms, both verbally and in written form, that once preparatory orthodontic treatment has started the patient's bite will become worse very quickly, and should they change their mind regarding their desire to have surgery, they will be in a worse situation than when they started, which is disastrous. It is important not to begin orthodontic treatment until the patient is fully committed to completing the whole treatment.

Box 10-2 Pretreatment information leaflet

Patient Information Leaflet

Orthognathic Surgery

This leaflet contains useful information if you have expressed an interest in combined orthodontics (braces) and orthognathic (corrective jaw) surgery.

Purpose of orthognathic surgery:
In some people, the jaw bones may be out of alignment to the extent that orthodontics alone cannot correct the tooth positions and provide a functioning bite. The purpose of combined orthodontics and jaw surgery is to move the jaws into a better position in order to improve the bite of your teeth (so that the teeth will meet correctly) and to improve the proportions and symmetry of your jaws and facial appearance.

Orthodontic braces:
Before the jaws can be repositioned with surgery, fixed orthodontic braces are used to place the teeth into the best position for their own jaw. This will allow the teeth to meet properly after surgery. Sometimes removable braces are also required, but fixed braces permit the most accurate positioning of the teeth. The braces stay on the teeth during the operation as they help the surgeon reposition the jaws and for some months after the operation in order to help the orthodontist improve the tooth positions and bite further.

Length of treatment:
The duration of this treatment is prolonged. It can take *approximately* 2 to 3 years from the day the braces go onto the teeth until they are removed, although this is an estimate and will vary for each patient depending on a number of factors, such as how quickly your teeth move. The operation takes place at some point during this orthodontic treatment, usually about two-thirds of the way through. The scheduling of the operation is elective and may be carried out when it is convenient for you, though this may add to your overall treatment time.

The surgery:
You should not eat or drink anything from midnight the night before your operation. The majority of your jaw surgery is carried out from inside your mouth. The surgery is carried out under a general anaesthetic, so you will be fully asleep throughout the procedure. Small metal plates and screws are used to hold the jaw bones in their new positions while they are healing. These plates and screws are on the surface of the bone but beneath your skin and muscles. They are not required after 6 weeks when your bones have healed in their new position, but generally they remain in place forever. Occasionally they may need to be removed at a later date, which requires a small operation. Very rarely, your teeth will need to be wired together for up to 6 weeks after the surgery.

How long is the hospital stay for surgery?
The hospital stay for the surgery is usually about 2 to 3 nights, though this is an estimate and you will not be discharged home until your surgeon is happy and you feel ready. There must be at least one responsible adult to pick you up from the hospital (preferably by car) and to look after you when you return home.

How long is the recovery time after the operation?
The first week after the operation you will be resting and recovering at home. You will feel better for the second week, but still mainly resting. Some patients will gradually resume normal daily activity from the third to fourth week after the operation, as long as nothing physically strenuous is carried out. It will take up to 6 weeks for the bones to heal.

Eating and drinking before the operation
To avoid the orthodontic braces damaging your teeth, you must maintain a healthy diet throughout your treatment. You should avoid any foods or drinks that are high in sugar (chocolates or sweets) or acidic (for example, fizzy drinks or excessive amounts of fruit juice), as these may damage your teeth. You should also avoid any food that is too hard (for example, French bread) or sticky (for example, toffees or chocolate bars), as these may dislodge your braces. Healthy hard foods, like apples, can be cut up and chewed carefully with your back teeth.

Eating and drinking after the operation
All the previous information is still important, but for the first week after the operation you will not be able to chew solid food. You will be on an almost liquid diet. You will need a blender at home and a dietician will advise you about food intake after your operation. You will gradually build up the consistency of your food until you are back to a normal diet at about 6 weeks after the operation.

Oral hygiene and cleaning of your teeth and braces
Orthodontic braces will not be placed until your tooth cleaning is of a very high standard, otherwise this may damage your teeth. You will need to brush your teeth thoroughly at least three times per day. It is vital that your standard of oral hygiene remains very good throughout treatment.

Medications after the operation
You will usually need antibiotics, pain control medication and possibly nasal decongestants for a few days after your operation.

What is expected of you as the patient?
You will need frequent appointments with your orthodontist throughout the treatment for

adjustments to be made to your brace. These will be scheduled during school/work hours, but must be kept. You must try to be on time for your appointments so that all the planned adjustments can be carried out at each visit. Failed or cancelled appointments with your orthodontist or repeated breakages of your brace will add considerably to your overall treatment time.

You should keep your regular check-up appointments with your dentist throughout this treatment.

You should start walking very soon after your operation, but you should avoid physical exertion for a few weeks following your surgery and contact sports for approximately 3 months.

What are retainers?
Once the active phase of treatment has been completed, the fixed braces will be removed and you will be fitted with retainer braces, which are used to hold the teeth in their new positions. These retainer braces will need to be worn on a long term basis as teeth always maintain a tendency to move, although the amount of wear of these retainers will be reduced over time.

Possible risks of orthodontic treatment:
All forms of medical and dental treatment, including orthodontics, have some risks and limitations. Fortunately, in orthodontics complications are infrequent and when they do occur they are usually of minor consequence. Nevertheless, they should be considered when making the decision to undergo orthodontic treatment. The main risks involved in orthodontic treatment may include, but are not limited to:

1. DECALCIFICATION: *(Permanent enamel markings)* Tooth decay, gum disease, and permanent markings (decalcification) on the teeth can occur if orthodontic patients eat foods containing excessive sugar and/or do not brush their teeth frequently and properly. These same problems can occur without orthodontic treatment, but the risk is *greater* to an individual wearing braces.
2. ROOT SHORTENING: In some patients the length of the tooth roots may be shortened during orthodontic treatment. Some patients are prone to this happening, some are not. Usually this does not have significant consequences, but on occasion it may become a threat to the longevity of the teeth involved. X-ray pictures are taken during treatment to check for this possibility.
3. GOOD ORAL HYGIENE: The health of the bone and gums which support the teeth may be affected if bacterial plaque is not removed daily with good oral hygiene, leading to inflammation of the gums and loss of supporting bone.
4. RELAPSE TENDENCY: Teeth may have a tendency to change their positions after orthodontic treatment. This usually is only a minor change and faithful wearing of retainers as instructed should help reduce this tendency.
5. JAW JOINT PROBLEMS: Occasionally problems may occur in the jaw joints, i.e., temporomandibular joints (TMJ), causing joint discomfort. These problems may occur with or without orthodontic treatment. Any symptoms should be promptly reported to the orthodontist.
6. LOSS OF TOOTH VITALITY: Sometimes a tooth may have been traumatized by a previous accident or a tooth may have large fillings, which can cause damage to the nerve of the tooth. Orthodontic tooth movement may in some cases aggravate this condition and in rare instances a tooth may require root canal treatment.
7. POST-ADJUSTMENT PAIN: Sometimes orthodontic appliances may accidentally be swallowed or aspirated or may irritate or damage the oral tissues. The gums, cheeks and lips may be scratched or irritated by loose or broken appliances or by traumatic blows to the mouth. Usual tenderness after brace adjustments should be expected, and the period of tenderness or sensitivity varies with each patient and the procedure performed. Typical post-adjustment tenderness may last up to 3 days.

Possible risks of jaw surgery:
These will be discussed with you in some detail by the surgeon prior to starting any treatment. In summary, they include the following:

1. PAIN AND DISCOMFORT: As with any surgery, some pain is to be anticipated. You will be given pain control medication during and after your operation. Routine pain control medications are usually enough and likely to be needed for about 2 weeks after your operation.
2. TRISMUS (DIFFICULTY OPENING THE MOUTH WIDELY): You will usually only be able to open your mouth about 1 to 2 cm (10 to 20 mm) after the operation. If orthodontic elastic bands are placed between your upper and lower teeth, this will further limit your mouth opening. Normal mouth opening gradually resumes as your swelling reduces.
3. SWELLING: The degree of facial swelling is variable for each patient. The swelling tends to increase for about 3 days following surgery, but most of it resolves in the first 1 to 2 weeks. Some residual puffiness of the face may take several months to resolve.

4. BRUISING: A variable degree of bruising may occur, particularly around the lower jaw, neck and possibly even the upper parts of the chest. This will gradually resolve over the first few weeks after your operation.
5. NAUSEA AND VOMITING: This is quite common following surgery and you will be given medication to reduce this feeling if it occurs. If you do vomit, you should remain calm and sit up and forward to expel the liquid from your mouth. A suction device will be available at your bedside and the nurses are experienced at dealing with these situations.
6. MINOR BLEEDING: This is common from the mouth (usually blood-stained saliva) and the nose following jaw surgery, but usually stops within 2 days.
7. NASAL CONGESTION (STUFFINESS): This may occur from the breathing tube placed in the nose during the operation and also after upper jaw surgery. It often feels like having a heavy cold and will last about 1 week.
8. WEIGHT LOSS: Due to a reduction in appetite after the operation and no chewing of solid food, it is usual for patients to lose approximately 2 to 5 kg in body weight in the two weeks after the operation. Most patients will put this weight back on soon after resuming a normal diet.
9. WIRING TEETH TOGETHER: With modern surgical techniques, this is usually not required, but sometimes the upper and lower teeth will have to be wired together after the operation for up to 6 weeks.
10. BLOOD TRANSFUSION: The need for blood transfusion has reduced dramatically with modern surgical and anaesthetic techniques, but a blood transfusion will be administered if required during the operation.
11. REOPERATION: Occasionally, for a variety of reasons, a patient may need a further operation for an adjustment to the jaw positions. If this is required, it is usually in the early stages following the original operation.
12. ALTERED SENSATION OR LOSS OF SENSATION: The sensation to the lower lip, chin, tongue, roof of the mouth and gums may alter or diminish following surgery. This does not affect the movement of the lips or cheeks. Although the feeling often returns to normal, it can take many months. *In some patients, the loss of feeling in these regions may be permanent.* Some patients may also notice a change in their taste perception, which is often temporary.

Questions?

The information presented in this leaflet is to help in your decision-making process. Before starting the orthodontic brace treatment please make certain you are happy with the proposed treatment plan, and that you have had the potential risks of treatment explained to you. If, however, you require any further information prior to your appointment please do not hesitate to contact us.

If you have any further questions, please write them down here and bring them with you so that we can go through them at your next appointment:

Postoperative information leaflet (Box 10.3)

A dietician should see the patient and their family prior to discharge from the hospital, and the importance of oral hygiene issues should be discussed and reaffirmed by the surgeon or member of the team (see Chapter 15). The postoperative information leaflet reiterates general postoperative guidance to the patient and their family, including issues regarding oral hygiene and nutrition.

Note:

Postoperative depression

It is very common for patients to feel low in mood and even mildly depressed for the first postoperative week. Such elevated symptoms of depression are likely to be due to a number of factors, such as nutritional status (being starved beforehand and being unable to eat properly afterwards and thereby being low in energy), the effects of the general anaesthetic, the stress of preparing for and going through surgery, the feeling of facial swelling, paraesthesia (which exacerbates the feeling of being swollen), nasal congestion, pain and discomfort. Perioperative medications, particularly steroids given to reduce postoperative oedema, may exacerbate the potential for short-term depression. It is advantageous for both the patient and their carers to be aware of and prepared for this low mood, reducing any potential feelings of resentment on the part of the carer. Patients also often state that knowing the low mood will be temporary and will soon come to an end makes it easier to tolerate.

Audiovisual information

Audiovisual information may be useful for some patients. The British Orthodontic Society (BOS) have developed an information DVD ('A Patient Guide to Orthognathic Surgery') for prospective orthognathic

Box 10-3 Postoperative information leaflet

Patient Information Leaflet

Instructions following

Orthognathic Surgery

This leaflet contains useful information for the time period AFTER your jaw surgery.

Oral Hygiene

It is vitally important to keep your teeth, gums and mouth clean after surgery. The following will help:

- Use a small headed toothbrush (e.g. a children's toothbrush)
- Brush at least 3 times per day, and following every meal
- Rinse your mouth with salt water 3 times per day for the first 2 weeks following the operation – dissolve only a half-teaspoon of salt into a tumbler of warm water, rinse your mouth and spit out.
- You will be given Corsodyl® mouthwash (chlorhexidine digluconate), which is a strong antibacterial mouthwash to be used for only the first 2 weeks (keep the bottle out of reach of children).

Diet and Nutrition

After your operation you will have some swelling, which can limit how wide you can open your mouth. Your diet will have to adapt while your jaws heal in their new position. This involves an almost liquid diet for the first week following your operation, and then gradually moving to a soft consistency food with light chewing and eventually to normal chewing. The following information is to ensure that your food and liquid intake is optimal to allow good healing and reduce complications.

Monitoring your weight:

It is important to monitor your body weight during your recovery period to ensure you are receiving adequate nutrition. About 2 to 5 kilograms of weight loss in the few weeks after surgery is common. It may be useful to weight yourself once a week in the 6 to 8 weeks following surgery to monitor your body weight, at about the same time of day. If you notice a large change in your weight you should contact your surgeon or the dietician at the hospital.

Nutrition for health:

Despite the fact that you will be unable to chew normally for a few weeks after your operation, it is important that you maintain a healthy diet to ensure you get enough protein, energy and water for a good recovery.

Protein requirements

You should aim to take around 1 gram of protein for each kilogram (kg) of your body weight each day following surgery. For example, if you weigh 70 kg before your operation, you will need a minimum of 70 grams of protein per day during your recovery.

Useful examples of the amount of protein in various foods:

- Pint of milk (or soy milk) = 19 g
- 1 medium egg = 6 g
- $^1/_2$ cup of baked beans = 15 g

Fluid requirements

To remain adequately hydrated you should aim to take at least 30 ml of fluid per kilogram of your body weight. For example, if you weigh 70 kg, you will need (70 × 30 ml) 2100 ml fluid per day.

Useful examples:

- 1 pint = 570 ml
- 1 cup = 250 ml

Energy (calorie) requirements

You should aim to eat 6 to 8 small meals each day, supplemented with high energy and high protein drinks.

Week 1 following your operation – Liquid diet:

During this first week you should not chew any food at all. This will allow your jaw bones to heal in their new position. You will be on a liquid only diet, which is smooth and requires no chewing. It should be easy to swallow using a large feeding syringe with a soft wide bore tip placed into the corner of the mouth between your cheeks and back teeth. You should gradually progress to sipping from a tablespoon and eventually a cup.

You should use a blender/food processor to liquidize any food, to which you may add water, milk or yogurt (or vegan alternative) to smooth the consistency.

Examples include:

- Liquidized scrambled eggs with milk
- Fruit and milk or yogurt 'smoothies' and/or ice cream (or vegan alternatives)
- Soups – blended to remove lumps

Week 2 following your operation – Fork-mashable diet:

At this stage you should be able to start eating with a small fork or spoon, though still with minimal chewing. This may have to wait until week 3 (your surgeon or dietician will advise you on your review appointment).

Fork-mashable food refers to any food that may be easily mashed to remove lumps with the back of a fork. Examples include:

- mashed potato
- yogurt with banana
- inside of jacket potato with soft filling
- soft pasta or well-cooked rice
- scrambled eggs.

Weeks 3 to 6 following your operation – Soft food diet:
From weeks 3 to 6 you may gradually increase the consistency of your diet, though still maintaining a relatively soft diet. Tough and fibrous food or hard food should be avoided.

Examples include:

- Egg omelettes
- Soft pancakes
- Well-cooked casseroles
- Pasta

Extra nutritional support:
High protein and high energy drinks may be useful in the first 1 to 2 weeks following your operation. These may be taken between 1 to 3 times per day, *as recommended by your dietician*. Each bottle usually contains 320 kcal and 20 g of protein.

Swallowing safely:
This is important advice for eating, drinking and taking your medication in the weeks following your operation:

- Sit upright in bed or in a chair every time you eat or drink
- Remain seated upright for at least 30 minutes after you have eaten
- Only eat and drink when you are awake and alert
- Take only one mouthful of food or fluid at a time
- Swallow and clear your mouth before taking the next mouthful
- Don't rush – eat slowly and take some time between mouthfuls
- Take small sips of water between every few mouthfuls
- At the end of each meal check your mouth for any food in your cheeks, and clean your teeth and braces, and rinse your mouth
- If you feel something has 'gone down the wrong way', try to clear it with a cough

Managing Constipation
Constipation may be a problem after a general anaesthetic, a change in diet and reduced activity. Some pain control medications may also lead to constipation. In order to maintain regular bowel movements, the following information may be useful:

- Eat regular meals to stimulate the transit of food and wastes through your digestive system
- Include high fibre foods as far as possible every day, e.g. cereals, oats, fruit and vegetables (peeled and pureed)
- Drink plenty of water and fluids to stay well hydrated
- Begin walking as soon as possible, even in the hospital and at home, which will help to stimulate your bowels
- If a problem persists, contact the department, or your doctor or a pharmacist for a laxative.

Other Advice
You will have some dissolvable stitches inside your mouth after the operation. These will usually fall out by themselves after a few weeks.

Sleep with your head in an elevated position for the first 1 to 2 weeks following surgery, e.g. place an extra pillow under your head. This will allow excess fluid to drain away naturally from your face and neck.

It is very common to feel low in mood and even mildly depressed for the first week following your operation. Most patients feel much better after the first week.

How To Contact Us?
You may contact the Maxillofacial Surgery department at any time during the day or night.

Daytime contact number:

Night-time contact number (on-call registrar):

The Department of Nutrition and Dietetics (daytime contact only):

patients. The DVD has been found to contain valuable information and potentially to have a role in the decision making process, but it has been highlighted that some aspects of the DVD need to be improved upon.[19]

Videos of actual surgery are now available online, but these may potentially put patients off surgery. Patients should use their judgement as to what they watch, with guidance from the clinician.

World Wide Web

Information from the Internet and various websites related to orthognathic surgery is readily available. The advantages and disadvantages of such information should be openly discussed with prospective patients. It has been found that few websites hold the correct amount of valid information to be of use to prospective orthognathic patients.[20] Some patient blogs and websites may contain misleading information, and some websites may rank highly on a particular search engine but not necessarily provide useful information. Patients should be advised to view formal University websites as far as possible.

Conclusion

Different methods of delivering information may be used in orthognathic surgery. Audiovisual tools and written information leaflets are potentially useful methods of supplementing clear verbal information provided by clinicians. It is incumbent upon the orthognathic team to ensure that each patient understands and fully participates in their treatment.

References

1 Macgregor FC. After Plastic Surgery: Adaptation and Adjustment. New York: Praeger, 1979.
2 Naini FB. Negative terminology. Br Dent J. 2009;207:345.
3 Naini FB. Lip seals. Br Dent J. 2010;209:106.
4 Kiyak HA, Iseri H, Kayaalp F, Altug A. Informed consent in orthodontic and orthognathic surgery. J Dent Res 2002;81:Abstract 0159.
5 Brons S, Becking AG, Tuinzing DB. Value of informed consent in surgical orthodontics. J Oral Maxillofac Surg. 2009;67:1021–5.
6 Ley P, Spelman MS. Communicating with the Patient. London: Staples Press, 1967.
7 Godwin Y. Do they listen? A review of information retained by patients following consent for reduction mammoplasty. Br J Plast Surg. 2000;53:121–5.
8 Rittersma J. Patient information and patient preparation in orthognathic surgery: the role of an information brochure – a medical audit study. J Craniomaxillofac Surg. 1989;17:278–9.
9 Lazaridou-Terzoudi T, Kiyak HA, Moore R, Athanasiou AE, Melsen B. Long-term assessment of psychologic outcomes of orthognathic surgery. J Oral Maxillofac Surg. 2003;61:545–52.
10 Cunningham SJ, Hunt NP, Feinmann C. Perceptions of outcome following orthognathic surgery. Br J Oral and Maxillofac Surg. 1996; 34: 210–3.
11 Macgregor FC. Patient dissatisfaction with results of technically satisfactory surgery. Aesthetic Plast Surg. 1981;5: 27–32.
12 Lenz ER. Information seeking: a component of client decisions and health behavior. ANS Adv Nurs Sci. 1984;6: 59–72.
13 Miller SM. Monitoring versus blunting styles of coping with cancer influence the information patients want and need about disease: implications for cancer screening and management. Cancer 1995;76:167–7.
14 Stephens R, Ryan FS, Cunningham SJ. Information-seeking behavior of adolescent orthodontic patients. Am J Orthod Dentofacial Orthop. 2013;143:303–9.
15 Thomson AM, Cunningham SJ, Hunt NP. A comparison of information retention at an initial orthodontic consultation. Eur J Orthod. 2001;23:169–78.
16 Patel JH, Moles DR, Cunningham SJ. Factors affecting information retention in orthodontic patients. Am J Orthod Dentofacial Orthop. 2008;133:61–7.
17 Broder HL, Phillips C, Kaminetzky S. Issues in decision making: should I have orthognathic surgery? Semin Orthod. 2000;6:249–58.
18 Ryan F, Shute J, Cedro M, Singh J, Lee E, Lee S, Lloyd TW, Robinson A, Gill D, Hunt NP, Cunningham SJ. A new style of orthognathic clinic. J Orthod. 2011;38:124–33.
19 Flett AM, Hall M, McCarthy C, Marshman Z, Benson PE. Does the British Orthodontic Society orthognathic DVD aid a prospective patient's decision making? A qualitative study. J Orthod. 2014;41:88–97.
20 Aldairy T, Laverick S, McIntyre GT. Orthognathic surgery: is patient information on the Internet valid? Eur J Orthod. 2012;34:466–9.

Chapter 11

Consent and Medicolegal Considerations

Robert A.C. Chate

Introduction

Paternalism: The policy of restricting the freedom and responsibilities of one's subordinates or dependents in their supposed best interests.
Autonomy: The possession or right of self-government; freedom of action. (O.E.D).

The process of acquiring a patient's agreement to undergo any clinical procedure essentially polarizes into following either a **paternalistic** or an **autonomous** approach. One or the other will prevail depending on each particular country's societal norm but this can change over time as cultural beliefs and values emerge and evolve.

Within each culture there will also be individuals who are either inherently passive or assertive and who will prefer to have decisions about their healthcare managed in either a paternalistic or an autonomous way, respectively.

Regardless of the style of consent that predominates in any particular society, when there is a contrast between personal preferences and societal norms as specified in legal statute, the clinician responsible for gaining consent should act with sensitivity and mindfulness of the patient's particular needs, while continuing to practice within the law of the land.

In most developed countries consent follows an autonomous model. Even so, within different countries the specifics can vary from nation to nation or from state to state. For example, within the United Kingdom the law on gaining consent for either children or for adults who lack capacity to give consent is different in England as compared to the law in Scotland.[1–3]

Similarly, in the United States of America, different state laws apply different standards for adequate disclosure in the process of gaining consent.[4,5,14]

UK perspective

In English speaking countries, consent begins with the tort of battery. This consists of intentional, unpermitted contact with another person even if this does not result in bodily harm. A patient's medical consent therefore distinguishes permitted from unpermitted clinical contact but should neither be confused with medical malpractice, which relates to the provision of incompetent care, nor with the higher standard of informed consent that relates to a patient's right to self-determination in matters concerning their healthcare choices,[4] in the absence of which a claim of negligence rather than battery could be made.

Historically, in the United Kingdom the test for the standard of care has been based on the Bolam test, that is whether a clinician has acted in accordance with a practice accepted as proper by a responsible body of medical men skilled in that particular art.[6]

Orthognathic Surgery: Principles, Planning and Practice. Edited by Farhad B. Naini and Daljit S. Gill.

However, in relation to a clinician's duty of risk disclosure during informed consent, the test is the same as the test applicable to diagnosis and treatment as set out in the House of Lords decision of *Sidaway*.[7] In this regard the clinician has to act in accordance not only with a practice accepted at the time as proper by a responsible body of medical opinion, but also with the *Bolitho* modification,[8] that the body of opinion should be reasonable and responsible and the opinion should be logical.[9] Indeed, in 1999 the Court of Appeal ruled that it is the responsibility of clinicians to divulge any significant risk which would affect the judgment of a reasonable patient.[10]

In 2004, Lord Steyn in *Chester* also stated that, 'In modern law, medical paternalism no longer rules and a patient has a *prima facie* right to be informed by a surgeon of a small, but well established, risk of serious injury as a result of surgery.'[11] There is little doubt that case law from other Commonwealth countries will set examples for other courts to follow, as was likely the case in the latter two rulings above.

Here, precedent was set by the High Court of Australia in 1992 when it ruled that, 'A risk is material if in the circumstances of the particular case, a reasonable person in the patient's position, if warned of the risk, would be likely to attach significance to it.'[12]

The problem is that there is a huge variation in the risks which judges deem to be acceptable, and so the standard of informing patients about risks is evolving as it shifts from those which are considered to be relevant to a responsible dentist to those of a reasonable patient.[13] Indeed, this evolution from the perspective of a prudent clinician to a prudent patient and now to each particular patient continues, with the term **'enlightened consent'** being proposed to encapsulate the concept that the patient needs to be placed in a position from which they can understand the key issues that will influence their willingness, or otherwise, to undergo a particular procedure.[1]

International perspective

In the United States, informed consent has evolved largely through case law, but in recent times, about half of the states have defined the doctrine by statute and many have provided statutorily for the standard to be applied in measuring the adequacy of the information provided to the patient.[14] In this regard, individual state courts either apply a patient-oriented standard of risk disclosure, that is, information that a reasonably prudent patient in those circumstances would wish to know (20/50 states), a practitioner-oriented standard, those which the responsible practitioner would reasonably provide to a patient in the same circumstances (22/50 states), or a hybrid approach that combines both the patient and practitioner-oriented standards (8/50 states).[4,5,14]

Therefore, a US clinician seeking to satisfy informed consent requirements needs to check both the statutory and case law in their particular state, recognizing that staying current can be challenging while health care systems continue to evolve.[14]

In many other countries of the world, a paternalistic standard applies especially in cultures that value strong vertical and inter-generational relationships, where extended families live under the same roof and where important decisions are made with reference to the family unit.[15] This is seen to be the case in Asia and Japan,[15,16] Pakistan,[17] Central Africa,[16] Central America,[16] Latin America and the Middle East.[18] Additionally, in some southern European countries such as France, Italy and Spain, significant but potentially distressing information is commonly withheld from patients by clinicians applying the responsible practitioner standard.[18]

With modern travel, many Western countries have become multicultural and so even though an autonomous standard for informed consent may legally prevail, trying to impose this approach on an immigrant may itself be paternalistic, because the practitioner otherwise might be trying to force upon them something which is counter to their deepest values.[15,17]

However, while sensitivity in these circumstances is laudable, it should not be presumed that all patients from a family-centred culture hold the same values. Cultural references should remain general because patients from a particular heritage may still have diverse values that are influenced by their education, income, religion and the length of time they have lived in their new adopted country.[15]

Nevertheless, in all cases the overarching principle when planning treatment is to act in the patient's best interests and such beneficence would apply equally in societies where either a paternalistic or an autonomous standard of risk disclosure legally exist.

Informed consent essential requirements

In those countries where individual autonomy prevails, for a patient to consent to a clinical intervention the clinician must explain:

- The risks and benefits of the proposed treatment;
- The risks and benefits of any alternative treatments; and
- The consequences of remaining untreated.[3,14]

Of equal importance, the clinician must also judge if the patient has capacity to give their consent by ensuring the information that was given to them was:

- Understood;
- Retained; and
- Weighed up by the patient before making their decision.[3]

However, in the United States, just as patients are entitled to have information about their healthcare, they are equally entitled not to have such information when they think they would be unduly distressed by it. Patients can waive their right to information, but a waiver of information must be knowing and voluntary to be effective. Therefore, the clinician must provide enough information that the patient knows the general nature of what they are forgoing. For example, the clinician could tell the patient that there are risks inherent in the procedure under consideration. Then, if the patient chooses not to have complete information on the risks that would be a legitimate election and the requirement of informed consent would be deemed satisfied. Obviously, any such waiver should be fully documented and one way to manage such a situation would be to create a two-part consent form. In the first part, the recommended treatment would be named and outlined, noting that there were risks, consequences and possible alternatives. The form would then recite that the patient is entitled to full information and the clinician stands ready to provide it. The patient would then sign the form, either to indicate that they choose not to have a more complete explanation, or that they do, in which case the second part would provide the full details.[14]

Informed consent for orthognathic surgery

Cases involving both orthodontics and an associated discipline such as maxillofacial surgery need special management. Only clinicians who are experienced in combined orthodontic and surgical care and are therefore capable of outlining and discussing the various options, the risks and benefits, the required patient commitments and any treatment limitations that may be anticipated should normally seek consent. This is often achieved in a joint clinic setting where the orthodontist and the maxillofacial surgeon simultaneously participate in managing orthognathic patients.

The consent process may take a number of visits over an extended period of time in order that the patient may review any simulated model or computer predictions of potential outcomes, consider the treatment choices, their respective implications and return for any clarifications before making a decision.

Of key importance in acquiring consent is the information that is given to the patient, as has been outlined in the preceding chapter. One could argue that for elective treatment where an improved quality of life is the desired primary outcome rather than an extended life expectancy or an improvement in ill health, the standard of risk disclosure should be such that each particular patient receives enough information on the risks and benefits to be sufficiently enlightened to make a decision on what they consider to be in their best interests.

A familiar dilemma for a clinician applying a paternalistic 'responsible practitioner' standard of risk disclosure when seeking consent for orthognathic surgery is what a patient should be told about the risks of general anaesthesia. Although an undeniably catastrophic consequence, the risk of anaesthetic death in a patient of good health remains a miniscule risk. Nevertheless, it would clearly be one that a reasonable patient would want to know about and perhaps more so because of the elective rather than the life-saving nature of the procedure involved.

The argument put forward by paternalistic practitioners in favour of withholding such information is that the disclosure could otherwise result in a refusal by the patient to undergo the treatment they would clearly benefit from.[4]

A counter argument in favour of patient enlightenment is that with specific knowledge of the minute scale of the anaesthetic risks involved, especially if set in context with the probabilities of other routine life-event risks that are accepted on a daily basis,[19] contrary to such information acting as a disincentive many patients find it reassuring.

Who may legally give consent?

In order to protect children, laws exist in many countries that define the age an individual can normally be considered capable of making their own decisions. In the United Kingdom, the legal age at which an individual can consent to medical or dental treatment is 16. In England and Wales, the relevant legislation is contained within the Family Law Reform Act of 1969, while in Scotland the issue is governed by the Age of Legal Capacity (Scotland) Act of 1991.[1,2]

However, in both of these nations, children under the age of 16 who are judged by a clinician as having capacity to consent may also legally do so on their own.[1,2] In relation to combined orthodontic treatment and orthognathic surgery, while this may be irrelevant for maxillofacial osteotomies that are usually undertaken after the cessation of pubertal growth and by which time the patient will have reached the age of majority, this may not be the case for either distraction osteogenesis or for the onset of pre-surgical orthodontic therapy. In such a situation where there might be discord between a capable minor who wants to proceed with the preparatory orthodontic aspect of the combined treatment and the adult with parental responsibility who may wish them not to undergo any of the treatment at all, while there is no legal requirement in the UK to dally it would be prudent to encourage the dissenting parent and the consenting minor to try and reach an amicable consensus.[1,2]

In contrast, when a minor who is deemed capable declines receiving such treatment that decision cannot be overridden by a person with either legal or parental responsibility, that is unless the child would otherwise be at risk of grave or irreversible mental or physical harm.[3] Clearly, this latter stipulation would not apply to such an elective procedure as combined orthodontic and orthognathic surgical treatment.

In England and Wales, the Children Act 1989 defines who has parental responsibility and the consequent right to give consent to a child's treatment, while in Scotland this is defined by the Children (Scotland) Act 1995. In both nations, all mothers have automatic parental responsibility, however, understanding whether a father also holds parental responsibility is not always straightforward and differences in the child's date of birth may mean that a father holds parental responsibility for one of his children but not for another. Parental responsibility rests with both parents, provided they are named on the birth certificate and regardless of whether they are married or not, for children whose births were registered from:

- 15 April 2002 in Northern Ireland
- 1 December 2003 in England and Wales
- 4 May 2006 in Scotland.

For children whose births are registered prior to these dates, the father would only have parental responsibility in the following circumstances:

- If he and the mother were married at the time of the conception, birth or sometime after.
- If he and the mother were never married, but he has parental responsibility agreement with the mother or a parental responsibility order from the court.[1,2]

In the United States, federal law does not legally define the age of a minor. The laws of each state govern this instead and as children become adults, they gain different legal rights at different ages with respect to issues such as acquiring a driving license, getting married, voting and buying alcohol etc. It seems that among the 50 states, the age of majority ranges between 18[14] to 21 years of age but with variable younger ages on occasions being legally prescribed for allowing consent to be given for medical or dental treatment.[20] Most states have provisions for 'emancipated' minors, those living on their own and not dependent on their families for support, to make their own health care decisions. Also, in many states a 'mature' minor, that is, one of sufficient age and discretion to be able to understand their situation, the proposed treatment and the consequences likely to flow from the treatment or its alternatives, is authorized to make treatment decisions in a situation when care is urgently needed and the minor's parent cannot be involved in the process. Generally, such exceptions are recognized in case law rather than statutory law, but it is common for statutes to provide that a minor is treated as an adult for the purpose of consent if the minor is either married or pregnant.[14]

As such, American clinicians wishing to gain consent from minors for the correction of their facial deformity would need to abide by the legislation of the particular state concerned, especially in relation to who may consent and at what age someone is considered legally capable.[14]

Adults who lack capacity

The issue of adult patients who lack capacity to give consent for combined orthodontic treatment and orthognathic surgery is one that rarely arises. Their special needs are such that many are likely to be precluded from receiving such complex and prolonged treatment on the basis that with or without the support of their carer, they may not be able to cooperate while having treatment, comply with instructions nor maintain a satisfactory standard of oral health throughout the course of their treatment.

On the other hand, when sufficient cooperation is anticipated and where there are unequivocal benefits to be gained in an individual's oral health and function through orthodontics and orthognathic surgery, the fact that an adult patient is incapable of consenting should not exclude them from receiving treatment that would otherwise be considered to be in their best interests. Some clinical examples of this would include severe Class II malocclusions of skeletal origin with increased traumatic overbites (Figure 11-1), complete buccal scissor bites where masticatory

(a) (b)

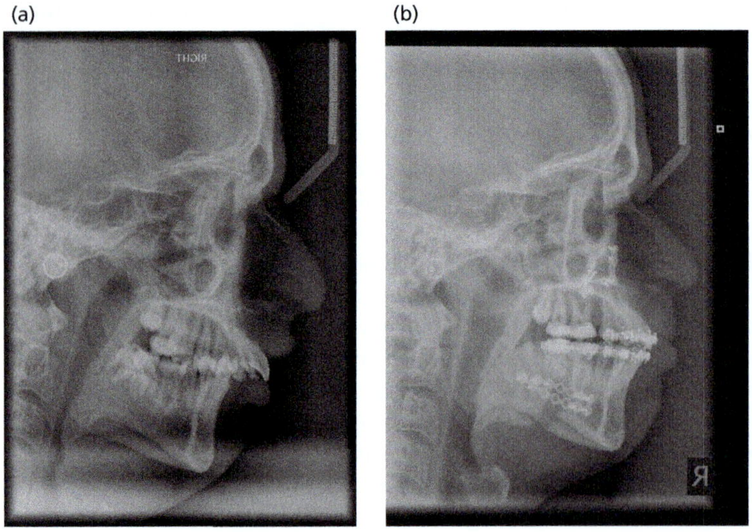

Fig. 11-1 (a) Pre-treatment lateral cephalometric radiograph illustrating the skeletal Class II base, the pronounced antegonial notches and the Class II division I malocclusion. (b) Postoperative lateral cephalometric radiograph illustrating the 6 mm vertical maxillary surgical repositioning, the 10 mm mandibular advancement and the maxillo-mandibular titanium fixation plates.

efficiency is significantly compromised and extensive anterior open bites which may attract social ridicule and rejection through aspects such as the appearance of their grossly incompetent lips, salivary dribbling and antisocial open-mouthed eating.

The Mental Capacity Act (MCA) 2005[21] that came into effect in October 2007[22] is the legislation that prescribes how adults who lack capacity to give consent must be managed in England and Wales. The majority of the MCA 2005 Act applies to those aged 16 years and over. It specifies that if an adult lacks capacity, no one else can give or withhold consent for that person and any subsequent treatment must remain in the person's best interest. Clinicians must have a 'reasonable belief' that capacity is lacking before treatment can be lawfully carried out without a patient's consent.

Under the Act, assessments of capacity still require discussions with those directly involved in the patient's care, namely family members, lay and professional carers, but where treatments may be complex or have long term effects, or where capacity is in dispute, referral to a consultant psychiatrist or psychologist for a capacity assessment may be appropriate. Ultimately though, it is the treating clinician who has to determine capacity with all of the others cited above merely acting in an advisory role.[22]

To determine what treatment is in the patient's best interests, the clinician should take into account and, if appropriate, consult anyone named by the patient as a person to be consulted, any carer or person interested in their welfare, any donee of a lasting power of attorney, any court 'deputy' appointed by the Court of Protection, and any Independent Mental Capacity Advocate (IMCA) who would be appointed by an NHS body where serious treatment is being considered and where there is no other person other than the paid carer to determine what would be in the patient's best interests. Nevertheless, where disputes between clinicians and, for example, a donee of lasting power of attorney arise as to what treatment does constitute a patient's best interests, referral to the Court of Protection may be required to resolve the conflict.[22]

With regard to a 16 to 17-year-old incapable child, there is a degree of overlap between the provisions of the MCA 2005 which applies to over 16-year-olds, and the exercise of parental responsibility under the Children Act 1989, which applies to under 18-year-olds.[23]

This overlap is recognized under section 21 of the MCA 2005, where the Lord Chancellor may 'by order make provision as to the transfer of proceedings relating to a person under 18, from the Court of Protection to a court having jurisdiction under the Children Act 1989 and *vice versa*.' This is particularly relevant where a dispute exists between the mother and the clinician as to what constitutes treatment that is in the young person's best interests. Where no such conflict exists, then under the provision of the Children Act 1989, the mother can legally give consent on behalf of her 16 to 17-year-old incapable child.

In Scotland, the Adults with Incapacity (Scotland) Act 2000 is the overarching legislation which deals with the issue of capacity to consent and is intended to safeguard the welfare and finances of adults who lack capacity to consent due to a mental disorder or inability to communicate.

For the purposes of the Act, an adult is considered to be an individual aged 16 and over and the Act allows other people to make decisions on behalf of such adults, subject to various safeguards, although the law in Scotland generally presumes that adults are capable of making decisions for themselves and it is important to recognize that simply because an individual has an illness, such as dementia, this does not necessarily mean that the person cannot make decisions for him or herself.

Under the Act, an individual can appoint a welfare attorney while that individual still has capacity, to act on their behalf in the event that capacity is lost at some point in future. Additionally, following an application to Court, a guardian can be appointed with healthcare decision making powers. Where either a welfare attorney or a guardian have been appointed, any treating medical or dental practitioner must seek the consent of that welfare attorney or guardian where it is practical and reasonable to do so. Where the adult has no such proxy in place, a doctor is authorized to provide medical treatment, subject to certain safeguards and exceptions.

For the purposes of the Act, incapacity means incapable of:

- Acting on decisions; or
- Making decisions; or
- Communicating decisions; or
- Understanding decisions; or
- Retaining the memory of decisions.

The aim of the Act is to protect those persons who lack capacity but also to support their involvement in making decisions as far as an individual is able to do so.

The Act provides principles that must be followed, as follows:

1. Any action or decision taken must benefit the person.
2. Any action or decision taken should be the minimum necessary to achieve the purpose.
3. Account must be taken of the present and past wishes and the feelings of the individual concerned as far as this may be ascertained.
4. Account must be taken of the views of others with an interest in the person's welfare, such as primary carer, nearest relative, named person, attorney or guardian.

Additionally, in some cases, even when there is a guardian or welfare attorney, medical or dental practitioners who are primarily responsible for the treatment of the adult and who have undergone specific training on *The Adults with Incapacity (Requirements for Signing Medical Treatment Certificates) (Scotland) Regulations 2007*, can sign a Section 47 certificate which states the person is unable to make a decision and details the proposed treatment. The practitioner then retains the certificate and carries out the necessary treatment. However, where serious or irreversible treatment may be needed, such as orthognathic surgery, prior approval by the Court of Session, would be required.[2]

In the United States, the management of an adult who lacks capacity to consent is similar to the UK. That is, next of kin may not consent on behalf of an incapable adult. Instead, either someone granted a durable power of attorney when the patient was previously competent[14] or a judicial appointment by a state court of a guardian who is legally designated as the surrogate decision-maker may do so.[24]

The legal systems of the American states historically have treated guardianship as an all-or-nothing proposition, global findings of incompetence being accompanied by virtually complete disenfranchisement of the ward of court, that is, the person whom the court has declared to be incompetent to make decisions. However, more latterly states have amended their statutes to recognize the concept of limited or partial guardianship, which accounts for the decision-specific nature of mental capacity and the ability of some people rationally to make certain choices but not others.

Because creating total guardianship entails an extensive deprivation of an individual's basic rights, the 'least restrictive/intrusive alternative' doctrine makes limited or partial guardianship preferred. The modern trend in surrogate decision-making has been toward the substituted judgment standard. Under this approach, the guardian is required to make the same decisions that the patient would make, if the patient currently were able to make and communicate competent decisions. The substituted judgment standard is highly consistent with respecting patient autonomy and when it cannot be reasonably ascertained what the patient would have decided if competent, the guardian would be expected to rely on the traditional best interests standard. This standard mandates that from the patient's perspective, decisions should be made in a manner that would confer the most benefit and the least burden on the ward.[24]

American clinicians therefore wishing to provide combined orthodontic treatment and orthognathic surgery in such circumstances should therefore consult and follow the relevant state legislation.

Conclusions

Consent is essentially a process of communication and of a transfer of knowledge and understanding from clinician to patient. As such, it is pertinent to note that the documentation of the discussions that leads to a patient's consent is more important than actually obtaining a signed consent from. While this is not a legal requirement in the United Kingdom, written confirmation of consent may offer an improved defence in a case of subsequent litigation, but the fact that one exists in writing does not necessarily demonstrate that the consent that was obtained was valid.

Nevertheless, written consent is recommended whenever a proposed treatment is complex and or involves significant risks and side effects. In relation to treatments to be undertaken with either conscious sedation or general anaesthesia, the UK General Dental Council stipulates that written consent must be obtained.[25]

Equally, consent should be considered a continuous process rather than a single event. In this regard, should a change of plan be needed during the patient's course of treatment, the patient should be fully informed of the circumstances and be given a further opportunity to reaffirm their consent. Alternatively, with or without a change of plan, the patient may withdraw their consent at any time, even right up to the point of having their orthognathic surgery upon completion of their preparatory orthodontic treatment. In such circumstances, the patient should be advised of the likely adverse consequences of terminating their treatment prematurely and these should be documented in the patient's case notes. Additionally, a disclaimer should be prepared that the patient may sign to clearly indicate they accept responsibility for the consequences of their action. Thereafter, the patient may be given further time to reflect upon the implications of terminating their treatment but if they remain adamant the clinician is obliged to comply. However, in these circumstances, the clinician would still retain a continuing responsibility for the patient's welfare and any measures that might help to maintain the partially improved outcome, such as retention appliances, should still be offered if likely to be beneficial.

In summary, clinicians should look beyond the specifics of the consent requirements as discussed above and always be mindful of the larger goal; respect for the dignity and autonomy of each individual patient and a commitment to assist them to participate fully and meaningfully in any decisions that affect their being and their lives.[14]

References

1 Consent. Suitable for UK excluding Scotland. Dental Protection Limited. www.dentalprotection.org/Default.aspx?DN=927506dc-8fdd-4f40-91a7-62f7f8606524: Accessed 22 December 2013.

2 Consent. Information suitable for Scotland. Dental Protection Limited. www.dentalprotection.org/Default.aspx?DN=61c91ac5-17ea-4a18-b2ec-07799e15f1ab: Accessed 22 December 2013.

3 Chate RAC. An audit of the level of knowledge and understanding of informed consent amongst consultant orthodontists in England, Wales and Northern Ireland. Br Dent J. 2008;205:665–73.

4 Raab EL. The parameters of informed consent. Trans Am Ophthalmol Soc. 2004;102:225–30.
5 Guideline on informed consent. Clinical Guidelines. Am Acad Pediatric Dent. 2009;35(6):301–303. www.aapd.org/media/Policies_Guidelines/G_InformedConsent.pdf#xml=http://pr-dtsearch001.americaneagle.com/service/search.asp?cmd=pdfhits&DocId=393&Index=F%3a%5cdtSearch%5caapd%2eorg&HitCount=26&hits=14+1f+3d+4c+4f+7b+80+c2+123+16d+184+19a+217+2df+2e1+330+3bf+43b+43d+524+560+597+636+65d+6bb+6fd+&hc=469&req=Guideline+on+Informed+Consent Accessed 22 December 2013.
6 Bolam v Friern Hospital Management Committee. [1957] 1 WLR 582.
7 Sidaway v Board of Governors of the Bethlem Royal Hospital. [1985] AC 871.
8 Bolitho v City and Hackney Health Authority. [1998] AC 232.
9 Boynton S. Don't just sign here. Dent Protect Servicematters. 2006;4:1–3.
10 Pearce v United Bristol Healthcare NHS Trust [1999] 48 BMLR 118.
11 Chester v Afshar [2004] UKHL 41.
12 Roger v Whitaker [1992] HCA 58; (1992) 175 CLR 479.
13 Brands WG. The standard for the duty to inform patients about risks: from the responsible dentist to the reasonable patient. Br Dent J. 2006;201:207–210.
14 LeBlang TR, Rosoff AJ, White C. Informed consent to medical and surgical treatment. In: Legal Medicine. 6th ed. Philadelphia, PA: Mosby, 2004, pp.343–51.
15 Ho A. Family and informed consent in multicultural setting. Am J Bioeth. 2006;6(1):26–28.
16 Levine RJ. Informed consent: Some challenges to the universal validity of the Western model. J Law Med Ethics. 1991; 19(3–4):207–213.
17 Jafarey A M, Farooqui A. Informed consent in the Pakistani milieu: the physician's perspective. J Med Ethics. 2005;31: 93–6.
18 Baile WF, Lenzi R, Parker PA, Buckman R, Cohen L. Oncologists' attitudes toward and practices in giving bad news: An exploratory study. J Clin Oncol. 2002;20(8):2189–96.
19 Lack JA, Rollin AM, Thoms G, White L, Williamson C. Raising the standard: Information for patients. www.rcoa.ac.uk/system/files/PI-Raising_2003.pdf Accessed 22 December 2013.
20 Goldfarb NM. Age of consent for clinical research. J Clin Res Best Pract. 2008;4(6). www.firstclinical.com/journal/2008/0806_Consent_Age.pdf Accessed 22 December 2013.
21 Mental Capacity Act 2005. London: The Office of Public Sector Information, UK government. www.legislation.gov.uk/ukpga/2005/9/pdfs/ukpga_20050009_en.pdf Accessed 22 December 2013.
22 Emmett C. The Mental Capacity Act 2005 and its impact on dental practice. Br Dent J. 2007;203:515–21.
23 The Chidren Act 1989. London: The Office of Public Sector Information, UK government. www.legislation.gov.uk/ukpga/1989/41/contents Accessed 22 December 2013.
24 Kapp MB. Geriatric patients. In: Legal Medicine, 6th edn. Philadelphia, PA: Mosby; 2004, pp.541–5.
25 Standards for the Dental Team. General Dental Council 2013. www.gdc-uk.org/Dentalprofessionals/Standards/Documents/Standards%20for%20the%20Dental%20Team%20FINAL.pdf Accessed 22 December 2013.

Chapter 12

Preparatory and Postoperative Orthodontics: Principles, Techniques and Mechanics

Farhad B. Naini and Daljit S. Gill

'Fast is fine, but accuracy is everything.'

Xenophon (430 BC–354 BC)[1]
Cyropaedia
Greek historian, student of Socrates, and biographer of Cyrus the Great

Introduction

'The desire to have things done quickly prevents their being done thoroughly.'

Confucius (5th century BC)[2]
Analects

Treatment time for the patient undergoing orthognathic surgery is *prolonged*. However, attempts by the orthodontist to cut corners in order to reduce treatment time, or by the surgeon to undertake surgery without adequate preoperative orthodontic preparation, will inevitably lead to problems, for the patient and the clinicians. Clearly, time should not be wasted by the orthodontist in the preparatory phase of preoperative orthodontics, but accuracy in placing the teeth of both arches into the desired positions far outweighs the speed of treatment, and may well reduce the overall treatment time by reducing the length of postoperative orthodontics.

The purpose of this chapter is to describe the five stages of orthodontic treatment required for the patient undergoing orthognathic surgery, which are:

1. Preoperative orthodontics.
2. Immediate preoperative appointment.
3. Intraoperative orthodontic requirements.
4. Immediate postoperative appointment.
5. Postoperative orthodontics.

Orthognathic Surgery: Principles, Planning and Practice. Edited by Farhad B. Naini and Daljit S. Gill.

Note:

Prior to undertaking any form of orthodontic treatment, it is incumbent upon the orthodontist to ensure that the patient has optimal oral hygiene, and the absence of gingival inflammation, active periodontal problems, or any other dental disease, such as caries. Any such issues must be managed prior to initiating orthodontic treatment. Good communication between the orthodontist and the general dental practitioner is important at this stage, and throughout treatment.

Preoperative orthodontics

'By failing to prepare, you are preparing to fail.'
Benjamin Franklin (1706–1790) (attributed)

The amount of preparatory orthodontic treatment required for the orthognathic patient is quite *variable*. It depends on the complexity of tooth movements required and the type of surgery being planned. For example, dental extractions and subsequent space closure are likely to be more time-consuming than non-extraction treatment. Dental midline corrections often can be rather time-consuming, whereas a dental midline deviation planned to be corrected with rotation of the respective jaw requires less preoperative orthodontic preparation. Inevitably, this preparatory phase is the most prolonged phase of treatment. Nevertheless, attempts to rush this stage will lead to potentially avoidable problems at the time of surgery. The time quoted to patients should be realistic, but, as a general rule, *it is better to overestimate than underestimate the treatment time required*, as patients are apt to remember!

Types of orthodontic appliance

The type of appliance used is essentially down to the preference of the orthodontist, though usually some form of preadjusted edgewise appliance is likely to be employed. The fixed orthodontic appliance is not only employed to achieve the desired tooth movements before and after surgery, but is also used by the surgeon to stabilize the jaws intraoperatively with intermaxillary fixation (IMF).

Preadjusted edgewise appliance

The former standard edgewise appliance employed relatively similar brackets on the teeth, and thereby required the orthodontist to place bends in the archwire to individually position each tooth in terms of their relative horizontal 'in–out' positions, their crown angulation (mesiodistal crown 'tip') and crown inclination (buccolingual crown 'torque'). This prepared archwire then engaged the brackets in an 'edgewise' manner, hence the name. In the mid-1970s, the American orthodontist Lawrence F. Andrews introduced the 'Straight-wire appliance',[3,4] which modified the standard edgewise system such that the information for the in-out position of each tooth, its crown tip and crown torque was incorporated into the respective bracket for each individual tooth, i.e. the details of the *final* tooth position is incorporated in each 'preadjusted' bracket. This was achieved by varying the thickness of each bracket base (for the in-out position of the respective tooth), and by varying the angulation of each bracket slot relative to the long axis of each tooth in the mesiodistal plane (for the crown angulation) and contouring the base of the bracket occlusogingivally (for the crown inclination). Therefore, when the teeth are in their correct three-dimensional positions, there is a level bracket slot line-up, i.e. the bracket slots in each arch are at the same height, and there are no offset bends in the archwire. These preadjusted bracket systems have reduced the requirement for wire bending dramatically. Nevertheless, accurate tooth positioning in preparation for surgery and effective postoperative finishing and detailing of tooth positions will almost always require some degree of wire bending (Table 12-1). Much of the artistic flair in orthodontic finishing still emanates from the orthodontist's ability to bend wire.

Bracket slot size

In this context, the *bracket slot size* refers to the dimensions of the horizontal channel within a

Table 12-1 Classification of orthodontic archwire bends (after Tweed)

Type of bend	Archwire type required	Tooth movement generated
First-order bend (also termed 'in-out' or horizontal 'offset' bends; vertical step bends that do not alter the tooth's angulation are also in this category) (Figure 12.1a and b).*	Round or rectangular stainless steel.	Buccolingual offset of a tooth crown in the horizontal plane; or vertical translation of a crown *without* a change in angulation.
Second-order bend (also termed 'tip bends' or 'angulation bends') (Figure 12.1c).	Round or rectangular stainless steel.	Mesiodistal angulation of the tooth crown and/or root.
Third-order bend (also termed 'torquing bends' or 'inclination bends') (Figure 12.1d).	Rectangular stainless steel or TMA (titanium-molybdenum alloy).	Buccolingual crown and/or root inclination.

*Clinicians should be aware that the Tweed system, described by the pioneering American orthodontist Charles H. Tweed (1895–1970), describes first-order bends as horizontal adjustments only, and second-order bends for any vertical adjustment, i.e. vertical bodily extrusion or intrusion bends are classified as second-order according to Tweed.

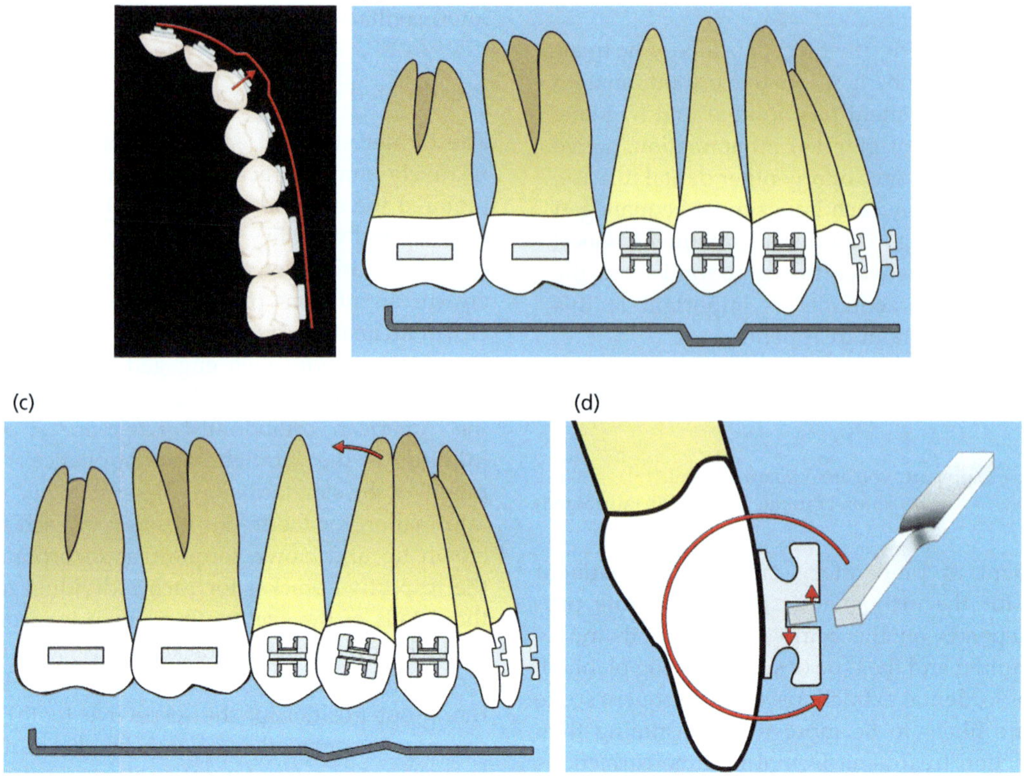

Fig. 12-1 (a) First-order bend to buccally offset a maxillary canine tooth. (b) First-order bend to vertically extrude a maxillary first premolar. (c) Second-order bend to correct the angulation of a maxillary first premolar. (d) Third-order bend to apply palatal root torque to a maxillary central incisor.

bracket that receives the orthodontic archwire. The most commonly used bracket slot sizes are the 0.018 × 0.025-inch (0.46 × 0.64 mm) and the larger 0.022 × 0.028-inch (0.56 × 0.7 mm). The type used is dependent on the preference of the orthodontist, but the 0.022 × 0.028-inch bracket slot does allow the use of heavier stainless steel archwires, which make dental arch levelling potentially easier (Figure 12-2).

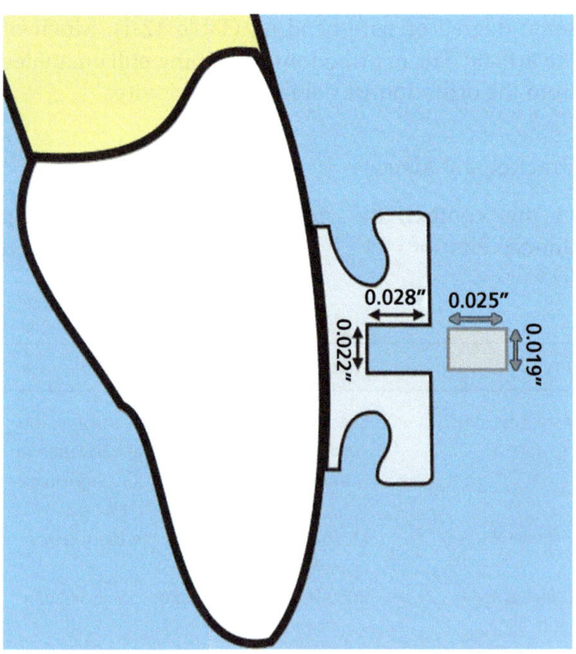

Fig. 12-2 Bracket slot dimensions and rectangular archwire dimensions in cross-section. A 0.022 × 0.028-inch bracket slot is shown, with a 0.019 × 0.025-inch rectangular archwire.

Note:

Pronouncing bracket slot size and archwire dimensions

To avoid long-winded terms in clinical practice, user-friendly abbreviations may be used at the chair side. The 0.018 × 0.025-inch bracket slot size is abbreviated and pronounced an '18-slot', and the 0.022 × 0.028-inch bracket slot a '22-slot'. A round archwire, e.g. a 0.018-inch stainless steel, is pronounced '18-steel', whereas a rectangular stainless steel archwire with the dimensions 0.019 × 0.025-inch is pronounced '19–25 steel'.

Banding vs. bonding of molar teeth

In modern orthodontics, bonded brackets are the norm for all the teeth, although molar bands are occasionally used, particularly when transpalatal arches or tooth-borne rapid maxillary expanders are required. Some surgeons prefer the molar teeth to be banded, particularly the final tooth in each arch, which is usually the second molar. The reasoning is that should this tooth be bonded rather than banded, and thereby debond during surgery, it may be a potential problem. Alternatively, it may be argued that a loose band may not be noticed for some time.

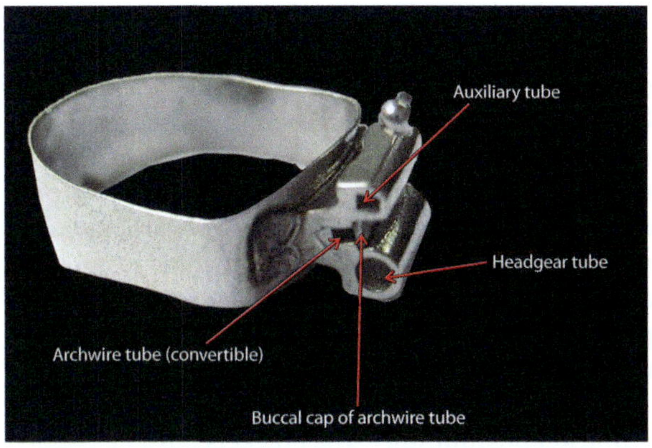

Fig. 12-3 A convertible maxillary right molar band. The buccal cap of a convertible tube on the first molar band may be removed, transforming the tube into a bracket.

Molar bands are also required *if a band tube needs to be converted into a bracket*, e.g. if a maxillary second molar tooth needs to be buccally offset or individually intruded, an archwire with the appropriate bend will not pass through a normal buccal tube on either a molar band or bonded buccal tube on the maxillary first molar. In such cases, the buccal cap of a convertible tube on the first molar band is removed, transforming the tube into a bracket (Figure 12-3). More recently, self-ligating molar tubes have been introduced, which may be used instead of a convertible tube.

A second, or auxiliary, archwire tube can be incorporated into a molar bond or band. This is useful in cases requiring segmental surgery, if an auxiliary wire needs to be constructed for placement into the auxiliary tubes to stabilize the segments immediately after segmental repositioning.

The use of *lingual and palatal cleats* on molar bands for attachment of elastics may be required in either the preoperative or postoperative phases; however, where bonded molar tubes have been used rather than molar bands, lingual or palatal buttons may be bonded directly onto the teeth if required.

Labial vs. lingual appliance

Labial orthodontic appliances are superior to lingual appliances in orthognathic patients for a number of reasons:

- **Intraoperative IMF placement** – Lingual appliances cannot be used by the surgeon intraoperatively for application of temporary intermaxillary fixation, and some form of labial attachment will be required, e.g. buttons or brackets bonded onto the labial aspects of the teeth, or temporary anchorage devices (e.g. microscrews) in the labial alveolar bone (see Figures 42.4–42.6).
- **Debonding brackets** – If a lingual bracket debonds during or immediately after surgery, it is very difficult to rebond in the immediate postoperative period, as the patient has discomfort, an inevitable degree of trismus leading to limited mouth opening, and often a mouth laden with blood-stained saliva.
- **Postoperative oral hygiene** – The same factors may potentially make it more difficult for the patient to keep the teeth and appliances clean if the brackets are lingual.
- **Anterior open bites** – An upper lingual appliance may also interfere with complete overbite correction in anterior open bite cases.

Use of aesthetic brackets

Some patients may demand labial 'aesthetic' brackets, in which case informed consent is essential. However, routine stainless steel brackets and bands/tubes are superior to aesthetic labial brackets in patients undergoing orthognathic surgery, for a number of reasons:

- **Susceptibility to fracture** – Ceramic brackets are brittle and thereby vulnerable to fracture intraoperatively, particularly during placement of IMF. They also often shatter into pieces, in which case parts may potentially enter open surgical sites.
- **Tooth wear** – Ceramic brackets may also lead to serious tooth wear from abrasion with the enamel of teeth in the opposing arch, which may be a serious problem in orthognathic patients at the start of treatment due to the variety of presenting malocclusions, particularly deep bites, and may also become a problem during the preoperative period as the teeth align and decompensate.
- **Plastic or resin composite type brackets** – These are often difficult to see and may impede or reduce tooth movement due to problems of increased friction. They are also usually rather weak, and prone to fracture, which is again an intraoperative problem for which the surgeon will not be thankful.

Objectives of preoperative orthodontics

'A rock pile ceases to be a rock pile the moment a single man contemplates it, bearing within him the image of a cathedral.'
Antoine de Saint-Exupéry (1900–1944)[5]
French writer, poet and aviator

Note:

If the 'rock pile' described by Saint-Exupéry can be compared to the teeth, which may be crowded, spaced, rotated, incorrectly positioned, incorrectly angulated and inclined with respect to their basal bone, then the contemplation described is the process of diagnosis and planning prior to the preoperative phase of preparatory orthodontics, which forms the basis of the *preparatory road map*, required to reach the ultimate goal. The orthodontist must have the precise destination in mind, in terms of where the teeth should be positioned in relation to the three planes of space, the three axes of rotation, and the eventual occlusion with the opposing dental arch; i.e. to have the 'image of the cathedral' in mind before a single bracket is bonded.

The aspiration of the orthodontist and overall purpose of preoperative orthodontic treatment is to place the teeth into the correct position for their respective jaw, so that on repositioning the jaws, the surgeon may attain the desired skeletal movements *and* obtain the best possible dental occlusion. *The preparatory orthodontic tooth movements should be determined in relation to the proposed surgical movements of the jaws* (see Chapter 6). The intended tooth movements may be described in relation to the **six objectives of preparatory preoperative orthodontic treatment:**

- Alignment
- Levelling
- Decompensation
- Incisor inclination preparation
- Arch coordination
- Elimination of occlusal interferences.

There is a seventh objective if *segmental surgery* is required:

- Creating interdental space for osteotomy cuts. This will be described under the 'alignment' section below.

Note:

These objectives of orthodontic preparation are not always achieved in the same order. For example, decompensation may occur prior to arch levelling, or maxillary arch expansion to coordinate the arches may be required at the beginning of treatment. In certain circumstances, some of these phases occur together. They are described separately below for enhanced descriptive clarity.

Alignment

Note:

Some authorities say that the best orthodontists of the past were those best at wire-bending, and that the best orthodontists of the present are those best at bracket positioning. Such statements, however well-intentioned, are rather misleading. Accurate bracket positioning is vitally important, but some degree of wire-bending, particularly in the final stages of finishing orthodontics, is inevitably required. The best orthodontists of the past, present (and future) are those who understand and apply the principles of accurate diagnosis and reasoned treatment planning, and develop technical finesse in undertaking logically applied and biologically sound orthodontic mechanics.

Alignment is usually, though not always, the first step in preoperative orthodontics (arch expansion is sometimes undertaken prior to alignment). Some arch levelling also begins at the same time as alignment, i.e. when the initial archwire is engaged into the brackets the teeth will begin to level. However, for the purpose of clarity, levelling will be described separately in the next section. The purpose of alignment is to correctly angulate ('tip') the crowns of the teeth into the correct position for their respective jaw and to correct tooth rotations.

- **Bracket positioning** – The brackets must be bonded into the correct position for each tooth. Time taken to accurately position the brackets at this stage is never wasted. Minor variations in bracket positioning may be required in some orthognathic patients:
  - **Maxillary canines** – In orthognathic patients, the coordination of the maxillary and mandibular labial segments, i.e. the canine-to-canine region, is paramount. Often, interference may occur between the tip of the mandibular canine and the mesio-palatal aspect of the maxillary canine, which prevents the intercuspation of the teeth. Therefore, it is advisable to *bond the maxillary canine bracket approximately $1/2$ to $3/4$ of a millimetre mesial to the long axis of the tooth*, leading to slight mesio-labial rotation of the tooth, and better ultimate interdigitation of the labial segment (Figure 12-4).
  - **In-standing maxillary lateral incisors** – Inverting the brackets provides labial/buccal root torque when the patient eventually has rectangular archwires placed, helping to prevent the 'proclined' appearance of the lateral incisor crown, which is a common problem in such cases.
  - **Maxillary second molars** – In many instances, these teeth should not be bonded, in order to prevent their extrusion, which will become a major interference in attempting arch coordination. If they must be bonded/banded, e.g. to derotate, then care should be taken to bonding the brackets somewhat occlusally (Figure 12-5). If a convertible tube is placed onto the first molar, steps can be added to an archwire to also minimise extrusion of the second molar (see Figure 12-46).
  - **Segmental surgery** – In preparation for segmental surgery, some interdental space is required, both *between the crowns and roots* of the teeth on either side of the planned osteotomy, to permit space for the surgical cuts *without damaging the teeth.* The crowns of the teeth on either side of the planned osteotomy may be separated using active coil spring, but root divergence may be achieved by either having the brackets in the correct positions and placing second-order bends in the archwire, or bonding the brackets at an angle to diverge the roots, and rebonding them in the correct position postoperatively (Figure 12-6). If the surgical

(a)

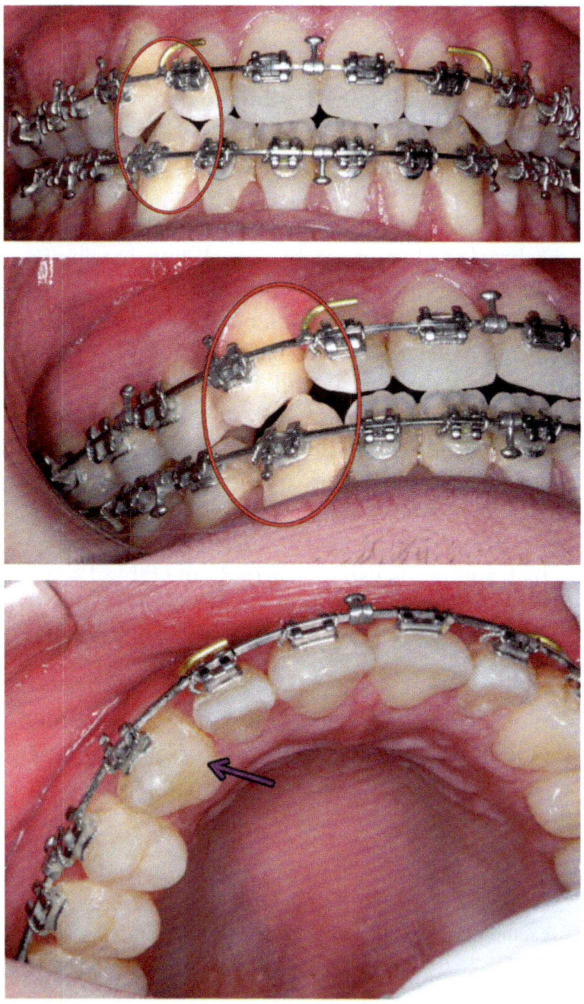

(b)

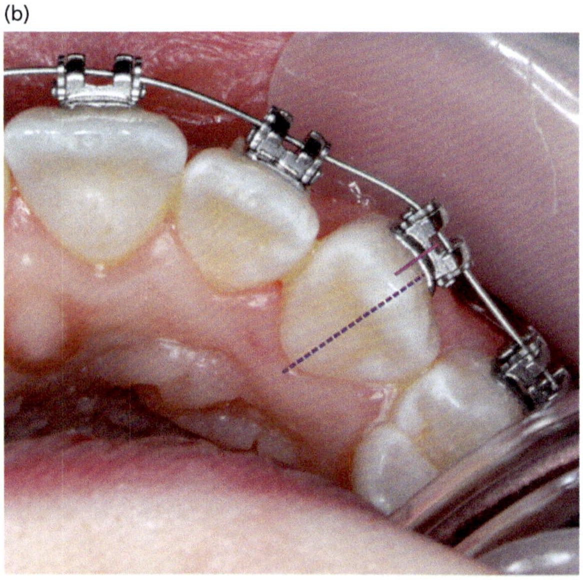

Fig. 12-4 (a) If the mesiopalatal aspect of the maxillary canine teeth is slightly prominent, it may prevent intercuspation of the anterior dentition, as in this postoperative Class III patient. (b) This may be prevented by bonding the maxillary canine bracket $^1/_2$ to $^3/_4$ of a millimetre mesial to the long axis of the maxillary canine in orthognathic patients with potentially reduced maxillary intercanine width. The slight mesio-labial rotation of the canine crown aids interdigitation.

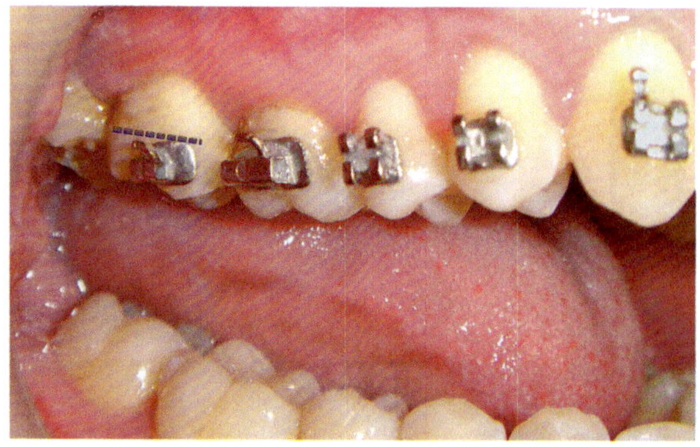

Fig. 12-5 If maxillary second molars have to be bonded/banded, care should be taken to bond the brackets somewhat occlusally in order to prevent their extrusion.

cut is planned distal to the canine teeth, contralateral canine brackets may be bonded, which reverses the tip in the brackets and angulates their roots mesially. Following surgery, the correct brackets may be bonded to correct the canine angulations.

- **Archwire size, shape and material** – A thin, round archwire is ideal for initial alignment, producing little binding and friction, and permitting relatively free tipping of the tooth crowns. The *forces should be as light as possible*, whilst permitting tooth movement. Nickel–titanium alloy (NiTi) is the initial aligning archwire material of choice, having both *shape memory* (i.e. it returns to its original form following plastic deformation, e.g. being ligated to a malpositioned tooth) and *superelasticity* (i.e. a flat 'superelastic' plateau in the middle of the force-deflection curve, allowing appreciable distortion of the wire in order to engage brackets on considerably displaced teeth whilst maintaining acceptable force levels) (Figure 12-7). The preliminary archwire is usually a round 0.014-inch, followed by a 0.016-inch NiTi or 0.018-inch copper NiTi after 1 to 2 visits of religation.

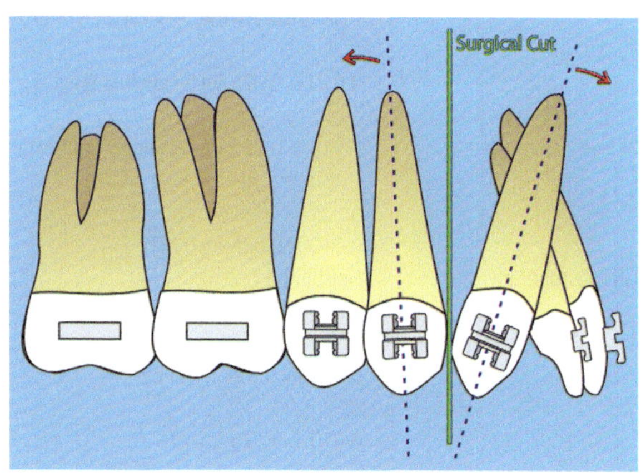

Fig. 12-6 Root divergence prior to segmental surgery.

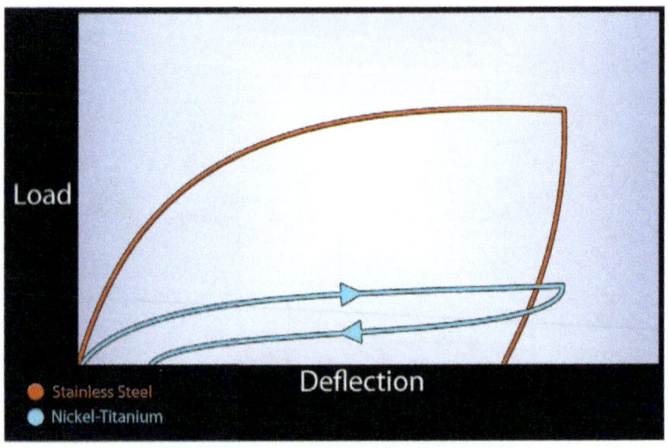

Fig. 12-7 The force-deflection curve comparing a nickel-titanium (NiTi) archwire with stainless steel. The almost horizontal plateau on the NiTi graph means that the wire will deliver approximately the same force over a large range of deflection. This highly desirable characteristic, known as **superelasticity**, is unique to NiTi archwires. In addition, the deactivation plateau is lower than the activation plateau, i.e. less force is delivered on unloading than is required to activate the wire (a property known as **hysteresis**), allowing the use of light forces for initial alignment of the dentition.

Note:

Archwire sequencing in orthognathic surgery
Typical sequencing of archwires for an orthognathic patient is variable, depending on the desired goals of treatment. Assuming a 0.022 × 0.028-inch bracket slot, the initial aligning archwire is usually 0.014-inch NiTi, moving onto 0.018-inch copper NiTi. If sliding mechanics are required, e.g. to correct a dental midline shift, a working archwire of 0.018-inch stainless steel may be used, though a working wire should always be ligated into the brackets for at least a month, allowing levelling of the bracket slots, prior to any sliding mechanics being undertaken. This helps to make the archwire passive and thereby avoids binding of the brackets onto the archwire. The 0.018-inch stainless steel archwire is also very useful for correcting the inclination of incisor teeth, as the teeth rotate round the transverse axis. If such movements are not required, then an interim 0.019 × 0.025-inch NiTi archwire is used to help prepare for the ligation of the 0.019 × 0.025-inch stainless steel archwires, on which surgery is usually carried out (Table 12-2).

Levelling

Dental arch levelling refers to the stage of orthodontic treatment which aims to flatten (or almost flatten) the curve of Spee, by permitting the relative vertical movement of the teeth in each arch to bring their

Table 12-2 Typical archwire sequencing in relation to stage of treatment (assuming a 0.022 × 0.028 bracket slot)

Stage of treatment	Archwire dimension and material	Examples of dental movements required
Early preoperative	0.014-inch NiTi	Alignment
Early preoperative	0.016-inch NiTi or 0.018-inch copper NiTi	Alignment (and very useful for derotation of severely rotated teeth)
Mid-preoperative	Rectangular NiTi, e.g.: 0.017 × 0.025-inch NiTi 0.018 × 0.025-inch NiTi 0.019 × 0.025-inch NiTi	Transitional archwire, mainly to level the bracket slots and begin torque, in preparation for rectangular steel archwires.
Mid-preoperative*	0.018-inch stainless steel	This archwire has many uses, including: • Sliding mechanics, e.g. dental midline correction • Retroclination or proclination of incisors • Levelling • Arch expansion/contraction
Mid to late preoperative	Rectangular stainless steel: 0.019 × 0.025-inch stainless steel (This is usually the surgical archwire)	• Levelling of dental arches • Arch expansion/contraction • Retraction of incisors • Space closure
Early postoperative	0.019 × 0.025-inch stainless steel	Usually maintained to allow stabilization of bony segments during initial healing phase; Useful if further expansion required.
Mid-postoperative	0.019 × 0.025-inch braided (multistrand) stainless steel or 0.019 × 0.025-inch NiTi	Permits vertical movement of teeth whilst maintaining torque, e.g. closing a lateral open bite.
Late-postoperative	Finishing: 0.019 × 0.025-inch stainless steel or 0.018-inch stainless steel or 0.019 × 0.025-inch TMA	Finishing and detailing of the dental occlusion and individual tooth positions.

*This stage, with a round steel archwire, is only required if any of the specific tooth movements described are required.

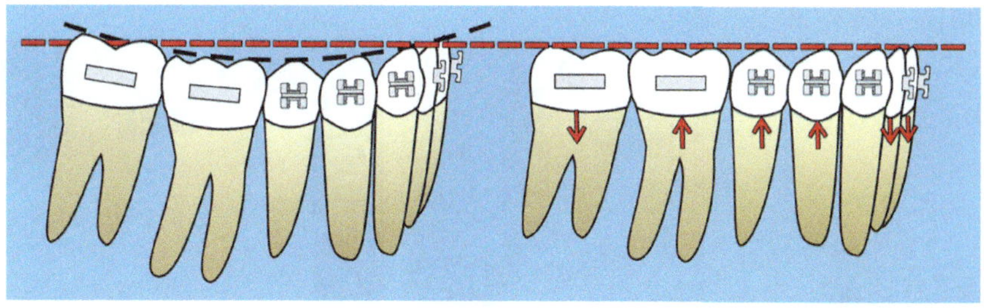

Fig. 12-8 Total continuous arch levelling.

marginal ridges to lie approximately in the same horizontal plane. A relatively flat (i.e. 'level') curve of Spee is one of the prerequisites to a normal dental occlusion.

In the orthognathic patient, levelling may be undertaken at different stages of treatment, depending on the requirements of the respective case:

- Preoperatively – In the majority of patients most or all the levelling may be undertaken prior to surgery.
- Intraoperatively – The preoperative phase is used to segmentally align 'segments' of each dental arch and the segments are subsequently surgically levelled.
- Postoperatively – Some or most of the levelling is undertaken following surgery, e.g. a **3-point landing** (interarch tooth contact at the incisors and terminal molars only) used to increase the lower anterior face height and reduce the incisor overbite (see below).

The decision on how to level in the maxillary arch is predominantly based on the final desired position of the maxillary incisors in relation to the upper lip and face. Once the desired postoperative position of the maxillary incisors has been planned, the decision on how to level the mandibular arch depends on the planned postoperative position of the mandibular incisors in relation to the maxillary incisors *and the effect of this position on the lower anterior face height* (LAFH). If no increase in LAFH is desired, the mandibular arch is levelled preoperatively by incisor intrusion. However, if an increase in LAFH is desired, the mandibular arch curve of Spee is either partially levelled if only a small increase in LAFH is desired, the curve is maintained if already present at the required depth, or the curve is accentuated if a significant increase in LAFH is desired, i.e. the degree of preoperative levelling depends on how much of an increase in LAFH is desired. *As the mandible is advanced, the degree of anterior-inferior movement of the mandibular incisors will determine the increase in LAFH* (see Figure 6-24).

In the preoperative phase of treatment, the levelling of each individual dental arch may be total, partial or segmental.

- **Total continuous arch levelling** – In most cases, total arch levelling will occur as the orthodontist moves through the archwire sequence into the flat, heavy rectangular stainless steel archwires. These will lead to extrusion of premolar and canine teeth, and intrusion of incisor and to a small extent terminal molar teeth, though the extrusive effect is always greater (Figure 12-8). However, if mandibular incisor intrusion is specifically desired, e.g. in a patient with an already increased LAFH, some form of orthodontic intrusion arch mechanics (e.g. Burstone mechanics) may be required, or temporary anchorage devices may be used to directly intrude the incisors.
- **Partial continuous arch levelling** – e.g. maintenance of a degree of curve of Spee in preparation for a 3-point landing. There is some controversy over how great a lateral open bite may be closed

(a)

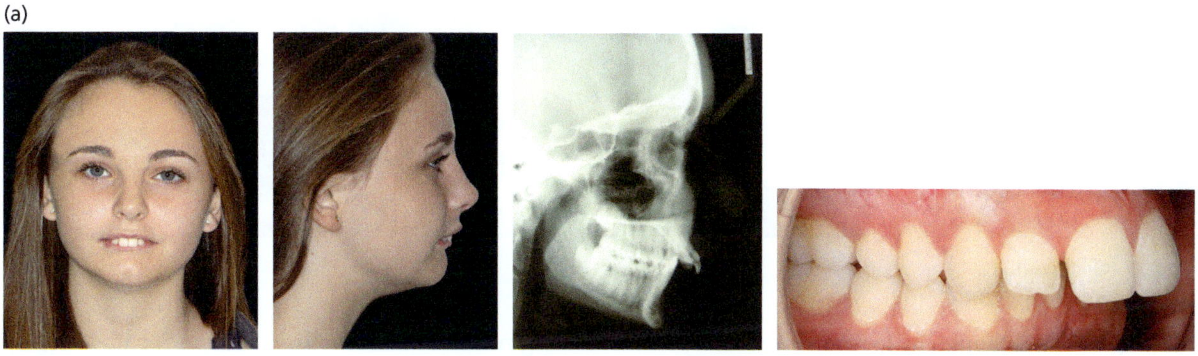

Fig. 12-9 3-point landing. (a) Preoperative images, demonstrating a Class II division 1 incisor relationship on a Class II skeletal pattern with mandibular retrognathia, a reduced lower anterior face height (LAFH) and increased curve of Spee. (b) Preoperative lateral cephalometric radiograph and mandibular model, demonstrating maintenance of the increased curve of Spee. (c) Postoperative result with a 3-point landing, with contact at the incisors and terminal molars bilaterally. The mandibular 0.019 × 0.025-inch stainless steel surgical archwire is still ligated in position. (d) A 0.017 × 0.025-inch flexible NiTi mandibular archwire is placed and box elastics are placed bilaterally to close the lateral open bites. (e) 12-weeks postoperative views, with lateral open bites essentially closed with postoperative levelling of the mandibular arch, and increase in LAFH.

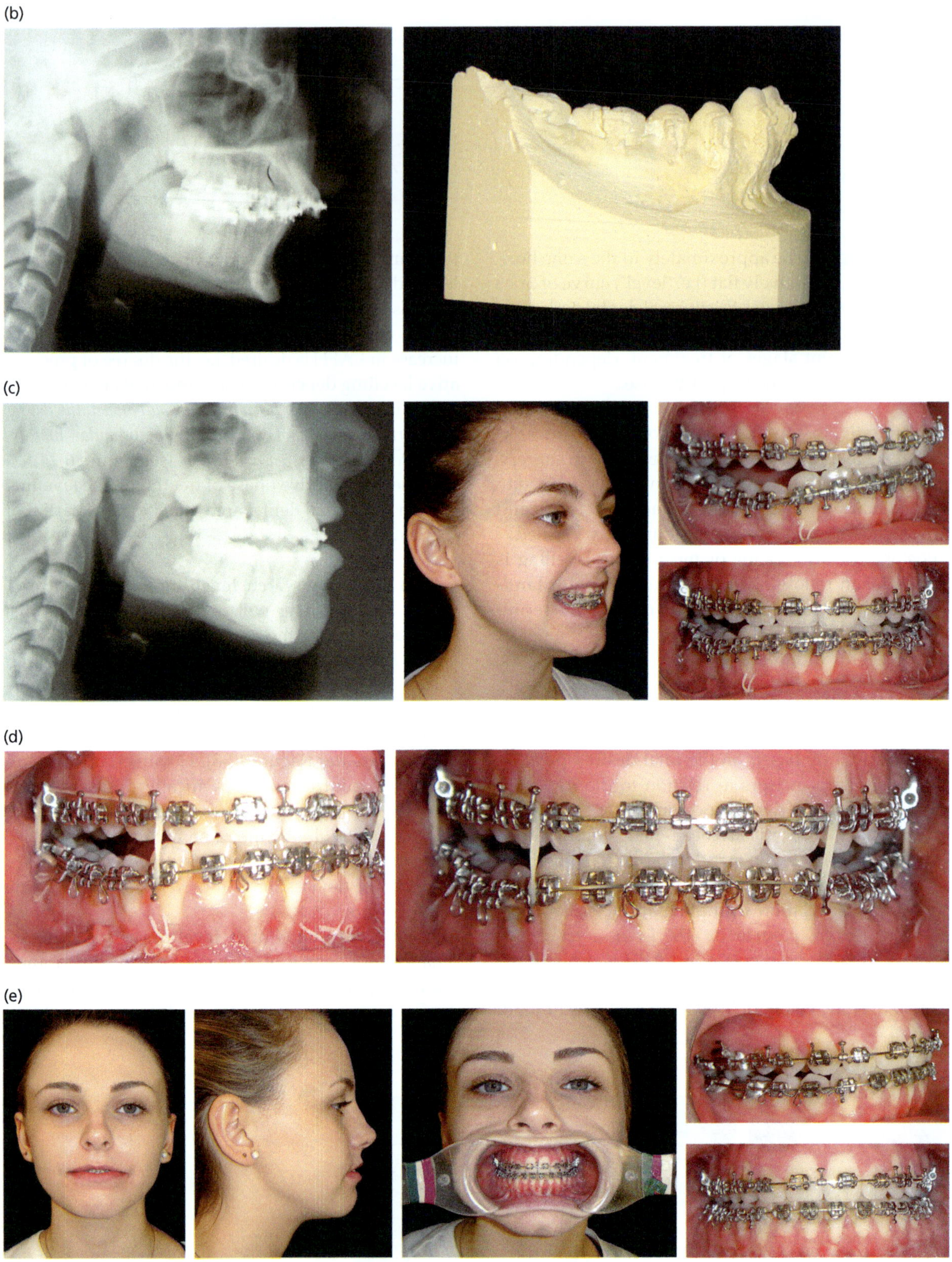

Fig. 12-9 (*Continued*).

postoperatively, though up to 5 mm is relatively routine, and up to 10 mm has been achieved clinically (Figure 12-9). There is a space requirement for levelling, as described below. An increased curve will need to be 'wiped' into the mandibular steel archwire to maintain or accentuate the curve of Spee preoperatively (Figure 12-10).

- **Segmental arch levelling** – For a patient being prepared for segmental surgery requiring levelling, the differential vertical movements required for each segment will depend on aesthetic and occlusal factors. In such cases the segments are aligned and levelled intra-segmentally, avoiding continuous initial aligning archwires. Subsequent stainless steel

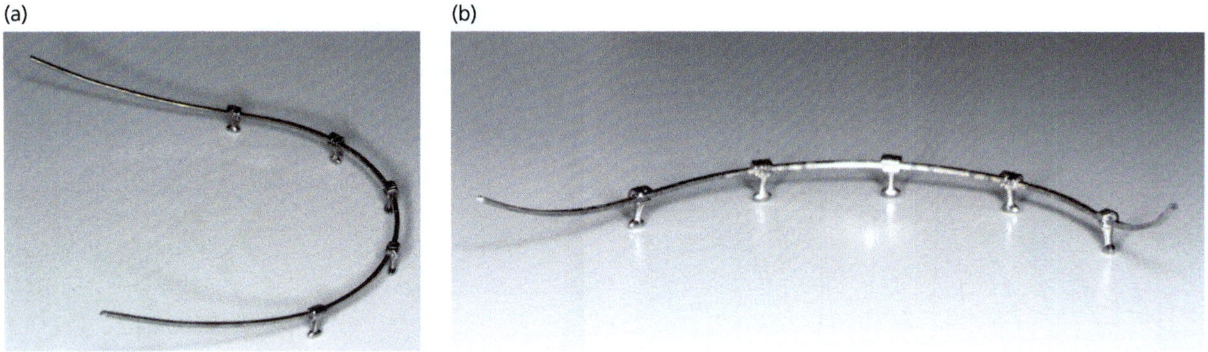

Fig. 12-10 An increased curve has been 'wiped' into the mandibular 0.019 × 0.025-inch stainless steel archwire in order to maintain the mandibular curve of Spee prior to surgery.

archwires may either remain segmental, or if continuous archwires are desired, they will require appropriate vertical bends placed between the segments (Figure 12-11). Such continuous archwires will need to be cut intraoperatively to permit surgical manipulation of the segments. Stabilization of the segments will be required with a continuous archwire, perhaps placed into auxiliary molar tubes, immediately following surgical repositioning of the segments.

Note:

Space requirement for levelling – It is important to bear in mind that some space within each dental arch is required for orthodontic levelling. A space of approximately 1mm is required to level a 3 mm depth curve of Spee.[6] Therefore, if the maximum depth of the curve of Spee in the mandibular arch is 3 mm, then 1 mm of space should be maintained in the mandibular arch to permit postoperative levelling by extrusion of the mandibular premolars and canines. More space is required for a greater depth of curve. Space may be acquired by interdental enamel reduction or maintained from space closure following dental extractions. Alternatively, this space for levelling may be acquired by proclination of the mandibular incisors, which is the alternative to space creation in the mandibular arch, particularly in non-extraction cases (Figure 12-12).

Decompensation

The discrepancy between the jaws in all three planes of space has an indirect yet considerable influence on the dental occlusal relationship as a result of **dentoalveolar compensation**. Dentoalveolar compensation describes the *variations in the positions of the teeth, in the sagittal, vertical and transverse dimensions, that may compensate for variations in the skeletal pattern*, i.e. it is nature's way of trying to get the teeth to meet when the jaws are growing away from one another.[7] In the normal situation, the erupting maxillary and mandibular teeth are guided towards each other by the surrounding **soft tissue envelope** of the tongue, lips and cheeks; hence, they erupt into a position of **soft tissue equilibrium** between the opposing forces of the tongue and lips/cheeks (Figure 12-13). Therefore, in the presence of *sagittal* or *transverse* skeletal discrepancies, alterations in the inclination of the teeth *compensate* for the skeletal discrepancy (Figure 12-14). In such cases, the occlusal discrepancy will appear less

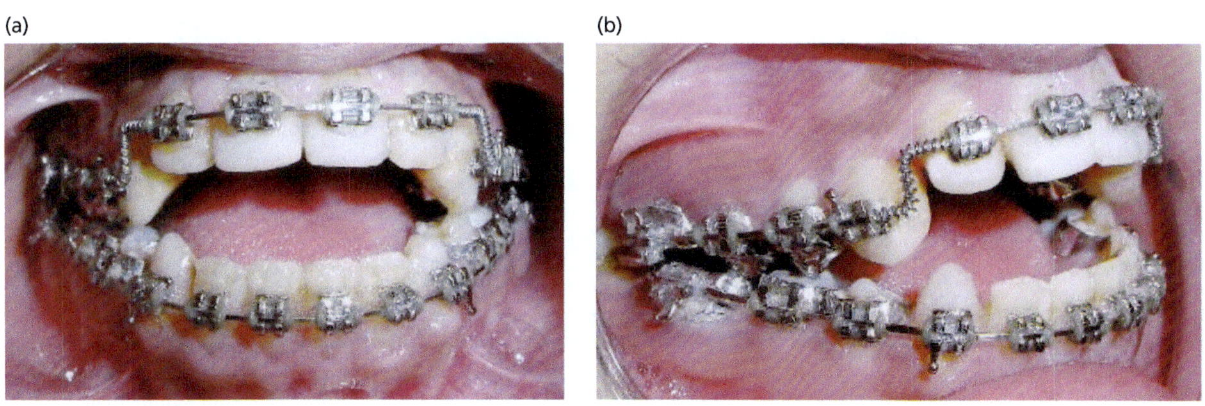

Fig. 12-11 Segmental arch levelling in preparation for segmental surgery. Continuous stainless steel archwires with appropriate vertical bends placed between the segments. The active coil springs ('pushcoil') is cut to a length larger than the interbracket distance between the maxillary lateral incisors and canines that need to be slightly separated at their crowns. The pushcoil is compressed prior to insertion, generating the forces required.

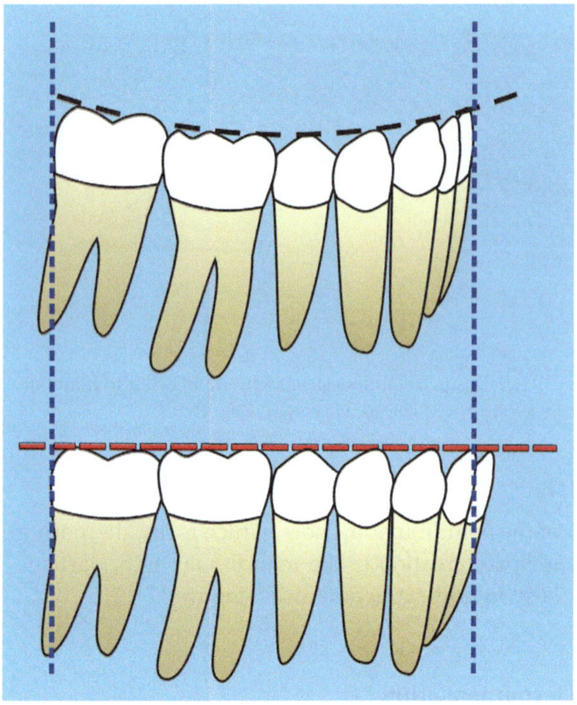

Fig. 12-12 Space requirement for arch levelling. Levelling an increased curve of Spee requires space. This may be gained by incisor proclination as demonstrated. If mandibular incisor proclination is to be avoided, space may need to be created by interdental enamel reduction, or a small degree of extraction space may be maintained preoperatively. In practice, the degree of space required is relatively small; approximately 1 mm of space (i.e. 0.5 mm per side) is required to level a 3 mm depth curve of Spee.

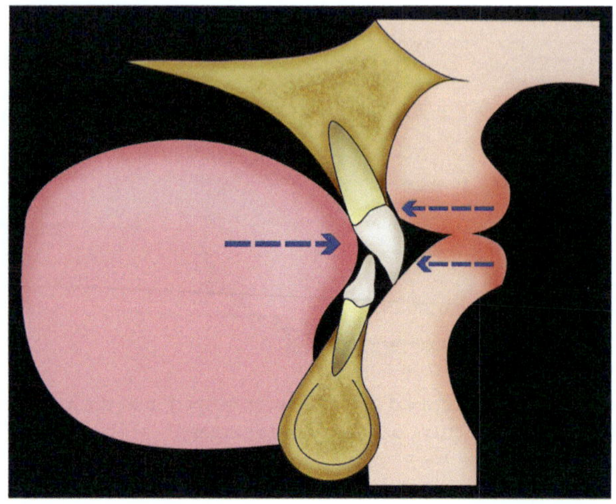

Fig. 12-13 The soft tissue envelope of the tongue, and lips/cheeks; the teeth are in a position of soft tissue equilibrium between the opposing forces of the tongue and lips/cheeks. (From: Naini FB. Facial Aesthetics: Concepts and Clinical Diagnosis. Oxford: Wiley-Blackwell, 2011. Reprinted with permission.)

severe than the underlying skeletal discrepancy. For example, in a patient with a severe Class III skeletal pattern, the dentoalveolar compensation involves proclination of the maxillary incisors and retroclination of the mandibular incisors (Figure 12-15). This compensatory mechanism may be unsuccessful either because the skeletal discrepancy is too severe or because the soft tissue pattern is unfavourable. For example, in a Class II skeletal discrepancy, if the soft tissues are unfavourable and the lower lip is unable to control the labial aspect of the maxillary incisors and instead falls behind them it will lead to their proclination and thereby magnify rather than compensate for the skeletal discrepancy. In the *vertical* plane, the incisors will tend to overerupt to compensate for increasing lower anterior face height, unless a forward tongue position prevents their overeruption. If the face height is dramatically increased, the incisors may not be able to fully compensate and an anterior open bite (AOB) will ensue.

Orthodontic preparation for orthognathic surgery requires **orthodontic decompensation** of the dental arches in *all three planes of space*, i.e. the process of removing the dentoalveolar compensations that may be present in the sagittal, transverse and vertical planes, and re-establishing the correct position of the teeth with regard to their own skeletal base thereby permitting adequate surgical correction of skeletal discrepancies.

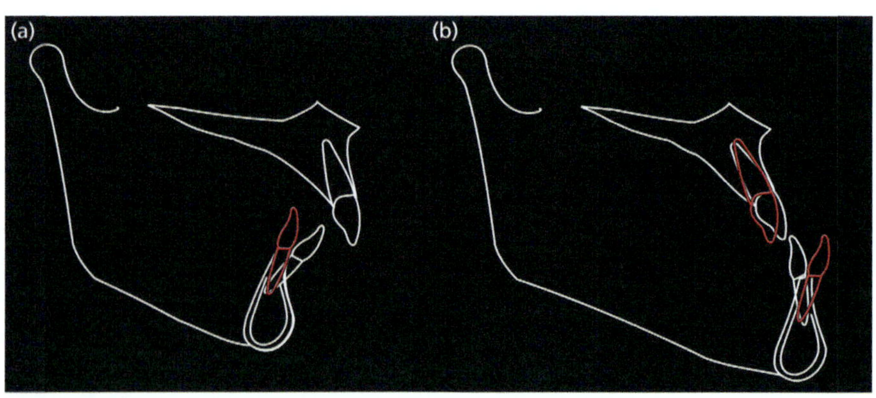

Fig. 12-14 Dentoalveolar compensation in the sagittal plane. (a) Proclination of the mandibular incisors often occurs to compensate for a Class II skeletal relationship; decompensation in preparation for mandibular advancement surgery would require their retroclination to a correct inclination for the mandibular skeletal base. (b) Proclination of the maxillary incisors and retroclination of the mandibular incisors may occur to compensate for a Class III skeletal relationship. Decompensation requires maxillary incisor retroclination and mandibular incisor proclination. (From: Naini FB. Facial Aesthetics: Concepts and Clinical Diagnosis. Oxford: Wiley-Blackwell, 2011. Reprinted with permission.)

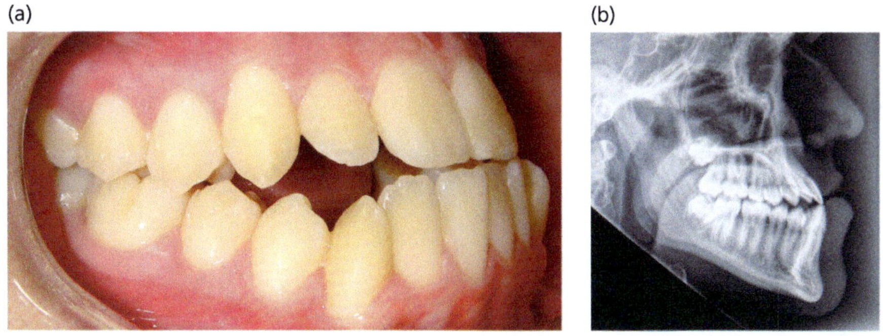

Fig. 12-15 Dentoalveolar compensation for a severe Class III skeletal discrepancy, with maxillary incisor proclination and mandibular incisor retroclination.

- **Decompensation and the planes of space and axes of rotation** – Compensatory tooth movements may have occurred in relation to all three planes of space and round the three axes of rotation. It thereby follows that decompensation of the teeth is required in relation to the three planes of space and the three axes of rotation. Decompensation in the transverse dimension is particularly important in patients with buccal crossbites, often associated with a hypoplastic maxilla and a Class III skeletal discrepancy. If the dental compensation is mild, orthodontic expansion may be all that is required, though this is only possible for expansion up to 4–5 mm, and buccal root torque is required to prevent further buccal flaring of the maxillary molars. If there has already been considerable dental compensation for the underlying skeletal discrepancy, this usually results in buccally flared maxillary molars and lingually inclined mandibular molars. Decompensation involves repositioning of the maxillary molars over basal bone, which increases the extent of the crossbite (Figure 12-16). In such cases, surgical expansion of the maxilla may be required, together with only partial decompensation of the mandibular molars. Alternatively, a bilateral posterior crossbite may be accepted (see Figure 6-29).
- **Total vs. partial decompensation** – Total decompensation is usually required, in order to position the teeth correctly in relation to their respective skeletal base. However, in some situations, it may be prudent to partially decompensate only, in order to reduce the extent of skeletal movements required where stability and relapse would be issues postoperatively. For example, when smaller skeletal movements are desired for facial aesthetic reasons, e.g. it may be planned to limit the extent of mandibular incisor proclination in preparation for a mandibular set-back procedure, in order to limit the degree of set-back.

  Another clinical situation where partial decompensation may be required is the maintenance or partial decompensation of lingually inclined mandibular molars in Class III patients. If the lingual inclination, i.e. dentoalveolar compensation, is maintained, crossbite correction will be easier (see Figure 12-16).

  Morphological reasons may also dictate partial decompensation in some instances, e.g. insufficient alveolar bone thickness and/or a thin gingival biotype prone to gingival recession. This may be a particular problem in the mandibular incisor region (Figure 12-17). Though free gingival grafts have been proposed prior to surgery in order to facilitate decompensation, their use is questionable, as the major problem is not lack of labial gingival tissue, but lack of labial alveolar bone. Consideration may be given to a free gingival graft *following* orthognathic treatment, for aesthetic reasons and to provide some protection to exposed root surfaces.
- **'Worsening' effect on dental occlusion and facial profile** – Just as dentoalveolar compensation tends to mask the extent of the underlying skeletal discrepancy, *orthodontic decompensation unmasks/unveils the true extent of the underlying skeletal discrepancy*. For example, a patient with a Class III skeletal discrepancy will often have retroclined mandibular incisors and possibly some proclination of the maxillary

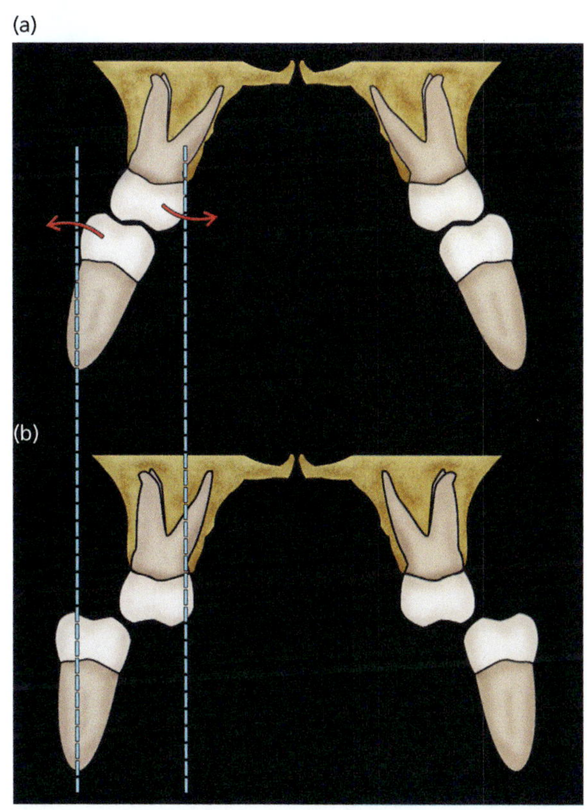

Fig. 12-16 (a) Dentoalveolar compensation in the transverse plane of space. (b) Decompensation in the transverse plane will increase the relative transverse discrepancy.

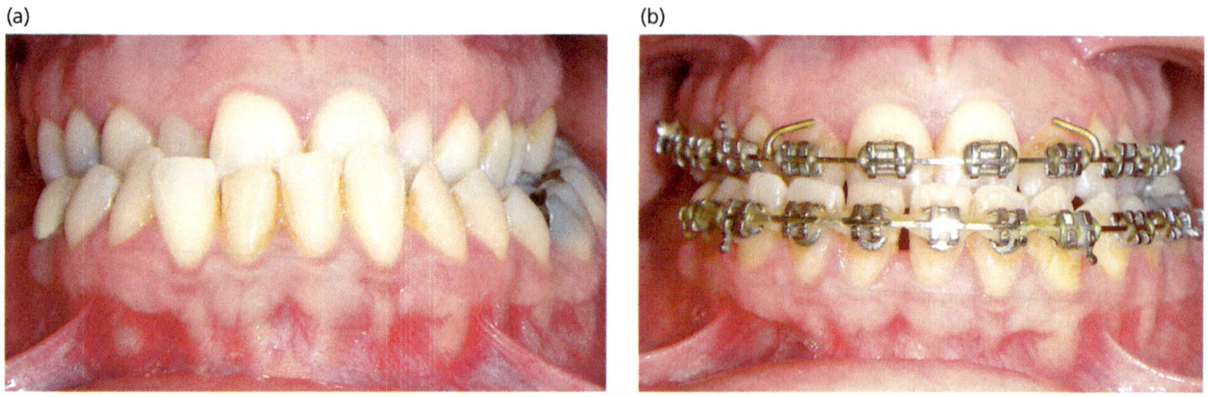

Fig. 12-17 (a) Pretreatment views of a Class III patient with thin gingival biotype, demonstrating 'washboard' appearance of the anterior tooth roots in the mandibular incisor and canine region. (b) Partial decompensation undertaken to limit the potential gingival recession and dehiscence as the mandibular incisors procline through thin labial alveolar bone.

incisors. As such, orthodontic decompensation results in retroclination of the maxillary incisors and proclination of the mandibular incisors, thereby increasing the reverse incisor overjet and making the lower lip more prominent (Figure 12-18). This is one aspect of treatment that may displease patients a great deal. As such, it is extremely important that patients are made aware of this issue prior to embarking on treatment, and as part of informed consent.

- **Retraction vs. retroclination of incisors** – Orthodontic retraction and retroclination are not the

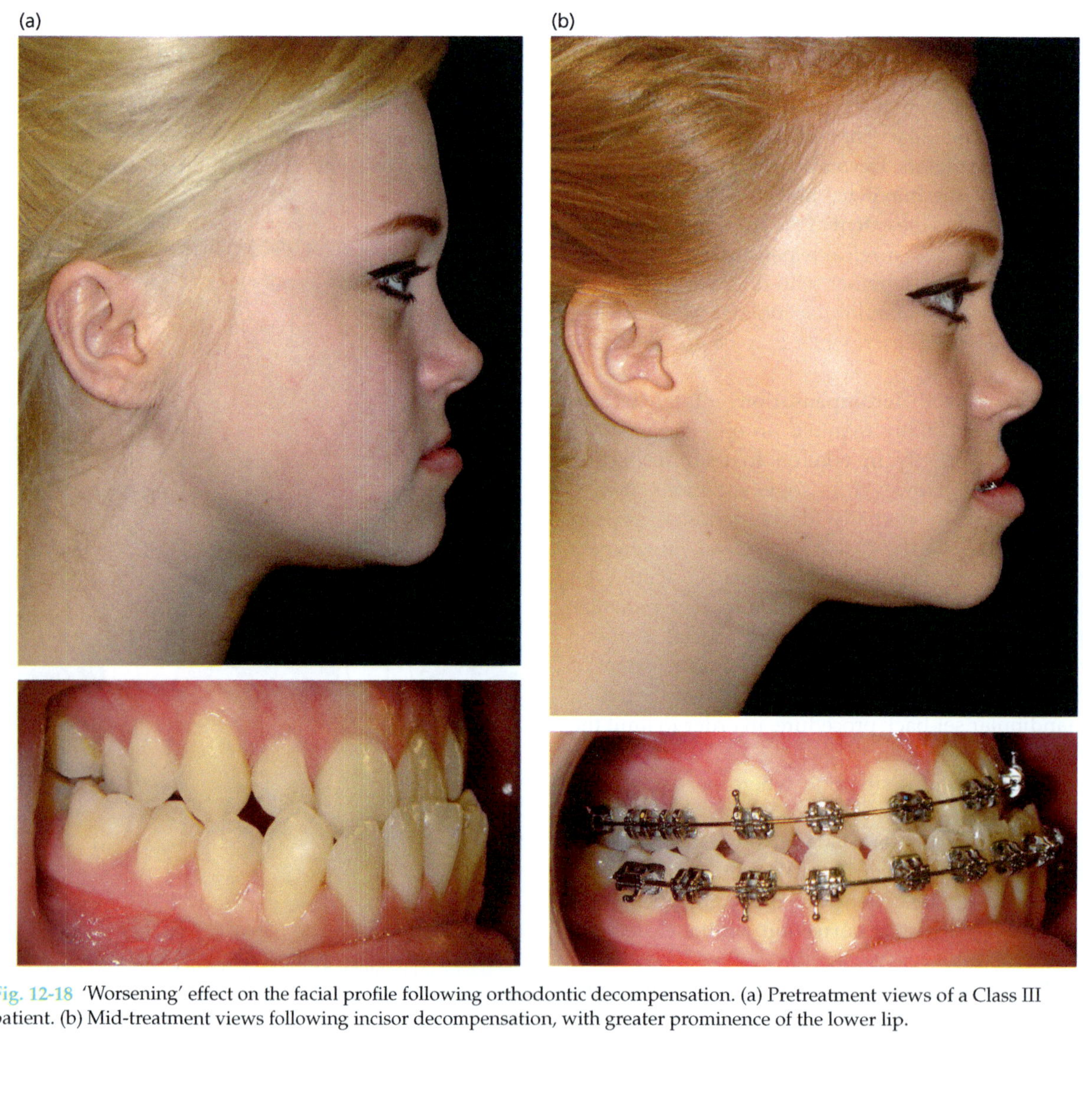

Fig. 12-18 'Worsening' effect on the facial profile following orthodontic decompensation. (a) Pretreatment views of a Class III patient. (b) Mid-treatment views following incisor decompensation, with greater prominence of the lower lip.

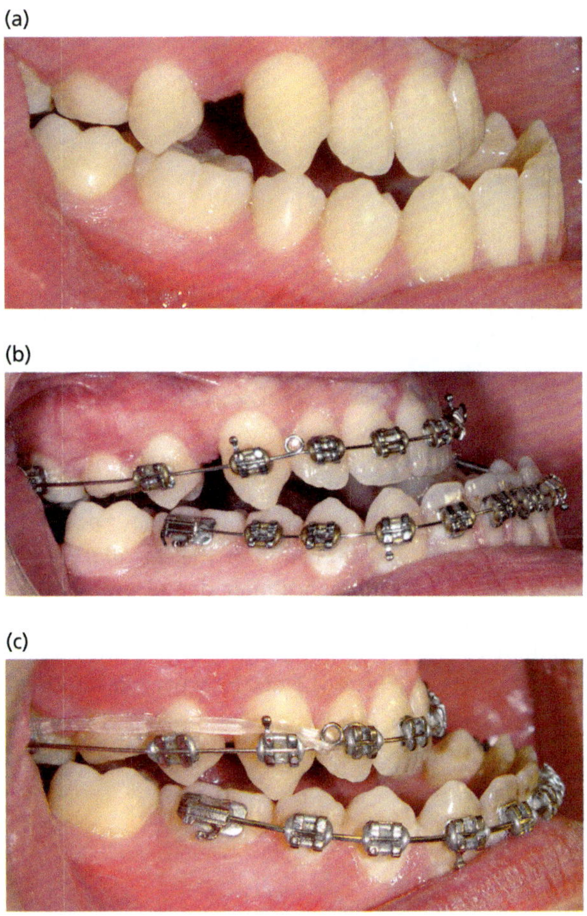

Fig. 12-19 Retroclination is undertaken on round stainless steel archwires. (a) Pretreatment view. (b) Mid-treatment view, following initial alignment and some decompensation of the mandibular arch. An upper 0.018-inch round stainless steel archwire is placed, with circle loops positioned between the lateral incisors and canines in order to provide a point of attachment for elastic intra-arch traction. (c) Retroclination of the maxillary incisors using the described mechanics.

same thing, and are not achieved with the same mechanics. Retraction describes the bodily translation of the incisor teeth in a lingual/palatal direction. Retroclination describes the rotation of the incisor teeth round the transverse axis of rotation, with the crown moving lingually/palatally. These movements arise from different orthodontic mechanics, which must be accurately planned. If the incisors are protruded, then they are retracted within the limits of the surrounding alveolar bone; if the incisors are proclined, they are retroclined to the correct or required inclination. Retroclination of incisors is undertaken on *round* stainless steel archwires, with elastomeric chain around the incisor brackets if there is interdental spacing, and intratraction (Figure 12-19). Retraction of incisors is undertaken with *rectangular* archwires. In some situations, the incisors may need to be retroclined to the correct inclination, then retracted to the correct sagittal position, in which case the former is carried out on a round stainless steel archwire (usually 0.018-inch) and the latter with a rectangular stainless steel archwire (Figure 12-20).

- **Interarch elastics** – Either Class II or Class III elastics may be required in order to help incisor proclination/retroclination. However, *their use is the opposite to a conventional orthodontic case*, i.e. in a patient with a Class III skeletal pattern, Class II elastics are used to retrocline/retract the maxillary incisors and procline the mandibular incisors. Conversely, in a patient with a Class II skeletal pattern, Class III elastics are often required to retrocline the mandibular and, if necessary procline the maxillary incisors, thereby increasing the incisor overjet in preparation for surgery (Figure 12-21).
- **Extraction patterns** – Dental extractions, when required, will be so as to permit the maximum extent of decompensation achievable, and thereby allow the desired extent of surgical movement of

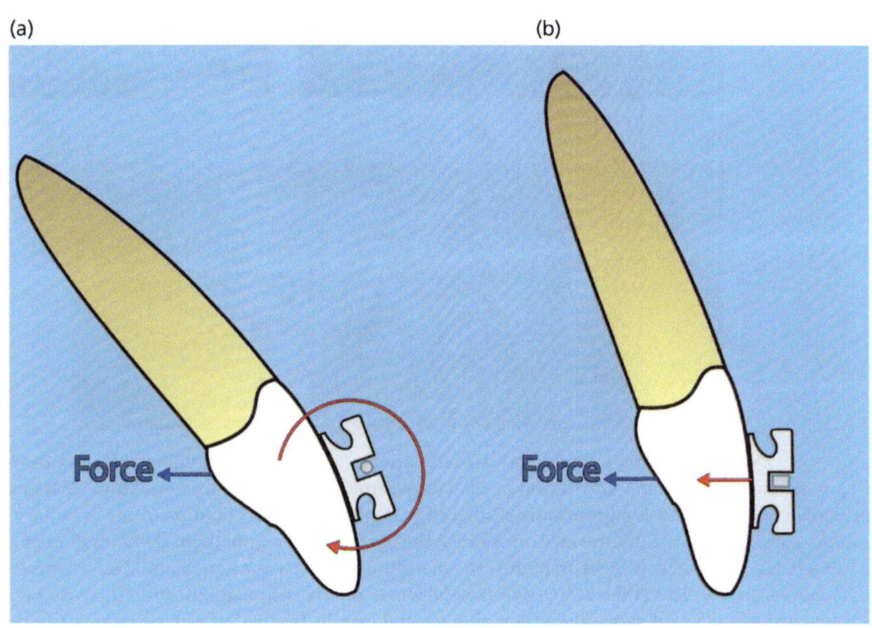

Fig. 12-20 Comparison of incisor retroclination and retraction. (a) Incisor *retroclination* should be undertaken on a *round* archwire, which permits rotation of the tooth, in order to correct its inclination. (b) Incisor *retraction* should be undertaken on a *rectangular* archwire, which permits bodily translation of the tooth with minimal change in inclination.

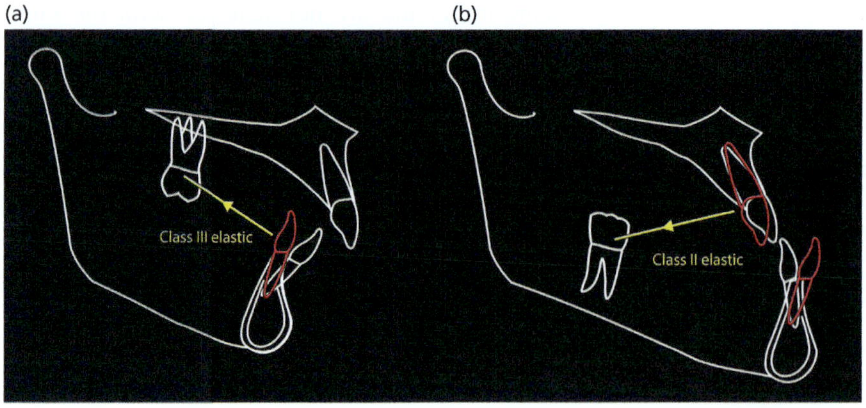

Fig. 12-21 (a) In a Class II patient, Class III elastics may be used to help incisor decompensation. (b) In a Class III patient, Class II elastics may be used to help incisor decompensation.

the jaws. *In preparation for orthognathic surgery dental extraction patterns are usually the opposite of those used in conventional orthodontics.* The Class II orthognathic patient with proclined mandibular incisors often requires extraction of mandibular first premolar teeth, to permit maximum retroclination and retraction of the mandibular incisors. In a Class III orthognathic patient, the extraction pattern is usually maxillary first premolars only to allow retroclination and retraction of the maxillary anterior dentition. The mandibular dental arch is usually treated on a non-extraction basis, as proclination of the mandibular incisors provides space for alignment (Figure 12-22). However, if required,

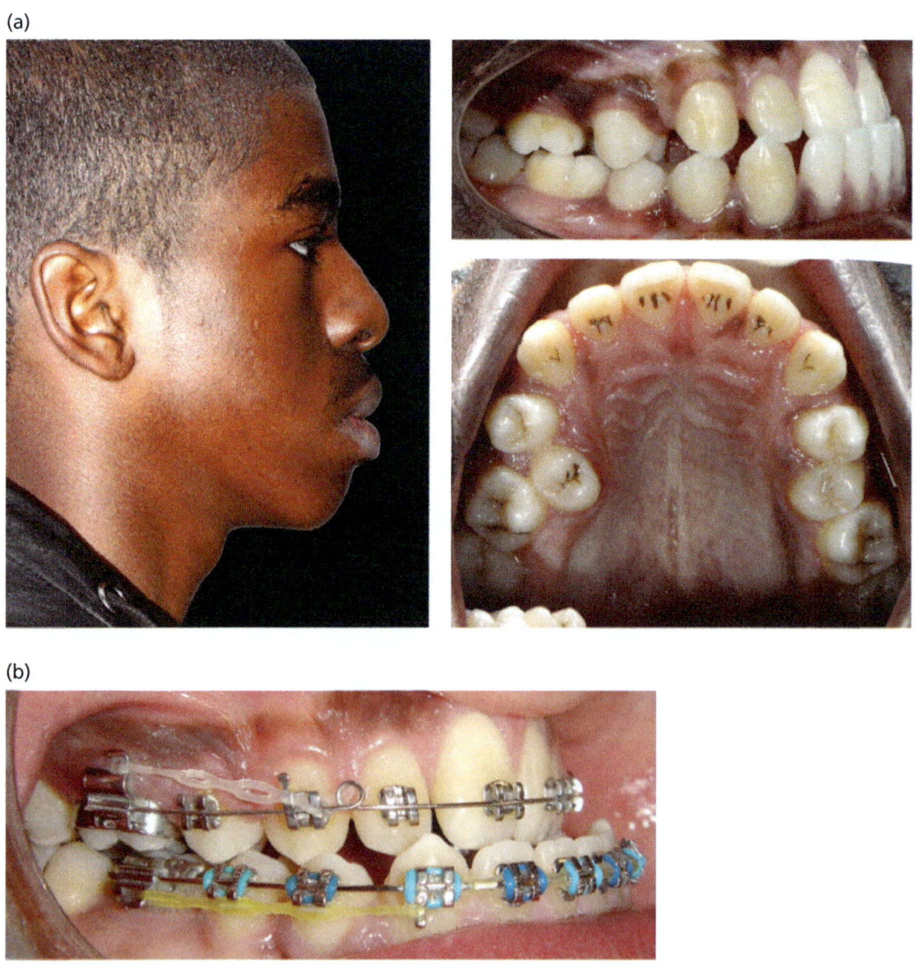

Fig. 12-22 Dental extraction pattern in a Class III patient. (a) Pretreatment views. The incisors are compensated for the skeletal Class III jaw relationship. Orthodontic decompensation required extraction of a premolar in each maxillary quadrant (right second premolar was extracted as significantly displaced palatally). (b) Retroclination of the maxillary incisors on a round 0.018-inch stainless steel archwire until the incisors were of the correct inclination, then: (c) Retraction of the incisors on a rectangular 0.019 × 0.025-inch stainless steel archwire. The mandibular arch was aligned and decompensated on a non-extraction basis. Incisor inclinations are correct to their respective skeletal bases and there is a significantly increased reverse incisor overjet in preparation for surgery. (d) The effect of decompensation on the facial profile, particularly lip prominences, may be observed. (e) Pretreatment lateral cephalometric radiograph compared with (f) preoperative radiograph, demonstrating incisor decompensation.

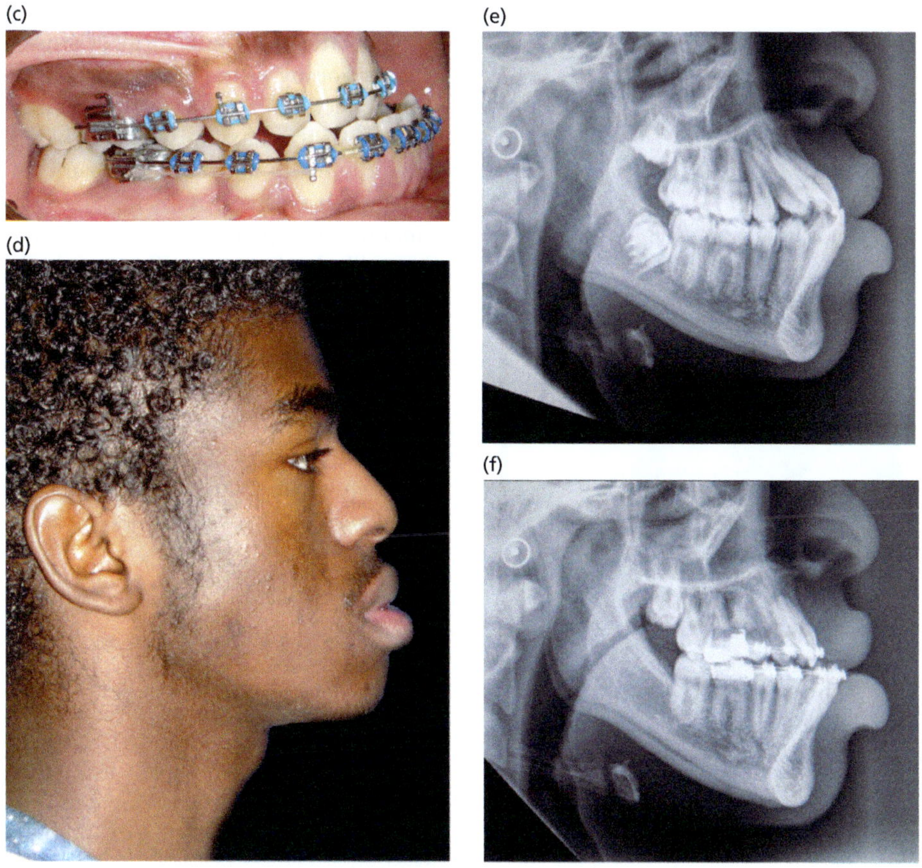

Fig. 12-22 (*Continued*).

mandibular second premolars may need to be extracted to create space to contract a broad mandibular arch. All extraction patterns should be planned after undertaking a comprehensive space analysis.

- **Anchorage requirements** – In a Class II orthognathic patient, the greatest anchorage requirement is usually in the mandibular arch, for retroclination and retraction of the mandibular incisors. In the Class III orthognathic patient, the maximum anchorage requirement is usually in the maxillary dental arch, for retroclination and/or retraction of the maxillary incisors.

Incisor inclination preparation

'... I always know the end from the beginning ... '
Charles Dickens (1812–1870)[8] (Figure 12-23)

The orthodontic treatment required to prepare the maxillary and mandibular incisor inclinations for surgery often occurs as part of incisor decompensation (see above). However, preoperative incisor inclination changes are not always, by definition, strictly speaking decompensation. For example, Class II patients with mandibular retrognathia often develop a lower lip trap, i.e. the lower lip gets caught behind the maxillary incisors, and leads to their proclination. This is not a compensatory proclination, but the inclination of the maxillary incisors needs to be corrected prior to mandibular advancement surgery.

Incisor inclination preparation for orthognathic surgery depends on whether surgery is being planned for a jaw, and whether that surgery involves rotation of the jaw round the transverse axis. If surgery is not being planned, then the incisor inclination for that jaw should be corrected prior to surgery, e.g. proclined maxillary incisors should be corrected preoperatively when only mandibular advancement surgery is being planned. If surgery is being planned for either jaw that will only entail sagittal bodily translation of the jaw, or if only vertical maxillary movement is required, then the incisor inclination for that jaw should again be corrected prior to surgery. However, *if either jaw is being planned for surgery that will involve the rotation of the jaw round the transverse axis*, such as differential posterior impaction of the maxilla, or autorotation of the mandible, which thereby alters the inclination of the incisors, then *the incisor inclination should be prepared preoperatively to take into account the change in incisor inclination that will occur as part of the surgical repositioning of the respective jaw.*

- **Differential posterior maxillary impaction** – In patients with an anterior open bite, the preparation for a Le Fort I differential posterior impaction of the maxilla requires the creation or maintenance of a *predetermined amount of maxillary incisor proclination.* As the posterior maxilla is superiorly repositioned by a greater amount than the anterior maxilla, the maxillary incisors are effectively retroclined to the correct inclination (see Chapter 29 for detailed description of planning in such cases) (Figure 12-24).[9]

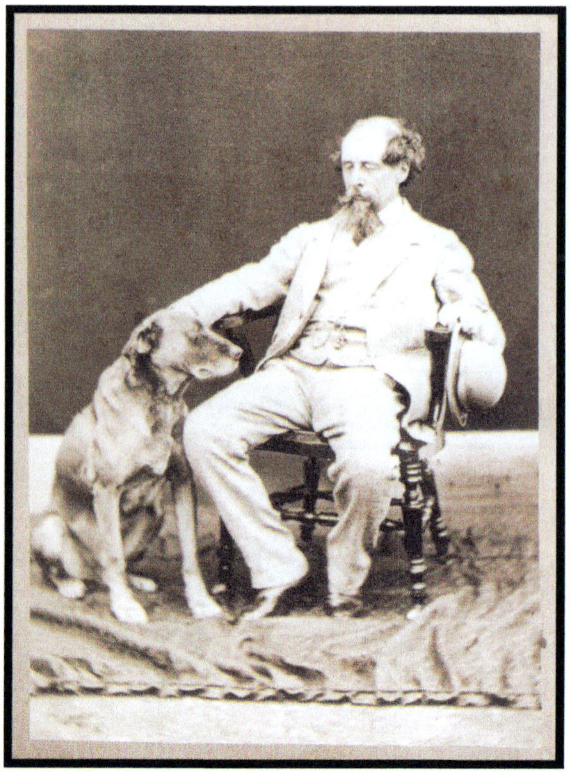

Fig. 12-23 Charles Dickens (1812–1870). By the 1860s, Dickens was the most famous and best-loved author in the English-speaking world. He often worked on more than one book at a time, with each chapter published in monthly instalments. The key formula to doing this, other than genius, was his meticulous planning and preparation. When asked how he was able to work on more than one book, his reply was 'I always know the end from the beginning.' *Note*: Dickens is pictured here with one of his beloved dogs. He was an avid dog-lover and kept a large number of dogs at his home. In 1862, Dickens wrote an article (published in the popular magazine *All The Year Round*), on the subject of abandoned and starving dogs in London, and the responsibility of decent people with a social conscience in the benevolent society that he longed for, to care for dogs and support the then much-ridiculed Home for Lost and Starving Dogs, established by the incredible Mrs Mary Tealby (1801/2–1865) in a disused stable yard in North London in 1860. As the most eminent Victorian writer, his words were hugely influential in changing public attitude, and Battersea Dogs and Cats Home recently celebrated its 150th anniversary. (Courtesy of the Dickens House Museum, London, UK.)

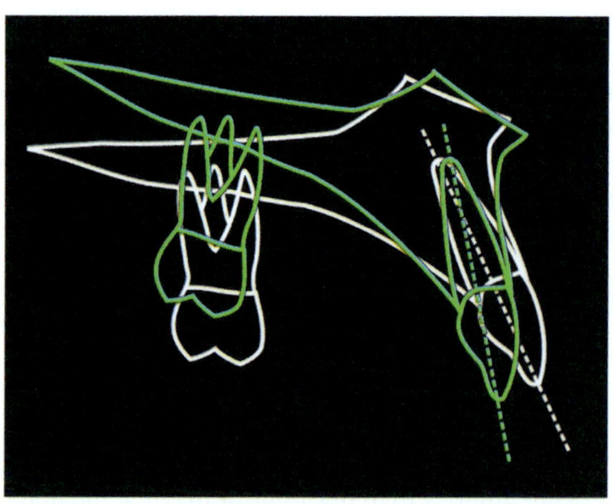

Fig. 12-24 Maxillary incisor inclination alters with differential impaction of the maxilla.

- **Mandibular incisor inclination and mandibular autorotation** – If any form of superior or inferior repositioning of the maxilla is being contemplated, the effect on the mandible should be borne in mind. As the maxilla is superiorly repositioned, the mandible will **autorotate forward** (in the direction of mouth closing), reducing the inclination of the mandibular plane. In preparation for this, the mandibular incisors will often need to be slightly proclined prior to surgery (the opposite is true in preparation for inferior repositioning of the maxilla). A useful guideline is that the inclination of the mandibular incisors to the mandibular plane should be approximately 120°; therefore, as the mandible autorotates forward, reducing the mandibular plane inclination, the mandibular incisor inclination increases, and vice versa (see Figure 6-14).

Arch coordination

'Orthodontics can help a lot but it can also make the necessary surgery almost impossible.'[10]

Hugo L. Obwegeser

Dental arch coordination refers to the aspects of orthodontic treatment which ensure that the maxillary and mandibular dental arches will fit well together in occlusion, with maxillary and mandibular arch forms that correspond to one another, and with normal incisor, canine and buccal segment overjet.

Of all the parameters that must be dealt with in orthodontic preparation, the coordination of the maxillary arch with the mandibular arch is often the most important, commonly the most challenging, and usually the most likely to cause problems at the time of surgery and in the postoperative phase of treatment.

Ideally, the dental arches should be as well-coordinated as possible prior to surgery. However, in some patients, if the occlusion is so well-interdigitated as to make expansion difficult, particularly in low angle patients, glass ionomer cement blocks may be placed on the occlusal surface of the maxillary first or second molars to disclude the arches, and permit easier expansion. Conversely, some of the posterior buccal segment expansion (perhaps 3–4 mm, i.e. no more than 2 mm per side) may be completed postoperatively. However, *the coordination of the canine-to-canine region of the maxilla to that of the mandible is the single most important preparatory requirement of preoperative orthodontics*. Good preoperative coordination of this region is mandatory.

The aims of preparatory orthodontic treatment in relation to arch coordination are twofold:

1. To expand or contract the maxillary and mandibular dental arches as required, so they will adequately conform to one another at the time of surgery; and
2. To prevent undesirable expansion or contraction in either arch.

Prior to initial orthodontic appliance placement, the pretreatment diagnostic study models should be hand

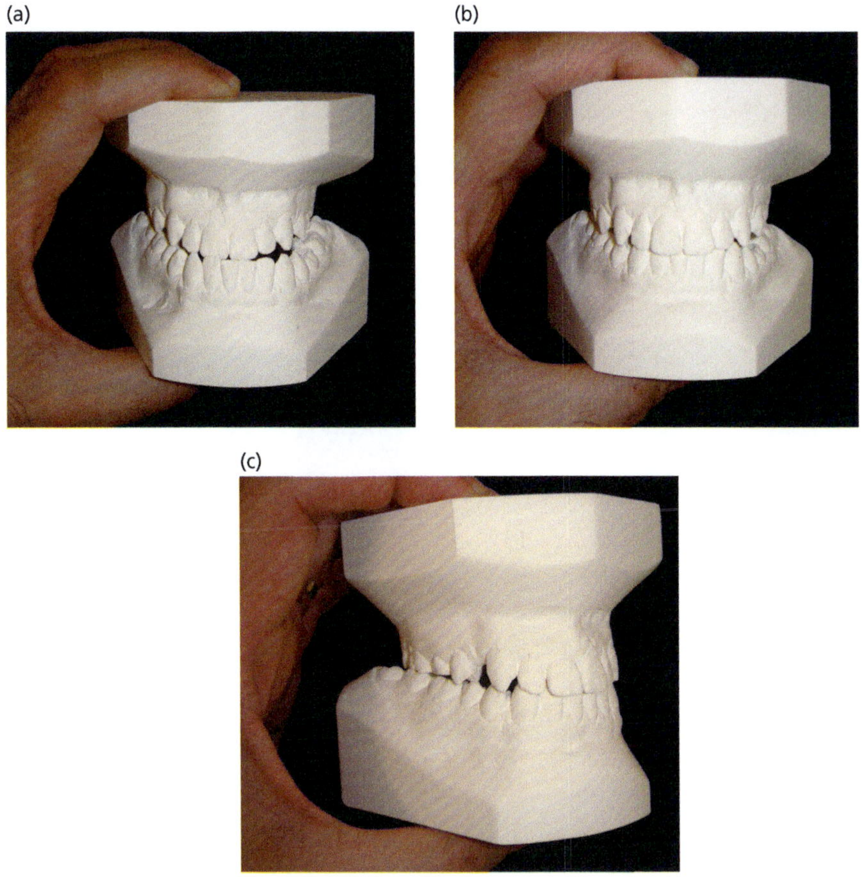

Fig. 12-25 (a) Pretreatment study models in pretreatment occlusion. (b, c) Hand articulated pretreatment study models in the approximate postoperative position of the skeletal bases. Hand articulating pretreatment study models in the approximate proposed postoperative position for the skeletal bases will provide an idea of the degree of arch coordination that will be required.

articulated such that they are held in the *approximate* proposed postoperative position of the skeletal bases. This will provide some idea of the degree of arch expansion or contraction that may be required (Figure 12-25).

Additionally, the *buccolingual inclination of the molar and premolar teeth relative to their respective skeletal base* should be observed:

- **Maxillary dental arch** – If the maxillary molars and premolars are at a correct inclination relative to the skeletal base, but the arch is narrow, it will need to be expanded whilst preventing buccal flaring. However, if the buccal segment teeth are already flared, their inclination will need to be corrected, and thereby the maxillary arch is likely to require even greater overall expansion (Figure 12-26).
- **Mandibular dental arch** – If the mandibular molars and premolars are lingually inclined, particularly in Class III cases with broad mandibular arches, their inclination may need to be maintained, by using transversely contracted round archwires or contracted rectangular wires with lingual crown torque in the buccal segments. Placement of regular rectangular archwires will very quickly lead to buccal crown movement of these teeth, increasing the mandibular intermolar width and making arch coordination difficult (Figure 12-27). The alternative is to allow the torque expression in these teeth to occur, but to accept a bilateral posterior crossbite at the end of treatment.

If preoperative maxillary arch expansion is required, a number of methods are available:

- **Expanded archwires** – In many cases, expansion in the maxillary dental arch, and the coordination of the maxillary and the mandibular arches to one another, may be best accomplished using coordinated archwires (Figure 12-28). The initial aligning archwires cannot be coordinated, but expanded arch forms in NiTi archwires will help expand where necessary – this effect is more pronounced with lower friction type bracket systems, such as self-ligating

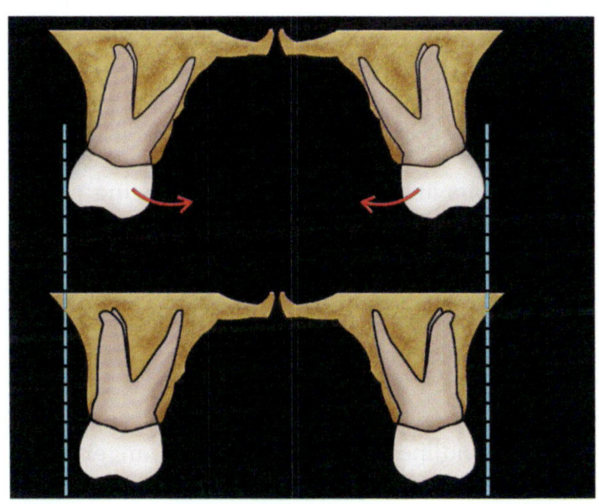

Fig. 12-26 If the maxillary posterior dentition is already buccally inclined, correcting their inclination will increase the amount of overall expansion required in the maxillary arch.

(a)

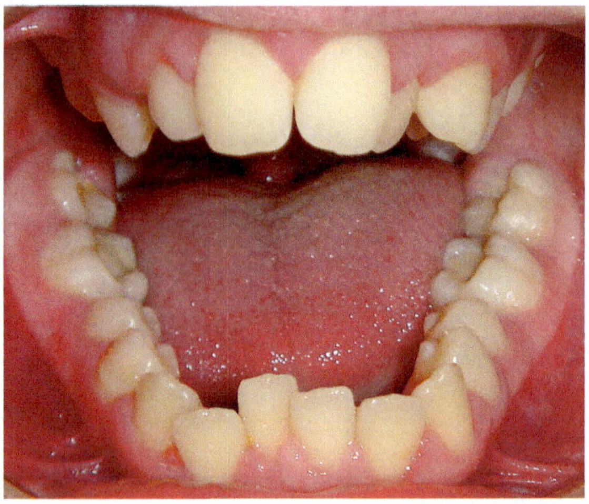

(b)

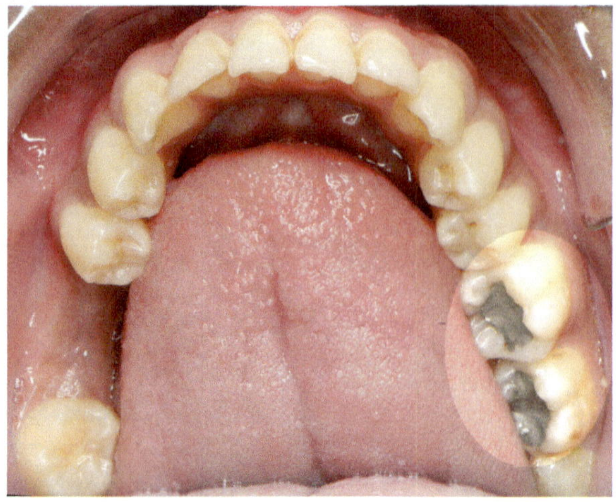

(c)

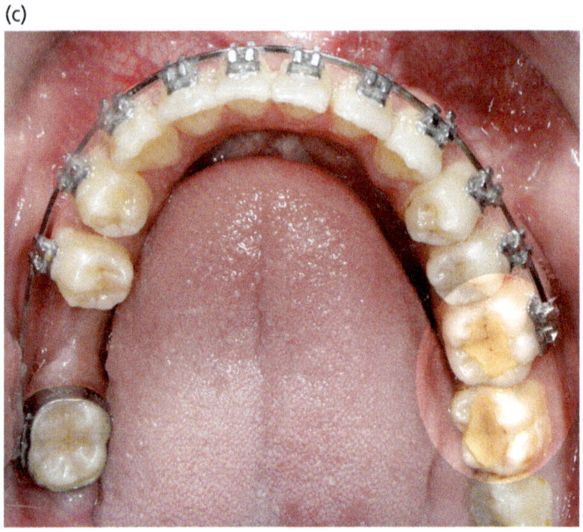

Fig. 12-27 (a) Lingually inclined (lingually 'rolled') mandibular molars (this represents dentoalveolar compensation in the transverse plane). (b) Pretreatment occlusal view of the mandibular arch demonstrating lingually inclined mandibular molars. (c) Placement of a mandibular rectangular archwire demonstrates the degree of buccal inclination and increase in intermolar width that will occur; compare the position of the first molar, which has moved buccally, and the obvious step with the second molar, which is still in the pretreatment position.

brackets (possibly due to the broader arch forms of the initial archwires), or the tying of brackets loosely with stainless steel ligatures. Tight elastomeric ligatures may limit such movement due to increased friction. However, as soon as stainless steel wires are used, their widths may be coordinated. Though round archwires may be useful in particularly difficult cases, e.g. an expanded 0.020-inch stainless steel, their downside is to buccally flare the maxillary molars and potentially cause hanging palatal cusps. As such, coordinated rectangular stainless steel archwires will eventually be required as the buccal root torque expression helps to limit buccal flaring, to elevate hanging palatal cusps and correct the inclination of the posterior teeth relative to their basal bone.

- **Removable appliances** – A removable appliance with a midline expansion screw is an excellent method of maxillary arch expansion (Figure 12-29). The authors prefer Adams clasps on the maxillary first molars and first premolars for retention. An expansion protocol of $^{1}/_{4}$ turn of the jackscrew per week, which equates to a 0.2 mm of expansion, may be used in adults. Clinical experience with this method appears to suggest reduced buccal flaring

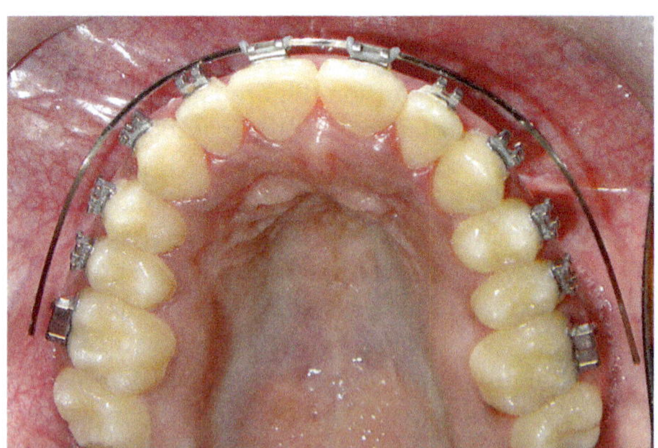

Fig. 12-28 A maxillary 0.019 × 0.025-inch rectangular expanded archwire prior to ligation, demonstrating degree of expansion per side.

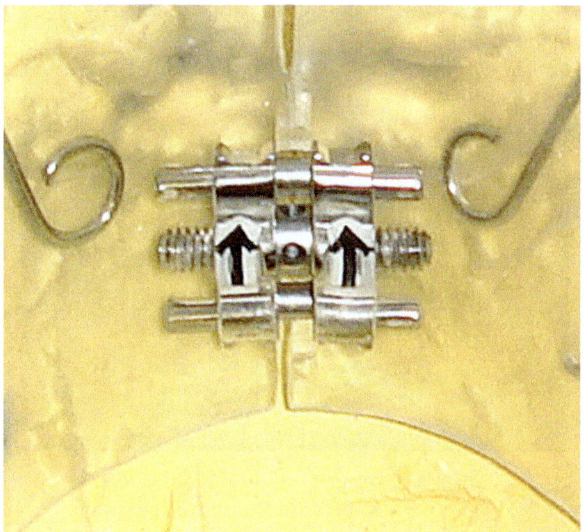

Fig. 12-29 An expansion jackscrew embedded in the acrylic of a removable appliance.

of the maxillary molars, compared to other types of expansion, though this is not an evidence-based statement. It is important to maintain the expansion while moving into the fixed appliance. Once the maxillary arch has been expanded, the Adams clasps may be removed from the first premolar teeth and the removable appliance wear continued, and the upper arch, excluding the molars, is bonded and aligned. Once into a round 0.018-inch stainless steel archwire, which is sturdy enough to maintain the expansion, the removable appliance is discarded and the molars bonded and aligned.

Note:

The orthodontic (or orthopaedic) jackscrew (see Figure 12-29) consists of a threaded cylinder. The pitch of the screw thread is set so that a complete 360° turn of the screw will produce a separation of 0.8 to 1.0 mm. A small key may be inserted into the holes in the centre of the screw allowing for one-quarter turn incremental adjustments. Therefore, each turn of the screw equates to 0.2 to 0.25 mm.

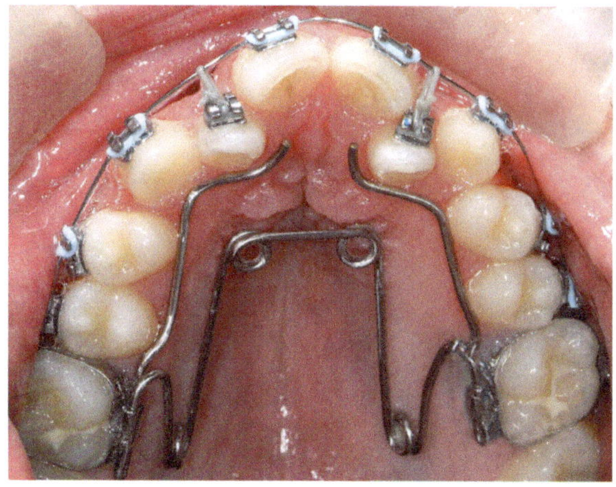

Fig. 12-31 Quadhelix appliance with palatal arms incorporated.

- **Auxiliary archwires** – Also known as jockey arches, these auxiliary wires may be easily constructed at the chair side and incorporated into a fixed appliance during treatment. They can also be used to maintain arch width after rapid maxillary expansion. The expansion arch, which can be made from 0.019 × 0.025-inch stainless steel or a larger round steel wire with a diameter of 1–1.13 mm, runs over the main archwire and is inserted into the headgear or auxiliary tubes of the first molar bands posteriorly and secured anteriorly with a ligature (Figure 12-30). Some operators prefer to bend the wire into the buccal sulcus in order to reduce its visibility. Expansion is likely to be produced by a degree of buccal molar flaring and this may be reduced by incorporating molar buccal root torque into the main rectangular archwire.
- **Quadhelix** (or trihelix in cleft patients or severely narrow maxilla) – This is a modification of Coffin's W-spring, which incorporates four helices to increase flexibility and range of activation. The length of the palatal arms may be altered, depending on which teeth other than the first molars need to be expanded (Figure 12-31). The majority of expansion in an adult will be due to buccal molar flaring. In patients with a very narrow palate and maxilla, a

(a) (b)

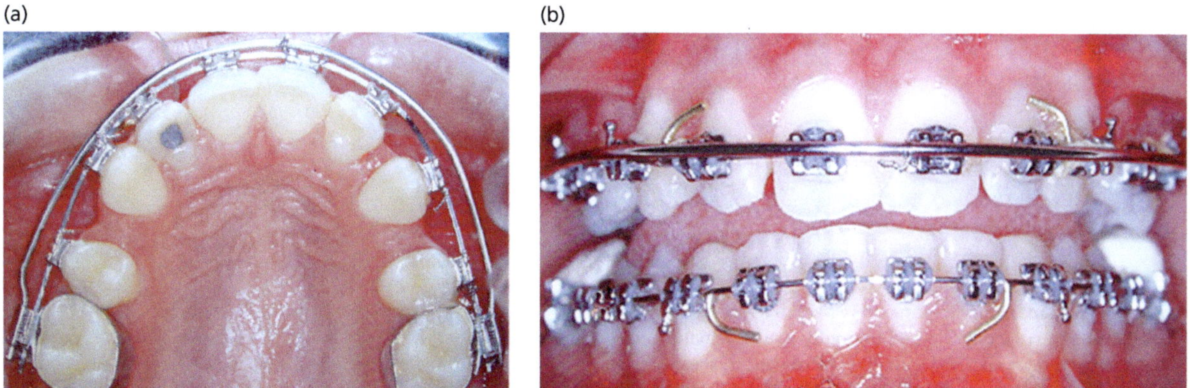

Fig. 12-30 An auxiliary archwire has been ligated over the main archwire.

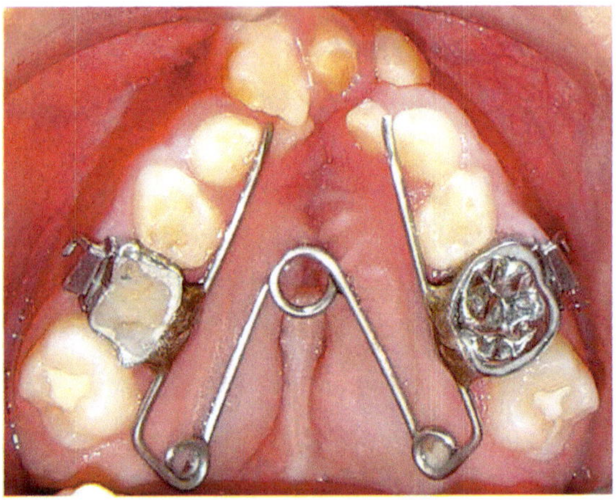

Fig. 12-32 Trihelix appliance for expansion of a severely narrow maxilla in a patient with cleft palate.

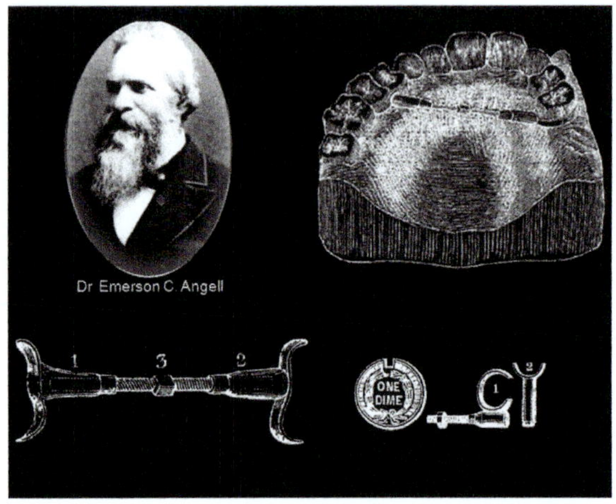

Fig. 12-33 Emerson C. Angell (1822–1903) expanded the maxilla by bony separation across the midpalatal suture.

trihelix may be used (Figure 12-32). An overall activation of 8 mm (i.e. 4 mm per side) provides approximately 400 grams of force for expansion.

- **Rapid maxillary expansion (RME)** – Rapid maxillary expansion was first described by the American dentist Emerson C. Angell (1822–1903) in 1860,[11] to laterally expand the maxilla by bony separation (*Dental Cosmos* mistakenly printed his second initial as *H*) (Figure 12-33).[12] The technique was later re-popularized by the orthodontist Andrew Haas. The aim of this technique is to improve the ratio of skeletal to dental lateral movement by producing sutural expansion at the midpalatal suture. This is achieved by using a rigid appliance, which will limit buccal flaring of the molars, expanding the midpalatal suture rapidly using high forces to limit the time allowed for dental movement and carrying out treatment during or before the pubertal growth spurt. Following puberty, there is greater interlocking of the maxillary sutures which may limit their separation.[13] As a general rule, rapid maxillary expansion is indicated in cases with a transverse discrepancy equal to or greater than 4 mm, and where the maxillary molars are already buccally inclined to compensate for the transverse skeletal discrepancy.[14] Approximately 40% of the expansion achieved may be attributed to skeletal changes.[15] The ratio between anterior (intercanine) to posterior (intermolar) skeletal expansion has been found to be approximately 2:1 and the greatest skeletal response is achieved when treatment is carried out before or during puberty (Figures 12-34 and 12-35).

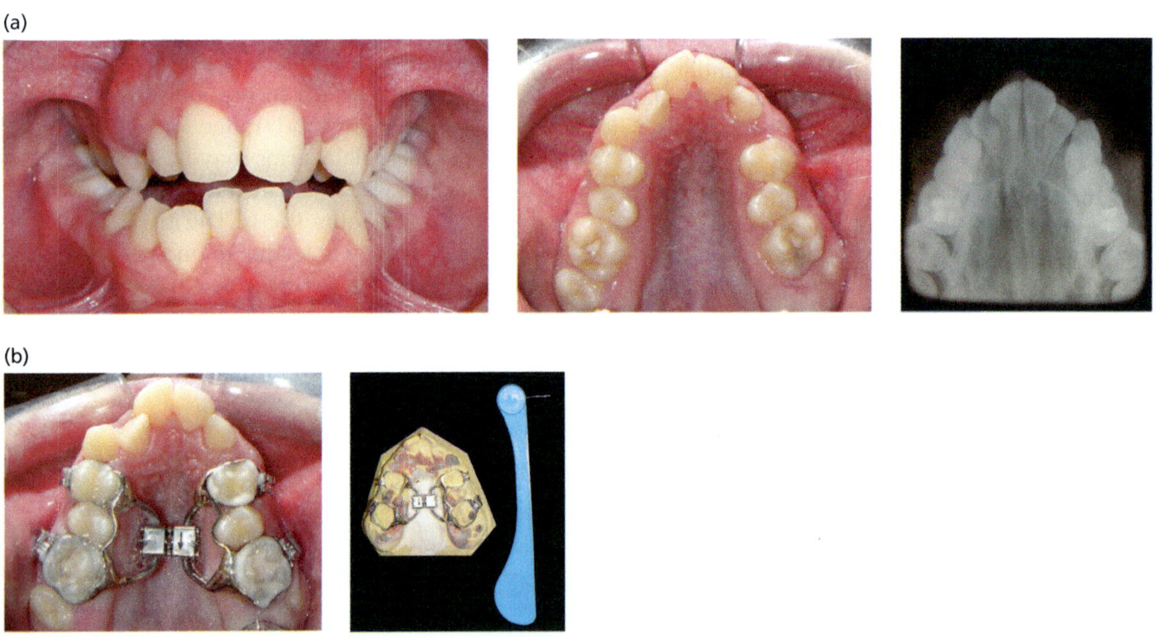

Fig. 12-34 Rapid maxillary expansion (RME) in a patient planned for eventual orthognathic surgery. (a) Pretreatment views demonstrating narrow maxilla and lingually inclined mandibular molars. (b) Banded RME appliance in situ; an expansion screw key is used to turn the Hyrax (Hygienic Rapid Expansion) screw. (c) 3 weeks review demonstrating expansion and formation of a maxillary midline diastema. The maxillary standard occlusal radiograph demonstrates opening of the midpalatal suture. To prevent the screw from turning backwards it is stabilized with glass ionomer cement. (d) Removal of the RME appliance after 3 months and placement of a transpalatal arch (TPA) with arms to maintain the expansion. The midline diastema has closed spontaneously due to the action of the transseptal fibres.

(c)

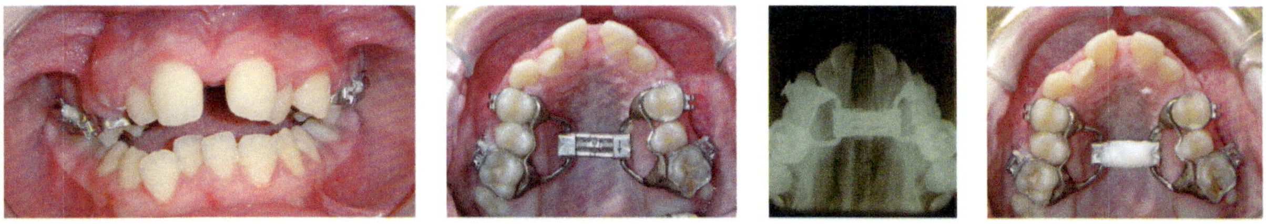

(d)

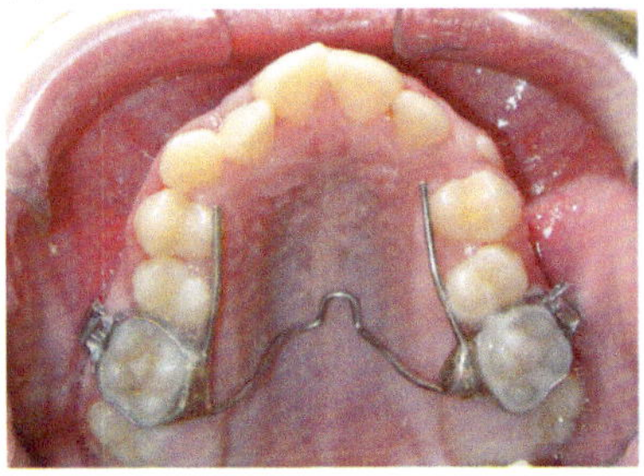

Fig. 12-34 (*Continued*).

(a)

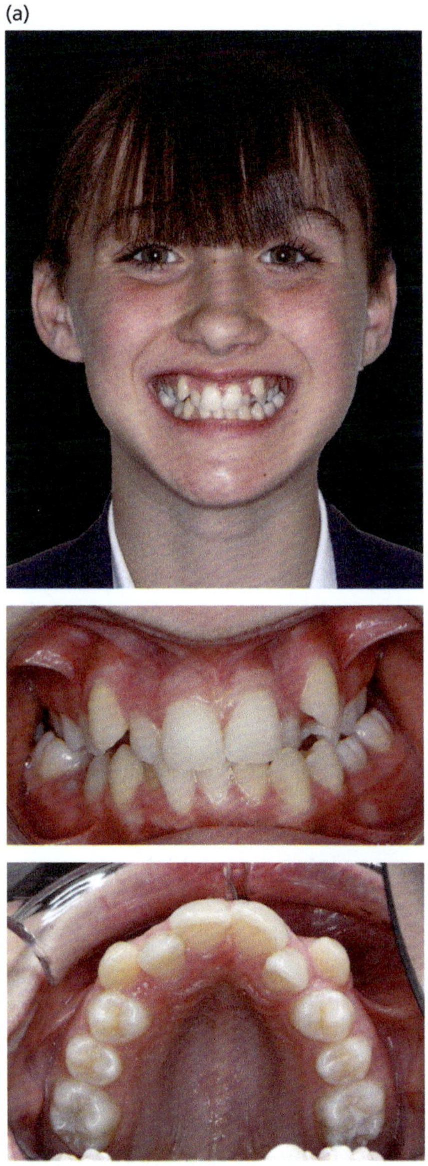

(b)

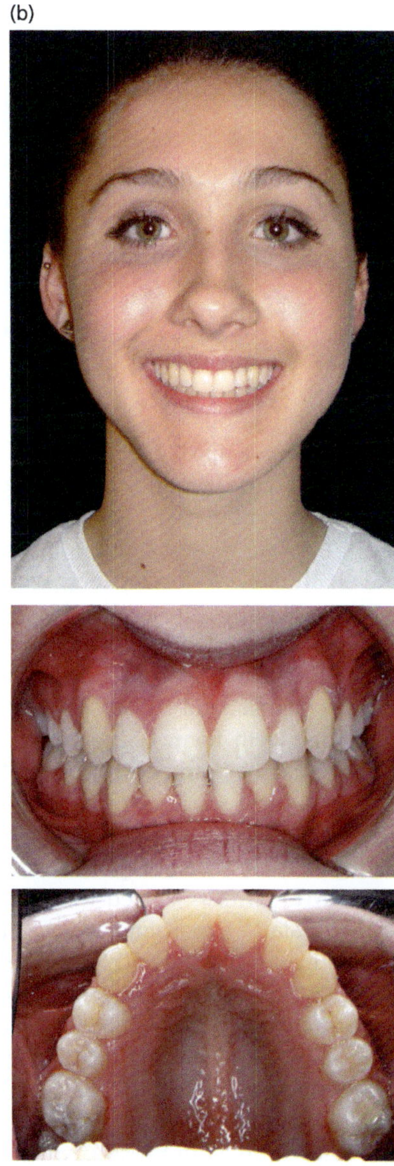

Fig. 12-35 RME in an orthodontic patient with narrow maxillary arch and crowding. (a) Pretreatment. (b) Following RME and fixed orthodontic appliance treatment. As well as creating a broader smile, space is created by the RME for alignment.

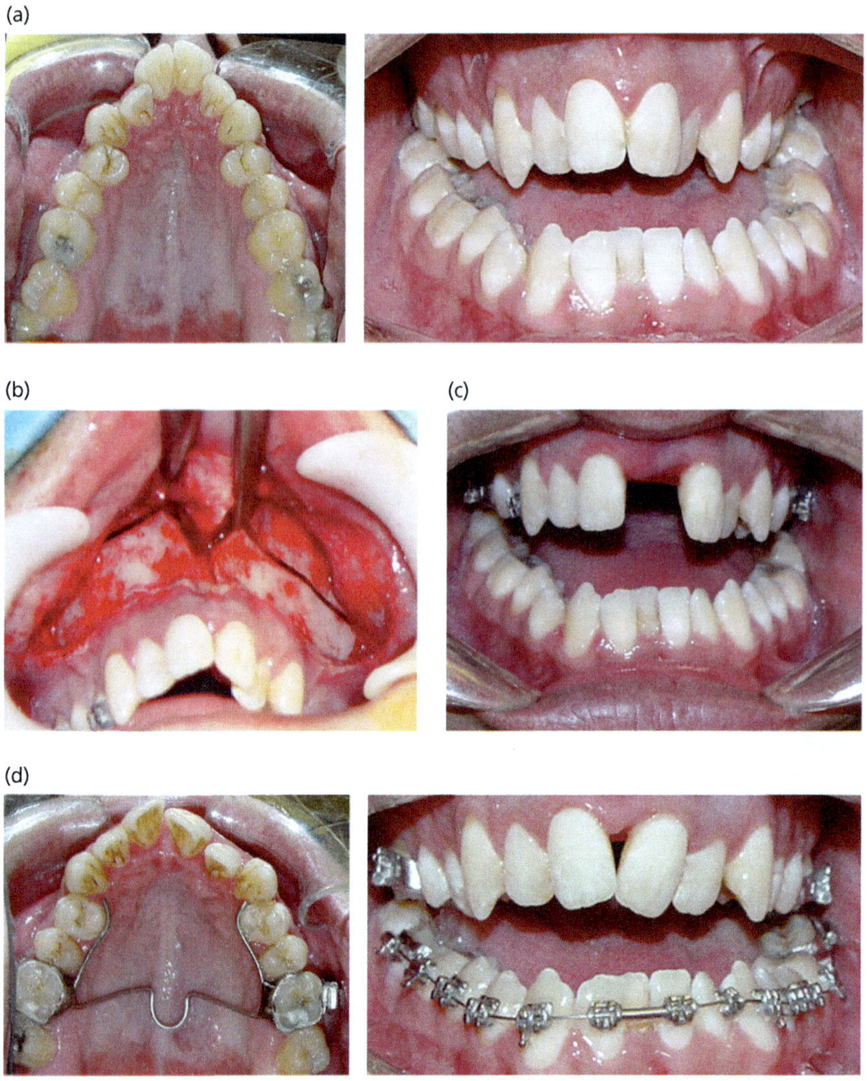

Fig. 12-36 Surgically-assisted rapid maxillary expansion (SARME). (a) Pretreatment views demonstrating severe transverse maxillary deficiency. (b) Intraoperative view showing Le Fort I surgical cuts before the midline maxillary cut is made to mobilize the maxilla. (c) A 10 mm diastema was created during SARME. (d) Spontaneous closure of the diastema during the retention period.

The posterior maxilla expands less readily because of the resistance produced by the zygomatic buttress and pterygoid plates.

In a *growing* patient with an already significant Class III skeletal discrepancy, where the need for orthognathic surgery is already evident, and where the maxilla is hypoplastic, with inevitable crowding, RME may be carried out. This will increase the width of the maxilla, and create space to align otherwise crowded teeth. Some bite opening is likely to occur, which may be detrimental in a tall face patient, but is a relatively short-term problem if the patient is planned for orthognathic surgery in the future.

- **Surgically assisted rapid maxillary expansion (SARME)** – (also referred to as surgically assisted rapid palatal expansion or SARPE) – This technique may be considered in skeletally mature individuals with significant transverse discrepancies. The main resistance to maxillary skeletal expansion comes from the buttressing effect of the zygomatic and sphenoid bones at their point of attachment to the maxilla and from the integrity of the midpalatal suture. With SARME, these attachments are surgically severed, which allows expansion to be easily achieved using a conventional RME appliance. Fixed appliances can be used to move apart the roots of the central incisors before surgery to avoid their damage by the midline maxillary cuts. Expansion is typically carried out at a rate of 0.4 mm per day (one turn of the screw in the morning and one turn in the evening) and patients develop a significant midline diastema, about which they must be warned beforehand (Figures 12-36 and 12-37). The diastema will close spontaneously by mesial tipping of the maxillary incisors, and root alignment and final space closure is accomplished with subsequent fixed orthodontic appliances. Surgical expansion has a high relapse tendency, probably because of the inelasticity of the palatal mucoperiosteum, and a degree of over-correction is valuable.

Note:

Coordination of the maxillary and mandibular dental arches is achieved by a combination of expansion of one arch (usually the maxillary) and/or contraction of the opposing dental arch.

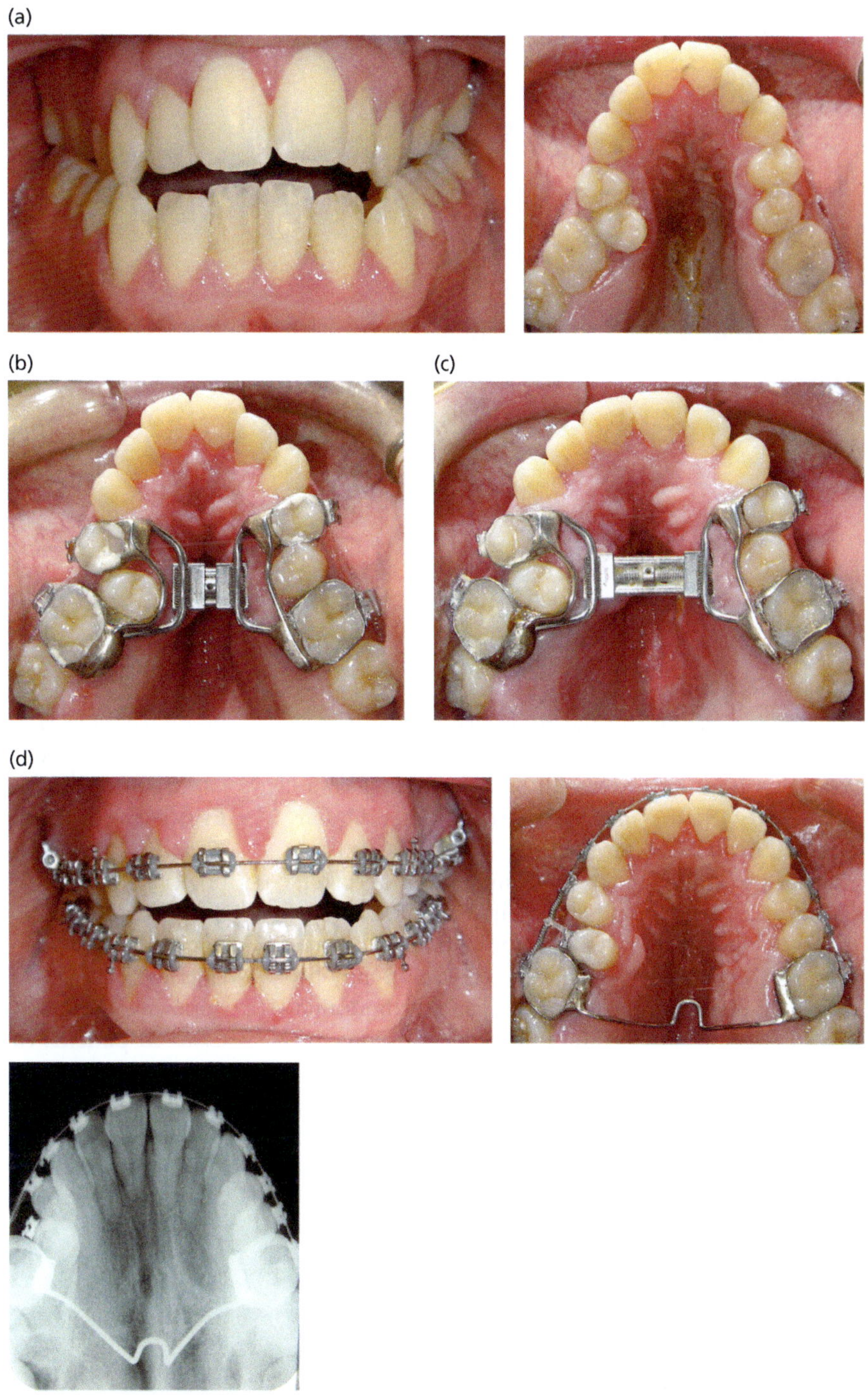

Fig. 12-37 Surgically-assisted rapid maxillary expansion (SARME). (a) Pretreatment. (b) RME appliance in situ prior to surgery. (c) 3-months following surgery. (d) 9-months following surgery and fixed orthodontic appliance treatment, with transpalatal arch (TPA) to help maintain the expansion. The patient is being prepared for bimaxillary surgery. A maxillary standard occlusal radiograph demonstrates bony infill of the midpalatal region.

- **Arch form** – The pretreatment arch forms may be acceptable, or may need to be altered. In Class III orthognathic patients with a retrusive maxilla, the maxilla tends to be hypoplastic as well. As such, the maxillary dental arch often needs to be expanded. In the Class II orthognathic patient, the maxillary arch form may be tapered and narrow in the premolar and canine regions (Figure 12-38). In such cases, the archwires will inevitably expand the canine-premolar regions due to their arch form. When intermolar width is constricted, expansion with archwires is usually not sufficient, and other forms of arch expansion should be considered, as discussed above.
- **Effect of sagittal jaw movement on transverse arch coordination** – It is important to bear in mind that sagittal movement of the maxillary arch in relation to the mandibular arch has an effect on their mutual transverse relationship, i.e. one is moving the broader posterior aspect of the maxillary arch forward relative to a narrower aspect of the mandibular arch. Therefore, in a Class II orthognathic patient, the broader posterior aspect of the mandibular arch is advanced against a narrower part of the maxillary arch (Figure 12-39). Conversely, in a Class III orthognathic patient, a broader part of the maxillary arch is often advanced relative to a narrower part of the mandibular arch.

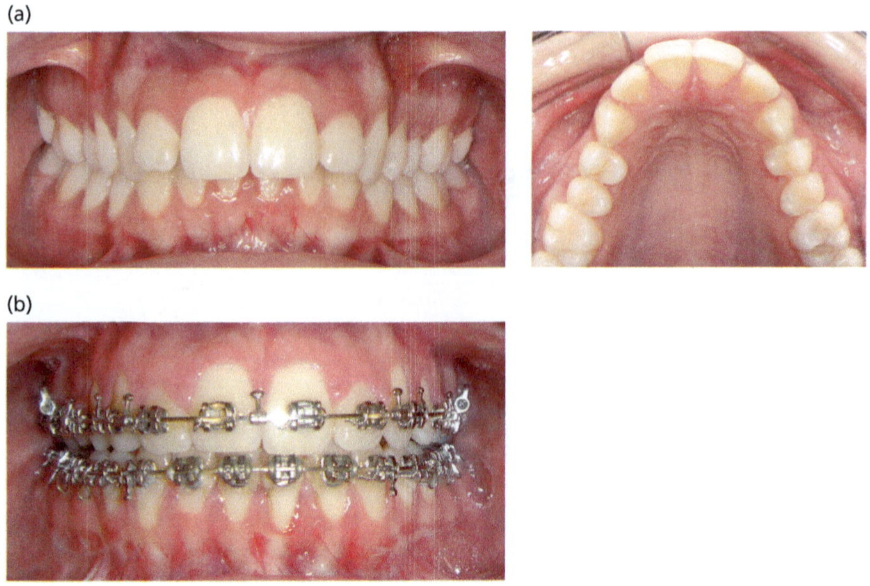

Fig. 12-38 (a) In this Class II orthognathic patient, the maxillary arch form is tapered and narrow in the premolar and canine regions, sometimes referred to as a V-shaped arch. (b) Postoperative view following orthodontic treatment and mandibular advancement surgery, demonstrating expansion and 'rounding out' of the maxillary arch, creating a U-shaped arch.

- **Extraction patterns** – As far as possible, it is better to avoid extracting in the maxillary arch in Class III cases, as the inevitable contraction of the arch resulting from reduced tooth tissue can make coordination with the inevitably broader mandibular arch difficult. Conversely, occasionally the extraction of second premolar teeth may be undertaken in the excessively broad mandibular arch to provide space for arch contraction. If the maxillary canine teeth are excessively ectopic, consideration may be given to their surgical removal, and orthodontic space closure, moving the first premolars into the canine space (Figure 12-40). Additionally, if the maxillary lateral incisors are missing, the canines may be placed in the lateral incisor positions and masked, so long as their crown height is not excessively increased, and their colour is not too dark (Figure 12-41). *As a general guideline, teeth may be orthodontically repositioned away from their normal locations in the dental arch as long as arch coordination may be maintained and smile aesthetics is not adversely affected.*
- **Evaluating arch coordination during treatment** – The Class II orthognathic patient may be asked to posture their mandible forward, to get an idea of the labial segment (canine-to-canine) interdigitation. The intermolar and interpremolar widths may be estimated visually, as these teeth will not meet their opposing arch by mandibular anterior posturing. Class III patients cannot posture in such a fashion, but assessing coordination is just as important. A relatively simple technique is to take an impression of the mandibular arch and from it to create an acrylic model of the cusp tips, which may be held against the maxillary arch to check arch coordination

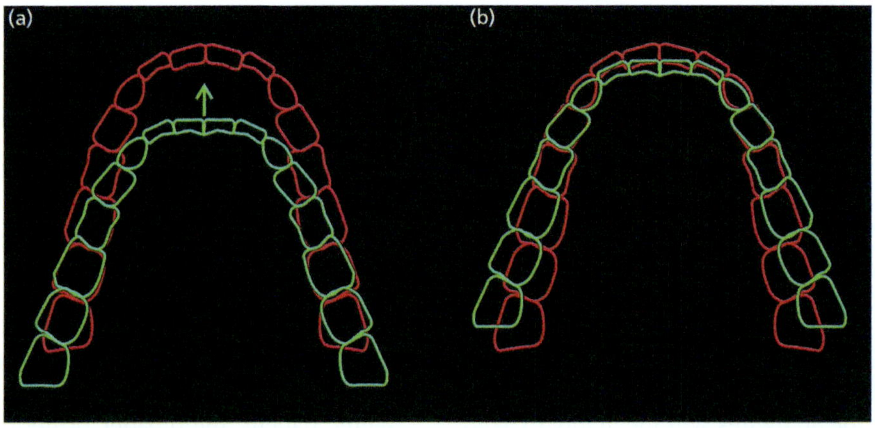

Fig. 12-39 Sagittal movement of the maxillary arch relative to the mandibular arch has an effect on their mutual transverse relationship, i.e. the broader posterior aspect of one arch is advanced relative to a narrower aspect of the opposing arch. As such, arch coordination should always be undertaken in relation to the desired postoperative sagittal position of the skeletal bases. (a) Position of the mandibular arch (green) relative to the maxillary arch (red) in a Class II patient. (b) Following mandibular advancement the broad posterior aspect of the mandibular arch moves forward relative to a narrower part of the maxillary arch. In such cases, the maxillary arch should be expanded preoperatively, and the arches coordinated.

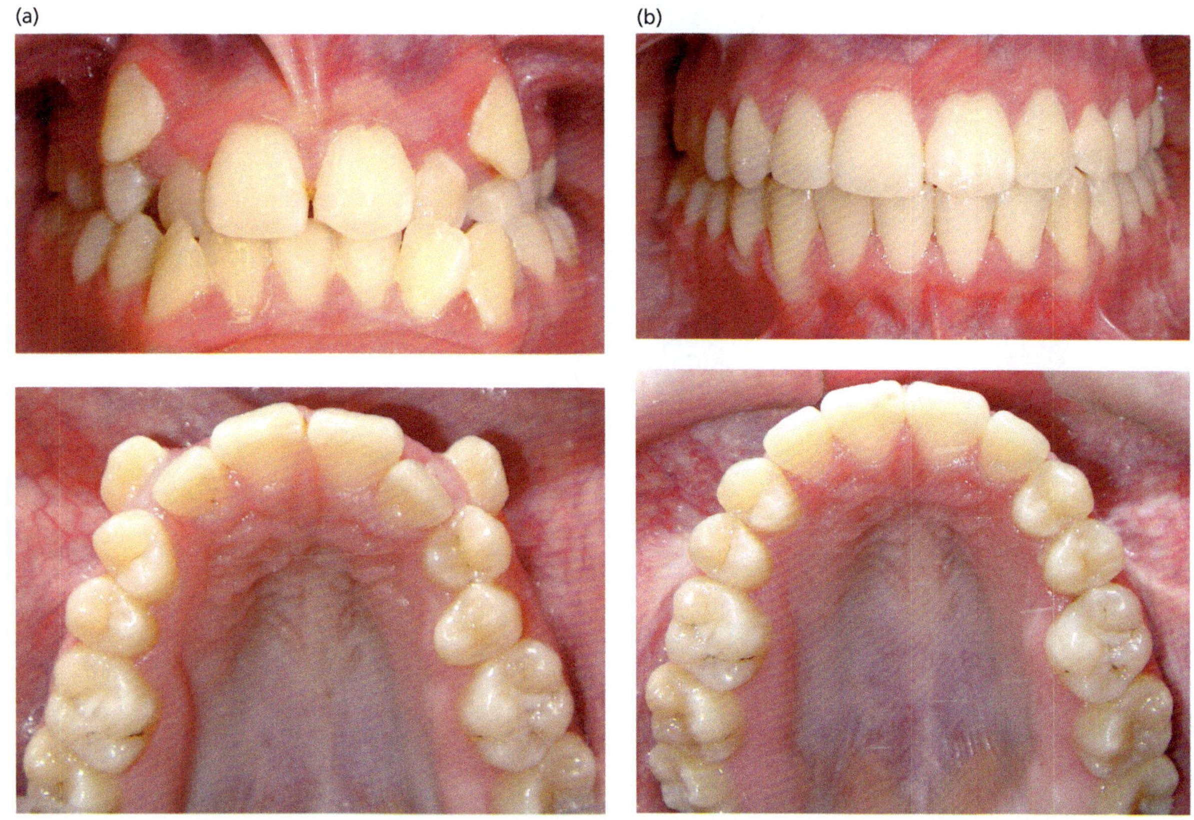

Fig. 12-40 Extraction of ectopic maxillary canines and orthodontic repositioning of the first premolars into the canine position. (a) Pretreatment views. Following decompensation the patient underwent a maxillary advancement. (b) End of treatment views.

(Figure 12-42).[16] Towards the end of treatment, the ideal way to check arch coordination is to remove the final archwires and take a set of impressions, from which may be cast the so-called 'snap models' or 'snaps'. These are then hand articulated to assess the potential postoperative 'fit' of the teeth.

Elimination of occlusal interferences

Planning to prevent occlusal interferences begins before a single bracket is bonded. Additionally, during treatment the dental arches should be checked at every visit, in order to continue preventing the formation of potential interferences, and eliminating them when they occur.

It is vitally important to check the patient's individual dental arches and their occlusion with keen observation and with interim 'snap models' when required, in order to detect potential occlusal interferences (Figure 12-43). The most common potential interferences in orthognathic patients are the following:

- **Coordination of intercanine width** – As already mentioned in the above section on arch coordination, the coordination of the canine-to-canine

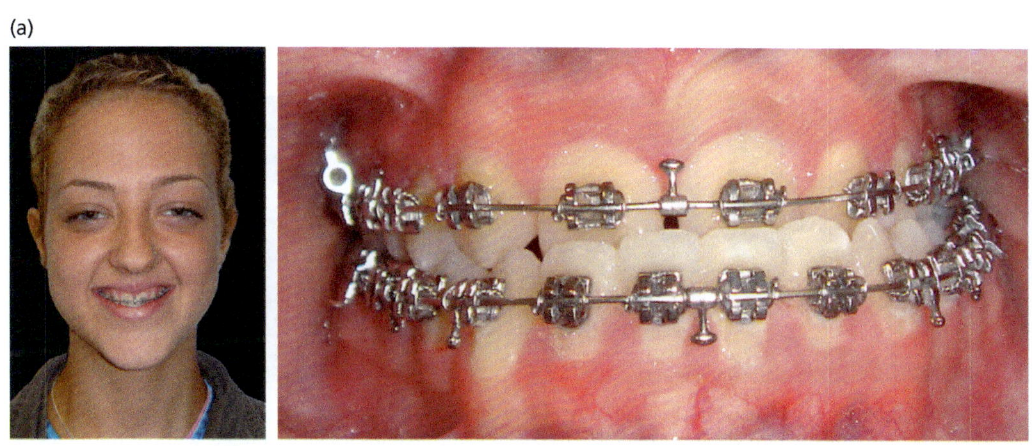

Fig. 12-41 Missing maxillary lateral incisors and orthodontic repositioning of the canines into the lateral incisor positions, and reshaping of the canines. (a) Preoperative views. (b) End of treatment views, following maxillary advancement and slight mandibular set-back.

(b)

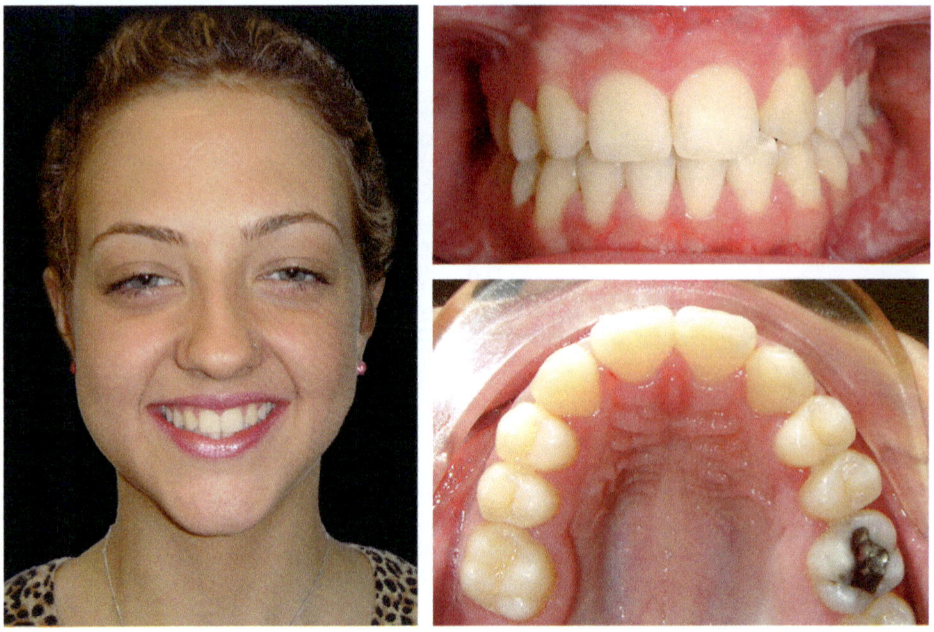

Fig. 12-41 (*Continued*).

(a) (b)

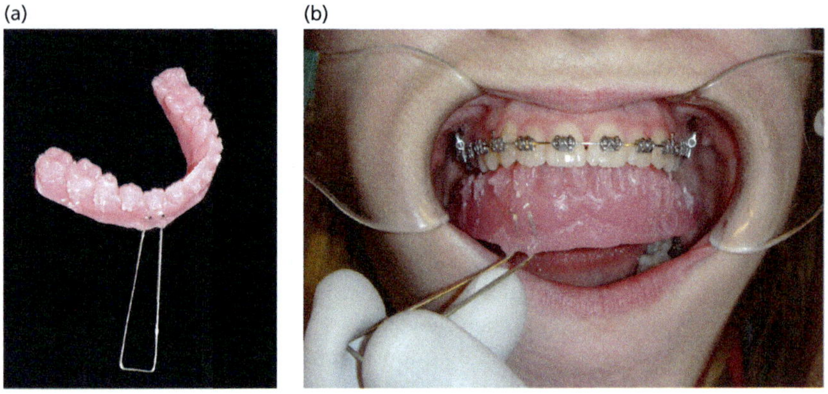

Fig. 12-42 Checking arch coordination in the Class III patient mid-treatment may be accomplished by creating an acrylic model of the mandibular arch. (From: Naini FB. The 'acrylic technique' to check arch coordination in orthognathic surgery patients. Br J Oral Maxillofac Surg. 2013;51:e9–10. Reprinted with permission.)

(a) (b) (c) (d) (e)

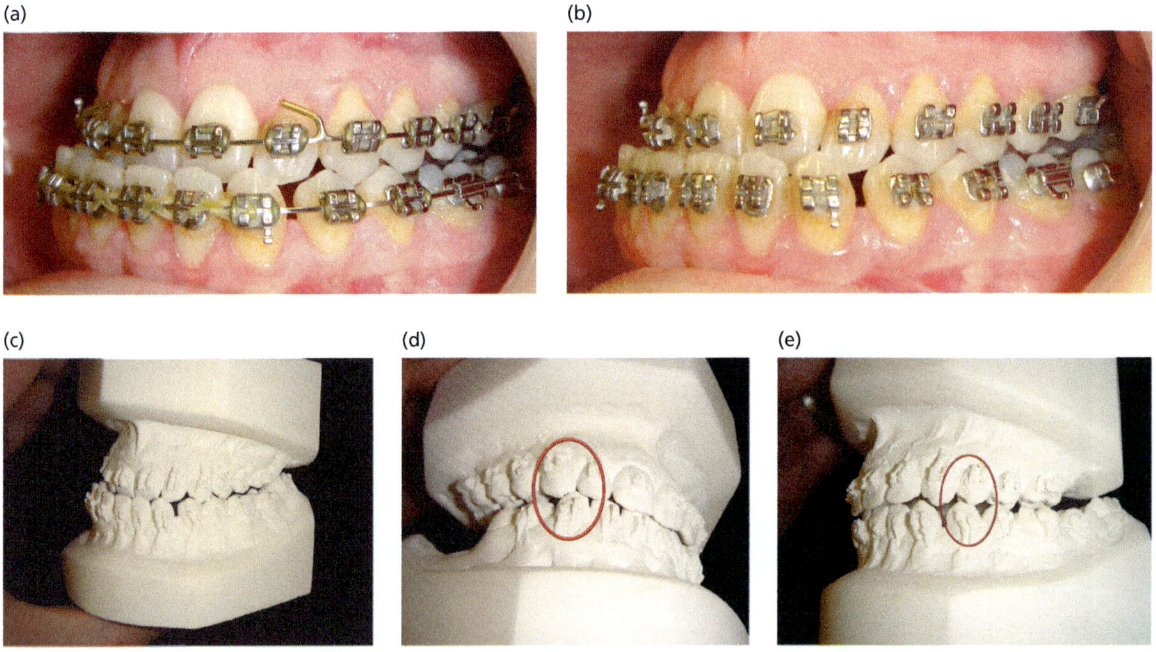

Fig. 12-43 'Snap' dental models may be used to check for any potential occlusal interferences during the preparatory stages of orthodontics, and particularly preoperatively. It is preferable to take the impressions for snap models without the archwires, which permits better visualization of the dentition on the models. (a) Preoperative view of a Class III patient. (b) Archwires are removed prior to taking impressions for snap models. (c) Snap models in preoperative occlusion. (d) Snap models are hand articulated into the proposed postoperative position, demonstrating potential interferences (d) in the right canine region and (e) the left premolar region.

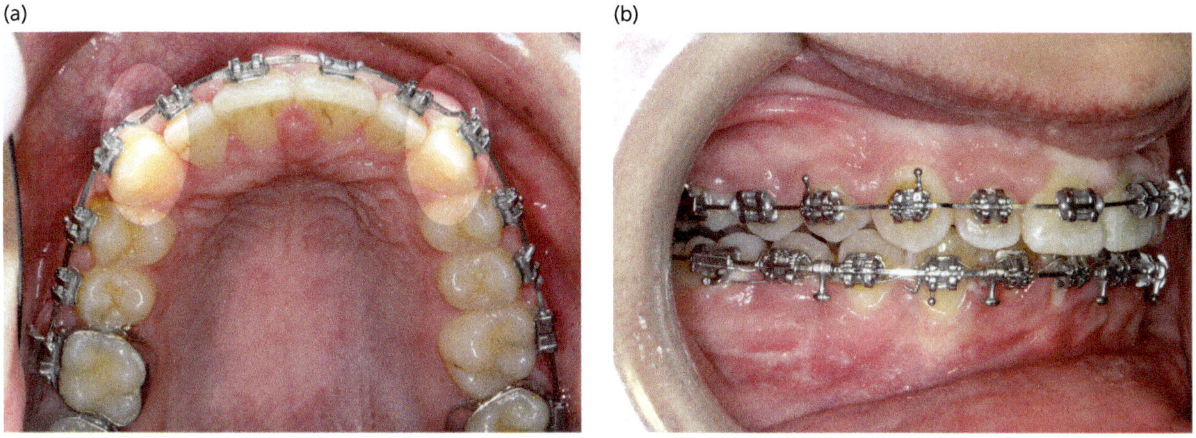

Fig. 12-44 (a) Canine offset bends in the archwire to permit better coordination of the anterior dentition. (b) Postoperative occlusion.

regions is paramount. In the Class III orthognathic patient with maxillary hypoplasia or mandibular macrognathia, coordinating the labial segments is often difficult. The orthodontist may use expanded arch forms for the anterior maxilla and contracted arch forms for the archwires in the anterior mandible. If this not enough, **canine offsets** may be placed in the maxillary archwire (Figure 12-44). Alternatively, some pushcoil may be used between the maxillary lateral incisors and canines, to expand the maxillary intercanine width. The space created can be closed postoperatively. Another important parameter is the *morphology of the mesiopalatal region of the maxillary canine*. If this region is pronounced, the maxillary canine bracket should be bonded $1/2$ to $3/4$ of a millimetre mesially, in order to *rotate the maxillary canine teeth mesiobuccally* (see Figure 12-4).

- **Extrusion of maxillary second molars** – It is vitally important to avoid extrusion of maxillary second molar teeth. If they are already extruded, a small amount of glass ionomer cement on their occlusal surface will lead to their slight intrusion (Figure 12-45); the material may be removed postoperatively. Alternatively, if they must be included in the appliance, they should be bonded slightly occlusally (see Figure 12-5). If a **convertible band** is used on the first molar, a step-up bend may be placed to intrude the second molar (Figure 12-46). When necessary, temporary anchorage devices, such as microscrews, may also be used to help intrude maxillary second molars.
- **Buccal flaring of maxillary molars** – Maxillary arch expansion tends to cause buccal flaring of the molars and resultant dropping down of their palatal cusps (Figure 12-47). It is important to avoid buccal flaring of maxillary molars by not expanding too quickly, particularly with quadhelices, and using rectangular archwires with buccal root torque. Occasionally, the rather prominent palatal cusp tips of maxillary second molars may be reduced in height using a dental handpiece.
- **Avoidance of premolar extrusion** – Accurate bracket positioning is always important, but its significance is magnified in orthognathic patients. Premolar extrusion usually results from incorrect bracket positioning (Figure 12-48). It is vital to avoid the relative extrusion of the premolar teeth, and if required, it is more cautious to bond these teeth slightly occlusally, and reposition them postoperatively.
- **Overeruption** – Any tooth may potentially overerupt. This is particularly true of maxillary posterior teeth when their antagonist is missing (Figure 12-49). These teeth should be re-intruded and levelled in

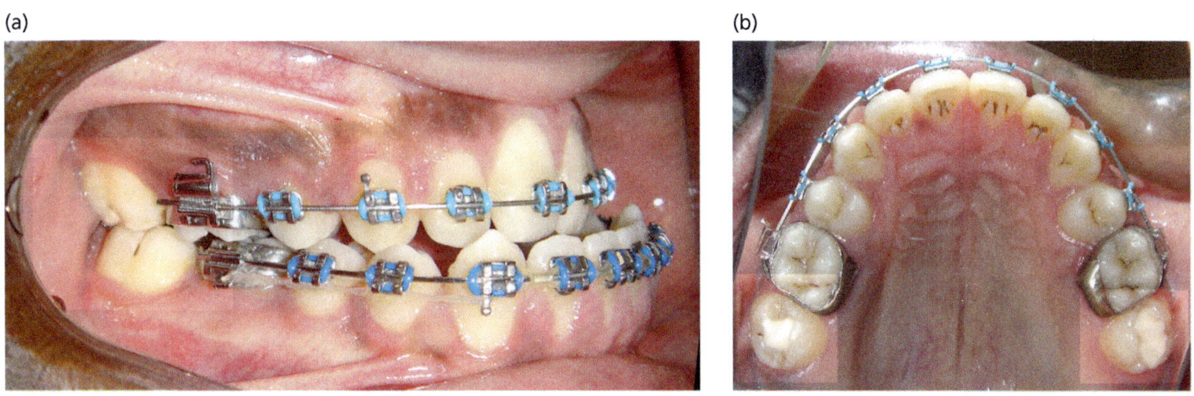

Fig. 12-45 Glass ionomer cement has been placed on the occlusal surface of the maxillary second molar teeth in order to intrude them.

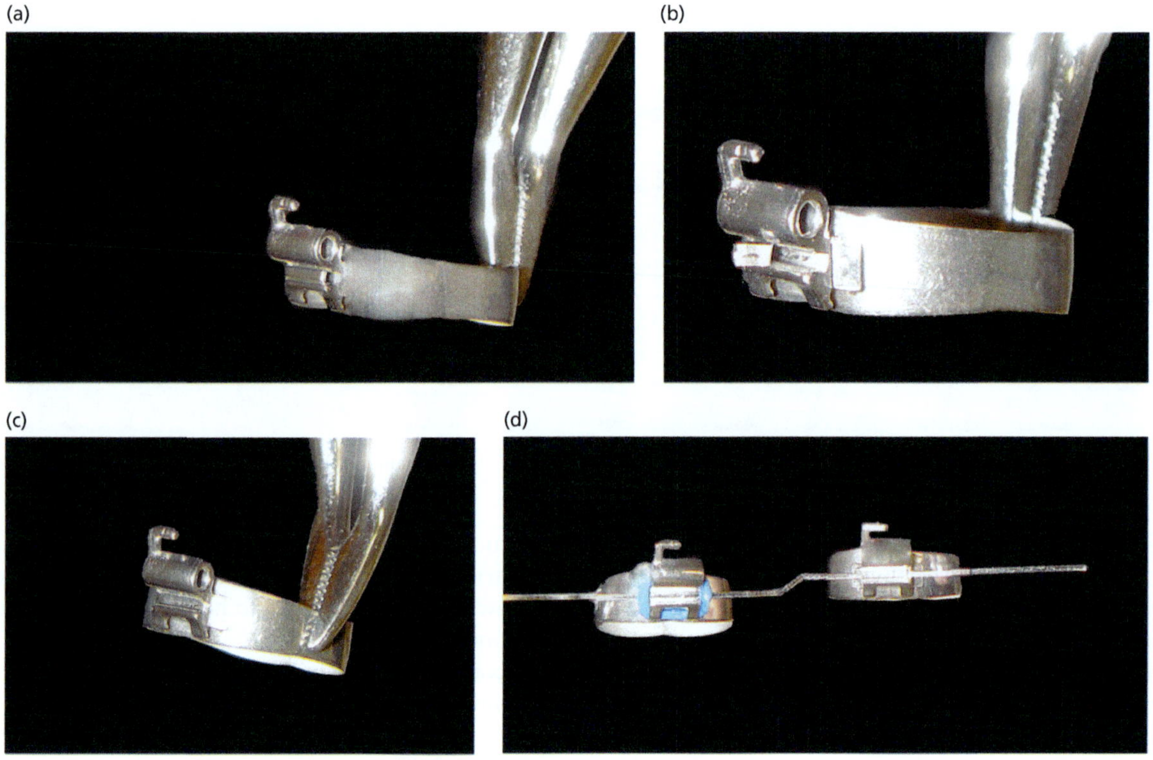

Fig. 12-46 Converting a molar tube into a bracket. (a) Molar band with convertible buccal tube. (b) The buccal cap of the convertible tube is being removed; ligature cutters may be used to peel back the cap. (c) Buccal tube converted into a bracket. (d) Convertible tubes on the maxillary first molars are useful in situations in which continuous archwire mechanics are required to align or reposition malpositioned second molars. Converting the first molar tube into a bracket permits insertion of a continuous archwire with a step between the first and second molars, which would otherwise not be possible.

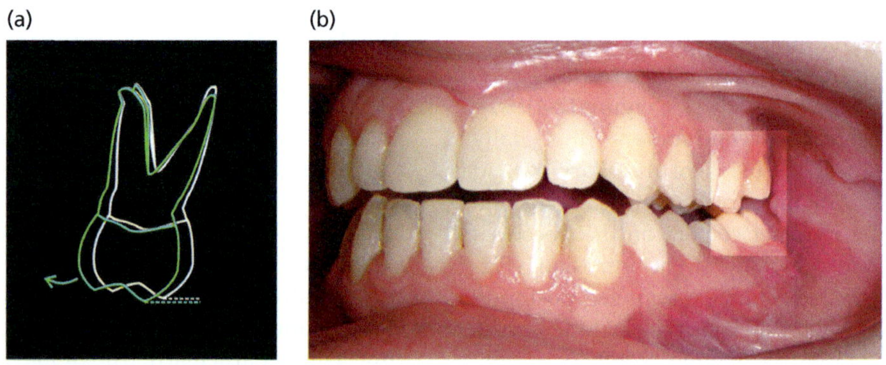

Fig. 12-47 (a) Buccal flaring (excessive buccal inclination) of maxillary molars may result in dropping down of their palatal cusps, which may cause an occlusal interference. Geometrically, the palatal cusp will only drop down after a small degree of rotation, following which it will elevate. Therefore, in clinical practice, what is likely to occur is overeruption of the molar following a small degree of buccal flaring. The combined buccal flaring and overeruption leads to an occlusal interference. (b) A buccally inclined maxillary second molar with hanging palatal cusp acting as an occlusal interference.

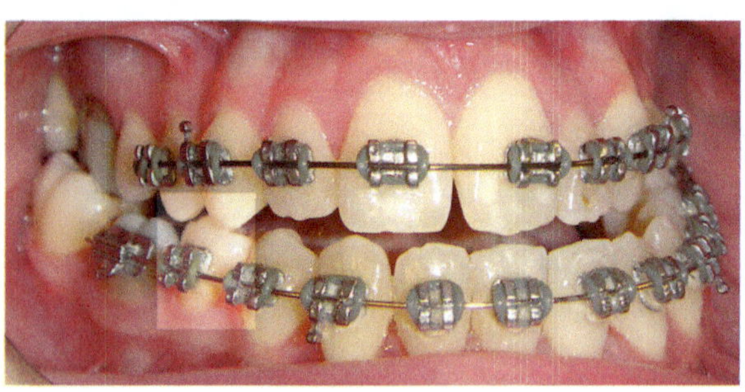

Fig. 12-48 Mandibular right second premolar is extruded relative to the rest of the mandibular arch. If uncorrected, this will lead to an occlusal interference.

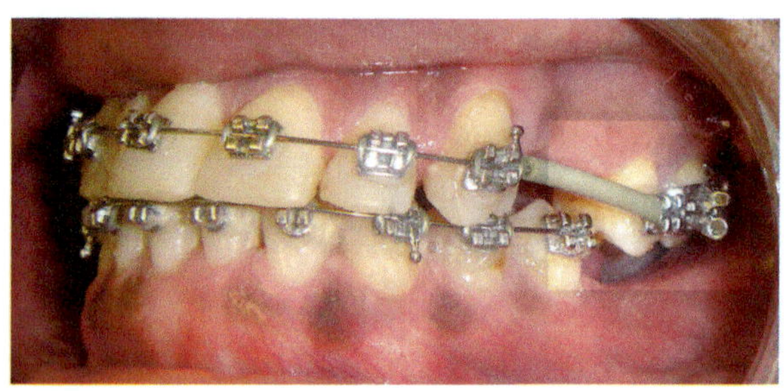

Fig. 12-49 Unopposed maxillary second premolar and molar are excessively over-erupted. The patient is being prepared for segmental maxillary surgery. As such these teeth must be levelled either with preoperative orthodontics or intraoperatively with a segmental relative dentoalveolar impaction.

relation to the rest of the arch as far as possible. Temporary anchorage devices, such as microscrews, may prove particularly useful under these circumstances. Where significant overeruption has occurred, occasionally surgical repositioning of the dentoalveolar segment at the time of surgery may be required.

- **Premolar–canine substitution** – If tooth positions have to be substituted, e.g. severely ectopic maxillary canine removal and mesialization of the first premolar into the canine position, the premolar palatal cusp may have to be reduced in height.
- **Canine-lateral incisor substitution** – If the maxillary lateral incisor is missing or has to be extracted, consideration may be given to substitution with the maxillary canine. Aesthetically, the parameters to consider are the gingival margin height on the canine, its colour and morphology, though the tip may be reduced and the shape of the tooth made more incisiform. However, the palatal surface of the canine, which is more prominent than a lateral incisor, may also need to be reduced to permit occlusion with the mandibular incisors (see Figure 12-41).
- **Prominent cusp tips** – The morphology of some teeth is such that their cusps may be long and pointed. Additionally, in some Class III patients normal attrition may not have occurred, so mandibular canines are often rather pointed and a potential interference. Minor enameloplasty of prominent canine tips will help achieve a better occlusion and is often an aesthetic enhancement.

Note:

When interferences are discovered, the orthodontist should resist the temptation of ignoring them, and would be ill-advised to abandon it to be dealt with postoperatively. Interferences can make the operative attainment of a good occlusal result impossible, and worse still, may impede accurate surgical repositioning of the jaws. Delaying surgery while potential interferences are eliminated is the right course of action, and will almost certainly reduce the length of postoperative orthodontics.

Preparation for the preoperative 'joint clinic'

When the active phase of preoperative orthodontics has been completed, and the final preoperative archwires have been in position long enough to become passive (at least 4 weeks), the patient will have an appointment to obtain the preoperative records:

- **Preoperative radiographs** – These should be taken only as required (OPT and lateral cephalometric radiograph are mandatory; periapical radiographs may be desired of regions where the surgical cuts for segmental surgery are planned; posteroanterior radiographs or 3D scans may be desired for complex asymmetries). Some clinicians prefer to take these radiographs *without the archwires in situ*, enhancing visualization of the teeth, particularly on cephalometric radiographs, and permitting better **cephalometric prediction tracings** to be undertaken (see Chapter 6).[17]
- **Preoperative photographs** – A complete set of facial and intraoral photographs are required.
- **'Snap' models** – The impressions for these study casts should be taken *without the archwires in situ*, to allow better visualization of the teeth in three dimensions.
- **Planning predictions** – If any form of prediction planning is used, it should be available for the surgeon to view at the joint clinic.

Once these records have been taken, the patient will be seen on the preoperative 'joint clinic' for planning by the surgeon and orthodontist, together with the preoperative records. Having analysed the patient and their records, and agreed on the surgical plan, the patient is then booked two appointments with either the treating clinician or the maxillofacial technologist (see Chapter 13):

1. For impressions (usually with the archwires in situ, to prevent the potential for the impression material moving the teeth), and facebow record as required, in order to undertake model surgery and make the surgical wafer splints – *The completed model surgery should be checked by both the surgeon and the orthodontist, ideally together, before the final splints are made by the maxillofacial technologist.*
2. Checking of wafer splints preoperatively for fit – These should be *checked by the surgeon (or orthodontist) to ensure a good fit and no rocking*. It is also useful to *check the final wafer on the preoperative study models to check the proposed final occlusion.*

Following the joint clinic and with the operation date set, the patient may also be booked for the immediate preoperative appointment with the orthodontist.

Immediate preoperative appointment

This appointment should be ideally no more than 2–3 weeks prior to the date of the operation. The purpose of this appointment is:

- **Checking brackets and bands** – It is important to ensure that the brackets and bands are all secure.
- **Ligate brackets with stainless steel ligatures** – All the brackets should be tied securely with stainless steel ligatures (Figure 12-50), except for self-ligating brackets, where ligatures are only required on a specific bracket if the orthodontist is concerned that the specific archwire engaging mechanism may not hold intraoperatively. Elastomeric ligatures are not acceptable, as they may dislodge intraoperatively and lodge into open surgical sites. Additionally,

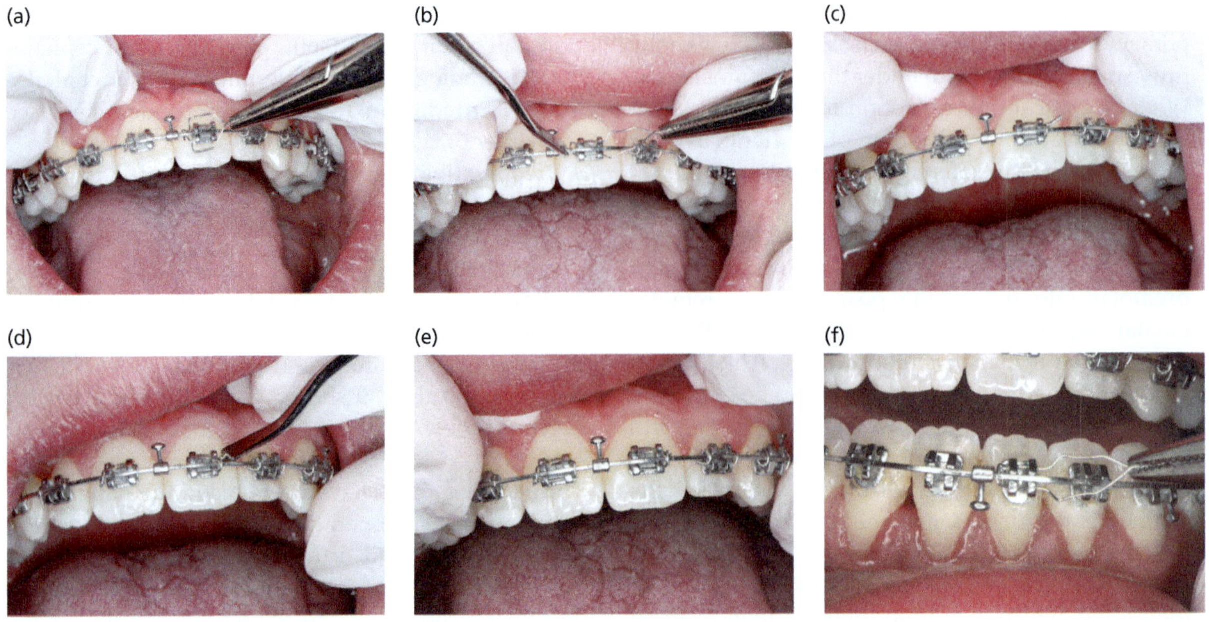

Fig. 12-50 Ligating brackets with stainless steel ligatures in the immediate preoperative orthodontic appointment. (a) A stainless steel ligature, either 0.008 or 0.012-inch (0.2 or 0.3 mm) diameter, is used to tie each bracket by engaging under the tie-wings. (b) It is pulled using the Mathieu pliers and simultaneously pushed with a ligature tucker from the opposite side. (c) It is twisted until tight around the bracket, thereby holding the archwire securely in position. The excess wire is cut. (d) The twisted end is tucked under the archwire and bracket wings, using the ligature tucker, for patient comfort and to prevent catching the surgeon's fingers intraoperatively. (e) There should be no sharp points evident. (f) The mandibular incisor brackets should be ligated *after* placement of the midline surgical hook, otherwise placement of the hook will be difficult in this small region.

when the surgeon places the intermaxillary fixation on the archwire hooks, steel ligatures prevent the archwire being pulled out of the bracket slot because of their inelasticity.

- **Placement of surgical hooks** – A number of bracket systems have **integrated hooks** on some (usually the canine brackets) or all of the brackets. These are primarily for the use of the orthodontist in placement of elastics, and should be avoided by the surgeon intraoperatively while placing wire intermaxillary fixation, as this may debond the respective bracket. Intermaxillary fixation should be placed on appropriately placed surgical hooks, either **crimpable** or **soldered** directly onto the archwire. When placing a crimpable surgical hook onto the archwire, it is important to *gently squeeze the hook onto the archwire without any upward or downward movement of the wrist*, in order to avoid debonding the brackets on either side, or inadvertently placing torque into the rectangular archwire (Figure 12-51). Alternatively, the archwire may be marked intraorally, and removed to have hooks crimped or soldered (Figure 12-52). Soldering of hooks is particularly useful if round archwires have to be used rather than rectangular archwires, e.g. in a patient prone to root resorption. Usually, each arch requires one midline hook and a hook between the premolars bilaterally. However, some surgeons prefer a greater number of hooks. The maxillary midline hook sometimes catches the patient's upper lip, and patients should always be provided with vegetable wax to place over this area if required. In the postoperative phase, both surgical hooks on the archwire and integrated hooks on brackets will be employed by the orthodontist for placement of both guiding and working elastics.
- **Kobayashi ligatures** – These specific ligatures are fabricated from either 0.012-inch (0.3 mm) or 0.014-inch (0.35 mm) annealed stainless steel wire, with the legs welded onto one another forming a

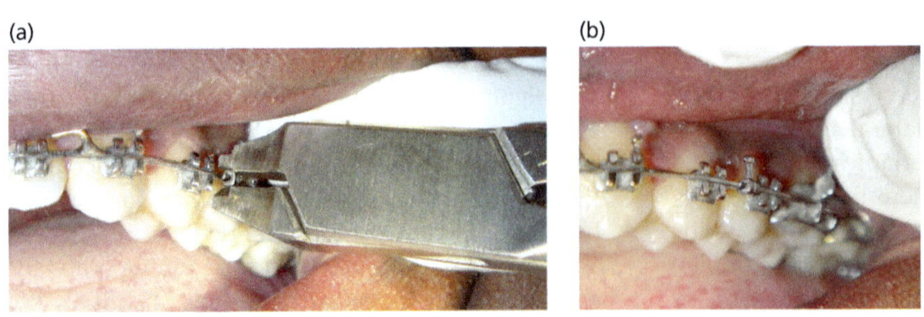

Fig. 12-51 When placing a crimpable surgical hook onto the archwire, it is important to gently squeeze the hook onto the archwire *without any upward or downward movement of the wrist*, in order to avoid debonding the brackets on either side, or inadvertently placing torque into the rectangular archwire.

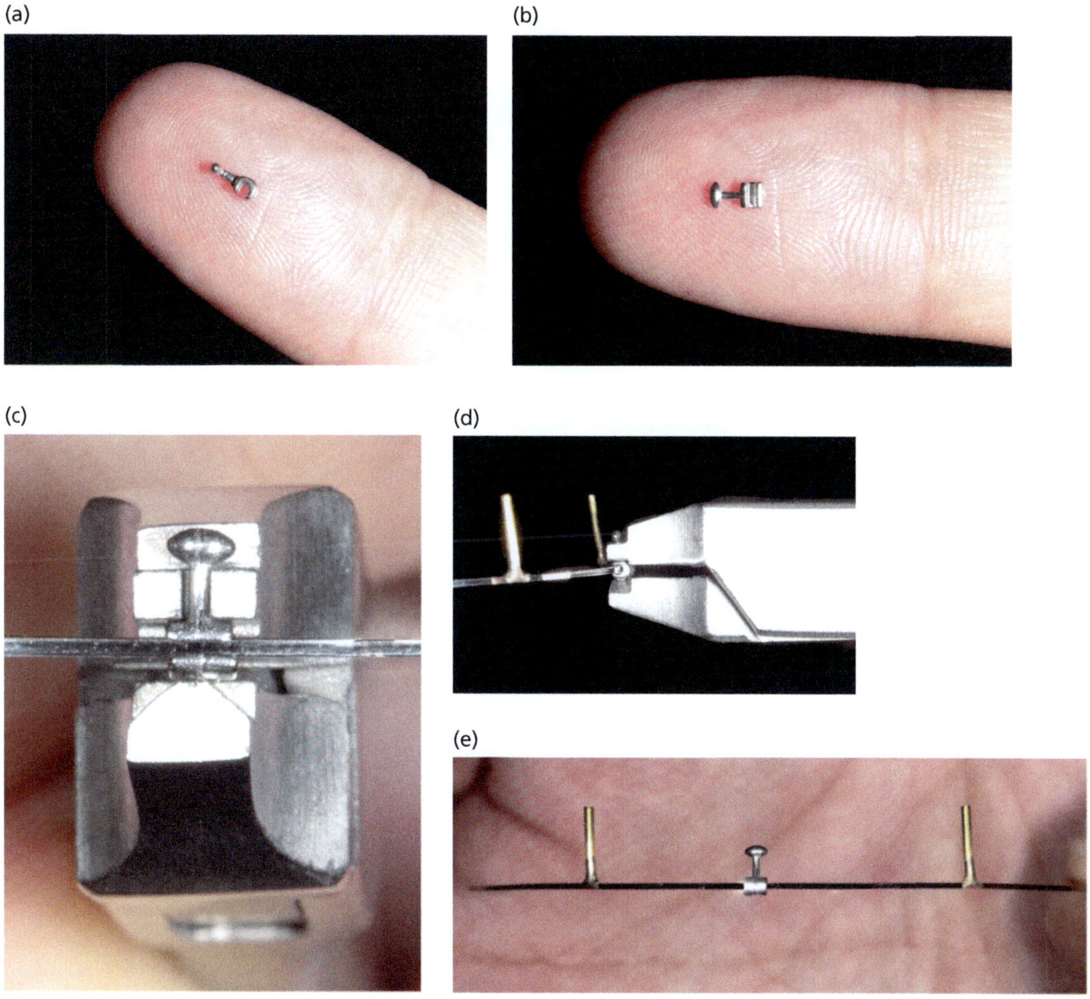

Fig. 12-52 (a, b) A crimpable surgical hook. (c) A crimpable hook held in the beaks of crimpable hook pliers. (d) Crimping a hook on a rectangular archwire. (e) A midline crimpable hook and bilateral soldered hooks on the surgical archwire.

helical hook at the end (Figure 12-53). Placement is as with conventional stainless steel ligatures, but the hook may be employed for elastic attachment by the orthodontist postoperatively. In some cases, where the inter-bracket span in the mandibular central incisor region is markedly reduced and a surgical hook cannot be crimped onto the archwire, or if a round archwire has to be used in place of a rectangular archwire (e.g. a patient prone to root resorption where rectangular archwires have to be avoided), Kobayashi ligatures may be used in place of the inter-bracket surgical hook. The surgeon will need to take extra care not to debond the mandibular incisor brackets intraoperatively while placing the IMF. Otherwise, these ligatures are for the use of the orthodontic elastics, not IMF.

Note:

It is also important for the orthodontist to put aside enough time to discuss any final issues with the patient. Despite previous information provision, patients may still have some questions at this stage. Finally, patients will be understandably anxious at this close stage to the operation, and the orthodontist should reassure the patient that they will be in the safe hands of an experienced surgeon and anaesthetist.

Intraoperative orthodontic requirements

Surgical finesse is vital, and excessive surgical force in placement of intermaxillary fixation may debond brackets. Nevertheless, debonds do occur intraoperatively, and can usually be ignored (hence the importance of reliable ligation) and repaired by the orthodontist postoperatively. However, if a band which is part of an RME appliance becomes loose, it may need to be repaired intraoperatively. Additionally, in segmental surgery, continuous archwires may need to be placed intraoperatively, or over tied to the segmented archwires, once the jaw has been surgically segmented and repositioned (see Figure 12-30). Therefore, the presence of an orthodontist may occasionally be required in the operating theatre.

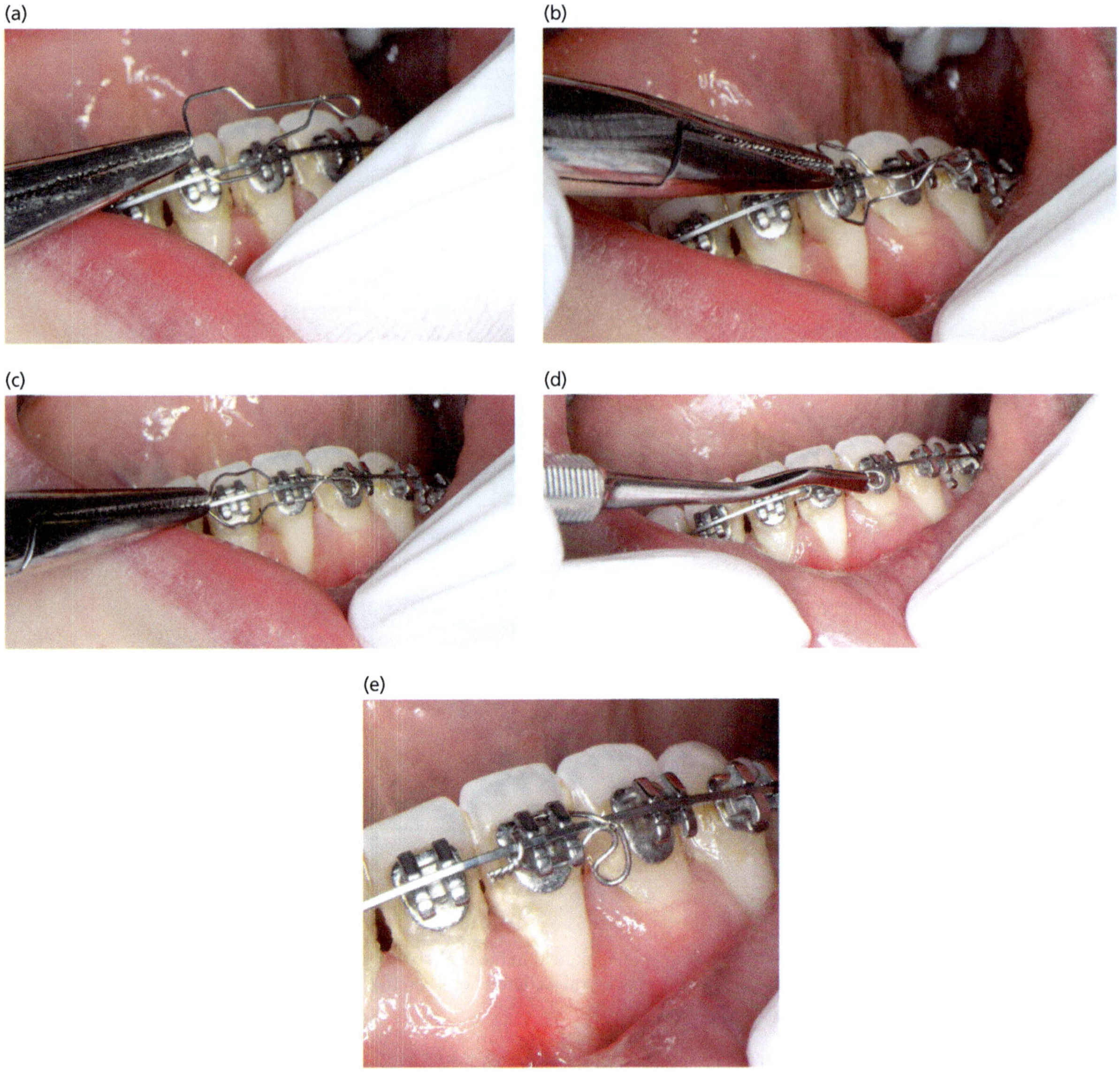

Fig. 12-53 Placement of a Kobayashi ligature.

A number of inaccuracies may occur during splint wafer construction, and, as such, the fact that a patient is occluding well into the surgical wafer is no guarantee that they will occlude well once the wafer has been removed. Wafers should be removed at the end of the operation, and the dental occlusion checked.

Immediate postoperative appointment

The patient should be seen by the orthodontist, together with the surgeon, on the day following surgery. It is important for patients to be mobilized as soon as possible following surgery. As such, it is better for patients to come from the ward to the maxillofacial department, walk and sit in the dental chair to be examined.

At this stage, the vast majority of patients feel absolutely terrible. Though they should have been informed preoperatively, it is important to reiterate to the patient that the first few days are always the worst, and that they will feel much better soon. Despite feeling dispirited, this encouraging information will hearten the patient and their parents/carer.

The main purpose of this appointment is *to check that the skeletal and dental-occlusal aims of the surgery have been achieved* (see Table 12-3). Despite the obvious facial soft tissue oedema, it is also important to check that potential untoward soft tissue changes have been minimal. Prior to clinical evaluation, the patient should be reassured by the clinician that they will be very gentle in their oral examination. Blood-stained saliva may be gently aspirated as far as possible, and any intermaxillary elastics placed intraoperatively may be removed. The patient's mandible may then be gently guided by light finger pressure in order to check the dental occlusion with the maxillary arch or into the wafer if it has not been removed.

Table 12-3 Checklist for one day postoperative evaluation

Clinical evaluation	
Vertical parameters	
Vertical facial proportions	Have the vertical facial proportions been corrected as planned?
Maxillary incisor exposure in repose	Is the maxillary incisor display in relation to the upper lip correct?
Occluding into wafer/occlusion with opposing arch	Is the patient occluding together well (or into the wafer if this has not been removed)? Are there any obvious interferences?
Transverse parameters	
Maxillary dental midline	Is this coincident with the mid-philtrum of the upper lip and facial midline?
Mandibular dental midline	Is this coincident with the maxillary dental midline?
Transverse canting	Is the transverse maxillary occlusal plane level (e.g. in relation to interpupillary plane or a true horizontal plane)? Has any preoperative transverse canting been corrected? Has any transverse canting been inadvertently introduced?
Nasal alar base width	Has this been adequately controlled (measure and compare to preoperative value)?
Sagittal parameters	
Columella inclination	Has this been adequately controlled (compare to preoperative clinical photograph)?
Relationship of upper lip, lower lip, mentolabial fold and chin to one another	Are these parameters in the desired relationship to one another?
Relationship of upper lip, lower lip, mentolabial fold and chin to facial profile	Are these parameters in the desired relationship to the facial profile?
Radiographic evaluation	
OPT (mandatory)	Are the condyles in the same position as the preoperative OPT? Are the bony segments well-aligned across the inferior border of the mandible? Is there any root damage evident if segmental surgery has been undertaken?
Lateral cephalometric radiograph (if required)	Are the condyles in the same position as the preoperative radiograph? Is the bony chin position correct (post genioplasty)? Check profile parameters as with clinical evaluation.

Note:

When to remove the wafer?

Traditionally, prior to the advent of rigid internal fixation (RIF), postoperative immobilization of the bimaxillary complex was required during the 6-8 week bone healing phase. Therefore, the final wafer was maintained in position, with the patient in intermaxillary fixation (IMF), while the wire osteosynthesis maintained the bone segments together until bony union occurred. Since the introduction of RIF, some authorities continue to advise the maintenance of the wafer tied to one or other arch, for up to one month, in order to reduce the risk of movement between the bone segments and potential risk of fibrous union. Placing heavy intermaxillary elastics in the first few weeks postoperatively may risk fibrous union, and should be avoided (see below). However, maintaining the wafer in situ has a number of downsides:

- Patients dislike them – When a wafer is removed postoperatively, the look of relief on a patient's face says it all.
- Oral hygiene hazard – Dental plaque and food debris is trapped between the teeth and wafer, and the stench of the wafer when removed even after one week can be nauseating.
- The actual occlusal result is unknown – The clinician only knows that the patient is occluding well into the wafer (see below).

For these reasons, unless segmental maxillary surgery has been undertaken, it may be advisable to remove the wafer in theatre at the end of the operation, and check the dental occlusion. Light intermaxillary guiding elastics may be placed as required. As long as untoward forces are not placed in the first few weeks postoperatively, the RIF maintains the bone segments together permitting bony union, and the patient is far more comfortable.

The patient is then sent for postoperative radiographs prior to returning for placement of intermaxillary guiding elastics as required.

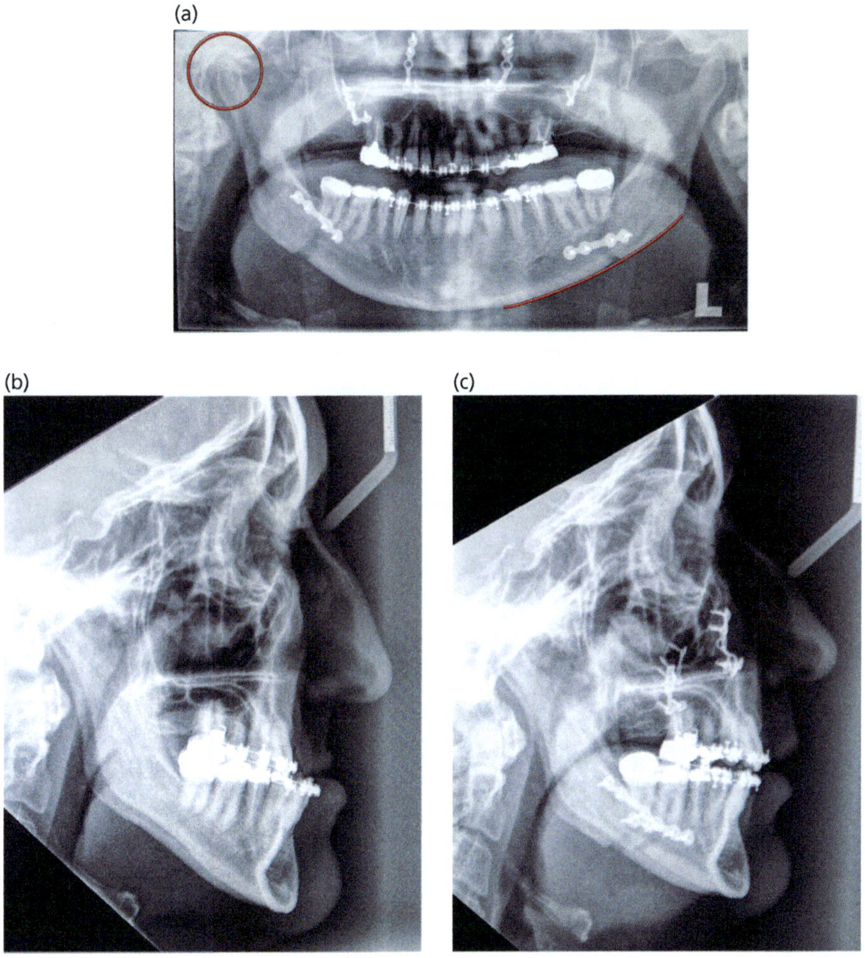

Fig. 12-54 One day postoperative radiographs. (a) OPT to check alignment of the bony borders in the surgical regions and the position of the condyles in the glenoid fossae bilaterally. (b) Preoperative lateral cephalometric radiograph may be compared with the (c) postoperative lateral cephalometric radiograph, again checking for bony alignment and condylar positions.

Postoperative radiographs

Following the clinical examination, the patient should have an orthopantomograph (OPT) and possibly a lateral cephalometric radiograph taken and critically compared with the preoperative radiographs. These radiographs are used to check:

- Postoperative condylar positions (Figures 12-54 and 12-55).
- The alignment of the bony borders in the surgical regions.
- Chin position after a genioplasty (Figure 12-56).

The fact that a patient is occluding well into the splint wafer is no guarantee that their dentition will be occluding well together when the wafer has been removed. In fact, maintenance of the final splint in situ potentially hides a bad occlusion (Figure 12-57). Therefore, ideally the wafer should be removed in the operating theatre at the end of the operation, and the dental occlusion checked (unless segmental maxillary surgery has been undertaken, in which case a longer period of immobilization is required with the wafer in situ). However, some surgeons prefer to maintain the wafer initially, usually ligated to the maxillary fixed appliance. As soon as the wafer is removed in the postoperative period, the dental occlusion should be checked. At this stage, a mild deviation (no more than 2–3 mm) of the mandibular dental arch, either anteriorly or laterally, may result from:

- altered proprioception in the immediate postoperative phase;
- minor dental interferences not picked up preoperatively;
- swelling of the intraoral soft tissues, particularly in the retromolar regions.

In these situations, light intermaxillary **guiding elastics**, also known as **training elastics**, may be placed to override the proprioceptive impulse of minor dental or soft tissue interference and gently guide the patient's teeth into occlusion (Figure 12-58). However, if a major discrepancy in the position of the jaws is observed, the patient will almost certainly need to return to the operating theatre for surgical adjustment as required. *Attempting excessive intermaxillary elastic placement with heavy forces, almost akin to intermaxillary fixation, is inappropriate, and should be avoided.* If the jaws have been rigidly fixed in an incorrect position, no amount of orthodontic elastics will correct this position, and one is simply delaying the inevitable. Additionally, immediate return to surgery, though unwelcome news for the patient, will be preferable to reoperating after a few weeks, both psychologically

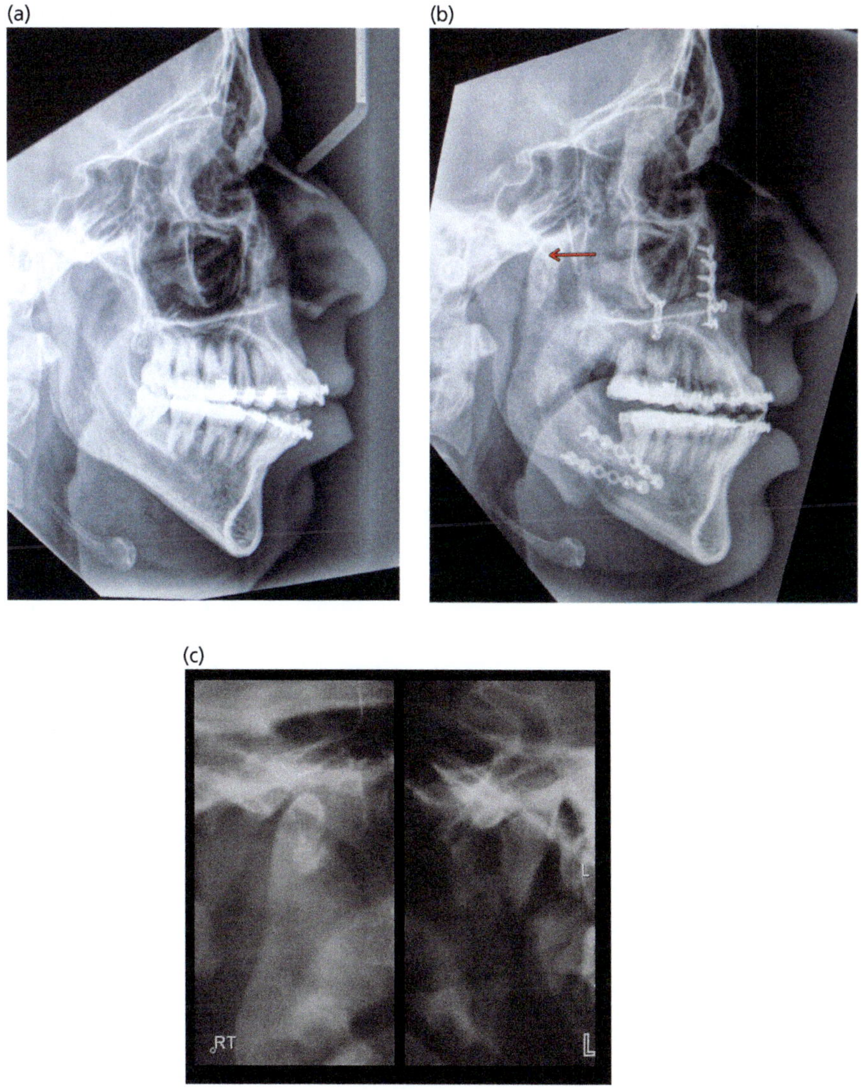

Fig. 12-55 (a) Preoperative lateral cephalometric radiograph prior to bimaxillary surgery. The patient left the operating theatre still intubated due to intraoperative complications. (b, c) On the day following surgery the patient was occluding but with a lateral displacement. Postoperative radiographs demonstrated that the right condyle was dislocated, and the patient was taken back to theatre. Recovery was uneventful, but this case highlights the importance of accurate postoperative radiographs.

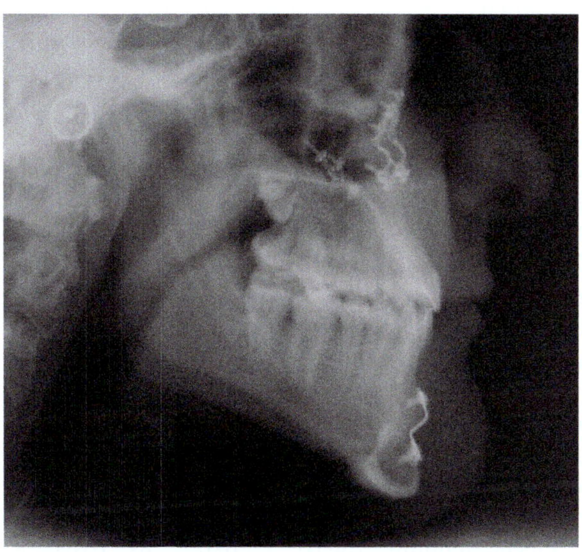

Fig. 12-56 Lateral cephalometric radiograph taken 1 day postoperatively to check chin relationships following a set-back genioplasty.

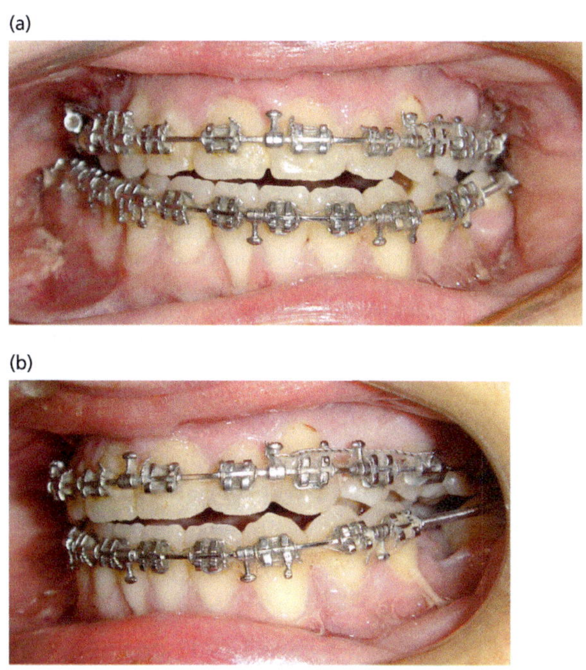

Fig. 12-57 One day postoperatively the wafer has been removed to reveal a poor dental occlusion and an occlusal interference on the left canine and premolar region.

(a)

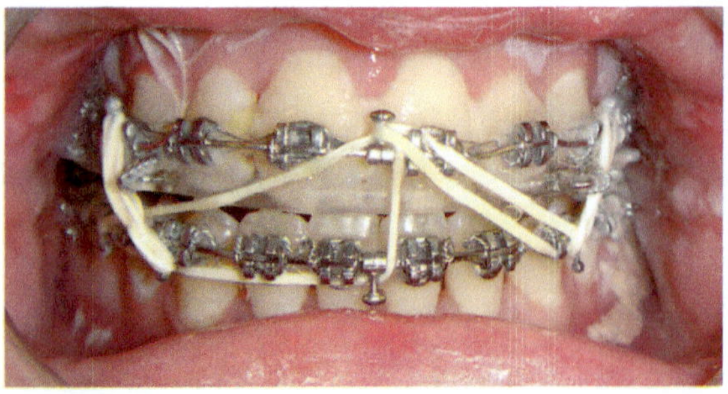

(b)

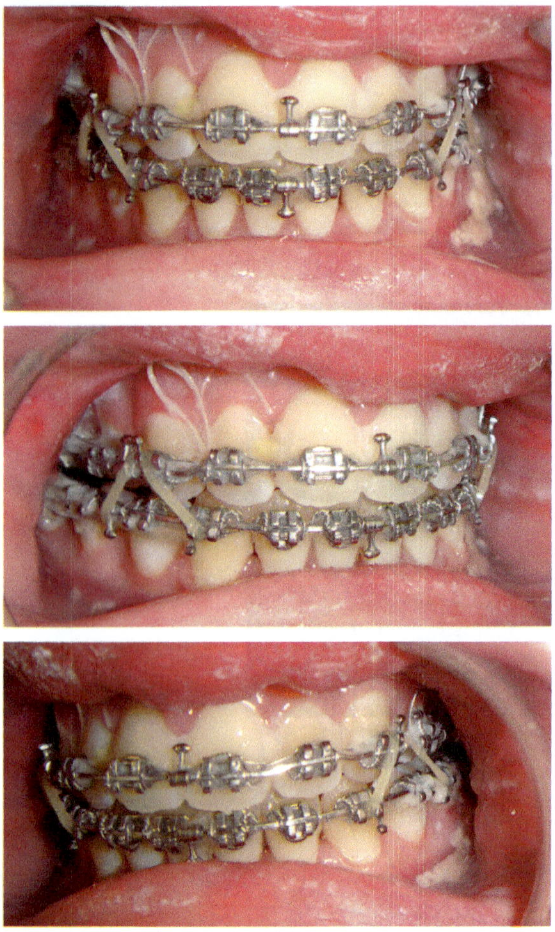

Fig. 12-58 (a) One day postoperative assessment reveals wafer in situ and rather overzealous intraoperative intermaxillary elastic placement. (b) The wafer is removed and light intermaxillary **guiding elastics**, also known as **training elastics**, are placed to override the proprioceptive impulse of minor dental or soft tissue interference and gently guide the patient's teeth into occlusion. Ideally, this should have been carried out at the end of the operation.

for the patient, and for the clinician, as bone healing may occur very quickly in a young healthy adult, as any surgeon attempting to reoperate after a few weeks will testify.

Postoperative orthodontics

Whether the wafer is removed early or not, active orthodontic treatment is usually delayed for 2 weeks, until the patient feels up to having treatment. During this time the patient will usually be wearing *light* intermaxillary guiding elastics, which help to guide the patient into the planned dental occlusion. These should be worn full time, and the patient should be seen by the surgeon and orthodontist weekly for the first 2 weeks, for close observation of any changes to the dental occlusion. Some patients will have an obvious, well-interdigitated dental occlusal result postoperatively. However, others may need closer observation, with variations in the intermaxillary elastic vectors made as required during this time (see below).

> **Note:**
>
> Repairs to the orthodontic appliance should be made as soon as practically possible during this initial period. If a bracket has debonded or a band is loose, it should be repaired or removed.

If full thickness stainless steel archwires had been placed prior to surgery, i.e. 0.0215 × 0.025-inch archwire in a 0.022 × 0.028 bracket slot, then these **stabilizing archwires** will need to be replaced with **working archwires**. However, most orthognathic surgeons are happy to operate with a larger dimension stainless steel working archwire, e.g. 0.019 × 0.025-inch stainless steel archwire, so long as it has been placed at least 4 weeks prior to the maxillofacial technologist's impressions in preparation for surgery. If a working archwire is already in place, there is no requirement to change it at this stage.

Working archwires

The type of working archwire required in either the maxillary or mandibular arch depends on the tooth movements desired. Often the most important initial movement is to guide the teeth vertically into a better dental occlusion. The orthodontist must decide on the teeth they would like to extrude, and in which arch. For example, if the maxillary arch is level, the 0.019 × 0.025-inch stainless steel archwire may be maintained in position. If the mandible has been advanced to a 3-point landing, the mandibular canines and premolars need to be extruded by elastic force; therefore a flexible mandibular archwire is required. The dimensions and material of the **flexible archwire** depend on the other types of movement that may be required, e.g. torque control, but the following are commonly used postoperatively:

- Braided (multistrand) stainless steel – 0.017, or 0.018 or 0.019 × 0.025-inch (Figure 12-59).
- TMA (titanium-molybdenum alloy) – 0.017, or 0.018 or 0.019 × 0.025-inch.
- Nickel–titanium (NiTi) – 0.017, or 0.018 or 0.019 × 0.025-inch.

If further lingual inclination of mandibular molars is desired, a flexible round archwire may be used, or a

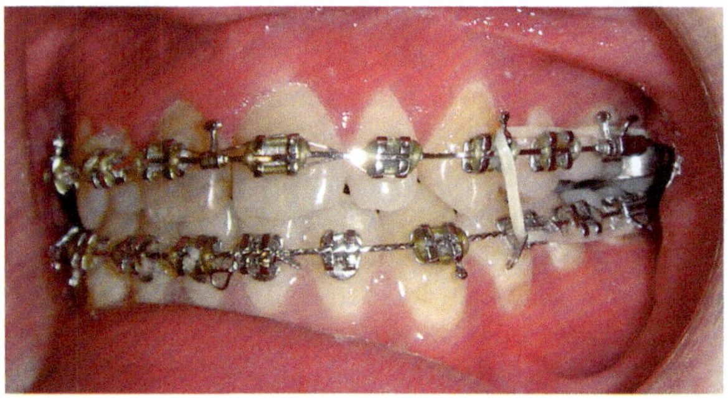

Fig. 12-59 A braided (multistrand) stainless steel archwire has been placed in the mandibular arch postoperatively. The dimension of the archwire is 0.019 × 0.025-inch and, as such, the rectangular wire will maintain the torque. However, unlike the rigid surgical archwire, this braided steel wire is flexible, and box type elastics against the rigid stainless steel maxillary archwire will permit extrusion of the mandibular dentition and improvement of the occlusion.

smaller dimension round stainless steel archwire (e.g. 0.018-inch).

In the transverse plane, further arch coordination may be required, as may further buccal root torque of the maxillary molars.

Kobayashi ligatures

As described previously, these are very useful means of attachment for orthodontic elastics, and should be placed as required (see Figure 12-53).

(a)

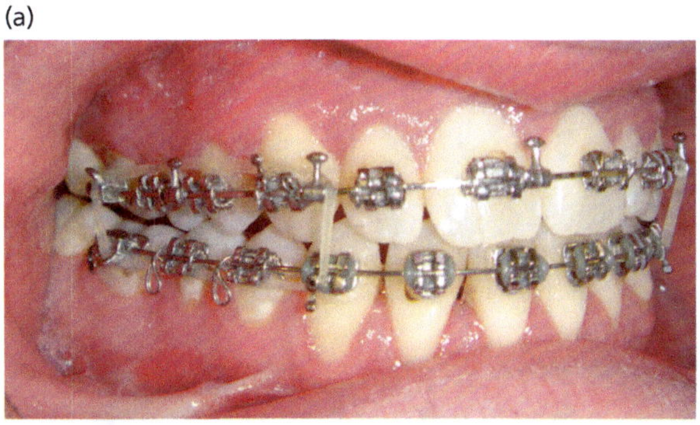

(b)

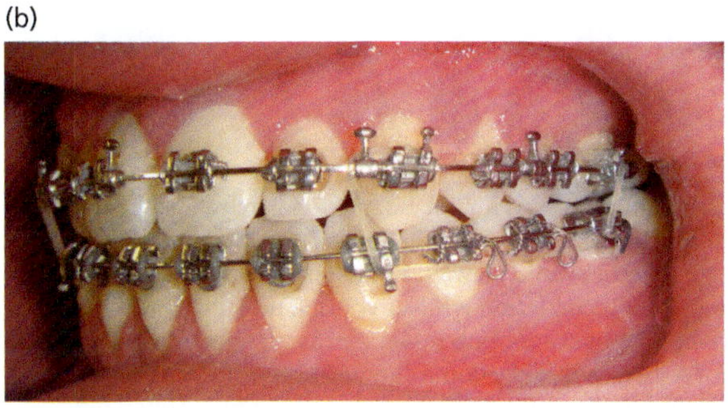

Fig. 12-60 Vertical tooth movement in the buccal segments may be facilitated with **box elastics**, maintaining a vertical vector as far as possible. The position of surgical hooks, integrated hooks on brackets and Kobayashi ligatures allows the orthodontist to vary the elastic vectors as required.

(a)

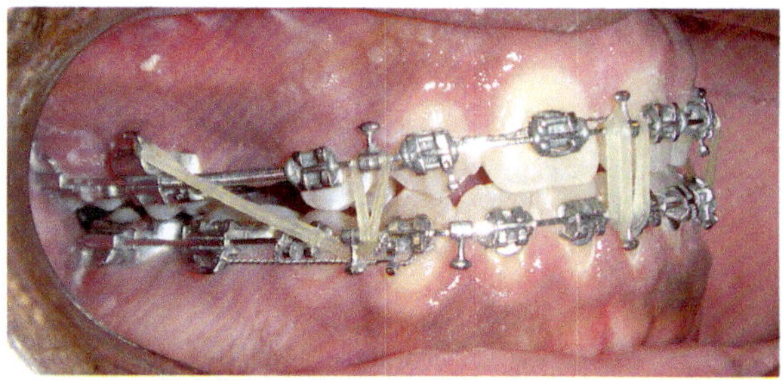

(b)

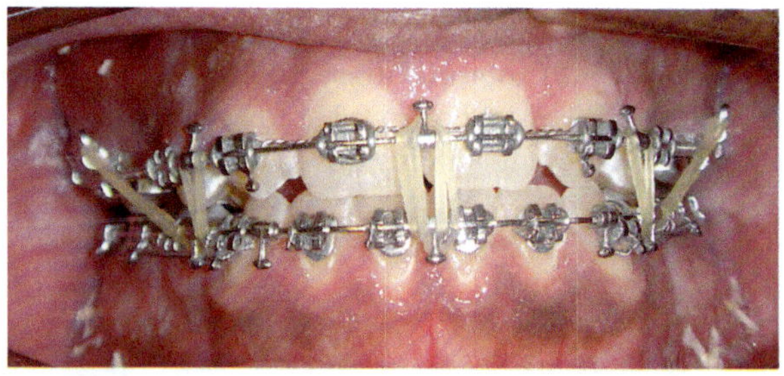

(c)

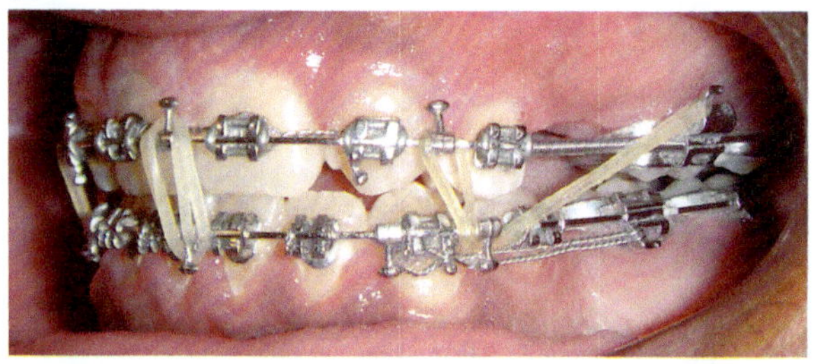

Fig. 12-61 Following maxillary advancement and mandibular set-back for a Class III patient with an anterior open bite, Class III elastics are placed with an anterior vertical vector.

Intermaxillary working elastics

The configuration of the working intermaxillary elastics depends on the type and direction of desired tooth movement. Incorrectly placed elastics will result in undesirable tooth movement; therefore, every effort must be made to ensure that patients do not incorrectly position them. A drawing demonstrating exactly which teeth should engage the elastics may be provided to the patient as a reminder.

Configurations and vectors for intermaxillary working elastics

Vertical tooth movement in the buccal segments is usually facilitated with **box elastics**, maintaining a vertical vector as far as possible (Figure 12-60). Vertical intermaxillary elastics, whether box type or triangular in configuration, aim at extrusion of selected teeth to improve the interdigitation of the dental arches. Box elastics are required to level a mandibular curve of Spee (see Figure 12-9). If necessary, a Class II or Class III vector may be advisable on one or both sides, depending on the desired tooth movements.

Class II or Class III elastics may be placed with an additional vertical vector, which is particularly useful

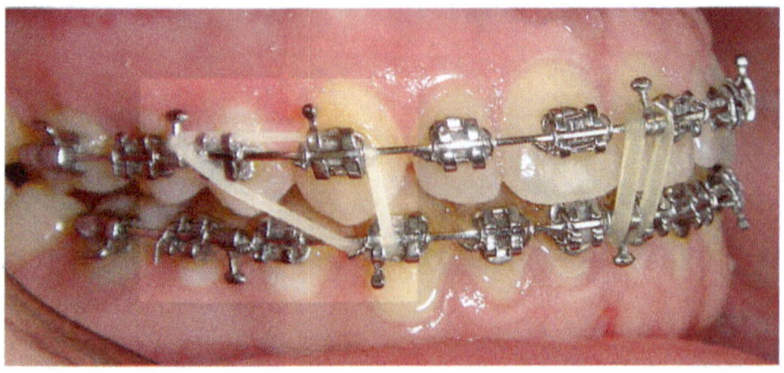

Fig. 12-62 Short triangular intermaxillary elastic with a Class III vector.

following surgery to correct an anterior open bite (Figure 12-61). **Short intermaxillary elastics**, either Class II or Class III, may be useful, providing the Class II or III vector but limiting the potential detrimental vertical eruption of the maxillary or mandibular molars from routine Class II or III intermaxillary elastics. These may also be placed in a triangular configuration (Figure 12-62).

Persistent dental midline deviations may require a Class II elastic vector on one side and Class III on the contralateral side. Sometimes an **anterior diagonal elastic** may also be added (usually just night times). In such situations, care must be taken not to cause transverse canting of the maxillary occlusal plane by extruding the teeth attached to these elastics; theoretically temporary anchorage devices may be used in one arch as a means of elastic attachment instead of the teeth, though in practice this is rarely required.

Variations of postoperative working elastic configurations are demonstrated in Figure 12-63.

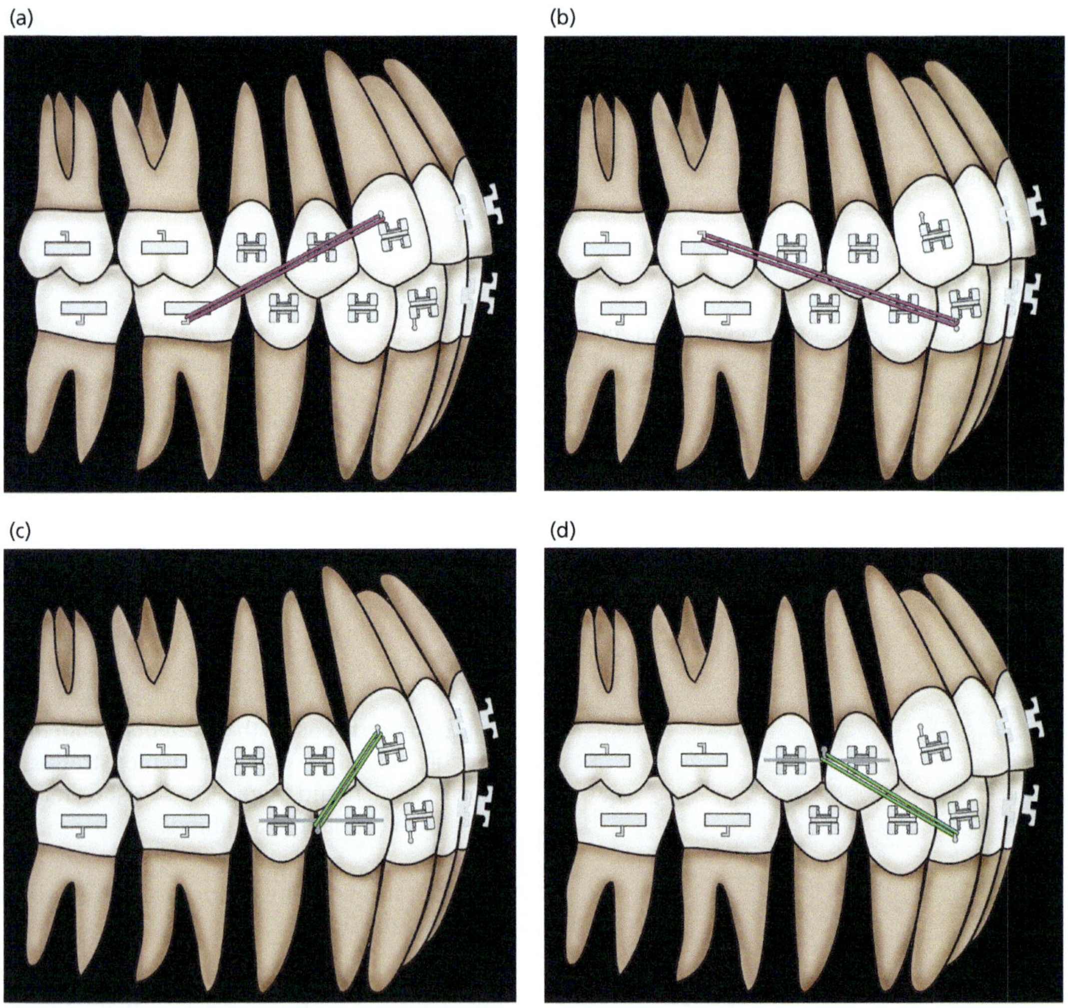

Fig. 12-63 Examples of commonly required postoperative working elastic configurations for elastic traction. Archwires are not shown to improve clarity, except partially where archwire hooks are shown. It should be noted that elastics may be placed around archwire hooks or integrated bracket hooks as required. Various other combinations and configurations may be used as required. (a) Class II elastic. (b) Class III elastic. (c) Short Class II elastic –useful for Class II correction whilst avoiding molar extrusion and anterior bite opening. (d) Short Class III elastic –useful for Class III correction whilst avoiding molar extrusion and anterior bite opening. (e) Class II elastic with vertical element (Delta Class II) – useful for Class II correction following anterior open bite correction. (f) Class III elastic with vertical element (Delta Class III) – useful for Class III correction following anterior open bite correction. (g) Box elastic – useful for closure of lateral or posterior open bites, and active occlusal 'settling'. (h) Box elastic with Class II vector – as with (g), but when Class II element required. (i) Box elastic with Class III vector – as with (g), but when Class III element required. (j) Triangular elastic – these may be used as guiding elastics postoperatively, or as working elastics, and placed between any group of opposing teeth, as required. (k) Anterior diagonal elastic, with Class II and Class III elastic traction, which is a combination commonly used for dental midline correction.

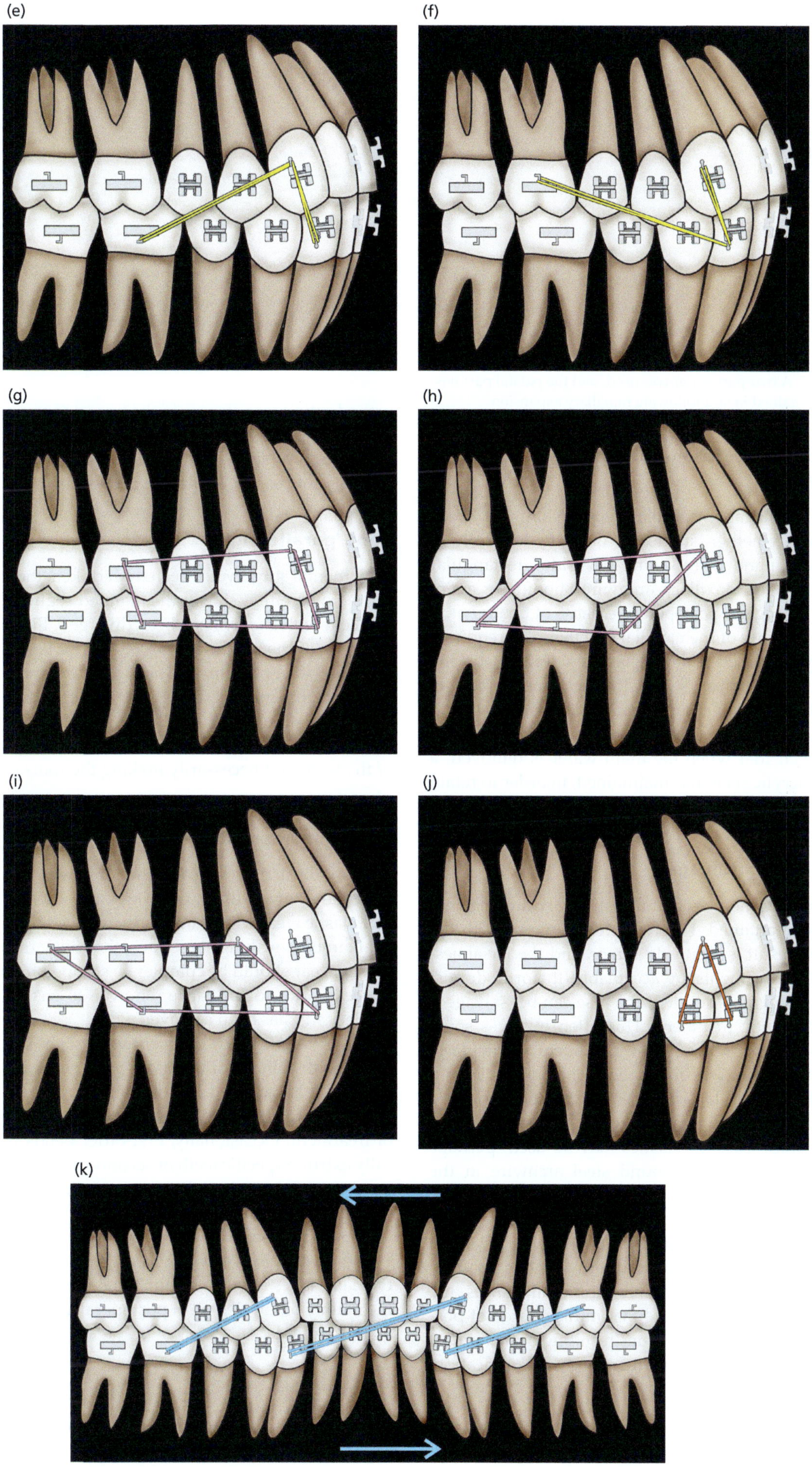

Fig. 12-63 (*Continued*).

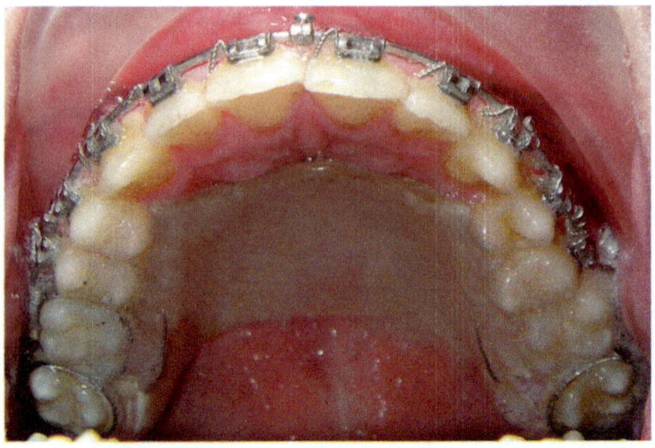

Fig. 12-64 A two-part wafer was used, and the palatal part has been maintained in situ following maxillary expansion.

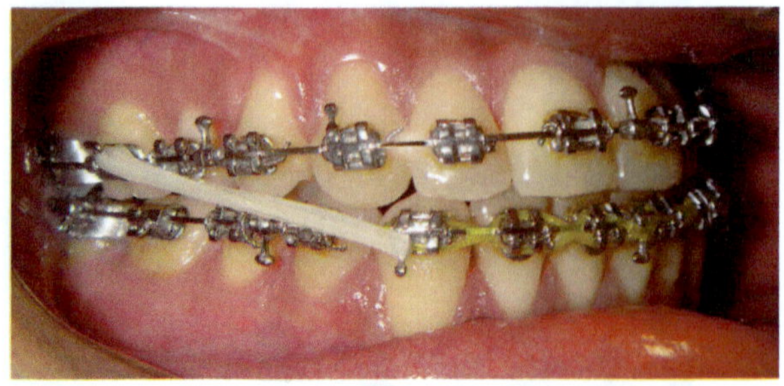

Fig. 12-65 Following a mandibular set-back, a slightly edge-to-edge incisor relationship was corrected with Class III elastics.

Specific considerations following maxillary expansion

When significant maxillary expansion has been achieved, whether surgically or orthodontically, a slightly expanded (~3 mm per side) rectangular stainless steel maxillary archwire should be maintained during the postoperative phase of treatment. If vertical settling of the maxillary teeth is also required, a heavy expanded wire may be tied over the working archwire, and placed into the headgear tubes, in order to maintain the expansion (see Figure 12-30). Alternatively, a two-part maxillary wafer may be used, such that when the main wafer is removed, a palatal acrylic section is maintained, in order to retain the expansion (Figure 12-64).

Orthodontic 'salvage'

Occasionally, the exact planned surgical result may not have been attained. Where the discrepancy with the planned result is relatively minor, and the facial aesthetic improvements are acceptable, the orthodontist and surgeon may decide if the case can be 'salvaged' by orthodontic treatment. This often involves some form of compensatory tooth movement, particularly in relation to incisor inclinations. For example, if a Class II mandibular advancement has been slightly over-advanced, with an edge-to-edge type incisor relationship, Class III elastics may be used, perhaps in conjunction with a round steel archwire in the mandibular arch, to improve the incisor relationship. Alternatively, if a Class III case has a slightly edge-to-edge incisor relationship postoperatively, Class III elastics may be beneficial in improving this relationship (Figure 12-65). Whatever the circumstances, the clinicians need to be aware that miracles are not possible, and significant problems resulting from surgical shortcomings may need further surgical modification.

Space closure

In some patients, particularly low angle, deep overbite patients with strong masseter muscles and a well-interdigitated dental occlusion, preoperative orthodontic space closure in the buccal segments may be extremely difficult and time-consuming. However, completion of space closure postoperatively may be considerably easier, as the bite is opened.

Root 'paralleling'

If segmental surgery has been undertaken, the roots of the teeth on either side of the planned segmental surgical cut will usually have been diverged. Either repositioning of the brackets or second order bends in the archwire will be required to achieve correct root angulation postoperatively. This is sometimes referred to as 'root paralleling', though the term is somewhat of a misnomer as the objective is correcting the angulations of the teeth, not necessarily making the roots parallel.

Orthodontic settling and finishing

Much of the active vertical orthodontic settling occurs with the intermaxillary working elastics. Intermaxillary elastic wear will be markedly reduced, if required at all, in the finishing stages of orthodontic treatment. Elastic wear should be completely stopped for at least 6 weeks prior to appliance removal, to ensure that a stable result has been achieved.

Minor variations in tooth crown morphology combined with minor variations in bracket position will mean that some tooth repositioning by 'artistic' wire bending is likely to be required in the finishing stages of treatment. Occasionally, first-order bends to vertically extrude specific teeth or second-order angulation bends for the incisor teeth may be required, as is labial or lingual root torque for specific teeth (usually maxillary lateral incisors).

The postoperative phase of orthodontic treatment typically takes anything from 3 to 6 months, depending mainly on the degree of postoperative tooth movement required.

Retention

There is an often-quoted aphorism in orthodontics:

> 'Stability is not *a* problem in orthodontics; it is *the* problem in orthodontics.'

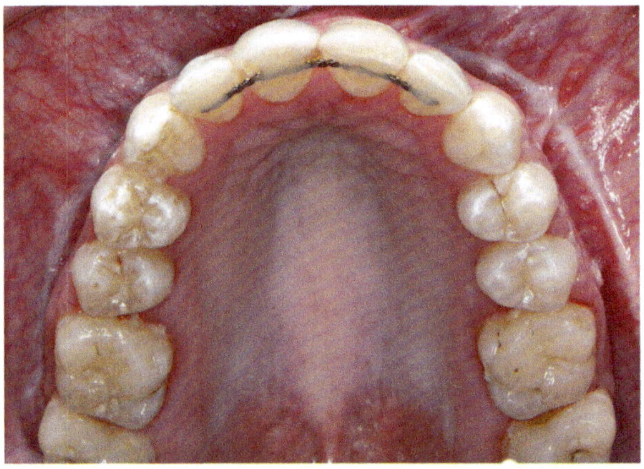

Fig. 12-66 A palatal bonded retainer.

Certain orthodontic tooth movements, e.g. significant derotation of teeth or closure of a maxillary midline diastema, are known to be relatively unstable and thereby potentially problematic in the long-term. In such cases the orthodontist may decide to place a lingual or palatal **bonded retainer** (Figure 12-66), in addition to removable retainers. However, the fact remains that the results of treatment in some patients are more stable than others, and we have no way of knowing who is in which camp. Therefore, all patients require some form of long-term retention, and this must be explained right at the beginning of treatment, and emphasized in the process of obtaining informed consent. Over time patients will realise the stability of their own dentition, and as long as retainer wear is reduced very gradually, whenever the patient places their retainer and it feels a little tight, they know their teeth have moved a little and they can increase their retainer wear for some time before reducing wear again.

Retention protocol

Retention protocols and regimes vary from unit to unit. Retainers should ideally be made and fitted on the same day as appliance removal, or at least within 1–2 days. Retainer wear begins close to full time, except for eating and cleaning of the teeth and retainers. This first 3–4 months of close to full time wear is to permit time for reorganization of the periodontal ligament and supporting tissues.[18,19] Wear may be reduced to evening and nights only after 3–4 months, and gradually onto nights only, which may be continued for between 12 to 24 months. Certain orthodontic tooth movements will require a longer period of full time retention, e.g. derotation of teeth, and may even require bonded retention. Realistically, many patients reduce retainer wear gradually to every other night, and eventually down to a few nights per week, which should then be maintained on a long term basis. However, for many patients the degree of stability of their orthodontically repositioned teeth is difficult to know with any degree of certainty; as such, the orthodontists' advice is usually for patients to continue their night time retainer wear *indefinitely*.

Types of retainer

Bonded retainers have been described above. Patients may be given some choice as to the type of removable retainer. Vacuum-formed, **Essix type retainers** (introduced by the American orthodontist Dr John Sheridan) have superior aesthetic qualities, but the patient's oral hygiene must be excellent, otherwise decalcification may result. They are often not particularly sturdy and may crack, wear and have to be remade after some variable interval.

When maxillary expansion has been undertaken, **Hawley type retainers,** introduced by Charles A. Hawley (1861–1929) in 1908, are preferable as the palatal acrylic helps to maintain the expansion and prevent transverse relapse. An alternative is a combined retainer, the **Hawlix or 'aesthetic' retainer**, which combines the anterior aesthetic advantage of the Essix retainer and the palatal acrylic of the Hawley retainer.[20] This retainer is particularly useful following treatment in cleft lip and palate patients in order to improve the aesthetics of anterior maxillary dentoalveolar cleft defects.

If mild relapse is predicted, features may be built into the retainers to help provide **'active' retention**. For example, if maxillary arch expansion has been undertaken and the transverse buccal relationship is tenuous, with a risk of developing a posterior crossbite, a midline expansion jackscrew can be placed in the Hawley retainer, in case it is required to deal with post debond relapse in the retention period (Figure 12-67). In cases where Class III relapse of the incisor relationship is predicted, hooks may be placed on the Adams clasps for the maxillary molars in a Hawley retainer, and some form of hook either on a lower Hawley retainer in the canine regions or on a lower

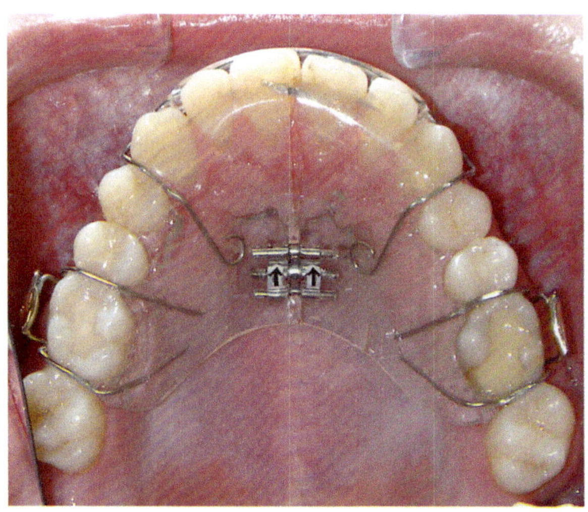

Fig. 12-67 'Active' retention – a midline Hyrax-type jackscrew has been placed in the Hawley retainer in case transverse expansion is required.

(a)

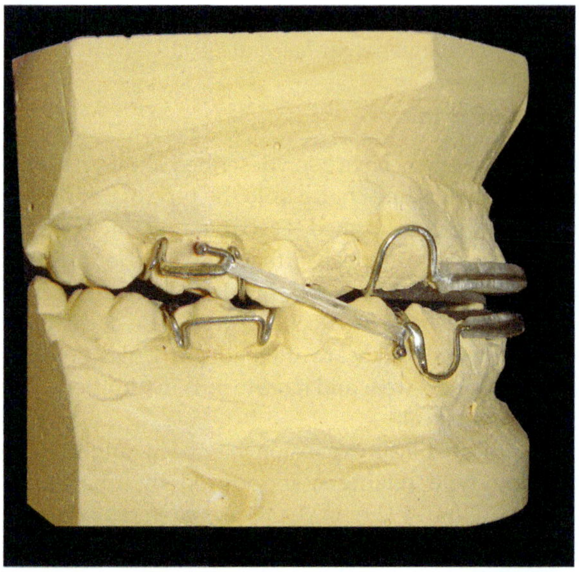

(b)

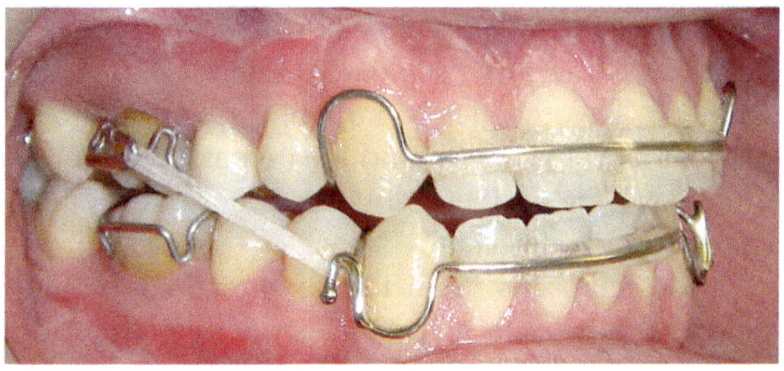

Fig. 12-68 'Active' retention – The Hawley retainers have been modified with hooks to allow placement of Class III elastic traction in this post-treatment patient in case of Class III relapse.

Essix retainer, for attachment of Class III elastics as required (Figure 12-68).

Natural vertical settling continues when retainer wear is reduced to part time, particularly with retainers that do not employ occlusal coverage. This is why the dental occlusion sometimes looks even better at the 1-year review appointment than at appliance removal.

Concluding remarks

> '... mechanics will be the science of motions resulting from any forces whatsoever, and of the forces required to produce any motions, accurately proposed and demonstrated.'
>
> Sir Isaac Newton (1642–1727)[21]
>
> English mathematician and physicist

The principles of orthodontic mechanics must be well-understood to permit accurate and timely positioning of the teeth in relation to their respective skeletal basal bone prior to orthognathic surgery. The type of tooth movement and mechanics required for orthognathic surgery is oftentimes different to standard orthodontics. It is imperative that the treating orthodontist is conversant with the principles and technical mechanical requirements in the management of the orthognathic patient. Surgeons should also have a working knowledge of modern orthodontics and what is realistically achievable.

References

1 Xenophon. Cyropaedia: Books 1–4 (Loeb Classical Library). London: William Heinemann Ltd., 1914.
2 Confucius. The Analects or The Conversations of Confucius With His Disciples and Certain Others. Trans. Soothill WE. Oxford: Oxford University Press, 1945.
3 Andrews LF. The straight-wire appliance, origin, controversy, commentary. J Clin Orthod. 1976;10:99–114.
4 Andrews LF. The straight-wire appliance. Explained and compared. J Clin Orthod. 1976;10:174–95.
5 Saint-Exupéry A. Flight to Arras (Pilote de Guerre). New York: Harcourt Publishing Co., 1942.
6 Lee R, Kirschen R. Space planning for the dentition (Space analysis). In: Gill DS, Naini FB (Eds).Orthodontics: Principles and Practice. Oxford: Wiley-Blackwell, 2011.
7 Naini FB. Dental-Occlusal Relationships: Terminology, Description and Classification. In: Naini FB. Facial Aesthetics: Concepts and Clinical Diagnosis. Oxford: Wiley-Blackwell, 2011.
8 Collins P. (Ed.). Dickens: Interviews and Recollections. Volume 2. New York: Barnes and Noble Books, 1981.
9 Naini FB, Hunt NP, Moles DR. The relationship between maxillary length, differential maxillary impaction, and the change in maxillary incisor inclination. Am J Orthod Dentofacial Orthop. 2003;124:526–9.
10 Obwegeser HL. Mandibular Growth Anomalies. Berlin Heidelberg: Springer, 2001.
11 Angell EC. Treatment of irregularity of the permanent or adult teeth. Dent Cosmos 1860;1:540–4, 599–600.
12 Timms DJ. The sawn of rapid maxillary expansion. Angle Orthodont. 1999;69:247–50.
13 Melsen B. Palatal growth studied on human autopsy material. A histologic microradiographic study. Am J Orthod. 1975;68:42–54.
14 Gill D, Naini F, McNally M, Jones A. The management of transverse maxillary deficiency. Dent Update. 2004;31:516–23.
15 Wertz RA. Skeletal and dental changes accompanying rapid midpalatal suture opening. Am J Orthod. 1970;58:41–66.
16 Naini FB. The 'acrylic technique' to check arch coordination in orthognathic surgery patients. Br J Oral Maxillofac Surg. 2013;51(1):e9–10.
17 Naini FB. Clinical Diagnostic Records, Natural Head Position and Craniofacial Anthropometry. In: Naini FB. Facial Aesthetics: Concepts and Clinical Diagnosis. Oxford: Wiley-Blackwell, 2011.
18 Reitan K. Tissue rearrangement during retention of orthodontically rotated teeth. Angle Orthod. 1959;29:105–13.
19 Reitan K. Principles of retention and avoidance of post-treatment relapse. Am J Orthod. 1969;55:776–90.
20 Collins JM, Witcher TP, Jones VS, Noar JH, Naini FB. An alternative retainer design for cleft patients: the 'aesthetic' retainer. Cleft Palate Craniofac J. 2010;47(6):597–9.
21 Newton I. Philosophiae Naturalis Principia Mathematica (1686). The Third Edition (1726) with Variant Readings. Cambridge: Cambridge University Press, 1972.

Chapter 13

Model Surgery

Farhad B. Naini, James McInnes, Daljit S. Gill and Andrew Stewart

'To measure is to know.'
Ernst Werner von Siemens (1816–92) (attributed)
German inventor

Introduction

The treating surgeon and orthodontist should have a thorough understanding of the principles of orthognathic model surgery. The technical aspects will vary depending on the background and training of the maxillofacial technologist and each maxillofacial technologist will eventually find their own preferred articulator/facebow system and method of undertaking model surgery. The method employed may vary quite considerably between technologists, even when using the same or similar instruments.[1–4] Therefore, the purpose of this chapter is to describe the principles and limitations of model surgery, which tend to be universal, and with which clinicians should be conversant. The technical aspects will also be described, but these are using one particular articulator system. Clinicians should aim to understand the principles and limitations, and it is useful for all senior trainees to help with and/or undertake model surgery under the supervision of an experienced maxillofacial technologist for a number of patients during their higher training.

Definitions

Facebow: The facebow (also 'face-bow' or 'face bow') is a device used to record the relationship of the maxillary dental arch to the transverse horizontal condylar hinge axis of the temporomandibular joints, used for orthognathic patients requiring *maxillary* surgery. The facebow allows the maxillary dental model to be placed in an equivalent relationship on an articulator.

Articulator: A mechanical device that represents the temporomandibular joints, to which the maxillary and mandibular dental models may be attached, with the intention of simulating some or all mandibular movements. The information is transferred from the patient to the articulator using a **facebow transfer**.

There are different types of articulator:

- **Simple hinge (plane line) articulator** – an articulator with a simple hinge joint preventing any lateral or sliding movements.
- **Anatomical articulator** – attempts to reproduce the various movements of the mandible during mastication.
- **Adjustable articulator** – an articulator which may be adjusted to accommodate the various positions and movements of the mandible relative to the maxilla.

Orthognathic Surgery: Principles, Planning and Practice. Edited by Farhad B. Naini and Daljit S. Gill.

- **Semi-adjustable articulator** – an articulator that allows adjustments that reproduce mandibular movements in the sagittal plane only.
- **Fully adjustable articulator** – allows replication of three-dimensional movement of recorded mandibular motion.
- **Arcon articulator** – (a contraction of the words 'articulator' and 'condyle') an articulator that differs from the usual anatomical articulator in that the condylar analogue is in the mandibular portion of the articulator and the glenoid fossa equivalent in the upper component.

Surgical wafer splint: Rigid interocclusal custom-made splints used in orthognathic surgery to guide intraoperative repositioning of the jaws, consisting of an acrylic resin prosthesis wired to the fixed orthodontic appliance/teeth in the maxilla (or mandible) and joined intraoperatively with stainless steel ligatures or elastics to keep the segments immovable while repositioning the jaws.

Model surgery – principles

Model surgery is an extremely important and intricate process, which permits the preoperative preparatory orthognathic surgical 'work up' to be undertaken by the maxillofacial technologist using models of the patient's dental occlusion.

The model surgery can be categorised by its complexity, which is directly related to the complexity of the planned surgical procedure. The simplest type of model surgery is for a planned bilateral sagittal split osteotomy (BSSO) of the mandible. The degree of difficulty increases for a bimaxillary Le Fort I osteotomy and BSSO, and the highest degree of complexity is for a multi-segment maxillary osteotomy with differential movement of the segments combined with a mandibular symphyseal osteotomy and BSSO.

Stages of model surgery

There are essentially four sequential stages in model surgery:

1. Dental impressions, facebow record (if required) and occlusal registration.
2. Articulation – transfer of the dental models and registration information to the articulator.
3. Model surgery – to evaluate and verify the feasibility of the planned surgery and to fabricate the wafer splints.
4. Wafer splint construction.

Each stage will vary somewhat depending on the type and complexity of the proposed surgical procedure.

Isolated mandibular surgery

If isolated mandibular surgery is being performed, it is usually possible to hand articulate the dental models into the desired occlusion. A simple hinge articulator will suffice for articulator mounting, and the wafer splints may then be made from the articulator. If there is an obvious and well-interdigitating proposed postoperative dental occlusion, a wafer splint is not absolutely essential. The osteotomized mandible may be secured intraoperatively into the postoperative position using the dental occlusion as the guide to the new position. However, most surgeons still prefer a final splint to be prepared for surgery.

Isolated maxillary or bimaxillary surgery

The principal role of model surgery in preparation for isolated maxillary surgery or bimaxillary surgery is to reproduce the correct maxillary repositioning determined at the preoperative clinical and cephalometric planning stages. Ultimately, it is the accurate repositioning of the maxilla that will dictate the subsequent mandibular repositioning. If a maxillary osteotomy is being performed, the dental models should be mounted on a semi-adjustable articulator using a facebow transfer and accurate registration of the patient's occlusion. Minimizing errors at all of these stages is important as inaccuracies will be transmitted to the interocclusal surgical splints and subsequently affect the accuracy of the final surgical outcome.[5,6]

In order to measure the proposed surgical moves on the models, some form of measuring instrument is required. Either a **model repositioning instrument** may be used (see below) or a model measuring block, such as the **Erickson Model Platform and Block** (Great lakes Orthodontics, Tonawanda, New York), may be used to measure the current position of the maxillary central incisor edges, canine cusp tips, and the mesiobuccal cusp tips of the maxillary first molars.[7] These three-dimensional measurements may be used to reproduce the maxillary model's exact location and to determine the proposed new position. The distances the maxilla will move in the three planes of space and in relation to the three axes of rotation will have been determined at the clinical and cephalometric planning stages.

The occlusal portion of the maxillary cast is separated from its base using a saw. As much plaster is removed from the cast as is required to accommodate the new position of the maxilla. Soft wax is inserted in the gap between the base of the cast and the occlusal portion. The wax will permit slight adjustments of the occlusal portion of the model. The tooth cusps are measured in three dimensions until they match the planned postoperative position of the maxilla. Once the measuring device verifies the maxilla to be in the new position, the model is secured with sticky wax or plaster to the mounting ring and placed on the articulator. At this stage, the maxillofacial technologist will have a mounting of the postoperative maxilla related to the preoperative position of the mandible. An acrylic splint is fabricated at this point – the **intermediate splint** – and is used intraoperatively to determine the new sagittal and transverse position of the maxilla to the preoperative position of the mandible. A second mounting with the dental models in the desired postoperative occlusion is used to fabricate the **final splint** that represents the new position of the mandible to the repositioned maxilla.

Model surgery – technique

Dental impressions, facebow record and occlusal registration

Ideally the final preoperative orthodontic archwire should be ligated with stainless steel ligatures several weeks prior to taking the dental impressions, and the impressions should not be taken any more than a month prior to surgery. This is to minimize the possibility of residual tooth movement, which may result in ill-fitting splints at the time of surgery and potentially compromise the postoperative position of the dental occlusion.

It is advisable to maintain the archwires in situ when taking the impressions in order to prevent the possibility of minor unwanted tooth movements during the taking of the impressions and during the replacement of the archwires.

A wax strip is flattened between the fingers and slid underneath the archwire and brackets, and moulded in position in order to prevent the impression material flowing underneath the archwire. However, with the wax in place, the occlusal aspect of the brackets should be visible, and not covered by the wax (Figure 13-1).

When choosing the size of the impression tray it is essential that all the teeth within the respective dental arch fit inside the boundary of the tray. It is easy to take the impression such that the second and third molars remain inadvertently outside the posterior part of the impression tray, which means that when the impression is cast, the alginate impression material will deform in that region and potentially result in an incorrect dental occlusion and an ill-fitting splint. It is also important that the alginate material does not lift out of the impression tray. If there are deep fissures in the occlusal surfaces of the posterior dentition, it is advisable to smear some alginate along these surfaces with a finger just prior to taking the impression. This will reduce the chance of air blows in the alginate, which would otherwise compromise the postoperative position.

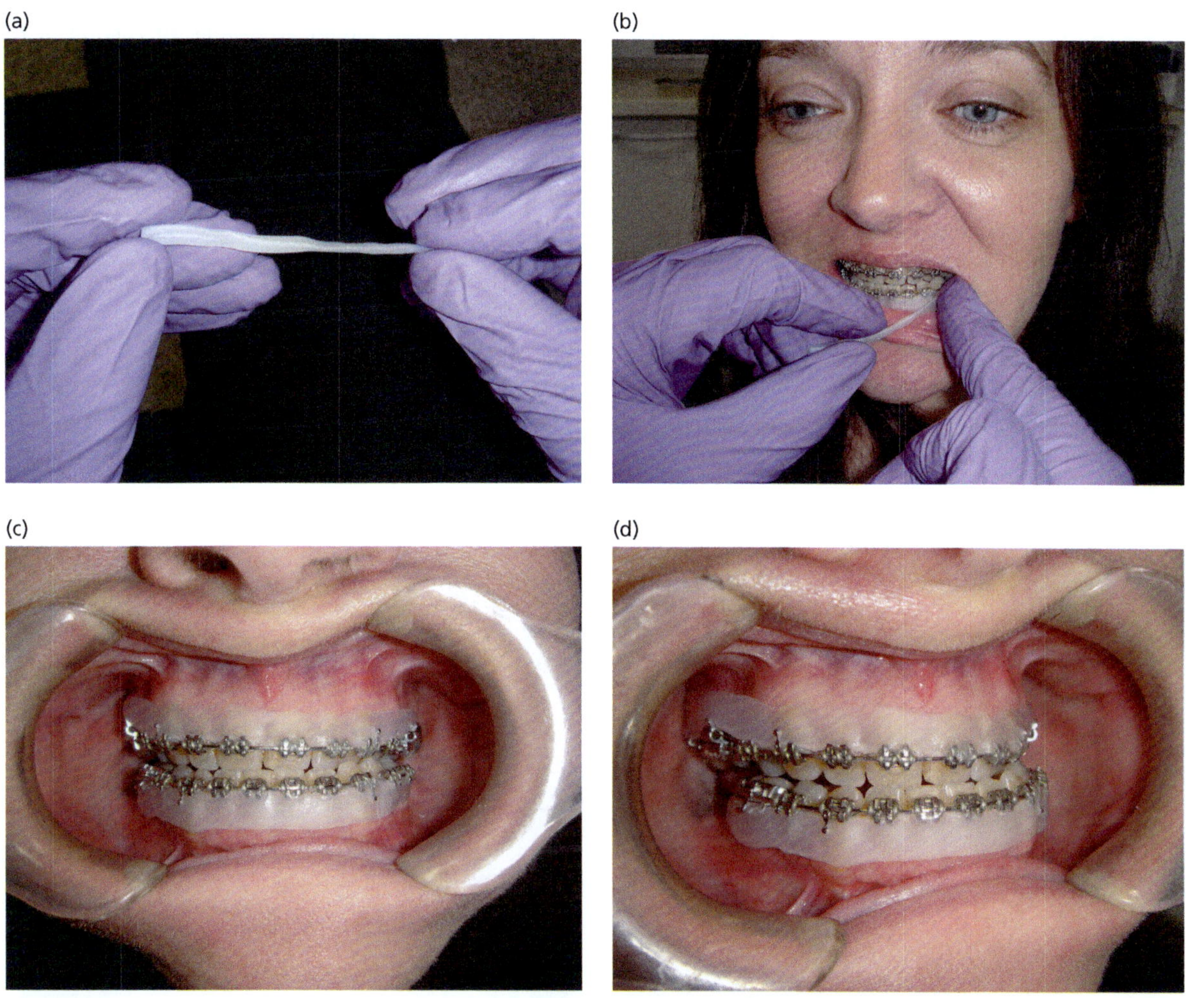

Fig. 13-1 A wax strip is flattened between the fingers and slid underneath the archwire and brackets, and moulded in position in order to prevent the impression material flowing underneath the archwire.

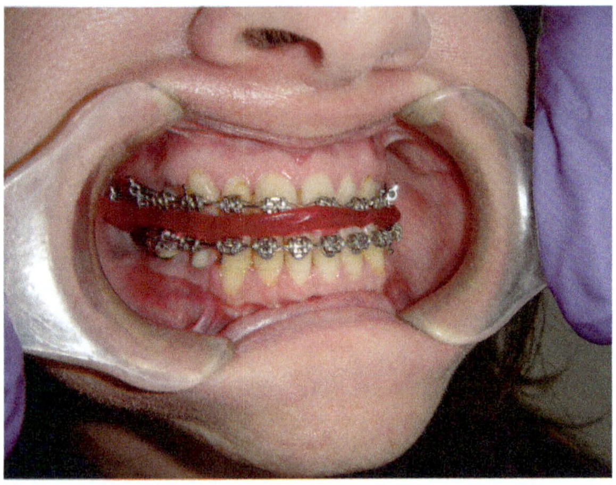

Fig. 13-2 Occlusal registration using interocclusal wax.

It is easy to underestimate the importance of the **occlusal registration**, which is a registration of the patient's dental occlusion. Occlusal registration is sometimes referred to as 'jaw registration', 'bite registration' or 'bite record' (Figure 13-2). In the laboratory the maxillofacial technologist is working to a tolerance of 0.3 mm. If the jaw relationship is incorrect, it will create imprecision in the maxillary movement. For example, if the patient has an anterior open bite, with perhaps tooth contact only on the second molars, it is easy for the mandible to slide laterally to the left or right. Patients with a significant incisor overjet sometimes posture their mandible anteriorly when taking the bite registration; the patient will feel the resistance in the wax as they bite together, and subsequently posture their mandible forward. If is easy for the clinician or maxillofacial technologist not to detect such movements. For example, a patient with an 8 mm incisor overjet may posture their mandible 2 mm anteriorly when the jaw relationship is being recorded, thereby reducing the overjet to perhaps only 6 mm. If this is not detected either in the laboratory or subsequent clinical stages, it will result in a discrepancy of 2 mm in the jaw movements. It is therefore vital for the clinician to actively look for anterior or lateral mandibular displacements or habitual posturing of the mandible (e.g. 'Sunday' bites), and for this information to be relayed to the maxillofacial technologist.

The following description is for the technical use of the SAM 3 articulator system (SAM Prazisionteck-nik GmbH, Germany). Other articulator systems (e.g. Denar, Dentatus, Hanau, KaVo) will vary to some extent from this account. The various component parts of the system are required to successfully undertake orthognathic model surgery. The following equipment descriptions will include the product codes for each item.

Ideally, each articulator system has its own **facebow** and **bite fork** assembly and these should not be interchanged between systems. The Axioquick transfer bow (ATB 303) and the Axiomatic transfer fork assembly (ATB 395) with a universal clamping mechanism and removable transfer fork are used to take the facebow recording and transfer the data to the SAM articulator (Figure 13-3). A facebow record is usually not required for isolated mandibular surgery, but will be required for isolated maxillary or bimaxillary surgery.

Casting the dental impressions

Due to the possibility of damage to the models, plaster of Paris is no longer advisable for casting of the impressions. A polyurethane resin (Hit Model, Euro Resina, Italy) produces a scratch resistant model, and metal retention rings (Retention Washers, Skillbond Direct Ltd. UK) are placed in the resin as it sets to allow for the retention of the plaster (Figure 13-4).

Transferring the maxillary model to the articulator

The Axiomatic transfer fork assembly is attached to the articulator using the Transfer Stand AX (ATB 398). The telescopic transfer support (ATB 336) is used to support the fork assembly (Figure 13-5). The maxillary

(a)

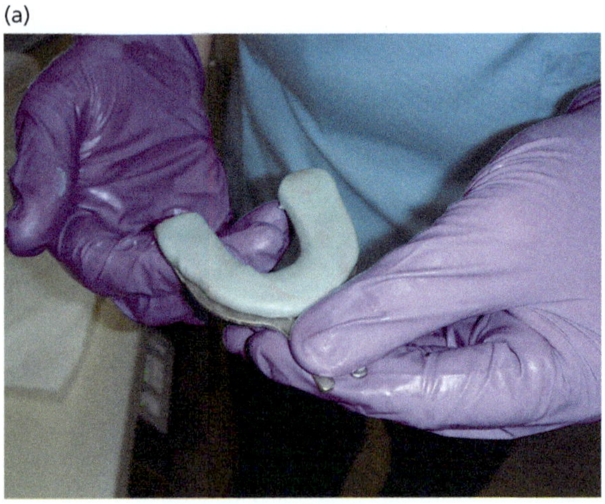

(b)

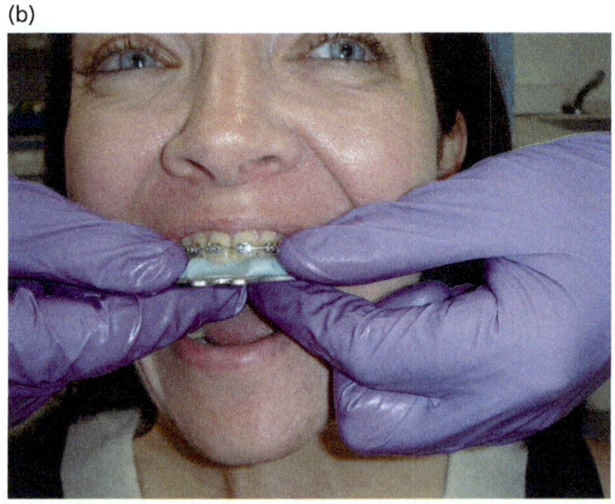

Fig. 13-3 (a) Bite fork with putty; (b) bite fork with putty on maxillary dental arch; (c, d, e) facebow registration; (f) facebow removed from patient and ready to be transferred to the articulator.

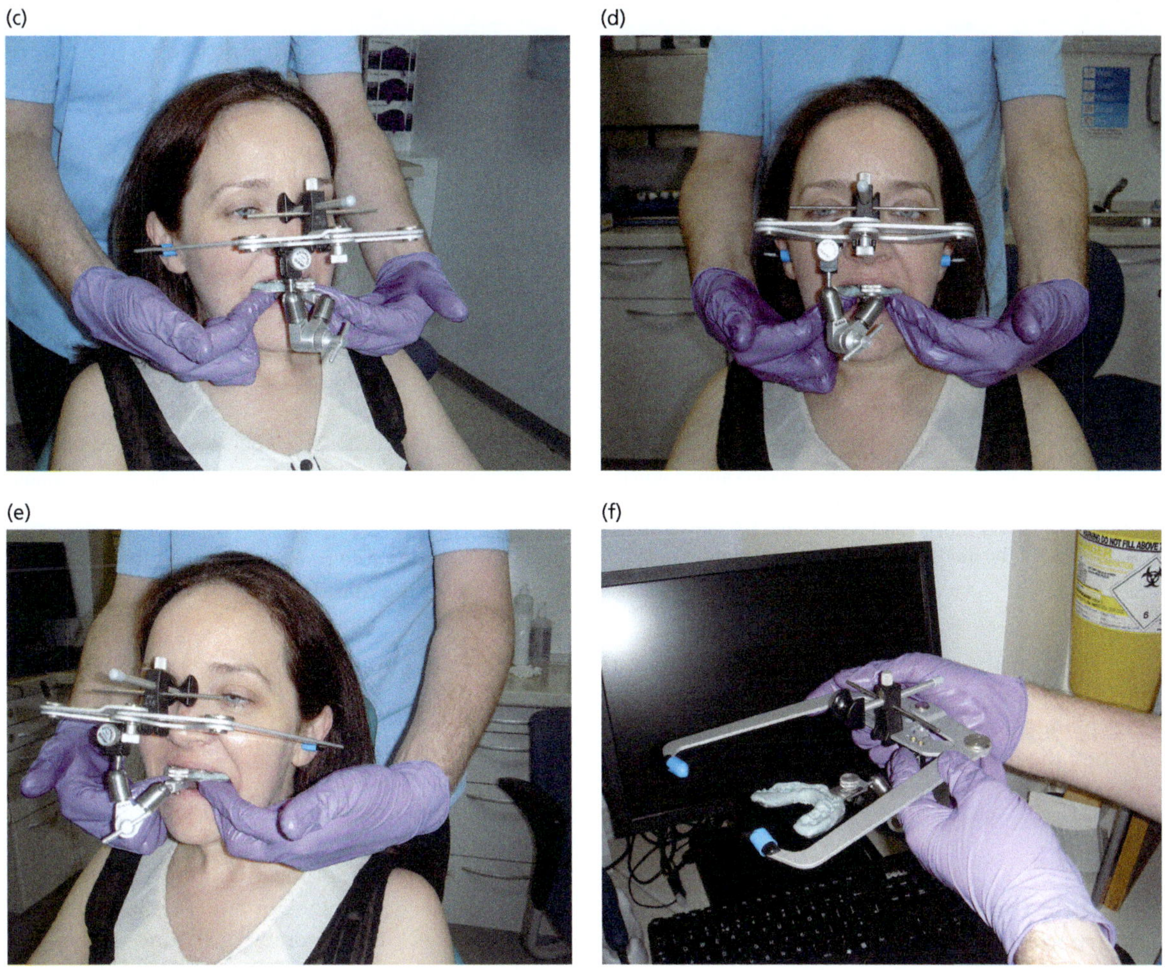

Fig. 13-3 (*Continued*).

model is placed onto the bite fork and secured in place using plaster.

Once the plaster has set, the base of the model is trimmed parallel to the true horizontal plane (the Frankfort plane if it is horizontal). Magnets are placed into the base of the model (Eclipse Magnets, UK), which allows the sections to be freely removed and repositioned (Figure 13-6), and grooves are cut into the base of the model to stop rotational movement. A plaster separator is used as an insulating material to prevent the plaster surfaces sticking together, (Ease Release 200, Bentley Advanced Materials, UK).

There has to be an easily recognizable colour difference between the preoperative and postoperative positions. For example, a peach colour may be used for the preoperative position and blue for the postoperative position. The peach plaster '**spacer**' is trimmed to a specific thickness, in this case 10 mm. The maxillary model and the plaster spacer are placed back onto the bite fork and articulated to the upper arm of the articulator using a zero expansion articulating

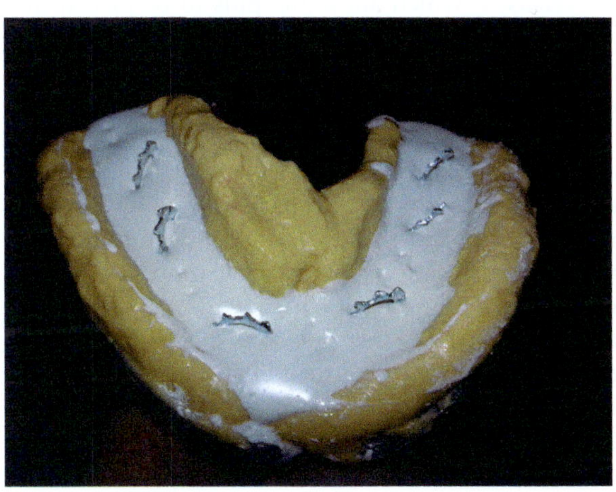

Fig. 13-4 Metal retention rings placed in the resin as it sets to allow for the retention of the plaster.

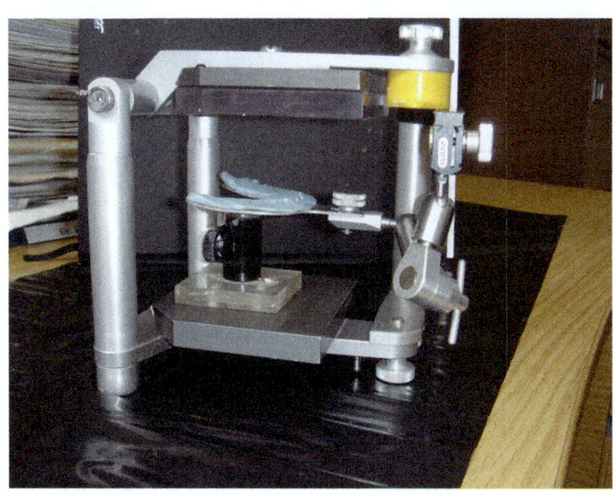

Fig. 13-5 The bite fork assembly placed onto the articulator.

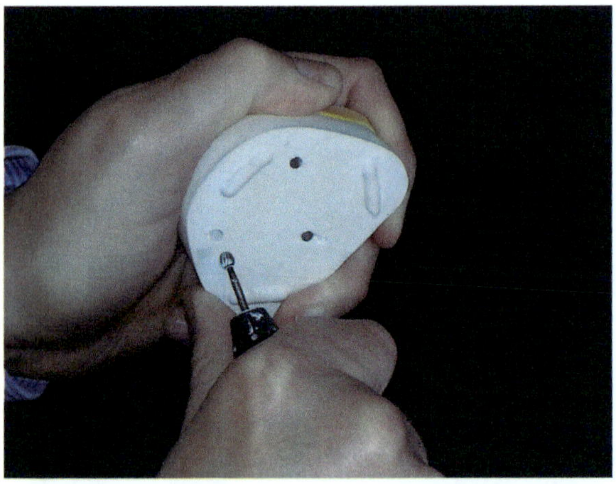

Fig. 13-6 Holes drilled into the base of the models and magnets secured in place using plaster, glue or a combination, allowing the sections to be freely moved and repositioned. Grooves are cut into the base of the model to prevent rotational movement of the segments.

plaster (Zero Arti Quick, Dentona AG, Germany) (Figure 13-7).

If the planned surgical procedure is a mandibular BSSO, then the maxillary model can be articulated to the upper arm of the articulator arbitrarily as no face-bow record is required.

Articulating the mandibular model to the maxillary model

Using the occlusal registration, the maxillary and mandibular models should be held together to check the relationship. Once satisfied that the position is correct and that there are no premature contacts, the mandibular model can be articulated to the maxillary model using the same process as previously described for articulating the maxillary model (Figure 13-8).

If the planned surgical procedure is an isolated maxillary Le Fort I osteotomy, then the mandibular model can be articulated to the maxillary model without the need for a removable plaster spacer as there will be no movement of the mandible.

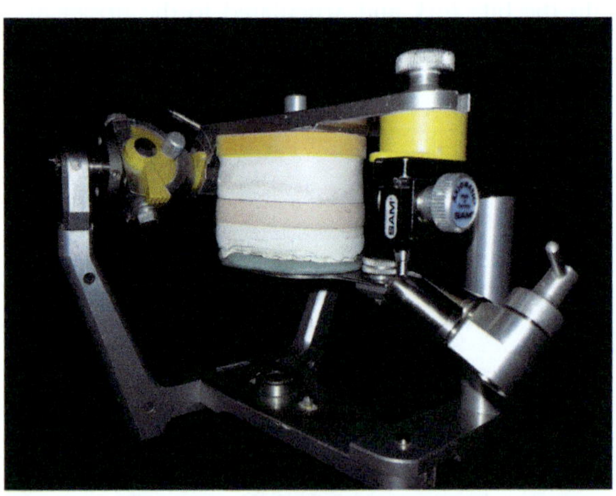

Fig. 13-7 A peach coloured plaster spacer is trimmed to a specific thickness, in this case 10 mm. The maxillary model and the plaster spacer are placed back onto the bite fork and articulated to the upper arm of the articulator using a zero expansion articulating plaster.

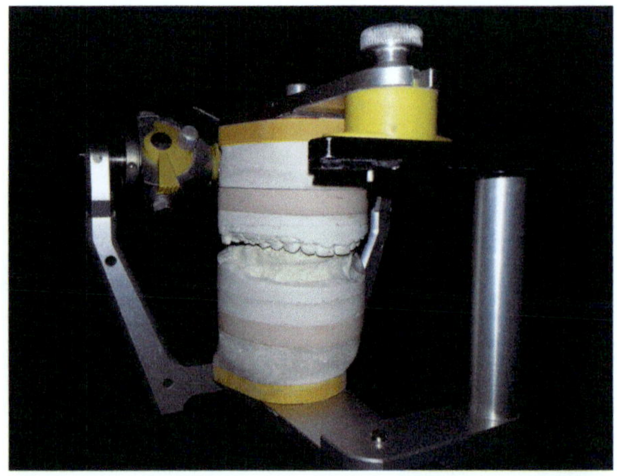

Fig. 13-8 Mandibular model articulated to the maxillary model.

Maxillary movement

The planned maxillary movement is carried out using the **model repositioning instrument** (MRI 300), which is specific to this articulator system. The alternative is to use the Erickson Model Platform and Block or similar alternative (see above). Additionally, even when using the model repositioning instrument, the Erickson measuring block or equivalent may be used to double check the accuracy of the movements (Figure 13-9). Holes are drilled into the maxillary model using the drill bit (MRI 311) in the area of the mesiobuccal cusp of the first molars bilaterally, with an additional hole drilled in the anterior region, in line with the midline of the maxillary central incisors. Plastic sleeve inserts (MRI 210) are placed into the holes using the insert tool (MRI 212).

The maxillary model is placed back onto the articulator ensuring that it is in the correct position in relation to the mandibular model. The mandibular model and articulating plate are then removed and the model repositioning instrument attached to the lower arm of the articulator. The repositioning unit has three pins, one right, one left and one central. The locking nuts are released, which allow the pins to be placed into the maxillary model. Once secure, the locking nuts are tightened and the plaster spacer between the model and articulating plate can be removed (Figure 13-10).

The arms on the model repositioning instrument are calibrated in millimetres; the reading for each arm should be noted prior to repositioning the maxillary model. The MRI will allow the full range of movement: superior repositioning (impaction), inferior repositioning (set-down), advancement, set-back, and rotation round the three axes of rotation, such as a differential impaction for the correction of a maxillary cant. The maxillary model may now be repositioned to the movement requested by the surgeon and orthodontist. When satisfied that the position is correct, plaster is used to secure the model in place, using magnets to retain the segments.

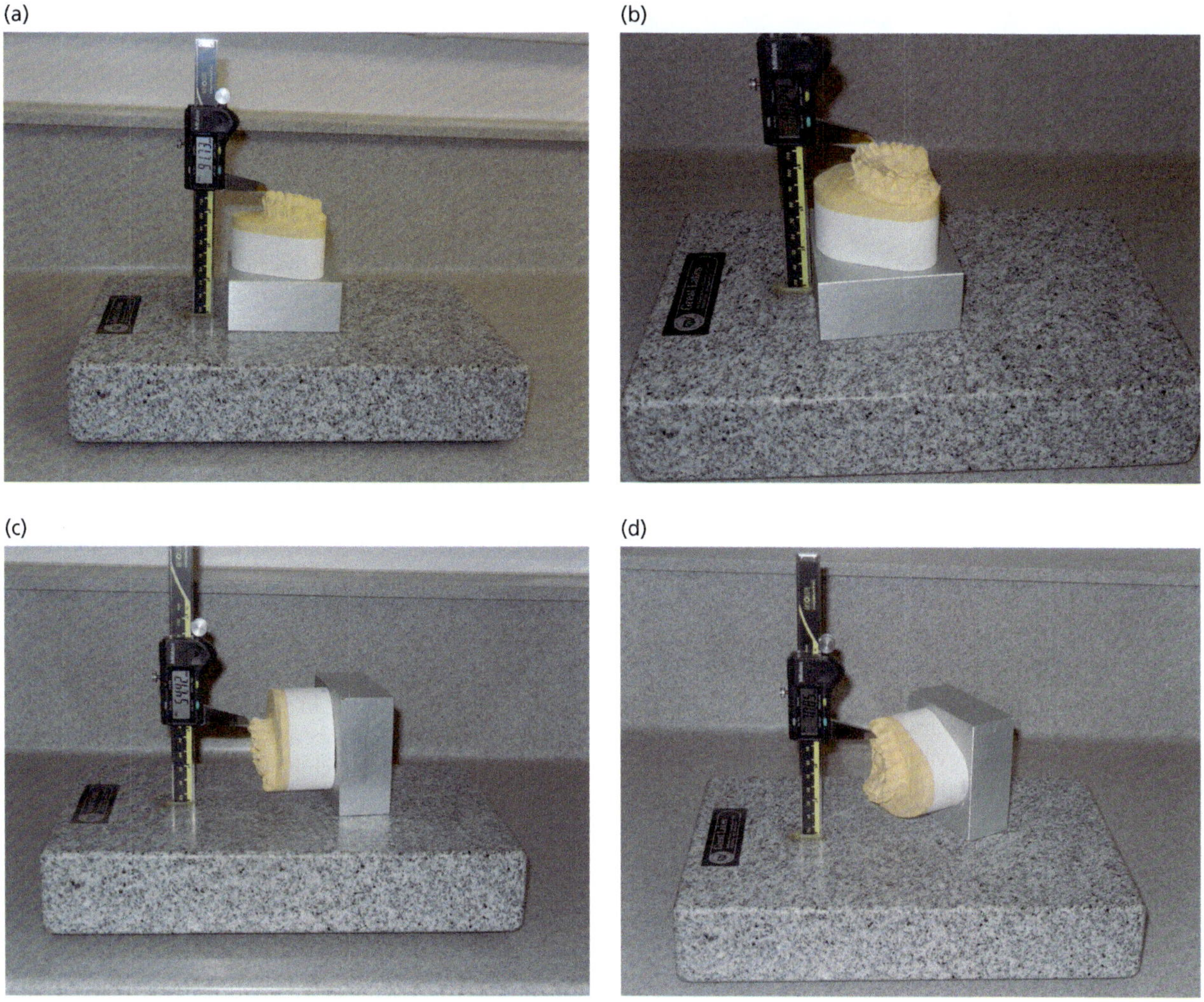

Fig. 13-9 The facebow-mounted maxillary model is placed on the Erickson Model Block and Platform which incorporates a vertically mounted digital Vernier calliper permitting precise measurement (to 0.01 mm) of the maxillary movement in the (a, b) vertical, (c) sagittal and (d) transverse planes.

Mandibular movement

The maxillary and mandibular models are secured together in the postoperative position using wax (Figure 13-11) and placed back onto the articulator. This postoperative position should be determined by

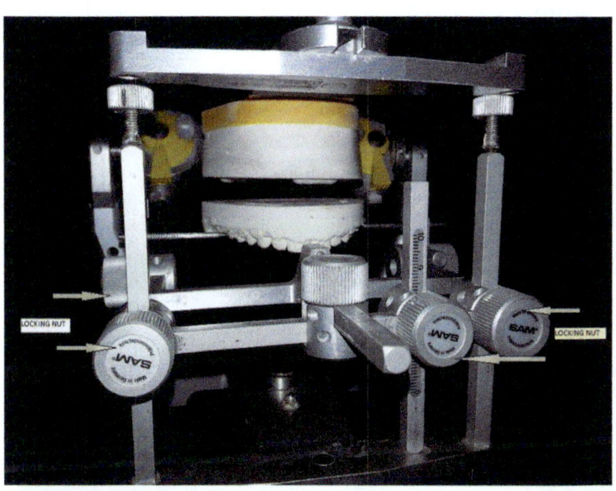

Fig. 13-10 Model repositioning instrument (MRI) in position attached to the lower arm of the articulator. The repositioning unit has three pins, one right, one left and one central. The locking nuts are released, which allow the pins to be placed into the maxillary model. Once secure, the locking nuts are tightened and the plaster spacer between the model and articulating plate is removed.

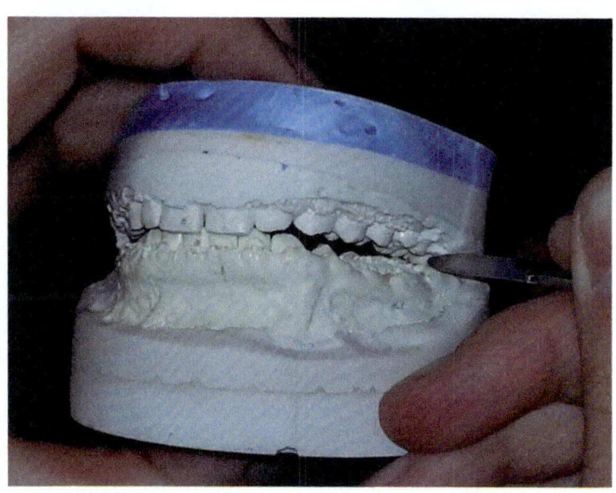

Fig. 13-11 The maxillary and mandibular models are secured together in the postoperative position using wax.

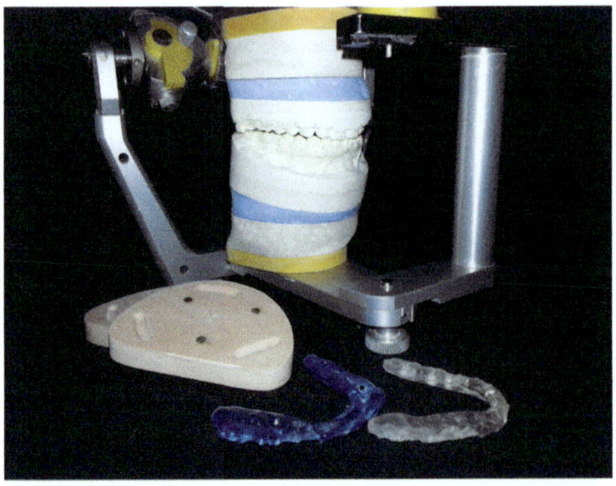

Fig. 13-12 Mandibular model secured in position using plaster.

the orthodontist and surgeon. The maxillofacial technologist subsequently secures the mandibular model in place using plaster (Figure 13-12).

Occasionally the surgeon may perform a mandibular symphyseal split in order to constrict the mandible and correct a crossbite. A maximum of 8 mm, i.e. 4 mm in each segment is achievable. Technically this is not a difficult procedure for the maxillofacial technologist, but the fulcrum point for the constriction should be between the mandibular central incisors as viewed from above, and it is important not to torque either of the segments as this will leave a triangular space between the central incisors (Figures 13-13).

Construction of the occlusal wafer splints

Once the model surgery has been completed, the occlusal splints may be fabricated. As described earlier, the facebow record and jaw registration are used to transfer the patient's preoperative position to the dental articulator. The constructed occlusal splints are then used to transfer the postoperative position to the patient at the time of surgery. With bimaxillary surgery there will be a requirement for two splints. An **intermediate splint** is used to reposition the maxilla relative to the unmoved mandible, and this splint forms the prescription for the repositioning of the mobilized maxilla to the unmoved mandible in the sagittal and transverse planes (the vertical position of the maxilla is decided using some form of skeletal reference guide intraoperatively). A **final splint** is used to reposition the mandible relative to the new maxillary position. *This technique allows one jaw at a time to act as the stable reference structure for the repositioning of the surgically mobilized opposing jaw.* The intermediate splint uses the initial, preoperative position of the mandible in relation to the maxilla to transfer the maxillary movement. This is why it is imperative that the preoperative position on the articulator is identical to the patient's preoperative position. Any discrepancy will result in the maxillary movements being incorrect. The intermediate and final splints may be colour coded to avoid intraoperative confusion.

The intermediate position is when the maxillary model is in the postoperative position and the mandibular model still in the preoperative position. Orthoresin (MP2, Orthocare, UK) may be used to construct the splints, which is an autopolymerizing acrylic that can produce the splints within an hour. It is important to block out the undercuts on both models using wax (Figure 13-14) in order to prevent the acrylic from locking into the undercuts, which will result in damage to the model when removing the splints. A separator is used to prevent the acrylic from sticking to the models (Ease Release 200, Bentley Advanced Materials, UK), which must be sprayed on both models to allow the acrylic to be freely removed from the models once cured. The acrylic is then placed on the dental occlusal surface of both the maxillary and mandibular models and the articulator arms closed together into the intermediate position. An elastic band is wrapped tightly round the articulator arms to stop any expansion of the acrylic during the setting process (Figure 13-15). The articulator is then placed into a

(a) (b)

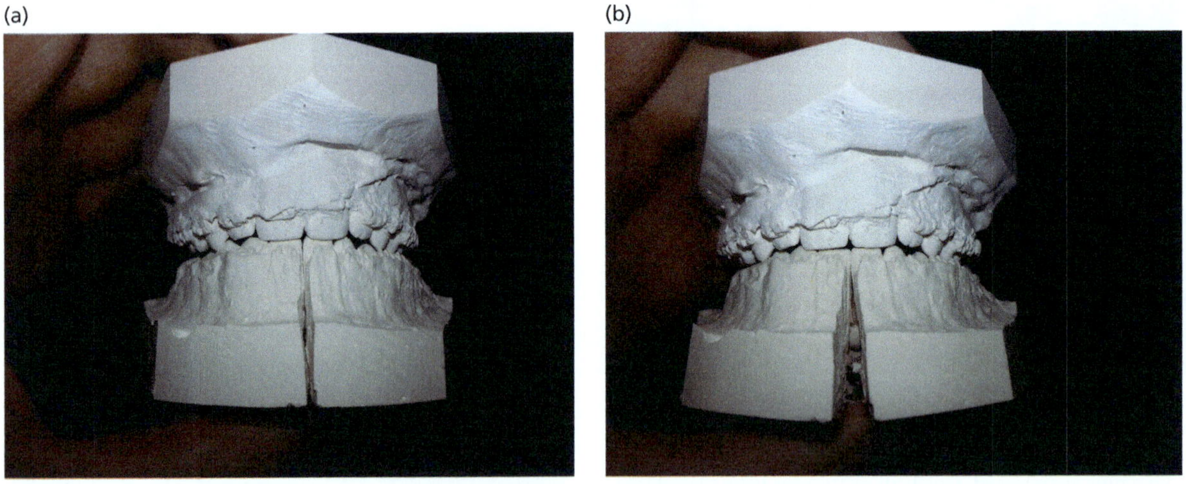

Fig. 13-13 (a) Correct preparation for a mandibular symphyseal split in order to constrict the mandible. (b) Incorrect technique, which will torque either of the segments and will leave a triangular space between the central incisors.

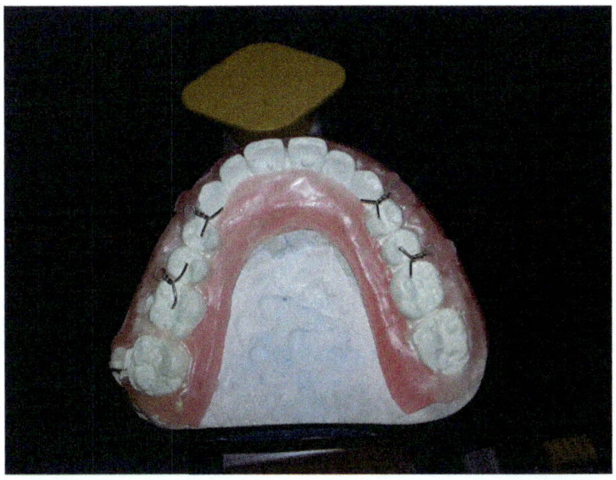

Fig. 13-14 Blocking out the undercuts on the dental models using wax in order to prevent the acrylic from locking into the undercuts, which will result in damage to the model when removing the splints. Wire loops in position, which may be used intraoperatively to ligate the splints to the orthodontic archwires.

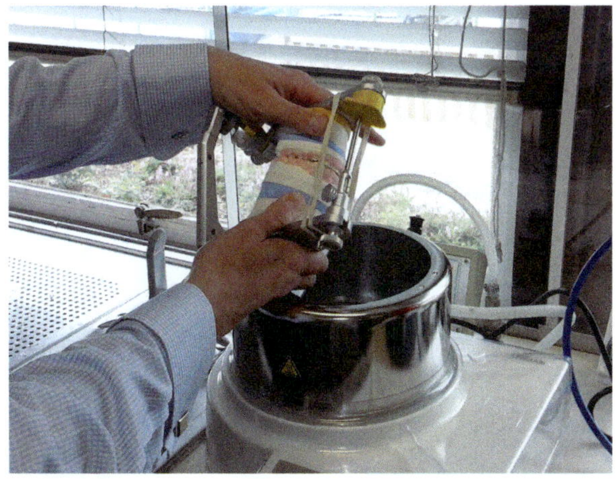

Fig. 13-15 An elastic band is wrapped tightly round the articulator arms to stop any expansion of the acrylic during the setting process.

pressure vessel for 30 minutes at 3 bars or 43.5 psi to cure the acrylic. The same procedure is carried out with the mandibular model in the postoperative position. Wire loops may be placed in the acrylic to allow the splint to be wired into place intraoperatively, though this is down to the personal preference of each individual surgeon. Once set, the acrylic splints are removed from the articulator and trimmed and polished.

The splints should be tried in on the patient to ensure accuracy and allow any minor adjustments to be undertaken prior to surgery. The splints should fit securely and passively on the patient's dental arches without rocking (Figure 13-16). However, in cases where there has been a mandibular constriction the splint cannot be tried on the mandible preoperatively.

The movements should be written clearly on the models, including the direction of the movement, and whether rotational movement or bodily movement has been undertaken. An example is provided in Figure 13-17.

Due to the instability of the acrylic at medium to high temperature it is not possible to sterilise the splints, though they can be disinfected.

Note:

Splint wafer modifications for partially dentate or edentulous patients.

In partially dentate patients missing their posterior dentition, or in the uncommon situation that an edentulous patient requires orthognathic surgery (e.g. for treatment of sleep apnoea), modifications to the surgical wafer splints are required. Use of a modified Gunning-type splint, originally described for use in maxillofacial trauma, is a potential possibility, in which case the occlusal-vertical dimension (OVD) must be determined (Figure 13-18). The Gunning splint is an eponym for a device fabricated from casts of edentulous maxillary and mandibular arches to aid in the reduction and fixation of a jaw fracture, named after the English-born American dentist Thomas Brian Gunning (1813–89).[8]

(a) (b)

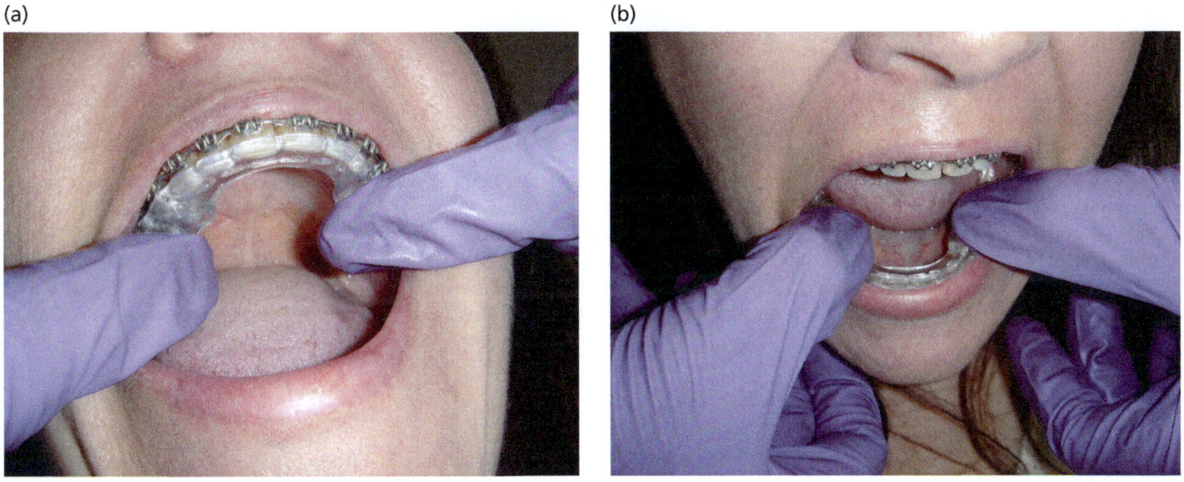

Fig. 13-16 (a, b) The splints being tried in to ensure a secure and passive fit on the patient's dental arches without rocking.

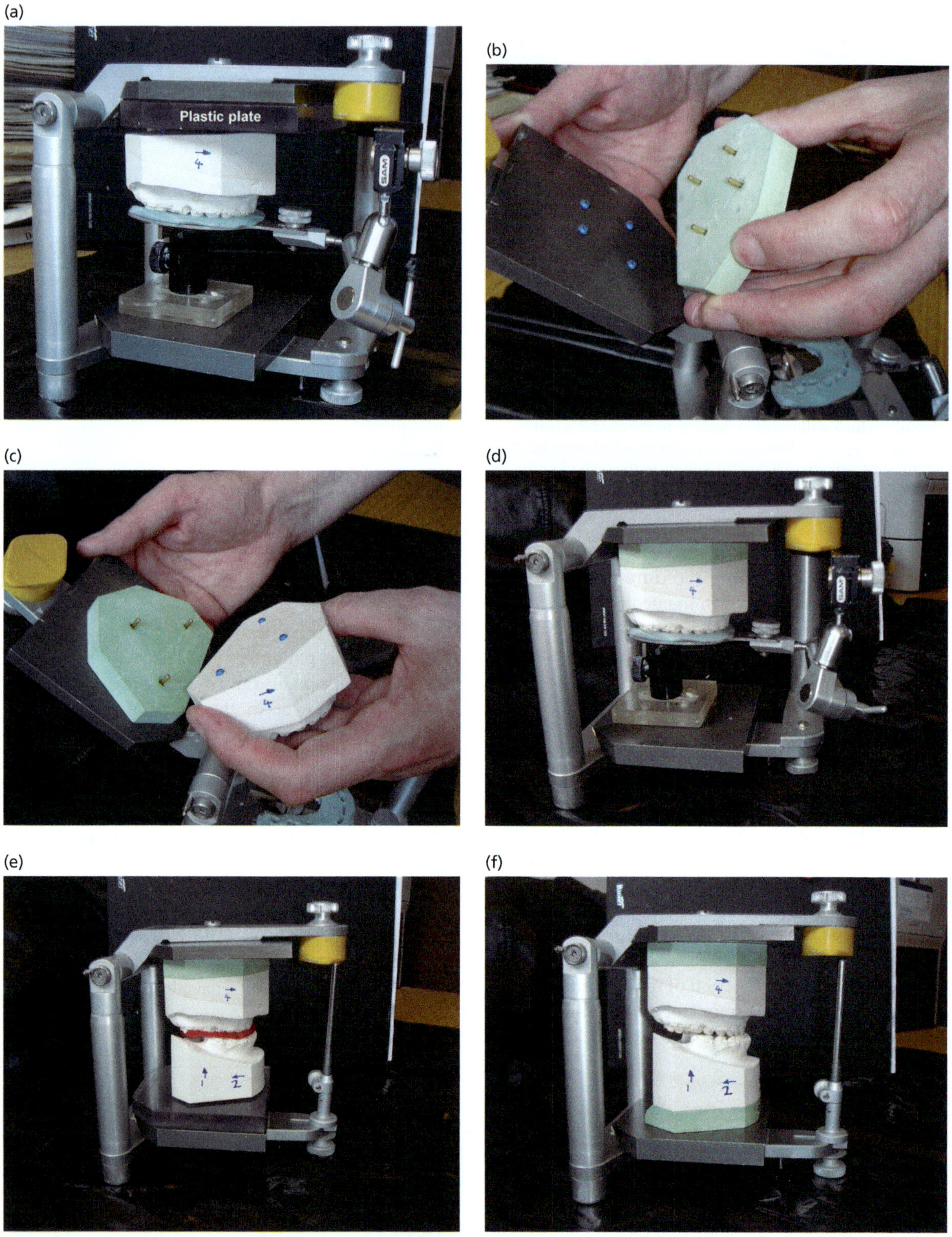

Fig. 13-17 (a) Maxillary model positioned on the bite fork on the articulator; 12 mm plastic plate in position, which will provide space for the preoperative plaster spacer; (b) a pin and sleeve system may be used to position the spacers to the articulator and (c) the models to the spacers; (d) plastic plate removed and preoperative plaster spacer in position (coloured green); (e) mandibular model articulated in preoperative position using the wax occlusal registration; (f) preoperative position with preoperative spacers (coloured green); (g) postoperative position of the maxilla with postoperative maxillary spacer (coloured peach); (h) postoperative position of mandible and maxilla with postoperative spacers (coloured peach); (i) interocclusal putty used to create the intermediate and final acrylic wafer splints.

(g)

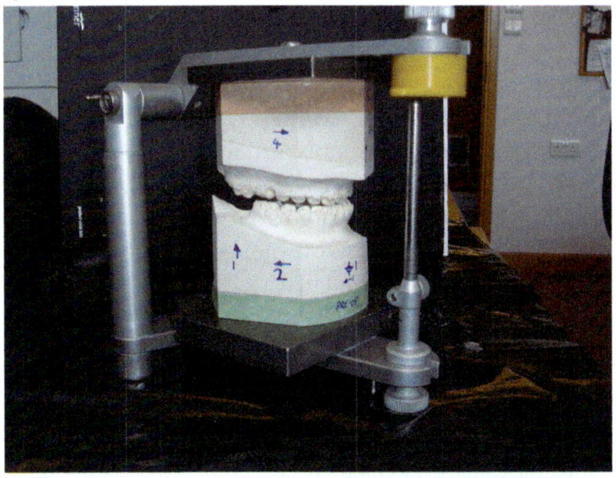

(h)

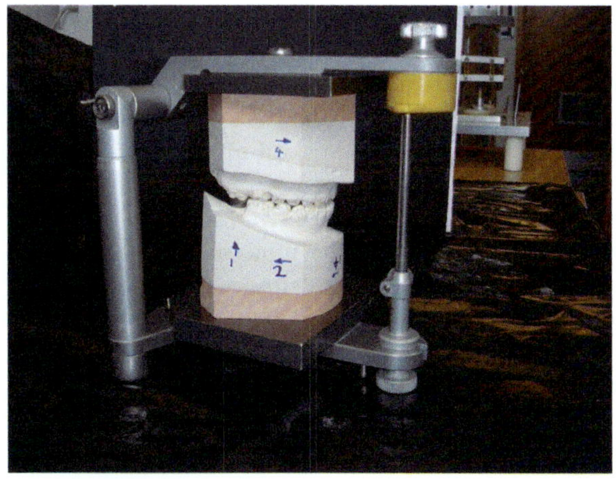

(i)

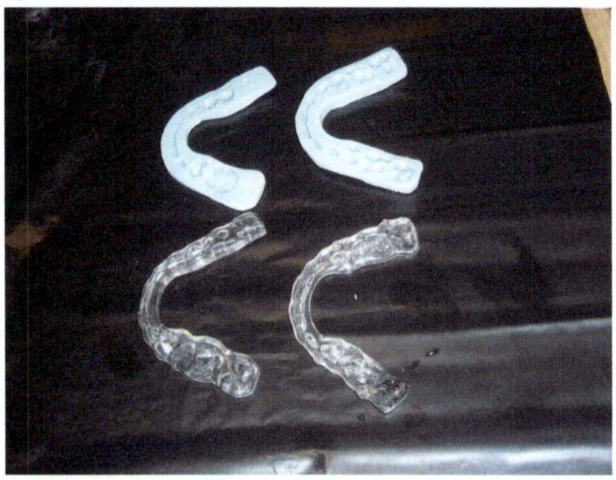

Fig. 13-17 (*Continued*)

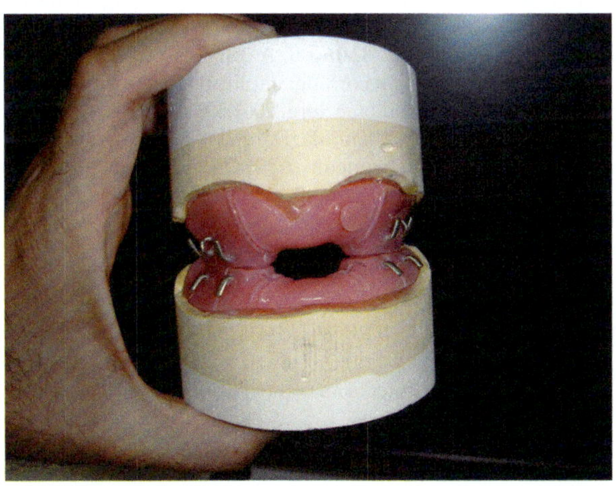

Fig. 13-18 Gunning-type splint.

Virtual model surgery

Traditional model surgery techniques have obvious drawbacks. First, dental models mounted on an articulator do not depict the body of the jaws; therefore, the clinician has to visualize the potential skeletal changes in relation to the movement of the dental models. The second issue is inaccuracy in facebow transfer. The dental models should be mounted on the articulator such that they replicate the position of the patient's dentition. However, significant differences have been found between the inclinations of the occlusal plane on mounted models compared with the occlusal plane on the lateral cephalometric radiographs of patients.[9,10] Third, there is the accuracy of mandibular autorotation simulation. There is evidence that even the initial rotational movement of the condyles in mouth opening involves a small element of condylar translation as well. That is, the movement is not a simple rotation around the condylar hinge axis.[11] Although this is likely to be a minor issue in orthognathic surgical planning, nevertheless, it does add an element of inaccuracy in model surgery on a semi-adjustable articulator.

Modern computer-aided surgical simulation may help to overcome some of these issues, though clinicians should always heed Albert Einstein's warning of technology creating 'a generation of idiots'. Computers are only as useful as the information they receive combined with the clinician's understanding of the information they provide, including potential drawbacks.

Computer-aided surgical simulation techniques have been described using a CT model of the skull incorporating a preformed bite-jig on which the patient is biting.[12,13] A separate accurate scan of the patient's dental models creates a digital model of the patient's dentition and occlusion, which is transferred and registered onto the CT skull. This creates a computerized composite model of the dentoskeletal structures. This composite skull model may be used to simulate the planned surgery, or to compare different procedures. The computerized skull may be sectioned and moved as many times as required, simulating a number of different surgical procedures. The computerized surgical plan may then be transferred to the patient via computer-aided design and manufacture of the surgical splints. Digital splints may be sent to a rapid prototyping machine to generate the physical splints, which may be sterilized and used intraoperatively (see Chapter 42).

Rapid technological advances are part of modern life. As computerized techniques evolve, improve and get to be more user-friendly, they are likely to become better accepted and eventually form the mainstay of model surgery.

Conclusions

Model surgery is an important step in the orthognathic surgical pathway. The predictability of orthognathic surgery is partly related to the accuracy of the technique of preoperative model surgery. However, the number of stages involved and the intricacy of the segmentation and repositioning required inevitably leads to potential sources of error. These are usually minor and the checking procedures undertaken clinically and cephalometrically in the preoperative planning stages, together with intraoperative checks by the surgeon, mean that the intraoperative surgical process is usually relatively seamless. However, from time to time it becomes evident *intraoperatively* that some error has arisen in the model surgery or the fabrication of the splints. This is an unfortunate and irritating eventuality that nevertheless sometimes arises. In such situations the surgeon will need to use all their critical faculties and surgical finesse to hand position the jaws.

Acknowledgements

We extend our gratitude to the maxillofacial technologists in the Maxillofacial Unit at St George's Hospital and Medical School, London, UK: Ian Muir-Nelson, Natalie Short and Pam Sandhu. Thanks to Ed Payne, Chief Orthodontic and Orthognathic technologist at the Eastman Dental Hospital, London, UK. To the memory of Brian Conroy, Head of Maxillofacial Technology at the former Norman Rowe Maxillofacial Unit, Queen Mary's University Hospital, Roehampton, UK (now at St George's Hospital), and the late Professor Norman Rowe, a pioneer of Oral and Maxillofacial Surgery in the UK.

References

1 O'Malley AM, Milosevic A. Comparison of three facebow/semi-adjustable articulator systems for planning orthognathic surgery. Br J Oral Maxillofac Surg. 2000;38:185–90.
2 Bamber MA, Harris M, Nacher C. A validation of two orthognathic model surgery techniques. J Orthod. 2001;28:135–42.
3 Walker F, Ayoub AF, Moos KF, Barbenel J. Face bow and articulator for planning orthognathic surgery: 1 face bow. Br J Oral Maxillofac Surg. 2008;46:567–72.
4 Walker F, Ayoub AF, Moos KF, Barbenel J. Face bow and articulator for planning orthognathic surgery: 2 articulator. Br J Oral Maxillofac Surg. 2008;46:573–8.
5 Ellis E 3rd. Accuracy of model surgery: evaluation of an old technique and introduction of a new one. J Oral Maxillofac Surg. 1990;48:1161–7.
6 Nattestad A, Vedtofte P. Pitfalls in orthognathic model surgery. The significance of using different reference lines and points during model surgery and operation. Int J Oral Maxillofac Surg. 1994;23:11–5.
7 Erickson K. An Instructional Manual for the Model Platform and Model Block. Great Lakes Tonawanda, NY: Orthodontics Ltd, 1990.
8 Gunning TB. The Treatment of Fractures of the Lower Jaw by Interdental Splints. New York Med. J. 1866;3:433.
9 Ellis E 3rd, Tharanon W, Gambrell K. Accuracy of face-bow transfer: effect on surgical prediction and postsurgical result. J Oral Maxillofac Surg. 1992;50:562–7.
10 Gateno J, Forrest KK, Camp B. A comparison of 3 methods of face-bow transfer recording: implications for orthognathic surgery. J Oral Maxillofac Surg. 2001;59:635–40.
11 McMillan AS, McMillan DR, Darvell BW. Centers of rotation during jaw movements. Acta Odontol Scand. 1989;47:323–8.
12 Xia J, Ip HH, Samman N, Wang D, Kot CS, Yeung RW, Tideman H. Computer-assisted three-dimensional surgical planning and simulation: 3D virtual osteotomy. Int J Oral Maxillofac Surg. 2000;29:11–7.
13 Hsu SS, Gateno J, Bell RB, Hirsch DL, Markiewicz MR, Teichgraeber JF, Zhou X, Xia JJ. Accuracy of a computer-aided surgical simulation protocol for orthognathic surgery: a prospective multicenter study. J Oral Maxillofac Surg. 2013;71:128–42.

Chapter 14

Perioperative Considerations and Anaesthesia for Orthognathic Surgery

Anne S. Blyth and Jelena Devic

Introduction

Orthognathic surgery aims to enhance the facial proportions and to improve the functional symptoms that arise from severe jaw discrepancies. As the indications for surgery vary from cosmetic to functional (although in many patients there is an element of both) it is important to consider the anaesthetic implications for this group of patients.

In general, the patients are young and healthy (ASA 1 physical status), thus it is imperative that anaesthesia should be safe and not cause any long-term complications.[1]

Anaesthesia, though carrying a risk of mortality and morbidity, is extremely safe.[2,3] Catastrophic complications are rare but potentially devastating. Complications tend to arise from intraoperative events such as hypoxia, anaphylaxis, hypotension and bleeding. Long-term complications may result from intraoperative adverse events, postoperative drug regimes and lack of nutrition. Thus it is important that all measures are taken to prevent these potential sequelae. Considering the possible complications, blood loss is likely to have the most profound common effect on the patient as it leads to fatigue and lethargy. This in turn can lead to depression, lack of nutrition, infection, poor bone union and a poor surgical result as well as impacting negatively on the patient's personal life.

Preoperative assessment

All patients in the UK should be pre-assessed following the Association of Anaesthetists of Great Britain and Ireland guidelines.[4]

Cardiovascular status should be assessed with particular reference to the presence of hypertension, cardiomyopathies and cardiac dysrhythmias. These chronic conditions should be medically optimized preoperatively. Cardiac ischaemia and symptoms of cardiac failure should be considered major risk factors for orthognathic surgery and are considered relative exclusion criteria. Patients with corrected congenital cardiac disease and those with pacemakers

Orthognathic Surgery: Principles, Planning and Practice. Edited by Farhad B. Naini and Daljit S. Gill.

or implantable cardioverter defibrillators would not be excluded provided they do not have functional limitation.

Respiratory pathology such as asthma and chronic obstructive airways disease should be well controlled bearing in mind that smokers are at an increased risk of infection (oral and lower respiratory tract) and poor healing. Long-term respiratory complications may result in raised intra-thoracic pressures and suboptimal ventilation through a nasal endotracheal tube leading to carbon dioxide retention. Raised carbon dioxide levels cause vasodilation and increased bleeding. Therefore preoperative assessment in respiratory patients should include lung function tests, chest radiographs and if required arterial blood gas analysis to determine the severity and chronicity of the condition as well as the presence of compensation (pH, pO_2, CO_2, bicarbonate levels). Any patient with severe hypoxia, carbon dioxide retention or a high bicarbonate level would not be a good candidate for orthognathic surgery.

Asthmatic patients, having been assessed, should be optimized. Preoperative optimization may include nebulized bronchodilators and oral steroids for several days before surgery. Dexamethasone is routinely used intraoperatively and in the immediate postoperative period asthmatic symptoms may diminish. In patients in whom symptoms can be triggered by seasonal factors the use of anti-histamines preoperatively may be beneficial. Bronchospasm associated with asthma leads to hyper-inflated lungs and raised intrathoracic pressures. This can lead to decreased venous return, hypotension and cardiovascular collapse as well as respiratory complications such as pneumothoraces.

Smokers and patients with chronic lung disease tend to have irritable airways and are more likely to cough during and after extubation, as well as in the immediate postoperative period. Coughing increases the risk of bleeding at the operative site.

Renal pathology should be excluded by measuring the urea, electrolytes and glomerular filtration rates. Renal impairment can lead to electrolyte imbalance, peripheral oedema and prolonged excretion of drugs. Renal dysfunction can preclude the use of analgesics, particularly non-steroidal anti-inflammatory drugs, which have an important role in the management of postoperative pain. Excessive blood loss and associated hypotension can result in an increase in urea and worsening of renal function.

Gastrointestinal pathology may affect the upper or lower gastrointestinal tract. The major concerns with the upper tract are hyperacidity and reflux. Hyperacidity will be worsened by surgical stress. Pre-existing anxiety is common in these patients and tends to be heightened around the time of surgery.

Hepatic disease may cause clotting disorders, thus it is essential to check the international normalized ratio (INR) and prothrombin time at pre-assessment. Patients with significant chronic liver disease resulting in poor synthetic function may have low albumin levels and this will contribute to more facial swelling postoperatively, poor healing and will increase the risk of infection.

Haematological disorders need to be addressed aggressively. All patients must be weighed in order to estimate the blood volume. Chronic anaemia needs investigation and may have many causes, although menorrhagia is common in young women.

The average blood loss for orthognathic procedures ranges from 200 mL to up to 800 mL. If patients lose more than 10% of their blood volume they feel fatigued and this can seriously influence their lifestyles. If we consider a 70 kg person with a blood volume of 70 mL/kg (= 4900 mL) a blood loss of 500 mL will affect the patient. Thus in a 50 kg patient a maximum of 350 mL blood loss is acceptable. In certain patients with pre-existing anaemia (e.g. eating disorders) it may be difficult to increase the haemoglobin, while iron therapy can cause constipation and diarrhoea. Consideration should be given to intravenous iron therapy and autologous transfusion.

Thrombocytopenia needs to be treated as it may significantly affect clotting. A normal platelet count is reassuring, but does not ensure normal platelet activity. Platelet function should be measured if there is a strong suspicion of a disorder or the patient gives a history of bruising easily.

White blood cells should be in the normal range and function. In patients with human immunodeficiency virus (HIV) infection it is essential to ensure that the oral anti-retroviral therapy is continued. Any sign of infection would preclude the operation.

Blood transfusion should be discussed at pre-assessment. The rare but possible risks of blood transfusion include allergic reactions, fluid overload, viral and bacterial infection and lung injury. In general blood transfusion should be avoided if at all possible especially in the young female population of reproductive age.

A blood group sample should be taken preoperatively and saved in case a blood transfusion is required.

Patients who do not accept blood transfusions (e.g. Jehovah's witnesses), should be fully informed of all the surgical and anaesthetic risks. Local hospital protocols should be adhered to.[5] Many centres organize preoperative meetings with the patient and the surgeon, the haematologist and the anaesthetist. This allows information to be shared, risks to be discussed and patient's wishes to be documented.

Sickle cell disease should be tested for in the African-Caribbean population. Sickle cell trait is not usually a problem and most carriers are asymptomatic. However, patients with sickle cell disease are at risk of sickle cell crises perioperatively.

A crisis can be precipitated by hypoxia, hypothermia, pain, dehydration and hypovolaemia. Pain is a major factor in a crisis and postoperative facial swelling may impede oral intake of analgesia. Chronic opioid use is common in patients with sickle cell disease and this can make pain management particularly challenging. Sickle cell patients often require a lot of opioids and if a crisis occurs they may need to go to the High Dependency Unit to meet their analgesic requirements. Sickle patients often have psychological issues relating to their chronic disease and must be carefully profiled for orthognathic surgery.

These patients are usually under the care of the haematology team and their input into perioperative management is vital. A multidisciplinary team approach including the acute pain team is advised in the management of this group of patients.

Obesity presents several challenges to the anaesthetic team. Obese patients are more likely to have co-morbidities as a result of being overweight such as hypertension, obstructive sleep apnoea and diabetes. They tend to have difficult venous access and specialized monitoring and positioning equipment may be required (extra large blood pressure cuffs, operating table size etc.) They are also more difficult to move once anaesthetized and as such should be anaesthetized in the operating theatre once they have positioned themselves on the table. Extra staff may be needed to move the patient at the end of procedure.

Obese patients have a heightened demand for ventilation, increased work of breathing and diminished respiratory compliance. These pathophysiological changes coupled with a decreased functional residual capacity and expiratory reserve volume predispose these patients to hypoxaemia, especially at induction of anaesthesia and emergence from anaesthesia, as well as during the operation in the supine position.

Obese patients are at an increased risk of aspiration of gastric contents at induction and emergence of anaesthesia. Intraoperatively they require higher ventilation pressures through a nasal endotracheal tube. This in turn can cause CO_2 retention, vasodilation and increased blood loss.

Psychological screening is occasionally recommended for anxious patients or those with a personality disorder. General anxiety issues can usually be alleviated by good preoperative assessment including topical anaesthesia for induction, preoperative anxiolytics and good postoperative analgesia. Patients with psychiatric conditions should continue with their regular medications bearing in mind potential drug interactions. An example of a potential drug interaction is between selective serotonin re-uptake inhibitors (SSRIs) and tramadol, which should be avoided in these patients. Some patients may still be taking monoamine oxidase inhibitors, and these medicines may potentiate the effect of epinephrine containing local anaesthetics, which are used in significant quantities during orthognathic surgery.

Airway assessment

Several papers have shown that in most orthognathic patients, airway management is uncomplicated.[6] However, a full airway assessment must be conducted which should include the modified Mallampati classification (to assess the size of the tongue relative to the oropharynx), inter-incisor distance, jaw protrusion, neck extension, mento-hyoid and thyromental distance as well as presence of airway symptoms. Any available imaging of the airway should be reviewed.

Several syndromes such as Apert, Crouzon and Treacher–Collins syndromes are associated with orthognathic problems, but these are often unilateral.

There are recognized markers that point to a potentially difficult intubation such as limited mouth opening, retrognathia, a modified Mallampati class 3 and 4 and reduced mandibular mobility.[7,8]

Medication

Ideally all conversations regarding medications should be conducted with the patient without the parents present but accompanied by a chaperone, as young adults are often reluctant to discuss oral contraception, alcohol and nicotine intake with a parent present. This is particularly true when trying to obtain an accurate history of illicit drug use. Patients who have a high alcohol intake often require a higher dose of anaesthetic drugs as they have increased metabolism due to enhanced liver function.

Nicotine patches in heavy smokers can help agitation especially postoperatively on the ward. Patients who use regular cannabis often emerge from anaesthesia agitated and can exhibit decerebrate posturing before they are fully awake.[7] Cannabis is often inhaled and these patients may suffer from chronic respiratory symptoms. A chest radiograph is often helpful as shadowing may indicate the severity of the impurities they have inhaled over the years. Regular use of cannabis from a young age while the brain is still developing (until 25 years of age) increases the risk of psychosis.[9,10]

Patients taking narcotic drugs will require more narcotic analgesia, but are also at a greater risk of respiratory depression. Homeopathic drugs (e.g. Arnica) should be taken at the time 'of injury', thus if a patient requests them they should be given immediately in the postoperative period and not prior to surgery. Vitamin supplements can cause perioperative problems, especially fish oil products, which can enhance bleeding. These substances should be stopped 2 weeks prior to surgery.

Oral contraceptives and hormone replacement therapy are continued, bearing in mind the increased venous thromboembolic risk. In these patients and the obese, graduated compression stockings or intermittent pneumatic compression boots should be used depending on the predicted length of surgery (intermittent pneumatic compression boots for procedures longer than 4 hours). All patients should be risk assessed prior to surgery and NICE guidelines on Deep Vein Thrombosis Prevention should be followed.[11]

Postoperative nausea and vomiting may lead to ineffective contraception as many of the oral contraceptives lose their efficacy outside 24 hours. Patients should be reminded that they may need to take other precautions.

Regular medication should in general be continued. However it is important to consider the half-life and maximal concentrations of drugs, e.g. atenolol has its maximal effect 6 hours post-ingestion and this could potentiate intraoperative hypotension.

It is recommended that anti-arrhythmics, thiazide diuretics and calcium channel blockers are continued, but certain antihypertensive agents such as ACE inhibitors ought to be omitted on the day of surgery. The decision regarding which medications should be taken or omitted should be discussed with the anaesthetist at pre-assessment.

Oral hypoglycaemic agents should be avoided and insulin dependent diabetics commenced on a sliding scale to continue into the postoperative period until adequate oral intake is resumed.

Consent should be obtained for per rectum administration of medication, which provides an alternative route when oral medication may not be easy to administer.

Patients are fasted for 6 hours preoperatively for solid food and 2 hours for clear fluids.[4] In accordance with the Enhanced Recovery Programme, a high calorie drink is recommended 2 hours preoperatively.[12]

The importance of a full drug history, both prescribed and illicit, is demonstrated by the possibility of serotonin syndrome. If patients taking serotonin releasing drugs are given certain drugs (e.g. tramadol or fentanyl), the syndrome may develop. Symptoms range from mild to major; severe cases may require intensive care. The symptoms are commonly described as a triad: cognitive effects (headache, agitation, mental confusion), autonomic effects (sweating, hyperthermia, hypertension, tachycardia, diarrhoea) and somatic effects (myoclonus, hyperreflexia, tremor). Some serotonin releasing drugs have a long half-life, e.g. fluoxetine. Other drugs, which may precipitate the syndrome are St John's wort, ginseng, ecstasy and cocaine.

Premedication

Premedication is recommended, as these patients are often anxious. An anxiolytic helps reduce endogenous cathecholamine release, and therefore vasoconstriction and hypertension. Diazepam in the following doses should be considered: 5 mg for patients weighing up to 70 kg, 7.5 mg for 70–100 kg and 10 mg for patients weighing >100 kg. Diazepam is long-acting benzodiazepine (half-life 40–100 hours) and is a useful adjunct in smoothing emergence and reducing anxiety in the immediate postoperative period, especially in patients with a high alcohol intake.

Needle phobic patients should have topical anaesthesia applied to an appropriate site, e.g. Amethocaine gel. If this is not possible inhalation of Entonox (a mixture of nitrous oxide 50% and oxygen 50%) in the anaesthetic room may be a useful adjunct. This allows venous cannulae to be sited in areas with topical anaesthesia.

Gastric protection is essential for the previously mentioned reasons and should be initiated preoperatively if possible. Proton pump inhibitors, e.g. omeprazole 20 mg daily for 7 days has been advocated in the past; however recently the link with proton pump inhibitors and the emergence of *Clostridium difficile* suggests that H_2 antagonists should be used in preference.[13]

Chlorhexidine mouthwash is given 30 minutes before surgery, while the other medication should be taken one hour prior to surgery with a small amount of water.

Intraoperative care

Airway management

Orthognathic surgery requires complete exposure of the facial features that allows the surgeons to assess facial symmetry and profile (Figure 14-1).

As with all airway surgery, the anaesthetic implications of shared airway procedures need to be considered.

It is better to encourage patients to preoxygenate themselves with deep diaphragmatic breathing and supplemental oxygen, prior to induction, rather than depending on hand ventilation post-induction, as mask ventilation can cause gastric distension and increase the risk of postoperative nausea and vomiting.

Endotracheal intubation is the gold standard. Laryngeal mask airways could be easily displaced during jaw manipulation; they do not provide a complete seal against aspiration of blood or gastric contents and may restrict surgical exposure.

Intubation can be oral, nasal or sub-mental. Most intubations are a Cormack-Lehane grade 1 but may be

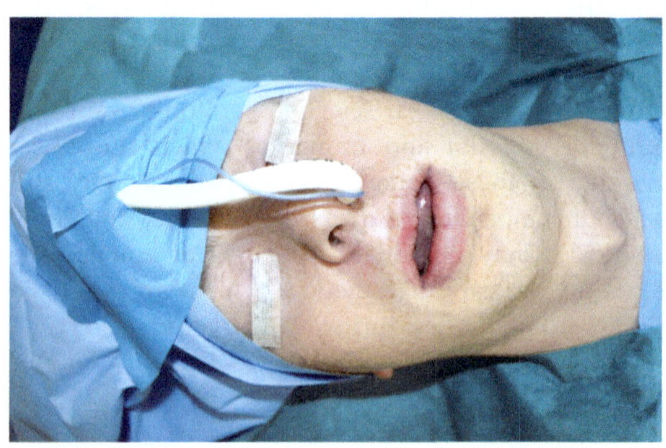

Fig. 14-1 Intubated patient (via nasal route), ETT secured ensuring facial features exposed.

more difficult in patients with severe retrognathia and some congenital syndromes. TMJ pathology or revision orthognathic surgery may restrict mouth opening which is unlikely to improve as a result of relaxation post induction of anaesthesia. In this context, an awake technique to secure the airway should be considered (e.g. awake fibreoptic intubation).

If an awake technique to secure the airway is required, the patient's comfort is of paramount importance. Local anaesthesia alone or in combination with sedation can be used.

If the procedure is to be carried out under local anaesthesia, maximum safe doses of local anaesthetics should be calculated. The calculation should take into account LA to be used intraoperatively by surgeons to minimize the risk of LA toxicity.[14,15] Adequate topicalization of the airway is a key element of smooth and comfortable awake intubation. Phenylephrine and lignocaine are sprayed into both nares, then 10% lignocaine is sprayed into the pharynx. Amethocaine lozenges can also be sucked, but these take longer to take effect. If more vasoconstriction of the nares is required Moffat's solution can be used: 1 mL :1000 adrenaline, 2 mL 10% cocaine, 2–4 mL sodium bicarbonate made up to 20 mL with saline solution. Topical anaesthesia of the vocal cords can be obtained by two routes:

1. Via an epidural catheter inserted into the fibreoptic scope using the 'spray-as-you-go' technique; or
2. A trans-tracheal injection of local anaesthetic.

Remifentanil is a potent short-acting synthetic opioid with very fast onset and rapid metabolism. It provides analgesia, sedation and suppression of airway reflexes. These properties have seen remifentanil increasingly used to facilitate awake fibreoptic intubation. The use of remifentanil may reduce the requirement for topical anaesthesia.[16]

Most intubations are nasal, but the submental route allows better access to the jaws. For submental intubation it is essential to have a reinforced endotracheal tube with a detachable connector. The pilot tube and balloon should be of a size that will pass through the submental incision (Figure 14-2).

Complications of the submental route are aspiration of blood if the cuff is damaged which can occur as it passes through the sub mental incision. Other complications include misplacement of the endotracheal tube, i.e. migration into a bronchus or as it curves in the pharynx it can spring out of the trachea leading to loss of airway. The endotracheal tube should be checked by direct vision after it has been placed through the submental incision.

Apnoeic oxygenation is often used while performing nasal intubations. Apnoeic oxygenation can provide invaluable extra time of adequate oxygenation (up to 10 minutes) in difficult airway problems.

A throat pack should be inserted at the start of surgery. Throat packs reduce the amount of blood entering the stomach and provide an element of stability and security of the tracheal tube. The throat pack should be inserted in theatre and it should be part of the swab count. All team members need to be aware that a throat pack is in situ and throat pack insertion/removal times should be documented in full view of all theatre staff.

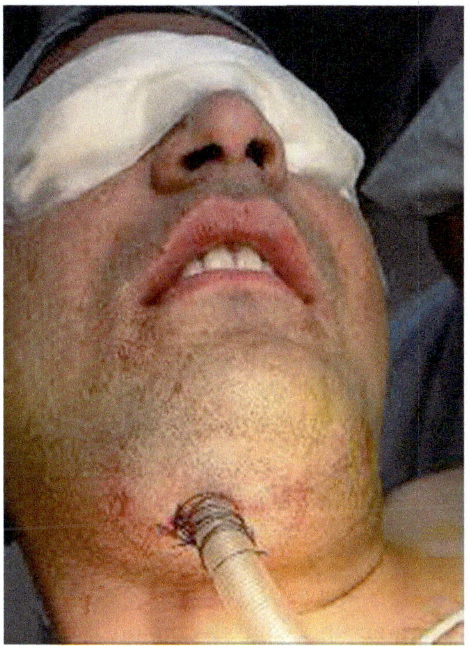

Fig. 14-2 Submental intubation.

Patient positioning

The aim of optimal positioning during surgery is to ensure ideal surgical conditions while minimizing risks to the patients. Anaesthetized patients are unable to position themselves into the most comfortable position or alert us to compromised positions. The responsibility of ensuring safe positioning lies with the surgical and anaesthetic teams.[17]

The head draping of the patient should expose the face ensuring pressure areas are adequately padded (Figure 14-3).

In the photograph there is no fixation of the endotracheal tube around the nares, but care should be taken

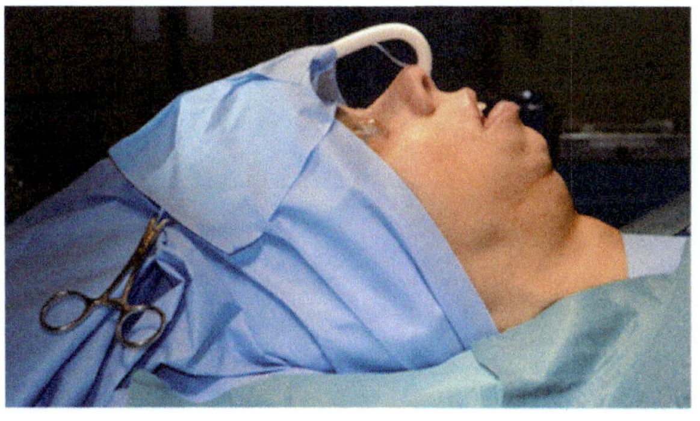

Fig. 14-3 Nasally intubated patient with surgical drapes in position.

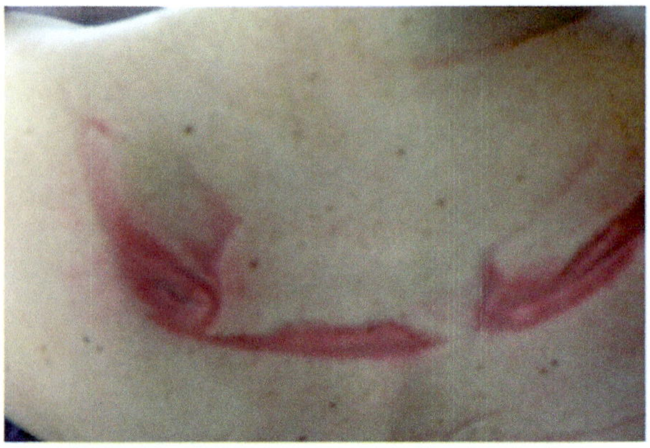

Fig. 14-4 Pressure sore arising from horseshoe head ring.

to prevent any drag of the tube on the nares as this can lead to pressure necrosis of the tip of the nose. The endotracheal tube must be supported at the head of the table with tracheal tube holders. Adequate fixation of the tube is ensured with tape and pressure relieving gauze/sponge on the upper end of the forehead. The tape is secured over the ears taking care to ensure the ears are aligned with the side of the head and free from pressure. Sweating and face creams impair the stickiness of most tapes. This can lead to loosening of the endotracheal fixation and displacement. Care should also be taken with surgical drapes that are taped to the endotracheal tube as these can inadvertently extubate the patient as they are removed at the end of surgery. A small gauze interface between the surgical drapes and the endotracheal tube/anaesthetic circuit can minimize the risk of accidental extubation.

There are many causes of pressure ulcers in maxillofacial surgery ranging from pressure sores such as may develop due to positioning of the head in a horseshoe head ring to peripheral nerve injuries (Figure 14-4).

If the drapes are too tightly stretched across the endotracheal tube pressure areas on the forehead may develop.

The patients are often completely covered with surgical drapes and with prolonged surgery pressure areas are more likely to occur over arms, hands, sacrum and heels (Figure 14-5).

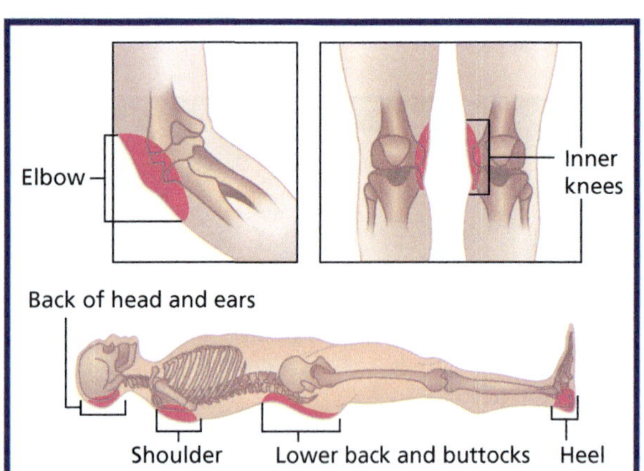

Fig. 14-5 Vulnerable pressure areas.

Thus care to protect these areas must be taken prior to the start of surgery as intraoperative hypotension will increase the risk of pressure sores in vulnerable areas. The legs should be flexed slightly at the knees to protect the lower back.

The patient should be actively warmed due to temperature loss associated with prolonged surgery. The patient's temperature should be monitored with a skin temperature probe.

Anaesthetic technique

Anaesthetic drugs

Induction of anaesthesia may involve a single agent or co-induction with another agent such as midazolam. Propofol is the most commonly used induction agent along with a short-acting narcotic such as fentanyl. Total intravenous anaesthesia (TIVA) with propofol and remifentanil is also a popular choice due to a good recovery profile after prolonged surgery, but the ultimate choice comes down to anaesthetic preference. Paralysis for intubation is achieved with a short-acting muscle relaxant (e.g. rocuronium or atracurium), both of which will have been metabolized by the time alignment of jaws is required.

All the induction agents cause a decrease in systemic vascular resistance (SVR) and in under-filled patients a reflex tachycardia will occur. A drop in SVR will result in hypotension, which may be treated with vasoconstrictors in the short-term, but the correct intervention is fluid optimization. Stroke volume optimization by increasing the pre-load will reduce the tachycardia due to stretch receptors in the atria and pulmonary arteries slowing the heart rate and decreasing the stroke volume (Figure 14-6).

If the blood pressure drops due to hypovolaemia and induction agents, the baroreceptors in the carotid sinus and aortic arch will respond by increasing the sympathetic output.

Tachycardia and increased stroke volume, particularly in the young patient, are the main causes of bleeding. The blood pressure does not have the maximal effect on blood loss. It is the heart rate and stroke volume increase that cause more bleeding. Thus drugs that reduce tachycardia are most helpful intraoperatively. Beta-blockers along with alpha and beta-blockers (e.g. labetalol) will reduce the heart rate (beta effect) and vasodilate (alpha effect). The patient must be adequately preloaded in order for these drugs to be used. A continuous infusion of remifentanil cab be used to reduce the heart rate and blood pressure thus achieving desired hypotensive conditions. Avoiding drugs which increase the heart rate, such as anticholinergics and cyclizine, as well as reducing the patient's own cathecholamine production, e.g. with anxiolytic premedication, is important.

Maintenance of anaesthesia is achieved with either inhalational agents (e.g. isoflurane) or TIVA. Both aid hypotension. Remifentanil will have no analgesic

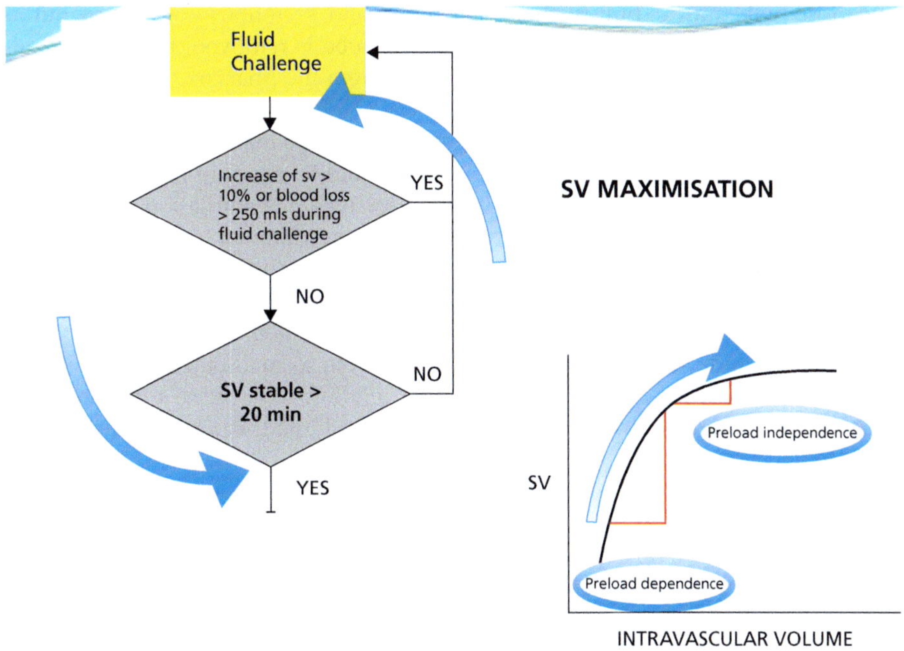

Fig. 14-6 Stroke volume optimization and the Frank-Starling mechanism (length-tension relation).

effect in the immediate postoperative period, therefore an adequate dose of morphine needs to be administered prior to the end of surgery. The dose of morphine should be carefully titrated at emergence to allow the patient to have adequate ventilation yet be pain and anxiety free.

When the osteotomies take place, it is helpful to deepen anaesthesia and this can be achieved with a bolus of propofol. Maintaining a normal arterial CO_2 or low/normal CO_2 throughout the procedure reduces vasodilation and thus reduces the blood loss. It can also assist ventilation as it suppresses the patient's own respiratory effort reducing the need for repeated doses of muscle relaxant and the chances of the patient spontaneously breathing through the nasal tube.

It is not necessary, in most orthognathic procedures, to insert an arterial line, a central venous catheter or a urinary catheter. These devices are invasive and increase the risk of infection; thus there must be a valid indication to insert them, e.g. using an arterial line in an obese patient where blood pressure reading are unreliable would be justifiable.

Induced hypotension

Minimizing blood loss intraoperatively is important and the anaesthetic technique plays a vital role in orthognathic surgery.

In addition to already mentioned measures, simple methods such as head-up positioning, ensuring unobstructed venous drainage and epinephrine-containing local anaesthesia aid in minimizing blood loss.

Hypotensive anaesthesia reduces the bleeding at the operative site and has been shown to reduce the need for blood transfusion.[18,19] However, this technique should only be employed in a carefully selected patient group. The mean arterial pressure (MAP) should be reduced by no more than 30% of the patient's normal MAP. This technique should not be considered for patients with ischaemic heart disease, uncontrolled hypertension, diabetes, severe anaemia, haemoglobinopathies (e.g. Sickle cell disease), cerebrovascular disease and hepatic and renal impairment.[20]

Other drugs, previously used for induced hypotension but much less popular now, are glyceryl trinitrate (GTN) and sodium nitroprusside (SNP).

Tranexamic acid

Tranexamic is a synthetic analogue of the amino acid lysine. It is an antifibrinolytic that competitively inhibits the activation of plasminogen to plasmin. It is useful in orthognathic surgery and 1 g should be given prior to the surgical incision. It should be given slowly as rapid injection may cause hypotension. It should be also used in patients on oral contraceptives or hormone replacement therapy; however one should consider its use in patients with a history of thromboembolic disease as it will increase the risk of venous thrombosis.

Anti-emetics

The incidence of postoperative nausea and vomiting is relatively high following orthognathic surgery. Literature suggests an incidence of PONV of 7–40%.[21]

A combination of anti-emetics with different modes of action should be given, e.g. ondansetron and dexamethasone. Ondansetron is a very effective anti-emetic and the drug of choice. Usually a single intraoperative dose will suffice but further doses may be required postoperatively and should be prescribed. Ondansetron can lengthen the Q-T interval so care should be taken if the patient has any cardiac abnormality. Dexamethasone is usually given for surgical reasons to decrease postoperative swelling, but its concomitant effect is efficacious anti-emesis. Cyclizine and prochlorperazine are the most effective anti-emetic for nausea due to opiates. Cyclizine commonly causes a tachycardia and should be diluted prior to administration and given as a slow intravenous bolus. Metoclopramide is less effective in orthognathic cases, but can be used if nausea is caused by delayed gastric emptying. This may occur secondary to constipation.

Despite the presence of a throat pack a small amount of blood ooze from the surgical site can enter the oesophagus/stomach and contribute to postoperative nausea and result in haematemesis. This risk can be reduced by inserting an Argyll catheter into the oesophagus at the end of the procedure and suctioning gastric contents. The catheter is not long enough to pass through the oesophageal sphincter, which in young patients is usually tight and therefore blood tends to pool above the sphincter. If the patient has had a sub-mental intubation it is more likely that blood will accumulate, so suctioning pre-extubation is strongly recommended. If there is ongoing oozing of blood in recovery, a topical vasoconstrictor to the nose (e.g. phenylephrine) or a further dose of tranexamic acid may help. Patients with impaired liver and renal function should be monitored closely as continued bleeding and ingestion of the blood will increase the protein load in the gut.

Emergence and extubation

The aim of emergence is to ensure an ideal environment for safe extubation to take place. The patient should be normotensive with no active bleeding. Check laryngoscopy should ensure that the oropharynx is dry of secretions and blood. The throat packs should be removed and there should be no coughing. Any residual muscle paralysis should be reversed with neostigmine and adequate spontaneous ventilation ensured. Doxapram is a respiratory stimulant and can be used in patients with suboptimal respiratory effort. The patient should be sitting head up at 35 degrees as this will also encourage blood to drain into pharynx where it can be suctioned. These measures provide the optimal conditions for a safe extubation. The patient can be extubated as soon as they are awake and co-operative and therefore able to protect their own airway.

A Guedel airway of the appropriate size should be inserted into the oropharynx providing a conduit for suction or oxygen. The presence of two conduits for suction and oxygen is useful, e.g. one via the endotracheal tube as it is withdrawn and the other through the Guedel airway. Laryngospasm is less likely to occur if blood and secretions are sucked out as the endotracheal tube is removed, but this will also suck out oxygen from the pharynx. Therefore a source of oxygen via a Hudson mask connected to a high flow oxygen source helps maintain adequate oxygenation. All effort should be made to minimize the need for positive pressure hand ventilation with a bag and mask, as this can be detrimental to the surgical result.

Continuing high flow oxygen for the next hour can help to dry secretions in the oropharynx.

The patient should leave theatre sitting up at 35 degrees, able to maintain and protect their own airway. High flow oxygen via a Hudson mask should be administered into the postoperative period.

Postoperative care

At the end of the operation all members of the team should discuss and document any untoward intraoperative events, estimated blood loss, any potential issues in recovery and any specific instructions for postoperative care.

It is worthwhile noting that the risk of bleeding into the airway leading to airway obstruction remains a threat, even in the awake patient in recovery. Recovery staff must maintain a high degree of vigilance while caring for patients who have had orthognathic surgery.

Patients should stay a minimum of 2 hours in the recovery room and should remain on a trolley in case there are any acute airway problems.

A recovery nurse should ensure that the patient is comfortable and there is no ongoing bleeding.

The patient may be given a small drink of water to encourage swallowing and to assist with speech. Patients often find it difficult to drink due to swelling and residual effects of local anaesthesia. The Enhanced Recovery Programme encourages patients to resume oral intake as soon as possible including high calorie/protein drinks in order to offset the catabolic triggers of surgery.

Intravenous fluids should be continued until a good oral intake is established.

Intravenous opiates should be used in recovery to ensure patients are comfortable. There are many preparations combining paracetamol and codeine, also in a dispersible form. The ideal analgesic combination should be tailored to the patient taking into account their age, weight, allergies and presence of liver/renal impairment. Multi modal analgesia should be administered regularly for the first 48–72 hours. If there is a problem with the oral route alternative routes of drug delivery should be considered such as patches (e.g. fentanyl), sublingual drug preparations as well as the rectal route. In recent times, pregabalin has established a role in the multimodal management of acute postoperative pain.[22]

Intraoperatively patients are given steroids and postoperatively steroids and non-steroidal analgesics, both of which can cause gastric ulceration.

Regular gastric protection and laxatives are an important part of the postoperative regime. Salt and chlorhexidine mouth wash should be prescribed. Many preparations are available in liquid form in case the patient has difficulty with ingestion.

Constipation is common in the postoperative period due to fasting, opioids and decreased oral intake.

Antibiotics

Gram-positive and Gram-negative antibiotic prophylaxis is required, e.g. co-amoxiclav. In case of penicillin allergy, clindamycin may be used. Choice of antibiotic prophylaxis and dosage regimes vary between hospitals, therefore local guidelines should be followed. Our current practice is three intravenous doses followed by 5 days of oral antibiotics. This may need to be reviewed and adjusted within certain patient groups, e.g. diabetics.

Conclusions

Thus the key points to good anaesthetic management for orthognathic surgery are:

Pre-assessment	Premedication	Detailed understanding of surgical technique
Airway management and positioning	Fluid loading	Hypotensive anaesthesia
Minimizing blood loss	Fibrinolysis inhibitor	Smooth emergence
Analgesia	Gastrointestinal care	Communication and team work

Finally, as Plato said, 'success in any endeavour requires single minded attention to detail and total concentration.'

References

1 American Society of Anaesthesiologists. New classification of physical status. Anaethesiology. 1963;24:111.

2 Pedersen T, Eliasen K, Henriksen E. A prospective study of mortality associated with anaesthesia and surgery: risk indicators of mortality in hospital. Acta Anaesthesiol Scand. 1990;34:176–82.

3 Bodlander FMS. Deaths associated with anaesthesia. Br J Anaesth. 1975;47:36–40.

4 Association of Anaesthetists of Great Britain and Ireland. Pre-operative Assessment and Patient Preparation – The Role of the Anaesthetist 2. London: AAGBI, 2010.

5 The Royal College of Surgeons of England. Code of Practice for the Surgical Management of Jehovah's Witnesses. 2002.

6 Wong P, Parrington S. Difficult intubation in ENT and maxillofacial surgical patients: a prospective survey. Int J Anesth. 2008;21: 1.

7 Shiga T, Wajima Z, Inoue T, Sakamoto A. Predicting difficult intubation in apparently normal patients: a meta-analysis of bedside screening test performance. Anesthesiology. 2005;103;429–37.

8 Tse JC, Rimm EB, Hussain A. Predicting difficult endotracheal intubation in surgical patients scheduled for general anesthesia: a prospective blind study. Anesth Analg. 1995; 81:254–8.

9 Flisberg PI, Paech MJ, Shah T, Ledowski T, Kurowski I, Parsons R. Induction dose of propofol in patients using cannabis. Eur J Anaesthesiol. 2009;26:192–5.

10 Mills PM, Penfold N. Anaesthesia. Cannabis abuse and anaesthesia. Anaesthesia. 2003;58:1125.

11 National Institute for Health and Care Excellence. Reducing the risk of venous thromboembolism (deep vein thrombosis and pulmonary embolism), Jan 2010.

12 Delivering Enhanced Recovery. NHS Enhanced Recovery Partnership Programme. DH, London, March 2010.

13 MacLaren R1, Campbell J. Cost-effectiveness of histamine receptor-2 antagonist versus proton pump inhibitor for stress ulcer prophylaxis in critically ill patients. Crit Care Med. 2014;42:809–15.

14 Haldar R, Gyanesh P, Samanta S. Lignocaine toxicity from topical anaesthesia of airway during awake fibreoptic intubation. J Neuroanaesthesiol Crit Care. 2014;1:146–7.

15 N. M. Woodall*, R. J. Harwood and G. L. Barker. Complications of awake fibreoptic intubation without sedation in 200 healthy anaesthetists attending a training course. Br J Anaesth. 2008;100:850–5.

16 Mingo OH1, Ashpole KJ, Irving CJ, Rucklidge MW. Remifentanil sedation for awake fibreoptic intubation with limited application of local anaesthetic in patients for elective head and neck surgery. Anaesthesia. 2008;63:1065–9.

17 Knight D, Mahajan R. Patient positioning in anaesthesia Contin Educ. Anaesth Crit Care Pain. 2004;4:160–3.

18 Ervens J, Marks C, Hecler M, Plat T, Hansen D, Hoffmeister B. Effect of induced hypotensive anaesthesia vs. isovolaemic hamodilution on blood loss and transfusion requirements in orthognathic surgery: a prospective, single-blinded, randomized, controlled clinical study. Int J Oral Maxillofac Surg. 2010;39:1168–74.

19 Choi WS, Samman N. Risks and benefits of deliberate hypotension in anaesthesia: a systematic review. Int J Oral Maxillofac Surg. 2008;37:687–703.

20 Beck J, Johnston K. Anaesthesia for cosmetic and functional maxillofacial surgery. Contin Educ Anaesth Crit Care Pain. 2014;14:38–42.

21 Chegini S, Johnston KD, Kalantzis A, Dhariwal DK. The effect of anaesthetic technique on recovery after orthognathic surgery, a retrospective audit. Anaesth Prog. 2012;59:69–74.

22 Zhang J, Ho K-Y, Wang Y. Efficacy of pregabalin in acute postoperative pain: a meta-analysis. Br J Anaesth. 2011;106:454–62.

Chapter 15

Postoperative Care, Nutritional Support and Oral Hygiene in the Orthognathic Surgical Patient

Richard Cobb, Kelly Wade-Mcbane and Mehmet Manisali

Postoperative care of the orthognathic surgical patient

Introduction

Postoperative patient management is critical for high quality patient treatment and predictable patient outcomes in orthognathic surgery. An insufficient understanding of the care of the postoperative patient by surgeon or orthodontist can lead to potentially catastrophic results. In order to provide consistent, high quality outcomes for patients a thorough understanding and ability to implement postoperative management protocols and strategies must be gained.

Adequate postoperative care involves pre-emptive management, regular re-assessment, selective monitoring and timely documentation.

Once a technically successful operation has been performed the patient will be transferred from the operating theatre to the recovery ward. This is a safe postoperative environment, which allows for immediate surgical/anaesthetic complications to be rapidly identified and managed. The patient should only be discharged from the recovery room once specific criteria have been met:[1]

- The patient is fully conscious, responding to verbal or light touch and is able to maintain a patent airway with a normal cough reflex.
- Respiration and oxygen saturation rates are within acceptable limits (12–14 breaths per minute, SpO_2 >94% in a patient with no respiratory co-morbidity).
- The cardiovascular system is stable with no unexplained arrhythmia and no ongoing bleeding. The patient should have a heart rate and blood pressure that are closely aligned to their preoperative values.
- Pain and emesis should be controlled and suitable analgesic and anti-emetic regimens should be prescribed.
- Temperature should be within acceptable limits.

Orthognathic Surgery: Principles, Planning and Practice. Edited by Farhad B. Naini and Daljit S. Gill.

- Oxygen and fluid therapy should be prescribed when required.

If the patient does not achieve these criteria then they should be urgently seen by the anaesthetist/surgeon responsible for the patient's care and consideration given to escalation to a level 2 or 3 environment for further management.

On discharge from the recovery room there should be clear documentation from both the anaesthetic and surgical team regarding any intraoperative difficulties or complications, any specific postoperative instructions and any specific prophylaxis that is required (e.g. antibiotics, thromboprophylaxis, fluid, etc.).

The essential consideration for the maxillofacial patient is the operative involvement of structures surrounding the airway. Therefore, there should be a high index of suspicion for the possibility of airway compromise by the postoperative care team. In modern orthognathic practice, planned intermaxillary fixation (IMF) is rare; however, there may be occasions where resorting to this may be a necessity. In these circumstances, appropriate instructions together with appropriate instrumentation (such as wire cutters) may need to be provided for the recovery staff. Whilst the application of formal intermaxillary fixation is a rarity, some surgeons are keen to apply guiding elastics whilst the patient is in recovery. A measure such as this requires appropriate communication between surgical staff and postoperative care staff.

The postoperative care of the patient may take place in a number of different locations, depending on the level of monitoring or organ support that the patient requires. The Intensive Care Society recommends a classification that reflects the level of care required by the patient rather than the historical classification by location (e.g. ward, high dependency unit (HDU), intensive care unit (ICU):[2]

- **Level 0** (formerly ward)
  Patients whose needs can be met through normal ward care (e.g. intravenous fluids, 4-hourly observations).
- **Level 1** (formerly ward, with outreach assistance)
  Patients in need of additional monitoring/clinical interventions (e.g. those requiring boluses of intravenous fluid but without the need for central venous pressure [CVP] monitoring, those with a tracheostomy, those on established intermittent renal support). These are patients at risk of clinical deterioration who may require escalation to level 2.
- **Level 2** (formerly HDU)
  These are patients requiring single organ support or are stepping down from a higher level of care.
- **Level 3** (formerly ICU)
  Patients who require advanced respiratory support alone or the support of two or more organ systems.

The vast majority of patients undergoing elective orthognathic surgery are young and with few co-morbidities; consequently it is unusual for these patients to require levels of care greater than Level 0–1. However, it is essential that the surgical team identify patients who are developing physiological changes early and escalate them to an appropriate level of care.

Ward-based care

The initial clinical assessment

The initial assessment of the patient should take place directly after the patient has been transferred to the ward environment. This provides an opportunity to reassess the physiological markers and set a baseline against which the patients' condition can be subsequently assessed. The assessment should be made by the surgical team responsible for the patient's postoperative care.

The initial assessment should review the intraoperative course, postoperative plan, prophylaxis requirements, past medical history, medications and allergies. Any information regarding clinical deterioration or complications during the patient's transit from theatre to ward should be handed over by the recovery team. Some departments choose to utilize a formal, structured care plan to aid the transfer of information between different healthcare teams.[3] This has been shown to be useful in minimizing error (Table 15-1).

The physical examination of the early postoperative patient can be considered using a similar framework to that used in the emergency setting. The standard 'Airways, Breathing, Circulation' or ABC is often followed and serves a useful purpose in assessing the orthognathic patient. As previously described all maxillofacial patients have the potential for airway compromise. A clear assessment of the airway must always be undertaken, with frequent reassessment. A respiratory and circulatory system assessment must also be made.

It is essential to assess the patient's conscious/cognitive level following surgical procedures. There are a number of reasons for patients to suffer with postoperative delirium and it is important to adequately assess their neurological function early.

Common causes for postoperative delirium include:

- Hypoxaemia
- Hypercarbia
- Sedative drugs
- Sepsis (unlikely in the early postoperative phase)
- Hypoglycaemia
- Acute urinary retention
- Acute neurological event
- Myocardial infarction
- Alcohol/drug withdrawal
- Biochemical abnormality (e.g. electrolytes, liver function, thyroid function, etc.)

Table 15-1 Checklist for the first postoperative assessment

Review intraoperative history and postoperative instructions
- ☐ Past medical history
- ☐ Medications
- ☐ Allergies
- ☐ Intraoperative complications
- ☐ Postoperative instructions
- ☐ Prophylaxis guidance

A complete airway and respiratory examination
- ☐ Ensure patent airway
- ☐ Oxygen saturations
- ☐ Effort of breathing/use of accessory muscles
- ☐ Respiratory rate
- ☐ Tracheal position
- ☐ Symmetry of chest expansion
- ☐ Breath sounds
- ☐ Percussion

A complete cardiovascular and volume assessment
- ☐ Hands: warm/cool, pink/pale
- ☐ Capillary refill time
- ☐ Pulse: volume, character and heart rate
- ☐ Blood pressure
- ☐ Conjunctival pallor
- ☐ Jugular venous pressure (JVP)
- ☐ Heart sounds and added sounds
- ☐ Urine colour and rate of production
- ☐ Drainage from surgical drains/wounds

A mental/cognitive assessment
- ☐ AVPU (alert, responds to verbal or painful stimuli, unresponsive)
- ☐ Glasgow Coma Scale
- ☐ Abbreviated Mental Test Score (AMTS)
  - ➢ If abnormal ensure to check blood glucose level.

Early assessment of the maxillofacial complex
- ☐ Airway patency
- ☐ Dental occlusion assessment
- ☐ Surgical site assessment
- ☐ Presence and position of guiding elastics
- ☐ Adequate pain control
- ☐ Appropriate prophylaxis prescribed (antibiotics, thromboprophylaxis, etc.)

The initial assessment is often too early to accurately assess specific orthognathic parameters. However, the occlusion should be checked to ensure stability, position and engagement of any splint/wafer that may be being used. Also, the presence/position of any guiding elastics should be checked. The advent of miniplate fixation means that rigid intermaxillary fixation is usually unnecessary, which benefits the patient in terms of airway management, early function and comfort. Finally, if any drains have been used, they should be inspected for contents and volume.

Local guidelines should be consulted and followed with respect to specific treatment and prophylaxis options.[4–6] This includes adequate pain control, venous thromboembolism (VTE) prophylaxis, use of corticosteroids, antibiotic prophylaxis, diabetic control requirements, prophylaxis for postoperative nausea and vomiting, and oral hygiene.

A clear assessment and management plan should be comprehensively documented in the notes, detailing any specific problems, concerns or necessary further investigations. The time interval before the next assessment of the patient should also be recorded.

The daily clinical assessment

The daily clinical assessment is an opportunity to regularly assess the patient and their progress through to discharge. Orthognathic patients should be nursed 'head up' at 45 degrees. The regular monitoring of core physiological parameters (heart rate, blood pressure, temperature, respiration rate and oxygen saturation) should be undertaken at appropriate time intervals by nursing staff and should be routinely assessed by the surgical team. Most hospitals in the UK utilize an Early Warning Score (EWS), which is a simple physiological scoring system aimed at identifying the deteriorating patient early and ensuring the appropriate healthcare professionals are called to manage that patient.[7]

Fluid balance, haemoglobin level, biochemical parameters, nutritional intake, analgesic requirements and swelling should all be assessed on the surgical ward round. Specific attention should be paid to the occlusion and its stability. This is also an appropriate time to assess sensory nerve function of the relevant anatomy.

Daily clear and contemporaneous notes should be made each time a patient is reviewed. The daily ward round is the most complete opportunity to ensure that the patient is improving in a satisfactory manner.

The anticipated inpatient stay for a typical orthognathic patient is expected to be 24–48 hours. This period also allows close observation of the patient for common early postoperative complications such as pain, swelling, bleeding and respiratory compromise.

Orthognathic surgery is considered to produce clean-contaminated wounds. Infecting microorganisms are often part of the normal mixed, endogenous flora of the oral cavity/paranasal sinuses. Infections following intraoral approaches are usually due to anaerobic Gram-positive cocci, anaerobic Gram-negative rods and streptococci.[8] The use of postoperative prophylactic antibiotics following orthognathic surgery remains controversial, and there is concern about their potential to lead to resistance and superinfection.[9] If used, postoperative oral antibiotics appear to be superior to intravenous in terms of associated morbidity and cost without increased rates of infection.[5]

Preoperative glucocorticoid therapy has been shown to be effective in reducing postoperative swelling in orthognathic surgery.[10] However, the dose and duration remain contentious and the additional value of postoperative doses remains uncertain.[6]

It is common after maxillary procedures for there to be some nasal and pharyngeal bloody drainage.

Patients can find this concerning, however, it usually arrests 6–12 hours postoperatively. Blood filling the sinuses may continue to clear over the first two weeks following surgery, presenting as blood stained drainage from the nose.

Early in the postoperative phase, the patient can be mobilized to the outpatient setting for a thorough dental occlusal assessment. This is best achieved utilizing a dental chair and optimal lighting, under the guidance of the orthodontist. This also provides an opportunity for a postoperative orthopantomograph (OPT) to be taken for reassurance of the condylar position and the position of plates/screws.

Nutritional support

There is a wealth of evidence in the surgical field demonstrating that a poor nutritional status in the preoperative period is associated with poorer outcomes, such as an increased risk of infection and hospital length of stay.[11–31] Interestingly, specific to orthognathic surgery, preoperative nutritional optimization is rarely indicated. It would be plausible to suggest that this is due to the nature of the patient group (young adults with minimal co-morbidities) alongside the type of surgery being performed.

Orthognathic surgery presents many physiological challenges that may compromise nutritional status including catabolism, postoperative facial swelling and increased nitrogen requirements to promote wound healing. The provision of adequate macro and micronutrients in conjunction with sufficient hydration is therefore essential.

The degree of movement of the mandible is restricted following orthognathic surgery, principally secondary to postoperative facial swelling and pain. An adequate nutritional and fluid intake can therefore be challenging, given an adult patient's daily nutritional needs (Table 15-2).

Dietary adaptation to maintain nutritional and hydration status is crucial to promote wound healing and to minimize postoperative complications. A patient's mood is often seldom discussed, but it is an important feature in the patient pathway. Evidence suggests that adequate nutritional provision and sufficient fluid to minimize dehydration helps to improve mood, thereby diminishing postoperative irritability or depression.[32]

Table 15-2 Recommended postoperative dietary and fluid requirements for patients over the age of 16 years undergoing orthognathic surgery[40]

	Energy (kcals)	Protein (g)	Fluid (mL)
Male	2500	1 g/kg/day	35 mL/kg/day
Female	2000	1 g/kg/day	35 mL/kg/day

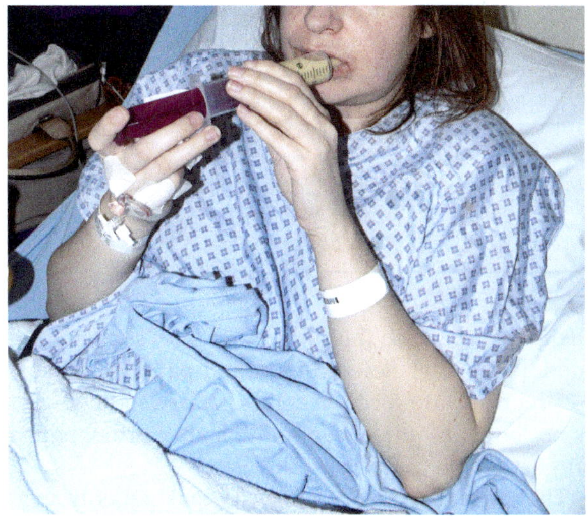

Fig. 15-1 An example of a patient administering oral liquid nutrition support via a 60-mL syringe one day following bimaxillary orthognathic surgery.

Dietary modification is recommended as a staged process, with efforts to minimize the masticatory forces being transmitted to the underlying healing bone, and optimizing the conditions for adequate healing. Initially, during the first seven days of the postoperative period, an energy and protein dense liquid diet is recommended to increase calorie density, whilst minimizing stress on the plates and screws. A liquid diet consists of foods that have been blended using a food processor or liquidizer to form a smooth consistency. Foods can then be swallowed easily using a teaspoon, a straw or a large syringe, eradicating the need for chewing (Figure 15-1). During this period, extra nutritional support is often indicated to supplement dietary intake to prevent malnutrition. A nutritional assessment by a specialist maxillofacial dietitian is therefore needed to ensure that the patient is meeting their calorie, protein and fluid requirements. This is particularly important, as evidence has demonstrated that the provision of high energy, high protein oral liquid nutritional support can result in weight maintenance, improved nitrogen retention and protein sparing in orthognathic surgical patients.[33–35]

There is little in the literature on the postoperative nutritional management of orthognathic patients. However, in view of the body of evidence on enhanced recovery after surgery with postoperative nutritional support,[36–42] it would be plausible to suggest that similar outcomes could apply to the present day in the field of orthognathic surgery.

During the second week of the postoperative recovery period, patients should be able to start eating with a small spoon or fork. Minimal chewing is still advised and thus, a high energy, high protein fork mashed diet is recommended. This consists of soft, moist foods that can be easily mashed with the back of a fork.

From week three onwards, a soft diet with some light chewing is advised. Patients may notice that

Table 15-3 Recommended progression of oral diet in the postoperative period following orthognathic surgery

Week	Recommended diet consistency
Week 1	Liquid diet
Week 2	Fork mashed diet
Weeks 3–8	Soft diet
Weeks 8 +	Normal diet

their jaw tires easily, but the jaw muscles soon accommodate for their new position and patients are able to progress onto a softer, solid diet. A modified diet is no longer required two months after orthognathic surgery (Table 15-3).

The current evidence suggests that patients who undergo orthognathic surgery will lose between 3.1 kg–6.8 kg during the 6-week recovery period secondary to difficulties achieving an adequate nutritional intake.[32] This thereby increases the risk of morbidity and the possibility of other postoperative complications.

All patients should have access to a specialist maxillofacial dietitian at the time of their preoperative medical consultation. The dietitian can then undertake a thorough nutritional assessment and provide dietary advice for both the pre and postoperative stages of the orthognathic surgery care pathway. Managing a patient's expectations is also important and the dietitian can provide written information and guidance on the impact of orthognathic surgery on eating and drinking. Furthermore, high energy, high protein oral liquid nutritional support can be provided during the preoperative consultation if indicated. This would help overcome many of the physiological barriers often incurred in patients who undergo orthognathic surgery, thereby enhancing postoperative recovery.

Taking into consideration the patient group, there is scope for two avenues of patient follow-up, the first being a designated dietetic clinic and the second being through a means of telephone communication. Orthognathic patients are usually independent, young adults and thus, they should be encouraged to take ownership of their nutritional and hydration status. Patients should monitor their weight weekly and if they notice a significant drop in weight or are struggling with their dietary intake for a prolonged period they should have access to both surgical and dietetic review (Figure 15-2).

Orthognathic surgery presents many physiological challenges that may compromise nutritional status. The provision of adequate macro and micronutrients in conjunction with sufficient hydration is essential. This can be achieved through the development of a robust orthognathic surgical care pathway, with a specialist maxillofacial dietitian involved at each stage of the patient pathway. This will reduce postoperative morbidity and minimize the risk of postoperative complications associated with a poor nutritional and hydration status.

Oral hygiene measures

Introduction

Following orthognathic surgery the maintenance of good oral hygiene is essential in order to avoid oral health issues such as dental caries and periodontal disease. This patient cohort is at particular risk as they will have fixed orthodontic appliances and will often be experiencing reduced mouth opening and postoperative pain. Orthognathic patients must be advised to re-start their oral hygiene regimen as soon as possible following surgery. The effective removal of dental plaque, a firmly adherent mass of bacteria in a mucopolysaccharide matrix, can occur using mechanical or chemotherapeutic techniques.

Brushing techniques for the orthognathic patient

An effective brushing technique for patients wearing fixed orthodontic appliances involves the separate

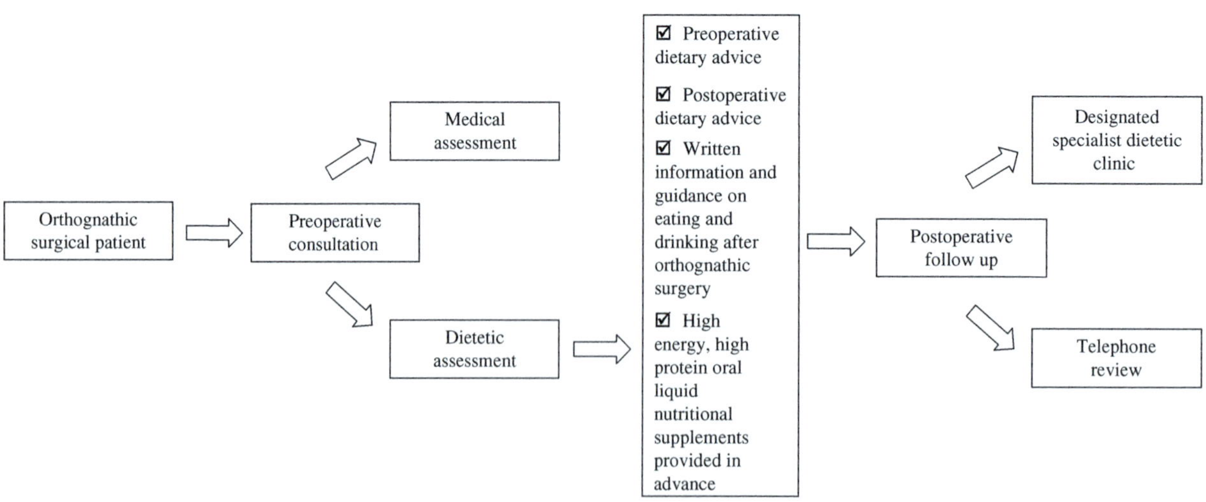

Fig. 15-2 Flow diagram illustrating the role of the specialist maxillofacial dietitian in the nutritional management of patients undergoing orthognathic surgery.

brushing of tooth surfaces lying occlusal and cervical to the orthodontic archwire. Often patients will neglect the cervical region, which can lead to plaque accumulation and gingivitis.

It is thought that patients with fixed appliances should apply more force than usual when brushing. This greater force causes a reduction in plaque accumulation with minimal risks of tooth wear.[43]

Interdental brushes are a useful adjunct to routine brushing. They have the advantage of removing subgingival plaque to a depth of 2.0–2.5 mm.[44] These brushes are particularly useful for cleaning around the fixed appliances of orthognathic patients.

Manual vs. electric toothbrushes

Electric toothbrushes are becoming more commonplace and they now take up a substantial proportion of the oral hygiene market. A Cochrane review comparing manual and powered toothbrushes in relation to the removal of plaque, the health of the gingivae, staining and calculus accumulation has shown that brushes with a rotation-oscillation action removed plaque and reduced gingivitis more effectively than manual toothbrushes.[45] Rotation-oscillation powered toothbrushes specifically designed for use with fixed orthodontic appliances now exist and may be beneficial in orthodontic patients.

It has previously been thought that the use of a powered toothbrush in orthodontic patients may lead to a greater risk of debonding brackets. This in fact appears to be untrue and may actually improve oral hygiene whilst having minimal effect on bracket adhesion.[46]

Adjunctive chemotherapeutic agents

There are a number of chemotherapeutic agents which inhibit bacterial plaque formation in common use. Chlorhexidine acts against Gram-negative/Gram-positive bacteria and yeasts making it one of the most effect chemotherapeutic agents available.[47] It binds to both soft and hard tissues, enabling it to maintain effective concentrations for extended periods of time, a process known as substantivity.[48] However, if used for extended periods it can alter taste and cause discolouration of teeth/orthodontic bracket adhesive materials as well as parotid swelling.[49]

Other chemotherapeutic agents in use include Triclosan and Listerine. Triclosan is a non-ionic antiseptic, which has moderate plaque inhibiting effects. Listerine is an essential oil/phenolic mouthwash that also has moderate plaque inhibiting and anti-gingivitis effects. Chlorhexidine is considered to be significantly more efficacious than Listerine or Triclosan in inhibiting plaque formation.[50]

Conclusions

Good postoperative care of the orthognathic patient is essential in order to achieve high quality results and predictable patient outcomes. This process begins as the patient leaves the operating theatre and continues through until discharge.

The regular assessment and re-assessment of the patient is essential to safe surgical practice. The daily clinical assessment provides an ideal opportunity to track the patient's progress and for early identification of medical/surgical issues that may arise.

Orthognathic surgery presents particular physiological challenges that may compromise nutritional status. All patients should have access to a specialist maxillofacial dietician in order to optimize their nutritional intake. Written information and the use of high energy, high protein, oral liquid nutritional supplements is beneficial for this cohort of patients (see Chapter 10).

Orthognathic patients are potentially at risk of dental disease due to the combined presence of fixed appliances, postoperative pain and trismus. They should receive specific advice regarding appropriate mechanical and chemotherapeutic techniques and their dental health should be regularly reviewed.

References

1 Association of Anaesthetists of Great Britain and Ireland (AAGBI) Safety Guideline. Immediate Post-Anaesthetic Recovery. Anaesthesia. 2013;68: 288–97.

2 The Intensive Care Society Standards. Levels of Critical Care for Adult Patients (2009).

3 Karakaya A, Moerman AT, Peperstraete H, François K, Wouters PF, De Hert SG. Implementation of a structured information transfer checklist improves postoperative data transfer after congenital cardiac surgery. Eur J Anaesthesiol. 2013:1.

4 Williams B, Indresano AT, O'Ryan F. Venous thromboembolism in oral and maxillofacial surgery: a review of the literature. J Oral Maxillofac Surg. 2011;69: 840–4.

5 Tan SK, Lo J, Zwahlen RA. Are postoperative intravenous antibiotics necessary after bimaxillary orthognathic surgery? A prospective, randomized, double-blind, placebo-controlled clinical trial. Internat J Oral Maxillofac Surg. 2011;40:1363–8.

6 Chegini S, Dhariwal DK. Review of evidence for the use of steroids in orthognathic surgery. Br J Oral Maxillofac Surg. 2012;50:97–101.

7 Subbe CP, Kruger M, Rutherford P, Gemmel L. Validation of a modified Early Warning Score in medical admissions, Q J Med. 2001;94:521–6.

8 Spaey YJE, Bettens RM, Mommaerts MY, Adriaens J, Van Landuyt HW, Abeloos JVS, De Clercq CAS, et al. A prospective study on infectious complications in orthognathic surgery. J Cranio-maxillo-fac Surg.2005;33: 24–9.

9 Chow LK, Singh B, Chiu WK, Samman N. Prevalence of postoperative complications after orthognathic surgery: a 15-year review. J Oral Maxillofac Surg. 2007;65:984–92.

10 Dan AEB, Thygesen TH, Pinholt EM. Corticosteroid administration in oral and orthognathic surgery: a systematic review of the literature and meta-analysis. J Oral Maxillofac Surg. 2010;68:2207–20.

11 Busby GP, Mullen JL, Mathews DC, Hobbs CL, Rosato EF. Prognostic nutritional index in gastrointestinal surgery. Am J Surg. 1980;139:160–7.

12 Klidjian AM, Foster KJ, Kammerling RM, Cooper A, Karran SJ. Relation of anthropometric and dynamometric variables to serious postoperative complications. Br Med J. 1980;281:899–901.

13 Warnold I, Lundholm K. Clinical significance of preoperative nutritional status in 215 noncancer patients. Ann Surg. 1984;199:299–305.
14 Detsky AS, Baker JP, O'Rourke K, Johnston N, Whitwell J, Mendelson RA, Jeejeebhoy KN. Predicting nutrition associated complications for patients undergoing gastrointestinal surgery. J Parent Ent Nutrit. 1987;11:440–6.
15 Von Meyenfeldt MF, Meijerink WJHJ, Rouflart MMJ, Buil-Maassen MTHJ, Soeters PB. Perioperative nutritional support: a randomised clinical trial. Clin Nutrit. 1992;11:180–6.
16 Shaw-Stiffel TA, Zarney LA, Pleban WE, Rosman DD, Rudolf RA, Bernstein LH. Effect of nutrition status and other factors on length of hospital stay after major gastrointestinal surgery. Nutrition. 1993;9:140–5.
17 Lassen K, Coolsen MME, Slim K, Carli F, de Aguilar-Nascimento JE, Schafer M, Parks RW, Fearon KCH, Lobo DN, Demartines N, Braga M, Ljungqvist O, Dejong CHC. Guidelines for perioperative care for pancreaticoduodenectomy: enhanced recovery after surgery (ERAS) society recommendations. Clin Nutrit. 2012;31:817–30.
18 McAleese P, Odling-Smee W. The effect of complications on length of stay. Ann Surg. 1994;220:740–4.
19 McWhirter JP, Pennington CR. Incidence and recognition of malnutrition in hospital. Br Med J. 1994;308:945–8.
20 Sagar PM, MacFie J. Effect of preoperative nutritional status on the outcome of cardiac valve replacement. Nutrition. 1994;10:490A.
21 Lennard-Jones JE, Arrowsmith H, Davison C, Denham AF, Micklewright A. Screening by nurses and junior doctors to detect malnutrition when patients are first assessed in hospital. Clin Nutrit. 1995;14:336–40.
22 Reilly HM, Martineau JK, Moran A, Kennedy H. Nutritional screening–evaluation and implementation of a simple nutrition risk score. Clin Nutrit. 1995;14:269–73.
23 Gallagher-Allred CR, Coble Voss C, Finn SC, McCamish MA. Malnutrition and clinical outcomes: the case for medical nutrition therapy. J Am Dietetic Ass. 1996;96:361–9.
24 Giner M, Laviano A, Meguid MM, Gleason JR. In 1995 a correlation between malnutrition and poor outcome still exists. Nutrition. 1996;12:23–9.
25 Lumbers M, Driver L, Howland RJ, Older MWJ, Williams CM. Nutritional status and clinical outcome in elderly female surgical orthopaedic patients. Clin Nutrit. 1996;15:101–7.
26 Tucker HN, Miguel SG. Cost containment through nutrition intervention. Nutrit Rev. 1996;54:111–21.
27 Beattie AH, Baxter JP, Prach AT, Pennington CR. An evaluation of the use of enteral nutritional supplements postoperatively in malnourished surgical patients. Proc Nutrit Soc. 1999;58:112A.
28 Corish CA, Flood P, Mulligan S, Kenned NP. Prevalence of undernutrition and weight loss changes during the course of hospitalization among patients admitted to two Dublin hospitals. Proc Nutrit Soc. 1998;57:10A.
29 Corish CA. Symposium on 'Nutrition and surgical practice' pre-operative nutritional assessment. Proc Nutrit Soc. 1999;58:821–9.
30 Gregg JR, Cookson MS, Phillips S, Salem S, Chang SS, Clark PE, Davis R, Stimson CJ Jr, Aghazadeh M, Smith JA Jr, Barocas DA. Effect of preoperative nutritional deficiency on mortality after radical cystectomy for bladder cancer. J Urol. 2011;185:90–6.
31 Todorovic VE, Micklewright A. A pocket guide to clinical nutrition: the parenteral and enteral nutrition group of the British Dietetic Association, 2011.
32 Robinson RC, Holm RL. Orthognathic surgery for patients with maxillofacial deformities. Assoc Periop Regist Nurs 2010;92:28–52.
33 Kendell BD, Fonseca RJ, Lee M. Postoperative nutritional supplementation for the orthognathic surgery patient. J Oral Maxillofac Surg. 1982;40:205–13.
34 Olejko TD, Fonseca RJ. Preoperative nutritional supplementation for the orthognathic surgery patient. J Oral Maxillofac Surg.: official journal of the American Association of Oral and Maxillofacial Surgeons 1984;42:573–7.
35 Chidyllo SA, Chidyllo R. Nutritional evaluation prior to oral and maxillofacial surgery. New York State Dent J. 1989;55:38–40.
36 Kehlet H. Multimodal approach to control postoperative pathophysiology and rehabilitation. Br J Anaesthes. 1997;78:606–17.
37 Fearon KC, Luff R. The nutritional management of surgical patients: enhanced recovery after surgery. Proc Nutrit Soc. 2003;62:807–11.
38 Younis J, Salerno G, Fanto D, Hadjipavlou M, Chellar D, Trickett JP. Focused preoperative patient stoma education, prior to ileostomy formation after anterior resection, contributes to a reduction in delayed discharge within the enhanced recovery programme. Internat J Colorect Dis. 2011;27:43–7.
39 Aarts MA, Okrainec A, Glicksman A, Pearsall E, Victor JC, McLeod RS. Adoption of enhanced recovery after surgery (ERAS) strategies for colorectal surgery at academic teaching hospitals and impact on total length of hospital stay. Surg Endosc. 2012;26:442–50.
40 Gustafsson UO, Scott MJ, Schwenk W, Demartines, N, Roulin D, Francis N, McNaught CE, MacFie J, Liberman S, Soop M, Hill A, Kennedy RH, Lobo DN, Fearon K, Ljungqvist O. Guidelines for perioperative care in elective colonic surgery: enhanced recovery after surgery (ERAS) society recommendations. Clin Nutrit. 2012;31:783–800.
41 Larsson J, Akerlind I, Permerth J, Hornvist JO. The relation between nutritional state and quality of life in surgical patients. Eur J Surg. 1994;160:329–34.
42 Nygren J, Thacker J, Carli F, Fearon KCH, Norderval S, Lobo DN, Ljungqvist O, Soop M, Ramirez J. Guidelines for perioperative care in elective rectal/pelvic surgery: enhanced recovery after surgery (ERAS) society recommendations. Clin Nutrit. 2012;31:801–16.
43 Laing E, Ashley P, Gill D, Naini F. An update of oral hygiene products and techniques. Dental Update. 2008;35:270–79.
44 Waerhurg J. The interdental brush and its place in operative and crown and bridge dentistry. J Oral Rehab. 1976;3:107–13.
45 Robinson PG, Deacon SA, Deery C, et al. Manual versus powered toothbrushing for oral health. The Cochrane Database of Systematic Reviews 2005, Issue 2.
46 Gheewalla E, Perry R, Kugel G. Effects of three electric toothbrushes on orthodontic bracket retention. J Clin Orthod. 2002;36:85–7.
47 Emilson CG. Effect of chlorhexidine treatment on *Stretococcus mutans* population in human saliva and dental plaque. Scand J Dent Res. 1981;89:239–46.
48 Rölla G, Löe H, Schiöt C. Retention of chlorhexidine in the oral cavity. Archiv Oral Biol. 1971;16:1109–16.
49 Addy M. Chlorhexidine compared with other locally delivered antimicrobials. J Clin Periodontol. 1986;13:957–64.
50 Deasy MJ, Battista G, Rustogi KN, Volpe AR. Anti-plaque efficiency of a triclosan/co-polymer pre-brush rinse: a plaque prevention clinical study. Am J Dent. 1991;5:91–4.

Chapter 16

The Soft Tissue Effects of Orthognathic Surgery

Daljit S. Gill, Farhad B. Naini and Maarten Koudstaal

Introduction

It is important to understand the relationship between the movement of the facial soft tissue envelope and the underlying skeletal bases during orthognathic surgery, as it is largely the final soft tissue form and position that determines the aesthetic outcome of treatment. One can go as far as saying that so important is the position of the soft tissues that during orthognathic planning one should consider the proposed final position of the soft tissues first and then plan skeletal movements accordingly, albeit taking into consideration the importance of a well-interdigitated dental occlusion (see Chapter 6). This **'aesthetic-centred'** approach to treatment planning has now superseded earlier **'occlusion-centred'** approaches even in orthodontic treatment. However, in orthognathic surgery, it is even more important that 'the teeth are made to fit the face, and not vice versa'.[1]

Orthognathic surgery has both effects on the static and dynamic soft tissue position(s) but the dynamic relationships, in particular, has been poorly studied. Evidence would suggest that there is no deterioration of soft tissue movement, due to intraoperative soft tissue dissection, following orthognathic surgery.[2]

Concerning the static soft tissue effects, one must take into consideration the immediate and longer term soft tissue changes to gain a full understanding of the changes that may be seen following treatment. The longer term effects are complex and are influenced by factors such as relapse, remodelling and the ageing process. To date, research has only focused on the shorter term (6–12 months post-surgery) soft tissue changes and these will be the focus of this chapter.

As well as positive changes, certain orthognathic surgical procedures can have detrimental effects on the soft tissues of the face, particularly in the nasal and submental regions. It is important that these are anticipated and minimised, but also that they are discussed during the planning and consenting stages of treatment as it is important for patients to fully understand the implications of treatment. Also, adjunctive soft tissue procedures may be considered to help reduce these negative changes, although there is a paucity of evidence available about the benefits of such procedures particularly in the longer term.

As well as effects on the soft tissue facial drape, orthognathic surgery can have important effects on

Orthognathic Surgery: Principles, Planning and Practice. Edited by Farhad B. Naini and Daljit S. Gill.

the soft tissues that determine the size and shape of the pharyngeal and nasal airway. These effects may be positive or negative, depending on the type of surgery, and should also be considered during the planning stages. Chapter 44 discusses these effects in more detail.

Research into the soft tissue effects of orthognathic surgery has largely been hampered by a past lack of tools for evaluating changes in all three dimensions, small sample sizes and the involvement of many different surgeons within any given series. These drawbacks can be tackled with use of three-dimensional imaging techniques such as stereophotogrammetry, laser scanning and cone beam computed tomography (CBCT), and improved research study designs to reduce confounding variables.

Before reading the remainder of this chapter, it is essential that the reader appreciates that there is tremendous **individual variation** in the soft tissue response to orthognathic surgery. Therefore, *it is impossible to predict the exact changes that may occur within any given individual.*[3] This chapter will describe the mean changes but is it important to remember that a large standard deviation may be associated with these means. Surgical prediction software utilises algorithms, which may be based upon linear or non-linear movement models, with average changes, and therefore cannot give precise predictions for any given individual. Another limitation of prediction software is that most packages only provide an idea of the changes typically seen in one dimension – the profile view. The possible reasons for the individual variation in soft tissue response are complex and diverse and may include factors such as:

1. Variation in the thickness of the facial soft tissues between individuals. Thicker soft tissues may have a greater ability to support themselves so that the changes may not be as great.[4]
2. Variation in muscular tone between individuals. Where there is greater muscular tone, there may be a closer relationship between hard and soft tissue movements. It is well established that with ageing the tissues become thinner and there is a loss of muscle tone.[5]
3. Anatomical variations in the position of muscular attachments to skeletal structures. The soft tissue responses at sites of muscular attachment are probably greater than at sites of non-attachment.[6]
4. The size of the skeletal movement. It is generally accepted that there is a non-linear relationship between the size of the hard and soft tissue movement. Larger skeletal changes may not induce proportionally larger changes within the soft tissues.
5. The surgical technique employed. The amount of soft tissue dissection, position of the osteotomy cuts (e.g. subspinal Le Fort I) and method of fixation are some factors that may influence the soft tissue responses.

The immediate response to orthognathic surgery

The immediate soft tissue response to orthognathic surgery is largely determined by the magnitude of the inflammatory response to surgical injury. This has been studied by Kau et al. (2007)[7] and Day and Lee (2006),[8] where a small number of patients were followed up prospectively using three-dimensional facial scanning before and after surgery, including both bimaxillary and single jaw procedures. Although the sample sizes were small some interesting general trends were found that may be informative:

1. There is large individual variation in the immediate (<6 months) soft tissue oedema (swelling).
2. Peak swelling typically occurs approximately 48 hours after surgery.
3. The swelling may be asymmetrical in nature. Patients and their carers should be reassured that this is normal; otherwise it can become a matter of concern in the postoperative period.
4. There is a vertical gradient in the reduction of swelling with resolution being quicker in the maxillary region compared to the mandibular region, possibly owing to the effects of gravity on the tissue fluids.
5. Approximately 60% of the swelling had resolved by 1 month following surgery with 100% resolution taking up to 6 months. These figures are useful to remember for the purposes of informed consent. It is possible that studies with larger sample sizes may show that swelling can take longer to resolve.
6. Resolution of swelling is also not symmetrical with one side often settling quicker than the other.

From the results of these two studies it is clear that the final soft tissue response, ignoring longer term soft tissue changes due to skeletal relapse, cannot be evaluated until at least 6 months following surgery. It is important that patients are informed of this during the consenting stages of treatment and that any fine tuning, secondary, adjunctive surgical procedures, for example rhinoplasty, are ideally planned following this period.

Soft tissue changes with maxillary surgery

The Le Fort I osteotomy

The Le Fort I osteotomy can be used to reposition the maxilla anteriorly, posteriorly to a small degree, superiorly and inferiorly. Maxillary advancement, and bimaxillary (maxillomandibular) advancement, has important effects on the soft tissues of the airway that can result in an improvement of the symptoms of obstructive sleep apnoea.[9]

The major facial soft tissue effects are seen within the nasolabial region although three-dimensional studies have also documented changes in the paranasal soft tissues.[6] Vertical repositioning of the maxilla also has an important secondary effect on the position of the mandible, due to autorotation, which will not be considered within this section in any detail but must be borne in mind (see Chapter 6). The major effects of Le Fort I surgery is on the following structures:

- Nose (nasolabial angle, alar bases, nasal tip, supratip depression and dorsal hump);
- Upper lip;
- Paranasal regions.

In almost all cases, a Le Fort I osteotomy results in widening of the alar bases.[10] The significant factor contributing to these changes is the soft tissue dissection rather than the skeletal movements themselves. Periosteal elevation will sever important muscular attachments (zygomaticus major, levator labii superioris, levator labii superioris alaeque nasi and nasalis) leading to muscular retraction, alar flaring and shortening, and flattening and thinning of the upper lip.[11,12] As a guideline the alar base width should ideally equal the intercanthal distance in Caucasians (see Chapter 5). The alar base is wider in African Americans and further widening must often be undertaken with great care. The alar cinch suture, first described by Millard (1980),[13] has been proposed as a method to control alar flaring at the time of surgery, however, some controversy remains as to the effectiveness of this procedure.[14] There is some evidence to suggest that an extraoral alar base cinch suture is more effective in maintaining alar base width, at least in the short-term (<9 months after surgery), compared to the classically described intraoral nasal suture.[15]

Maxillary advancement

Maxillary advancement is most commonly undertaken for the management of maxillary retrognathia, in Class III correction, and occasionally for the correction of bimaxillary retrusion. There is variability in the reported hard to soft tissue movement ratios within the literature,[16] and Table 16-1 summarizes some of the reported changes.

Table 16-1 Range of reported ratios for soft tissue to hard tissue movements in Le Fort I maxillary advancement surgery

Measurement	Ratio
Maxillary incisor to upper lip (stomion superius)	57%[20]
	86%[21]
	70%[6]
	82%[22]
	69%[23]
Alar base widening	9%[24]
Elevation and advancement of nasal tip	34%[20]
	29–34%[6]
	35%[22]
Paranasal area	74–79%[6]

The Le Fort I advancement leads to alar base widening and there is an elevation and widening of the nasal tip, leading to an increase in the supratip depression, and a lowering of the columella. In patients with an already upwardly inclined nasal columella, elevation of the nasal tip can result in an increase in nostril exposure,[17] which may be detrimental to facial aesthetics. If the nasal dorsum is convex in shape, nasal tip elevation can lead to accentuation of this convexity. Conversely, if there is a nasal dorsal hump before surgery, elevation of the nasal tip may improve the nasal appearance. There is no evidence at present that a subspinal osteotomy is superior to a conventional Le Fort I osteotomy in minimising changes at the nasal tip.[18]

Changes to the upper lip include advancement, which may increase the nasolabial angle if subnasale advances more than labrale superius, and shortening due to periosteal dissection. As the nasolabial angle is determined by both the inclination of the upper lip and the columella, the overall change in this angle is dependent upon the change within its individual components which increases the variability of the response.[1,16]

Soncul and Bamber (2004),[6] in a study using three-dimensional surface scans, found that the upper lip at subnasale (80%) followed the skeletal movements more closely than the upper lip at stomion superius (70%) and the upper lip in the supracommissural region (45%). This suggests that there is a vertical and a horizontal gradient in the movement of the upper lip with the biggest changes occurring at subnasale, which is a major area of muscle attachment. The horizontal gradient in the movement of the upper lip may be explained because areas of muscle attachment (incisive and mental slips of orbicularis oris) also occur in the midline, which may also help to explain why the soft tissues follow the hard tissues more closely in these regions.

Advancement of the paranasal soft tissue region appears to closely follow the advancement of the hard tissue.[6] There is evidence to suggest that the soft tissue effects of a high level Le Fort I osteotomy extend further laterally within the face, compared to a conventional Le Fort I osteotomy, to include the zygomatic region,[19] which may be of benefit to those with a degree of malar deficiency.

Maxillary superior repositioning (impaction)

Maxillary impaction is most commonly undertaken for the treatment of vertical maxillary excess, to reduce the lower anterior facial height, close an anterior open bite (posterior maxillary impaction) and reduce incisor or gingival display (anterior impaction). It is very difficult to study the effects of maxillary impaction alone because there is often also a planned anterior-posterior movement of the maxilla.

With maxillary impaction, similar changes occur to those with maxillary advancement such as widening of the alar bases, elevation and widening of the nasal tip and deepening of the supratip nasal depression. Also, secondary to the effects of soft tissue dissection, there may be thinning, shortening and flattening of the upper lip, which can lead to a reduction in vermillion exposure. As a more anterior portion of the maxillary incisor crown comes to lie against the upper lip with impaction, the degree to which flattening of the upper lip occurs will depend on the pretreatment inclination of the maxillary incisors. Where they are proclined, the lip support may increase and when they are more average in inclination the increase in support may be minimal. More research is required to clarify if the V-Y closure method helps to maintain upper lip height following orthognathic surgery.[16]

Maxillary impaction will also result in anticlockwise (or forward) autorotation of the mandible, which will reduce the lower anterior facial height and move the chin point further forward. This not only increases the prominence of the chin point, relative to the forehead, but also increases the prominence relative to the lower lip. This occurs because the lower lip is positioned closer to the centre of rotation of the mandible and moves forward less than pogonion.

Maxillary inferior repositioning (setdown)

The maxilla may be inferiorly repositioned when there is vertical maxillary deficiency, leading to reduced maxillary incisor display and a reduction in the lower anterior facial height. Inferior maxillary repositioning can also help to reduce the prominence of the chin point by causing clockwise (or backward) autorotation of the mandible.

Inferior maxillary movement may lead to drooping of the nasal tip, alar base and columella. Care has to be taken that drooping of the nasal tip does not lead to a 'parrot beak' deformity.[10] The upper lip may flatten and thin with downward movement of the maxilla. This effect is accentuated as a posterior portion of the maxillary incisor crown repositions against the upper lip. The degree of the latter effect will depend again on the inclination of the maxillary incisors. Finally, setting down the maxilla will cause autorotation of the mandible with a resultant increase in lower anterior facial height and posterior movement of the chin point relative to the forehead and lower lip.

Maxillary set-back

Maxillary set-back, at the Le Fort I level, can be undertaken to a small degree for the management of maxillary protrusion during Class II correction. The effects of a set-back may include a reduction of nasal tip and upper lip support. This may lead to a reduction of the supratip depression and an increase in the nasolabial angle. There may be widening of the alar bases due to soft tissue dissection.

Soft tissue changes with mandibular surgery

Bilateral sagittal split osteotomy (BSSO)

The main indications for the BSSO are for the correction of mandibular retrognathism, prognathism and asymmetry. A recent systematic review on the profile changes after BSSO advancement concluded that there was poor evidence on the short and long term effects of advancement.[25] Studies tend to have small sample sizes, no power calculation and a mixture of surgical procedures performed on the study subjects.

Mandibular advancement

With mandibular advancement alone, one can expect a downward and forward repositioning of soft tissue pogonion with a resultant reduction in facial convexity, increase in the lower anterior facial height and increase in throat length. The increase in lower anterior facial height will be influenced by the maxillary occlusal plane inclination, with a steeper plane resulting in a greater increase in lower facial height. The reported short-term (<2 years) and long-term (>2 years) ratios with rigid fixation are summarized in Table 16-2.[25]

The figures in Table 16-2 generally suggest that a vertical gradient in effects exists with the greater proportional changes occurring at soft tissue pogonion with reducing changes as one moves up to the upper lip. In the short-term the upper lip can be affected by oedema and the upper lip may also follow the lower lip movement to some degree. Longer term changes to the upper lip may be related to relapse and the ageing process with gradual thinning and inferior movement of labrale superius.[26] The changes at soft tissue pogonion may be more predictable as there is close attachment of the facial muscles onto this bony region.

With mandibular advancement, one may also expect a reduction in facial convexity, an increase in submental length, reduction in any submental soft tissue sag, and a reduction of the lower lip-chin-submental plane angle. There may also be an uncurling effect on the lower lip, particularly if the preoperative lower facial height was reduced.[27] Although mandibular advancement had no effect on absolute nasal dimensions,

Table 16-2 Range of ratios for soft tissue to hard tissue movements for mandibular advancement, without genioplasty, with rigid internal fixation[25]

	Short-term (<2 year) ratios	Long-term (>2 year) ratios
Upper lip to incisor inferior	−2% to 29%	−10% to −67%
Lower lip to incisor inferior	35% to 108%	31% to 60%
Mentolabial fold to B-point	88% to 111%	86% to 111%
Soft tissue pogonion to hard tissue pogonion	90% to 124%	102% to 127%

Table 16-3 Range of ratios for soft tissue to hard tissue movements for mandibular set-back, without genioplasty, with rigid internal fixation.[28]

	Short-term (<2 year) ratios	Long-term (>2 year) ratios
Soft tissue pogonion to hard tissue pogonion	–94% to 128%	94% (after 3 y)
Mentolabial fold to B-Point	106% to 108%	106% (after 3 y)
Labrale inferius to incision inferius	73% to 90%	100% (after 3 y)
Labrale superius to hard tissue pogonion	–1% to 23%	35% (after 3 y)

advancement of the chin point may reduce the relative prominence of the nose in relation to the forehead and chin point.

Mandibular set-back

The reported short-term (<2 years) and long-term (>2 years) soft tissue ratios for mandibular set-back are summarized in Table 16-3.[28]

The figures in Table 16-3 suggest a vertical gradient in effects occurring, with the greatest proportional changes occurring at soft tissue pogonion, and with reducing changes as one moves up to the upper lip. The upper lip may move forwards slightly in a number of cases, possibly because it is not trapped by the lower lip following mandibular set-back. Again, the changes at soft tissue pogonion may be more predictable as there is close attachment of the musculature onto this region.

With mandibular set-back, one may also expect a reduction in facial concavity, a reduction in submental length, increase in submental soft tissue sag, and an increase of the lower lip-chin-submental plane angle. Although mandibular set-back has no effect on absolute nasal dimensions, setting back the chin point may increase the relative prominence of the nose in comparison to the forehead and chin point. Particular attention should be paid to the effects of mandibular set-back on submental aesthetics during the planning stages of treatment. Submental-cervical surgical procedures may be required as adjunctive procedures. For example, submental liposuction may be used to attempt to reduce these negative changes. However, there are no clinical trials evaluating the effectiveness of this procedure.

Genioplasty

Genioplasty is a versatile surgical procedure that allows sagittal, vertical and transverse changes to be made to the chin without affecting the dental occlusion. It can be undertaken in isolation or in combination with other more extensive mandibular procedures.

With advancement genioplasty the reported ratio of hard to soft tissue changes range from 1:0.6 to 1:1.[29–35] Effects also include an increase in the submental length, a reduction in submental soft tissue sag, a decrease in the lower lip-chin-submental plane angle, deepening of the labiomental fold, a reduction in facial convexity and a reduction in relative nasal prominence. Because genioplasty involves dissection of the mentalis muscle, which is important in elevating the lower lip, there may be an increase in lower incisor exposure following surgery.[36]

There are fewer reported studies on the soft tissue effects of set-back genioplasty and sample sizes tend to be smaller. The opposite changes may be expected with set-back genioplasty and a recent study suggested a soft tissue:hard tissue movement ratio of 1:1 at menton, 0.7:1 at pogonion and 0.9:1 at B-point.[37] Effects also may include a decrease in the submental length, a possible increase in submental soft tissue sag, an increase in the lower lip-chin-submental plane angle, a reduction of the mentolabial fold, an increase in soft tissue thickness,[37] an increase in facial convexity and a relative increase in perceived nasal prominence.

Conclusions

Orthognathic surgery can lead to significant alteration in the position of the soft tissues. These changes are not restricted to the soft tissues of the face but also the soft tissues forming the airway. There is large individual variability in how the soft tissues respond to changes in the underlying hard tissues making precise prediction planning difficult. It is important that potential detrimental effects of surgery are discussed with the patient early on such that realistic expectations are achieved and, if necessary, adjunctive surgical procedures are carried out to minimize any undesirable changes.

References

1 Naini FB, Cobourne MT, McDonald F, Wertheim D. The aesthetic impact of upper lip inclination in orthodontics and orthognathic surgery. Eur J Orthod. 2015;37:81–6.
2 Nooreyazdan M, Trotman CA, Faraway JJ. Modeling facial movement: II. A dynamic analysis of differences caused by orthognathic surgery. J Oral Maxillofac Surg. 2004;62:1380–6.
3 Kaipatur NR, Flores-Mir C. Accuracy of computer programs in predicting orthognathic surgery soft tissue response. J Oral Maxillofac Surg. 2009;67:751–9.
4 Mobarak KA, Espeland L, Krogstad O, Lyberg T. Soft tissue profile changes following mandibular advancement surgery: Predictability and long-term outcome. Am J Orthod Dentofacial Orthop. 2001;119:353–67.
5 Zoumalan RA, Larrabee WF Jr. Anatomic considerations in the aging face. Facial Plast Surg. 2011;27:16–22.
6 Soncul M, Bamber MA. Evaluation of facial soft tissue changes with optical surface scan after surgical correction of Class III deformities. J Oral Maxillofac Surg. 2004;62:1331–40.
7 Kau CH, Cronin AJ, Richmond S. A three-dimensional evaluation of postoperative swelling following orthognathic surgery at 6 months. Plast Reconstr Surg. 2007;119:2192–9.

8 Day CJ, Lee RT. Three-dimensional assessment of the facial soft tissue changes that occur postoperatively in orthognathic patients. World J Orthod. 2006;7:15–26.
9 Holty JE, Guilleminault C. Maxillomandibular advancement for the treatment of obstructive sleep apnea: a systematic review and meta-analysis. Sleep Med Rev. 2010;14:287–97.
10 Schendel SA, Carlotti AE Jr. Nasal considerations in orthognathic surgery. Am J Orthod Dentofacial Orthop. 1991;100:197–208.
11 Altman JI, Oeltjen JC. Nasal deformities associated with orthognathic surgery: analysis, prevention, and correction. J Craniofac Surg. 2007;18:734–9.
12 O'Ryan F, Schendel SA Jr. Nasolabial Esthetics and Maxillary Surgery. In: Bell WH, ed. Modern Practice in Orthognathic and Reconstructive Surgery. St Louis: W.B. Saunders, 1992.
13 Millard Jr DR. The alar cinch in the flat, flaring nose. Plast Reconstr Surg. 1980;65:669–72.
14 Howley C, Ali N, Lee R, Cox S. Use of alar base cinch suture in Le Fort I osteotomy: is it effective? Br J Oral Maxillofac Surg. 2011;49:127–30.
15 Ritto FG, Medeiros PJ, Moraes M, Ribeiro DPB. Comparative analysis of two different alar base sutures after Le Fort 1 osteotomy: randomised double-blind controlled trial. Oral Surg Med Oral Pathol Oral Radiol Endod. 2011;111:181–9.
16 Khamashta- Ledezma L, Naini FB. Systematic review of the changes in maxillary incisor exposure and upper lip position with Le Fort I type osteotomies with or without cinch sutures and/ or VY closures. Int J Oral Maxillofac Surg. 2014;43:46–61.
17 Dann JJ 3rd, Fonseca RJ, Bell WH. Soft tissue changes associated with total maxillary advancement: a preliminary study. J Oral Surg. 1976;34:19–23.
18 Mommaerts MY, Lippens F, Abeloos VS, Neyt LF. Nasal profile changes after maxillary impaction and advancement surgery. J Oral Maxillofac Surg. 2000;58:470–5.
19 Kim Y, Park S, Son W, Hwang D. Midfacial soft-tissue changes after advancement of the maxilla with Le Fort I osteotomy and mandibular setback surgery: Comparison of conventional and high Le Fort I osteotomies by superimposition of cone-beam computed tomography volumes. J Oral Maxillofac Surg. 2011;69:e225–e33.
20 McCollum AG, Dancaster JT, Evans WG, Becker PJ. Sagittal soft tissue changes related to the surgical corrections of maxillary deficient class III malocclusions. Semin Orthod. 2009;15:172–84.
21 Conley RS, Boyd SB. Facial soft tissue changes following maxillomandibular advancement for treatment of obstructive sleep apnoea. J Oral Maxillofac Surg. 2007;65:1332–40.
22 Lin S, Kerr WJ. Soft and hard tissue changes in Class III patients treated by bimaxillary surgery. Eur J Orthod. 1998;20:25–33.
23 Jensen AC, Sinclair PM, Wolford LM. Soft tissue changes associated with double jaw surgery. Am J Orthod Dentofacial Orthop. 1992;101:266–75.
24 Betts NJ, Vig KW, Vig P, Spalding P, Fonseca RJ. Changes in the nasal and labial soft tissues after surgical repositioning of the maxilla. Int J Adult Orthodon Orthognath Surg. 1993;8:7–23.
25 Joss CU, Joss-Vassalli IM, Kiliaridis S, Kuijpers-Jagtman AM. Soft tissue profile changes after bilateral sagittal split osteotomy for mandibular advancement: a systematic review. J Oral Maxillofac Surg. 2010;68:1260–9.
26 Behrents RG. Growth in the aging craniofacial skeleton. In McNamara JA (Ed.) Monograph 17, Craniofacial Growth Series. Ann Arbor, University of Michigan, 1985.
27 Maal TJJ, de Koning MJJ, Plooij JM, Verhamme LM, Rangel FA, Berge SJ and Borslap WA. One year postoperative hard and soft tissue volumetric changes after a BSSO mandibular advancement. Int J Oral Maxillofac Surg. 2012;41:1137–45.
28 Joss CU, Joss-Vassalli IM, Berge SJ and Kuipers-Jagtman AM. Soft tissue profile changes after bilateral sagittal split osteotomy for mandibular setback: A systematic review. J Oral Maxillofac Surg. 2010;68:2792–801.
29 McDonnell JP, McNeill RW, West RA. Advancement genioplasty: A retrospective cephalometric analysis of osseous and soft tissue changes. J Oral Surg. 1977; 35:640–7.
30 Park HS, Ellis E, Fonseca RJ, Reynolds ST, Mayo KH. A retrospective study of advancement genioplasty. Oral Surg Oral Med Oral Pathol. 1989;67:481–9.
31 Davis WH, Davis CL, Daly BW. Long term bony and soft tissue stability following advancement genioplasty. J Oral Maxillofac Surg. 1988;46:731–5.
32 Nishioka GJ, Mason M, Van sickels JE. Neurosensory disturbance associated with the anterior mandibular horizontal osteotomy. J Oral Maxillofac Surg. 1988;46:107–10.
33 Polido WD, Regis LDC, Bell WH. Bone resorption, stability and soft-tissue changes following large chin advancements. J Oral Maxillofac Surg. 1991;49:251–6.
34 Talebzadeh N, Pogrel MA. Long-term hard and soft tissue relapse rate after genioplasty. Oral Surg Oral Med Oral Pathol Oral Radiol Endod. 2001; 91:153–6.
35 Reddy PS, Kashyap B, Hallur N, Sikkerimath BC. Advancement genioplasty – cephalometric analysis of osseous and soft tissue changes. J. Maxillofac. Oral Surg. 2011;10: 288–95.
36 Soydan SS, Cubuk S, Pektas ZO, Uckan S. The extent of chin ptosis and lower incisor exposure changes following the osseous genioplasties. J Craniofac Surg. 2013;24:e445–58.
37 Park J, Kim MJ, Hwang SJ. Soft tissue profile changes after setback genioplasty in orthognathic surgery patients. J Cranio-Maxillo-Facial Surg. 2013;41:657–64.

Chapter 17

Early Orthognathic Surgery: Considerations for Surgical Management

Pushkar Mehra and Larry M. Wolford

Introduction

Growing patients can present with significant dentofacial deformities that may require early surgical intervention for specific functional, aesthetic, and psychosocial factors. Although there is extensive literature regarding the effects and stability of orthognathic surgical correction of dentofacial deformities in adults, there are few studies in reference to paediatric and adolescent growing patients. Not as much is known about the predictability of orthognathic surgical procedures performed during growth, and the effects that such procedures have on subsequent facial growth and development. The dilemma for orthodontists and surgeons who may consider early treatment revolves around the following main areas:

a) What is the appropriate timing for orthognathic surgery in growing patients?
b) What differences exist in anatomy?
c) What alterations in surgical technique will be required?
d) Will there be any adverse effects of such surgery on subsequent growth?

This chapter discusses some common dentofacial deformities, the surgical techniques applicable for each, and the earliest age (in our experience) at which these can be performed with predictable results. There are, of course, exceptions to these general guidelines, based on individual patient characteristics, hormonal or other factors affecting growth, the presenting deformity, temporomandibular joint (TMJ) pathology, other local or systemic factors, and the orthodontist's and surgeon's clinical abilities.

Orthognathic Surgery: Principles, Planning and Practice. Edited by Farhad B. Naini and Daljit S. Gill.

Diagnostic considerations

General considerations

Facial appearance is an important factor in child growth and development.[1,2] It is well documented that aesthetics plays a major role in determining interpersonal relationships. Orthognathic surgery is often performed for functional and aesthetic reasons, but when performed during growth may hold important psychosocial implications for some younger patients. Teenage patients with significant dentofacial deformities are often perceived as less attractive by their friends and others. This difference of behaviour towards attractive and unattractive people has been well-documented. Delaying orthognathic surgery until growth is complete or alternatively choosing non-surgical treatments (e.g. myofunctional therapy, or orthodontic and dental camouflage) may not always be acceptable options. In some cases, they could be damaging to the patient's self-image and adversely affect a child's social development. Delaying treatment until adulthood can also potentially exacerbate problems related to occlusion, mastication, TMJ function and dysfunction, speech, airway, and the psychosocial component.

Jaw growth considerations

Determination of growth rate and vector can be challenging. As the jaws grow in all three dimensions, growth disturbances can occur in one or more dimensions. Generally, females have about 98% of facial growth complete by age 15 years and males by the age of approximately 17 years.[3,4] An understanding of facial growth tendencies of the specific anatomical facial types (e.g. brachycephalic, normocephalic, dolicocephalic) provides important information about subsequent growth. Evaluation of the patient's medical and family history, as well as serial clinical and radiographic examinations are helpful to identify growth imbalances of the jaw structures. Comparison of serial lateral and posteroanterior (PA) cephalometric radiographs, as well as dental models can be helpful in growth assessment relative to skeletal and occlusal changes. Specialized radiography (e.g. CT scans, MRI, nuclear scintiography) may be indicated in certain cases, especially for identification of TMJ pathology. Hand-wrist films or other such comparisons may be useful in determining the growth potential in some patients, but are not usually beneficial for skeletal Class III patients, especially those with condylar hyperplasia. The effects of orthognathic surgery on subsequent facial growth and development also require understanding so that timing of required surgery will minimize adverse affects on jaw growth.

TMJ considerations

Two-thirds of all TMJ pathologies begin during the teenage years, particularly during the pubertal growth phase. TMJ pathology can create dentofacial deformities, develop as a result of the dentofacial deformity, or the two conditions can develop independently. If the TMJs are not healthy and stable, orthognathic surgical results may be unstable with resultant increased TMJ dysfunction, pain, and relapse of the surgical and orthodontic results.[5] Therefore, it is very important to evaluate the TMJs in growing patients prior to any contemplated surgical intervention clinically, radiographically, and with MRI when indicated.

The most common TMJ disorder seen in orthognathic surgery patients is the displaced TMJ articular disc, which can be identified clinically by the presence of clicking and popping, but only if the disc is anteriorly displaced with reduction on opening. Patients may have displaced TMJ discs but exhibit no clicking or popping in conditions such as: anterior disc displacement without reduction; medial, lateral, and posterior disc displacements; certain pathologies that cause thickening of the bilaminar tissues; or previous treatment with growth appliances or 'disc recapturing' splints where the bilaminar tissues have thickened so there is a smooth transition onto the displaced disc on opening. These 'silent' joints increase the difficulties in identifying the presence or absence of TMJ disc displacement. It has been documented that post-surgical complications can occur when orthognathic surgery (especially anticlockwise rotation with mandibular advancement) is performed in the presence of TMJ articular disc displacement that is left unrepaired, such as initiation or increased TMJ pain, headaches, myofascial pain, skeletal and occlusal instability, condylar resorption, etc. Thus, we recommend an MRI examination to adequately evaluate the TMJ and associated areas prior to surgery in cases where TMJ pathology is suspected.

Progressive changes in jaw position and occlusion or the development of facial asymmetry are usually related to TMJ pathology. TMJ pathologies that may create these changes and affect treatment outcomes include condylar hyperplasia, condylar hypoplasia, adolescent internal condylar resorption (AICR), idiopathic condylar resorption, reactive arthritis, osteochondroma, juvenile idiopathic arthritis (JIA), connective tissue/autoimmune diseases, traumatic injuries, and various other arthritides. These conditions are usually associated with bone morphology changes and although some of these conditions may not be readily apparent on plain fims (e.g. panoramic radiographs), they may be identified with specialized imaging investigations including MRIs, CT scans with 3-dimensional reconstructions and nuclear scintigraphy scans.

Habitual considerations

Children and teenagers with dentofacial deformities may have associated habits such as thumb sucking, tongue thrusting, etc. The tongue is an important factor in jaw growth and development. The tongue usually reaches its approximate adult size by the age of 8 years.[6] An evaluation of the tongue should include clinical and functional assessments relative to interference with speech, mastication, airway, and treatment stability. Microglossia can cause underdevelopment of the jaws with lingual collapse of the dentoalveolar structures. Macroglossia can result in overdevelopment of the jaws, especially the dentoalveolus. The most common cause of macroglossia is muscular hypertrophy. When indicated, a speech and swallowing (dysphagia) specialist can be consulted and proper tongue posture and movement corrections achieved prior to surgery. Surgical reduction of the tongue size may be indicated in patients with true macroglossia to improve treatment outcomes.[7]

It is not uncommon to encounter habitual posturing of the mandible anteriorly with hyper-extension of the head in significant Class II cases as a secondary response to open the constricted oropharyngeal airway obstruction or an intentional response to improve unfavourable aesthetics, thus causing a significant centric relation-centric occlusion shift. In growing patients with significant skeletal Class II relations, a triad of associated factors may be present: (1) TMJ pathology; (2) Nasal airway obstruction (hypertrophied turbinates, deviated septum, etc.) and (3) Constricted oropharyngeal airway (hypertrophied nasopharyngeal adenoids and tonsils, retruded mandible posteriorly displacing the tongue and soft palate, etc.) creating the potential for obstructive sleep apnoea in these young patients. For these patients additional evaluations may include polysomnography, TMJ evaluation, 3-D airway evaluation, etc. Some patients may benefit from pre-orthognathic surgery treatment such as tonsillectomy, adenoidectomy, splint therapy, appliances, muscle weakening and strengthening, physical therapy, CPAP, etc.

Mandibular deformities

Mandibular hypoplasia/retrognathism

These patients usually present with Class II skeletal and dental relationships. An important aspect in diagnosis is to determine whether the mandibular growth pattern is normal (proportional growth) or deficient (disproportional growth). In the former, the maxilla and mandible are growing at normal and congruent rates while in the latter the mandible is slower in development than the opposing maxilla. Thus, the overjet and Class II relationships would be relatively stable during the subsequent growth years in normal/proportional growers as compared to deficient/disproportional growers, where the Class II relationship would worsen during the remaining growth years as the mandible lags behind the normally growing maxilla. This interruption of normal mandibular growth is commonly related to TMJ pathologies or congenital deformities.

Two common TMJ disorders occurring in this younger patient population include disc displacement and AICR. AICR is a common condition seen predominately in teenage females, with onset between the ages of 11 to 15 years, where the discs become anteriorly displaced and the mandibular condyles slowly but progressively resorb, creating a retruded mandible, high occlusal plane angle facial morphology, with or without clicking/popping or pain. Other less common TMJ pathologies include reactive arthritis, ankylosis, and JIA. These TMJ conditions need to be addressed or the treatment outcomes may be significantly compromised.

Surgical considerations

Patients with normal harmonious growth patterns and healthy TMJs can be treated relatively early with mandibular orthognathic surgery with predictable and stable results.[8–10] The aim of the surgery is to spatially advance the mandible forward into alignment with the maxilla. If maxillary and mandibular growth is normal at equal rates, maintenance of the surgical results can be expected, especially relative to occlusion. Contrastingly, in patients with deficient mandibular growth, a surgical mandibular advancement would be expected to redevelop a Class II relationship as the maxilla continues to grow normally and the mandible maintains its deficient growth rate.[11] Surgery during growth may be indicated in cases of disproportional growth, especially in cases of severe deformities with adversely affected function (e.g. malnutrition secondary to masticatory dysfunction, airway compromise, and speech disorders) or for psychosocial factors. In these circumstances, surgery during active growth may improve the quality of life, however, the patient and parents must be made aware that additional surgery may likely be necessary at a later stage.

The bilateral mandibular ramus sagittal split osteotomy is the procedure of choice for surgical management of these patients. With healthy TMJs and proper use of routine surgical techniques, the rate of growth should be unaltered by surgery since the surgical procedure is performed in the mandibular body and ramus areas. The post-surgical vector of facial growth may be altered by proximal segment rotation and final repositioning during the mandibular osteotomy fixation.[12]

In patients with excessive vertical growth of the maxilla, a skeletal Class II tendency with deficient chin projection (convex facial profile) may be seen at growth completion despite maintenance of the occlusion relationships; this occurs as even though the advanced mandible and unoperated maxilla grow proportionally post-surgically, the downward vector from the increased vertical maxillary growth pushes the chin in a downward and backward direction. In cases of repositioned TMJ discs the mandible should continue to grow normally as long as the condyles are not damaged during surgery. Figure 17-1 shows the clinical course with long-term follow up of a Class II

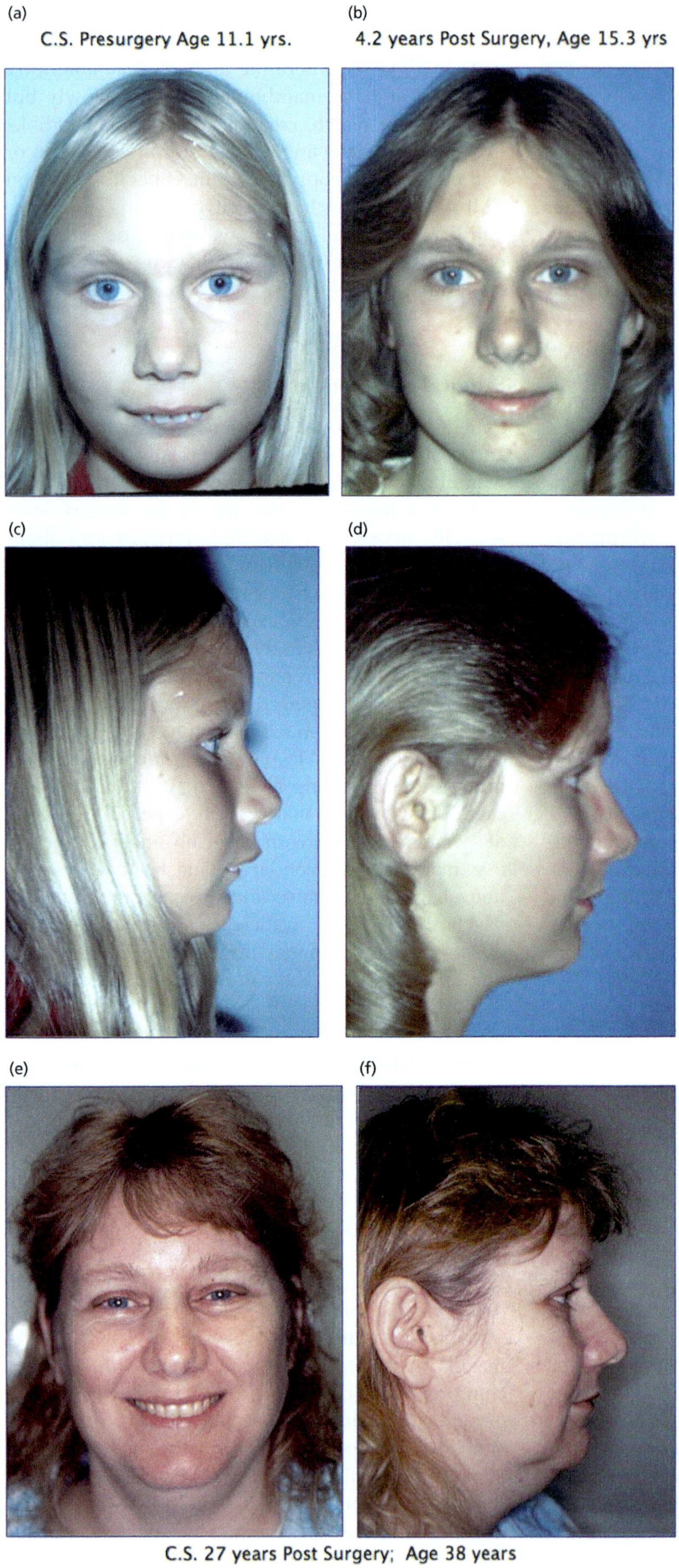

Fig. 17-1 (a) Preoperative frontal view of an 11.1-year-old actively growing female patient with mandibular retrognathism. (b) Four years postoperative frontal view of same patient at age 15.3 years. The patient was a 'proportional' grower and the mandible was advanced with bilateral mandibular ramus sagittal split osteotomies at age 11.1 years. (c) Preoperative profile view at age 11 years. (d) Postoperative profile at age 15 years. (e) Frontal view at age 38 years (27 years post-surgery). (f) Profile view at age 38 years (27 years post-surgery). (g–i) Intraoral photographs taken at the 27-year postoperative interval demonstrating maintenance of occlusion and stability of surgical results. (j) Preoperative cephalometric tracing at 11.1 years of age demonstrating Class II skeletal relationship. (k) Postoperative cephalometric tracing at 15.3 years of age demonstrating surgical movements performed (mandibular advancement). (l) Superimposition of the 5-month and 8.7-year postoperative radiographs, demonstrating the postoperative facial growth vector in a downward and forward direction.

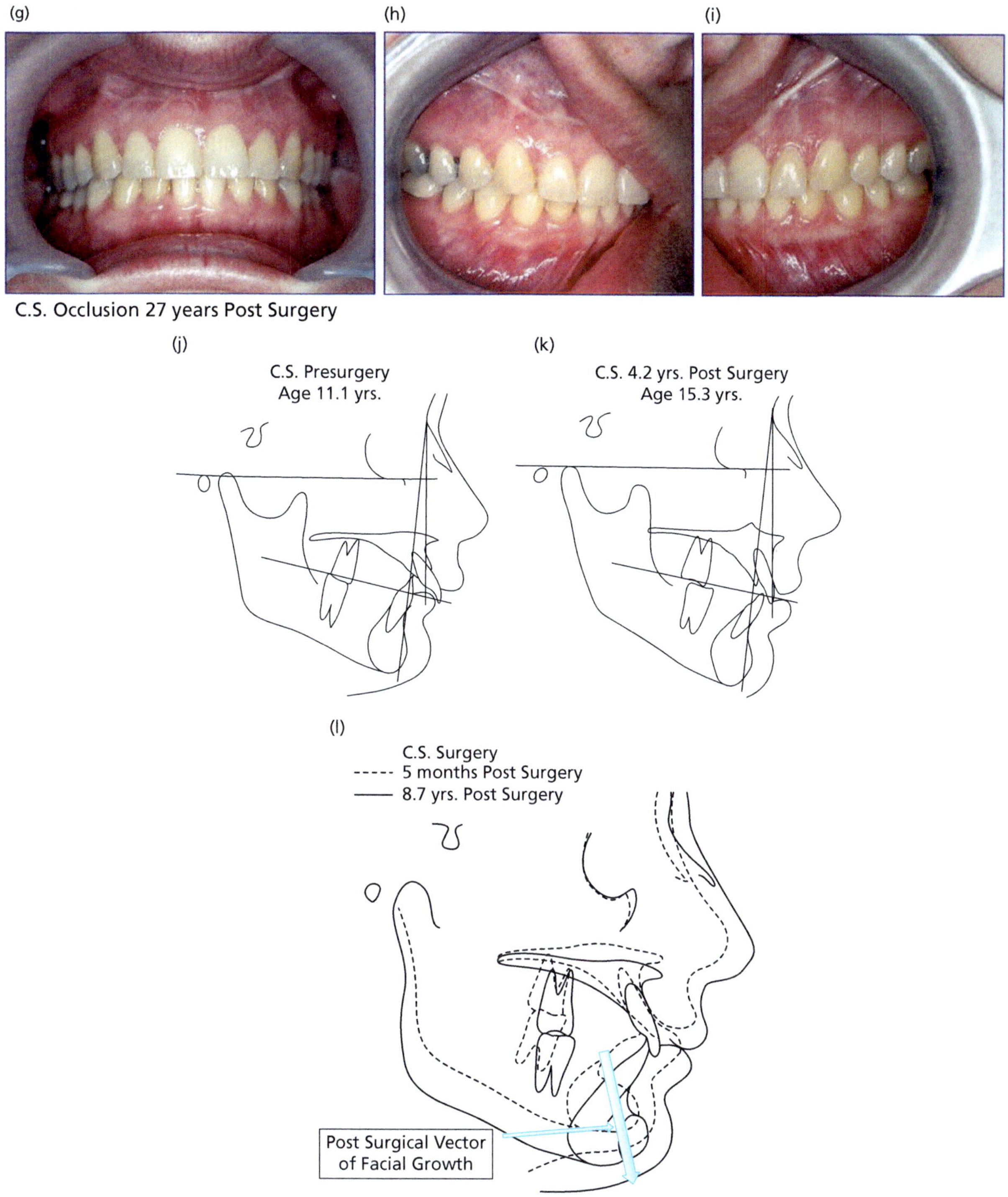

Fig. 17-1 (*Continued*).

patient who underwent early orthognathic surgery during growth.

Mandibular retrognathism with TMJ disorders[13–16]

TMJ pathologies require treatment to provide stable orthognathic outcomes. For patients requiring TMJ surgery, it is performed first as either a separate procedure prior to the orthognathic surgery or it can be done concomitantly in the same operation depending on the surgeon's preference and expertise.

If surgical repositioning of the displaced discs is necessary (*salvageable discs*), it is best accomplished by open TMJ surgery. Various techniques exist in the literature for surgical disc repositioning but in the authors' research based experience, use of a bone anchor (Mitek mini anchors with 0-Ethibond suture as artificial ligaments) to secure the discs to the condyles provides for the most optimal outcomes. Our studies have demonstrated that there is generally a 4 to 6-year window from the onset of the disc displacement to where the repair outcomes are highly predictable. Beyond this time frame, the disc is often morphologically and structurally altered, and repositioning surgery may have a significantly lower success rate.

One of the authors of this chapter (LMW) has recently published a report of successful treatment of AICR cases with concomitant TMJ and orthognathic surgery with arrest of the condylar resorption using the Mitek anchor disc repositioning technique. In younger treated patients with residual growth potential, the condyles have been shown to even begin to grow relatively normally again until normal cessation of growth is complete. More clinical data and multicentre studies are required to document the long-term predictability of these promising reports.

In cases where the discs are non-salvageable (often seen in JIA, ankylosis, reactive arthritis, or long-standing disc dislocation conditions), TMJ reconstruction is required. Autogenous TMJ reconstruction with costochondral and sternoclavicular grafts are traditionally accepted options for TMJ reconstruction in growing patients. Patient-fitted total joint prostheses are our preferred method for TMJ reconstruction for these end-stage conditions in growing patients from 10 years old or older. Many surgeons elect to wait until growth is complete and then perform TMJ reconstruction with patient-fitted total joint prostheses. Use of these prostheses allows for large mandibular advancements, minimizes operating room time, besides eliminating donor site morbidity. With the use of total joint alloplastic prostheses, no postoperative anteroposterior (A-P) growth of the mandible will occur. Thus, when used at a younger age, secondary surgery may be indicated such as orthognathic surgery procedures and possibly replacement of the mandibular components with longer length components.

Mandibular hyperplasia/prognathism[14–16]

Growing patients with Class III skeletal and occlusal relationships require careful assessment to determine the aetiology of their deformity. In treating mandibular prognathism, tongue size and position must be carefully evaluated presurgery. The most common tongue related factors affecting surgical results are macroglossia and habitual tongue posture. When the mandible is surgically moved posteriorly, the volume of the oral cavity decreases and the tongue displaces posteriorly. An enlarged tongue or abnormal tongue posturing habit may create post-surgical relapse by causing forward posturing of the condyle relative to the fossa, lead to shifting between segments that are wire fixated, or cause forward protrusion of the mandibular and maxillary dentoalveolus. This condition may present with a normal or accelerated mandibular growth rate.

Condylar hyperplasia (CH) is a relatively common condition of various aetiologies that causes enlargement of the mandibular condyle, neck, and mandibular body resulting in dentofacial deformity and malocclusion, usually developing during pubertal growth in the teenage years. A new proposed classification system based on occurrence rate and aetiology is as follows: CH type 1 identifies enlargement of the condyle and mandible by an accelerated rate of condylar growth of the 'normal' condylar growth mechanism and can occur bilaterally (CH type 1A) or unilaterally (CH type 1B) with predominately a horizontal mandibular growth vector creating symmetrical or asymmetrical mandibular prognathism. CH type 2 identifies a unilateral condylar enlargement related to a benign tumour (osteochondroma) that develops in the condyle usually causing unilateral vertical elongation of the mandible, maxilla, and face as well as a malocclusion. The condylar growth can occur predominately vertically (CH type 2A) or the tumour can grow horizontal extensions off the condyle (CH type 2B) that are sometimes quite large. CH type 3 covers other benign tumours, and CH type 4 consists of malignant tumours initiated in the condyle.

In mandibular prognathic patients with a normal proportionate growth rate with the maxilla, the mandible initiates its growth from a forward position relative to the maxilla, or the mandible is anatomically larger, but maintains the same Class III jaw relation throughout growth. This deformity can be corrected during growth with predictable and stable results using various mandibular ramus osteotomies. With these techniques, the rate of growth should be unaltered by surgery, and harmonious postoperative maxillary and mandibular growth can be expected, with maintenance of the surgical result.

In contrast, in patients with disproportional accelerated mandibular growth rate (CH type 1), the Class III skeletal and occlusal relationship becomes progressively more severe or begins as a Class I relationship and develops into a progressively worsening Class III relation. The accelerated mandibular growth is usually initiated during pubertal growth and outpaces the normal maxillary growth in this condition. However, it is important to note that maxillary growth deficiency with normal and/or accelerated mandibular growth can create the Class III jaw and occlusal relationship, thus, these maxillary deficient patients must be clearly differentiated from the patients with accelerated mandibular growth but normal maxillary growth.

The increase in mandibular growth rate occurs as a result of the accelerated 'normal' growth mechanism (growth plate) in the mandibular condyles (CH type 1). Patients with this pathological condition present with a radiographic picture usually demonstrating elongation of the condylar head, neck, and mandibular body, leading to subsequent development of dental compensations (lingual inclination of the mandibular incisors and excessive labial inclination of the maxillary incisors), especially in long-standing cases. The condition usually begins during the pubertal growth phase, and rarely precedes or succeeds it. The growth can continue far beyond the normal growth period (15 years old for females, 17 to 18 years old for males) into the early and middle twenties but the growth condition is self-limiting. Growth may be accelerated bilaterally (CH type 1A) or unilaterally (CH type 1B), and usually in a horizontal vector, but it can occasionally grow in a vertical direction.

Age considerations

The following are three options regarding the timing of surgery relative to growing Class III patients with active CH type 1:

Treatment Option 1: Defer surgery until growth is complete

The maxilla and mandible in most patients with dentofacial deformities stop growing at predictable times; usually about age 15 years for females and 17 to 18 years for males. However, jaws in Class III patients with CH type 1 may grow into the mid-20s. A significant advantage of delaying surgery until growth is complete is that only orthognathic surgery will be required unless there is an associated TMJ articular disc displacement that requires surgical disc repositioning. Potential disadvantages include prolongation of functional problems (mastication, speech), aesthetic disfigurement, pain, and psychosocial stigmata associated with a significant facial deformity. Additionally, the magnitude of the deformity will worsen, including deformity of the mandible, significant dental compensations, and increased volume of skin and soft tissue, making the surgery more complex, and may preclude an ideal result. Compensatory changes are likely to occur in the maxilla particularly with dentoalveolar compensations. CH type 1B, because it is unilateral, can generate significant mandibular asymmetry creating warpage of the mandible, additional dental compensations, and unilateral increase in skin and soft tissue volumes adding additional difficulties to the treatment including the increased risk of developing TMJ internal derangements.

Treatment Option 2: Perform surgery to posteriorly position the mandible during growth, with over-correction of the mandible (based on estimation)

The accelerated growth should be expected to continue after surgery, and repeat surgery will be necessary if the overcorrection was insufficient or excessive. Early intervention may benefit the patient, relative to function, aesthetics, and psychosocial concerns. If this alternative is chosen, surgery is best performed after the majority of maxillary growth is complete to better facilitate the estimation of over-correction necessary. The authors do not recommend use of this 'guessing' approach.

Treatment Option 3: Surgically eliminate further mandibular growth with open joint surgery for high condylectomies (Figure 17-2), with concomitant or delayed correction of the jaw deformity using standard orthognathic surgery techniques

The high condylectomy procedure surgically removes the active growth centre(s), and thus prevents further mandibular growth. If orthognathic and TMJ surgery are performed concomitantly at one operation, the mandibular sagittal split ramus osteotomy (SSRO) is the procedure of choice since it maintains maximal soft tissue attachments, and thus vascularity to the proximal segment. Other commonly used techniques to set the mandible posteriorly include the inverted 'L' osteotomy (ILO) and the vertical ramus osteotomy (VRO), but require increased stripping of periosteum, may lead to vascular compromise of the proximal segment, cause difficulties with positional control of the condyle, and may require intermaxillary (maxillomandibular) fixation, that may increase the risk of adhesions and ankylosis development when performed with concomitant TMJ surgery. Figure 17-3 shows a growing patient with a Class III malocclusion who was treated for CH with high condylectomies and concomitant orthognathic surgery.

(a) (b)

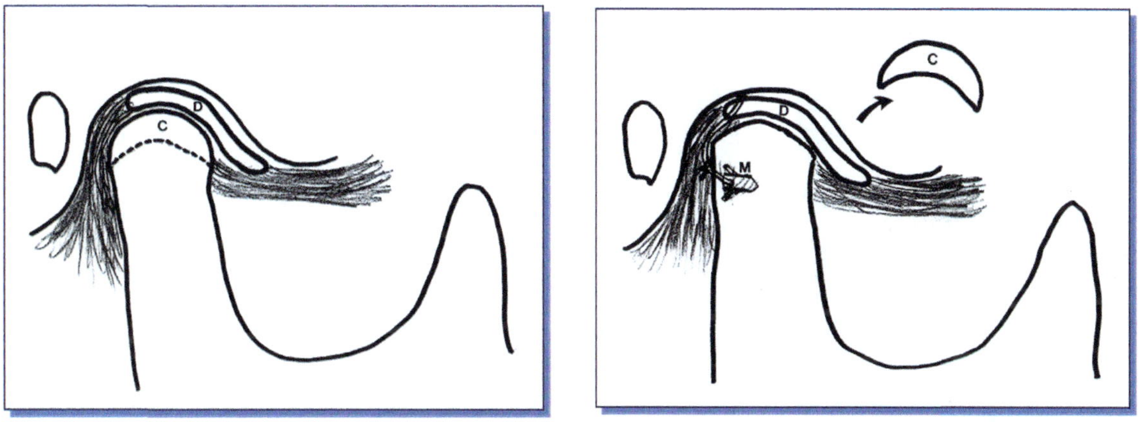

Fig. 17-2 The high condylectomy procedure (dotted line) involves removal of the superior 3–5 mm of the cartilaginous cap and associated head of the mandibular condyle. The bone is then recontoured to reform a condylar stump and usually the articular disc repositioned and stabilized to re-establish a normal condyle–disk relationship. It is an invasive yet predictable method to stop mandibular growth.

(a) (b) (c) (d) (e) (f)

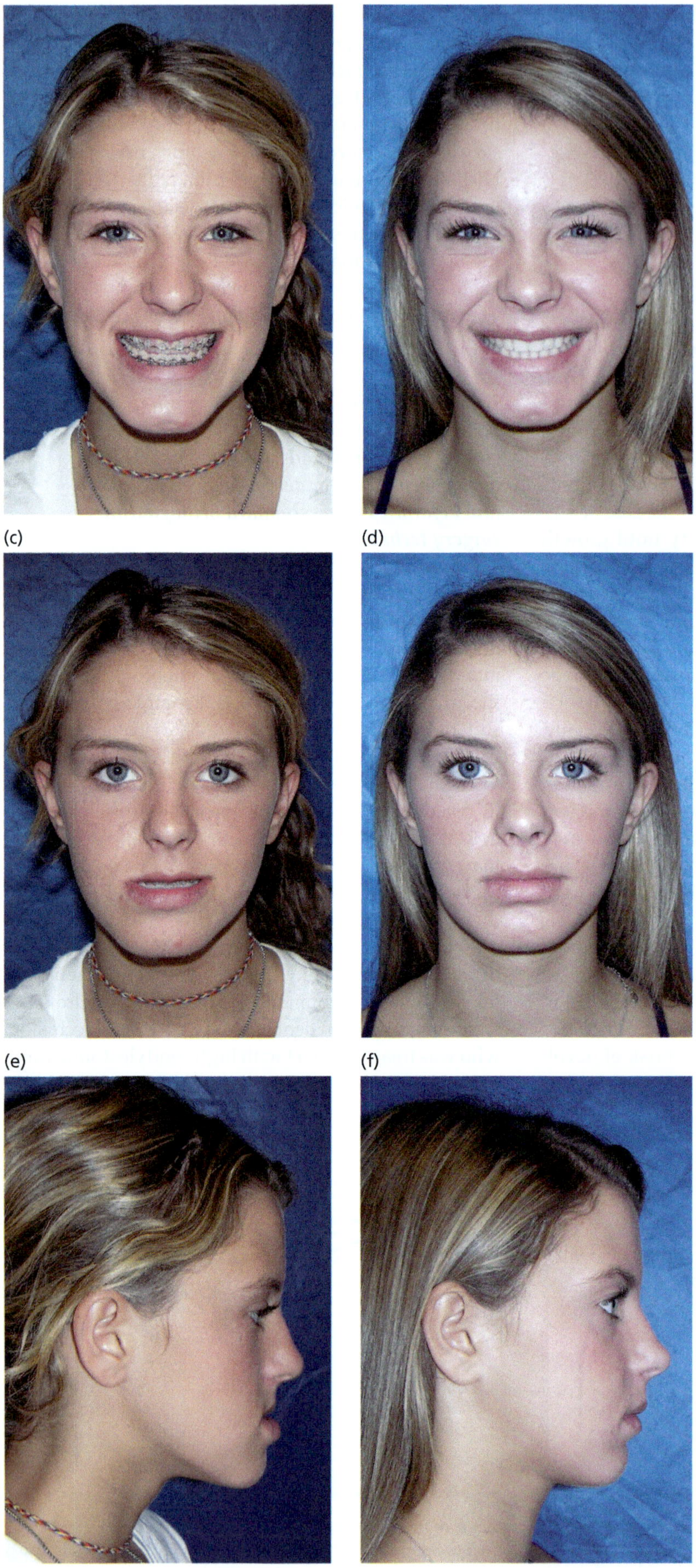

Fig. 17-3 (a) Preoperative frontal (smiling) view of a 13.8-year-old female patient with mandibular prognathism due to bilateral condylar hyperplasia. The patient underwent bilateral high TMJ condylectomies to arrest the mandibular growth at the same time as orthognathic surgery. Orthognathic surgery included bilateral mandibular ramus osteotomies for a set-back with anticlockwise rotation to decrease occlusal plane angulation. The Le Fort I maxillary osteotomy was performed in 3-pieces for segmental widening and advancement. (b) Postoperative frontal (smiling) view of same patient at age 16 years. (c) Preoperative frontal (repose) view at age 13.8 years. (d) Postoperative frontal (repose) view at age 16 years. (e) Preoperative profile view at age 13.8 years. (f) Postoperative profile view at age 16 years. (g–i) Intraoral preoperative photographs showing Class III occlusion, immediately prior to surgery. (j–l) Intraoral postoperative photographs demonstrating maintenance of surgically established occlusion after completion of jaw growth at 16+ years of age. (m) Preoperative cephalometric tracing at 13.8 years of age demonstrating Class III skeletal relationship due to bilateral condylar hyperplasia. (n) Surgical treatment objective (prediction tracing) demonstrating planned surgical movements and procedures (Bilateral TMJ high condylectomies and maxillary advancement and mandibular set-back with anticlockwise rotation of the maxillomandibular complex).

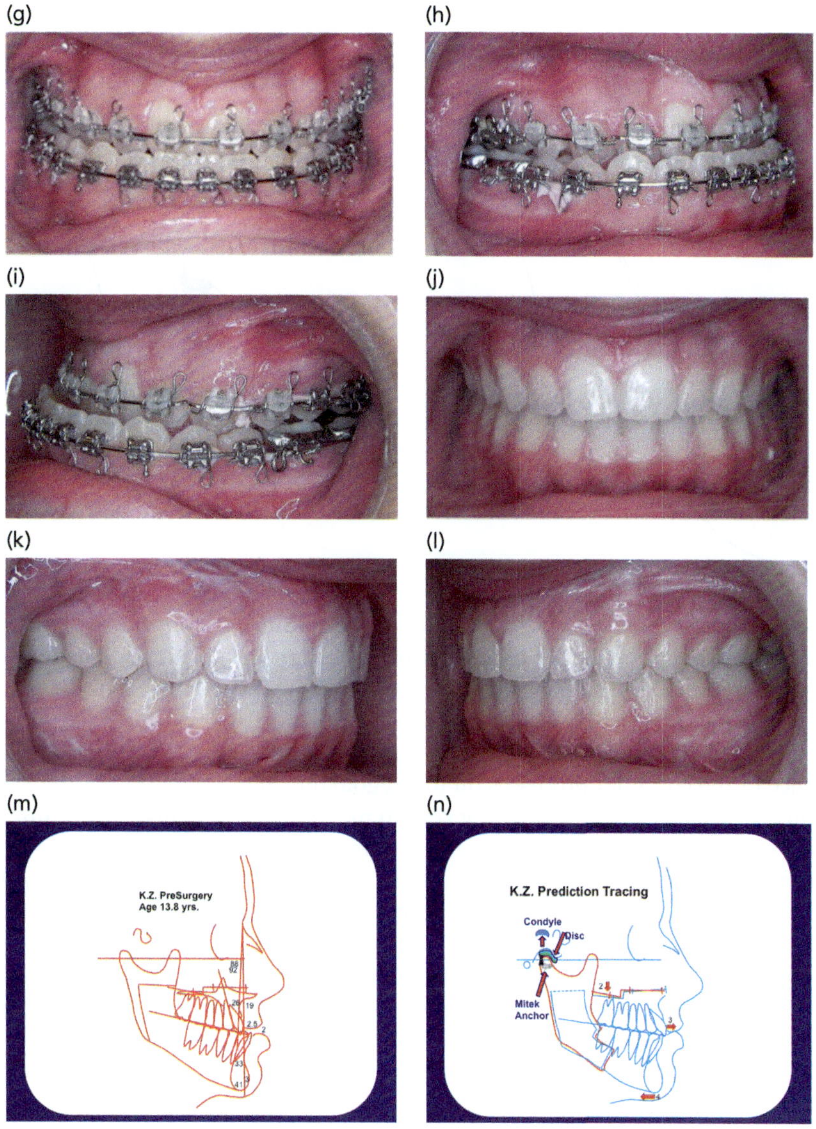

Fig. 17-3 (*Continued*).

Mandibular osteotomy techniques for growing patients

With the following mandibular surgical procedures used in growing patients, the preoperative rate of mandibular growth should neither be stimulated nor hindered postoperatively providing that the TMJs are healthy and the growth centres of the condylar heads are not damaged by the surgery. The vector of facial and mandibular growth, however, may be altered by a change in the orientation of the proximal segment, and thus the condyle.[12] With any of the following techniques, if the proximal segment is rotated forward due to surgery as compared to the presurgical position, an increased vertical growth vector may be seen post-surgery. Likewise, rotation of the proximal segment backward will result in a more horizontal growth vector post-surgically.

Sagittal split ramus osteotomy (SSRO)

The SSRO (Figure 17-4) is technically more difficult to perform on younger patients due to greater bony elasticity, the thinness of the cortical bone, the presence of unerupted molar teeth, and the relatively shorter posterior vertical mandibular body height, as compared to adults. It does have the advantages of easy application of rigid fixation as well as better positional control of the proximal segment.

Age considerations

SSRO is best reserved for patients over the age of 12 years, i.e., after the eruption of the permanent second molars, so as to avoid damage to these teeth during surgery.

Inverted 'L' osteotomy (ILO), and vertical ramus osteotomy (VRO)

The ILO (Figure 17-5) can be used to advance or set-back the mandible and/or vertically lengthen the ramus but may require bone grafting to control the positional orientation of the proximal segment and to fill the bony voids between segments.

The VRO (Figure 17-6) is more commonly employed to set-back the mandible but can also be used to advance the mandible with appropriate bone grafting

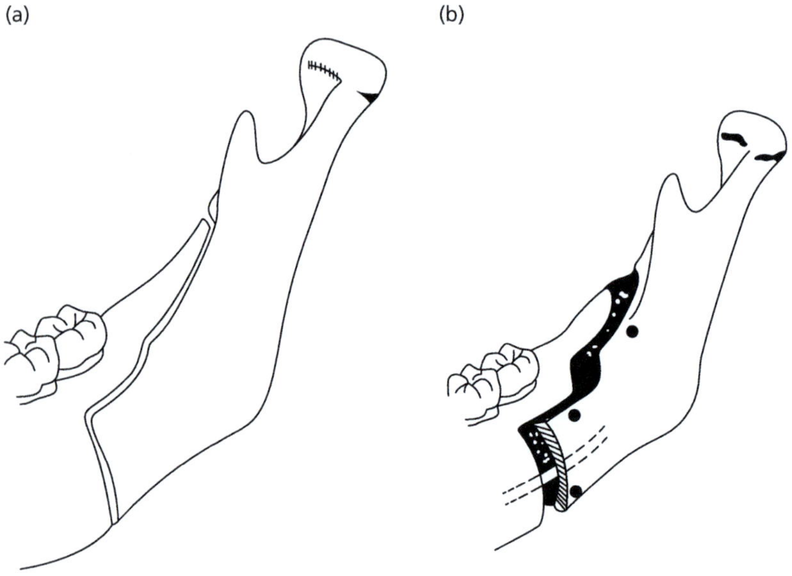

Fig. 17-4 The SSRO procedure (a) can be used to advance the mandible, or (b) to reposition it backward. Rigid fixation (conventional metallic or bioresorbable) is used to stabilize and fixate the osteotomized segments.

and internal fixation. The amount of mandibular advancement or set-back possible with this technique may be limited by the temporalis muscle attachment (advancement or set-back cases and especially in vertical posterior facial lengthening cases) and/or interference of the coronoid processes on the zygomatic arch (in advancement cases). Thus, for certain movements, a coronoidectomy may be needed or the surgeon may need to revert to other surgical options such as the SSRO or ILO where the coronoid process remains in its original position.

The application of rigid fixation of the bony segments may be technically difficult for ILO and VRO osteotomies, particularly from an intraoral approach. Without rigid fixation, intermaxillary fixation (wiring the teeth and jaws together) will be required, but this is difficult in children due to mixed dentition and compliance issues. Additionally, condylar position control may be less than exact, which can result in difficulties with the post-surgical occlusion.

Age considerations

The ILO and VRO can be performed at virtually any age, since the design of the osteotomies avoids developing teeth. However, care must be taken to avoid damage to developing teeth if any internal rigid fixation is being applied in the tooth bearing areas.

TMJ high condylectomy[15,16]

This procedure involves open TMJ surgery for removal of the superior 3–5 mm of the condylar head (Figure 17-2) with repositioning of the articular disc over the remaining condyle, and will stop any further A-P growth of the mandible by removing the active growth centre in CH type 1. Appositional mandibular growth and dentoalveolar growth should not be affected by this surgical procedure. TMJ function after surgery can be expected to remain unchanged.

Age considerations

This surgery should be performed only in cases of confirmed CH type 1 where mandibular growth is accelerated and continues beyond the normal expected time of growth cessation. The surgery should not be performed before maxillary A-P growth is complete since post-surgically, the mandible will not grow

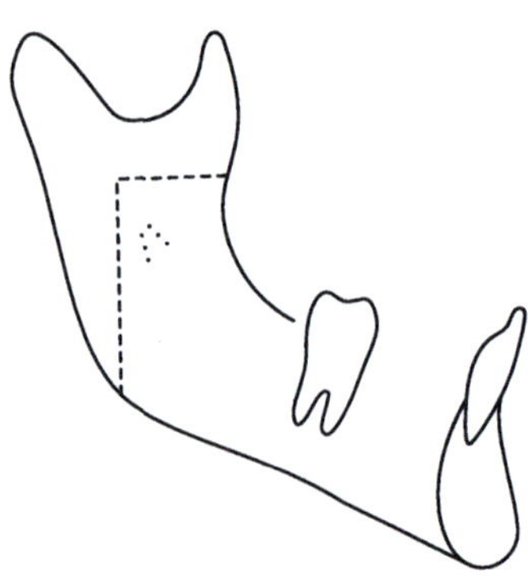

Fig. 17-5 The ILO procedure can be used to advance the mandible or to reposition it backward. When used to advance the mandible, the bone gap created between the proximal and distal segments requires grafting.

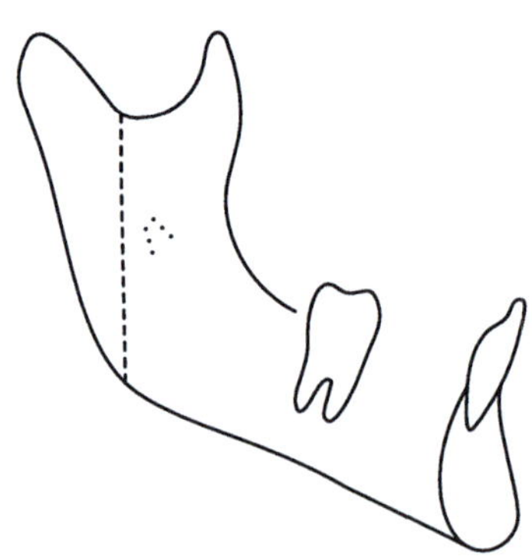

Fig. 17-6 The VRO procedure can be used to advance the mandible or to reposition it backward. The coronoid process may limit the extent of movement. When used to advance the mandible, the bone gap created between the proximal and distal segments requires grafting.

when performed bilaterally and any residual maxillary A-P growth may cause a Class II relationship to develop. The severity of the deformity may warrant earlier surgery in some severe cases. However, since no further A-P growth of the mandible occurs after this procedure, continued maxillary A-P and vertical alveolar growth will result in subsequent downward and backward rotation of the maxillomandibular complex, with the chin point more posteriorly positioned at the end of growth as compared to the immediate post-surgery position. With continued A-P maxillary growth, a Class II occlusion could develop. If maxillary surgery is concomitantly performed, then the surgery can be done at an earlier age (14 years for females, 16 years for males) since Le Fort I maxillary osteotomies will arrest any further A-P growth of the maxilla so that the occlusion will remain stable since neither the maxilla or mandible will exhibit further A-P growth, although the subsequent growth vector will be somewhat downward and backward since only vertical alveolar bone growth remains.

In CH type 1B cases, where the high condylectomy is performed unilaterally, the unoperated contralateral condyle will maintain normal growth, and could cause shifting of the mandible towards the operated side until cessation of growth. Generally, it is best to delay surgical treatment for CH type 1B until the age of 15 years for females and 17 to 18 years for males when the maxillary growth is close to completion.

TMJ low condylectomy[16,17]

CH type 2 is a unilateral enlargement of the mandibular condyle caused by an osteochondroma. There is controversy regarding the pathogenesis of this entity and although historically regarded as a benign tumour, some clinicians consider it a reactive process. Two-thirds of these cases begin in the teenage years. This condition usually causes excessive vertical growth and elongation of the ipsilateral side of the jaws and face. Facial asymmetry develops as well as a transverse cant of the occlusal plane and in more rapidly developing tumours an ipsilateral posterior open bite can develop. This condition is not self-limiting and can continue indefinitely with progressive worsening of the facial deformity. This condition is best treated by open joint surgery, performing a low condylectomy to remove the lesion with repositioning of the articular disc over the remaining condylar stump with concomitant or delayed orthognathic surgery to correct the facial asymmetry.

Age considerations

The low condylectomy and disc repositioning surgery should be performed in cases of CH type 2 when the disc is still salvageable. Ideally, the surgery should not be performed before maxillary A-P growth is complete. The severity of the deformity may warrant earlier surgery in some cases. However, since no further ipsilateral A-P or vertical growth of the mandible occurs after this procedure, continued contralateral mandibular growth and maxillary A-P and vertical alveolar growth may result in subsequent downward and backward rotation of the maxillomandibular complex with the mandible shifted toward the ipsilateral side as the contralateral mandible continues to grow. Generally, it is best to delay surgical treatment until the age of 15 years for females and 17 to 18 years for males when the maxillary and contralateral mandibular growth is closer to completion.

Maxillary deformities[18]

Similar to mandibular cases, an in-depth understanding of normal facial growth is invaluable in properly managing growing patients with maxillary deformities. Maxillary transverse growth is usually 85% complete by 8 years of age and almost all expected growth to be complete by the age of 12 years.[1,9] Anteroposterior and vertical maxillary growth is usually 98% completed in females by age 15 years and in males by age 17 to 18 years.[20–26] Factors that can significantly affect the direction and rate of maxillary growth include genetics, developmental conditions, hormonal stimulants, and nasal/oropharyngeal airway obstruction. Serial clinical, radiographic, and dental model analyses are helpful in determining the rate and direction of facial growth. Surgical management of the growing patient with maxillary deformities remains even more controversial as evident by the reasons discussed below.

Maxillary anteroposterior hypoplasia

Maxillary deficiencies can occur in the A-P, transverse, and/or vertical planes. The most common maxillary orthognathic procedure for correction of these deformities is the Le Fort 1 osteotomy (Figure 17-7). During this surgical procedure, the surgeon separates the maxilla from its bony skull buttresses and the nasal septum. This surgical separation (termed as downfracture of the maxilla) effectively stops further maxillary A-P growth.[27,28] Thus, if surgery is performed during the growth years, post-surgical recurrence of the Class III skeletal relationship would occur as the mandible continues to grow normally. If earlier surgery is indicated for functional, aesthetic, and psychosocial reasons, the Le Fort I osteotomy for maxillary advancement must take into consideration some overcorrection to allow the growing mandible to naturally grow and develop into it. If this surgery is performed during growth, the patient and parents must be informed that future surgery will likely be necessary.[18]

Alternatively, the surgeon can choose the 'Horseshoe' maxillary osteotomy (complete dentoalveolar osteotomy) (Figure 17-8). This osteotomy maintains the septal and vomer attachment to the maxilla since only the dentoalveolus is mobilized. The objective is to hopefully have post-surgical maxillary growth

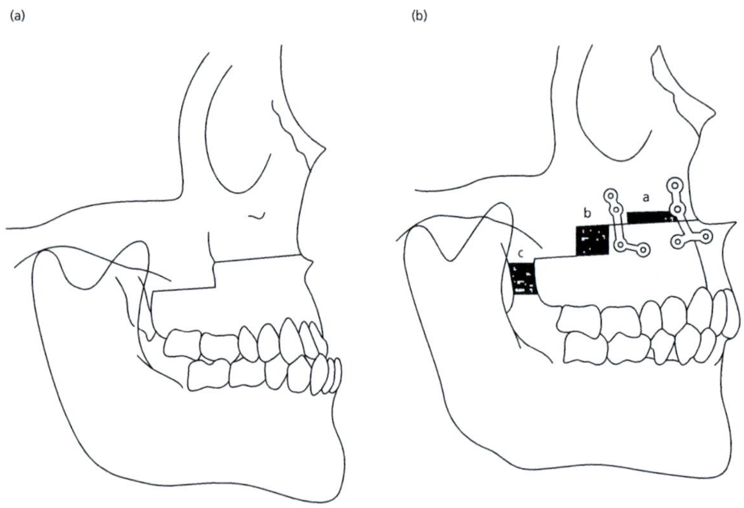

Fig. 17-7 The Le Fort I osteotomy with segmentalization allows repositioning of the maxilla in all three planes of space. The maxillary step osteotomy modification is illustrated which allows for grafting of bone defects.

continue at a normal rate since the nasal septum and vomer remain attached to the mid-palatal bone of the maxilla. It is important to remember that for patients requiring maxillary advancement, the maxillary growth is deficient and following Le Fort I osteotomy, there will be no further A-P growth, but the vertical maxillary growth will continue post-surgery at the same presurgical rate,[28–30] with the normal mandibular growth resulting in a Class III relationship.

Maxillary anteroposterior hyperplasia

This dentofacial deformity is less common and may present with a Class II skeletal and occlusal relationship. No studies exist regarding facial growth after maxillary orthognathic surgery in these patients. The deformity may be genetically related or the result of excessive dentoalveolar growth. Post-surgical growth in this deformity may be dependent on the procedure selected to correct it, as well as the rate of dentoalveolar growth presurgery, but normal A-P growth of the maxilla will likely be arrested. The horseshoe osteotomy, although technically difficult to perform, particularly when repositioning the maxilla posteriorly, may be the procedure of choice when surgery is performed on growing patients as it may have the least effect on post-surgical maxillary growth.

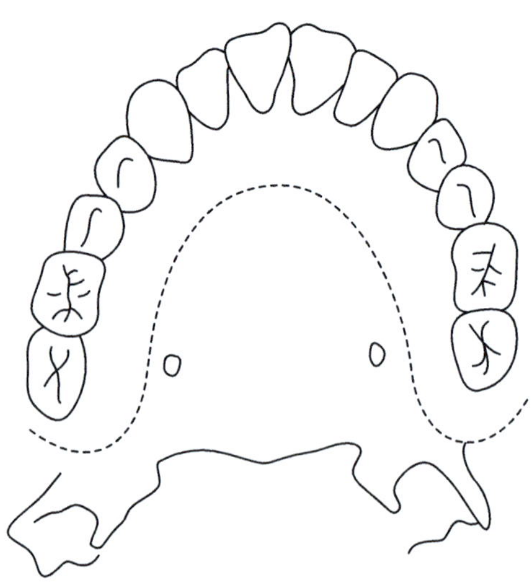

Fig. 17-8 The horseshoe osteotomy maintains the attachment of the horizontal palate to the vomer and lateral nasal walls. Only the dentoalveolus is mobilized.

Maxillary vertical deformities

Vertical maxillary excess (VME) is a common deformity, frequently associated with nasal airway obstruction, usually related to an excessive rate of vertical dentoalveolar growth, and it may or may not present with an anterior open bite. This deformity can be corrected during growth, with reasonably predictable results. However, vertical maxillary dentoalveolar growth can be expected to continue postoperatively at the same rate as before surgery until growth cessation. It has been reported that the vertical alveolar growth can continue into the 20s. While the maxilla continues to grow downward after surgery and the mandible continues to grow at a normal rate, the postoperative occlusal result should be maintained. The vector of facial growth will continue to be downward and backward due to the maxillary alveolus growing downwards. Anteroposterior maxillary growth cannot be expected after surgery if a Le Fort I osteotomy is used, but may be preserved with a dentoalveolar 'horseshoe' osteotomy.

Maxillary osteotomy techniques for growing patients

A. Le Fort I maxillary osteotomy

The Le Fort I osteotomy when performed during growth, effectively inhibits any further anterior growth of the maxilla. Vertical maxillary growth, however, can be expected to continue postoperatively at the same rate as before surgery. If interdental and midline osteotomies are performed, then transverse maxillary growth may be inhibited. The use of rigid fixation will optimize outcomes.

B. Horseshoe maxillary osteotomy (dentoalveolar osteotomy)[31,32]

With this surgical procedure, the nasal septum and vomer remain attached to the stable palate, and only the dentoalveolar structures are mobilized. Thus, some A-P maxillary growth may be expected to occur postoperatively although there are no studies to confirm this. In maxillary hypoplasia, the growth rate will remain deficient, resulting in the redevelopment of a skeletal Class III deformity if performed during the growth years. This maxillary dentoalveolar osteotomy is technically much more difficult to perform in this patient type.

Age and other considerations for the Le Fort I osteotomy and horseshoe osteotomy
For both techniques, the most predictable outcome can be expected if performed near to or after completion of mandibular growth (approximately 15 years in females and 17+ years in males). Serial lateral cephalographs are helpful in documenting cessation of mandibular growth.

Severe functional or psychosocial factors may indicate earlier treatment. Either maxillary procedure can technically be performed in the late first decade, provided that sufficient space exists above the apices of the developing permanent teeth, to place the osteotomies, and apply rigid fixation. Although vertical maxillary growth is likely unaffected by this procedure, damage to developing tooth roots may cause dento-osseous ankylosis, and localized dentoalveolar growth impairment.

C. Surgically assisted rapid palatal expansion (SARPE)

This procedure usually involves performing Le Fort I osteotomies without mobilization or downfracture of the maxilla. It is used in cases where the deficiency exists in the transverse dimension. There are no evidence-based studies available in the literature regarding growth after this procedure. This procedure may be contraindicated in most growing patients as the mid-palatal suture usually has not closed, thereby making the less invasive, non-surgical orthodontic and/or orthopaedic expansion possible. Moreover, postoperative A-P maxillary growth may be inhibited by this procedure if the nasal septum is separated from the palatal bone as part of the surgical procedure (note: some surgeons do not perform this step in SARPEs).

Double jaw orthognathic surgery

The following maxillary and mandibular procedures can be combined and performed during growth with predictable and stable results post-surgery:

a) Orthognathic surgery for the correction of vertical maxillary hyperplasia can be performed with corrective mandibular surgery for retrognathia or prognathism, if the preoperative rate of mandibular growth is normal, and the TMJs are healthy. Use of the Le Fort I osteotomy will inhibit any further A-P maxillary growth, while still allowing vertical maxillary growth.
b) In cases of mandibular prognathism secondary to active CH type 1, surgery involving bilateral high condylectomies will arrest the pathological growth and can be combined with maxillary and mandibular osteotomies with predictable results, regardless of the presurgical growth rate of the mandible and maxilla. The high condylectomies should be performed first as the initial step in the same surgical setting or as a separate staged surgery depending on surgeon's preference, training and expertise. When properly performed, the high condylectomies stop further A-P growth of the mandible. In the presence of vertical maxillary excess, the vector of facial growth will be downward and backward. In cases of normal or deficient maxillary growth, the occlusion should remain stable since the mandible and maxilla will not exhibit any further A-P growth.

Conclusions

Management of the growing patient with dentofacial deformities requiring surgical correction presents a unique and challenging problem for orthodontists and surgeons. Paediatric and adolescent patients with dentofacial deformities may, at times, require surgical treatment during active growth due to functional, aesthetic, and psychosocial factors. Having a sound understanding of facial growth, available treatment options, and the effects of surgery on postoperative growth patterns while managing these patients should improve treatment outcomes. Serial clinical, dental model, and radiographic analyses are important in predicting growth rates and patterns for individual patients.

The type of facial deformity present and the specific growth vectors of the patient will affect the surgical outcome and must be carefully assessed prior to surgery. The patient and family must understand the expected results, potential risks, and possible complications that can occur as a result of early surgical intervention. Factors such as presence of mandibular disproportionate growth (excessive or deficient) and co-existing TMJ pathology may significantly affect post-surgical growth and treatment outcomes, and must be identified and treated appropriately.

The surgical procedures required for correction of the deformity may affect post-surgical growth and dentofacial development. Further, facial growth may continue postoperatively and negate the benefits of surgery performed, thereby resulting in less than ideal treatment outcomes. The material presented in this article is based on available research, literature information, and personal clinical experience. It is in no way meant to be absolute, but rather should serve as a guide to formulate a specific treatment plan for each individual growing patient with respect to the appropriate type and timing of corrective surgical procedures on the maxilla and mandible.

References

1 Broadbent BH Sr., Broadbent BH Jr., Golden WH. Bolton standards of dentofacial developmental growth. St. Louis: Mosby, 1975.
2 van der Linden F. Facial growth and facial orthopaedics. Surrey, U.K.: Quintessence Publishing, 1986.
3 Broadbent BH Sr., Broadbent BH Jr., Golden WH. Bolton standards of dentofacial developmental growth. St. Louis: Mosby, 1975.
4 Linden F. van der. Facial growth and facial orthopaedics. Surrey, U.K.: Quintessence Publishing, 1986.
5 Wolford LM, Reiche-Fischel O, Mehra P. Changes in temporomandibular joint dysfunction after orthognathic surgery. J Oral Maxillofac Surg. 2003;61:655–60.
6 Proffit WR, Mason RM. Myofunctional therapy for tongue-thrusting: Background and recommendations. J Am Dent Assoc. 1975;90:403–11.
7 Wolford LM, Cottrell DA. Diagnosis of macroglossia and indications for reduction glossectomy. Am J Orthod Dentofac Orthop. 1996;110:170–7.
8 Wolford LM, Schendel SA, Epker BN. Surgical-orthodontic correction of mandibular deficiency in growing children: Long-term treatment results. J Maxillofac Surg. 1979;7:61–72.
9 Schendel SA, Wolford LM, Epker BN. Mandibular deficiency syndrome: Part III. Surgical advancement of the deficient mandible in growing children: Treatment results in twelve patients. O Surg O Med O Path. 1978;45:364–77.
10 Snow MD, Turvey TA, Walker D, Proffit WR. Surgical mandibular advancement in adolescents: Post-surgical growth related to stability. Int J Adult Orthodon Orthognath Surg. 1991;6:143–151.
11 Huang CS, Ross RB. Surgical advancement of the retrognathic mandible in growing children. Am J Orthod. 1982;82:89–102.
12 Epker BN, O'Ryan F. Effects of early surgical advancement of the mandible on subsequent growth. II. Biomechanical considerations. In: McNamara JA, Carlson DS, Ribbens KA (Eds). The Effect of Surgical Intervention on Craniofacial Growth. Ann Arbor: University of Michigan, 1982, pp. 207–29.
13 Obwegeser HL, Makek MS. Hemimandibular hyperplasia – hemimandibular elongation. J Craniomaxillofac Surg. 1986;14:183–5.
14 Wolford LM, Karras SC, Mehra P: Considerations for orthognathic surgery during growth. Part I: Mandibular deformities. Am J Orthod Dentofacial Orthop. 2001;119:95.
15 Wolford LM. Mandibular asymmetry: temporomandibular joint degeneration. In: Bagheri SC, Bell RB, Khan HA (Eds). Current Therapy in Oral and Maxillofacial Surgery. St. Louis: Elsevier Saunders, 2012, pp. 696–725.
16 Wolford LM, Rodrigues DB. Orthognathic considerations in the young patient and effects on facial growth. In: Preedy VR (Ed.) Handbook of Growth and Growth Monitoring in Health and Disease. New York: Springer, 2012, pp. 1789–1808.
17 Wolford LM, Rodrigues DB. Temporomandibular joint (TMJ) pathologies in growing patients: effects on facial growth and development. In: Preedy VR (Ed.) Handbook of Growth and Growth Monitoring in Health and Disease. New York: Springer, 2012, pp. 1809–28.
18 Wolford LM, Karras SC, Mehra P. Considerations for orthognathic surgery during growth. Part II: Maxillary deformities. Am J Orthod Dentofacial Orthop. 2001;119:102.
19 Björk A, Skieller V. Growth of the maxilla in three dimensions as revealed radiographically by the implant method. Br J Orthod. 1977;4:53–64.
20 Savara BS, Singh IJ. Norms of size and annual increments of seven anatomical measures of maxillae in boys from three to sixteen years of age. Angle Orthod. 1968;38:104–20.
21 Sillman JH. Dimensional changes of the dental arches: Longitudinal study from birth to twenty-five years. Am J Orthod. 1964;50:824–42.
22 Björk A. Facial growth in man studied with the aid of metallic implants. Acta Odont Scan. 1955;13:9–34.
23 Scott JH. The analysis of facial growth from fetal life to adulthood. Angle Orthod. 1963;33:110–13.
24 Singh IJ, Savara BS. Norms of size and annual increments of seven anatomical measures of maxillae in girls from three to seventeen years of age. Angle Orthod. 1968:312–24.
25 Björk A, Skieller V. Facial development and tooth eruptions: An implant study at the age of puberty. Am J Orthod. 1972;62:339–83.
26 O'Reilly MT. A longitudinal growth study: Maxillary length at puberty in females. Angle Orthod. 1979;49:234–58.
27 Friehofer HP. Results of osteotomies of the facial skeleton in adolescence. J Maxillofac Surg. 1977;5:267–97.
28 Mogavero FJ, Buschang PH, Wolford LM. Orthognathic surgery effects on maxillary growth in patients with vertical maxillary excess. Am J Orthod Dentofac Orthop. 1997;111:288–96.
29 Epker BN, Schendel SA, Washburn M. Effects of early surgical superior repositioning of the maxilla on subsequent growth: III. Biomechanical considerations. In: The Effect of Surgical Intervention on Craniofacial Growth. McNamara JA, Carlson DS, Ribbens KA (Eds). Ann Arbor: University of Michigan, 1982, pp. 231–250.
30 Washburn MC, Schendel SA, Epker BN. Superior repositioning of the maxilla during growth. J Oral Maxillofac Surg. 1982;40:142–9.
31 Vig KW, Turvey TA. Surgical correction of vertical maxillary excess during adolescence. Int J Adult Orthod Orthognathic Surg. 1989;4:110–28.
32 Epker BN, Wolford LM. Dentofacial Deformities: Surgical-Orthodontic Correction. St. Louis: CV Mosby, 1980.

Chapter 18

Stability of Orthognathic Surgery

Tate H. Jackson and Brent A. Golden

Introduction

Patients who receive surgical-orthodontic correction of dentofacial problems expect aesthetic and functional outcomes that remain stable over time, and an understanding of the principles underlying surgical stability is needed to plan treatment that will, in fact, remain stable in the long term.

Aside from operative technique, two types of information can help oral and maxillofacial surgeons plan and execute orthognathic surgeries that will be stable. The first is an appreciation of the physiological rationale that dictates whether certain surgical movements will relapse or not. The second is an evidence-based understanding of the actual long-term results of specific surgical movements in the average patient, and more importantly, in the patients who experience clinically significant relapse.

Much of the available evidence to support clinical decision making in terms of planning and operating for stability comes from the database at the University of North Carolina at Chapel Hill. Since 1978, both the ongoing collection of stability data for patients undergoing orthognathic surgery and studies investigating the physiological basis for surgical stability have been continuously supported by funding from the National Institute of Dental Research and National Institute of Dental and Craniofacial Research. We are grateful to have access to this tremendous data source and to the study results generated by researchers at UNC over the past 35 years. We are especially thankful to Dr William Proffit, the seminal principal investigator and long-time steward of the stability database, as well as Dr Ceib Phillips and Dr Timothy A. Turvey for their commitment to furthering our understanding of surgical stability.

Perhaps the most recognized outcome from the UNC data is the classification of surgical movements into a **hierarchy of stability**. In this chapter, we draw heavily from UNC findings and emphasize Proffit's hierarchy of stability,[1] as well as critical reports from elsewhere. First, we briefly highlight the most important principles of craniofacial physiology that must be understood in order to rationally comprehend surgical stability. We then present the best evidence regarding the stability of surgical movements in the context of treatment planning.

The principles of stability

Why does relapse occur after orthognathic surgery? The very complex answer to this question begins with the very common assertion that 'form follows

Orthognathic Surgery: Principles, Planning and Practice. Edited by Farhad B. Naini and Daljit S. Gill.

function.' Long-term change following surgery is almost entirely the result of function overpowering the anatomical form created by the surgeon.

The most obvious example of the power of function after surgery comes from patients for whom normal function is simply not a possibility. Neurological issues that prevent normal muscle tone, such as cerebral palsy, make adaptation to surgical change impossible. For patients who have neurophysiological issues, a change in the patient's anatomy without a concomitant change in physiology is a recipe for almost certain relapse. The information that follows here is intended to be applied to clinical scenarios where the patient is neurophysiologically normal.

Growth

Perhaps the most apparent physiological process that can undermine the stability of surgical change is facial growth. The positive changes brought about by treatment can easily be diminished over time if the pattern of growth – which likely led to the need for surgery in the first place – continues over the long term. For example, the pre-pubertal prognathic patient who gains ideal positive overjet with surgical intervention at age 12 is likely to outgrow that change in relatively short order. Likewise, the patient who had successful growth modification to protract the maxilla at age eight has a significant risk of losing that gain in the coming years, even if efforts are made to retain the change.

Why is the correction lost? As a rule, neither orthopaedic growth modification nor orthognathic surgery changes growth potential overall, although surgery may affect the growth of the specific area operated. When normal growth potential remains, the pattern of growth tends to be constant. After growth is modified, either by inhibition or acceleration, a period of rapid catch-up growth or quiescence usually follows – and that catch-up growth or lack thereof, tends to erase the positive effects of treatment. In younger patients, this point is particularly salient. It is not efficient to attempt to surgically correct jaw relations in young patients with significant growth potential remaining.

Two situations exist, however, when the risk of post-surgical change is overwhelmed by the need to treat early: in especially severe cases (particularly syndromic patients with airway compromise or psychosocial detriment) and in cases of progressive aberrant growth. Severe cases necessitate treatment because the patient's quality of life is so reduced that the burden of multiple surgeries becomes insignificant by comparison. Progressive cases require early and possibly multiphase treatment because growth is not simply following an unfavourable pattern, but it is instead pathologically delayed or advanced. For example, cases of mandibular ankylosis that prevent normal growth of one side of the mandible require early surgery to encourage symmetrical growth.

Absent these uncommon situations, modern orthognathic surgical planning dictates that patients be operated when facial growth is essentially complete in order to avoid significant post-treatment change. It is important to point out, however, that hard and soft-tissue facial growth continues, albeit in much smaller increments, well beyond early adulthood and actually quite late into life. Although this late facial growth may not cause noticeable changes in dentofacial relationships for most patients, it is important to remember that facial growth should be considered when it comes to surgical stability in all patients, not just those under the age of 18.

Physiological adaptation after surgery

After the very real anatomical changes brought about by orthognathic surgery, physiological adaptation is not only inevitable but also necessary. Changes in the soft tissues of the head and neck, particularly the craniofacial musculature, can have a significant effect on post-treatment stability since their role in maintaining posture means nearly constant forces are applied to the facial skeleton.

Head posture tends to be unique and consistent for individuals and can be measured using cephalometric radiographs. By assessing the inclination of the cranial base (sella-nasion line, S-N) to an extracranial reference line with the patient in natural head position (NHP), that is with the patient in a relaxed position and focused on a visual point on the horizon – or looking into her own eyes in a mirror at eye level – one can visualize changes in head posture after orthognathic surgery. Investigators at UNC did just that and found that head posture changed in different ways depending on the surgical moves accomplished.[2] As seen in Figure 18-1, head posture changes occurred in

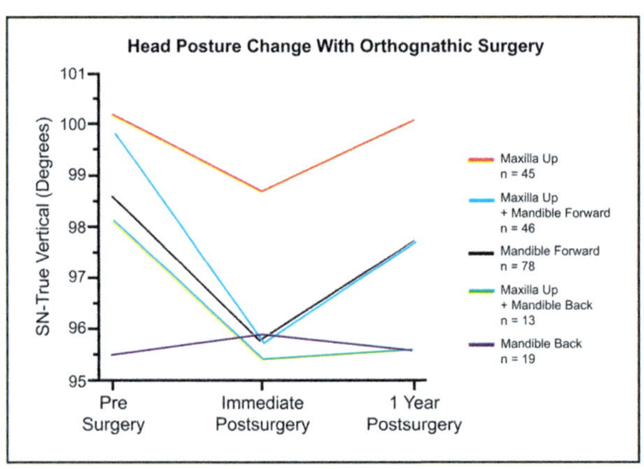

Fig. 18-1 Changes in head posture with orthognathic surgery. The angle of S-N to true vertical was measured on lateral cephalographs before and after surgery. Note that for most operations, that angle decreased after surgery, indicating that the patient tipped his or her head more downward at rest. Head posture tended to return to the pre-surgical position after one year for patients who had single jaw surgery, while patients who received bimaxillary surgery maintained their change in head posture.

opposite directions for those who had the mandible set back versus those who had the maxilla impacted. For both of these groups, however, head posture had returned to the pre-surgical position at 12 months after surgery. Those who had the mandible moved forward saw some short term change that was almost completely recovered at one year. For patients who had bimaxillary surgery, the immediate post-surgical adaptation in head posture was maintained at one year after surgery. In short, it appears that with single-jaw surgery, head posture is likely to change immediately following surgery, but return to the pre-surgical position in relatively short order. Patients who have two-jaw procedures are likely to see a more long-term change in head posture.

If changes in how patients hold their head at rest are seen after surgery, it should not be a surprise that changes in how patients hold their jaw may be seen as well. The resting position of the mandible is not to be confused with the postural position of the mandible. The resting position is achieved when minimal muscle activity allows the posterior teeth to be separated by a centimetre or more. The postural position, which tends to be the focus during surgical planning, is the position of the mandible where the normal freeway space of about 3 mm is present. The determinants of the postural position of the mandible are still poorly understood, but the position of the maxillary posterior teeth appears to play a significant role. When these teeth are extruded orthodontically, the mandible tends to rotate down and back to preserve the freeway space. With surgical repositioning of the maxilla upward, the upper molars are also repositioned superiorly, and the mandible follows, preserving the freeway space. Downward movement of the posterior maxilla can also move the upper molars into a position that eliminates the freeway space. Physiological adaptation will ensue that re-establishes the postural position of the mandible so that the freeway space returns, and that process can lead to a loss of surgical correction. So, although the interaction of the central nervous system with the proprioceptive mechanism responsible for the postural position of the mandible is not fully understood, it is evident that failure to consider the interaction of jaw posture with surgical movements can lead to post-surgical instability.

Intuitively tied to mandibular position is the consideration of bite force. After all, if the freeway space is invaded and the teeth are in occlusion but the patient is incapable of generating sufficient bite force, the potential for relapse could change. One might assume that increasing the mechanical advantage for the biting system by changing its geometry would be the rule, i.e. advancing the mandible should provide a less effective lever system, and the patient's bite force should decrease. In practice, that logic simply is not borne out. A study where bite force was measured both before and after surgery,[3] found it equally likely that bite force would increase, decrease, or remain unchanged when the mandible was either advanced or set-back when the patient's face height was normal. When long face patients are considered, bite force during function and swallowing as well as maximum bite force all increase significantly. In fact, the increase in bite force for these patients is much greater than predicted by geometry alone – and not just at maximum bite, but during function as well.[3] There is no doubt that physiological adaption in bite force occurs when it comes to bite force simply because the data cannot be explained by the change in jaw geometry and change in mechanical advantage alone. Changes in bite force after surgery illustrate physiological adaptation, but it is important that the role of bite force in post-surgical stability not be overestimated. After all, teeth are normally brought into occlusion for only minutes each day.[4] Of greater potential importance are the soft-tissue pressures surrounding the face, neck, and mouth that almost constantly provide a force against the skeletal and dental units affected by orthognathic surgery.

Orthodontists tend to be acutely aware of these pressures since an imbalance in soft-tissue forces is almost always a major causal factor of malocclusion. Lip and tongue pressure changes after surgery have been investigated using pressure transducers,[5] with the aim of understanding if these post-surgical changes could contribute to relapse. After surgical movements that allow the mandible to rotate upward significantly without operating the mandible itself (when the maxilla is moved upward, for example), there is a decrease in resting lip pressure against the lower incisors. That decrease is a logical response to the positional change of the mandible, and the incisor position in these cases tends to be more stable over time. When the mandible is moved forward or backward surgically, the lower incisors are either pushed forward into the lower lip or moved backward away from it. One would expect then that the lip pressure against these teeth would either increase or decrease postoperatively. Remarkably, for both advancement and set-back patients, post-surgical lip pressure remains almost identical to pre-surgical levels.

Perhaps for the surgeon, changes in lip pressure are of less concern than changes in the position and pressure of the tongue. Given the growing awareness of sleep apnoea and the systemic health implications of the condition,[6] there is particular interest in what happens to the tongue and pharyngeal tissues after orthognathic surgery, particularly with surgery to retrude the mandible. Fortunately for patients in the short term, when the mandible is moved posteriorly, the tongue tends to move downward rather than back, and the airway is maintained post-surgically in this way. Long-term data on whether these patients are more susceptible to developing sleep apnoea as they age are not yet available. Although recently there has been great enthusiasm for the use of three-dimensional data from cone beam computed tomography to evaluate changes in airway after orthognathic surgery, this type of information is simply

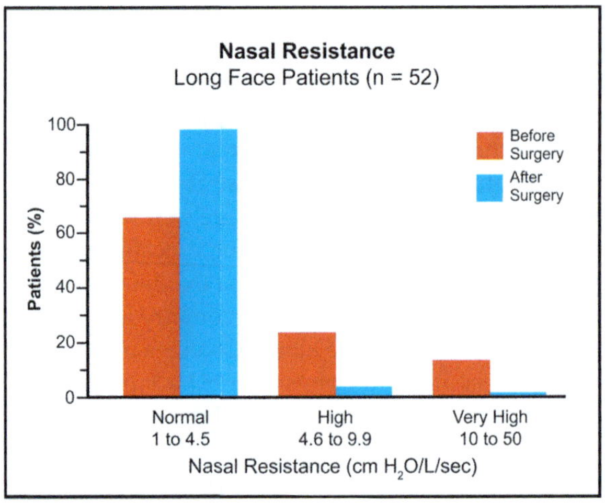

Fig. 18-2 Resistance to nasal airflow in long face patients who had surgery to impact the maxilla. The number of patients who had normal resistance to airflow increased with surgery, while the number who had high or very high resistance to airflow decreased. No patients who had normal resistance pre-surgically saw an increase in resistance. Only three of 52 participants had no improvement in nasal resistance to airflow.

inadequate to evaluate respiration and the causal factors of sleep apnoea. Studies using methods that effectively analyze airflow and include polysomnography are needed to better understand the long-term effects of mandibular set-back surgery on the risk for sleep apnoea (see Chapter 44).

Two studies analyzing airflow and nasal resistance have investigated the effect of maxillary surgery on respiration.[7,8] Nasal respiration generally tends to remain unchanged or increases after maxillary surgery, no matter what surgical moves were accomplished.[8] Interestingly, repositioning the maxilla superiorly, which would seem to limit nasal volume and interfere with respiration, does not actually have the expected effects. Instead, nasal resistance in long-face patients who had superior repositioning of the maxilla actually decreased post-surgically (Figure 18-2). Why? As the maxilla is moved up, the nares, which are the point of greatest possible constriction in the nasal airway, tend to widen and allow better airflow.

It is clear that the physiological response to surgery is complex and as yet not completely understood. Failure of the clinician, however, to have a basic appreciation of the interaction of physiological adaptation with anatomical surgical changes ultimately will limit his or her capacity to deliver an aesthetic and stable surgical outcome.

Rigid fixation

Although the use of wire osteosynthesis is occasionally still indicated in modern orthognathic surgery, rigid internal fixation (RIF) is used with such overwhelming frequency that it is easy to inappropriately limit one's consideration of how RIF affects stability. RIF enhances stability by allowing more precise and predictable stabilization of bony segments both intra-operatively and immediately after surgery.

Fixation with plates and screws also encourages faster bone healing. When bone heals under compression, it occurs by primary intent.[9] That is to say that there is no callus formation preceding the osteoblastic activity that is responsible for the deposition and remodelling of new bone. With wire osteosynthesis, callus formation occurs and makes the process of bone healing less efficient, and studies using animal models have demonstrated that bone strength is greater at six weeks when RIF is used to stabilize osteotomy sites rather than wire fixation.[10,11]

Both the greater stabilization and the faster healing allowed by RIF have obvious implications for stability – for the potential to fight the natural muscle and soft tissue pull during function that could encourage post-surgical relapse. Of course, RIF also allows an early return to function for patients. The interaction of RIF with early function must be considered – especially in terms of mandibular surgery and condylar remodelling.

When mandibular osteotomies – most often by bilateral sagittal-split – are performed, the condyle is torqued or twisted about the vertical axis of the ramus when the mandibular segments are approximated and rigidly fixated. The twisting of the condyle within the soft tissue capsule of the temporomandibular joint results in an environment where remodelling of the bony surface of the condyle is necessary to meet the physiological demands of the joint. In experiments with primates, condylar remodelling is precisely what occurs in the short term with RIF.[12] Evidence from human studies examining the return of function post-surgically suggests the same is true clinically. At six months after surgery, the number of RIF patients with clinically significant deficits in maximum opening was less than half that for those with wire osteosynthesis and intermaxillary fixation.[13] Prolonged immobility and soft tissue healing must be considered, but even then, the time to return to adequate opening after surgery is more closely associated with bone healing and condylar remodelling than the time for soft tissue healing. It is thought that RIF facilitates the condylar remodelling necessary to allow TM joint function to return to normal with the mandible in the desired position. With wire fixation, there likely is more accommodation of condylar position than condylar remodelling, and that movement of the mandible could contribute to a loss of surgical change.

Interestingly, as we will see in the following section, some single jaw surgeries, including mandibular advancement, tend to be stable whether RIF or wire osteosynthesis is used. Others, however, benefit significantly from the use of RIF.

Surgical planning using the hierarchy of stability

The UNC database

For the clinician, it is important to consider how data are presented and if research results translate to information that can be used to make clinical decisions. When it comes to surgical stability, the majority of relapse occurs in a minority of patients. That is to say that the data for relapse are not normally distributed. Accordingly, simply looking at mean or average changes, even in large samples, can be misleading.

Likewise, reporting post-surgical changes in relation to the magnitude of the surgical movements that occurred is not ideal. Why? Because that type of data tends to imply a linear relationship between surgical displacement and relapse potential (i.e. the farther you advanced the mandible, the less stable it will be). In reality, the magnitude of surgical movement is unrelated to stability up to a point. There is often a threshold at which relapse becomes more likely, but for the overwhelming majority of patients, that threshold lies within a narrow window and is not distributed evenly across the entire range of movement that is possible.

Although knowing the point at which a surgical move becomes inherently unstable is important, the hierarchy of surgical stability addresses another crucial piece of information that the clinician needs: what percentage of patients are likely to experience relapse of a clinically significant magnitude? For the UNC data reported here, the threshold for clinically significant post-treatment change is a 2 mm difference in cephalometric landmark location between time points. Less than 2 mm of change is within the error of the method for measuring relapse on cephalometric films. Change greater than 4 mm is considered highly significant in terms of clinical consequence to the patient.

In addition to this definition of clinical significance, the following categories have been developed from the UNC data to describe the relative stability of certain surgical moves:

- *Very stable*: Less than 10% of patients experience significant post-treatment change.
- *Stable*: Less than 20% of patients experience significant post-treatment change, and nearly none experience highly significant change.
- *Stable if modified in a certain way* (e.g. RIF only is used).
- *Problematic*: Considerable likelihood that highly significant post-treatment change will occur.

Note that the use of RIF warrants its own category to describe stability for some orthognathic procedures. In the discussion of stability that follows, data for relapse using rigid internal fixation will be emphasized.

The hierarchy of post-surgical stability

The classic hierarchy of stability represented by Figure 18-3 comes from data collected at one year following surgery on more than 1500 patients operated at UNC. Post-surgical skeletal change is likely to be greatest during this time period in the vast majority of patients. Bone healing, physiological adaptation, and post-surgical orthodontics all have the potential

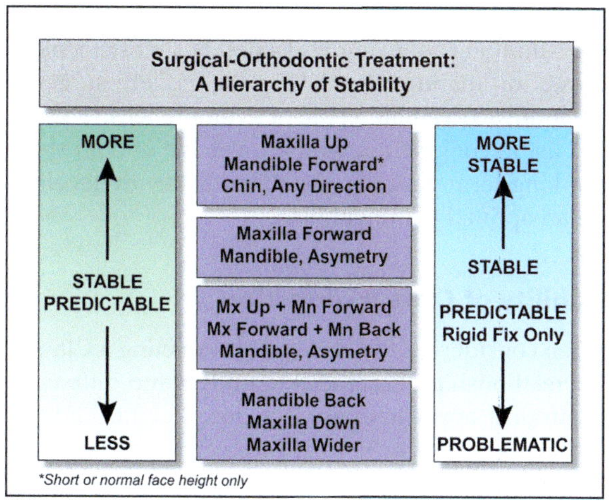

Fig. 18-3 The hierarchy of post-surgical stability for orthognathic surgical procedures. These data reflect stability at one year following surgery.

to affect stability during this initial period following surgery.

In the first year, three procedures are *Very Stable*, whether rigid or wire fixation is used. Upward movement of the maxilla is the most stable, followed by mandibular advancement of less than 10 mm (as long as the patient has a normal or short anterior face height). Genioplasty to move the inferior border of the bony chin in any direction is also very stable. For all three of these procedures, more than 90% of patients will experience essentially no relapse (<2 mm change in the position of cephalometric landmarks) and have an excellent clinical outcome in terms of post-surgical stability.

Advancement of the maxilla 8 mm or less is the only surgical move that falls into the category of *Stable*. Whether stabilized with wire osteosynthesis or rigidly, forward movement of the maxilla results in almost no post-surgical relapse in 80% of patients and in relapse less than 4mm in only 20% of patients. Almost no patients in this category experience relapse greater than 4 mm. These data hold true whether the maxilla is advanced symmetrically or asymmetrically as well.

Three procedures are *Stable Only with Rigid Fixation*: (1) bimaxillary surgery to simultaneously impact the maxilla and advance the mandible; (2) bimaxillary surgery to advance the maxilla and retrude the mandible; and (3) bimaxillary procedures to correct complex facial asymmetry. Only 20% of these patients see change greater than 2 mm post-surgically, and 90% achieve an excellent clinical result.

Isolated mandibular set-back, maxillary downgraft, and surgical expansion of the maxilla all may be classified as *Problematic* in terms of post-surgical stability. For each, 40–50% of patients experience 2–4 mm of post-surgical change, and 20% have more than 4 mm of change.

The hierarchy of post-surgical stability is a convenient reference tool for clinicians. It must be emphasized, however, that the pattern of long-term stability is different. It can also be misleading to limit one's thinking about surgical stability simply to 'maxilla up' or 'mandible back.' For the modern surgeon, the ability to evaluate a patient's comprehensive problem list in conjunction with knowledge of both short and long-term patterns of stability is key to developing an optimal treatment plan.

Stability of Class II correction

When considering the stability of correcting a Class II jaw relationship, it is crucial to understand difference in surgical approach based on face height. Patients with a short face or normal face height are best corrected with mandibular advancement alone. Patients with a long face and anterior open bite are corrected in a more stable fashion with a bimaxillary procedure that impacts the maxilla and advances the mandible. Why? The answer, not surprisingly, has a physiological rationale.

The posterior mandible and ramus are enveloped in a sling of musculature that work to move the mandible and, importantly, to elevate it. When the mandible is advanced in long face patients to increase posterior face height and decrease the anterior face height, the jaw is rotated in an anticlockwise fashion. With this rotation, the posterior ramus length increases, and the musculature surrounding that part of the jaw is stretched. Elongation of the pterygomandibular sling of muscles creates an environment where relapse is highly likely. As the muscles work hard to re-establish their pre-surgical length, the posterior ramus length does the same, and anterior open bite and mandibular retrusion return as the mandible rotates down and back.

How can elongation of the pterygomandibular sling of muscles be avoided? Surgery to impact the posterior maxilla such that the mandible rotates closed in a clockwise fashion (whether the mandible is simultaneously advanced or not) preserves the length of theses muscles and provides a more stable result. With this foundation, let us consider the best current evidence for stability of Class II correction.

The hierarchy of post-surgical stability indicates that for Class II patients with a short or normal face height, mandibular advancement is very stable. And that is true for both wire osteosynthesis and rigid fixation within the first year following surgery.

In the long-term (1–5 years post-treatment), about 25% of patients with mandibular advancement alone experience more than 2 mm relapse in mandibular length and height of the ramus (Figure 18-4). Interestingly, only 10% of these patients have an increase in overjet of 2–4 mm.[14] In other words, the skeletal change is not mirrored by dental change. That means that as remodelling of the mandible occurs (primarily at the condyles), the dentition frequently compensates to maintain a more ideal anterior-posterior relationship. That compensation occurs primarily by proclination of the lower incisors.

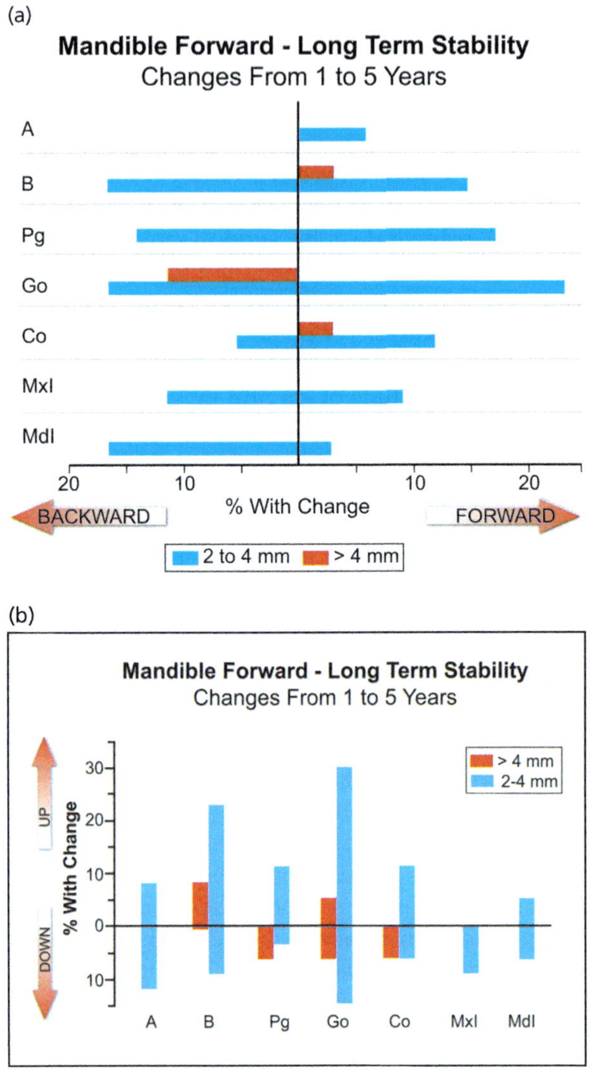

Fig. 18-4 Long-term stability of mandibular advancement for patients with a normal or short anterior face height. Changes in the (a) horizontal and (b) vertical dimensions. Note that 25% of patients saw a loss in mandibular length of 2 mm or more, although nearly the same percentage of patients had a net gain. The higher percentage of patients who had changes at gonion is no surprise since significant remodelling occurs at the angle of the mandible as muscle attachment is re-established shortly after surgery.

It is important to emphasize once again that these values do not represent an average expectation for patients. Note that both B point and pogonion were just as likely to move forward as back in the long term (Figure 18-4).

Also instructive is a comparison of long-term stability in surgery patients to patients with Class II skeletal problems who did not receive surgical treatment. Remember that post-treatment change is the result of physiological adaption, importantly growth. Do patients who do not have surgery experience a pattern of late craniofacial growth that affects their Class II skeletal relationship? Data for long-term recall of Class II orthodontic patients indicate that the answer is no.[15]

Not all Class II patients require mandibular advancement alone, and patients with a long face

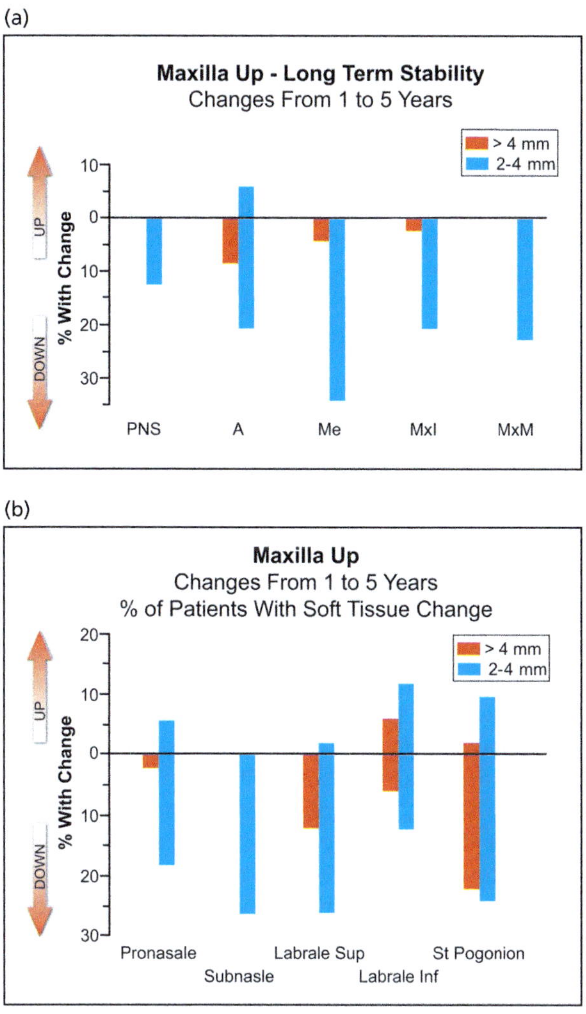

Fig. 18-5 Maxillary impaction, long-term stability data. For 80% of patients, skeletal landmarks did not change significantly in the vertical dimension (a). Note that changes in the hard tissues of the face are mirrored by soft-tissue changes (b).

Class II problem, as we have already noted, are often best treated with maxillary surgery, either with or without concurrent mandibular advancement.

Isolated superior repositioning of the maxilla is the most stable surgical procedure in the short term, and for 95% of patients with wire fixation and nearly 100% with rigid fixation, the maxilla essentially does not move in the first year after surgery.[16] At five years following surgery, 20% of patients experience 2–4 mm of change in the vertical position of the maxilla, and almost half as many have more than 4 mm of relapse (Figure 18-5). This long-term vertical change is seen in the soft tissues of the face as well and is not the result of unfavourable healing or fixation after surgery. Since relapse of the maxilla occurs in the same pattern of growth that almost certainly caused the patient's long face problem in the first place, it is logical to think that this long-term change might be the result of unfavourable facial growth. Despite these skeletal changes, overbite is maintained in these patients remarkably well, primarily because of compensatory eruption of the incisors.[17,18] Given the possible role of vertical maxillary growth in long-term relapse, when should these patients be operated? Should treatment be delayed? Data at this time suggest that as long as the adolescent growth spurt has been completed, patients with a long face problem can be treated surgically with superior repositioning of the maxilla with a good prognosis in terms of short and long-term stability.[19]

Waiting until the adolescent growth spurt has finished is an appropriate guideline for patients who receive two-jaw surgery for long face Class II problems as well. In the short term, superior repositioning of the maxilla combined with mandibular advancement is stable only with rigid fixation. 60% of patients with wire osteosynthesis have an excellent clinical result, but 21% actually relapse into open bite.[20] When RIF is employed, 90% of patients have a clinically excellent result, and almost never is there relapse to clinical open bite.[21]

In the first five years after surgery, changes in both the maxilla and mandible, when both are operated, are quite similar to the long-term changes seen for isolated osteotomies of each jaw (see Figure 18-6 and compare with Figures 18-4 and 18-5). That is to say that the maxilla behaves similarly in the long term whether or not the mandible is advanced as well. The same holds true for mandibular relapse. Again, note that despite unfavourable skeletal change in some patients, both overbite and overjet are more likely to increase than decrease in the long term.

When compared to long face Class II patients who did not receive surgery, those who did have bimaxillary surgery show greater long-term change in skeletal landmarks.[22] These changes are seen in a minority of patients, however. Of particular note in these patients are the changes seen at the condyle and reflected in a loss of ramus height. There has been some concern that patients with the long face skeletal pattern are at greater risk for long-term condylar resorption when they undergo two-jaw surgery. The UNC database reflects that long-term resorption is the same in patients who have isolated mandibular osteotomies as those who have bimaxillary surgery (10% for both). Very recent unpublished data from the UNC dataset examining more than 1200 records for long face patients shows that the condylar resorption seen in those who received two-jaw surgery occurs almost entirely in the first post-surgical year.

Data on the stability of correcting long face Class II problems using upward movement of the maxilla are extensive. Recently, data have become available regarding the long-term stability of correction using mandibular surgery alone and rigid fixation. Recall that this procedure rotates the mandible anticlockwise and elongates the mandibular sling of muscles. Early data on this procedure using wire osteosynthesis were so troubling that anticlockwise rotation of the mandible has been avoided at UNC, and the data reflect that fact. Is rotation of the mandible up in the anterior and down in the posterior more stable with

(a)

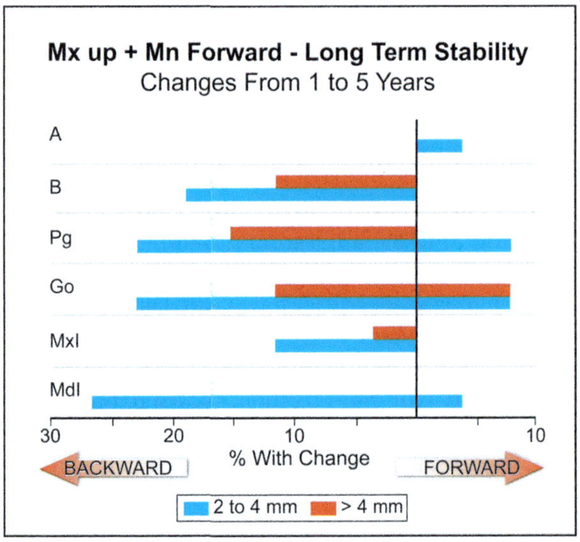

(b)

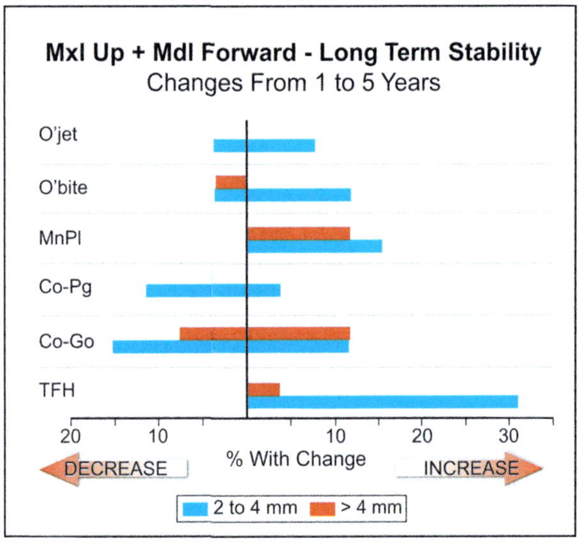

Fig. 18-6 Stability over the first five years after bimaxillary surgery for long face, Class II problems. One-third of patients experienced significant backward movement of horizontal landmarks (a), and about 15% had horizontal relapse greater than 4 mm. Vertical changes (b), including changes in mandibular plane angle (MnPl) and dental relationships. Again, one-third of patients experienced inferior movement of the maxilla greater than 2 mm. Dental compensation was evident as overjet (O'jet) increased significantly in only 8% of patients. Overbite (O'bite) was more likely to increase than decrease in these patients.

modern RIF? Work by Fontes et al. has generated data that may give some insight.[23] In their retrospective study that examined the records of 31 patients with an average of 4.5 years of follow-up data, 60% of the skeletal anticlockwise rotation of the mandible was lost. Only 10% of these patients actually relapsed to clinical open bite. Again, dental compensation is seen for skeletal relapse. It is important to note that the average open bite for this sample was –2.6 mm (SD, 1.1 mm).

So, is anticlockwise rotation of the mandible stable with modern rigid fixation techniques? There really is still not enough long-term information to answer that question confidently in the affirmative. Even for closure of mild to moderate open bites, 60% of the skeletal change is lost, and 10% of patients relapse to open bite, despite dental compensation. At this time, the best clinical recommendation remains that anticlockwise rotation should be avoided when possible and used with caution to correct Class II open bite and long face problems.

Stability of Class III correction

Less data are available concerning the stability of correcting Class III problems because historically fewer patients sought correction of that facial pattern at UNC, but that trend has changed in recent years.[24] The UNC dataset for surgical Class III correction is certainly adequate, however, and it is interesting that the pattern of stability for Class III patients is different than that seen for Class II patients.[25] Overall, Class III patients tend to experience greater change in the short term than Class II patients. After the first post-surgical year, however, Class III patients experience very little additional change.

In the first year post-surgically, maxillary advancement is stable, regardless of fixation technique, although that fact only holds if the maxilla is not moved downward as well[26]. In the long term, very little relapse is seen with maxillary advancement, and in only 10% of patients does the maxilla move posteriorly 2–4 mm.[27]

Double-jaw surgery to correct a Class III skeletal relationship is classified as stable in the short term only if rigid fixation is employed, with only 20% of patients seeing relapse of 2–4 mm, and almost none with greater than 4 mm change. In the long term, the UNC data reflect almost no change whatsoever of a significant magnitude. Interestingly, one-third of patients in this group had their anterior maxilla rotated down more than 2 mm. For these patients, in the first post-surgical year, the maxilla relapsed back to its original position in almost all of these patients. This point emphasizes the fact that downward movement of the maxilla is not a stable move.[28]

Moving the maxilla down is classified as problematic in terms of stability in the first post-surgical year. Even with rigid fixation, almost 50% of patients experienced relapse of 2–4 mm, and 20% had more than 4 mm relapse (Figure 18-7). Good long-term data do not exist for these patients, although the post-surgical data are discouraging enough to suggest down-grafting the maxilla, in absence of some modification, does not have a good stability prognosis. Simultaneously operating the mandible might improve stability,[29] but as we have already pointed out, vertical relapse of the maxilla is still possible with two-jaw surgery. Extreme rigid fixation measures and rigid alloplastic grafting techniques promote stability for this procedure,[30] but more data are still needed to evaluate these techniques.

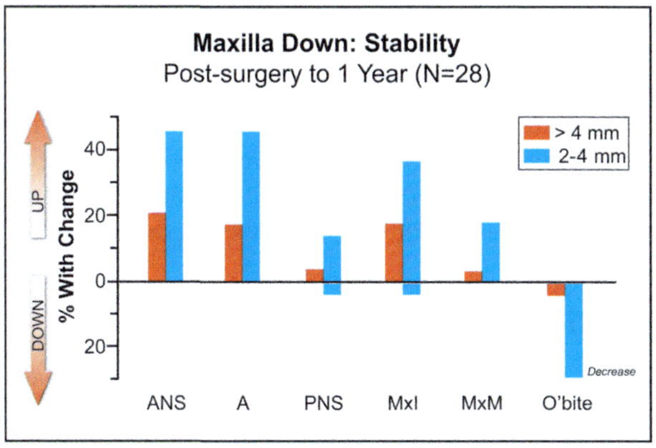

Fig. 18-7 Stability of maxillary downgraft in the first post-surgical year. Even with rigid internal fixation, almost two-thirds of patients experienced vertical relapse of 2 mm or more. Two-jaw surgery, robust rigid fixation, and rigid interpositional grafts all improve the stability of this procedure.

Isolated mandibular set-back to correct Class III malocclusion is classified as problematic in terms of post-surgical stability, with up to 50% of patients experiencing more than 2 mm of relapse. Quite interestingly, use of rigid fixation, especially with bilateral sagittal osteotomies, seemed to actually decrease the stability of the isolated mandibular set-back procedure in the 1990s at UNC. Why would rigidly fixating the mandible actually decrease stability? The answer revealed itself as a problem in surgical technique rather than physiological adaptation.[31] When the mandible is retruded in the operating room, the chin is pushed back towards the posterior border of the mandible. If the proximal segment of the mandible is also retruded (in other words if the ramus is forced backward and inclined distally), relapse is very likely after surgery. As the muscle sling that surrounds the ramus re-establishes itself, the pre-surgical inclination of the ramus returns, and the rigidly fixated distal segment moves forward resulting in relapse of prognathism (Figure 18-8). Even with this technical consideration addressed, post-surgical stability is low enough to be a real consideration in the planning for treatment of prognathic patients.

Long-term data for isolated mandibular set-back surgeries show that 20% of patients experience forward movement of the chin of 2–4 mm, and 10% have more than 4 mm of relapse (Figure 18-9). When compared to Class III patients who did not receive surgical treatment, the increased relapse of mandibular prognathism appears to indicate continued growth in these patients. This continued growth, however, only occurs in a relatively small number of patients (Figure 18-9).

Stability of early surgical treatment

The principles of growth and development might lead one to expect that post-treatment relapse, especially for patients treated at a younger age, would be a more prevalent problem for Class III patients than Class II patients. Ironically, it is Class II patients who experience a greater degree of post-treatment change (after

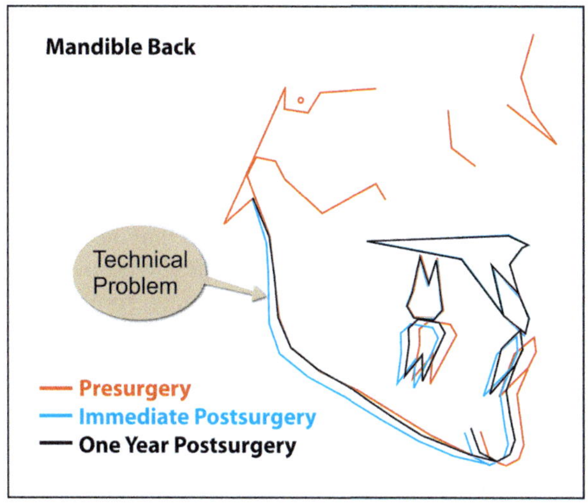

Fig. 18-8 Illustration of the technical operative problem for mandibular set-backs performed before 1995 at UNC. These composite superimpositions for 19 patients demonstrate that the ramus was distally inclined with surgery and self-corrected afterward, moving the chin forward.

the first post-surgical year). A study that examined changes in patients treated for mandibular deficiency early (less than age 16 for girls, 18 for boys) compared to patients treated as adults found that mandibular advancement was actually less stable in the younger group.[32] 50% of the younger patients saw relapse of 2–4 mm with isolated mandibular advancement, and 15% had more than 4 mm of relapse. Only 15% of adult patients had relapse of 2–4 mm, and none had more

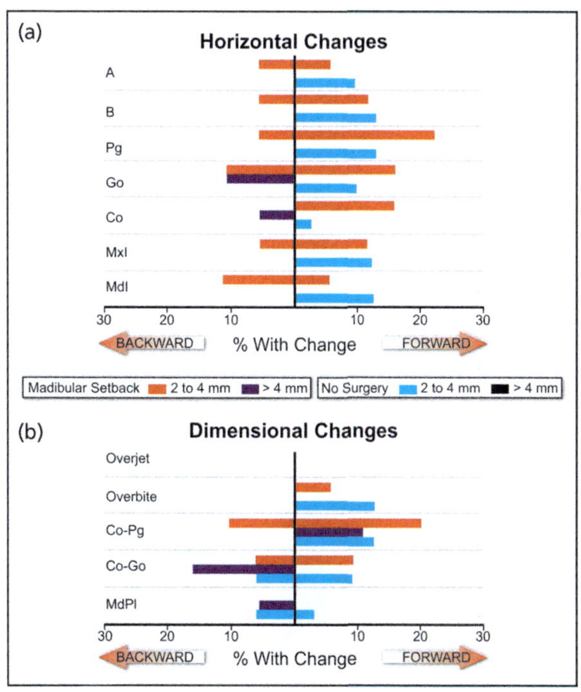

Fig. 18-9 Long-term data for patients with isolated mandibular set-back and for Class III patients treated with orthodontics only. Over the first five post-surgical years, mandibular length increased by 4 mm or more in only 10% of surgical patients (a). This relapse may represent post-treatment growth. Note that overjet was unchanged (b) for both groups over the same time.

than 4 mm. Backward movement of the mandible was even greater for young patients who received two-jaw surgery. It is particularly interesting to note that despite greater relapse, the younger group was actually slightly more satisfied with their treatment result than the older group whose advancement was more stable.

Good data also challenge the notion that most prognathic Class III patients, especially those who are operated at an earlier age, will experience more post-treatment growth of the mandible.[33,34] When stability for young patients treated for Class III problems (less than age 18 for females and 20 for males, who were selected for early treatment because serial cephalometric radiographs showed mandibular growth had essentially been completed) is compared to those who are treated later, almost no difference is seen. For both groups, nearly 25% of patients had a post-treatment loss in overjet of 2–4 mm, although none returned to negative overjet.[33]

Stability of transverse correction

Surgical expansion and constriction of both the mandible and maxilla are possible. Good data are only available, however, for expansion procedures for the maxilla, and the post-surgical stability data from UNC apply to segmental Le Fort I osteotomy for transverse correction.[35] In the short term this procedure is problematic. 30% of patients experienced more than 3 mm of relapse at the molars, although most patients actually experienced some expansion at the first premolars (Figure 18-10).

In young patients, orthopaedic expansion of the maxilla using tooth or mini-implant borne devices is possible and highly effective. For older patients, surgical expansion of the maxilla is possible by segmental osteotomy or surgically-assisted rapid palatal expansion (SARPE). SARPE has been advocated as being more stable than orthopaedic expansion or segmental osteotomy in older patients.[36–38] More recent and more extensive data indicate that the stability of SARPE is clinically equivalent to that of segmental Le Fort I osteotomy,[39,40] and provide good evidence that for patients who require widening and repositioning of the maxilla, two stages of surgery are not necessary to obtain surgical stability of maxillary expansion.

Stability of asymmetry correction

Asymmetry may exist in any component of the face and almost never can be fully corrected in an isolated fashion. In two jaw procedures with rigid fixation, maxillary repositioning for asymmetry tends to be stable in terms of both vertical and horizontal change, with 20% or less of patients showing relapse in the first post-surgical year. Changes at the gonial angles of the mandible appear large but are typical for any mandibular osteotomy. Other mandibular change tends to truly be less stable; up to 50% of patients experience more than 2 mm of change in vertical and horizontal landmarks (Figure 18-11). Genioplasty is stable

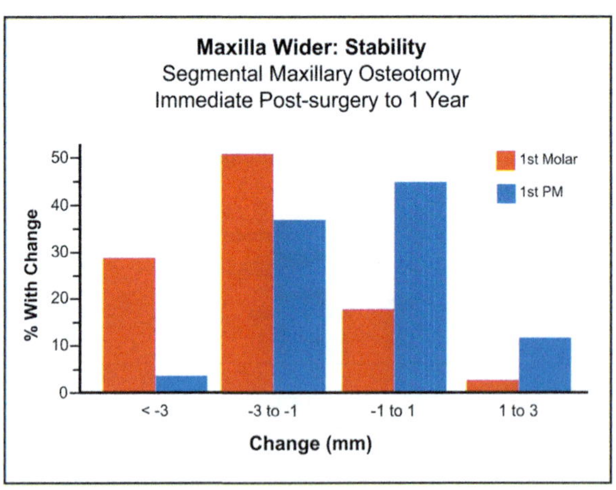

Fig. 18-10 Post-surgical stability of maxillary expansion with segmental Le Fort osteotomy. Note that greater relapse is likely more posterior, with 30% of patients experiencing more than 3 mm of relapse at the molars.

(a)

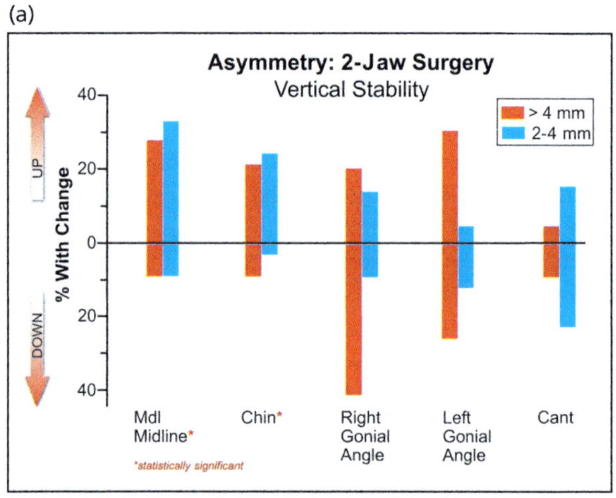

(b)

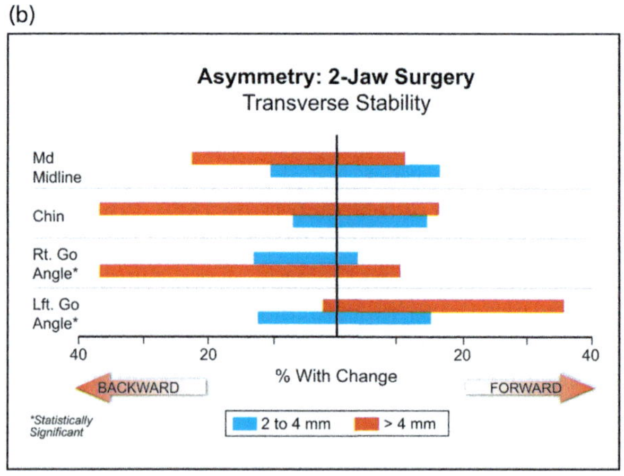

Fig. 18-11 Vertical (a) and transverse (b) changes in the first post-surgical year for patients receiving two-jaw surgery. Vertical correction of the maxilla was quite stable. Asymmetrical mandibular relapse of 2 mm or more was seen in one-third of patients. Remodelling of the gonial angles occurred symmetrically and did not exceed that which is expected for isolated mandibular osteotomy.

in any direction. Considered as a whole, correction of complex facial asymmetry is stable in the short term only if rigid fixation is used.

Conclusion

The hierarchy of surgical stability is an important clinical resource, but it is crucial for clinicians to remember that when it comes to orthognathic procedures, stability is influenced by factors that the surgeon may not be able to control. Indeed, the direction and magnitude of surgical moves, type of fixation, and operative technique all affect stability. But even with the finest surgical skill, significant short and long-term relapse occurs in some patients. Our understanding of the physiological adaptation that precipitates relapse in these patients remains incomplete. Nevertheless, in order to provide optimal treatment outcomes, it is important that clinicians understand the principles that affect stability, plan treatment with stability in mind, and appropriately communicate the risk of relapse to patients.

Acknowledgements

The studies carried out at UNC as well as the preparation of this chapter were supported in part by NIH grants DE-05221 and T90DE-021986-01 from the US National Institutes of Health. We thank Ms Debora Price for her long-time management of the Dentofacial Program Data Base.

References

1 Proffit WR, Turvey TA, Phillips C. The hierarchy of stability and predictability in orthognathic surgery with rigid fixation: an update and extension. Head Face Med. 2007;30;3:21.
2 Phillips C, Snow MD, Turvey TA, Proffit WR. The effect of orthognathic surgery on head posture. Eur J Orthod. 1991;13:397–403.
3 Proffit WR, Turvey TA, Fields HW, Phillips C. The effect of orthognathic surgery on occlusal force. J Oral Maxillofac Surg. 1989;47:457–63.
4 Proffit WR, Fields HW, Sarver DM, Ackerman JL. Contemporary Orthodontics. 5th ed. St. Louis, MO: Mosby, 2013.
5 Proffit WR, Phillips C. Adaptations in lip posture and pressure following orthognathic surgery. Am J Orthod Dentofacial Orthop. 1988;93:294–302.
6 Young T, Palta M, Dempsey J, Skatrud J, Weber S, Badr S. The occurrence of sleep-disordered breathing among middle-aged adults. N Engl J Med. 1993;328:1230–5.
7 Turvey TA, Hall DJ, Warren DW. Alterations in nasal airway resistance following superior repositioning of the maxilla. Am J Orthod. 1984;85:109–14.
8 Spalding PM, Vig PS, Lints RR, Vig KD, Fonseca RJ. The effects of maxillary surgery on nasal respiration. Int J Adult Orthodon Orthognath Surg. 1991;6:191–9.
9 Perren SM. Physical and biological aspects of fracture healing with special reference to internal fixation. Clin Orthop Relat Res. 1979;138:175–96.
10 Reitzik M. Cortex-to-cortex healing after mandibular osteotomy. J Oral Maxillofac Surg. 1983;41:658–63.
11 Frost DE, Koutnik AW. Alternative stabilization of the maxilla during simultaneous jaw-mobilization procedures. Oral Surg Oral Med Oral Pathol. 1983;56:125–7.
12 Boyne PJ. Osseous healing after oblique osteotomy of the mandibular ramus. J Oral Surg. 1966;24:125–33.
13 Buckley MJ, Tulloch JF, White RP, Jr, Tucker MR. Complications of orthognathic surgery: a comparison between wire fixation and rigid internal fixation. Int J Adult Orthodon Orthognath Surg. 1989;4:69–74.
14 Simmons KE, Turvey TA, Phillips C, Proffit WR. Surgical-orthodontic correction of mandibular deficiency: five-year follow-up. Int J Adult Orthodon Orthognath Surg. 1992;7:67–79.
15 Schubert P, Bailey LJ, White RP, Jr, Proffit WR. Long-term cephalometric changes in untreated adults compared to those treated with orthognathic surgery. Int J Adult Orthodon Orthognath Surg. 1999;14:91–9.
16 Proffit WR, Phillips C, Turvey TA. Stability following superior repositioning of the maxilla by LeFort I osteotomy. Am J Orthod Dentofacial Orthop. 1987;92:151–61.
17 Bailey LJ, Phillips C, Proffit WR, Turvey TA. Stability following superior repositioning of the maxilla by Le Fort I osteotomy: five-year follow-up. Int J Adult Orthodon Orthognath Surg. 1994;9:163–73.
18 Proffit WR, Bailey LJ, Phillips C, Turvey TA. Long-term stability of surgical open-bite correction by Le Fort I osteotomy. Angle Orthod. 2000;70:112–7.
19 Wolford LM, Karras SC, Mehra P. Considerations for orthognathic surgery during growth, part 2: maxillary deformities. Am J Orthod Dentofacial Orthop. 2001;119:102–5.
20 Turvey TA, Phillips C, Zaytoun HS, Jr, Proffit WR. Simultaneous superior repositioning of the maxilla and mandibular advancement. A report on stability. Am J Orthod Dentofacial Orthop. 1988;94:372–83.
21 Forssell K, Turvey TA, Phillips C, Proffit WR. Superior repositioning of the maxilla combined with mandibular advancement: mandibular RIF improves stability. Am J Orthod Dentofacial Orthop. 1992;102:342–50.
22 Miguel JA, Turvey TA, Phillips C, Proffit WR. Long-term stability of two-jaw surgery for treatment of mandibular deficiency and vertical maxillary excess. Int J Adult Orthodon Orthognath Surg. 1995;10:235–45.
23 Fontes AM, Joondeph DR, Bloomquist DS, Greenlee GM, Wallen TR, Huang GJ. Long-term stability of anterior open-bite closure with bilateral sagittal split osteotomy. Am J Orthod Dentofacial Orthop. 2012;142:792–800.
24 Proffit WR, Jackson TH, Turvey TA. Changes in the pattern of patients receiving surgical-orthodontic treatment. Am J Orthod Dentofacial Orthop. 2013;143:793–8.
25 Bailey LJ, Duong HL, Proffit WR. Surgical Class III treatment: long-term stability and patient perceptions of treatment outcome. Int J Adult Orthodon Orthognath Surg. 1998;13:35–44.
26 Proffit WR, Phillips C, Prewitt JW, Turvey TA. Stability after surgical-orthodontic correction of skeletal Class III malocclusion. 2. Maxillary advancement. Int J Adult Orthodon Orthognath Surg. 1991;6:71–80.
27 Busby BR, Bailey LJ, Proffit WR, Phillips C, White RP, Jr. Long-term stability of surgical class III treatment: a study of 5-year postsurgical results. Int J Adult Orthodon Orthognath Surg. 2002;17:159–70.
28 Severt TR, Proffit WR. The prevalence of facial asymmetry in the dentofacial deformities population at the University of North Carolina. Int J Adult Orthodon Orthognath Surg. 1997;12:171–6.
29 Proffit WR, Phillips C, Dann C,4th, Turvey TA. Stability after surgical-orthodontic correction of skeletal Class III malocclusion. I. Mandibular setback. Int J Adult Orthodon Orthognath Surg. 1991;6:7–18.
30 Perez MM, Sameshima GT, Sinclair PM. The long-term stability of LeFort I maxillary downgrafts with rigid fixation to correct vertical maxillary deficiency. Am J Orthod Dentofacial Orthop. 1997;112:104–8.

31 Schardt-Sacco D, Turvey TA. Minimizing relapse after sagittal osteotomy for correction of mandibular prognathism. J Oral Maxillofac Surg. 1997;55 (suppl 3) (85).
32 Proffit WR, Phillips C, Turvey TA. Long-term stability of adolescent versus adult surgery for treatment of mandibular deficiency. Int J Oral Maxillofac Surg. 2010;39:327–32.
33 Bailey LJ, Phillips C, Proffit WR. Long-term outcome of surgical Class III correction as a function of age at surgery. Am J Orthod Dentofacial Orthop. 2008;133:365–70.
34 Bailey LJ, Dover AJ, Proffit WR. Long-term soft tissue changes after orthodontic and surgical corrections of skeletal class III malocclusions. Angle Orthod. 2007;77:389–96.
35 Phillips C, Medland WH, Fields HW, Jr, Proffit WR, White RP, Jr. Stability of surgical maxillary expansion. Int J Adult Orthodon Orthognath Surg. 1992;7:139–46.
36 Northway WM, Meade JB, Jr. Surgically assisted rapid maxillary expansion: a comparison of technique, response, and stability. Angle Orthod. 1997;67:309–20.
37 Silverstein K, Quinn PD. Surgically-assisted rapid palatal expansion for management of transverse maxillary deficiency. J Oral Maxillofac Surg. 1997;55:725–7.
38 Stromberg C, Holm J. Surgically assisted, rapid maxillary expansion in adults. A retrospective long-term follow-up study. J Craniomaxillofac Surg. 1995;23:222–7.
39 Chamberland S, Proffit WR. Closer look at the stability of surgically assisted rapid palatal expansion. J Oral Maxillofac Surg. 2008;66:1895–1900.
40 Chamberland S, Proffit WR. Short-term and long-term stability of surgically assisted rapid palatal expansion revisited. Am J Orthod Dentofacial Orthop. 2011;139:815–22.e1.

Chapter 19

Management of Select Complications in Orthognathic Surgery

David S. Precious

Introduction

The surgeon who performs orthognathic surgery must also be able to manage the complications of that surgery. This statement seems almost so obvious and basic as to preclude the necessity to utter it. Nevertheless, in my opinion, it requires a much wider skill-set and significantly broader surgical experience to be able to effectively and efficiently manage the complications of orthognathic surgery. As the surgeon becomes more experienced in the management of complications, the intellectual exercise of reflection bubbles up from below and almost without announcement, the surgeon assumes a new, more important role of developing a strategy of *prevention* of complications and unwanted events. It is at this point that (s)he becomes the true advocate of the patient.

There are three principal aspects of orthognathic surgery where we encounter the possibility of complications:

1. Diagnosis and planning
2. During surgery
3. After surgery.

Orthodontic factors

(i) Poor and/or inadequate bracket placement

This not only leads to increased operating time but also causes inadequate fixation and uncontrolled intra-arch forces (Figure 19-1). The orthodontist must be made aware of the need for proper bracket placement to prevent this problem.

(ii) Bolton discrepancy

A Bolton discrepancy or Bolton-like circumstance can arise due to missing teeth, space loss from restorations as well as failure to establish and maintain lost space from missing or small lateral incisors (Figure 19-2). If the orthodontist closes all space prior to surgery, the occlusion will never be realized such that at the end of surgery a Class I molar/canine relationship is

Orthognathic Surgery: Principles, Planning and Practice. Edited by Farhad B. Naini and Daljit S. Gill.

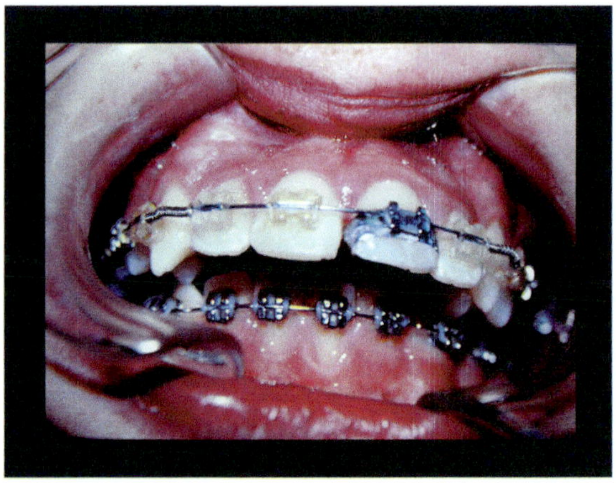

Fig. 19-1 Tentative bracket condition which looks at high risk for bracket loss during the procedure.

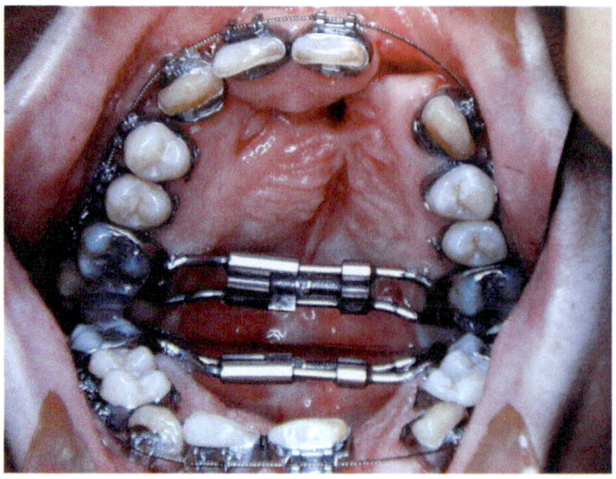

Fig. 19-3 Careful planning and patient supervision must be exercised when increasing the transverse dimension of the maxilla.

achieved. This problem frequently results in unnecessary surgical segmentalization of the maxilla and should be avoided.

(iii) Inappropriate transverse therapy

Great care must be taken by the orthodontist to avoid maxillary transverse expansion by lateral flaring of teeth beyond the alveolar apical base (Figure 19-3). This action almost always results in orthodontic relapse, which depending on the original deformity also induces failure to maintain the surgically achieved occlusion.

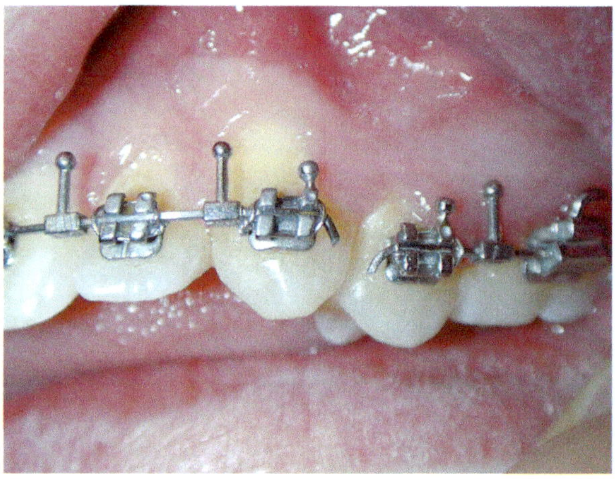

Fig. 19-4 Segmental archwires can be very helpful to the surgeon particularly in management of open bite.

(iv) Segmental vs. continuous archwire (Figure 19-4)

Failure to consider the use of segmental orthodontic archwire mechanics can contribute to 'building in' orthodontic tooth relapse, particularly in certain cases of vertical deformity and open bite.

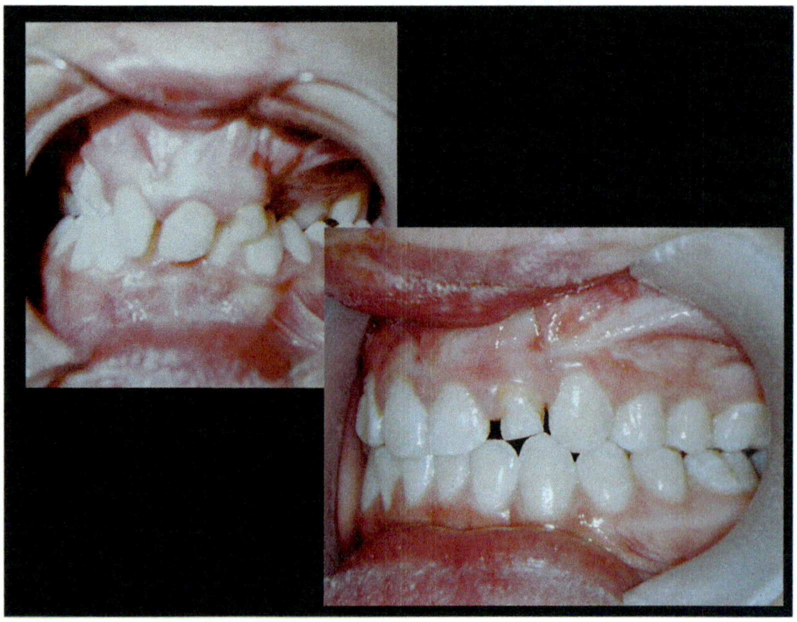

Fig. 19-2 Before and after Le Fort I osteotomy. Note the creation and maintenance of space between the central incisor and maxillary canine which allowed the surgeon to achieve the correct maxillary position.

(v) Communication between the orthodontist and the surgeon

Both the orthodontist and the surgeon must communicate with each other during the planning phase of case management. In particular the surgeon must be made aware of the orthodontic treatment limitations just as the orthodontist must be made aware of the surgical limitations. Most important of all is that the patient be made aware of all of the treatment limitations, before accepting the treatment plan. If possible, for this consultation with the patient, both the surgeon and the orthodontist should be present.

Maxillary surgery

Complications from maxillary osteotomies include instability of the osteotomized parts, infections, vascular, neural and ophthalmic injuries, and psychosocial problems.

Haemorrhage following Le Fort I osteotomy can be severe and potentially life-threatening. The incidence of this very rare complication is estimated to be less than 1%. Post-orthognathic surgery vascular complications include arterio-venous fistulae, carotid-cavernous fistulae and pseudoaneurysms. In spite of the rarity of such complications, oral and maxillofacial surgeons must be familiar with techniques involved in their diagnosis and management.

Ramping in maxillary advancement surgery

It is well-known that when one surgically advances the maxilla using a straight cut osteotomy the vertical dimension of the anterior maxilla can be difficult to control. Several solutions exist to deal with this problem the most popular of which is to use a stepped osteotomy design. We prefer to use a reverse step osteotomy design because in our view this design results in better bone contact of the new position of the maxilla (Figures 19-5 and 19-6).

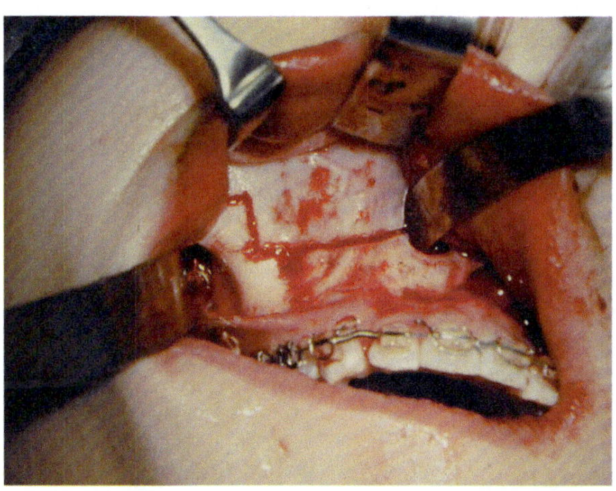

Fig. 19-5 Reverse step osteotomy design gives excellent bone contact in maxillary advancement surgery while at the same time prevents 'ramping'.

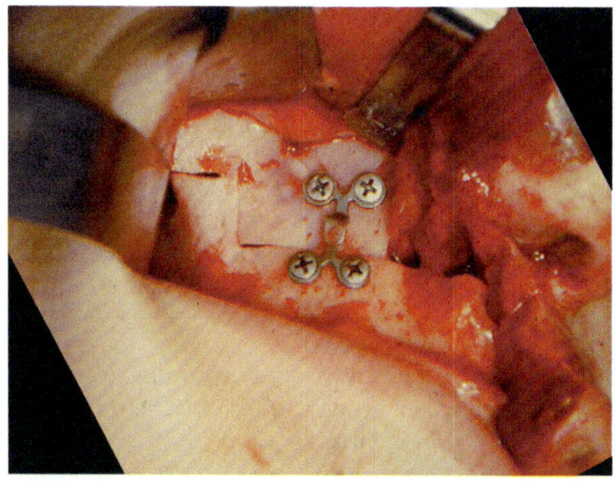

Fig. 19-6 Note overlap of bony parts of maxilla in advanced position.

Avoidance of the use of large pterygoid chisel to achieve pterygomaxillary separation

Pterygomaxillary separation can be predictably and safely achieved using only Tessier spreaders and Rowe disimpaction forceps by first spreading the Le Fort I osteotomy cut using the Tessier spreader to its maximum vertical opening followed by easy pterygomaxillary separation using the Rowe forceps. This technique offers maximum maxillary mobility without threat to the integrity of the descending palatine vessels, a particular benefit in the case of Le Fort I osteotomy in a patient with cleft lip and palate.

Serious bleeding after Le Fort I osteotomy

Delayed severe epistaxis after Le Fort osteotomy, although rare, is potentially life-threatening. This complication may be associated with other vascular complications such as pseudoaneurysm or arteriovenous fistula. Many authors suggest that one possible cause of haemorrhage after Le Fort I osteotomy is fracture of the pterygoid plates, although good evidence is lacking on this hypothesis. CT studies by Rennick[1] (12 patients), Precious et al.[2] (58 patients) and Lanigan[3] (16 patients) have demonstrated variable frequency of intraoperative fracture of the pterygoid plates, but of the 86 cases reported, none of the patients had clinical bleeding.

A representative selection of four patients who experienced delayed (7–10 days post-surgery) serious epistaxis serves to illustrate the variability of findings regarding fractured pterygoid plate and clinical bleeding (Table 19-1).

Overall our observed rate of bleeding was 9 in 5401. We used this cross-sectional data with the Fisher's exact test to determine if delayed severe epistaxis was independent of pterygoid fracture. At the 0.05 level there was no association between pterygoid plate fracture and postoperative epistaxis. Indeed to demonstrate a reduction in frequency of bleeding to 3/4501,

Table 19-1 Representative selection of four patients who experienced delayed (7–10 days post-surgery) serious epistaxis

Patient	Epistaxis	Angiography	Pterygoid plate
1	Yes, bilateral nostril	Pseudoaneurysm	Fractured, bilateral
2	Yes, bilateral nostril	Normal	Fractured bilateral
3	Yes, bilateral nostril	Normal	Normal
4	Yes, right nostril only	Normal	Normal right Fractured left

we would need a study of two groups of 25,000 patients each when testing at traditional alpha level of 0.05 with a power of 90%.

Accordingly, there is no strict causal relationship between pterygoid plate fracture and epistaxis after Le Fort I osteotomy.

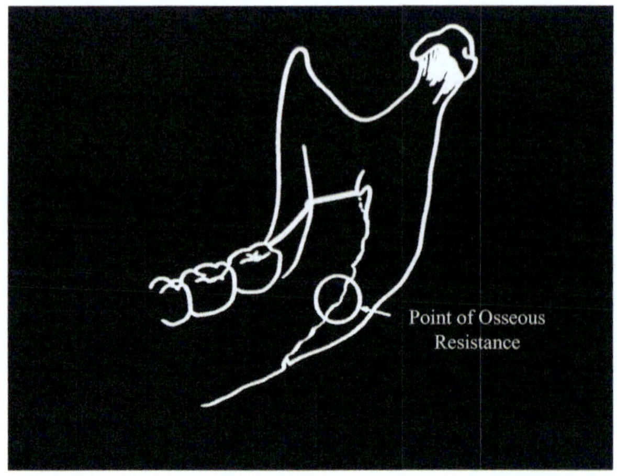

Fig. 19-8 The point of common osseous resistance, which is why it is safer to open the sagittal split from above down rather than from anterior to posterior.

Mandibular surgery

Mandibular body ostectomy

The surgeon must not overlook the possibility of using mandibular body osteotomy/ostectomy if planning shows that this is occlusally feasible. Mandibular body surgery has been shown to be one of the most stable orthognathic procedures (Figure 19-7).

Sagittal split ramus osteotomy (SSRO)

There are several important technical aspects of the SSRO which can enhance the safety and accuracy of this operation. First the lingual horizontal osteotomy must be sufficiently deep to communicate with the bony trough just supero-posteriorly to the entrance of the inferior alveolar neurovascular bundle. Second, the vertical osteotomy must engage half the thickness of the inferior border of the mandible. Third the sagittal osteotomy must follow the contours of the external oblique ridge. When the osteotomies have been carried out in this fashion one can complete the split without using a chisel and by opening the bone from the top down, thus avoiding the more dangerous act of opening the bone from anterior to posterior. The point of osseous resistance on the lingual aspect of the mandible yields more predictably, in our experience, when one uses this top–down approach (Figure 19-8). When the surgeon uses the 'top–down' technique the inferior alveolar neurovascular bundle can be seen much earlier in the split and as a result can be very effectively protected.

The clinical maxim germane to the SSRO is that prevention of an unwanted split or fracture is much preferable to having to deal with a 'bad split'.

SSRO and third molars (Figure 19-9)

There is controversy about the presence or absence of third molars during sagittal split osteotomies (SSOs) on the frequency of unfavourable fractures, degree of entrapment and manipulation of the inferior alveolar nerve.

In our own research we have conducted a number of studies, the most recent of which was a prospective cohort study of 339 (670 SSRO) patients who underwent SSOs to correct mandibular deformities. The primary predictor variable was the status of the mandibular third molar at the time of SSO, and it was divided into two levels, present at the time of SSO (group I) or absent at the time of SSO (group II). The primary outcome variable was unfavourable splits. The secondary outcome variables were the degree of

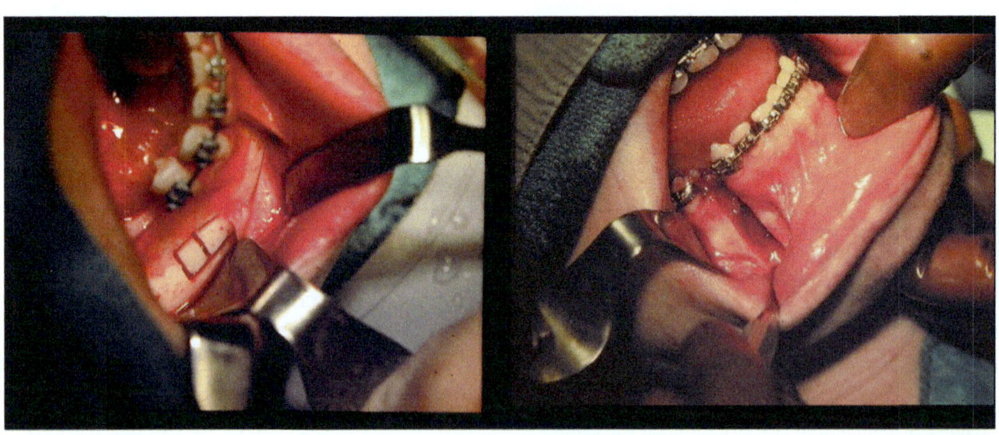

Fig. 19-7 Body ostectomy is among the most stable procedures in orthognathic surgery.

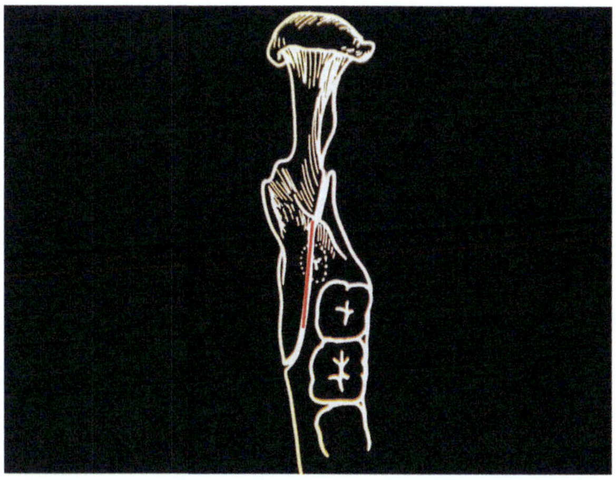

Fig. 19-9 When the third molar is present the surgeon should make the sagittal osteotomy according to the position of the external oblique ridge and cut right through the tooth, removing it through the split when it is complete.

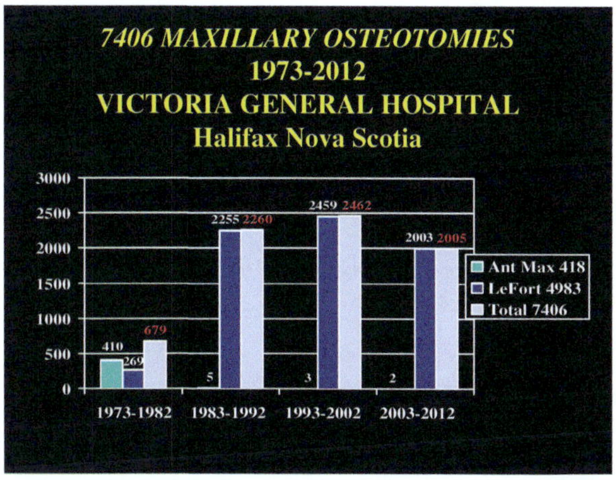

Fig. 19-10 Log of maxillary surgery over 40 years at Dalhousie.

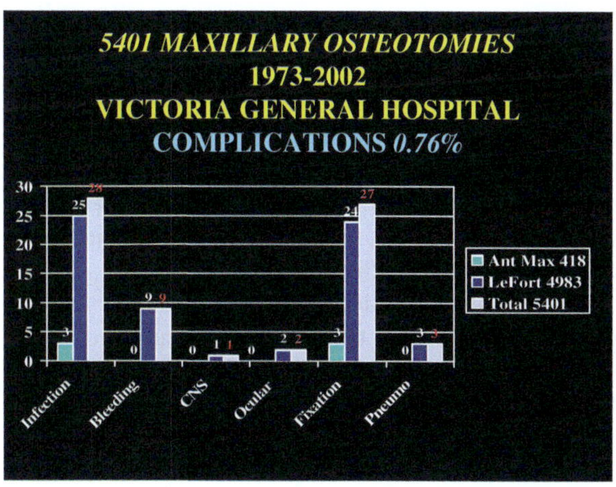

Fig. 19-11 Summary of complications associated with maxillary surgery over 30 years.

entrapment/manipulation of the inferior alveolar nerve and the procedural time.

The presence of third molars during SSOs did not appear to be associated with an increased frequency of unfavourable fractures. Concomitant third molar removal in SSROs also decreases proximal segment inferior alveolar nerve entrapment.

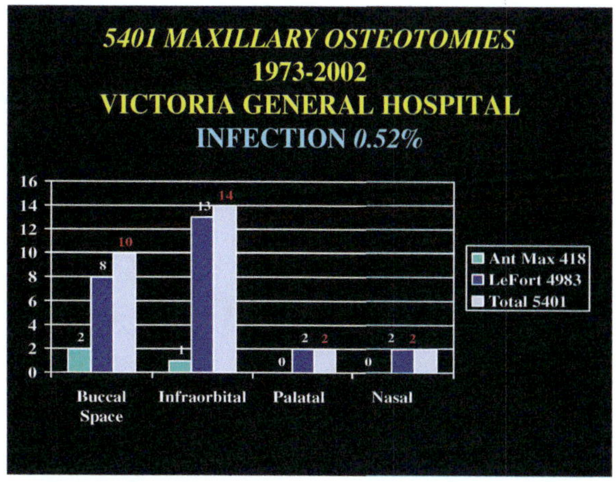

Fig. 19-12 Anatomical distribution of maxillary infections over 30 years.

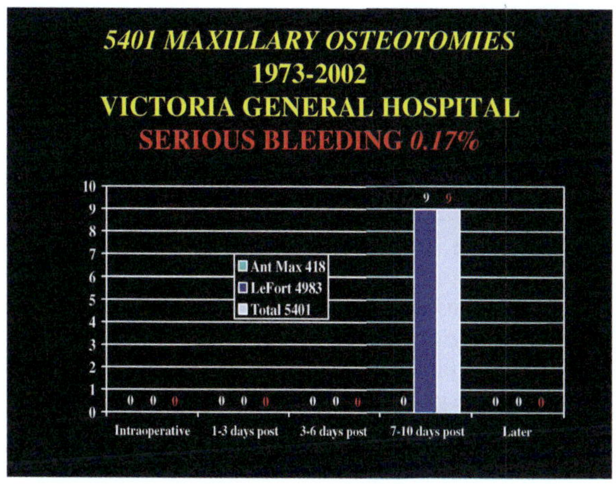

Fig. 19-13 Serious bleeding post-surgery occurred in every observed case between 7 and 10 days after Le Fort procedure.

Summary of orthognathic surgery complications

1. Orthognathic surgery is relatively safe (Figures 19-10 to 19-13).
2. Complications related to factors in play before surgery can be minimized by careful planning and close collaboration between the orthodontist and the surgeon.
3. Complications during and after surgery are rare.
4. The precise aetiology of rare events is difficult to determine.

References

1 Renick BM, Symington JM. Postoperative computed tomography study of pterygomaxillary separation during the Le Fort 1 osteotomy. J Oral Maxillofac Surg. 1991;49:1061–10.

2 Precious DS, Goodday RH, Bourget L, Skulsky FG. Pterygoid plate fracture in Le Fort I osteotomy with and without pterygoid chisel: A computed tomography scan evaluations of 58 patients. J Oral Maxillofac Surg. 1993;51:151–3.

3 Lanigan D, Loewy T. Postoperative computed tomography scan study of the pterygomaxillary separation during the Le Fort I osteotomy using a micro-oscillating saw. J Oral and Maxillofac Surg. 1995;53:1161–6.

Chapter 20

Patient Satisfaction and Patient-Centred Outcome Measures in Orthognathic Surgery

Ceib Phillips and Caitlin Magraw

Introduction

Clinicians who treat patients with a dentofacial disharmony know that the aesthetic and functional changes that result from orthognathic surgery can have profound long-lasting benefits for patients: improved function; improved quality of life; improved self-concept; decreased fear of negative evaluation; and improved psychological well-being.[1–7] Likely the most influential consideration in a person's decision to have orthognathic surgery is their level of anticipation, 'the feeling of looking forward, usually excitedly or eagerly, to something that is going to happen.' And a person's expectations, 'a mental image of something expected, often compared to its reality,' likely influence their perception and experiences during recovery.[7] For the clinician, one of the most difficult jobs is to be able to 'read' and correctly 'interpret' a patient's clues or cues with respect to their motivation for surgery, their understanding of the process and procedures, and their recovery experience. Although published as a three-stage, conceptual model for assisting oncologists,[8] the communication stages of Recognition, Exploration, and Therapeutic action can be adapted to any clinical encounter where the patient may be confused over treatment options, anxious, worried, or distressed.

How patient–clinician communication affects patient perception of treatment outcomes and recovery is an important field of research given the importance of patient-reported outcomes as a component of patient-centred outcomes research (PCOR). The first Methodology Committee report written for the PCOR Institute provided a working definition as 'PCOR helps people and their caregivers communicate and make informed healthcare decisions, allowing their voices (patients) to be heard in assessing the value of healthcare options.'[9] Perhaps a more simplistic definition is that PCOR assesses the outcomes that

Orthognathic Surgery: Principles, Planning and Practice. Edited by Farhad B. Naini and Daljit S. Gill.

Box 20-1 A relevance problem related to questions and endpoints

Clinicians generally choose questions and endpoints that they consider to be of interest and importance to the clinical outcome. Although the 'success' of the surgery is important to patients, patients are frequently anxious about more personal problems or issues that may occur during recovery and appreciate the clinician's recognition that these concerns are real and who engage in supportive communications, and if necessary, therapeutic actions.

Clinician concern examples	Patient concern examples
Immediate post-op:	
Serious complications	Extent of nausea and vomiting experienced
Stability	Difficulty breathing
Short-term post-op:	
Infection	Resolution of swelling and difficulties eating normal diet
	Ability to return to work/normal activities
Long-term post-op:	
Hardware failure	Persistent altered sensation
Relapse	

are important, relevant, and valued by the patients undergoing the treatment (Box 20-1). In this chapter, we will explore outcomes following orthognathic surgery that patients notice and care about using comments from orthognathic surgery patient blogs available on the internet for illustration. Immediate postoperative disturbances will be addressed first and include postoperative nausea/vomiting, overall patient comfort, and weight loss. Next, long-term disturbances and physical impacts including complications, temporomandibular joint disorder and functionality, will be discussed. Finally, long-term patient satisfaction and perception of improvement will be addressed including psychosocial effects, aesthetics and regret. The last section will provide general recommendations for improving patient satisfaction with an emphasis on improving provider pre-surgical communication.

Immediate postoperative disturbances

Postoperative nausea and vomiting

Nausea and vomiting that occurs after surgery but prior to discharge (PONV) can negatively impact a patient's recovery, increase morbidity, delay discharge, and increase hospital costs,[10] while nausea and vomiting that occurs after discharge (PDNV) can increase a patient's and caregiver's anxiety and

Box 20-2 PONV/PDNV comments from patient blogs on the internet

'The next thing I remember is throwing up. I had tons of blood in my stomach and I can't tolerate that.'

http://rearrangemyface.blogspot.com/2007_03_01_archive.html

'So far the worst part has been the nausea.'

http://brandysjawjourney.blogspot.com/2007_05_01_archive.html

'This was the day I was discharged.... This 2 days before the hell of nausea broke out. The nausea for me was worse than the surgery.'

www.jenrowsell.ca/2010/02/jaw-surgery-recovery-pictures.html

'Hey there, I'm 9 days post op with double jaw surgery... I had nausea that kept me from sleeping sometime, then I threw up like 5–6 times, all the liquids I had taken earlier came out.'

www.jawsurgeryblog.com/forums/viewtopic.php?f=5&t=2705 by sweetrock » Mon Aug 29, 2011 12:39 pm

agitation and result in unplanned hospital department/practice visits (Box 20-2). Interestingly, patients before surgery have reported that PONV is of greater concern than the expected postoperative pain.[11,12] And short-term patient dissatisfaction has been significantly associated with the occurrence of PONV.[13,14]

PONV and PDNV is a frequent complication of orthognathic surgery. According to reports, 40[10] to 60%[15] of patients experience nausea and 25% vomiting within the first 24 hours after surgery. These estimates are considerably higher than the 8 to 30% reported for general surgical populations, despite application of conventional antiemetic therapies.[10,16] After discharge, approximately 50% of patients who completed a structured medical diary reported experiencing nausea and 25% reported episodes of vomiting.[17,18] Vomiting post-discharge was significantly more frequent in patients who had undergone a two jaw procedure (43%) versus a maxillary osteotomy only (16%) or a mandibular osteotomy alone (5%).[15]

Multiple factors have been associated with PONV including the type of general anaesthetic, particularly nitrous oxide,[15] the length and type of surgery, postoperative analgesics given, and patient risk factors that predispose a patient to PONV with all general anaesthetics.[10] Preoperative patient characteristics that may increase a patient's risk of PONV include:

1. Non-smoking status. Cigarette smoking tends to inhibit emesis, likely through an increase in hepatic enzymes.[10,19]
2. Being female. Women have an increased risk of PONV that is 2–3 times greater than that of men.[20–22]

3. Being young (15–25 years).[10]
4. A prior history of motion sickness, PONV, vertigo, or migraine headaches.

Operative factors also play a role in the risk for PONV and PDNV. Research has shown that PONV occurred in a significantly higher frequency in patients who experienced a longer operation time,[16] which is likely related to the type of procedure performed. Patients who undergo two jaw procedures report the highest frequency of PONV and PDNV, followed by those undergoing maxillary osteotomy only, and then those with mandibular osteotomy only. These associations with length of surgery and type of procedure may be related to increased blood loss, which may subsequently increase the amount of blood in the stomach, the strongest peripheral emetogenic stimuli.[10] Postoperative factors can also contribute to the occurrence of PONV/PDNV. Pain is frequently treated by opioid analgesics. It is unclear whether pain itself plays a role in initiating emesis via the sympathetic nervous system,[10] or opioids via sensitization to motion of both the vestibular and otic areas cause PONV,[16,23] or both mechanisms work in concert. Use of longer-acting opioids (e.g., morphine, meperidine) has been related to a higher frequency of PONV than short-acting opioids (e.g., fentanyl, remifentanil).[24]

PONV/PDNV prevention for orthognathic surgery patients is an under-investigated domain of clinical care. As more orthognathic surgical procedures are performed on an ambulatory basis (often outside of the hospital setting), tactics to reduce the high incidence of PONV/PDNV in this surgical population become important to maximize patient safety and satisfaction, and to potentially contain costs. A multimodal protocol has been introduced that shows promising results for decreasing the frequency of postoperative nausea and vomiting in patients undergoing a Le Fort I osteotomy.[15] Approximately 25% of patients who had a two jaw procedure and were given the multimodal protocol had postoperative nausea compared to 74% of those who did not. The decrease in the frequency of postoperative vomiting was as striking: 11% of those who had the multimodal protocol vs. 33% of those who did not.[15] Decreasing PONV is valuable clinically, but understanding and controlling PDNV is particularly important if surgery is performed in an ambulatory care setting which requires patients and their caregivers to cope with postoperative sequelae in the absence of direct medical supervision. Post-discharge nausea and vomiting is increasingly recognized as a separate entity that may require different management strategies than does PONV and has received little attention.[12]

Postoperative discomfort

Convalescence after orthognathic surgery is a complex process requiring the resolution of pain, swelling, and difficulty with eating. Although pain from orthognathic surgery is often partially masked by altered sensation, almost one-third of patients describe their pain as 'severe' even after discharge from the hospital.[4] The degree of postoperative pain correlates with the length of the operation.[4] Pain/discomfort persists for 2 to 3 weeks after surgery for the majority of patients. By 30 days after surgery, less than 5% of patients report experiencing 'substantial' pain at some time during the day, but approximately 20% report still taking medication for pain/discomfort.[18] Although the vast majority of patients believe that their pain is managed effectively by the analgesics they were prescribed, many patients report that their pain persists longer than expected after surgery.[4]

Swelling is a well-known side effect of orthognathic surgery, but patients are often not prepared for the extent of the swelling or how long the resolution of the swelling will take (Box 20-3). Resolution of swelling takes approximately 1 to 2 weeks longer than other immediate post-surgery sequelae such as nausea, bruising, bleeding, or food collection in the soft tissue incision. The average number of days until patients perceive swelling has resolved (no or only slight concern) is 10 and 75% of patients report no/slight concern by day 22 after surgery.[18] Difficulty breathing is primarily related to postoperative oedema. Although the majority of patients recovering from orthognathic surgery do not experience difficulty breathing, it is a troubling sensation for those that do (Box 20-3). Individuals that undergo bimaxillary or maxillary surgery report more difficulty breathing in the postoperative period than individuals undergoing single-jaw mandibular surgery.

Difficulty eating after orthognathic surgery is compounded by several factors including pain, oedema, altered sensation, and physical limitations associated with the procedure itself (i.e., intraoral splints, wires, rubber bands, and maxillomandibular fixation). Problems with eating, chewing, and mouth opening take the longest to resolve, approximately 6 to 8 weeks. Seventy-five percent of the subjects report no or only a slight problem with chewing by day 70.[18] Bimaxillary surgery tends to produce more difficulty eating than single-jaw surgery, although average weight loss for patients with single-jaw and bimaxillary surgery is approximately the same (~6.5%).[5] It takes approximately 4 to 6 weeks for patients to regain lost weight.[4]

Substantial clinical research evidence indicates that patients who are psychologically distressed before surgery tend to have a slower post-surgical recovery, report more pain, and use more pain medication.[5,6,25] These findings highlight the importance of improving patient management strategies for orthognathic surgery patients who display symptoms of psychological distress pre-surgery. Clinicians should be aware of the potential negative effect on recovery and satisfaction of pre- or post-surgery distress and consider ways to provide appropriate counseling.[4]

Box 20-3 Short-term recovery comments from patient blogs on the internet

Swelling

'There's a lead-like heaviness on the front of my face, like there's a good 10 lbs hanging off my nose and chin.'
http://roxsjawsurgery.wordpress.com/2013/03/06/day-3-home-to-stay/

'... my face felt like a pressure-cooker. If I swelled any more I'd burst! Everyone tells me that some people swell more than this, but it's just this feeling in the skin on my face – there's just no more stretch, my skin is at max capacity, like patent leather!'
http://roxsjawsurgery.wordpress.com/2013/03/06/day-3-home-to-stay/

'10 days post-op... and not looking very happy. I'd smile if I could!'
http://realityalwaysbites.wordpress.com

'Day 15 ... and I've hit the wall. Can't sleep. Eating is annoying. Swelling doesn't seem to be going away. Verge of tears at any minute.'
http://crazyjaw.blogspot.com/2007_02_01_archive.html

'4 Weeks Post: I still have quite a bit of swelling. I am working really hard on trying to hold my lips closed as it is a bit disturbing to me that my right lower lip droops down a bit.'

'6 Weeks Post-op: I'm still trying to get used to my new face. The swelling is still there. It is pretty bad today... Some days I just feel like it's not me and this chubby face is just weird looking.'
http://aimeesfunkyjaw.blogspot.com/

'3 months: NOT used to my face yet. Some days I feel like a wildebeest, some days I feel just fine. It's an adjustment.'
http://iagreedtoorthognathicsurgery.blogspot.com/search?updated-max=2009-08-25T19:03:00-07:00&max-results=7

Breathing

'My nose gets really stuffed and my throat is sore from the intubation and coated in thick saliva. It's very hard to breathe. When I start to fear that I won't be able to breathe, I start to panic and start crying and it makes it so much harder to breathe.'
http://roxsjawsurgery.wordpress.com/2013/03/05/day-2-codeine-sleep-mask-and-clear-liquids/

'I remember not being able to breathe.'
http://steffies-orthognathic-surgery.blogspot.com/2012/11/waking-up-in-recovery-after.html

Eating

'I'm wondering if I'll ever eat normally again.'
http://megsjaw.blogspot.com

Return to everyday life

'I didn't have any motivation to get up and face another day of slurping foods, not talking properly and feeling the many discomforts of jaw surgery.'
http://roxsjawsurgery.wordpress.com/2013/03/27/day-21-something-to-talk-about/

Depression is a known side effect of surgery, including orthognathic surgery, which involves lengthy general anaesthetics. Multiple studies have indicated postoperative depression may be more common than clinicians realize.[26,27] Because orthognathic surgery is an elective procedure and patients are generally in good health, depression can be particularly troubling to patients. Alerting patients in advance that feeling anxious or depressed may occur after surgery gives the patient 'permission' to discuss these problems if they occur. Clinicians often are uncomfortable discussing personal issues such as family, mental health or emotional issues. But practitioners can easily establish a rationale for this discussion by explaining that there are two main reasons for addressing personal topics as part of the pre-surgery evaluation or during a post-surgery follow-up. The first is that a change in facial appearance can be stressful, even when it is aesthetically pleasing. Some patients may find this surprising, so it is important to emphasize that any change, good or bad, may produce stress, and that stress management is an important component of good medical care. The second is the stress related to the time, physiological responses, and recovery issues associated with treatment, especially the surgery. These explanations will help the patient appreciate why the practitioner needs information about the 'whole' patient, not just the mouth and face. Most patients appreciate an interest in the non-technical side of their care, and this sets the stage for questions about marital status, available social support, history of drug/alcohol abuse, psychological counselling (current or past), and current life satisfaction.

Return to everyday life

Recovery from orthognathic surgery frequently takes longer than patients anticipate. It has been estimated that 5 to 7 days are necessary for generalized adaptation,[4] but returning to 'normal', (i.e. no problems sleeping, talking, taking part in their everyday routine and social life) generally takes two to three weeks which mirrors the resolution of discomfort/pain.[18] The median time taken off school or work is 4 weeks which should be sufficient for the majority of patients to recover, although consideration should be given to the type of surgery since individuals who have bimaxillary surgery take approximately 1 week longer to recover than those who have single jaw surgery.[4] When questioned, many patients (34%) report that they were given insufficient preoperative information regarding postoperative return to normal life (Box 20-3).[5]

Long-term disturbances and physical impacts

Complications

Neurosensory injury is a well-known complication of orthognathic surgery and is often unavoidable. Direct injury is caused by surgical instrumentation, whereas indirect injury is related to oedema and haematoma formation. Altered sensation after orthognathic surgery includes hypoaesthesia, paraesthesia, and dysaesthesia.[28,29] Recovery from neurosensory injury varies from patient to patient but generally occurs more rapidly in the first 6 weeks postoperatively and more slowly thereafter.[30] Although sensation recovers in the majority of patients over time, it can be permanent.[28]

The most commonly affected nerve is the inferior alveolar nerve (IAN) and sensory changes most frequently occur in the chin and lower lip region.[28] Injury has been related to the type of mandibular osteotomy, rigid fixation placement, concomitant procedures, and surgeon experience.[31–33] Cranial nerve involvement outside of the trigeminal nerve is much less common but can have dramatic consequences, including facial palsy and blindness.[34]

Altered sensation can create difficulties in day-to-day life (Box 20-4). Tactile sensation, location, and two-point discrimination tend to be more affected than thermal sensation.[32] Consequences of altered sensation include lip biting and difficulties with food mastication, awareness of food on the lip, and talking.[32,35] Patients who are aware of their altered sensation all the time reported greater distress in their everyday life.[35] Patients with persistent altered sensation tend to report more difficulties with orofacial function and with daily activities long-term after surgery.[4,5,28,35,36] Reassuringly, the majority of patients are disappointed when altered sensation persists, but few are angry, upset, or consider the sensory deficit as disabling.[32,35]

Sensory retraining or sensory re-education, consisting of a set of simple facial exercises performed daily with only an inexpensive cosmetic brush and a mirror, has been shown to be an effective cognitive behavioural therapy for reducing subjects' perceptions of the burden associated with negative altered sensations in the short term after mandibular osteotomy.[37] At 6 months after surgery, subjects who performed the sensory retraining exercises reported fewer problems related to residual numbness and loss of lip sensitivity than those subjects who performed only the standard of care mouth opening exercises.[38] This difference between the two exercise groups appears to be related to the difference in how the 'retrained' individual experiences or interprets tactile stimuli rather than any difference in nerve recovery or repair.[39,40] The positive effect of the sensory retraining persisted even after the exercises were stopped. At two years after surgery, patients who performed only the opening exercises were significantly more likely to report the presence of an altered facial sensation than those who used both the sensory retraining exercises and the opening exercises.[41] Sensory retraining is not a cure but rather an aid in helping patients' accommodate to any residual sensory deficit and desensitizing the patient to the impact of an altered sensation.[37]

Dental complications of orthognathic surgery include gingival recession, tooth devitalisation, and tooth loss. Overall, dental injuries during orthognathic surgery are rare and occur in approximately 1% of patients.[42] Interestingly, treatment for tooth devitalization should be delayed until symptoms arise since there is evidence that many of the dental pulps

Box 20-4 Long-term recovery comments from patient blogs on the internet

Altered sensation

'My chin is completely numb. I don't like it. I hope the feeling comes back soon.'

http://aimeesfunkyjaw.blogspot.com/search?updated-max=2009-05-10T11:06:00-07:00&max-results=7&start=14&by-date=false

'The only thing that is annoying to me now is the numbness. It's a constant tingling in my chin and lower lip. I've started snapping at people when they tell me I have food on my face ('I KNOW! I CAN'T FEEL IT!'), and putting on lipstick is a joke.'

http://melissanm.blogspot.com/search?updated-max=2009-10-04T16:10:00-06:00&max-results=7

'My chin is still quite numb. I find that there are weeks (like right now) that it drives me NUTS – it tingles, it tickles, it twitches, it feels like I have two inches of dried wax sitting on it... '

http://theteethofsteph.blogspot.com

'I'm almost 2 years post-op... still have some numbness on my lower lip – which can be pretty embarrassing when I wonder why my lip feels cold but then realize I've drooled.)'

'I wasn't so bothered about how I looked straight after but I did get upset a couple of times fretting about the amount of numbness I had in my face and whether the feeling would come back! Most people probably have some degree of feeling like they regret it straight after but it doesn't last long!'

'The only problem I have is that my mouth starts hurting since the weather is getting colder. Once in a while I have shooting pains but nothing too major; just glad it's over with!'

www.facebook.com/groups/2233483630

will heal spontaneously over time. Although there has been some concern in the past that multi-segmentation of the maxilla involving interdental osteotomies may lead to increased dental complications, recent reports have demonstrated that this is not necessarily true.[43] Gingival recession tends to occur when procedures are performed in direct proximity to mucogingival tissues. Physical effects of gingival recession include tooth sensitivity, increased susceptibility to root caries, and tooth loss. The greatest predictor of gingival recession is the angle between the long axis of the maxillary central incisors and the sella-nasion plane (i.e. the degree of maxillary incisor proclination).[44] Recession can be associated with either pathological or non-pathological bone loss. Non-pathological bone loss can be influenced by anatomical factors, orthodontic tooth movement, tooth position, plaque retention, and mechanical trauma.[45] Predisposing anatomical factors include narrow width of keratinized gingiva, abnormal frenum attachment, and decreased bone height. Pathological bone loss is related to periodontal disease and smoking.[44]

Infection following orthognathic surgery is uncommon but prolongs the healing period and can cause significant patient discomfort when it occurs. More infections arise in the mandible than in the maxilla, likely secondary to vascular supply.[42] While most postoperative infections are relatively benign, they can potentially become severe and enter the mediastinum.[34] Maxillary sinusitis is an uncommon postoperative infection after a maxillary osteotomy, with incidence reported ranging from 0.24 to 20%. Clinicians should screen patients carefully preoperatively for sinus infections, which may increase the likelihood of developing acute sinusitis in the postoperative period.[46] Overall, most infections following orthognathic surgery are related to a bony sequestrum or loosened internal rigid fixation hardware.[47] Localized infections near hardware may necessitate hardware removal requiring the patient to undergo an additional procedure with the potential for increased morbidity.[48]

Condylar resorption is a late and irreversible complication of orthognathic surgery, which often arises only several years after surgery.[49] Classically, condylar resorption occurs in young women with mandibular retrognathia, a steep mandibular plane angle, and a history of temporomandibular joint disorder.[49] Preoperative condylar deformities and atrophy are associated with progressive condylar resorption.[50,51] Those undergoing posterior condylar displacement and anticlockwise rotation of the mandible are also at risk.[50] Not surprisingly, when condylar resorption occurs and results in relapse, patient dissatisfaction will likely increase.

Function

Aside from improving aesthetics and occlusion, orthognathic surgery has the potential to affect the airway, mastication, and speech. Patients with maxillary skeletofacial deformities often have septal deviation, turbinate enlargement, and nasal valve constriction. Most studies have found nasal airway function after maxillary surgery improves. Those with greater nasal airway resistance experience the most improvement.[52] Additionally, it has been well-documented that bimaxillary advancement can also be used to improve the airway of individuals with obstructive sleep apnoea (see Chapter 44).[53,54]

Approximately one quarter of patients who seek orthognathic surgery report difficulty chewing secondary to malocclusion.[55] The vast majority of patients who undergo orthognathic surgery report improvement in mastication postoperatively (Figure 20-1).[55,56] In fact, improved masticatory capacity is frequently the most enhanced functional component.[56] These results support the notion that ideal occlusion makes physiological functions more harmonious. However, not all patients report improvement. Elderly

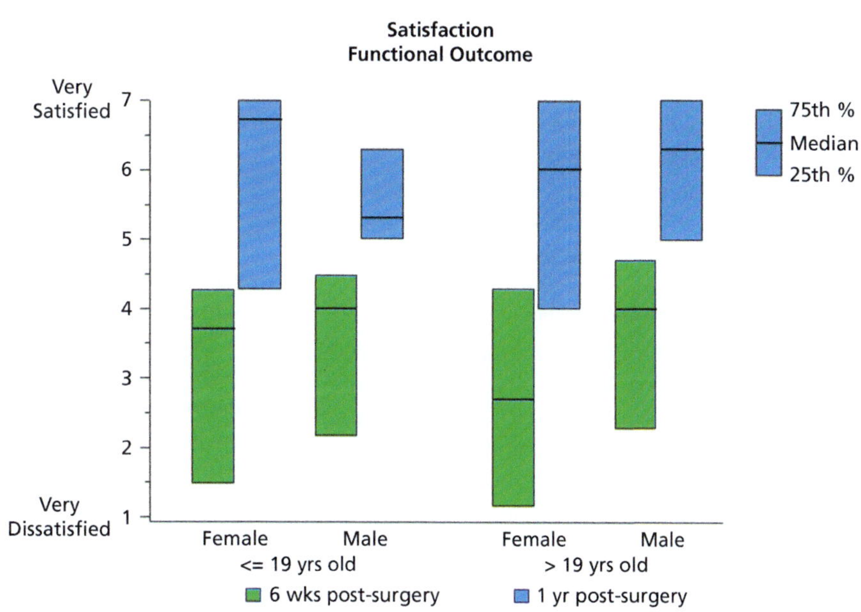

Fig. 20-1 Responses from 147 patients who had surgery between 2003 and 2012 at 6 weeks and 1 year after two jaw orthognathic surgery with respect to their satisfaction with the functional outcome of their surgery. Satisfaction with Function was calculated as the average of 3 items related to eating, chewing, and biting into foods rated on a 1 (very dissatisfied) to 7 (very satisfied) scale.

patients tend to have more difficulty adapting to their new occlusion compared to younger patients and are more likely to report reduced masticatory capacity after surgery.[55]

Long-term satisfaction and perception of improvement

Self-confidence

A negative body image can lead to pronounced psychiatric problems, especially in regards to self-confidence. Teenagers are very vulnerable to emotional difficulties and appearance during puberty, a major period of mental development. Research has demonstrated significant changes after orthognathic surgery with a positive influence on psychosocial aspects, including self-confidence (Box 20-5).[57] Patients report decreased psychological discomfort and social disability after orthognathic surgery.[58] Females tend to report greater improvement in self-confidence and diminished depressive symptoms compared to their male counterparts.[59]

> **Box 20-5** Long-term satisfaction and perception of improvement
>
> 'If I'm honest, the main reason I wanted to get this surgery done was because I hated the effect my jaws had on my appearance and I wanted to look better… So, am I happy with my new face? 100% yes. I love my new face. At the early stages after surgery there were a few times when I had doubts, but I can safely say I'm happy with my new face and I'm 100% happy that I went through with this surgery. I no longer have a gummy smile, a long face, a wonky top jaw, a recessed chin and a big nose.'
>
> http://jawsurgerystory.blogspot.com/search?updated-max=2012-11-27T04:41:00-08:00&max-results=7&start=14&by-date=false
>
> 'My previous lack of self-confidence and self-worth held me back. But since I had the surgery I am a different person. I love my face. I no longer avoid cameras. I thrive in the centre of attention whereas before I would run a mile.'
>
> http://jawsurgery-journey.blogspot.com
>
> 'It's been one year since I went under the knife and emerged with a new face and a new life. This past year has changed me as a person, inside and out.'
>
> http://rearrangemyface.blogspot.com
>
> 'Truthfully, looking back and reading my entries I know it was terrible. But a year later, I don't remember much about it – in fact, the whole month of July 2009 is a bit hazy (probably all the Demerol and lack of a sleeping schedule). I'm really glad I did it. So, know that a year after surgery you'll think it 'wasn't THAT bad.'
>
> http://theteethofsteph.blogspot.com

Because there are significant psychosocial benefits of orthognathic surgery and patients seeking surgery often have psychological needs, these factors should be acknowledged during consultation in addition to morphological and functional indications for surgery.[55] Females have more interest in improving self-confidence than males who may often be more interested in improving functionality.[59]

Interpersonal support and relationships

Interpersonal support has been shown to have a positive effect on a patient's ability to cope with illness and recovery from orthognathic surgery is no exception. Interestingly, individuals with greater support reported increased satisfaction in the early postoperative period. Reactions of significant others and close friends is crucial in forming a patient's opinion of the treatment result.[60] In fact, reactions have more influence than perceived level of general support. Negative reactions also impair the patient's ability to adapt in the postoperative period.

To optimize treatment satisfaction, good support should continue through the postoperative orthodontic treatment period until the treatment result is clear. There is a tendency for support to decrease after the initial postoperative period once the physical effects of surgery have stabilized. This is a concern specific to orthognathic surgery because while undergoing orthodontic treatment, the psychological healing is not yet complete.[60]

A negative body image also leads to difficulties in socialization. After orthognathic surgery, the vast majority of patients report improvement in their relationships with friends and relatives (Figure 20-2).[5] The positive effects on social life and relationships as well as self-confidence are likely related to the patient's overall improvement in psychological status, body image, and appearance.[61]

Quality of life

The World Health Organization defined Quality of Life (QoL) as 'an individual's perception of their position in life in the context of culture and value systems in which they live and in relation to their goals, expectations, standards and concerns'.[58] Skeletofacial deformities have been shown to negatively affect patient QoL.[59] Interestingly, individuals that identify as 'self-conscious' before surgery tend to report improved QoL postoperatively.[58]

QoL changes can be categorized as general and condition-specific health-related. The psychosocial aspects of general health-related QoL including social interaction, communication, and emotional behaviour, all improve following orthognathic surgery.[3] Likewise, sleep and rest, recreation and pastimes, and overall general health also improved following surgery.[3] Condition-specific health-related QoL also improved including general oral health, oral

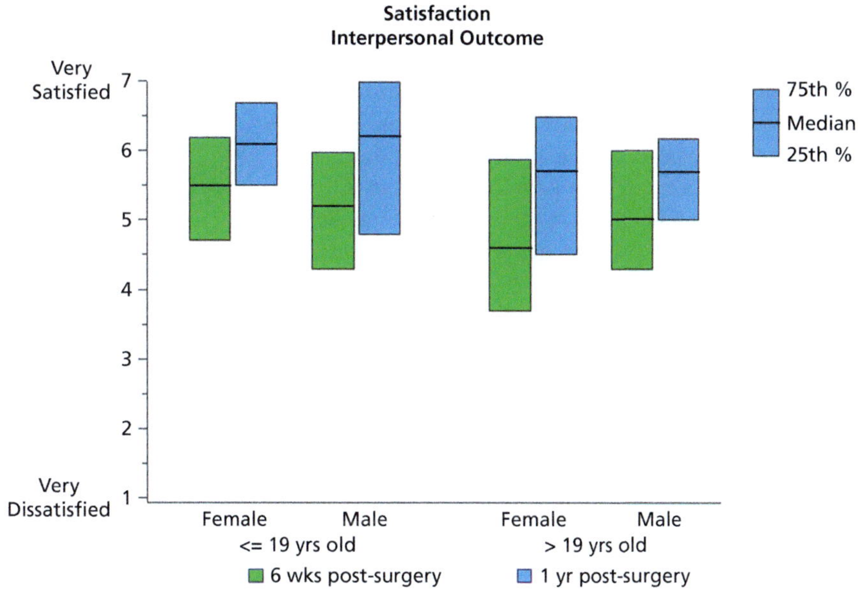

Fig. 20-2 Responses from 147 patients who had surgery between 2003 and 2012 at 6 weeks and 1 year after two jaw orthognathic surgery with respect to their satisfaction with their interpersonal relationships after their surgery. Satisfaction with Interpersonal Relationships was calculated as the average of six items related to positive comments and change in appearance rated on a 1 (very dissatisfied) to 7 (very satisfied) scale.

function, sensitivity, and aesthetics.[57] Many patients feel that they benefited from orthognathic surgery despite long-term side effects.[4] Postoperative QoL improvements have been shown to be stable and satisfaction maintained for 5 years after surgery.[3] Not surprisingly, improvement in facial aesthetics is associated with improvement in QoL.[62]

Aesthetics

Aesthetic improvement and related psychosocial benefits are major motivators for patients undergoing orthognathic surgery.[57] The change in appearance secondary to orthognathic surgery is considered an improvement by the vast majority of patients. This perception of improvement is seen as early as 2 months after surgery.[63] Men and older patients tend to experience more difficulty adapting to a new body image after surgery.[57]

The clinical impact of improved perception of appearance has been found to be greater than the impact on functionality.[64] In fact, the primary determinant of patient satisfaction in orthognathic surgery is aesthetic outcome.[59] Self-concept has been identified as an independent predictor of postoperative satisfaction with appearance.[65]

Overall satisfaction

The vast majority of patients report they would undergo orthognathic surgery again if they were faced with the same situation (Box 20-5). Similarly, the majority of patients also report they would recommend surgical treatment to a person with skeletofacial deformities.[5] Only approximately 5% of patients undergoing orthognathic surgery report dissatisfaction and regret despite having clinically acceptable treatment outcomes.[66] Dissatisfied patients identified inadequate pre-surgical explanations and lack of advice regarding side effects as problems that negatively affected their satisfaction (Figure 20-3).[67]

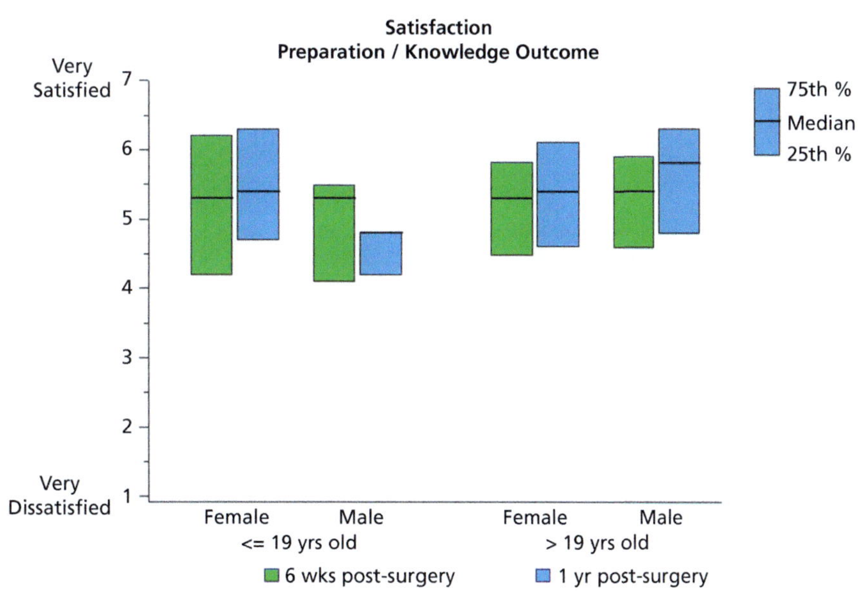

Fig. 20-3 Responses from 147 patients who had surgery between 2003 and 2012 at 6 weeks and 1 year after two jaw orthognathic surgery with respect to their satisfaction with the preparation and information they received prior to and after their surgery. Satisfaction with Preparation and Information was calculated as the average of 10 items related to expectations, explanations provided, feeling of preparation rated on a 1 (very dissatisfied) to 7 (very satisfied) scale.

Recommendations

1. Improve preoperative communication with patients to appropriately manage immediate and long-term postoperative expectations. Even if a good surgical outcome is achieved, poor communication between the provider and patient can lead to dissatisfaction. In general, patients with realistic expectations are generally more satisfied with treatment.
2. Altered sensation is almost universal in the immediate postoperative period and can be permanent. Thus, although it remains a critical aspect of the informed consent process, it rarely significantly influences patient satisfaction.
3. Shorten orthodontic treatment, both pre- and postoperatively. Cooperation between orthodontists and oral and maxillofacial surgeons is essential to reduce treatment time and improve patient satisfaction.
4. Supportive family and friends should be involved in preoperative planning, postoperative surgical care, and postoperative orthodontic treatment, to maximize adaptation and improve treatment satisfaction.
5. General health-related quality of life, oral health-related quality of life, and psychosocial function including self-confidence and interpersonal relationships have shown significant and stable improvements after orthognathic surgery.
6. Aesthetic outcome is frequently the primary predictor of patient satisfaction, especially in females.
7. Discuss the patient's motivation for orthognathic surgery. Function, aesthetics, and psychological impact should all be taken into consideration when treatment planning.

Acknowledgements

Funding: Research reported in this publication was supported by NIDCR of the National Institutes of Health under award number R01DE005215. The content is solely the responsibility of the authors and does not necessarily represent the official views of the National Institutes of Health.

References

1 Hunt OT, Johnston CD, Hepper PG, Burden DJ. The psychosocial impact of orthognathic surgery: a systematic review. Am J Orthod Dentofacial Orthop. 2001;120:490–7.
2 Lazaridou-Terzoudi T, Kiyak HA, Moore R, Athanasiou AE, Melsen B. Long-term assessment of psychologic outcomes of orthognathic surgery. J Oral Maxillofac Surg. 2003;61:545–52.
3 Motegi E, Hatch JP, Rugh JD, Yamaguchi H. Health-related quality of life and psychosocial function 5 years after orthognathic surgery. Am J Orthod Dentofacial Orthop. 2003;124:138–43.
4 Williams RW, Travess HC, Williams AC. Patients' experiences after undergoing orthognathic surgery at NHS hospitals in the south west of England. Br J Oral Maxillofac Surg. 2004;42:419–31.
5 Kim S, Shin SW, Han I, Joe SH, Kim MR, Kwon JJ. Clinical review of factors leading to perioperative dissatisfaction related to orthognathic surgery. J Oral Maxillofac Surg. 2009;67:2217–21.
6 Hatch JP, Rugh JD, Clark GM, Keeling SD, Tiner BD, Bays RA. Health-related quality of life following orthognathic surgery. Int J Adult Orthodon Orthognath Surg. 1998;13:67–77.
7 Phillips C, HL Broder, and M.E. Bennett, Dentofacial disharmony: motivations for seeking treatment. Int J Adult Orthodon Orthognath Surg. 1997;12:7–15.
8 Dean M, Street, Jr. RL. A 3-stage model of patient-centered communication for addressing cancer patients' emotional distress. Patient Educat Counsel. 2014;94:143–8.
9 PCORI, M.C., Draft Methodology Report: 'Our questions, our decisions: Standard for patient-centered outcomes research', 2012.
10 Silva AC, O'Ryan F, Poor DB. Postoperative nausea and vomiting (PONV) after orthognathic surgery: a retrospective study and literature review. J Oral Maxillofac Surg. 2006;64:1385–97.
11 Gan T, Sloan F, Dear Gde L, El-Moalem HE, Lubarsky DA. How much are patients willing to pay to avoid postoperative nausea and vomiting? Anesth Analg. 2001;92:393–400.
12 Macario A, Weinger M, Truong P, Lee M. Which clinical anesthesia outcomes are both common and important to avoid? The perspective of a panel of expert anesthesiologists. Anesth Analg. 1999;88:1085–91.
13 Lehmann M, Monte K, Barach P, Kindler CH. Postoperative patient complaints: a prospective interview study of 12,276 patients. J Clin Anesth. 2010;22:13–21.
14 Myles PS, Williams DL, Hendrata M, Anderson H, Weeks AM. Patient satisfaction after anaesthesia and surgery: results of a prospective survey of 10,811 patients. Br J Anaesth. 2000;84:6–10.
15 Dicus Brookes C, Rich J, Golden BA, Blakey G, Turvey TA, Kopp V, Phillips C, Anderson J. Multimodal protocol reduces incidence of postoperative nausea and vomiting in patients undergoing maxillary osteotomy: a preliminary report. J Oral Maxillofac Surg. 2013;71:e19–e20.
16 Tabrizi R, Eftekharian HR, Langner NJ, Ozkan BT. Comparison of the effect of 2 hypotensive anesthetic techniques on early recovery complications after orthognathic surgery. J Craniofac Surg. 2012;23:e203–5.
17 Phillips C, Blakey G 3rd. Short-term recovery after orthognathic surgery: a medical daily diary approach. Int J Adult Orthodon Orthognath Surg. 2008;37:892–6.
18 Phillips C, Blakey G 3rd, Jaskolka M. Recovery after orthognathic surgery: short-term health-related quality of life outcomes. J Oral Maxillofac Surg. 2008;66:2110–5.
19 Wrighton SA, Stevens JC. The human hepatic cytochromes P450 involved in drug metabolism. Critical Rev Toxicol. 1992;22:1–21.
20 Ku, C.M. and B.C. Ong, Postoperative nausea and vomiting: a review of current literature. Singapore Med J. 2003;44: 366–74.
21 Koivuranta M, Läärä E, Snåre L, Alahuhta S. A survey of postoperative nausea and vomiting. Anaesthesia. 1997;52: 443–9.
22 Apfel CC, Läärä E, Koivuranta M, Greim CA, Roewer N. A simplified risk score for predicting postoperative nausea and vomiting: conclusions from cross-validations between two centers. Anesthesiology. 1999;91:693–700.
23 Watcha MF, White PF. Postoperative nausea and vomiting. Its etiology, treatment, and prevention. Anesthesiology. 1992;77:162–84.
24 Kamath B, Curran J, Hawkey C, Beattie A, Gorbutt N, Guiblin H, Kong A. Anaesthesia, movement and emesis. Br J Anaesth. 1990;64:728–30.
25 Phillips C, Kiyak HA, Bloomquist D, Turvey TA. Perceptions of recovery and satisfaction in the short term after orthognathic surgery. J Oral Maxillofac Surg. 2004;62:535–44.

26 Scott AA, Hatch JP, Rugh JD, Hoffman TJ, Rivera SM, Dolce C, Bays RA. Psychosocial predictors of satisfaction among orthognathic surgery patients. Int J Adult Orthodon Orthognath Surg. 2000;15:7–15.
27 Stewart TD, Sexton J. Depression: a possible complication of orthognathic surgery. J Oral Maxillofac Surg. 1987;45: 847–51.
28 Kim YK, Kim SG, Kim JH. Altered sensation after orthognathic surgery. J Oral Maxillofac Surg. 2011;69:893–8.
29 Phillips C, Essick G, Zuniga J, Tucker M, Blakey G 3rd. Qualitative descriptors used by patients following orthognathic surgery to portray altered sensation. J Oral Maxillofac Surg. 2006;64:1751–60.
30 Travess HC, Cunningham SJ, Newton JT. Recovery of sensation after orthognathic treatment: patients' perspective. Am J Orthod Dentofacial Orthop. 2008;134:251–9.
31 Choi BK, Lo LJ, Oh KS, Yang EJ. The influence of reduction mandibuloplasty history on the incidence of inferior alveolar nerve injury during sagittal split osteotomy. Plast Reconstr Surg. 2013;131:231e–237e.
32 Gianni AB, D'Orto O, Biglioli F, Bozzetti A, Brusati R. Neurosensory alterations of the inferior alveolar and mental nerve after genioplasty alone or associated with sagittal osteotomy of the mandibular ramus. J Craniomaxillofac Surg. 2002;30:295–303.
33 Kobayashi A, Yoshimasu H, Kobayashi J, Amagasa T. Neurosensory alteration in the lower lip and chin area after orthognathic surgery: bilateral sagittal split osteotomy versus inverted L ramus osteotomy. J Oral Maxillofac Surg. 2006;64:778–84.
34 Kim YS, Oh ES, Hong JW, Roh TS, Rah DK, Paik HC. Descending necrotizing mediastinitis and facial palsy as serial complications in orthognathic surgery. J Craniofac Surg. 2011;22:559–61.
35 Lee EG, Ryan FS, Shute J, Cunningham SJ. The impact of altered sensation affecting the lower lip after orthognathic treatment. J Oral Maxillofac Surg. 2011;69:e431–45.
36 Lemke RR, Clark GM, Bays RA, Tiner BD, Rugh JD. Effects of hypesthesia on oral behaviors of the orthognathic surgery patient. J Oral Maxillofac Surg. 1998;56:153–7; discussion 158–60.
37 Phillips C, Blakey G 3rd, Essick GK. Sensory retraining: a cognitive behavioral therapy for altered sensation. Atlas Oral Maxillofac Surg Clin North Am. 2011;19:109–18.
38 Phillips C, Essick G, Preisser JS, Turvey TA, Tucker M, Lin D. Sensory retraining after orthognathic surgery: effect on patients' perception of altered sensation. J Oral Maxillofac Surg. 2007;65:1162–73.
39 Essick GK, Phillips C, Turvey TA, Tucker M. Facial altered sensation and sensory impairment after orthognathic surgery. Int J Adult Orthodon Orthognath Surg. 2007;36:577–82.
40 Essick GK, Phillips C, Kim SH, Zuniga J. Sensory retraining following orthognathic surgery: effect on threshold measures of sensory function. J Oral Rehabil. 2009;36:415–26.
41 Phillips C, Kim SH, Essick G, Tucker M, Turvey TA. Sensory retraining after orthognathic surgery: effect on patient report of altered sensations. Am J Orthod Dentofacial Orthop. 2009;136:788–94.
42 Kim SG, Park SS. Incidence of complications and problems related to orthognathic surgery. J Oral Maxillofac Surg. 2007;65:2438–44.
43 Kahnberg KE, Vannas-Lofqvist L, Zellin G. Complications associated with segmentation of the maxilla: a retrospective radiographic follow up of 82 patients. Int J Oral Maxillofac Surg. 2005;34:840–5.
44 Zhu S, Chen Z. Association between gingival recession and proclination of maxillary central incisors near the cleft in patients with unilateral cleft lip and palate: A retrospective case–control study. Am J Orthod Dentofacial Orthop. 2013;143:364–70.
45 Weinspach K, Staufenbiel I, Günay H, Geurtsen W, Schwestka-Polly R, Demling AP. Influence of orthognathic surgery on periodontal tissues: short-term results. J Orofac Orthop. 2011;72:279–89.
46 Pereira-Filho VA, Gabrielli MF, Gabrielli MA, Pinto FA, Rodrigues-Junior AL, Klüppel LE, Passeri LA. Incidence of maxillary sinusitis following Le Fort I osteotomy: clinical, radiographic, and endoscopic study. J Oral Maxillofac Surg. 2011;69:346–51.
47 Panula K, Finne K, Oikarinen K. Incidence of complications and problems related to orthognathic surgery: a review of 655 patients. J Oral Maxillofac Surg. 2001;59:1128–36; discussion 1137.
48 Ho MW, Boyle MA, Cooper JC, Dodd MD, Richardson D. Surgical complications of segmental Le Fort I osteotomy. Br J Oral Maxillofac Surg, 2011;49:562–6.
49 de Santana Santos T, Albuquerque KM, Santos ME, Laureano Filho JR. Survey on complications of orthognathic surgery among oral and maxillofacial surgeons. J Craniofac Surg. 2012;23:e423–30.
50 Gill DS, El Maaytah M, Naini FB. Risk factors for post-orthognathic condylar resorption: a review. World J Orthod. 2008;9:21–5.
51 Kobayashi T, Izumi N, Kojima T, Sakagami N, Saito I, Saito C. Progressive condylar resorption after mandibular advancement. Br J Oral Maxillofac Surg. 2012;50:176–80.
52 Williams BJ, Isom A, Laureano Filho JR, O'Ryan FS. Nasal airway function after maxillary surgery: a prospective cohort study using the nasal obstruction symptom evaluation scale. J Oral Maxillofac Surg. 2013;71:343–50.
53 Zinser MJ, Zachow S, Sailer HF. Bimaxillary 'rotation advancement' procedures in patients with obstructive sleep apnea: a 3-dimensional airway analysis of morphological changes. Int J Adult Orthodon Orthognath Surg. 2013;42:569–78.
54 Raunio A, Rauhala E, Kiviharju M, Lehmijoki O, Sándor GK, Oikarinen K. Bimaxillary advancement as the initial treatment of obstructive sleep apnea: five years follow-up of the pori experience. J Oral Maxillofac Res. 2012;3:e5.
55 Pahkala RH, Kellokoski JK. Surgical–orthodontic treatment and patients' functional and psychosocial well-being. Am J Orthod Dentofacial Orthop, 2007;132:158–64.
56 Trovik TA, Wisth PJ, Tornes K, Bøe OE, Moen K. Patients' perceptions of improvements after bilateral sagittal split osteotomy advancement surgery: 10 to 14 years of follow-up. Am J Orthod Dentofacial Orthop. 2012;141:20–12.
57 Kim, S.J., Kim MR, Shin SW, Chun YS, Kim EJ. Evaluation on the psychosocial status of orthognathic surgery patients. Oral Surg Oral Med Oral Pathol Oral Radiol Endod. 2009;108: 828–32.
58 Rustemeyer J, Gregersen J. Quality of Life in orthognathic surgery patients: post-surgical improvements in aesthetics and self-confidence. J Craniomaxillofac Surg. 2012;40: 400–4.
59 Rustemeyer J, Eke Z, Bremerich A. Perception of improvement after orthognathic surgery: the important variables affecting patient satisfaction. Oral Maxillofac Surg. 2010;14:155–62.
60 Holman AR, Brumer S, Ware WH, Pasta DJ. The impact of interpersonal support on patient satisfaction with orthognathic surgery. J Oral Maxillofac Surg. 1995;53:1289–97; discussion 1297–9.
61 Turker N, Varol A, Ogel K, Basa S. Perceptions of preoperative expectations and postoperative outcomes from orthognathic surgery: part I: Turkish female patients. Int J Oral Maxillofac Surg. 2008;37:710–5.
62 Sadek H, Salem G. Psychological aspects of orthognathic surgery and its effect on quality of life in Egyptian patients. East Mediterr Health J. 2007;13:150–9.
63 Kavin T, Jagadesan AG, Venkataraman SS. Changes in quality of life and impact on patients' perception of esthetics after

orthognathic surgery. J Pharm Bioallied Sci. 2012;4(Suppl 2):S290–3.
64 Murphy C, Kearns G, Sleeman D, Cronin M, Allen PF. The clinical relevance of orthognathic surgery on quality of life. Int J Oral Maxillofac Surg. 2011;40:926–30.
65 van Steenbergen E, Litt MD, Nanda R. Pre-surgical satisfaction with facial appearance in orthognathic surgery patients. Am J Orthod Dentofacial Orthop. 1996;109:653–9.
66 Posnick JC, Wallace J. Complex orthognathic surgery: assessment of patient satisfaction. J Oral Maxillofac Surg. 2008;66:934–42.
67 Cunningham SJ, Crean SJ, Hunt NP, Harris M. Preparation, perceptions, and problems: a long-term follow-up study of orthognathic surgery. Int J Adult Orthodon Orthognath Surg. 1996;11:41–7.

Part II: Clinical Practice and Techniques

Section 1: Orthognathic Surgical Planning and Techniques

Section 3: Orthognathic Surgery in the Cleft Patient and Orthognathic Aspects of Craniofacial Surgery

Section 4: Appendix

Section 1: Orthognathic Surgical Planning and Techniques

Chapter 21

Introduction: Perspectives on Treatment Planning

Harvey M. Rosen

Throughout my surgical career, I made a point of reviewing my initial patient consultation the night before the orthognathic surgical procedure was performed. Because I encouraged my referring orthodontic colleagues to have the patient seen prior to the commencement of presurgical orthodontic treatment, the time elapsed from consultation to procedure was, more often than not, a fairly long interval, usually in the range of 9–15 months in the fully grown patient. During the initial visit with the patient, I endeavoured to commit to a preliminary surgical treatment plan (whether one or both jaws were to be repositioned, the vectors of movement, an estimate of the magnitude of movement and the need for a genioplasty) without the benefit of reviewing radiographs, cephalometric tracings or study models that may have been available at the time. I wanted to simply look at the individual and examine the face. My observation during a 28-year period was this: my initial treatment plan rarely differed from the procedure that was eventually executed save for modest changes in the magnitude of movement and the requirement for maxillary segmentation. *The obvious lesson is that the evaluation of facial appearance through the simple act of the physical exam is, without exception, the most important aspect of the treatment planning process.*

How then does one evaluate appearance and how does this evaluative process lead to a cogent surgical philosophy? Although certain quantitative measurements can be made (for instance, the height of the lower face relative to the midface, the extent of incisal and gingival exposure or the measurement of soft tissue asymmetries), one must employ concepts of facial appearance, all of which are interrelated, interdependent and all relying on qualitative judgments.

The first concept is that of visual perception versus clinical reality. This means that the visual perception of certain morphological facial features may be disparate from its quantitative measurement and that the perception must always take precedence. This concept most frequently applies to the perception of excessive sagittal projection of the lower face and excessive height of the lower face.

For instance, the appearance of certain Class III patients due to mandibular excess is visually objectionable, not because of the excessive anterior facial divergence but because of the concavity of the midsagittal and parasagittal profiles and the abnormal relationship of the lips. These are the visual cues one automatically associates with this deformity. If one restores facial convexity and normal labial relationships with maxillary advancement without reducing anterior facial divergence, the appearance becomes visually acceptable. Correction of the visual cues eliminates the perception of excessive anterior divergence and excessive projection of the lower face.

Similarly, the appearance of certain long face patients due to vertical maxillary excess is visually objectionable not because of the presence of excessive lower face height but because of the perioral lip strain needed to achieve oral competence and excessive incisal and gingival exposure, the visual cues with which one automatically associates with this deformity. If one can correct these visual cues yet leave the lower face long, the appearance becomes visually acceptable because the perception of excessive facial height will have been eliminated.

By invoking the concept of visual perception versus clinical reality, one can argue that facial disproportion (excessive projection and/or excessive height

Orthognathic Surgery: Principles, Planning and Practice. Edited by Farhad B. Naini and Daljit S. Gill.

of the lower face) can be visually acceptable. One can further posit that facial disproportion can, in fact, be rather attractive under the right aesthetic circumstances. This then is the second concept of facial appearance: beauty versus normalcy. This concept implies that facial attractiveness and facial disproportion can coexist provided none of the visual cues with which we associate excessive projection and height are present. In other words, beauty is not necessarily synonymous with normalcy.

How frequently have we all observed images of models' faces that have excessive projection and/or excessive height and yet we all would agree that they are extremely attractive. The aesthetic circumstances under which this can occur for excessive facial projection are: it must be accompanied by overall convexity of the midsagittal profile and the parasagittal profile (the relationship of the infraorbital to the paranasal to the parasymphyseal region) and normal sagittal relationships between the upper and lower lip. In addition, there must be an adequately projecting nasal dorsum and tip to counterbalance the projection of the lower face.

The aesthetic circumstances under which this can occur for excessive facial height are: there must be an absence of lip strain with lip closure, an absence of excessive gingival exposure with full smiling and an absence of excessive incisal exposure with the lips relaxed. The conventional wisdom of 2–3 mm of incisal show being the ideal is no longer operative. In female patients, exposure of 5, 6 or even 7 mm can potentially be very attractive. In addition, the morphology of the labiomental fold is critical to the perception of facial height. The fold must be of normal depth and height. Since the fold is perpendicular to the long axis of the lower face it interrupts this axis and, therefore, mitigates the perception of excessive facial height. Strict adherence to these aesthetic conditions justifies treatment plans that create facial disproportion.

The third concept of appearance is that of facial countenance, that is, what is the emotional expression of the face in the unanimated state? This is important since observers of dentofacial deformity patients will, more often than not, attribute them with negative emotional characteristics. These most frequently include sadness or sullenness and anger or discontent.

In addition to the periorbital soft tissues having the ability to convey emotion, so too, do the perioral soft tissues. What are the potential changes in the perioral soft tissues that may accompany jaw surgery and which can influence facial countenance? They include the width of the mouth, inclination of the oral commissures, fullness of the lips, procumbency of the lower lip and depth of the labiomental fold. It is my belief that these changes are due to obligatory alterations in the resting tone of the perioral musculature that must occur to accommodate changes in skeletal volume. As skeletal volume is increased by adding projection and height to the lower face, resting musculature tone increases to maintain oral competency. As this occurs the mouth narrows, the inclination of the oral commissures shifts superiorly, the lips become fuller, the lower lip becomes less procumbent and the labiomental fold becomes less deep. The greater the increase in skeletal volume, the greater the change in perioral soft tissues. These morphological changes mitigate the negative emotional expressions of sadness and anger and provide for a beneficial change in facial countenance. In addition, they create a more youthful look.

The final concept of facial appearance is the evaluation of the qualities of the soft tissue. Long ignored, it is now generally accepted that the appearance of the soft tissues is a critical factor in determining the aesthetic success or failure of orthognathic surgery. In this context, certain facts are indisputable. First, increases in skeletal volume (skeletal expansion) by adding projection and height enhance skeletal support to the soft tissues. Second, decreases in skeletal volume (skeletal contraction) by reducing projection and height reduces skeletal support to the soft tissues. Third, the soft tissues have a very limited and finite ability to contract secondary to reduction in skeletal volume and support. Accordingly, skeletal contraction risks creating a volume discrepancy between skeletal and soft tissue masses or worsening a pre-existing one.

Inadequately supported soft tissues can appear thick, redundant, fleshy, and, in the extreme, rather amorphous. The zygomatic complex and inferior border of the mandible may be poorly defined. Jowls and submental fullness may be present. The subtle suggestion of a submalar depression may be absent. Adequately supported soft tissues appear more angular and highlighted. There is the sense of lightness and elegance. The zygomatic complex and inferior border of the mandible are well defined. There is an absence of jowls and submental fullness. A submalar depression may be present.

The treatment planning implications of these soft tissue concepts are profound:

1. If an aesthetic option exists, always choose an expansive procedure. For instance, advancing the maxilla in modest cases of mandibular excess;
2. Have a low threshold to use a double jaw procedure when a better soft tissue result can be achieved since this eliminates the aesthetic constraints of establishing a normal occlusion; and
3. Utilize the concept of facial disproportion to achieve well supported soft tissues.

In summary, a surgical philosophy has evolved dependant on the concepts of facial appearance: to utilize the principles of visual perception versus clinical reality, and beauty versus normalcy, to achieve the aesthetic goals set for the facial soft tissues and a favourable change in facial countenance. This may require creating excessive projection and/or height of the lower face. Ironically, in what is a skeletal surgical discipline, soft tissue goals may dictate facial proportions.

Orthognathic surgery represents a unique surgical opportunity. It is the only instance in all of plastic surgery in which the following three parameters coexist: the option to create facial disproportion, the ability to favourably alter emotional expression and the capability to profoundly affect the qualities and attributes of the facial soft tissues. It is a surgical opportunity that must not be wasted; it must be planned to achieve its full aesthetic potential.

Chapter 22

Le Fort I Osteotomy and Maxillary Advancement

Helen Witherow and Farhad B. Naini

Introduction

Orthognathic surgery is generally very safe, with high levels of patient satisfaction. However, excellent results may only be achieved with a combination of careful patient evaluation, comprehensive treatment planning, meticulous surgery, and excellent communication between all involved, in a multidisciplinary setting.

Living with significant facial disproportions can have adverse functional and psychological effects on a person. The Le Fort I advancement osteotomy, particularly a high level Le Fort I osteotomy, is capable of producing profound aesthetic change to an individual's facial appearance.

Many studies have been undertaken reviewing 'ideal' facial proportions, which should be age-, gender- and ethnicity-specific.[1] Clinicians involved in orthognathic surgery need to be aware of the impact of different facial proportions and gender differences. A straight profile is often considered attractive in both sexes; however, gender stereotypes would suggest that a mildly Class III profile with a 'strong chin' (i.e. mildly prominent chin) may be deemed attractive in a male profile, whereas a mildly Class II profile may be more acceptable in a female profile.[2]

Facial proportions also need to be in keeping with the patient's body frame, standing height and stature. For example, it would be inappropriate to reduce excessively the height of a tall thin face if the patient was also tall and thin.[3]

History of the Le Fort I osteotomy

The historical background to the Le Fort I osteotomy has been covered in Chapters 1 and 2. However, it is important to reiterate that prior to the development of the midface osteotomy, the scope for altering the facial profile was confined to adjusting the mandible. Whilst an acceptable dental-occlusal result could be achieved, the facial aesthetic result was often disappointing.[4]

Orthognathic Surgery: Principles, Planning and Practice. Edited by Farhad B. Naini and Daljit S. Gill.

Development of the Le Fort I osteotomy has revolutionized the treatment of dentofacial deformities. The procedure was first described by Von Langenbeck in 1859 and was subsequently used by Wassmund in 1927 for correction of midfacial deformity. Axhausen and Schuchardt later described the separation of the pterygomaxillary suture using an osteotome. Further modifications were made by Moore and Ward in 1949 and finally Obwegeser in 1962. Modification of the Le Fort I osteotomy has resulted in a technique that has become overwhelmingly the technique of choice for the treatment of all midfacial retrusion and maxillary hypoplasia. 'In treatment planning for facial anomalies, consider first the profile and then the occlusion' is one of Obwegeser's maxims (see Chapters 1 and 2).

It is possible to combine the Le Fort I osteotomy with other augmentation techniques such as zygomatic osteotomies or implants, thus achieving similar result to the higher level Le Fort II and Le Fort III osteotomy, whilst potentially avoiding the higher morbidity.

Awareness of the facial soft tissue changes that occur as a result of the dentoskeletal movements and the effects on the nose and lips that can occur following maxillary advancement are essential when deciding the surgical movements required.

Recent advances using the submental technique for endotracheal intubation enable direct observation of the changes that occur during the osteotomy. This enables easy visualization of transverse maxillary occlusal plane cants, dental midlines and adjustment to the nose to be undertaken during the surgery, potentially enhancing facial aesthetics (Figure 22-1).

Assessment of the maxilla

Clinical evaluation has been described in Chapter 5. A maxillary deformity may be described in the three planes of space, sagittal, vertical and transverse. Sagittal deficiency tends to produce a concave facial profile, retrusive upper lip, acute nasolabial angle, ptotic nasal tip, narrow nasal alar base and inadequate maxillary incisor exposure. The vertically deficient/short face has an edentulous appearance with a concave facial profile, reduced facial height, increase in alar base width and reduced maxillary incisor exposure, which is viewed as a feature of aging (Figure 22-2).

The hypoplastic maxilla often gives inadequate support for the surrounding soft tissues. Therefore inadequate support at the orbital rim level may produce a proptotic appearance (exorbita) and increased scleral exposure (Figure 22-3). This is noted most dramatically in those patients with craniofacial dysostosis where shallow orbits predispose to such severe exorbitism that inability to close the eyelids may result in corneal damage and dislocation of the orbit. Inadequate maxillary vertical height may not support the nasal tip, resulting in an acute nasolabial angle and a ptotic nasal tip (Figure 22-4).

The characteristics of sagittal maxillary excess are a convex facial profile, and an obtuse nasolabial angle. Vertical maxillary excess is demonstrated by a tall face, increased lower face height, obtuse nasolabial angle, excessive incisor exposure, incomplete lip seal with increased mentalis activity required to maintain a lip seal, and a relatively tall, retruded chin, due to posterior rotation of the mandible.

(a) (b)

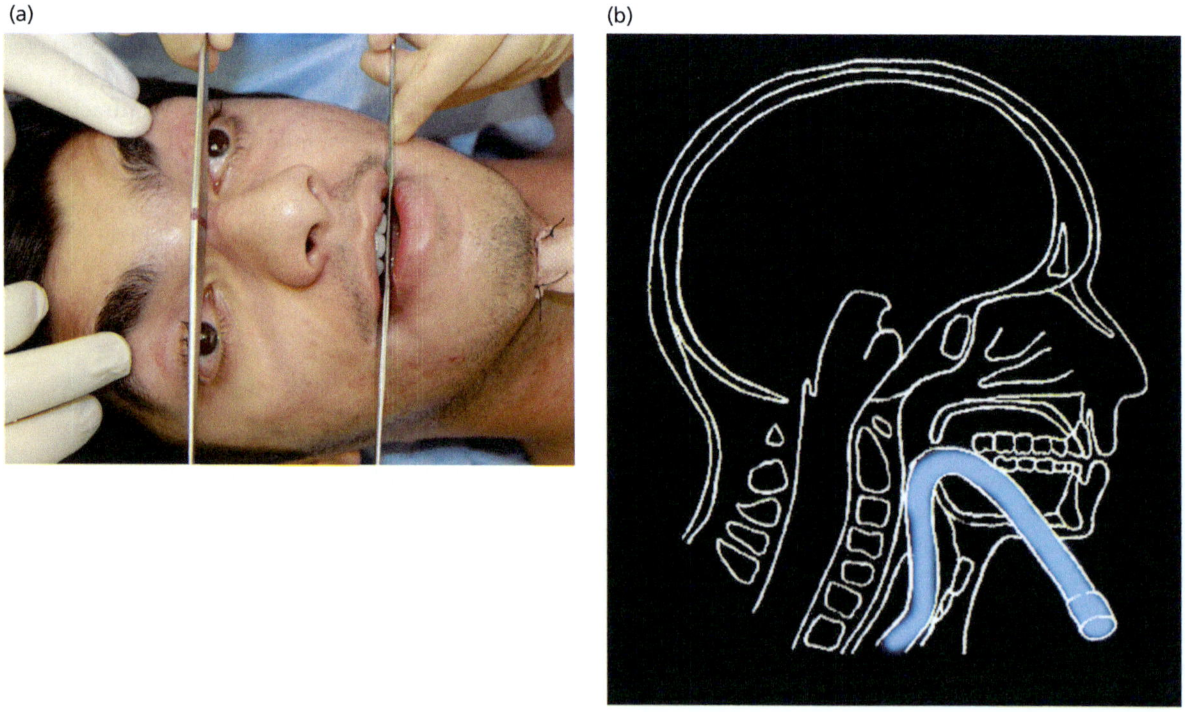

Fig. 22-1 (a) Showing the access to the face with submental intubation. The unimpeded view of the face ensures that dental midlines, maxillary incisor exposure and transverse occlusal plane cants can be more easily assessed. (b) Diagram showing the position of the endotracheal tube in submental intubation.

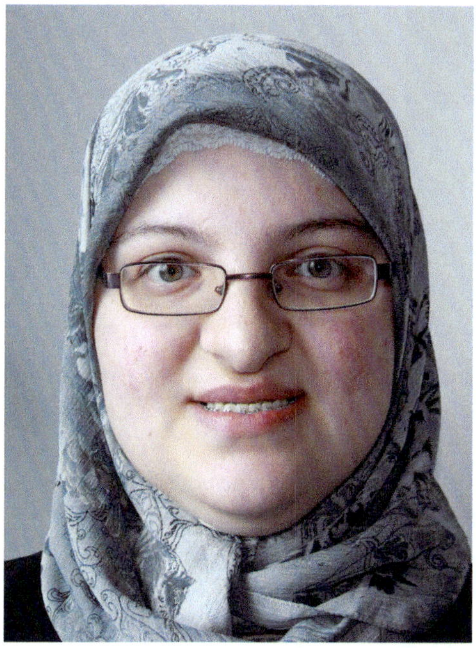

Fig. 22-2 Reduced maxillary incisor exposure in a patient with vertical maxillary deficiency.

Transverse maxillary deficiency may result in posterior crossbites and unattractive dark buccal corridors on smiling. A narrow maxilla may also be associated with a narrow nasal airway. Many patients report improvement in airway following a maxillary advancement.[5]

Anatomy

The Le Fort I osteotomy is a relatively safe operation with low morbidity and mortality. However, anatomically it is a complex area, close to the skull base and

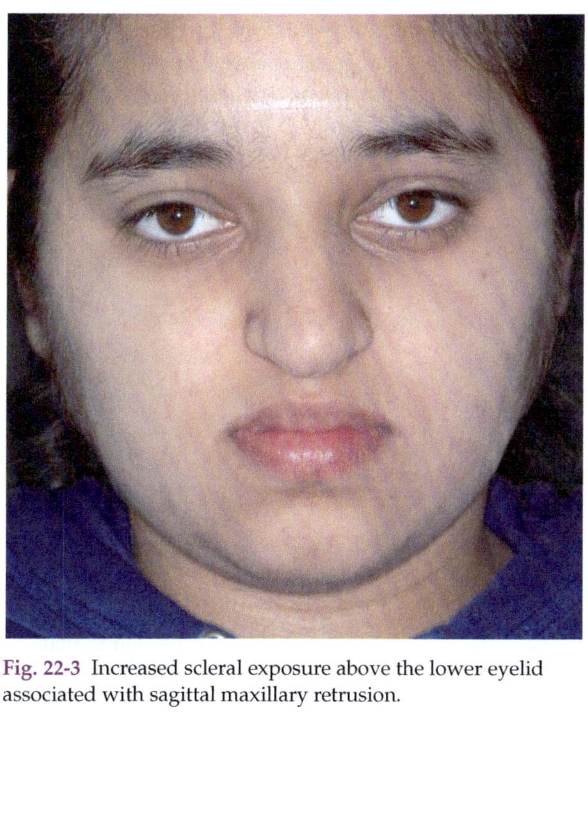

Fig. 22-3 Increased scleral exposure above the lower eyelid associated with sagittal maxillary retrusion.

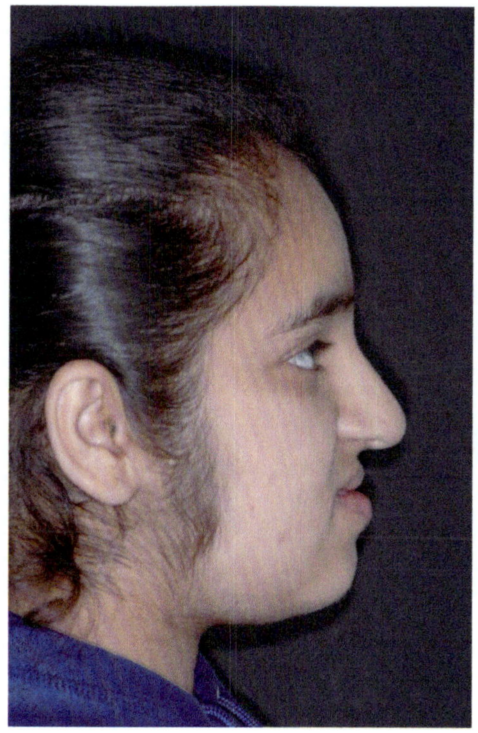

Fig. 22-4 Ptotic nasal tip, and an acute nasolabial angle as a result of a hypoplastic maxilla.

airway. It is paramount that the anatomy of the area is understood to ensure a safe operation.

The maxilla has an integral relationship with the orbits, cheekbones and the nose, and should not be considered in isolation. It consists of the tooth bearing dentoalveolar bone, the bilateral maxillary air-filled sinuses, and forms the orbital floor. The maxillary bone articulates with the bilateral zygomatic bones (cheek bones) and the nasal bones. Above the sinus lies the orbital floor, and within its floor lies the infraorbital nerve (V2 of the trigeminal nerve). Superiorly and medially is located the nasolacrimal system, and posteriorly the pterygoid plates, which lead to the cranial base.

Blood supply

A comprehensive understanding of the vascular blood supply to the maxilla is crucial in osteotomy surgery, both to avoid haemorrhage and maintain the vascularity of the mobilized maxillary bone. The arterial blood supply to the maxilla comes from four primary sources (Figure 22-5):

1. The descending palatine branch of the maxillary artery.
2. The ascending palatine branch of the facial artery.
3. The anterior branch of the ascending pharyngeal artery from the external carotid.
4. The alveolar branches of the maxillary artery.

With complete mobilization of the maxilla, the descending palatine vessels are frequently disrupted

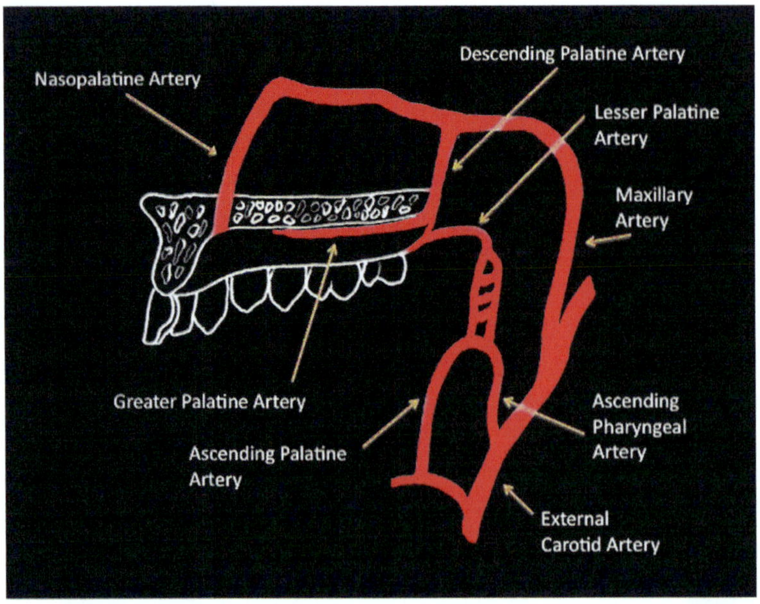

Fig. 22-5 Schematic diagram showing the arterial blood supply to the maxilla. The main blood supply following Le Fort I osteotomy is from the ascending pharyngeal and ascending palatine arteries.

and the mobilized maxilla derives its vascularity from the remaining sources, primarily the ascending palatine and pharyngeal vessels. The main blood supply to the maxilla is maintained through the buccal pedicle.[6,7] It is therefore essential that this pedicle is preserved. An incision curving upwards in front of the parotid papilla reduces the chance of the pedicle tearing posteriorly, which would reduce the size of the pedicle and jeopardize the blood supply to the maxilla (Figure 22-6).

The descending palatine/greater palatine artery, whilst not an essential vessel for the viability of the maxilla in a non-cleft patient, is an important vessel. Its partial division may occasionally be the cause of severe postoperative haemorrhage. This can be particularly dangerous as it remains occult in the hypotensive patient, but becomes very evident when the patient becomes normotensive often following extubation. It is sometimes necessary to divide this artery, particularly when large posterior impactions of the maxilla are necessary. If this is the case then haemostasis with bipolar forceps is essential outside the bony channels. The vessels may then be safely divided (Figure 22-7).

Knowledge of the position of the maxillary artery within the pterygomaxillary fissure is important when the pterygoid disjunction is undertaken. The artery lies at least 1.5 cm above the most inferior point of the pterygomaxillary junction. The risk of damaging the artery can be minimized by ensuring the pterygoid osteotome is directed downwards towards the palate and is less than 1.5 cm above the inferior part of the fissure.[8,9] The pterygoid venous plexus of veins in another potential source of haemorrhage. Haemorrhage from this area can be minimized by subperiosteal dissection in the posterior maxillary region and avoiding fractures of the pterygoid plates.

Blood loss is variable but rarely requires transfusion. A review of over 500 osteotomies concluded an average loss of just under 300 mL greater for bimaxillary osteotomies and less for single jaws surgery.[10] A number of recent papers have questioned the need to cross match patients or even group and save patients

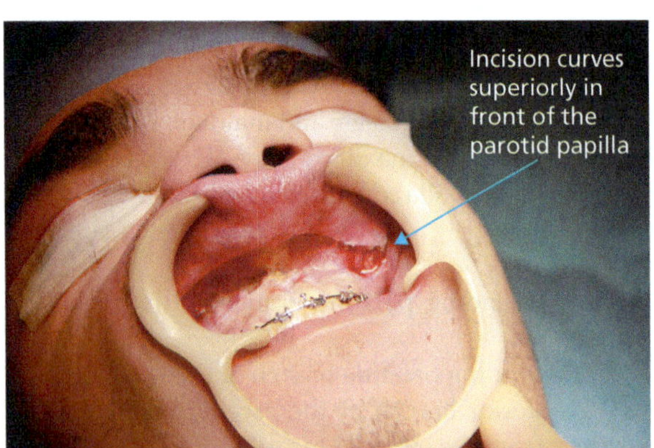

Fig. 22-6 The initial incision for the Le Fort I osteotomy. The incision curves superiorly and protects the buccal pedicles, which is the main blood supply to the maxilla following osteotomy.

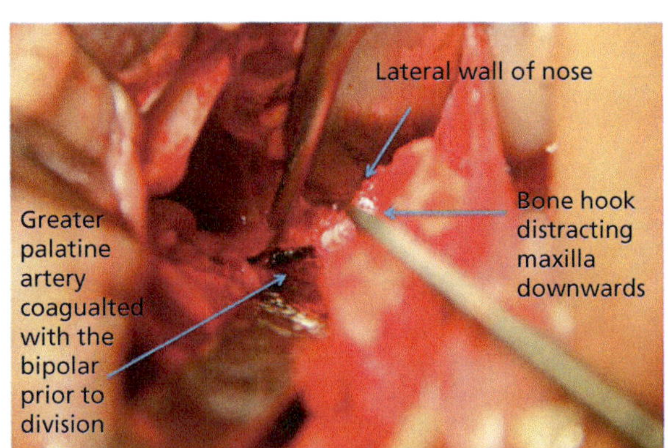

Fig. 22-7 The greater palatine artery at the posterior medial aspect of the maxilla, demonstrating deliberate bipolar diathermy prior to its division.

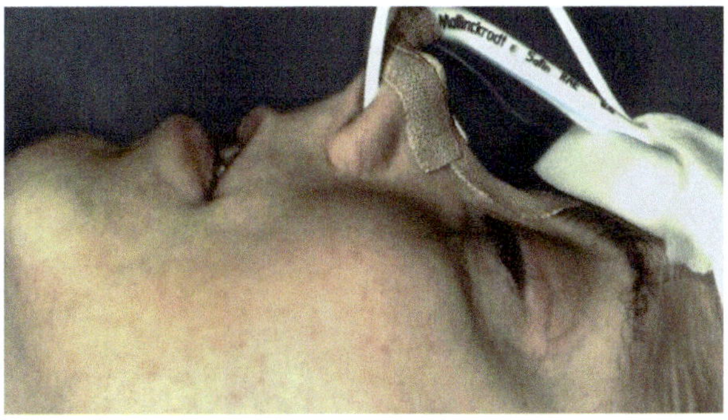

Fig. 22-8 The distortion of the upper lip and nose often produced by nasal intubation.

prior to orthognathic surgery as the incidence of major bleeding requiring transfusion is so low.[10–12]

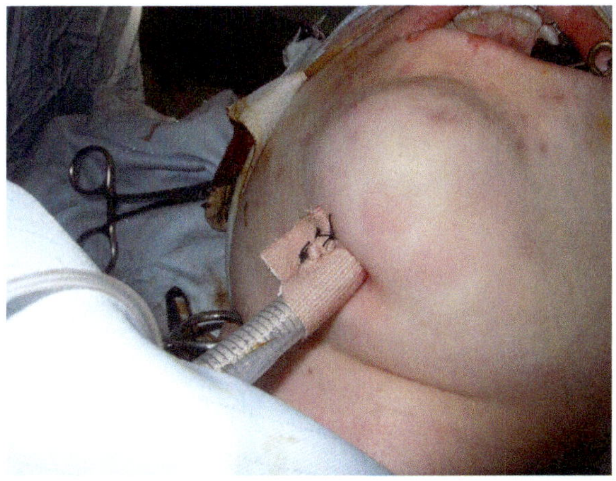

Fig. 22-9 Photograph showing submental intubation. Here the endotracheal tube exits not via the nose but under the chin. The tube is well secured with surgical tape and sutures.

Surgical technique

Submental intubation

Many different techniques have been developed to ensure that the planned surgical moves are those achieved during surgery. A nasal tube, no matter how carefully placed, distorts the nose making assessment of dental midlines, incisor exposure, upper lip height, maxillary occlusal plane cant and the nasolabial angle difficult (Figure 22-8). Simultaneous rhinoplasty to correct a crooked nose or nasal adjustments to prevent adverse changes to the nose is not possible using a nasal endotracheal tube.

With a nasal tube in place other techniques such as placement of a K-wire into the glabellar region need to be employed to attempt to surgically deliver the planned move.[13]

We use the submental intubation technique for the majority of our patients undergoing Le Fort I osteotomy. The benefits of this technique are that it produces an unimpeded view of the whole face and the results of the bony moves can be seen immediately (Figure 22-1). Assessment of cants, incisor exposure, upper lip height, dental midlines and nasal changes can be easily undertaken. It also enables unwanted changes to the nose to be modified at the time of the osteotomy.

Submental intubation is an airway technique that places the endotracheal tube (traditionally placed via the nose), directly under the chin (Figure 22-9). The residual scar is virtually invisible, and being under the chin, it is in a place not usually seen (Figure 22-10).

The technique was initially developed for the trauma patient as an alternative to the tracheostomy, by Hernandez Altemir in 1986.[14] It was designed specifically for patients with base of skull fractures (where nasal intubation is contraindicated) and a deranged dental occlusion. Until submental intubation was described, a temporary tracheostomy was the only solution, a technique that carries both morbidity and an obvious unattractive scar.

A number of orthognathic surgeons have used submental intubation,[15] and we now use it for the majority of our Le Fort I osteotomies.[16] It also enables simultaneous rhinoplasty to straighten the crooked nose and allows excellent access to the nasal septum from an inferior approach (Figures 22-11 and 22-12).

Submental intubation is a simple technique with a low complication rate, provided communication between the surgical and anaesthetic teams is good. The surgical or anaesthetic team has complete control of the airway at all times, and the endotracheal tube is either held or taped to the face. Loss of airway control during surgery or at the end is potentially life-threatening.

The important features of the endotracheal tube are that it is armoured to prevent compression and that the connectors need to be removable.

We use the intubating tube of the Laryngeal mask (LMA/Fastrach ETT oral single use) (Figure 22-13).

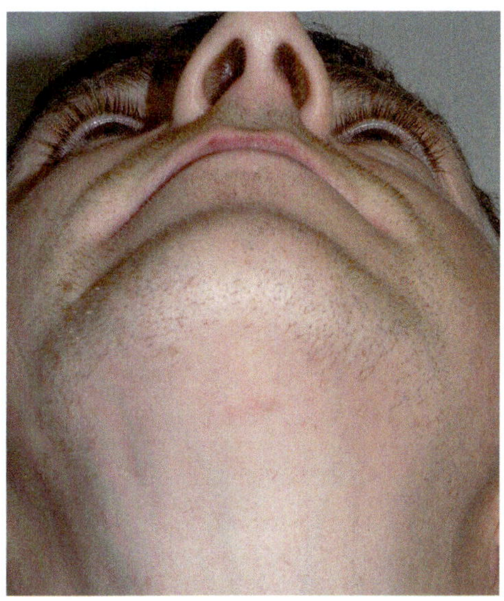

Fig. 22-10 Image showing the typical appearance of a submental scar one year postoperatively.

(a) (b)

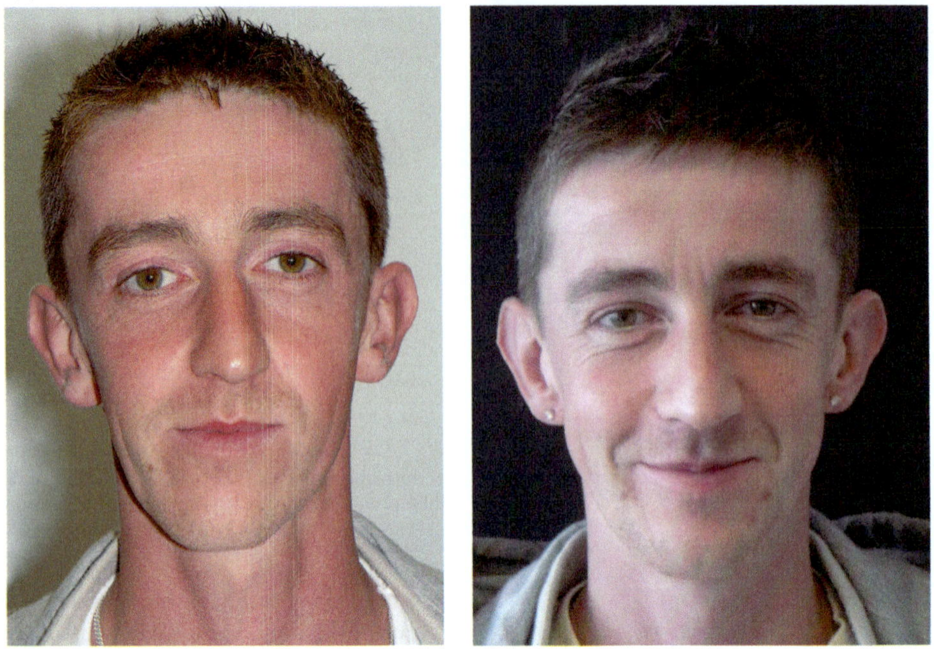

Fig. 22-11 Demonstrating deviated nose (a) preoperatively and (b) improved nasal symmetry postoperatively, following simultaneous bimaxillary osteotomy and rhinoplasty.

The patient is intubated orally by the anaesthetist. The tube is temporarily secured with tape and a note is made of the centimetres intubated to the incisors (Figure 22-14).

Positioning of the patient

It is helpful to have the patient's head slightly extended either by placing a sandbag under the shoulders or by extending the head of the table. This helps with access to the submental region. Local anaesthetic with adrenaline is infiltrated into the area. An incision under the chin is made through the skin and subcutaneous tissue (Figure 22-15). A mouth prop is placed between the teeth. A long clip is used to blunt dissect from the extraoral incision through to the floor of the mouth (Figures 22-16 and 22-17). It is important that the forceps enter the mouth anterior to the submandibular ducts and behind the mandibular incisor teeth to prevent damaging the ducts. There are no important anatomical structures in this area other than a few small blood vessels. The pilot tube is grasped with the tip of the forceps, ensuring that the cuff is not deflated accidentally with the tip of the forceps. The endotracheal tube is then pulled through the same track from the intraoral to the submental extraoral region (Figures 22-11(a) and 22-9).

It is important to avoid extubating the patient accidentally, by pulling the tube too far out of the skin. As a guideline the same centimetre mark should be showing as the tube comes through the skin in the submental region as was recorded at the level of the incisor teeth at oral intubation.

When the surgeon is happy the tube is in the correct place the anaesthetist will listen to the chest to make sure both sides of the lung are being ventilated. It is relatively easy to push the tube too far down resulting in ventilation of the right lung only. It is then essential to secure the tube well to prevent any movement of the tube during surgery. The tube is secured with

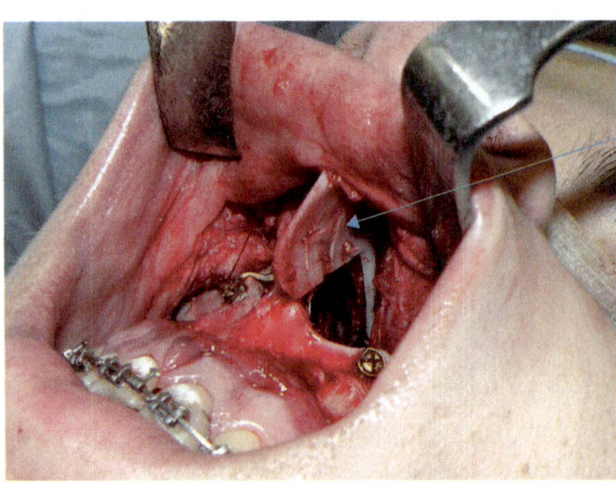

The Le Fort I osteotomy gives excellent access to the septum allowing septoplasty to help straighten a crooked nose. The distal part of the septum has been removed and used to splint and help straighten the remaining septum.

Fig. 22-12 Demonstrating access to the nasal septum from an inferior approach.

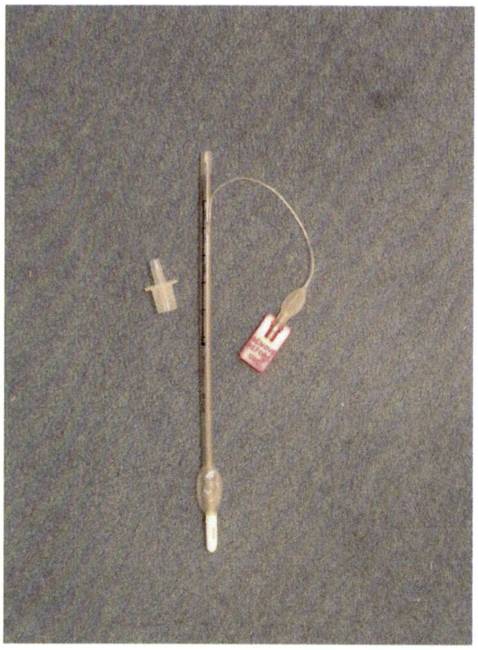

Fig. 22-13 The intubating tube of the laryngeal mask (LMA/Fastrach ETT oral single use, manufactured by The Laryngeal Mask Company Limited, Le Rocher, Victoria, Mahe, Seychelles, distributed by intravent, Orthofix LTD, www.intraventorthofix.com.)

surgical tape and sutured to the skin at the side of the tube (Figure 22-9).

A throat pack is placed to further protect the airway and prevent large volumes of blood irritating the stomach.

Reversal of the submental tube prior to extubation

At the end of the procedure when haemostasis has been achieved, the post-pharyngeal space throat pack

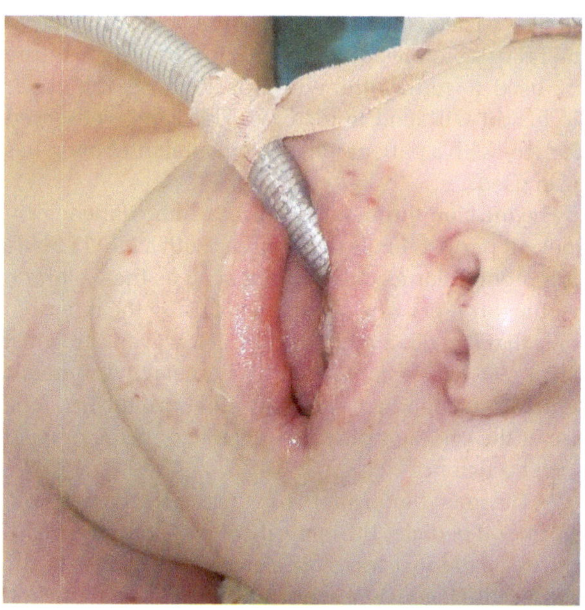

Fig. 22-14 The patient is intubated orally by the anaesthetist and the endotracheal tube is secured by tape.

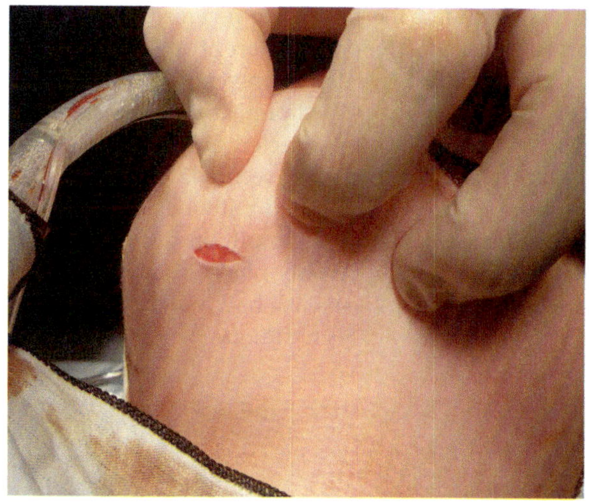

Fig. 22-15 A 1 cm incision is made in the midline under the chin.

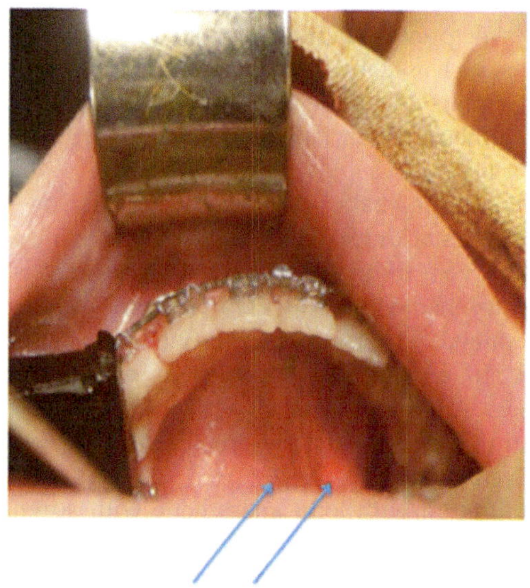

Fig. 22-16 A long clip is used to blunt dissect from the extraoral incision through to the floor of the mouth. It is important that the forceps enter the mouth anterior to the submandibular ducts and behind the mandibular incisor teeth to prevent damage to the ducts.

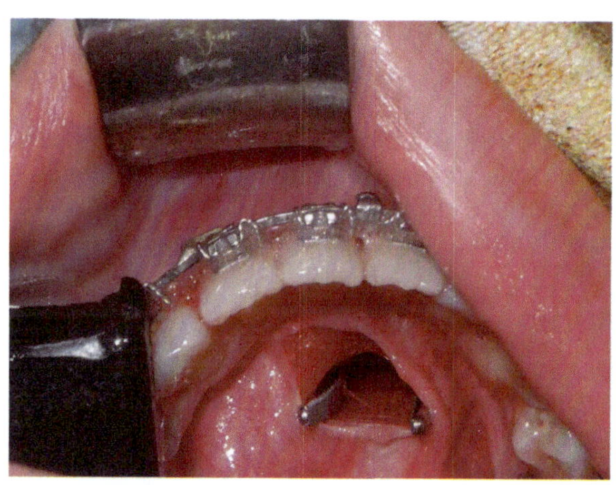

Fig. 22-17 The clip is used to widen the tract for the endotracheal tube.

is removed and the procedure reversed. The mouth prop is placed. The oral section of the tube is held securely with a heavy clip to prevent it being accidentally extubating the patient prematurely. The external part of the tube is disconnected, pushed intraorally, and then reconnected and re-secured.

The skin incision is sutured with 6-0 Vicryl rapide. No sutures are placed intraorally in the floor of the mouth. This is to allow any blood to drain out and prevent airway problems. We have had no significant complications using this technique.[16]

Surgical technique – Le Fort I osteotomy

Technique

Positioning of the patient

It is important to spend some time ensuring the position of the patient on the operating table is optimal. This will prevent morbidity from pressure to bony points, such as elbows and heals. Ensure that if a nasal tube is placed the tube is supported to prevent damage to the nasal rim and too much distortion to the upper lip.

Either pneumatic compression boots or anti-embolism stockings are placed to reduce the incidence of deep vein thrombosis. A warming blanket is also used to ensure the body temperature is optimally maintained. The eyes are protected with adhesive strips to prevent any inadvertent damage to the cornea. Antibiotics are given on induction (Augmentin 1.2 grams) and Dexamethasone (8 mg), both intravenously.

Infiltration with local anaesthetic with adrenaline or Tumescent solution produces a relatively bloodless field. Approximately 100 mL of tumescent solution is infiltrated.

Recipe for Tumescent solution

- 500 mL normal saline of Hartman's
- 10 mL Marcaine 0.25%
- 1 mL 1:1000 adrenalin
- 1 vial Hyalase
- 8 mg Dexamethasone

Dose: 7 mL/kg.

Hypotensive anaesthesia is also important in contributing to a bloodless field. It is important to place a good throat pack to prevent blood being swallowed, which will be a gastric irritant postoperatively.

Retraction of the lips

Use of a photographic retractor is extremely helpful in preventing trauma to the lips that can occur by stretching the lips or direct trauma from instruments, drills or from thermal injury caused by accidental conduction from the monopolar to metal instruments (Figure 22-18).

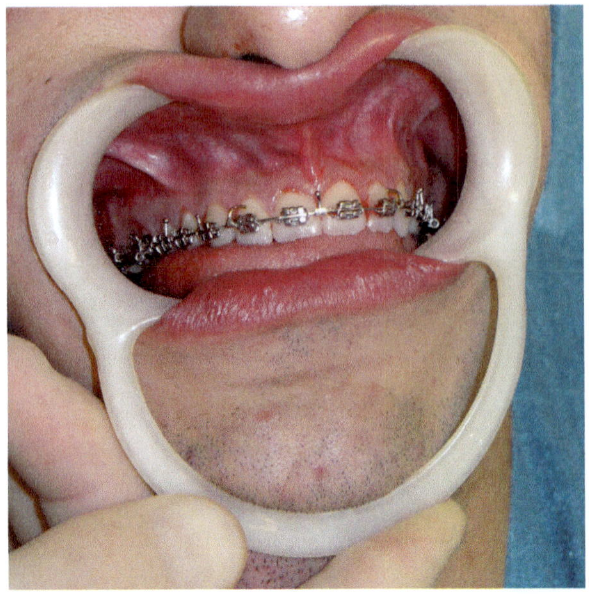

Fig. 22-18 Use of the photographic retractor to protect the lips and aid retraction.

Incision

A number of different incisions have been described. All incisions have in common the ability to maintain the blood supply to the maxilla, whilst allowing adequate access to make safe cuts to the bone and enable the mucosa to be carefully closed at the end. Other factors to consider when making the incision are lip height and thickness, and whether V-Y lengthening of the upper lip would be desirable. Although traditionally the teaching is that the upper lip will be advanced only half the distance of the anterior skeletal move, this is a generalization and depends on the individual soft tissue morphology and thickness, and the suturing techniques used when the Le Fort I incision is closed. Maxillary incisor exposure will increase when the maxilla is advanced. The height of the upper lip also varies with the width of the nose, such that if lateral osteotomies of the nose and/or a cinch suture are used to reduce the width of the nose, the upper lip height will tend to increase. This can be observed directly with a patient when submental intubation has been used.

The incision through the mucosa, subcutaneous tissue and periosteum is made either with a No. 15 blade or a monopolar electrode point such as the Colorado needle (Stryker). The advantage of using the monopolar is that it is relatively bloodless. However, care must be taken to avoid contact with any metal instruments, which could conduct electricity and burn the lips. The use of the photographic cheek retractor helps prevent such occurrences.

As the main blood supply to the maxilla comes from the buccal pedicles the integrity of these must be maintained. If the incision slopes cranially anterior to the parotid ducts any tearing of the flap due to retraction will occur superiorly and not posteriorly, compromising the buccal pedicles (Figure 22-6).

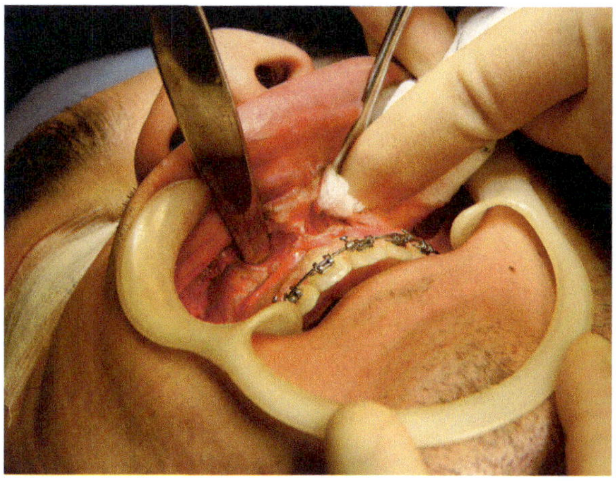

Fig. 22-19 The use of a swab with digital pressure superiorly to strip the periosteum from the bone.

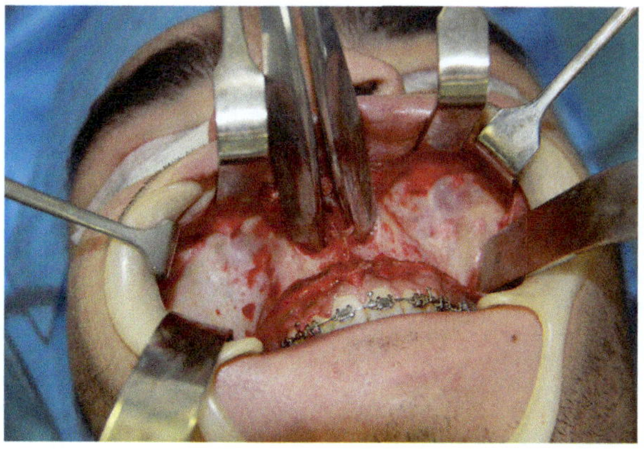

Fig. 22-21 The subperiosteal dissection required with a high level quadrangular Le Fort I osteotomy and good retraction.

Dissection

Once the initial incision is made the periosteum is elevated off the underlying bone, superiorly as far as the infraorbital nerve. This can be achieved easily and quickly using a swab and the periosteal elevator (Figure 22-19). Depending on the height of the osteotomy cut, sharp dissection of the masseter muscle attachments over the zygoma may be necessary in order to expose the inferior portion of the zygoma (Figure 22-20).

Posteriorly dissection should be sub-periosteal up unto the pterygomaxillary fissure. This is particularly important as inadequate dissection in this area can lead to bleeding from the pterygoid venous complex. Subperiosteal dissection up onto the zygomatic arch may be necessary particularly if a high Le Fort I osteotomy is planned. Sharp dissection of the masseter muscle is required with a scalpel or the Obwegeser periosteal elevator.

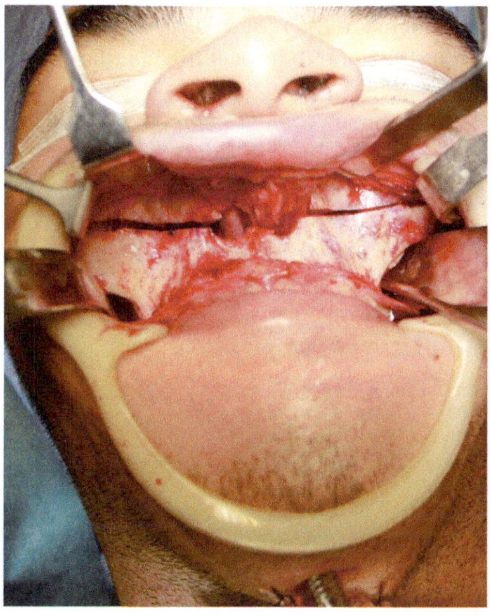

Fig. 22-20 The bone is exposed as far as the zygomatic arches. Sharp dissection of the masseter muscle is required to expose the zygoma. The osteotomy cuts are demonstrated for a quadrangular osteotomy.

Careful dissection of the nasal mucosa using a Ward periosteal elevator, or Mitchell's trimmer and Howarth periosteal elevator is another important step in minimizing blood loss during the downfracture.

Retraction

A useful tip is to bend a Lax tongue depressor so that the tip bends behind the maxillary tuberosity and fits into the pterygomaxillary fissure. It is important to ensure it is placed sub-periosteally.

Howarth periosteal elevators are placed submucosally along the lateral nasal lining. Two Langenbeck retractors are used to elevate the buccal mucosa and protect the infraorbital nerves (Figure 22-21). Care should be used in retraction of this area to prevent temporary neuropraxia of these nerves.

Design of the osteotomy

General considerations

The position of the maxilla should produce the best aesthetic and functional results and will have been pre-determined in the planning stage. However, the benefit of having the face exposed without an endonasal tube is that the immediate effects of the move may be assessed intraoperatively, altered if necessary, and any unwanted changes addressed at the time of the surgery. The maxillary incisors support the upper lip and should be positioned such that incisor exposure is 2–5 mm in repose.

The osteotomy cut can be made at a variety of levels from just above the apices of the maxillary teeth to just beneath the infraorbital nerve, and extended laterally if necessary to improve malar prominence. The sagittal inclination of the osteotomy cut can also be altered, to either move the maxilla superiorly or inferiorly while advancing, without removing bone or bone grafting, as described below.

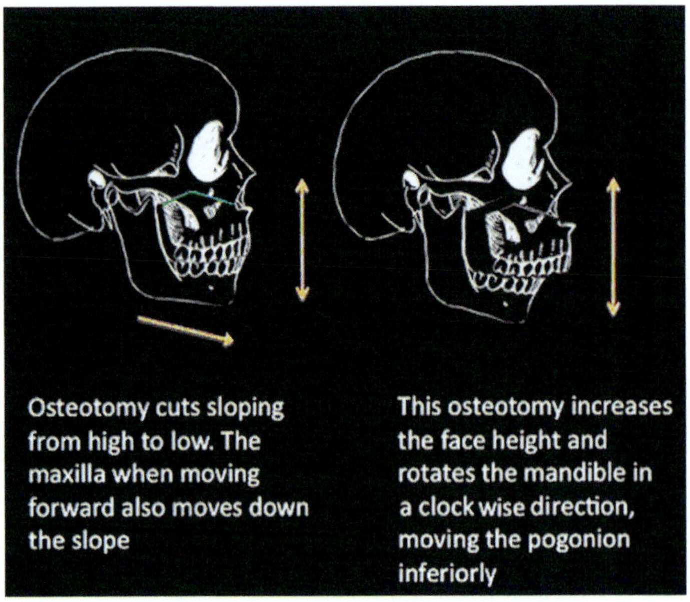

Fig. 22-22 Diagram showing effects of the inclination of the osteotomy cut when advancing the maxilla – osteotomy inclination to increase incisor exposure and potentially increase lower face height.

Effect of changing the inclination (slope) of the osteotomy cut

If the osteotomy cut is made parallel to the occlusal plane and the maxilla advanced, the maxillary incisor exposure will increase but the face height will not change. However, if the osteotomy cut starts high posteriorly and slopes downwards towards the piriform aperture, the maxilla will move down the slope as it is advanced, thus increasing the maxillary incisor exposure. The mandible will subsequently rotate in a clockwise direction and the lower anterior face height will increase (Figure 22-22). The opposite is true for the osteotomy cuts that start low posteriorly and slopes upwards toward the piriform aperture (Figure 22-23).

Technique – making the bone cuts

Bone is usually cut using a reciprocating sagittal saw. To produce a maxillary advancement which will neither result in the maxilla moving up (ramping effect) or moving down, the bony cut should be parallel to the maxillary occlusal plane. The osteotomy cut extends from the pterygomaxillary fissure to the pyriform fossa, avoiding damage to the apices of the maxillary canine teeth. The bone thickness varies considerably, thickest in the zygomatic and pyriform regions and thinnest in between these two zygomatic buttresses. Back cuts are made against the Lax retractor to ensure the posterior wall of the maxillary antrum is divided (Figure 22-24). The back cuts are very important as they reduce the possibility of fractures propagating through the pterygoid plates superiorly to the cranial base during the pterygomaxillary disjunction. Anteriorly the cut extends through the lateral wall of the nose. The Howarth periosteal elevator is used to protect the nasal mucosa.

The height of the Le Fort I osteotomy cut needs to be planned to achieve the required result. Any reduction in height of the bone to impact the maxilla needs to be

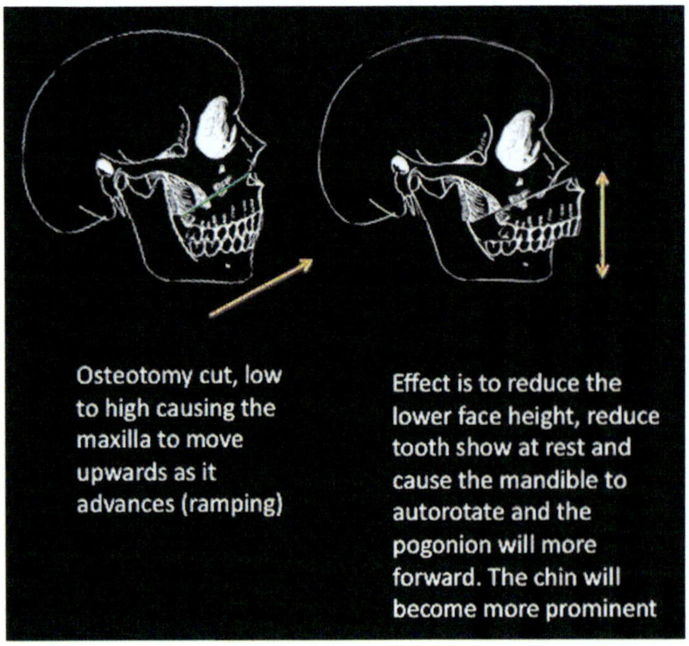

Fig. 22-23 Diagram showing effects of the inclination of the osteotomy cut when advancing the maxilla – osteotomy inclination to reduce incisor exposure and potentially reduce lower face height.

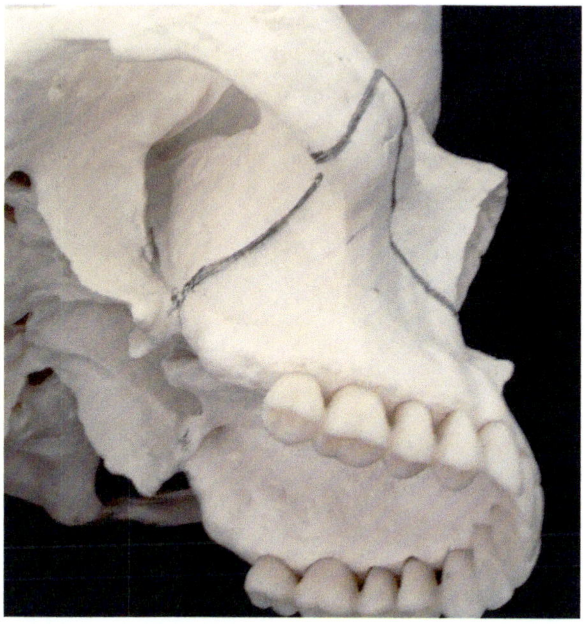

Fig. 22-24 Showing the posterior cuts towards the pterygoid plates in a high Le Fort I osteotomy. These important cuts reduce the risk of uncontrolled fractures cranially towards the cranial base.

undertaken prior to the downfracture. Although the dentoalveolar occlusal result will be the same whatever the level and direction of the Le Fort I osteotomy cut, the aesthetic result on the facial profile will be very different. Low level cuts just above the level of the teeth will advance the dentoalveolar area alone and will have a more profound effect on rotating the nasal tip upwards, but will do little to change the zygomatic, infraorbital and paranasal regions. A higher level osteotomy including the lower part of the zygomatic arch, cutting just below the infraorbital nerves and crossing the lateral part of the nose, will increase the support for the infraorbital rims, reduce scleral exposure below the corneas, improve the appearance of midfacial retrusion and flattening, and have less of an effect on nasal tip rotation.

Detachment of the nasal septum and lateral nasal wall

The anterior part of the nasal septum is cartilaginous and the posterior part is bony (the vomer). To enable the maxilla to be mobilized, both the bony and cartilaginous parts of the septum need to be detached. This may be achieved using the notched septal chisel. The assistant places a finger intraorally behind the soft palate to ensure the chisel does not go further than the back of the hard palate.

The osteotomies of the lateral nasal walls are achieved using a fine osteotome. There is an audible change of note heard on tapping the osteotome when it hits the perpendicular plate of the palatine bone. It is important to stop at this point as this is the region where the descending/greater palatine vessels are and it is desirable to avoid division of these at this stage.

Division of the maxilla from the pterygoid plates

This manoeuvre is probably the stage of the operation associated with the highest morbidity, as fractures of the pterygoid plates may be inadvertently propagated cranially, towards the cranial base. The scientific literature cites examples of damage to each of the cranial nerves during the Le Fort I osteotomy.[17–20]

A number of techniques have been developed in an attempt to reduce complications during the pterygomaxillary disjunction. Usually, a curved Obwegeser osteotome is used with a blind approach to the pterygomaxillary fissure. Some surgeons have modified this by using the Swan's neck osteotome and ultrasonic bone curettes. Some use a technique where leverage alone is used with the aid of Tessier's spreaders or using Smith's three pronged spreaders.[21] The important technique to reduce this possibility are to make sure there is a good 'back cut' from the maxilla to the pterygoid plate (Figure 22-24), to ensure the pterygoid osteotome is sub-periosteal and to direct the pterygoid osteotome caudally rather than cranially. The assistant places their index finger intraorally at the position of the pterygoid hamulus palatally and can feel when the disjunction has occurred. This, together with the change in resonance when hitting the osteotome with the mallet, indicates disjunction. The procedure is repeated on the contralateral side.

Due to the risk of serious postoperative haemorrhage during the pterygomaxillary split, some surgeons have developed techniques to reduce this incidence by using the tuberosity osteotomy.[21]

Downfracture of the maxilla

This is the point at which excessive bleeding can occur. Therefore, close communication with the anaesthetist is essential to ensure hypotensive anaesthesia has been attained. Downfracture is achieved by firm digital pressure. Alternately, the surgeon may place the bone hook in the piriform rim and pull caudally. At the same time a large osteotome can be used to leaver the maxilla downwards. This should only be used where the bone is thick, posteriorly at the zygomatic buttress, otherwise part of the maxilla may fracture. During this controlled displacement downwards the nasal mucosa should be carefully elevated to prevent tearing and bleeding.

Full mobilization of the maxilla is essential. Downward and lateral traction with the bone hook placed anteriorly, together with the pterygoid osteotome positioned behind the maxillary tuberosity, leavers the maxilla forward and demonstrates any areas where the bone is still attached. It is also an excellent technique for demonstrating the greater palatine vessels (Figure 22-7). The greater palatine vessels should be identified. Whilst these vessels are not essential to maintain the blood supply of the maxilla, and may be divided without compromising blood supply, inadvertent division, not recognized intraoperatively, is responsible for some of the postoperative bleeding

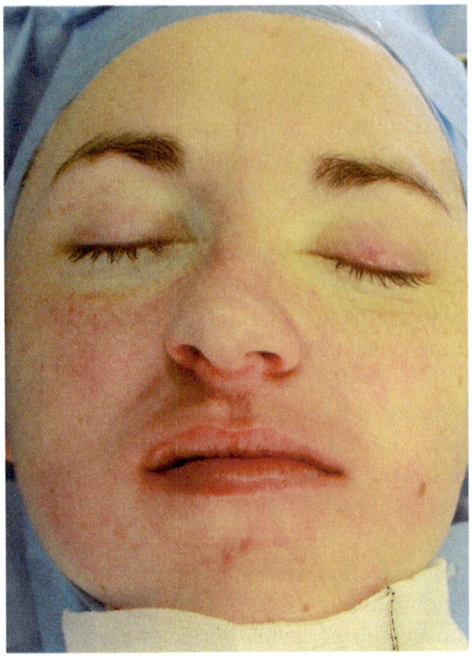

Fig. 22-25 Inadequate nasal septal reduction inferiorly can cause nasal septal deviation and nasal asymmetry postoperatively.

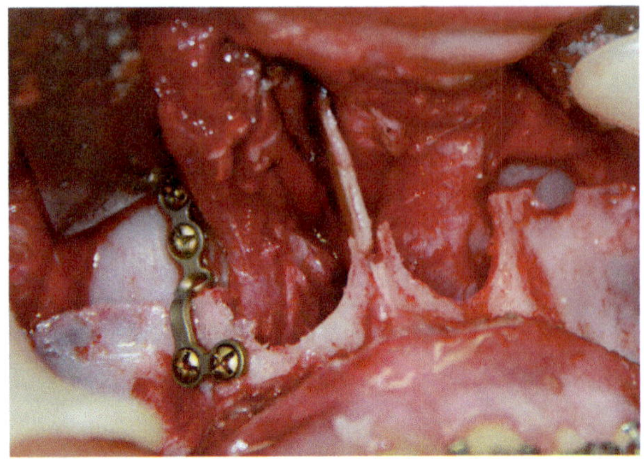

Fig. 22-26 A groove can be cut in the anterior nasal spine to secure the septum.

that can occur. Sometimes the vessels need to be divided if a significant impaction is required. Good haemostasis with bipolar diathermy is essential.

The intermediate wafer splint is placed using power chain or 0.35 mm wire. It is important to make sure the teeth are occluding into the wafer and that there is nothing trapped between the teeth, such as the tongue or the throat pack.

Nasal changes – specific considerations and minimizing undesirable changes

Exposure of the inferior part of the nasal septum, and sometimes the anterior part of the septum, is achieved using an Obwegeser–Freer periosteal elevator. The septum needs to be reduced inferiorly if the maxilla is going to be impacted. Failure to do this will result in nasal deviation postoperatively (Figure 22-25).

A groove can to be made for the septum along the palate and into the anterior nasal spine (Figure 22-26). The septum can be sutured centrally through a hole in the anterior nasal spine. Bone needs to be removed around the piriform fossa to help avoid nasal widening and unwanted changes to the nasolabial angle (Figure 22-27).

If a maxillary impaction, particularly without advancement, is required, bone may need to be removed in many areas including the area where the greater palatine vessels enter the bony channel in the maxilla. A decision must be made either to preserve the vessels or to deliberately use bipolar diathermy and divide the vessels. If the vessels are to be preserved great care should be taken in removing the bone above them. This may be achieved by using a bone rongeur and crushing the bone above the vessel, and then carefully removing the pieces of bone. Another technique is to use a small osteotome above the vessels. Bone needs to be removed from wherever it prematurely touches, thereby preventing the seating of the mobile maxilla.

(a) (b)

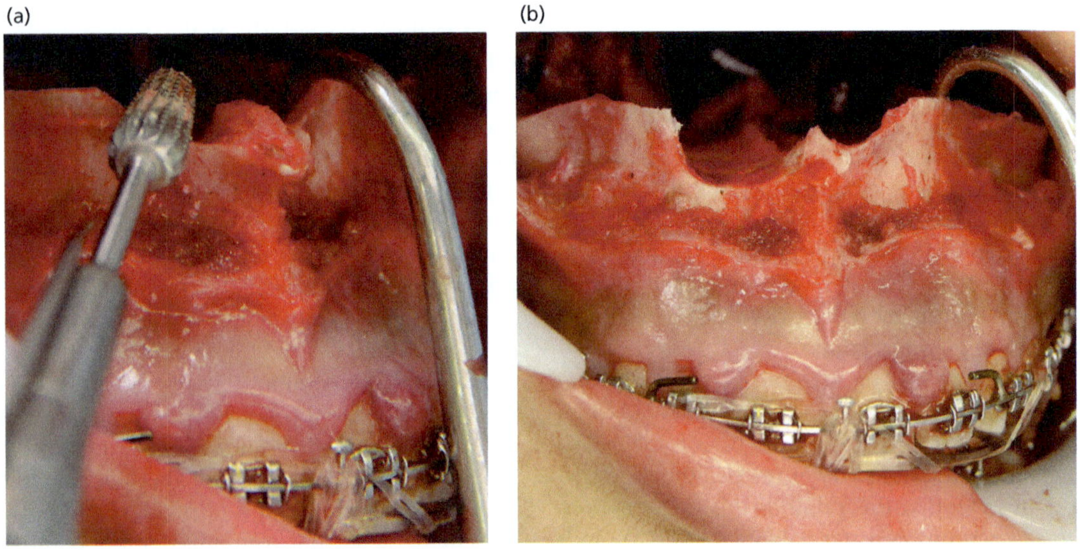

Fig. 22-27 (a, b) Widening and increasing the depth of the piriform aperture helps control the nasal base widening.

Occasionally the inferior turbinates need to be removed to permit adequate superior repositioning of the maxilla. These are vascular structures; from a practical aspect the blood supply comes from the posterior aspect of the turbinates and travels anteriorly. Therefore haemostasis either with the Colorado needle or bipolar haemostasis is essential in this region. Removal of the turbinates may change nasal air flow and therefore they should not be removed unless necessary.

Nasal changes related to the Le Fort I osteotomy

The advantage of submental intubation is most apparent in assessing the nasal changes at the time of the Le Fort I osteotomy and adjusting the hard and soft tissues to reduce any unwanted effects. Conventional endonasal tubes prevent this intraoperative advantage.

The nose is one of the most important elements in facial profile aesthetics, but it is one of the most variable facial structures in terms of bone, cartilages and soft tissue coverage. It has been demonstrated that patients with very similar cephalometric skeletal measurements and dental occlusions may have very different facial profiles based on their nasal morphology.[22]

Conventional belief is that advancement of the maxilla often produces elevation of the nasal tip and shortening of the dorsum of the nose, nasal hump reduction and an increase in the nasolabial angle predominantly due to the tip elevation.[23]

However, the nasolabial angle is reported as sometimes increasing and sometimes decreasing with maxillary advancement. This variation is explained by the different structure of the septum and prominence of the anterior nasal spine. In some patients, where the nasal septum is well-developed and the anterior nasal spine is prominent, advancement of the maxilla results in a more obtuse nasolabial angle (Figure 22-28), whereas if the septum and anterior nasal spine is less well developed, maxillary advancement will result in less nasal tip elevation and a more acute nasolabial angle (Figure 22-29).

Attempts to study the nasal changes resulting from maxillary movements have demonstrated very variable results. The general consensus is that nasal changes are unpredictable after Le Fort I osteotomy.[22]

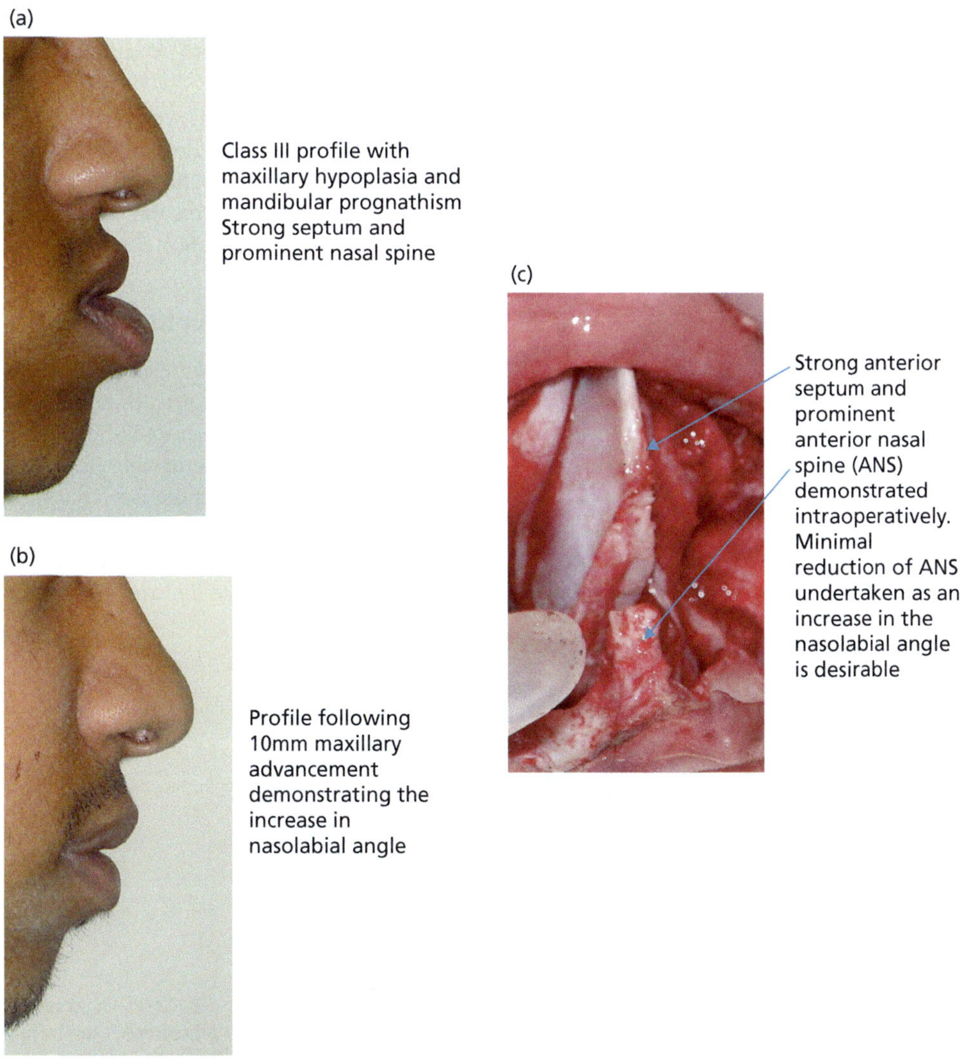

Fig. 22-28 Demonstrating nasolabial changes with a Le Fort I advancement osteotomy with a well-developed nasal septum and anterior nasal spine.

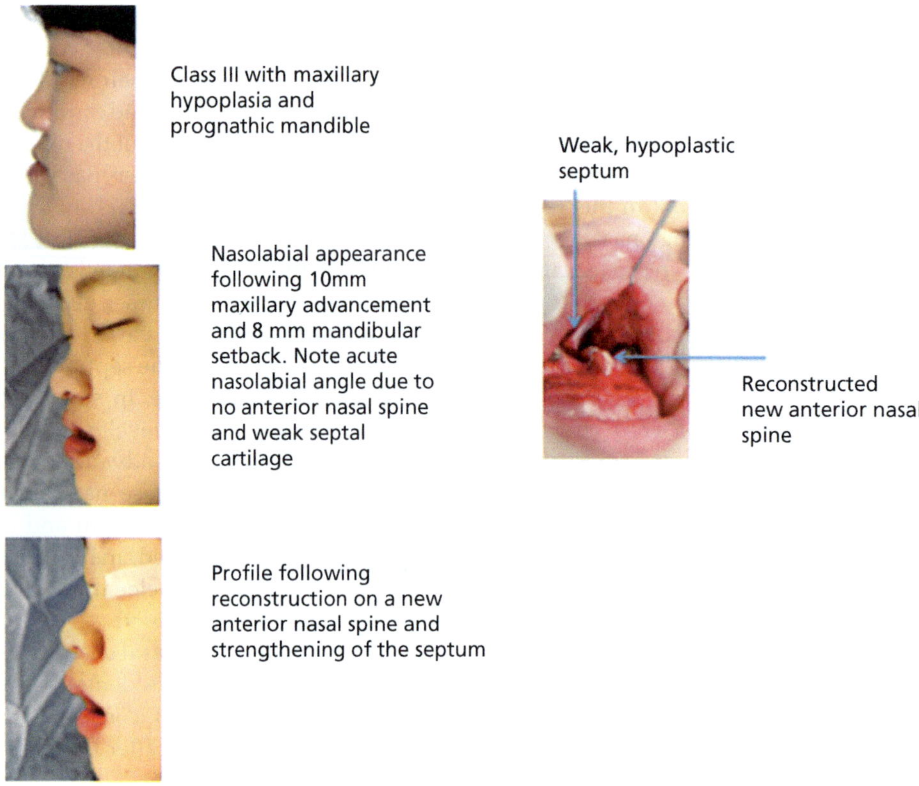

Fig. 22-29 Demonstrating nasolabial changes with maxillary advancement osteotomy with a poorly developed septum and anterior nasal spine. In this patient with a poorly developed septum and anterior nasal spine, a significant advancement of the maxilla does not increase the nasolabial angle. Only when the septum is reinforced and a new anterior nasal spine reconstructed can the increase in the nasolabial angle be demonstrated.

Techniques to reduce unwanted changes to the nasal profile

Unwanted nasal tip rotation can be controlled by a combination of reduction to the anterior nasal spine, piriform aperture sculpting (particularly the lateral nasal wall) and adjustments to the inferior part of the nasal septum (Figures 22-27 and 22-30).

Adjustment to the anterior nasal spine and piriform aperture

Mommaerts et al. reported that the anterior nasal spine is an important component of nasal tip projection and may need to be reduced to limit the degree of nasal tip rotation.[24] Betts et al. emphasized that changes in the lateral portion of the piriform aperture have a significant effect on the soft tissue of the nasal base and nasal tip projection.[25]

Changes to the nasal septum

It is possible to control some of the unwanted changes to the nasal profile by careful adjustment of the inferior aspect of the septum (Figure 22-30). The effect of this can be observed intraoperatively if submental intubation has been used and there is no nasal tube in place. It is important not to remove too much of the septum as this can produce a retracted columella, which is a potentially unattractive feature.

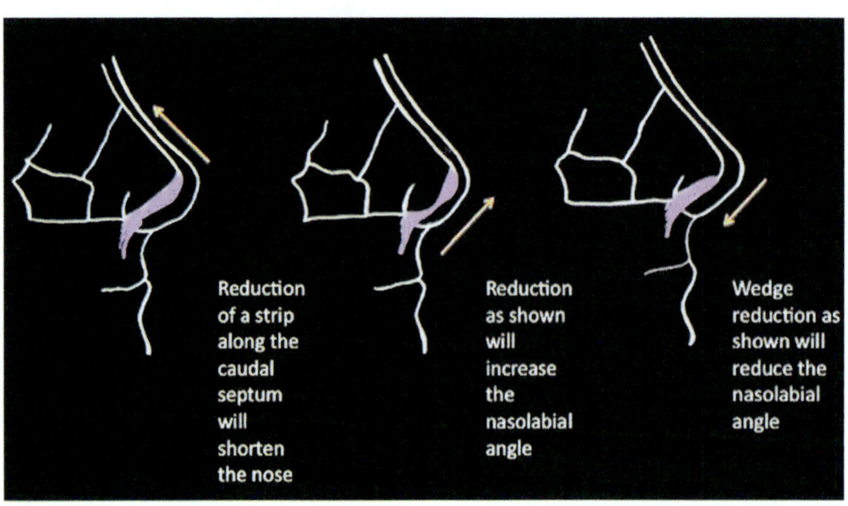

Fig. 22-30 Diagram showing how adjustments can be made to the nasal tip rotation and nasolabial angle by adjusting the caudal aspect of the nasal septum.

Deviated nose

The 'crooked' nose often detracts from a person's facial symmetry, affects breathing and may distort the philtrum of the upper lip. This may make attempts to ensure the coincidence of the maxillary dental midline with the philtrum and face difficult. It is possible with the submental intubation technique that closed rhinoplasty at the time of the maxillary osteotomy can be undertaken to straighten the nose and septum (Figure 22-11). Access to the whole of the nasal septum is easily achieved from an inferior approach (Figure 22-12).

The width of the alar base should be approximately the same as the intercanthal distance. In patients with tall faces, the alar width is often narrow; conversely, the alar width if often wide in patients with a vertically deficient maxilla. There is also ethnic variability.

Any procedure that elevates the periosteum around the nasal base is likely to result in widening of the alar base, particularly with advancement or impaction of the maxilla.

Sometimes this nasal widening may be an advantage, particularly if the nasal alar base width is found to be narrow presurgery; but often it is not. Techniques such as piriform aperture widening and cinch suturing can reduce the unwanted widening.

Cinch suture

The alar base cinch suture was first described by Millard in patients with clefts, following which Collins and Epker described it in non-cleft patients.[26] Traditionally, the suture is secured to the anterior nasal spine. This has the frequently unwanted effect of elevating the nasal tip, thereby increasing the nasolabial angle. However, if the technique is adapted to pass the suture directly under the septum rather than to the anterior nasal spine, it results in narrowing but with fewer adverse effects on the nasolabial angle (Figure 22-31).

The long-term stability of the cinch suture has been evaluated. Stewart et al. found that it is a useful

(a) (b) (c) (d)

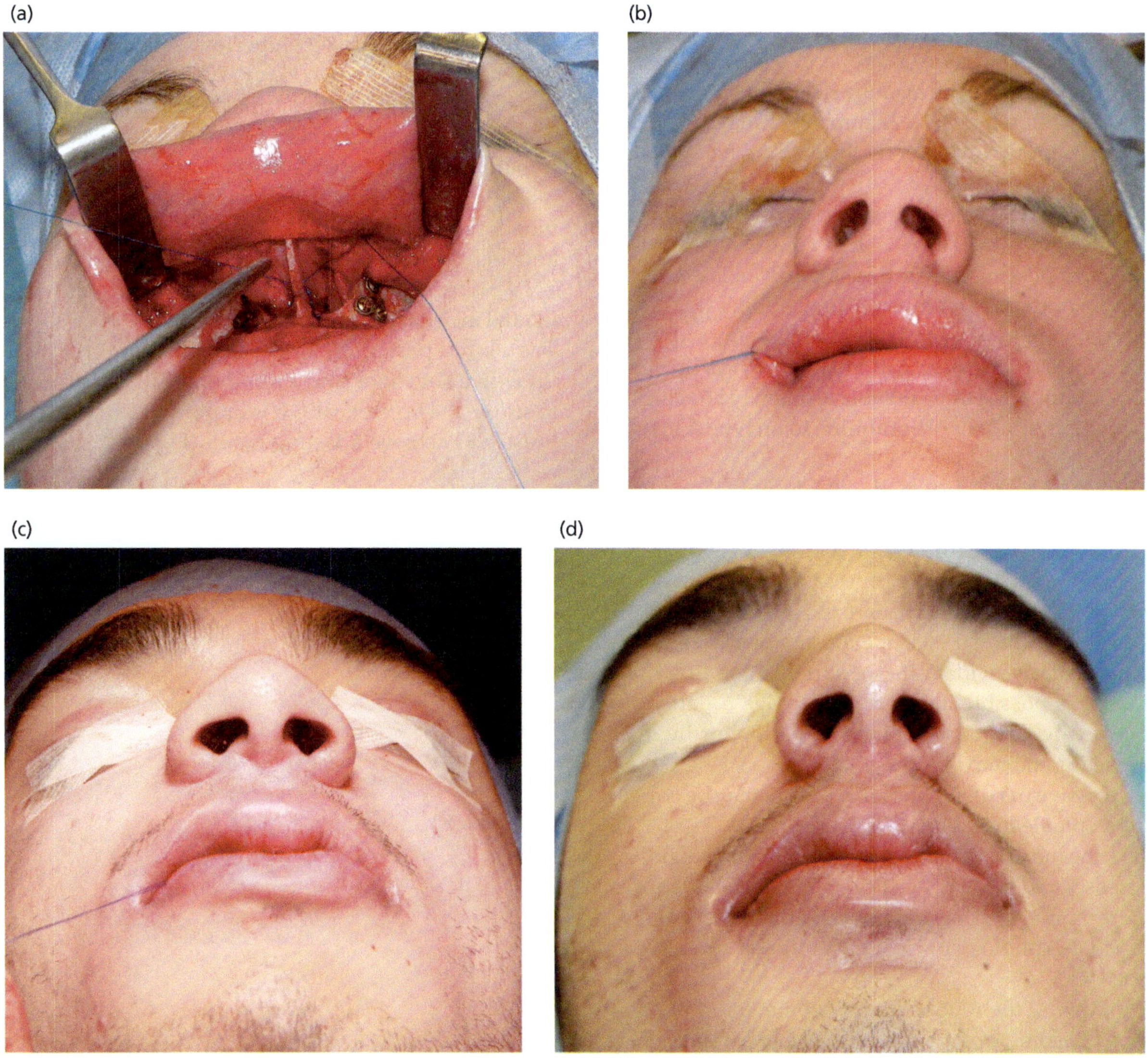

Fig. 22-31 The alar cinch suture; (a) 3-0 Prolene suture travelling below the nasal septum rather than to anterior nasal spine in order to reduce the nasal tip elevation that may occur with the cinch suture. (b) The effect of the cinch suture on the width of the nose on the patient's left side compared to the width on their right side without the cinch effect. (c) Pre-cinch suture and (d) post-cinch suture, demonstrating significant reduction in nasal alar base width.

technique in controlling the width of the alar base, but relapse of 10–20% should be expected.[27] They suggested that over-correction in reducing the nasal width should be undertaken, in order to take the aforementioned relapse into account. Another study used three-dimensional optical surface scanning pre- and postoperatively, but found little benefit in the technique.[28] As with all scientific literature, caution is advised in the interpretation of results, as techniques, sample sizes and confounding variables may have been issues in the design of the studies.

Rhinoplasty

Increases of nasal alar base width which cannot be controlled by the above techniques may require wedge resection of the nasal base or alar base (see Chapter 48).

Upper lip height and lip support

The appearance and morphology of the upper lip, and the amount of maxillary incisor exposure in repose and smiling are some of the key areas to optimize in maxillary surgery. These are age, gender and ethnicity-specific. The average height of the upper lip in a Caucasian female is 22 mm and a male is 24 mm, which is approximately one-third of the height of the lower face.

Maxillary incisor exposure at rest should be approximately 2–5 mm. There is less control over incisor exposure on smiling, as this is partly related to the activity of the levator muscles of the upper lip. Whilst it is possible to weaken these muscles surgically, it is unpredictable and may lead to asymmetrical lip elevation on smiling. A more reliable result may be achieved by regular injections of botulinum toxin type A to these levator muscles.

Fuller lips are considered to be desirable in women and certain ethnic groups, such as the African-Caribbean/African-American tend to have fuller lips.

As a result of the ageing process, the upper lip height increases, maxillary incisor exposure reduces (conversely, mandibular incisor exposure increases, which is particularly evident in speech) and the lips thin.[1] Thus it is possible inadvertently to age a patient by excessively 'lengthening' their upper lip, or by over-impacting the maxilla.

Excessive maxillary incisor exposure may be equally unacceptable to a patient.

As the maxilla advances, maxillary incisor exposure increases and the effective upper lip thickness reduces. There is however considerably variation depending on the morphology of each patient's soft tissue envelope.

Following the routine use of submental intubation, it has become apparent that there is a relationship between the nasal alar base width and upper lip height. Widening of the alar base appears to result in shortening of the upper lip, and the narrowing of the nose with a cinch suture 'lengthens' the upper lip. Changes to the upper lip morphology, in terms of thickness and height, may be achieved with suturing techniques (Figure 22-32). A degree of relapse is inevitable, but long term changes are achievable.

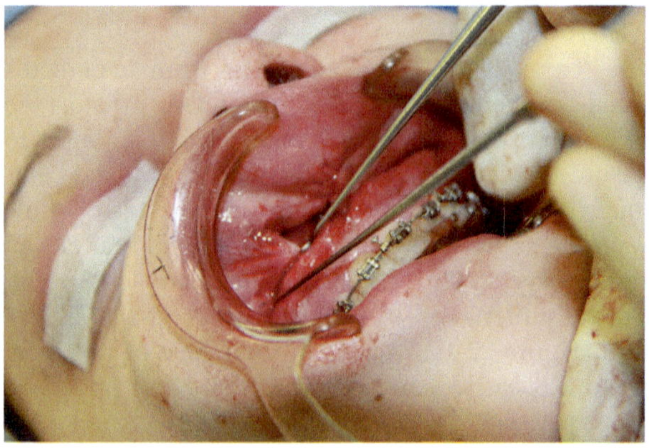

Fig. 22-32 Increasing the volume and height of the upper lip can be achieved by closing the Le Fort I incision in such a way that the posterior, superior part of the incision is advanced.

Increasing the volume and height of the upper lip can be achieved by closing the Le Fort I incision in such a way that the posterior, superior part of the incision is advanced as shown in Figure 22-32. This produces a thicker and 'longer' upper lip. The initial appearance can be unnaturally swollen, but over a few weeks this unnatural appearance resolves.

The upper lip height may be increased by a combination of reducing the alar width (if appropriate), and using the above suturing technique together with a VY-plasty. This is a technique where the straight horizontal incision below the lip is converted to a Y-shape. The central part of the upper lip (philtrum) is picked up with a skin hook and a number of sutures are used to suture the lip vertically. It is important to include the muscle to achieve a lasting result (Figure 22-33). The

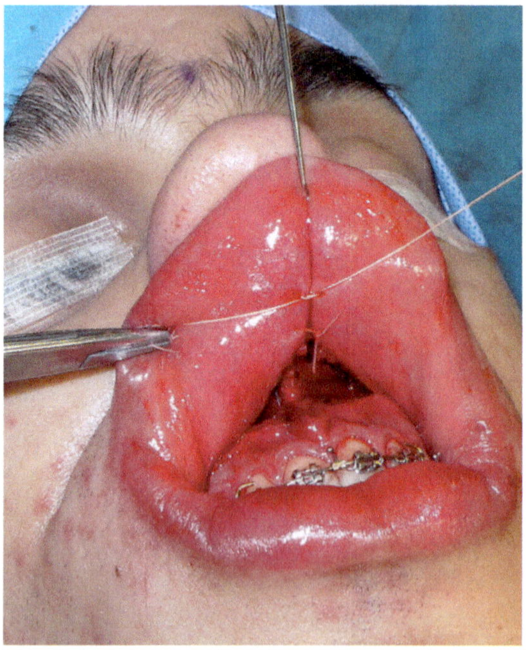

Fig. 22-33 A V-Y closure of the upper lip.

initial result can often look un-natural but this settles within a few weeks producing a natural appearance and upper lip height increase by a few millimetres.

Thus adjustments at this final stage of incision closure are very important and attention to detail is imperative, as changes to the appearance of the upper lip can be made at this point in order to optimize the final aesthetic result.

Before fixing the maxilla it important to check that the maxillary dental midline is coincident with the facial midline, usually taken as the mid-philtrum of the upper lip.[1] It is also important to check there is no transverse cant of the maxillary occlusal plane (Figure 22-1), no nasal deviation, and that nasal alar base width and maxillary incisor exposure is optimal.

Checks to be made before plate fixation of the maxilla

- Ensure there are no bony interferences.
- Check the teeth are occluding into the wafer correctly (particularly posteriorly, ensure the tongue is out of the way) and the condyles are seated correctly.
- Check there are no soft tissue/septal interferences.
- Check the nasal septum is central (suture or cut groove into anterior nasal spine).
- Check any septal adjustment and piriform aperture bony adjustments have been made.
- Make sure the maxillary dental midline, and transverse maxillary occlusal plane cant are correct.
- Ensure facial appearance, incisor exposure and aesthetics are optimal.

Plates and screw fixation

L-shaped plates are used to fix the maxilla at the piriform region and 1.5 mm plates (Synthes®) placed in the zygomatic buttress regions, as these are the thickest parts of the bone. The plates are carefully moulded and contoured to shape, and 4 or 6 mm screws are used. 4 mm should be used where the roots of the teeth are close. It is important to use good irrigation to avoid over-heating or burrning the bone.

It is also important, as far as possible, that the plates and screws are placed such that they cannot be palpated postoperatively by the patient. However, this can occasionally occur in the infraorbital regions with the most superior part of the plates around the piriform aperture.

Variations of the Le Fort I osteotomy

Quadrilateral (quadrangular) osteotomy

This variation of the Le Fort I osteotomy is a high level osteotomy which extends up to the inferior part of the zygoma and just below the infraorbital nerve bilaterally (Figures 22-20, 22-21, 22-24, 22-34, 22-35).

The indications for this osteotomy are midface retrusion, including excessive scleral exposure above the lower eyelid, and hypoplastic zygomas (Figures 22-2 and 22-3). Therefore, the benefits of the quadrangular osteotomy are that it improves the appearance of midfacial retrusion and flattening, improves zygomatic prominence and support for the lower eyelid. If the cuts are made from high to low (Figure 22-22), a significant inferior movement of the maxilla can be achieved thus reducing the necessity for an interpositional bone graft (which would be required following a maxillary setdown) and alloplastic onlay grafts for the zygomatic regions. It is more stable than conventional inferior positioning of the maxilla as there is good bone contact with native bone and no bone graft. This osteotomy also produces less nasal tip rotation than the conventional Le Fort I osteotomy.

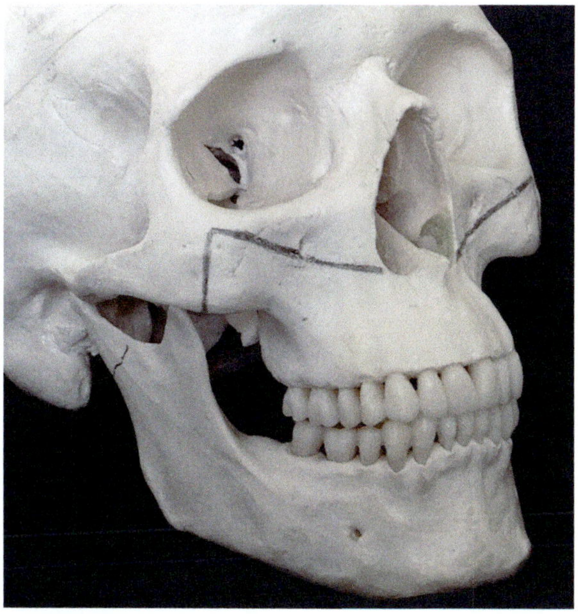

Fig. 22-34 Diagram showing effects of the inclination of the osteotomy cut when advancing the maxilla – osteotomy inclination to increase incisor exposure and potentially increase lower face height.

However, is important to recognize that if there is a mild facial asymmetry in the maxillary region, this asymmetry can be emphasized with this high level cut as the maxilla is advanced.

The surgical technique is as described above for a standard Le Fort I osteotomy, but significant sharp dissection of the masseter muscle from the zygoma is required to expose the prominence of the zygomatic bone. The bony cuts are demonstrated in (Figure 22-35). The cuts are made just below the infraorbital nerves. It is important to recognize that the floor of the orbit is not far from this area and therefore the cut should not be deep in this region. The bone over the zygomatic prominence is thick and control over the shape of the cuts is easier using a burr and a saw.

A crucial step is demonstrated in (Figure 22-35). This ensures that the bony cut does not propagate upwards to the cranial base, but instead is directed downwards to the normal pterygomaxillary disjunction level. The

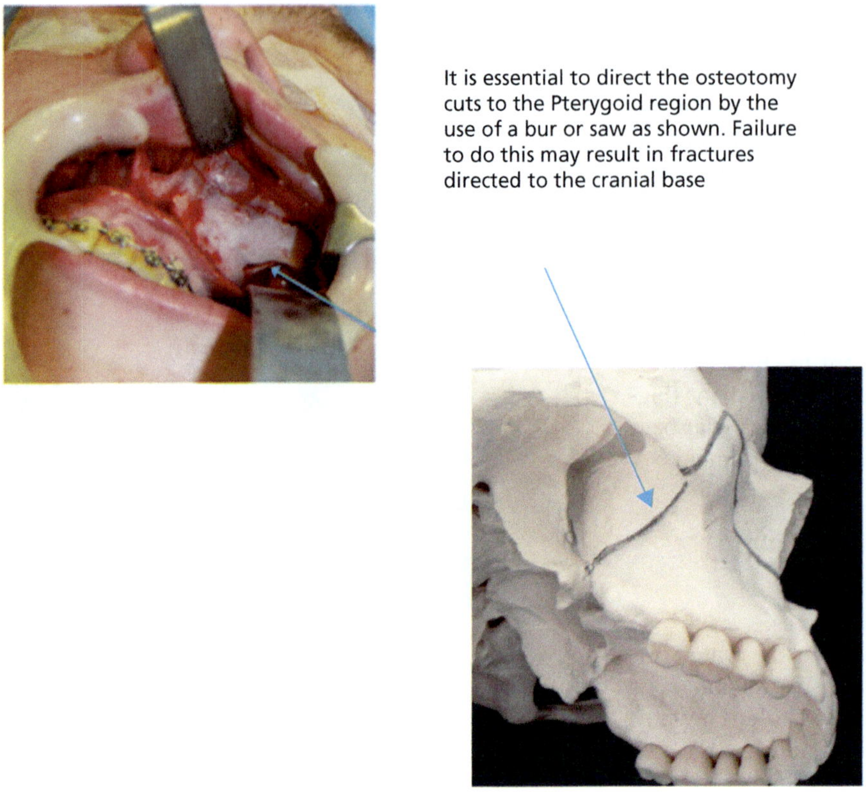

Fig. 22-35 It is important to continue the saw or cut with a fissure burr through the inferior part of the zygomatic arch and extend it inferiorly and posteriorly to enable the important back cut to the pterygoid plates. This reduces the possibility of unwanted propagation of fractures to the cranial base.

other steps to complete the bony cuts and downfracture the Le Fort I cut are made as above. Fixation is with miniplates. However, care must be taken to ensure the plates are not palpable in the infraorbital regions.

Subspinal osteotomy

This osteotomy was described by Mommaerts to in an attempt to minimize the nasal changes that can occur following a conventional Le Fort I osteotomy. However, it is only appropriate for very low level osteotomies. It avoids dissection around the nose and takes the bony cuts below the anterior nasal spine.[24]

Complications associated with the Le Fort I osteotomy – occurrence, prevention and management

No surgical procedure is without risk. However, orthognathic surgery is elective surgery, usually on young healthy individuals, and thus complications should be kept to an absolute minimum.

Complications may be classified as local or general, and early, intermediate and late. The most serious and devastating complication, death, is most likely to occur in the perioperative period due to bleeding, airway problems or a previously undiagnosed medical condition. Deaths can occur in the intermediate period due to, for example, pulmonary embolus. However, this is extremely rare in otherwise fit and healthy patients. The exact number of deaths attributed to orthognathic surgery is unknown; however, a survey of maxillofacial consultants in the UK reported 7 deaths out of 6625 (single jaw), and 9024 (bimaxillary osteotomies) over a 5-year period. This would give a risk rate of 0.16% for a single jaw and 0.23% for a bimaxillary osteotomy. However, these results are based on a response rate of only 47%.[29]

In general, serious complications are extremely low despite operating in an anatomically complex neurovascular region close to the skull base and the patient's airway. Bays and Bouloux cite serious complications in less that 0.1% of all osteotomies,[17] as a result of airway problems, aspiration, anaphylaxis or serious haemorrhage.

Careful assessment of the patient, optimizing health, balancing risk and benefit, and good communication with the patient and their family, between the medical team, the anaesthetist, and the patient's medical practitioner at all stages helps to minimize problems. Time spent listening to the patient and exploring their specific concerns is time well spent, and can prevent an ultimately dissatisfied patient.

A thorough patient medical history is vitally important. Orthognathic surgery is usually elective, and thus the risks and benefits need to be assessed carefully. In some patients, the risks may outweigh the benefits, in which case orthognathic surgery should not be undertaken.

Other factors also need to be taken into consideration. Smoking increases the risk of infection and either an abnormally high or low Body Mass Index (BMI) will increase the risk of potential complications. The ethics of subjecting a patient to an elective procedure which carries risks to their health if they are not in generally good health is questionable. A patient's religious views may also influence treatment, e.g. a Jehovah's Witness may refuse blood transfusion. A formal meeting with all those involved, including the hospital haematology team, should be arranged before undertaking any treatment. Blood products are rarely required now in orthognathic surgery and refusal to accept blood products should not necessarily prevent someone having an osteotomy. However, a clear plan needs to be agreed before commencing treatment.

Serious, life-threatening risks also relate to general anaesthesia. The risks of an apparently fit and healthy patient dying under general anaesthesia are quoted as 1 in 100,000.[30] Such occurrences may be related to previously undiagnosed cardiomyopathies, or anaphylactic reactions to pharmaceutical drugs. However, the major life threatening causes in orthognathic surgery are related to airway and bleeding problems. It has been estimated that 0.5% of patients undergoing orthognathic surgery have some sort of airway problem. This may be related to the initial intubation, or the airway becoming dislodged or damaged during the procedure.[31]

Intubation dislodgement is particularly dangerous if it occurs at the time of the maxillary downfracture, as bleeding may make re-intubation particularly difficult. Time spent in ensuring the airway is in the correct place and that it is secured well is essential. Other airway problems include damage to the tube or pilot during the procedure by the surgeon, or kinking of the tube. Immediately postoperatively, the surgeon must ensure that the throat pack is removed and that the post-pharyngeal space is free of blood clots, which could drop down into the airway in the early recovery period. Aspiration is another serious risk in the intraoperative and postoperative period. There have been recorded cases where the throat pack has been swallowed as the patient began to regain consciousness towards the end of the procedure.

Specific complications related to the Le Fort I osteotomy and advancement will now be described.

Haemorrhage

Serious complications in orthognathic surgery are rare. However, they can be life-threatening. With orthognathic surgery both the anaesthetist and the surgeon share the same airway and therefore close co-operation and communication is essential.

The head and neck region is highly vascular and uncontrolled bleeding is a potential serious complication. If excessive bleeding occurs, clotting factors will become depleted and a *hypocoagulation state* may ensue, leading to bleeding from all the incisions. In the past, blood transfusions were common with this type of surgery. However, more recently techniques have improved to the extent that the necessity for even grouping a patient preoperatively has been questioned.[11]

Positioning of patient with their head upwards, the injection of tumescence, local anaesthetic with adrenaline and the use of an antifibrinolytic agent (tranexamic acid, 25 mg/kg orally, or 0.5–1 g by slow intravenous injection) all help to reduce bleeding.

The vasculature of the midfacial region is excellent, which is one of the main reasons that the area heals so well. However, the disadvantage is that bleeding may be excessive. If excessive bleeding occurs, a coagulopathy may ensue, resulting in a haematological picture of disseminated intravascular coagulopathy (DIC). This should be avoided at all costs as bleeding from all mucosal surfaces occurs and blood loss can be excessive.

The reported incidence of serious haemorrhage requiring blood transfusion with a Le Fort I osteotomy has been cited as approximately 1%.[32]

The most serious haemorrhage occurs usually as a consequence of the pterygomaxillary separation. In the maxilla the specific areas that may result in excessive bleeding are the pterygoid venous plexus, the maxillary artery within the pterygopalatine fossa, the greater palatine vessels and the mucosa of the nose and maxillary sinus.

To prevent bleeding from the pterygoid venous plexus it is important to ensure subperiosteal dissection is maintained and the pterygoid plates are not fractured.

To ensure that the maxillary artery is not damaged, the pterygoid osteotome needs to be directed inferiorly towards the pterygoid hamulus. The maxillary artery is at least 1.5 cm above the base of the pterygoid fissure.[6] If the artery is damaged then the best course of action is packing of the pterygoid region, temporary closure of the osteotomy and returning the following day to complete the operation. Interventional radiology is occasionally required, as is ligation of the maxillary artery.

Whilst the greater palatine vessels are not absolutely necessary for the vascular maintenance of the maxilla, inadvertent partial damage may be responsible for extensive postoperative bleeding. Recognition of bleeding may only become apparent in the postoperative recovery stage when the blood pressure normalizes. This is a potentially dangerous time, as re-intubation at this point is particularly difficult. Therefore, it is essential that if there is a chance the greater palatine vessels are damaged, haemostasis using bipolar diathermy is undertaken prior to fixing the osteotomy.

Other very rare vascular complications reported have included false aneurysm of the sphenopalatine artery, carotid-cavernous fistula and false aneurysm of the maxillary artery.[33]

Ischaemic changes in non-segmental Le Fort I osteotomies and in non-cleft patients are extremely rare. Although the blood supply of the maxilla has been studied extensively, there are a number of consequences that can occur due to ischaemia. There has been no correlation between division of the descending palatine artery and ischaemia. However, maintaining the buccal vascular pedicles is imperative. Minor ischaemic complications include loss of tooth vitality, periodontal defects, and bone necrosis. Kramer reported minor complications attributed to ischaemia in 0.8% of patients undergoing maxillary osteotomy and found the complications were higher in maxillary moves greater than 9 mm, or associated with segmental surgery.[17]

Nerve damage

Nerve damage may occur to varying degrees, as described by the Seddon classification (1942):

- Type I – Neuropraxia – is 'bruising' to the nerve, and likely to recover from between 2 weeks to several months post-injury.
- Type II – Axonotmesis (*Greek* tmesis signifies 'to cut') – is a crush or significant stretch injury and may take 3 months to 2 years to recover.
- Type III – Neurotmesis – The most severe injury, where the nerve is inadvertently divided. Recovery is unpredictable.

There are reports in the literature of every cranial nerve being damaged during the osteotomy process. However, the commonest nerves to be affected in the Le Fort I maxillary osteotomy are the infraorbital, and the descending/greater palatine nerve. Transient paraesthesia of the infraorbital nerve can occur through traction by retractors. The incidence of infraorbital nerve sensory deficits at 12 months following surgery has been reported to be as high as 6% when tested objectively.[19] However, it rarely persists or is a subjective problem.

Age is a strong indicator for potential complications, particularly for permanent nerve damage.

Descending/greater palatine nerve injury

During the Le Fort I osteotomy the nasopalatine, posterior, middle and anterior superior alveolar nerves are all divided. The descending/greater palatine vessels can also be divided. Despite their division, sensation does appear to return.[34]

Much more rarely, other cranial nerves have been damaged, including the optic nerve, resulting in loss of vision. The method by which this may occur is variable. In some cases, the pterygoid fracture may propagate through to the orbital floor and cause retrobulbar bleeding or distortion of the optic canal.[35]

In others, occipital intracranial bleeding is thought to be the cause.

Isolated oculomotor (III) nerve palsies have also been described.[36] Isolated abducens (VI) nerve palsy has also been described.[37]

Positioning

The positioning of the maxilla is potentially more complex that the mandible because it can be moved in the three planes of space and rotated round the three axes of rotation.

It is important to ensure that the position of the maxilla in relation to all planes of space and axes of rotation is correct prior to plating. Submental intubation makes assessment at this stage easier than with conventional nasal intubation. Any pre-existing facial asymmetry or inadvertent rotation of the maxilla will be more noticeable with the higher level osteotomies when the maxilla is advanced. Whilst small maxillary dental midline deviations (2–3 mm) may be corrected by rotation of the maxilla round the vertical axis, larger moves of the maxilla attempting to correct dental midline problems may affect the position of the condyles as well as the intercuspation of the posterior dentition, and should be avoided.

Stability

There have been a number of studies reviewing the stability of the main Le Fort I movements: maxillary advancement, superior 'impaction' and inferior 'set-down' movements. The studies have looked at the stability of the main movement, whilst recognizing movement may be in a number of different vectors (see Chapter 18).

Rigid fixation with plates provides the initial stability until bone has united. Bone first unites in the pterygoid region.[38]

Following bony union the plates become redundant and stability then results from stable buccal dental relationships and the soft tissue muscle balance.

The most stable maxillary movement is superior repositioning, followed by advancement and the least stable is inferior repositioning. However, the studies looking at the inferior positioning of the maxilla have been based on the need for bone grafting. The technique described above, quadrilateral osteotomy with anterior–inferior sloping maxillary osteotomy cuts, theoretically may result in better stability as no gaps are produced. Studies have reported relapse rates for maxillary superior repositioning of the maxilla ranges from a mean of 0–18% for the anterior maxilla and 6–7% for the posterior maxilla.[19] Relapse rates for maxillary advancement range from 5–15%.[19] As with most orthognathic surgery, the greater the maxillary advancement, the greater the relapse. With inferior maxillary repositioning (using bone grafts), there may be 28% anterior relapse and up to 70% posterior relapse.[19]

Non-union

Non-union is rare and probably associated with failure of the initial plate fixation and poor bony contact. If this persists for greater than 6 months, further surgery with rigid fixation and autogenous bone grafting is recommended.[39]

Infection

Severe infections are rare in orthognathic surgery. Overall, the incidence of postoperative infection has been reported as 0–18% when antibiotics are given antibiotics.[19] Protocols that include intravenous antibiotics at induction, two further postoperative doses at 8-hour intervals and 5 days of oral antibiotics are often used. Some units give only perioperative antibiotics. Rates of infection between 0% and 53% have been described in patients without antibiotics. The evidence in reducing infection by giving a postoperative course of antibiotics is marginal.[19] Smoking increases the risk of infection, as does poor oral hygiene. Septic complications in 1.1% of osteotomy operations have been recorded.[17] These have included abscess formation, and maxillary sinusitis. Low-grade infections related to plate infections can occur several months or years after the initial operation.

Undesirable nasal changes

The nose is a complex structure that is of profound importance in assessing the face. Adverse change in its appearance is probably the single most important reason for patient dissatisfaction following maxillary orthognathic surgery, where patient satisfaction is otherwise generally very high. All midface surgery will affect the nose. Some of these changes may be beneficial and some adverse.

An understanding of the anatomy of the nose, the consequences of maxillary movement on the nasolabial angle and nasal width is vital in treatment planning and informed consent with the patient. The use of submental intubation which allows an unimpeded view of the face has enabled corrective techniques to minimize any adverse changes.

The nose behaves like a tripod. The columella supported by the alar cartilages forms the central strut together with the septum and the lateral alar cartilages the side struts.

Nasal asymmetry may occur as a result of inadequate resection of the inferior part of the nasal septum. Superior repositioning of the maxilla, if inadequate cartilage has been resected, will result in buckling of the septum and deviation of the nasal tip (Figure 22-25). If this occurs it must be addressed as soon as possible.

Other potentially undesirable nasal changes are widening of the nasal alar base and nasal tip rotation in a cephalic direction.

Ideally the nasal width should be the same as the intercanthal width. Any detachment of the nasal soft tissues from the underlying bone will result in widening of the nose.

In some patients with a 'tall adenoidal type face', widening of the nasal base can be advantageous. In others with an already wide nose further widening should be reduced and the patient should be informed preoperatively that they may need further surgery in terms of alar wedge resection to reduce the potential widening at the nasal alar base. Impaction and advancement of the maxilla will also result in widening of the nasal base.

The cinch suture and widening of the piriform aperture are both useful techniques for reducing nasal widening. Modifying the technique to pass the suture below the septum reduces the cephalic rotation of the nose. Burring the lateral wall of the piriform aperture will reduce the forward movement of the alar cartilage which contributes to the cephalic rotation of the nasal tip.

Dental problems

Tooth vitality and viability should be considered in orthognathic procedures. Innervation of the maxillary teeth and gingivae is provided by the infraorbital nerves and the superior alveolar nerves running on the inner side of the lateral and posterior walls of the maxilla. As a result of the osteotomy cut the maxillary teeth lose their nerve supply. Generally the nerve supply is re-established after 18 months to 2 years.[39] The teeth maintain their viability from the collateral blood supply. Patients should be warned that their teeth and gingivae may be 'numb' for up to 2 years.[40] Osteotomy cuts should be a minimum of 4 mm above the root apices to avoid complications.

Periodontal problems, gingival recession, and tooth devitalization can occur if cuts are too close to the teeth and if the vascular blood supply is compromised. They are however rare in uncomplicated Le Fort I osteotomies.

Case examples

Case 1 (Figure 22.36)

19-year-old female patient presented with a Class III skeletal and occlusal relationship. The features of maxillary retrognathia are: increased scleral exposure above the lower eyelid, a ptotic nasal tip, reduced maxillary incisor exposure at rest and poor upper lip support.

A submental airway approach was used to enable optimal assessment of the nose, nasolabial angle, lip support and volume and incisor show.

A high level quadrilateral osteotomy was performed. The maxilla was advanced 8 mm in an anterior–inferior direction, thereby improving incisor exposure. The anterior movement of the maxilla advanced the lateral aspects of the nasal wall and anterior nasal spine. No tissue was removed from the anterior nasal spine. A cinch suture was used to reduce the nasal alar base width and the volume of the lip was increased by the above suturing technique and a small VY-plasty.

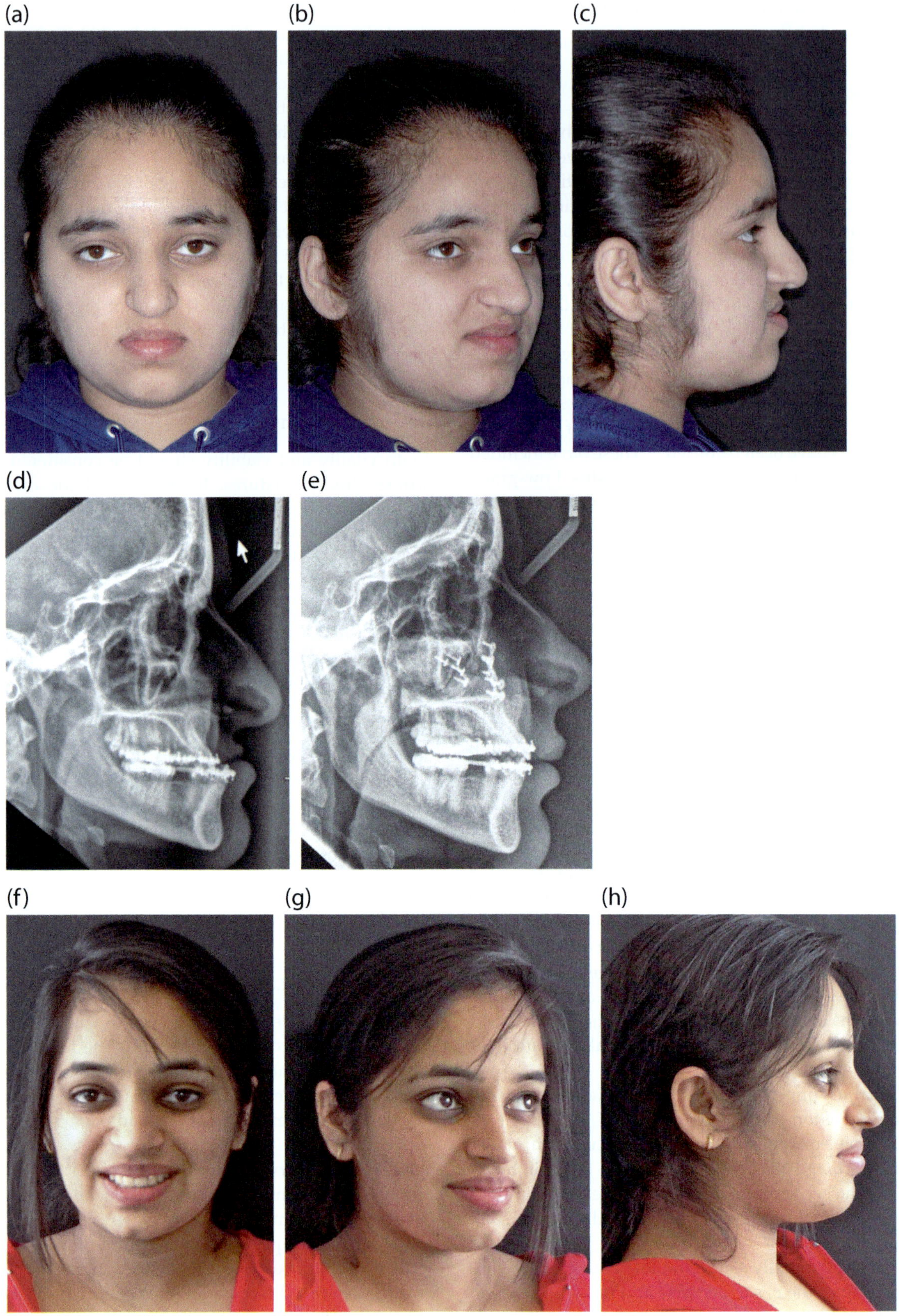

Fig. 22-36 Pre- (a–d) and postoperative (e–h) images and lateral cephalometric radiographs for a Class III patient with both sagittal maxillary retrognathia and vertical deficiency, treated with a quadrilateral high level advancement Le Fort I osteotomy.

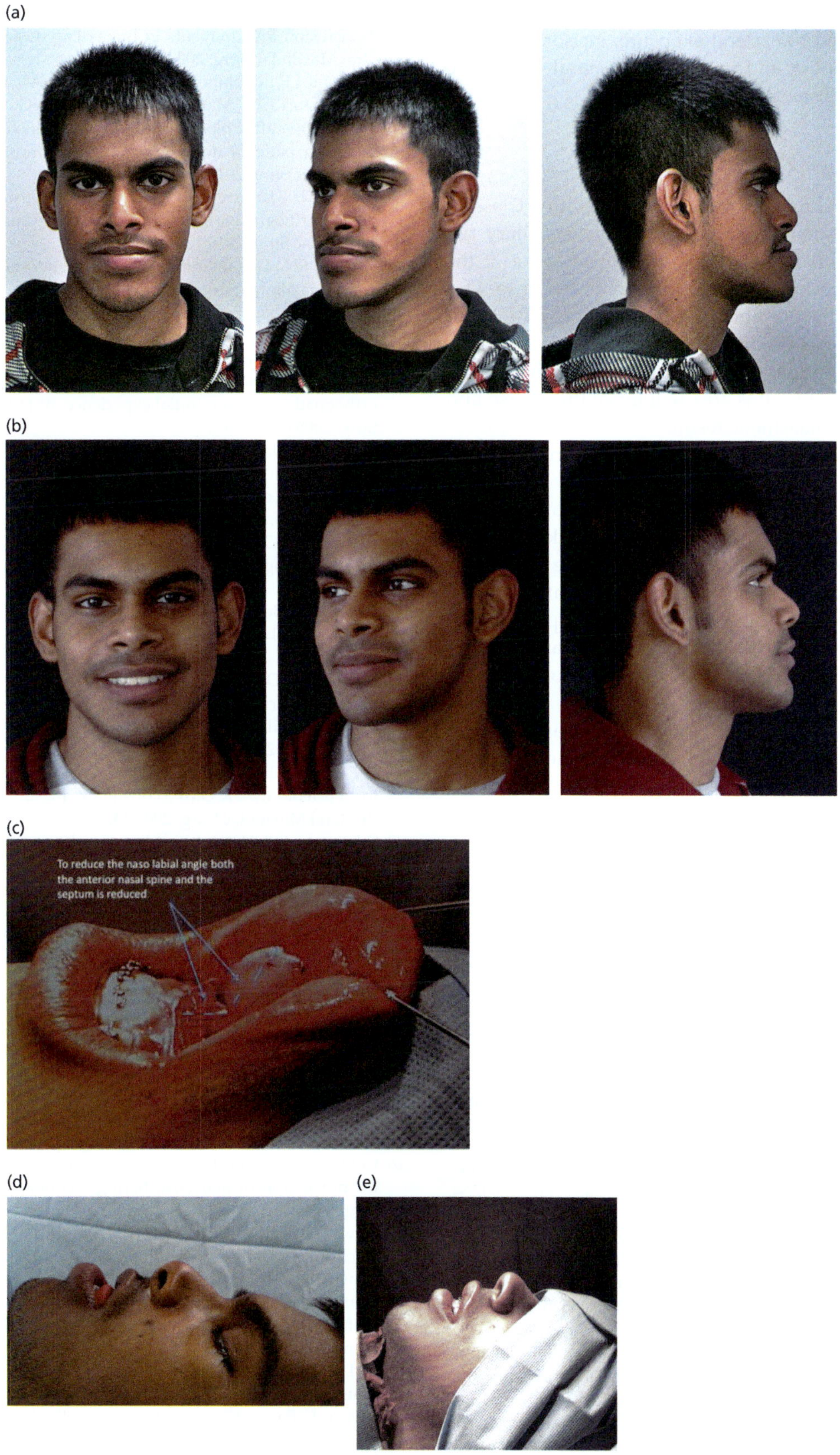

Fig. 22-37 (a) Preoperative images showing hypoplastic maxilla and prognathic mandible. Note the preoperative obtuse nasolabial angle and the 'hanging columella'. (b) Postoperative images following a bimaxillary osteotomy. The nasal septum was reduced to prevent the nasolabial angle becoming more obtuse. (c) Image showing the prominent anterior nasal spine and caudal part of the septum. This is reduced as shown by the dotted line to prevent unwanted changes to the nose following the maxillary advancement. (d) Image showing the nasolabial angle after Le Fort I advancement before reduction of the anterior nasal spine and caudal part of the columella. (e) Image demonstrates the reduced nasolabial angle, and correction of the 'hanging columella' following the septal reduction and removal of the anterior nasal spine.

The Le Fort I quadrangular advancement osteotomy has improved the scleral exposure, incisor exposure, and lip support, and improved the nasal ptosis. No mandibular osteotomy was performed.

Case 2 (Figure 22.37)

A 25-year-old male patient presented with a Class III skeletal and dental relationship due to maxillary retrognathia and mandibular prognathism. One of the most difficult areas to manage here is the nose. Preoperatively the prominent caudal septum and anterior nasal spine has produced an obtuse nasolabial angle and a hanging columella. Advancement of the maxilla without adjusting this area will make this worse and produce an unaesthetic result.

A bimaxillary osteotomy was performed using a submental airway. A quadrangular Le Fort I osteotomy was advanced 7 mm. A bilateral sagittal split osteotomy was used to set back the prognathic mandible. The caudal part of the nasal septum was exposed and the septum and anterior nasal spine reduced (as shown). The piriform aperture was increased in depth and width to reduce any adverse tip rotation and a cinch suture used to help control the nasal widening.

Postoperatively incisor show at rest has increased and facial proportions are improved, without adverse effects on the nasolabial angle.

References

1 Naini FB. Facial proportions. In: Naini FB. Facial Aesthetics: Concepts and Clinical Diagnosis. Oxford: Wiley-Blackwell, 2011.

2 Naini FB, Donaldson AN, McDonald F, Cobourne MT. Assessing the influence of lower facial profile convexity on perceived attractiveness in the orthognathic patient, clinician, and layperson. Oral Surg Oral Med Oral Pathol Oral Radiol. 2012;114:303–11.

3 Naini FB, Cobourne MT, McDonald F, Donaldson AN. The influence of craniofacial to standing height proportion on perceived attractiveness. Int J Oral Maxillofac Surg. 2008;37:877–85.

4 Obwegeser JA. Maxillary and midface deformity: characteristics and treatment strategies. Clin Plast Surg. 2007;34: 519–33.

5 Hsieh YJ, Liao YF, Chen NH, Chen YR. Changes in the calibre of the upper airway and the surrounding structures after maxillomandibular advancement for obstructive sleep apnoea. Br J Oral Maxillofac Surg. 2014;52:445–51.

6 Bell WH: Biological basis for maxillary osteotomies. Am J Phys Anthropol. 1973;38:279–89.

7 Bell WH, et al. Bone healing and revascularization after total maxillary osteotomy. J Oral Surg. 1975;33:253–60.

8 Choi J, Park H. The anatomy of the maxillary artery in the pterygopalatine fossa. American Association of Oral and Maxillofacial Surgeons 2003:72–78.

9 Turvey TA, Fonseca RJ. The anatomy of the internal maxillary artery in the pterygopalatine fossa: Its relationship to maxillary surgery. J Oral Surg. 1980;38:92–5.

10 Moenning JE, Bussard DA, Lapp TH, Garrison BT. Average blood loss and the risk of requiring perioperative blood transfusion in 506 orthognathic surgical procedures. J Oral Maxillofac Surg. 1995;53:880–3.

11 Dhariwal DK, Gibbons AJ, Kittur MA, Sugar AW. Blood Transfusion Requirements in Bimaxillary Osteotomies. Br J Oral Maxillofac Surg. 2004; 42:231–5.

12 Faverani LP, Ramalho-Ferreira G, Fabris AL, Polo TO, Poli GH, Pastori CM, Marzola C, Assunção WG, Garcia-Júnior IR. Intraoperative blood loss and blood transfusion requirements in patients undergoing orthognathic surgery. Oral Maxillofac Surg. 2013 Apr 26.

13 Bouchard C, Landry PÉ. Precision of maxillary repositioning during orthognathic surgery: a prospective study. Int J Oral Maxillofac Surg. 2013;42:592–6.

14 Altemir FH. The submental route for endotracheal intubation. J Maxillofac Surg. 1986;14:6–65.

15 Nyárády Z, Sári F, Olasz L, Nyárády J. Submental endotracheal intubation in concurrent orthognathic surgery: a technical note. J Craniomaxillofac Surg. 2006;34(6):362–5.

16 Chandu A, Witherow H, Stewart A. Submental intubation in orthognathic surgery: initial experience. Br J Oral Maxillofac Surg. 2008;46:561–3.

17 Kramer FJ, Baethge C, Swennen G, Teltzrow T, Schulze A, Berten J, Brachvogel P. Intra- and perioperative complications of the Le Fort I osteotomy: a prospective evaluation of 1000 patients. J Craniofacial Surg. 2004;15:971–9.

18 Aldridge T, Gulati A, Baker N. Theories of acquired blindness following Le Fort 1 osteotomy. Br J Oral Maxillofac Surg. 2013;51:e86.

19 Bays RA, Bouloux GF. Complications of orthognathic surgery. Oral Maxillofac Surg Clin North Am. 2003;15;229–42.

20 Richardson D. Avoiding surgical complications in orthognathic surgery. In: Ward-Booth P, Schendel S, Hausamen J (Eds). Maxillofacial Surgery. (2nd Ed.) London: Churchill Livingstone, 2006, pp.1259–74.

21 O'Regan B, Bharadwai G. Pterygomaxillary separation in Le fort I osteotomy UK OMFS consultant questionnaire survey. Br J Oral Maxillofac Surg. 2006;44:20–23.

22 Schendel SA Carlotti AE. Nasal considerations in orthognathic surgery. Am J Orthod Dentofacial Orthop. 1991;100:197–208.

23 Esenlik E, Kaya B, Gülsen A, Çukurluoğlu O, Özmen S, Yavuzer R. Evaluation of the nose profile after maxillary advancement with impaction surgeries. J Craniofac Surg. 2011;22:2072–9.

24 Mommaerts MY, Abeloos JV, De Clercq CA, Neyt LF. The effect of the subspinal Le Fort I-type osteotomy on interalar rim width. Int J Adult Orthodon Orthognath Surg. 1997;12:95–100.

25 Betts NJ, Vig KW, Vig P, Spalding P, Fonseca RJ. Changes in the nasal and labial soft tissues after surgical repositioning of the maxilla. Int J Adult Orthod Orthognath Surg. 1993:8:7–23.

26 Collins PC, Epker BN. The alar base cinch: a technique for prevention of alar base flaring secondary to maxillary surgery. Oral Surg Oral Med Oral Pathol. 1982;53:549–53.

27 Stewart A, Edler RJ. Efficacy and stability of the alar base cinch suture. Br J Oral Maxillofac Surg. 2011;49:623–6.

28 Howley C, Ali N, Lee R, Cox S. Use of the alar base cinch suture in Le Fort I osteotomy: Is it effective? Br J Oral Maxillofac Surg. 2011;49:127–30.

29 Farmah S, Ali Z, Rao J, Clark S. Survey of mortality rates and consent practices for orthognathic surgery in UK OMFS units. Br J Oral Maxillofac Surg. 2013;51:e127.

30 Jenkins K, Baker AB. Consent and anaesthetic risk. Anaesthesia. 2003;58:962–84.

31 Valentine DJ, Kaban LB. Unusual nasoendotracheal tube damage during Le Fort I osteotomy Case report. Int J Oral Maxillofacial Surg. 1992;21;333–4.

32 Posnick JC, Al-Qattan MM, Pron G. Facial sensibility in adolescents with and without clefts 1 year after undergoing Le Fort I osteotomy. Plast Reconstr Surg. 1994;94:431–5.

33 Lanigan D, Hey J, West R. Major vascular complications of orthognathic surgery: false aneurysm and arteriovenous

fistulas following orthognathic surgery. J Oral Maxillofacial Surg. 1991;49;571–7.
34 Bouloux G, Bays R. Neurosensory return after ligation of the descending palatine neurovascular bundle during Le Fort 1 osteotomy. J Oral Maxillofacial Surg. 2000;58:841–5.
35 Girotto JA, Davidson J Wheatley M, Redett R, Muehlberger T, Robertson B, Zinreich J, Iliff N, Miller N, Manson PN. Blindness as a complication of Le Fort osteotomies: role of atypical fracture pattern and distortion of the optic canal. Plast Reconstr Surg. 1998;102:1409–21.
36 Carr R, Gilbert P. Isolated partial third nerve palsy following Le Fort I osteotomy in a patient with a cleft lip and palate. Br J Oral Maxillofac Surg. 1986:24;206–11.
37 Reiner S, Willoughby JH. Transient abducens nerve palsy following a Le Fort I maxillary osteotomy: report of a case. J Oral Maxillofac Surg. 1990;28:306–8.
38 Eley KA, Witherow H, Hayward R, Evans R, Young K, Clark A, Dunaway D. The evaluation of bony union after frontofacial distraction. J Craniofac Surg. 2009;20:275–8.
39 Gulabivala K, Naini FB. The orthodontic-endodontic interface. In: Gulabivala K, Ng YL (Eds.). Endodontics (4th Ed.). Mosby (Elsevier), 2014.
40 El Deeb M, Wolford L, Bevis R. Complications of orthognathic surgery. Clinics in Plastic Surgery Vol 16 No 4 October 1989. Clin Plast Surg. 1989;16:825–40.

Chapter 23

Total Maxillary Set-Back Osteotomy

Joel Ferri and Romain Nicot

Introduction

True maxillary prognathism is not classically recognized as a specific entity. So in many centres, Class II patients are treated by sagittal splitting and advancement of the mandible whatever the position of the maxilla. This treatment is inappropriate in cases of true maxillary protrusion. In some patients, advancing the mandible to an already prominent maxillary position may lead to an unattractive facial profile due to the very anterior position of the lower facial skeletal structure. In our opinion, true maxillary protrusion is an indication for maxillary set-back (push-back) osteotomy.

Human facial anatomy has undergone much change with evolution, from the muzzle of animals to our own faces. Many factors have played a role in establishing the current human face. Today it is accepted that the face has a specific position under the cranial base. Many elements are involved during the embryological life and growth period to set up the maxillary position.[1]

When considering embryological development of the craniofacial structures we must keep in mind that the chondrocranium plays an important role in the development of craniofacial structure and morphology. This cartilaginous entity has an important genetic origin and little environmental dependence. The chondrocranium is situated at the origin of the anterior cranial base of the skull and the deep part of the nose, including the bone and cartilage of the septum.[2]

The shape of this structure, even in non-syndromic cases, has a great deal of variability.[3–6]

In terms of the craniofacial structures, the position of the maxilla under the skull base is relatively well-defined.[7] The maxillary position in the maxillofacial balance depends on the development of the cranial base, and so has an important genetic pattern.

If the anterior cranial base has excessive sagittal development, there is a risk of developing maxillary protrusion and thereby an associated Class II malocclusion, due to the fact that the face is positioned under the skull. This link between the anterior cranial base and the maxilla is essential to understand.

The sagittal position of the maxilla may be assessed using a variety of cephalometric analyses.

In the Delaire cephalometric analysis, it is clearly stated that the vertical 'craniofacial balance line' (CF1 line) normally runs from the FM point (where the frontal process of the maxilla articulates with the lacrimal bone) through the Cnp (nasopalatine foramen) to the menton. Maxillary prognathism is present when the patient's Cnp point is positioned anterior to the CF1 line (Figure 23-1).

It is important to differentiate such maxillary prognathism from proclination of the dentoalveolar processes, or from maxillary dentoalveolar protrusion, which are separate entities. Often there is confusion

Orthognathic Surgery: Principles, Planning and Practice. Edited by Farhad B. Naini and Daljit S. Gill.

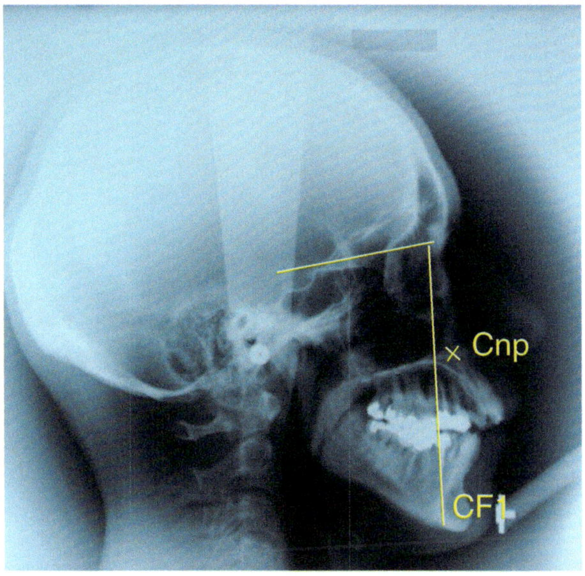

Fig. 23-1 True maxillary prognathism is clearly established in Delaire's analysis by a Cnp point in forward position of the CF1 line.

between these entities leading to inappropriate treatment (see below).

In adults, the maxillary protrusion is a specific entity which cannot be treated except by osteotomy, in order to separate the maxilla from the skull base.

Treatment planning

The presurgical orthodontic phase is not specific for this osteotomy. The orthodontist needs to align and decompensate the teeth. The preoperative study models must be checked to be sure that there is a stable occlusion, which is the guarantee of safe and reliable surgery.

Surgical technique and considerations

The osteotomy itself doesn't have any particular features. It was described by Bell in 1975, and there has been no change in the method of performing it.[8] However, space must be found in order to set-back the maxilla. This space is generally achieved by sectioning of the pterygoid process (Figure 23-2). The cut pterygoid is not removed; it remains attached to the pterygoid muscles. It is important to respect the anatomical elements in this region, particularly the posterior palatal bundle, which is protected with retractors.

Some difficulties can arise:

1. Technically speaking the section is undertaken in the deep part of the face, and it is not always easy to carry out this procedure in such a reduced space.
2. Venous bleeding can be observed due to damage to the pterygoid plexus. Such bleeding may lead to problems, but generally it stops spontaneously.

We recommend undertaking the pterygoid section with surgical pliers, in order to avoid radiating fractures that could appear when other methods are used. Once the pterygoids are sectioned, the maxillary push-back is relatively straightforward. When the maxilla has been positioned correctly, it is fixed with miniplates. In some cases, insufficient sectioning of the medial part of the pterygoid process can be a source of interference, and can limit the required maxillary movement. When such difficulty occurs it can be resolved simply by removing more bone in the posterior region.

In a pure backward movement, the orientation of the occlusal plane does not change. In some cases the push-back can be associated with other movements (anterior impaction, posterior downward displacement, etc.), which will alter the occlusal plane inclination.

The pterygoid section is a straightforward procedure for experienced orthognathic surgeons. When the section is done, the maxillary push-back is easy to carry out (Figure 23-3).

General remarks

1. Posterior repositioning of the entire maxilla at the Le Fort I level is not a classical surgical movement. Among the Class II malocclusions, true maxillary prognathism is not a very common deformity. In many centres, these deformities are treated by mandibular advancement. This type of

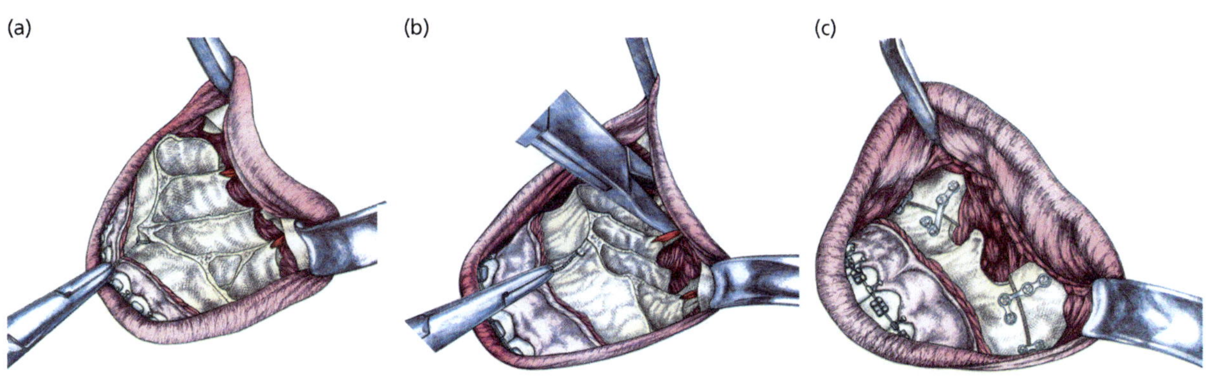

Fig. 23-2 Section of the pterygoid process: There is nothing specific or different in undertaking the Le Fort I osteotomy (a). The section of the pterygoid process is undertaken with surgical pliers (b). The maxilla is then fixed in its new position (c).

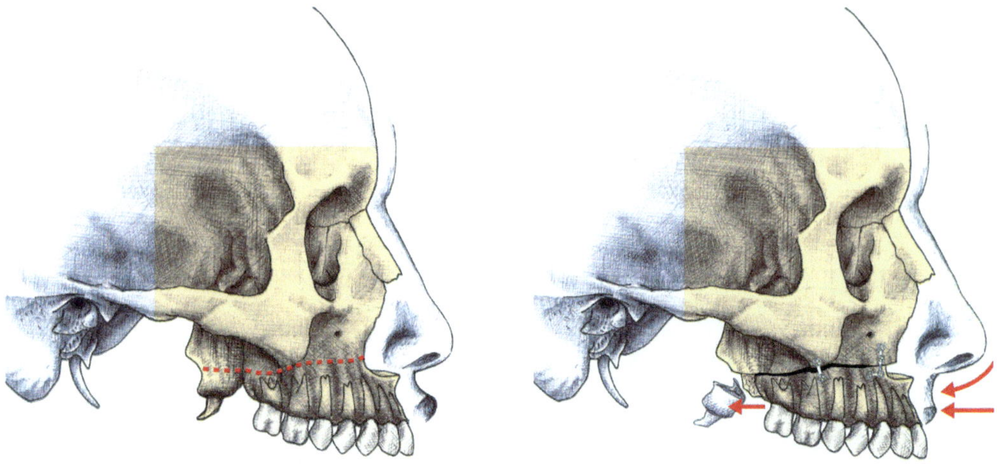

Fig. 23-3 The posterior set-back of the maxilla is easy when the pterygoid processes are sectioned.

treatment, undertaken irrespective of the type of Class II skeletal relationship, may provide acceptable results in some cases, but it may also lead to an unattractive facial result. When the maxilla is already forward in position, an advancement of the mandible induces a very protrusive facial profile (simian-like face). It may also result in an enlargement of the posterior part of the face (bigonial distance).

2. The advancement of the face could also induce a source of instability of the occlusion. Because the original problem is not the mandible, to correct a maxillary protrusion by mandibular advancement may be a source of instability and relapse. Indeed the mandible has functional units which are required for normal function. In a well-balanced situation, these different units are proportionally related to one another.[9] Six units have been identified and two are particularly involved in orthognathic surgery: the corpus and the ramus-condyle. An orthognathic procedure must restore these proportions and not damage them when normal. The advancement of the mandible, if incorrectly performed, disrupts the balance between the different units. The corpus is longer than it was originally and, above all, longer than it should have been if we consider just the mandible itself. This imbalance is a source of occlusal instability. Backward positioning of the maxilla is the way to conserve the proportion of the different units of the mandible, and so reduce the risk of relapse. When the malocclusion is due to a combination of maxillary protrusion and mandibular retrusion, a bimaxillary osteotomy is required. It is also important to point out that in these situations the reduction of the maxillary projection reduces the required advancement of the mandible, and so minimizes the risk of condylar overloading.
3. The backward displacement of the maxilla also has some limitations, particularly from an aesthetic point of view. Indeed the posterior displacement of the maxilla changes the upper lip. In some cases this movement can modify the nasolabial angle by retrusion of the upper lip, which appears flatter and thinner. Eventually the result can be unaesthetic and may prematurely 'age' the face, with increase in the nasolabial folds, and retrusion of the upper lip.[10] This may also be seen in incorrect orthodontic treatment, in which maxillary premolars have been extracted and incisor retraction has been undertaken.
4. One must differentiate the different protrusive processes of the maxilla involved in Class II malocclusion:
   - Dentoalveolar protrusion: In cases of pure dentoalveolar protrusion, the maxilla itself is in the correct sagittal position but the dentoalveolar elements are in a prominent position (Figure 23.4). In these situations teeth extractions solve the anomaly by reducing the alveolar mass. The teeth extractions reduce the alveolar bony mass and so

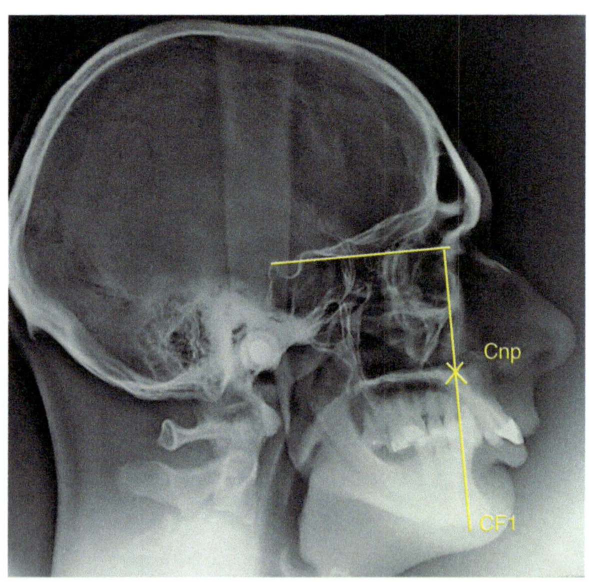

Fig. 23-4 In Delaire's analysis, the maxillary dentoalveolus is characterized by an anterior position of the alveolar process, with the Cnp point in the correct position.

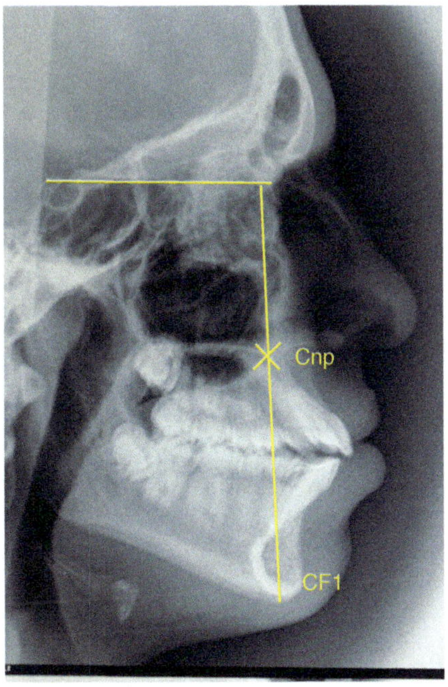

Fig. 23-5 Proclination of the incisors: The Cnp point and the alveolar processes are in normal positions, but the incisor axis is inclined labially.

reduce the alveolar protrusion and the dental discrepancy.

- Incisor proclination: In case of pure incisor proclination, it is the incisor teeth which are inclined labially, but the alveolar processes and the maxilla are in normal positions (Figure 23-5). In cases of incisor proclination it is orthodontic treatment which will normalize the position of the teeth.

Of course these anomalies can be found together in the same patient, but it is mandatory to make the distinctions between them in order to avoid incorrect application of the maxillary set-back osteotomy.

It is important to point out that the only indication for total maxillary set-back is maxillary prognathism. Indeed, if dentoalveolar protrusion is treated by maxillary set-back, it will not resolve the problem and could result in retrusion of the upper part of the upper lip. It is the same issue with proclination of the incisor teeth, which leads to a retrusion of the maxilla if treated by maxillary set-back.

Appropriate treatment should be adapted to appropriate deformities.

5. It should be emphasized that the indication for total maxillary set-back is uncommon. The decision to perform the procedure must take into account many elements (true maxillary prognathism, the soft tissue contour etc.).

Case report

A female patient presented at the age of 26 years with a classical Class II open bite malocclusion. She had maxillary protrusion, with the upper lip somewhat protrusive, and the lower part of the face was retrusive (Figures 23-6 and 23-7). She wanted to improve her dental occlusion and facial appearance. She attended the clinic after 1.5 years of orthodontic treatment.

The lateral cephalometry showed a true protrusion of the maxilla without either significant dentoalveolar protrusion or proclination of the maxillary incisors. The corpus of the mandible was short (Figure 23-8).

She was diagnosed with a Class II bite due to maxillary protrusion and mandible retrusion.

(a) (b)

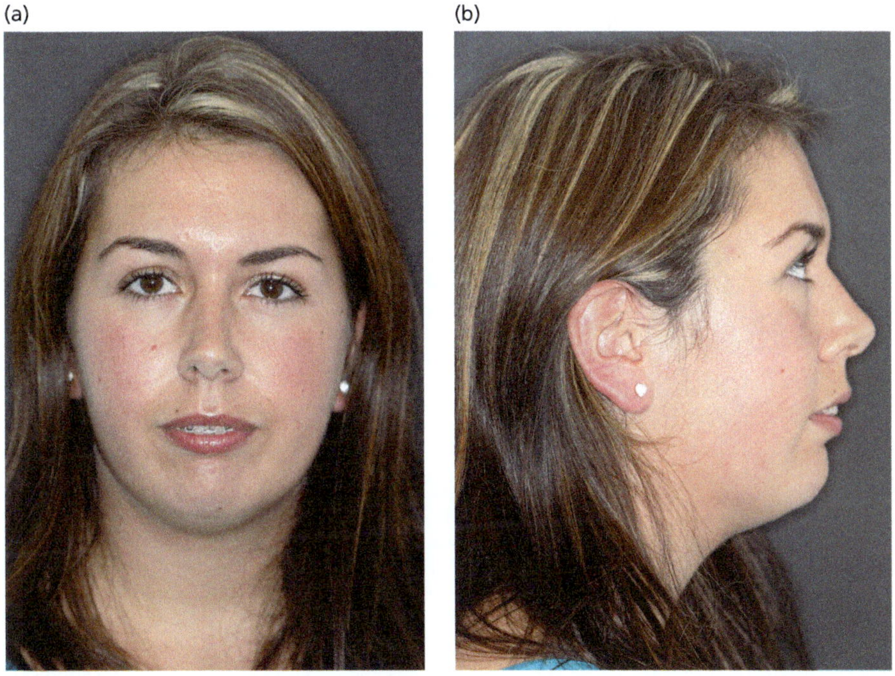

Fig. 23-6 (a face; b profile): Facial images of a Class II case due to maxillary prognathism and mandibular retrognathism. Note the retrusion on the profile of the lower part of the face.

(a) (b)

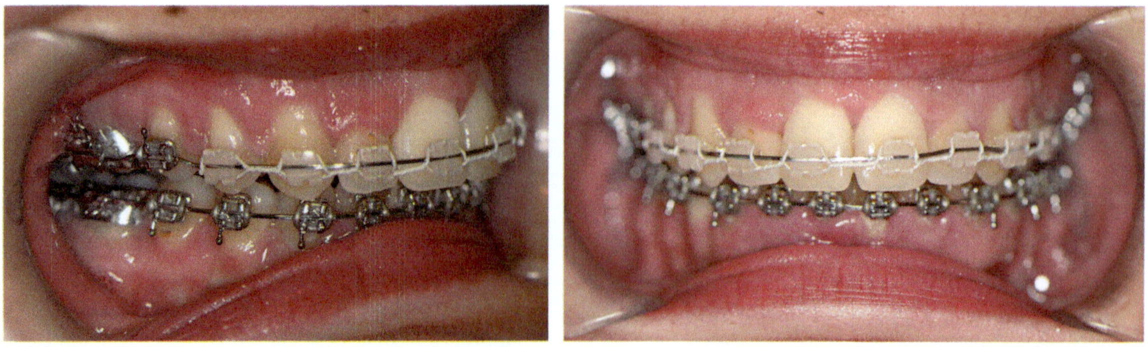

Fig. 23-7 (a right lateral view; b frontal view). The occlusion was complete Class II.

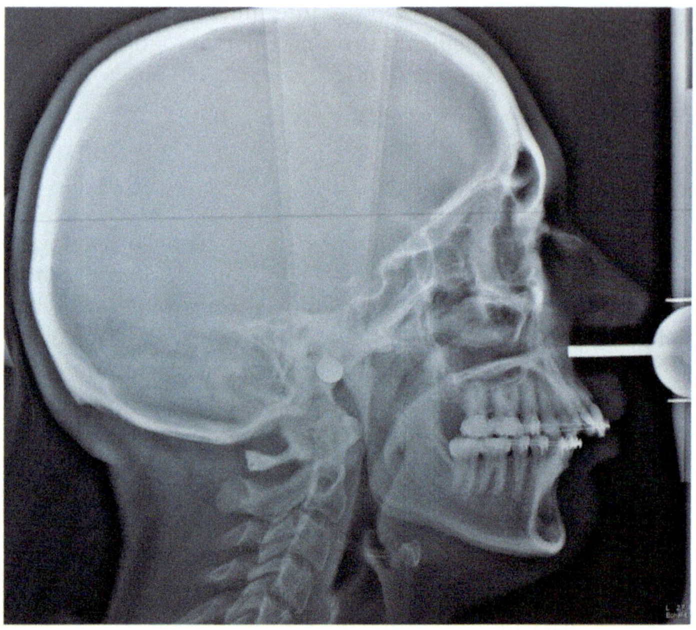

Fig. 23-8 (lateral view). The lateral cephalograph before surgery shows a complete Class II maxillomandibular relationship due to maxillary protrusion and mandible retrusion.

(a) (b)

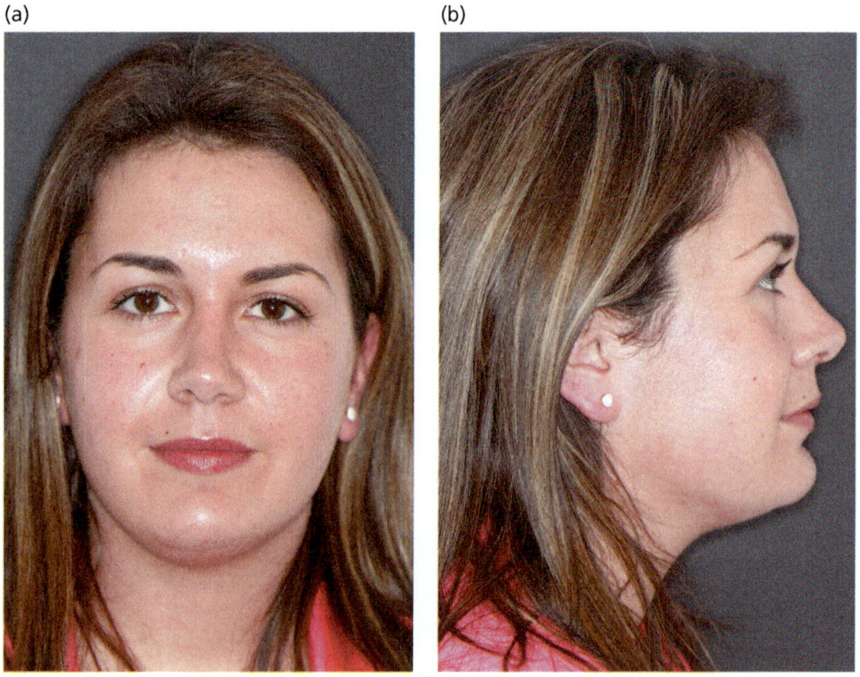

Fig. 23-9 (a face; b profile). Facial images of the patient 2.5 years after the surgery, 2 years after removal of the orthodontic appliances. The facial aesthetics were dramatically improved: the upper lip is normalized (due to the maxillary set-back), and the projection of the chin is better (due to the mandible advancement and the chin surgery).

(a) 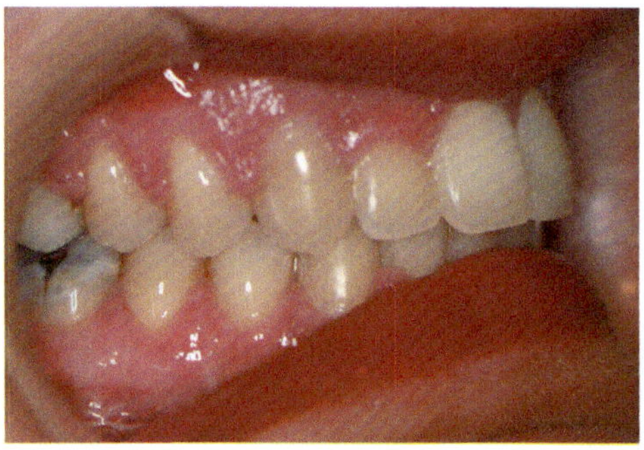 (b) 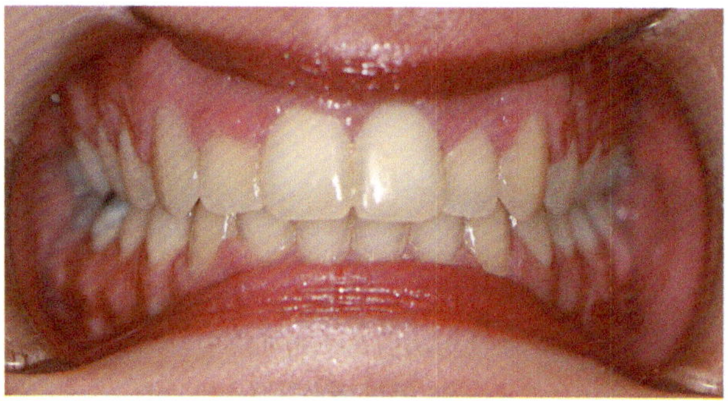

Fig. 23-10 (a right lateral view; b frontal view): The occlusion is Class I.

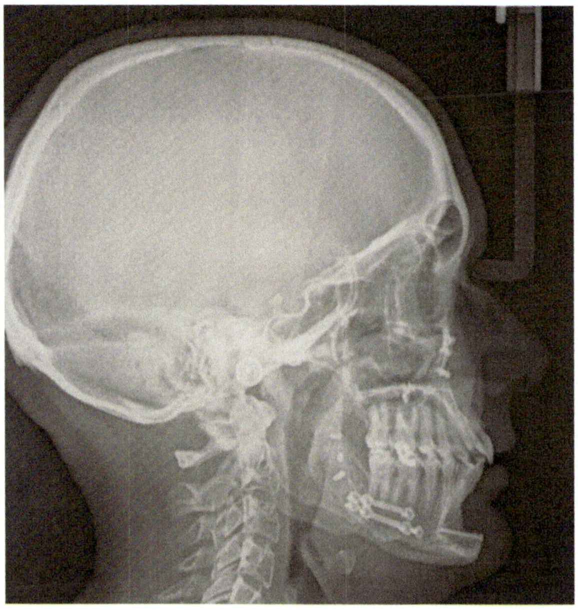

Fig. 23-11 Lateral cephalograph shows a normalization of the maxillomandibular relationship.

The treatment undertaken was Le Fort I set-back osteotomy of the maxilla, sagittal split mandibular osteotomy advancement, and advancement genioplasty.

After the surgery she had a further 6 months of orthodontic treatment. She was followed up for 2 years after the removal of the orthodontic appliances.

The clinical appearance of the patient was improved with a reduction of the upper lip protrusion in the frontal view, an improved facial profile and a stable occlusion. The lateral cephalometric radiograph shows a normalization of the maxillomandibular relationship (Figures 23-9 to 23-11).

Acknowledgements

Our thanks go to Sandra Villet for drawing the illustrations in this chapter.

References

1 Enlow DH. Handbook of facial growth. Philadelphia: Saunders, 1982.
2 Meikle MC. Craniofacial development, growth and evolution. Bressingham, Norfolk, England: Bateson Publishing, 2002.
3 Björk A. Cranial base development. A follow up X-ray study of the individual variations in growth between the age of 12 and 20 years and its relation to brain case and face development. Am J Orthodont. 1955;41:198–225.
4 Brodie A. The behavior of the cranial base and its component as revealed by serial cephalometric roentgenograms. Angle Orthodont. 1955;25:148–60.
5 Knott VB. Ontogenic change of four cranial base segments in girls. Growth. 1969;33:123–42.
6 Knott VB. Change in cranial base measures of human males and females from age 6 years to early adulthood. Growth. 1971;35:145–58.
7 Enlow DH, McNamara JA Jr. The neurocranial basis for facial form and pattern. Angle Orthod. 1973;43:256–70.
8 Bell WH. Le Fort I osteotomy for correction of maxillary deformities. J Oral Surg. 1975;33:412–26.
9 Dixon DA. Muscles, soft tissues, and craniofacial growth. In: Dixon A, Hoyte DAN, Rônning O. Fundamentals of craniofacial growth. New York: CRC Press LLC, 1997.
10 Schouman T, Baralle MM, Ferri J. Facial morphology change after total maxillary setback osteotomy. J Oral Maxillofac Surg. 2010;68:1504–11.

Chapter 24

Sagittal Split Osteotomy and Mandibular Advancement

Christoph Huppa and Gavin Mack

Introduction

The **bilateral sagittal split osteotomy (BSSO)** is the mainstay of mandibular orthognathic surgical procedures. This procedure is versatile and can be used to achieve mandibular movements that include forward and backward sliding osteotomies, as well as corrective surgery for mandibular asymmetries.

The historical development of the procedure has been described comprehensively in Chapters 1 and 2. One of the first types of mandibular ramus osteotomies was publicized by Georg Perthes in 1907,[1] performed via an extraoral approach (see Figures 2.50 and 2.51).

In 1942 Karl Schuchardt suggested undertaking the same osteotomy via an intraoral approach.[2] This procedure included an osteotomy of the condylar base which was done in a transversally oblique rather than horizontal way. In a lingual–buccal direction, the osteotomy plane was pointing downwards laterally. This was a very important modification of the previously horizontal osteotomies to increase stability and bone healing.

Rigid fixation methods like plates and screws were not available at the time. The oblique osteotomy increased bony contact surfaces between the proximal and distal segments and avoided medial displacement of the proximal segments by traction of the lateral pterygoid muscles, which had been a risk with horizontal osteotomies (see Figures 2.52 and 2.53).

To increase the surface area of the bone contact and improve consolidation during the healing period Hugo Obwegeser introduced in 1957 the sagittal split osteotomy.[3] This technique allowed a significant increase in the size of the buccal plate of the proximal osteotomy segment as it included a much larger proportion of the mandibular ramus area (see Figure 2.56). This principle was developed further by G. Dal Pont in 1959 (see Chapters 1 and 2) who suggested increasing the surface of the buccal plate even more by extending it into the proximal mandibular body area (see Figure 2.56).[4]

Nowadays many surgeons use the Hunsuck/Epker modification (Figure 24-1), which differs from the Obwegeser/Dal Pont procedure in the extent of the lingual osteotomy.[5,6] The lingual plate osteotomy is

Orthognathic Surgery: Principles, Planning and Practice. Edited by Farhad B. Naini and Daljit S. Gill.

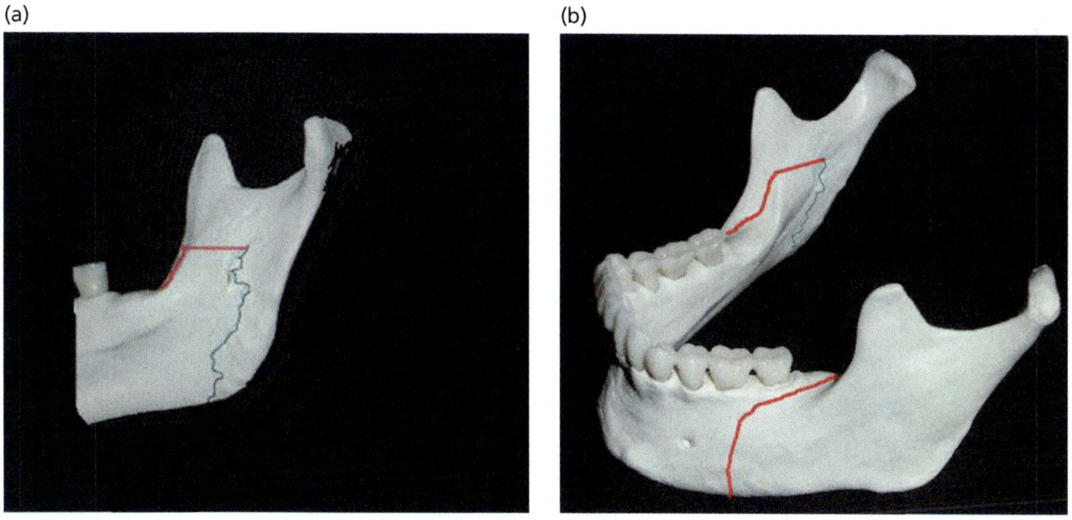

Fig. 24-1 Hunsuck/Epker modification of the Obwegeser osteotomy; osteotomy lines in red and lingual fracture line in grey.

extended to the area just posterior to the lingula rather than the whole width of the ramus. This technique has the advantage of reduced soft tissue dissection lingually but it can cause difficulties when used for a backward sliding osteotomy.

Indications

A forward sliding BSSO is indicated for surgical advancements of the mandible to correct Class II malocclusions which are based on a skeletal Class II relationship that is due to mandibular retrognathia.

The BSSO can be carried out as a single jaw procedure or as part of a bimaxillary procedure. Bimaxillary advancement surgery may be used to increase the airway in the treatment of obstructive sleep apnoea (see Chapter 44). In severe mandibular retrognathia, particularly in male patients, a simultaneous advancement genioplasty is sometimes indicated depending on the aesthetic concerns of the patient. Occasionally, a patient with mandibular retrognathia and a relatively excessive chin prominence will be suitable for a simultaneous mandibular advancement procedure and a reduction genioplasty. This is more likely to be indicated in female patients (Figure 24-2). Alternatively, a total subapical osteotomy with isolated advancement of the dentoalveolar segment could be considered (see Chapter 39).[7–9]

In the case of a mandibular asymmetry, one side may need further advancement than the other (see Chapter 34).

There is a limit to the magnitude of mandibular advancement that can be achieved safely, with predictable long-term stability, with a conventional BSSO. Surgical forward movements of up to 10 mm are relatively predictable. If there is a need for mandibular advancement surgery well beyond 10 mm other techniques like distraction osteogenesis may be considered.[10,11]

The indication for surgery can be functional. This could be related to an increased overjet resulting in reduced anterior occlusal contacts, to aid the

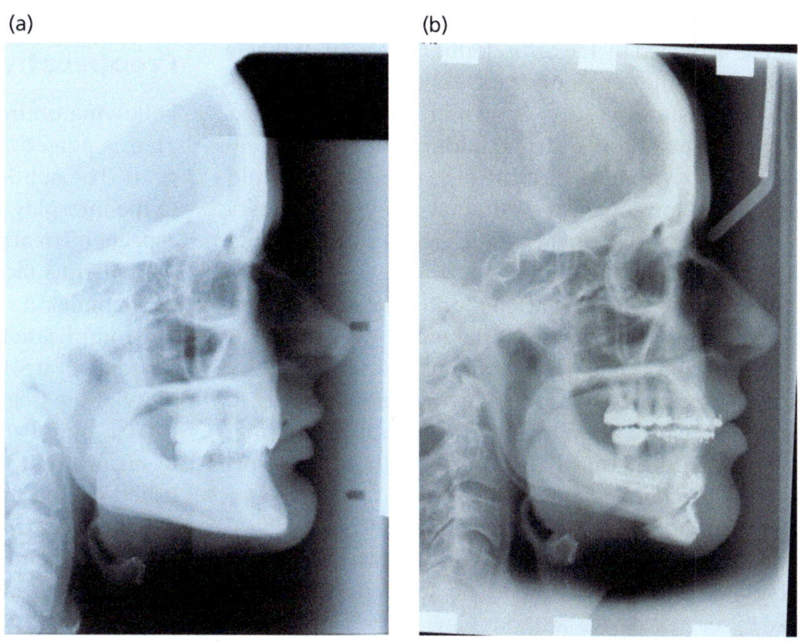

Fig. 24-2 Lateral cephalometric radiographs of a patient with (a) Class II division 2 malocclusion who benefited from (b) incisor decompensation followed by simultaneous mandibular advancement and reduction genioplasty.

correction of increased and traumatic incisor overbites or to improve lip competence. In certain cases the indication can be purely aesthetic to improve the patient's profile, but in the majority of cases it is a combination of both.

Temporomandibular joint dysfunction (TMD) is not on its own an indication for orthognathic surgery as there is no clear evidence that the disorder improves by correcting the dental-occlusal relationships, and occasionally TMD may even worsen during or following orthognathic surgery.[12–16]

Treatment planning

Prior to the commencement of the preoperative orthodontic treatment the patient should be seen jointly by the Orthodontist and the Oral and Maxillofacial Surgeon. It is recommended to follow a thorough and systematic clinical and radiological assessment protocol when the patient is seen at this first 'joint clinic' appointment.

During this appointment the decision should be taken if single or two-jaw surgery is necessary.

Factors which would preclude the patient from having single jaw surgery include the presence of a skeletal cant of the maxillary occlusal plane, a midline discrepancy between the maxillary dental and the facial midline which cannot be resolved orthodontically, vertical discrepancies with significant anterior open bites and bimaxillary retrognathia.

With regards to the clinical assessment of the mandible, it is fundamental to establish if the mandibular dental midline and the midpoint of the chin are coincident as this may influence orthodontic and surgical treatment decisions significantly. It is also important to check if the chin is coincident with the facial midline or if there is an asymmetry of the chin position.

If the chin point and mandibular dental midline are not coincident it has to be decided if their alignment can be achieved by the orthodontic treatment. If that is not the case the decision has to be taken if the postoperative occlusion is set up with a discrepancy of the maxillary and mandibular dental midlines in order to preserve chin symmetry or if the dental midlines should be aligned intraoperatively. In that case a genioplasty needs to be carried out to compensate for the resulting chin asymmetry.

If there is a concurrent chin and mandibular dental midline asymmetry and the midline is coincident with the chin point, both problems can be solved by an asymmetrical mandibular advancement leading to a mandibular rotation to align the mandibular dental midline with the maxillary, and simultaneously correcting the chin position.

An orthopantomograph (OPT) and a lateral cephalometric radiograph should be available at the first joint clinic appointment and some surgeons also like to see a posterior–anterior view of the mandible to assess the thickness of the bone. Radiological assessment should of course include dental and periodontal fitness for orthodontic and surgical treatment, but also establish if it is necessary to remove third molars prior to the mandibular surgery, as this procedure should be scheduled as early as possible in the orthognathic treatment pathway. Any bone pathology has to be excluded or investigated further before the onset of orthodontic treatment. Particular emphasis should be placed on the radiological assessment of the mandibular condyles to rule out pathology such as idiopathic condylar resorption. This would be especially important in patients who complain about a deteriorating anterior open bite and present with a Class II malocclusion. In the presence of this condition BSSO surgery may not be appropriate and other options such as occlusal correction with total temporomandibular joint replacement surgery should be considered depending on the patient's symptoms (see Chapter 35).

Prediction tracing of the lateral cephalometric radiograph can be undertaken manually, using tracing paper, or digitally, using one of the available computer systems. The prediction tracing should be carried out before the patient presents in the first joint clinic to facilitate decision-making.

In the case of severe asymmetries, which require complex surgical movements and three-dimensional planning, it can be beneficial to arrange for the patient to have a computerized tomograph (CT), be it a conventional or a cone beam scan. The scan can be processed with the relevant software and virtual 3D planning can help to define the most appropriate surgical movements. This allows more detailed surgical preparation than conventional planning with prediction tracing of the lateral cephalometric radiograph, clinical assessment and model surgery. If necessary a stereolithographic model can be produced, which can also be a very helpful adjunct to the treatment planning of complex cases.

Preoperative orthodontics

Following on from the joint consultation, a treatment plan is agreed by the patient, orthodontist and surgeon. The subtleties of the treatment plan will relate to the interplay between the orthodontic and surgical aspects of treatment and the anticipated response of the patient's facial soft tissues to the repositioning of the dental and skeletal tissues. These interactions will have implications for the dental and facial aesthetic outcome of treatment, and are also relevant to the stability of the treatment delivered.

At a simplistic level, the surgical plan is agreed to ensure that optimal facial proportions are established by the treatment, and the orthodontic plan is developed to facilitate the optimal surgical repositioning of the mandible and or maxilla, and to ensure a stable dental occlusion is achieved on completion of treatment.

Anteroposterior orthodontic preparation

The orthodontic repositioning of the maxillary and mandibular labial segments will be of primary importance in ensuring the ideal mandibular procedure can be undertaken. During orthognathic treatment the optimum anterior occlusion is achieved when the incisors are ideally inclined relative to the underlying skeletal bases. This may require premolar extractions both to relieve dental crowding and provide space in the arch for dental decompensation to be achieved.

Compensation can occur in patients with mandibular retrognathia as a result of the tongue applying pressure to the mandibular incisors, causing them to be relatively advanced and proclined in relation to the underlying mandible basal bone. Whilst the natural process of compensation can partially reduce the magnitude of the incisor overjet that would reflect the true anteroposterior discrepancy that exists between the upper and lower jaws, the compensation limits the scope for surgically advancing the mandible and addressing the retrognathia. The orthodontic process of decompensation allows the mandibular incisors to be retroclined and/or retracted into an ideal position relative to the basal bone and ensures that the surgical procedure to advance the mandible results in a Class I incisor relationship, a functional dental occlusion and an ideal improvement in the patient's facial appearance.

Conversely, in patients presenting with a skeletal Class III discrepancy, the mandibular incisors can undergo compensatory retroclination under the retractive pressure exerted by the lower lip, which may also lead to mild crowding. If this crowding in the mandibular arch is mild, it is often possible to avoid premolar extractions, as the process of orthodontically decompensating the mandibular incisors can provide sufficient space in the arch for the dentition to be ideally aligned.

Patients should be fully advised of the effects of decompensation during the preoperative stage of treatment. This is because the process of undoing the natural effects the soft tissues have had on the dentition typically results in the malocclusion and skeletal discrepancy appearing to be more severe.

Another consideration that relates to the orthodontic positioning of the teeth in the mandibular labial segment is the relationship the dentition has to the shape and relative protrusion of the patient's chin. It may be necessary to consider a genioplasty procedure either at the time of surgery, or as a secondary procedure, to optimise the support provided to the lower lip by the dental and skeletal tissues, ensuring a balanced facial profile is established.

Transverse orthodontic preparation

In relation to the preoperative orthodontic transverse preparation for a BSSO procedure, the key considerations relate to the coordination of the maxillary and mandibular arch forms, and the ideal positioning of the dental midlines.

The surgical procedure of advancing the mandible has an impact on the transverse coordination of the maxillary and mandibular arches. As the mandible is advanced it is important to ensure the forward translation of the mandible does not result in a bilateral crossbite tendency. This can be avoided by systematically coordinating the maxillary and mandibular arch forms during the preoperative orthodontic stage – usually attempting to maintain the mandibular arch form and intercanine width if appropriate. Arch form guides are available to assist the uniform shaping of stainless steel arch wires and the selected choice of arch from can be documented in the clinical records. Also, a review of the transverse dimensions of the maxillary and mandibular dental arches can be undertaken throughout treatment by assessing the buccal occlusion when the patient postures the mandible forward into a Class I occlusion, or more accurately by taking snap impressions to allow the fabrication of mid-treatment study models.

Difficulties in achieving an ideal coordination of the arch forms can be experienced in preparation for mandibular advancement surgery and this often is due to the established occlusion limiting the ideal orthodontic positioning of the buccal dentition. Typically it is the terminal molars that can be particularly challenging to accurately position as they can be locked in an undesirable position by the existing malocclusion. In these instances slight overcorrection of the transverse dimension is advised if possible, as after surgery the settling of the buccal dentition in the transverse dimension is more predictably achieved after the anteroposterior discrepancy has been addressed.

In relation to dental midlines, as previously outlined in the assessment section, the ideal positioning of the mandibular incisor teeth is with the mandibular dental midline coincident with the midpoint of the chin. This will ensure that as long as the maxillary dental midline is coincident with the mid-facial axis, as the mandible is advanced in to an ideal position, an ideal anterior occlusion is established with optimal facial symmetry.

A mandibular dental midline discrepancy can complicate the preoperative phase of orthodontic treatment, and asymmetric extractions or the use of temporary anchorage devices may be indicated to ensure the discrepancy is addressed in preparation for surgery.

Vertical orthodontic preparation

The implications of the vertical dimension for preoperative orthodontics relate to the technique of planning for a **'three-point landing'** to reduce an increased overbite and increase the lower anterior facial height, and for intruding teeth in preparation for surgery to close an anterior open bite.

The technique of preparing a patient for a three-point landing mandibular advancement procedure involves maintaining an increased curve of Spee in the mandibular arch during the preoperative orthodontic stage of treatment. This will mean the surgical plan will deliver stable contacts between the incisors and terminal molars, with the mid-buccal dentition being out of occlusal contact at the time of surgery. By avoiding the mandibular arch being levelled during the preoperative preparation the lower anterior dental height is maintained and the mandibular advancement procedure translates into a normal overbite and a maximum increase in the lower anterior facial height. The postoperative orthodontic stage of treatment is then used to extrude the mid-arch buccal dentition into occlusion, using interarch elastics, extrusion bends and possibly sectioning the archwires. As an increased curve of Spee in the mandibular arch represents a series of slipped interproximal contacts, a space requirement to level the arch postoperatively exists and this should be considered during the treatment planning process. The theoretical benefit of preparing for a three point landing is that by avoiding the complete levelling of the mandibular arch, the scope for maximally increasing the lower anterior facial height exists. In practice, it is often challenging to fully level the curve of Spee in a patient with an increased overbite and a significantly reduced lower facial height, and so planning for a three point landing can also represent a pragmatic approach to progressing a patient's treatment.

In relation to the vertical preparation of the dentition for a mandibular advancement procedure undertaken to reduce an anterior open bite, a procedure that typically also involves a differential posterior maxillary impaction,[17] the relative intrusion of the maxillary and mandibular incisors can confer a theoretical enhancement to the stability of the corrected occlusion. This is due to the intrusion of the maxillary and or mandibular incisors during the preoperative stage of treatment, either by positioning the brackets more incisally on the anterior teeth, or by wiping bite opening curves into the working stainless steel archwires, increasing the anterior open bite in preparation for the surgical repositioning of the skeletal bases. This type of vertical decompensation allows for the open bite correction to be primarily delivered through the surgical procedure, and avoids or at least limits the orthodontic extrusion of the anterior teeth, which is accepted as being a relatively unstable orthodontic tooth movement.

Surgical technique

The mucosal incision extends from the retromolar region lateral to the ascending ramus (avoiding the risk of lingual nerve damage by not incising medial to the ramus) to the buccal aspect of the second premolar, leaving a couple of millimetres of mobile unattached gingiva. In the presence of an erupted third molar, which is to be extracted, the incision has to be planned with a crevicular segment in the buccal area of that tooth. Otherwise a small mucosal bridge will be created which is likely to become necrotic.

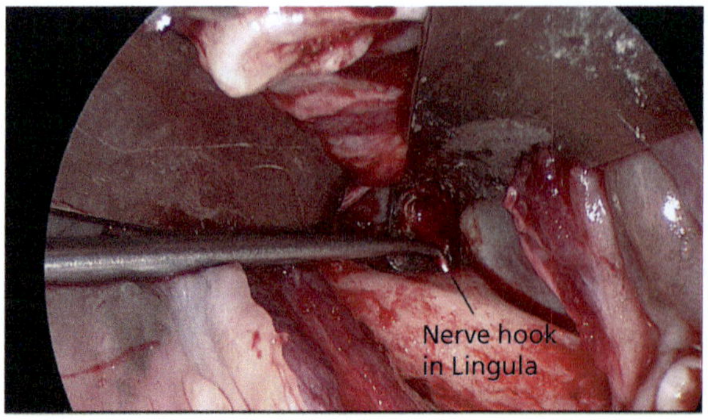

Fig. 24-3 Blunt nerve hook in situ.

The buccal mandibular bone is now exposed by subperiosteal dissection. The dissection can be limited to the molar and premolar region but has to include the mandibular margin, thus minimizing the extent of periosteal and muscular detachment from the mandibular ramus buccally, allowing excellent healing potential to be preserved. In mandibular advancement surgery it is crucial to detach all muscle attachments in the anterior body area to control relapse potential. Particular care has to be taken by dissecting the mental foramen to preserve the mental nerve function. The foramen lies in the area between the apices of the first and second premolar teeth.

The next step is the dissection of the anterior ridge of the ascending ramus cranially to the coronoid process and retraction of soft tissues with a forked ramus retractor. A clamp can be applied to the coronoid process to facilitate soft tissue retraction.

After checking the OPT for the anatomical level of the lingula the dissection of the lingual aspect of the ramus has to be carried out with upmost care and is strictly subperiosteally cranial to the lingula with the use of a sharp and slightly curved periosteal elevator.

The position of the lingula can be confirmed using a blunt nerve hook in order to identify and preserve the inferior dental (ID) nerve (Figure 24-3). To prevent any damage to the nerve a channel retractor can be introduced just cranial to the neurovascular bundle (Figure 24-4).

To increase surgical access and enhance visibility a small groove can be cut into the lingual aspect of the mandible a few millimetres cranial to the lingula. The easiest way to do this is to use a rotating burr with a

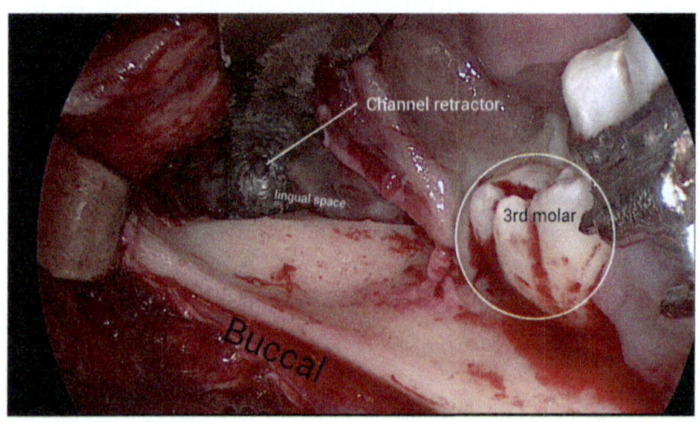

Fig. 24-4 Cranio-lingual dissection of the mandibular ramus with channel retractor inserted cranial to the lingula.

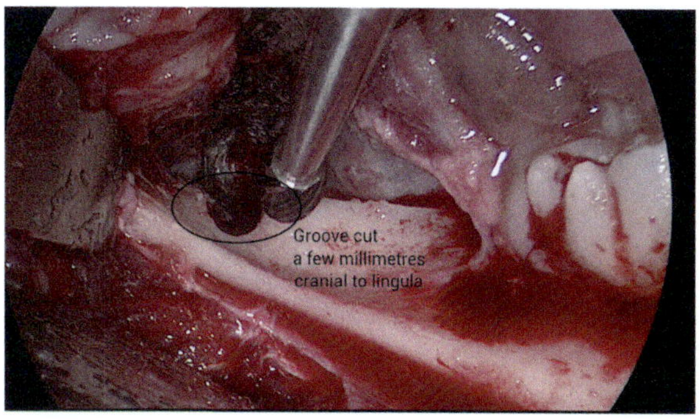

Fig. 24-5 Groove cut cranial to lingula level for better visualization of the lingual osteotomy line and inferior alveolar nerve.

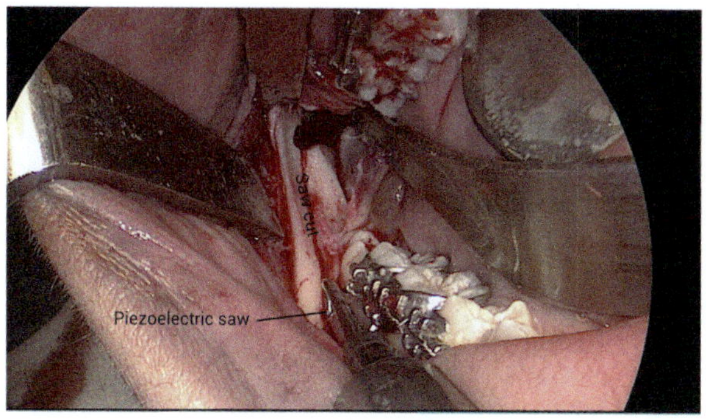

Fig. 24-7 Saw cut of the anterior surface of the ascending mandibular ramus

diameter of about 4–5 millimeters. This helps to visualize the nerve and the necessary extent of the lingual osteotomy line (Figure 24-5).

Classically, the ramus osteotomy is carried out with a fissure burr drilling multiple holes next to each other in the line of the proposed osteotomy along the lingulo-anterior aspect of the ramus (postage-stamp osteotomy) and then buccally down to the mandibular margin in the area of the first molar tooth.

An incomplete osteotomy of the mandibular margin is often an obstacle to a smooth splitting procedure. Care has to be taken to limit the osteotomy to the mandibular cortex in order to avoid any damage to the ID nerve.

A much quicker and very precise osteotomy can be achieved with the help of a reciprocating saw. There are a number of different saws and blade shapes available but a rigid blade with a slightly round cutting edge seems to be safer than a straight one as the tip of a straight blade can accidentally dive in deep and damage the nerve (Figure 24-6).

The most controlled but also slightly slower type of saw is the piezo-electric saw which carries out ultrasonic micro-movements and tends to be less traumatic when it comes into contact with soft tissues (Figure 24-7).

For the buccal osteotomy a rosehead burr or similar seems to be advantageous as the depth of the cut is easier to control, which is essential in that area as the ID nerve can be quite superficial (Figure 24-8). A channel retractor has to be inserted to protect the soft tissues. Accidental damage to the facial vessels could lead to severe haemorrhage which is difficult to control in that area. The osteotomy is strictly restricted to the cortical bone and it is complete when the first bleeding points of the underlying cancellous bone come into sight. Due to the fine cut of a saw, gauging its depth is much more difficult.

After the osteotomy is completed the split is carried out with two Lexer osteotomes, which are introduced into the osteotomy slit and slowly rotated in parallel until the split is completed. Alternatively Smith spreaders can be used for this procedure (Figure 24-9).

If great care is not taken, an unfavourable split (bad split) may occur and the buccal plate can fracture. If this happens the damage has to be repaired using miniplates. If a repair is not possible the patient has to be put into rigid intermaxillary fixation (IMF) for approximately 6 weeks until the bone has healed.

In the horizontal plane the anatomical shape of the mandible is similar to the letter 'V'. This has surgical implications particularly for advancement surgery as the advancement in the areas of the posterior ends of the distal segment will lead to a rotational movement or even a lateral displacement of the condyles if the buccal plates of the proximal segments are forced into complete alignment with the distal segment after advancement. This problem can be solved by osteotomizing the retromolar part of the lingual plate as suggested by Edward Ellis III.[18]

After intraoperative IMF is established using an acrylic wafer as a positioning splint, fixation of the three segments can be carried out either with positioning screws or fixation plates. Usually three positioning

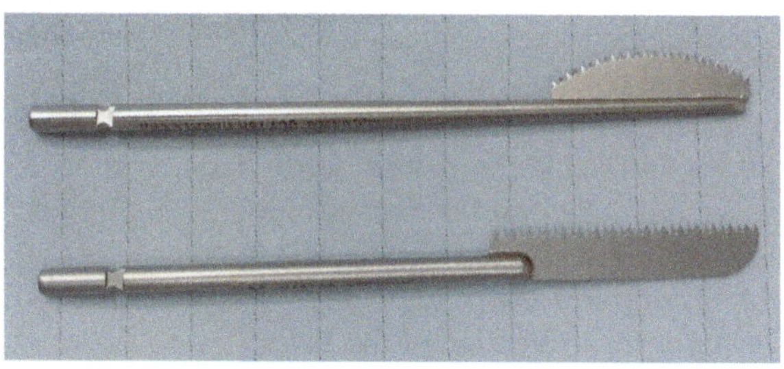

Fig. 24-6 Curved rigid blade for the osteotomy of the anterior surface of the ramus and straight rigid blade to complete the osteotomy in the lingual groove.

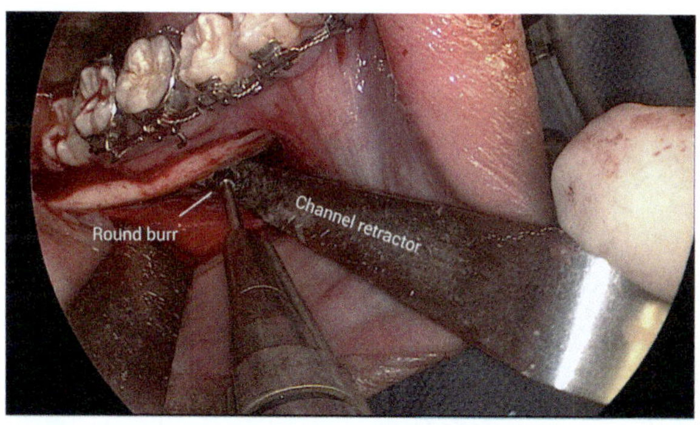

Fig. 24-8 Buccal osteotomy with round burr and inserted channel retractor to protect soft tissues and facial vessels.

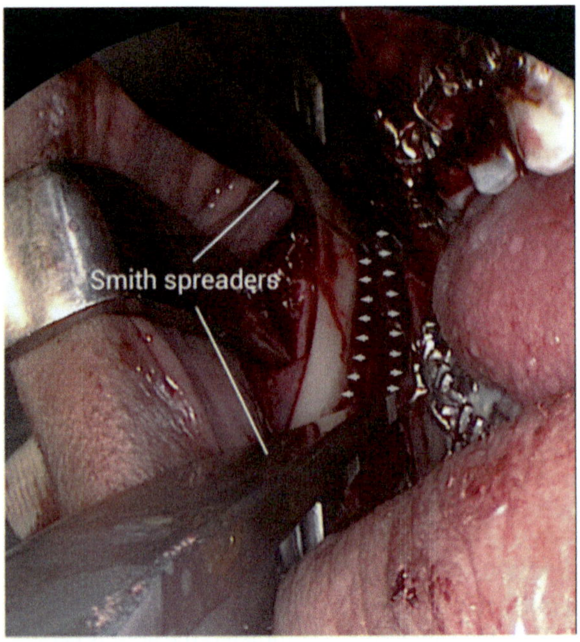

Fig. 24-9 Two Smith spreaders inserted to complete the sagittal split osteotomy.

screws or one four-hole positioning plate per side is sufficient.

Nowadays a trans-buccal approach to insert the fixation screws is avoided. Right angle drills and screw drivers are available and widely used to avoid facial scar formation, which is inevitable when a trans-buccal system is used (Figures 24-10 and 24-11). Although in most cases these scars are not very obvious they can show as dimples when the patient is smiling.

In mandibular advancement surgery it is essential to push the proximal segments backwards and upwards to position the condyles in the most retro-cranial position. Otherwise an 'early relapse' could occur, which is entirely due to slipping of the condyles back into their natural position postoperatively. This is not a skeletal relapse but a surgical error.

In mandibular set-back surgery slightly more anterior positioning of the condyle supports the mandibular set-back.

Postoperatively light elastic traction can be helpful to improve the patient's comfort in the first few days and may be beneficial for orthodontic reasons.

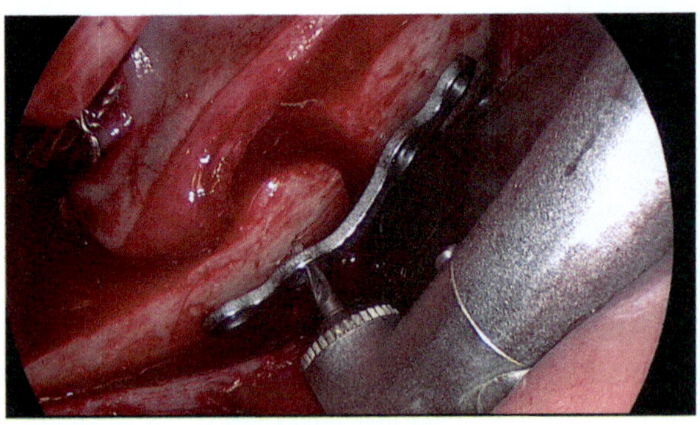

Fig. 24-10 Right angle drill.

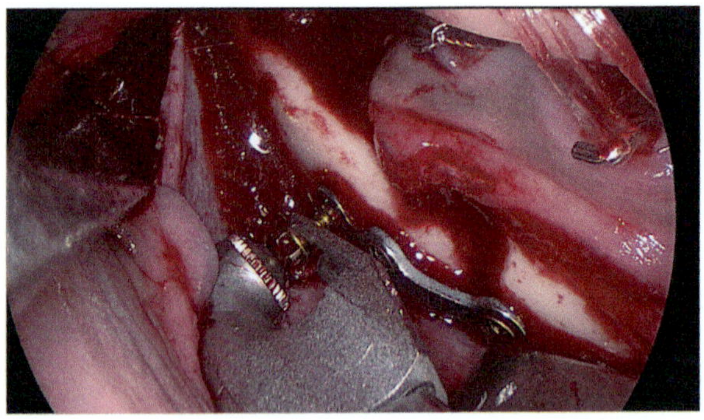

Fig. 24-11 Insertion of screw with the right angle screw driver.

Third molars and mandibular osteotomies

The question whether or not to remove mandibular third molar (wisdom) teeth in preparation for a BSSO is still controversial. Many surgeons prefer to remove mandibular third molars well in advance of the mandibular surgery as the presence of wisdom teeth could lead to an unfavourable split.[19]

Other surgeons do not see a benefit in the removal of wisdom teeth prior to surgery and argue that the split gives the best access to the tooth. Some surgeons even suggest that the risk for an unfavorable split is lower when the third molar had been left in situ.[20]

Most surgeons would, however, agree that if the decision has been taken to remove wisdom teeth this should happen at least 6 to 9 month before the split osteotomy to make sure that the regenerative bone is mature enough to avoid complications.

It seems to be practical to take a decision about the wisdom tooth removal in every individual case at the beginning of the preparatory orthodontic treatment. The size and position of these teeth may influence the decision and the surgery should be scheduled for the early stages of the orthodontic treatment to avoid unnecessary delays prior to the jaw surgery.

Osteosynthesis

There has been discussion about how rigid the fixation of the mandibular segments should be.[21–23] The spectrum of available fixation systems range from simple wire fixation and 6 weeks IMF to variably rigid plating systems to very rigid 3-point fixation with bicortical positioning screws or even lag screws, which do not allow any movement of the segments postoperatively. The use of lag screws leads inevitably to a lateral displacement of the condyles.

Correct intraoperative condylar positioning is crucial for immediate and long term stability and displacement of the condyles has to be avoided. The more rigid fixation systems, like bicortical screws, are very unforgiving and less rigid plating systems may be beneficial for the protection of the TMJs.

This problem did not arise until wire fixation was replaced in favour of plates and screws to improve patient comfort by avoiding fixed IMF for 6 weeks postoperatively. Wire fixation allowed the condyles to re-position into their habitual position during the healing period.

In the mid-1990s Joos developed an adjustable plate, which was very rigid when bent over its edge but quite soft when bent over its plane.[24] This system gave good stability controlling the vertical forces of the mandible, and allowed some lateral movement of the segments, giving the condyles some leeway for postoperative repositioning in a medio-lateral direction. The system also allowed for an intraoperative check of the occlusion before definitive fixation was applied.

Subsequently, several similar plating systems have been developed with the intention of avoiding postoperative condylar resorption and temporomandibular joint dysfunction. Currently there is a lack of evidence to support the clinical effectiveness of these systems.

Previously, screws were inserted via a trans-buccal approach leaving tiny scars on the skin of the cheeks. These scars were usually unnoticeable but in some patients caused cosmetic concern. The surgeon always tries to avoid scars on the face and therefore many surgeons nowadays use right angled drills and screw drivers to perform the surgery entirely intraorally without the need for a trans-buccal approach, as suggested by Luhr and Fritzemeier.[25]

Complications

Neurosensory deficit

The most common complication of sagittal split osteotomies is temporary or permanent neurosensory deficit in the distribution area of the inferior alveolar nerve. Reports in the literature about the frequency of this complication vary quite significantly and can reach up to 85%.[26] The literature suggests that sensory deficit is more likely to have a higher incidence in older patients, in patients undergoing large advancements or if the sagittal split osteotomy is combined with a genioplasty.[27,29,29–31]

Disturbances to the facial nerve can also occur but they are much less common and are reported to be well below one percent by most authors in the scientific literature.[32] Injuries to the facial nerve can occur by direct trauma in the retromandibular space if the classical Trauner/Obwegeser technique is applied. There can also be indirect nerve weakness by excessive postoperative swelling.

Haemorrhage

Life-threatening haemorrhage, which requires a blood transfusion, is very rare in isolated BSSO procedures. The vessels that can be traumatized and lead to severe haemorrhage are mainly the retro-mandibular vein, the facial artery and its concomitant vein. Severe haemorrhagic complications have been reported in up to 2.2% of cases.[33] Small postoperative haematomas and bruising are quite common but rarely lead to severe problems such as infections or abscesses. Perioperative systemic anticoagulation therapy can, however, aggravate this problem and therefore it is advisable not to commence any anticoagulation with heparin or similar medications for 24 hours postoperatively if medically justifiable.

Unfavourable split

An unfavourable split can occur when osteotomies are not complete and the split is forced despite increased resistance. The problems lie mostly in incomplete osteotomies of the inferior border of the mandible as this area is composed of thick cortical bone. The osteotomy should include a few millimetres of the lingual surface of the mandibular margin to facilitate an uncomplicated split. Bad splits most often occur at the inferior and anterior buccal cortex of the proximal segment, keeping the continuity of the mandible intact. In this case the spit has to be completed and the fractured buccal cortex can be fixed to the proximal segment with two miniplates and the procedure can be continued as planned. It is also possible but less frequent that the coronoid process is fractured, particularly if the mandibular ramus is very thin and the osteotomy is carried out too buccally in the ramus area. In this case the surgery can also be salvaged by completing the split in the correct way and fixing the coronoid process to the proximal segment as described above.[30]

In very rare cases the bad split can be very high and it can involve the condylar process, which is much more difficult to fix. Depending on the surgical situation a trans-oral repair with endoscopic support is sometimes possible but otherwise a trans-cutaneous approach or conservative management with wire IMF for 6 weeks can be considered.

Plate breakage

In rare cases fixation plates can break due to a mechanical overload. Plates can either be under-designed or the mechanical load can be excessive as in patients with habitual bruxism. A rare reason for mechanical overload of fixation material can be repeated forced vomiting if patients suffer from bulimia.

Airway obstruction

Airway obstruction is a life-threatening complication but fortunately it is extremely unlikely in single jaw surgery. It can occur as a result of severe haematoma or surgical oedema. It can be aggravated by postoperative IMF and should this be the case, release of the IMF can solve the problem. In the first 12 to 24 hours after surgery, partial airway obstructions can be overlooked as patients may just be agitated. In this scenario application of sedatives by the nursing team can have life-threatening consequences and it is advisable to closely monitor orthognathic patients in the immediate postoperative phase.

Relapse

Within the range of possible orthognathic surgical procedures, a forward sliding BSSO, where the anterior facial height is maintained, is considered to be relatively stable and more stable than a backward sliding BSSO.[34] Relapse can occur, but does not occur immediately postoperatively and is a slow process, which can develop over years. The first two postoperative years are the most vulnerable as the majority of the postoperative bony remodelling takes place during this time. It is, however, possible that relapse may occur even later than two years after the surgery. There are different factors which have an influence on the relapse, such as the degree of intraoperative mobilization of the perimandibular muscles, tongue thrust (which is associated with the relapse of an anterior open bite) and the quality of the postoperative occlusion.

If the mandible slips back in the first few days after the intervention this cannot be seen as a relapse but may be due to a surgical error if the condyles are not seated in the glenoid fossae. Therefore, it is crucial to send the patient for an OPT on the first day postoperatively to check if the condyles are in the correct position.

Breakage of the fixation plates can also cause an 'early' relapse.

Fibrous union of the bone

A fibrous union of the mandibular segments is extremely rare and is usually due to inadequate fixation of the segments or reduced healing capacity of the bone and surrounding soft tissue. Underlying causes can be malnutrition with depletion of vitamin C and D, or imbalances of calcium metabolism. Previous radiotherapy is also a possible cause for reduced bone healing capacity. Breakage of the fixation system which goes unnoticed can also lead to a fibrous union.

Treatment of this complication may involve the application of rigid IMF for about 6 weeks or surgical intervention with excision of the fibrous tissue and re-fixation of the segments, with or without an autogenous bone graft.

Infection

Infections after BSSO procedures are very rare as the mandibulo-myo-mucosal complex has an extremely good healing potential. Infections can be due to haematomas, which can develop into abscesses, or generally reduced healing capacity due to underlying medical conditions such as general or local immunosuppression due to conditions like AIDS, previous radio- or chemotherapy, bisphosphonate therapy, or similar conditions. Exposure of the mandibular bone after mucosal wound dehiscence can also lead to an infection and in rare cases a mandibular osteomyelitis with the formation of bony sequestra, developing particularly in the area of the osteotomized buccal plate.

Postoperative orthodontics

It is good practice for the orthodontist and surgeon to jointly review the patient shortly after the surgery has been undertaken, following which the patient is closely reviewed during the following 6 to 8 weeks as bony healing occurs.

During the first 4 weeks postoperatively, if surgery has proceeded uneventfully and as planned, and the occlusion is stable, intervention can be limited to the use of light supportive interarch elastic traction, and reinforcing dietary advice and oral hygiene instructions.

If during the first 4 weeks postoperatively an unfavourable change in the occlusion is noted the vectors and the magnitude of the interarch elastic traction can be varied as required.

Beyond the 4 week postoperative stage, the healing process is still progressing and typically the swelling has reduced considerably and patient comfort has increased to the extent that simple archwire adjustments can be made to assist in the settling of the occlusion. The typical rectangular stainless steel archwires used to ensure stability and control during the surgical procedure can be sectioned to allow settling, or changed to small diameter stainless steel archwires, or even flexible multistrand archwires. The advantages of these lighter archwires is that they allow some vertical settling of the occlusion, are amenable to the introduction of artistic finishing bends and still allow for arch form control to be maintained.

When the best possible occlusion has been established with postoperative orthodontics, it is advisable to withdraw the use of the interarch elastics for at least 1 month prior to debonding the fixed appliances. This allows the operators to carefully monitor the occlusion for any unplanned changes to the bite that can be masked by the ongoing use of elastic traction, and would ideally be addressed as required before the fixed appliances are removed.

Retention regimes are determined at the outset of treatment and communicated to the patient as part of the consent process. Typically a significant change to a pre-existing arch form is more securely maintained through the ongoing use of a retainer consisting of an acrylic baseplate, such as a modified Hawley retainer. However, if the arch forms have been largely maintained during treatment, vacuum formed retainers can be used and are likely to be more readily accepted by the older patient group that typically undergo orthognathic treatment.

Case report

Initial presentation

A 21-year-old female patient presented with a Class II division 1 incisor relationship and an underlying skeletal Class II base that was due to mandibular retrognathia. The presenting malocclusion was complicated by crowding in the maxillary and mandibular

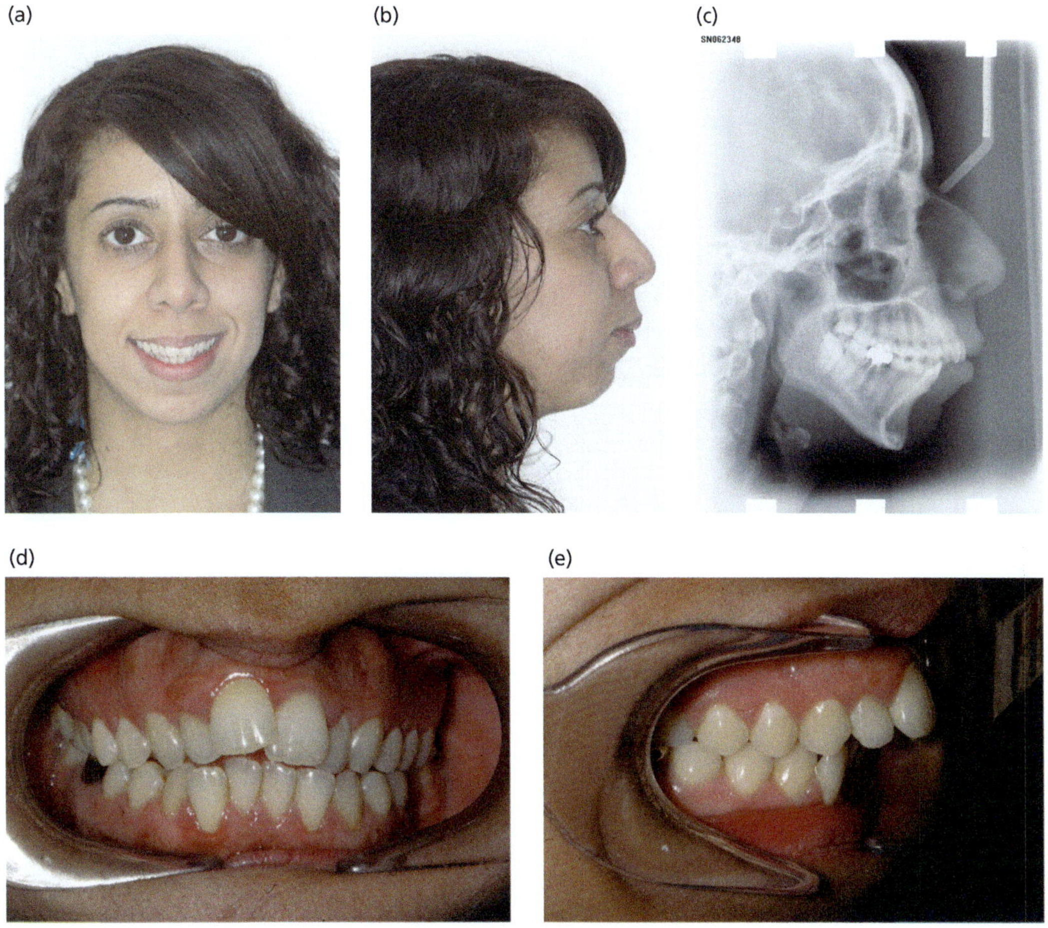

Fig. 24-12 (a–e) Initial presentation.

labial segments. There had been the previous extraction of mandibular left first molar tooth, and mandibular right first molar tooth was root filled and had a guarded long-term prognosis.

Treatment plan

Preoperative orthodontics (Treatment time = 21 months)

1. Extraction of maxillary second premolars and mandibular right first molar.
2. Upper and lower fixed appliance treatment using the MBT prescription.
   a) Align the upper and lower arches
   b) Coordinate the upper and lower arches
   c) Decompensate the proclined mandibular labial segment.

Surgical treatment plan

Bilateral sagittal split osteotomy and mandibular advancement to a Class I incisor relationship and a Class II molar relationship.

Postoperative orthodontics (Treatment time = 4 months)

Detail occlusion.

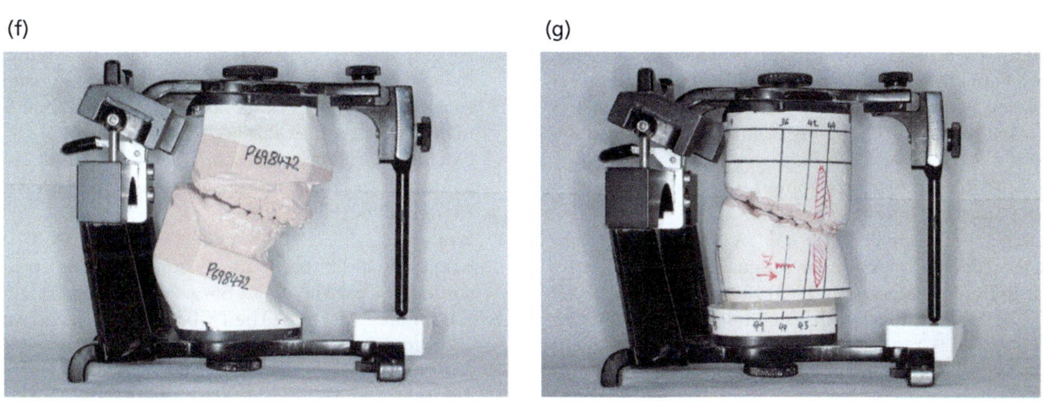

Fig. 24-12 (f,g) Model surgery.

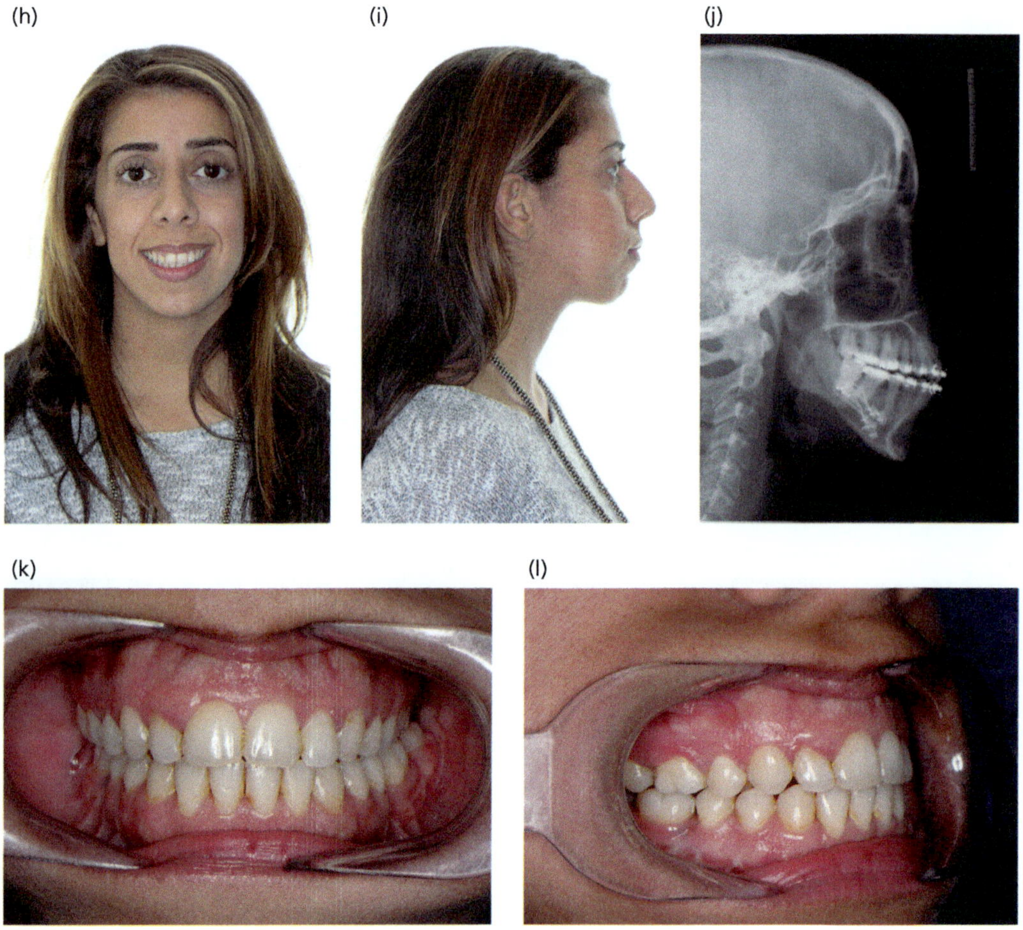

Fig. 24-12 (h–l) End treatment.

Retention

Upper Hawley and lower vacuum formed retainers gradually reducing to occasional night-time only use.

References

1 Perthes G. Verletzungen und Krankheiten der Kiefer. Deutsche Chirurgie 33a, Stuttgart, 1907; 2nd Edition by Eduard Kurt Borchers, 1932 (Injuries and diseases of the jaw).

2 Schuchardt K. Ein Beitrag zur chirurgischen Kieferorthopädie unter Berücksichtigung ihrer Bedeutung für die Behandlung angeborener und erworbener Kieferdeformitäten bei Soldaten. Dtsch. Zahn-, Mund- u. Kieferheilk. 1942;9:73–89.

3 Trauner R, Obwegeser H. The surgical correction of mandibular prognathism and retrognathia with consideration of genioplasty: Part II. Operating methods for microgenia and distoclusion (Cont'd). Oral Surg Oral Med Oral Pathol. 1957;10:899–909.

4 Dal Pont G. Retro-molar osteotomy for correction of prognathism. Minerva Chirurg. 1959;14:1138.

5 Hunsuck EE. A modified intraoral sagittal splitting technic for correction of mandibular prognathism. J Oral Surg. (American Dental Association: 1965) 1968;26:250–3.

6 Epker BN. Modification in the sagittal osteotomy of the mandible. J Oral Surg. 1977;35:157–9.

7 Boye T, Doyle P, McKeown F, Sandler J. Total subapical mandibular osteotomy to correct class 2 division 1 dentofacial deformity. J Cranio-Maxillofac Surg. 2012;40(3):238–42.

8 Köle H. Surgical operations on the alveolar ridge to correct occlusal abnormalities. Oral Surg Oral Med Oral Pathol. 1959;12:277–88.

9 Hofer O. Operation der prognathie und mikrogenie. Dtsch Zahn Mund Kieferheilkd. 1942;9:121.

10 Joss CU, Vassalli IM. Stability after bilateral sagittal split osteotomy advancement surgery with rigid internal fixation: a systematic review. J Oral Maxillofac Surg. 2009;67:301–13.

11 Joss CU, Thüer UW. Stability of the hard and soft tissue profile after mandibular advancement in sagittal split osteotomies: a longitudinal and long-term follow-up study. Eur J Orthodont. 2008;30:16–23.

12 Borstlap WA, Stoelinga PJW, Hoppenreijs TJM, van't Hof, M A. Stabilisation of sagittal split advancement osteotomies with miniplates: a prospective, multicentre study with two-year follow-up: Part III – Condylar remodelling and resorption. Internat J Oral Maxillofac Surg. 2004;33:649–55.

13 Flynn B, Brown DT, Lapp TH, Bussard DA, Roberts WE. A comparative study of temporomandibular symptoms following mandibular advancement by bilateral sagittal split osteotomies: rigid versus nonrigid fixation. Oral Surg Oral Med Oral Pathol. 1990;70(3):372–80.

14 Obwegeser H, Trauner R. Zur Operationstechnik bei der Progenie und anderen Unterkieferanomalien. Dtsch Zahn Mund Kieferheilkd. 1955;23:2.

15 Wolford LM, Reiche-Fischel O, Mehra P. Changes in temporomandibular joint dysfunction after orthognathic surgery. J Oral Maxillofac Surg. 2003; 61:655–60.

16 Karabouta I, Martis C. The TMJ dysfunction syndrome before and after sagittal split osteotomy of the rami. J Maxillofac Surg. 1985;13:185–88.

17 Bell WH, Creekmore TD, Alexander RG. Surgical correction of the long face syndrome. Am J Orthodont. 1977;71:40–67.

18 Ellis III E. A method to passively align the sagittal ramus osteotomy segments. J Oral Maxillofac Surg. 2007;65:2125–30.
19 Beukes J, Reyneke J P, Becker PJ. Variations in the anatomical dimensions of the mandibular ramus and the presence of third molars: its effect on the sagittal split ramus osteotomy. Internat J Oral Maxillofac Surg. 2013;42:303–307.
20 Precious DS. Removal of third molars with sagittal split osteotomies: the case for. J Oral Maxillofac Surg. 2004;62:1144–6.
21 Cutbirth M, Van Sickels JE, Thrash WJ. Condylar resorption after bicortical screw fixation of mandibular advancement. J Oral Maxillofac Surg. 1998;56:178–82.
22 Dolce C, Hatch JP, Van Sickels JE, Rugh JD. Rigid versus wire fixation for mandibular advancement: skeletal and dental changes after 5 years. Am J Orthodont Dentofac Orthoped. 2002;121:610–19.
23 Pereira Filho VA, Iamashita HY, Monnazzi MS, Gabrielli MFR, Vaz LG, Passeri LA. In vitro biomechanical evaluation of sagittal split osteotomy fixation with a specifically designed miniplate. Internat J Oral Maxillofac Surg. 2013;42:316–20.
24 Joos U. An adjustable bone fixation system for sagittal split ramus osteotomy: preliminary report. Br J Oral Maxillofac Surg. 1999;37:99–103.
25 Luhr HG, Kubein-Meesenburg D, Schwestka-Polly R. [The importance and technic of temporomandibular joint positioning in the sagittal splitting of the mandible]. Fortschr Kieferorthopad. 1991;52:66–72.
26 August M, Marchena J, Donady J, Kaban L. Neurosensory deficit and functional impairment after sagittal ramus osteotomy: a long-term follow-up study. J Oral Maxillofac Surg. 1998;56:1231–5.
27 Al-Bishri A, Dahlberg G, Barghash Z, Rosenquist J, Sunzel B. Incidence of neurosensory disturbance after sagittal split osteotomy alone or combined with genioplasty. Br J Oral Maxillofac Surg. 2004;42:105–11.
28 Rodella LF, Buffoli B, Labanca M, Rezzani R. A review of the mandibular and maxillary nerve supplies and their clinical relevance. Arch Oral Biol. 2012;57:323–34.
29 Van Sickels JE, Hatch JP, Dolce C, Bays R A, Rugh JD. Effects of age, amount of advancement, and genioplasty on neurosensory disturbance after a bilateral sagittal split osteotomy. J Oral Maxillofac Surg. 2002;60:1012–17.
30 Teltzrow T, Kramer, FJ, Schulze A, Baethge C, Brachvogel P. Perioperative complications following sagittal split osteotomy of the mandible. J Cranio-Maxillofac Surg. 2005;33:307–13.
31 Westermark A, Bystedt H, Von Konow L. Inferior alveolar nerve function after mandibular osteotomies. Br J Oral Maxillofac Surg. 1998;36:425–8.
32 de Vries K, Devriese PP, Hovinga J, van den Akker HP. Facial palsy after sagittal split osteotomies: A survey of 1747 sagittal split osteotomies. J Cranio-Maxillofac Surg. 1993;21: 50–3.
33 Turvey TA. Intraoperative complications of sagittal osteotomy of the mandibular ramus: incidence and management. J Oral Maxillofac Surg. 1985;43:504–9.
34 Proffit WR, Turvey TA, Phillips C. Orthognathic surgery: a hierarchy of stability. Internat J Adult Orthodont and Orthognath Surg. 1995;11:191–204.

Chapter 25

Mandibular Set-Back Procedures

Manolis Heliotis and Shamique Ismail

Introduction

The majority of mandibular set-back procedures are undertaken to address Class III skeletal patterns. There are broadly three clinical scenarios giving rise to such an anteroposterior skeletal disproportion:

1. The majority are a combination of maxillary retrognathism/hypoplasia and mandibular prognathism.
2. A not uncommon aetiology is an isolated maxillary retrognathism/hypoplasia, giving the false impression of mandibular prognathism. The patient, and occasionally inexperienced clinician, will often incorrectly consider the resolution of this problem, being addressed by a single mandibular set-back procedure.
3. In a minority of patients the mandible is the sole causative reason for the Class III appearance. Assessment and recognition of this less usual presentation is therefore important in planning the correct procedure and achieving the correct aesthetic result.

Clearly in relation to such an anteroposterior discrepancy, there may also be superimposed dentoskeletal variations in the vertical and transverse planes of space.

Not to be dismissed in management of these cases are the circumstances relating to patient choice and preference, which may indicate a mandibular set-back procedure in isolation, even if there is a combination of maxillary retrognathism and mandibular prognathism. This is particularly so in patients seeking a Class II feminized appearance (see Chapter 41). Very careful assessment of such cases is required and possible prosthetic midface enhancement or other interventions may be necessary to complete the desired effect.

Clinical assessment and planning

Below are the hallmarks particular to mandibular prognathism as the sole aetiology of a Class III appearance, which the authors use. The diagnosis is based on excluding a midface deficiency:

1. The presence of a harmoniously positioned nasomaxillary soft tissue complex in profile (defined from the supratip break of the nose to upper lip stomion):
   a) This is usually accompanied by a visibly pleasant nasolabial angle of 85 to 110 degrees.
   b) A gentle curvature is noted to run in a convex manner from below the lateral canthus of the eye down the cheek in its maximum convexity and inferiorly backwards behind the upper lip.
2. Another guide in determining this would be to block out the mandible during clinical examination of the patient, or on the photographs, and examine

Orthognathic Surgery: Principles, Planning and Practice. Edited by Farhad B. Naini and Daljit S. Gill.

the position of the nasomaxillary soft tissue complex relative to the oculo-nasal complex and forehead, as described above.

3. Carrying out a prediction tracing by hand or using software methods to model the optimal facial appearance, profile and facial proportions is a reasonably good indicator of whether an isolated mandibular set-back procedure is applicable in any given case.

From a cephalometric viewpoint, measurements such as maxillary and mandibular unit lengths can assist in determining the treatment modality for anteroposterior skeletal disproportion using a mandibular set-back procedure alone.

Measurement of the mandibular dentoalveolar height on the lateral cephalometric radiograph may also be of some assistance in cases of mandibular prognathism where the clinical presentation also includes an anterior open bite. In such a scenario it would be quite common for the patient to also have a reduced labiomental angle.

It is well acknowledged that a degree of dentoalveolar compensation will be present in patients with mandibular prognathism. An element of incisor retroclination in the mandible, along with the maxillary incisors proclining would be expected as a result of dentoalveolar compensation. The extent of compensation of these incisors often masks the degree of true skeletal disproportion.

In summary, the presence of a correctly positioned maxilla betrays the isolated prognathic mandible being the sole cause of a Class III appearance. The physical examination, basic cephalometric measurements and the above hallmarks are a guide.

The treatment plan is then moulded with cephalometric based predictive profile manipulation methods and shared between the patient, surgeon and orthodontist to determine the best functional and aesthetic outcome suitable to the individual patient. This dictates the operative facial movements, which in turn will dictate the accompanying orthodontic plan necessary to facilitate the desired surgical outcome.

Preoperative orthodontic treatment

The orthodontic preparation for a combined orthognathic case, requiring a mandibular set-back procedure, is focused initially on addressing the aforementioned preexisting dental compensation, whilst acknowledging the biological and physiological boundaries of the tissues in the area.

Conversely borderline surgical patients that present in their early teenage years for orthodontic correction of their dentition with a mild skeletal disproportion will often undergo a degree of further orthodontic compensation of their incisor inclinations to establish their final dental occlusion. This may well involve the extraction of permanent premolar teeth from the mandibular dental arch to facilitate this objective.

In the instance where such a patient has historically undergone unsuccessful orthodontic 'camouflage' and presents in later years requiring combined orthognathic treatment, it would be necessary to correct the resultant dental compensation from this erroneous orthodontic treatment, over and above the expected 'natural' dental compensation occurring in an untreated skeletal III case. Whilst it is an uncommon phenomenon, if previous mandibular arch extractions have taken place as part of an orthodontic 'camouflage' treatment in adolescence, it may also be necessary to consult a prosthodontist to factor in the need for subsequent prosthetic replacement of these extracted teeth. Whilst the placement of these prosthetic teeth would normally take place after completion of the orthognathic treatment, the prosthodontic consultation should occur at the initial treatment planning stage.

The orthodontic decompensation of the preexisting incisor inclinations that takes place as part of the preoperative orthodontics must respect the viability of the gingival tissues, in particular labial to the mandibular incisors. The root profiles of the mandibular incisors are often visible and palpable within this labial gingival tissue, and as such are prone to recession of their gingival attachments. Appropriate care is important with decompensation in such a scenario as possible dehiscence of the teeth through the gingivae may result if not carefully managed.

If it is felt that the risk of significant recession is of concern, then consideration should be given to the opinion of a periodontist prior to starting orthodontic treatment. Alternatively it may be more suitable to consider extractions in the mandibular arch, or alternatively to only partially decompensate the mandibular incisor inclination, in order to limit the anterior movement of the mandibular incisors.

The preoperative orthodontic decompensation is likely to have both functional and aesthetic effects on the patient. It is therefore imperative that the patient is made aware of not only a temporary deterioration in their occlusion, as the dentition is decompensated, but also have an understanding of the impact on their facial appearance that this preoperative orthodontic phase will have (Figures 25-1 and 25-2). The likelihood is the degree of mandibular prominence will visibly increase, such that the patient and those around them will be aware of the facial change. Reference should also be made to the fact that as the dentition is decompensated there may also be deterioration in speech as well as mastication.

It is not uncommon for a patient with a significant anteroposterior discrepancy to also exhibit signs of poor transverse maxillomandibular arch coordination, with or without the influence of the tongue musculature on the mandibular arch.

In such a scenario, the use of surgical planning models is of benefit to ascertain the degree of transverse correction required, and therefore determining the means by which this correction should be

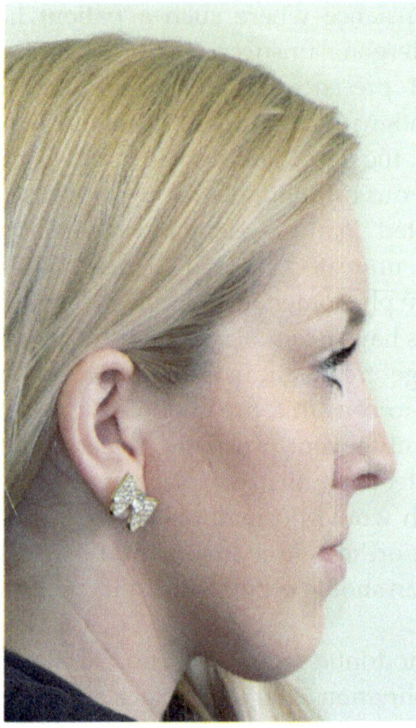

Fig. 25-1 Pretreatment facial profile view.

undertaken. This may be through orthodontic means alone, purely surgical treatment, or a combination of the two.

Surgical techniques

The most common operation for a mandibular set-back procedure is the **bilateral sagittal split osteotomy (BSSO)**. However, it has become increasingly recognised that if a large set-back is required, the most stable procedure in terms of surgical outcome that can be offered is the **intraoral vertical subsigmoid osteotomy (IVSSO)**. The historical development of these procedures is described in Chapter 2.

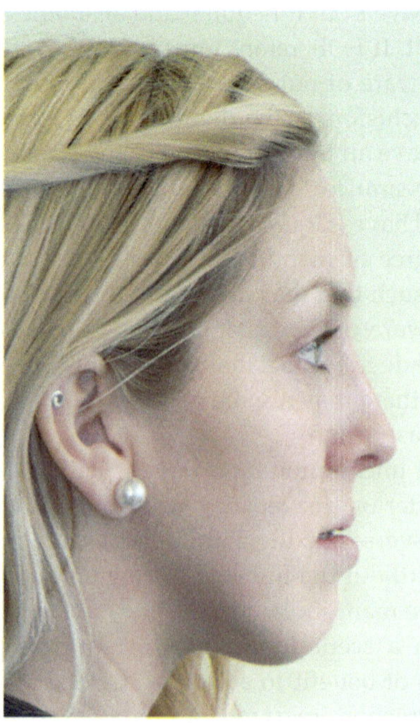

Fig. 25-2 Preoperative facial profile view.

Bilateral sagittal split set-back osteotomy versus the intraoral vertical subsigmoid osteotomy

The advantage of a bilateral sagittal split osteotomy (BSSO) is that once the mandible has been set-back it can be fixed by using bicortical screws or plates depending on operator preference, negating lengthy postoperative intermaxillary fixation (IMF).

The advantage of the IVSSO is the much smaller possibility of inferior alveolar nerve damage. The major disadvantage of this osteotomy is that postoperative IMF is required for approximately six weeks. We feel, however, that for the large mandibular set-back osteotomies this is probably the better of the two methods in terms of surgical outcome.

Bilateral sagittal split set-back osteotomy

The procedure is carried out under hypotensive general anaesthesia using naso-endotracheal intubation. The soft tissues are injected intraorally with lignocaine (2% with 1 in 80,000 adrenaline) inferior alveolar nerve blocks and buccal infiltration around the external oblique ridge and ramus for analgesia and vasoconstriction, ten minutes before the incisions are executed. In addition 0.5% chirocaine blocks and infiltration are used at the onset for postoperative analgesia lasting hours. The surgical field is prepared and draped as per the operator's preference but it is well advised to always be able to see the whole face from forehead to neck.

Intraoperatively, a photographic retractor is placed for exposure of the operative field, retraction and protection of the lips. A mouth prop is placed in the contralateral side and the tongue gently retracted with a Lax retractor.

Intraorally the incision is carried out up the anterior bony border of the ascending ramus of the mandible and forward opposite the second molar buccally with a 5mm soft tissue mucosal cuff to enable closure.

Ideally we ensure that mandibular third molar (wisdom) teeth have been removed at least nine months preoperatively. If not, the procedure can still be executed with the wisdom teeth in situ, however there has to be caution in several respects:

1. There is an increased risk that the retromolar lingual bony plate may fracture.
2. There is an increased risk of inferior alveolar nerve damage.
3. There is an increased risk of infection.
4. There is an increased risk in failure of optimal bone contact and therefore healing.

Following the incision, a subperiosteal dissection takes place buccally, stripping as little of the masseter muscle as possible. Excessive stripping of the masseter will result in larger haematomas and excessive swelling postoperatively. In addition, detachment of the muscle from the proximal fragment increases the possibility of poor positioning of the proximal segment during fixation and the risk of bone necrosis.

The subperiosteal dissection buccally must proceed inferiorly in front of the antegonial notch, exposing the inferior border of the mandible.

The dissection then proceeds upward against the external oblique ridge as high up as the coronoid process. A notched ramus retractor is placed against the external oblique ridge as it courses to the anterior border of the ramus. The notched retractor is pulled up against the anterior border of the ascending ramus, stripping as much of the temporalis muscle attachment, going high up, as close onto the coronoid process as possible. With the cutting diathermy, the temporalis fibres are cut away from the ascending ramus as high as possible. The notched retractor is replaced by a curved Kocher retractor to retract the tissue superiorly by an assistant.

The lingual (medial) subperiosteal dissection proceeds superior to inferior. The subperiosteal dissection is done with a small Obwegeser. It is imperative that the elevator remains subperiosteal at all times. The dissection proceeds from superior to inferior along the lingual aspect of the ramus, until the lingula is reached. A yellow/white hue subperiosteally at this point indicates the inferior alveolar nerve before entering the lingula. It is important to avoid levering or stretching of the tissues and inferior alveolar nerve as prolonged anaesthesia of the lower lip may follow.

The medial (lingual) ramus osteotomy, also known as the horizontal part of the osteotomy is done with a fissure burr or a Lindemann burr. The burr is placed parallel to the occlusal plane, above and just behind the lingula. This point is critical. If the cut terminates anterior to the lingula, the alveolar canal will remain attached to the proximal segment (the segment with the ramus and condyle). This is one of the commonest errors, with difficulty in splitting the superior and posterior aspect of the osteotomy and increased damage to the nerve.

With ample irrigation the cut is made through the medial cortex into the medullary bone. As a guide, we know this has been achieved when blood is seen to ooze from the bone. In set-back procedures, it is advisable to remove a small segment of bone from the superior part of the osteotomy.

The vertical section of the osteotomy starts from the medial osteotomy superiorly and ends inferiorly opposite the second molar. We ensure the burr has gone through the cortex, about 5 mm deep and again this is verified by seeing blood coming through the medullary bone. Ideally there are no wisdom teeth, but if there are, do not make the error of going buccally between the crown of the tooth and buccal bone; instead the cut is continued through the tooth in line with the osteotomy, as if this was bone and the tooth did not exist.

The buccal osteotomy is performed next. For this, the curved Kocher is removed from the ramus and a channel retractor is placed in the lower border of the mandible, in front of the antegonial notch. The osteotomy aims to be in front of the antegonial notch posteriorly: the channel retractor positioned correctly in front of the notch will indicate this. Another guide is to be roughly between the roots of the lower second molar when making the cut. The author (MH) uses a Lindemann burr cutting through the buccal cortex from below to above. We know the correct depth is achieved once blood is again seen to appear from the medullary bone. The buccal osteotomy and the vertical osteotomy are joined.

At this stage the mouth props are removed, the two jaws approximated as close as possible with the dentition almost touching, and with the channel retractor in situ, we aim to cut the lower border through and through from buccal to lingual with the burr at a depth of about 5 mm to ensure the buccal osteotomy has extended through the lower border and captured the lingual cortex. This manoeuvre is critical in ensuring the split will run from the lower border, lingually up and behind the lingula. The most common cause of difficulty in initiating the split, or giving rise to a 'bad split' is failure to complete this step.

Caution must be exercised in patients with mandibular prognathism, unilateral condylar hyperplasia and the excessive side of mandibular asymmetries, because the neurovascular bundle in these cases is usually situated very buccally and very inferiorly in relation to the lower border of the mandible.

Splitting of the mandible

With a 10 mm wide chisel we proceed along the external oblique ridge (the vertical cut) aiming the chisel in a buccal direction such that we see a slight separation of the buccal and lingual fragments, but not attempting to completely separate the segments.

With a 7 mm width chisel placed at the junction of the buccal cut and the vertical cut (external oblique ridge), the chisel is levered so that the buccal (proximal) segment starts separating from the dentoalveolar supporting segment (the lingual or distal segment). The Smith's spreader is used to take up the slack, and never to split the segments. The dissection proceeds from anterior to posterior peeling the bone backwards and separating the buccal from the lingual fragments as we proceed.

Care is taken to ensure that the inferior alveolar nerve remains in the lingual or dentoalveolar (distal) segment. Separation of the segments is demonstrated by independent movement of the proximal and distal segments not only in an anteroposterior but also in a superior to inferior fashion to ensure complete detachment.

With set-back osteotomies, a segment of bone requires removal from the proximal segment of the buccal osteotomy in order to set-back the body of the mandible. The amount of bone removed will depend on the amount of the set-back required. This is carried out next.

We ensure the detachment of the medial pterygoid muscle on the lingual aspect so that there is easy uninterrupted set-back of the mandible with no interference of the medial musculature.

The same procedure is carried out on the contralateral side of the mandible. Using the final wafer the jaws are placed in the planned occlusal position with temporary IMF using an elastomeric chain.

The fixation of the mandible is carried out using transbuccal bicortical screws.

A 4 mm external incision opposite the angle of the mandible is carried out. A transbuccal trocar is introduced. The mandibular proximal fragment is palpated inferiorly so that it sits in line with the distal mandibular fragment. The condyles are positioned passively in Class III cases and are not pushed or encouraged hard into the condylar fossae. This is an extremely important step. The proximal segment is positioned passively and a transbuccal bicortical screw is placed following bicortical drilling with ample irrigation. Three such screws are placed, usually two superior to the inferior alveolar nerve and one inferior to it.

Once the bicortical screws are placed on both sides the intermaxillary fixation is removed, and the occlusion checked and tested. The author usually waits at least five minutes to ensure that the bite remains in the predetermined position and there is no evidence of any condylar sag or change. The wafer is removed.

The internal mucosal wounds are closed with 4/0 Vicryl Rapide interrupted and the external skin wound closed with 6/0 Nylon.

We place the patient in one or at most two light intermaxillary elastics overnight, which act as a simple splint to support the mandible in the new position so that the patient's mouth with the swelling does not hang open. The patient is given standard preoperative and postoperative analgesia consisting of paracetamol and an anti-inflammatory of choice. Opioids postoperatively are seldom if ever used. The patient also receives two postoperative doses of dexamethasone.

Intraoral vertical mandibular ramus osteotomy

The second procedure available for the set-back osteotomy is the intraoral vertical subsigmoid osteotomy (IVSSO).[1] Anaesthesia, local analgesia, preparation and draping are as described for the BSSO set-back procedure.

An incision is carried out along the external oblique ridge mid-way up the ramus and opposite the second molar. A subperiosteal dissection is carried out buccally stripping the musculature including the masseter this time cleanly off the buccal aspect of the ramus of the mandible and identifying the sigmoid notch.

Two Bauer retractors are now placed, one in the sigmoid notch superiorly and one in the antegonial notch inferiorly. We now look for our landmarks to place the vertical subsigmoid cuts. The antilingula is now identified as a slight bony protuberance on the lateral (buccal) surface of the ramus. It *roughly* corresponds buccally to the position of the lingula, which is found medially on the ramus of the mandible. In addition this protuberance is thought to be approximately 10 mm above the occlusal plane. There is some controversy in the use of the antilingula as a reference mark, as it may not correspond to the actual position of the lingula. Another easier way to mark the vertical cuts from the sigmoid notch to the antegonial notch is to estimate approximately a safe line 6 to 7 mm anterior to the posterior border of the mandibular ramus.

A line is drawn therefore 7 mm in front of the posterior aspect of the mandible buccally from the sigmoid notch down to the antegonial notch. A second vertical line is drawn approximately 2 mm behind this line (Figure 25-3).[1]

With an oscillating saw a cut is made first on the posterior of the two vertical lines going from the sigmoid notch downwards into the antegonial notch. A second cut is now carried out from the superior opposite the sigmoid notch downward again to the antegonial notch. Both cuts must be aimed not only medially but also angled posteriorly. Once these cuts are made the proximal and distal segments are mobilized. With a subperiosteal elevator, the medial part of the proximal segment musculature is mobilised from inferior to superior and all the musculature including the medial pterygoid muscle and pterygomandibular ligaments are stripped in order to have the proximal segment free. The procedure is repeated on the contralateral side.

The patient is placed in fixed intermaxillary fixation in the desired occlusion for 6 weeks.

Integral to this procedure is that following release of the intermaxillary fixation active physiotherapy is carried out in order to allow for normal return to function and good mouth opening.

Postoperative management

With either of the above surgical procedures, the orthodontist will review the patient prior to discharge from the hospital the following day. Prior to discharge from the hospital the patient is also given dietary and oral hygiene advice.

At this early postoperative stage, the orthodontist will assist the seating of the occlusion with appropriate intermaxillary guiding elastics if required. Further orthodontic review will take place on a weekly basis for the first month. By the end of this period the occlusion should ideally be showing suitable interdigitation, however it is often necessary to assist the detailing of the occlusion. This may involve sectioning

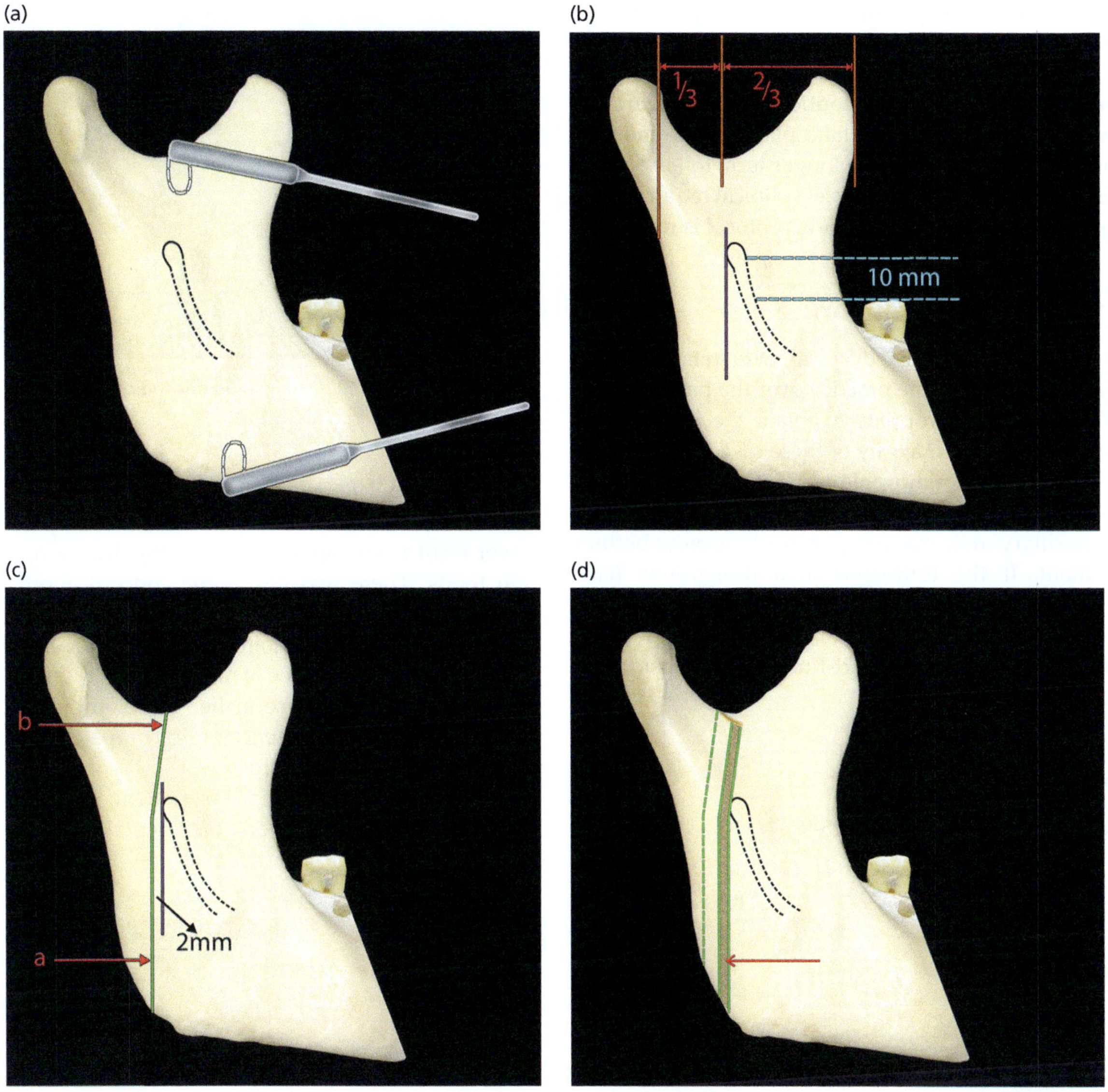

Fig. 25-3 (a) Two curved Bauer retractors are placed on the lateral surface of the ramus, one hooked around the antegonial notch and another hooked over the sigmoid notch. On the figure, the path of the inferior alveolar nerve and its entry via the lingula is marked with dotted lines, representing the approximate position on the medial aspect of the mandible, which cannot be directly viewed with this operation. (b) The antilingula eminence found on the lateral aspect of the ramus corresponds to the approximate position of the lingula and entrance of the inferior alveolar nerve found on the medial aspect. We find the antilingula eminence by using the following intersecting two lines: A horizontal line running 10 mm above the mandibular occlusal plane, and a vertical line two-thirds of the way from the anterior aspect of the ramus. Their intersection marks the antilingula eminence on the lateral aspect of the ramus. This point may be marked on the bone with a sterile marker or a Colorado needle using diathermy. We proceed to mark a vertical reference line (purple line in figure), 2 mm posterior to the antilingula eminence, down towards the antegonial notch, with a sterile marker or a Colorado needle as above. (c) An osteotomy cut (green line) is made 2 mm posterior to the reference line (shown as 'a'). A second osteotomy (shown as 'b') is angulated slightly anteriorly towards the sigmoid notch. Note that the osteotomy cut (green line) is a total of 4 mm behind the antilingula eminence and therefore clear of the inferior alveolar nerve, which remains medial to it. A round oscillating saw is used for the osteotomy cut. (d) The osteotomy cut is mobilized and completed with curved osteotomes. The distal segment is now mobilized and the osteotomized surface of the proximal segment may be seen (red arrow). We then proceed to dissect off the medial pterygoid and stylomandibular ligaments from the medial aspect of the proximal (ramus) segment. The distal segment (tooth bearing) is then mobilised and placed medially to the proximal segment of the ramus so that the segments overlap. The distal segment is set-back and intermaxillary fixation applied into this final position. (After Reyneke[1].)

the mandibular archwire, or by using light force and smaller dimension archwires in the mandible, whilst maintaining a rigid rectangular steel wire for the maxillary dentition. Again the appropriate use of intermaxillary elastics will aid this process.

If associated transverse occlusal discrepancies were evident pretreatment, then an awareness of possible transverse relapse should be borne in mind. If this eventuality arises, then to resolve this may require the wearing of inter-arch cross elastics or appropriate modification of the archwire dimensions to resolve this.

A joint clinical review takes place with the orthodontist and the surgeon a week postoperatively. The dental panoramic tomograph taken prior to discharge from the hospital department will be available for review. A lateral cephalometric radiograph may be requested at this initial postoperative review, or if not clinically required, would be delayed until the time of removing the orthodontic appliances. Further joint orthognathic reviews take place at one month, 3 months and 6 months, with longer-term follow up on an annual basis for 5 years, unless clinical requirement is such that an alternative review protocol is required.

Orthodontic retention

The use of anterior fixed spiral wire retainers has become a fairly routine practice over the past decade, and would be appropriate to retain the incisor and canine teeth in the majority of these cases.

The use of a removable acrylic upper Hawley retainer would be recommended in cases where the maxillary arch was comparatively narrow before treatment. If the transverse arch dimensions had not required any modification, then vacuum formed retainers would be appropriate. In either case, the long term use of retainers on a part-time basis is considered appropriate.

Case report

(See Figures 25-1, 25-2, 25-4–25-9.)

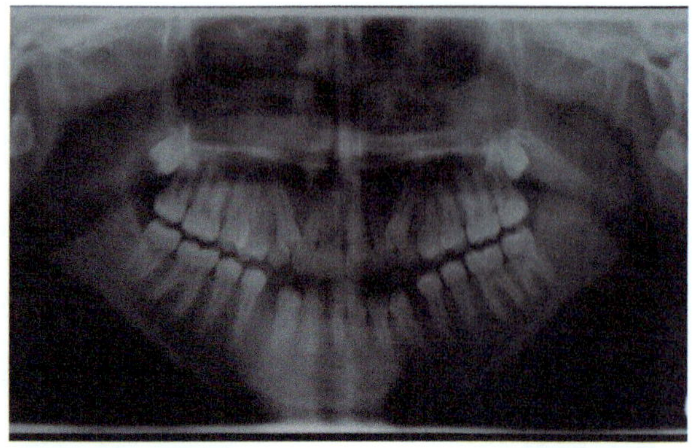

Fig. 25-5 Pretreatment dental panoramic tomograph.

A 17-year-old female patient attended the department complaining of the gap between her upper and lower front teeth and associated difficulty eating certain foods. There was also some concern about the prominence of her lower lip.

On assessment on a joint orthognathic clinic the patient exhibited a degree of mandibular prognathism as well as slight increase in her lower anterior face height. There was an absence of lip competence, with an eversion of her lower lip at rest.

From the radiographic assessment, there was no evident pathology on the dental panoramic

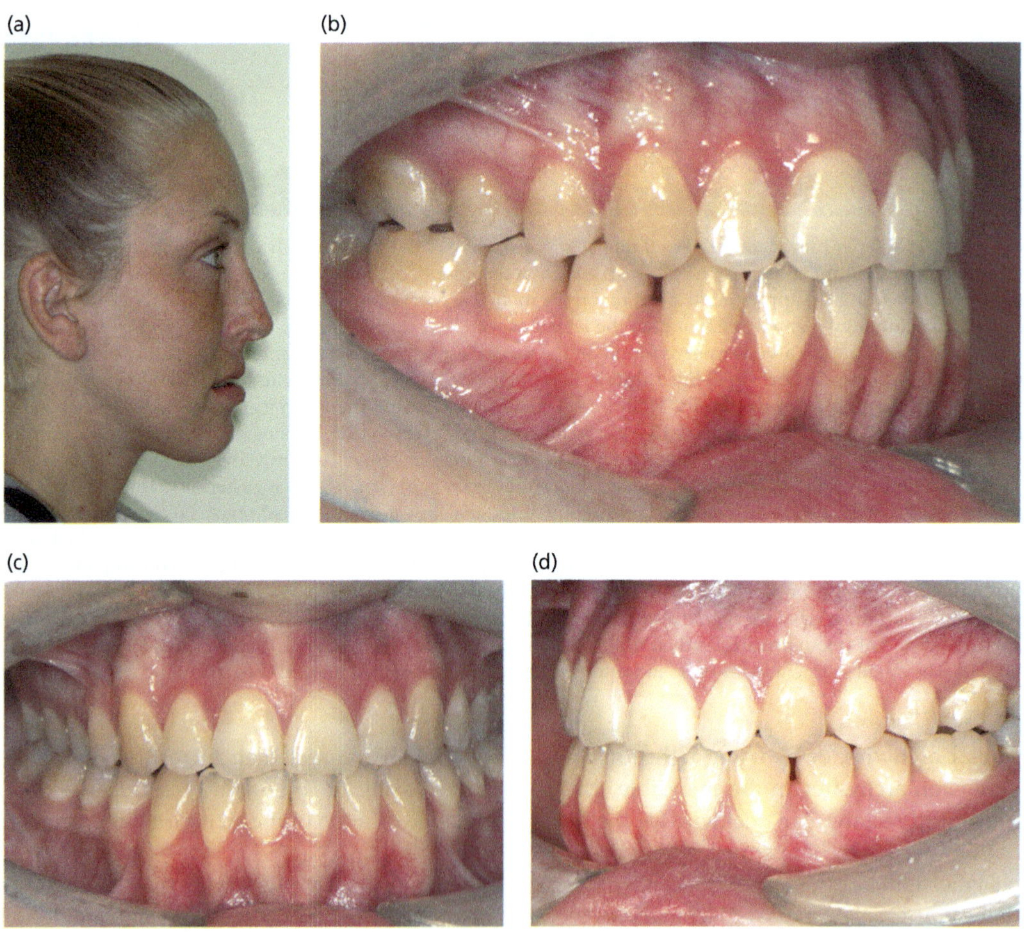

Fig. 25-4 (a) Facial profile view one year post-treatment. (b) Intraoral right lateral view one year post-treatment. (c) Intraoral anterior view one year post-treatment. (d) Intraoral left lateral view one-year post-treatment.

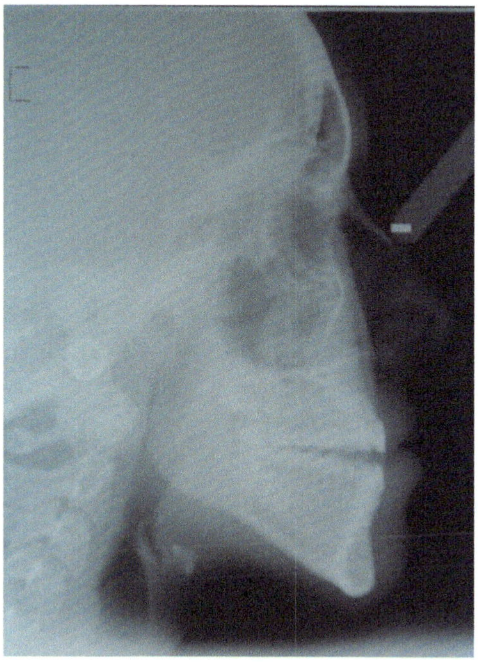

Fig. 25-6 Pretreatment lateral cephalometric radiograph.

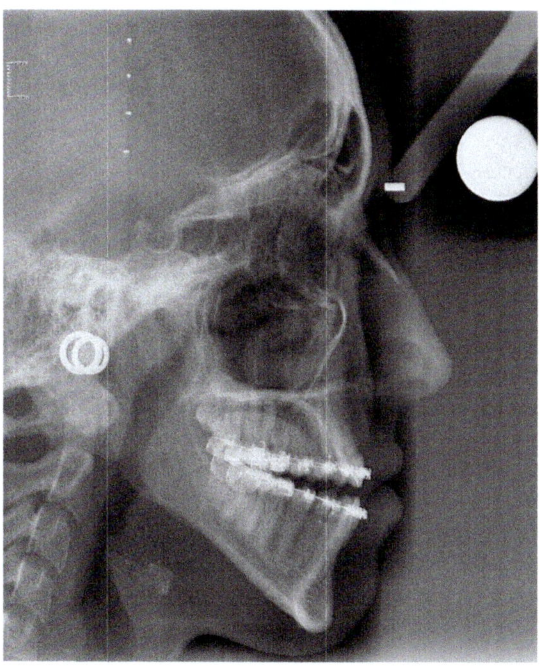

Fig. 25-7 Preoperative lateral cephalometric radiograph.

tomograph, and the lateral cephalograph confirmed both the anteroposterior skeletal III discrepancy, as well as the increased lower face height.

The treatment was planned around correction of the mild mandibular prognathism and anterior open bite through a combined orthognathic plan involving an isolated mandibular bilateral sagittal split osteotomy set-back procedure.

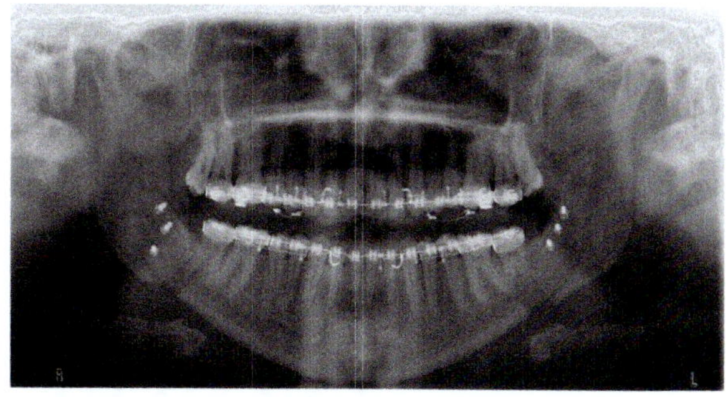

Fig. 25-8 Postoperative dental panoramic tomograph.

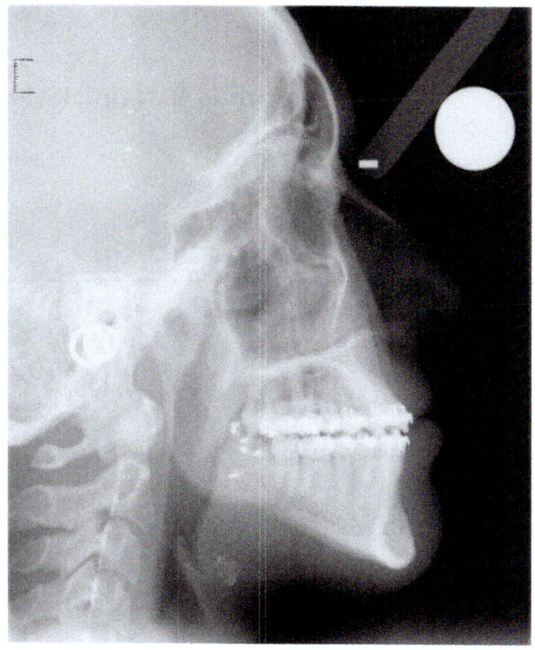

Fig. 25-9 Lateral cephalometric radiograph prior to removal of fixed appliances.

The orthodontic decompensation resulted in the facial changes expected as outlined above. The dental decompensation in the mandibular incisor region is exhibited when comparing this area in the lateral cephalometric radiographs in Figures 25-6 and 25-7. These images also illustrate the maintenance of the open bite in this case, which is important to minimize the potential of orthodontic relapse in the vertical plane.

After an uneventful surgical procedure, and subsequent orthodontic detailing of the occlusion, a pleasing dental and facial appearance resulted. At the one year review appointment the facial and dental appearance was seen to be maintained.

Reference

1 Reyneke JP. Essential of Orthognathic Surgery (2nd Ed.). Hanover Park, IL: Quintessence Publishing Co., 2010.

Chapter 26

Surgical Correction of Vertical Maxillary Excess (VME)

Farhad B. Naini, Helen Witherow and Daljit S. Gill

Introduction

'Measure several times, cut once.'
Pür Sina (Avicenna) (AD 980–1037), Persian physician–scholar
Canon Medicinae (*The Canon of Medicine*)

Planning and preparation in a careful and thorough manner are of paramount importance in surgical practice. Avicenna's advice appears to be particularly apt for orthognathic surgery, where the actual operative jaw movements need to be re-checked a number of times, based on clinical evaluation, cephalometric analysis and planning, model surgery and, finally, judicious intraoperative assessment in the operating theatre. Although much of the planning for orthognathic surgical procedures is undertaken prior to the patient reaching the operating theatre, vertical repositioning of the maxilla requires a number of accurate intraoperative measurements to be taken, making the surgical correction of dentofacial deformities associated with vertical maxillary excess challenging and the resultant aesthetic changes often very rewarding.

Diagnosis and aetiology

Vertical maxillary excess (VME) may be defined as excessive maxillary development in the vertical plane. VME may involve the posterior maxilla only (**posterior VME**), the anterior dentoalveolus only (**anterior VME**) or the entire maxilla (**total VME**) (Figure 26-1). Patients with VME tend to exhibit a *predominantly vertical facial growth pattern*, sometimes termed a **tall (or 'long') face deformity**.

Presenting features of VME[1]

Anterior face height

There is an increased total anterior face height (TAFH), almost entirely due to an increased lower anterior face height (LAFH).

Vertical maxillary development

There is excessive inferior maxillary skeletal development (VME). There may be up to 10–15 mm of bone between the nasal floor and the root apices of the

Orthognathic Surgery: Principles, Planning and Practice. Edited by Farhad B. Naini and Daljit S. Gill.

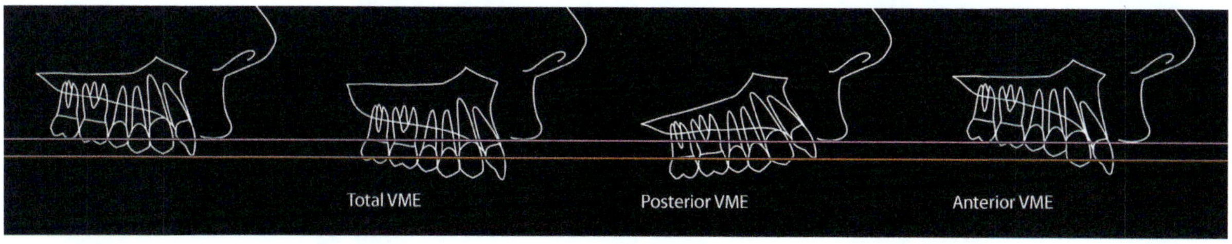

Fig. 26-1 Schematic drawing comparing total VME, posterior VME and anterior VME.

maxillary teeth (Figure 26-2). Vertical maxillary excess (VME) may be:

- **Total VME:** There is excessive vertical development of the entire maxilla, both anteriorly and posteriorly. The maxillary incisor exposure in relation to the upper lip in repose is increased, and on smiling there is increased gingival exposure, or 'gummy smile,' both anteriorly and posteriorly (Figure 26-3).
- **Posterior VME:** There is excessive vertical development of the posterior maxilla and posterior maxillary dentoalveolus (Figure 26-4). There is likely to be increased gingival exposure in the premolar and molar regions. There is inferior rotation of the posterior maxilla, i.e. the maxillary plane is canted downward posteriorly. Anterior vertical maxillary dentoalveolar development may be impeded by a forward resting tongue position; therefore, the maxillary incisor exposure in relation to the upper lip at rest may be normal or even reduced. Alternatively, there may be increased VME anteriorly as well, but less than the degree of posterior VME.
- **Anterior dentoalveolar VME:** This, by definition, is not a skeletal basal problem, but a dentoalveolar problem. Excessive overeruption of the maxillary incisors leads to a 'gummy smile,' but only anteriorly, i.e. increased anterior gingival exposure on smiling (Figure 26-5). Anterior segmental maxillary impaction or intrusion of the maxillary incisors and associated gingivae will correct this problem.

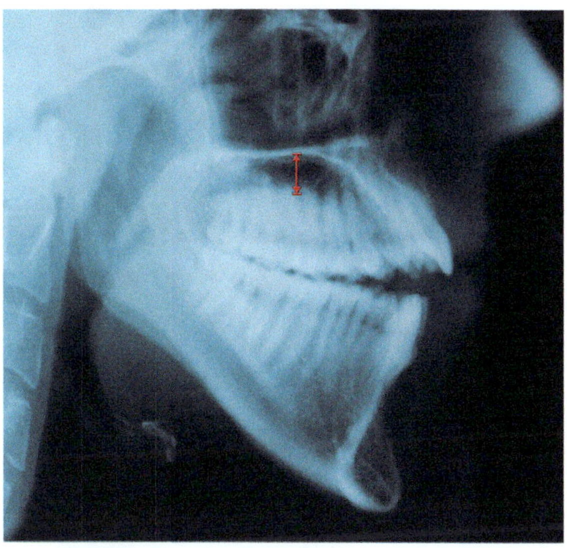

Fig. 26-2 There may be up to 10–15 mm of bone between the nasal floor and the root apices of the maxillary teeth if there is excessive inferior maxillary skeletal development; in this case the excessive development in the posterior maxilla exceeds that in the anterior region. (From: Naini FB. Facial Aesthetics: Concepts and Clinical Diagnosis. Oxford: Wiley-Blackwell, 2011; used with permission.[1])

Upper lip–maxillary incisor relationship

- Increased exposure of the maxillary incisors in relation to the upper lip in repose, i.e. excessive upper incisor display (Figure 26-6).
- Increased dentogingival exposure on smiling, i.e. a 'gummy smile'.

Posterior mandibular rotation

There is posterior (downward and backward) mandibular rotation. This will affect the apparent sagittal prominence of the chin. If the mandible is large, the otherwise prominent chin may be rotated to a more normal position in the sagittal plane (skeletal Class III rotated to a skeletal Class I (Figure 26-7); conversely, and more commonly, if the mandible is of normal or reduced size, the chin will rotate downward and backward to an even less prominent position (skeletal Class I rotated to a skeletal Class II).

Mandibular plane angle

There is an increased mandibular plane angle; hence the terms **high angle** facial type or **hyperdivergent** face.

Lip posture

There is usually an incomplete lip seal (lip incompetence), though the extent depends on the upper and lower lip heights, the degree of increase in LAFH, and the degree of downward and backward rotation of the mandible. The greater the LAFH and the downward and backward rotation of the mandible, and the shorter the lips, the greater will be the interlabial distance in repose and the degree of lip incompetence.

Nasal morphology

There is a tendency towards a narrow nose, with a narrow alar base and some paranasal hollowing. It is common for Class II, 'long face' patients to also have a prominent nasal dorsum.

(a)

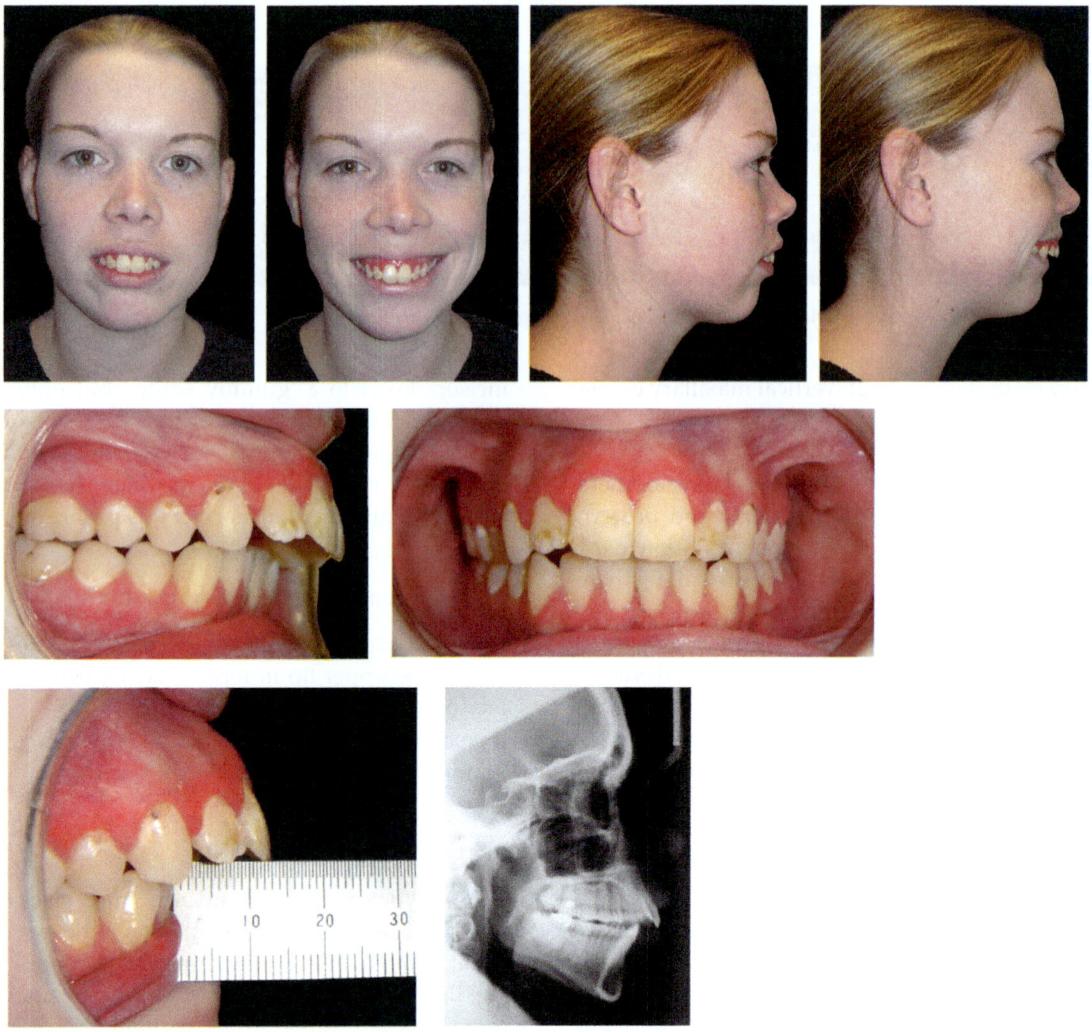

(b)

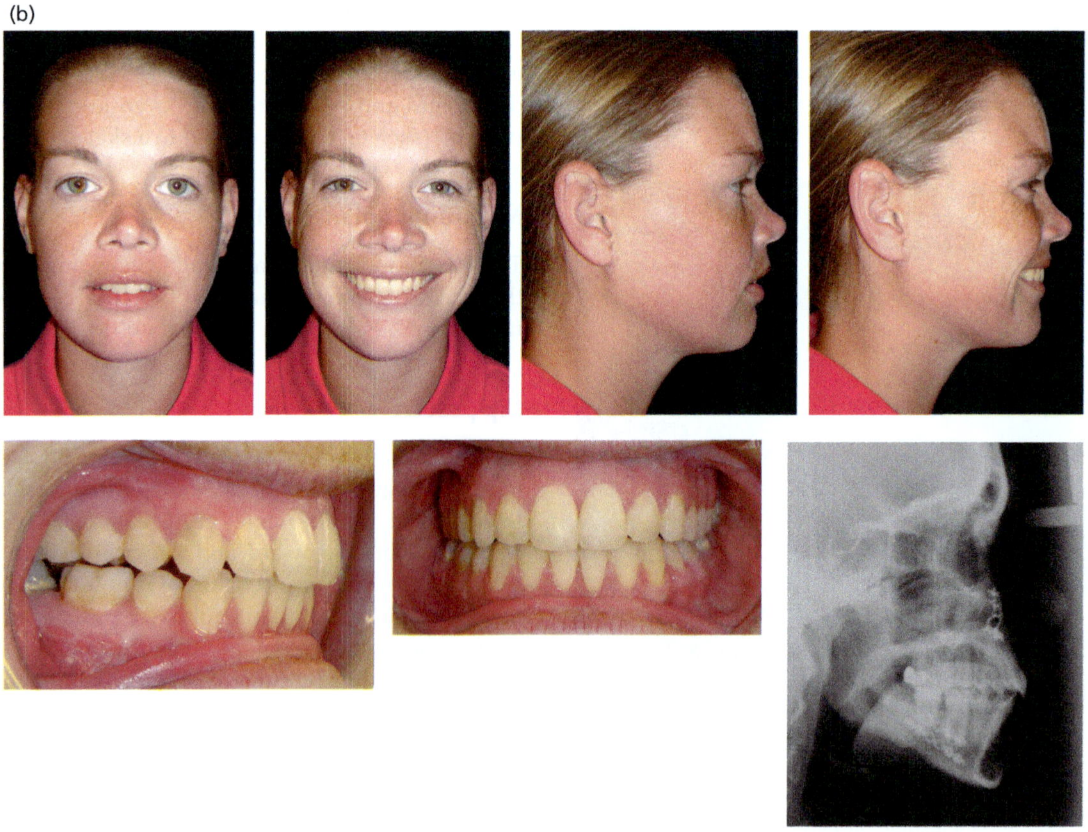

Fig. 26-3 Total VME. (a) Pretreatment views of a patient with total VME. Maxillary incisor exposure is increased in repose and gingival exposure is increased on smiling. The patient underwent preparatory orthodontics, followed by maxillary impaction (5 mm anteriorly and 7 mm posteriorly). The mandible autorotated forward and was advanced. (b) End of treatment views.

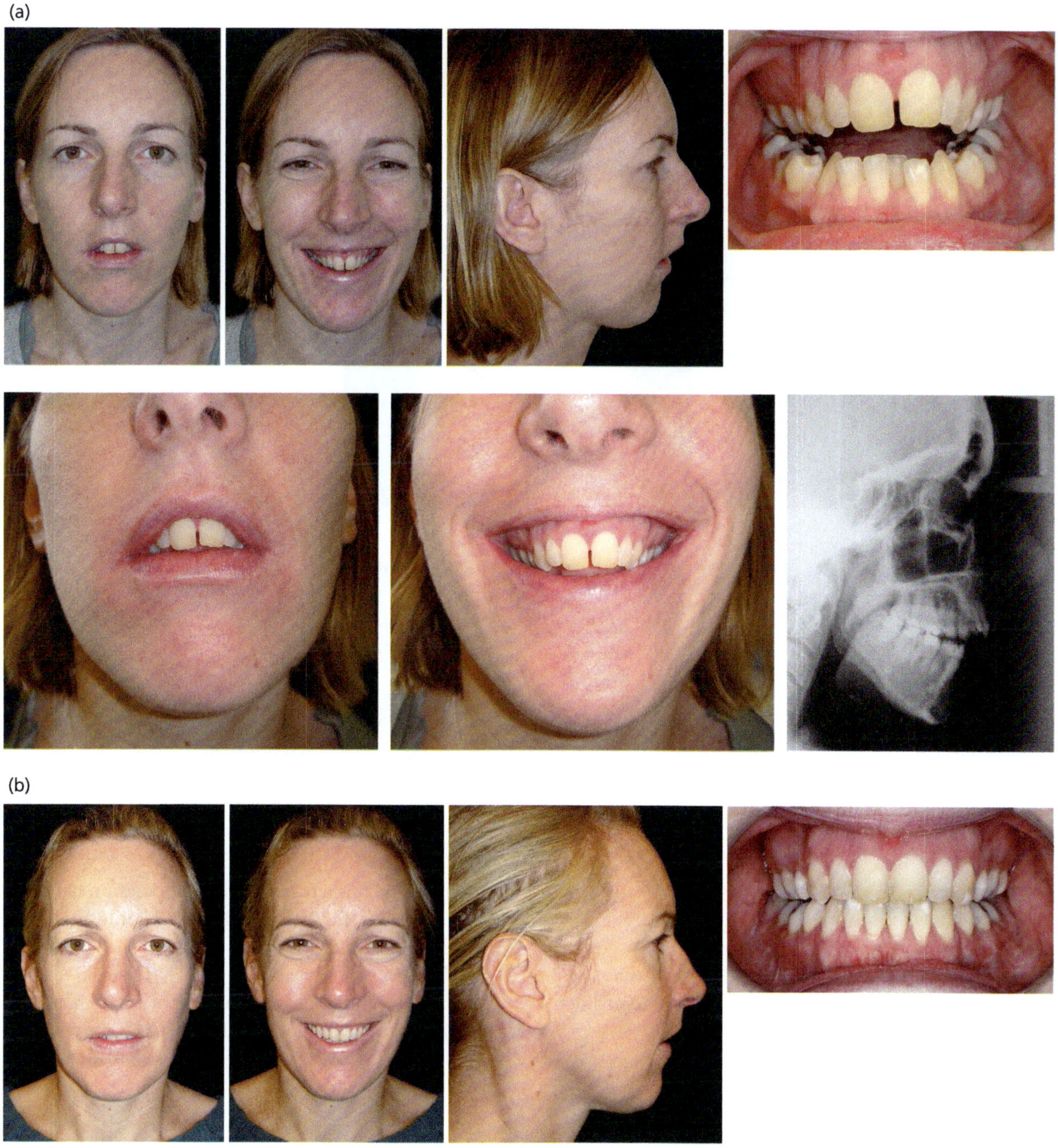

Fig. 26-4 Posterior VME. (a) Pretreatment views of patient with VME, which is more pronounced posteriorly. (b) End of treatment views, demonstrating the result following differential impaction of the maxilla (more posteriorly than anteriorly), forward mandibular autorotation and mandibular repositioning to a Class I incisor relationship. The maxillary arch is level and maxillary incisor-gingival exposure improved.

Palatal vault morphology

There is a tendency towards a high and narrow palatal vault. This may be due to a lower tongue position and compensatory overeruption of the maxillary dentition due to the increased LAFH. Therefore, there is a tendency to posterior dental crossbite.

Incisor overbite

VME may be associated with **anterior open bite (AOB)**. *When the primary aetiological factor in the presence of an anterior open bite is the excessive face height, it is termed a* **skeletal open bite**. The extent of an anterior open bite will depend on the LAFH, the degree of compensatory overeruption of the incisor teeth and the resting tongue position.

- If the LAFH is increased and the tongue does *not* have a forward resting position between the incisor teeth, the incisors will overerupt either until they meet, or until they cannot erupt any further. In this situation, the presence of an AOB depends on the LAFH. If the LAFH is excessively increased and the incisors are unable to meet, there will be an AOB, but an increased curve of Spee in the mandibular dental arch and a reverse curve in the maxillary arch (Figure 26-8).

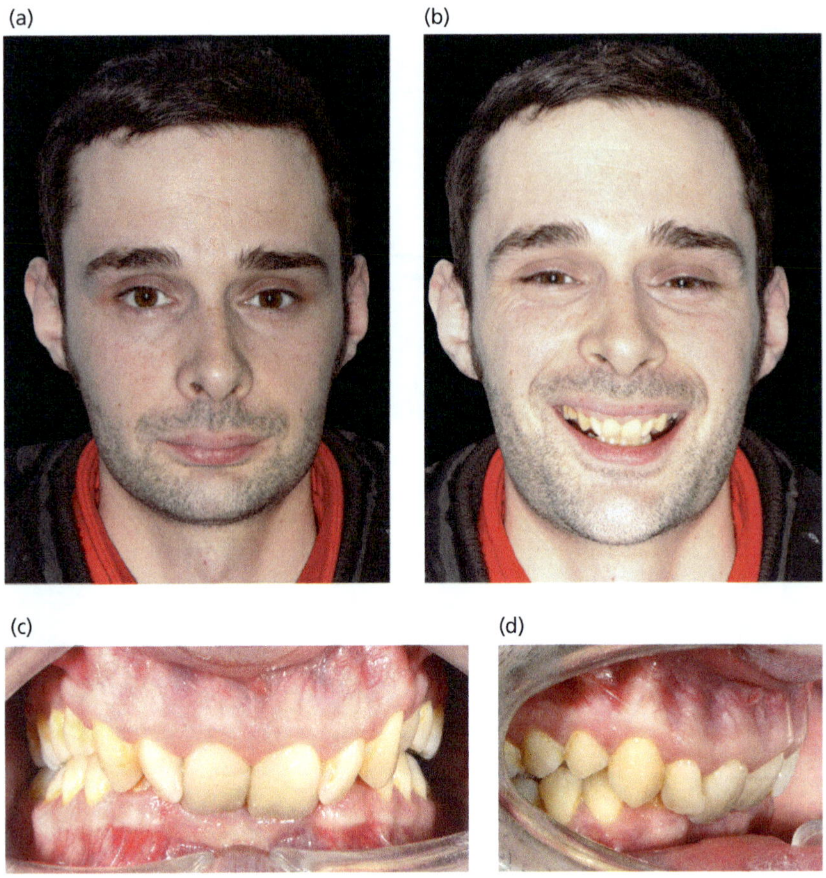

Fig. 26-5 Anterior VME. This patient has a reduced lower anterior face height, but excessive maxillary gingival exposure anteriorly on smiling due to anterior VME, resulting from overeruption of the maxillary incisors and associated gingivae. This is common in Class II division 2 type malocclusions.

Note:

If the incisor teeth are able to vertically compensate for the increased LAFH, there may be a normal or even an increased incisor overbite (Figure 26-9).

- If the tongue has a forward resting position between the incisor teeth, there will be an anterior open bite. In this situation, the presence of the AOB does not depend directly on the LAFH. There is often a reverse curve of Spee in the mandibular arch and an increased curve in the maxillary arch (Figure 26-10).

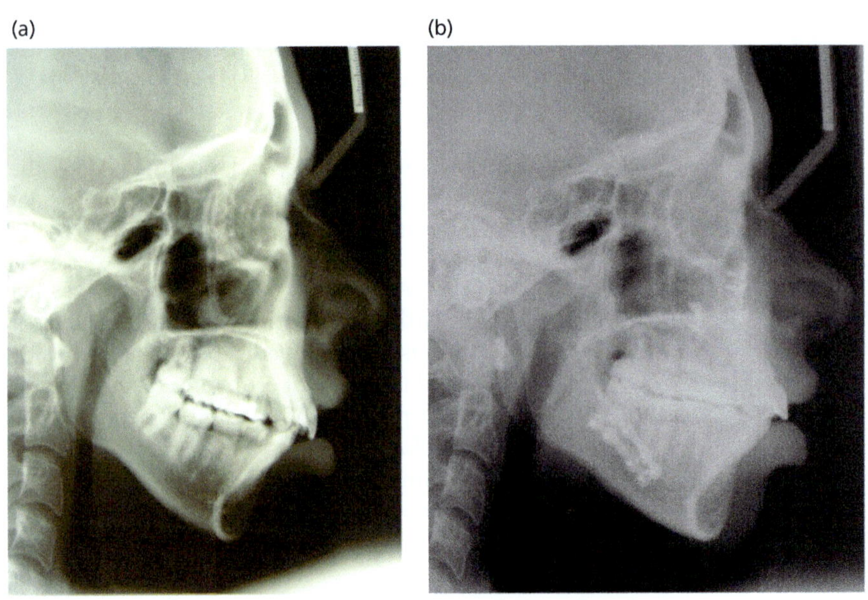

Fig. 26-6 Maxillary incisor exposure in relation to the upper lip. (a) Pretreatment. (b) Following superior repositioning of the maxilla.

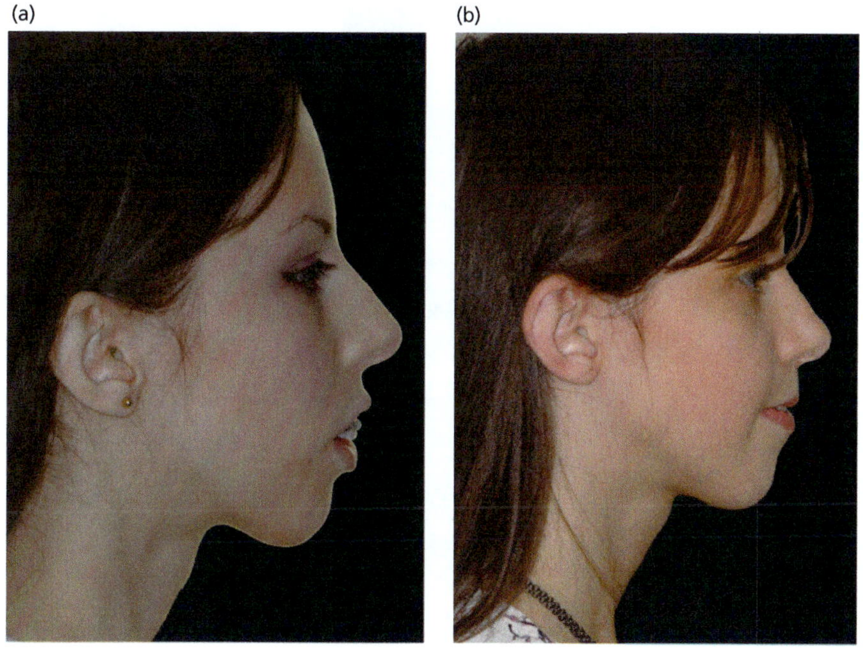

Fig. 26-7 (a) Posterior mandibular rotation, secondary to posterior vertical maxillary excess, moves the chin downward and backward. (b) Superior repositioning of the maxilla allows forward autorotation of the mandible, and upward and forward movement of the chin.

Principles in planning the surgical correction of vertical maxillary excess

Excessive vertical facial growth has a very strong genetic determination (see Chapter 3).[2] The extent and direction of surgical repositioning of the maxilla depends on the extent and direction of the original deformity. *The foundation for treatment planning is the desired upper lip-incisor relationship.*

The surgical management of VME often involves the following (Figure 26-11):

- Vertical (superior) repositioning of the maxilla – This should always be planned in relation to the degree of maxillary incisor exposure with the lips in repose.
- Vertical (by forward autorotation) and sagittal (by osteotomy) repositioning of the mandible.
- Vertical and sagittal repositioning of the bony chin.

The Le Fort I type downfracture osteotomy of the maxilla permits the removal of bone between the nasal floor and maxillary dental root apices (Figure 26-12 and 26-13), allowing superior repositioning (impaction) of the maxillary dentoalveolus. The amount of bone removal for a patient with total VME will be the same anteriorly and posteriorly. Alternatively, the amount of bone removal anteriorly and posteriorly may be altered, e.g. greater bone removal posteriorly permits a greater *differential impaction* of the posterior maxilla.[3] Alternatively, the posterior maxilla may be segmentally impacted. Following superior repositioning of the maxilla, the mandible will *autorotate* anteriorly around the condylar hinge axis, and the chin thereby moves forward and upward. If this forward autorotation of the mandible brings the mandibular body into a good sagittal relationship and provides an acceptable dental occlusion, then no mandibular surgery may be required, or perhaps only

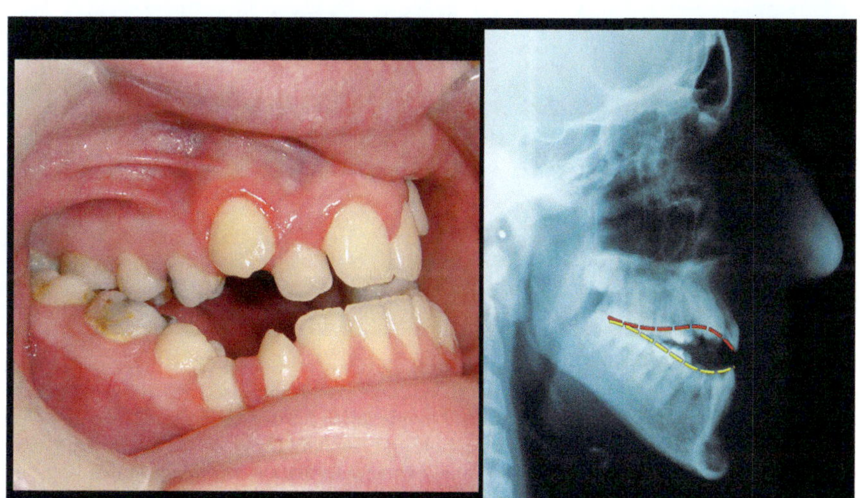

Fig. 26-8 A predominantly skeletal aetiology to the anterior open bite, with an increased curve of Spee in the mandibular dental arch and a reverse curve in the maxillary arch. (From: Naini FB. Facial Aesthetics: Concepts and Clinical Diagnosis. Oxford: Wiley-Blackwell, 2011; used with permission.[1])

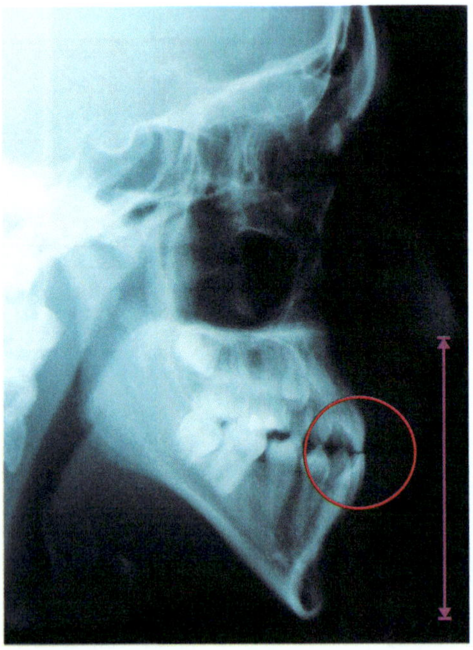

Fig. 26-9 Vertical dentoalveolar compensation (incisor overeruption) for the increased lower anterior face height. (From: Naini FB. Facial Aesthetics: Concepts and Clinical Diagnosis. Oxford: Wiley-Blackwell, 2011; used with permission.[1])

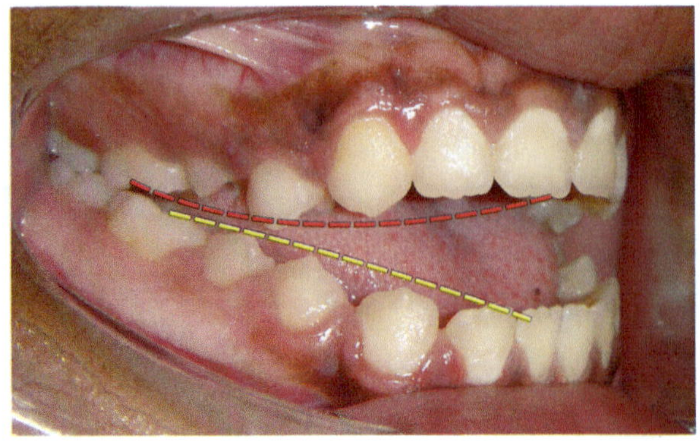

Fig. 26-10 A predominantly soft tissue aetiology to the anterior open bite, with a slightly reverse curve of Spee in the mandibular arch and an increased sagittal curve in the maxillary arch. (From: Naini FB. Facial Aesthetics: Concepts and Clinical Diagnosis. Oxford: Wiley-Blackwell, 2011; used with permission.[1])

a relieving osteotomy of the mandible. However, if the mandibular body is inherently deficient or excessive in size, it may need to be repositioned in the sagittal plane following autorotation. The sagittal and vertical position of the chin may be determined following mandibular autorotation and sagittal repositioning of the mandibular body, in order to determine the potential requirement for an osseous genioplasty. As well as VME, patients with a tall face deformity often have excessive vertical chin height, and thereby may benefit from vertical reduction genioplasty.

The most important determining factors when planning the extent of maxillary impaction are the resultant upper lip–incisor relationship, which is the mainstay of treatment planning, and the lower anterior facial height.[1]

Lower anterior face height

Reduction of the lower anterior face height (LAFH) requires taking into consideration the face height ratios, so that the LAFH is proportionate to the total face height and standing height, and the facial height to width ratio. These proportional relationships are important and excessive reduction of the LAFH should be avoided.

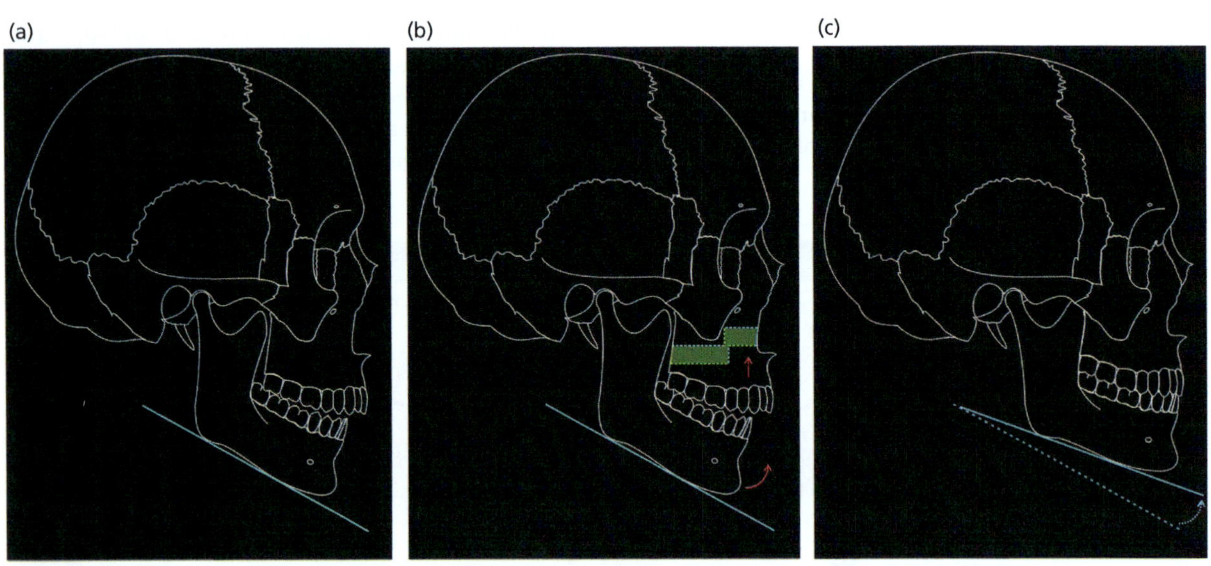

Fig. 26-11 (a) Schematic representation of vertical maxillary excess (VME), with posterior rotation of the mandible, moving the chin downward and backward. The mandibular plane inclination is increased. (b) The surgical management of VME often involves superior repositioning of the maxilla (planned in relation to the degree of maxillary incisor exposure in relation to the upper lip, and the LAFH), forward autorotation of the mandible and resultant forward and upward movement of the chin. Any sagittal repositioning of the mandible is undertaken following autorotation, as required, as is vertical and sagittal repositioning of the bony chin. (c) Postoperative position, demonstrating reduced mandibular plane inclination towards a more average inclination.

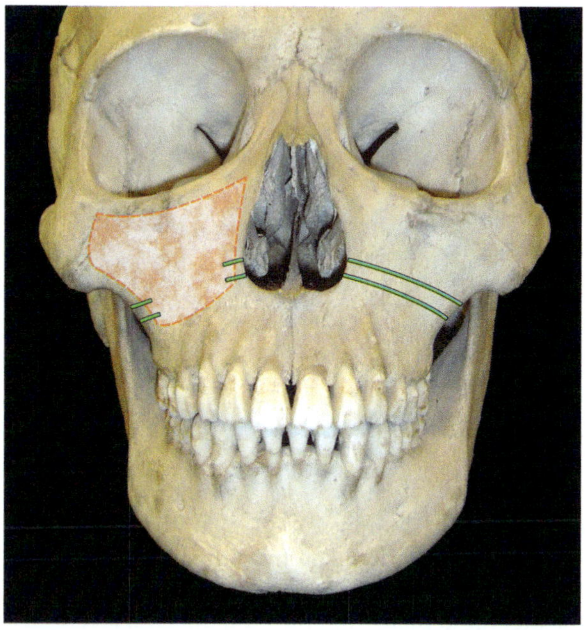

Fig. 26-12 The Le Fort I type downfracture osteotomy of the maxilla permits the removal of bone between the nasal floor and maxillary dental root apices, allowing superior repositioning of the maxillary dentoalveolus.

Upper lip–maxillary incisor relationship

This important relationship has been described in detail in Chapters 5 and 6. The degree of maxillary incisor display in repose is accepted as *approximately* 2–3 mm for young adult men (as a minimum) and 4–5 mm in young adult women (as a minimum). When deciding on the degree of superior repositioning of the maxilla and improving the upper lip-incisor relationship, a number of factors must be borne in mind:

Patient's age and gender

The facial soft tissues tend to descend or 'sag' with age. Therefore, maxillary incisor exposure inevitably reduces and mandibular incisor exposure increases with advancing age. This is a significant factor, as it may be prudent to maintain a slightly increased degree of maxillary incisor exposure in a young adult, bearing in mind the reduction in incisor display that inevitably occurs with advancing age. This is particularly important in women, where maxillary incisor exposure of up to 6–7 mm may be an advisable objective of treatment. As a general guideline, it is better to under-impact the anterior maxilla, than to over-impact and risk 'burying the incisors' behind the upper lip and causing a prematurely aged appearance.

Sagittal repositioning of the maxilla

Advancement of the maxilla tends to increase maxillary incisor exposure. Therefore, when planning maxillary impaction, the effects of concomitant maxillary advancement or set-back must also be taken into consideration.

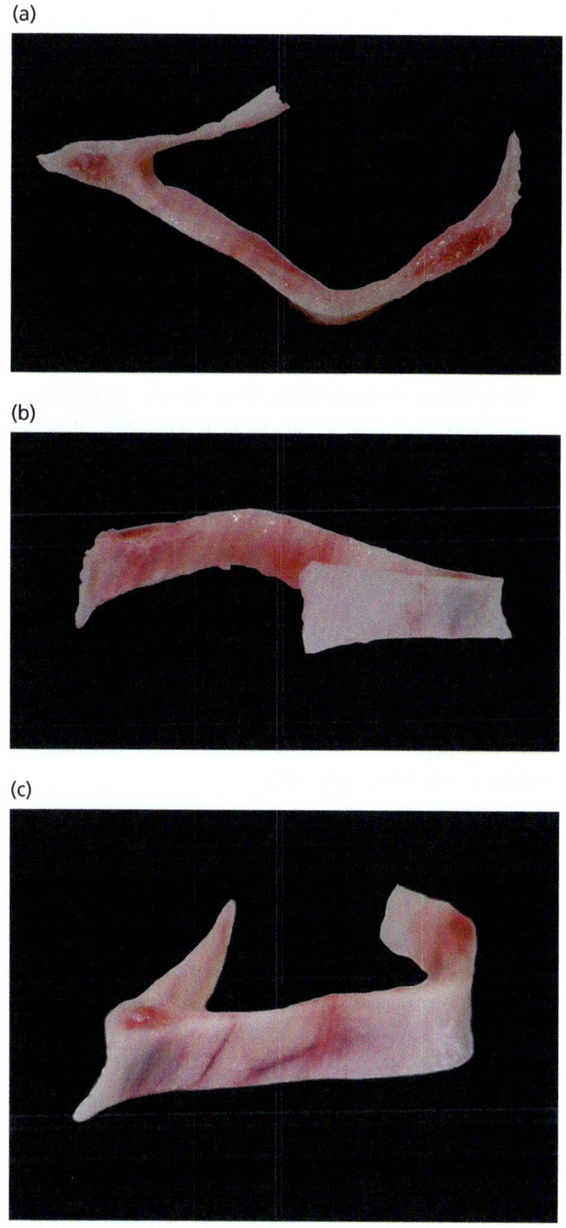

Fig. 26-13 Bone removed from patient's left side prior to superior maxillary repositioning. (a) Superior view. (b) Antero-medial view. (c) Antero-lateral view.

Smile curtain

If maxillary incisor exposure in repose is almost correct but there is excessive elevation of the upper lip on smiling, this may either have to be accepted, or an alternative management strategy sought, e.g. to reduce the hyperelevation of the upper lip (see below).

Undesirable sequelae of excessive maxillary impaction

Maxillary impactions of up to 5–6 mm produce desirable changes to the maxillary incisor display with little untoward facial aesthetic changes. However, excessive maxillary impactions should be avoided as they may lead to broadening of the nasal alar base, elevation of the nasal tip and potentially a vertically over-compressed 'bunched-up' appearance of the midfacial soft tissues. The potential soft tissue consequences of vertical skeletal reduction may be deepening of the nasolabial folds, creation of jowls, deepening of the mentolabial fold, reduction in height and thinning of the vermilion of the upper lip and a general reduction in skeletal support for the overlying facial soft tissues. In such cases a calculated compromise may be required. Rosen[4,5] has suggested the following treatment planning guidelines to mitigate these undesirable soft tissue consequences of vertical skeletal reduction:

- Undercorrect in the vertical dimension – particularly in relation to maxillary impaction for VME; it is better to leave a patient with slightly increased maxillary incisor display rather than over-impacting the maxilla.
- Overcorrect in the sagittal dimension – expansion of the facial skeleton in the sagittal dimension may be used to compensate for undercorrection in the vertical dimension. In a tall face patient *without* excessive maxillary incisor exposure or excessive lip strain to achieve a complete lip seal, the increased face height may be accepted, albeit with some sagittal skeletal expansion (see Chapter 21).

Orthodontic preparation

Preparatory orthodontics has been described in detail (see Chapter 12). However, there are a number of specific points to consider in preparation for maxillary impaction and subsequent mandibular autorotation.

When the LAFH is to be reduced, the mandibular arch should be levelled as far as possible in the preoperative stage. If the reduction in facial height is to be maximized, the lower arch should be levelled by incisor intrusion rather than premolar/molar extrusion. Maintenance of any degree of curve of Spee in the mandibular arch preoperatively will lead to a requirement for postoperative levelling, making surgical reduction in face height more difficult. In terms of the planned autorotation of the mandible, the relative inclination of the mandibular incisors will tend to reduce as the mandible autorotates forward. Therefore, a degree of proclination of the mandibular incisors may need to be a part of the preparatory orthodontics. One word of caution is required, as a reduced labial alveolar bone thickness coupled with thin gingival biotype in the mandibular labial gingival region may lead to gingival recession if the mandibular incisors are proclined. This may be exacerbated by contraction of scar tissue following a vestibular incision if an osseous genioplasty is also being planned.

Specific planning issues related to the surgical correction of anterior open bites in tall face patients will be described in Chapters 28 and 29.

Surgical technique

Le Fort I osteotomy of the maxilla has been described in detail in Chapter 22. A vestibular incision

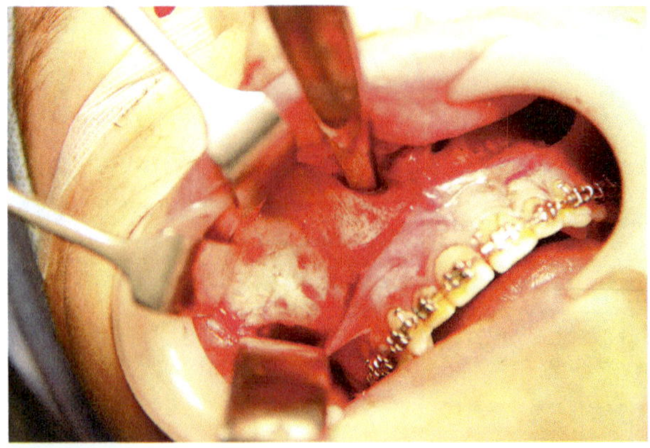

Fig. 26-14 Access for maxillary Le Fort I-type osteotomy.

approximately 5 mm superior to the mucogingival junction is undertaken from the first molar to the first molar. The mucoperiosteum is tunnelled towards the pterygoid plates and the nasal mucosa is reflected from the nasal floor, providing access for osteotomy and downfracture of the maxilla from the lateral maxillary and nasal walls, nasal septum and separation from the pterygoid plates (Figure 26-14). The amount of bone to be removed will have been determined and confirmed during the preoperative planning, including clinical evaluation, cephalometric planning and model surgery. Inferior turbinectomy may be required, as well as nasal septal straightening and removal of the required amount of the inferior aspect of the septum to prevent septal deviation following maxillary impaction. An intermediate splint wafer will have been prepared during model surgery, for repositioning of the mobilized maxilla in the sagittal and transverse planes, and the splint is indexed to the unoperated mandible.

The vertical position of the maxilla has to be determined from a stable superior reference structure, in order to determine the correct amount of bone removal and degree of impaction. Some surgeons use an **external reference marker** (e.g. in the glabellar region, or the medial canthus of each eye), though it is easier to create **internal reference marks** on the bone of the maxilla above the proposed osteotomy line, from which to measure vertical alterations in the maxillary position. The advantage of the submental intubation technique (described in Chapter 22) is that the relationship of the incisor display at rest in relation to the upper lip can be directly viewed without a nasal endotracheal tube distorting the upper lip.

There are two techniques used to determine the marking of maxillary bone to be removed. The first technique involves using callipers to measure the amount of bone to be removed at the level of the maxillary first molar tooth (above the apices of the teeth), at the required height, and also anteriorly (Figure 26-15). The position of the points of the calliper may be marked on the bone by tapping the calliper with a mallet such that the points indent the bone (Figure 26-16). An alternate technique involves the monopolar haemostatic point touching the metal

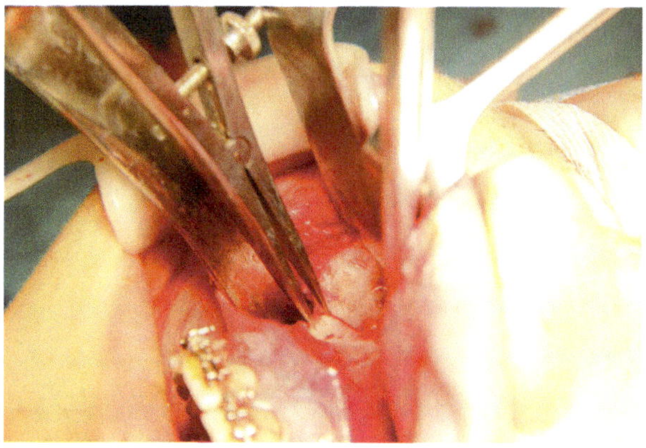

Fig. 26-15 Using callipers to measure the amount of bone to be removed at the level of the maxillary first molar tooth.

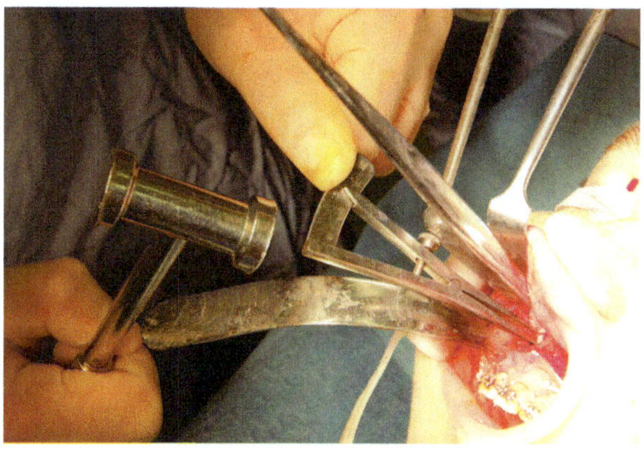

Fig. 26-16 The position of the points of the calliper being marked on the bone by tapping the calliper with a mallet such that the points indent the bone.

calliper and transmitting a small 'burn mark' to the bone (Figure 26-17). It is essential, if using the latter technique, that the callipers do not touch any part of the soft tissues, as these will also burn. The amount of bone to be removed is thereby marked on the maxilla (Figure 26-18).

Once the section of bone from the anterior wall of the sinus is removed (Figure 26-19) and the Le Fort I osteotomized maxilla is downfractured, any further areas of interference will need to be removed.

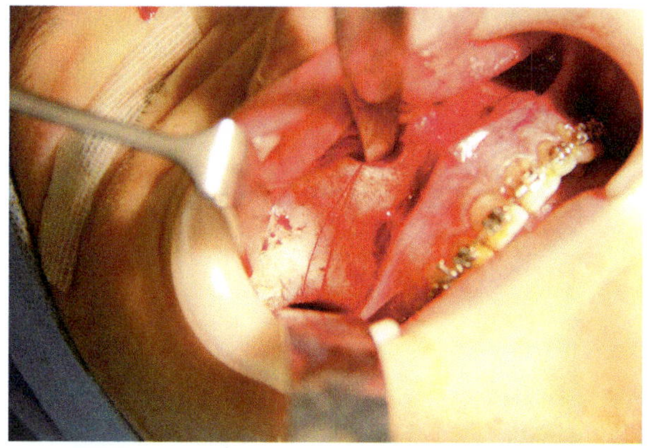

Fig. 26-18 The predetermined amount of bone to be removed is marked on the maxilla. In this case, more bone is being removed posteriorly than anteriorly.

These are usually the area where the greater palatine neurovascular bundle lies, the nasal turbinates, and lateral nasal wall (see Chapter 22). The nasal turbinates have important physiological functions, warming and humidifying the nasal air, together with trapping foreign particles. They are also highly vascular. They should not be excised completely and if partially excised the soft tissue should be haemostatically divided before resection to prevent haemorrhage.

The intermediate (if undertaking a bimaxillary osteotomy) or final wafer splint is then placed using elastic intermaxillary fixation (Figure 26-20). The maxilla is offered up and any initial interference removed. The relationship of the maxillary incisor display in relation to the upper lip is reviewed. Once the internal skeletal reference marks have been placed, it is possible to measure directly the changes in these reference marks after the maxilla has been repositioned in order to accurately determine whether the planned vertical change has been accomplished.

Prior to fixation of the maxilla, particularly with large impactions, the nasal width at the alar base and the nasolabial angle should be reviewed. The piriform rim should be adjusted, and the septum reduced to prevent iatrogenic nasal asymmetry. It is also

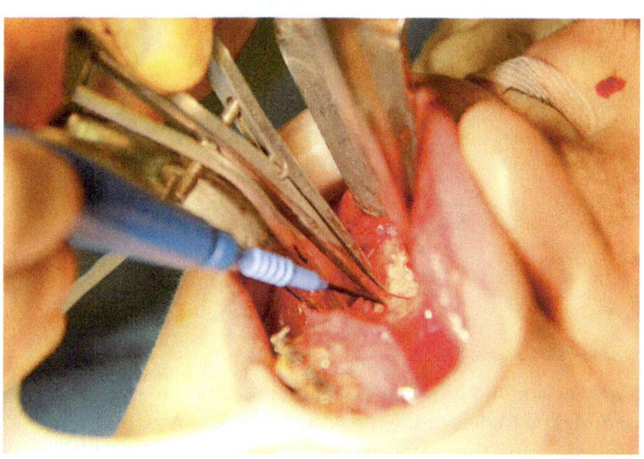

Fig. 26-17 Using the monopolar haemostatic point to touch the metal calliper and transmitting a small 'burn mark' to the bone.

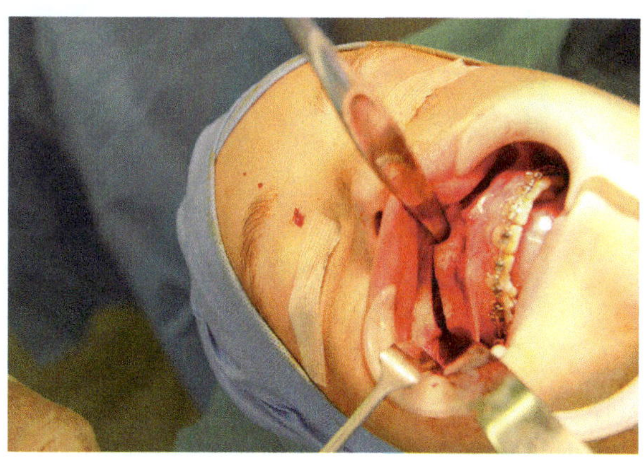

Fig. 26-19 The predetermined, measured section of bone has been removed.

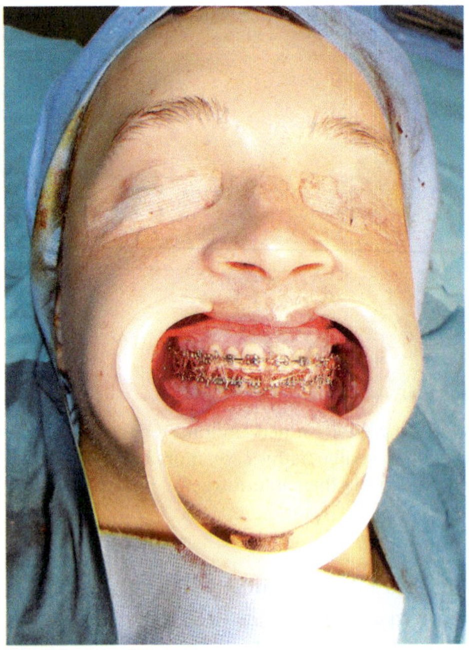

Fig. 26-20 Wafer splints and elastic intermaxillary fixation.

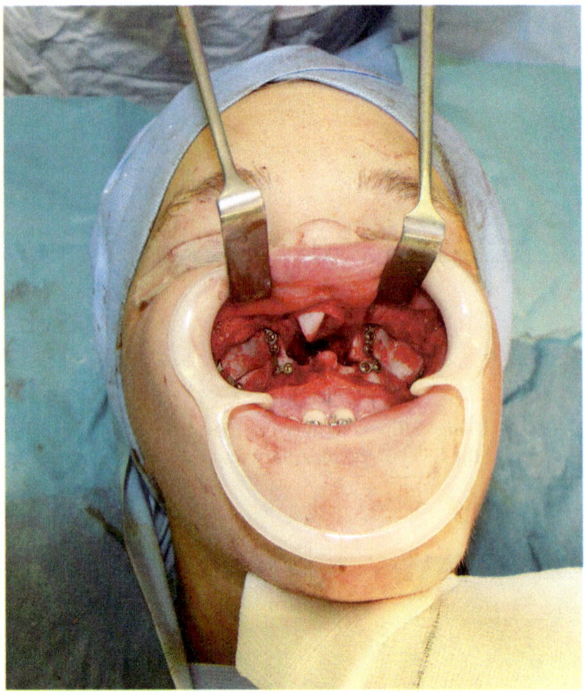

Fig. 26-21 The mobilized, superiorly repositioned maxilla is stabilized in the desired position with 1.5 mm plates.

necessary to reduce undesirable nasolabial angle changes by adjustment of the septum (see Chapter 22).

Once the mobilized maxilla is stabilized in the desired position with 1.5 mm plates (Figure 26-21), intraoperative checks should be undertaken to determine the accuracy of this new position, particularly the degree of maxillary incisor exposure in relation o the upper lip and the maxillary dental midline in relation to the mid-philtrum of the upper lip (Figure 26-22). Unless submental intubation has been employed, the nasal tube will make such checks more difficult, in which case they will need to be undertaken as best as possible, and rechecked following nasal tube removal. The mandible will be operated and stabilized with a final splint in relation to the new position of the maxilla.

Postoperative orthodontics

Postoperative orthodontics has been described in detail (see Chapter 12). As arch levelling tends to be completed in the preparatory stage of orthodontics, the dental occlusion should be relatively acceptable postoperatively, with only minor occlusal settling and finishing required. If maxillary expansion has been achieved either preoperatively or intraoperatively, the

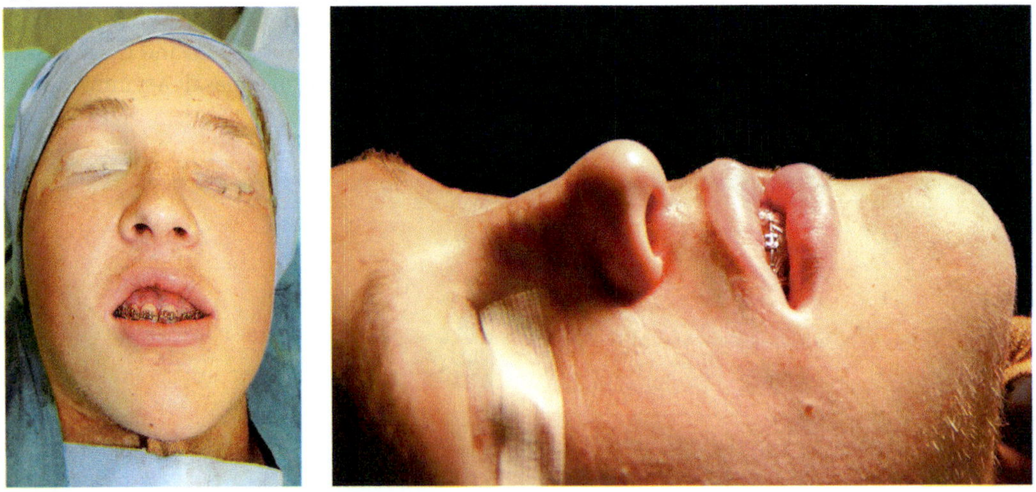

Fig. 26-22 (a) Preoperative assessment, demonstrating degree of maxillary incisor and gingival exposure in relation to the upper lip. (b) Having repositioned the maxilla, intraoperative checks should be undertaken to determine the accuracy of this new position, particularly the degree of maxillary incisor exposure in relation to the upper lip and the maxillary dental midline in relation to the mid-philtrum of the upper lip. Such intraoperative checks are easier when using submental intubation.

expansion will need to be maintained in the postoperative period. A large dimension stainless steel maxillary archwire with some expansion is often enough, though an auxiliary expanded archwire may be placed in the headgear tubes and over-tied. On debonding of the appliances, a modified Hawley retainer with a midline expansion screw may be used, allowing some activation of expansion should this become necessary in the retention phase of treatment.

Case examples

Case 1

Case 1 is presented in Figure 26-23.

Case 2

Case 2 is presented in Figure 26-24.

Alternative treatment options

In some patients the incisor exposure in repose is almost correct, and their concern is excessive dentogingival exposure in animation, particularly smiling, hence the term 'gummy smile'. Alternatively, a patient may have an element of VME but not desire orthognathic surgery. In such situations, an alternative is to reduce the mobility of the levator muscles of the upper lip. This may be accomplished by injecting botulinum toxin type A into these levator muscles and other circumoral muscles, i.e. the levator labii superioris and levator labii superioris alaeque nasi muscles, complemented with applications in the depressor septi nasi, levator labii superioris, zygomaticus minor, or orbicularis oris.[6–8]

The contribution of each muscle to the elevation of the upper lip and to other aspects of facial expression is individually variable. These muscles affect a person's smile and some, such as orbicularis oris, are important in speech. The orbicularis oris is important in forming the lip seal required for the plosive sounds 'p' and 'b'. It is therefore essential to warn the patients that it may require several attempts to produce the optimal result and that for several weeks they may notice alteration in facial expression and occasionally alteration in their speech. However, patients may be reassured that this is temporary and will resolve after a few weeks.

An initial injection (e.g. 20 units of Dysport®; it should be noted that 'units' are not interchangeable between different products, and manufacturer's

(a)

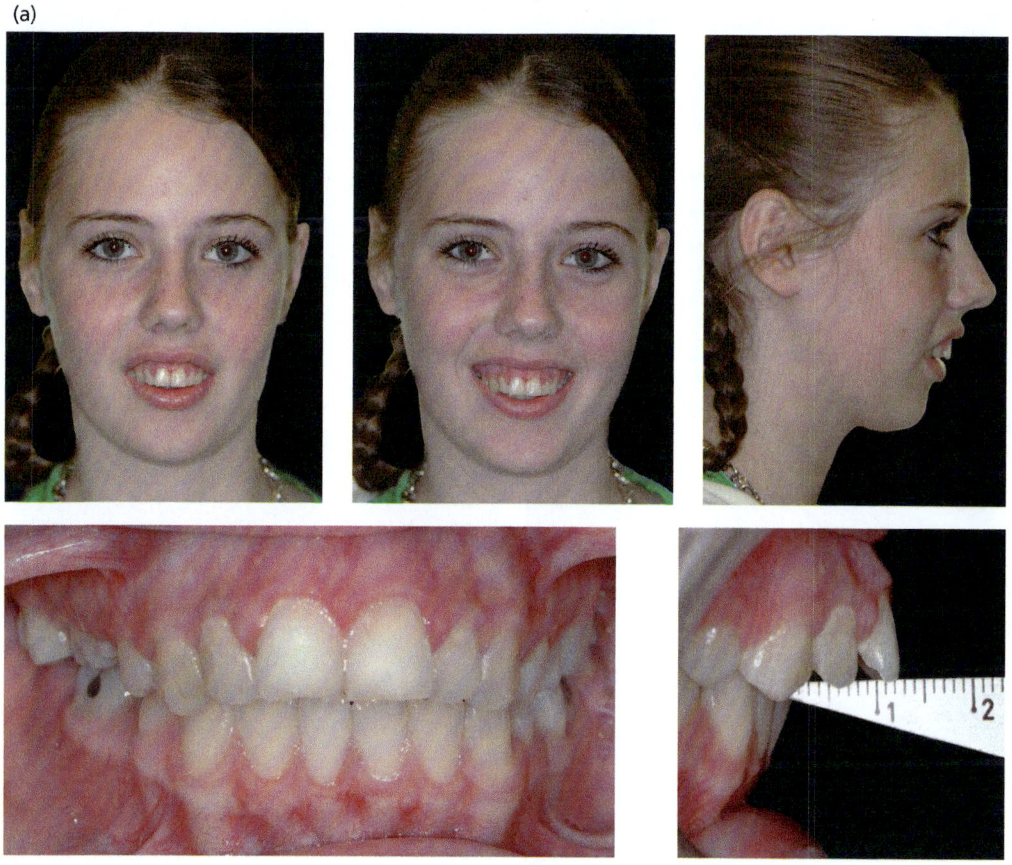

Fig. 26-23 Case example of a female patient aged 19 years. (a) Pretreatment views demonstrate total vertical maxillary excess with excessive maxillary incisor and gingival exposure at rest and on smiling. Upper lip height was average (20 mm at mid-philtrum). Sagittal relationship was Class II, with posterior (clockwise) mandibular rotation, mandibular retrognathism and a 12 mm incisor overjet. (b) Following preparatory orthodontics, the patient underwent a 5 mm maxillary impaction, forward mandibular autorotation and advancement to a Class I incisor relationship.

(b)

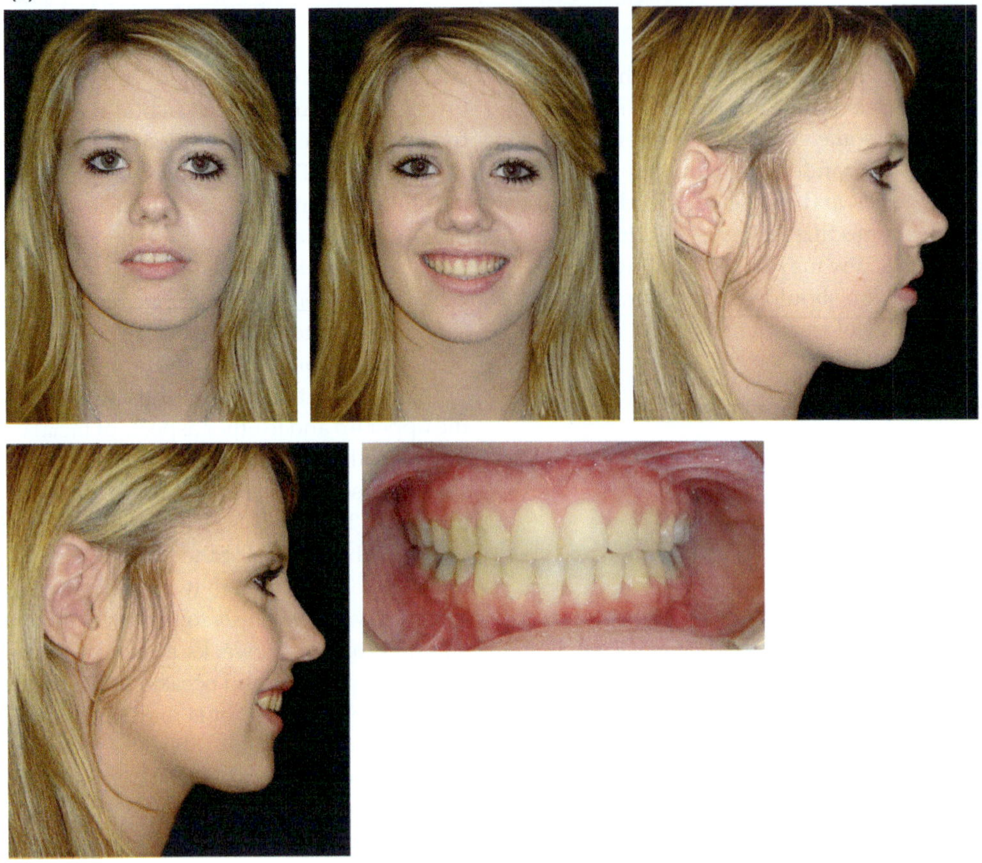

Fig. 26-23 (*Continued*).

(a)

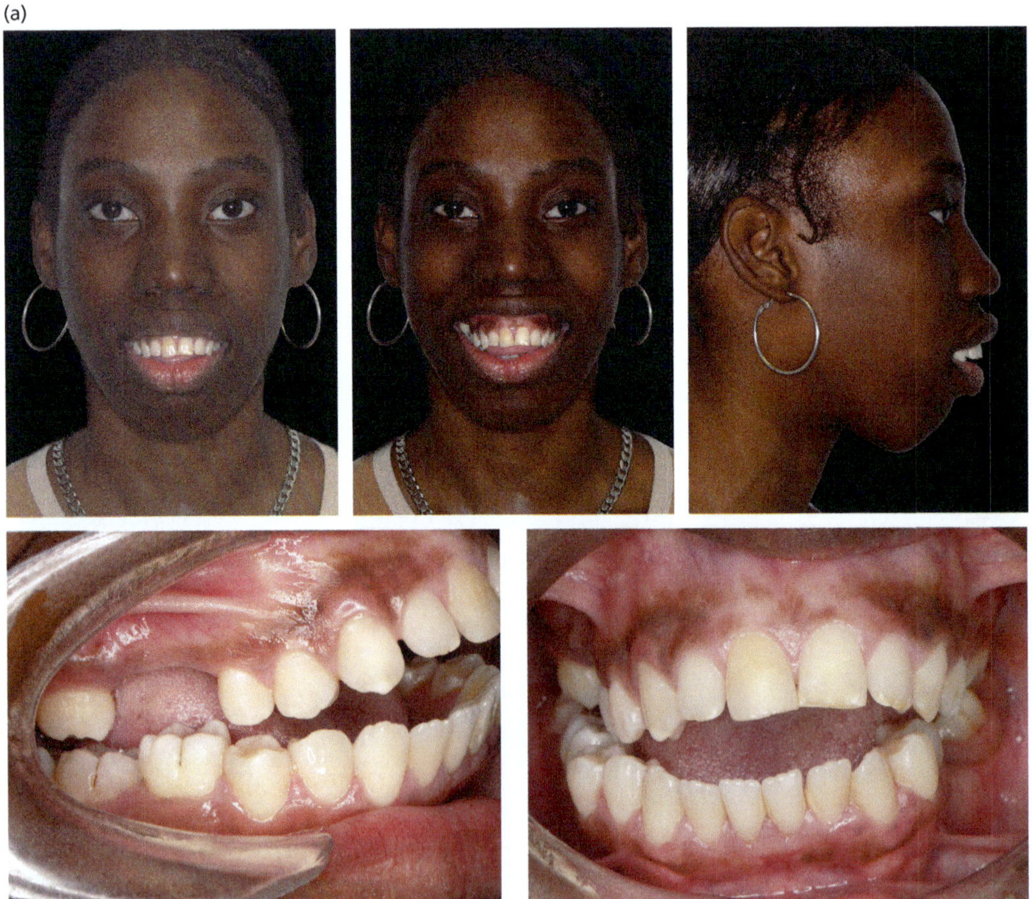

Fig. 26-24 Case example of a female patient aged 20 years. (a) Pretreatment views demonstrate vertical maxillary excess anteriorly, and even more so posteriorly. There is maxillary dentoalveolar protrusion, a Class II skeletal pattern with posterior mandibular rotation, mandibular retrognathism and retrogenia. (b) Preoperative views demonstrating degree of dentoalveolar protrusion, as well as VME. (c) End of treatment views – the patient underwent maxillary impaction, forward mandibular autorotation and advancement to a Class I incisor relationship, and advancement genioplasty.

(b)

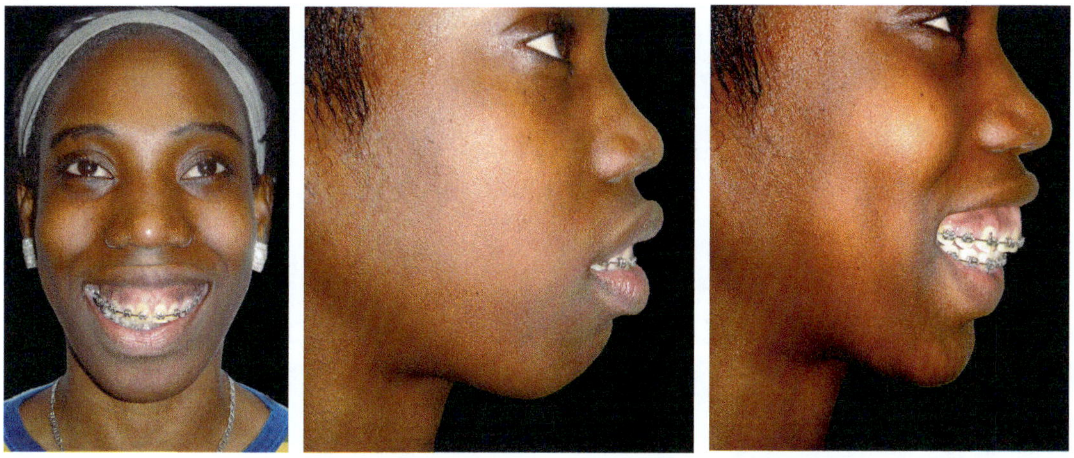

(c)

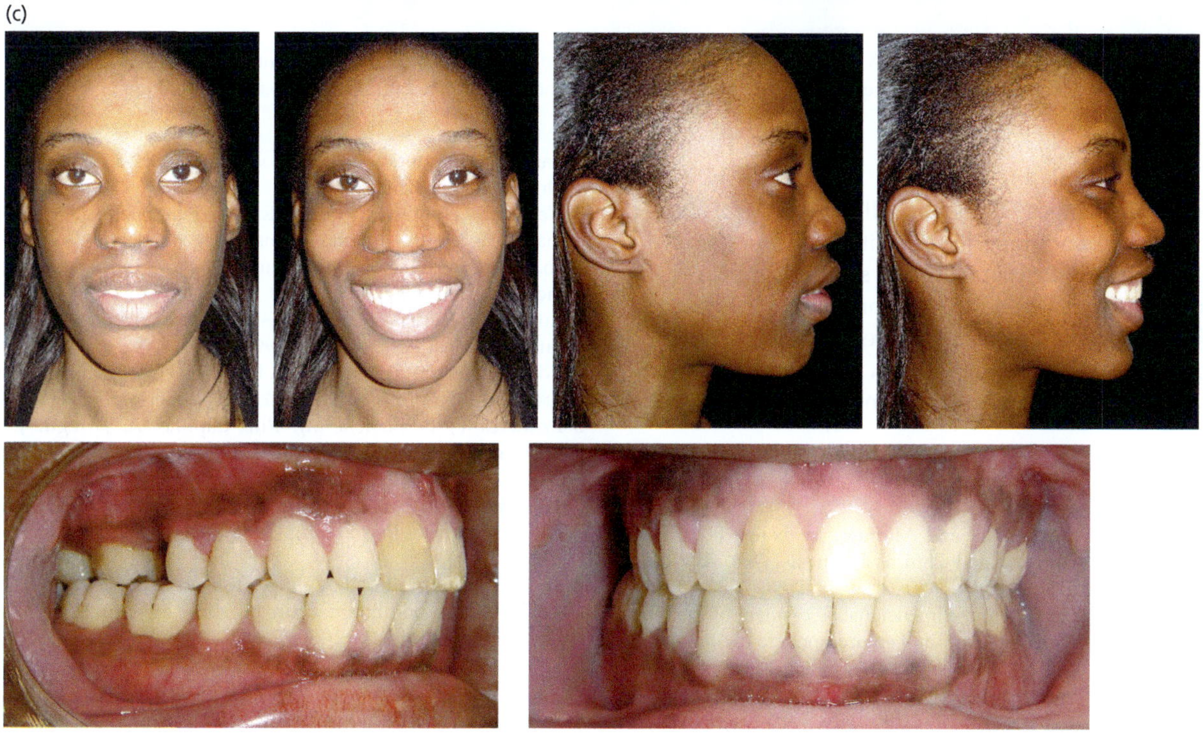

Fig. 26-24 (*Continued*).

guidelines should be followed) injected into the levator labii superioris (either side of the nose, approximately 1 cm below the inferior orbital rim, below and slightly lateral to the medial canthus) is the initial choice (total injection 40 units) (Figure 26-25). The patient should be reviewed two to three weeks after the injection, as the botulinum toxin often takes one to two weeks to be effective.

Electromyography (EMG) may be useful if available to allow accurate injection of the individual muscles. This, however, is rarely necessary. The position of the injection should be recorded accurately to allow modifications in the future.

Injection of the superior (cephalic) fibres of orbicularis oris will lower the vertical position of the upper lip and may affect speech temporarily. The muscle fibres affected will result in a reduction in thickness of the injected part of the lip and an 'apparent thickening' of the lip below the affected fibres.

The botulinum toxin is effective for approximately 3 months. Frequent injections at intervals of less than 3 months are likely to result in antibody production to the botulinum toxin and tolerance. This makes the toxin less likely to work in the future.

Injections over several years can lead to atrophy of the muscle fibres and a more permanent 'lengthening' of the upper lip.

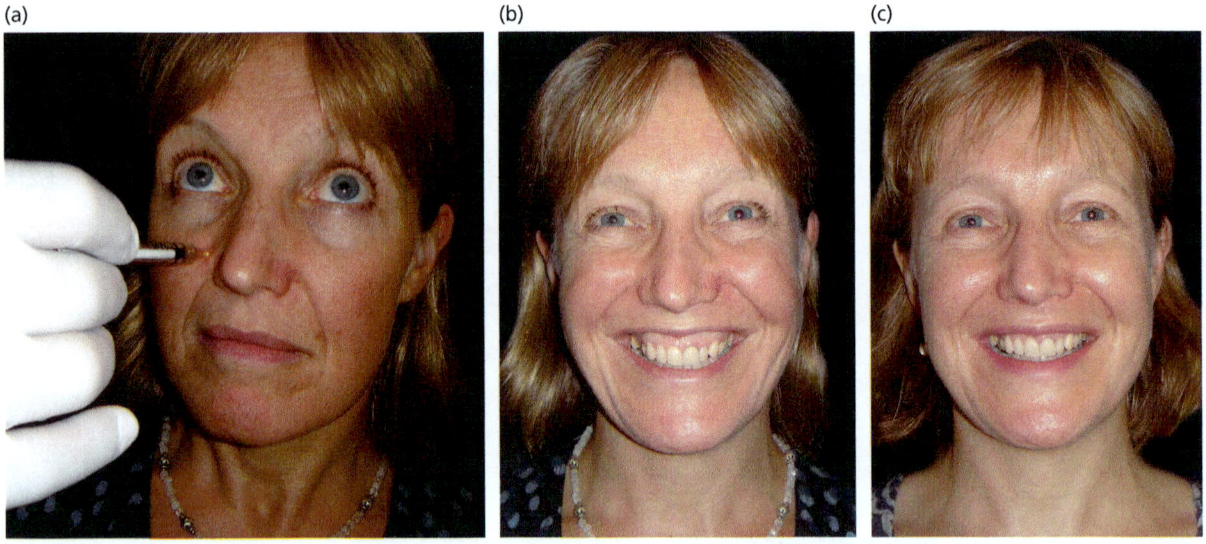

Fig. 26-25 (a) Botulinum toxin type A injection into the levator muscles of the upper lip. (b) Pretreatment smiling view. (c) 3-weeks following injections, demonstrating reduced elevation of the upper lip and a reduction in gingival exposure on smiling.

Conclusion

Vertical changes in the maxilla through Le Fort I osteotomy and superior repositioning and concomitant forward autorotation and sagittal surgical repositioning of the mandible may produce quite dramatic facial aesthetic and functional results. The importance of accurate diagnosis, thorough planning and meticulous surgical technique should not be underestimated.

References

1 Naini FB. The Maxilla and Midface. In: Naini FB. Facial Aesthetics: Concepts and Clinical Diagnosis. Oxford: Wiley-Blackwell, 2011.

2 Naini FB, Moss JP. Three-dimensional assessment of the relative contribution of genetics and environment to various facial parameters with the twin method. Am J Orthod Dentofacial Orthop. 2004;126:655–65.

3 Naini FB, Hunt NP, Moles DR. The relationship between maxillary length, differential maxillary impaction, and the change in maxillary incisor inclination. Am J Orthod Dentofacial Orthop. 2003;124:526–9.

4 Rosen HM. Facial skeletal expansion: treatment strategies and rationale. Plast Reconstr Surg. 1992;89:798–808.

5 Rosen HM. Vertical facial excess. In: Rosen HM. Aesthetic Perspectives in Jaw Surgery. New York: Springer-Verlag, 1999.

6 Ezquerra F, Berrazueta MJ, Ruiz-Capillas A, Arregui JS. New approach to the gummy smile. Plast Reconstr Surg. 1999;104:1143–50; discussion 1151–2.

7 Tamura B. Facial anatomy and the application of fillers and botulinum toxin: Part 2. Surg Cosmet Dermatol. 2010;4:291–303.

8 Sucupira E, Abramovitz A. A simplified method for smile enhancement: botulinum toxin injection for gummy smile. Plast Reconstr Surg. 2012;130:726–8.

Chapter 27

Surgical Management of Vertical Maxillary Deficiency (VMD)

David J. David

Introduction

The maxillae occupy the keystone of the middle third of the face and articulate with bones in three dimensions, hence the terms 'maxilla' and 'midface' are not synonymous. This and other distinctions need to be made at the beginning of this chapter because the terms often used to describe vertical maxillary anomalies have been used as synonyms of short face syndrome.[1,2] Freihofer[3] described four categories of short faces of which groups 3 and 4 involve deficiency of the maxilla, his category 3 being a sagittally deficient maxilla which may or may not have an element of vertical deficiency, in which there is a Class III malocclusion and overclosure of the mandible. Category 4 he describes as having a vertically deficient maxilla alone but associated with a Class III malocclusion. Others (Ortiz-Monasterio,[4] Rosen,[5] and Naini,[6]) describe a square short face with a deep bite where the maxillary deficiency is in the lower maxilla. These deformities are often referred to as idiopathic short faces. The brief of this chapter is to discuss the management of vertical maxillary deficiency (VMD), and so in the author's view, being from a craniofacial background, it is important to discuss the other pathologies that present with vertical maxillary deficiency and their management to a lesser degree, and focus on the so called *idiopathic vertical deficiency of the maxilla* in the context of multidisciplinary team management. The craniosynostosis syndromes, cleft lip and palate, isolated cleft palate, post trauma of the middle third of the face and iatrogenic causes often from overzealous correction of the 'long face syndrome' warrant some attention but are always three dimensional, complex problems the management of which may extend over decades.

Pathology

The idiopathic deformity

Figure 27-1 is a good example of a patient with a deep bite and vertical maxillary deficiency, with the curved lower border of the mandible, and a short distance

Orthognathic Surgery: Principles, Planning and Practice. Edited by Farhad B. Naini and Daljit S. Gill.

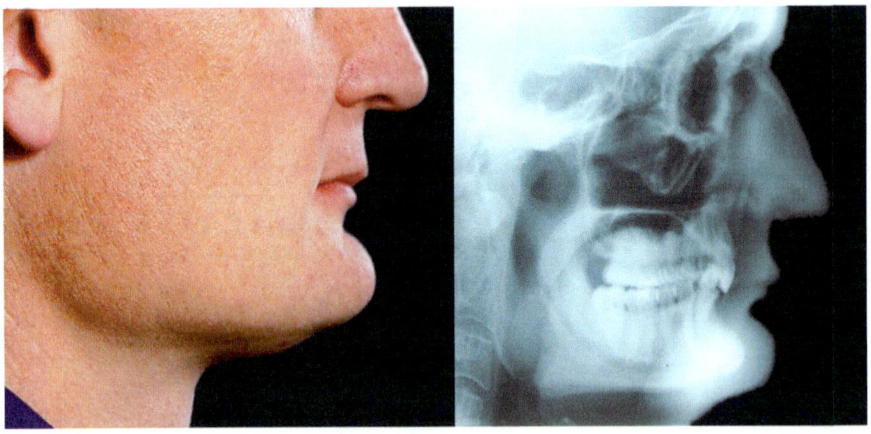

Fig. 27-1 An example of a patient with vertical maxillary deficiency, with forward (anterior, anticlockwise) rotation of the mandible. (From: Naini FB. Facial Aesthetics: Concepts and Clinical Diagnosis. Oxford: Wiley-Blackwell, 2011; used with permission.[6])

between the nasal spine and the maxillary tooth roots. The lips are pouting and there is a deep labiomental fold. The presenting symptom is often deficient tooth show at rest and on smiling.

Cleft lip and palate

Figure 27-2 shows the vertical maxillary deficiency in a cleft lip and palate patient. The bone is usually short in two or three dimensions. The severity of the deformity depends on the severity of the original cleft as well as the nature of the surgery used for closure. The soft tissues are, of course, affected and contribute to the pathology.

The short and sagittally retruded maxilla will need to be advanced and inferiorly repositioned by Le Fort I osteotomy and bone graft. Secondary surgery to the lip, nose and chin completes the result.

Syndromal

A 15-year-old girl with untreated Crouzon Syndrome is shown in Figure 27-3. She exhibits maxillary deficiency in three dimensions, exorbitism and Class III malocclusion with overclosure of the mandible.

Craniosynostosis syndromes e.g. Crouzon, Apert and Pfeiffer, have the genetic problems driving three dimensional maxillary constrictions around the upper airway. The cranial base is short, influencing the midface growth and complicating the attempts to use conventional measuring tools such as cephalometrics.

Binder syndrome affects the part of the midface that develops from the nasal capsule. There is deficiency of bone around the pyriform aperture and the upper lip is long with a typical absent nostril sill. It too can cause vertical maxillary deficiency, and has other systemic manifestations as well (vide infra).

Post-trauma

Fractures of the middle third of the face, even when repaired appropriately, can result in scarring and movement of fragments such that there is a shortening and retrusion of the middle third and each fracture pattern has different consequences. The maxilla may be concertinaed up, the lip and nose are scarred, and any and every pattern is possible (Figure 27-4).

(a) (b)

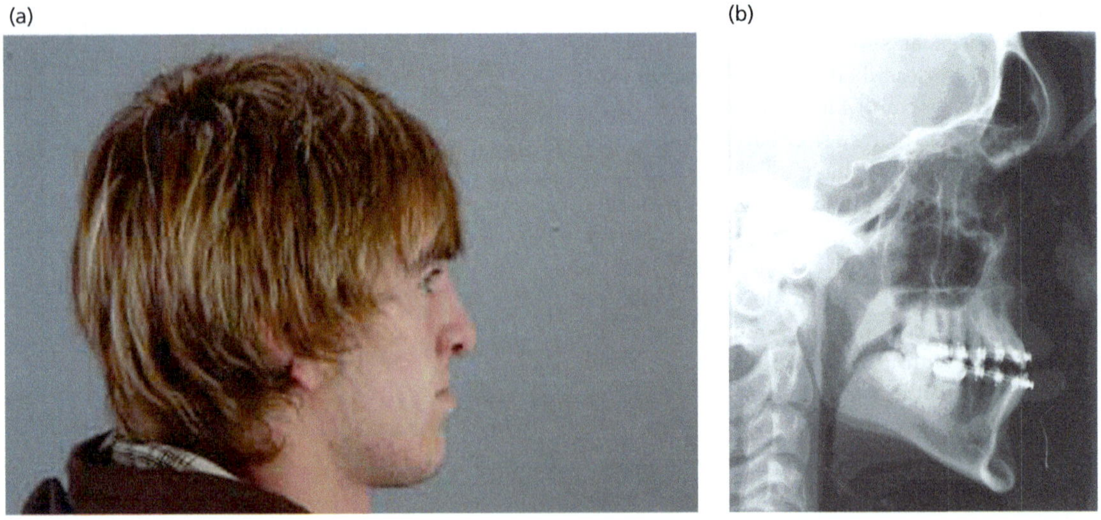

Fig. 27-2 A patient with unilateral cleft lip and palate. The vertical maxillary deficiency is associated with a reduction in the other dimensions. There is a Class III malocclusion with overclosure of the mandible as well as soft tissue anomalies.

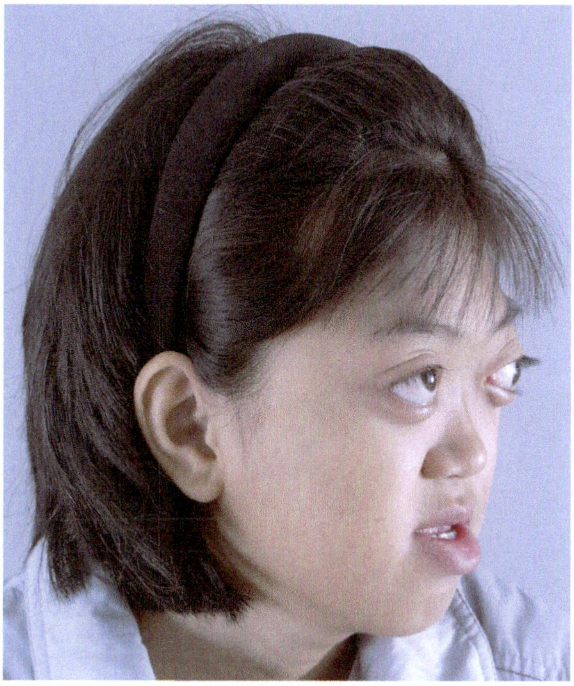

Fig. 27-3 This 15-year-old girl with untreated Crouzon syndrome exhibits maxillary deficiency in three dimensions, exorbitism, Class III malocclusion with overclosure of the mandible. She has premature fusion of her cranial sutures and a short cranial base.

A relatively simple unreduced Le Fort I fracture can present with a short face and open bite.[7] More insidious is the comminuted fracture where in spite of a good occlusion, the multiple fragments and the contracting scar shortens and distorts the face over the healing time.

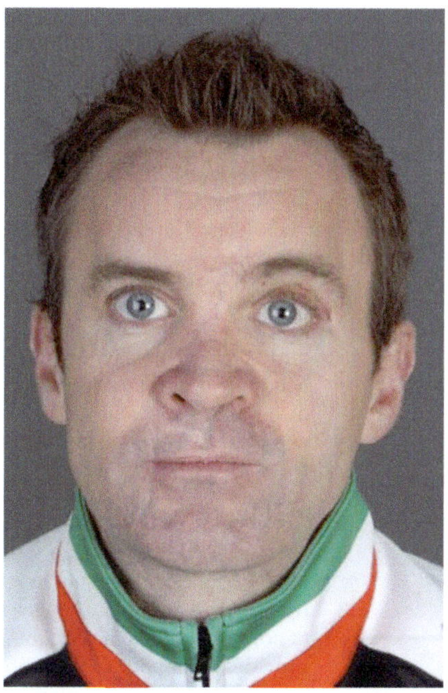

Fig. 27-4 A cyclist who suffered a compound comminuted fracture of all elements of the middle third of the face. Post reduction he is left with a shortened and retrusive face that is scarred.

Iatrogenic

A distressing example of overzealous shortening of the 'long face' patient producing a wide mouth, wide nasal alae, and shortened maxilla. The smile is absent (Figures 27-5).

Changes such as these are often psychologically very distressing. The orthodontic preparation which widened the upper arch, as well as the overcorrection of the vertical dimension has contributed to the iatrogenic problem.

Treatment planning

Management implies investigation and treatment. It is the author's view that the investigation is based on a thorough history and complete examination before proceeding to any special investigations. This is best done in a multidisciplinary setting where all aspects of the problem and necessary care can be elicited. Patients presenting to have changes to their face may come for aesthetic reasons, which in themselves may have social, cultural and psychological implications. Therefore, the social worker becomes an essential member of the team.

The maxillae form part of the resonating cavities of the upper airway and any alteration to volume and structure of the oral and nasopharyngeal cavities as well as relative tooth position can significantly alter the quality of speech.

Otorhinological assessment and examination is necessary to detect any abnormalities of the sinuses and internal nasal structures. Patients with maxillary hypoplasia frequently have obstructive sleep apnoea.

The orthodontic /surgical team is, of course, central to the treatment planning.

Once it has been determined that the indication for treatment is an aesthetic one, the first and best approach depends on a thorough physical examination that enables an accurate description of the patient's facial morphology and how this might be altered to produce the best possible aesthetic outcome (Figure 27-6), taking into account the patient's presenting symptoms and requests. It is a less than satisfactory approach to make a treatment plan primarily on the basis of the dental occlusion, the facial anthropometrics or the cephalometric analysis.[4] Rosen[5] goes further in advocating that normative cephalometric and anthropometric measurements be ignored in surgical planning. Freihofer[3] takes a more moderate view with which this author agrees, viz. '… the measurements on cephalometric radiographs and calculations such as facial proportion index will only give a general idea. The clinical impression plays a very significant role'.[8,9]

An analysis of the soft tissues is vital to the success of any surgical correction of maxillary insufficiency. No consistent, clinically significant correlation has been made between the soft tissues and the underlying bony skeleton. When one adds to this the wide

(a)

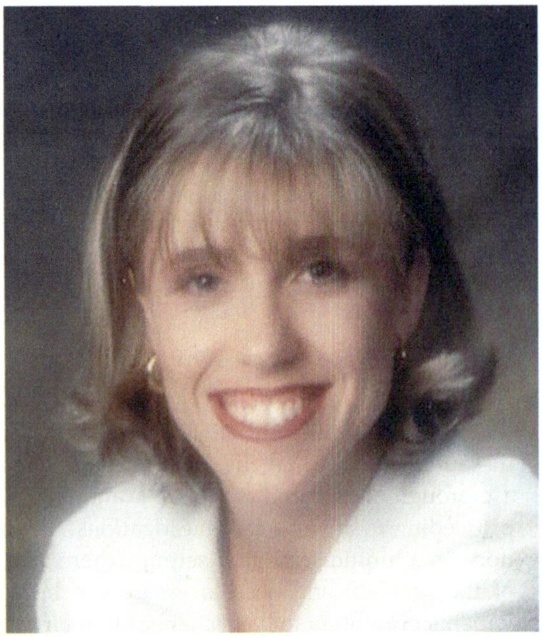

(b)

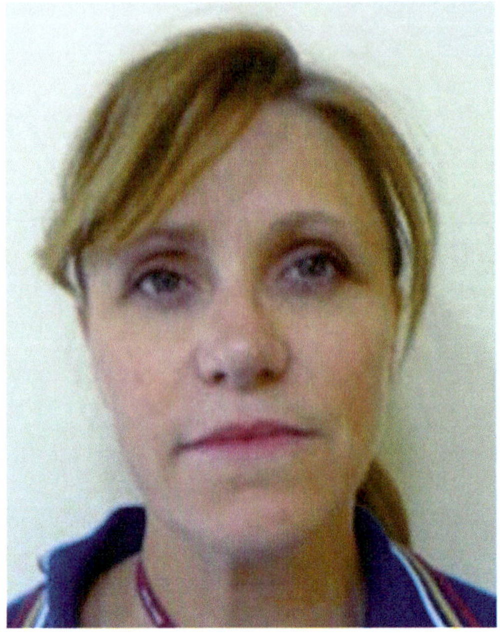

Fig. 27-5 (a and b) Overzealous correction of the 'long face' can produce all the negative features of vertical maxillary deficiency. The face is shorter, squarer, with absent smile and much altered nose.

variety of facial norms and aesthetic perceptions of various ethnic groups, the need for very careful multidisciplinary assessment is obvious.

Idiopathic vertical maxillary deficiency

In the case of idiopathic vertical maxillary deficiency the facial appearance is clinically recognisable showing a square looking face from the front view, with an overclosed mandible. There is reduced exposure of the upper incisors, and at rest there is no tooth show and this may persist even when smiling. The lips may appear squashed and the mouth wide. The alar base of the nose may be flared and the chin may be prominent with a deep mentolabial fold. It is therefore vital to assess the quality of the soft tissues.

(a)

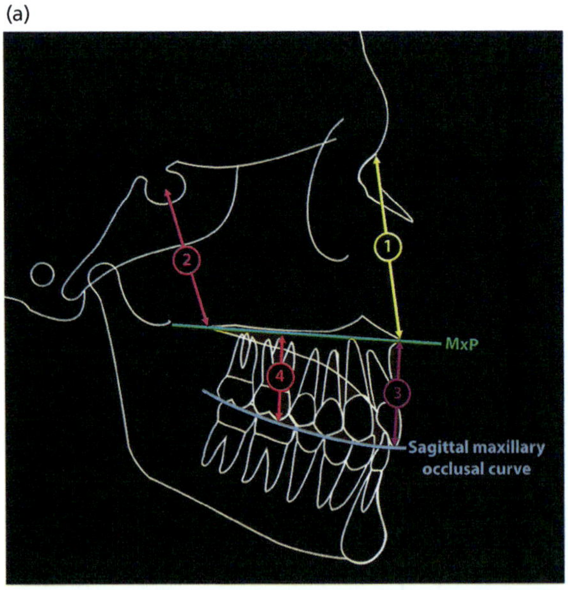

(b)

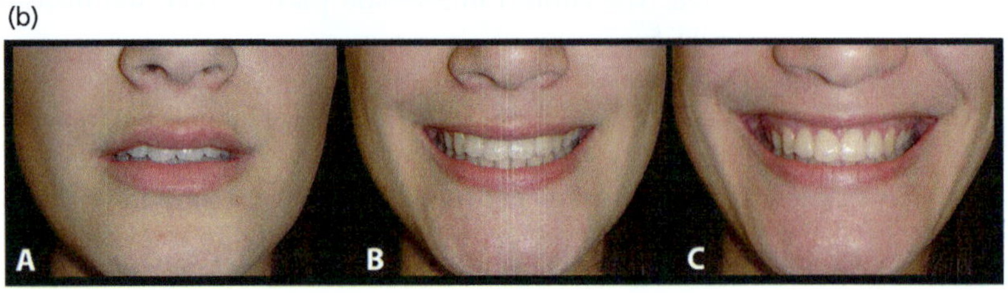

Fig. 27-6 (a) Maxillary dentoalveolar heights (3 and 4) are reduced, and the distance from the nasal spine to the maxillary incisor tooth roots is much reduced. (From: Naini FB. Facial Aesthetics: Concepts and Clinical Diagnosis. Oxford: Wiley-Blackwell, 2011; used with permission.[6]) (b) Maxillary incisor exposure in relation to upper lip: (A) In repose – in the presence of normal upper lip height, this provides an important indication of the vertical position of the anterior maxilla. (B) Posed smile. (C) Spontaneous smile. (From: Naini FB. Facial Aesthetics: Concepts and Clinical Diagnosis. Oxford: Wiley-Blackwell, 2011; used with permission.[6])

Radiological analysis shows a deficiency of bone between the pyriform aperture and the apices of the maxillary teeth. It is paramount to consider the aesthetics of the whole face as a patient presenting for aesthetic reasons may warrant more than a one-dimensional skeletal manoeuvre. The nose being the centre piece of the face must be considered as it will change with midface surgery. The adjacent zygomas must be harmonious, and the chin shape, size and consistency taken into consideration. Anthropometric, cephalometric and model analyses provide confirmation of the clinical plan.

Following the thorough history including determining the patient's aesthetic expectations, the examination, anthropometric, cephalometric and model studies, a treatment plan can be formulated. Usually there is a short square face with reduced tooth show, broad alar bases, and a prominent chin point associated with a deep labiomental fold. Cephalometric analysis show a plethora of deviations from normal but from the surgical planning point of view the decreased vertical maxillary height, large freeway space, and low mandibular plane angle are most significant. The principal maxillary pathology is the reduced distance between the nasal floor and the apices of the maxillary teeth. In this particular deformity the vertical maxillary deficiency is mostly associated with a Class II malocclusion. The supraorbital, palatal, occlusal and mandibular planes tend to be horizontal and parallel. The palatal vault may be flat and broad.

Preparing for the surgical treatment of this deformity involves orthodontic preparation of the arches. In general the orthodontic management before surgery aims to position the teeth over their bases so that the maxilla can be surgically so positioned in order for post-surgical orthodontic finishing to be completed. In some cases the aesthetics of the face cannot be managed by a simple elongation of the maxilla and consideration will then be given to bimaxillary surgery to achieve the final result (Figures 27-7–27-9).

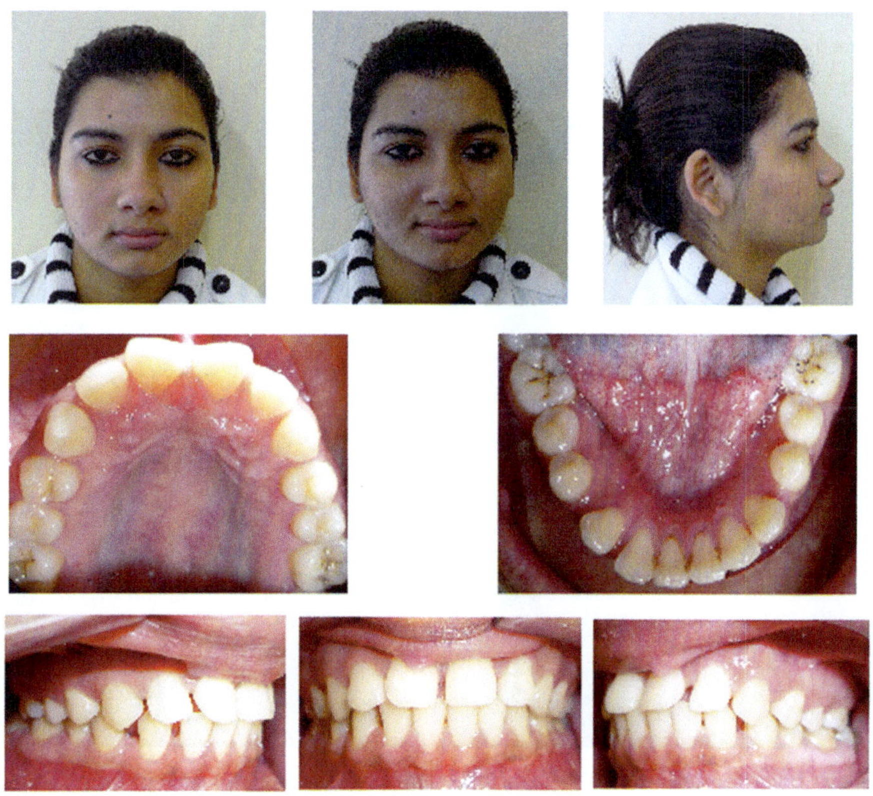

Fig. 27-7 A 26-year-old woman who presented to her orthodontist with the chief concern of decreased incisor display on smiling. On examination she had a mildly convex facial profile with decreased lower face height and her chin deviated to the right. Intraoral examination revealed generalized dental spacing with the upper midline 2 mm right of facial. The aim of treatment was to align the dentition and achieve a good occlusion as well as improve tooth display at rest and on smiling. In order to address these issues upper and lower full fixed appliances were placed to level and align the occlusion and close spaces in preparation for a downfracture of the maxilla. The sequence of archwires for treatment was as follows: At placement of upper and lower braces 0.014-inch Copper wires were used to commence tooth movement. 12 weeks later upper and lower 19 x 25 Copper wires were placed to commence to torque the roots and in preparation to start space closure. 12 weeks later upper and lower 19 x 25 stainless steel wires were placed and spaces begun to be closed. Space closure was then continued over the following visits.

Following space closure impressions were taken to construct the wafer for surgery. Surgical hooks were also placed throughout the arches to assist in wafer placement. Approximately 12 months after the initial consultation surgery was performed. She had a 7 mm downfracture of the maxilla, as one piece with interpositional hip graft fixed with miniplates.

Following orthognathic surgery strong anterior box elastics were placed 4 mm (3/4") heavy 4 oz to encourage settling of the occlusion.

Towards the end of treatment these were converted to straight box elastics on the right and left buccal segments with a Class II vector. 6 months after surgery full fixed appliances were removed and retention wires placed.

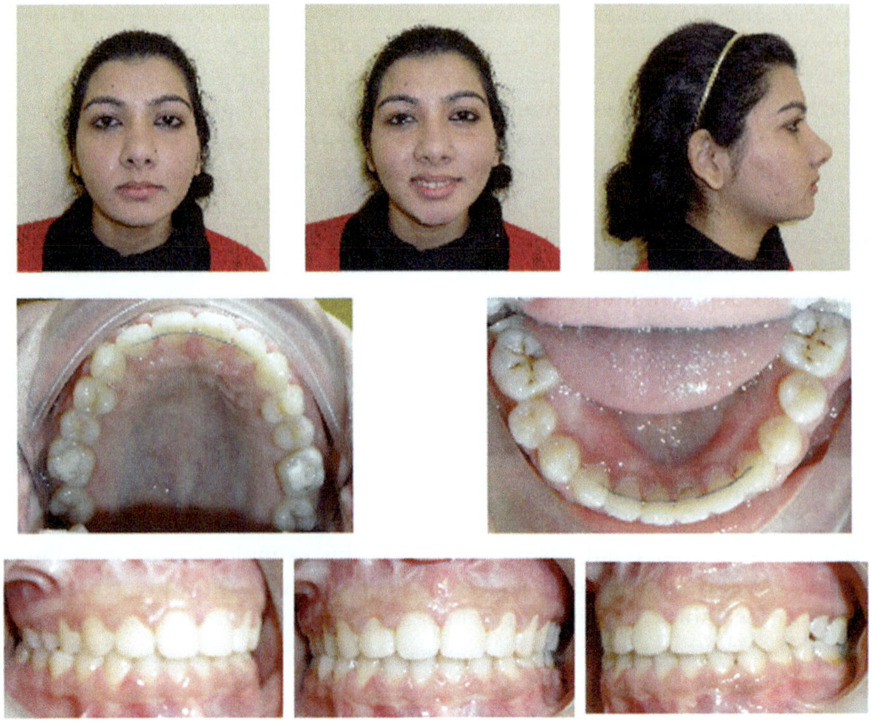

Fig. 27-8 Patient currently displays 4–5 mm on smiling and 2–3 mm at rest.

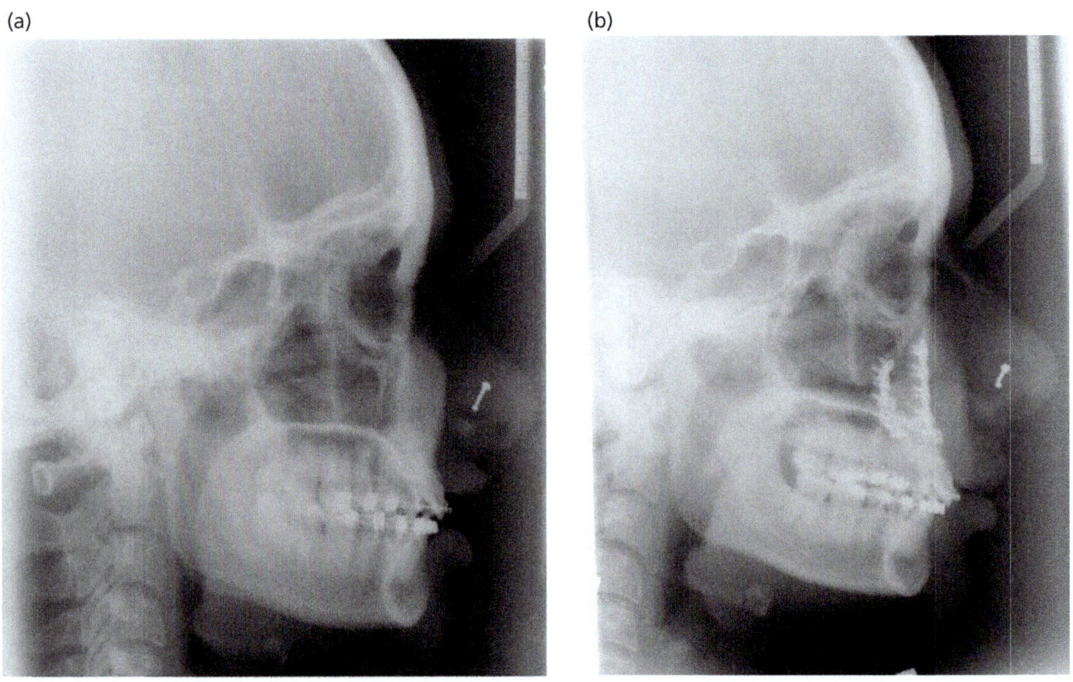

Fig. 27-9 (a) Preoperative lateral cephalometric radiograph. (b) Postoperative lateral cephalometric radiograph.

The following planning decisions need to be made for the idiopathic shortening:

1. When there is anterior maxillary vertical deficiency reflected in minimal or absent maxillary incisal show and a normal upper lip then the maxilla needs to be 'lengthened'. However, a decision is needed as to whether, after orthodontic preparation, mandibular autorotation will produce the aesthetic result, or whether genioplasty needs to be added or indeed whether the mandible needs to be advanced as well.

With a Class I occlusion the mandible will undergo clockwise rotation and it is likely that the chin will need to be advanced to give adequate projection of the lower face.

With Class II malocclusion and a deep bite the lengthening of the maxilla will make the lower facial appearance worse as the mandible rotates downwards and backwards necessitating the need for a bimaxillary approach.

Vertical maxillary deficiency with Class III malocclusion is most commonly associated with abnormalities in the other dimensions of the maxillae and indeed of the overall facial skeleton and integument (vide infra).

2. How much do you 'lengthen' the face to get a 'nice smile'? This is difficult; it is well-known that the ideal relationship of approximately 3 mm of maxillary incisor exposure with the upper lip at rest is the aim of treatment. Cut outs of radiographs and tracings[9] are interesting, however it is naive to think that human tissue reacts to changes in the same way as reassembled tracings. Even the modern computer programmes that predict changes in face shape are prone to wide variations in interpretation and outcome (vide infra). This is predominantly a clinical judgement. In the idiopathic case the robust normal lip will move a little with the lengthening of the maxilla; some degree of relapse postoperatively can be expected although this is much reduced with modern fixation devices. Taking these factors into account adds up to the need for some degree of overcorrection. The situation with damaged soft tissue such as post trauma or cleft lip and palate is vastly different as the soft tissue movement with respect to bone is very difficult to predict. Speaking in terms of a few millimetres with respect to surgical changes that a human face has to undergo such as swelling, healing, scar contracture and re-establishment of function, accurate prediction is in itself optimistic.
3. Ancillary aesthetic manoeuvres: In some cases the lengthening of the maxilla alone will achieve the desired result, however it is simplistic to imagine that this is always so. If the cheeks or periorbital region need augmenting, this is best done at the time of maxillary osteotomy through the same surgical exposure, similarly, with the perialar grafting. In the authors practice the need to advance the chin, in order to adjust the chin, nose, lip relationship is best assessed and performed at least 12 weeks after moving the basal bones as the final aesthetic relationships can only be assessed after swelling has abated, bone healed and muscles started to function normally. At that time genioplasty and rhinoplasty can be most successfully performed.

Cleft lip and palate

A significant number of cleft cases present at the later stages of their protocol management, when growth is complete, with maxillary hypoplasia, which can occur in three dimensions (Figures 27-10 and 27-11).[10] Correction of function and form is necessary to remove the stigma of the cleft. In the usual protocol the maxillary segments have been expanded, the teeth aligned, and the cleft alveolus bone grafted. Invariably the maxillary lengthening is combined with sagittal

(a) (b) (c)

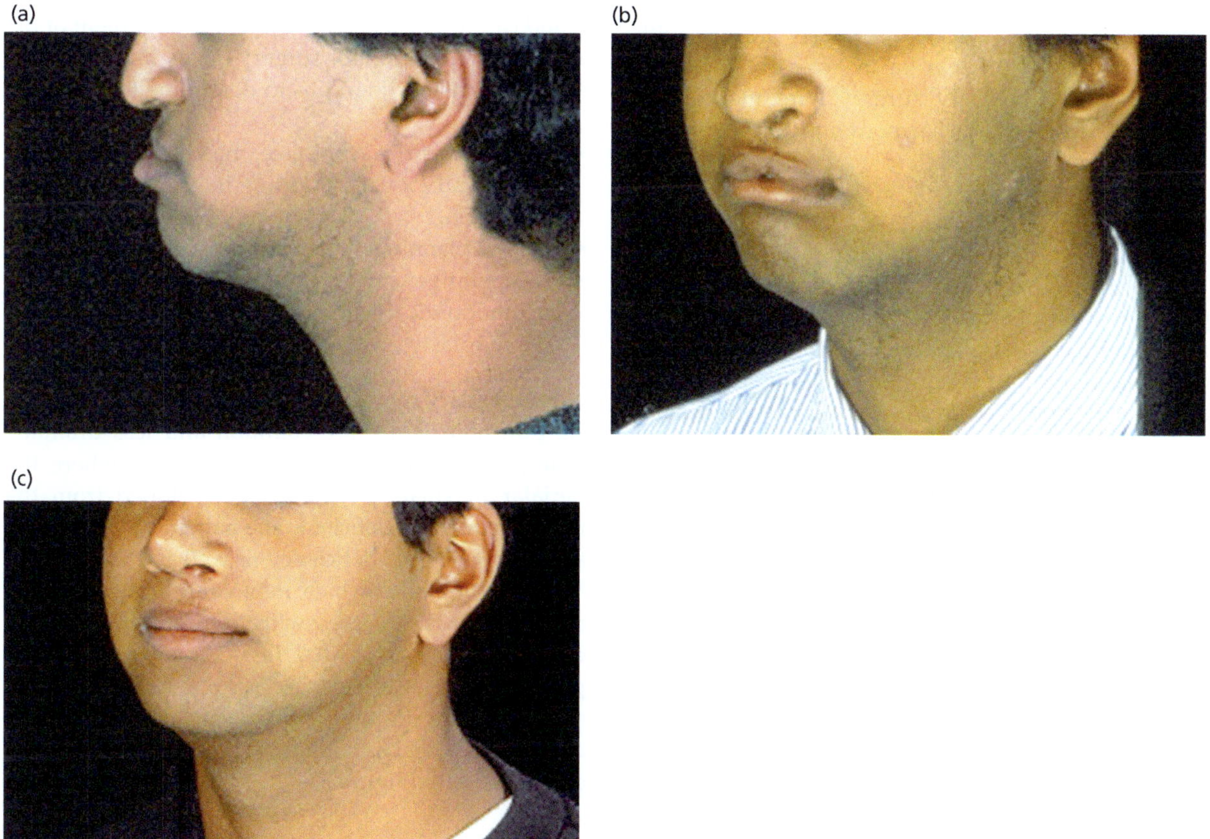

Fig. 27-10 A unilateral cleft lip and palate patient with severe dish face deformity, who is orthodontically prepared (a), has had midface osteotomy with over correction and orthodontic finishing (b). However it is only when the nose and chin are corrected that the stigma of the cleft is reverted (c).

(a) (b)

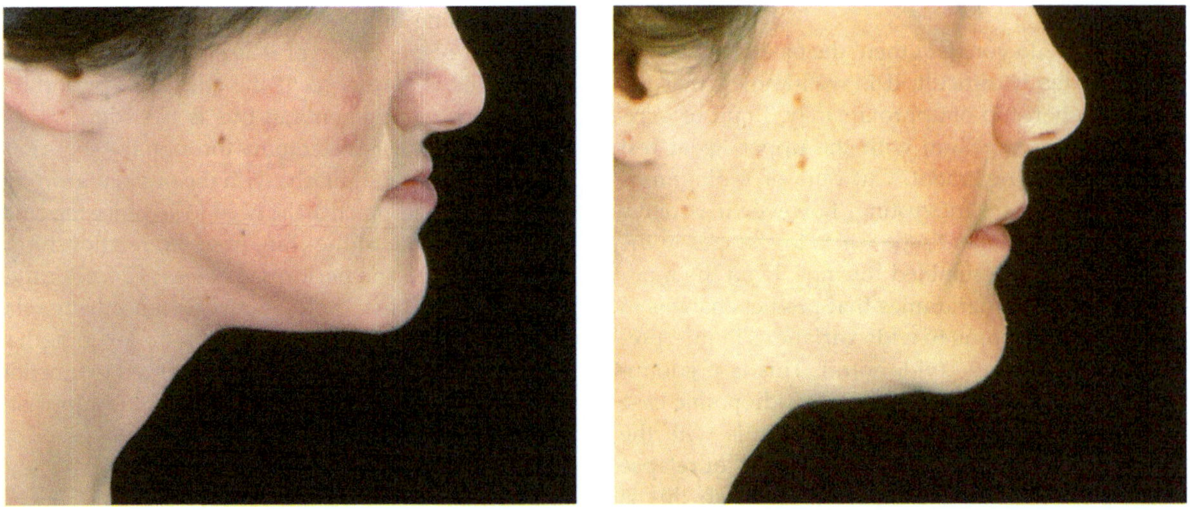

Fig. 27-11 (a) An adult female patient with an isolated cleft palate, flat middle third of face, Class III malocclusion and overclosure of the mandible. (b) The maxilla has been advanced and inferiorly repositioned by Le Fort I osteotomy; her speech exhibited velopharyngeal incompetence post-operatively and she needed a pharyngoplasty.

advancement. A number of other considerations must be taken into account; viz. the need for bimaxillary surgery; flat cheekbones often asymmetrical in the case of unilateral clefts and the need for secondary lip, nose and chin correction as a secondary procedure. Paul Tessier is reputed to have said that the role of maxillary osteotomies is to provide a platform for the nose! In cleft cases with a repaired and scarred lip and palate, the lip–incisor relationship is difficult to establish. Speech can also be seriously affected with advancements of the maxilla in excess of 11 mm,[11] necessitating bimaxillary surgery with mandibular set-back to achieve facial harmony and avoid a serious speech defect.

Syndromes

The craniosynostosis syndromes pose extreme examples of vertical deficiency of the maxilla and as such may require extensive treatment of the whole craniofacial skeleton in a programme extending from birth to maturity and beyond.[12] Attention to the maxillary deficiency, often gross and in four dimensions – growth having prematurely ceased - forms only part of the complex care pathway. These conditions warrant inclusion in this discussion because the techniques of assessment and treatment are essentially the same when it comes to the final management of the maxillary position and the functions that revolve around its restoration.

The protocol management involves calvarial surgery in infancy, and all other problems apart, ideally prepared at the end of growth for subcranial Le Fort III osteotomy having had frontal advancement in infancy. The treatment plan is set out in the usual way and dental models assist in establishing the occlusion but the basis of the advancement is usually determined by the position of the infraorbital margin. The preoperative orthodontic preparation aims to expand the contracted maxillary arch and align the teeth as best as can be done as the correction of the facial dimensions, especially in relation to the eyes, is the primary goal (Figure 27-12).

The surgical treatment plan for the patient in Figure 27-12 was as follows:

- Cranial vault reshaping (aged 3 months).
- Banding using brackets with hooks on the premolars and canines to achieve orthodontic alignment of the teeth in reparation for surgery (takes 18 months).
- Hand/wrist radiographs to determine the status of growth.
- When growth is complete, heavy archwires are placed (0.019×0.025), adding intermaxillary hooks for fixation.
- Surgical planning: Le Fort III osteotomy.
- Postoperative:
  - Orthodontic finishing
  - Genioplasty.

Nasomaxillary hypoplasia of Binder (chondrodysplasia punctata) is a more common and less dramatic example of vertical maxillary deficiency where the perialar maxillary bone – that developed from the nasal capsule – is deficient. The patient has a long lip, alar and nostril sill deficiency, as well as a wider spectrum of anomalies which may complicate the management. In those cases with demonstrable vertical deficiency of the maxilla, Tessier's saying becomes particularly relevant because it is the nasal projection, as well as the lip-tooth relationship that is required after the maxilla has been repositioned, that gives the aesthetic result (Figure 27-13).

Post-trauma

This is one of the most common presentations to the craniomaxillofacial team of patients with vertical

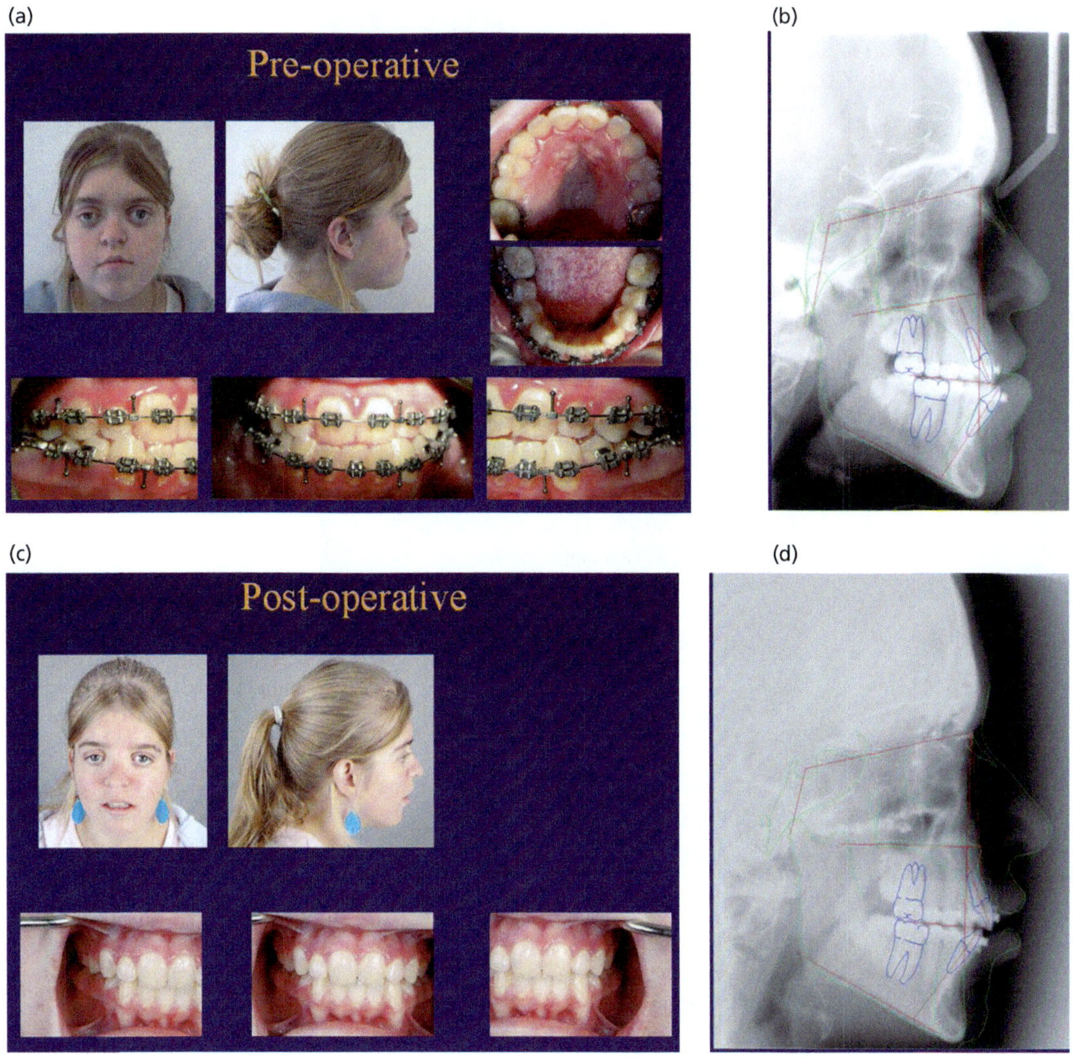

Fig. 27-12 A case study of a patient with Crouzon syndrome of moderate severity. Cranial surgery has been done according to protocol in infancy. (a,b) She presents at maturity, with exorbitism, three-dimensional contracture of the maxilla, and Class III malocclusion. (c,d) She has been treated by orthodontic preparation of the arches, subcranial Le Fort III osteotomy with advancement and lengthening of the whole middle third of the face together with interpositional and onlay bone grafting.

maxillary deficiency. The established post traumatic deformity may arise from displacement of the midface bones, loss of bone, and/or soft tissue, loss of specialized structures such as teeth, or any combination of these. The result is a loss of form, function and aesthetic appearance.[7]

The aim of aesthetic and functional restoration is measured against the pre-traumatic situation, and may be impossible to restore. The complex anatomy of the region, interwoven with vital functions, and the need for aesthetic acceptability make secondary surgical correction of deformity in the middle third of the face very challenging, and nowhere are the needs for precise planning more evident.

The most common deformity caused by a comminuted fracture of the upper jaw is flattening of the profile and shortening of the vertical dimension. There is often associated perialar flattening, widening of the alar base of the nose and flattening of the nasal bridge. The result is often a significant change from the pre morbid appearance even if the primary correction restores the occlusion the contracture between the fragments plus or minus the scarring in the integument produces this result which is most distressing to the patient (Figure 27-14).

Iatrogenic

With the advent of orthognathic treatment of the long face syndrome (gummy smile, idiopathic long face), together with the rules of thumb and latterly computer programmes for predicting the results of surgery, there has been an increased number of overcorrected and mal-corrected faces. This situation presents a difficult planning, technical, psychosocial and potentially medicolegal situation (Figure 27-15). In the author's experience a major contribution to this iatrogenic situation is firstly the attempt to correct multiple problems in the one surgical intervention, and secondly the over enthusiastic attempts to correct the long face utilising a combination of poor planning and poor technique.

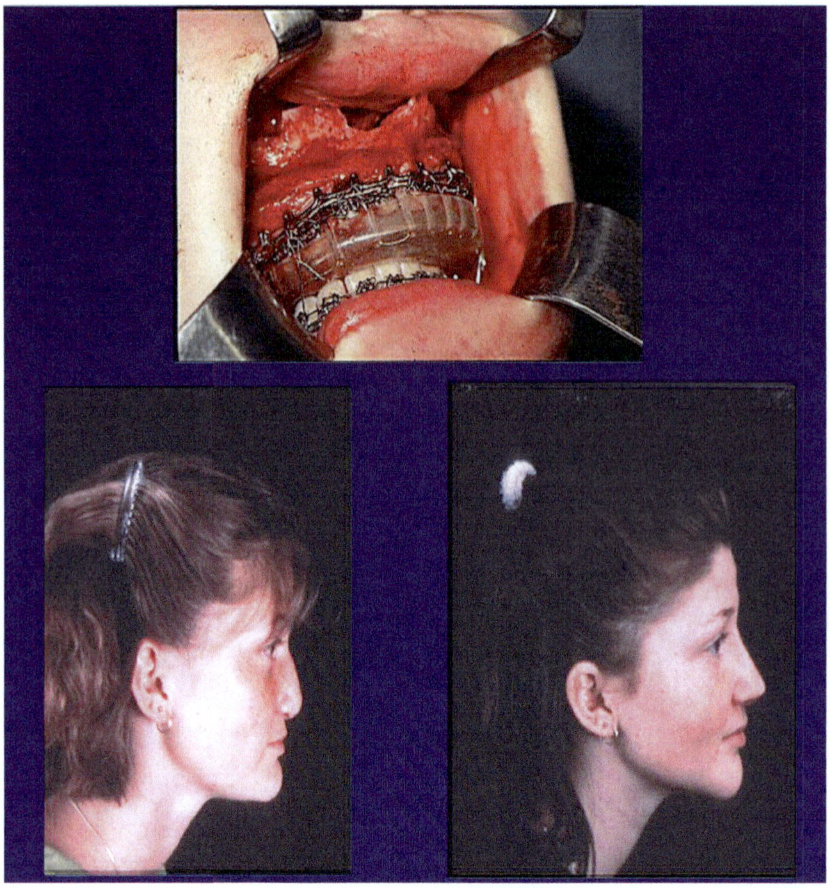

Fig. 27-13 The typical facial appearance of Binder syndrome is corrected by a Le Fort I osteotomy which advances and lengthens the maxilla and at a second stage the depressed nose is augmented with a costochondral graft and the chin advanced to regularize the nose–lip–chin relationship.

(a) (b) (c)

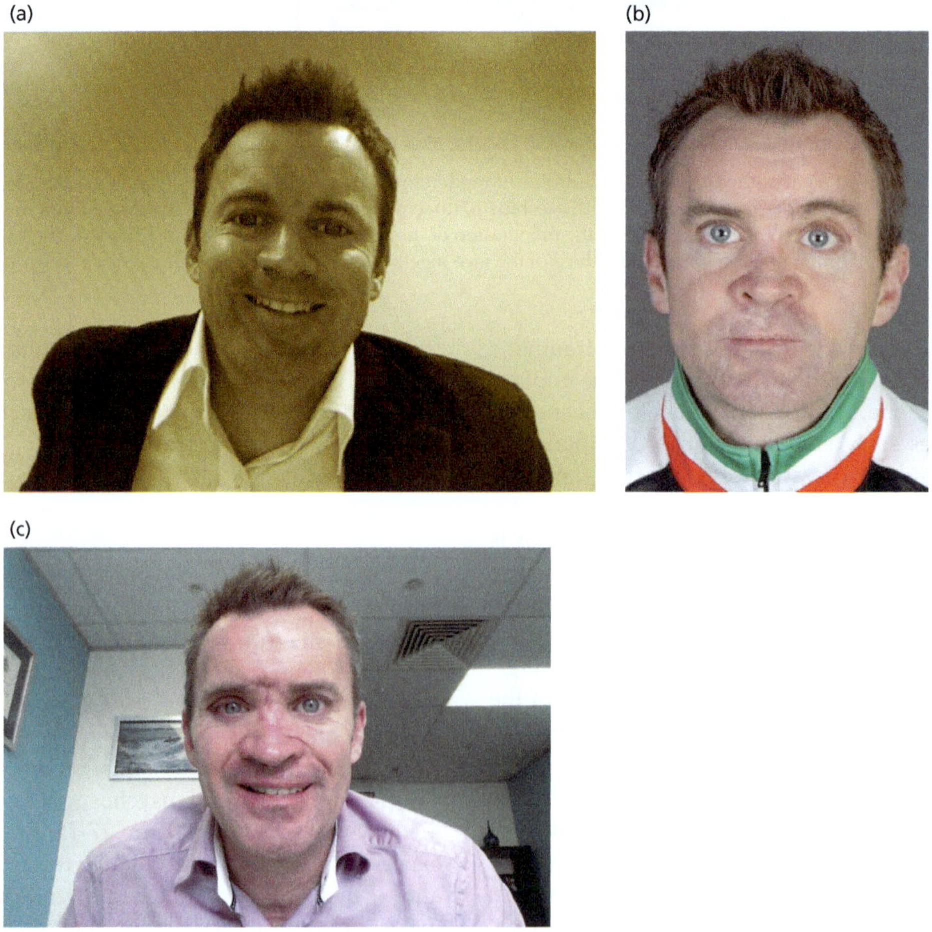

Fig. 27-14 The comminuted compound case: (a) pre trauma; (b) at the pre reduction phase; (c) post open reduction and internal fixation; with a foreshortened middle third of face, long lip, no smile; after vertical lengthening by Le Fort I osteotomy and bone graft.

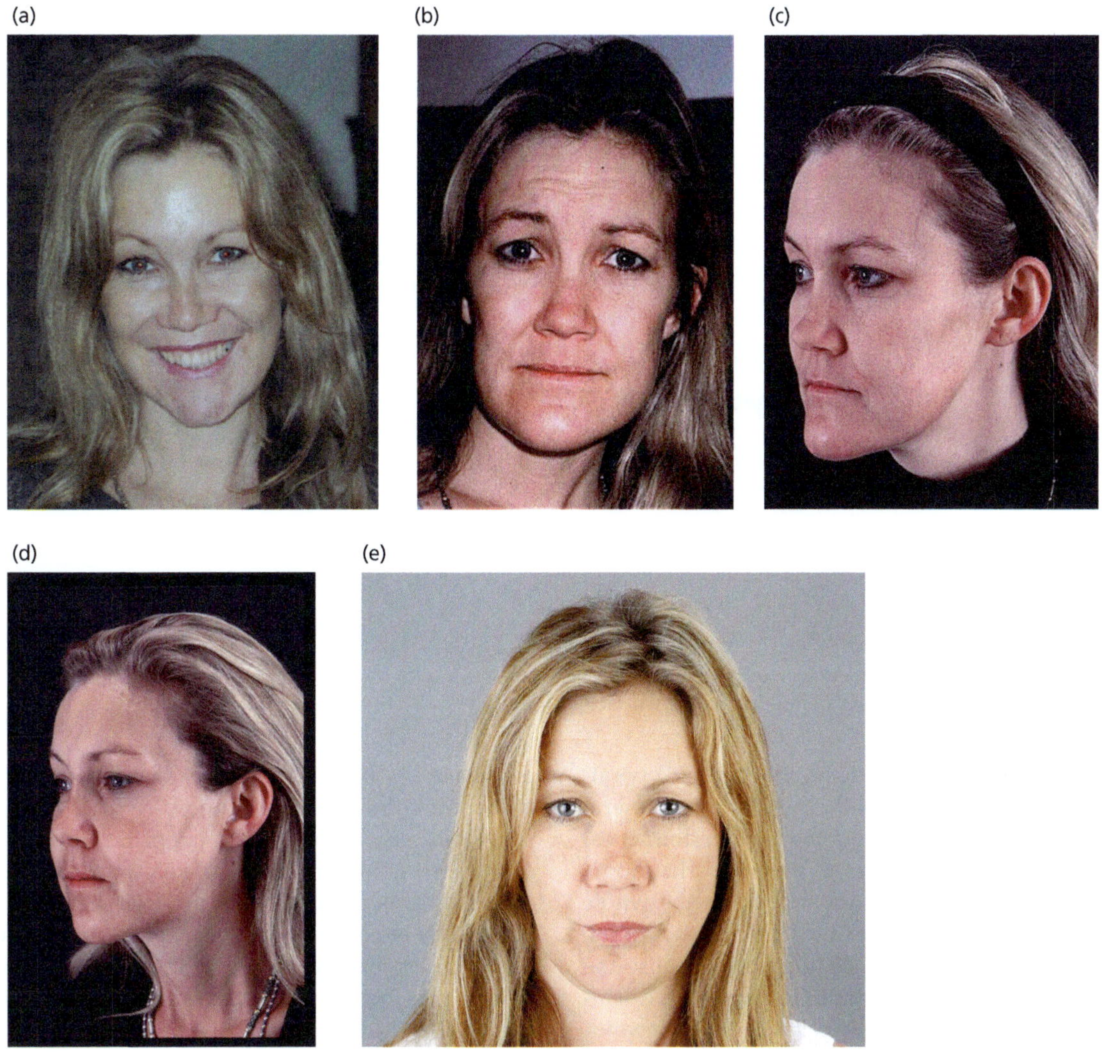

Fig. 27-15 (a) Initial view of a patient with a 'long' face. (b, c) Overzealous correction of 'long' face where the occlusal plane was flattened with assisted maxillary expansion. The face was shortened too far. The mandible was advanced and the chin advanced producing an unaesthetic result. The patient was severely disturbed and it took several surgical interventions to approach the original situation. (d, e) The ultimate restoration involved lengthening of the midface, reducing the mandible, reducing the chin and redraping the integument.

Surgical techniques

The basic surgical technique for lengthening the maxilla is the Le Fort I osteotomy (Figure 27-16). There are many modifications to the basic surgical procedure that can be used to produce the desired result. The maxilla can be osteotomized in various ways to produce movements in three dimensions, and some authors have described using segmental osteotomies in this context.[1] It has been the author's experience that this is rarely necessary in the presence of experienced orthodontic treatment. For the sake of stability, for example in cleft patients, it is best to have the maxillary segments bone grafted into a single unit and where possible have a tooth or teeth erupt into the grafted area. Planning and preparation for the surgery may need to commence as part of treatment protocol many years in advance. The Le Fort I osteotomy can be performed at various levels, low and parallel to the more horizontal occlusal plane in the case of the idiopathic vertical maxillary deficiency with a deep bite. Starting the osteotomy higher posteriorly will produce some lengthening as well as advancement when there is a flat face and Class III elements to the problem. Similarly taking the osteotomy as high as possible up to the level of the infraorbital foramen sloping to include the lower third of the margin of the pyriform aperture in cases such as clefts or other 'dish face' deformities that need support for the alar bases.

The pattern of the osteotomy depends on the nature of the deformity. In the case of iatrogenic vertical deficiency of the maxilla the patient comes to the operating theatre together with the articulated planning models, the measurements and radiology from which the treatment plan was produced and the acrylic wafer fashioned to secure the precise occlusion. The patient's orthodontic appliances are augmented with appropriately stout archwires and have hooks attached to facilitate intermaxillary fixation.

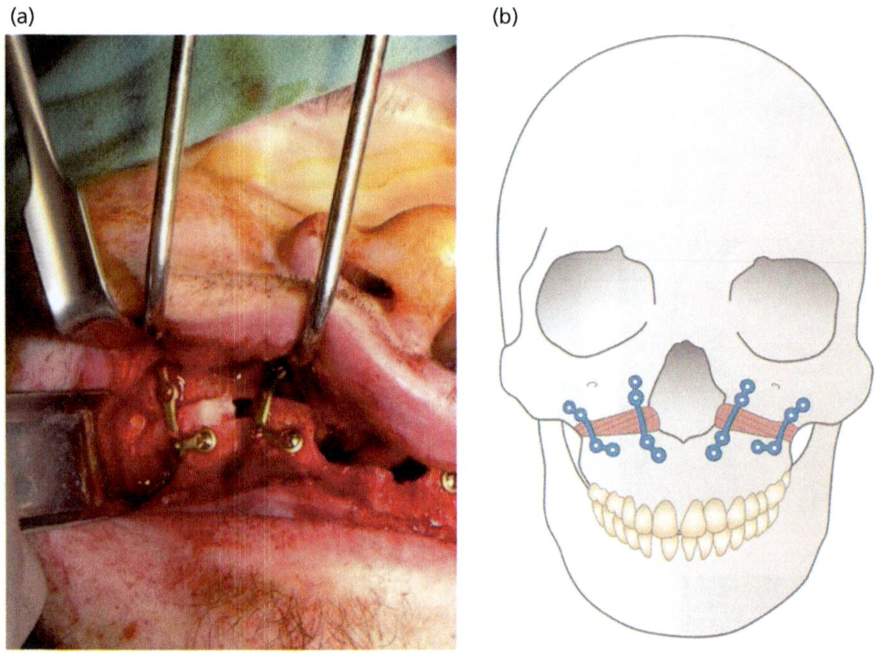

Fig. 27-16 (a) A horizontal osteotomy with interpositional iliac crest bone fixed with titanium miniplates. (b) Diagrammatic representation of the interpositional bone graft after downfracture and fixation with titanium miniplates and four buttresses.

The patient is positioned supine on the operating table in a slightly head up position. General anaesthesia is delivered through a naso-endotracheal tube securely fixed by suture to the nose. The face is draped with head towels so as to expose the whole face as the surgeon needs to be able to measure the facial height during the procedure and visualise the effects of the surgery. In order to facilitate this a temporary tattoo is place in the glabella region in the midline using blue ink, a calliper is used to measure the distance to the central incisal edge, the distance that is planned for lengthening (i.e. inferior repositioning) is added and the calliper changed and fixed, thus giving a further check to the accuracy of the maxillary lengthening.

The right hip is exposed and draped as bone graft is used to fill the gap in the maxilla after lengthening. When the planning indicates the need for augmentation to the malar eminences or the orbital rims, this grafting takes place at this operative intervention. It is usual in the authors practice to have two teams working simultaneously, as the hip graft can be harvested in time for its use in the face thus reducing the length of anaesthesia. Other authors[5] prefer non autologous material for this purpose.

The maxillary vestibular mucosa is infiltrated with a solution of lidocaine 2% and 1:80,000 adrenaline, delivered through a dental syringe. The technique is to infiltrate the subperiosteal plane ballooning up the integument, similarly in the nasal septum and lateral nasal walls. Not only is there vasoconstriction but also an element of hydro-dissection.

The maxilla is exposed through a horizontal buccal sulcus incision extending from first molar to first molar and leaving a 3 mm cuff of mucosa inferiorly for ease of suture. The cut exposes the margins of the periosteum which is dissected superiorly to the level of the infraorbital foramen and posterolaterally to the pterygoid region. When dissecting the lateral aspect of the pterygoid plate care is taken to stay under the periosteum as annoying bleeding can occur if it is breeched. Medially the pyriform aperture is dissected, the mucosa being elevated from the medial wall of the maxilla and the tube of mucosa surrounding the nasal airway – and indeed the naso-endotracheal tube – is elevated as far back as possible.

Once the maxilla is exposed the proposed osteotomy line can be drawn with a bone marking pencil; it is helpful to then mark, using a fine drill, a spot above and one below the line at the medial buttress adjacent to the pyriform aperture for reference purposes, and a smaller calliper can be used to measure the elongation. Metallic brain strips are now inserted medially in the pyriform aperture to protect the mucosa and the endotracheal tube. Laterally they protect the elevated periosteum just beyond which is the pterygoid plexus of veins. A reciprocating power saw is used to make the cuts which are above the apices of the teeth and go through the lateral nasal wall, and the anterior wall of the maxillary antrum. The septum is separated from the nasal floor with a periosteal elevator or a fine osteotome. Finally, the pterygomaxillary junction is separated by inserting a fine curved osteotome around the back of the maxillary tuberosity into the junction.

The initial manoeuvre is a downfracture performed by pressing on the anterior maxilla - not the teeth. Good vision of the posterior osteotomies is achieved enabling any further mobilisation to be achieved under vision. There are a number of effective spreading forceps now available that can be inserted into the osteotomy gaps in the areas of the buttresses to gently mobilise the segment without the trauma of tools like disimpaction forceps. At this stage any bleeding can be controlled by coagulation under direct vision, pressure or application of various types of haemostatic foam or gauze.

The occlusal wafer is now attached to the maxillary fragment and secured with fine wires to the orthodontic hooks. Temporary intermaxillary fixation is then carried out with loops of wire around the maxillary and mandibular hooks. The desired lengthening can then be determined by autorotation of the mandible with its attached maxillary segment referring to the two points marked on the anterior maxilla and checked by the calliper measurement taken at the start of the procedure. The bone graft is fashioned to fit the defects and secured with four titanium plates at the buttresses and incorporating the graft with one screw at least. If additional bone grafting is planned it can now be placed in the desired location – malar prominence, orbital rim, or perialar, and fixed with a single screw. The oral mucosa is closed with a running absorbable suture.

The intermaxillary fixation is removed and light elastics attached to support the jaws. Postoperatively the patient sits up, has some ice packs to the face and is able to take fluids and soft diet as soon as able. The acrylic wafer stays in place with the elastic band support for several days until swelling is on the way down and the patient can easily locate the occlusal grooves in the wafer. It is important to keep close contact postoperatively with frequent visits to surgeon and orthodontist in the first few weeks.

Variations in technique are necessary for *cleft osteotomies.* The basic planning and technique is the same, however there are two major considerations with respect to the planning. Cleft maxillae that are short are invariably misshapen and retruded. They are all associated with the scarring of previous surgery and over correction of advancement of about 25% are necessary. However, when lengthening care needs to be taken in planning because of the abnormal and scarred lip so some degree of unsightly overcorrection may occur. One must be aware that with the maxilla in clefts there is a limit to the degree of advancement before there is a problem with increased velopharyngeal incompetence even when the preoperative speech is acceptable, thus necessitating two-jaw surgery to achieve the aesthetic goal of removing the stigma of the cleft.

From the technical point of view the cleft maxilla should be grafted, expanded, and the arches prepared for surgery in the usual way. The osteotomy cuts are different in that they are higher coming further up the pyriform aperture, and right up to the foramen of the infraorbital nerve. Four fixation plates are used; bone supports the osteotomy and is invariably used to augment the flat cheeks.

When two jaw surgery is planned two wafers are used; the first is used as with the maxillary osteotomy as described, the second to locate the repositioned mandible following the bilateral osteotomy. Intermaxillary fixation is implemented, the fragments fixed with bicortical triangulated screws and the intermaxillary fixation replaced with light elastics as above. The postoperative management remains the same.

The planning and execution of surgical technique may become more complex with *syndromal cases.* An example of this is Binder syndrome (Chondrodysplasia punctata),[13] where the short face and overclosed mandible is associated with the need for nasal, and perinasal augmentation as well as genioplasty. The essential lengthening of the maxilla is basically the same as described above.

By way of contrast the more severe deformities of Crouzon, Apert or Pfeiffer syndrome have multiple dimensions of deformity and complex protocols for delivery of care which are beyond the scope of this chapter (see Chapters 57 and 58). However, some idea can be gained by considering two examples of vertical maxillary deficiency in such cases. The first is the situation in a relatively mild case of Crouzon syndrome whose cranial vault has been expanded in infancy and who presents at maturity with some exorbitism, Class III malocclusion and three dimensional contraction of the maxilla with all the facial stigmata of the syndrome (see Figure 27-12). The contracted upper arch is expanded orthodontically, the teeth aligned in the arches, and the planning tools used as above. However, the use of many cephalometric analyses is severely limited in view of the foreshortened and distorted cranial base. The key measurement is the distance from the inferior orbital rim to the convexity of the globe in the mid-pupillary line when planning a Le Fort III osteotomy. This movement will invariably produce a malocclusion which must be predicted in the model planning and dealt with orthodontically or by further orthognathic surgery at a Le Fort I level at a later date. Shape adjustments to the advanced maxilla are achieved with onlay bone grafts. The author's technique for this surgery is to expose the orbits and middle third of the face via the coronal approach, insert bone grafts into the gaps created in the lateral orbital walls, and zygomatic arches. The osteotomies are fixed with titanium plates. The intermaxillary fixation is released as before and the advancement supported with light elastics.

The second example comes from the other end of the severity spectrum, a case of Apert syndrome where the vertical maxillary deficiency is but part of such a severe midface constriction that the eyes are threatened with exposure and the airway is compromised. The indication for surgery in these circumstances is functional and basic viz. creating the ability to breathe and see. Whilst ultimately important in its own right the occlusion takes second place in this scenario.

If the patient is a child or if a young adult who has been operated before the method of choice for achieving the lengthening and advancement of the middle third of the face is a Le Fort III osteotomy using distraction devices to achieve a forward and downward

(a) (b)

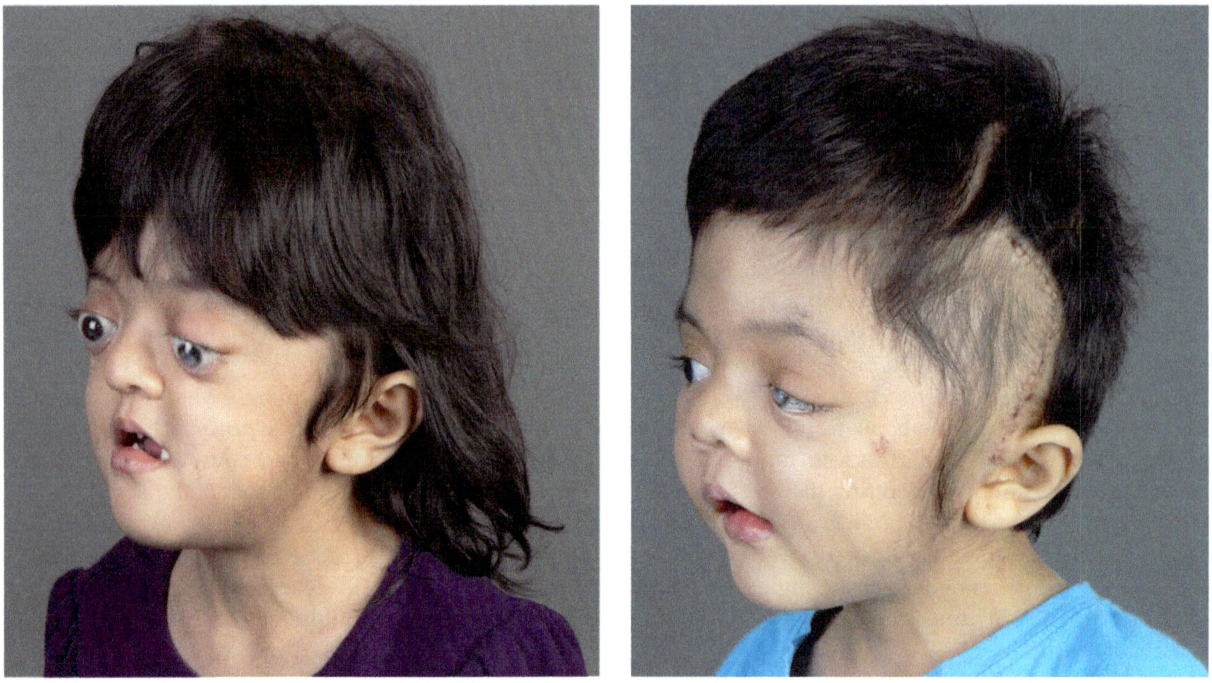

Fig. 27-17 A case of Apert syndrome previously unoperated; she has gross exorbitism and corneal damage, chronic airway obstruction and a severe Class III malocclusion. Full frontofacial advancement in a monobloc has been achieved with distraction devices, relieving the exorbitism and airway obstruction as well as changing the facial aesthetics.

movement. If time and clinical circumstances allow the dental arches are prepared as before (Figure 27-17).

The patient shown was treated with a monobloc osteotomy which includes the midface and brow in one piece and the frontal bone attached by plates. This result has been achieved by using internal distraction devices. Note that the lengthening and advancement of the midface has autorotated the mandible to such a degree as to expose a sagittal mandibular deficiency.

In the case of vertical deficiency of the maxilla resulting from *trauma* the multidisciplinary approach is even more essential as the trauma causing the vertical midface deficiency may affect the teeth, oral cavity and nasal cavities thus altering speech and mastication. Neurological deficit should be taken into account as a result of the head injury. Generally prosthodontic and orthodontic treatment is necessary, following the restoration; surgical planning can proceed with clinical assessment, radiology and model surgery. More than ever when deciding the desired vertical dimensions of the impacted maxilla, problems with overlying scarred tissue must be considered; when the lips are scarred the soft tissue will not readily follow the bone, and an ideal maxillary restoration may expose too much tooth and gum.

The pattern of osteotomy depends on the pattern of the fracture and the nature of the deformity. To re-establish normal occlusion and premorbid dimensions of the maxilla the surgeon must be prepared to and capable of moving all the segments in order to achieve the result as planned. However, the commonest surgical manoeuvre is the Le Fort I osteotomy as described but with the added emphasis of restoring adjacent structures such as the pyriform aperture, and the supporting buttresses of the middle third of the face using bone graft where and when necessary[7] (Figures 27-14 and 27-18).

With the advent of, and enthusiasm for correction of the long face came a number of *iatrogenic vertical maxillary deficiencies*. This can result from misdiagnosis, over enthusiastic reduction of the midface height, or by attempting to correct multiple lengths and angles using predictive computer models at one operation. It is the author's experience that reversing the series of procedures is not always a simple matter (Figure 27-15).

Ancillary surgical techniques

The bone grafting, inlay and onlay, is performed at the stage of midface osteotomy for lengthening (Figure 27-16). The other ancillary surgical procedures that need to be considered to enhance the final aesthetic result are genioplasty, rhinoplasty and the manipulation of soft tissues. It is the author's view that these procedures are best performed at least three months after the original major surgery as a more precise idea of the nature and extent of the surgery can be gained and is not dependent on second guessing how previous movements will turn out. For example, the Ricketts E-line can be achieved in a suitable case by a combination of genioplasty, rhinoplasty and soft tissue reduction or augmentation of the lips (see Chapter 5).

In the Caucasian population the relationship of lip, nose and chin as described by Ricketts is a consistent

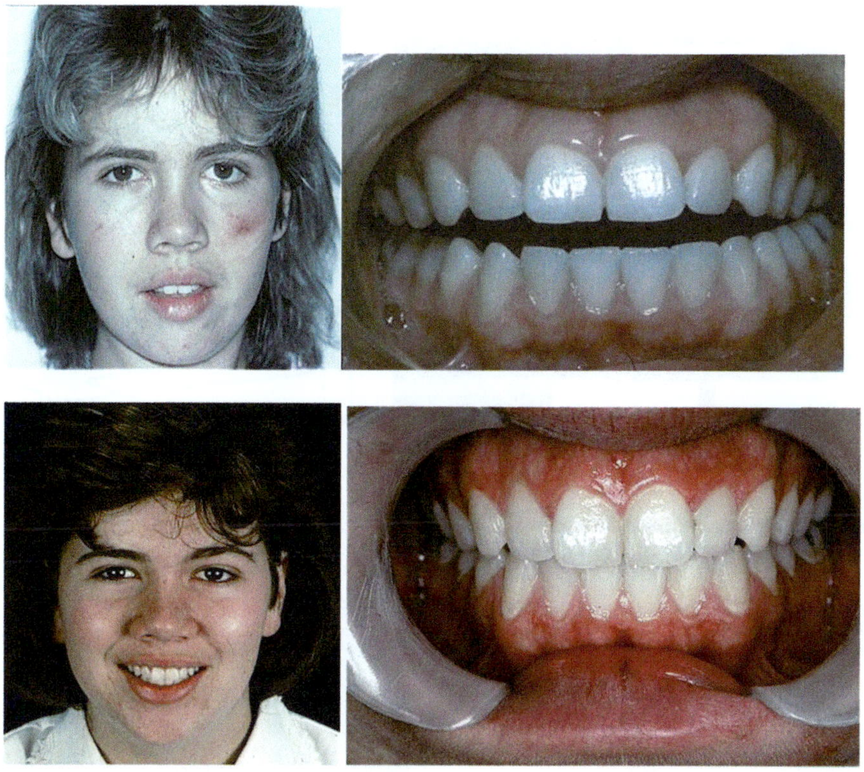

Fig. 27-18 An uncorrected fracture with open bite and short face corrected by a simple Le Fort I osteotomy. (From: David DJ, Simpson DA. Craniomaxillofacial Trauma. Churchill Livingstone, 1995; used with permission.[7])

standard. However, the patients desired end result is best achieved if these 'touch up' procedures are done after the basal bone has been moved and the aesthetics reassessed.

It is beyond the scope of this chapter to go into the details of rhinoplasty and soft tissue surgery. However, osseous genioplasty is a very versatile and successful operation and gives excellent results when appropriately performed (Figure 27-19). In this context the manipulation of the chin needs to be versatile and this means that chin implants have little use. The chin consists of bone and soft tissue, and correct examination of the patient is important, paying attention to the proportions that each contributes. These patients are presenting in most cases with a small chin and the need to have the lip, nose tip, chin relationship aesthetically improved. The osseous genioplasty can be advanced and rotated to improve a labiomental groove, shortened and moved from side to side if required. It is important to understand that the overlying soft tissue must not be completely disconnected from the underlying bone as it will not follow the bony movement and can produce the 'witch's chin', which is a very distressing complication that is difficult to correct.[14]

Caution is also necessary when planning the surgery to not over correct, and certainly not to do so at the same time as the primary surgery.

The surgical technique can be performed at the same time as the corrective rhinoplasty and lip adjustment. The patient has general anaesthesia via an oral endotracheal tube; the lower buccal mucosa is infiltrated with local anaesthetic and adrenaline as above, not only infiltrating beneath the periosteum but also into the submental muscles at their attachment to the chin where bleeding can occur. A slightly curved incision is made in the labial mucosa and deepened obliquely through the mentalis muscle leaving a robust cuff to ensure easy and water tight closure. The incision extends through the periosteum, which is elevated but care is taken not to deglove the soft tissue attachments to the symphysis. The dissection is carried well back beneath the mental foramina to the region of the first molar. The bone cut is performed with a reciprocating saw introduced into the subperiosteal tunnel. The cut is started as far back as possible to ensure a smoother and less noticeable step, and should clear the mental foramen by 5 mm as suggested by Ousterhout's studies to avoid injuring the nerve as it dips down before exiting the foramen. It is the authors practice to secure the fragment relatively loosely with a 26 G wire, the desired position is then fixed with two titanium monocortical plates. Closure is achieved in two layers with absorbable sutures.

Outcomes and complications

With respect to the *idiopathic* category of vertical maxillary deficiency there has been considerable concern about stability, relapse being attributed to resorption of the interposed grafted bone, or indeed bone substitutes.[3,5,15] It is the author's experience that use of rigid fixation using miniplates and blocks of iliac crest bone graft produces a stable and predictable result.

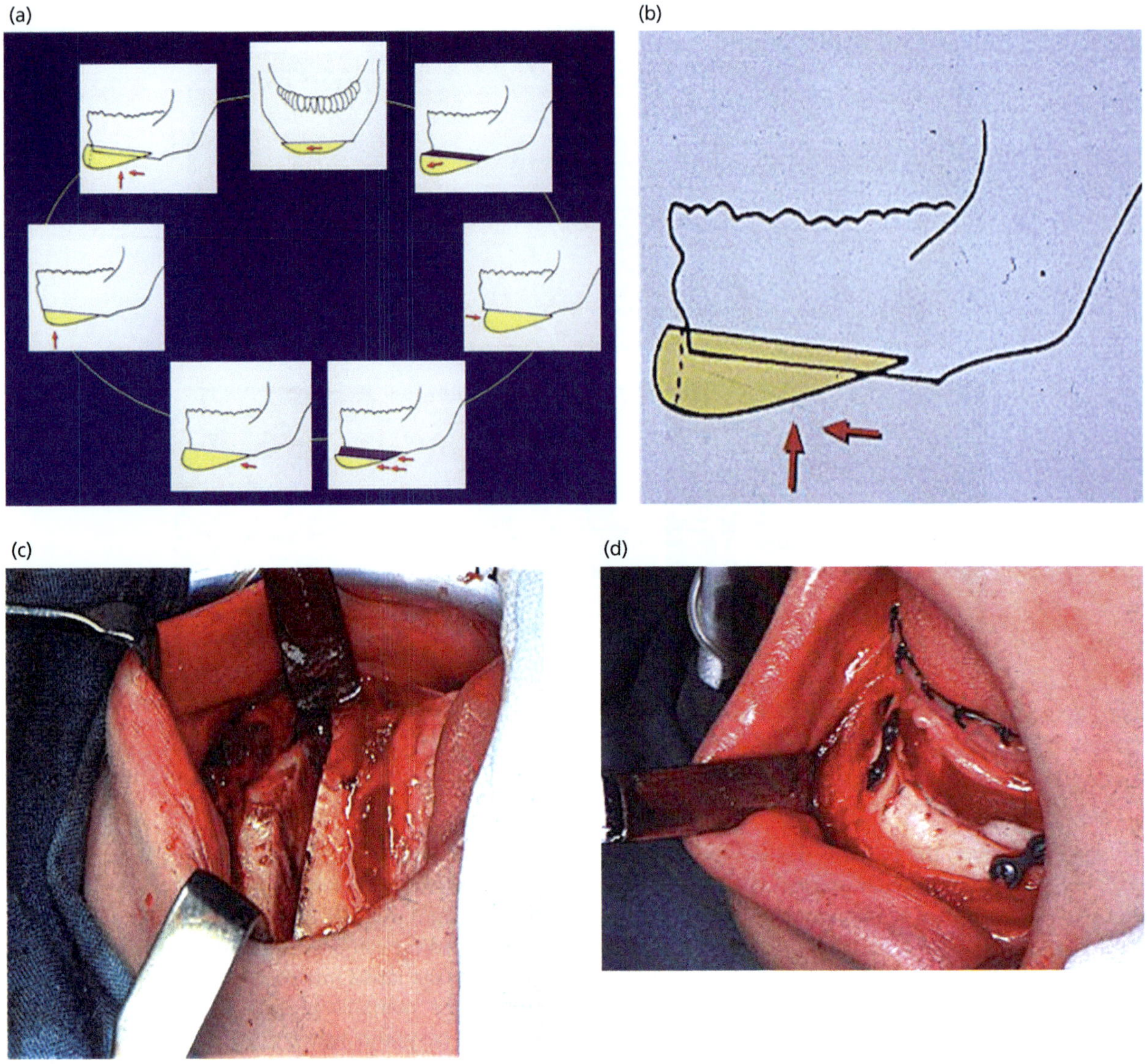

Fig. 27-19 The value of the osseous genioplasty is that it can be moved in three dimensions. It carries the attached soft tissue with the movement. These attributes are not available with implants.

The same stable situation exists whether or not bimaxillary surgery is necessary, however adding a rhinoplasty and or genioplasty at the one operation is in the authors experience courting the possibility of an unacceptable result.

The situation becomes more unstable and complex the more severe the initial pathology. The cleft lip and palate patient is prone to relapse due to the deficient bone and soft tissue integral to the disease process combined with the scarring of previous repairs that occurs even in the most carefully performed protocols. Relapse of 25% to 30% can occur and needs to be taken into account in the planning. This is not as easy as the aim of the maxillary lengthening is to give good aesthetic tooth show and this may be compromised by the quality of the cleft lip repair. The vertical stability can be enhanced by bevelling the Le Fort I osteotomy cut as suggested by Ortiz-Monasterio[4] to give greater bone to bone contact in smaller vertical movements.

The more general complications of haemorrhage and wound infection are rare. Damage to the inferior dental nerves as they exit the bone during genioplasty is possible but rare. One of the most significant problems is when the surgical outcome fails to meet the patient's expectations. This is obviated by extensive preoperative preparation in a multidisciplinary setting.

The outcomes and complications of treatment of *syndromic* and *post trauma* cases are best dealt with in articles specific to those disease processes.

Conclusions

Altering the proportions of the human face for aesthetic and or functional reasons is best done in a multidisciplinary setting that is patient-focused. Psychosocial considerations must be given equal weight to surgical and orthodontic considerations to avoid failure. Technological advances in imaging, fixation and surgical techniques mean that it is now possible to treat the patient with vertical deficiency of the maxilla in a stable fashion. When other dimensions of the face require change, or the shape needs altering, then technology is still the servant of clinical judgement based on a good history and thorough examination. The treating team should always give consideration to staged procedures in more complex cases which involve the lip, nose, chin relationship.

Acknowledgements

Michael Nugent, BD Sc (Qld), D ORTH, RCS (Eng), MS (Roch NY), FRACDS.

Neena Chisholm, BD Sc (Adel), BSc (Hons), Grad, Dip. Adel M Orth (Edin), Doc Clin Dent (Orth) Adel.

References

1 Bell WH. Correction of the short face syndrome in vertical maxillary deficiency: A preliminary report. J Oral Surg. 1977;35:110–20.
2 Bell WH, Creekmore TD, Alexander RG. Surgical correction of the long face syndrome. Am J Orthod.1977;71:40–67.
3 Freihofer HP. Surgical Treatment of the Short Face Syndrome. J Oral Surg. 1981;39:907–11.
4 Ortiz Monasterio F. The Short and Broad and the Long and Narrow Face. In: Ousterhout DK (Ed.). Aesthetic Contouring of the Craniofacial Skeleton. Little Brown and Co, 1991.
5 Rosen HM. Aesthetic Perspectives in Jaw Surgery. Springer Verlag, 1991.
6 Naini FB. Facial Aesthetics: Concepts and Clinical Diagnosis. Oxford: Wiley-Blackwell, 2011.
7 David DJ, Abbott JR et al. In: David DJ, Simpson DA (Eds.). Craniomaxillofacial Trauma. Churchill Livingstone, 1995.
8 Watted N, Witt E, Bill J. A Therapeutic Concept for the Combined Orthodontic Surgical Correction of Angle Class II Deformities with Short-face Syndrome: Surgical Lengthening of the Lower Face. Clin Orthod Res. 2000;3:78–93.
9 David DJ, Nugent MAC, Moore MH. Maxillary and Mandibular Surgery: Aesthetics verses the Occlusion; in Aesthetic Contouring of the Craniofacial Skeleton. In: Ousterhout DK (Ed.). Aesthetic Contouring of the Craniofacial Skeleton. Little Brown and Co, 1991.
10 Schnitt DE, Agir H, David DJ. From birth to maturity-a group of patients who have completed their protocol management. Part 1: Unilateral cleft lip and palate. Plast Reconstr Surg. 2004;113:805–17.
11 Maegawa J, Sells RK, David DJ. Pharyngoplasty in patients with cleft lip and palate after maxillary advancement. J Craniofac Surg. 1998;9:330-5; discussion 336–7.
12 David DJ, Poswillo D, Simpson DA. The Craniosynostoses. Springer-Verlag, 1982.
13 Sheffield LJ, White J, David DJ, Nugent MAC. Chondrodysplasia punctata (mild type) presenting as Binder's Syndrome (Abstract). Pathology. 1984;16:107.
14 Ousterhout DK. Mandibular width reduction including the surgical treatment of benign masseteric hypertrophy: in Aesthetic contouring of the craniofacial skeleton. In: Ousterhout DK (ed.) 451-469 Little, Brown and Company, 1991.
15 Major PW, Phillippson GE, Glover KE, Grace MG. Stability of maxilla downgrafting after rigid or wire fixation. J Oral Maxillofac Surg. 1996;54:1287–91.

Chapter 28

Surgical Correction of Skeletal Anterior Open Bite: Segmental Maxillary Surgery

Johan P. Reyneke and Carlo Ferretti

Introduction

The term open bite describes a section of the occlusion where no dental contact or overlap occurs and may be anterior or lateral. Open bite deformities have aesthetic and functional implications for patients and thus physicians are often called upon to rectify this malocclusion. The successful correction of this malocclusion can be elusive particularly if inappropriate treatment attempts are made. The latter scenario will result in aesthetic facial compromise and tendency to relapse to the pretreatment situation. Although no treatment has the support of strong research data this chapter will highlight the fundaments of open bite correction moderated with the authors' personal philosophies to present an approach to the correction of this malocclusion which has proven to be routinely successful.

Development of the open bite malocclusion

How an anterior open bite malocclusion develops is still subject to debate and discussion and although it may be considered of abstract clinical relevance, an appreciation of the developmental mechanisms will assist the treating physician to identify the offending jaw/s and in growing patients institute interventional therapies. Two theoretical mechanisms have a modicum of backing from research findings: *the morphogenetic theory* and *the adaptive theory*. The former theory proposes that the anterior open bite may be the

Orthognathic Surgery: Principles, Planning and Practice. Edited by Farhad B. Naini and Daljit S. Gill.

result of aberrant genetic control of growth patterns producing abnormal occlusal morphology, whilst the latter theory suggests that the open bite develops as a secondary maladaptation to functional anomalies of the naso-oropharyngeal apparatus. It has proven difficult to separate these two causative mechanisms, and the question remains incompletely answered.[1] Complicating the issue is the fact that there is a wide racial variation in the incidence of anterior open bite, which suggests a modulating effect of genetic control of skeletal proportions. The on-going research challenge is unravelling correlation from causation and the quality of the data to support causative theories is weak. Nevertheless an overview of our generally accepted view in this field is appropriate.

Non-nutritive sucking is a normal phenomenon whose frequency decreases with age but whose persistence beyond the age of 6 years is strongly associated with open bite malocclusion.[2] Nasopharyngeal and oropharyngeal obstruction as a result of one of several conditions, such as allergic rhinitis, enlarged adenoids, and enlarged tonsils, has been associated with anterior open bite deformity.[3] Any obstruction to normal nasal breathing triggers an adaptive neuromuscular response that results in open rotation of the mandible, inferior and anterior repositioning of the tongue, and extended head posture giving rise to the classical 'adenoidal facies.' These functional adaptations may produce permanent morphological changes in the craniofacial skeleton. First, a change in the direction of mandibular growth from horizontal to vertical results in increased lower facial height. Second, inferior and anterior repositioning of the tongue has several dental effects, including narrowing of the maxillary dental arch caused by the unopposed action of the buccinator muscles, retroclination of the upper incisors caused by the unopposed actions of orbicularis oris, and proclination of the lower incisors caused by increased tongue pressure.

Support for this mechanism has been strengthened by the finding that early removal of the obstruction and return to nasal breathing often results in normalization of anterior height.

Increased vertical development of the maxilla also has been associated with several muscle weakness syndromes. Weakness of the mandibular elevators and decreased biting force allow the posterior teeth to over erupt and the mandible to rotate downward. It has been stated that the biting force of patients with long faces is below normal, although the bite force of preadolescent patients with long face characteristics is normal. The role of decreased bite force as an aetiological factor in the development of vertical maxillary excess and anterior open bite is not clear, however.[4,5]

Tongue thrust or abnormal tongue activity during speech has also been blamed for the development of anterior open bite malocclusion and poor stability after treatment. Various attempts to change patients' swallowing patterns, such as speech therapy and removable appliance with a crib have been used to control anterior open bite problems. Contemporary research has shown that tongue thrust swallow is a physiologic adaptation to an anterior open bite rather than the cause of it. An abnormally large tongue or true macroglossia should first be differentiated from pseudomacroglossia and only then considered as an etiologic factor in the development of an anterior open bite. A large tongue also may be the cause of poor stability after treatment.[6]

Diagnosis

As with all malocclusion, it is important to identify the cause of the anterior open bite. Thus the diagnostic process has two important goals: to identify the anatomical location of the discrepancy, i.e. maxilla, mandible, or both, and identification of a cause. The latter is pertinent in younger patients where intervention to guide growth or interfere with a habit may result in correction of the malocclusion. The open bite as a result of thumb sucking is usually limited to the anterior region, with a narrow palate, often posterior crossbites, and relatively normal facial proportions.

Skeletal anterior open bite malocclusion in adults is a vertical dentofacial problem caused by excessive vertical development of the maxilla, shortening of the mandibular ramus, or a combination of both (Figure 28-1). The clinical signs often associated an open bite malocclusion due to maxillary posterior vertical excess are increased vertical facial height, paranasal flattening, narrow nasal base, convex facial profile and increased interlabial gap. Anterior open

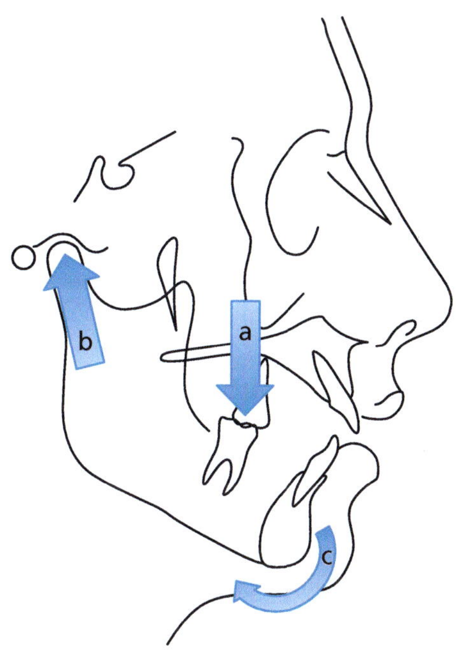

Fig. 28-1 Open bite malocclusion is mostly secondary to a disturbance in the vertical dimension, either posterior maxillary vertical excess (a), decreased mandibular ramus/condyle height (b) or both resulting in clockwise rotation of the mandible (c) resulting in an open bite. The open bite is often combined with transverse maxillary deficiency.

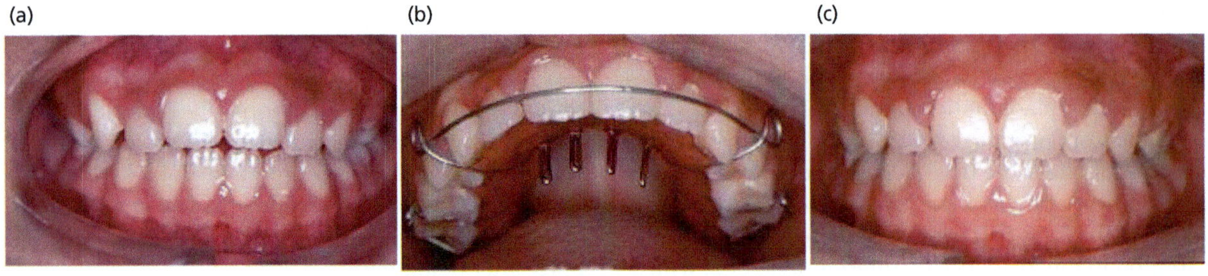

Fig. 28-2 Open bite adaptive to long-term thumb sucking in a child with mixed dentition (a). The use of a removable appliance to interrupt the habit (b), results in spontaneous correction (c)

bite due to decreased mandibular ramus height has subtly different clinical features: convex facial profile and increased interlabial gap without a markedly increased lower facial height, paranasal flattening and narrow nasal base.

Radiographic evidence of condylar deformation or resorption points to the shortened ramus as the site of the malocclusion and increased mandibular plane angle with a normal maxillary occlusal plane angle. Open bite due to maxillary posterior vertical excess will have an increased mandibular plane angle and a decreased maxillary occlusal plane angle and often a reversed occlusal curve.

Treatment of growing patients

Anterior open bite in children with mixed dentition and good facial proportions is usually caused by prolonged thumb sucking (beyond the age of 6 years) or other environmental influences, and the most important corrective measure in these patients is cessation of the habit. It is often accompanied by posterior cross bite due to maxillary transverse deficiency. Removable and fixed appliances can be effective in the correction. Maxillary dental expansion not only corrects the cross bite but also assists in closing the anterior open bite and should be combined with habit control (Figure 28-2). By the time adolescence is reached, environmental causes become less important. A poor response to habit control and maxillary expansion increases the likelihood that an aberrant growth pattern may co-exist.[7]

Treatment of skeletally mature patients

Orthodontic correction of anterior open bite

The correction of the anterior open bite by means of orthodontic treatment alone is achieved with the following: (1) extrusion of upper and lower incisor teeth; (2) intrusion of molar teeth; and (3) expansion of the maxillary dental arch. This requires predominantly the deployment of vertical mechanics. Extrusion of incisor teeth can be accomplished in three ways: (1) the use of anterior elastics; (2) using a continuous arch wire from molar to molar to level a reverse occlusal curve in the maxillary arch; and (3) levelling a reverse curve of Spee in the mandibular arch in the same manner. The mechanics to intrude the molars include intrusion of molars with temporary anchorage devises,[8] high-pull headgear and Class III elastics,[9] titanium screw anchorage,[10] a rapid molar intruder appliance,[11] reverse headgear combined with Class III and anterior box elastics,[12] zygomatic anchorage,[13] and bite blocks with repelling magnets.[14] The increasing use of temporary anchorage devices has increased reports of orthodontic correction of open bite.

Expansion of the maxillary posterior teeth in adult individuals with skeletal transverse deficiency usually results in dental tipping and has doubtful stability.[15,16]

Most of the reports in the literature regarding orthodontic correction of skeletal anterior open bite are case reports that discuss specific orthodontic techniques or introduce new orthodontic mechanics. There is, however, a paucity of studies regarding results after orthodontic correction of anterior open bite malocclusions to draw any evidence-based conclusions.[17–19] Few studies have reported on the pretreatment aesthetic considerations and facial aesthetic outcomes. Regardless of the specific mechanism used to achieve the tooth movements, stability is unpredictable and in many cases results in compromised aesthetics.[20,21] In cases in which the anterior open bite is associated with increased incisor inclination (as may be found in cases with bimaxillary protrusion), correction of the incisor inclination by retroclination of the incisors towards the correct inclination has a relative extrusive effect (see Figure 5-43), thus closing the bite.

Combined orthodontic and surgical treatment

Vertical maxillary excess – orthodontic preparation

Presurgical orthodontic mechanics should avoid attempting to correct vertical, transverse, or anteroposterior skeletal discrepancy. The goal of presurgical orthodontic treatment should be to align the maxillary teeth (either in segments or as one piece) and resist the temptation to close the bite. Segmental surgery is indicated when: (1) the maxillary dental arch has a natural step as a result of vertical discrepancy between anterior and posterior segments; (2) the upper arch requires surgical expansion due to skeletal transverse deficiency; and (3) surgical closure of inter dental spaces are planned following tooth extraction. Levelling within a segment is desirable and intrusion of the incisors or maintaining their pretreatment height is recommended. Opening the bite before surgery improves stability as relapse of incisor intrusion serves to further close the bite after surgery. Orthodontic alignment of the maxilla in segments can be done with or without extractions. The need for extractions in these cases is dictated by the amount of crowding and the dental movements necessary to place the upper and lower incisors in their desired inclination and in the central trough of bone. The inclination of the incisor and posterior teeth can be altered with segmental surgery and this must be taken into account during the preparation. In cases in which segmental surgery is contemplated, care should be taken to coordinate the arch form of the maxillary segments with the mandibular arch and deviate the roots of the teeth adjacent to the intended inter dental osteotomy sites. Although the mandible may require surgical advancement or set-back, the lower dental arch serves as the 'template' and ultimately dictates the symmetry and form of the upper arch. The presurgical orthodontic treatment goals are to place the lower dentition symmetrically in the ideal anteroposterior, vertical, and transverse positions in relation to its supporting bone.

Planning the position of the interdental osteotomies

Pretreatment planning for segmental surgery is important and will influence the pre-surgical orthodontic preparation in several ways:

- Deviation of the roots of teeth adjacent to the planned interdental osteotomies. In cases requiring only vertical adjustment between segments the root deviation should be less than in cases requiring closure of interdental spaces.
- Orthodontic tipping of the molar teeth in the posterior segments should be avoided. Hanging palatal cusps will increase the amount of skeletal expansion during surgery and increase the possibility of transverse relapse (see Figure 28.15 a-d).
- The authors prefer to perform the interdental osteotomies between the maxillary lateral incisor and canine teeth for several reasons: (1) The surgical sight is anterior in the mouth and easily accessible during surgery; (2) The alveolar bone is thin in this area; (3) The anterior segment containing the four upper incisors forms a near straight line which allows for surgical tipping of the segment and so changing the inclination of the incisor teeth (Figures 28-3a and 28-4); (4) The final orthodontic finishing of the canine tooth requires the root to be slightly distally angulated. With an interdental osteotomy

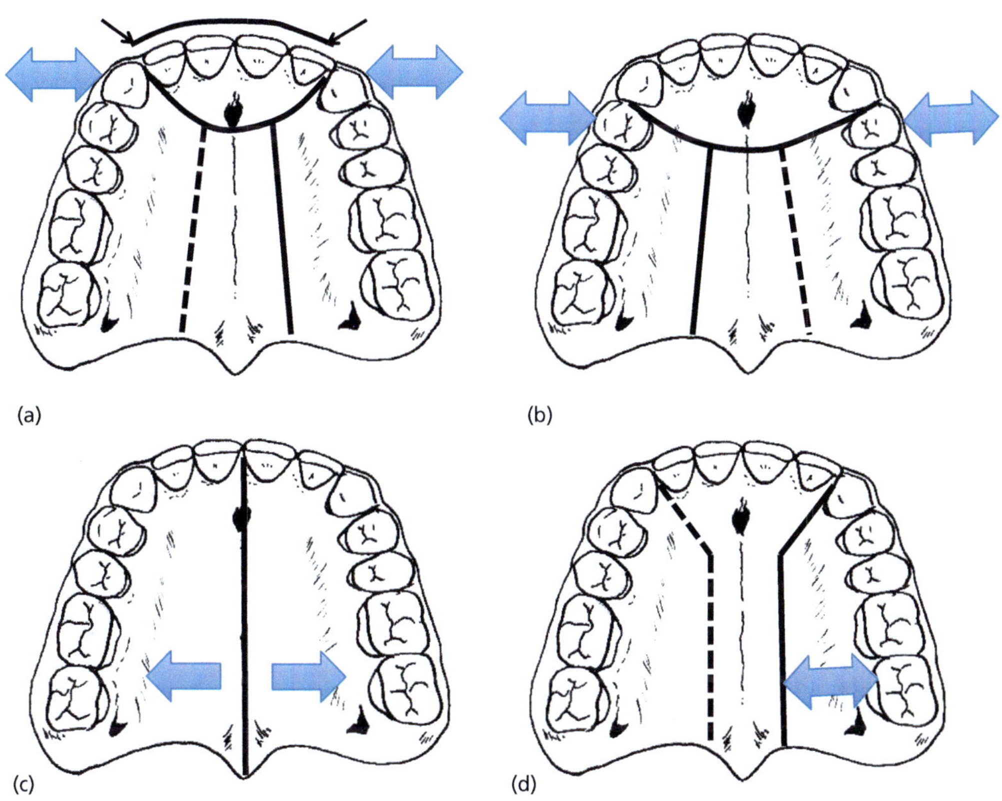

Fig. 28-3 Segmental surgery design (a) To expand the intercanine width osteotomy is performed between canines and lateral incisors. Note the four incisor teeth in the anterior segment are almost in a straight line (black arrows). (b) If the intercanine width is appropriate the interdental osteotomy can be positioned between the canine and first premolar. (c) A midline osteotomy is an option if the transverse deficiency is due top a 'V' shaped arch (d) A unilateral cross bite can be corrected with a unilateral osteotomy.

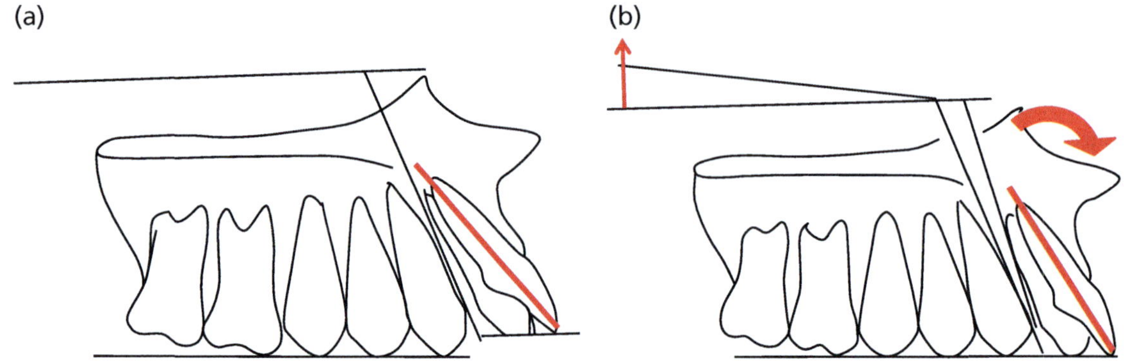

Fig. 28-4 Orthodontic preparation for segmental surgery allows for surgical differential impaction of the anterior and posterior segments (a). By rotating the anterior segment containing the upper four incisor teeth the inclination of the incisors is altered (b).

anterior to the canine tooth the root will already be close to its final angulation. However, when the osteotomy is planned between canine and first premolar the canine root needs to be moved mesially before surgery and again distally following surgery (Figure 28-3b). This will increase the treatment time. With the canine teeth situated in the distal segments it allows the surgeon to control the intercanine distance and achieve an ideal canine position in all three dimensions at the time of surgery (Figure 28-3a).

Patients presenting for surgery following orthodontic attempts to close a skeletal anterior open bite pose a dilemma. It is imperative that the surgeon obtain the pretreatment orthodontic records to quantify the orthodontic bite closure that has been achieved and the potential for relapse. It is recommended to discontinue all vertical mechanics and allow vertical relapse by placing light sectional arch wires to maintain alignment and rotations. Once no further vertical opening of the bite occurs, the patient can be re-evaluated for appropriate orthodontics and surgery.

Surgery

The vertical deformity often occurs in conjunction with either a primary or secondary sagittal deformity. During treatment planning three factors should be considered: (1) the amount of superior repositioning of the maxilla (anterior and posterior); (2) the position of the mandible after autorotation; and (3) the need for surgical correction of a transverse discrepancy.

The amount of superior repositioning of the maxilla

The amount of superior repositioning of the anterior and posterior maxilla is influenced by two aspects: (1) the planned ideal maxillary incisor/upper lip relationship determines the amount of vertical and anteroposterior repositioning of the anterior maxilla (1–4 mm) (Figure 28.5). In most cases the incisor teeth require

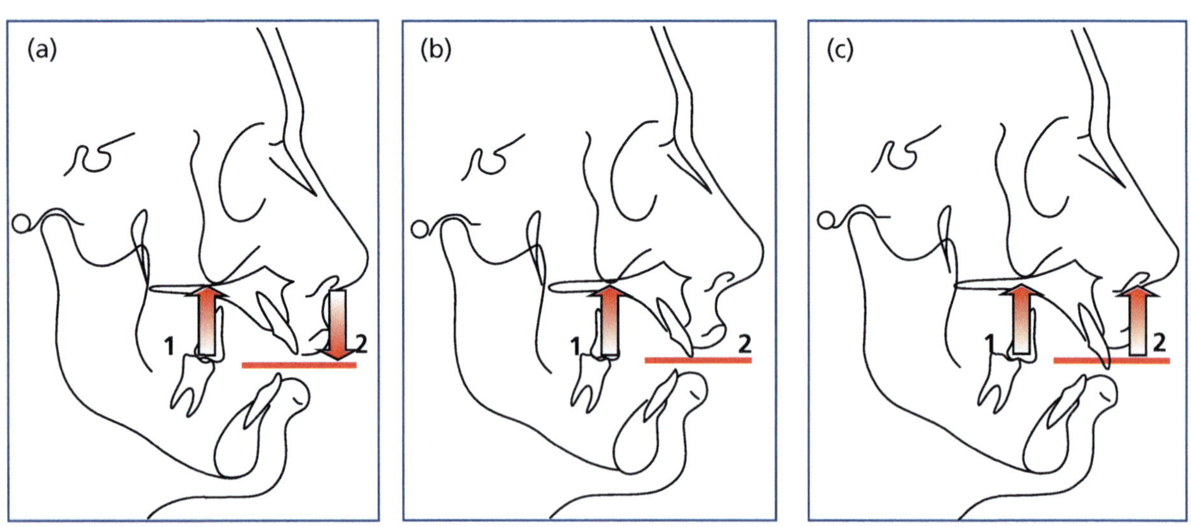

Fig. 28-5 Open bite malocclusion with anterior vertical maxillary deficiency is corrected with a combination of anterior downgraft (2) and if required posterior maxillary impaction (1) (a). Open bite malocclusion with adequate upper incisor show is corrected by posterior maxillary impaction only (1) maintaining the vertical incisor/lip relationship (2) (b). Open bite malocclusion with excessive incisor show is corrected with (1 & 2) differential maxillary impaction (c).

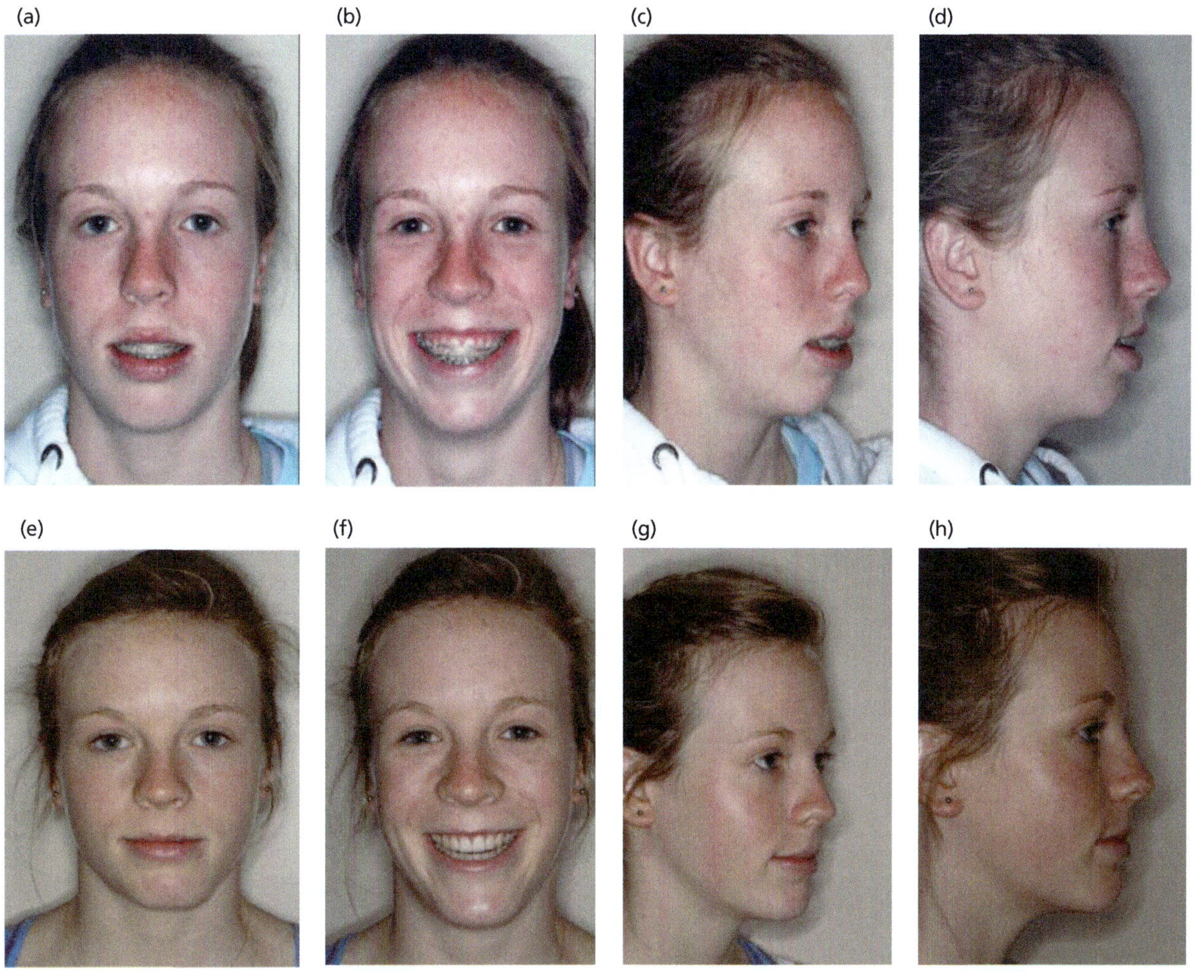

Fig. 28-6 Case 1: Open bite malocclusion due to posterior and anterior vertical maxillary excess (a–d). Impaction of the entire maxilla (more posterior than anterior) closed the open bite and corrected the anterior vertical maxillary excess (e–h). The aesthetics are enhanced by advancing the chin by means of a genioplasty.

superior repositioning (Figures 28-6–28-8: CASE 1). In some cases, however, the incisor height may need to be maintained (Figures 28-9–28-11: CASE 2), whereas in other cases the anterior maxilla may have to be inferiorly repositioned (Figure 28-12: CASE 3). The final anteroposterior and vertical position of the maxillary incisors is the key to treatment planning (Figure 28-5);[22,23] The final occlusal plane is determined by the mandibular occlusal plane after autorotation of the mandible. (2) The amount of superior repositioning

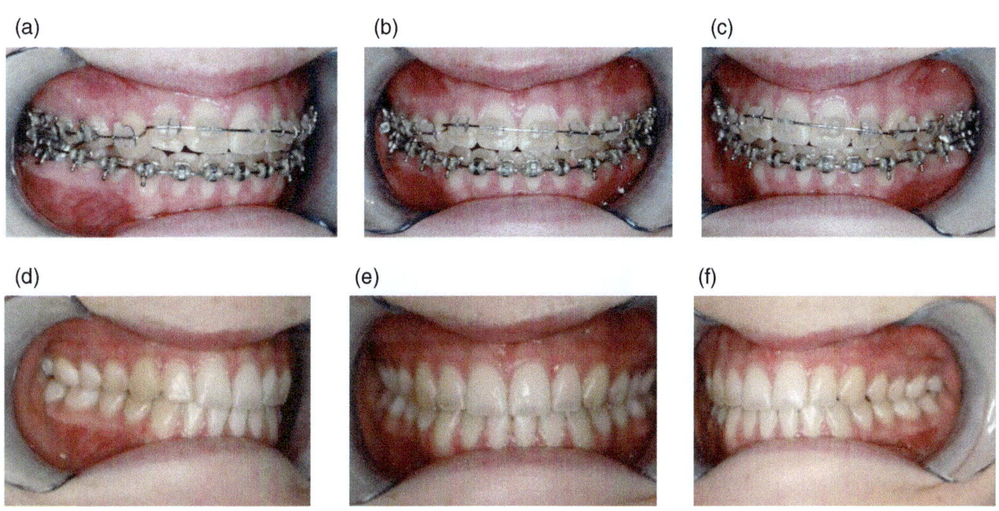

Fig. 28-7 Case 1: Preoperative orthodontic preparation in segments (a–c) shows preparation of stepped occlusal plane to allow for segmental surgery and differential maxillary impaction. Post-treatment occlusion (d–f)

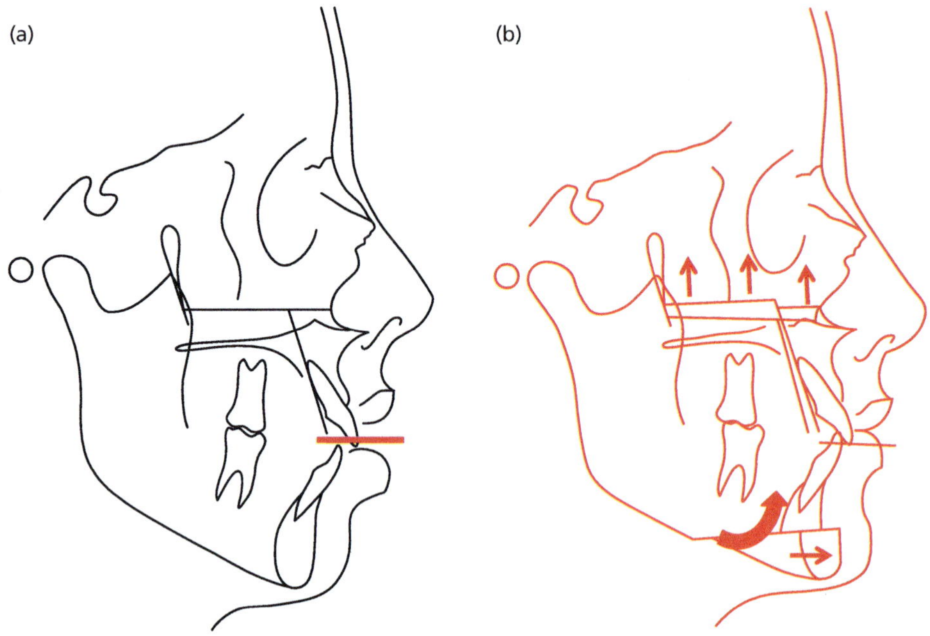

Fig. 28-8 Case 1: Treatment planning for patient with open bite and anterior vertical maxillary excess. The vertical position (horizontal red line) of the upper incisor is selected (a). The surgical visual treatment objective shows the planned differential maxillary impaction with segmental surgery, mandibular counterclockwise rotation into a Class I molar relationship. The aesthetic result is enhances by means of an advancement genioplasty (b).

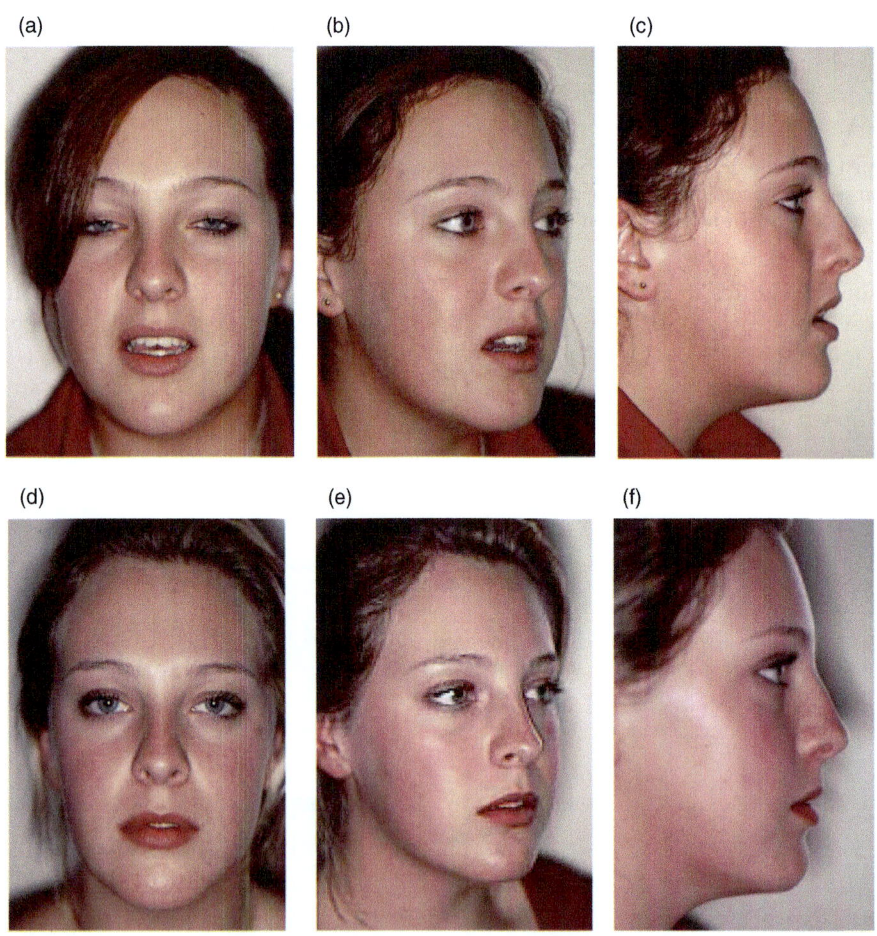

Fig. 28-9 Case 2: Patient with posterior vertical maxillary excess and adequate upper incisor show (a–c). Impaction of only the posterior maxilla closes the open bite whilst maintaining an aesthetically pleasing upper incisor show (d–f)

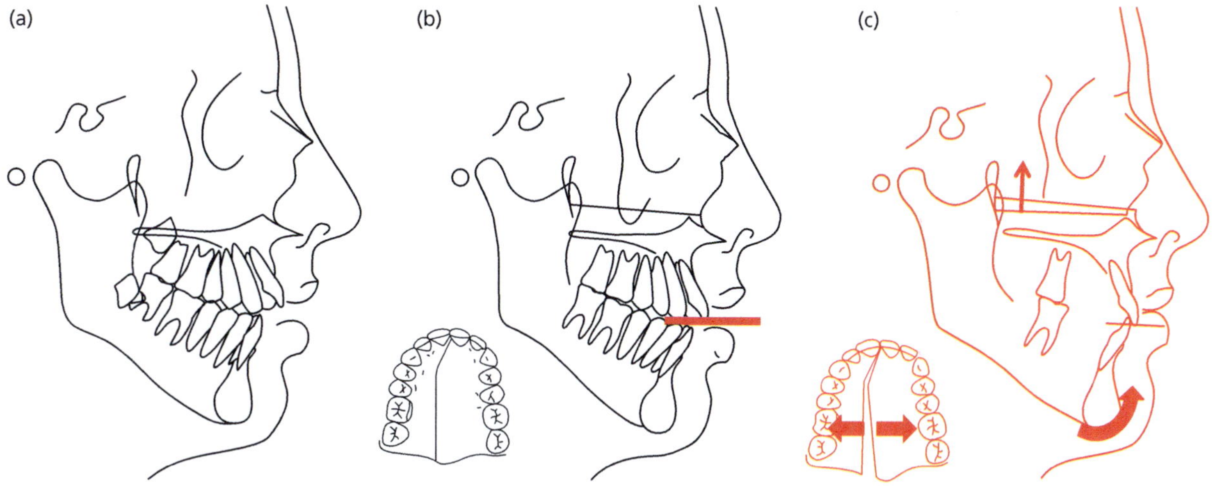

Fig. 28-10 Case 2: The lateral cephalometric tracing of a patient with an anterior open bite and adequate upper incisor upper lip relationship (a). The immediate pre surgical tracing following orthodontic preparation. The narrow upper dental arch requires surgical expansion (b). The surgical VTO maintains the upper incisor vertical position, the posterior maxilla is impacted, and expanded (c).

of the posterior maxilla is determined by the height of the mandibular posterior teeth after autorotation (Figure 28-13). An exception to this is for very large open bites where the amount of posterior impaction of the maxilla is not technically achievable or aesthetically favourable. In this situation the bulk of the anterior open bite correction is obtained with the maxillary posterior impaction and the residual open bite is corrected with counterclockwise mandibular rotation.

Mandibular position after autorotation (Figure 28-14)

The anteroposterior position of the lower incisor after autorotation determines whether mandibular surgery

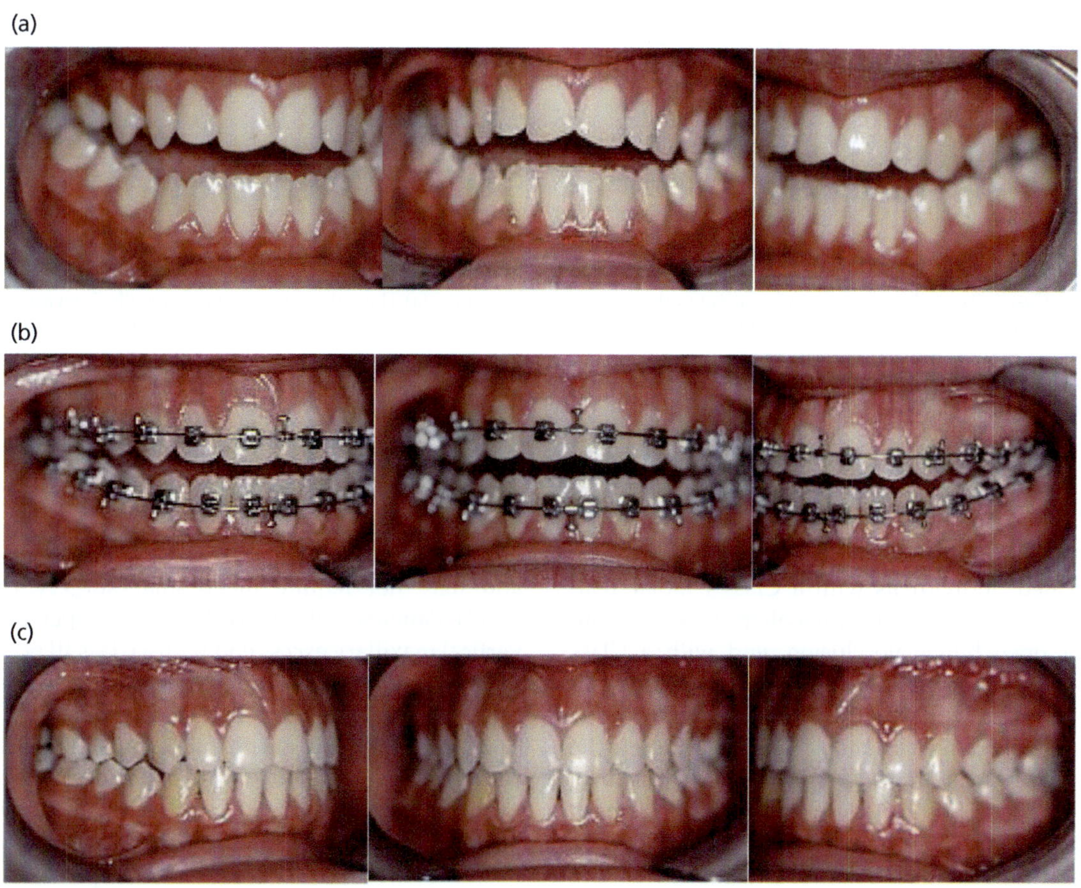

Fig. 28-11 Case 2: Pretreatment occlusion showing anterior open bite and maxillary transverse deficiency (a). Orthodontic preparation of a single level occlusal plane and deviation of the central incisor roots (b). Post-surgery occlusion (c).

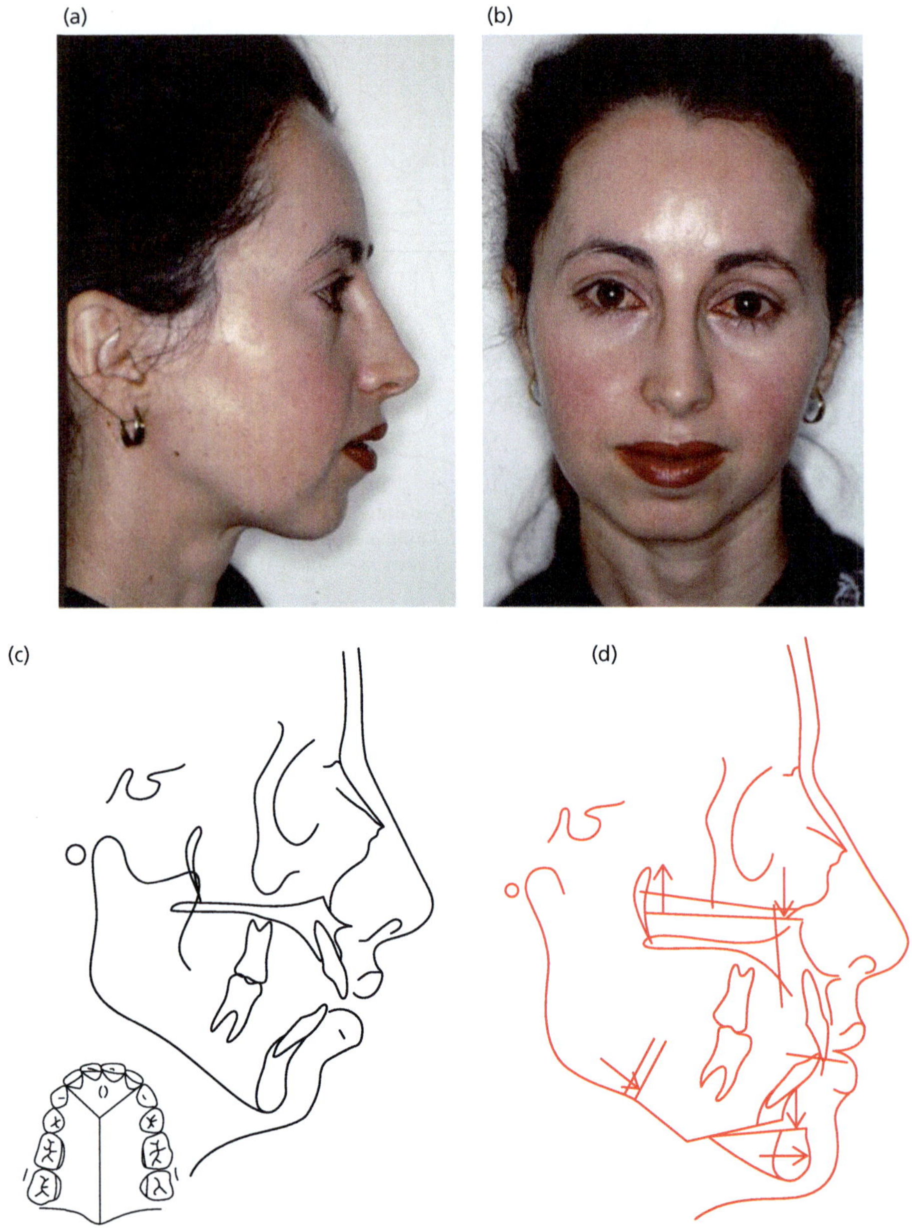

Fig. 28-12 Case 3: Typical appearance of a patient with an open bite deformity. (a) The patient has a convex profile, increased lower facial height, mandibular AP deficiency and labial incompetence. (b) Frontal view reveals narrow nasal base with subtle paranasal flattening.

Treatment planning for the patient in Figure 28-12 (Case 3). Lack of incisor show requires downgrafting of the anterior maxillary segment, autorotation and advancement of the mandible to correct the AP mandibular discrepancy, and finally positioning of the posterior maxillary segment to reveal the magnitude of posterior maxillary impaction required to close the bite. Final aesthetic refinement is achieved with a vertical and horizontal augmentation genioplasty Preoperative frontal view (e) and post-operative frontal view (f). Preoperative occlusion (g) and post-operative occlusion (h). Preoperative profile view (i) and post-operative profile view (j).

is indicated. Individuals with a Class I molar relation, combined with vertical maxillary excess and an anterior open bite malocclusion, end with a Class III dental relationship after maxillary superior repositioning. Based on the aesthetic requirements of the case, the clinician must decide whether the Class III dental relationship should be corrected by advancement of the maxilla or mandibular set-back (Figure 28-14).

In patient with vertical maxillary excess and a Class II occlusion, the mandible will rotate to a Class I relation after superior repositioning of the maxilla and may not require mandibular surgery (Figure 28-14). Patients with a Class III anterior open bite and vertical maxillary excess end with a Class III occlusion of increased severity after vertical correction of the maxilla and anterior rotation of the mandible. These cases most probably need a mandibular set-back procedure in conjunction with maxillary advancement. This decision is based on the aesthetic requirements of each case. Patients with open bite due to posterior vertical maxillary excess complicated by a severe Class II malocclusion will end with a Class II occlusal relationship after maxillary superior

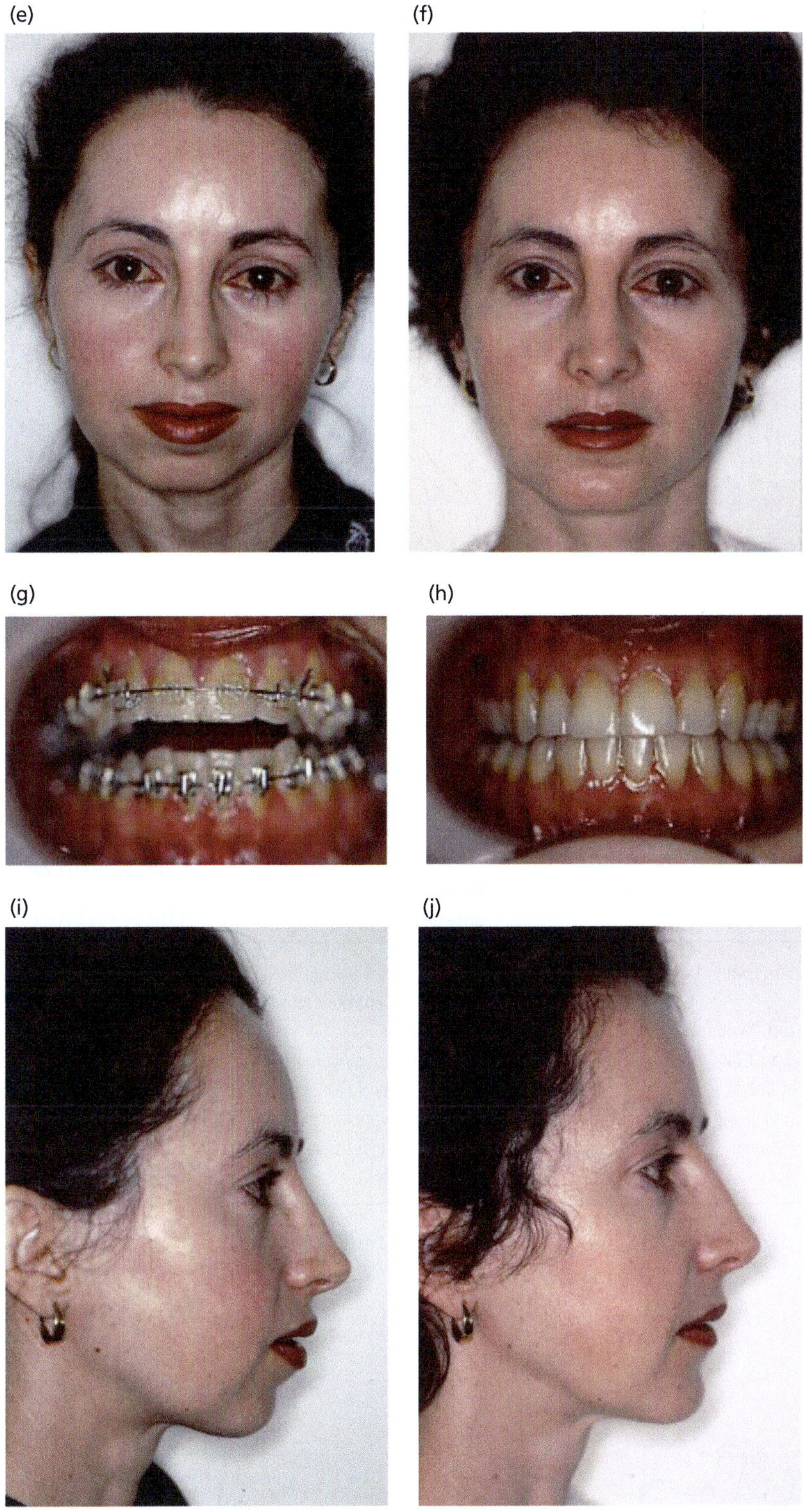

Fig. 28-12 (*Continued*)

repositioning. To establish a Class I occlusion mandibular advancement is often required (Figure 28-14 and Table 28-1). The temptation to set-back the maxilla to correct the anteroposterior discrepancy should be resisted as this often results in poor midface aesthetics. A combination of maxillary superior repositioning and set-back will compromise the aesthetics further. The mandible should rather be advanced in these cases, and the maxilla superiorly repositioned and preferably slightly advanced. The slight advancement (2–3 mm) has the added technical advantage that the posterior maxilla is moved away from the pterygoid plates. Due to the disproportionate vertical excess of the posterior maxilla in open bite deformities more bone removal in the posterior maxilla is needed than in correction of non–open bite deformities with vertical maxillary excess. In all of these treatment scenarios the chin contour and

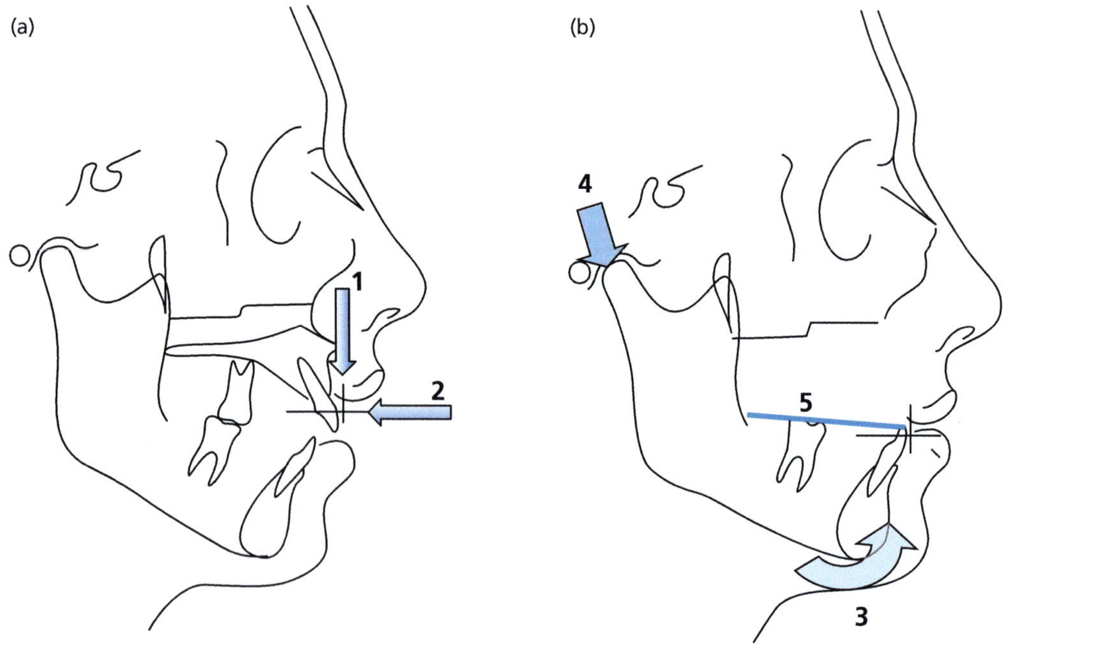

Fig. 28-13 As always, treatment planning is commenced by selecting the ideal anteroposterior (1) and vertical (2) upper incisor position (a). The mandible then autorotates (3) around the condyle (4) until the lower incisor overlaps the selected vertical upper incisor position by about 2 mm. The position of the maxillary molars is dictated by the (5) mandibular molars after autorotation (b).

Table 28-1 Secondary anteroposterior problems following open bite correction (Where will the mandible be after autorotation?)

Occlusion following the correction of vertical maxillary excess	Correction of secondary anteroposterior problems
Class I will rotate to a Class III	Mandibular set-back/maxillary advancement/genioplasty
Class II will rotate to a Class I	Genioplasty
Super Class II will rotate to a Class II	Mandibular advancement/ genioplasty
Class III will rotate to a super Class III	Maxillary advancement/ mandibular set-back/ genioplasty

position should be evaluated to enhance the aesthetic outcome.

Correction of transverse discrepancies

The open bite malocclusion due to posterior maxillary vertical excess is often accompanied by a transverse maxillary skeletal deficiency. Correction is achieved by means of segmental maxillary surgery. Surgical expansion of the maxilla is one of the most unstable orthognathic procedures, and transverse relapse is a common postsurgical complication and inevitably leads to recurrence of the anterior open bite. Incorrect preoperative diagnosis, inappropriate presurgical orthodontics, poor surgical management, and poor

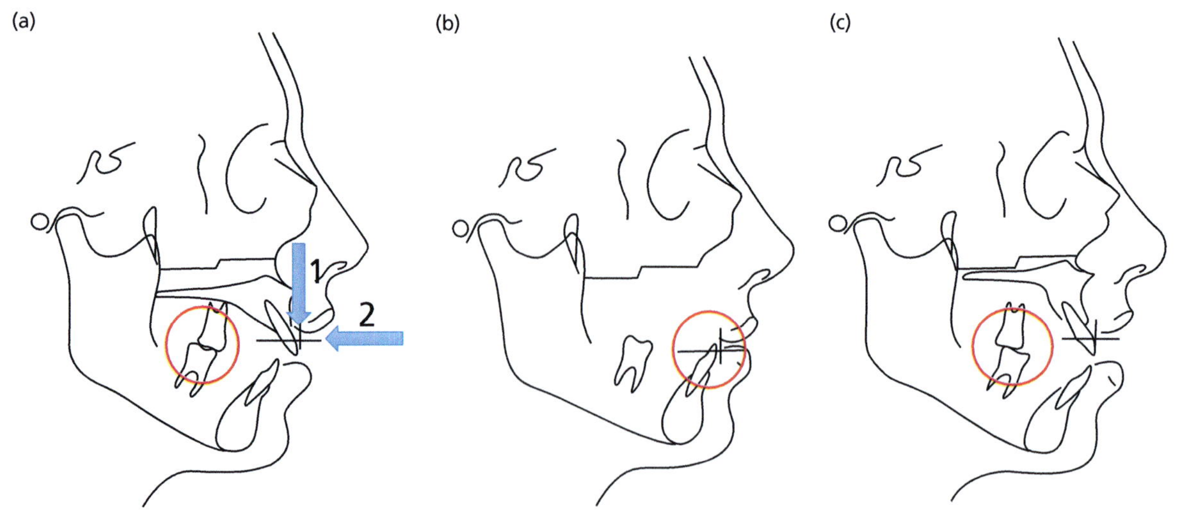

Fig. 28-14 Rotational changes of the mandible will alter the molar relationship. Following the selection of horizontal (1) and vertical (2) position of the upper incisor a patient with a Class II molar relationship (a) will rotate counterclockwise thus advancing the mandible sufficiently to allow single jaw correction (b). A patient with an initial Class I molar relationship (c) will rotate into a negative incisor overjet (d) thus requiring mandibular set-back surgery. A patient with a large Class II molar relationship (e) will remain with a large incisor overjet (f) and thus require mandibular advancement surgery.

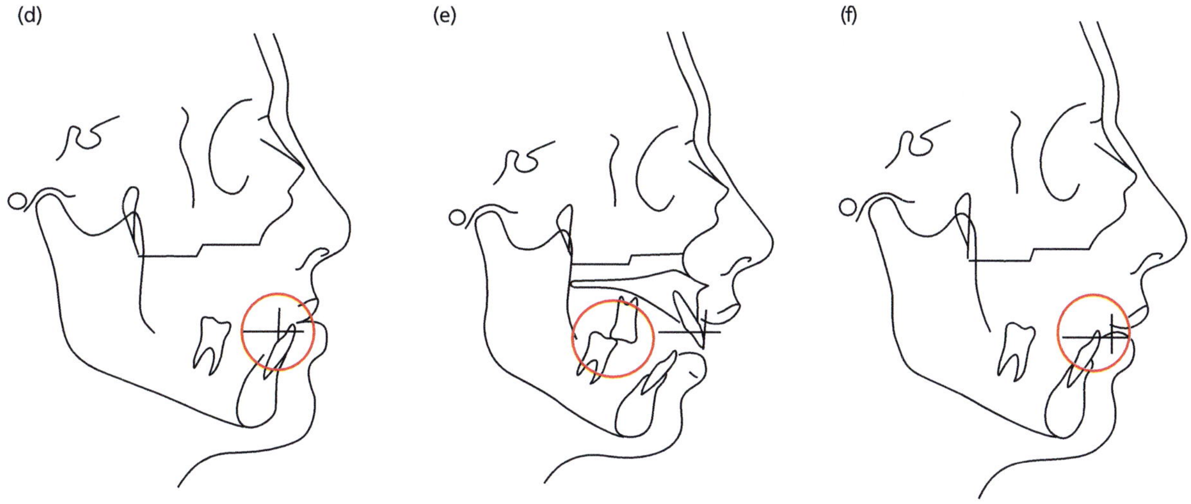

Fig. 28-14 (*Continued*)

post-surgical orthodontic control all contribute to transverse relapse.[24] Naturally, the first step in the diagnostic algorithm is to ascertain whether the discrepancy is skeletal or dental in nature and whether it is relative or absolute. Elucidation of the latter is achieved by observing the transverse relationship of dental casts held in the correct sagittal relationship with the canines in a Class I occlusion. If the cross bite is obviously skeletal in nature, compensatory dental expansion, headgear, archwires or through-the-bite elastics should be avoided. These dental changes have a high potential for relapse that may only manifest long after treatment.[25] Presurgical orthodontic tipping of molar teeth that leaves the lingual cusps hanging below the occlusal plane creates additional surgical problems. Hanging palatal cusps of the molars increase the amount of surgical expansion of the palate that is required (Figure 28-15). Surgical palatal expansion in these cases would involve expansion of the bony base and an element of up righting of the molar teeth. The increased amount of expansion leads to increased potential for relapse. Transverse stability can be enhanced by placing a bone graft in the palatal defect. Stabilization of the bone graft can be facilitated by performing the palatal osteotomy in the midpalate, where the bone is thickest. The disadvantage is that the mucosa in this area of the palate is at its thinnest. A tear in the palatal mucosa exposes the graft to the oral environment and eventually leads to loss of the graft. Performing bilateral osteotomies in the palate assists larger expansion; however, grafting these areas where the bone is thin is more difficult. The use of a splint during surgery and maintaining the splint in position for at least 6 weeks after

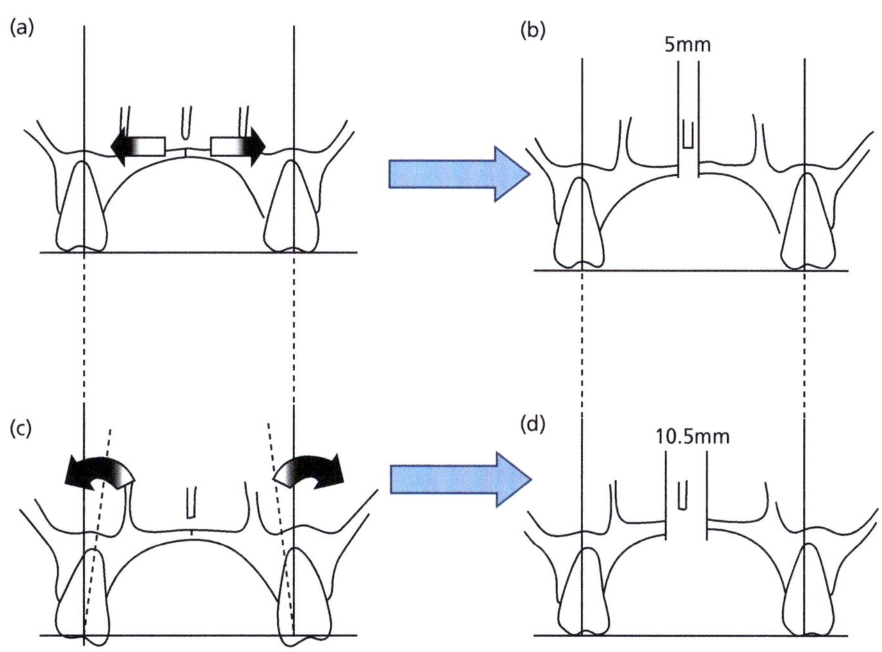

Fig. 28-15 Surgical expansion is increased if orthodontic preparation is inappropriate. The same maxillary alveolar arch width in (a) & (c), however, buccal flaring with hanging palatal cusps in (c) it will require a larger surgical expansion to correct the occlusion (b) & (d).

surgery allow stabilization during bone healing and may enhance skeletal stability. Obtaining immediate postsurgical orthodontic control by placing a palatal bar or a strong arch wire or both to support the palatal expansion further enhances stability of the result.

Patients with macroglossia may benefit from tongue reduction concurrent to orthognathic surgery. An abnormally large tongue does not adjust to the decreased oral volume after surgical correction and plays an important role in relapse. A normal-sized tongue with forward posturing does adjust to the smaller volume after surgery. Pretreatment tongue thrust swallowing disappears after correction of the anterior open bite because the physiological necessity for tongue thrust has been eliminated.

Open bite secondary to short mandibular ramus with a normal condyle: mandibular surgery

Orthodontic preparation

In general, avoidance of pre-surgical bite-closing mechanics also applies in these cases. A transverse discrepancy between the upper and lower arch may exist. The absolute or true transverse discrepancy can be measured by holding the models in the desired Class I relation. The potential crossbites should be corrected orthodontically if the discrepancy falls within the range of stable orthodontic movement. When an absolute crossbite exists because of a transverse maxillary deficiency that is not the result of dental tipping, three surgical options should be considered: (1) surgically assisted orthodontic expansion of the maxillary dental arch;[26] (2) narrowing of the mandibular arch by an osteotomy through the symphysis;[27,28] and (3) two-jaw surgery with surgical expansion of the maxilla by means of segmental surgery.[29]

Surgery

Aesthetic and functional correction in these cases demands a different surgical approach, and consideration should be given to correcting this type of dentofacial deformity by means of mandibular surgery. Surgical closure of an anterior open bite by mandibular surgery involves counterclockwise rotation of the mandible at the posterior teeth. Historically this surgical movement of the mandible has been considered to be unstable.[30] Reports in the literature identify three main factors that may influence the stability after orthognathic surgical procedures: (1) stretching of soft tissue; (2) neuromuscular adaptation; and (3) alteration of the muscle orientation.[30] These factors are particularly important when closing an open bite by counterclockwise rotation of the mandible. These factors have been reviewed in detail but a synopsis of the current understanding is that modern sagittal split design obviates pterygomasseteric sling lengthening and thus obviates its influence on postoperative stability. Moreover the influence of the lengthening of the suprahyoid musculature has proven to be less important in postoperative relapse.

Changes in the inclination of the mandibular ramus alter the orientation of the mandibular elevators. Few studies have assessed the long-term post-operative stability after surgical closure of anterior open bite dentofacial deformities by surgical counterclockwise rotation of the mandible. However, skeletal stability after counter clockwise rotation of the mandible as part of the rotation of the maxillomandibular complex was studied and reported by Reyneke[31] and Chemello et al.[32] With this surgical design, an anterior open bite is created by surgical counterclockwise rotation of the maxillary occlusal plane. The counterclockwise rotation of the maxilla is followed by the surgical rotation of the mandible. Long-term postoperative stability in both studies was found to be comparable to other mandibular surgical procedures (Figure 28.16: CASE 4).

Open bite secondary to a combination of vertical maxillary excess and short mandibular ramus

Many individuals with anterior open bite may display a combination of the clinical, dental, and cephalometric features of excessive vertical development of the maxilla and deficient development of the mandibular rami. In these cases the treatment objectives should be aimed at addressing the specific skeletal, soft tissue and dental problems as discussed for each of the two groups.

Open bite secondary to short mandibular ramus with condylar resorption

Any process of resorption of the condyle alters the morphology of the condyle and its position in the glenoid fossa. Resorption of the condyles and consequent shortening of the mandibular rami lead to the development of a Class II anterior open bite malocclusion. When considering correction of an anterior open bite caused by resorption of the condyle, the clinician should differentiate between idiopathic condylar resorption, degenerative joint disease, and rheumatic arthritis with destruction of the condyle.

Idiopathic condylar resorption

Although it may occur in any patient population, idiopathic condylar resorption often presents in relatively young Caucasian women with high mandibular and occlusal plane angles and develops into a Class II anterior open bite malocclusion. The anterior open bite usually develops progressively with no TMJ pain or hypomobility. The process is usually self-limiting and may last from 6 months to 2 years. It is thought

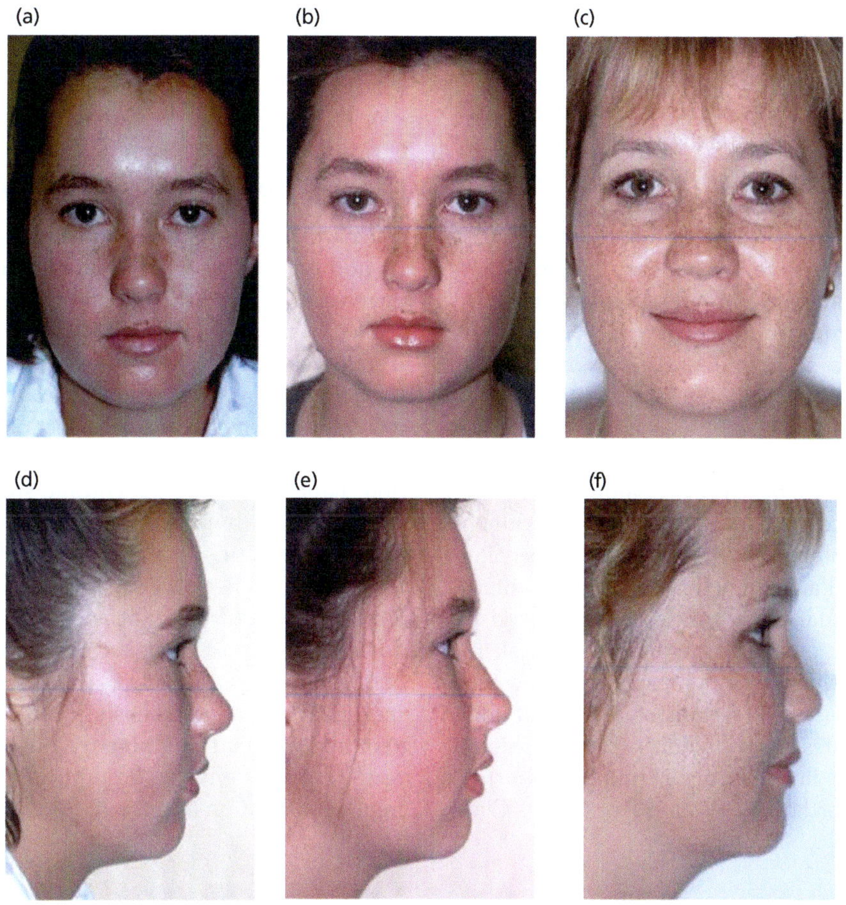

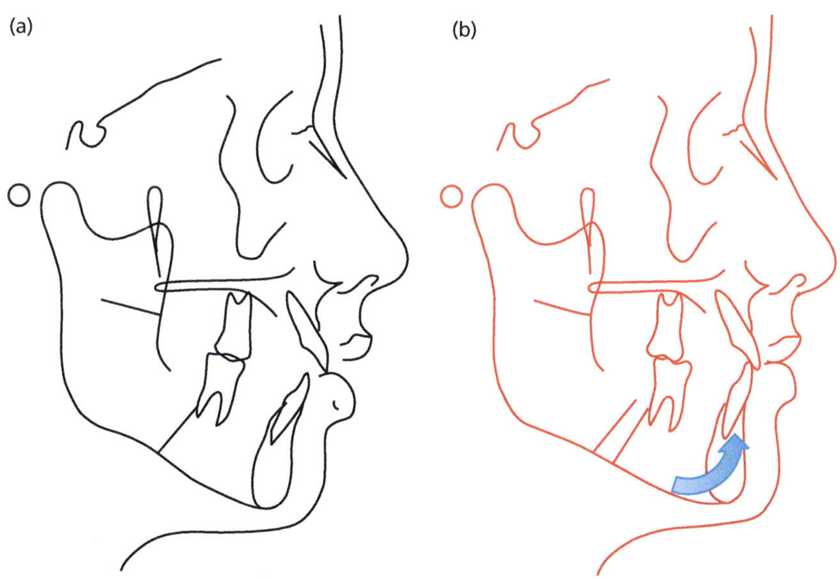

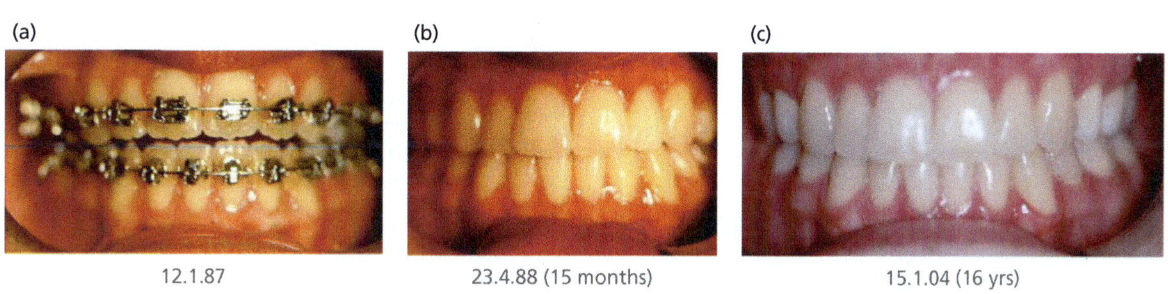

Fig. 28-16 Case 4: CASE 4. Pretreatment frontal view (a), one year post-operatively (b), and sixteen years after treatment (c). Pretreatment profile view (d), one year post-operatively (e), and sixteen after treatment (f).

The lateral cephalometric tracing of CASE 4. The Class II anterior open bite is evident (a). The Class II anterior open bite is corrected by means of a bilateral sagittal split mandibular ramus osteotomy with counterclockwise rotation of the distal segment (b). CASE 4. The presurgical occlusion (a), one year post-treatment (b), and sixteen years after treatment (c).

that the resorption may be related to chronic excessive loading of the mandibular condyle, which produces progressive remodelling of the condyle. There are two important aspects when planning the correction of the existing dentofacial deformity: (1) ensuring that the resorption process is inactive and (2) treating the deformity in such a way that the loads on the condyles are not increased. To establish whether the condition is still active, the patient's previous dental records, cephalometric radiographs, and occlusal models can be compared with current records. A radioisotope bone scan of the temporomandibular joints may help to detect the presence of any resorptive activity in the condyle. Surgical correction by traditional orthognathic surgery must await a period of quiescence (confirmed by serial cephalometry). Moreover, the residual condyle must be of adequate dimension. In these instances the open bite is corrected by posterior maxillary impaction. Secondary anteroposterior mandibular discrepancies are corrected by sagittal split osteotomy. The unquantifiable risk for post-surgical reactivation of the resorptive process is a source of concern. The option of alloplastic joint replacement obviates this problem and is increasingly considered a first line therapy in many cases (see Chapter 35). Any orthodontic treatment, such as Class III elastics, that increases the loading of the condyles (and could reinitiate the condylar resorption process) should be avoided.

Degenerative joint disease (osteoarthrosis)

Osteoarthrosis of the temporomandibular joint is not an acute entity but rather a progressive degenerative disease that alters the position, morphology, and physiology of the bony joint structures. It involves the progressive uncontrollable degeneration of the mandibular condyle, and unfortunately, the diagnosis and treatment selection are complicated by the variability of the rate of progression of resorption. Patients experience chronic signs of joint pain, crepitus, and hypomobility with periods of acute exacerbations. It may be possible to obtain short-term relief of the symptoms by conservative partial reconstruction of the joint and orthognathic surgery; however, in most patients the natural progression of the degenerative process leads to recurrence of the open bite and increasing joint symptoms. Total joint replacement combined with orthognathic correction of the dentofacial deformity is often the final treatment solution (Figure 28.17: CASE 5).

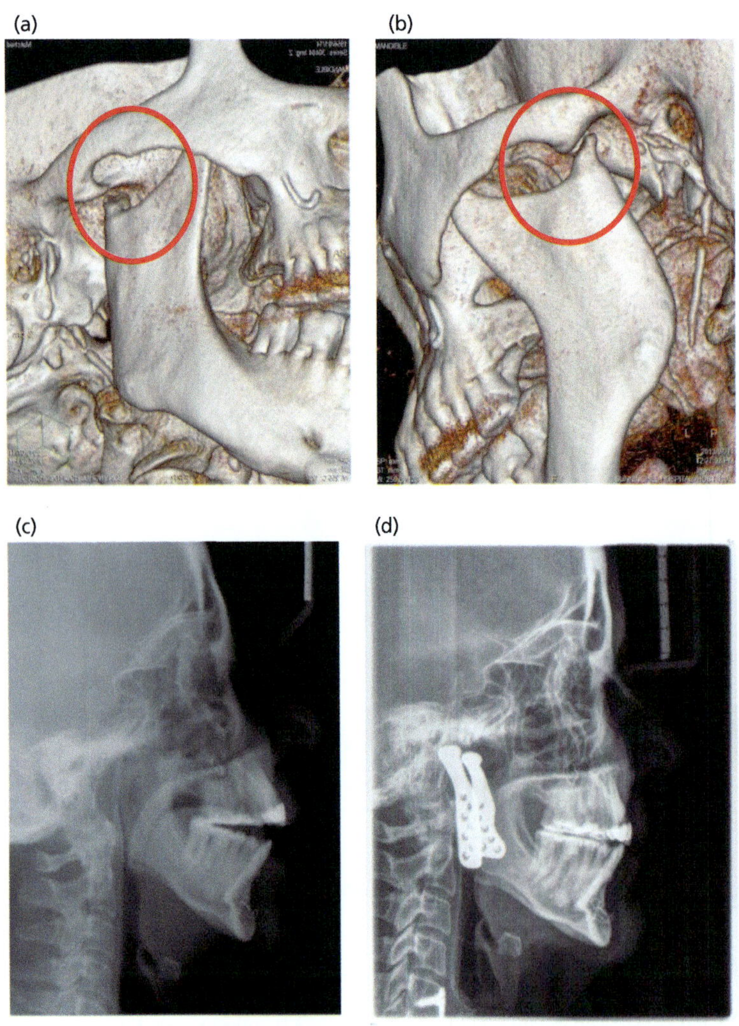

Fig. 28-17 Case 5: 3D CT of patient with advanced condylar resorbtion (circles) causing open bite deformity (a & b).

Presurgical cephalometric radiographs. (c) showing open bite due to reduction in mandibular ramus height. Post-surgical cephalograph (d) of the corrected occlusion following alloplastic joint replacement. Note the change in hyoid position and airway space which resulted in a marked improvement in the patient's sleep apnoea symptoms.(e–g) Patient with open bite due to condylar resorbtion has no typical midface signs. Clinical signs limited to increased lower facial height, decreased chin-throat length and mandibular anteroposterior deficiency. Both temporomandibular joints were reconstructed with titanium joint prosthesis and fossae. Post-surgical correction (h–j) reversal of the clinical signs and correction of the open bite

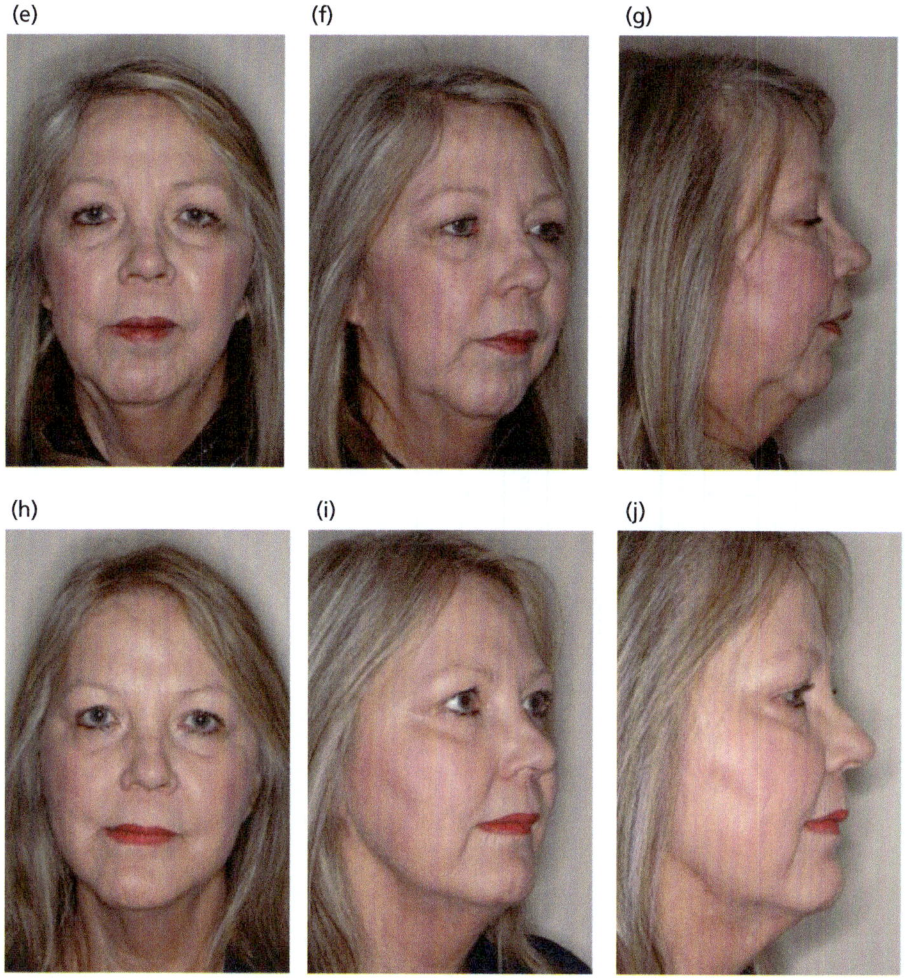

Fig. 28-17 (*Continued*)

Treatment planning for combined orthognathic surgery and total joint replacement does not differ from conventional orthognathic treatment planning. There is, however, a limited amount of mandibular advancement that can be obtained by the placement of a joint prosthesis. To maintain satisfactory contact between the implant and the mandibular ramus, the advancement should be limited to 7 to 8 mm.

Conclusions

The development of an anterior open bite in adolescence with mixed dentition may develop as a result of an upper airway obstruction and/or a thumb sucking habit and is usually managed by addressing the airway problem, habit control and dental expansion. An altered vertical growth pattern during and after adolescence are the predominant etiological factor in the development of a skeletal anterior open bite mal occlusion. Altered growth in these individuals results in either excessive vertical growth of the maxilla, lack of vertical growth of the mandibular ramus or a combination of both. Most of these patients, especially those with vertical maxillary excess will also have a tendency to have transverse maxillary deficiency. Successful management of patients with skeletal anterior open bite dentofacial deformities requires careful assessment of the specific anatomical location of the discrepancy, the aesthetic and functional demands and an understanding of the factors that may influence the long term stability of the treatment results. The authors present a flowchart (Figure 28-18) summarizing the suggested principles of surgical orthodontic treatment of anterior open bite dentofacial deformities.

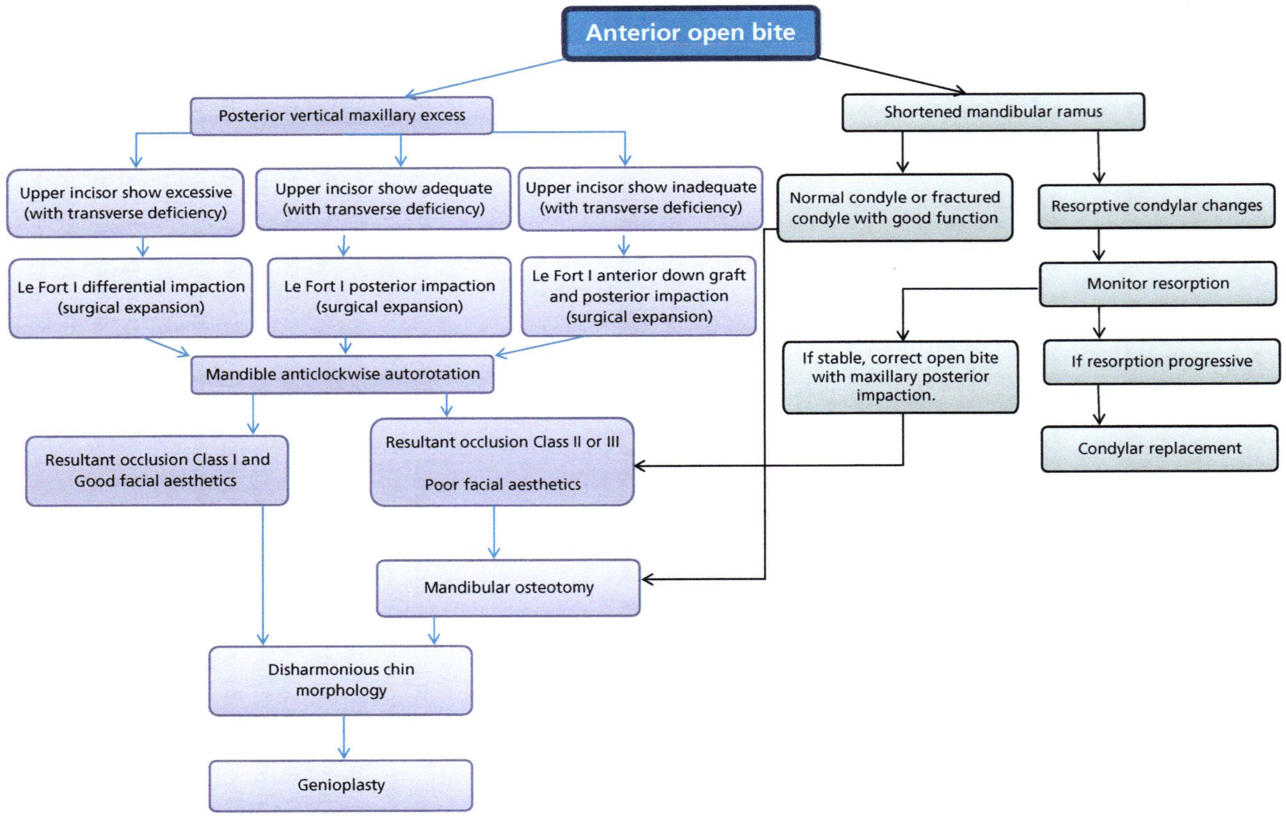

Fig. 28-18 Suggested principles of surgical orthodontic treatment of anterior open bite dentofacial deformities.

References

1 Lentini-Oliveira D, Carvalho FR, Qingsong Y, Junjie L, Saconato H, Machado MA, Prado LB, Prado GF. Orthodontic and orthopaedic treatment for anterior open bite in children. Cochrane Database Syst Rev. 2007 Apr 18;(2):CD005515. Review.

2 Haryett RD, Hansen FC, Davidson PO. Chronic thumb sucking. Am J Orthod. 1970;57:164–78.

3 Linder-Aronson S, Woodside D. Factors affecting the facial and dental structures in excess face height: malocclusion, etiology, diagnosis, and treatment. Chicago: Quintessence Pub Co; 2000, pp. 1–33.

4 Proffit WR, Fields HW, Nixon WL. Occlusal forces in normal and long face adults. J Dent Res. 1983;62:566–70.

5 Proffit WR, Fields HW. Occlusal forces in normal and long face children. J Dent Res. 1983;62:571–4.

6 Turvey TA, Journot V, Epker BN. Correction of anterior bite deformity: a study of tongue function, speech changes, and stability. J Max Fac Surg. 1976;4:93–101.

7 McNamara JA. Early intervention in the transverse dimension: is it worth the effort? Am J Orthod Dentofacial Orthop. 2002;121:572–4.

8 Sherwood KH, Burch JG, Thomson WJ. Closing open bites by intruding molars with titanium miniplate anchorage. Am J Orthod Dentofacial Orthop. 2002;122:593–600.

9 Siato I, Amaki M, Hanada K. Non-surgical treatment of adult open bite using edgewise appliance combined with high-pull headgear and class III elastics. Angle Orthod. 2005;75:277–83.

10 Kuroda S, Katayama A, Takano-Yamamoto T. Severe anterior open-bite using titanium screw anchorage. Angle Orthod. 2004;74:558–67.

11 Carano A, Siciliani G, Bowman SJ. Treatment of skeletal open bite with a device for rapid molar intrusion: a preliminary report. Angle Orthod. 2005;75:736–46.

12 Hamamci N, Basaran G, Sahin S. Non-surgical correction of an adult skeletal class III and open-bite malocclusion. Angle Orthod. 2006;76:527–32.

13 Erverdi N, Usumez S, Solak A. New generation open-bite treatment with zygomatic anchorage. Angle Orthod. 2006;76:519–26.

14 Kuster R, Ingervall B. The effect of treatment of skeletal open bite with two types of bite-blocks. Eur J Orthod. 1992;14:489–99.

15 Mao JJ. Mechanobiology of craniofacial sutures. J Dent Res. 2000;81:810–6.

16 Handelman CS, Wang C, BeGole EA, et al. Nonsurgical rapid maxillary expansion in adults: report on 47 cases using the Haas expander. Angle Orthod. 2000;70:129–44.

17 de Freitas MR, Beltrao RT, Janson G, et al. Longterm stability of anterior open bite extraction treatment in the permanent dentition. Am J Orthod Dentofacial Orthop. 2004;125:78–87.

18 Janson G, Valarelli FP, Henriques JF, et al. Stability of anterior open bite nonextraction treatment in the permanent dentition. Am J Orthod Dentofacial Orthop. 2003;124:265–76.

19 Cozza P, Mucedero M, Baccetti T, et al. Early orthodontic treatment of skeletal open-bite malocclusion: a systematic review. Angle Orthod. 2005;75:707–13.

20 Behrents RG. Growth in the aging facial skeleton-Monograph #17: Craniofacial Growth Series. Ann Arbor: The University of Michigan, Centre for Human Growth and Development, 1985.

21 Fotis V, Melsen B, Williams S. Vertical control as an important ingredient in the treatment of severe sagittal discrepancies. Am J Orthod. 1984;86:224–32.

22 Reyneke JP. Vertical variation in skeletal open bite: a classification for surgical planning. J Dent Ass S Africa. 1988;43:465–72.

23 Arnett GW, Bergman RT. Facial keys to orthodontic diagnosis and treatment planning. Part I. Am J Orthod Dentofacial Orthop. 1993;103:299–312.

24 Jacobs JD, Bell WH, Williams C, et al. Control of the transverse dimension with surgery and orthodontics. Am J Orthod. 1980;77:284–306.

25 Bell WH, Jacobs JD, Quejada JG. Simultaneous repositioning of the maxilla, mandible and chin. Am J Orthod. 1986;89:28–50.

26 Koudstaal MJ, Poort LJ, Van der Wal KGH, Wolvius EB, Prahl-Andersen B, Schulten AJ. Surgically assisted rapid maxillary expansion (SRME): a review of the literature. Int J Oral Maxillofac Surg. 2005;34:709–14.

27 Bloomquist DS. Mandibular narrowing: advantage in transverse problems. J Oral Maxillofac Surg. 2004;62:365–8.

28 Alexander CD, Bloomquist DS, Wallen TR. Stability of mandibular constriction with a symphyseal osteotomy. Am J Orthod Dentofacial Orthop. 1993;103:15–23.

29 Phillips C, Medland WH, Fields HW, et al. Stability of surgical maxillary expansion. Int J Adult Orthodon Orthognath Surg. 1992;7:139–46.

30 Proffitt WR, Turvey TA, Phillips C. Orthognathic surgery: a hierarchy of stability. Int J Orthod Orthog Surg. 1996;11:191–204.

31 Reyneke JP. Rotation the maxillomandibular complex: an alternative surgical design in orthognathic surgery academic dissertation. Tampere, Finland: University of Tampere, Institute of Regenerative Medicine, 2006.

32 Chemello PD, Wolford LM, Buchang PH. Occlusal plane alteration in orthognathic surgery. Part II: long term stability of results. Am J Orthod Dentofacial Orthop. 1994;104:434–40.

Chapter 29

Surgical Correction of Anterior Open Bite: Differential Posterior Maxillary Impaction

Farhad B. Naini, Andrew Stewart and Daljit S. Gill

'... a gap in nature.'

William Shakespeare (1564–1616)
Antony and Cleopatra (c.1606)[1]

Introduction

There are two extremes in the vertical relationship of the incisor teeth, namely the anterior open bite (AOB) and the 'deep' overbite. In anterior open bite, there is a vertical space between the maxillary and mandibular incisor teeth when the posterior teeth are in occlusion.

The aetiology of the degree of incisor overbite may involve skeletal, and/or dental and/or environmental factors, which may combine to determine the degree of incisor overbite. However, the extent to which these various aetiological factors are responsible for the vertical discrepancy is variable. The dentofacial morphological relationships often point to the major component in the aetiology, though in many cases the clinician may remain uncertain as to the degree of influence of each aetiological factor.[2]

If the primary aetiology of an anterior open bite is a **hyperdivergent facial growth pattern**, which refers to an excessive divergence of the maxillary, occlusal and mandibular planes in relation to each other and to the anterior cranial base, the terms **skeletal open bite**,[3] or **apertognathia** (Latin *apertus*: open; Greek *gnathos*: jaw) may be used.[4]

The potential for attempting to restrict vertical maxillary development in an adolescent, growing patient with vertical maxillary excess has been discussed in Chapter 3. However, there are three principal methods to surgically correct an anterior open bite of primarily skeletal aetiology in a non-growing adult patient:

1. **Segmental impaction of the posterior maxilla**
   The Le Fort I osteotomized maxilla is vertically segmentalized, either distal to the canines or distal to the lateral incisors. The posterior and anterior segments, which will have been preoperatively aligned and levelled independently, will be moved separately. The posterior segment is

Orthognathic Surgery: Principles, Planning and Practice. Edited by Farhad B. Naini and Daljit S. Gill.

superiorly repositioned, allowing forward autorotation of the mandible to close the AOB, and the anterior segment is repositioned vertically to obtain the ideal maxillary incisor exposure in relation to the upper lip. This approach is described in detail in Chapter 28.

2. **Differential posterior impaction of the Le Fort I osteotomized maxilla**
   Rotation of the maxillary occlusal plane round the transverse axis with differential posterior impaction permits forward autorotation of the mandible to close an AOB. Orthodontic preparation requires an element of proclination of the maxillary incisors, as the effect of surgical posterior impaction is relative retroclination of the maxillary incisors. Therefore, the orthodontic preparation for this approach is significantly different to the maxillary segmental surgical approach described above. This second approach is described in this chapter.
3. **Isolated mandibular surgery**
   Anterior rotation (in the direction of mouth closing) of the distal segment of the mandible following a bilateral sagittal split osteotomy may be used to close an AOB in appropriately selected cases. This approach is discussed in detail in Chapter 30.

Ideally, the choice of procedure should be determined based on the diagnostic features of the individual patient. For example, an obvious and potentially convenient step in the maxillary occlusal plane between the anterior and posterior segments may be better approached with segmental surgery, though surgeon preference for a technical option is also a factor.

Diagnosis and aetiology

'The knowledge of anything, since all things have causes,
is not acquired or complete unless it is known by its causes.'
Pür Sina (Latinized Avicenna) (AD 980–1037)
Canon Medicinae (The Canon of Medicine)

Understanding the aetiology of every malocclusion and dentofacial discrepancy is critical, but the significance of understanding the aetiology of anterior open bites is more consequential, as it will have a direct bearing on the choice of treatment strategy and will fundamentally influence its potential stability. It should be noted that an anterior open bite is not a diagnosis per se, but a clinical sign that may be present in a number of dentofacial configurations, with an array of potential causes.

The various possible aetiological factors in the development of an AOB are presented in Table 29-1, though it should be remembered that the aetiology may be multifactorial, involving several aetiological factors.[4]

Table 29-1 Aetiology of anterior open bite with presenting features

Aetiology	Presenting features
Skeletal: increased LAFH	Excessive increase in LAFH (usually due to posterior VME), with the incisors unable to erupt to such an extent that they fully compensate for the face height, resulting in an AOB. Usually correlated with an increased mandibular plane angle and increased gonial angle, but these are only a correlation, and depend on the posterior face height.
Skeletal: reduced ramus height	Vertical deficiency in mandibular ramus height, leading to an increased anterior to posterior face height ratio, a steep mandibular plane angle, a clockwise rotation of the mandible and an AOB.
Soft tissue: tongue size, resting position and/or activity	**Resting tongue position** A *forward resting* tongue position (between the incisor teeth) may impede anterior vertical dentoalveolar development, leading to an AOB with the incisors at a different vertical level to the posterior dentition (Figure 29.1). **Adaptive swallowing pattern** There is an atypical *adaptive* swallowing pattern – i.e. an anterior oral seal is formed by contact between the lower lip or the tongue and the anterior palatal mucosa. *This is likely to be an adaptation to the AOB, not its cause.* **Endogenous tongue thrust** The rare condition known as an endogenous tongue thrust will be associated with:[5] • bimaxillary incisor proclination • symmetrical AOB • an almost constant presence of a significant portion of the tongue between the anterior teeth • a reverse curve of Spee in the mandibular arch and an accentuated curve in the maxillary arch • significant sigmatism (sibilant lisping) *Note*: As the aetiology of an AOB is due primarily to the activity of the tongue in this rare condition, the vertical skeletal height relationships may well be normal.
Nasorespiratory function and head posture	**Postural changes to the head** (extending the head back by tilting it around the transverse axis of rotation) due to **partial nasal airway obstruction** and excessive long-term **mouth breathing** allow downward and backward posturing of the mandible, downward positioning of the tongue and overeruption of the posterior teeth in both dental arches. Such changes were *previously assumed* to be the main aetiological factors resulting in skeletal AOB in tall face individuals.[6–10] The facial appearance of such individuals was formerly, and erroneously, referred to as **'adenoid facies'**.[11]

(continued)

Table 29-1 (*Continued*)

Aetiology	Presenting features
	Note: It appears to be more likely that the skeletal pattern and vertical facial growth tendency are predominantly genetically determined, but that environmental influences may result in additional changes, perhaps in some cases exacerbating the effects, e.g. worsening an AOB.
Habit: digit sucking	Non-nutritive sucking behaviour is very common in the infant, who appears to derive comfort from the habit, and is of little importance in the deciduous dentition. Intensity and prolonged duration into the permanent dentition are likely to cause dentoalveolar discrepancies: • Usually asymmetrical AOB (Figure 29.2) • Impeded maxillary incisor eruption • Narrowing of the maxilla and concomitant buccal crossbite(s) ± lateral mandibular displacement (Figure 29.3)
Pathological	**Idiopathic condylar resorption** Significant risk factors identified for post-orthognathic condylar resorption include being female with mandibular retrognathia associated with an increased mandibular plane angle, the presence of pretreatment condylar atrophy, and undergoing posterior condylar displacement and upward and forward rotation of the mandible at the time of surgery.[12] **Neuromuscular conditions** E.g. cerebral palsy or muscular dystrophy, where the severe reduction in muscle tone may lead to significant posterior rotational growth of the jaws and a significant anterior open bite. **Systemic conditions** Condylysis may also be related to systemic conditions, such as systemic lupus erythematosus (SLE).
Traumatic	Bilateral condylar fractures, particularly in a growing patient, potentially leading to temporomandibular joint ankylosis.
Iatrogenic	Poorly controlled extrusive orthodontic forces on the posterior dentition, leading to their extrusion and thereby opening of the bite anteriorly.

AOB, anterior open bite; VME, vertical maxillary excess; LAFH, lower anterior face height.

(a)

(b)

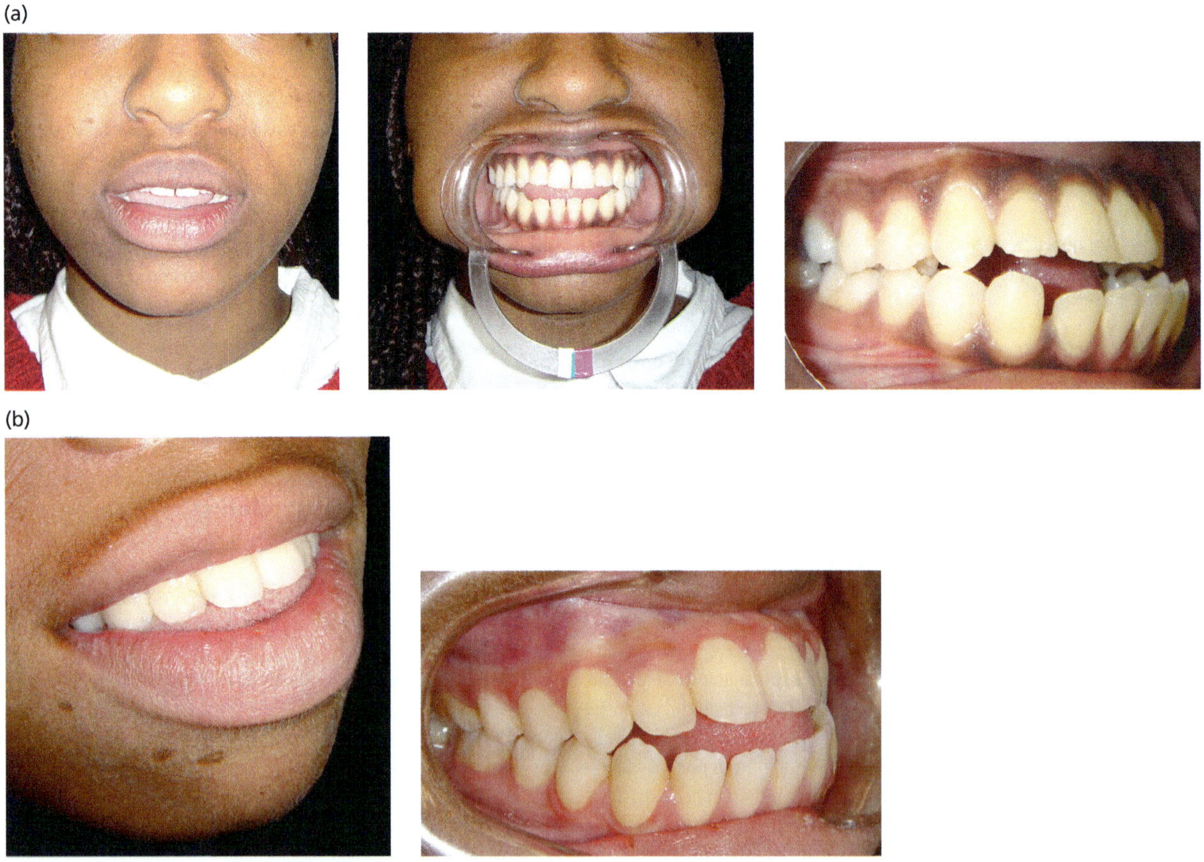

Fig. 29-1 A forward resting tongue position may be evident with a patient in repose. The incisors will be at a different vertical level to the posterior dentition, and are usually proclined. (a) Example of a skeletal Class III patient with predominantly soft tissue AOB. (b) Example of a skeletal Class I patient with predominantly soft tissue AOB.

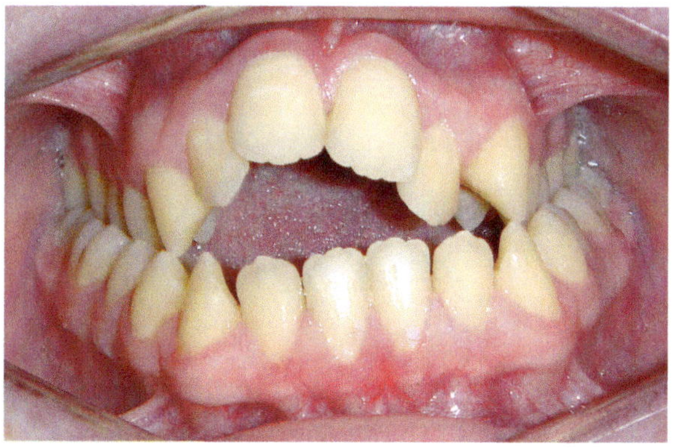

Fig. 29-2 Asymmetrical AOB in a patient aged 17 years with a continued thumb sucking habit. Narrowing of the maxillary arch is common in such cases.

Presenting features[4]

Lower anterior face height

In a patient with an average posterior face height (i.e. average mandibular ramus height), a skeletal anterior open bite may occur due to a significant increase in the lower anterior face height (LAFH), often related to posterior vertical maxillary excess. In such patients, the lower anterior face height will be significantly greater than the midfacial height. If the incisor teeth are unable to erupt in relation to the increased LAFH, an AOB ensues (Figure 29-4).

Anterior to posterior face height ratio

It is possible that a patient may present with an average lower anterior face height, but significantly reduced posterior face height (i.e. reduced mandibular ramus height). Therefore, the anterior to posterior face height ratio will be significantly increased (Figure 29-5).

Relative inclination of the maxillary, occlusal and mandibular planes (Sassouni analysis)

In a well-proportioned face, the maxillary, occlusal and mandibular planes should converge symmetrically toward an approximate area of intersection

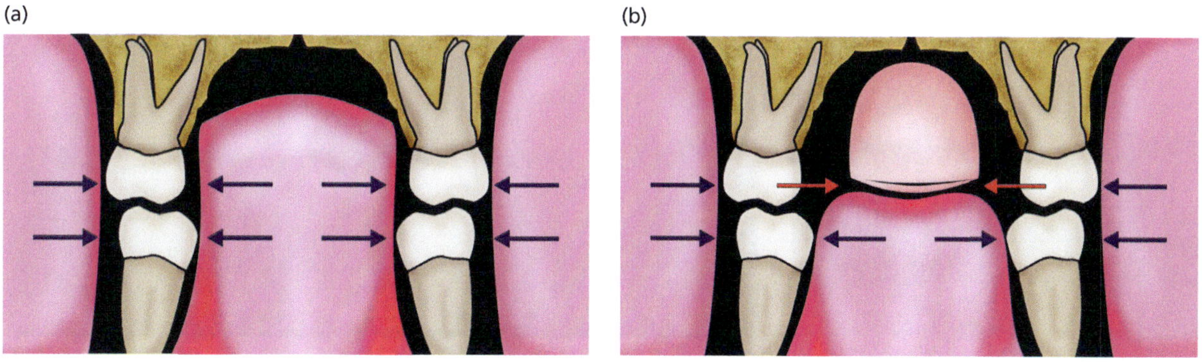

Fig. 29-3 (a) Schematic representation of the average patient, with the teeth in a zone of soft tissue equilibrium between the pressure from the soft tissue forces of the cheeks and tongue. (b) In a patient with a prolonged digit sucking habit, the digit (e.g. thumb) displaces the tongue inferiorly. The excessive buccal forces from the cheek musculature due to forces generated by sucking pressure will be offset by those from the highly muscular tongue situated between the mandibular dentition, but lead to narrowing of the maxillary dentition where they are unopposed.

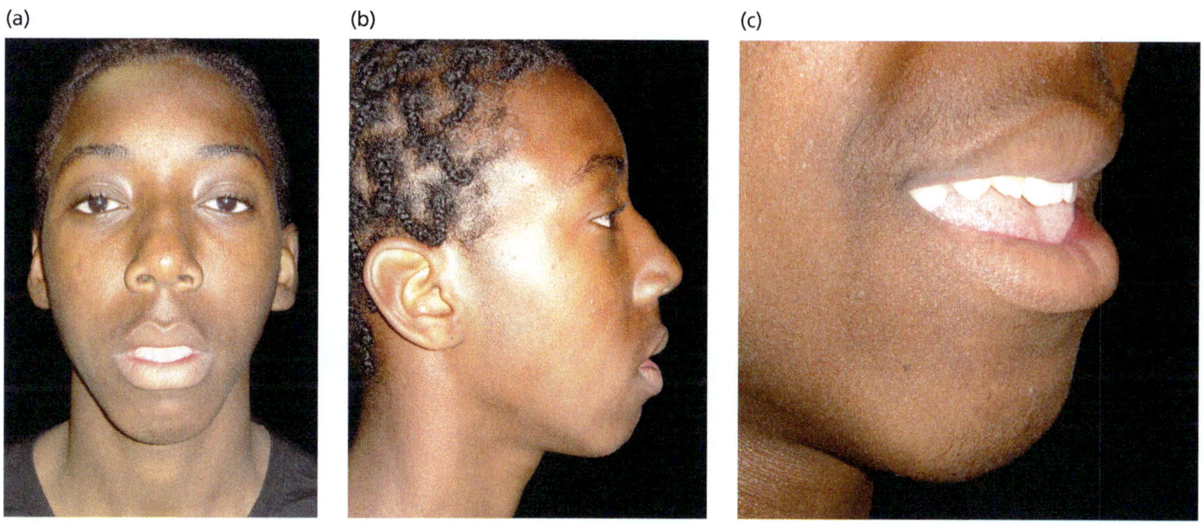

Fig. 29-4 Skeletal anterior open bite due to increased lower anterior face height. The mandibular ramus height is average. There is posterior vertical maxillary excess, which has led to a posterior rotation of the mandible, moving the chin downward and backward relative to the face. There is an adaptive forward position of the tongue.

(d) (e) (f) (g)

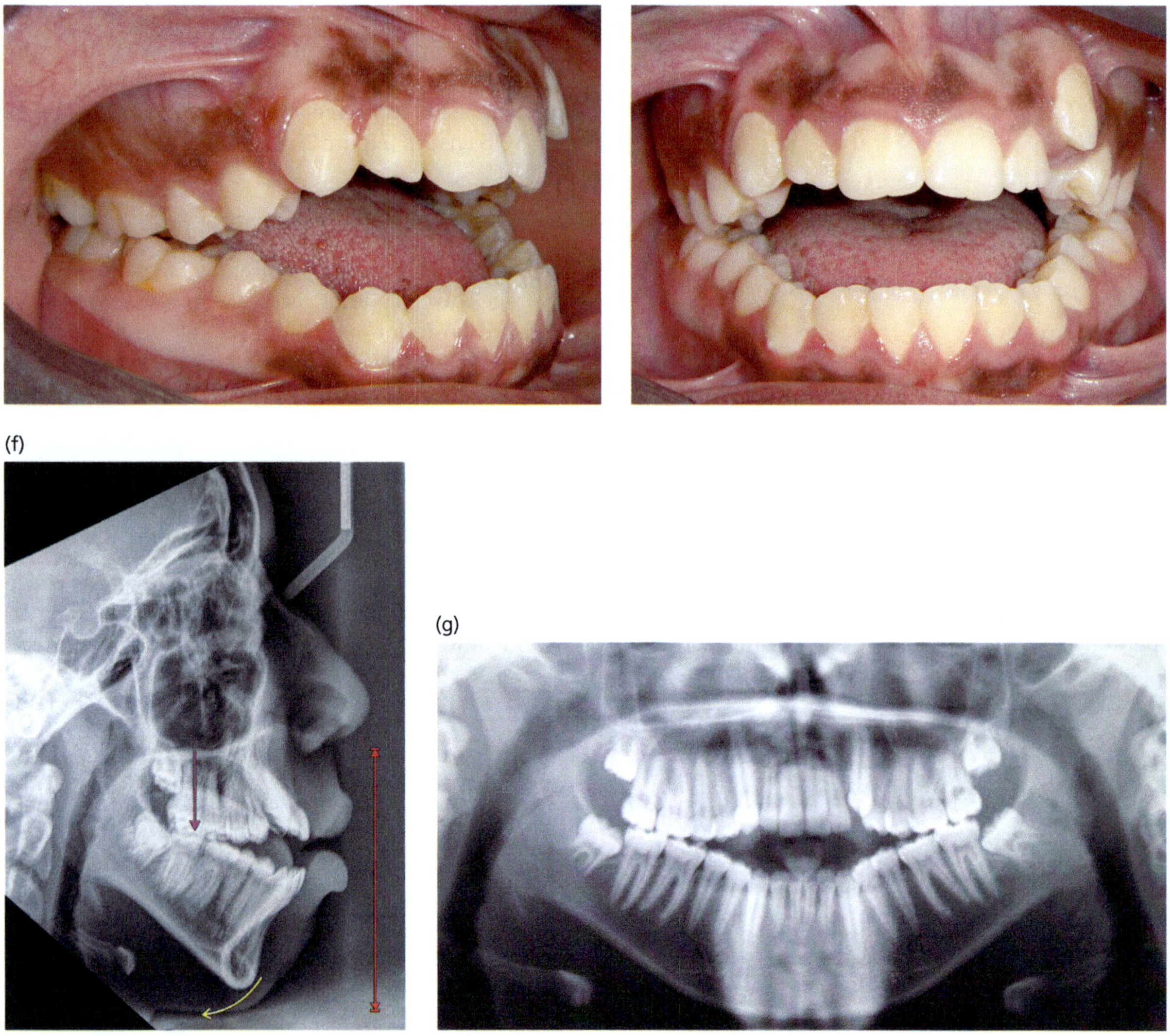

Fig. 29-4 (*Continued*).

located near the occiput (back of the skull) (see Figure 5-54a). If either jaw is vertically disproportionate, its associated plane will not converge with the others. If the area of convergence of these planes is positioned in front of the occiput, towards the face, the planes will diverge anteriorly (see Figure 5-54c). This skeletal pattern is associated with markedly different anterior and posterior facial heights, and correlates with an anterior open bite tendency, which Sassouni classified as a 'skeletal open bite'.[3,13]

(a) (b) (c)

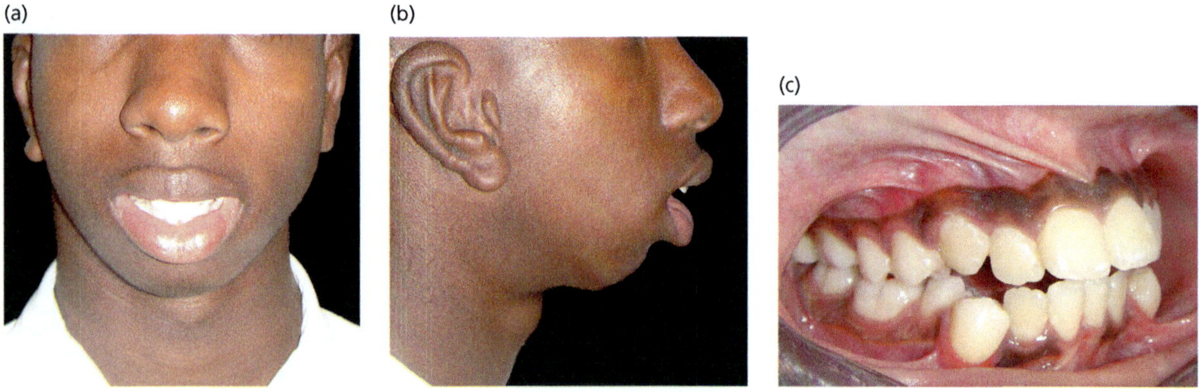

Fig. 29-5 Skeletal anterior open bite due to reduced ramus height. The vertical position of the maxilla is average, as is the lower anterior face height. The mandible is rotated posteriorly, and there is a pronounced antegonial convexity in the morphology of the mandible.

(d)

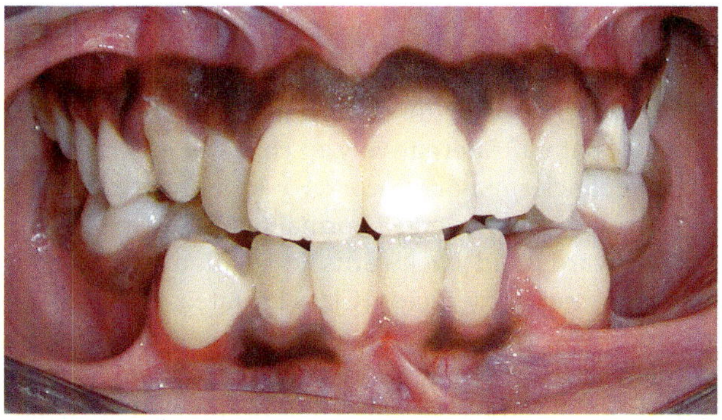

(e)

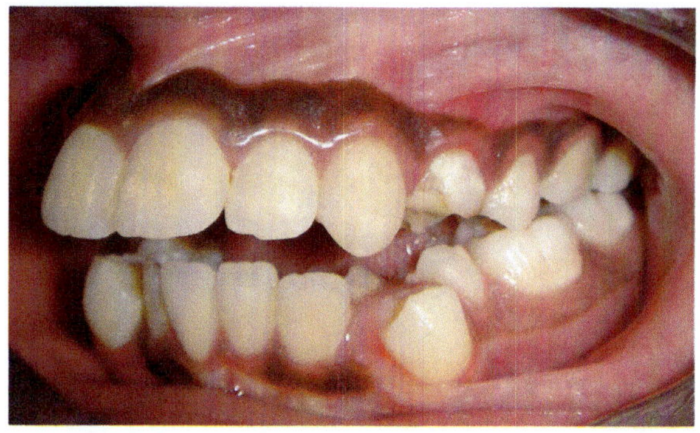

(f)

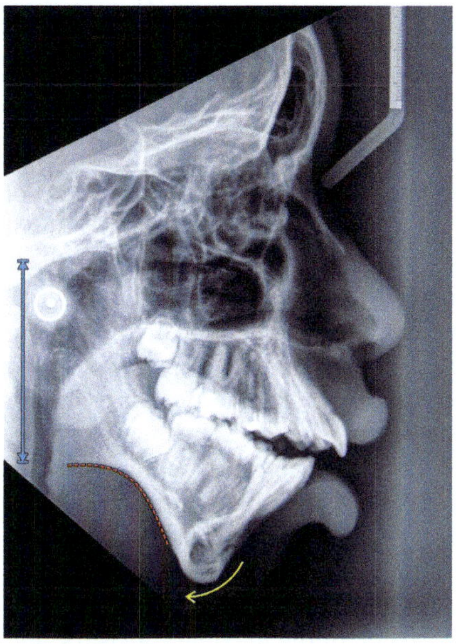

(g)

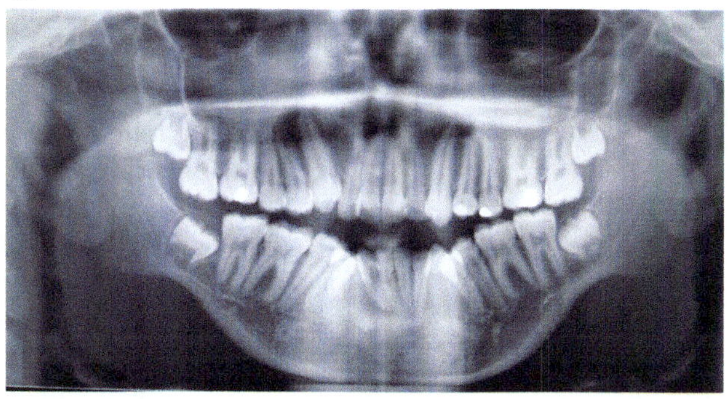

Fig. 29-5 (*Continued*).

Pattern of rotational development of the jaws

The pattern of rotational growth of the jaws in relation to each other and the craniofacial complex has a direct influence on the morphological characteristics of vertical skeletal discrepancies and thereby to the development of anterior open bites of predominantly skeletal aetiology.

Abnormal **bimaxillary posterior rotational growth** leads to *divergent rotational growth of the maxilla and mandible*. The maxilla will be tilted down posteriorly, as will the maxillary occlusal plane, resulting in an anticlockwise rotation of the maxilla observed in right profile view. A posterior (backward, clockwise) growth rotation of the mandible also results. This pattern of mandibular growth rotation may be indicated by Björk's seven structural signs (Table 29-2 and Figure 29-6).

Björk's facial polygon is a useful method of analysing the effects of various cranioskeletal angular relationships on the jaws in the sagittal and vertical planes.[14] An obtuse 'saddle angle' formed between the anterior and middle cranial fossae may be found in patients with skeletal open bite, and this angle is set relatively early in life (Figure 29-7). Richardson[15] compared the craniofacial morphology of 110 AOB individuals with the same number of deep overbite individuals (matched in respect of age and sex), and found that the LAFH was considerably greater, on average, in AOB cases compared with deep overbite. However, the difference could not be directly

Table 29-2 Björk's seven structural signs indicating a posterior pattern of mandibular growth rotation (Numbers refer to Figure 29-6)

	Structural signs	Backward (posterior) mandibular growth rotation
1	Inclination of the condylar head	Backward
2	Curvature of the mandibular canal	Straight canal
3	Shape of the lower border of the mandible	Convex lower border and antegonial notch
4	Inclination of the mandibular symphysis (bony chin)	Backward inclination, reduced chin projection
5	Interincisal angle	Reduced
6	Intermolar and interpremolar angle	Reduced
7	Lower anterior face height	Increased

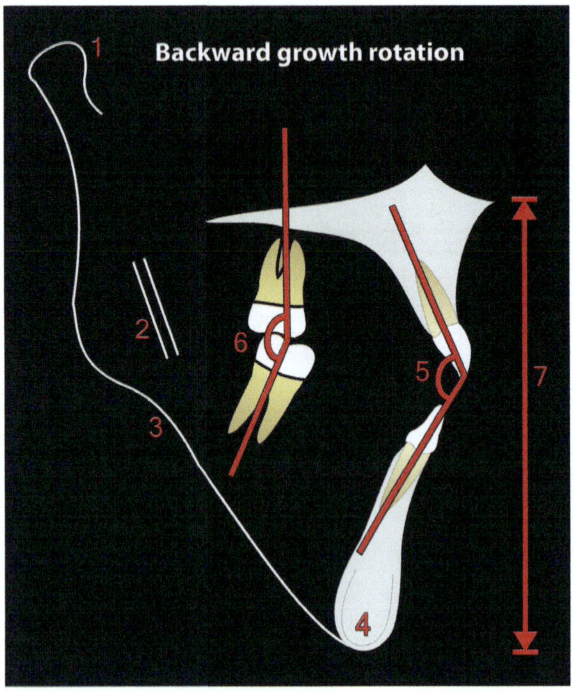

Fig. 29-6 Björk's seven structural signs, which may be used to indicate the pattern of posterior (backward) mandibular growth rotation (For an explanation of the numbers, refer to Table 29-2.) (From: Naini FB. Facial Aesthetics: Concepts and Clinical Diagnosis. Oxford: Wiley-Blackwell, 2011; used with permission.[20])

attributed to differences in linear values for Björk's facial polygon, but seemed to be related more to the obtuse gonial and articular angles, i.e. *a question of cranioskeletal shape rather than size.*

Sagittal skeletal base relationship

Sagittal discrepancies may be primary but present with a skeletal AOB, e.g. sagittal mandibular excess or deficiency due to mandibular macrognathia or micrognathia. Alternatively, or concomitantly, sagittal discrepancies may be secondary to the vertical skeletal growth pattern, e.g. a normal mandible may rotate downwards and backwards in relation to posterior vertical maxillary excess (Class I rotated to a Class II). Either way, posterior maxillary impaction will result in forward autorotation of the mandible, i.e. the position the mandible would have occupied had it not been for the posterior VME. The sagittal position of the mandible subsequently may be corrected by mandibular repositioning.

Upper lip–maxillary incisor relationship

The degree of maxillary incisor exposure is of paramount importance in diagnosis and treatment planning. In a skeletal anterior open bite, the maxillary incisors may have reached their eruptive potential, but have been unable to meet the opposing mandibular incisors due to the excessive increase in lower anterior face height. Therefore, the maxillary incisor exposure in relation to the upper lip may be average or even increased. In such cases, as the maxillary incisors are already in a reasonable position relative to the upper lip, any extrusion of the maxillary incisors may appear very unsightly, as well as being prone to relapse. Preparatory orthodontics should aim at alignment without extrusion of the maxillary incisors, and

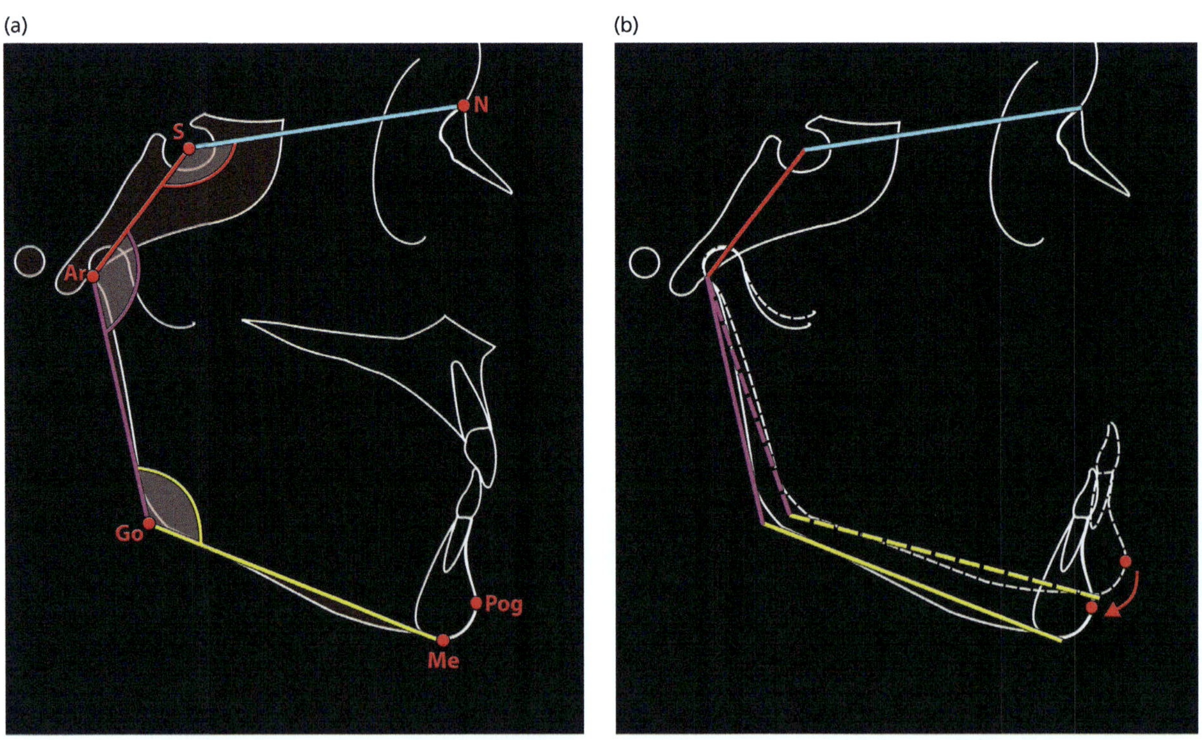

Fig. 29-7 (a) Björk's polygon, demonstrating the saddle angle, articular angle and gonial angle. (b) An increase in the articular angle will lead to downward and backward movement of the mandibular incisors (and chin), and potential opening of the bite. (Modified from: Naini FB. Facial Aesthetics: Concepts and Clinical Diagnosis. Oxford: Wiley-Blackwell, 2011; used with permission.[20])

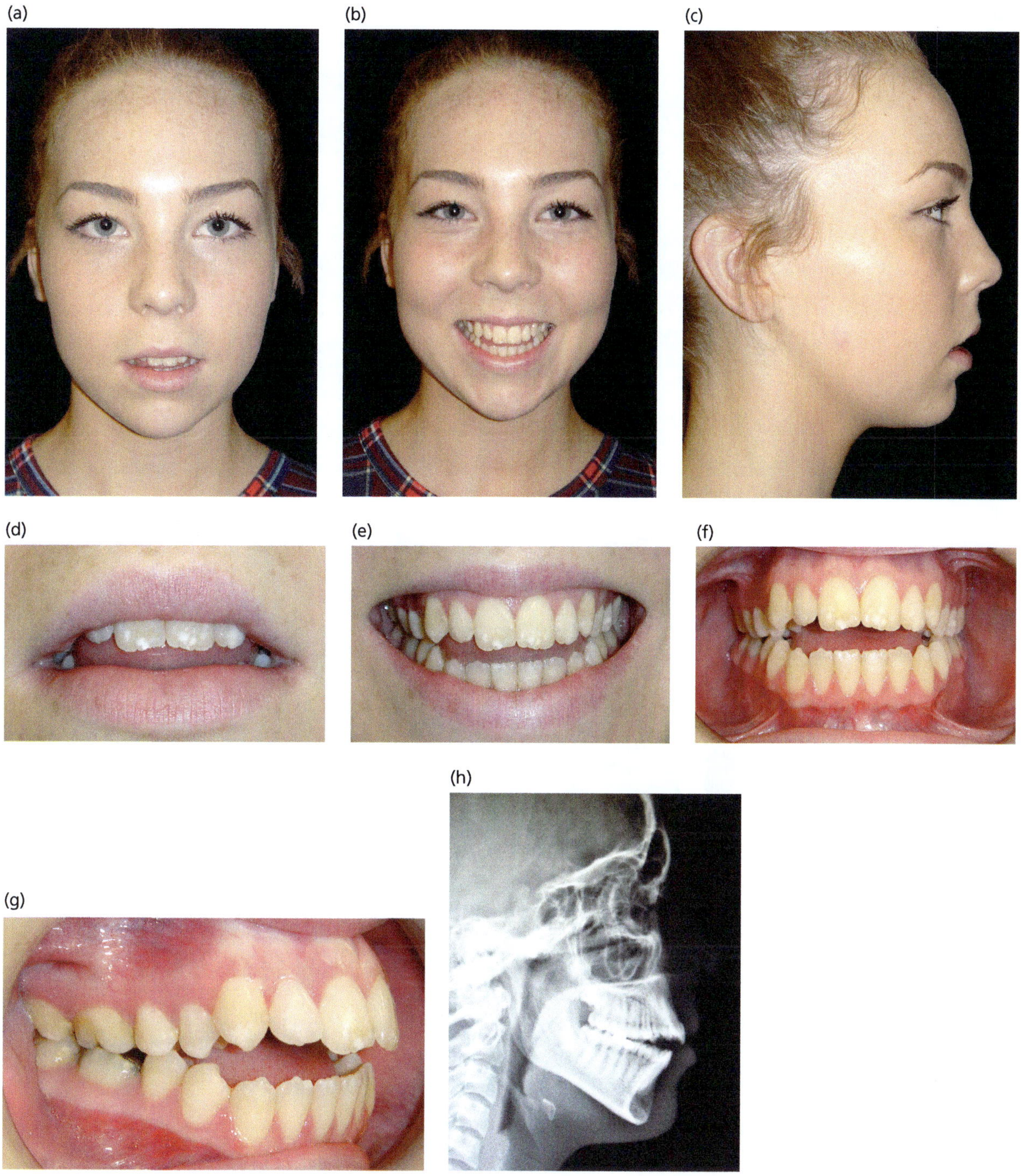

Fig. 29-8 Skeletal AOB with adaptive tongue posture (and very mild lisp), with good lip-incisor relationship at rest and smiling. Therefore, the problem is entirely posterior VME and posterior mandibular rotation. There is excess bone in the posterior maxilla between the root apices of the molars and the palate as seen on the cephalometric radiograph. LAFH is slightly increased, and there is a mild incomplete lip seal. Preparatory orthodontic treatment should aim to maintain the lip–incisor relationship, and impact the posterior maxilla.

the open bite will be closed by elevation of the posterior maxilla and subsequent forward autorotation of the mandible (Figure 29-8).

Conversely, if there is a significant additional soft tissue element to the aetiology of a skeletal anterior open bite, the forward resting tongue position may well have impeded the eruption of the maxillary incisors. In frontal view, the posterior maxillary dentition will be at an inferior level to the anterior dentition, and there will either be an increased sagittal curve to the maxillary arch or an obvious vertical step between the posterior and anterior maxillary dentition. The anterior dentoalveolar vertical maxillary deficiency due to the restrictive effect of the forward positioned tongue will often lead to a reduced maxillary incisor display or in extreme cases a 'no tooth show' smile (Figure 29-9). In such situations, a degree of levelling by extrusion of the maxillary incisors in the preparatory orthodontics is likely to remain stable postoperatively, as the tongue will re-adapt

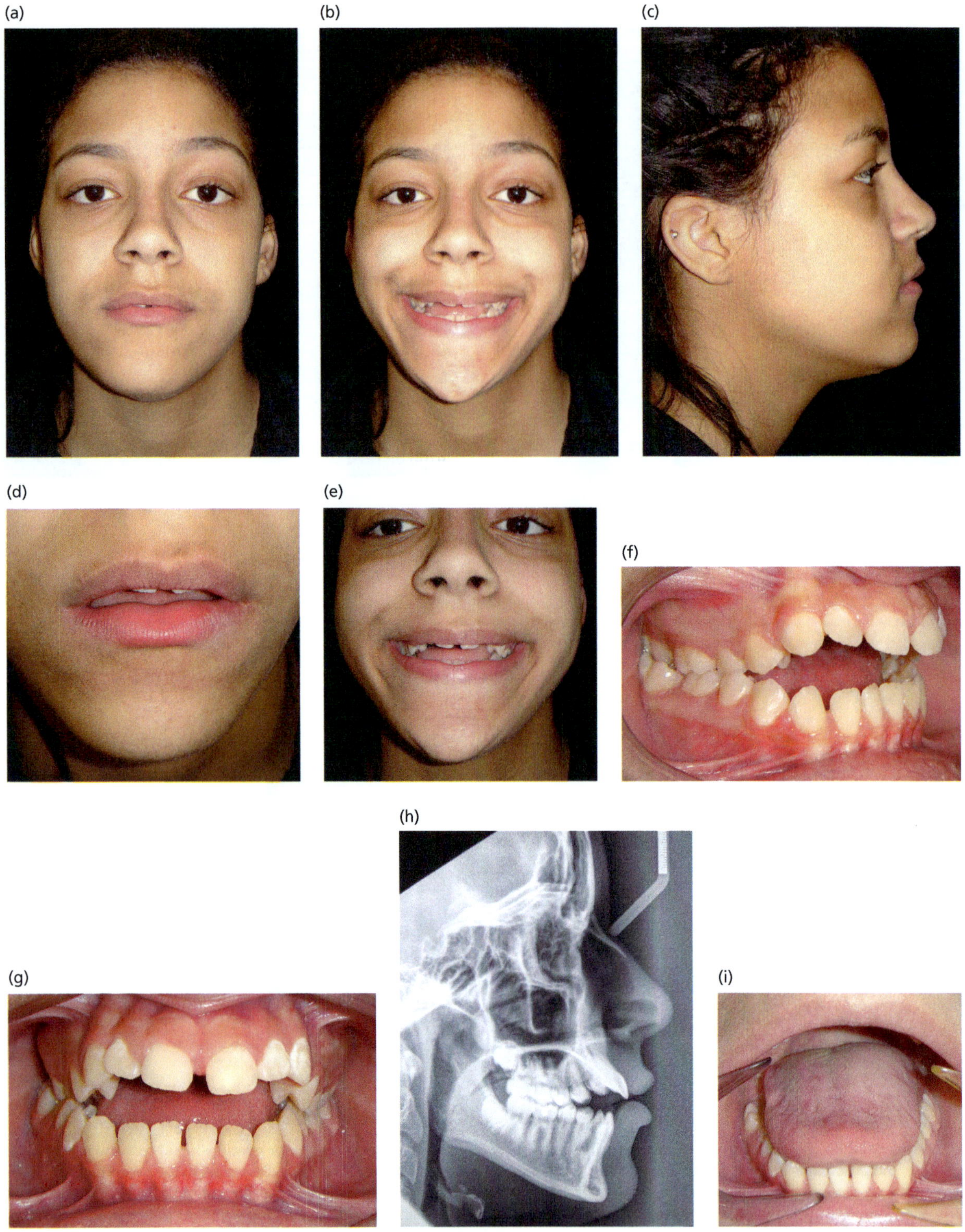

Fig. 29-9 Anterior open bite with a significant soft tissue (tongue) aetiology. Maxillary incisor exposure is reduced at rest and on smiling. An important treatment aim should be to increase the maxillary incisor exposure.

to the new anterior dentolabial relationships. Alternatively, an anterior segmental maxillary setdown may be required in addition to posterior maxillary impaction.

Nasolabial angle

The upper and lower components of the nasolabial angle should be evaluated separately, as they vary independently (see Figure 5-12).[16] In tall face patients with a skeletal anterior open bite, particularly those with a Class II skeletal pattern, the nasolabial angle tends to be obtuse, and the upper lip posteriorly inclined (Figure 29-10).[17] The clinical relevance is that following a posterior maxillary impaction, there is likely to be a requirement for a maxillary advancement as well, otherwise there is risk of exacerbating an already obtuse nasolabial angle.

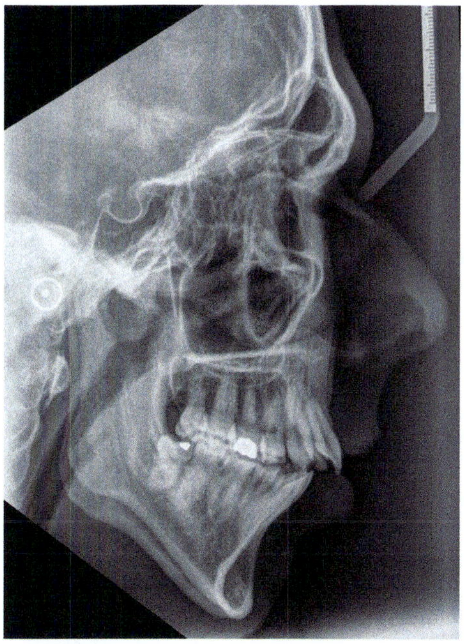

Fig. 29-10 A Class II patient with increased lower anterior face height and a skeletal anterior open bite. The nasolabial angle is obtuse and the upper lip posteriorly inclined.

The tongue

The role of the tongue in the aetiology of anterior open bite must be a matter for consideration during diagnosis and treatment planning. If there is an *abnormally* large tongue, for example in a Class III AOB patient (Figure 29-11), or abnormal tongue function, surgical correction of an anterior open bite may be prone to relapse. If the tongue is significantly enlarged (e.g. Beckwith–Wiedemann syndrome) on clinical examination (**true macroglossia**), consideration may need to be given to **tongue reduction surgery (reduction glossectomy)**, though this is uncommon. If required, a useful technique, described by Egyedi and Obwegeser (1964),[18] involves the resection of an anterior V-shaped wedge and an oval midline excision from anterior to the vallate papillae (Figure 29-12).

An anterior open bite predominantly due to the action of the tongue is extremely rare. This so-called **endogenous tongue thrust** is associated with obvious sigmatism (lisping) and symmetrical AOB with bimaxillary dentoalveolar proclination, usually with a normal face height. This condition is likely to be due to an underlying abnormality in the neuromuscular control of the tongue and is thereby difficult to correct and any treatment is likely to be highly unstable. However, in most patients with a part soft tissue aetiology to their AOB, the forward tongue position and atypical swallowing behaviour is **adaptive** to the AOB, often *secondary* to a prolonged digit-sucking habit. Adaptive tongue postures and adaptive swallowing patterns will often re-adapt to the new dentolabial relationship following orthognathic surgery, and in general do not impose limitations on surgical correction of an AOB.

Principles in planning the surgical correction of skeletal anterior open bite

The surgical correction of anterior open bite includes patients whose treatment may involve a differential impaction of the maxilla. This includes cases of skeletal anterior open bite and vertical maxillary excess, with greater posterior than anterior vertical maxillary growth. The maxillary plane is canted down posteriorly. The treatment for such conditions involves Le Fort I downfracture of the maxilla and **differential posterior maxillary impaction**, i.e. moving the posterior maxilla superiorly more than the anterior maxilla, often referred to as a 'posterior impaction'. The mandible may then autorotate forward, thereby

(a)

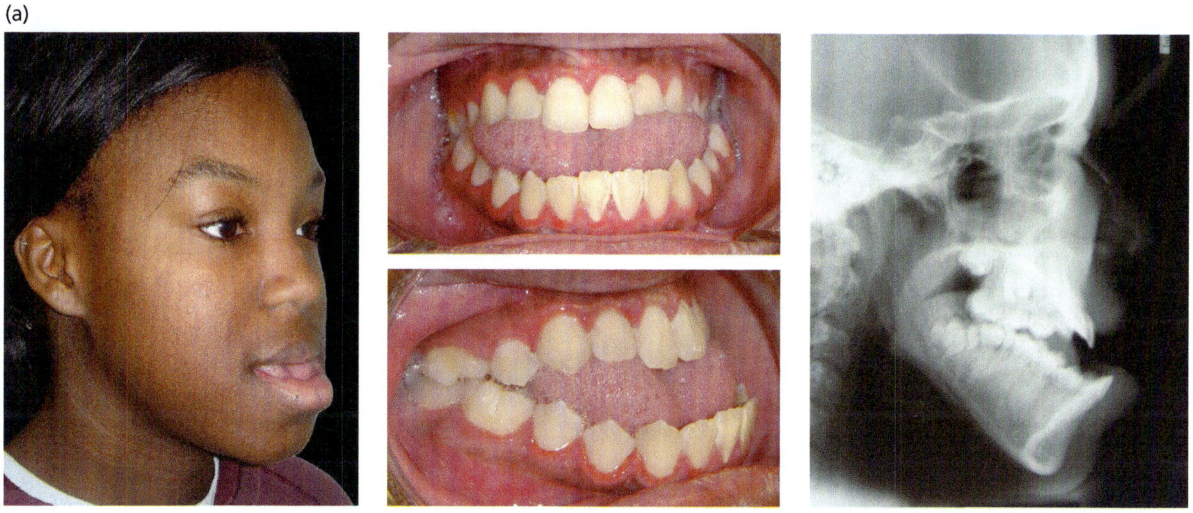

Fig. 29-11 Female patient with severe Class III skeletal pattern and anterior open bite, and a large tongue. (a) Pretreatment views demonstrate the enlarged tongue. (b) Preoperative views. Arches have been levelled in preparation for differential posterior maxillary impaction and advancement, and mandibular forward autorotation and set-back. (c) End of treatment views. In the initial postoperative period, the patient complained of a feeling of 'not enough space for my tongue', though she appeared to adapt within a few weeks. Although consideration was given to a tongue reduction, the patient declined. Her occlusion has been stable at 2 years postoperative review.

(b)

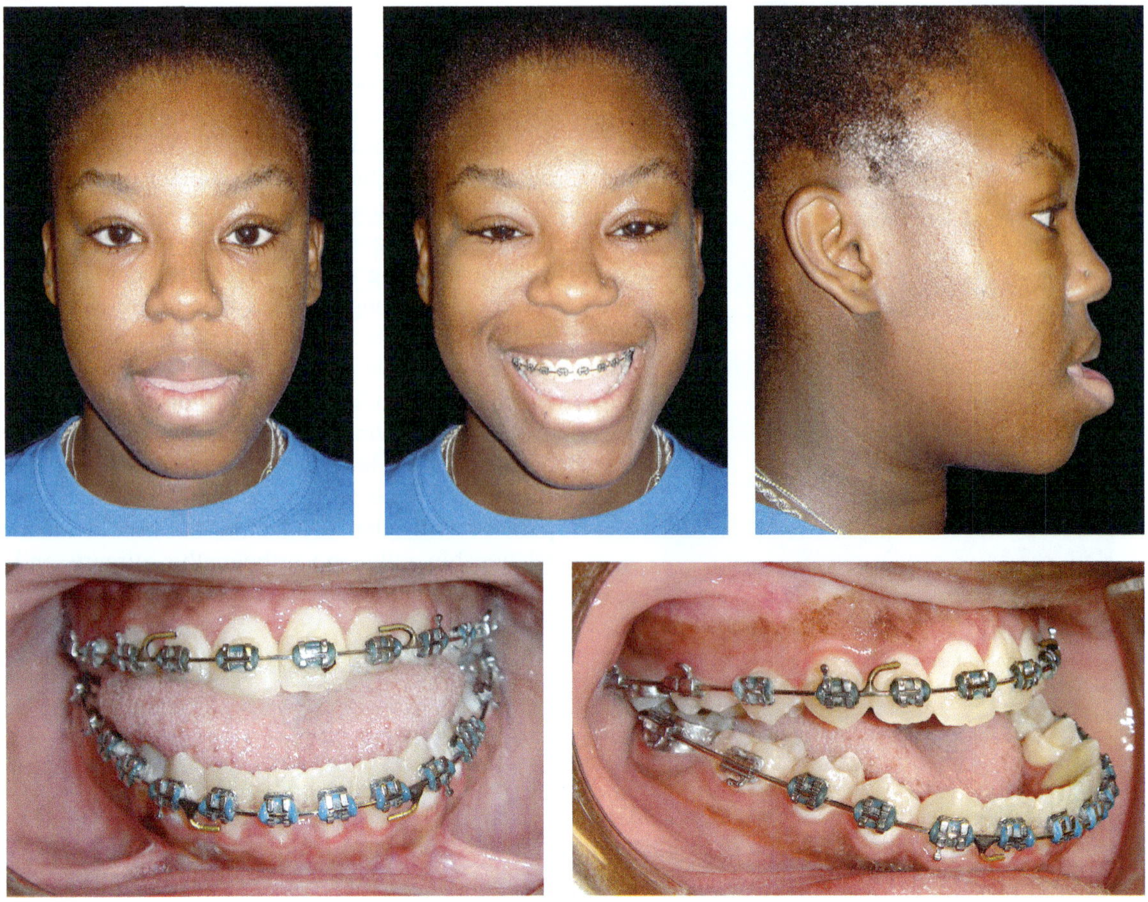

(c)

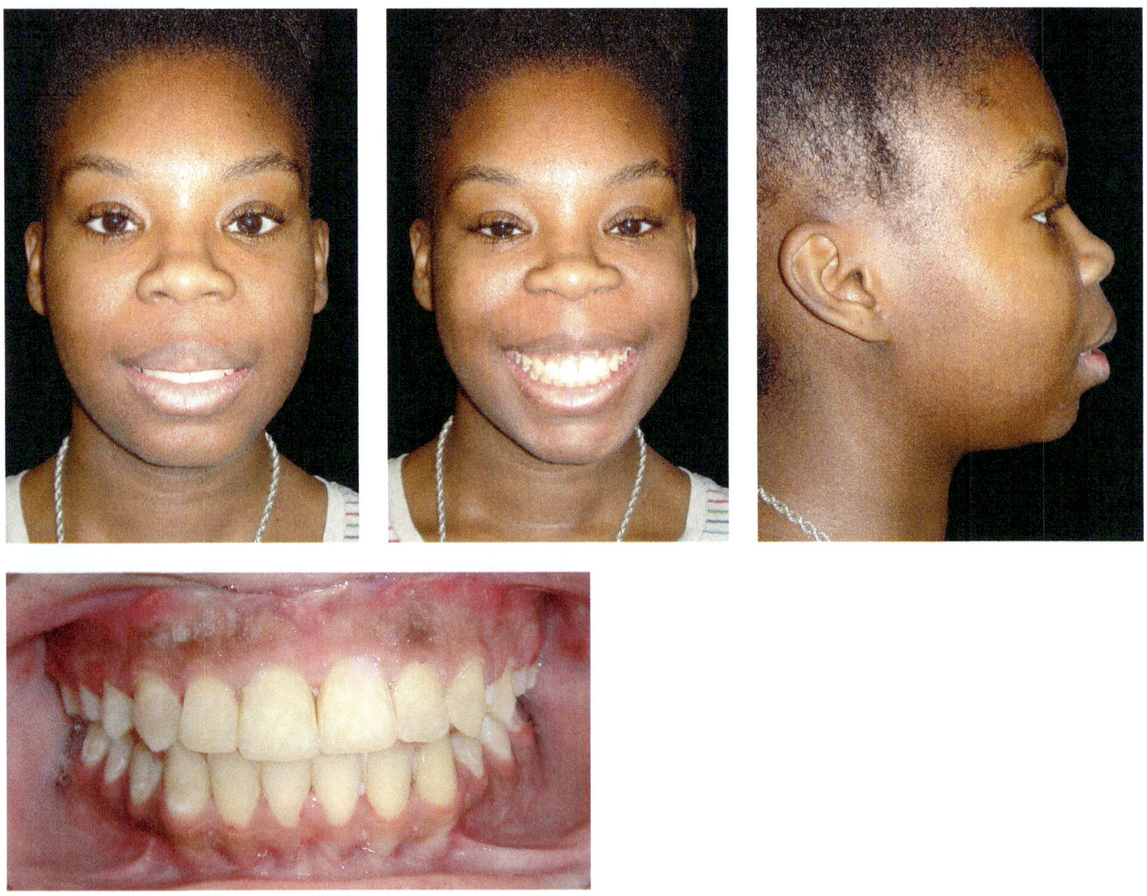

Fig. 29-11 (*Continued*).

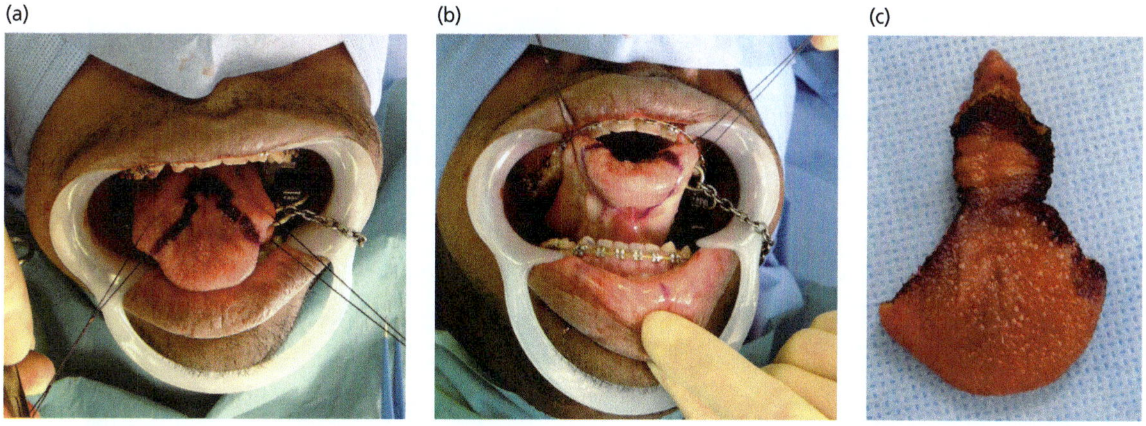

Fig. 29-12 Reduction glossectomy.

helping to correct the lower anterior face height. The vertical exposure of the maxillary incisors in relation to the upper lip may be correct or may require reduction. Alternatively, the anterior maxilla may need to be repositioned inferiorly if necessary.

The two most significant parameters in planning the surgical correction of an anterior open bite are the maxillary incisor relationship to the upper lip (the 'lip–incisor' relationship), and the lower anterior face height (LAFH). The correction of an AOB and the reduction in LAFH are both achieved by superior repositioning of the posterior maxilla and the subsequent forward autorotation of the mandible. The degree of posterior maxillary impaction required essentially will be dictated by the size of the AOB and the initial LAFH.[4]

Incisor inclination preparation for posterior maxillary impaction

In association with a differential posterior impaction of the maxilla, the maxillary incisors will retrocline. The amount of retroclination is important in surgical planning, as *a compensatory degree of incisor proclination must be built into the preoperative orthodontic preparation, such that the maxillary incisors will return to their correct inclination with surgery*.[19] If insufficient proclination is built into the preoperative orthodontics, the maxillary incisors will become excessively retroclined with surgery. Alternatively, if too much proclination is built into the preoperative orthodontics, or the degree of planned surgical posterior maxillary impaction is not achieved, then the incisors will remain somewhat proclined following surgery (Figure 29-13).

The amount of change in inclination of the maxillary incisors depends on the amount of differential posterior impaction of the maxilla. However, the ratio of both these variables also depends on the sagittal length of the maxilla, and the geometrical relationship between these three variables has been described (see Figure 7.4).[19] The anatomical length of the maxilla is usually measured from anterior to posterior nasal spine. However, the effective length of the maxilla is from the maxillary incisors to the first molar cusp tip, from where the posterior impaction is usually measured. For example, a differential posterior impaction of 6 mm will lead to a retroclination of the maxillary incisors of almost 10 degrees if the effective maxillary length is 35 mm, and 6 degrees if the maxillary length is 55 mm. The greater the differential impaction and the shorter the length of the maxilla, the greater will be the change in inclination of the maxillary incisors.[19]

Orthodontic preparation for mandibular autorotation

The mandibular incisors usually will have been retroclined by the lower lip as the mandible rotated posteriorly during growth. In preparation for forward autorotation of the mandible, the mandibular incisors will need to be proclined such that their inclination effectively corrects with the mandibular autorotation (see Figure 6-14). This needs to be planned cephalometrically pretreatment and checked preoperatively.

Planning the sagittal position of the mandible and chin

Finally, the autorotated sagittal position of the mandible and chin need to be considered, in addition to the dental-occlusal relationship. In the autorotated position, if the mandible is in a good sagittal position and the dental occlusion is acceptable, either no mandibular surgery or perhaps a relieving bilateral sagittal split osteotomy only will be required. Alternatively, the body of the mandible may need to be advanced or set-back in the sagittal plane to improve the facial aesthetic appearance and/or dental occlusion. Advancement or reduction genioplasty may also need to be considered depending on the morphology and prominence of the soft tissue chin and the morphology of the mentolabial fold. This may need to be considered as a secondary procedure.

The pterygomasseteric sling

Elongation of the mandibular ramus against the pterygomasseteric investing tissues (the so-called 'pterygomasseteric sling'), in particular the masseter

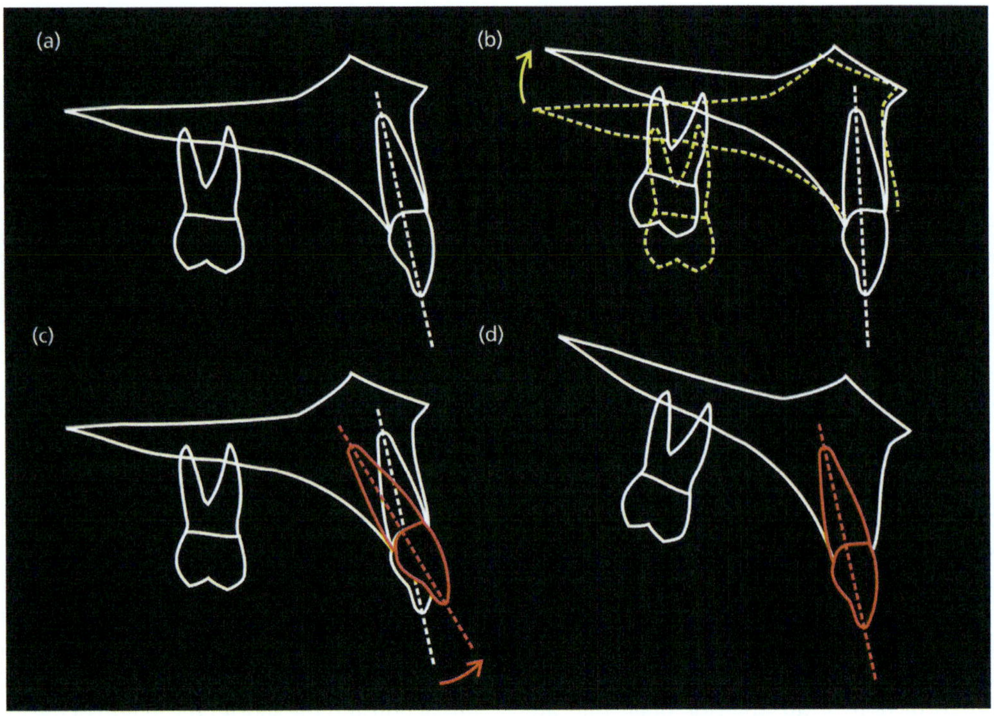

Fig. 29-13 Incisor inclination preparation for differential posterior maxillary impaction. (a) In the preoperative position, with the maxillary incisors at an average inclination. (b) In association with a differential posterior impaction of the maxilla, the maxillary incisors will retrocline. They are now excessively retroclined. (c) Therefore, a compensatory degree of incisor proclination must be built into the preoperative orthodontic preparation. (d) As such, the maxillary incisors will effectively retrocline as the maxilla rotates with the posterior impaction, thereby correcting their inclination with surgery.

and medial pterygoid muscles, should usually be avoided, due to the potentially high risk of postoperative relapse. Any rotation of the mandibular body around a pivot in the mandibular second or third molar region, downwards posteriorly and upwards anteriorly, may vertically stretch the musculofascial sling, the relapse of which leads to reoccurrence of an anterior open bite. Mild anterior open bites (perhaps up to 4 mm, in the absence of excessive occlusal plane inclination) may be treated with such a rotation following a bilateral sagittal split osteotomy with rigid internal fixation, as long as certain precautions are taken (see Chapter 30).

Approximate rules of thumb to aid chair side planning

It is important to iterate that these guidelines are *approximate* rules of thumb, which may aid preliminary chair side treatment planning. Accurate planning will require careful clinical evaluation, cephalometric planning and model surgery to confirm the degree of desired movements.

Maxillary incisor inclination change in relation to degree of posterior impaction

Based on the formula already described above, and assuming an approximately average maxillary length, the following may be used as an *approximate guideline* for chair side planning:[19]

> 1 mm posterior impaction leads to *approximately* 1.5° of maxillary incisor retroclination.

Relationship of size of AOB and degree of required posterior impaction

> For every 1.5 mm of AOB, *approximately* 1 mm of posterior impaction will be required.

Therefore, a 3 mm AOB will require *approximately* 2 mm of posterior impaction (measured from the mesiobuccal cusp of the maxillary first molar); a 6 mm AOB will require approximately 4mm of posterior impaction etc.

Orthodontic preparation

Preparatory orthodontics has been described in detail (see Chapter 12). However, there are a number of specific points to consider in preparation for differential posterior maxillary impaction and subsequent mandibular autorotation.

Incisor inclination preparation

In preparation for maxillary posterior impaction and forward mandibular autorotation, the incisor teeth will need to be proclined to the appropriate extent, such that their inclinations will correct with the surgery, in order to achieve ideal incisor inclinations and an ideal interincisal angle after surgery. The degree of required incisor proclination is calculated with pretreatment cephalometric planning, using a Ballard-type conversion (Figure 29-14). With preadjusted edgewise bracket systems, much of the proclination of the incisors occurs due to the mesial angulation or 'tip' in the canine brackets. This needs to be

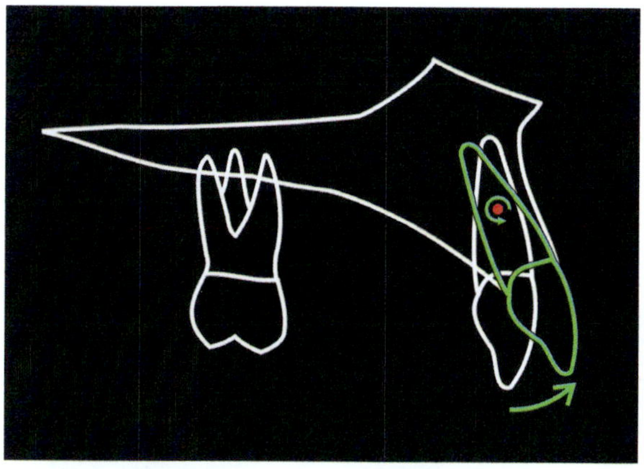

Fig. 29-14 Calculating the degree of required incisor proclination with pretreatment cephalometric planning, using a Ballard-type conversion. The incisor is rotated around the root centroid (centre of rotation), located approximately one-half of the root length from the apex.

carefully controlled to obtain the desired preoperative incisor inclination.

Levelling of the arches

There are three potential scenarios, based on the presenting features and thereby presumed aetiology of the anterior open bite:

Predominantly skeletal aetiology with mild adaptive soft tissue aetiology

In the ideal situation, both the maxillary and mandibular occlusal planes will be levelled (flattened) in the preparatory orthodontic phase of treatment. Therefore, the maxillary posterior impaction will permit forward mandibular autorotation and a relatively good dental occlusion. This is possible if a predominantly skeletal anterior open bite has some adaptive soft tissue (tongue) aetiology, which permits a small degree of maxillary incisor extrusion and thereby arch levelling preoperatively, without a risk of post-treatment relapse (Figure 29-15).

(a)

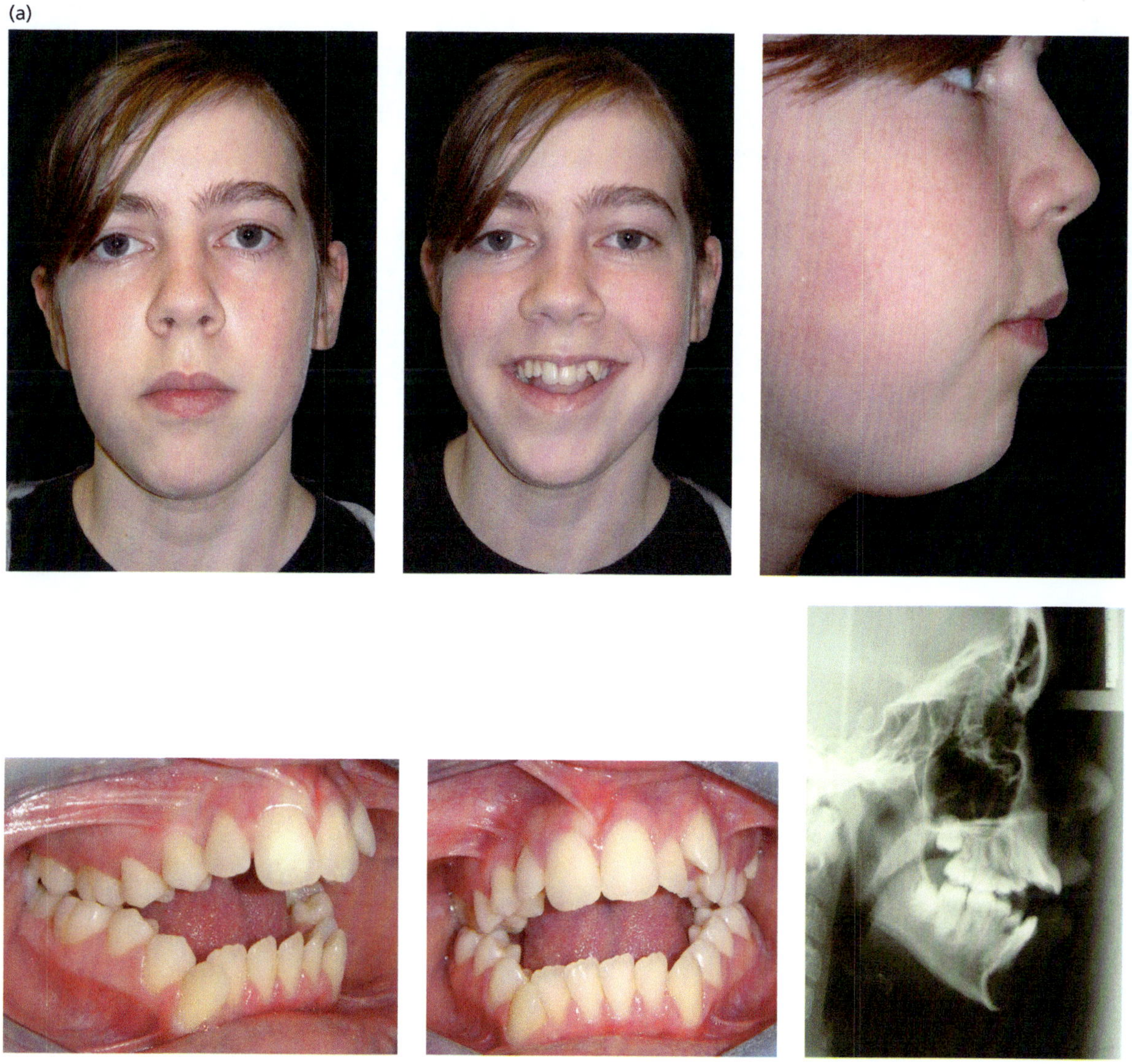

Fig. 29-15 (a) Pretreatment views. (b) Preoperative views, demonstrating levelling (flattening) of the maxillary and mandibular dental arches. (c) End of treatment views.

(b)

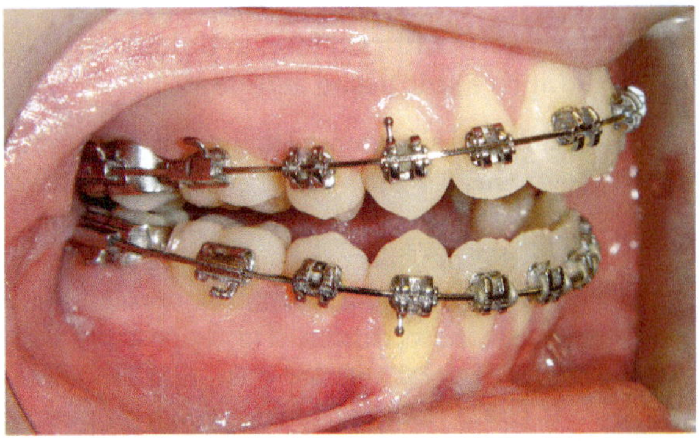

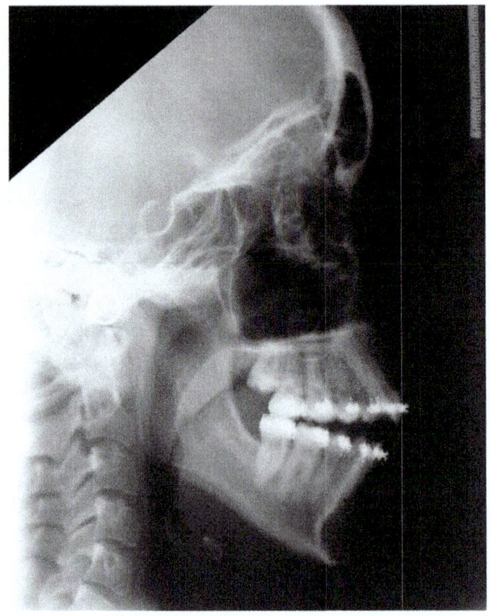

(c)

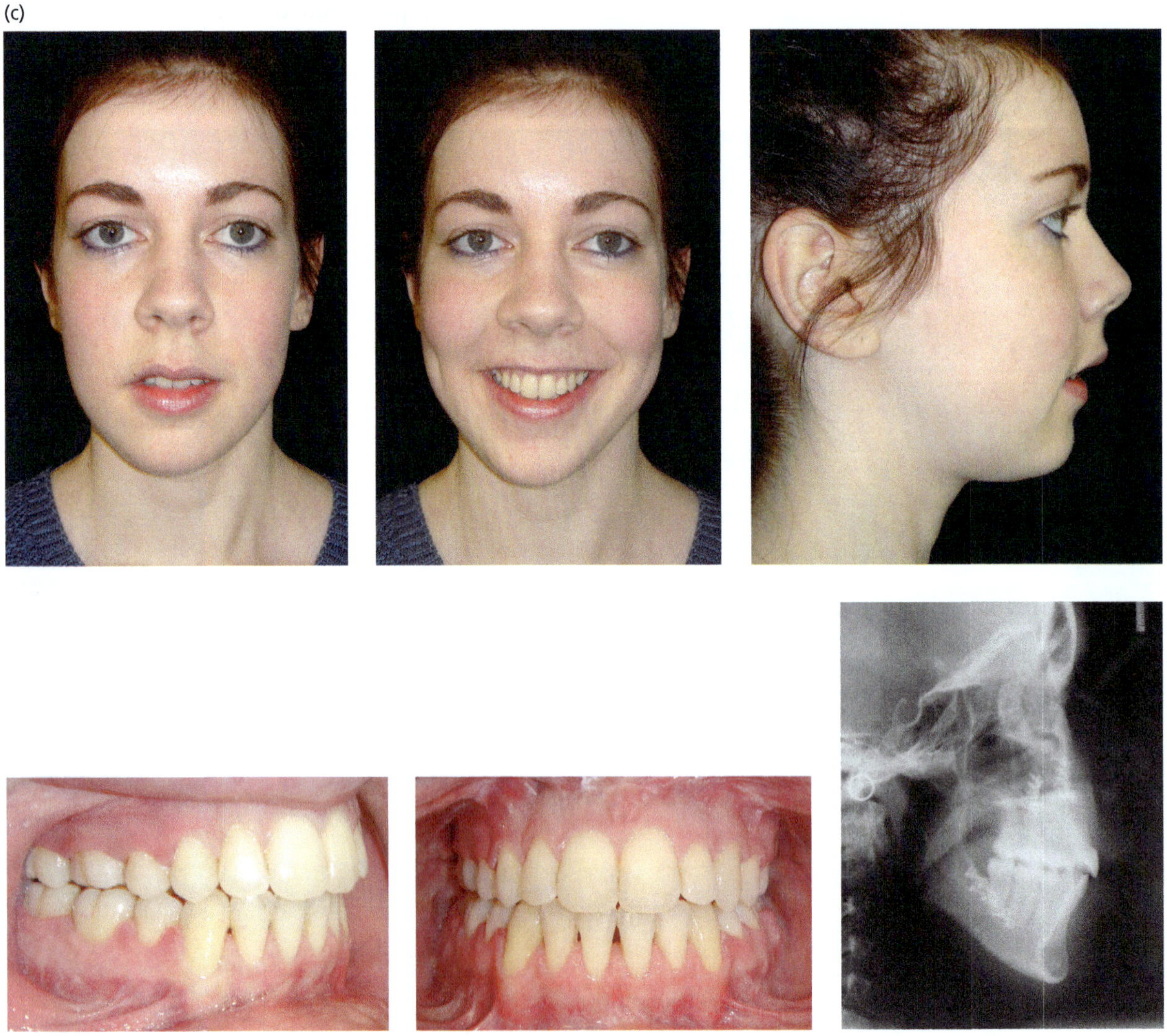

Fig. 29-15 (*Continued*).

Combined skeletal and soft tissue aetiology

Alternatively, if there is a marked increased sagittal curve in the maxillary arch, it may be prudent to maintain the accentuated curve in the maxillary arch by placing a curve in the archwire, though this will inevitably lead to a postoperative posterior open bite (Figure 29-16). In such cases, preoperative orthodontic levelling of the maxillary arch may lead to excessive extrusion of the maxillary incisors, producing a relapse tendency. Relapse of the maxillary incisors in an apical direction when the orthodontic appliances are removed will tend to reopen the bite anteriorly. The alternative is to align and level the anterior and posterior segments independently and undertake segmental posterior impaction of the maxilla (see Chapter 28).

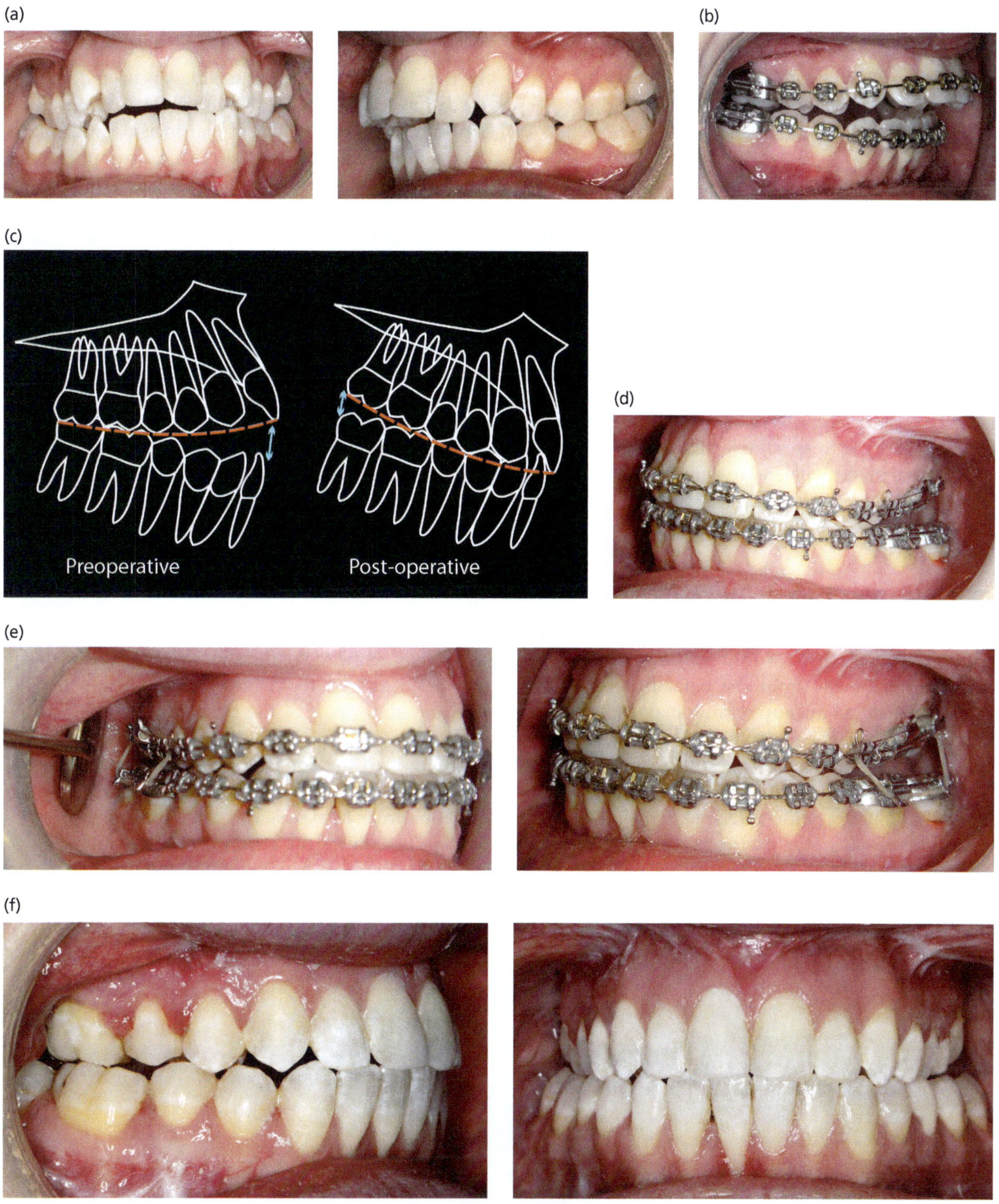

Fig. 29-16 (a) Pretreatment views, demonstrating an increased sagittal occlusal curve in the maxillary arch. (b) Preoperative views, demonstrating maintenance of the sagittal curve using an accentuated curve in the maxillary archwire. (c) Closure of the anterior open bite will result in a posterior open bite. (d) Postoperative view, demonstrating closure of the anterior open bite, but resultant posterior open bite. (e) Flexible rectangular archwires placed, and posterior box elastic to extrude the posterior maxillary molars and the level the arch. (f) End of treatment views. The patient asked for debond prior to completion of treatment, for personal reasons; therefore a posterior open bite remains on her left side.

Predominantly skeletal aetiology

In a patient with a skeletal open bite *without* a soft tissue element, there will often be an accentuated curve of Spee in the mandibular dental arch and a reverse curve in the maxillary arch. This is due to the incisors having erupted as far as possible in the unsuccessful attempt to meet the opposing incisors, compensating for an increased lower anterior face height. In such cases, levelling of the dental arches should occur by some degree of intrusion of the incisor teeth. The postoperative relapse tendency of the intruded incisors will be for occlusal eruption, which will help to maintain the corrected incisor overbite.

Maxillary occlusal plane inclination and the smile curvature

The **smile curvature**, alternatively termed the **smile arc**, may be defined as the relationship of the curvature of the incisal edges of the maxillary anterior dentition (**incisal edge curvature**) to the curvature of the upper border contour of the lower lip (**lower lip curvature**) in a posed smile.[20] Differential posterior impaction of the maxilla following a Le Fort I osteotomy, which elevates the posterior maxilla relative to the anterior maxilla and thereby increases the inclination of the maxillary occlusal plane, will tend to improve the smile curvature (smile arc) relationship (see Chapter 7 for more detail) (Figure 29-17).

Transverse maxillary deficiency

In patients with a skeletal anterior open bite the tongue will often have a low position in the floor of the mouth, away from the palatal vault, which may exacerbate an already narrow maxilla. No more than approximately 4-5mm of orthodontic maxillary arch expansion is possible without buccal flaring of the molar teeth and resultant postoperative occlusal problems, together with a relapse tendency of the expansion. As such, the pretreatment dental models may be hand articulated in a Class I occlusion to evaluate the approximate amount of maxillary expansion required, and consideration should be given to either preliminary surgically assisted rapid maxillary expansion, or alternatively a segmental approach to the maxillary surgery with concomitant expansion of the posterior segments, if significant maxillary expansion is required.

Surgical technique

Le Fort I osteotomy of the maxilla has been described in detail in Chapter 22. The maxilla is exposed by the standard sublabial vestibular incision and subperiosteal dissection (Figure 29-18a). A saw cut is made at the Le Fort I level from the zygomatic buttress forwards to the piriform aperture (Figure 29-18b–d). A back cut is then made from the buttress in a posterior direction to the pterygomaxillary fissure. In accordance with the preoperative planning, marks are made above this osteotomy line at the buttress and the piriform rim (Figure 29-18e–g). These indicate the position of the upper osteotomy cut and therefore the amount of bone to be removed in the vertical dimension posteriorly and anteriorly (Figure 29-18h–k). Differential posterior impaction of the maxilla requires the removal of a tapering bone strip of appropriate width, greater posteriorly than anteriorly.

After separation of the nasal septum from the maxillary crest, osteotomies of the lateral nasal walls and pterygomaxillary disjunction (Figure 29-18l), the maxilla is downfractured and mobilized in the normal way. The successful outcome of the operation depends greatly upon the meticulous removal of bone between the osteotomized tooth bearing part of the maxilla and the upper part of the maxilla so as to allow the impaction/superior repositioning as planned.

Downward traction is applied to the osteotomized maxilla with a bone hook in the incisive (nasopalatine) canal in order to expose its upper surface (Figure 29-18m). This allows the removal of the wedge shaped

(a) (b)

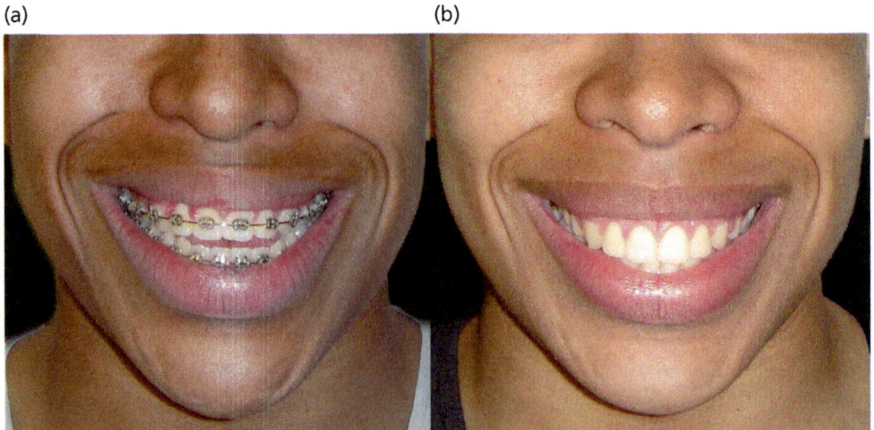

Fig. 29-17 (a) Preoperative view, demonstrating a flat smile curvature (smile arc) relationship. (b) Following differential posterior impaction of the maxilla and the increase in the maxillary occlusal plane inclination, there is an improved smile arc relationship.

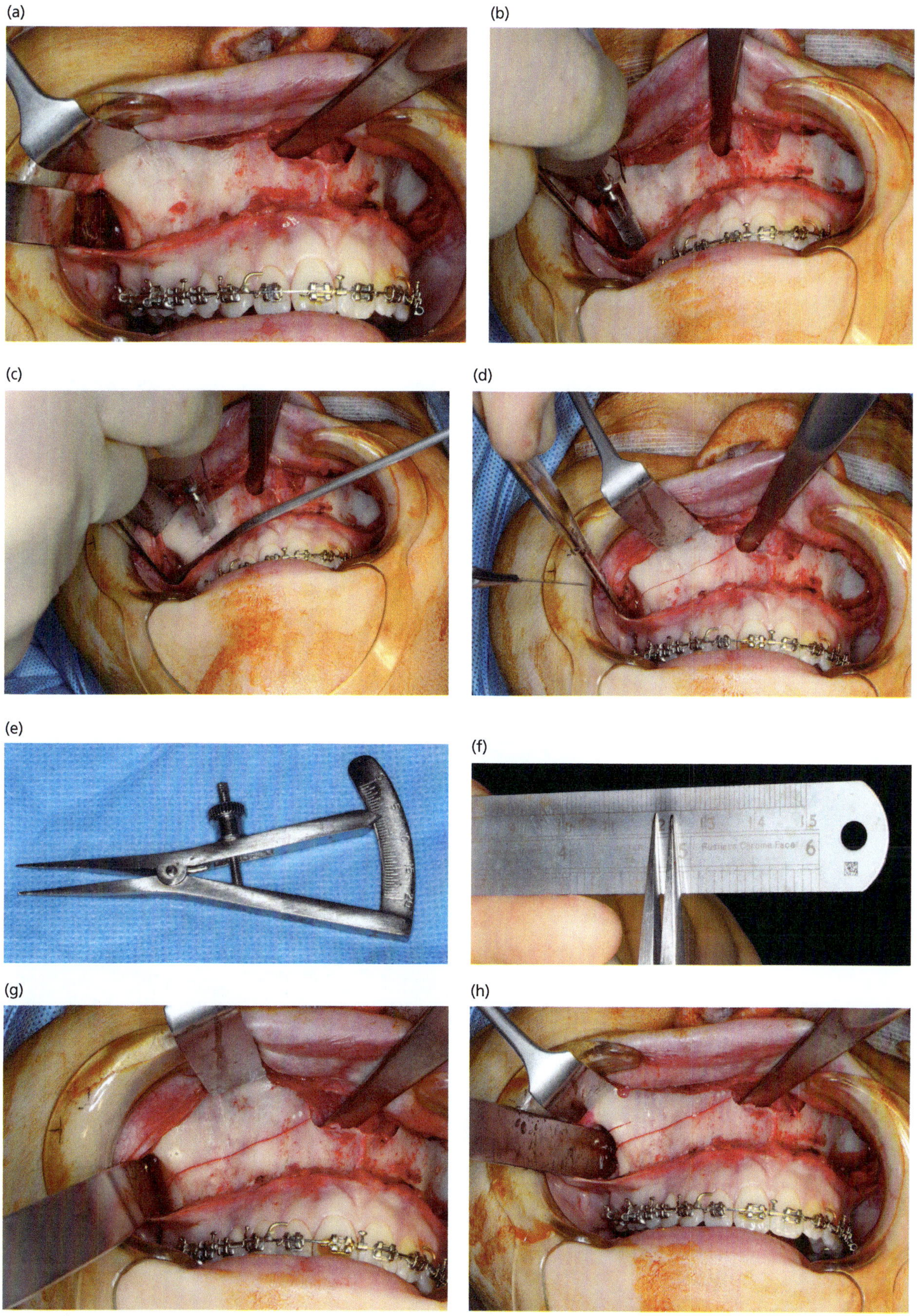

Fig. 29-18 Surgical technique (see main text for full explanation and description).

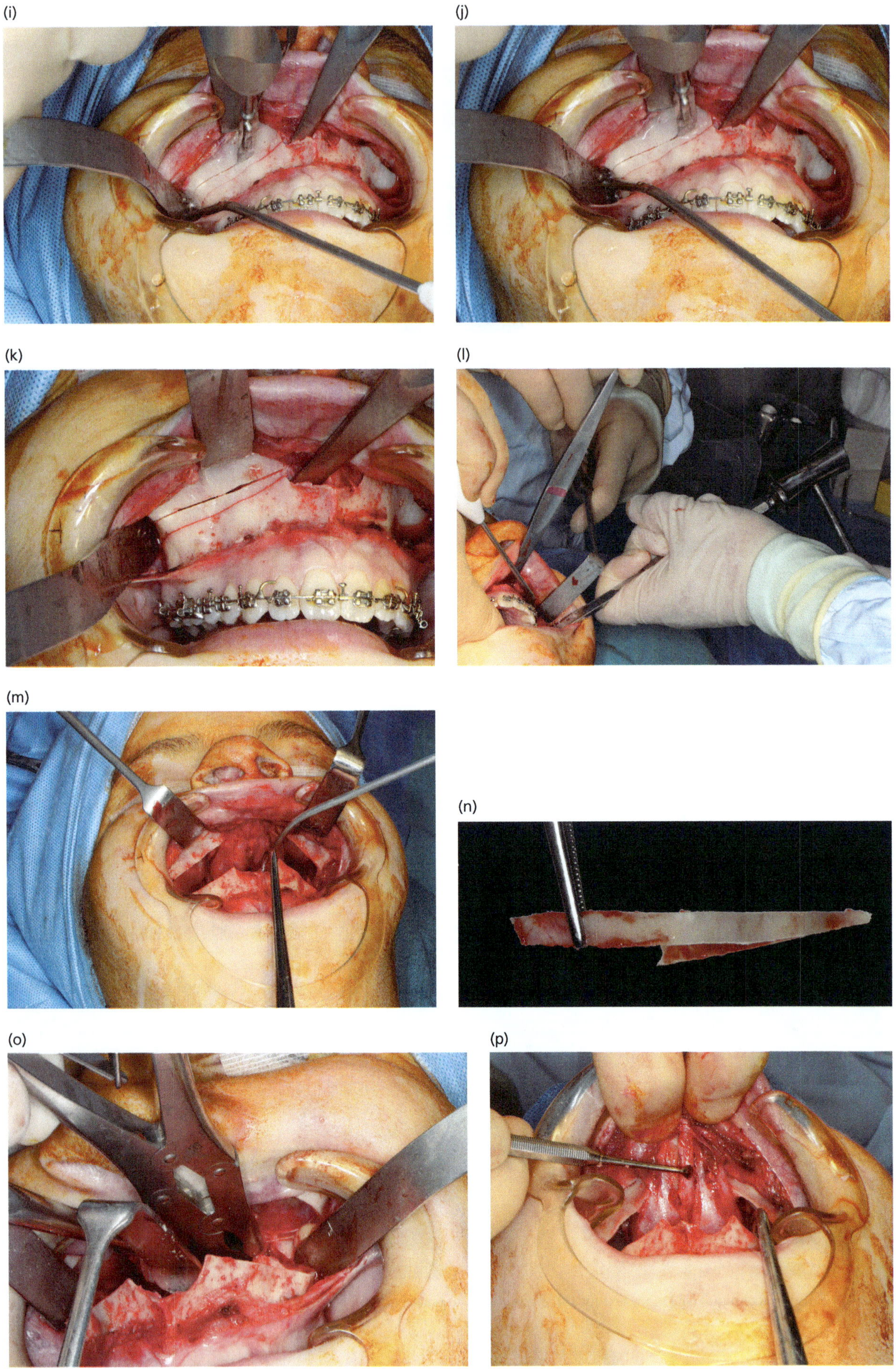

Fig. 29-18 (*Continued*).

(q)

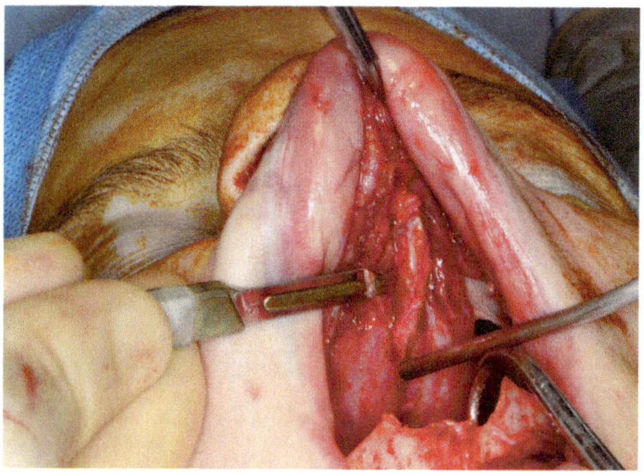

(r)

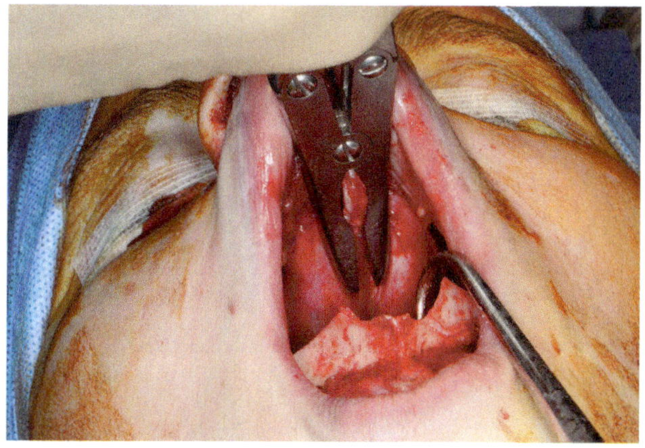

(s)

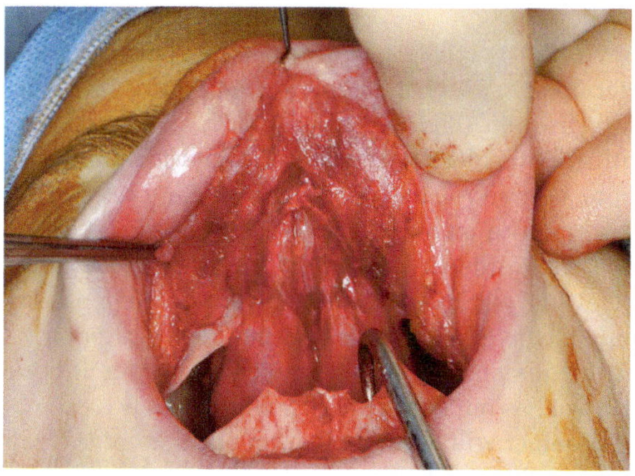

(t)

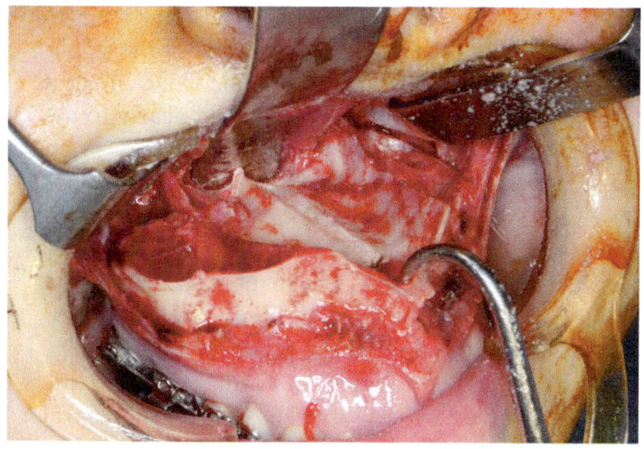

(u)

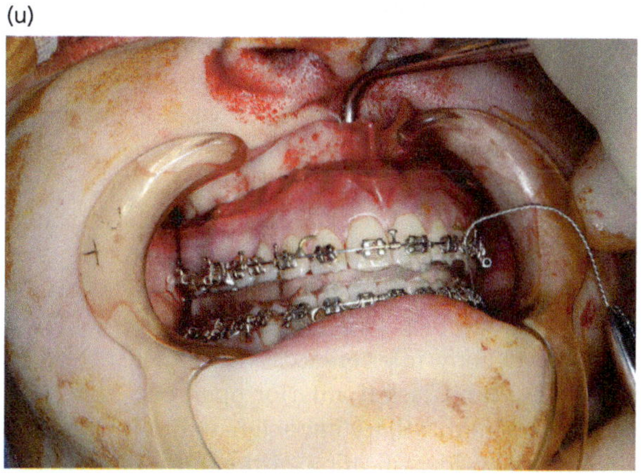

(v)

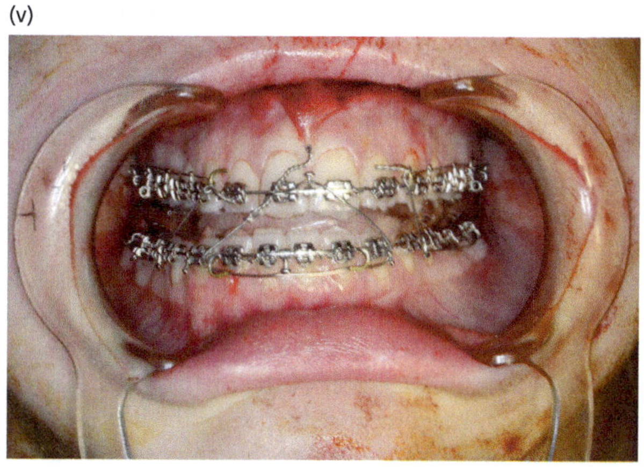

(w)

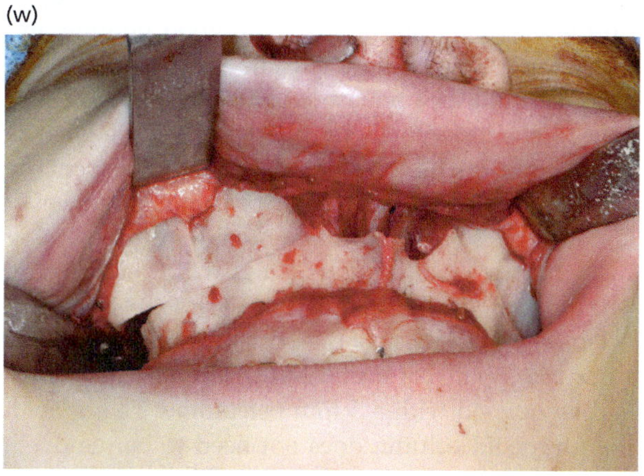

(x)

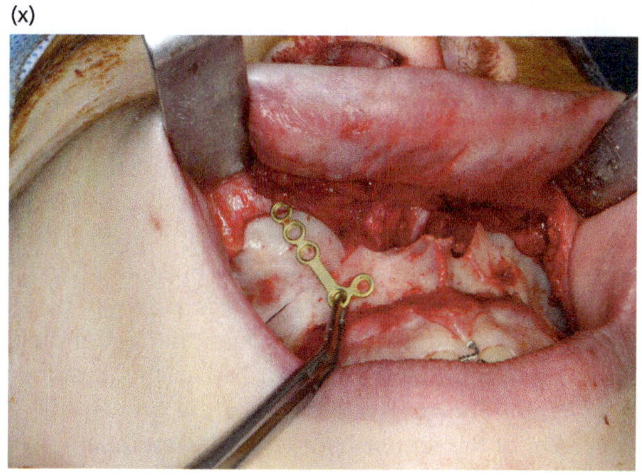

Fig. 29-18 (*Continued*).

(y)

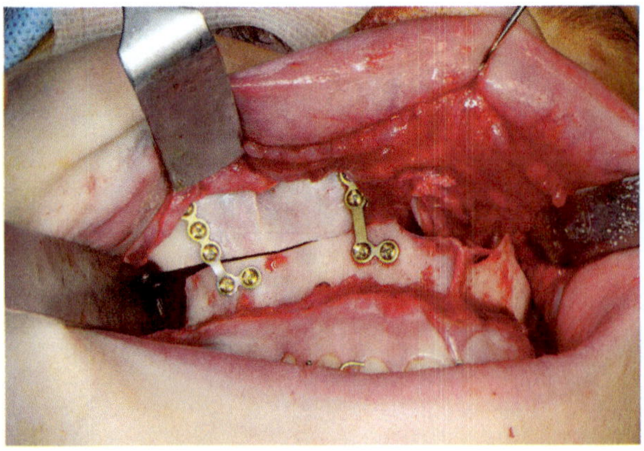

(z)

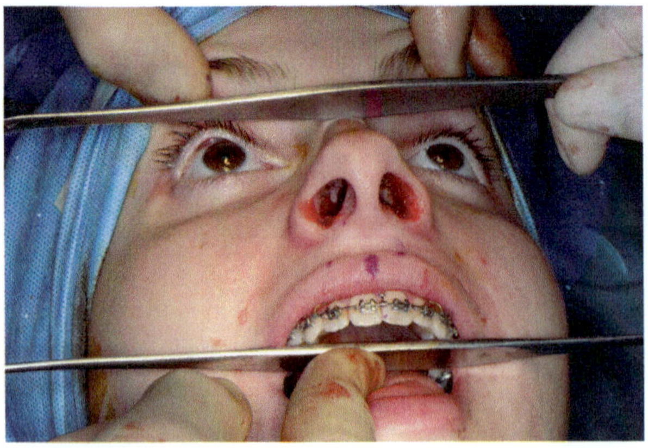

Fig. 29-18 (*Continued*).

piece of bone of the lateral maxilla between the upper and lower saw cuts (Figure 29-18n). The vertical height of the lateral nasal walls is then reduced nearly to the level of the floor of the nose with rongeurs and/or an acrylic burr in an anterior to posterior direction (Figure 29-18o). As the greater palatine artery comes into view the vertical plate of the palatine bone is carefully removed down to the level where the vessel enters the posterior aspect of the maxilla. Bone removal is continued at this level around the posterior aspect of the tuberosity and then forwards towards the zygomatic buttress. The vertical height of the bone of the lateral aspect of the maxilla from the buttress to the piriform rim must be preserved as it is this that determines the vertical dimension of the maxilla in accordance with the preoperative planning. Bone is then removed from the corresponding sites of the superior part of the osteotomized maxilla.

The caudal aspect of the nasal septum must be reduced vertically by the same amount as the planned maxillary impaction to prevent its distortion and buckling as the maxilla is superiorly repositioned. Subperiosteal dissection of the vomer is extended forwards on both sides into the subperichondral plane to expose the caudal aspect of the cartilaginous septum. This enables vertical reduction of the septum in such a way as to correspond to the impaction of the maxilla (Figure 29-18p–s). The maxillary crest is the midline ridge of bone in the floor of the nose, extending from the anterior to the posterior nasal spine and represents the site of insertion of the nasal septum. Using an acrylic bur, the crest is removed and a midline groove is fashioned in the floor of the nose instead extending from anterior to posterior nasal spine (Figure 29-18t). This groove will eventually receive the nasal septum as the maxilla is repositioned and fixed. Prior to mucosal closure, the septum is stabilised by a non-resorbable suture passed through the caudal cartilaginous septum and a hole drilled in the anterior nasal spine. The groove and the suture prevent displacement of the septum away from the midline.

After reduction of the nasal septum and the removal of bone between the two osteotomy cuts as described above, the maxilla is repositioned by inserting the intermediate wafer and applying temporary intermaxillary fixation (Figure 29-18u and v). The mandible, with the maxilla attached by the intermaxillary fixation, is manipulated by gentle finger pressure on the chin. The mandibular condyles are seated in the retruded position in the glenoid fossae as the mandible is elevated. At this stage there should be even bony contact between the tooth bearing lower fragment of the maxilla and the upper maxilla. However, if bone removal has not been completed adequately a premature contact will occur, preventing closure of the gap between the two fragments. This is usually due to a bony interference between the superior surface of the maxillary tuberosity and the dense pterygoid columns of the base of the skull. This type of interference is much less likely in cases when posterior impaction and advancement of the maxilla are combined as in the treatment of Class III anterior open bites. In these cases the upper surface of the tuberosity moves forwards and away from the pterygoid columns, thereby reducing the chance of interference as the posterior maxilla is impacted.

Posterior bony interferences are most likely to be encountered in Class II anterior open bite cases that need posterior maxillary impaction without maxillary advancement. Identification of the bony interference is achieved by depressing the mandible so as to open up the maxillary osteotomy. With good lighting and retraction, the mandible with the maxilla attached is elevated until the premature bony contact occurs and once the interfering bone has been identified, it is removed. It is usually easier to remove bone from the upper surface of the tooth bearing fragment, however it may be necessary to eliminate an interference arising from the pterygoid columns. This can be done with an acrylic bur or on occasions it is necessary to perform an osteotomy of the base of the pterygoid plates. A transverse osteotomy cut is made with a fissure bur which is then opened with a 5 mm osteotome. The bone of the pterygoid column does not need to be removed. It is simply displaced posteriorly to allow unimpeded posterior maxillary impaction.

In some patients, with posterior bony interferences, it may be possible to close the anterior gap between the osteotomy fragments by forcibly elevating the mandible with the maxilla attached. This should be avoided as although the gap between the two fragments will have been closed, this will have been achieved by downwards and forwards rotation of the posterior mandible and maxilla by distracting the condyles from the glenoid fossae. If the maxilla is fixed in this position, the posterior mandible will rotate backwards and upwards when the intermaxillary fixation is released so leading to premature contact between the molars, and it will be apparent that the anterior open bite has not been corrected.

Once the operator is satisfied that all bony interferences have been removed, the mandible is elevated to achieve even bony contact between the two parts of the maxilla (Figure 29-18w) and fixation is achieved with plates and screws in the normal way (Figure 29-18x and y). At this stage the new position of the maxilla is checked to ensure that the maxillary dental midline is coincident with the facial midline, there is correct lip support and incisor display and the maxillary occlusal plane is parallel to the interpupillary line (Figure 29-18z). This process is much easier when submental intubation has been used rather than traditional nasal endotracheal intubation because the latter tends to distort the nose and upper lip making judgements about incisor display and midline coincidence, in particular, rather difficult. If the new position of the maxilla is not correct, adjustments can be made at this stage and though not often needed this would imply errors had occurred in the preoperative planning and/or the model surgery.

There are three distinct components of the soft tissue repair. As mentioned above, the caudal part of the cartilaginous nasal septum is sutured to the anterior nasal spine with a non-resorbable suture to prevent its displacement away from the midline. The maxillary osteotomy will have increased the width of the nasal base, partly due to division of the transverse nasalis muscles and partly as a result of the bony movements. In patients in whom nasal width is normal or increased prior to surgery the placement of an alar base cinch suture may be needed to mitigate this change. This can be done by identifying and suturing together in the midline the cut ends of the transverse nasalis muscles so re-establishing their insertions. Following this the soft tissue repair is completed with a single V-Y vestibular mucosal closure using a resorbable suture. If submental intubation has been used, the effect of the osteotomy, the cinch suture and V-Y mucosal repair can be assessed by measuring nasal width before the osteotomy, after the osteotomy and fixation and then finally after soft tissue repair.

Postoperative orthodontics

Postoperative orthodontics has been described in detail (see Chapter 12). If the dental arches have been levelled (flattened) preoperatively, the dental occlusion should be relatively acceptable postoperatively, with only minor occlusal settling and finishing required (see Figure 29-15). If an accentuated sagittal occlusal curve has been maintained in the maxillary dental arch and rectangular stainless steel archwire, there is likely to be an element of posterior open bite present postoperatively. The maxillary archwire should be replaced with a more flexible flat archwire (usually a rectangular braided stainless steel archwire), and posterior box elastics used to gradually extrude the posterior maxillary molars into occlusion (see Figure 29-16).

If maxillary expansion has been achieved either preoperatively or intraoperatively, the expansion will need to be maintained in the postoperative period. A large dimension stainless steel maxillary archwire with some expansion is often enough, though an auxiliary expanded archwire may be placed in the headgear tubes and over-tied. On debonding of the appliances, a modified Hawley retainer with a midline expansion screw may be used, allowing some activation of expansion should this become necessary in the retention phase of treatment.

Conclusion

A significant anterior open bite is commonly a significant functional and aesthetic concern for patients. The usual multifactorial aetiology and range of relevant diagnostic factors and treatment planning concerns, as well as the diversity of surgical options available and potential long-term considerations regarding stability, make this one of the most challenging dentofacial deformities to treat.

References

1 Shakespeare W. Antony and Cleopatra (c.1606). London: New Penguin Shakespeare, 1973.
2 Naini FB. Facial Type. In: Naini FB. Facial Aesthetics: Concepts and Clinical Diagnosis. Oxford: Wiley-Blackwell, 2011.
3 Sassouni V. A classification of skeletal facial types. Am J Orthod. 1969;55:109–23.
4 Naini FB. The Maxilla and Midface. In: Naini FB. Facial Aesthetics: Concepts and Clinical Diagnosis. Oxford: Wiley-Blackwell, 2011.
5 Ballard CF. Oro-facial behaviour. Public Health. 1961;76:10–18.
6 Linder-Aronson S. Adenoids. Their effect on mode of breathing and nasal airflow and their relationship to characteristics of the facial skeleton and the dentition. A biometric, rhino-manometric and cephalometro-radiographic study on children with and without adenoids. Acta Otolaryngol (Suppl.) 1970;265:1–132.
7 Linder-Aronson S. Effects of adenoidectomy on mode of breathing, size of adenoids and nasal airflow. ORL J Otorhinolaryngol Relat Spec. 1973;35:283–302.
8 Linder-Aronson S. The relation between nasorespiratory function and dentofacial morphology. Am J Orthod. 1983;83:443–4.
9 Behlfelt K, Linder-Aronson S, Neander P. Posture of the head, the hyoid bone, and the tongue in children with and without enlarged tonsils. Eur J Orthod. 1990;12:458–67.

10 Woodside DG, Linder-Aronson S, Lundstrom A, McWilliam J. Mandibular and maxillary growth after changed mode of breathing. Am J Orthod Dentofacial Orthop. 1991;100: 1–18.
11 Vig KW. Nasal obstruction and facial growth: the strength of evidence for clinical assumptions. Am J Orthod Dentofacial Orthop. 1998;113:603–11.
12 Gill DS, El Maaytah M, Naini FB. Risk factors for post-orthognathic condylar resorption: a review. World J Orthod. 2008;9:21–5.
13 Naini FB. Cephalometry and Cephalometric Analysis. In: Naini FB. Facial Aesthetics: Concepts and Clinical Diagnosis. Oxford: Wiley-Blackwell, 2011.
14 Björk A. The face in profile: an anthropological X-ray investigation on Swedish children and conscripts. Svensk Tandl Tidskr. 1947;40(suppl 5B).
15 Richardson A. A cephalometric investigation of skeletal factors in anterior open bite and deep overbite. Rep Congr Eur J Orthod. 1967:159–71.
16 Naini FB. Regional Aesthetic Analysis: The Nose. In: Naini FB. Facial Aesthetics: Concepts and Clinical Diagnosis. Oxford: Wiley-Blackwell, 2011.
17 Naini FB, Cobourne MT, McDonald F, Wertheim D. The aesthetic impact of upper lip inclination in orthodontics and orthognathic surgery. Eur J Orthod. 2015;37:81–6.
18 Egyedi P, Obwegeser H. Zur operativen zungenverkleinerung. Dtsch Zahn Mund Kieferhlkd. 1964;41:16–25.
19 Naini FB, Hunt NP, Moles DR. The relationship between maxillary length, differential maxillary impaction, and the change in maxillary incisor inclination. Am J Orthod Dentofacial Orthop. 2003;124:526–9.
20 Naini FB, Gill DS. Smile Aesthetics. In: Naini FB. Facial Aesthetics: Concepts and Clinical Diagnosis. Oxford: Wiley-Blackwell, 2011.

Chapter 30

Surgical Treatment of Anterior Open Bite with Mandibular Osteotomies

Dale Bloomquist and Don Joondeph

Introduction

Significant instability of correcting anterior open bite with the use of mandibular osteotomies is a long-held and persistent belief among oral and maxillofacial surgeons, despite not having any support in the research literature. This reticence appears to be due to three factors: early experiences of relapse during the use of wire osseous and intermaxillary fixation, the initial well reported clockwise relapse pattern of the distal fragment in mandibular advancement using bilateral sagittal split osteotomies; and the strong belief that lengthening posterior facial height is not stable. The fact that maxillary osteotomies with posterior intrusion has clearly been shown to have notable relapse through the work of Denison in 1989,[1] which was later supported in a larger study by Hoppenreijs in 1999,[2] has not seemed to dampen the surgeon's enthusiasm for using these procedures. Both studies reported about a 20% incidence of no incisor overlap on long-term follow-up as well as the majority of patients having a significant decrease in overbite postoperatively. Despite the overwhelming confirmation of relapse occurring following posterior intrusion of the maxilla in the literature, individual surgeons seem to believe that their surgical treatments are stable. Confounding a clinician's decisions on whether to recommend orthodontics alone versus orthodontics with surgery have been review articles in the orthodontic literature describing similar rates of relapse in open bite of between 20–25%.[3,4] Although the authors admit to the deficiencies in making such comparisons, a cursory read by a clinician could result in inappropriate treatment decisions. In spite of the apparent confusion in the literature on treatment of anterior open bite, there are now a number of factors on which both experienced clinicians and research seem to agree. These factors will be reviewed especially in respect to what part the anticlockwise rotation of the mandible fits into the treatment alternatives.

Aetiology and description of skeletal anterior open bite

Potential causes of anterior open bite can be generally broken down into two categories: universally accepted or research proven and uncertain or disputed. The accepted aetiologies include congenital, developmental, trauma, pathology, digit sucking and other non-nutritive sucking habits.[5–7] Controversial are airway obstruction and muscular influence.[8–11] Primary among the disagreements about muscular effects is the pressures exerted by the tongue. It is generally accepted that tongue thrusting develops secondary to the presence of an anterior open bite.[7,12] Less clear is the effect of tongue posture as well as decreased tone in the muscles of mastication. Patients with

Orthognathic Surgery: Principles, Planning and Practice. Edited by Farhad B. Naini and Daljit S. Gill.

anterior open bite generally have decreased muscle tone of the masseter, medial pterygoid, and temporalis muscles.[9,12,13] As will be discussed further, surgery to decrease open bite in individuals with increased lower face height may increase muscle tone but probably not back to a normal range.[14,15] The theory that airway obstruction in early childhood was caused by enlarged tonsils and adenoids has resulted in many patients being referred for tonsillectomies. Trask[11] in her study of paired siblings with and without allergic rhinitis, found that the siblings with persistent rhinitis did have a greater degree of increased facial height and more obtuse gonial angle, but they did not have a greater chance of anterior open bite.

One problem in the treatment decision-making for anterior open bite is determining what cases can be treated with orthodontics alone and when would orthognathic surgery be most appropriate. Patients in whom surgery should be the treatment of choice then pose a further dilemma of whether maxillary, mandibular, or a combination of the surgeries is best. Orthodontists deal with anterior open bites routinely, especially in the mixed dentition, and most of those can safely be considered a dental rather than skeletal open bite. Difficulty, however, sometimes does exist in making that determination since patients successfully treated with orthodontics alone often have the visual and cephalometric features consistent with those associated with skeletal open bite.[16] Ellis has reviewed the features of anterior open bites in both Class II as well as Class III patients.[17,18] Both groups had similar findings, in that they generally exhibited an increase in anterior facial height, steeper mandibular plane, increased gonial angle, and a decreased maxillary plane. Individuals who have developed anterior open bite secondary to 'non-nutritive' sucking habits generally are considered to simply have dental changes and no skeletal deformities and thus amenable to conventional orthodontics.[19,20] However, children with prolonged habits can develop an increased anterior facial height which is consistent with a skeletal problem. Orthodontists can use growth modification techniques in children who do have cephalometric findings consistent with skeletal open bite and therefore are generally successful in their treatment. The decisions become much more difficult as the facial skeleton matures.[21] The mechanics necessary to close an open bite in an adult with conventional orthodontics unfortunately may result in dental instability which will result in treatment failure if surgery is then attempted. The two most common ways that this instability will happen is with extensive extrusion of incisors or tilting (buccal flaring) of posterior teeth in attempts to correct crossbites.[7]

Treatment decisions for surgery

Surgical closure of anterior open bite, as mentioned previously, has been traditionally limited to clockwise rotation of the maxilla preferably by intruding the molars. Mandibular osteotomies have also combined with the maxillary osteotomies, but only to correct anterior-posterior deformities as well as asymmetries. Interestingly, the combination surgeries have been slightly less stable than treating in the maxilla alone.[2,22] The reason for this discrepancy is unclear especially in light of our present thesis that mandibular osteotomies alone can be used to correct anterior open bites. Knowledge of the possibility that there seems to be greater relapse when open bite is treated with combination maxillary and mandibular osteotomies, would certainly dissuade a very experienced orthognathic surgeon knowledgeable with the research literature from attempting to rotate the mandible anticlockwise in bimaxillary surgery. Fortunately, we started using the mandibular bilateral sagittal osteotomy for the correction of anterior open bite in the late 1980s, which was well in advance of the research report by Hoppenreijs[2] who initially discussed the increased stability of using a maxillary Le Fort I alone.

Postoperative changes following intentional closing of an anterior open bite with anticlockwise rotation of the mandible in Class II patients was initially reported in the early 1970's. Poulton and Ware[23,24] and later McNeill[25] both demonstrated a clockwise relapse pattern through the use of case reports of patients who had significant preoperative open bites. Since much of this relapse occurred early and during the period of intermaxillary fixation, the patients did retain some anterior over bite during the short follow-up periods reported in these articles. Poulton and Ware proposed two methods of minimizing the possibility of bite reopening following surgery. First was planning a posterior open bite into the surgical splint. They then suggested that the patient continued to wear an occlusal splint after the fixation was released employing a gradual reduction of the posterior part of the splint allowing the molars to erupt as the muscles readapted to the new mandibular position and maintaining the incisor overbite. A more direct way of minimizing the early effects of soft tissue and muscle pull was the use of a neck brace. A later study failed to show that this latter technique was of any value for preventing relapse in mandibular advancements with the bilateral sagittal split osteotomies.[26] Surprisingly no study has been published looking specifically at the stability of mandibular advancements using bilateral sagittal split osteotomies stabilized with wire osseous fixation combined with intermaxillary fixation. MacIntosh[27] did claim to have over 30% relapse among the open bite patients in his review of 326 patients. Unfortunately, his methodology precluded a clear understanding of how many patients had open bite as well as how the relapse was measured. Kahnberg[28] did describe success in treating Class III patients with anterior open bite using a vertical ramus osteotomy (VRO) but this success has not been shown since. However, this chapter will address only closing anterior open bites with anticlockwise rotation of the distal segment in the BSSO. Clinicians evidently primarily based their belief that this was an unstable technique based on a few case reports and individual experience. Proffit, Turvey, and Phillips[29] admitted to this problem in their initial publication of the hierarchy of stability in orthognathic surgery. This bias against closing anterior open bites with mandibular osteotomies persists despite recent evidence in the literature, based both on research as well as reports by well recognized experts in orthognathic surgery, that this technique is as stable as the correction with maxillary osteotomies.

The first report of the stability of closing open bites in patients with mandibular retrognathia was somewhat hidden in a research article by Knaup comparing the use of three versus four bicortical screws for fixation.[30] This was closely followed by three articles reporting anticlockwise rotation of the mandibular body using a BSSO. Two of the articles were by Wolford, Chemello, Hilliard, and Buschang[31,32] and the third by Rosen.[33] In the first paper by Wolford et al., they reviewed their experience with altering the occlusal plane and the second followed with a more complete reporting of the stability of occlusal plane rotation in bimaxillary surgery. It must be emphasized that in some of the cases in this study there was decrease in the occlusal plane angle which was different from the anticlockwise rotation of the mandible that always occurs with posterior impaction of the maxilla. Maxillary impaction with 'autorotation' of the mandible is widely accepted as a very stable procedure.[29] However, in a number of Wolford's cases, the maxillary molar vertical position was held while the incisors were intruded essentially creating an anterior open bite that was closed with the mandibular osteotomy. Rosen at almost the same time reported the results of a small retrospective study of eleven patients who had been treated with bimaxillary osteotomies in which the bilateral sagittal split osteotomies were used to correct mandibular retrognathia along with an anterior open bite. His emphasis in discussing these cases was the dramatic amount of mandibular advancement that can occur with this purposeful movement.[33] Both sets of these authors emphasized the potential major benefit of anticlockwise rotation of the mandibular body in orthognathic surgery.

The question that remained to be answered was whether using a mandibular osteotomy alone would be an acceptably stable surgery. The possibility existed in the bimaxillary cases that some compensatory changes had occurred in the maxilla that helped in maintaining the closed bite. Rosen did not discuss any vertical measurements in his article while Wolford et al. did mention that there was further intrusion of maxillary molars postoperatively in those patients in which there was a decrease in the occlusal plane. Unfortunately, there was no breakdown of the results between those patients in whom there was simple autorotation of the mandible versus anticlockwise rotation of the mandibular body. The first report of an attempt to evaluate the stability of using the mandible alone to close open bite with rigid fixation was by Reitzik,[34] but he used an inverted 'L' osteotomy with bone graft through a skin incision. It wasn't until Oliveira and Bloomquist[35] published in 1997 on their retrospective study, that stability of anticlockwise rotation of the distal segment with a BSSO in order to close an anterior open bite was evaluated. Although there was no relapse to open bite of any of the patients at one year, there was a significant clockwise rotation of mandibular plane angle in the majority of the patients. The small size of this study precluded making any definitive statements about the practical use of closing open bites with mandibular osteotomies alone. Frey et al.[36] using the data generated from a much larger study found a similar skeletal relapse pattern in patients in which there was anticlockwise rotation of the mandible. This multicentre study compared rigid internal fixation versus wire osseous fixation. Similar to Oliveira they reported that patients who had a decrease in the mandibular plane angle at the time of surgery had both a small relapse in that angle as well as an increase in the distance from B point to a constructed 'Y' axis. These increases were small but statistically significant and different from changes seen in these measurements from patients in whom there was clockwise rotation of the mandible during the advancement surgery. Unfortunately there was no mention if this relapse had any clinical relevance such as opening of the bite. The problem that this was not mentioned along with two interesting items noted in this article makes it somewhat difficult to interpret this study when comparing it with other papers dealing with open bite treatment. First only minor skeletal relapse was found with the anticlockwise movement and was first noted to be significant only at the two year follow-up. Secondly only six of the 127 patients studied started with an anterior open bite. Interestingly, 70 of the 127 patients were found to have had a decrease in mandibular plane angle during surgery which put them in the anticlockwise rotation group. This apparent paradox may be related to the difficulty of using head films when there is movement along both vertical and horizontal axes especially when using measurements of mandibular plane angle. These measurements are effected both by gnathion which varies with distal segment movement, and gonion which generally only varies with the vertical ramus positioning. Noteworthy in this study was a statement that anticlockwise repositioning of the mandible results in the gonial angle moving down as the chin rotates up. Most surgeons now avoid having the sagittal split extend completely to the posterior border and therefore the gonial angle is not influenced by the distal fragment in mandibular advancements. The variations in surgical technique as well as research designs many times make comparison of different studies in orthognathic surgery difficulty and this is especially the case in the treatment of anterior open bites. Unfortunately, this fact does not provide the clinician with sufficient information for easy treatment decision making.

More recent studies of using bilateral sagittal split osteotomies alone to close anterior open bites have come from three different centers.[37–39] Although these studies had relatively small sample sizes, 12, 28, and 31 patients; and relatively short follow-up, at least one year with the larger study having an average of 4.5 years; the stability of the surgery appears to be very good with the largest percentage relapse to no overbite being 10%. Unfortunately no direct comparisons with the use of maxillary osteotomies in closing anterior open bite have been made in any of the studies of mandibular osteotomies. However, the mandible only studies that have been reported are extremely favourable and seem to lend credence to the use of the bilateral sagittal split osteotomy. This impression of comparability also appears to be supported by two recent articles, one a systematic review of surgical correction[40] and the second a meta-analysis of orthodontic alone and with surgical correction of anterior open bites.[3] The authors of both these reports however warned of the shortfalls of reviewing the literature in this area and cautioned against direct comparison of treatment efficacies based on this literature.

Evidence that closing anterior open bite with anticlockwise rotation of the distal segment in bilateral sagittal split osteotomies is becoming accepted is evidenced by recent publications by noted orthognathic surgeons. As noted earlier, Wolford and Rosen led the way with their description of this mandibular rotation in conjunction with maxillary osteotomies to close anterior open bites. More recently there have been articles by Reyneke,[7,41] Gunson and Arnett,[42] and Van Sickles[43] discussing their experience with and indications for using this procedure. While all these surgeons emphasize the potential aesthetic benefit of using mandibular anticlockwise rotation versus clockwise rotation of the mandible, only Reyneke[7] specifically identified other criteria for making this decision. He constructed a flow chart for surgical treatment of anterior open bite based on the patient either demonstrating a decrease in ramus height – indicator for considering mandibular osteotomy, versus increased maxillary vertical height – primary indicator for a maxillary osteotomy (see Chapter 28). An emphasis is made, however, in this paper, as well as others, supporting anticlockwise rotation of the occlusal plane, on the potential positive aesthetic effects of this rotation of the mandible especially by providing for greater projection of the chin. A more recent benefit of anticlockwise rotation of the occlusal plane has been the interest of using maxillomandibular advancement in treatment of obstructive sleep apnoea (OSA). Wolford noted an increase in anterior–posterior dimension of the oropharyngeal airway with a decreased occlusal plane angle,[31] but surprisingly it wasn't until Van Sickle's article in 2012[43] that OSA would be listed as an indication for anticlockwise rotation of the mandible in bimaxillary surgery. We have, in fact, found this type of rotation to be very valuable in patients who present with dentoskeletal deformities that do not seem amenable to traditional maxillomandibular advancements (Figures 30-1 and 30-2). The best example of this kind of patient is an individual with minimal anterior overjet who would not aesthetically tolerate a large maxillary advancement. With the increased acceptance of using this type of surgery in the treatment of OSA, a number of young, thin, and otherwise healthy individuals are being referred for surgery (Figure 30-3). Many of these patients are retrognathic and have had either orthodontic or natural dental compensations resulting in minimal anterior overjet. Although premolar extractions in the lower arch can be considered, it may not be possible due to previous orthodontic extractions or simple adult patient reluctance for even short-term appliance wear. Purposely creating an anterior open bite by an anticlockwise rotation of the maxillary occlusal plane and then closing it with the mandible can result in a large mandibular advancement with minimum maxillary incisor movement. This positive impact on the airway can be improved even further if the posterior part of the maxilla is downgrafted and thus increasing the nasopharyngeal airway. These types of movements, however, may seem heretical to a maxillofacial surgeon since they definitely violate traditional beliefs on minimizing relapse. Large mandibular advancements, closing anterior open bite with mandibular rotation, and increasing facial height, especially posterior facial height, have been reported to be unstable. The relative stability of closing anterior open bites with mandibular osteotomies alone has previously been discussed in this chapter. There is unfortunately only one study that looks specifically at anticlockwise rotation of the occlusal plane in bimaxillary surgery and compares it with two more traditionally accepted bimaxillary surgical movements. Reyneke[44] compared patients in whom the mandibular body was rotated anticlockwise with patients who either had anterior face height decreased based on autorotation of the mandible or had the mandibular facial height increased through clockwise rotation of both jaws. In this retrospective study of 88 patients, 41 of which had anticlockwise movement of the occlusal plane, no significant difference was noted in anterior posterior or vertical relapse between the study group and the two 'traditional' movement groups. The question that needs to be answered is: What is being done surgically that now seems to result in such good stability.

Techniques for maximizing stability when anticlockwise rotation of the mandible is used

The most significant change in orthognathic surgical techniques that has occurred since the introduction of the bilateral sagittal split and the Le Fort I osteotomy has been the introduction of rigid internal fixation. The perfection of these fixation techniques has

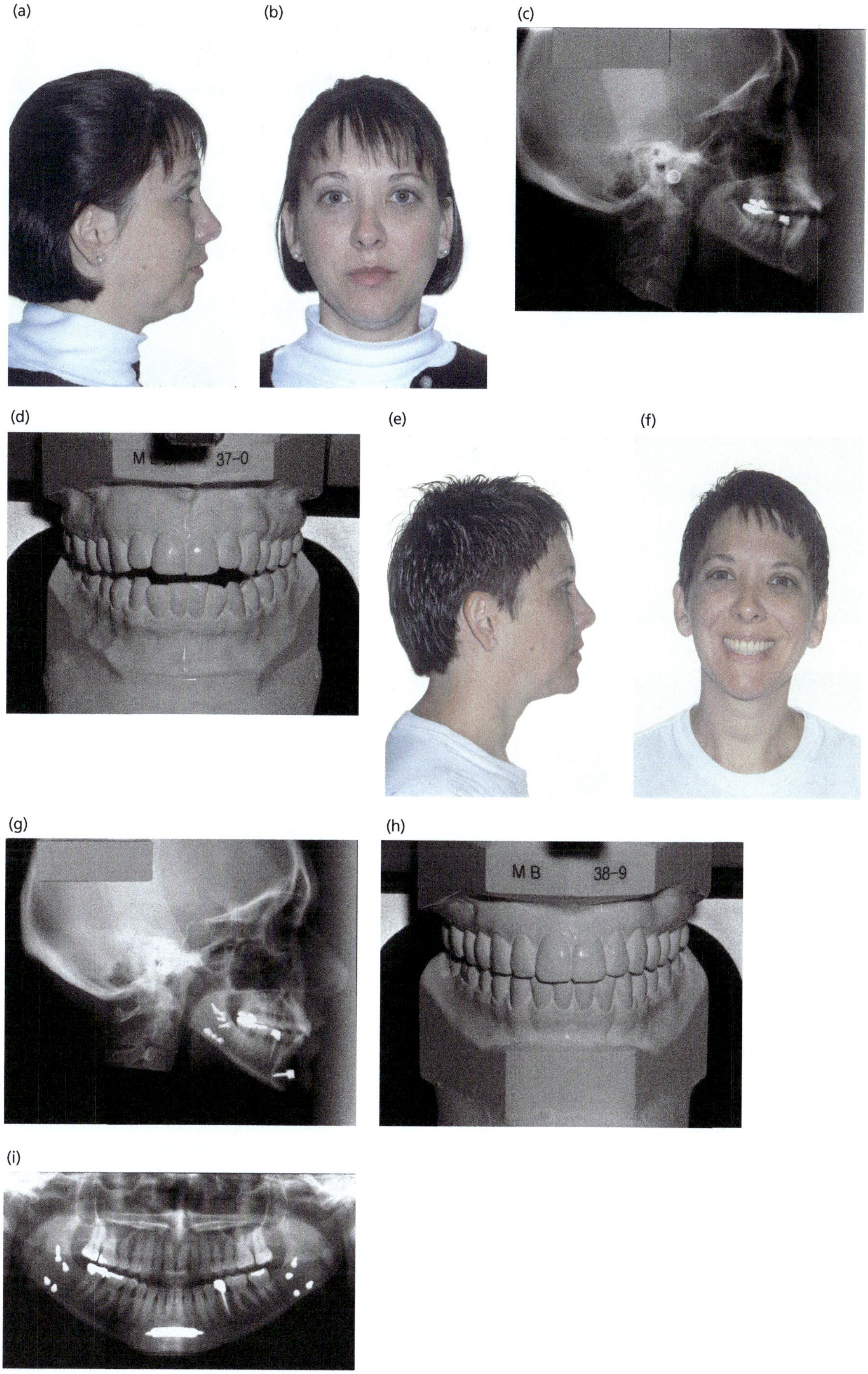

Fig. 30-1 (a–d) Pretreatment records for patient who had mandibular retrognathia with an anterior open bite. (e–i) One year post-orthodontic records.

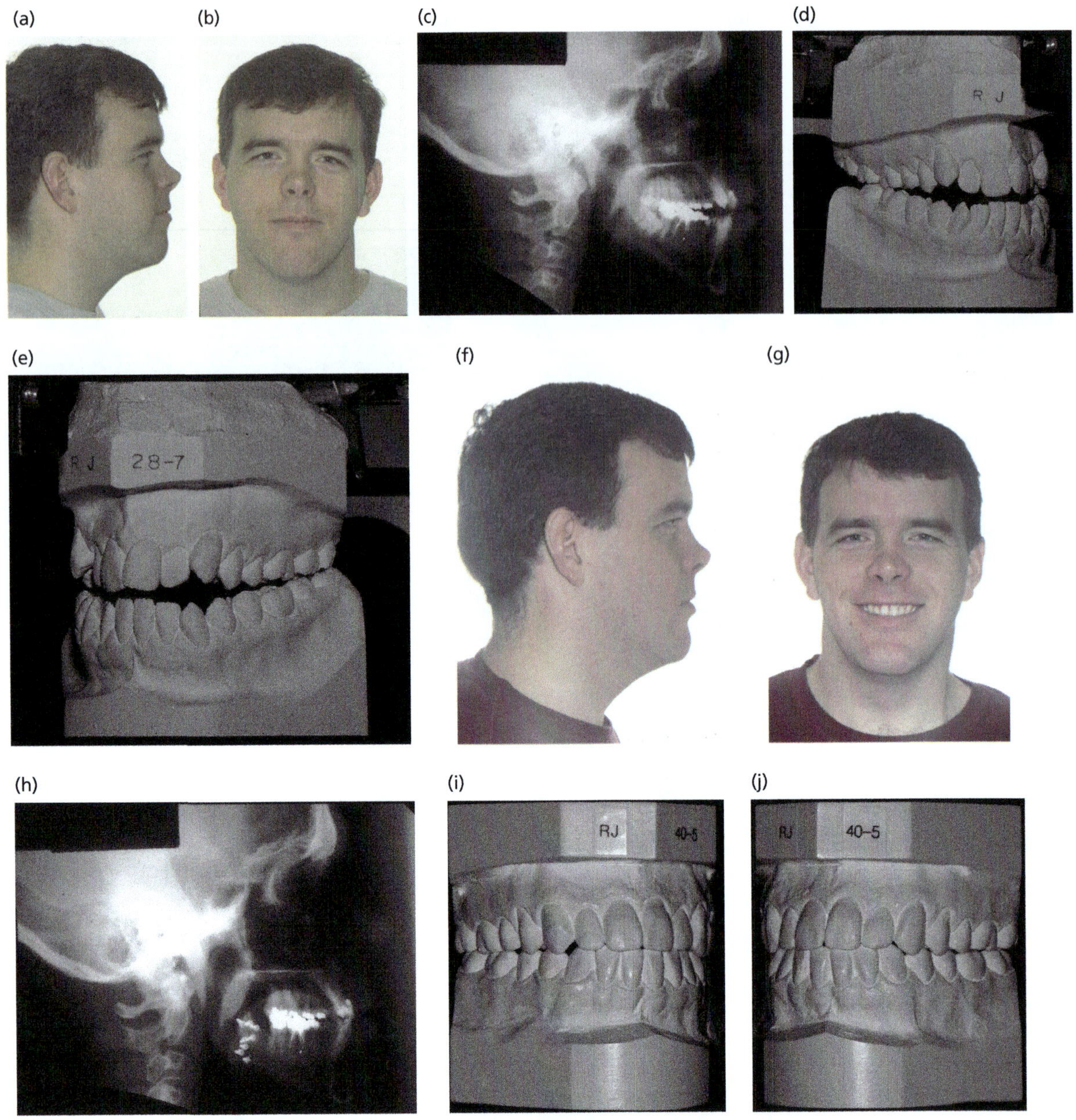

Fig. 30-2 (a–e) Pretreatment records for a patient with a Class I occlusion and anterior open bite, but had midface features that precluded a maxillary Le Fort I. He also had a SARPE to correct the transverse problem without negatively affecting facial aesthetics. (f–j) Ten year post-orthodontic records demonstrating stability of the treatment.

benefitted the patient not only by allowing earlier function, but by increasing stability. This increase in stability appears to be clearly demonstrated in the correction of anterior open bites.[2,36] The question then becomes what type and amount of fixation is preferable in stabilizing the mandible when closing anterior open bites. There has been only one study that appears to directly address that question. Knaup,[30] in her study comparing three versus four bicortical screws in large advancements found the only difference in stability between the two fixation techniques occurred in the anticlockwise rotation of the mandibular body. This use of four screws on each side was the method used in four of the previously mentioned studies (Figure 30-1). Methods of fixation that have been advocated for the achievement of increased stability by other surgeons have included the use of large fixation plates, skeletal wire fixation, and prolonged interarch elastic wear. The use of these techniques is based on some research but primarily on individual surgeon's experiences in treating large mandibular advancements.

The basic goal of all maxillofacial surgeons in minimizing relapse is focused on techniques that are intended to neutralize the perceived causes for these postoperative changes. Two generally accepted aetiologies are neuromuscular imbalance and soft tissue pressures. Primarily the suspected muscular components include the stretching of the pterygomasseteric sling and the suprahyoid muscles. However, another neuromuscular component, as noted earlier in discussing the aetiology of open bite, is an existing weakened muscle tone of the masseter, medial pterygoid and temporalis muscles. Therefore a possible conflict exists on the contribution of the muscles

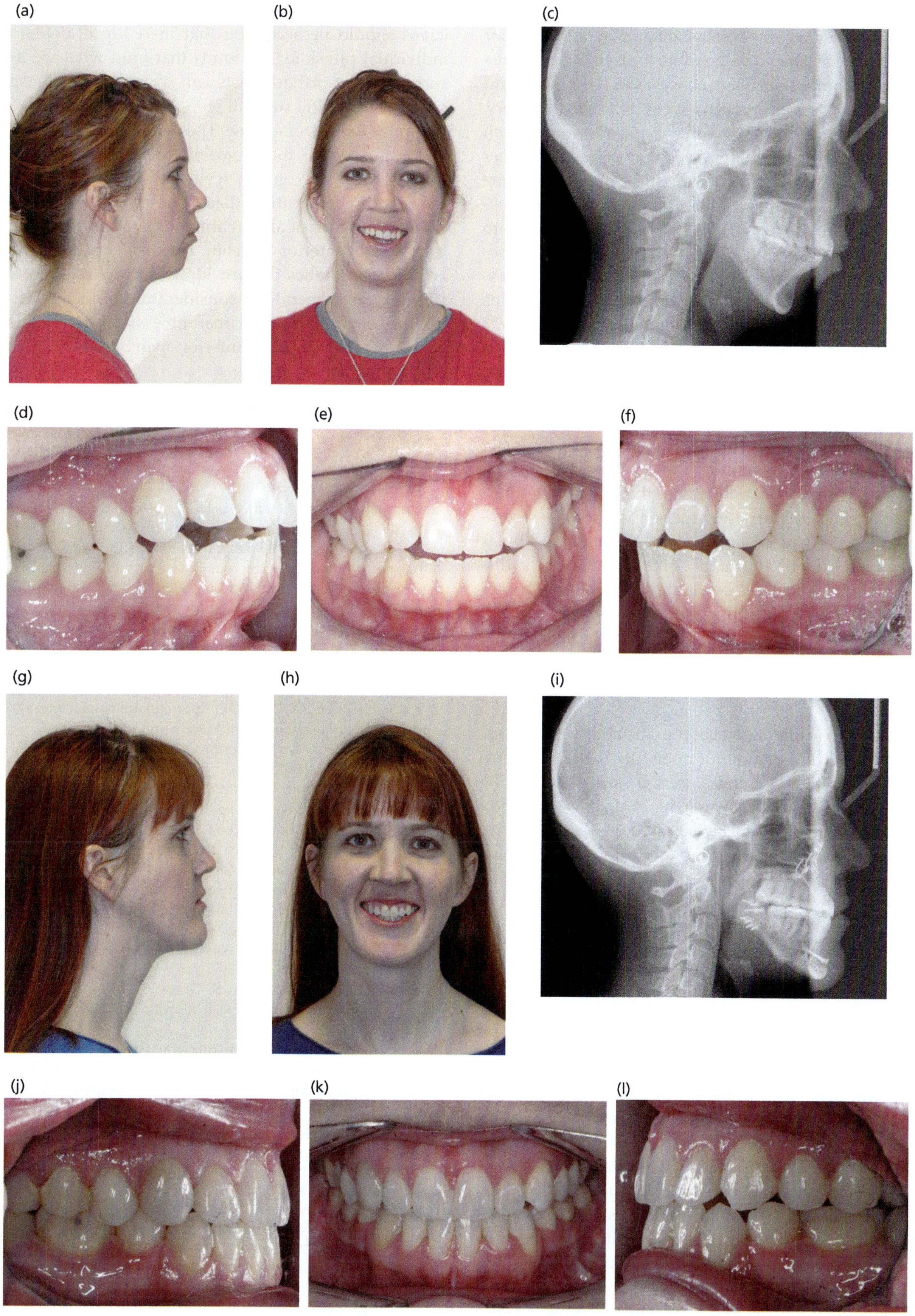

Fig. 30-3 (a–f) Pretreatment records of patient with obstructive sleep apnoea, mandibular retrognathia, and anterior open bite. (g–l) Final records of patient who had presurgical mandibular premolar extractions and then anticlockwise rotation of maxillary occlusal plane, closure of the open bite and mandibular advancement with a BSSO, and horizontal osteotomy with advancement (genioplasty advancement).

of mastication to relapse. One would suspect that if the muscle tone was weaker than normal in anterior open bites, it should be possible to stretch those muscles with minimal consequences. On the other hand if the muscle tone remains week following surgery, it could be hypothesized that opposing forces such as dental eruption, suprahyoid muscles, and other submandibular soft tissue pressures may lead to the reopening of the bite. This apparent paradox however may not be relevant in most cases. This is due to the fact that many times the posterior-inferior component of the sagittal split does not extend to the posterior border of the mandible, instead ending up as described by Dal Pont,[45] or as advocated by Epker.[46] *Thus these muscles remain attached primarily to the proximal segment and are minimally stretched, if at all, by the anticlockwise rotation of the mandibular body.*[7] The exception to this would occur if the split extended all the way to the posterior border especially if the posterior maxilla is downgrafted. In that case the suggestion by Wolford[31] and Reyneke[7] that the pterygomasseteric sling be purposely incised is strongly recommended. Finally, stripping of the sphenomandibular ligament from its attachment on the medial of the distal fragment has also been suggested although care needs to be given to the inferior alveolar nerve and vessels if this is attempted. The role of the suprahyoid muscles in relapse is unclear since studies on releasing these muscles when the mandible is advanced are equivocal.[26,47]

The fascinating fact related to instability of the surgical correction of anterior open bite is that the postoperative relapse changes are the same whether the deformity is corrected by maxillary clockwise rotation or mandibular anticlockwise rotation. These changes include increase in anterior facial height, anticlockwise rotation of the maxillary occlusal plane due to eruption of molars, and an increase in mandibular plane angle. This is consistent with the literature reviews of open bite relapse which have found similar relapse rates between the surgical techniques. A possible reason for this is the culpability of preexisting muscle tone weakness in the muscles of mastication. There have been studies that found closing open bite with maxillary surgery has increased muscle tone in some patients.[48] However, it can be expected that there are also patients who either have little or even no improvement in muscle tone and then, as was noted earlier, it is possible that opposing forces will result in relapse. Since it is still quite unclear as to the influence of these forces, we feel that research needs to be encouraged on exploring the possibilities of improving that tone. Well-designed, randomized, prospective studies also need to be emphasized both in the areas of osteotomy design as well as fixation techniques. There should be no question that multiple factors including methods of fixation, neuromuscular balance, and soft tissue pressures contribute to the stability or instability of the correction of anterior open bite with mandibular osteotomies. It is clear that the greater the movement the larger the relapse potential and clinicians should be accepting that there are ill-defined individual physiological limits that limit what we as surgeons and orthodontists can overcome. We have suggested specific surgical steps that can be taken to minimize the risk of relapse. The bottom line, however, for the surgeon is the choice of criteria to be used in making a decision on which surgical technique is best for an individual patient. Based on the present inconclusive evidence of any treatment's superiority in the treatment of anterior open bite, the answer in our mind is clear – aesthetics (Figure 30-2). For that reason we strongly recommend the consideration of using anticlockwise rotation of the mandible as an acceptable alternative in correcting anterior open bite.

References

1 Denison T, Kokich V, Shapiro P. Stability of maxillary surgery in openbite versus nonopenbite malocclusions. Angle Orthod. 1989;59:5–10.
2 Hoppenreijs TJM, Freihofer HPM, Stoelinga PJW, et al. Skeletal and dento-alveolar stability of Le Fort I intrusion osteotomies and bimaxillary osteotomies in anterior open bite deformities. Int J Oral Maxillofac Surg. 1997;26:161–75.
3 Greenlee GM, Huang GJ, Chen SS-H, Chen J, Koepsell T, Hujoel P. Stability of treatment for anterior open-bite malocclusion: a meta-analysis. Am J Orthod Dentofacial Orthop. 2011;139:154–69.
4 Huang GJ. Long-term stability of anterior open-bite therapy: A review. Semin Orthod. 2002;8:162–172.
5 Kwon HJ, Bevis RR, Waite DE. Apertognathia (open bite) and its surgical management. Int J Oral Surg. 1984;13:278–89.
6 Otuyemi, OD; Noar J. Anterior Open-bite: A Review. Saudi Dent J. 1997;9:149–57.
7 Reyneke JP, Ferretti C. Anterior open bite correction by Le Fort I or bilateral sagittal split osteotomy. Oral Maxillofac Surg Clin North Am. 2007;19:321–38.
8 Turvey TA, Journot V, Epker BN. Correction of anterior open bite deformity: A study of tongue function, speech changes, and stability. J Maxillofac Surg. 1976;4:93–101.
9 Ciccone de Faria T dos S, Hallak Regalo SC, Thomazinho A, Vitti M, de Felício CM. Masticatory muscle activity in children with a skeletal or dentoalveolar open bite. Eur J Orthod. 2010;32:453–8.
10 Solow B, Siersbæk-Nielsen S, Greve E. Airway adequacy, head posture, and craniofacial morphology. Am J Orthod. 1984;86:214–23.
11 Trask GM, Shapiro GG, Shapiro PA. The effects of perennial allergic rhinitis on dental and skeletal development: A comparison of sibling pairs. Am J Orthod Dentofac Orthop. 1987;92:286–93.
12 Proffit WR; Fields HW; Nixon WL. Occlusal forces in normal- and long-face adults. J Dent Res. 1983;62:566–70.
13 Proffit WR; Fields HW. Occlusal forces in normal- and long-face children. J Dent Res. 1983;62:571–4.
14 Proffit WR, Turvey TA, Fields HW, Phillips C. The effect of orthognathic surgery on occlusal force. J Oral Maxillofac Surg. 1989;47:457–63.
15 Breuel W, Krause M, Schneider M, Harzer W. Genetic stretching factors in masseter muscle after orthognathic surgery. Br J Oral Maxillofac Surg. 2013;51:530–5.
16 Arat ZM; Akcam MO; Esenlik E; Arat FE. Inconsistencies in the differential diagnosis of open bite. Angle Orthod. 2008;78:415–9.
17 Ellis E, McNamara JA, Lawrence TM. Components of adult Class II open-bite malocclusion. J Oral Maxillofac Surg. 1985;43:92–105.

18 Ellis E, McNamara JA. Components of adult Class III open-bite malocclusion. Am J Orthod. 1984;86:277–90.
19 MC Iz-III. Prevalence and factors associated with anterior open bite in 2–5 year old children in Benin city, Nigeria. African Heal Sci. 2012;12:446–51.
20 Lentinie-Oliveira DA, Carvalho FR, Ye Q, Luo J, Saconato H, Machado MAC, Prado LBF, Prado GF. Orthodontic and orthopaedic treatment for anterior open bite in children (Review). Cochrane Libr. 2007;18(2).
21 Phelan A, Franchi L, Baccetti T, Darendeliler MA, McNamara JA. Longitudinal growth changes in subjects with open-bite tendency: a retrospective study. Am J Orthod Dentofacial Orthop. 2014;145:28–35.
22 Proffit WR, Bailey LJ, Phillips C, Turvey TA. Long-term stability of surgical open-bite correction by Le Fort I osteotomy. Angle Orthod. 2000;70:112–7.
23 Poulton DR, Ware WH. Surgical-orthodontic treatment of severe mandibular retrusion. Am J Orthod. 1971;59:244–65.
24 Poulton DR, Ware WH. Surgical-orthodontic treatment of severe mandibular retrusion (Part II). Am J Orthod. 1973; 63:237–55.
25 McNeill RHJSR. Skeletal relapse during intermaxillary fixation. J Oral Surg (Chic). 1973;31:212–27.
26 Schendel, Stephen; Epker B. Results after mandibular advancement surgery: an analysis of 87 cases. J Oral Surg (Chic). 1980;38:265–82.
27 MacIntosh RB. Experience with the sagittal osteotomy of the mandibular ramus: A 13-year review. J Maxillofac Surg. 1981;9:151–65.
28 Kahnberg K-E, Widmark G. Surgical treatment of the open bite deformity. Int J Oral Maxillofac Surg. 1988;17:45–8.
29 Proffit W, Turvey T, Phillips C. Orthognathic surgery: A hierarchy of stability. Int J Adult Orthodonitics Orthognath Surg. 1996;11:191–204.
30 Knaup C, Wallen T, Bloomquist D. Linear and rotational changes in large mandibular advancements using three or four fixation screws. Int J Adult Orthodont Orthognath Surg. 1993;8:245–63.
31 Wolford LM, Chemello PD, Hilliard FW. Occlusal plane alteration in orthognathic surgery. J Oral Maxillofac Surg. 1993;51:730–40.
32 Chemello PD, Wolford LM, Buschang PH. Occlusal plane alteration in orthognathic surgery – Part II: Long-term stability of results. Am J Orthod Dentofac Orthop. 1994;106:434–40.
33 Rosen H. Occlusal plane rotation: aesthetic enhancement in mandibular micrognathia. Plast Reconstr Surg. 1993;91:1231–40.
34 Reitzik M, Barer PG, Wainwright WM, Lim B. The surgical treatment of skeletal anterior open-bite deformities with rigid internal fixation in the mandible. Am J Orthod Dentofac Orthop. 1990;97:52–7.
35 Oliveira J, Bloomquist D. The stability of the use of bilateral sagittal split osteotomy in the closure of anterior open bite. J Adult Orthod Orthognath Surg. 1997;12:101–8.
36 Frey DR, Hatch JP, Van Sickels JE, Dolce C, Rugh JD. Alteration of the mandibular plane during sagittal split advancement: short- and long-term stability. Oral Surg Oral Med Oral Pathol Oral Radiol Endod. 2007;104:160–9.
37 Bisase B, Johnson P, Stacey M. Closure of the anterior open bite using mandibular sagittal split osteotomy. Br J Oral Maxillofac Surg. 2010;48:352–5.
38 Stansbury CD, Evans C, Miloro M, BeGole E, Morris DE. Stability of open bite correction with sagittal split osteotomy and closing rotation of the mandible. J Oral Maxillofac Surg. 2010;68:149–59.
39 Fontes AM, Joondeph DR, Bloomquist DS, Greenlee GM, Wallen TR, Huang GJ. Long-term stability of anterior open-bite closure with bilateral sagittal split osteotomy. Am J Orthod Dentofacial Orthop. 2012;142:792–800.
40 Solano-Hernández B, Antonarakis GS, Scolozzi P, Kiliaridis S. Combined orthodontic and orthognathic surgical treatment for the correction of skeletal anterior open-bite malocclusion: a systematic review on vertical stability. J Oral Maxillofac Surg. 2013;71:98–109.
41 Reyneke, JP; Bryant, RS; Suuronen, R; Becker P. Postoperative skeletal stability following clockwise and counter-clockwise rotation of the maxillomandibular complex compared to conventional orthognathic treatment. Br J Oral Maxillofac Surg. 2007;45:56–64.
42 Gunson MJ, Arnett GW, Milam SB. Pathophysiology and pharmacologic control of osseous mandibular condylar resorption. J Oral Maxillofac Surg. 2012;70:1918–34.
43 Van Sickles J, Wallender A. Closure of anterior open bites with mandibular surgery: advantages and disadvantages of this approach. Oral Maxillofac Surg. 2012;16:361–7.
44 Reyneke JP, Bryant RS, Suuronen R, Becker PJ. Postoperative skeletal stability following clockwise and counter-clockwise rotation of the maxillomandibular complex compared to conventional orthognathic treatment. Br J Oral Maxillofac Surg. 2007;45:56–64.
45 Dal Pont G. Retromolar osteotomy for the correction of prognathism. J Oral Surg (Chic). 1961;19:42–7.
46 Epker B. Modifications of the sagittal split osteotomy of the mandible. J Oral Surg (Chic). 1977;35:157–9.
47 Ellis E, Carlson DS. Stability two years after mandibular advancement with and without suprahyoid myotomy: An experimental study. J Oral Maxillofac Surg. 1983;41: 426–37.
48 Hunt NP, Cunningham SJ. The influence of orthognathic surgery on occlusal force in patients with vertical facial deformities. Int J Oral Maxillofac Surg. 1997;26:87–91.

Chapter 31

Rotation of the Maxillomandibular Complex

Johan P. Reyneke

Introduction

Rotation of the maxillomandibular complex (MMC) as an alternative treatment design to conventional orthognathic treatment planning was first described as the 'rotation of the occlusal plane' or the 'manipulation of the occlusal plane' for the correction of Class II low angle mandibular plane cases.[1] Because of the possible confusion regarding the above mentioned misnomers as well as the difference between conventional treatment design and the surgical treatment design involving rotation of the maxillomandibular complex as treatment, it is important to discuss and to clarify the principles of the two treatment methods. Many dentofacial deformities can be corrected by means of conventional orthognathic treatment planning.[2,3] However, by adhering to conventional treatment planning principles optimal aesthetic outcomes may not always be achieved. In these cases alternative treatment designs such as the rotation of the maxillomandibular complex should be considered.

Principles of conventional treatment designs

Many dentofacial deformities can be corrected by surgery to one jaw only whereby either the mandible or the maxilla is repositioned. Repositioning of the mandible may involve surgical advancement or setback, and this horizontal movement will take place along the occlusal plane of the maxilla (the unoperated jaw).[3] When the maxilla is repositioned, either

Orthognathic Surgery: Principles, Planning and Practice. Edited by Farhad B. Naini and Daljit S. Gill.

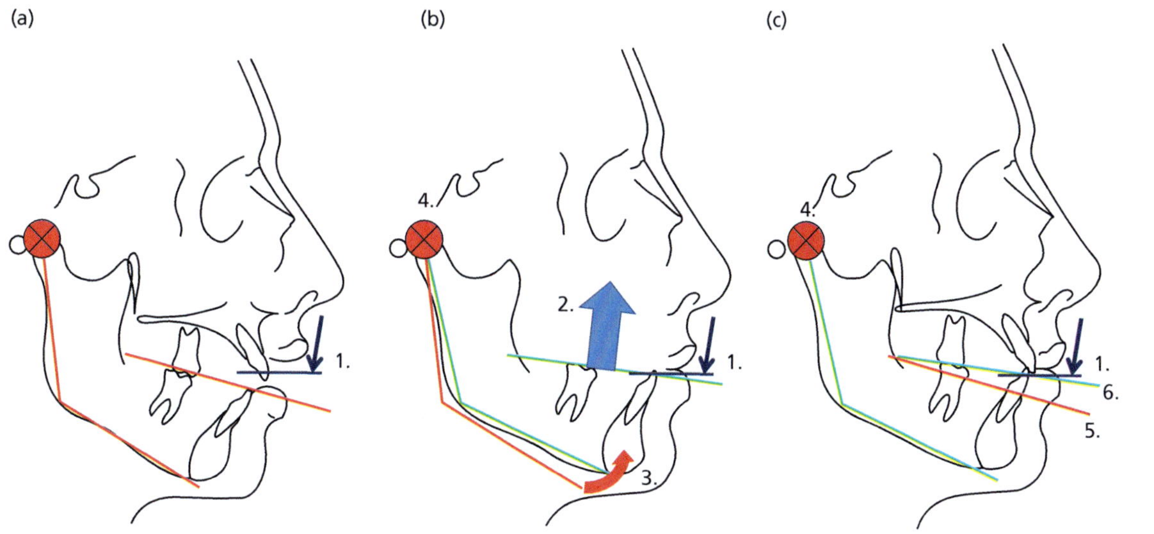

Fig. 31-1 Conventional treatment planning. **a.** A cephalometric tracing of a patient with vertical maxillary excess requiring superior repositioning of the maxilla. The ideal height of the upper incisor is indicated by line and arrow (1). **b.** Super repositioning of the maxilla (arrow (2)) will result in counterclockwise rotation of the mandible (arrow (3)) until an ideal overbite is achieved. The rotation takes place at the condyle (4). **c.** As a result of the counterclockwise rotation of the mandible the occlusal plane has changed from (5) to (6). An ideal occlusion and soft tissue relationship had been achieved.

anteriorly or posteriorly (albeit seldom), the horizontal movement will take place along the occlusal plane of the mandible (the unoperated jaw). Surgery to the maxilla however, allows the surgeon to also change the height of the lower face by either superiorly or inferiorly repositioning of the maxilla. Correction of vertical maxillary excess will require superior repositioning of the maxilla while for vertical maxillary deficiency the maxilla will need to be inferiorly repositioned. Vertical change of the maxilla will result in either clockwise rotation of the mandible when the maxilla is down grafted or counterclockwise rotation when the maxilla is superiorly repositioned. The rotation of the mandible will take place around a point at or just posterior to the condyle and the occlusal plane will change as a consequence of the autorotation (Figures 31-1 and 31-2).[4] Hence it is the position assumed by the mandible and the mandibular occlusal plane after autorotation that will dictate the final occlusal plane angle. A change in the anterior facial height has however also a significant effect on the horizontal relationship of the jaws as a result of forward (counterclockwise) and backward (clockwise) rotation of the mandible around the condyle. The consequent anteroposterior change of the mandibular lower incisors will require consideration. Small anteroposterior discrepancies can often be corrected by either advancing the maxilla or setting it back. The maxilla is however seldom setback due to poor aesthetic outcomes. In Figure 31-3 a case with vertical maxillary excess is demonstrated. The patient was treated according to conventional treatment principles. The

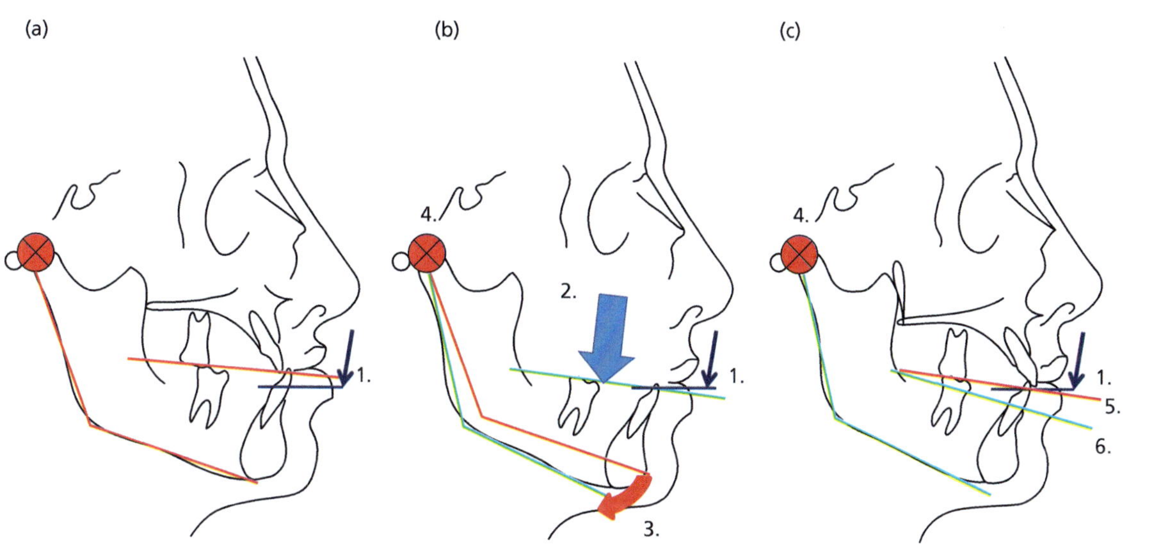

Fig. 31-2 Conventional treatment planning. **a.** A cephalometric tracing of a patient with maxillary vertical deficiency requiring maxillary downgraft. The ideal height of the upper incisor is indicated by line and arrow (1). **b.** Downgraft of the maxilla (arrow (2)) will result in clockwise rotation of the mandible (arrow (3)) until an ideal overbite is achieved. The rotation takes place at the condyle (4). **c.** As a result of the clockwise rotation of the mandible the occlusal plane has changed from (5) to (6). An ideal occlusion and soft tissue relationship has been achieved.

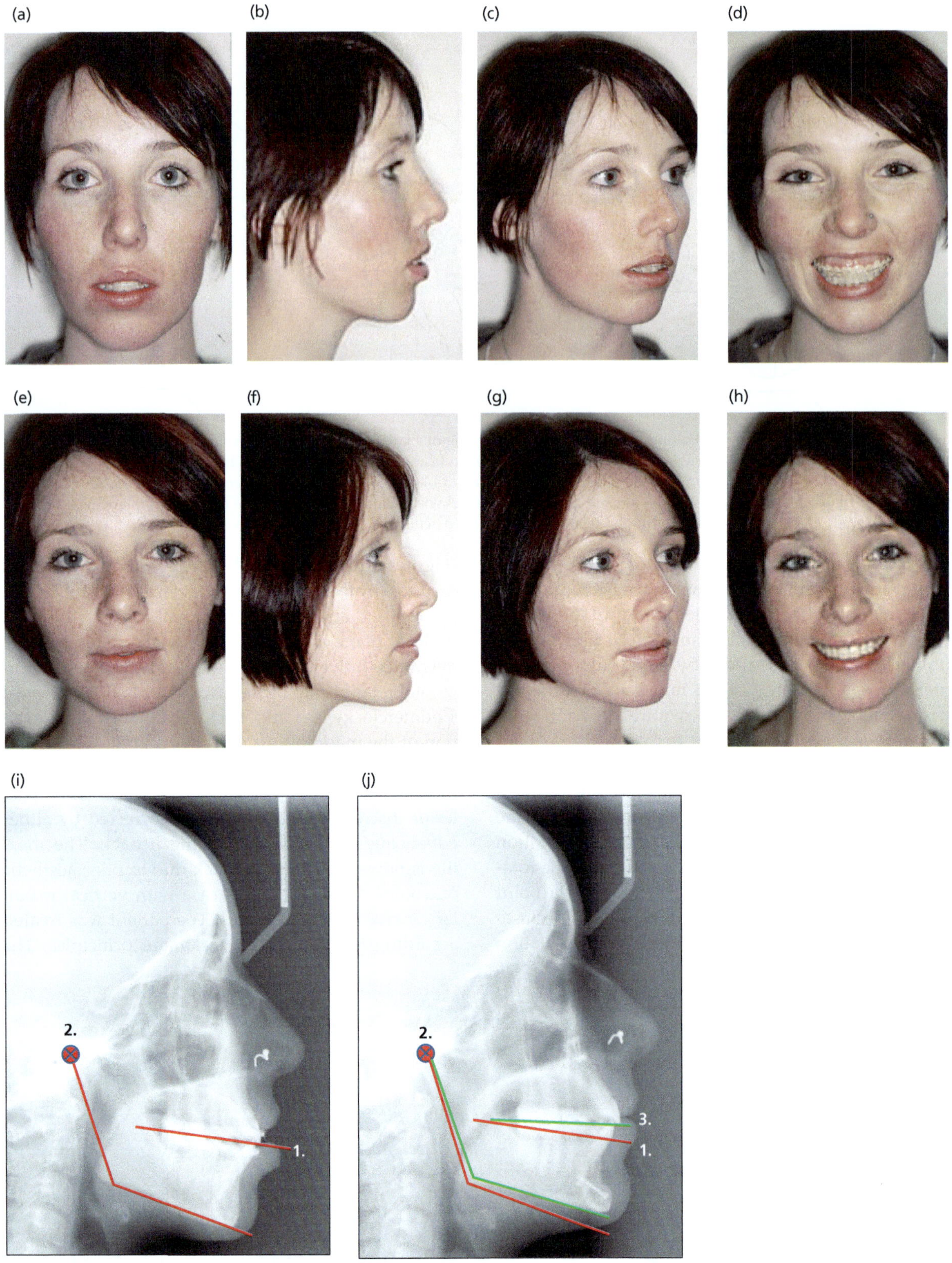

Fig. 31-3 A patient with vertical maxillary excess and microgenia was treated by means of conventional treatment planning. **a.** Frontal view; **b.** Profile view; **c.** Three quarter view; and **d.** Smile. The postoperative result following superior repositioning of the maxilla and genioplasty advancement is demonstrated in figures **e, f, g** and **h.** The pre surgical **(i)** and post-surgical **(j)** lateral cephalometric radiographs illustrate the counterclockwise rotation of the mandible at the condyle (2) and the occlusal plane change from (1) to (3).

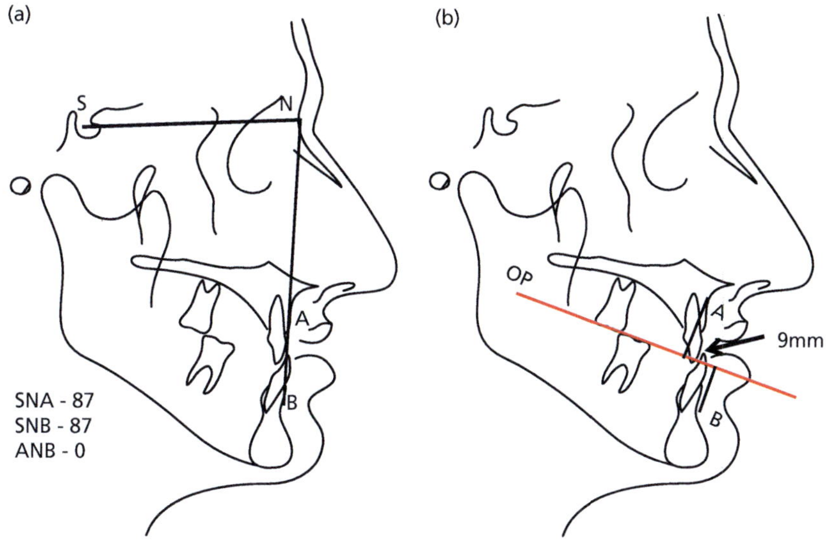

Fig. 31-4 Due to the high occlusal plane angle the Steiner and Wits cephalometric analysis reflect contradictory results in this case. In **(a)** the Steiner analysis indicates a mild anteroposterior discrepancy (ANB angle – 0 degrees) between the upper and lower jaws while in **(b)** the Wits analysis however indicates a severe discrepancy between the jaws (A-occlusal plane to B-occlusal plane 9 mm).

maxilla was superiorly repositioned and the mandible has rotated counterclockwise around the condyle. The occlusal plane has changed and the lower incisors advanced. When large anteroposterior discrepancies occur as a result of the autorotation of the mandible, surgery to both jaws should be considered and the discrepancy, or part of it, managed by mandibular surgery.

When corrective treatment require surgery to both jaws the same principles as discussed above will apply during treatment planning. When the final occlusal plane is dictated by the mandibular occlusal plane after autorotation.

It may however not be possible to achieve optimal aesthetic outcomes by adhering to conventional treatment methods, especially in very high of low mandibular- and occlusal plane angle cases. In these cases the aesthetic limitations may be overcome by rotating the maxillomandibular complex, also known as *alteration* or *manipulation of the occlusal* plane.[1] The latter two are however misnomers. The change in the occlusal plane angle is a consequence of the rotation of the maxillomandibular complex and by no means an attempt to treat or change an abnormal occlusal plane angle to an angle which is considered to be a cephalometric more normal angle. The occlusal plane angle however plays an important role in the aesthetic and cephalometric assessment of the face (Figure 31-4).

Principles of rotation of the maxillomandibular complex treatment design

By performing surgery to both jaws the surgeon is also enabled to rotate the lower face (maxillomandibular complex) in a clockwise or counterclockwise direction. This would either decrease the lower facial prominence (clockwise) or increase the prominence of the lower facial (counterclockwise). Facial types that would usually benefit from the rotation of the maxillomandibular complex are the high occlusal- and mandibular plane angle, leptoprosopic, dolichocephalic facial types and the low mandibular- and occlusal plane angle, europrosopic, brachicephalic facial types.[8]

The relationship between the vertical and anteroposterior dimensions of the face is influenced by the anterior cranial base length, the steepness of the cranial base and the occlusal plane angle. The profound effect that a high or low occlusal plane angle has on the cephalometric relationship between the bony apical base of the maxilla, the mandible and the skull base and to each other is well demonstrated in Figure 31-5. The occlusal plane should therefore always be an important consideration in orthodontic and orthognathic diagnosis and treatment planning.[8] When two-jaw surgery is planned and performed the interrelationship of important soft-tissue landmarks such as Subnasale (Sn), upper lip position (and its relation to the upper incisors), and soft tissue Pogonion (Pog′) are directly dependant on the position of the underlying dental and skeletal structures (ANS, upper incisors and bony Pogonion respectively). Key elements for good aesthetic outcomes are: (1) the vertical relationship among anterior nasal spine, upper incisor edge and Pogonion and influenced by: vertical skeletal deficiency, vertical maxillary excess, and deep- or open bite; and (2) the horizontal interrelationship between ANS, upper incisor edge and Pogonion is a consequence of the horizontal skeletal and dental relations (that is Class I, II or III). In some hypo- or hyperdivergent faces the hard tissue landmarks such as ANS, incisor edge and Pogonion may be well related; however the patient may still have an excessively convex or concave profile. The interrelationship between the above mentioned hard tissue landmarks in Figure 31-6 is identical; however owing to the difference in the occlusal plane angle in the three cases, the facial contours differ substantially.

Geometry and visualization of the rotation of the maxillomandibular complex

To facilitate an understanding of the concepts of MMC rotations and to visualize the treatment options a

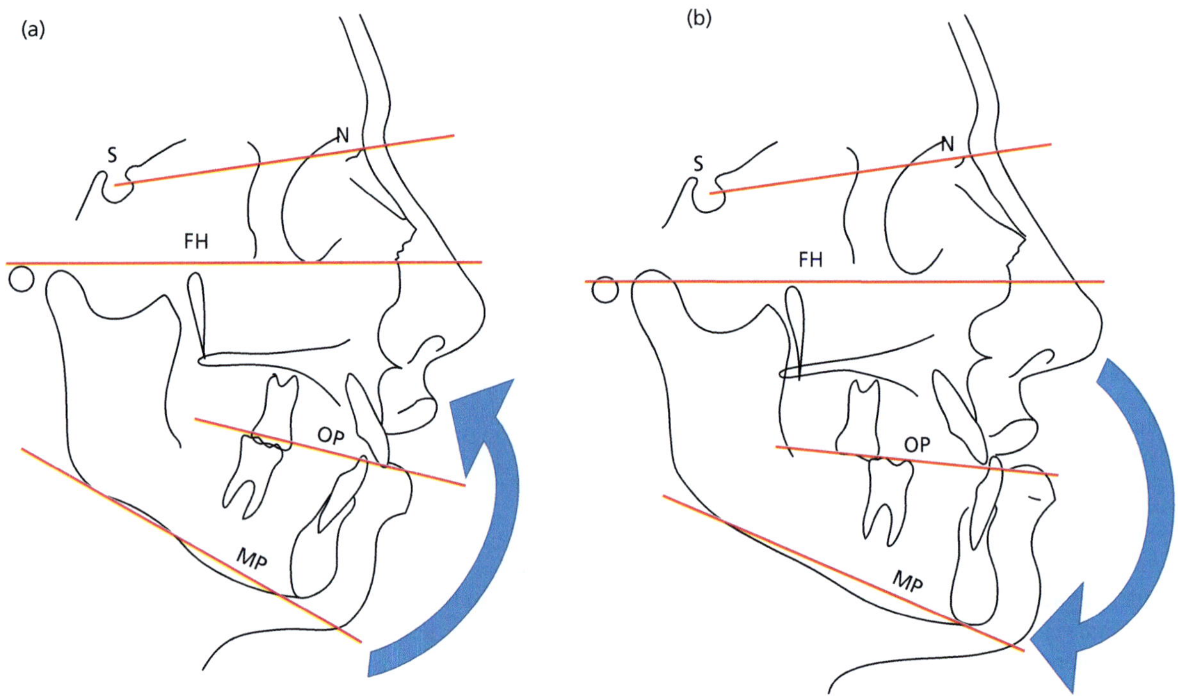

Fig. 31-5 The significant effect that a **(a)** high occlusal plane angle or **(b)** a low occlusal plane angle may have on the facial profile is well demonstrated. Counterclockwise rotation of the maxillomandibular complex (arrow) will enhance the mandibular advancement in **(a)**, while clockwise rotation (arrow) will enhance the correction and increase the convexity of the profile in the case demonstrated in **(b)**.

triangle representing the MMC is constructed. A cephalometric tracing of a patient with relatively normal soft- and hard tissue relationship and a Class I occlusion is demonstrated in Figure 31-7. A triangle is constructed by connecting ANS, PNS and Pogonion and is called the *maxillomandibular complex triangle*. This triangle will assist in predicting and visualizing the expected hard and soft tissue changes subsequent to surgical repositioning of the maxilla and the mandible as a complex but independent of the existing occlusal plane. Rotation of the MMC can take place in a clockwise or counterclockwise direction around ANS, Pog or PNS. However zygomatic buttress (BT) and upper incisor tip or any point along the lines of the triangle can also be used and is influenced by the aesthetic requirements of the case (Figure 31-7).[7–9]

By studying 40 adult human dry skulls, Reyneke[8] found that the average maxillary length (ANS to PNS – represented by the horizontal leg of the MMC triangle) was 47.6 mm while the average facial height (ANS to Pogonion – represented by the length of the vertical leg of the MMC triangle) was 66.5 mm (Figure 31-8a).

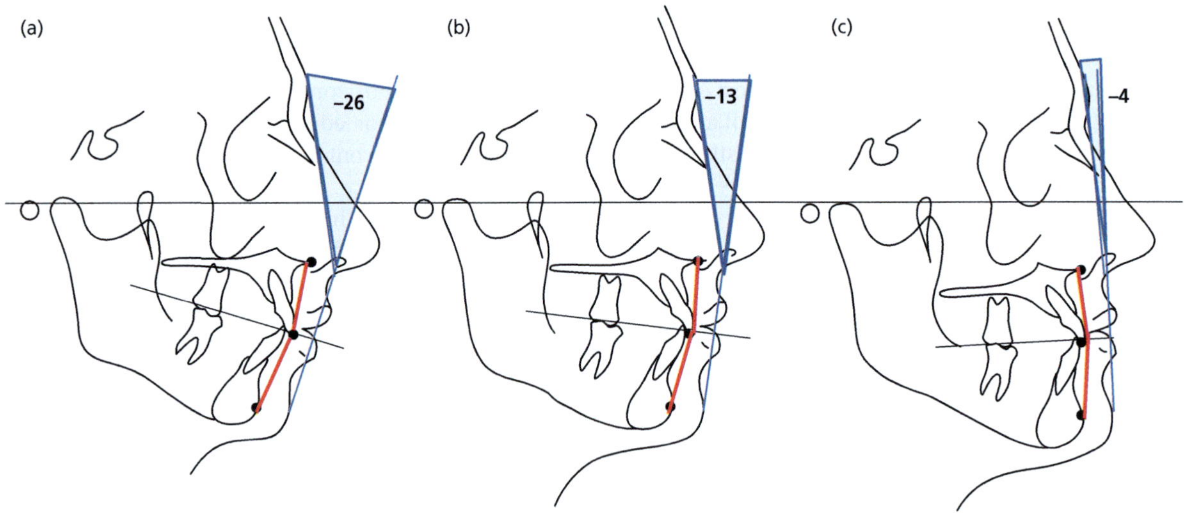

Fig. 31-6 The relationship between ANS, incisor edge and Pogonion is exactly the same in all three figures however due to the difference in the plane of occlusion the convexity differs. **(a)** A high occlusal plane results in a convex profile (facial contour angle –26 degrees), while in **(b)** a normal occlusal plane results in a straight profile (facial contour angle –13 degrees.). In **(c)** a low occlusal plane results in a concave profile (facial contour angle –4 degrees).

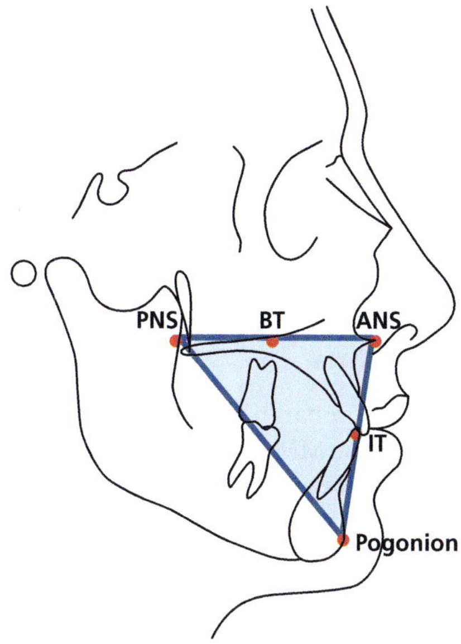

Fig. 31-7 To facilitate visualization of the treatment effects and to understand the geography of rotating the MMC, a triangle is constructed connecting ANS, PNS and Pogonion. Additional rotation points are indicated such as zygomatic buttress (BT) and incisor tip (IT).

The ratio between ANS-PNS AND ANS-Pog is 1:1.4. The fact that the horizontal leg of the triangle is shorter than the vertical leg enables the surgeon to use a 'gearing' effect of 40% when rotating the triangle. A small rotation at the posterior (PNS) of the horizontal leg (the Le Fort I osteotomy line) will result in a 40% larger change at the inferior of the vertical leg (Pogonion) (Figure 31-8b).

Indications and treatment designs using the constructed maxillomandibular triangle

Control of the aesthetic treatment effect

Many Class III dentofacial deformities will require maxillary advancement and mandibular setback procedures. As a result of the surgical correction the facial profile will change from concave to a straight profile. Clockwise rotation of the maxillomandibular complex will enhance the profile change while counterclockwise rotation will limit the change. The surgical correction of Class II dentofacial deformities often requires surgery to both jaws, i.e. superior repositioning of the maxilla and advancement of the mandible. Counterclockwise rotation of the maxillomandibular complex will allow the surgeon to increase the advancement of the mandible and thereby enhance the correction. Counterclockwise rotation will limit the mandibular advancement. The convexity of the face can therefore be controlled by either clockwise or counterclockwise rotation of the maxillomandibular complex (Figure 31-8).

Another important aspect to consider is the selection of a point around which the MMC should be rotated as it will certainly affect the outcome. By varying the points around which the complex is rotated, various soft tissue effects can be achieved. For descriptive purposes, ANS, upper incisor tip (IT), Pogonion,

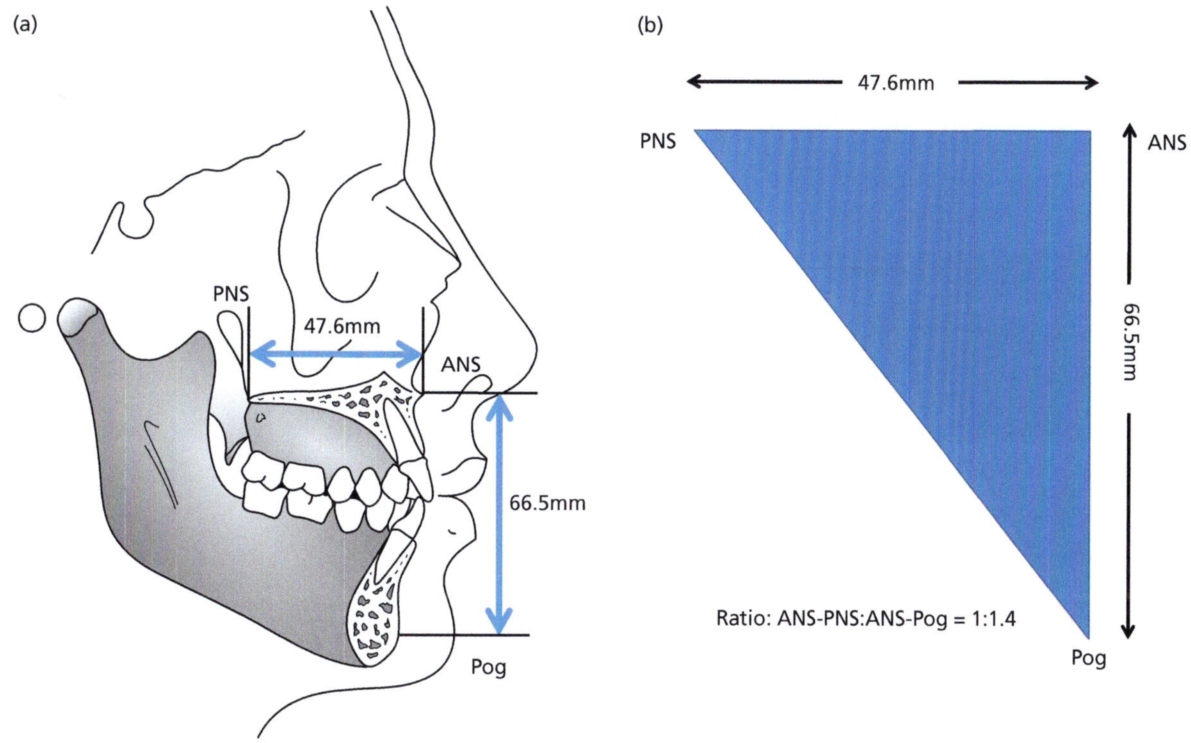

Fig. 31-8 **(a)** The average maxillary length (ANS to PNS) of 20 dry human skulls was 47.6 mm while the anterior facial height (ANS TO Pogonion) measured on average 66.5 mm. **(b)** If the vertical length of the of the MMC triangle is compared to the horizontal length of the MMC triangle, the ratio is: 66.5:47.6 = 1:1.4. The anterior facial height is 40% longer than the maxillary length.

PNS and the zygomatic buttress (BT) will be used as rotation points; however any anatomical point may be used and tested for the best aesthetic outcome (Figure 31-7). The selection of the rotation point and direction of rotation is primarily dictated by the aesthetic requirements of each case and the treatment plan can be designed and tested by a surgical cephalometric prediction tracing.

Surgical compromise for orthodontic compromise

Basic surgical orthodontic principles demand the early recognition of a skeletal component as aetiology of a malocclusion and it should be considered during treatment planning. Some mild to moderate skeletal discrepancies may be managed by orthodontic dental compensation or growth modification. However, conservative management of moderate to severe skeletal discrepancies and noticeable facial imbalance by dental compensation will have unacceptable aesthetic and functional outcomes and will often prove to have poor postoperative stability.

Early diagnosis of a dentoskeletal deformity allows the orthodontist and the surgeon to plan the appropriate dental decompensations and alignment of the teeth to achieve the best aesthetic and functional treatment results. The decision to follow a combined orthodontic/surgical route is however influenced by factors such as: the patient's preferences and main complaint, the orthodontist's experience and preferences, the orthodontist's previous experiences with orthognathic surgery, the availability of surgical skills and financial factors. Orthodontic treatment in some cases will be commenced with only orthodontic compensation as treatment plan. However, during treatment or at the end of orthodontic treatment it may be realized that a poor aesthetic result had been achieved. Dental decompensations, possible additional extractions and extended orthodontic treatment at this stage may not be acceptable to many patients. In these cases rotation of the maxillomandibular complex should be considered. The case demonstrated in Figure 31-10/Case 1a – Case 1 is an example of the above.

Orthodontic treatment considerations

The orthodontic preparation for cases planned for surgical rotation of the MMC is the same as for all orthognathic cases. However, the consequential change of the occlusal plane will result in a change in the inclinations of the incisor teeth (see Tables 31-1 to 31-7). In high occlusal plane angle cases a counterclockwise rotation of the MMC will result in a more acute occlusal plane angle and an increased upper incisor, and decreased lower incisor inclination after surgery. The opposite is true when the MMC is rotated in a clockwise direction (Figure 31-9). Although these changes are relatively small it is desirable to reconcile the expected change of the incisor teeth inclinations with the planned change in the occlusal plane angle.[9]

Rotation points and direction of rotation

Convex profiles require counterclockwise rotation while concave profiles require clockwise rotation. By changing the point around which the maxillomandibular complex will be rotated the aesthetic effect can be controlled. As in the treatment planning of all orthognathic surgery cases it is mandatory that the ideal vertical and anteroposterior relationship of the upper incisor and upper lip is established before the rotation of the MMC is planned.

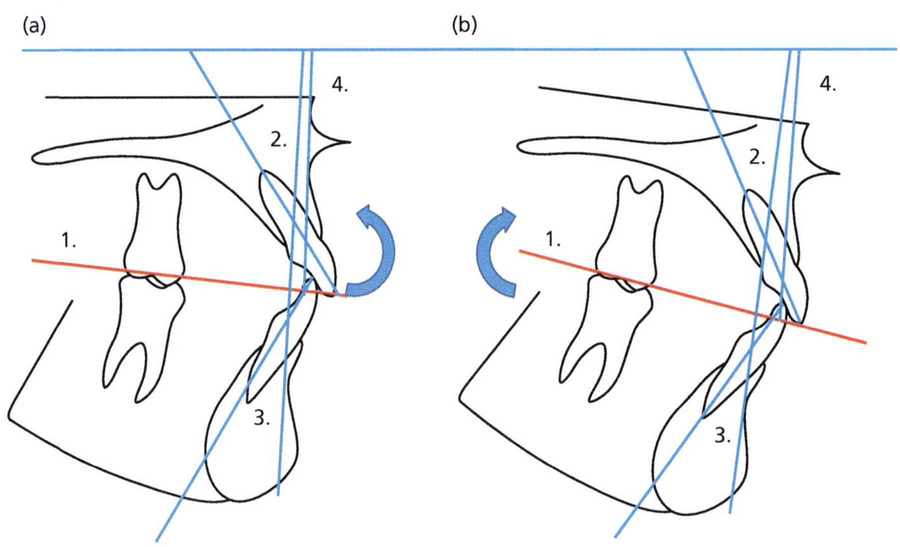

Fig. 31-9 **(a)** Counterclockwise rotation of the MMC will: (1) Decrease the occlusal plane angle; (2) Increase the upper incisor inclination; (3) decreased lower incisor inclination and (4) decrease the ANB angle. **(b)** Clockwise rotation of the MMC will: (1) increase the occlusal plane angle; (2) decrease the upper incisor inclination; (3) increase the lower incisor inclination and (4) increase the ANB angle.

Table 31-1 Clockwise rotation of the maxillomandibular complex with rotation point at ANS (Figure 31-10/Case 1a)

Dental changes	
Occlusal plane angle	Increase
Upper incisor angle	Slight decrease
Maxillary incisor tip	No change
Skeletal changes	
Posterior maxillary height	Decrease
Maxilla at ANS	Advance
Pog	Set back
Soft tissue changes	
Subnasale	Advance
Facial convexity (facial contour angle)	Increase
Upper lip support	No change
Mandibular prominence	Increase
Paranasal fullness	Increase
Nasolabial angle	Increase
Anterior facial height	No change
Chin–throat length	Decrease

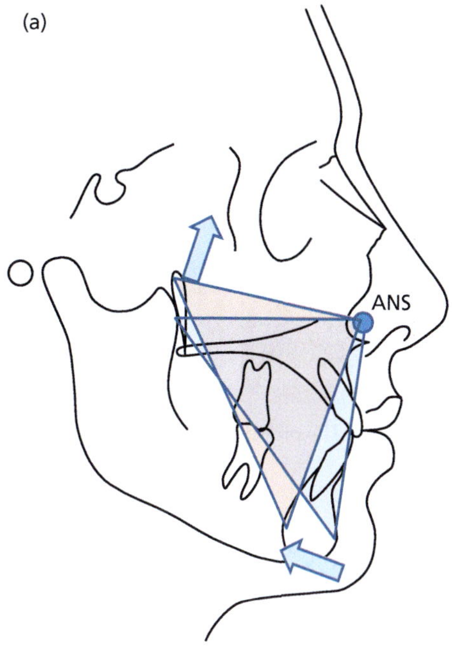

Fig. 31-10/**CASE 1a:** Clockwise rotation of the MMC with the rotation point at ANS. By selecting a rotation point superiorly on the vertical leg of the MMC triangle the mandibular set-back will be enhanced. The expected dental, skeletal and soft tissue changes are summarized in Table 31-1.

Clockwise rotation of the maxillomandibular complex

Clockwise rotation of the MMC is usually, but not exclusively, indicated for the treatment of patients with concave profiles and low mandibular and occlusal plane angles. Cases 1, 2 and 3 demonstrate clockwise rotation of the MMC and the variation of aesthetic effects that can be achieved by changing the point of rotation.

Centre of rotation at ANS

The posterior maxilla is superiorly repositioned allowing the maxilla to rotate clockwise around ANS. As a consequence, the mandible will follow this rotation (by means of a bilateral sagittal split osteotomy). The expected hard and soft tissue changes are summarized in Table 31-1 and illustrated in Figure 31-10/Case 1a. **Case 1** has a skeletal Class III relationship however the occlusion is orthodontically compromised for the relative skeletal discrepancy. The patient also suffers from vertical maxillary excess requiring surgical superior repositioning of the maxilla which will further increase the mandibular prominence due to autorotation. By increased superior repositioning of the posterior maxilla the MMC will rotate clockwise reducing the prominence of the lower jaw. To enhance the anteroposterior reduction of the mandible ANS is used as rotation point (Figure 31-10/Case 1a).

CASE 1

This patient showed a strong tendency to a Class III skeletal and dental relationship and a prominent lower jaw when she consulted the orthodontist at age

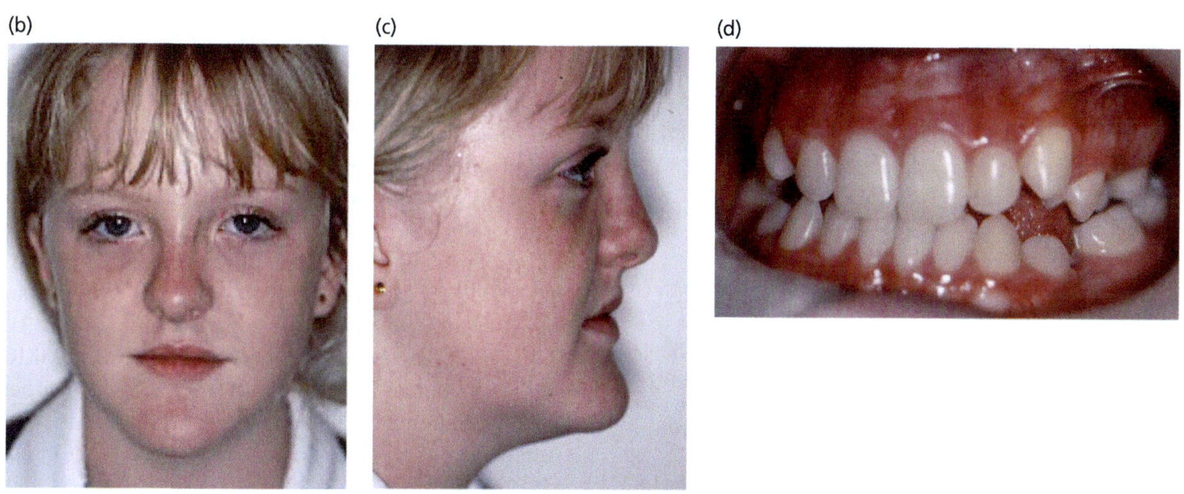

Fig. 31-10/**CASE 1:** The **(b)** frontal view, **(c)** profile view, and **(d)** occlusion at age 12 years.

(e) (f) (g) (h)

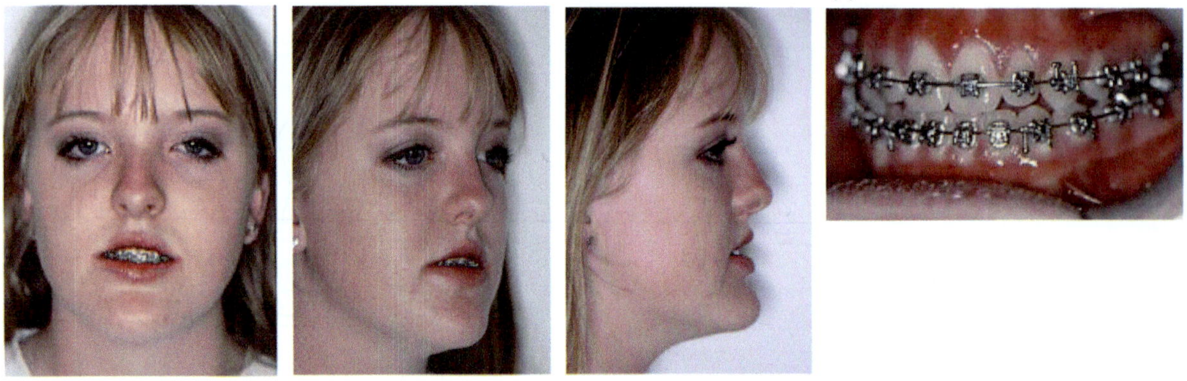

Fig. 31-10/**CASE 1:** The pre-surgical **(e)** frontal view, **(f)** three-quarter view, **(g)** profile view, and **(h)** occlusion.

(i)

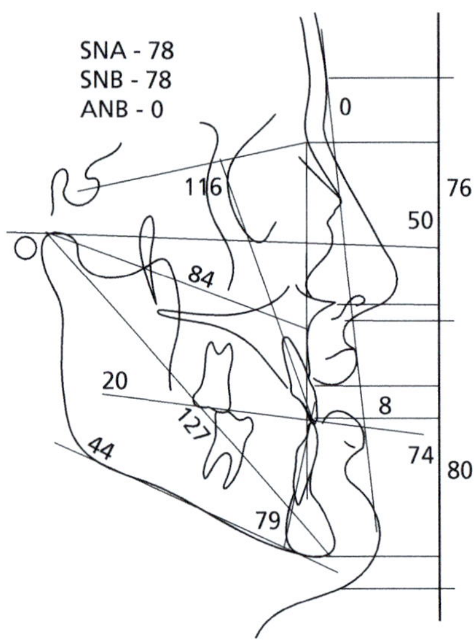

Fig. 31-10/**CASE 1i:** The cephalometric analysis of **CASE 1.**

(j)

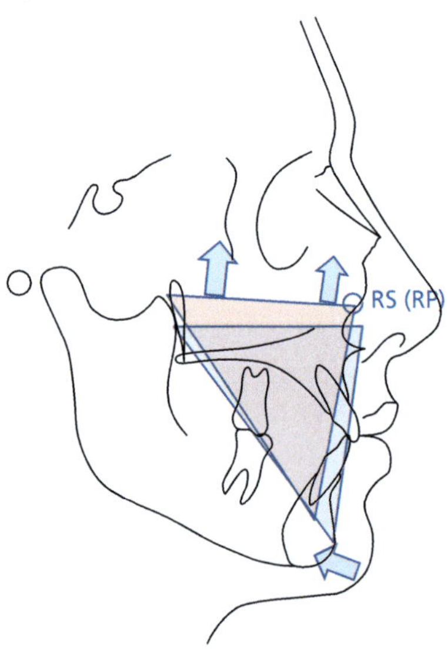

Fig. 31-10/**CASE 1j:** The surgical aesthetic objectives are limited by the mild pre-surgical Class III occlusion. The MMC triangle test however reveals the possibility to improve the severe convexity of the face by clockwise rotation of the MMC after correction of the vertical maxillary excess by superior repositioning the maxilla. ANS is selected as rotation point to maximize mandibular set-back.

(k)

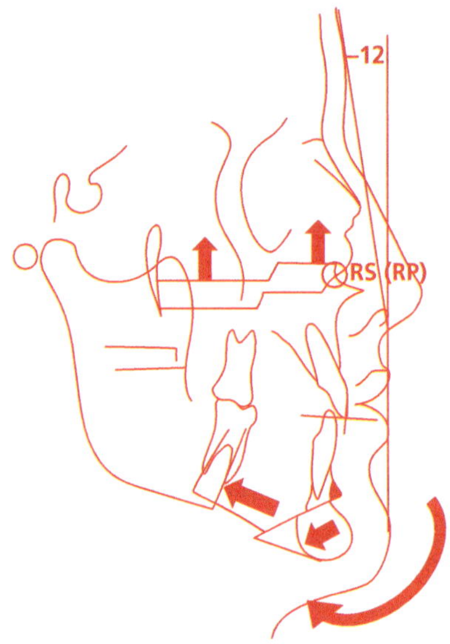

Fig. 31-10/**CASE 1k:** The final surgical visual treatment objective indicates the required surgical movements and the expected soft tissue outcome. The anterior maxilla should be superiorly repositioned to correct the upper incisor lip relationship. The posterior maxilla should however be repositioned more than anterior. The rotation point at surgery will be at ANS. The mandible will follow the rotation of the maxilla by setting it back. A reduction genioplasty is indicated to achieve good chin contour.

12 years (Figure 31-10/Case 1b–d). Orthodontic treatment commenced at age 14 years and the dentition was slightly compromised for the skeletal discrepancy (Figure 31-10/Case 1e–h). The patient was concerned about her prominent chin and the fact that she could not get her lips together without force. Her cephalometric analysis confirmed the following clinical problem list: (1) A Class III malocclusion; (2) vertical maxillary excess; (3) macrogenia; (4) mandibular anteroposterior excess; (5) a concave profile (Figure 31-10/Case 1i). The principle of the rotation of the MMC triangle in a clockwise direction after the ideal upper incisor relationship had been achieved is demonstrated. The ANS is used as rotation point to maximize the mandibular setback (Figure 31-10/Case 1j). The surgical prediction tracing indicate superior

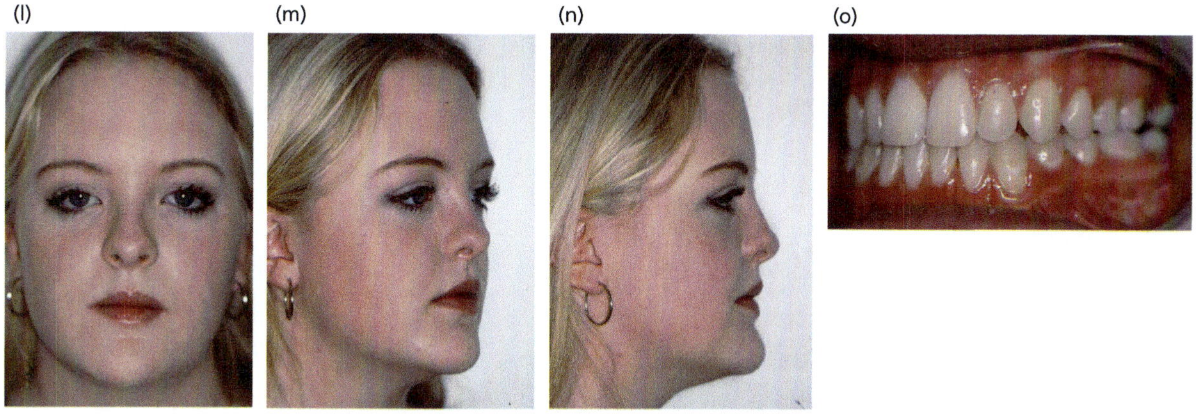

Fig. 31-10/**CASE 1:** The post-surgical **(l)** frontal view; **(m)** three-quarter view; **(n)** profile view; and Occlusion (o).

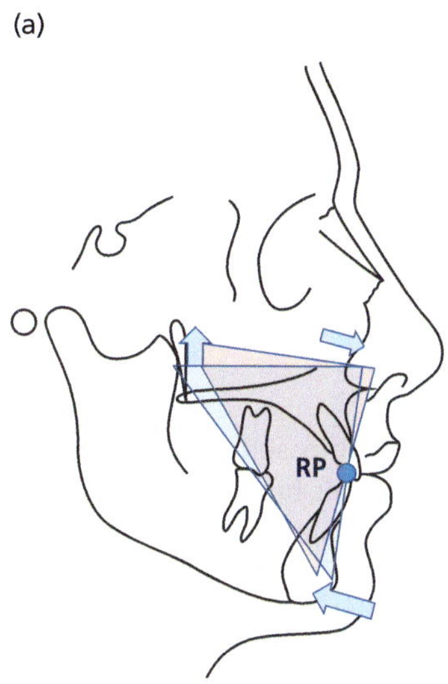

Fig. 31-10/**CASE 2a:** Clockwise rotation of the MMC with the rotation point at the incisor tip (IT). This surgical design allows the surgeon to enhance maxillary advancement and mandibular set-back. The dental, skeletal and soft tissue changes are summarized in Table 31-2b.

repositioning of the maxilla (more posterior than anterior), mandibular setback and reduction genioplasty (Figure 31-10/Case 1k). Surgery was performed at age 17 years and an improved soft tissue and occlusal result was achieved (Figure 31-10/Case1 l–o).

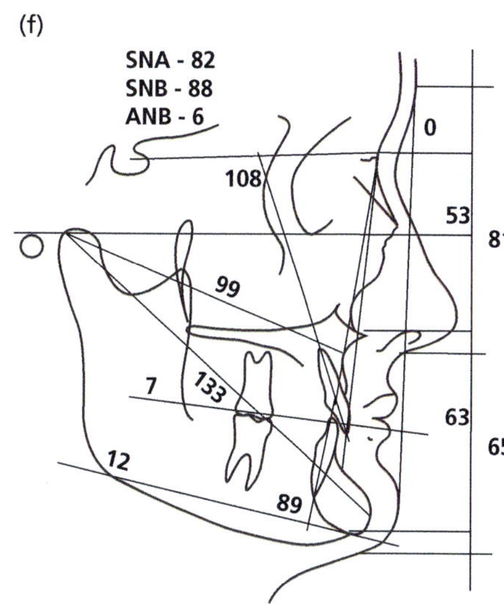

Fig. 31-10/**CASE 2f:** The pre-treatment cephalometric analysis.

CASE 2

A 32-year-old patient consulted her orthodontist with the main complaint of an uncomfortable bite and that her lower jaw appeared too strong. Her hard and soft tissue problem list included the following: (1) A Class II deep bite malocclusion; (2) low occlusal and mandibular plane angles with a dolicoprosopic facial pattern; (3) prominent chin; (4) a concave

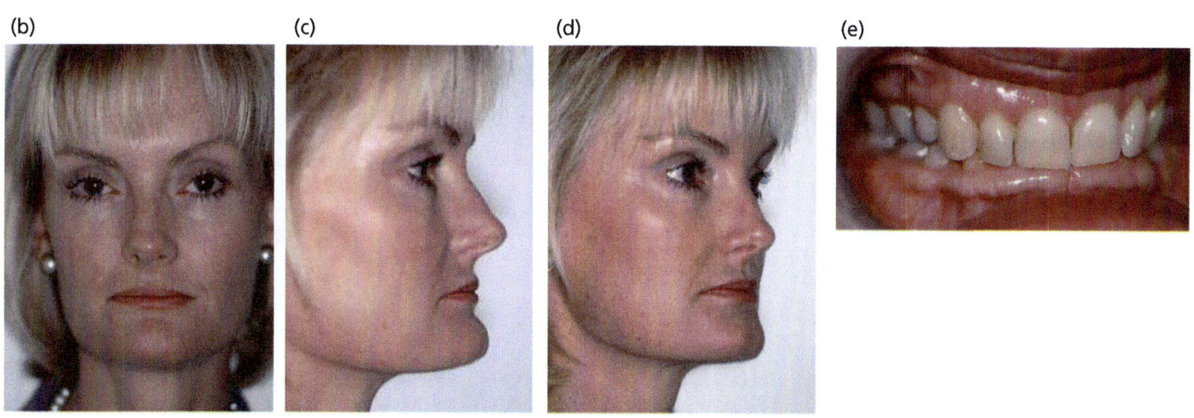

Fig. 31-10/**CASE 2:** The pre-treatment **(b)** frontal view; **(c)** profile view; **(d)** 3/4 view; and **(e)** occlusion. The patient has a Class II deep bite malocclusion however a concave profile and very prominent chin and square mandible.

(g)

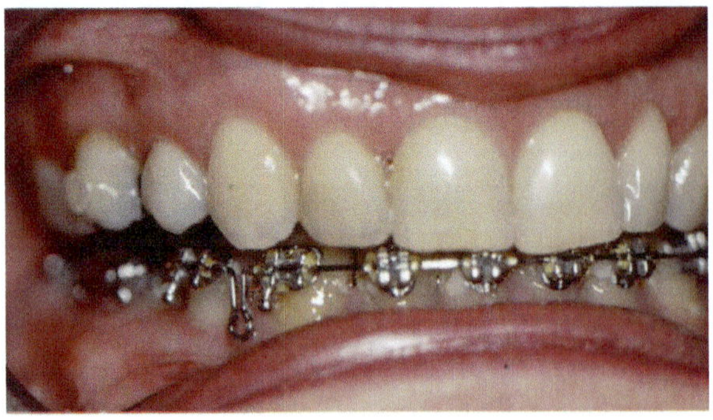

Fig. 31-10/**CASE 2g:** The pre-surgical occlusion.

(i)

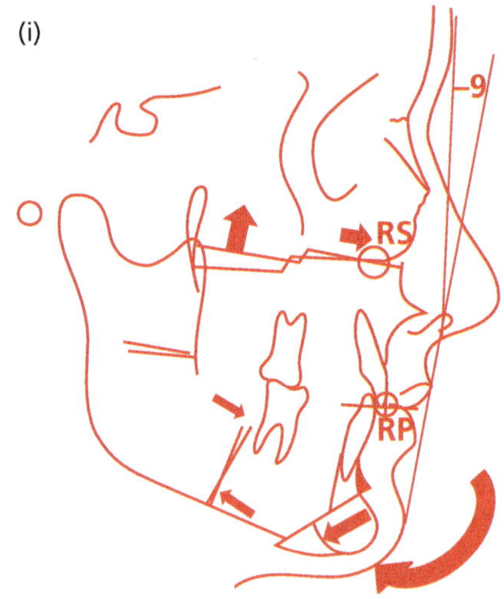

Fig. 31-10/**CASE 2i:** The final surgical visual treatment objective indicate the planned surgery and expected soft tissue outcome. The surgery would involve superior repositioning of the posterior maxilla and advancement of the maxilla. The rotation point at surgery would be 7 mm posterior of the anterior end of the Le Fort I osteotomy line. This rotation will be followed by the mandible with set-back. The chin deformity will be corrected by means of a reduction genioplasty taking care not to obliterate the labiomental fold.

(h)

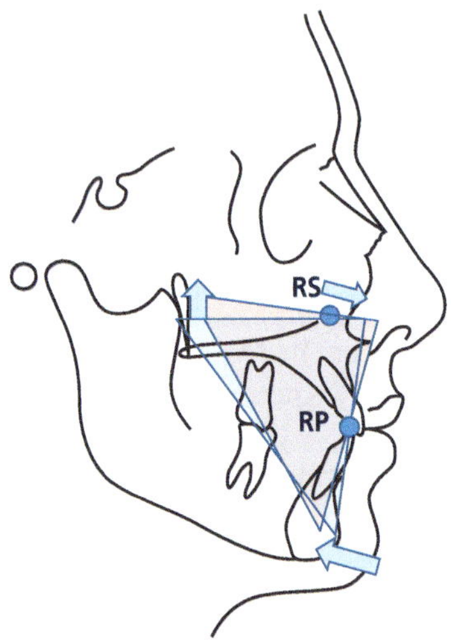

Fig. 31-10/**CASE 2h:** The MMC triangle test indicate that by rotating the MMC clockwise with rotation point (RP) at the incisor tip (IT) the surgeon would be able to advance the maxilla and set the mandible back. The rotation point at surgery will be at the anterior maxilla (RS). The prominent chin can be corrected by means of a reduction genioplasty.

profile and a Class II deep bite malocclusion (Figure 31-10/Case 2b–e). The lateral cephalometric analysis confirms the clinical assessment (Figure 31-10/Case 2f). The aesthetic objectives of the case required maxillary advancement combined with mandibular and chin setback. These surgical movements were however limited by the Class II deep bite malocclusion occlusion (Figure 31-10/Case 2g). The concept of the MMC triangles indicate the possibility of correcting soft and hard tissue problems by clockwise rotation of the MMC and selecting incisor tip as rotation point (Figure 31-10/Case 2h). The surgical visual treatment objective indicates that an acceptable soft tissue and occlusal result could be achieved by advancement of the maxilla and at the same time superior repositioning the posterior maxilla. This rotation will be followed by the mandible by means of a bilateral sagittal split osteotomy while the chin prominence could be managed by a reduction genioplasty (Figure 31-10/Case 2i). The post-treatment soft tissue and occlusal results are demonstrated in Figure 31-10/Case 2 j–m.

(j) (k) (l) (m)

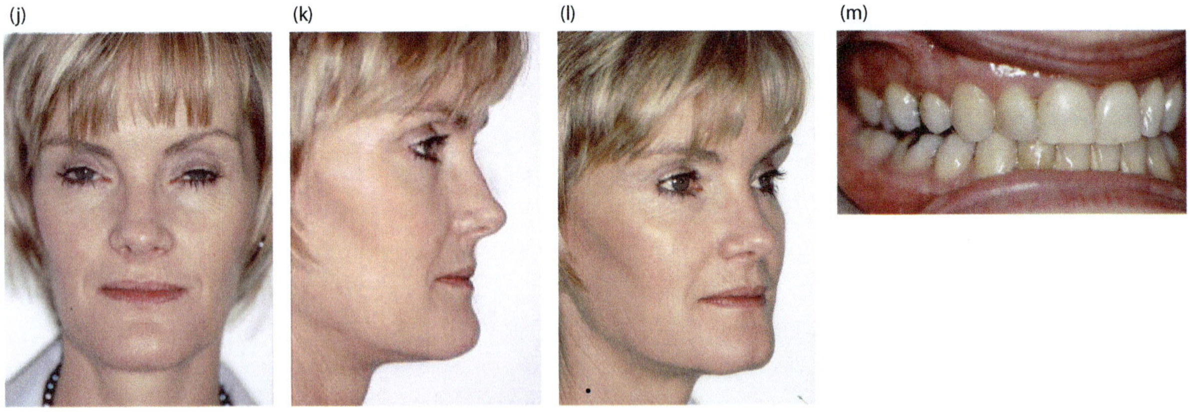

Fig. 31-10/**CASE 2:** The post-treatment **(j)** frontal view; **(k)** three-quarter view; **(l)** profile view; and **(m)** occlusion.

Table 31-2 Clockwise rotation of the maxillomandibular complex with rotation point at the incisor tip (Figure 31-10/Case 2a)

Dental changes	
Occlusal plane angle	Increase
Maxillary incisor tip	No change
Upper incisor inclination	Decrease
Skeletal changes	
Pogonion position	Set back
Maxilla at ANS	Advance
Posterior maxillary height	Decrease
Soft tissue changes	
Subnasale	Advance
Upper lip support	No increase
Facial convexity (facial contour angle)	Increase
Mandibular prominence	Decrease
Paranasal fullness	Increase
Nasolabial angle	Increase
Anterior facial height	No change
Chin–throat length	Decrease

Centre of rotation at the upper incisor tip

By moving the rotation point inferiorly to the maxillary incisor tip the clockwise rotation will result in maxillary advancement and mandibular setback. The expected hard and soft tissue changes are summarized in Table 31-2 and illustrated in Figure 31-10/Case 2. The dolicoprosopic facial pattern with prominent nose and chin, and poor lip support in **Case 2** required maxillary advancement and mandibular setback. The tendency to a Class II occlusion and deep bite incisor relationship, low occlusal plane and low mandibular plane inclination limited surgical correction. Clockwise rotation of the MMC with rotation point at incisor tip enabled the surgeon to achieve an improved aesthetic result (Figure 31-10/Case 2). **Case 3** had vertical maxillary excess requiring superior repositioning if the maxilla. The autorotation of the mandible following superior repositioning of the maxilla would however increase the mandibular prominence with a strong tendency to a concave profile. By rotating the MMC clockwise following superior repositioning of the maxilla with rotation point 8 mm above the incisor tip a more convex profile is achieved. This demonstrates the principle of first correcting the upper incisor lip relationship by superior repositioning of the maxilla, before rotating the MMC (Figure 31-10/Case 3).

CASE 3

A 17-year-old female patient started her orthodontic treatment at age 15 years. The four first bicuspids were removed and fixed orthodontic appliance placed. Orthognathic surgery was not contemplated at this stage. At the final stage of orthodontic treatment the patient was not happy regarding her appearance and complained about her gummy smile. The patient was referred for a surgical consultation. She had a Class I occlusion; however her diagnosis consisted of the following: (1) a tendency to bimaxillary dental protrusion; (2) vertical maxillary excess; (3) a low occlusal plane angle; (4) an increased lower facial height; (5) an increased interlabial gap; (6) a short upper lip; and (7) a straight to concave profile (Figure 31-10/Case 3a–e). Conventional surgical treatment planning would

(e)

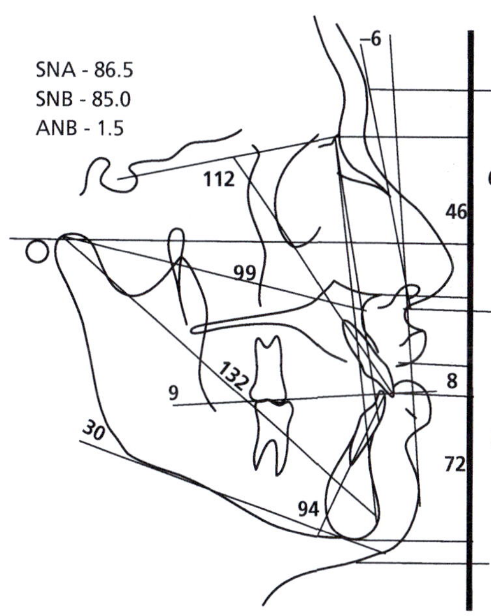

Fig. 31-10/CASE 3e: The pre-surgical cephalometric analysis.

(a) (b) (c) (d)

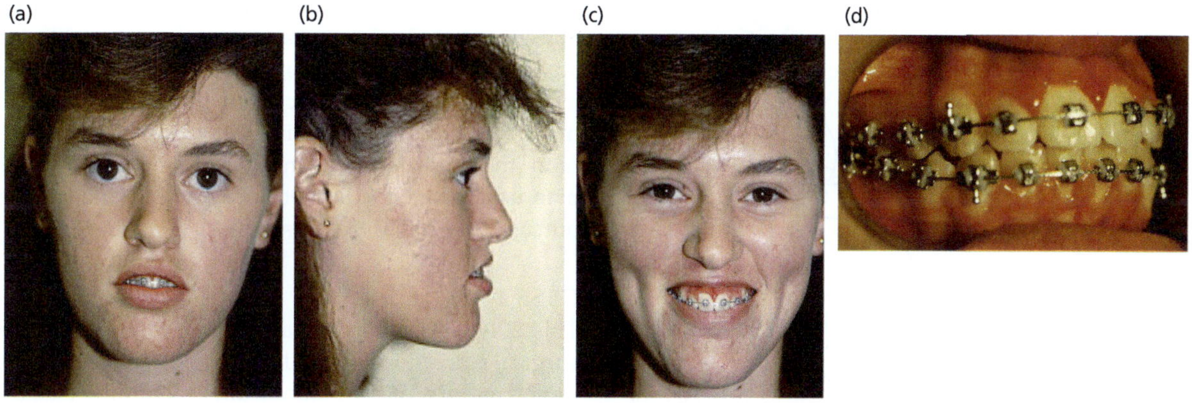

Fig. 31-10/**CASE 3:** Pre-surgical **(a)** frontal view; **(b)** profile view; **(c)** gummy smile; and **(d)** occlusion.

(f)

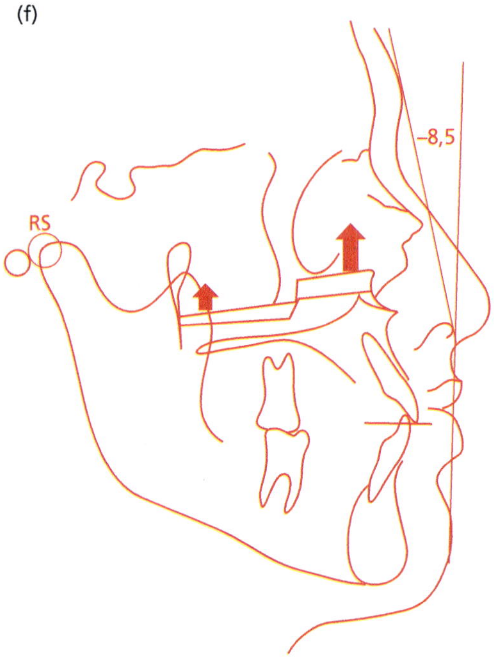

Fig. 31-10/**CASE 3f:** The conventional surgical treatment objective with superior repositioning of the maxilla and autorotation of the mandible (rotation point just posterior to the condyle) indicate a worsening of the aesthetics with increased mandibular prominence.

(h)

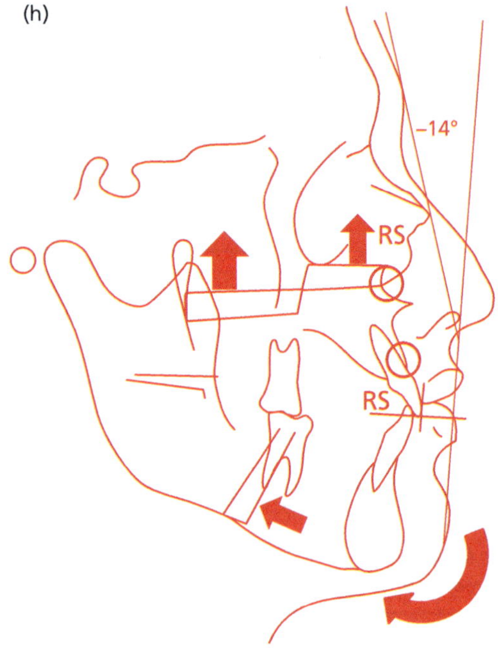

Fig. 31-10/**CASE 3h:** The final surgical treatment objective indicates the planned surgical correction and expected soft tissue outcome. The maxilla will be superiorly repositioned, more at the posterior than the anterior. The mandible will follow this rotation and will be set back. The rotation point at surgery will be at the anterior and of the Le Fort I osteotomy line **(RS)**.

require superior repositioning of the maxilla. However autorotation of the mandible (superior and forward with rotation at the condyle) will further increase the concavity of the face (Figure 31-10/Case 3f). Clockwise rotation of the MMC following superior

(g)

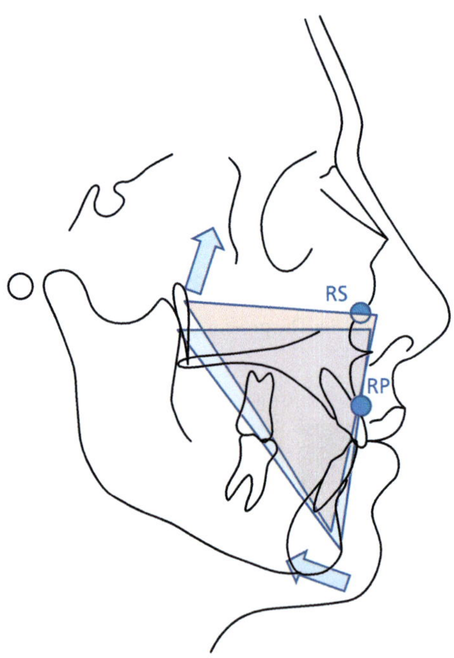

Fig. 31-10/**CASE 3g:** The MMC triangle test indicate that clockwise rotation of the MMC after superior repositioning of the maxilla would allow the surgeon to set the mandible back and improve the facial convexity. To enhance the amount of mandibular set-back a point 8 mm superior to the upper incisor is used as rotation point **(RP)**.

repositioning of the maxilla was investigated (Figure 31-10/Case 3g). The cephalometric surgical visual tracing indicated that an acceptable facial contour could be achieved by selecting a rotation point 8mm superior of the upper incisor tooth (Figure 31-10/Case 3h). The post treatment soft tissue and occlusion is demonstrated in Figure 31-10/Case 3i–l.

Centre of rotation at Pogonion

By using Pogonion as rotation point and rotating the maxillomandibular complex clockwise the maxilla, upper lip and lower incisors will be rotated forward while the chin is maintained in position. The expected hard and soft tissue changes are summarized in Table 31-3 and illustrated in Figure 31-10/Case 4. **Case 4** had a Class III skeletal relationship however a Class II dental relationship. The aesthetic treatment objectives required maxillary as well as mandibular advancement. Clockwise rotation of the MMC will facilitate the above surgical correction however by moving the rotation point inferior to just above Pogonion the maxillary advancement is enhanced and mandibular setback limited, improving the aesthetic outcome (Figure 31-10/Case 2).

CASE 4

This 20-year-old female patient was referred for the surgical correction of her Class II malocclusion following 12 months of orthodontic alignment of her teeth. The patient's main complaint was her prominent chin

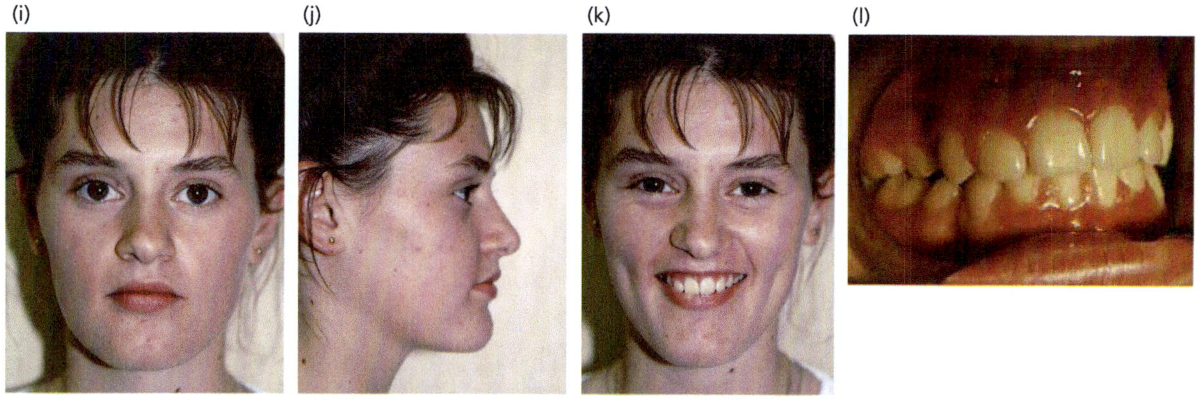

Fig. 31-10/CASE 3: The post-treatment frontal view (i), profile view (j), smile (k), and occlusion (l).

Table 31-3 Clockwise rotation of the maxillomandibular complex with rotation at Pogonion (Figure 31-10/Case 3)

Dental changes	
Occlusal plane	Increase
Upper incisor tip	Advance
Upper incisor inclination	Decrease
Skeletal changes	
Pogonion position	No change
Maxilla at ANS	Advance
Posterior maxillary height	Decrease
Soft tissue changes	
Subnasale	Advance
Upper lip support	Increase
Facial convexity (facial contour angle)	Increase
Mandibular prominence	No change
Paranasal fullness	Increase
Nasolabial angle	Increase
Anterior facial height	No change
Chin–throat length	Decrease

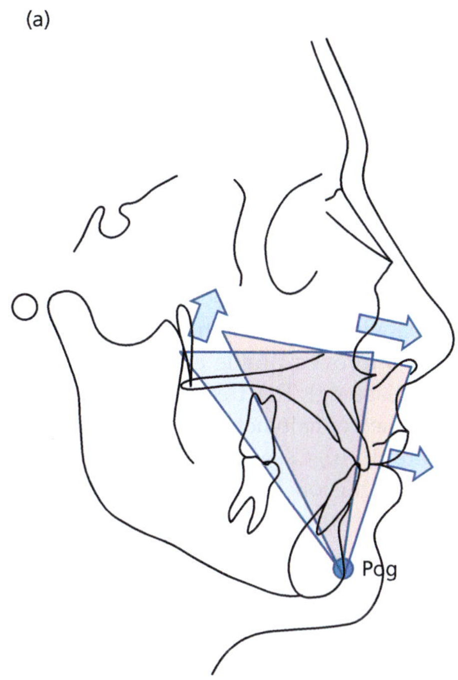

Fig. 31-10/CASE 4a: Clockwise rotation of the MMC with the rotation point at Pogonion (Pog). The dental, skeletal and soft tissue changes are summarized in Table 31-3.

and nose. Her clinical and cephalometric evaluation revealed the following: (1) a Class II malocclusion; (2) low occlusal and mandibular plane angles; (3) a straight to concave profile; (4) a prominent chin; (5) deficient lip support; and (6) a prominent nose (relative) (Figure 31-10/Case 4a–f). Although the surgical

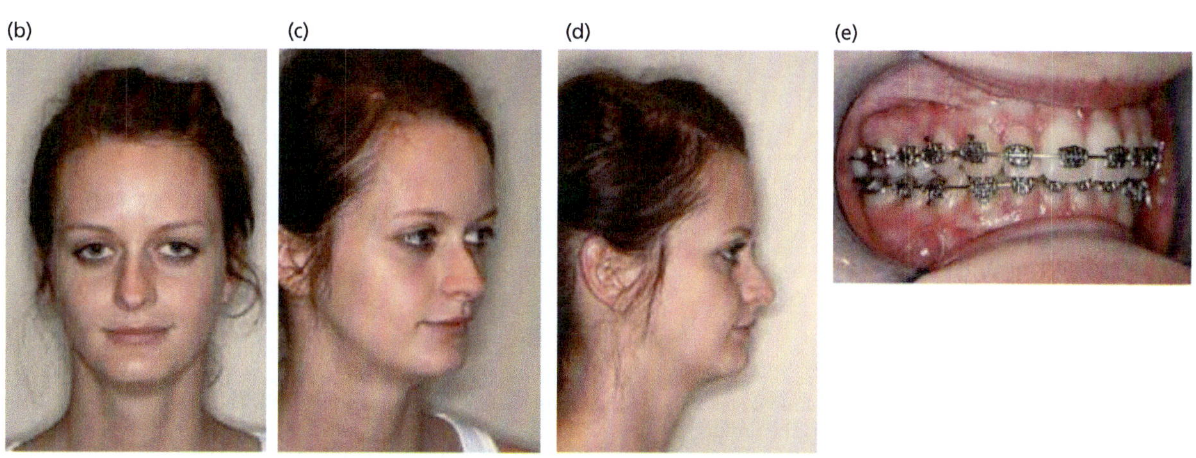

Fig. 31-10/CASE 4: The pre-surgical frontal view (b); three quarter view (c); profile view (d); and occlusion (e).

(f)

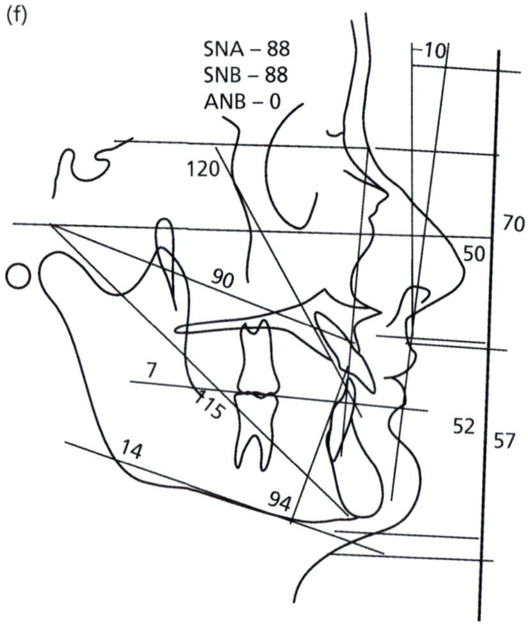

Fig. 31-10/CASE 4f: The cephalometric analysis of CASE 4.

(h)

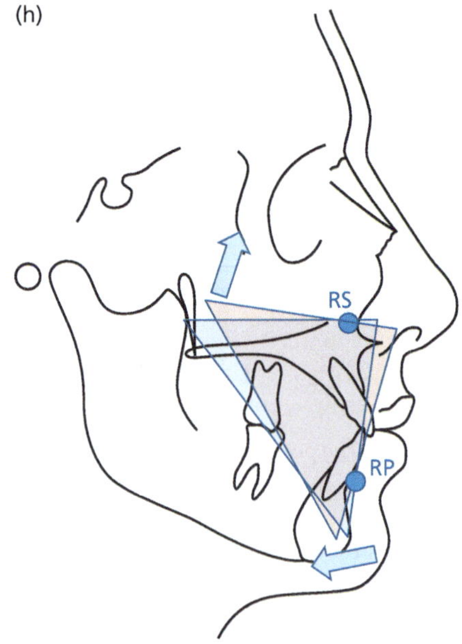

Fig. 31-10/CASE 4h: The MMC triangle test indicates an improved aesthetic result when the MMC triangle is rotated clockwise with rotation point at B-point **(RP)**. This rotation allows the maxilla to be advanced and the chin prominence is corrected by slight mandibular set-back.

advancement of her mandible would have corrected her malocclusion it would not have improved her profile. By clockwise rotation of the MMC with rotation at B-point an improved profile could be achieved (Figure 31-10/Case 4g) The treatment design was confirmed by the cephalometric visual treatment objective (Figure 31-10/Case 4h).The post treatment soft tissue and occlusion is demonstrated in Figure 31-10/Case 4i.

Centre of rotation at points posterior to ANS (i.e. zygomatic buttress or PNS)

By moving the rotation point to posterior of ANS a vertical component is introduced to the changes. Clockwise rotation of the MMC around any point posterior of ANS will increase the anterior facial height and increase the upper incisor exposure under the upper

(g)

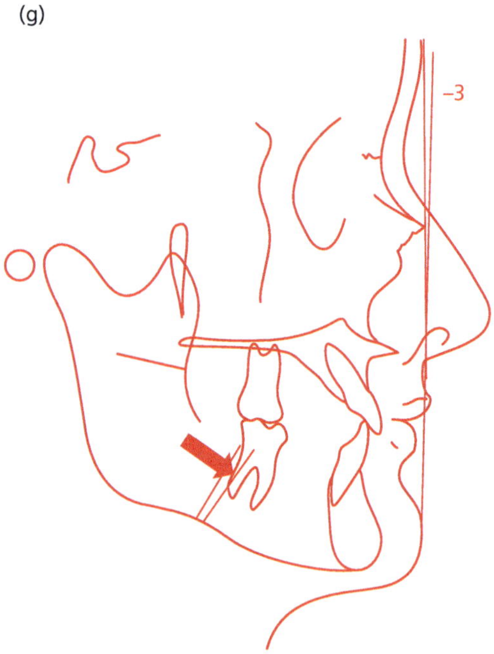

Fig. 31-10/CASE 4g: The surgical visual treatment objective according to conventional treatment design. The profile appears straight (facial contour angle –3 degrees) and the mandible too prominent.

(i)

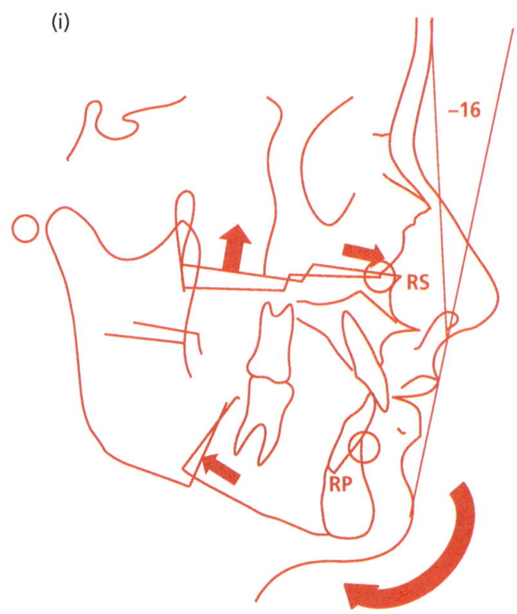

Fig. 31-10/CASE 4i: The final surgical treatment objective indicates the rotation point at surgery to be at the anterior end of the Le Fort I osteotomy line **(RS)**. The surgical plan indicates the posterior maxilla should be superiorly repositioned while the maxilla as a whole is advanced. The mandible will follow this movement by setting it back.

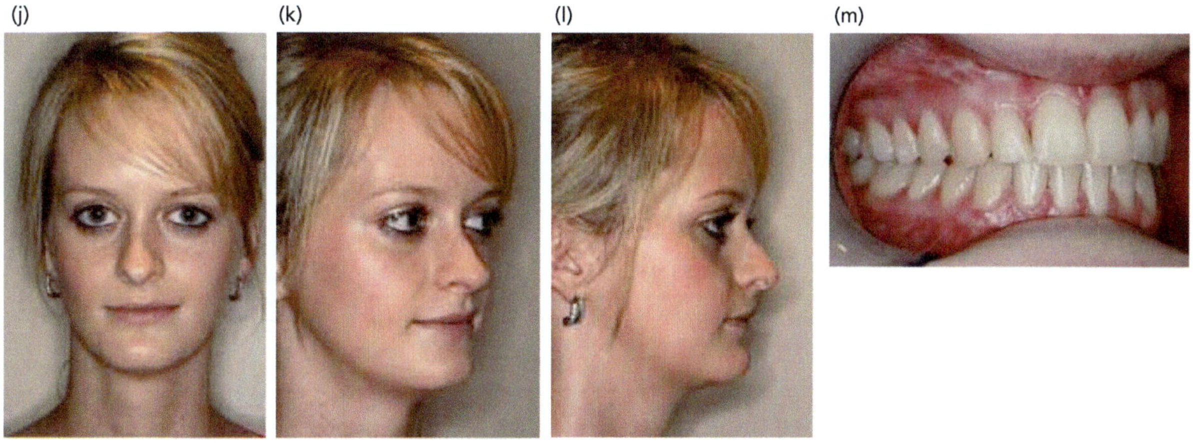

Fig. 31-10/**CASE 4:** The post-treatment **(j)** frontal view; **(k)** three-quarter view; **(l)** profile view; and **(m)** occlusion.

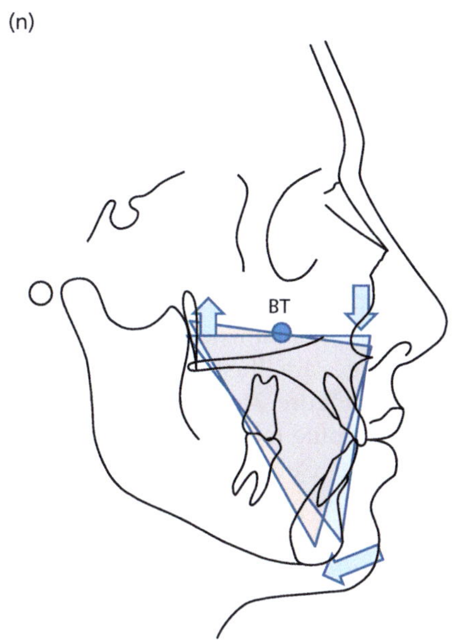

Fig. 31-10/**CASE 4n:** Clockwise rotation of the MMC with the rotation point at the zygomatic buttress (BT). The dental, skeletal and soft tissue changes are summarized in Table 31-4.

lip. The expected hard and soft tissue changes are summarized in Table 31-4 and illustrated in Figure 31-10/Case 4n.

Counterclockwise rotation of the maxillomandibular complex

Counterclockwise rotation of the MMC is usually but not exclusively indicated for the correction of patients with severe convex profiles and high mandibular and occlusal lane angles.

Centre of rotation at ANS

Counterclockwise rotation of the MMC around ANS will require downgrafting of the posterior maxilla. This rotation of the maxilla followed by the mandible (by means of a bilateral sagittal split osteotomy) will enhance the advancement of the mandible. The expected hard and soft tissue changes are summarized in Table 31-5 and illustrated in Figure 31-11/Case 5a.

Table 31-4 Clockwise rotation of the maxillomandibular complex with rotation point posterior to ANS (Zygomatic buttress to PNS) (Figure 31-10/Case 4a)

Dental changes	
Occlusal plane angle	Increase
Maxillary incisor tip	Inferior + slight retraction
Upper incisor inclination	Decrease
Skeletal changes	
Pogonion position	Inferior + slight set-back
Maxilla at ANS	Inferior + slight set-back
Mandibular plane angle	Increase
Posterior maxillary height (RP at Pog)	Decrease
Soft tissue changes	
Subnasale	No change
Upper lip support	Slightly decreased
Facial convexity (facial contour angle)	Increase
Mandibular prominence	Decrease
Paranasal fullness	No change
Nasolabial angle	Increase
Anterior facial height	Increase
Chin–throat length	Decrease

Table 31-5 Counterclockwise rotation of the maxillomandibular complex with rotation at ANS point (Figure 31-11/Case 5a)

Dental changes	
Occlusal plane angle	Decrease
Maxillary incisor tip	Advance
Upper incisor inclination	Increase
Skeletal changes	
Pogonion position	Advance
Maxilla at ANS	No change
Mandibular plane angle	Decrease
Posterior maxillary height	Increase
Soft tissue changes	
Subnasale	No change
Upper lip support	Increase
Facial convexity (facial contour angle)	Decrease
Mandibular prominence	Increase
Paranasal fullness	No change
Nasolabial angle	Decrease
Anterior facial height	No change
Chin-throat length	Increase

(a)

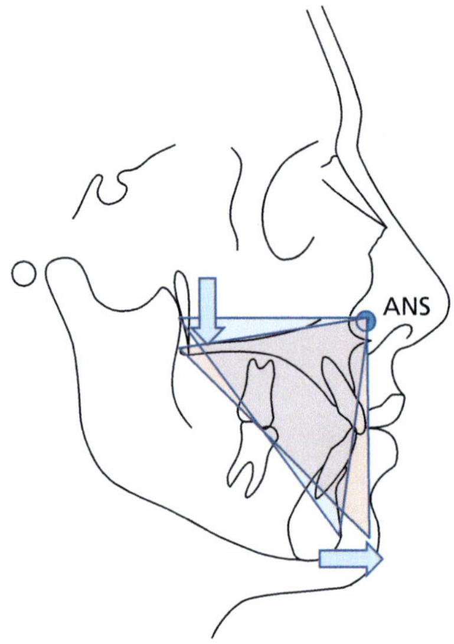

Fig. 31-11/**CASE 5a:** Counterclockwise rotation of the MMC with the rotation point at ANS. This will require down grafting of the posterior maxilla. The dental, skeletal and soft tissue changes are summarized in Table 31-5.

(b)

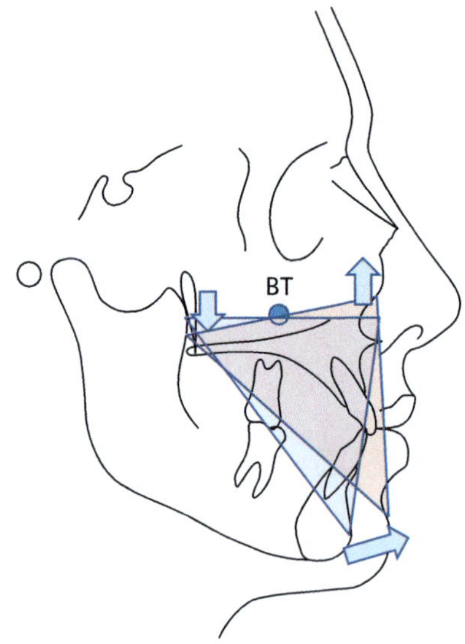

Fig. 31-11/**CASE 5b:** Counterclockwise rotation of the MMC with the rotation point at the Zygomatic buttress (BT). The anterior maxilla is superiorly repositioned while the posterior maxilla is down grafted. The dental, skeletal and soft tissue changes are summarized in Table 31-6.

Centre of rotation at the zygomatic buttress

With the rotation point posterior to ANS the posterior maxilla will be inferiorly repositioned while the anterior maxilla and upper incisor will move superiorly. The expected hard and soft tissue changes are illustrated and summarized in Table 31-6 and Figure 31-11/Case 5b.

Centre of rotation at the PNS

This point of rotation is usually selected to maximize mandibular advancement. The anterior maxilla is superiorly repositioned while the height of the posterior maxilla is maintained. The expected hard and soft tissue changes are illustrated and summarized in Table 31-7 and Figure 31-11/Case 5c. **Case 5** had a severe convex profile requiring substantial mandibular advancement. Counterclockwise rotation of the MMC with rotation point at PNS is used to maximize mandibular advancement (Figure 31-11/Case 5c).

CASE 5

In preparation for surgery, the orthodontic treatment of this 19-year-old male patients consisted of

Table 31-6 Counterclockwise rotation of the maxillomandibular complex with rotation point at Zygomatic buttress point (Figure 31-11/Case 5b)

Dental changes	
Occlusal plane angle	Decrease
Maxillary incisor tip	Advance + superior
Upper incisor inclination	Increased
Skeletal changes	
Pogonion position	Advance + superior
Maxilla at ANS	Superior
Mandibular plane angle	Decrease
Posterior maxillary height	Increase
Soft tissue changes	
Subnasale	Advance
Upper lip support	Increase
Facial convexity (facial contour angle)	Decrease
Mandibular prominence	Increase
Paranasal fullness	Increase
Nasolabial angle	Decrease
Anterior facial height	Decrease
Chin–throat length	Increase

Table 31-7 Counterclockwise rotation of the maxillomandibular complex with rotation point at PNS (Figure 31-11/Case 5c)

Dental changes	
Occlusal plane angle	Decrease
Maxillary incisor tip	Advance + superior
Maxillary incisor inclination	Increase
Skeletal changes	
Pogonion position	Advance + superior
Maxilla at ANS	Superior
Mandibular plane angle	Decrease
Posterior mandibular height	No change
Soft tissue changes	
Subnasale	Advance
Upper lip support	Increase
Facial convexity	Decrease
Mandibular prominence	Increase
Paranasal fullness	Increase
Nasolabial angle	Decrease
Anterior facial height	Decrease
Chin–throat length	Increase

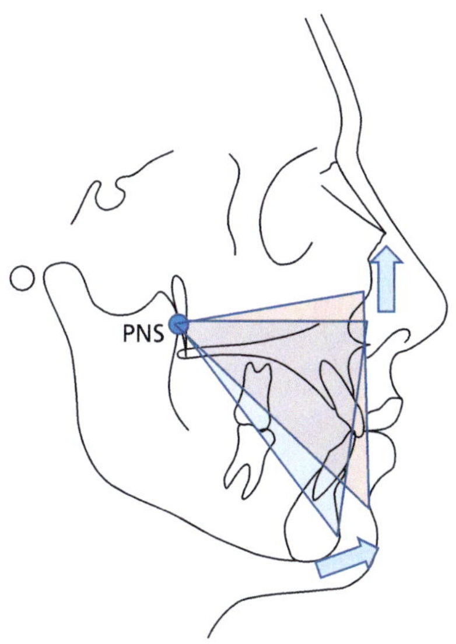

Fig. 31-11/CASE 5c: Counterclockwise rotation of the MMC with the rotation point at the posterior nasal spine (PNS). This surgical design will maximize the advancement of the mandible. The dental, skeletal and soft tissue changes are summarized in Table 31-7.

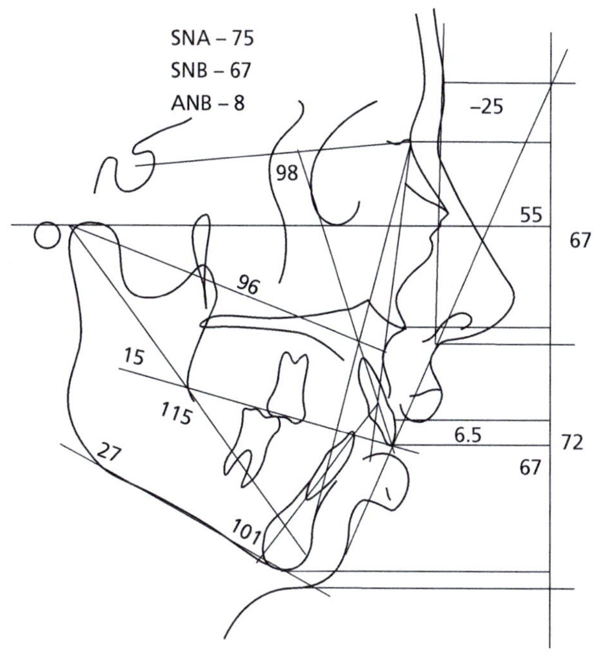

Fig. 31-11/CASE 5g: The cephalometric analysis.

extraction of lower first premolars, level and alignment of both dental arches and establishment of arch compatibility between the dental arches. His diagnosis before surgery consisted of the following: (1) a severe Class II malocclusion with a tendency to an anterior open bite; (2) a severe convex profile; (3) vertical maxillary excess; (4) microgenia; and (5) maxillary and mandibular anteroposterior deficiency (Figures 31-11/Case 5a–c). The cephalometric analysis confirmed the clinical hard and soft tissue assessment (Figure 31-11/Case 5d). The surgical visual treatment objective according to conventional treatment principles revealed that the profile would still be too convex (facial contour angle –18 degrees) (Figure 31-11/Case 5e). The principle of counterclockwise rotation with rotation point distal to the zygomatic buttress is demonstrated in Figure 31-11/Case 5f and the expected results are summarized in Tables 31-6 and 31-7. Testing the treatment outcome by rotating the MMC triangle in a counterclockwise direction revealed that by selecting a rotation point 10 mm anterior to PNS it would allow the surgeon to advance the mandible substantially more than with conventional treatment planning (facial contour angle –11 degrees) (Figure 31-11/Case 5g). The final surgical treatment plan consisted of superior repositioning of the maxilla with the surgical rotation point (RS) 10 mm anterior to PNS, advancement of the mandible and advancement of the chin. The treatment outcome is demonstrated in Figure 31-11/Case 5h–j.

(d)

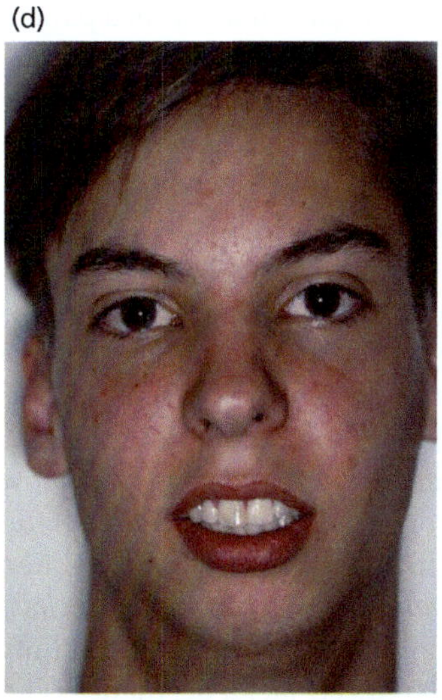

(e)

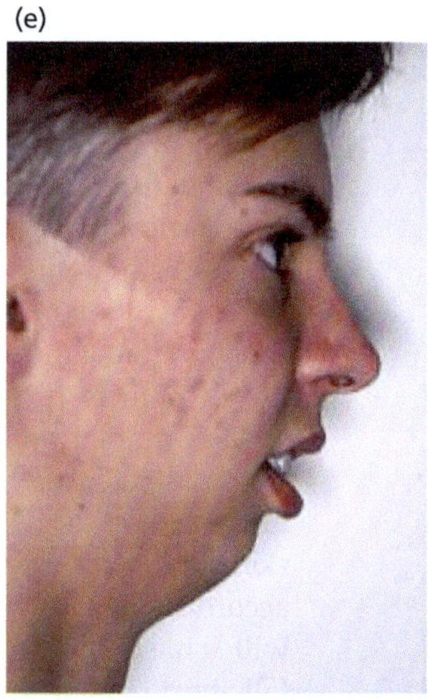

(f)

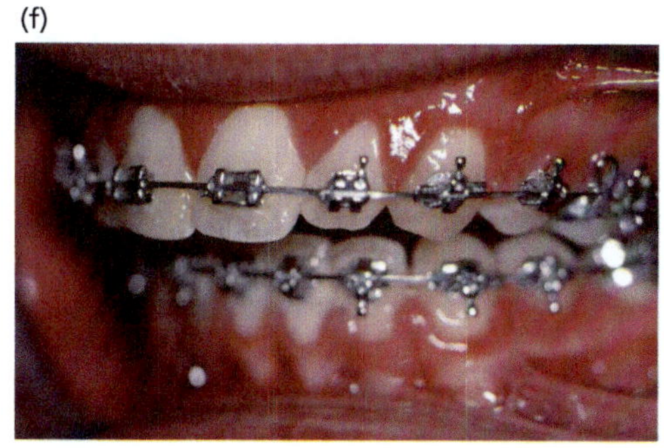

Fig. 31-11/CASE 5: The presurgical **(d)** frontal view; **(e)** profile view; and **(f)** occlusion.

(h)

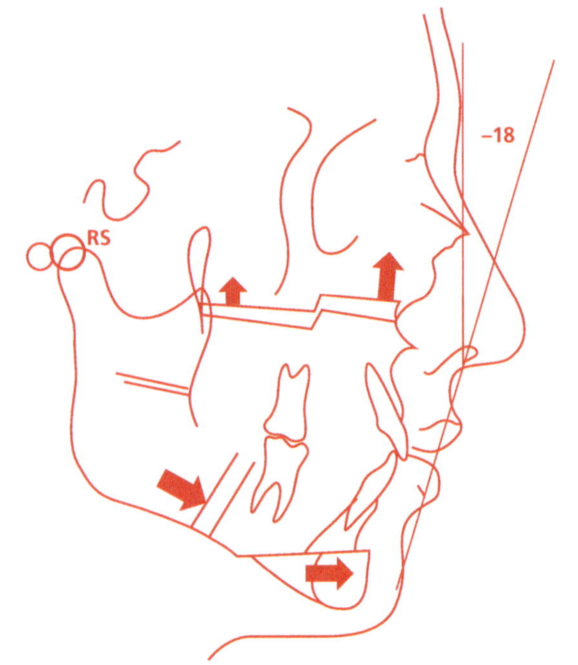

Fig. 31-11/**CASE 5h:** The surgical visual treatment objective according to conventional treatment principles. The maxilla is superiorly repositioned and the mandible will auto rotate around a point just posterior of the condyle. An advancement genioplasty is planned to improve the chin shape and projection. This treatment design would not adequately address the severe convex profile (facial contour angle −18 degrees).

(j)

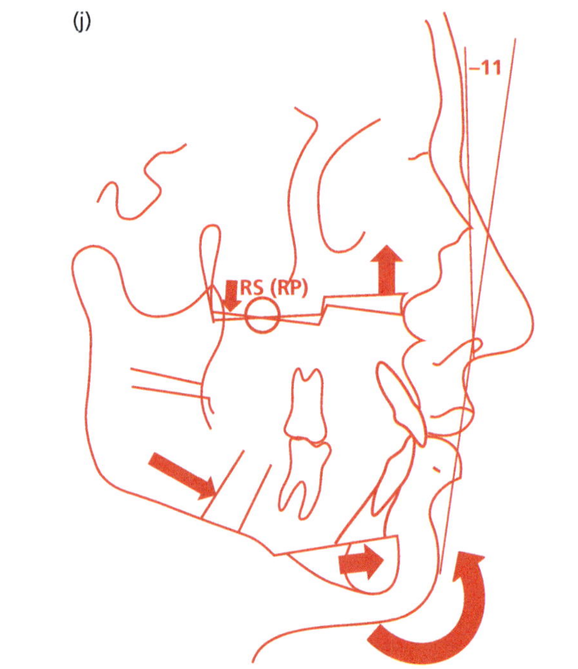

Fig. 31-11/**CASE 5j:** The final cephalometric surgical treatment objective using MMC rotation treatment principles indicates the expected soft and hard tissue treatment results. The anterior maxilla is superiorly repositioned rotating it counterclockwise at a point 10 mm anterior of the PNS **(RS)**. In this case the rotation point during planning **(RP)** and the rotation point at surgery **(RS)** coincide. This surgical movement is followed by the mandible by advancement and counterclockwise rotation. Final aesthetic chin contour is achieved by an advancement genioplasty. An improved aesthetic outcome is predicted (facial contour angle −11 degrees).

(i)

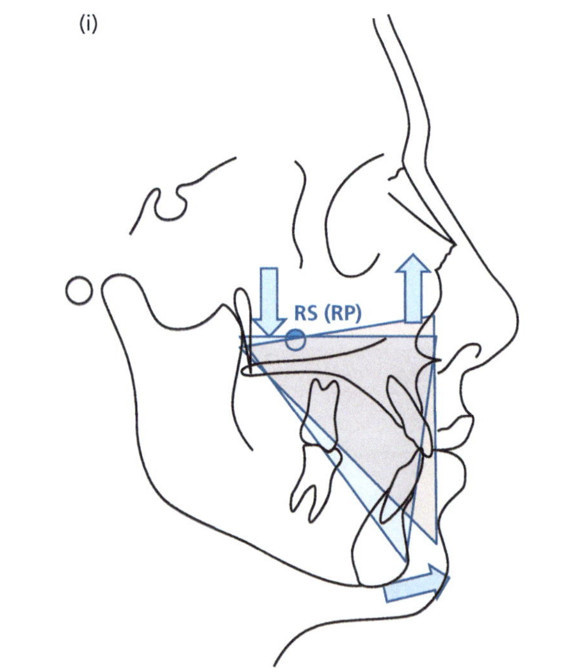

Fig. 31-11/**CASE 5i:** A treatment test using the MMC triangle concept indicates that counterclockwise rotation of the MMC triangle with rotation point just anterior to PNS would allow the surgeon to advance the mandible more than with conventional treatment planning.

Step-by-step development of a cephalometric surgical visual treatment objective

The development of a **cephalometric surgical visual treatment objective (VTO)** for the rotation of the MMC will differ from conventional orthognathic treatment designs.[9]

Figure 31-12a is a cephalometric analysis of a patient with an orthodontically compromised dentition for a Class III skeletal relationship. A concave profile (facial contour angle 0 degrees), maxillary anteroposterior deficiency, mandibular anteroposterior excess, and vertical mandibular excess is evident. The occlusion is orthodontically compensated for the skeletal problem by extraction of the upper first premolars, proclination of the upper incisors and retroclination of the lower incisors. There is an edge to edge incisor and a Class I molar and Class III canine relation present. The relatively small dental discrepancy does not allow for adequate surgical correction of the soft tissue and skeletal discrepancy. Although the surgical correction according to *conventional treatment planning principles* will achieve a functional occlusion it would certainly fall short in achieving balanced facial aesthetics (Figure 31-12b). The treatment possibility by rotating the

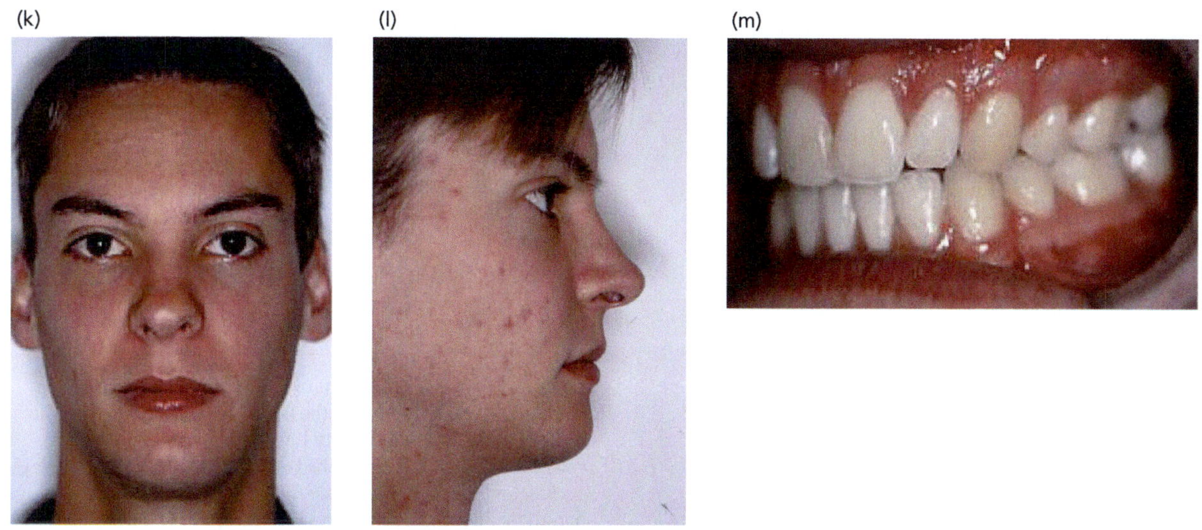

Fig. 31-11/**CASE 5:** The post treatment **(k)** frontal view; **(l)** profile view; and **(m)** occlusion.

MMC in a clockwise direction is tested by developing a surgical visual objective in a step by step fashion.

Step 1 (Figure 31-12**c**). Place a clean acetate tracing paper over the cephalometric tracing and construct the Le Fort I, mandibular sagittal split, and genioplasty osteotomy lines on the tracing. This tracing is called the *original tracing* **(OT)**.

Step 2 (Figure 31-12**d**). Lay a clean piece of tracing paper over the OT and trace all the hard and soft tissue structures (in red) that will not change as a result of the surgery – that is, all the structures above the Le Fort I osteotomy line and behind the vertical sagittal split osteotomy line. The soft tissue profile is traced to end at the supratip break. Use cephalometric parameters (i.e., the facial contour angle, ideal horizontal and vertical upper incisor lip relation, Holdaway's H-line, etc.) to indicate the ideal hard and soft tissue positions for the patient. This tracing is called the prediction tracing **(PT)**.

Step 3 (Figure 31-12**e**). *The construction of a maxillomandibular complex tracing*. Remove the PT from the OT and lay a clean tracing paper over the OT. Trace the bone and teeth of the maxilla below the Le Fort I osteotomy line. Then move the tracing paper to the left so that the upper and lower teeth are in the planned occlusion. As a result of previous extraction of upper first premolars, an ideal incisor and Class I canine relationship will be achieved,

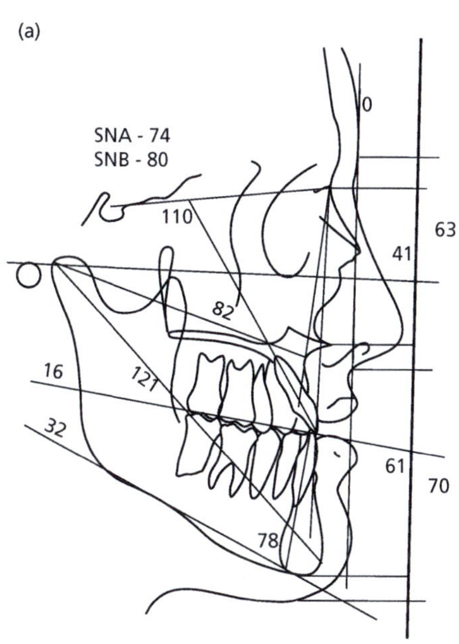

Fig. 31-12a A cephalometric analysis of a patient with a Class III skeletal relationship. The dentition has been compromised for the skeletal imbalance. The profile is concave and the mandible appears prominent while the upper lip support is deficient.

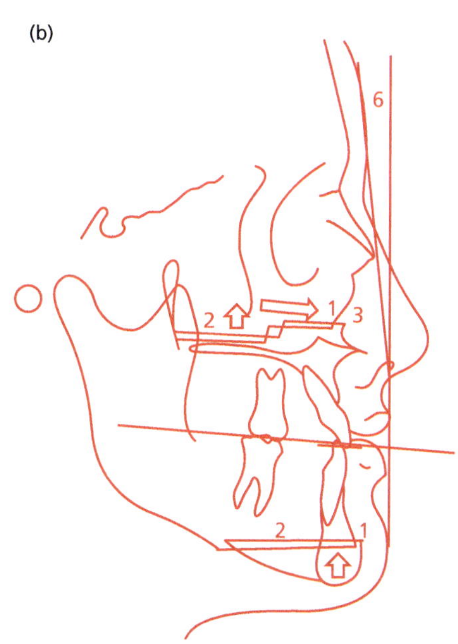

Fig. 31-12b The surgical visual treatment objective according to conventional treatment methods. Due to the dental compromise the surgical correction would be limited to maxillary advancement and reduction genioplasty. The predicted soft tissue outcome is not pleasing and would leave the patient with a straight profile (facial contour angle of 6 degrees).

(c)

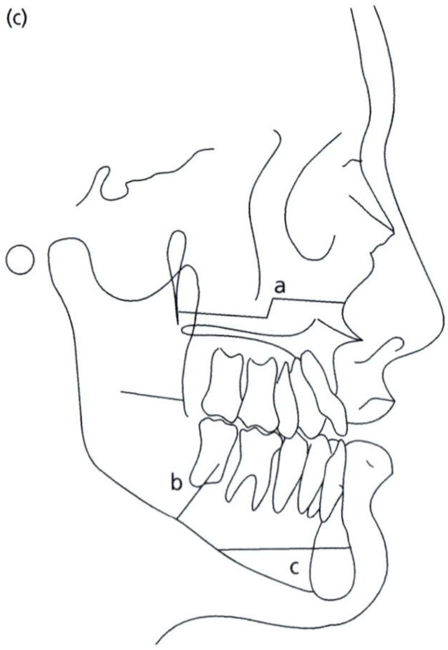

Fig. 31-12c Place a clean piece of acetate paper over the cephalometric analysis and trace all the hard and soft tissue structures. Now construct the Le Fort I (a), mandibular sagittal split osteotomy (b) and genioplasty (c) osteotomy lines on the tracing. This tracing is called the *original tracing* **(OT)**.

however a Class II molar relationship will result. Now, trace the bone and teeth of the mandible in front of the vertical sagittal split osteotomy line and above the genioplasty osteotomy line. This tracing is called the *maxillomandibular complex tracing* **(MMCT).**

Step 4 (Figure 31-12**f**)**.** Mark the important soft tissue landmarks (Subnasale, Pogonion, and stomion superius) on the MMCT. In cases requiring genioplasty for the improvement of the contour of the chin, the genioplasty and soft tissue prediction of the ideal chin shape should now be done on the MMCT. In this case a vertical reduction genioplasty with slight advancement is planned. Two important principles regarding genioplasty should be kept in mind: (1) Chin shape is more important than chin projection (position of Pogonion); and (2) Genioplasty is not a substitute for mandibular surgery. Mandibular deficiency or excess should not be compensated for by chin advancement or reduction to achieve ideal position of Pogonion. This will result in an unaesthetic deepening or reduction of the labiomental fold.

Step 5 (Figure 31-12**g and h**)**.** Place the PT over the OT so that all the traced objects coincide. Slide the MMCT between the OT and the PT. The MMCT can now be rotated and adjusted to fit the ideal guidelines as marked on the PT in Step 2. As with the planning of all orthognathic cases, the

(d)

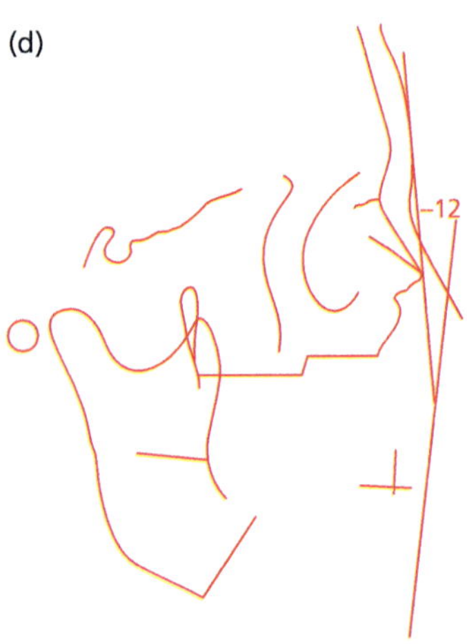

Fig. 31-12d The treatment outcome utilizing the rotation of the MMC is considered and tested. Place a clean tracing paper over the **OT** and use a red pencil to trace all the hard and soft tissue structures that will not change during surgery. An appropriate facial contour angle (i.e. –12 degrees) is constructed to serve as a guide during planning. Guidelines for the ideal maxillary incisor position are indicated by a vertical line (indicating the ideal anteroposterior position of the anterior incisor surface) and a horizontal line (indicating the ideal vertical position of the incisor tip). This tracing is called the *prediction tracing* **(PT)**.

(e)

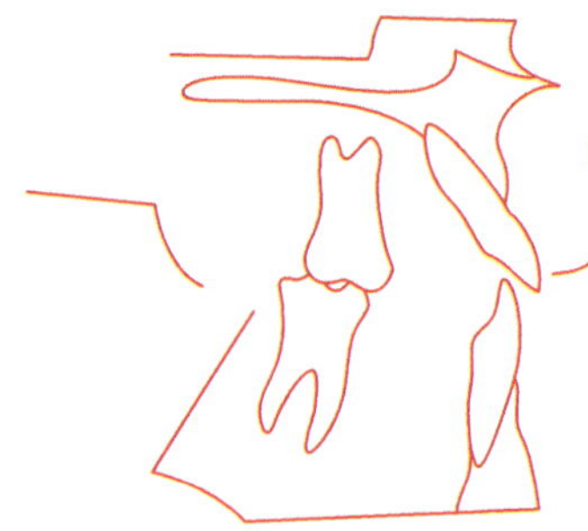

Fig. 31-12e The development of a MMC tracing. Use a clean tracing paper and first trace the bone and teeth of the maxilla below the Le Fort I osteotomy line. Also trace the Le Fort osteotomy line. Now move the tracing paper to achieve the best occlusal relationship and trace the bone and teeth of the mandible ahead of the vertical sagittal split osteotomy line and above the genioplasty osteotomy line. The soft tissue Subnasale point and Stomion inferius are marked on the tracing. This tracing is called the MMC tracing **(MMCT)**.

(f)

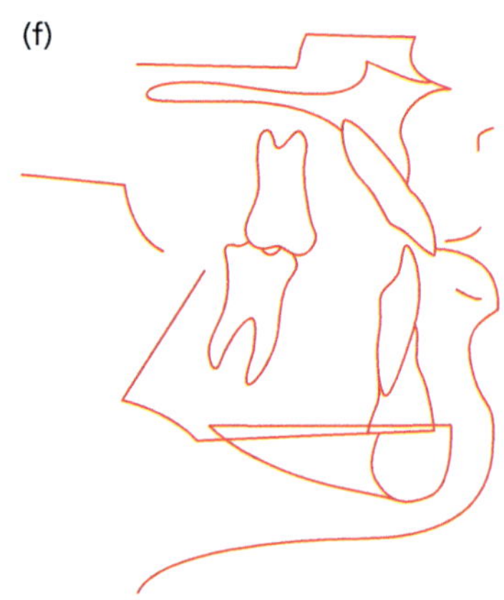

Fig. 31-12f Draw the ideal chin shape on the MMCT and adapt the bony genioplasty accordingly (soft tissue change to hard tissue change = 1:1 (0.9).

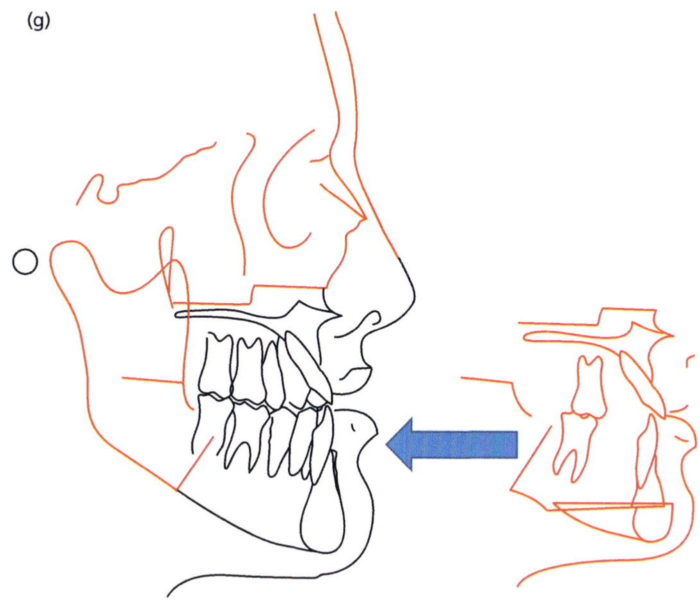

Fig. 31-12g The MMCT is now slipped between the OT and the PT.

upper incisor position remains a key and is positioned first. Due to the facial concavity of this case, the MMCT will be rotated in a clockwise direction. The case requires more maxillary advancement and mandibular setback, than what the compensated occlusion would allow according to *conventional treatment design* (see Figure 31-12b). To allow for increased maxillary advancement as well as increased mandibular setback the incisor edge is used as rotation point. The MMCT is rotated in a clockwise direction until Subnasale and Pogonion (marked in Step 3) coincide or the closest fit according the 'ideal' cephalometric guidelines constructed on the OT in Step 2.

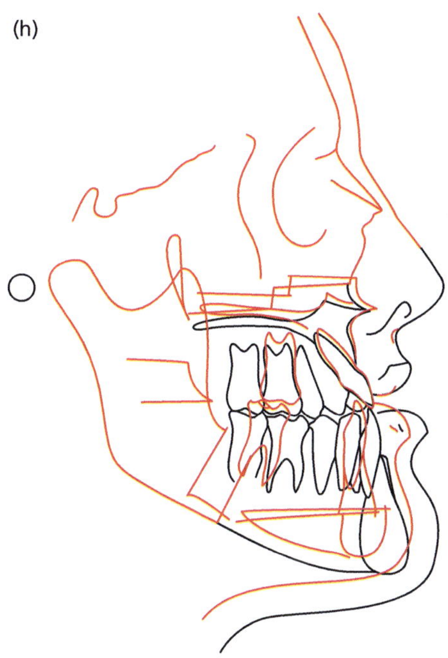

Fig. 31-12h The MMCT can now be rotated guided by the planned upper incisor position, and the ideal facial contour angle (Subnasale and Pogonion).

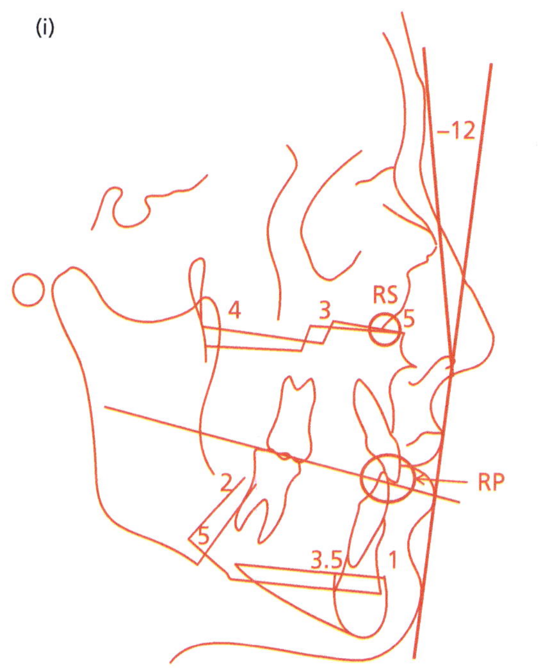

Fig. 31-12i Use a red pencil and complete the tracing by tracing all the hard and soft tissue structures of the maxilla and the mandible. Reconcile the rotation point at surgery by noting the point where the Le Fort I osteotomy lines cross (RS). Measure the required surgical movements. An improved facial contour can be achieved by clockwise rotation of the MMC (facial contour angle –12 degrees).

Step 7 (Figure 31-12**i**). The bone and teeth of the maxilla and the mandible are traced in and the soft-tissue changes predicted. The proximal segment of the mandible (ramus) can now be rotated around the condyle to align the lower borders of the mandibular proximal and distal segments. This may sound contradictory to the concept; however, it is often necessary to rotate the proximal segment a small amount to compensate for vertical changes and to align the lower border of the mandible.

The surgical changes can now be measured and noted.

Step 8 (Figure 31-12**i**). *Correlation of the rotation points.* It is obvious that it is not possible to rotate the MMC around random points such as Pogonion, ANS, incisor tip etc. at the time of surgery. The rotation point during surgery, in this case, is the maxillary incisor tip (**RP**). The rotation point at surgery will however, differ from the rotation point during the development of the surgical treatment objective. The rotation point at the time of surgery is identified by noting the point at which the Le Fort I osteotomy lines (of the OT and the PT) cross on the surgical treatment objective. In this case it is at **RS**, the anterior contact point on the Le Fort I osteotomy line.

Reconciling the cephalometric prediction rotation point with the surgical rotation point

At the stage when the surgical visual treatment objective is developed the MMCT can be rotated around any point, posterior or inferior of ANS and, in addition, the complex can be rotated in a clockwise or a counterclockwise direction to achieve the best facial balance. The rotation point during planning is called the **RP** point. Once the final cephalometric treatment objective is completed the planned surgical movements are measured and noted. At this stage the point where the Le Fort I osteotomy line on the OT and the osteotomy line on the PT crosses is noted. This point is called the **RS** point and will serve as the surgeons guide during model surgery and fabrication of an intermediate surgical splint. It also serves as an accurate reference point during surgery. In exceptional cases such as very large maxillary down graft procedures the lines will not cross on the PT and the surgeon will rely on the accuracy of the intermediate surgical splint.

Stability after clockwise and counterclockwise rotation of the maxillomandibular complex

There is a paucity of data in the modern literature regarding skeletal stability following clockwise or counterclockwise rotation of the maxillomandibular complex. In the past counterclockwise rotation of the mandible following bilateral sagittal split mandibular ramus osteotomy was considered to have poor postoperative stability.[10–12] It was postulated that counterclockwise rotation of the mandible would result in an increase in the posterior height of the mandibular ramus. This increase in height of the ramus would inevitably stretch the pterygomasseteric sling resulting in skeletal relapse. This would certainly occur when the osteotomy is performed as described by Trauner and Obwegeser in 1955[13] and Dal Pont in 1961[14] (Figure 31-13). However when performing a bilateral sagittal split osteotomy according to modern orthognathic surgical technique the distal osteotomy will split short of the posterior and inferior border of the mandible (Figure 31-14).[15] Counterclockwise rotation of the distal segment of the mandible would

(a)

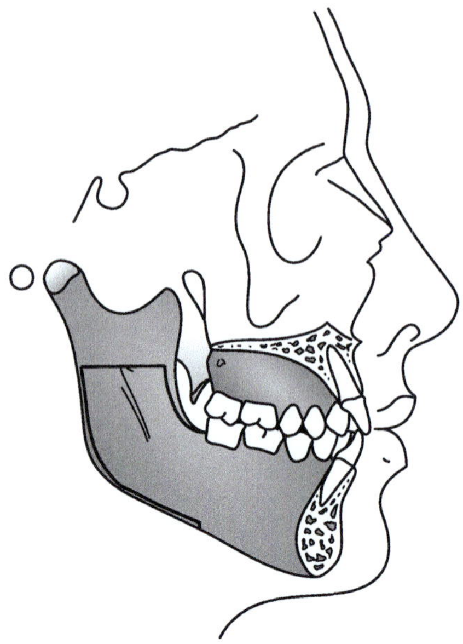

Fig. 31-13a When the sagittal split mandibular ramus osteotomy is performed as described by Trauner and Obwegeser[13] the horizontal osteotomy is carried backwards to the posterior border of the mandibular ramus. The mandible is then split along the lower and posterior border of the ramus to meet the horizontal osteotomy superiorly.

(b)

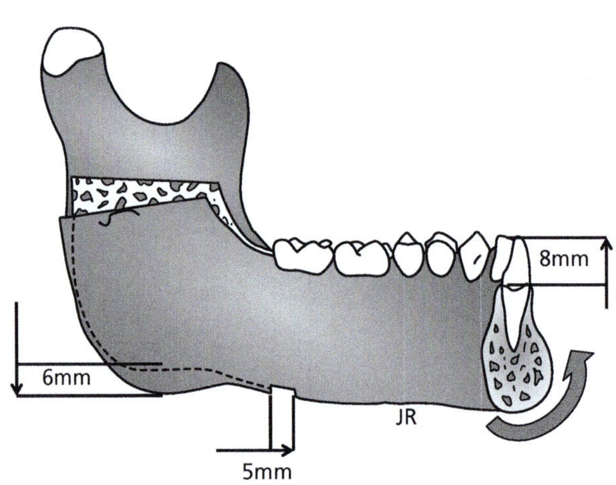

Fig. 31-13b When the osteotomy is performed according to Trauner and Obwegeser[13] and the distal segment is rotated counter clockwise the posterior height of the mandible is increased. This will certainly stretch the pterygomassetric sling. In this figure the distal segment of the mandible is advanced by 5 mm and the incisors rotated counterclockwise by 8mm. The height of the mandibular ramus has increased by 6 mm.

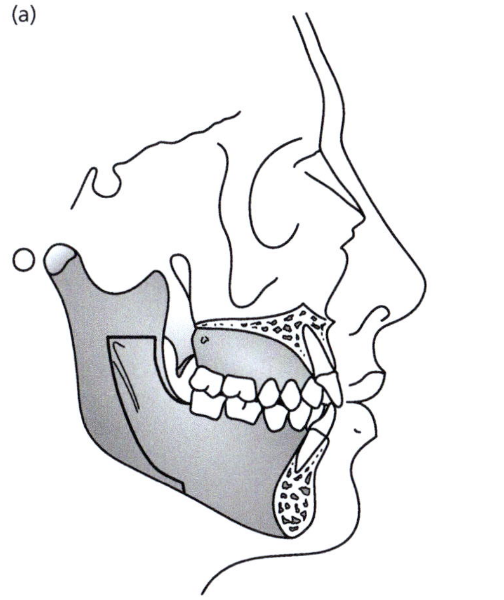

Fig. 31-14a The 'short split' technique described by Epker.[15] The horizontal osteotomy is carried to just past the lingula on the medial side of the mandibular ramus. The medial osteotomy will split anteriorly and downwards, well short of the posterior border of the mandible. The split will meet the vertical osteotomy on the lingual side of the corpus.

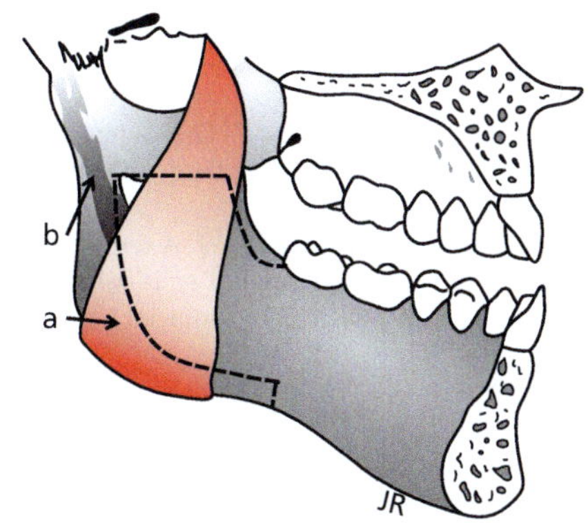

Fig. 31-15 According to Beukes and Reyneke[19] the attachments of the medial pterygoid muscle **(a)** and the stylomandibular ligament **(b)** may influence the control of the proximal segment and long-term skeletal stability. They recommend stripping of the muscle and ligament from the medial side of the mandibular angle during surgery.

not influence the posterior height of the mandible and therefore have no influence on postoperative stability. Subsequent studies have found that long term postoperative stability of the mandible following counterclockwise rotation is comparable to clockwise rotation or conventional mandibular advancement procedures.[16–18] Beukes and Reyneke have however found that the medial pterygoid muscle and stylomandibular ligament may influence postoperative stability following advancement of the mandible and recommend stripping of the muscle and ligament attachments during surgery (Figure 31-15).[19] This seems to also be advantageous with counterclockwise rotation of the mandible.

Rotation of the MMC is a valuable surgical design to improve aesthetic outcomes in orthognathic surgery. When conventional treatment planning does not render satisfactory aesthetic treatment outcomes, rotation of the MMC should be considered as an alternative treatment design.

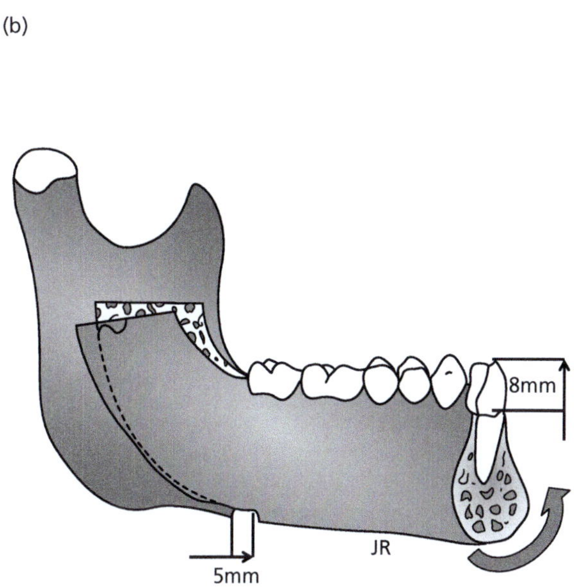

Fig. 31-14b The same movement of the distal segment of the mandible is carried out as in Figure 31-13b (5 mm advancement and 8 mm counter clockwise rotation at the incisors). It is evedent that there is no increase in the posterior height of the mandible.

References

1 McCollum AGH, Reyneke JP, Wolford LM. An alternative for the correction of the Class II low angle mandibular plane angle, Oral Surg Oral Med Oral Pathol. 1989;67:231–41.
2 Wolford LM, Hilliard F, Dugan DJ. Surgical treatment objective: a systematic approach to the prediction tracing. St Louis, 1985, Mosby.
3 Reyneke JP. Essentials in Orthognathic Surgery. (2nd Ed.) Chapter 3, Diagnoses and treatment planning. Carol Stream, IL: Quintessence Publishing, 2010.
4 Nattestad A, Vedlofte P. Mandibular autorotation in orthognathic surgery: a new method of locating the center of mandibular rotation and determining the consequence in orthognathic surgery. J Craniomaxillofac Surg. 1992;20:163–70.
5 Reyneke JP. Rotation of the maxillomandibular complex. In: Fonseca RJ, Marciani R, Turvey TA (Eds.). Oral and Maxillofacial Surgery. 2nd Ed. Vol III, Elsevier, 2009.
6 Reyneke JP, Evans WG: Surgical manipulation of the occlusal plane. Int J Adult Orthodon Orthognath Surg. 1990;5:99–110.
7 Reyneke JP. Surgical manipulation of the occlusal plane: new concepts in geometry. Int J Adult Orthodon Orthognath Surg. 1998;13:307–16.
8 Reyneke JP. Rotation of the maxillomandibular complex: an alternative in orthognathic treatment planning, Academic dissertation. Acta Univ Tamperensis. 2006;142:35.
9 Reyneke JP. Surgical cephalometric prediction tracing for the alteration of the occlusal plane by means of the rotation of the maxillomandibular complex. Int J Adult Orthodon Orthognath Surg. 1999;14:55–64.

10 Schendel SA, Epker BN. Results after mandibular advancement surgery: an analysis of 87 cases. J Oral Surg. 1980;38:265–82.
11 Proffit WR, Turvey TA, Phillips C. Orthognathic surgery: a hierarchy of stability. Int J Adult Orthodon Orthognath Surg. 1996;1:191–204.
12 Van Sickels JE, Larsen AJ, Thrash WJ. A retrospective study of relapse in rigidly fixated sagittal split osteotomies: contributing factors. Am J Orthod Dentofacial Orthop. 1988;93: 413–8.
13 Trauner R, Obwegwser H. Zur Operationstechnik bei der Proggenia und anderen Unterfieferanomalien. Dtsch Zahn Mund Kieferhlkd. 1955;23:11–25.
14 Dal Pont G. Retromolar osteotomy for correction of prognathism. J Oral Surg. 1961;19:42–7.
15 Epker BN. Modification in the sagittal osteotomy of the mandible. J Oral Surg. 1977;35:157–9.
16 Chemello PD, Wolford LM, Buschang PH. Occlusal plane alteration in orthognathic surgery – Part II: Long term stability of results. Am J Orthod Dentofacial Orthop. 1994;106:434–40.
17 Rosen HM. Occlusal plane rotation: aesthetic enhancement in mandibular microgenia. Plast Reconstruct Surg. 1993;91:1231–40.
18 Reyneke JP, Bryant RS, Suuronen R, Becker PJ. Post-operative skeletal stability following clockwise and counter clockwise rotation of the maxillomandibular complex compared to conventional orthognathic treatment. Brit J Oral Maxfac Surg. 2006;45:56–64.
19 Beukes J, Reyneke JP. Medial pterygoid muscle and stylomandibular ligament: the effects on postoperative stability. Int J Oral Maxillofac Surg. 2013;42:43–8.

Chapter 32

Specific Considerations in the 'Low Angle' Patient

Declan Millett

Introduction

Definition

The term 'low angle' refers to patients with a reduced Mandibular Plane Angle (MPA, measured relative to, and almost parallel with the true horizontal plane), associated usually with a reduced Lower Facial Height (LFH) and a deep overbite. Although these features are more commonly seen in association with a Class II skeletal pattern, they may also exist with Class III or Class I skeletal bases.[1]

Aetiology and consequences

The direction and amount of condylar growth, temporal fossa growth, vertical growth of the maxilla and tooth eruption determine vertical facial growth.[2] Individuals with reduced LFH exhibit more increase in posterior facial height than the combined sutural and alveolar growth of the maxilla and mandible; also evident is an upward and forward growth of the mandibular condyle with less eruption of the posterior teeth and reduced maxillary vertical growth.[1] All result in an anterior mandibular growth rotation which continues throughout life (Figure 32-1).

This leads to overbite increase and may be associated with flaring of upper incisors and periodontal breakdown.[3] The association of deep bite, particularly with retroclined upper incisors, and bruxism[4], signs and symptoms of temporomandibular joint dysfunction (TMD)[5] or as a risk factor for TMD[6] is controversial.

Common features of low angle cases

Those identified in low angle Class I, Class II and Class III cases are given in Table 32-1 and Figure 32-2.

Orthognathic Surgery: Principles, Planning and Practice. Edited by Farhad B. Naini and Daljit S. Gill.

(a)

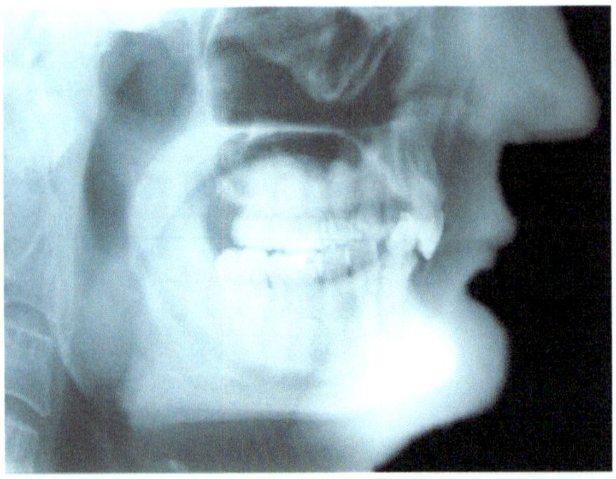

(b)

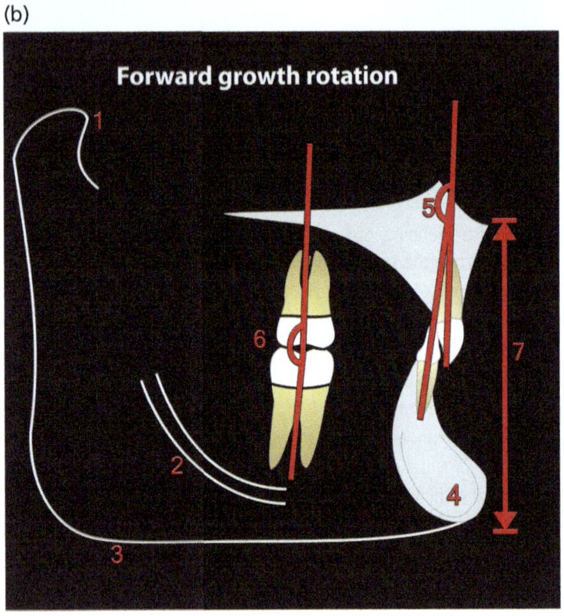

Fig. 32-1 Seven structural signs characterized by Bjork[2] diagnostic of an anterior mandibular growth rotation: (1) forward inclination of the condylar head, (2) increased curvature of the mandibular canal, (3) absence of an antegonial notch, (4) forward inclination of the mandibular symphysis with increased chin projection, (5) increased interincisal angle, (6) increased intermolar and interpremolar angles and (7) reduced lower face height. Shown on (a) a lateral cephalometric radiograph and (b) diagrammatically. (Modified and reprinted with permission from Naini FB. Facial Aesthetics: Concepts and Clinical Diagnosis. Oxford: Wiley-Blackwell, 2011. Chapter 19, pp. 298–9.)

Other features

Over 40% of adults with skeletal deep bite had fusion of cervical vertebrae (C2, C3) and morphological deviations of the cervical column have been found to be significantly more common compared to controls.[7]

Case assessment and treatment planning

General

A systematic approach to case assessment is essential. This includes appraisal of the patient's concerns with appropriate psychological assessment, clinical extra- and intraoral assessments supplemented with cephalometric and study model evaluation and other special investigations as required. These are addressed in Chapters 5 and 6. Elements particularly pertinent to the low angle case are highlighted here.

Table 32-1 Associated clinical facial features found with short facial form in Class I, Class II or Class III antero-posterior dental base relationships

Class I	Prominent chin
	Decreased anterior and posterior dentoalveolar heights
	Frequently retroclined upper and lower incisors (bi-dentoalveolar retrusion)
Class II	Most common associated a-p relationship
	Retruded mandible
	Adequate or excessive soft tissue chin
	Upper lip height usually normal
	Obtuse NLA
	Acute labio-mental fold
	Obtuse chin-throat angle
Class III	Prognathic appearing mandible
	Short upper lip (or normal height but somewhat compressed/'squashed up' from overclosed mandible)
	Acute NLA (mainly due to upper lip inclination)
	Obtuse labiomental fold

a-p = antero-posterior; NLA = Nasolabial Angle.
Note: Features common to all are thin and competent lips, deep Curve of Spee and excessive overbite.

Clinical and cephalometric assessments for a low angle case

A number of *clinical* and *cephalometric* parameters may be evaluated in order to analyse vertical facial form. The former are primarily soft tissue factors while the latter provide skeletal and dental information regarding hard tissue contribution.

Both clinical (Figure 32-3[8–11]) and cephalometric (Figure 32-7[12–16]) assessments must be undertaken with the patient in *natural head position* (NHP), which is adopted when relaxed and looking straight ahead at a distant object. This allows a true vertical and a true horizontal to be used for facial aesthetic analysis (see Chapter 5), as well as being standardised and reproducible over time.[17] The cant of all other reference lines, including the alternative use of the Frankfort plane, is subject to biological variation,[18,19] and likely to give inaccurate representation where facial skeletal discrepancies exist.[19]

Full face, frontal and profile, assessments should be performed. As short lower face height may accompany a Class I, Class II or Class III malocclusion and may be due to vertical mandibular deficiency, vertical maxillary deficiency allowing overclosure of the mandible or deficient vertical dentoalveolar development, the profile (Figure 32-4) must be examined with the *mandible rotated open in the rest position.*

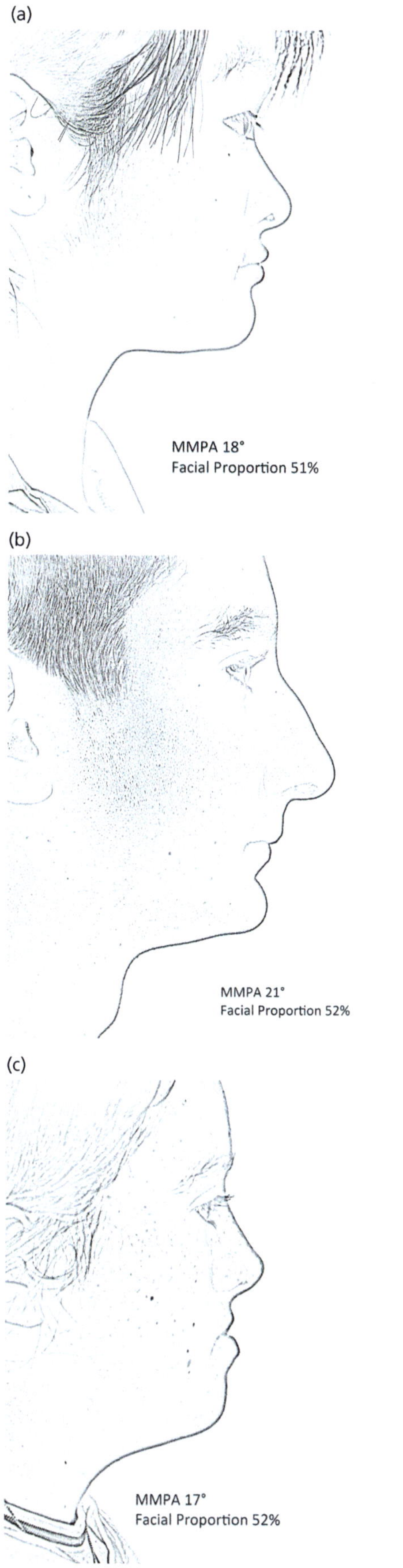

Fig. 32-2 Low mandibular planes angle associated with (a) Class I (b) Class II and (c) Class III skeletal bases.

Proportional assessment of the face is more important than those of linear and angular measurements as surgical correction aims to establish more normal proportions. The patient's ethnicity, gender and age must be considered in facial proportional assessments to help determine what aspects of the face are beyond the bounds of normal. Ideal normative values, however, should be regarded only as a guide (see Chapter 5).

Temporomandibular joint considerations

The presence of clicks, crepitus, deviations or displacements on closure should be noted along with any associated symptoms. No guarantee should be given that treatment of the malocclusion by combined orthodontic-surgical means will cure the problem.[20] Generally, where temporomandibular joint surgery is necessary in addition to maxillary and/or mandibular surgery, the former should be delayed until after the new joint and occlusal positions have been determined as the result is likely to be more certain (see Chapter 35).

Soft tissue factors and lip musculature

In addition to those factors given in Figure 32-2, the musculature tone should be assessed. Short face patients have a predominance of type II muscle fibres[21,22] and strong jaw closing muscles; this may lead to resorption of interpositional grafts after inferior positioning of the maxilla.[23] The patient must be advised of this pre-treatment.

Periodontal considerations

As deep overbite may be related to periodontal pathology, especially in the presence of poor oral hygiene,[24] the periodontal condition must be treated and stabilized before orthodontic treatment, with a maintenance plan put in place. Limited and low level evidence shows little difference in gingival recession between cases with proclined or non-proclined incisors, although cases treated by orthognathic surgery were not included.[25] Incisor proclination, however, is likely to lead to gingival recession in the presence of some or all of the following: pre-treatment gingival recession, poor oral hygiene, gingivitis and/or thin gingival biotype.[26] Where a narrow band of attached gingivae exists in relation to the lower incisors and levelling is to be undertaken on a non-extraction basis, a gingival graft may be considered. Additionally, grafting may be required before genioplasty or on teeth near other vestibular osteotomy cuts, especially if gingival recession is evident on posterior teeth,[27] to avoid recession from contraction of the incision line on healing.[28] However, it should be borne in mind that the problem with gingival recession in these situations is predominantly due to lack of alveolar bone; as such, placement of a gingival bone graft prior to decompensation of the incisors will not necessarily reduce the recession.[29]

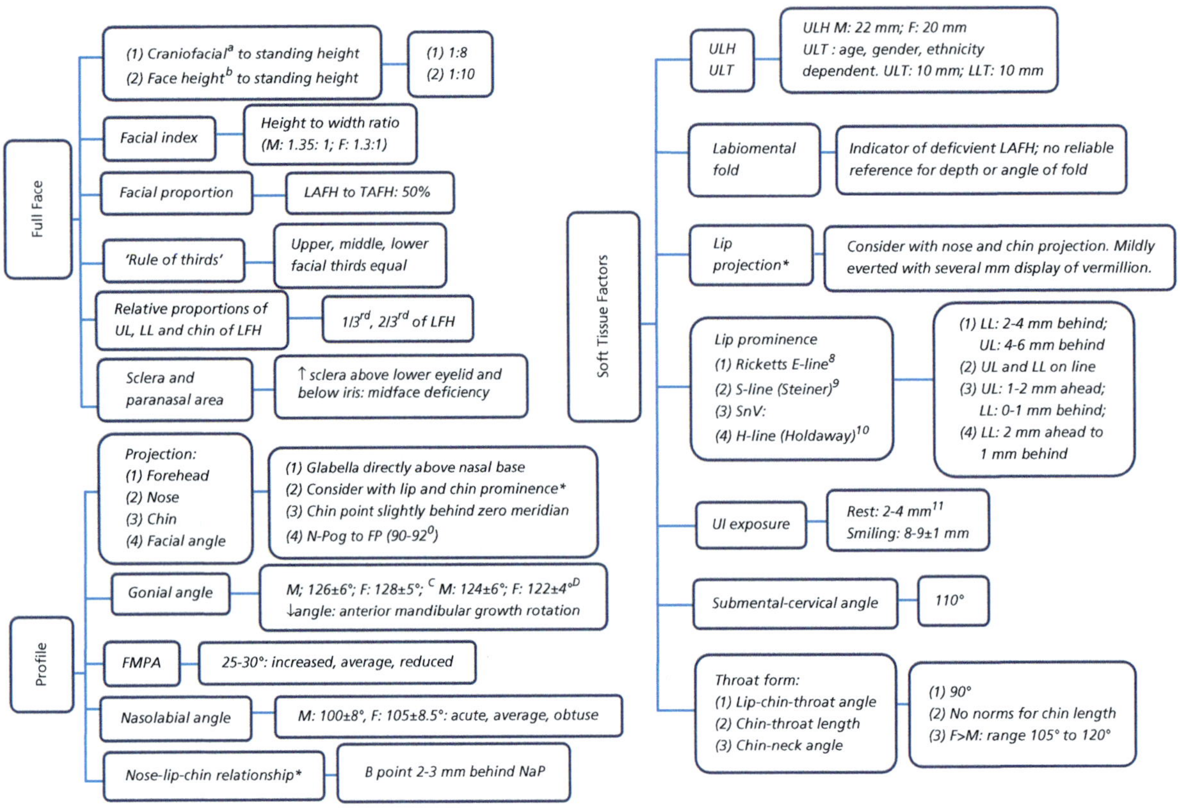

[a], Top of the head to base of chin; [b], from the hairline to base of chin; M, Male; F, Female; TAFH, Total anterior facial height; LAFH, Lower anterior facial height; UL, Upper lip; LL, Lower lip; LFH, Lower face height; ↑, increased; *, linked assessments; N-Pog, Nasion-pogonion; FP, Frankfort plane; [C], UK; [D], US; NaP, Nasion perpendicular; ULH, Upper lip height; ULT, Upper lip thickness; LLT, Lower lip thickness; SnV, True vertical through subnasale; LL, Lower lip; UL, Upper lip; UI, Upper incisor.

Fig. 32-3 Clinical full face, profile and soft tissue assessments to analyse vertical facial form.

Restorative considerations

Functional restorations should be placed to maintain patient comfort during treatment, with final occlusal rehabilitation completed post-surgery.

Cephalometric assessment

Aspects that should be considered, including normative vertical skeletal and dentoalveolar measurements for UK and US populations, are given in Figure 32-7[12–16] and Table 32.2[29–31] respectively. It is important to consider the *overall pattern of relationships* of linear and angular measurements, as well as soft tissue relationships, and not each in isolation. Firstly, drawing and assessing the relationship of Sassouni's horizontal planes allows immediate recognition of any rotations of the maxilla and/or mandible as well as vertical disproportions[14]. Then the anteroposterior jaw relationships and the relative positions of the upper and lower dentitions to their respective bases can be assessed using either the nasion-perpendicular as in the McNamara analysis[12] or by template (e.g. Bolton[16]) superimposition. Lastly, linear measurements e.g. face height, maxillary and mandibular lengths[13] or other specific components may be considered (Figure 32-8).

Treatment planning

Treatment planning is a team inter-disciplinary activity to ensure the best possible outcome to deal with the patient's concerns. Having identified the dentofacial area(s) that need correction, the changes necessary to create well-balanced facial soft tissue aesthetics are outlined; then the surgical movements required to achieve these are estimated before finally designing the orthodontic plan for these to occur (see Chapter 6).

In the low angle case, special attention must be paid to lengthening the lower face without increasing chin prominence and minimizing stretch of the suprahyoid musculature.[32] Repositioning the mandible vertically to assess its effect on the profile is key to thorough soft tissue analysis for treatment planning.[1] For 2D planning, the lateral cephalograph should be taken with the patient in natural head position (NHP). Care is needed to ensure that the Class II low angle patient is not postured forward and that the mandible is in the retruded contact position. For the Class III patient with overclosure and maxillary deficiency, the image should be recorded with the assistance of an interocclusal wax wafer to hold the mandible in the rest position; this is determined by asking the patient to say 'N' or 'Mississippi', wet the lips and bring them gently together.[33,34] (Figure 32-9). Each mm of vertical

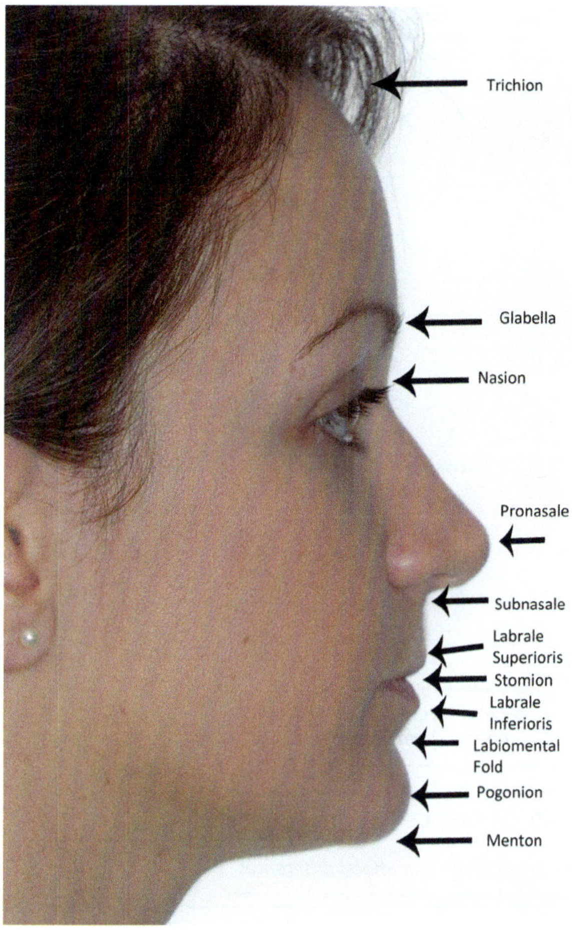

Fig. 32-4 Soft tissue facial landmarks in profile view: Trichion (hairline); Glabella (most prominent aspect of the forehead); Nasion (deepest concavity between forehead and nose); Pronasale (nasal tip); Subnasale (junction of nasal base and upper lip); Labrale superioris (vermillion border of upper lip); Stomion (mid-interlabial fissure); Labrale inferioris (vermillion border of lower lip); Labiomental fold (deepest concavity between labrale inferioris and menton); Pogonion (most prominent point on chin); Menton (most inferior point of chin).

opening reduces anteroposterior chin prominence by about 1 mm.[12]

A digital profile photograph ideally taken simultaneously or immediately after the radiograph with the soft tissues in the same position aided by the wax wafer, as required, can then be superimposed using proprietary software for planning purposes.[1,32] In sequence, and incorporating desired but realistic decompensation to achieve the target overjet, the maxillary and upper incisor positions are determined first; then, the mandibular and lower incisor positions incorporating any necessary maxillary and/or mandibular rotation to optimise the occlusion and lower facial height. Finally, consideration is given to the chin and the need to make anteroposterior and/or vertical surgical changes to produce the best profile aesthetics, followed by consideration of rhinoplasty to refine the nasal shape. The Class II short face patient benefits from both an increase in lower face height and forward positioning of the retruded mandible. Again digital photographs with the mandible postured forward to achieve a Class I incisor relationship can assist in determining the final plan (Figure 32-10).

Prediction of surgical outcome

Computer image prediction allows the patient to view the predicted outcome from each of the treatment options proposed, and in concert with discussion by the orthodontist and surgeon, so provides the patient with the information needed to make an informed decision regarding management. More accurate for profile than frontal views,[35] patients who view the prediction pretreatment may be more likely to be satisfied with the outcome.[36] Though 3D prediction software is available, integrating cone beam computed tomography (CBCT) and 3D stereophotogrammetric images, further refinement is required to improve the accuracy.[37,38]

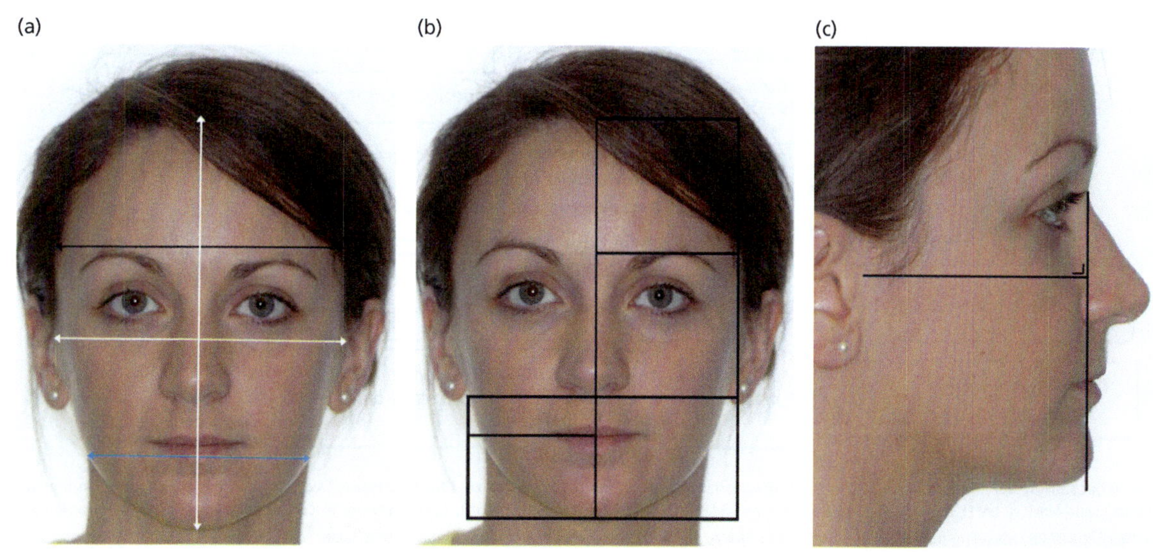

Fig. 32-5 (a) Facial index (height to width ratio); facial height and bizygomatic width (white; ~70% of vertical facial height); bitemporal width (black) and bigonial width (blue): ~80-85% and ~70-75% respectively of bizygomatic width. (b) Vertical facial proportions showing facial trisection and anterior lower facial third proportions; the anterior lower facial height is often slightly greater than the middle third, most commonly in males. (c) Zero-meridian line (true vertical from soft tissue Nasion).

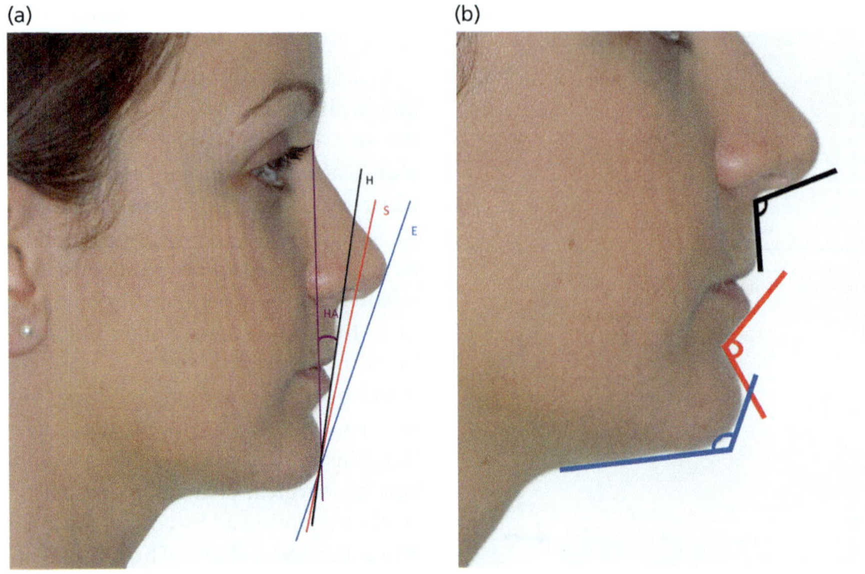

Fig. 32-6 (a) Profile lines: Ricketts E Line, S-Line, H Line and Holdaway angle; Soft tissue angles: Nasolabial, labiomental, chin-submental plane.

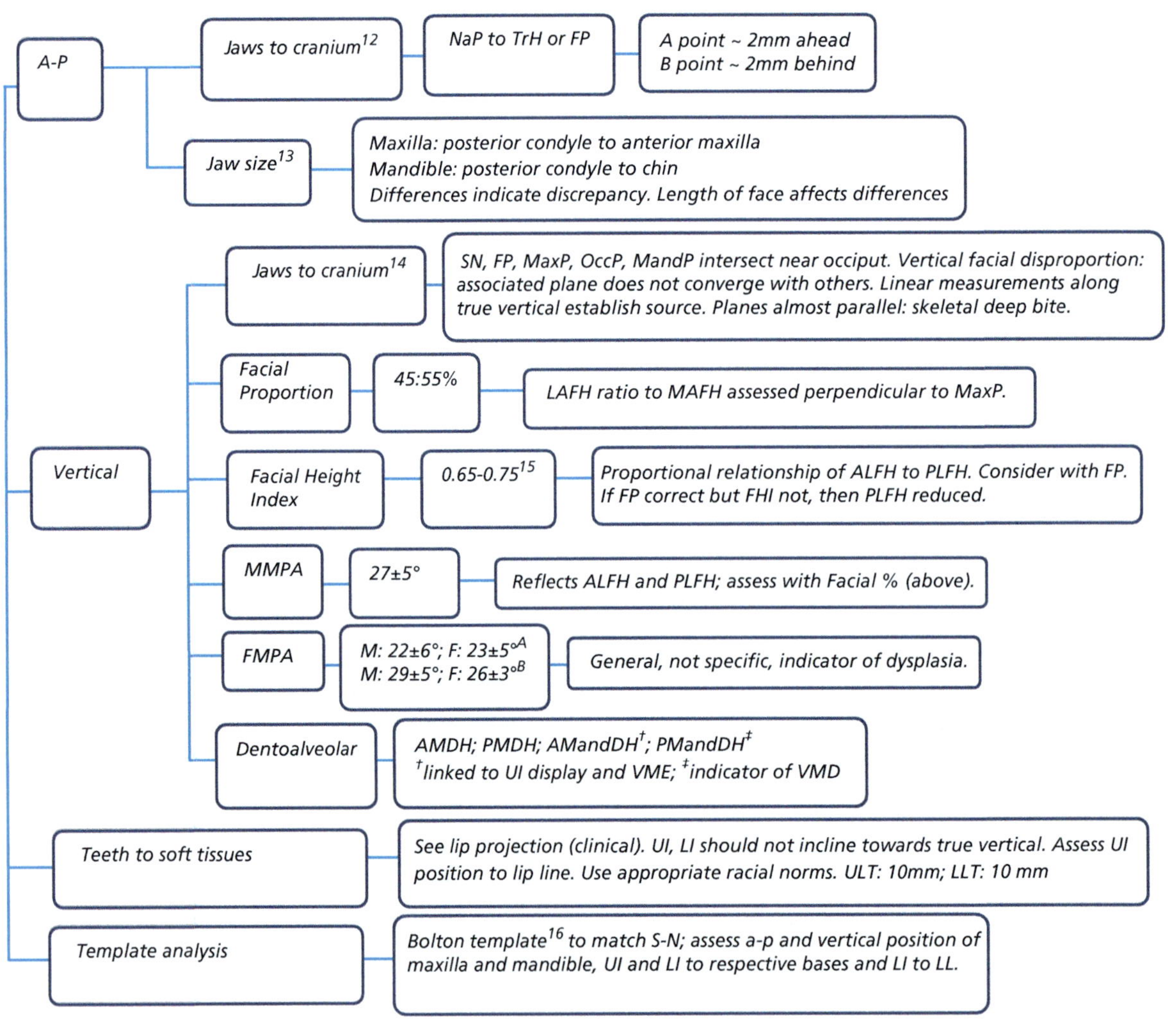

A-P, anteroposterior; NaP, Nasion perpendicular; TrH, true horizontal; FP, Frankfort Plane; MaxP, Maxillary Plane; OccP, Occlusal Plane; MandP, Mandibular Plane; SN, Sella-Nasion; LAFH, Lower anterior facial height; MAFH, Middle anterior facial height; ALFH, anterior lower facial height; PLFH, Posterior lower facial height; MMPA, maxillary-mandibular planes angle; FMPA, Frankfort-mandibular planes angle; M, Male;[A], UK;[B], US; F, Female; AMDH, Anterior maxillary dental height; UI, Upper incisor; VME, Vertical Maxillary Excess; PMDH, Posterior maxillary dental height; AMandDH, Anterior mandibular dental height; VMD, Vertical Maxillary Deficiency; PMandDH, Posterior mandibular dental height. ULT, Upper lip thickness; LLT, Lower lip thickness; LI, Lower incisor; LL, Lower lip;

Fig. 32-7 Cephalometric assessment to assist with analysis of vertical facial form.

Table 32-2 Normative cephalometric vertical linear and angular skeletal and dentoalveolar measurements for UK and US populations

		Normative value			
		UK[a]		US[b]	
Linear	**Parameter**	**mm**	**mm**	**mm**	**mm**
Anterior face height	N-Me	121 ± 7	112 ± 6	137 ± 8	123 ± 5
Anterior midface height	N-ANS	54 ± 2	51 ± 2	60 ± 4	56 ± 2
Midface height	N perpendicular to MaxP	53 ± 2	50 ± 3	Not provided	Not provided
Lower face height	ANS-Me	68 ± 6	63 ± 5	80 ± 6	69 ± 5
Lower face height	Me perpendicular to MaxP	67 ± 6	61 ± 5	76 ± 6	67 ± 4
Sella-point A		86 ± 4	78 ± 3	99 ± 5	91 ± 6
Sella-Gn		129 ± 5	117 ± 4	144 ± 7	131 ± 5
Posterior midface height	S-PNS	50 ± 2	45 ± 2	56 ± 4	51 ± 5
Posterior face height	S-Go	80 ± 4	72 ± 4	88 ± 6	79 ± 4
Lower posterior face height	Ar-Go	49 ± 4	44 ± 4	54 ± 4	50 ± 4
Anterior maxillary dental height	UI tip perpendicular to MaxP	28 ± 3	27 ± 3	33 ± 3	30 ± 3
Posterior maxillary dental height	Mesial cusp of U6 perpendicular to MaxP	27 ± 3	24 ± 3	28 ± 3	25 ± 2
Anterior mandibular dental height	LI tip perpendicular to MandP*	40 ± 3	38 ± 3	49 ± 3	42 ± 3
Posterior mandibular dental height	mesial cusp of L6 perpendicular to MandP	34 ± 3	33 ± 3	38 ± 3	33 ± 3
Angular		°	°	°	°
N-Sn-Gn		66 ± 5	68 ± 4	67 ± 4	66 ± 4
SN to Frankfort plane (Po-Or)		10 ± 3	11 ± 3	3 ± 4	5 ± 3
SN to maxillary plane (ANS-PNS)		6 ± 2	7 ± 3	7 ± 3	8 ± 2
SN to functional occlusal plane		15 ± 6	19 ± 3	14 ± 4	15 ± 3
SN to mandibular plane (Go-Me)		32 ± 7	34 ± 6	33 ± 5	31 ± 3
SN to posterior ramus plane (Ar-Go)		89 ± 6	89 ± 4	89 ± 5	89 ± 4
Frankfort mandibular planes angle (FMPA)	General indicator of vertical problem	22 ± 6	23 ± 5	29 ± 5	26 ± 3
Maxillary-mandibular planes angle (MMPA)	Reflects ALFH and PLFH	26 ± 7	26 ± 5	26 ± 5	23 ± 4

Adapted with permission from Naini FB. Facial Aesthetics: Concepts and Diagnosis. Oxford: Wiley-Blackwell, 2011.[29]; [a] UK data from Bhatia and Leighton[30]; [b] US data from Riolo et al.[31]; N, Nasion; Me, Menton; ANS, Anterior Nasal Spine; MaxP, Maxillary Plane; Gn, Gonion; S, Sella; PNS, Posterior Nasal Spine; Ar, Articulare; UI, Upper permanent central incisor; U6, Upper first permanent molar; LI, Lower permanent central incisor; MandP, Mandibular Plane; SN, Subnasale; Po, Porion; Or, Orbitale; *Also useful in evaluation of vertical skeletal chin height but depends on inclination and vertical eruption of the LIs; L6, Lower first permanent molar; ALFH, Anterior Lower Facial Height; PLFH, Posterior Lower Facial Height.

Orthodontic management

Sequence of treatment

While in selected cases it may be possible to achieve a satisfactory facial and occlusal outcome *without* any orthodontic intervention or instead to undertake *orthodontics post-surgery*, it is customary contemporary practice that orthodontics should coincide with pre-, peri- and post-surgical phases.

Pre-surgical orthodontics

This aims to align the arches, either wholly or in segments, locate the incisors in their desired

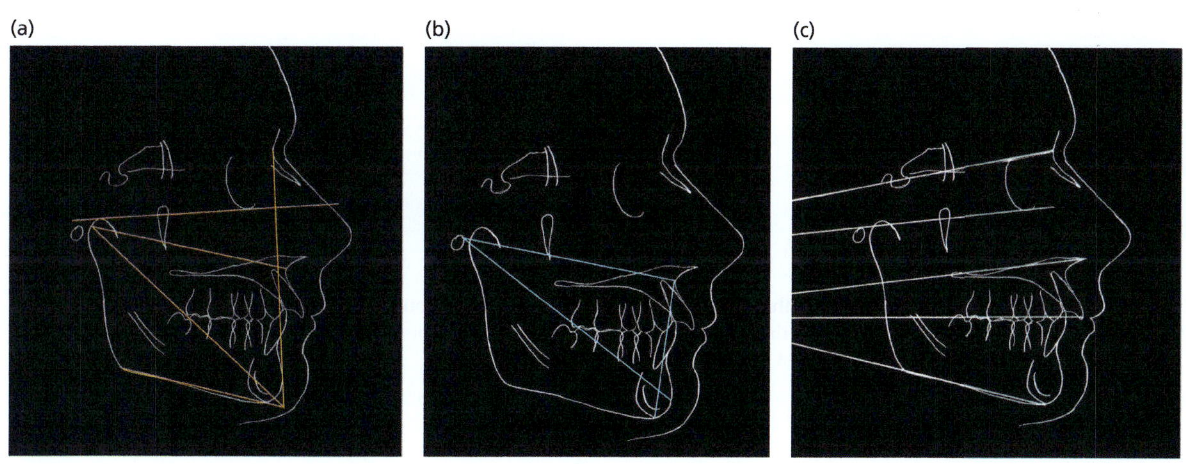

Fig. 32-8 (a) McNamara analysis; (b) Harvold analysis; (c) Sassouni analysis.

(a) (b)

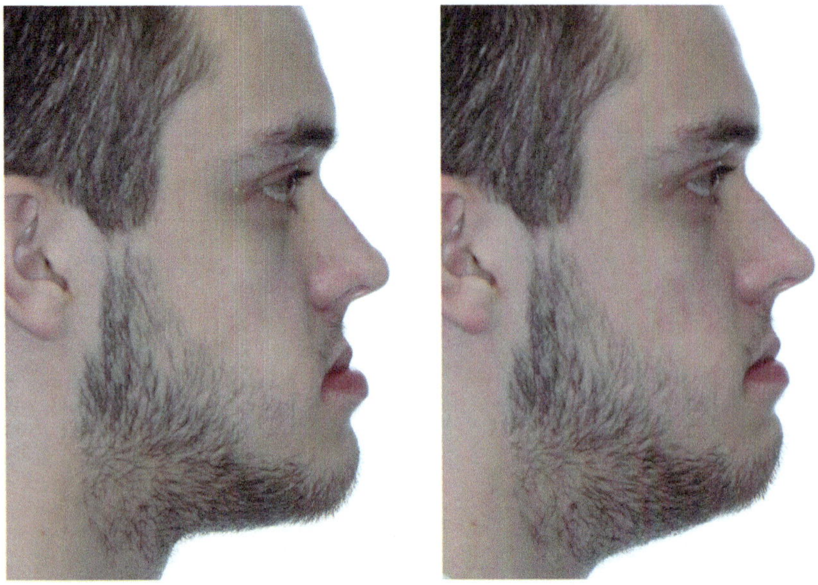

Fig. 32-9 Profile views of Class III deep bite malocclusion with (a) the teeth in maximum intercuspation and (b) the mandible rotated open to the rest position maintained with a wax wafer; the lateral cephalometric radiograph and profile photograph were recorded in this position for surgical planning.

(a) (b) (c) (d)

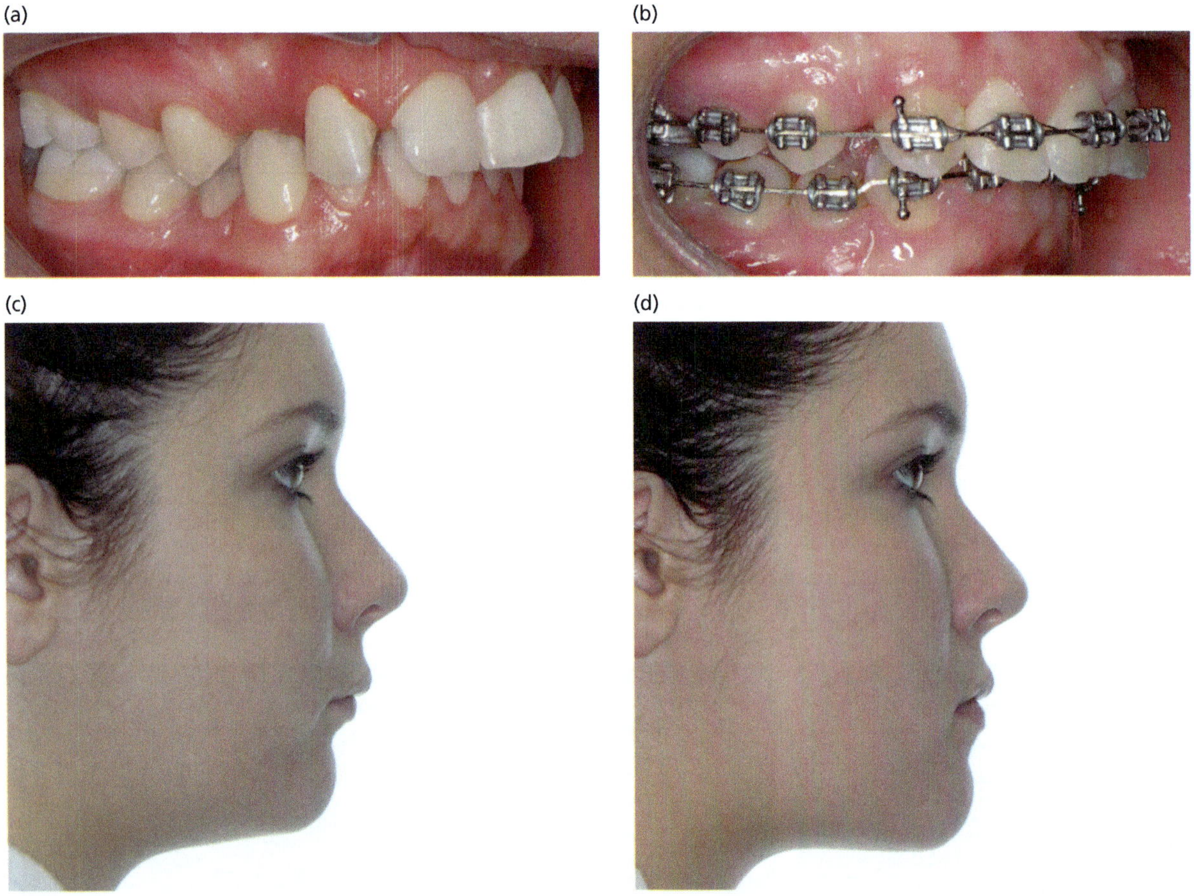

Fig. 32-10 Class II division 1 malocclusion with deep bite and reduced LFH (a) Right buccal occlusion pre-treatment; (b) stepped 19 × 25 in stainless steel archwire to maintain the increased Curve of Spee; (c) Profile pre-treatment and (d) with the mandible postured to Class I incisor relationship to assist surgical planning.

Table 32-3 Implications of lower face height for levelling the lower arch in Class II deep bite cases

Lower face height	Distance from lower incisal edge to base of chin	Implication for levelling the lower arch
Short	Normal or increased	Continuous arch mechanics with increased Curve of Spee, or set-up bend to incisors, in steel archwires. Extrude posterior teeth *post-surgery.*
Normal	Increased	Intrude incisors using sectional (anterior and posterior segments separately) arch mechanics *pre-surgically* or rarely by subapical osteotomy

anterior-posterior and vertical positions and coordinate arch widths. The incisor positions govern the amount the mandible can be moved forward, and determine the face height post-surgically. The desired final face height determines the decision to level an increased curve of Spee by incisor intrusion or premolar extrusion (Table 32-3).

Where the overbite is deep, usually from an excessive curve of Spee in the lower arch and sometimes an additional reverse curve in the upper arch, this must be levelled to allow an optimal occlusal result. Levelling by extrusion is done post-surgically using continuous arches whereas levelling by intrusion is accomplished pre-surgically and is best achieved using segmented arch mechanics. As levelling the lower arch moves the incisors labially, premolar extractions are often required especially when a marked curve of Spee exists in conjunction with incisor crowding. Rarely upper premolar extractions are required to provide space for incisor retraction as this is forthcoming from lateral arch expansion necessary for arch coordination with the mandible advanced. In the adult, maintenance of intermolar orthodontic expansion of more than 4 mm is unlikely and surgically assisted expansion may be required to give the best buccal segment occlusion. In Class III deep bite cases, upper first with or without lower second premolar extractions may be required to effect the desired decompensatory movements (Figure 32-11).

Upper and lower labial edgewise fixed appliances with an 018-inch or 022-inch slot are required; a self-ligating system that allows full size rectangular wire

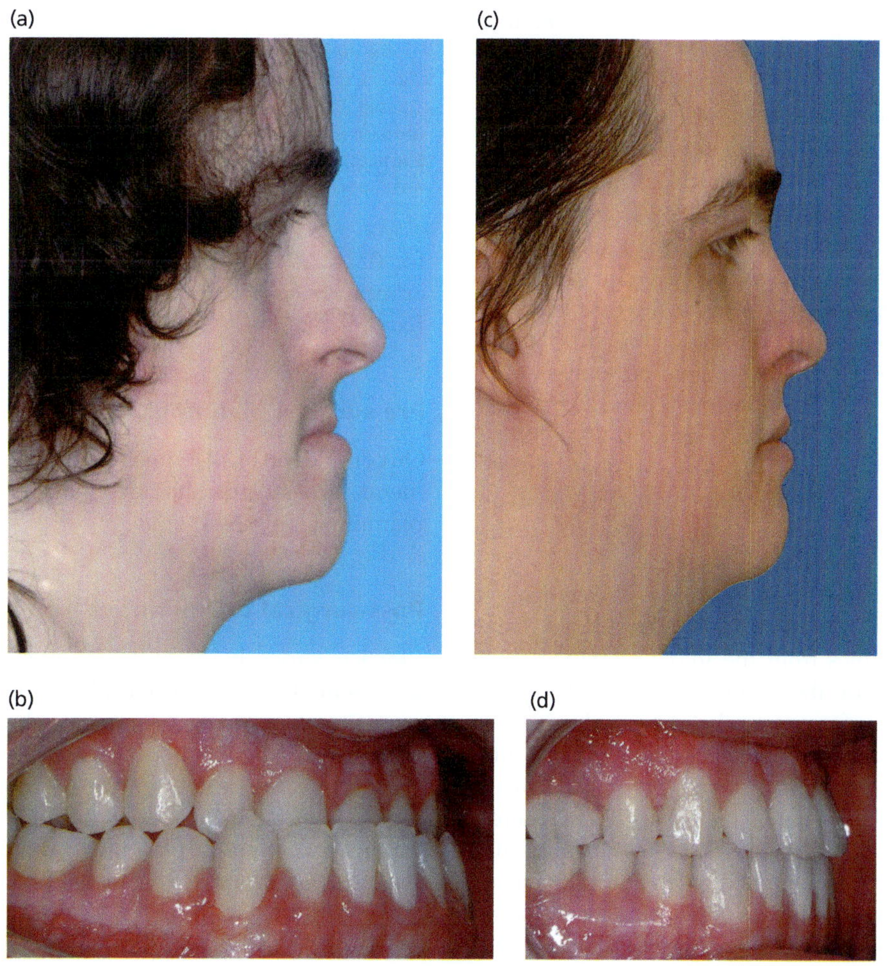

Fig. 32-11 Class III malocclusion with deep bite treated by Le Fort I osteotomy to move the maxilla forward and down with interpositional bone graft and slight BSSO mandibular setback. Pre-treatment (a) Profile and (b) Right buccal occlusion. Post-treatment (c) Profile and (d) Right buccal occlusion.

engagement for stabilization is an acceptable alternative. Bands, rather than bonded tubes, should be used on molars with buccal tubes for auxiliary archwires and welded lingual/palatal attachments to allow for elastic use post-operatively. Fully bonded appliances, however, are required for the periodontally involved dentition. Metallic, rather than ceramic, brackets are preferred due to the risk of bracket fracture with ceramics; if ceramic brackets are used, they should be confined to the upper labial segment. Brackets with integrated hooks may be considered for orthodontic elastic attachment, but attaching surgical hooks to the archwires will be required in preparation for the surgeon to place temporary intermaxillary fixation intraoperatively. Although, Invisalign or lingual appliances may be used for pre-surgical orthodontics, some form of labial attachment will have to be placed for surgery (see Chapter 12).

Where decompensation requires retroclination of the lower incisors and proclination of the upper incisors, the MBT prescriptions may confer some advantages over an alternative due to the –6° of lingual crown torque in the lower incisors and the increased palatal root torque in the upper incisors. If anterior segmental surgery is planned, space needed for the surgical cuts between the canines and premolars can be created by using contralateral canine brackets in the same arch to reverse the tip. Following surgery, however, they should be replaced in the correct position.

Initial alignment usually commences with a superelastic nickel titanium archwire with the specific choice of diameter depending on the degree of crowding. Because for most Class II patients, lower arch levelling will be accomplished by extrusion post-surgery, subsequent round and rectangular steel archwires should be flat in the upper arch but with an increased curve of Spee in the lower. Arch coordination and final anteroposterior incisor positioning should be completed on heavier archwires with the lower stepped to maintain the increased curve of Spee (Figure 32-10d). Where applicable, it is advisable to leave a small amount (1–2 mm) of lower premolar extraction spaces to avoid shifting the lower incisor position forward during post-surgical levelling.

When *pre-surgical incisor intrusion* is required to level the arches, this should be carried out using sectional mechanics from the initial alignment with separate wires for the anterior and posterior segments; intrusive forces can be delivered using an auxiliary depressing archwire. Alternatively a utility arch which pits the incisors versus the molars, avoiding the buccal segment teeth, may be considered. Palatal and/or lingual arches or bone anchors may be required for anchorage reinforcement. When levelling has been achieved, continuous heavier archwires are used to finalise the anteroposterior incisor positioning and coordinate the arches with closure of any premolar extraction spaces. Directly prior to surgery, rigid stainless steel archwires (usually 019 × 025 in for 022 in slot) should be placed with attachments, crimped or soldered, for intraoperative intermaxillary fixation.

Table 32-4 Records required for pre-surgical planning

Records	
Radiographs[a]	Lateral cephalometric film[a1] Panoramic film PA-cephalometric film (if asymmetry present or narrow maxilla) Periapicals of interdental osteotomy areas CBCT if jaw asymmetry to be corrected
Clinical photographs[a]	Facial (profile, $\frac{3}{4}$ profile, full-face (at rest and with natural smile) and intra-oral (anterior, right and left buccal occlusion, upper and lower occlusal) views
Upper and lower impressions[a] with/ without facebow record[b]	For model surgery and surgical occlusal wafer construction[c]

CBCT, Cone-beam computed tomography.

[a]A cone beam CT scan, 3D stereophotogrammetric facial images and intra-oral scans of the dentition (or digital images of the dental casts) may be used for 3D surgical planning[35,39] (see Chapter 8)

[a]Taken 1–2 weeks pre-surgery after removal of passive stabilizing archwires (should have been in place for ≥4 weeks). [b] Required to mount casts on semi-adjustable articulator if maxillary surgery planned but not necessary for mandibular surgery only.

[c]Where the lower arch is to be levelled post-surgically, *the wafer*: will be thicker in the premolar area than elsewhere; it should also be trimmed to facilitate oral hygiene and mandibular excursive movements, be as slim as possible but not fragile and be constructed with the mandibular cast advanced symmetrically to the agreed occlusion[a1].

[a1]Using the lateral cephalometric radiograph and digital profile image or CBCT, surgical movements can be simulated and the profile effects assessed. The final agreed plan is carried out on the models (or using CBCT) and reviewed preferably by the orthodontist and the surgeon before wafer construction. If necessary, minor adjustments may be incorporated in the wafer to allow for subsequent restorative treatment.

Pre-surgical planning

On completion of all requisite orthodontic tooth movements, full records should be taken for pre-surgical planning (Table 32-4).

Post-surgical orthodontics

Practice varies between teams regarding the need to retain the final occlusal wafer in the early post-operative period.[34] It is reasonable, however, that it be kept until the patient is reviewed on a combined clinic one-week post-surgery. An exception would be if the wafer is being used to hold surgical maxillary expansion, although placement of a 1 mm stainless steel expansion arch in theatre eliminates its need. Soft diet is recommended for 6–8 weeks, with gradual jaw exercises advised from 1 week post-surgery gradually increasing the range of motion from opening and closing to lateral excursions, so that by 2 months optimal jaw function has returned.

At one week post-surgery, it is customary to check the occlusion having removed the elastics supporting the surgical and occlusal correction and the removable wafer, if such was used. If the wafer is ligated in situ, there should be a consistent and reliable path of closure with no mandibular displacement. Medium strength elastics should then be worn during the healing phase for the next 6 weeks or so. Minor occlusal corrections can be made by adjusting the direction and force of the elastics applied. When healing is satisfactory, post-surgical orthodontics may begin. This phase aims to idealise the occlusion and is typically complete in 4–6 months. What follows relates primarily to Class II deep bite correction. Slight modifications will be necessary for Class I and Class III cases but the guiding principles remain the same.

Where the lower arch is to be levelled post-mandibular advancement surgery, there is normally only occlusal contact on the incisors and on a single terminal molar on each side, a so-called 'three-point landing'. These lateral open bites may be accompanied by a minor crossbite tendency, affecting the buccal segment teeth. In some cases, there may be residual extraction spaces in the lower arch following pre-surgical levelling. Not surprisingly due to the surgical trauma and reduced jaw activity, maximal bite force is reduced post-surgery but steadily increases over the first post-operative year.[40,41]

Where levelling is to be undertaken by extrusion, the rigid stabilizing archwires *must* be changed to working wires to commence occlusal settling; this may be simultaneous with wafer removal, if appropriate or may proceed seamlessly from a period of wear of lighter weight elastics only. Specifically, the selection of wires is determined by the nature and magnitude of tooth movement required. Often this means with near full size rectangular TMA in the maxillary arch and round 016-inch stainless steel in the mandibular arch. To assist with lateral open bite closure, light box elastics should be worn between the buccal segment teeth fulltime initially then gradually reducing to night only before stopping usually by the third month (see Chapter 12). The elastics should be directed to support the anteroposterior correction and should not be withdrawn until the teeth have settled into a reliable occlusion. Where a crossbite tendency exists, an expanded auxiliary stainless steel wire (036 or 040-inch) may be placed in the headgear tubes and tied loosely anteriorly between the central and lateral incisors; this may be placed with the usual flexible archwires and settling elastics. Rectangular steel archwires may be necessary for final detailing.

Retention

Following appliance removal, retention follows on similar lines to that of non-surgical deep bite cases. In Class II deep bite cases, an upper Hawley retainer incorporating a flat anterior bite plane and a lower vacuum formed retainer to be worn at night only long term, would be advisable. For Class I and Class III deep bite cases, upper and lower vacuum formed retainers will likely suffice, again with long-term wear at night recommended. If, however, surgical maxillary expansion was undertaken and a transpalatal arch adapted to all teeth fitted post-surgically during the completion of orthodontic treatment, this should remain in situ for the first postoperative year.[28] Otherwise full-time wear of a palate covering Hawley retainer for at least six months is advisable before moving onto long-term, part-time wear. With the skeletal and dental relationships achieved, final restorative and prosthetic treatment can be completed. Retainers may need to be modified or replaced to adapt for definitive restorative care.

Post-surgical review is recommended at 1, 2 and 5 years with appropriate clinical records taken at each stage to facilitate audit and research. A different recall schedule will be required to monitor any post-surgical complications.

Surgical aspects

Means of surgical correction to increase lower anterior face height in the Class II mandibular deficient patient are given in Table 32-5 along with those considered for low angle Class I and Class III correction. Details regarding the surgical procedures are provided in the relevant chapters of this book. For all surgical procedures, it is sensible to bear in mind that a moderately short face is preferred over a 'long' face.[42,43] To err on the side of a shorter than normal face may be, therefore, preferable to making the lower face excessively tall. Mandibular third molars should be removed a minimum of 6 months before surgery as they normally occupy the best site for placement of screws required for rigid internal fixation.

A bilateral sagittal split osteotomy (BSSO) to advance and rotate the mandible down anteriorly is the customary surgical means to address mandibular deficiency. Because with short face patients, the position of the chin needs careful consideration, it may be necessary to move the chin straight down in addition to mandibular advancement. This increases anterior face height by rotating the mandible within the ramus and moves the chin down; as the gonial angle moves up, this relaxes the elevator muscles. To *decrease chin prominence*, a simultaneous osseous genioplasty may be required. A subapical advancement is indicated when face height is only slightly short and overbite mildly increased with a prominent chin. It is less common that it would be deemed necessary to move the maxilla inferiorly to address a short face problem. As inferior movement of the posterior maxilla stretches the pterygomasseteric sling and creates instability, where maxillary incisor visibility is desired, the maxilla should be rotated so that inferior movement is confined solely to the incisors. Typically, where maxillary deficiency exists with a short face mandibular deficiency, bimaxillary surgery is required which in effect

Table 32-5 Surgical procedures that may be considered for correction of low angle Class II mandibular deficiency, Class I and Class III low angle cases

	Surgical procedure	Comments
Class II	Bilateral sagittal split osteotomy (BSSO) to advance the mandible (Figure 32-12)	Intra-oral approach Allows mandibular lengthening and increase in LFH Minimal alteration in mandibular musculature length Compatible with RIF Predictable outcome
Class II	Inferior border osteotomy ('sliding genioplasty') and BSSO May be modified to allow vertical chin augmentation with or without interpositional bone graft (Figure 32-13)	Provides additional mandibular length Controls for excessive a-p or vertical chin prominence Predictable outcome to improve lip function and aesthetics; 1:1 ratio of soft tissue changes to bony advancement; highly stable long-term with RF Improves chin-neck contour as tightens suprahyoid musculature Mental nerve trauma possible and lateral border 'notching', especially with >5 mm advancements
Class II	Inferior border osteotomy and BSSO with alloplastic chin augmentation	Rarely indicated Large chin and deficient LL, a-p reduction of inferior border may improve lip function but requires augmentation to improve aesthetic outcome
Class II	Total subapical mandibular advancement osteotomy (see Chapter 39)	Where limited advancement required; facilitates differential advancement of dentoalveolar segment; flattens labiomental sulcus with relative reduction in chin projection; reduces need for genioplasty
Class II	Extra-oral approach to mandibular advancement	Significant asymmetry present Mandibular lengthening >12 mm required
Class II	Distraction osteogenesis	Large asymmetric mandibular advancement required usually in syndromic patient
Class II	Maxillary surgery with mandibular advancement (Figure 32-14)	Mainly SARPE to widen maxilla (>4 mm expansion required) Le Fort I to rotate maxilla down anteriorly but not posteriorly when greater UI visibility relative to UL required*
Class II	Anterior mandibular/maxillary segmental osteotomy (Figure 32-15)	Sets down lower labial segment where excessive curve of Spee and decompensation to correct LI axial inclination not possible; facilitates a-p movement of mandible Sets up upper labial segment where VME with 'gummy smile'
Class II	Mandibulotomy (Figure 32-15)	Allows movement of lower anterior segment *and* lower border of mandible where risk of incisor root damage by short mandibular anterior height; similar uses to anterior segmental osteotomy (see above)
Class II	Inferior border osteotomy with interpositional bone graft alone	Only possible where camouflage has produced acceptable outcome for Class II malocclusion and vertical deficiency mild Allows vertical and/or a-p repositioning of chin to improve profile
Class I	Downward repositioning of maxilla with interpositional graft*	Vertical maxillary deficiency
Class III	Le Fort I osteotomy** alone to move maxilla down and forward	Vertical maxillary deficiency Also rotates mandible down and back, often eliminates need for mandibular surgery
Class III	Le Fort I osteotomy** to move maxilla down and forward with BSSO set back (Figure 32-11)	Vertical maxillary deficiency and mandibular excess

LFH, Lower Facial Height; RIF, Rigid Internal Fixation; a-p, antero-posterior; RF, Rigid Fixation; LL, Lower Lip; SARPE, Surgically Assisted Rapid Palatal Expansion; UI, Upper Incisor; UL, Upper Lip; LI, Lower Incisor; VME, Vertical Maxillary Excess; *Provided UL height within normal limits, maxilla should be moved down so 2–4 mm of UIs are visible at rest, keeping ≥ 2–3 mm freeway space. Consequent mandibular rotation will lessen chin prominence but chin repositioning with/without adjunctive surgery to the submental-cervical area possibly required for optimal facial aesthetics. **UI exposure at rest and on smiling determines amount maxilla is positioned inferiorly.

rotates both the maxillary and mandibular occlusal planes (Figure 32-14; see Chapter 31); this improves facial contours and smile aesthetics by reducing gonial angle prominence and optimizes labial positioning of the maxillary and mandibular dentitions.

Maxillary downgraft or mandibular subapical osteotomy that elongates the mandibular posterior teeth produces a downward and backward rotation of the mandible. The strong biting forces in short face subjects tend to lead to overbite relapse following a subapical osteotomy to advance the mandibular dentition (see Chapter 39). Where extrusion of the posterior teeth is used to increase face height, this tends to be lost to some extent in the settling phase.[1]

Where severe mandibular deficiency exists, a habit of posturing the mandible forward may become established. This may compromise the surgeon's ability to seat the condyles properly during surgery which in

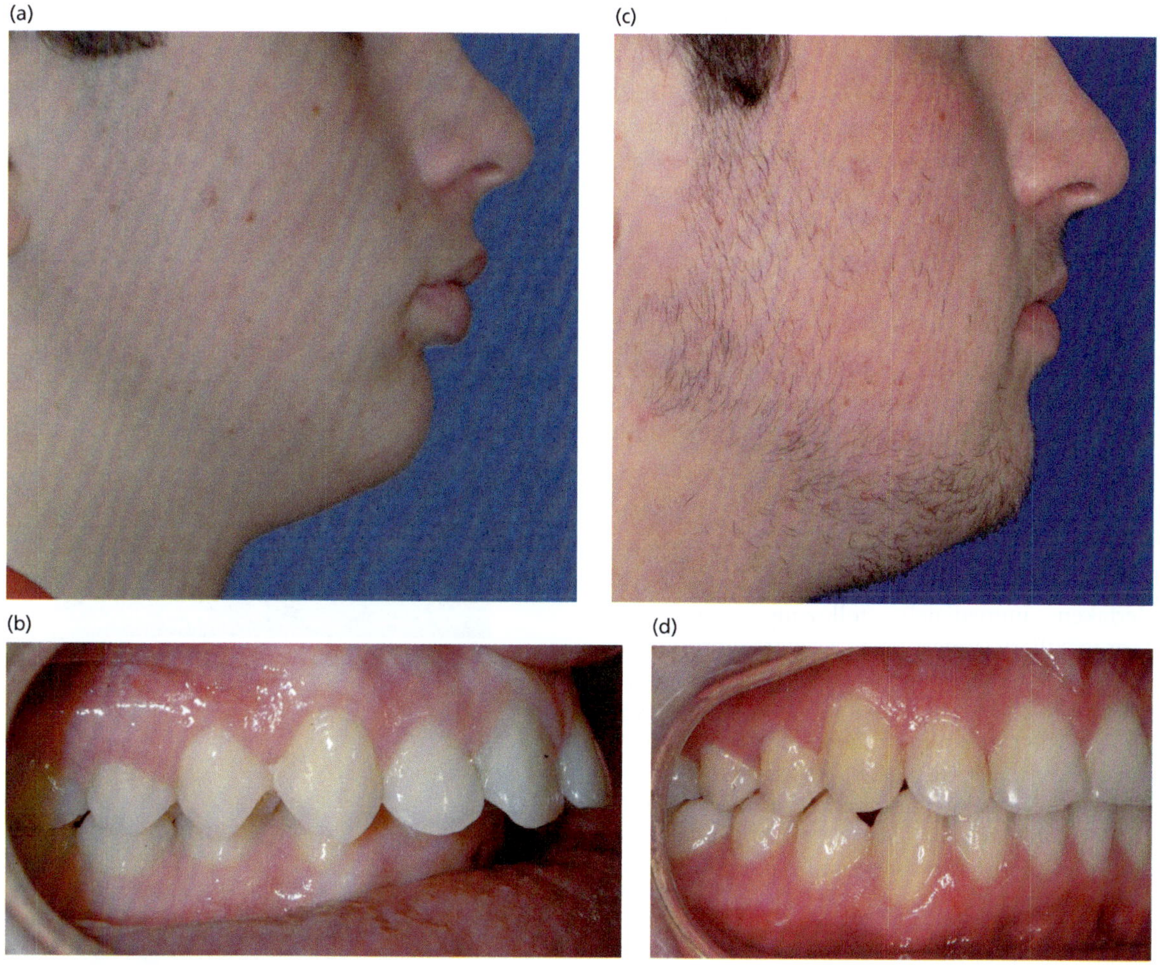

Fig. 32-12 Class II Division 1 malocclusion with reduced LFH and deep bite treated by BSSO mandibular advancement. Pre-treatment (a) Profile and (b) Right buccal occlusion. Post-treatment (c) Profile and (d) Right buccal occlusion.

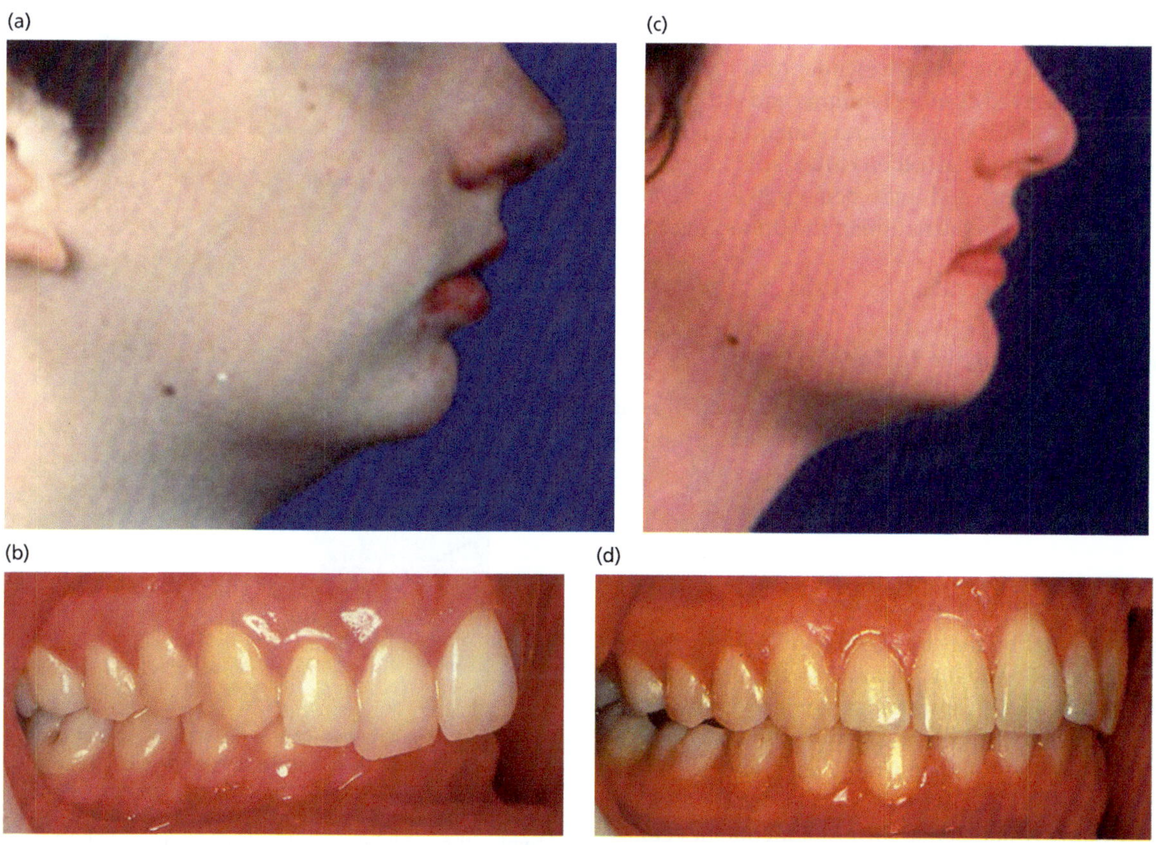

Fig. 32-13 Class II division 2 malocclusion with reduced LFH and deep traumatic overbite treated by BSSO mandibular advancement and genioplasty to increase LFH. Pre-treatment (a) Profile and (b) Right buccal occlusion. Post-treatment (c) Profile and (d) Right buccal occlusion.

turn will compromise the occlusal outcome; this must be explained to the patient pre-operatively. Splint therapy to establish centric condylar relation has been advised 4–6 weeks prior to surgery and1to eliminate any mandibular postural habit.[32]

Adjunctive procedures

Aside from genioplasty (see Table 32-5), several procedures may be performed to further enhance the soft tissue profile changes obtained with orthognathic surgery.

Rhinoplasty

Undertaken immediately following mandibular and/or maxillary surgery, or as a separate procedure, rhinoplasty may adjust the dorsal contour, tip shape or alar base width to provide optimal chin-nose balance.[27] The relative prominence of the nose may, however, have been reduced by an increase in lower facial height. This can be checked using the Rees aesthetic plane, which joins the nasal tip and the upper lip in profile view and should pass on or near skeletal pogonion.[46]

Mandibular re-contouring

In the East Asian female population, mandibular recontouring procedures have been employed to convert a square face with low gonial angle (perceived as coarse and unattractive) to a slender oval lower facial contour (perceived as more feminine and attractive).[47] Three sets of surgical procedures – mandibular V-line ostectomy, mandibular outer cortex split ostectomy, sliding genioplasty and inlay bone graft – have been used depending on the nature of the presenting facial features.[48]

Implants to improve facial contours

Where paranasal deficiency exists, onlay grafts using the patient's bone, freeze-dried cadaveric bone or alloplastic materials may increase soft tissue fullness and improve facial contours.

Lip and submental procedures

Lip augmentation may be carried out to improve projection and is normally separate to the orthognathic surgery. In cases of 'gummy smile', lip 'lengthening' with V-Y closure of the incision of the muco-buccal fold and lip mucosa may be considered. Although mandibular advancement and forward sliding genioplasty improve submental form, submental lipectomy and platsyma lift may be necessary when the submental tissues show sagging in older adults.

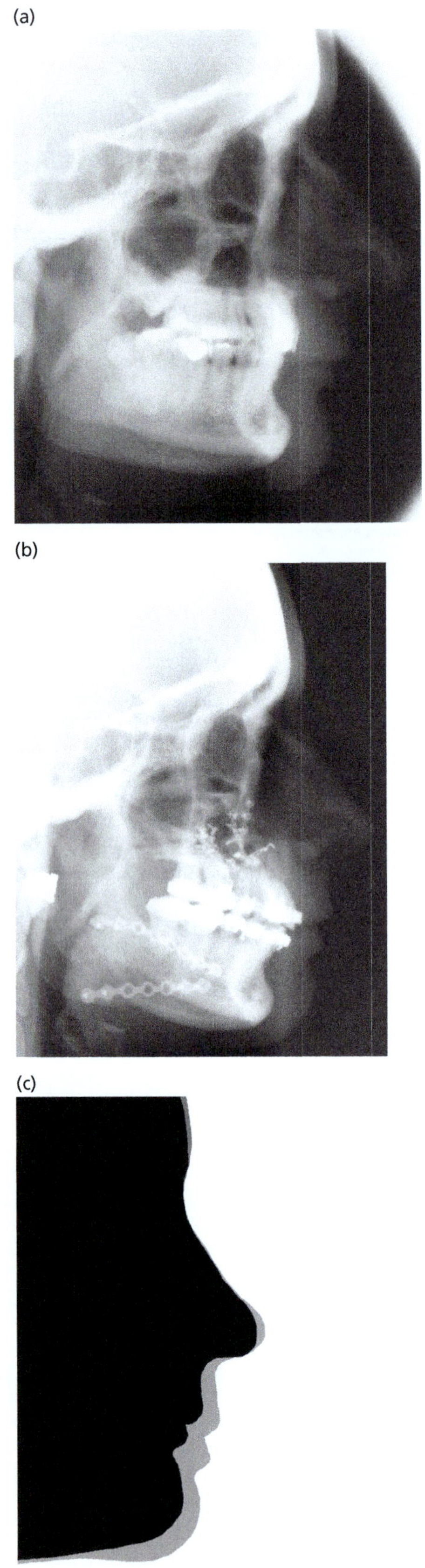

Fig. 32-14 Cephalometric films (a) Pre-treatment and (b) Post-treatment with profile superimposition (c) of a Class II division 2 malocclusion with deficient upper incisor show and reduced LFH treated by Le Fort I advancement and downfracture with interpositional bone graft and BSSO mandibular advancement.

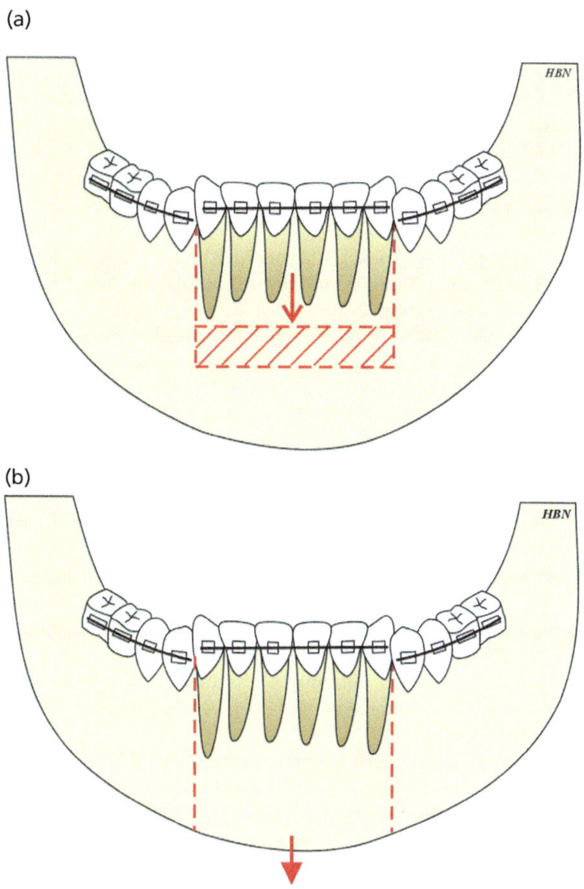

Fig. 32-15 Diagrammatic representation of (a) lower labial segment setdown subapical osteotomy and (b) mandibulotomy. Reprinted with permission from Naini FB, Gill DS, Sharma A, Tredwin C. The aetiology, diagnosis and management of deep overbite. Dental Update 2006;33:326–36.[44,45]

Post-surgical stability and evidence of effectiveness

Several factors including patient age, condylar positioning, extent of advancement, mandibular plane angle, residual mandibular growth, muscular and soft tissue forces and surgical skill influence relapse. In the short- and long-terms, moving the mandible forward with BSSO when the anterior facial height is maintained or increased seems very effective,[49,50] but appears less stable than BSSO set-back.[51] In the short term, skeletal stability is similar with bicortical screws (titanium, stainless steel, bioresorbable) or miniplates.[50] Assessed at point B cephalometrically, short–term relapse of BSSO with miniplate rigid internal fixation varied from 1.5–18% whereas long-term relapse was 1.5–8.9%.[51] Horizontal relapse is more likely with advancements of 6 to 7 mm and vertical relapse is greater with low mandibular planes angle.[52]

Greatest stability exists when the soft tissue stretch created by mandibular advancement is minimized by upward rotation of the mandible at the gonial angle and downward at the chin. Downward movement of the maxilla that results in downward and backward movement of the mandible is, however, problematic, but can be overcome somewhat by BSSO set-back which reduces occlusal forces applied to the maxilla by the mandible during closing. Interpositional grafting with hydroxyapatite increases the rigidity of the downgrafted maxilla and is currently the preferred method.[52] Both rigid and slow to remodel due to its internal structure, there are few postoperative problems.[53] Where SARPE is required, this is the least stable orthognathic procedure because of stretching of the inelastic palatal mucosa (see Chapters 18 and 36).

Due to the primarily retrospective nature of the studies undertaken on mandibular advancement BSSO and their inferior design coupled with the lack of standardized outcome measures, robust data are still lacking on both short-and long-term soft tissue profile changes.[51] Prospective or randomized clinical trials of short-term and long-term outcomes of BSSO advancement with rigid internal fixation excluding genioplasty or maxillary surgery are required.

Acknowledgements

Ms Niamh Kelly is thanked for her valued assistance with the figures and bibliography. The support of Dr S. McMorrow, Dr D. Morris, Dr E. Salloum, Dr D. Counihan, Dr T. McSwiney, Dr A. Downing and Dr F. Naini with clinical images and illustrations is gratefully appreciated.

References

1 Turley PK. Orthodontic management of the short face patient. Semin Orthod. 1996;2:138–53.
2 Bjork A. Facial growth in man studies with the aid of metallic implants. Acta Odontol Scand. 1955;13:9–54.
3 Turley PK. An American Board of Orthodontics case report. The surgical-orthodontic management of a Class I malocclusion with excessive overbite and periodontal bone loss. Am J Orthod Dentofacial Orthop. 1993;104:402–10.
4 Lobbezoo E, Ahlberg J, Manfredini D, Winocour. Are bruxism and the bite causally related? J Oral Rehab. 2012;39:489–501.
5 John MT, Hirsch C, Drangsholt MT, Mancl LA, Setz JM. Overbite and overjet are not related to self-report of temperomandibular disorder symptoms. J Dent Res. 2002;91:164–9.
6 Sonnensen L, Svensson P. Temperomandibular disorders and psychological status in adult patients with deep bite. Eur J Orthod. 2008;30:621–9.
7 Sonnensen L, Kjaer I. Cervical vertebral body fusions in patients with skeletal deep bite. Eur J Orthod. 2007;29:464–70.
8 Ricketts RM. A foundation for cephalometric communication. Am J Orthod. 1960;46:330–57.
9 Steiner CC. Cephalometrics for you and me. Am J Orthod. 1953;39:729–55.
10 Holdaway RA. A soft tissue cephalometric analysis and its use in orthodontic treatment planning. Part 1. Am J Orthod. 1983;84:1–28.
11 Vig RG, Brundo GC. The kinetics of anterior tooth display. J Prosthet Dent. 1978;39:502–4.
12 McNamara JA. A method of cephalometric evaluation. Am J Orthod. 1984;86:449–69.
13 Harvold EP. The Activator in Orthodontics. St Louis: The CV Mosby Co., 1974.
14 Sassouni V. A roentgenographic cephalometric analysis of cephalo-facio-dental relationships. Am J Orthod. 1955;41:735–64.

15 Horn A. Facial height index. Am J Orthod Dentofacial Orthop. 1992;102:180–6.
16 Broadbent BH Sr, Broadbent BH Jr, Golden WH. Bolton Standards of Dentofacial Developmental Growth. St Louis: Mosby, 1975.
17 Cooke MS, Wei SH. The reproducibility of natural head posture: a methodological study. Am J Orthod Dentofacial Orthop. 1988;93:280–8.
18 Downs WB. Analysis of the dentofacial profile. Angle Orthod. 1956;26:509–19.
19 Naini FB. The Frankfort plane and head positioning in facial aesthetic analysis – The perpetuation of a myth. JAMA Facial Plast Surg. 2013;15:333–4.
20 Luther F, Layton S, McDonald F. Orthodontics for treating temporomandibular joint (TMJ) disorders. Cochrane Database Syst Rev. 2010; Jul 7:CD006541.
21 Sciote JJ, Rowlerson AM, Hopper C, Hunt NP. Fibre type classification and myosin isoforms in the human masseter muscle. J Neurol Sci. 1994;126:15–24.
22 Hunt N, Shah R, Sinanan A, Lewis M. Northcroft Memorial Lecture 2005: muscling in on malocclusions: current concepts on the role of muscles in the aetiology and treatment of malocclusion. J Orthod. 2006;33:187–97.
23 Wessberg GA, Epker BN. Surgical inferior repositioning of the maxilla: Treatment considerations and comprehensive management. J Oral Surg Oral Med Oral Path. 1981;52:349–56.
24 Nasry HA, Barclay SC. Periodontal lesions associated with deep traumatic overbite. Br Dent J. 2006;200:557–61.
25 Joss-Vassalli I, Grebenstein C, Topouzelis N, Sculean A, Katsaros C. Orthodontic therapy and gingival recession: a systematic review. Orthod Craniofac Res. 2010;13:127–41.
26 Flores-Mir C. Does orthodontic treatment lead to gingival recession? Evid-Based Dent. 2011;12:20.
27 Proffit WR, White RP. Surgical-Orthodontic Treatment. St Louis: Mosby, 1991.
28 Proffit WR, Fields HW. Contemporary Orthodontics (3rd Ed.) St Louis: Mosby, 1999.
29 Naini FB. Facial Aesthetics: Concepts and Clinical Diagnosis. Oxford: Wiley-Blackwell, 2011.
30 Bhatia SN, Leighton BC. A Manual of Facial Growth: a Computer analysis of Longitudinal Cephalometric Growth Data. Oxford: Oxford University Press, 1993.
31 Riolo M, Moyers RE, McNamara J, Hunter WS. An Atlas of Craniofacial Growth. Ann Arbor, MI: University of Michigan Centre for Human Growth and Development, 1974.
32 Watted N, Bill JS, Witt EA. therapeutic concept for the combined orthodontic surgical correction of angle Class II deformities with short-face syndrome: surgical lengthening of the lower face. Clin Orthod Res. 2000;3:78–93.
33 Zachrisson BU. Aesthetics factors involved in anterior tooth display and the smile: vertical dimension. J Clin Orthod. 1998;32:432–45.
34 Ayoub A, Khambay B, Benington P, Green L, Moos K, Walker F. Handbook of Orthognathic Treatment – A team approach. Oxford: Wiley-Blackwell, 2013.
35 Smith JD, Thomas PM, Proffit WR. A comparison of current prediction imaging programs.Am J Orthod Dentofacial Orthop. 2004;125:527–36.
36 Phillips C, Kiyak HA, Bloomquist D, Turvey TA. Perceptions of recovery and satisfaction in the short term after orthognathic surgery. J Oral Maxillofac Surg. 2004;62:535–44.
37 Swennen GR, Mollemans W, Schutyser F. Three-dimensional treatment planning of orthognathic surgery in the era of virtual imaging J Oral Maxillofac Surg. 2009;67:2080–92.
38 Popat H, Richmond S, Drage NA. New developments in: three-dimensional planning for orthognathic surgery. J Orthod. 2010;37:62–71.
39 Cevidanes LHC, Tucker S, Styner M, Kim H, Chapuis J, Reyes M, et al. Three-dimensional surgical simulation. Am J Orthod Dentofacial Orthop. 2010;138:361–71.
40 Hunt NP, Cunningham SJ. The influence of orthognathic surgery on occlusal force in patients with vertical facial deformities. Int J Oral Maxillofac Surg. 1997;26:87–91.
41 Grunheid T, Langenbach GEJ, Korfage JAM, Zentner A, van Eijden TMGJ. The adaptive response of jaw muscles to varying functional demands. Eur J Orthod. 2009;31:596–612.
42 Johnston DJ, Hunt O, Johnston CD, Burden DJ, Stevenson M, Hepper P. The influence of lower face vertical proportion on facial attractiveness Eur J Orthod. 2005;27:349–54.
43 Naini FB, Cobourne MT, McDonald F, Donaldson AN. The influence of craniofacial to standing height proportion on perceived attractiveness. Int J Oral Maxillofac Surg. 2008;37:877–85.
44 Naini FB, Gill DS, Sharma A, Tredwin C. The aetiology, diagnosis and management of deep overbite. Dental Update 2006;33:326–36.
45 Naini FB. Deep overbite malocclusion. In: Gill DS, Naini FB (Eds.). Orthodontics: Principles and Practice. Oxford: Wiley-Blackwell, 2011.
46 Rees TD. Aesthetic Plastic Surgery. Vol 2. Toronto: WB Saunders, 1980.
47 Hsu Y-C, Li J, Hu J, Luo E, Hsu MS, Zhu S. Correction of square jaw with low angles using mandibular 'V-line' ostectomy combined with outer cortex ostectomy. Oral Surg Oral Med Oral Path Oral Radiol Endod. 2010;109: 197–202.
48 Li J, Hsu Y, Khadka A, Hu J, Wang Q, Wang D. Surgical designs and techniques for mandibular contouring based on categorisation of square face with low gonial angle in orientals. J Plast Reconstruct Surg. 2012;65:e1–e8.
49 Proffit WR, Turvey TA, Phillips C. The hierarchy of stability and predictability of orthognathic surgery with rigid fixation: an update and extension. Head Face Med. 2007;3:21.
50 Joss CU, Vassalli IM. Stability after bilateral sagittal split osteotomy advancement surgery with rigid internal fixation. J Oral Maxillofac Surg. 2009;67:301–13.
51 Joss CU, Joss-Vassalli IM, Kiliaridis S, Kuijpers-Jagtman AM. Soft tissue profile changes after bilateral sagittal split osteotomy for mandibular advancement: a systematic review. J Oral Maxillofac Surg. 2010;68:1260–9.
52 Rosen H. Aesthetic refinements in genioplasty: the role of the labio-mental fold. Plast Reconstruct Surg. 1991;88: 760–7.
53 Wolford LM, Moenning JE. Diagnosis and treatment planning for mandibular subapical osteotomies with new surgical modifications. Oral Surg Oral Med Oral Pathol. 1989;68:541–50.

Chapter 33

Osseous Genioplasty

Ali Totonchi, Sima Molavi and Bahman Guyuron

Introduction

The position, shape, and size of the chin are determining factors of lower face aesthetics and the labiomental fold. Attention to this area is an integral part of any establishment of facial congruity. In this chapter, we will discuss the anatomy of the chin area and ways to evaluate a patient's lower face and make a proper plan of action to correct chin deformities.

Anatomy

Bone

The bony part of the chin includes the anterior part of the mandible and symphysis. The midline ridge is representative of fusion of the two halves of the foetal mandible; caudally, the ridge divides to enclose a triangular, raised area called the mental protuberance. Between the first and second premolar teeth lies the mental foramen. The lower border of the symphysis near the median raphe presents a small, roughened depression called the *digastric fossa*. Cephalad to the symphysis is the alveolar segment, which includes the front portion of the mandibular arch. The deepest socket in this area belongs to the canine, roughly 25.5 mm from the occlusal surface to the caudal end of the root (Figure 33-1).

Muscles

The muscles anterior to the chin:

- ***Depressor anguli oris*** (angularis) originates from the oblique line of the mandible. It converges into a narrow fasciculus, blending with other muscles at the angle of the mouth. This muscle draws the angle of the mouth caudally and laterally in expressions of sadness and when the mouth is opened. It is supplied by the marginal mandibular branch of the facial nerve.
- ***Depressor labii inferioris*** is a quadrilateral muscle arising from the oblique line of the mandible and inserts into the skin of the lower lip and depresses the lower lip, drawing it laterally in mastication. It is supplied by the marginal mandibular nerve.
- ***Mentalis muscle*** is shaped conically, arises from the incisive fossa of the mandible, and is attached to the skin over the chin. It elevates and protrudes the lower lip. It is supplied by the marginal mandibular nerve (Figure 33-2).

The muscles attached to the lingual aspect:

- ***Anterior belly of digastric*** extends anteriorly and attaches to the caudal margin of the mandibular symphysis, close to the middle. It is innervated through the mylohyoid branch of the inferior alveolar nerve. The posterior belly of the muscle is innervated by the facial nerve. It generally depresses the mandible and elevates and advances the hyoid bone.
- ***Mylohyoid*** is a flat, triangular, and comparatively thin muscle that attaches anteriorly to the mylohyoid line of the mandible. It locates deep to the

Orthognathic Surgery: Principles, Planning and Practice. Edited by Farhad B. Naini and Daljit S. Gill.

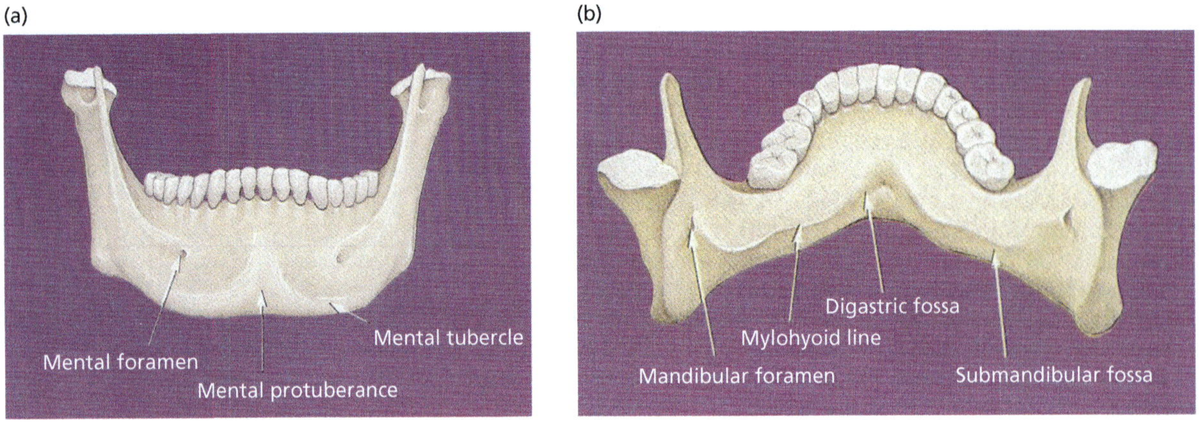

Fig. 33-1 Anterior and posterior view of the bony mandible. (From Genioplasty. Guyuron B. Little, Brown and Company, 1990.[3])

anterior belly of the digastric muscle and extends posteromedially, attaching to the inferior border of the hyoid bone. Mylohyoid receives its nerve supply from the mylohyoid branch of the third division of the trigeminal nerve. Its function is to elevate the floor of the mouth and raises and advances the hyoid bone to depress the mandible.

- ***Geniohyoid*** muscle is deep and located cephalad to the medial portion of mylohyoid. It extends from the inferior mental spine on the posterior aspect of the symphysis menti to the anterior surface of the body of the hyoid bone. It is innervated by the hypoglossal nerve through the first cervical spine nerve. It elevates the hyoid bone; when fixed, it depresses the mandible.
- ***Genioglossus*** is a triangular muscle that parallels the median plane. It originates from the upper genial tubercle and radiates in a fan fashion. The caudal fibres are attached by a thin aponeurosis to the cephalic part of the anterior surface of the body of the hyoid. The middle fibres pass posteriorly and the superior fibers pass upward and forward to enter the ventral surface of the tongue. This muscle protrudes the apex of the tongue from the mouth. Its motor nerve is a branch of the hypoglossal nerve (Figure 33-2).

Nerves

The inferior alveolar is a sensory nerve originating from the third division of the Trigeminal Nerve. It passes through the mandibular canal, exits from the mental foramen and terminals as the mental nerve. The mental nerve divides beneath the depressor anguli oris into three branches. One descends to the skin of the chin and two branches ascend to the skin and mucus membranes of the lower lip (Figure 33-3). Anterior cutaneous nerve of the neck is another source for sensory innervations of the chin. It arises from second and third cervical roots and encircles the posterior border of the sternocleidomastoid muscle cephaled to its midportion, then runs obliquely forward, deep to the external jugular vein toward the anterior border of the muscle. It divides beneath the platysma into ascending and descending branches. The ascending branch passes upward to the submandibular regions.

Blood supply

The labial branch of the facial artery is the major vascular supplier of the skin and muscle of the chin. The inferior alveolar artery is a branch of the maxillary artery and provides the primary supply to the bone.

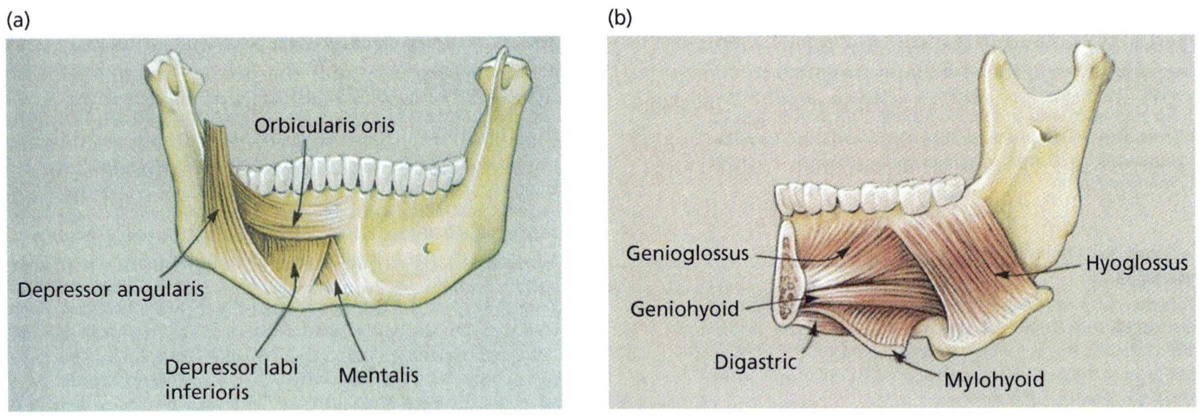

Fig. 33-2 Anterior and posterior view of chin muscles. (From Genioplasty. Guyuron B. Little, Brown and Company, 1990.[3])

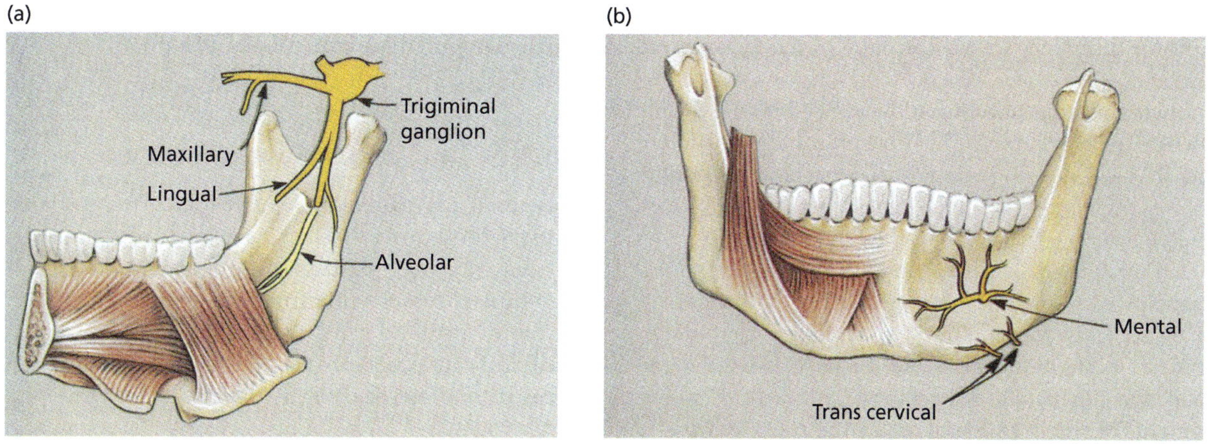

Fig. 33-3 Alveolar and mental nerves. (From Genioplasty. Guyuron B. Little, Brown and Company, 1990.[3])

It travels through the bone and mandibular canal and divides at the level of mental foramen. The periosteum and musculature attachments also provide some of the blood supply to the mandible. It is important to maintain these muscles in order to minimize the chance of avascular necrosis of the caudal segment when the inferior alveolar artery is interrupted (Figure 33-4).

Blood mostly drains to the labial, facial and external maxillary veins. It also drains through the mental vein to the pterygoid plexus, posterior and anterior facial veins and the jugular vein. Posteriorly, the chin drains through the ranine vein to the lingual vein.

Patient evaluation

Clinical examination

Evaluation of the patient starts with an extensive history and review of the patient's medical problems and past surgeries. Although we are not going to discuss the facial analysis in detail within this chapter (see Chapter 5), the entire face needs to be analyzed before focusing on the chin. The chin is defined by a graceful transition of the mandibular angles toward the midline. It results in a double light reflection in males and single light reflection in females. Both the examination and photographic analysis are used to evaluate chin deformities. The patient's entire face should be examined for any aesthetic imbalance. Either a simple chin asymmetry or a mandibular deformity can cause chin asymmetry. Upon examination of the lower face front view, the first part to note is the lips and commissural lineup. Except for facial paralysis, any distortion of commissural line usually indicates skeletal asymmetry. Therefore, genioplasty alone may not be an appropriate treatment. If the oral commissures are lined up horizontally and the occlusal plane is horizontal as well, but the chin is shifted, this asymmetry is considered an isolated chin deformity. However, a tilt of the oral commissure or occlusal plane or if the midline of the maxilla does not correspond to the midline of the mandible, would indicate a mandibular shift or maxillary–mandibular rotation. Again, it is critical to emphasize that while the underlying foundation is positioned abnormally, any surgery which only corrects the asymmetry of the chin will not result in an ideal aesthetic outcome.

The life size photographic facial analysis, coupled with clinical examination, can help to decide the number of millimeters advancement needed to achieve the aesthetic goals. Not only is hard tissue analysis on cephalometric radiographs essential, but also soft tissue analysis on life size photographs assists in detailed planning and ensures increased predictability. Small

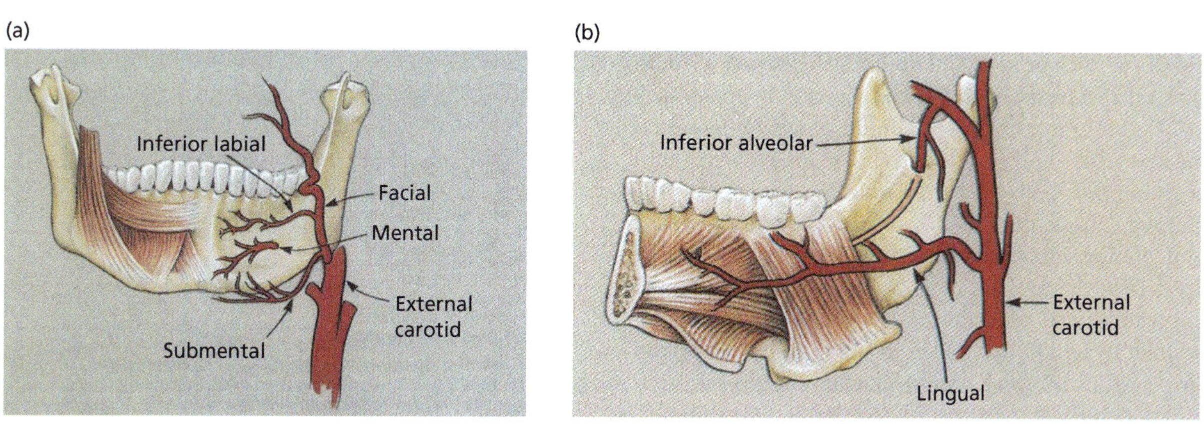

Fig. 33-4 Blood supply of chin area. (From Genioplasty. Guyuron B. Little, Brown and Company, 1990.[3])

fractions, such as 0.5 to 1.0 millimeters can make a significant difference in the harmony of the facial structures.[1]

The chin projection should be viewed on the profile picture for assessment. The most prominent portion of the chin is called pogonion. In an ideal chin projection, a line connecting the upper and lower lips will touch the pogonion – this is called the Riedel line.

An imaginary vertical line connecting the mid-glabella to the midline of the chin is the midline of face, which divides the chin into two equal parts. To determine any chin deformities, one needs to assess the vertical and horizontal dimensions. The cardinal determinants of chin harmony are its projection, symmetry and vertical height. The first step in full face evaluation is to divide the face into three equal portions, with four horizontal lines on the life size photograph in frontal view: one passing through the hair line, another passing through glabella, the next passing through the subnasale, and the last one passing through the most caudal portion of the chin, which is called menton. To assess the vertical dimension, the lower third is subdivided using a line passing through the stomion (see Chapter 5). The height between menton to stomion should be twice the distance from the stomion to subnasale. A vertical line passing through the mid-glabella and the tip of a straight nose determines any chin asymmetry. Projection of the chin is assessed on the profile view. There are several methods to evaluate the chin projection, the most practical being the Riedel line. This line connects the most prominent portion of the upper lip to the most prominent portion of the lower lip and continues caudally. The pogonion touches this line in an ideally balanced chin-to-lip relationship. The labiomental groove is probably one of the most underrated features of the lower face. Generally, it is about 4 mm deep in a female and 6 mm deep in a male profile.

The shape of the mandibular arch is also important. A very wide mandibular arch is the result of a wide mandibular body and would thus necessitate adjustment in chin osteotomy.

An overhead view and basilar view help evaluate the nasal and chin line-up and malar projection, especially in patients with minimal asymmetry.

No patient should undergo a genioplasty without an intraoral examination. Any disharmony between the upper incisors and the lip indicates an underlying skeletal abnormality. In a relaxed position, at least 2.0 to 2.5 mm of upper incisor should be visible between the lips. This exposure reaches to the full crown height of the upper teeth on a full smile. Any excess visible gingivae above the crowns or inadequate tooth show indicate abnormality of the underling maxilla or upper lip deficiency, and should be noted. One of the most important parts of intraoral examination is the dental occlusion, which has a role in the surgical planning. Any significant periodontal disease should be eradicated completely in the patient undergoing genioplasty. Both the clinical examination and this type of chin analysis make the surgery plan more precise, which is required for an optimal outcome.

Patient and procedure selection

In general, any patient being considered for aesthetic surgical procedures needs to be medically suitable, without any major medical conditions that may result in complications or suboptimal outcomes.

Chin deformities can be classified into seven main categories (Table 33-1): (1) Macrogenia, which can be horizontal, vertical, or a combination of the two; (2) Microgenia, which can be horizontal, vertical, or a combination of the two; (3) Combination of macrogenia and microgenia in different directions; (4) Asymmetrical chin; (5) Pseudomacrogenia; (6) Pseudomicrogenia; (7) Witch's chin deformity.

Asymmetry of the chin can be on a horizontal plane (side to side) or it can have a rotational element as well (clockwise or counterclockwise). It can be short or with increased anterior facial height. In pseudomacrogenia, the size of the chin is larger than normal and excess tissue is due to excess soft tissue with the size of the bone seeming to be normal. This condition also is seen in patients who undergone removal of chin implants. In pseudomicrogenia, patients have 'long face' deformity, causing clockwise rotation of the normal mandible. Witch's chin deformity is referred to soft tissue ptosis of the chin, which is usually seen in the patient with a long history of denture use after full dental extraction or purely due to the age. In a study by Guyuron et al.,[2] in an evaluation of 2879 patients, 684 patients were noted to have normal occlusion and some type of chin deformity. Among them 24.9% fell into group I, 63.6% group II, 7.9% group III, 0.6% group IV, 0.73 group V, 0.4% group VI and 1.9% group VII.

Table 33-1 Classification of chin deformities

I	Macrogenia • Horizontal • Vertical • Combination
II	Microgenia • Horizontal • Vertical • Combination
III	Combined micro and macrogenia • Vertical excess and horizontal deficiency • Vertical deficiency and horizontal excess
IV	Asymmetrical chin • Normal lower anterior facial height • Reduced lower anterior facial height • Increased lower anterior facial height
V	Pseudomacrogenia
VI	Pseudomicrogenia
VII	Witch's chin deformity

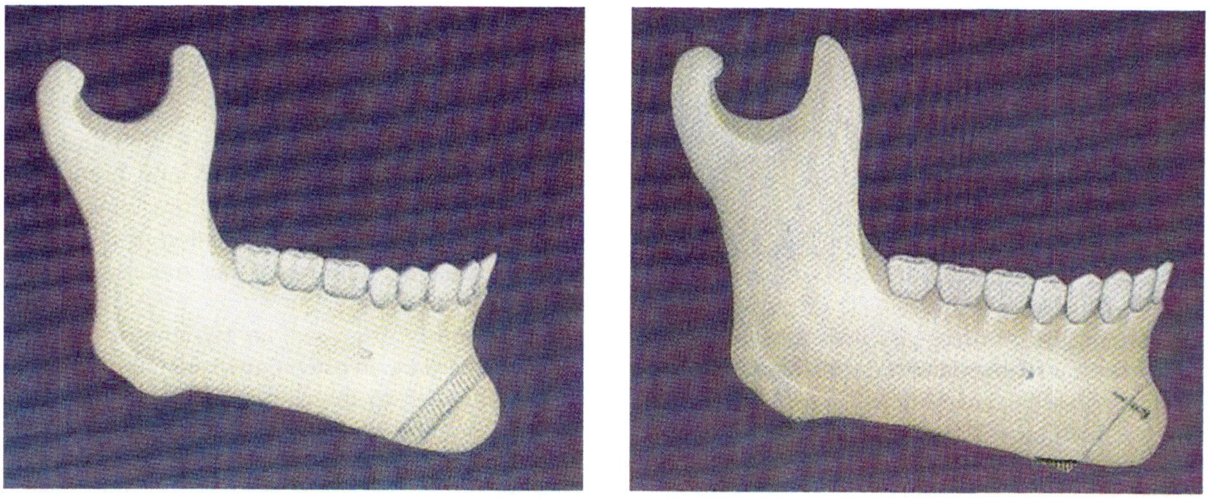

Fig. 33-5 Isolated horizontal excess treatment. (From Genioplasty. Guyuron B. Little, Brown and Company, 1990.[3])

Usually patients with **macrogenia** and asymmetry are not good candidates for alloplastic genioplasty, while osteotomy almost always provides predictable improvement or ideal outcome. Therefore patients with simple microgenia are potential candidates for the alloplastic genioplasty and among this group the patients with mild to moderate microgenia who are older (above age 50) are better candidates for alloplastic genioplasty, while the rest of the chin deformities can be treated with osseous genioplasty with greater success.

In patients with horizontal/vertical or oblique macrogenia (dependent on the deformity) osteotomy is performed by removing a segment of the bone and setting the chin back. Rarely, ostectomy by shaving of the bone using a wide burr can be accomplished (Figures 33-5 to 33-7) for horizontal macrogenia. It should be noted that there is a significant difference in the soft tissue response between patients undergoing osteotomy vs. ostectomy (Table 33-2). The inclination of the osteotomies can be changed to deal with combination of horizontal and vertical excess (Figure 33-8).

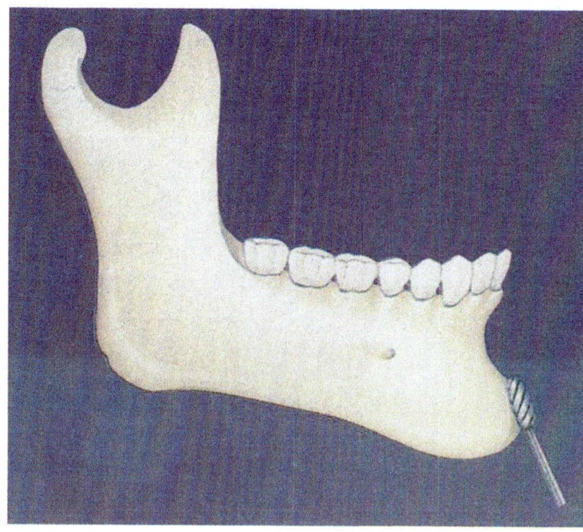

Fig. 33-7 Chin reduction with burr. (From Genioplasty. Guyuron B. Little, Brown and Company, 1990.[3])

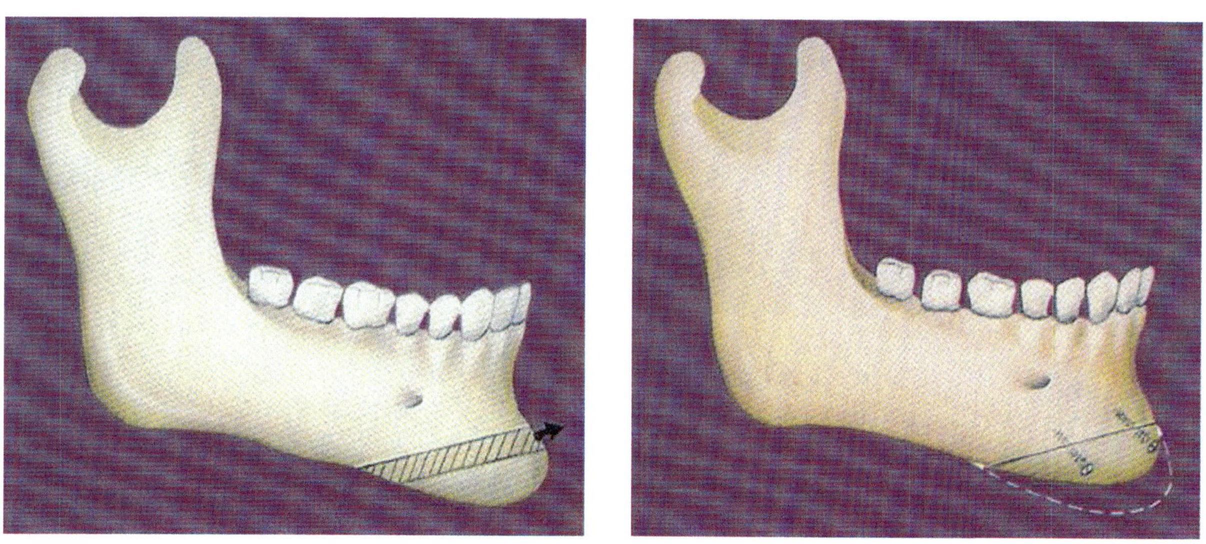

Fig. 33-6 Isolated vertical excess treatment. (From Genioplasty. Guyuron B. Little, Brown and Company, 1990.[3])

Table 33-2 Soft tissue response to bone adjustment

Osteotomy	Retraction	0.9 for 1.0
	Vertical reduction	0.8 for 1.0
	Advancement	0.9 for 1.0
Ostectomy	Horizontal	0.25 for 1.0
	Vertical	0.5 for 1.0
Augmentation	Augmentation	0.8 for 1.0

In dealing with **microgenia** there are more surgical options available. However, in this chapter we will focus on osteotomy. Sliding horizontal osteotomy, which is performed 4–5 mm below the mental foramen, is shown in Figure 33-9. For a combination of horizontal deficiency and vertical excess, the osteotomy travels posterior and caudal, and by advancing this segment, anterior height is usually decreased. A horizontal step osteotomy is also a possibility, this being more suitable for a wide-angle mandible with steep mandibular plane or patient who requires significant chin advancement. Two osteotomies are done and the segments are advanced overlapping each other (Figures 33-9 to 33-11). For severe vertical deficiencies a bone graft can be added between the segments, or if the distances of the two segments are within the osteoplastic jumping distance of 4–5 mm, it can be left without bone grafting. If a patient has vertical deficiency and horizontal excess, rotation of the caudal segment caudally, following a horizontal osteotomy can address the issue.

As previously discussed, an **asymmetrical chin** is best addressed by an osteotomy, as long as the asymmetry is limited to the chin area. For isolated chin asymmetry with normal height, a segment from the long side can be removed and added to the short side after wedge osteotomy. If the facial height is small after wedge osteotomy, a bone graft can be added to the short side. If the overall facial height is excessive, a wedge can be removed from the long side. Occasionally, asymmetry is due to horizontal displacement, which can be treated by a horizontal osteotomy and

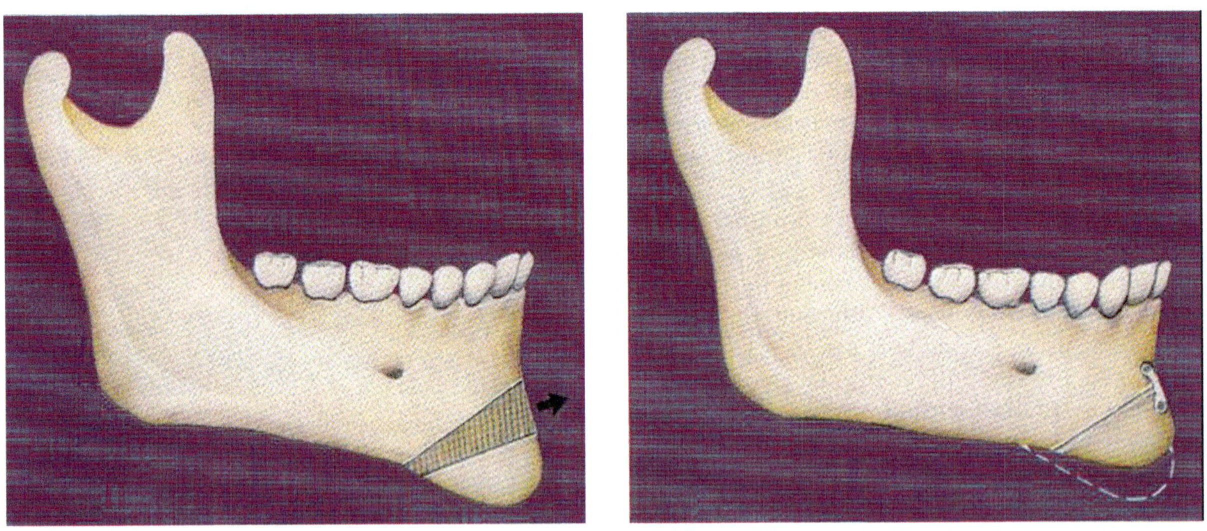

Fig. 33-8 Change of the inclination of resected bone. (From Genioplasty. Guyuron B. Little, Brown and Company, 1990.[3])

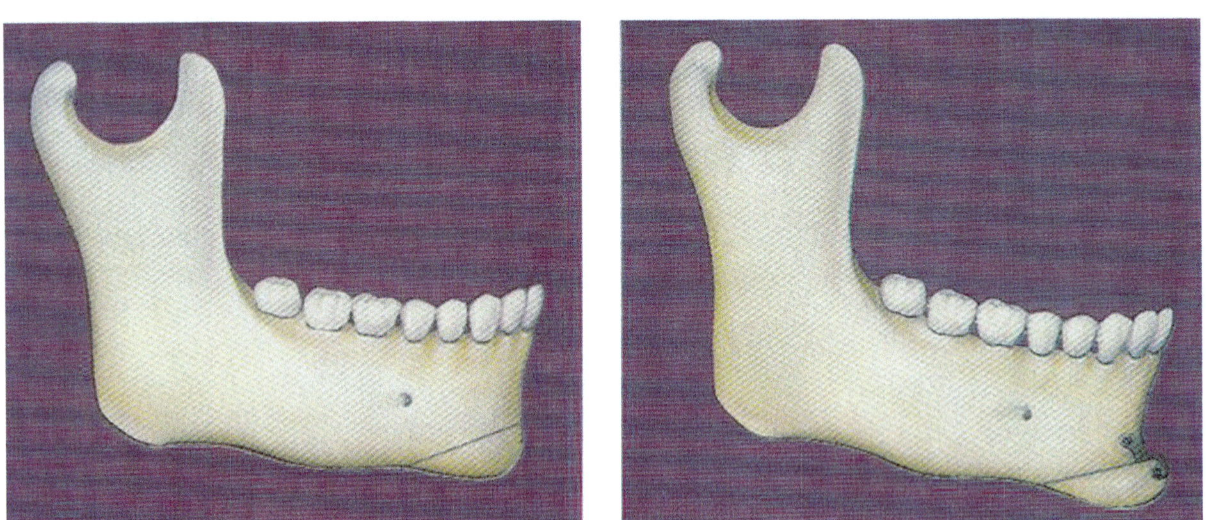

Fig. 33-9 Horizontal osteotomy. (From Genioplasty. Guyuron B. Little, Brown and Company, 1990.[3])

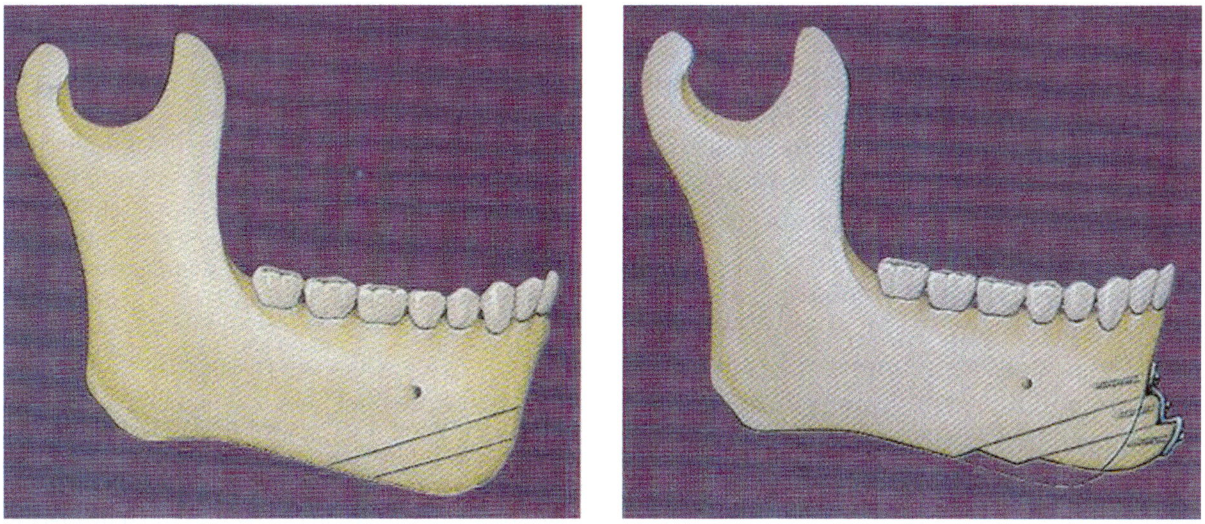

Fig. 33-10 Double step osteotomy. (From Genioplasty. Bahman Guyuron. Little, Brown and Company, 1990.)

repositioning of the segment in the horizontal plane sliding it side to side.

Pseudomacrogenia, or soft tissue excess, is treated by excision of the soft tissue through an elliptical incision in the submental area, including skin and subcutaneous layer without disruption of the mentalis muscle. **Pseudomicrogenia** patients require orthognathic surgery to correct the mandibular rotation. A Witch's chin deformity can be treated by combination of tissue excision using an elliptical incision and application of fat graft to the submental mental crease.

Surgical technique

Osseous genioplasty is usually undertaken under general anaesthesia with endotracheal intubation. After

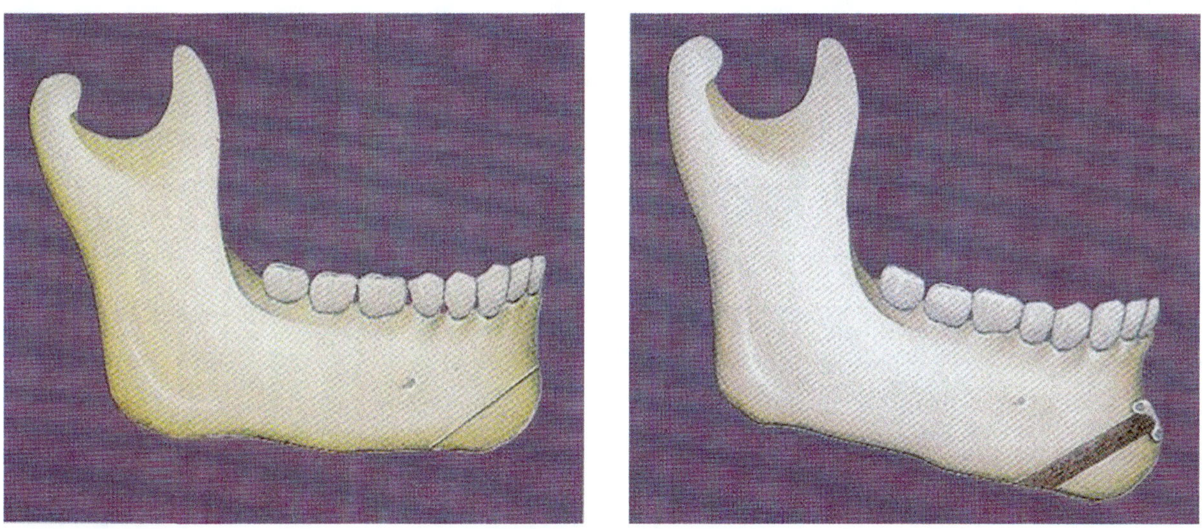

Fig. 33-11 Combination of vertical and horizontal deficiency managed with oblique osteotpmy and bone grafting. (From Genioplasty. Guyuron B. Little, Brown and Company, 1990.[3])

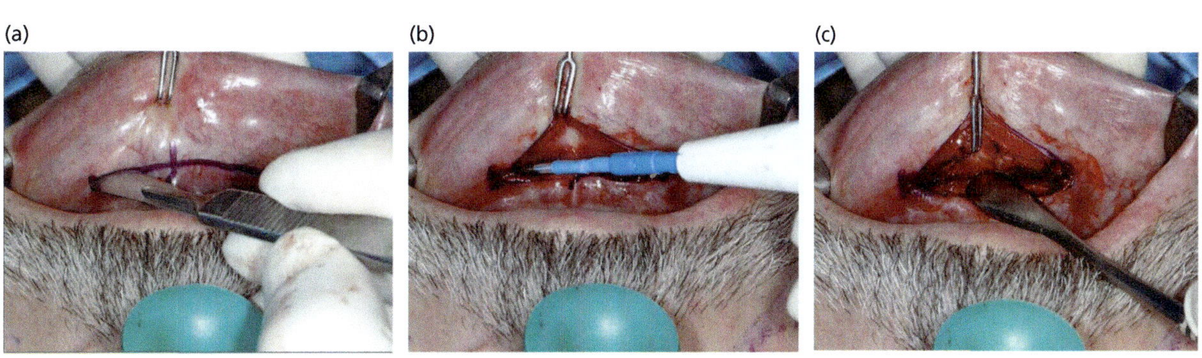

Fig. 33-12 (a–c) Chin exposure. (From Genioplasty. Guyuron B. Little, Brown and Company, 1990.[3])

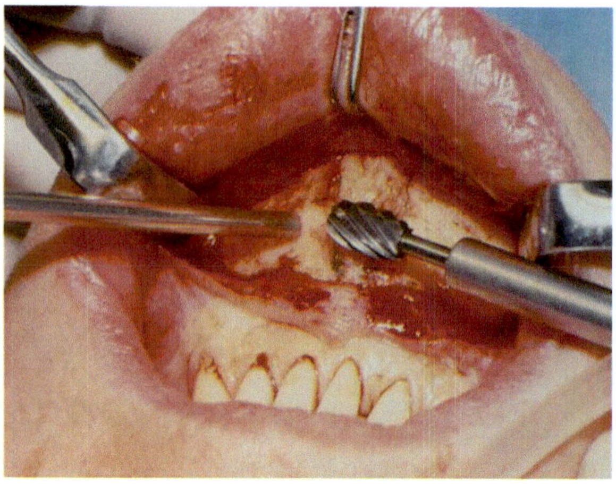

Fig. 33-13 Ostectomy. (From Genioplasty. Guyuron B. Little, Brown and Company, 1990.[3])

injection of local anaesthetic including 1/100,000 adrenaline (epinephrine), an incision is made 8–10 mm on the labial side of the sulcus to prevent the gingival retraction. Dissection is carried through the mucosa, mentalis muscle, and then to subperiosteal level. Next, dissection is carried caudally and laterally to expose the chin and mental nerves (Figure 33-12a–c). If the plan is to perform an ostectomy, the bone is removed using an oval burr. Each half is removed at the time to allow for precise measurement. The opposite side is then leveled (Figure 33-13). If the plan is to perform an osteotomy, it is achieved using a sagittal saw (Figure 33-14 a–g). Pre- and postoperative examples of osseous genioplasty combined with other procedures are shown in Figures 33-15 to 33-17.

Postoperative complications

Complications such as wound dehiscence and infection are rare after osseous genioplasty. If it occurs, a haematoma needs to be drained to prevent infection. Tooth devitalization can be prevented by placing the osteotomy at least 30.5 mm caudal to the occlusal edge. Dental root exposure manifests itself with caudal retraction of the gingivae, causing exposure of the sensitive part of the tooth, which is extremely painful. This can be prevented by leaving sufficient distance between the incision and the gingival line. Varying degrees of sensory loss may occur in more than 50%

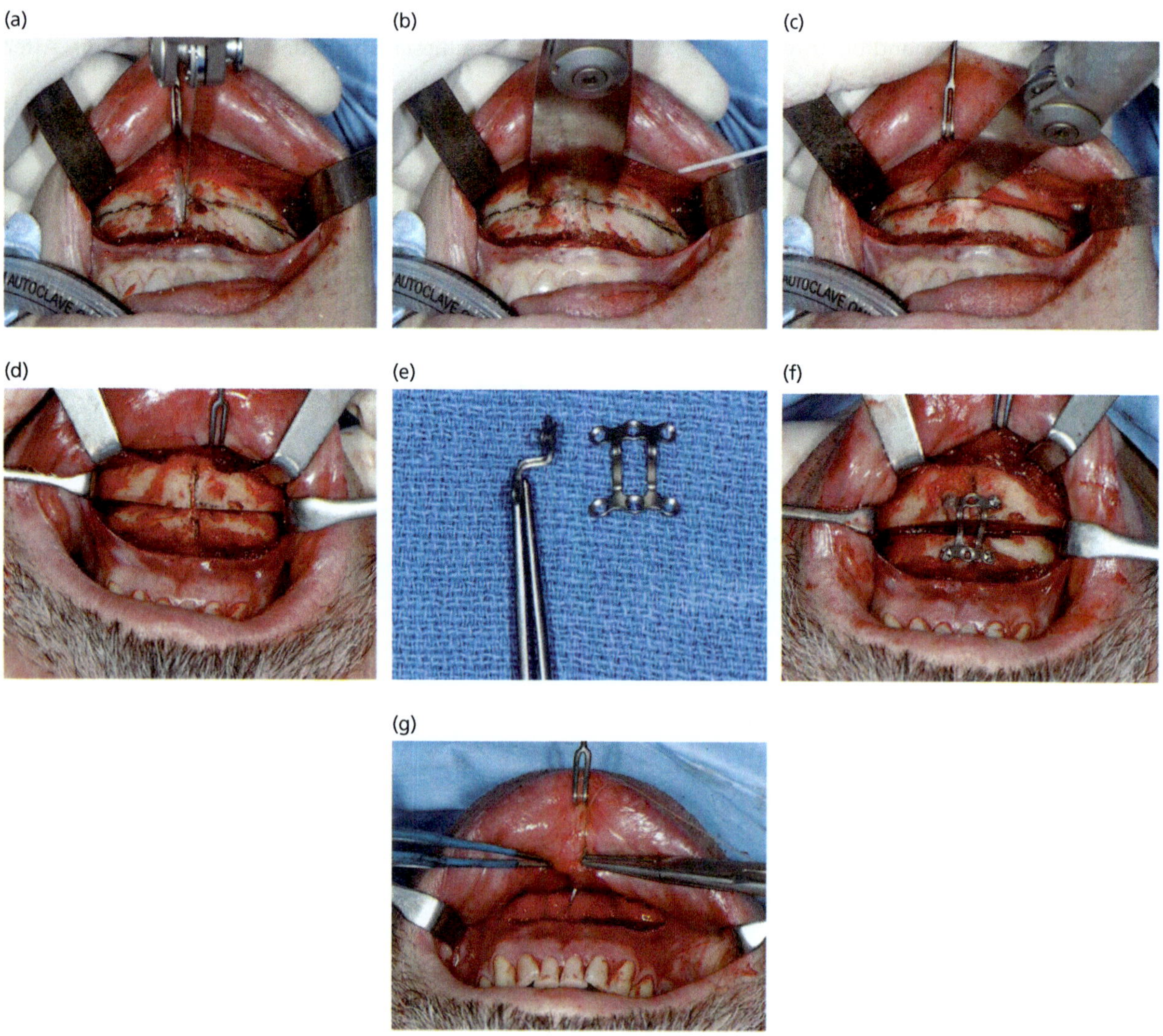

Fig. 33-14 (a–g) Sliding osseous genioplasty. (From Genioplasty. Guyuron B. Little, Brown and Company, 1990.[3])

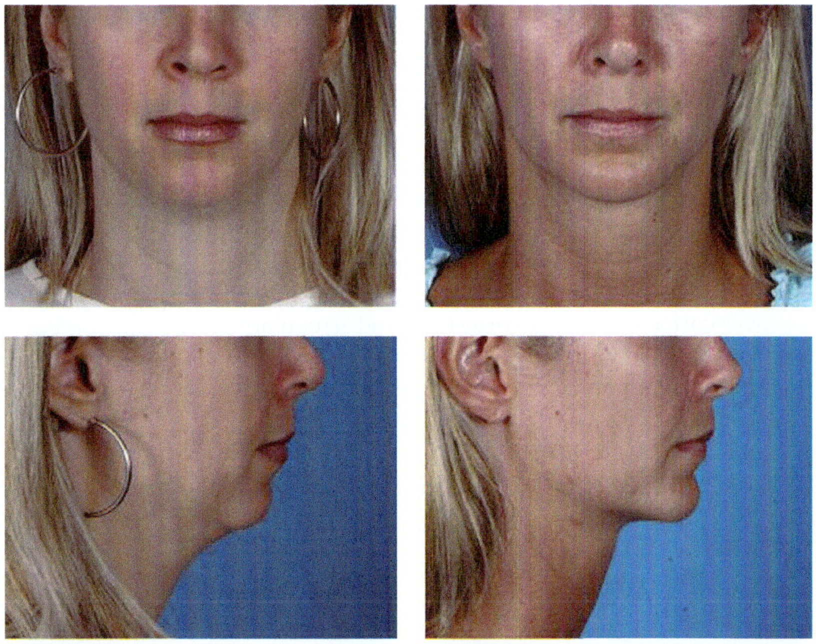

Fig. 33-15 A patient with horizontal micogenia before (left) and after advancement genioplasty, secondary rhinoplasty and submental lipectomy(right) on front view (above) and profile (below). (From Genioplasty. Guyuron B. Little, Brown and Company, 1990.[3])

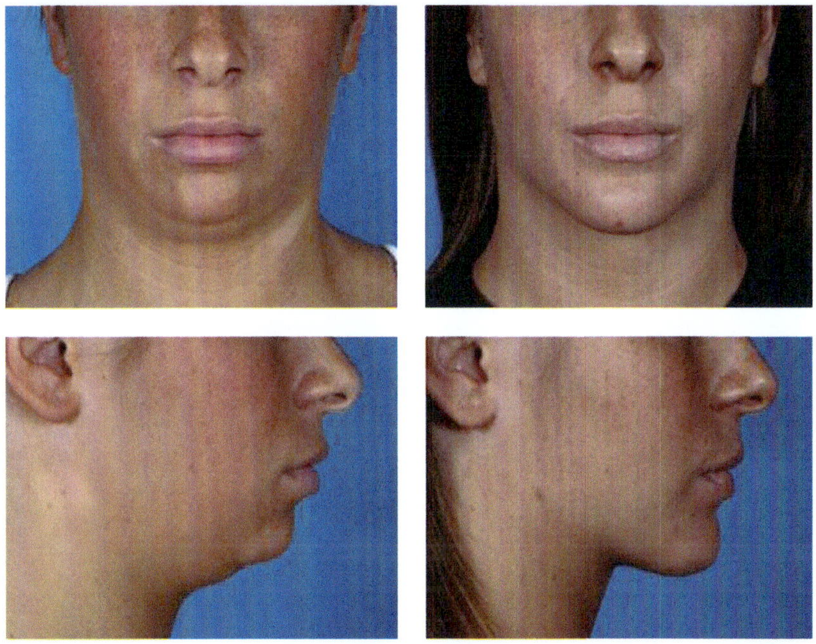

Fig. 33-16 A patient with combined horizontal and vertical micogenia before (left) and after osseous genioplasty and submental lipectomy(right) on front view (above) and profile (below). (From Genioplasty. Guyuron B. Little, Brown and Company, 1990.[3])

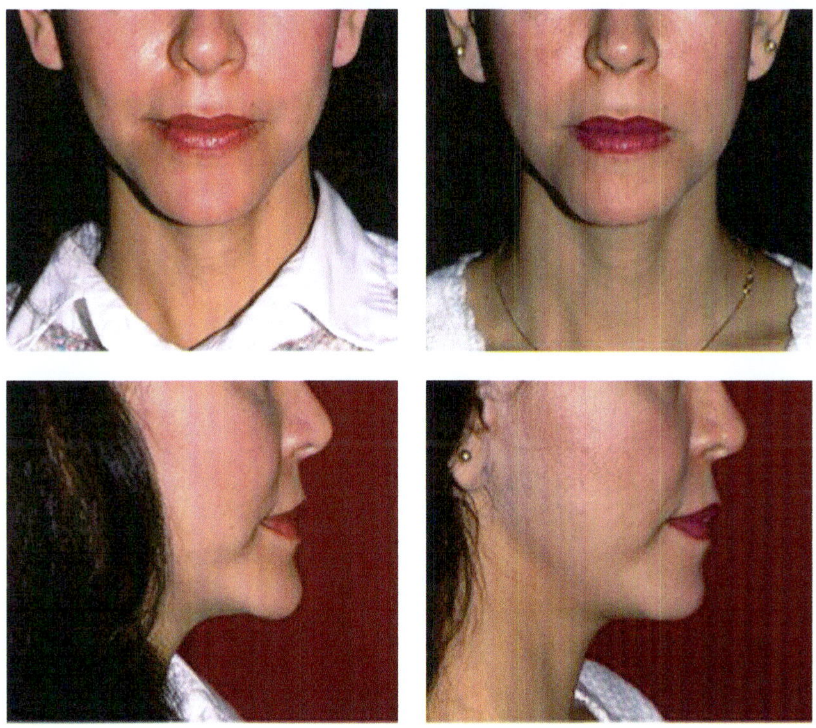

Fig. 33-17 A patient before (left) and after reduction genioplasty with ostectomy (right) on front view (above) and profile (below). (From Genioplasty. Guyuron B. Little, Brown and Company, 1990.[3])

of patients undergoing osseous genioplasty. The aetiology is usually traction of the nerve, which is transient, but avulsion of the nerve can occur as well. Ptosis of the soft tissue is due to over-reduction of the bony part or reduction genioplasty. Retraction of the lower lip is usually due to inadequate repair of the mentalis muscle. Other complications like asymmetry, over-correction, under-correction, and irregularities may occur after this surgery. Proper planning with precise execution and meticulous closure can minimize complications and displeasing results.

References

1 Guyuron B. Precision rhinoplasty. Part 1: the role of the life size photographs and soft tissue cephalometric analysis. Plast Reconstr Surg. 1988;81:489–99.
2 Guyuron B, Michelow BJ, Willis L. Practical classification of chin deformities. Aesthetic Plast Surg. 1995;19:257-64.
3 Guyuron B. Genioplasty. Boston: Little, Brown and Company, 1990.
4 Guyuron B, Eriksson E, Persing JA. Plastic Surgery, Indications and Practice. Saunders and Elsevier, 2009.

Chapter 34

Asymmetries of the Maxilla and Mandible

Farhad B. Naini, Mehmet Manisali and Daljit S. Gill

'The principles of symmetry result from proportion … Thus in the *well-proportioned* human body there is a kind of *symmetrical harmony*.'

Vitruvius (first century BC)[1]
Roman architect

Introduction

The word 'symmetry' literally means 'of like measure'. It entered the English language from the Old French 'symmétrie' (now: symétrie), from the Latin 'symmetria', from the Greek 'summetria', itself from súmmetros. The word is formed from the prefix 'sym' (similar, alike) and the suffix 'metron' (measure).

Symmetry may be defined as correspondence in size, shape and relative position of parts on opposite sides of a dividing line or median plane. **Asymmetry** is defined as a lack or absence of symmetry.[2] The application of this definition to the human face illustrates an imbalance or disproportionality between the right and left sides of the face. No human face exhibits perfect bilateral symmetry and a mild degree of asymmetry may be considered normal and acceptable in the average face. However, beyond this asymmetries are likely to be noticeable and thereby a potentially important parameter in perceptions of facial attractiveness,[3] and significant facial asymmetries have been correlated with clinical depression, low self-esteem and other health problems associated with poor quality of life, such as neurosis and inferiority complex.[4]

An investigation into the influence of different types of asymmetry affecting the mandible and chin point (i.e. horizontal, vertical and combined horizontal-vertical asymmetries) on perceived attractiveness found that mandibular/chin point asymmetry of 10 mm is perceived as significant; at 5 mm, and

Orthognathic Surgery: Principles, Planning and Practice. Edited by Farhad B. Naini and Daljit S. Gill.

thereby below 5 mm, it appears to be largely irrelevant to the observer in terms of desire for surgical correction.[3] The greater the degree of asymmetry past 10 mm, the more noticeable it becomes. From 10 mm of asymmetry upwards, patients desire treatment for correction of the asymmetry. It was also observed that horizontal asymmetry, akin to hemimandibular elongation (see below), appears to be perceived as the most unattractive type of lower facial asymmetry, though at greater degrees of asymmetry all types of asymmetry were rated as unattractive. It was also found that pretreatment orthognathic patients and clinicians were more critical than laypeople. The desire for surgical correction was negligible for 5 mm of mandibular or chin point asymmetry, but increased considerably at 10 mm of asymmetry and continued to increase with greater degrees of asymmetry. The highest rated images demonstrated bilateral symmetry and the lowest rated images demonstrated significant degrees of mandibular/chin asymmetry. Therefore, the clinical pursuit of attaining a result as close to bilateral facial symmetry as attainable appears to be a worthy treatment aim.

The aetiology and clinical management of severe panfacial and craniofacial asymmetries are described in Chapter 57. The purpose of this chapter is to describe the clinical diagnosis and management of asymmetries affecting the lower aspect of the midface/maxilla and the lower face.

Aetiology and classification

Facial asymmetry may result from discrepancies in the size, shape or relative position of individual bones in the craniofacial complex and/or the overlying soft tissues.[2] Due to the range of diverse aetiological factors that may affect the underlying facial skeleton and/or the overlying soft tissue envelope, and the various morphological presentations involved, asymmetries of the face have long defied rational classification. This explains why there are so many varying classification systems. A useful classification system involves broadly separating the causes of facial asymmetry into three groups: congenital, developmental and acquired (Table 34-1).[3,5,6]

Classification of maxillary asymmetry

A simple classification of developmental maxillary asymmetry may be based on aetiological-morphological characteristics (Table 34-2). The asymmetry may be categorized as **primary** if it is

Table 34-1 A classification of the aetiology of facial asymmetry

Aetiology		Examples	
Congenital (prenatal)	Malformations[I]	Cleft lip and palate (unilateral) Hemifacial microsomia Hemifacial hyperplasia Plagiocephaly	
	Deformations[II]	Mandibular deformation resulting from sharp lateral flexion of the head with the shoulder pressed against the mandible in late intrauterine growth.[6]	
	Disruptions [III]	Rare facial clefting	
Developmental (postnatal)	Intrinsic jaw growth anomalies	Hemimandibular elongation Hemimandibular hyperplasia Unilateral condylar hyperplasia	
	Secondary jaw growth anomalies	Hemifacial atrophy (Parry Romberg syndrome) Sternocleidomastoid torticollis (Figure 34-1) Duchenne muscular dystrophy Cerebral palsy	
	Functional	Lateral mandibular displacement	
Acquired	Traumatic	Condylar trauma	
		Maxillary/facial trauma	
	Pathological	Condylar resorption	Juvenile rheumatoid arthritis
			Adult onset rheumatoid arthritis
		Infection/inflammation	
		Cysts	
		Tumours	

I: A **malformation** is a morphological defect (of an organ, part of an organ, or a larger area of the body) resulting from an intrinsically abnormal developmental process, e.g. unilateral cleft lip. The earlier in embryogenesis such defects are initiated, the more complex the resulting malformation.

II: A **deformation** is an abnormal form or position of a part of the body caused by non-disruptive mechanical forces.

III: A **disruption** is a morphological defect (of an organ, part of an organ, or a larger area of the body) resulting from a breakdown of, or interference with, an originally normal developmental process.

(Reprinted with permission from Naini.[2])

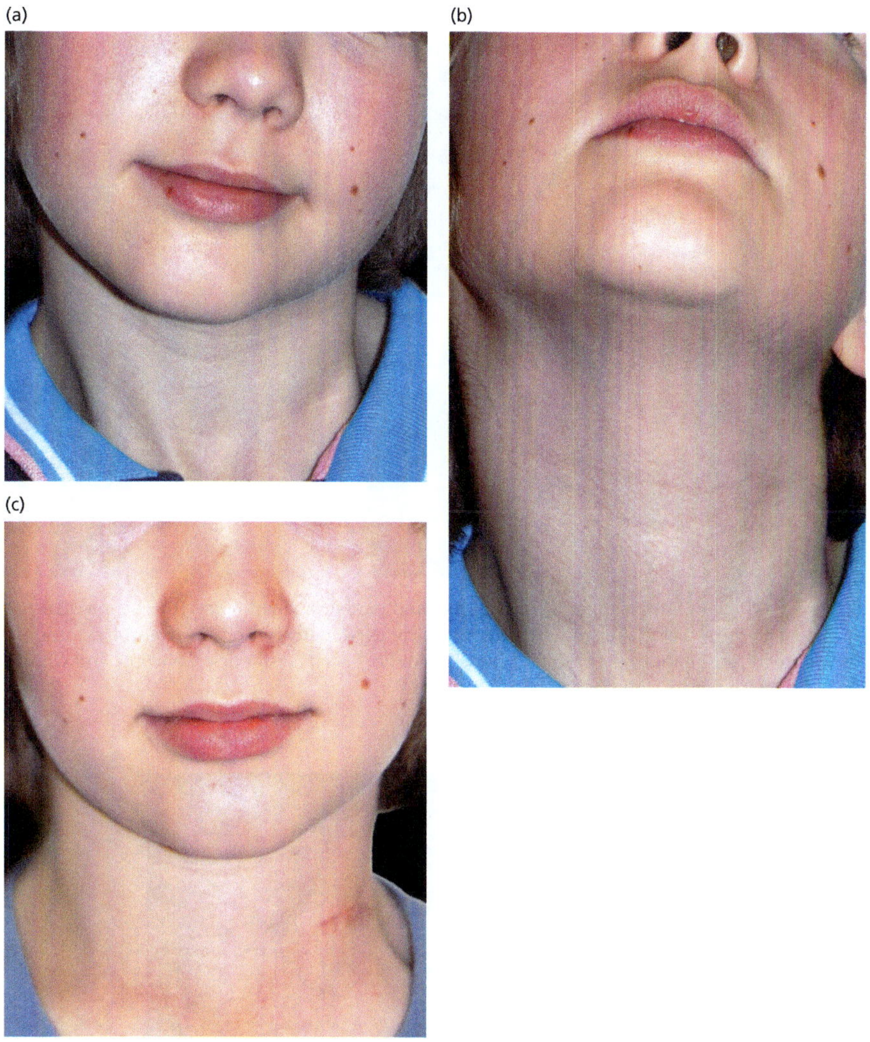

Fig. 34-1 (a, b) Left-sided sternocleidomastoid torticollis. (c) Postoperative view.

Table 34-2 Classification of developmental maxillary asymmetry

Developmental maxillary asymmetry	Type	Presenting features
Primary (i.e. due to an inherent developmental discrepancy of the maxilla)	Vertical	• Uncommon • Usually associated with a panfacial asymmetry and craniofacial syndromic conditions such as craniofacial/hemifacial microsomia (Figure 34-2). • Likely to present relatively early in age. • It may be due to unilateral overgrowth, unilateral undergrowth or a combination of both. • The infraorbital foramina will almost certainly be at different vertical positions, with a transverse cant of the infraorbital plane. • Usually associated with vertical orbital dystopia and a transverse cant in the orbital plane.
	Horizontal	• Skeletal translation of the maxilla and/or maxillary dentoalveolus to the left or right (Figure 34-3). • Associated with a severe panfacial asymmetry. • Rare
Secondary (i.e. as a response to a developmental discrepancy of the mandible or a dentoalveolar discrepancy)	Vertical	A unilateral maxillary dentoalveolar vertical response (overeruption of the teeth) to an ipsilateral lateral open bite in a patient with hemimandibular hyperplasia (Figure 34-4).
	Horizontal	A maxillary dental midline deviation, due to: • A localized dentoalveolar discrepancy, e.g. incisor lateral drift due to dental arch crowding, or unilateral ankylosis in the mid-arch region resulting in transseptal fibre pull on the incisors. • Maxillary skeletal rotation around the vertical axis (rare).

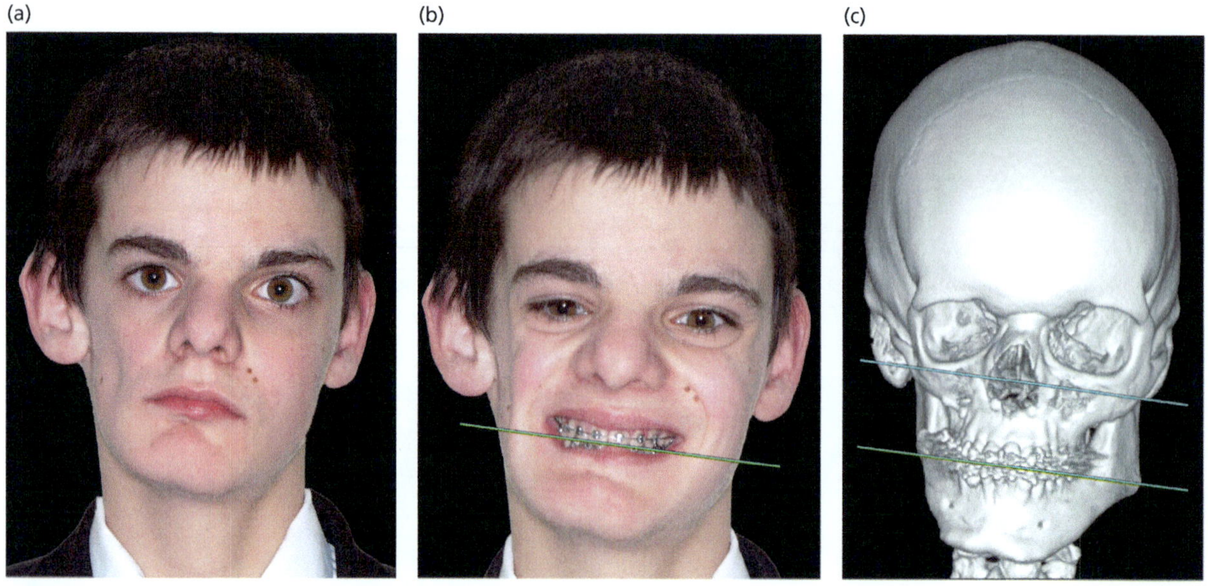

Fig. 34-2 (a) Patient with hemifacial microsomia and panfacial asymmetry. (b) The maxillary occlusal plane is canted down on the patient's left. (c) The entire maxilla exhibits a vertical asymmetry, with the infraorbital foramina at different vertical positions and a cant of the infraorbital plane. (Modified from: Naini FB. Facial Aesthetics: Concepts and Clinical Diagnosis. Oxford: Wiley-Blackwell, 2011; used with permission.[16])

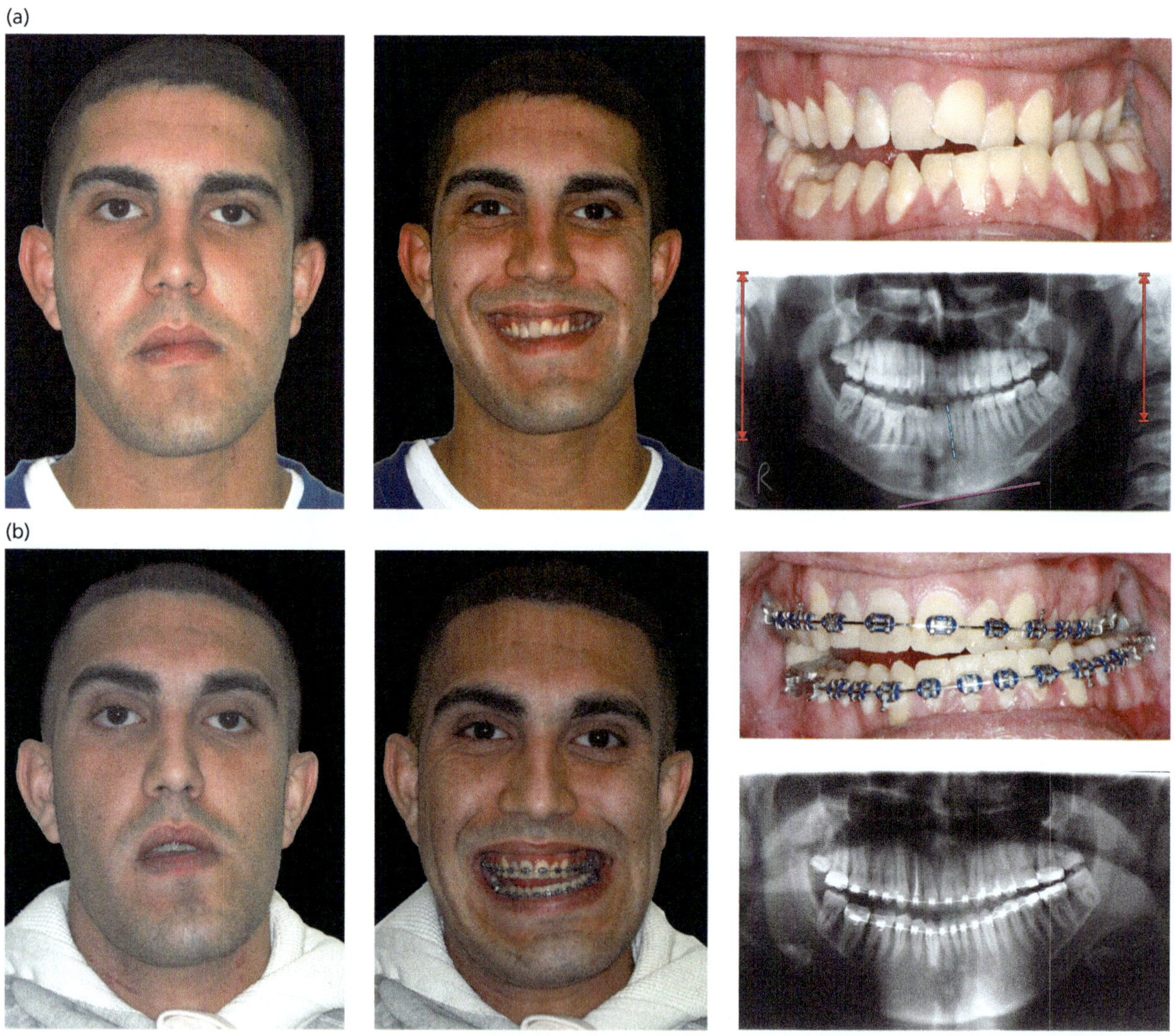

Fig. 34-3 (a) Severe panfacial asymmetry, with the maxilla to the patient's right, but minimal transverse cant. Hemimandibular hyperplasia and elongation on the patient's right. (b) Preoperative views. The maxilla was bodily repositioned towards the left, and minimal cant correction was required. Asymmetrical mandibular set-back osteotomy was employed to improve the symmetry of the mandible, chin point and dental occlusion. (c) Postoperative views.

(c)

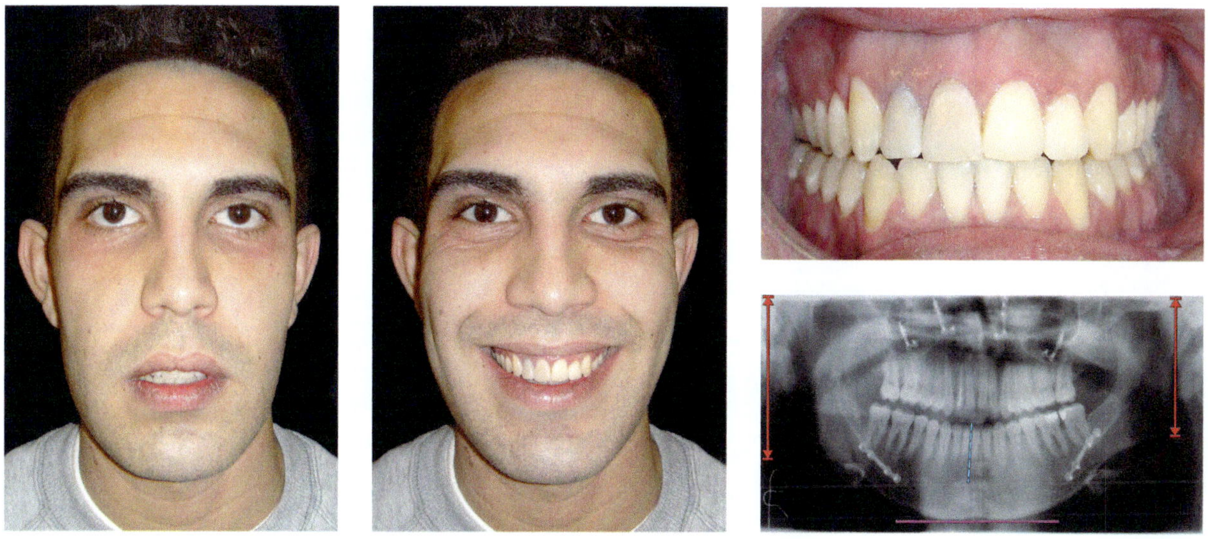

Fig. 34-3 (*Continued*).

likely to be due to an inherent developmental discrepancy of the maxilla, or **secondary** if it develops as a response to either a developmental discrepancy of the mandible or a dentoalveolar discrepancy.

Classification of mandibular asymmetry

Based on the classification described in Table 34-1, mandibular asymmetry may be classified as developmental, functional, traumatic or pathological. Significant facial asymmetry may result from *localized* aberrant growth patterns of the mandible itself. It is important to clinically distinguish true asymmetrical mandibular excess from *relative* excess, which may result from unilateral inhibition or arrest of growth. In such cases, the normal side will *appear larger* due to lack of growth on the affected side, e.g. unilateral temporomandibular joint trauma in childhood resulting in retarded ipsilateral growth, or a pathological condition such as unilateral fibrous dysplasia.

Many partially successful attempts were made to classify developmental mandibular asymmetries due to intrinsic jaw growth anomalies, e.g. Rushton (1944),[7] Waldron et al. (1946),[8] Cernea (1948),[9] Gottlieb (1951),[10] Hinds et al. (1960),[11] Rowe (1960),[12] and Bruce and Hayward (1968)[13]. The number of classifications demonstrates the considerable difficulty in developing an adequate, inclusive and user-friendly classification.

(a)

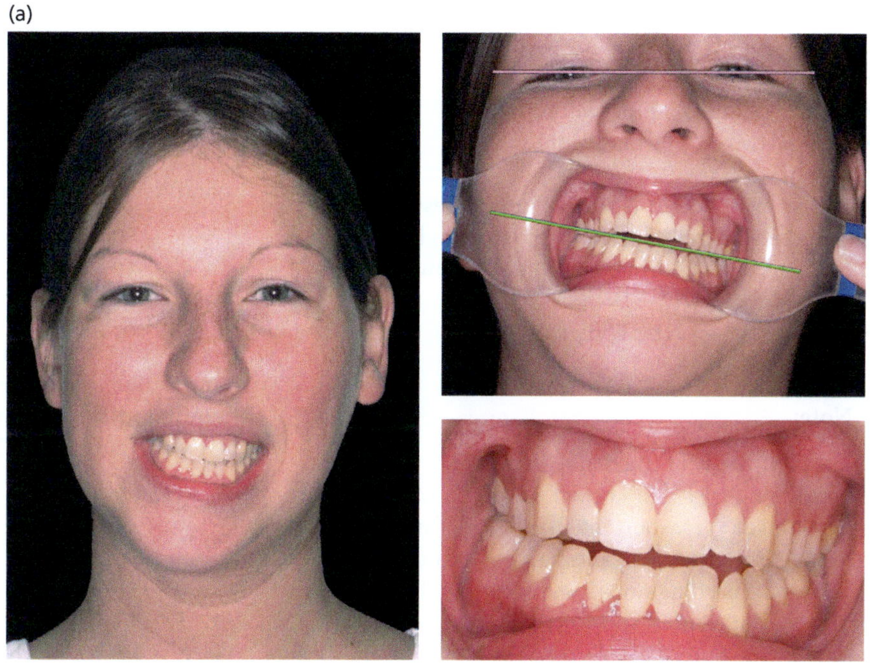

Fig. 34-4 (a) Patient with increased ramus height on her left and reduced ramus height on her right. The maxillary occlusal plane is canted down on her left due to overeruption of the maxillary dentition. (b) Preoperative view, demonstrating maintenance of the transverse cant. (c) Maxillary transverse cant correction by superior repositioning at the Le Fort I level on the patient's left and set down on her right.

(b)

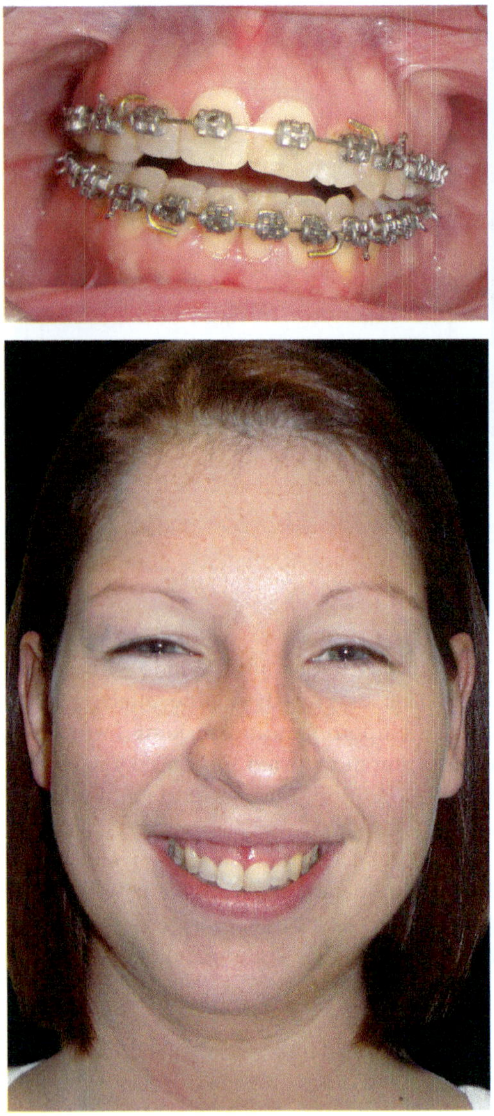

(c)

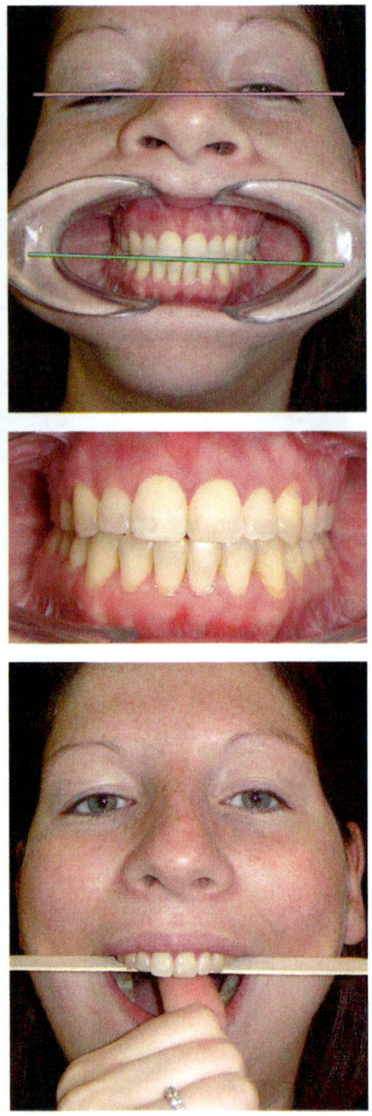

Fig. 34-4 (*Continued*).

However, a classic article by Obwegeser and Makek (1986)[14] classified mandibular asymmetry into three general groups (**Obwegeser classification**):

- Hemimandibular Hyperplasia (HH).
- Hemimandibular Elongation (HE).
- Hybrid (Mixed) forms of HH and HE.

To these was added a further group resulting from isolated unilateral hyperplasia of a condyle occurring after cessation of normal craniofacial growth:

- Unilateral Condylar Hyperplasia.

Note:

The aetiology of such developmental mandibular asymmetries is unknown. However, Obwegeser and Makek[14] reason that the steering mechanism for the growth of these anomalies is located entirely within the cartilaginous zone of the condylar head. This hypothesis is supported by the fact that in rapidly developing cases, the abnormal growth ceases after a high condylar resection has been performed.

The Obwegeser classification defines three forms of **condylar hyperactivity**, only two of which produce condylar hyperplasia; pure hemimandibular elongation (HE) does *not* produce condylar hyperplasia.

Asymmetry of the lower third of the face resulting from excessive asymmetrical growth of the mandible may be predominantly vertical in direction (**hemimandibular hyperplasia**), predominantly horizontal (**hemimandibular elongation**), or a combination of the two (Figure 34-5) (Table 34-3).[15]

Clinical evaluation

Before embarking on the clinical evaluation, a thorough **patient history** is required (see Chapter 5). However, the presence of a significant facial asymmetry

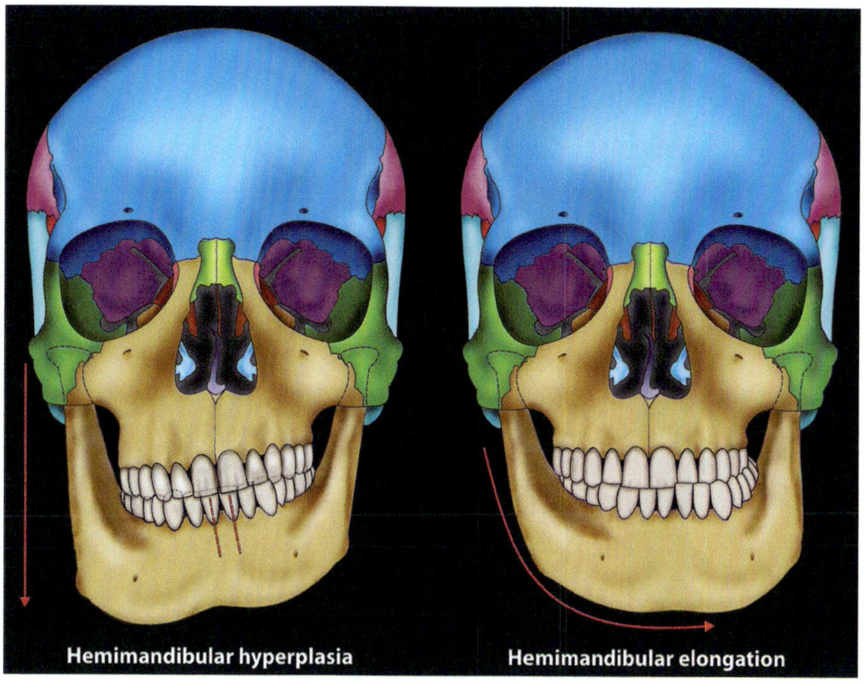

Fig. 34-5 Hemimandibular hyperplasia and hemimandibular elongation (see with Table 34-3). (From: Naini FB. Facial Aesthetics: Concepts and Clinical Diagnosis. Oxford: Wiley-Blackwell, 2011; used with permission.[16])

Table 34-3 Comparison between hemimandibular hyperplasia and elongation (see with Figure 34-5)[15]

Hemimandibular hyperplasia (HH)	Hemimandibular elongation (HE)
Unilateral three-dimensional enlargement of the mandible (hence the alternative term of hemimandibular hypertrophy), terminating exactly at the midline of the mandibular symphysis.	Unilateral horizontal increase in length of the affected side, mainly of the mandibular body.
Excessive asymmetrical growth is predominantly in a **vertical direction** (Figure 34-6).	Excessive asymmetrical growth is predominantly in a **horizontal direction** (Figure 34-7).
Condyle enlarged on the affected side.	Condyles of normal size, but the affected side of the mandible is thought to be elongated due to *unilateral condylar hyperactivity*.
Vertical ramus height is increased on affected side.	There is no height difference between the two sides of the face.
Inferior mandibular border *bows* excessively downward on affected side.	No bowing of the inferior mandibular border.
Mandibular canal bows down close to the inferiorly bowed mandibular lower border.	No downward bowing of mandibular canal.
Body of the mandible on the affected side has increased bone height, i.e. the distance between the tooth root apices and the inferior mandibular border is increased.	Normal bone heights.
Dental midlines tend to remain coincident, but the mandibular incisors are excessively angulated towards the affected side.	Mandibular dental midline (and chin point) move to the unaffected side; incisor angulations are normal.
The mandibular occlusal plane is oriented downward on the affected side (Figure 34-8), with compensatory overeruption of the maxillary dentoalveolus leading to a transverse cant of the maxillary occlusal plane.	No transverse canting of the maxillary or mandibular occlusal planes.
There is no posterior crossbite.	A posterior dental crossbite results on the unaffected side.
There may be a lateral open bite on the affected side depending on whether the extent of maxillary dentoalveolar compensation on the affected side has kept up with the increased vertical ramal growth, and whether or not the tongue has found a resting position between the posterior dental occlusion.	No lateral open bite.
Chin may be almost in the midline of the face, but with a transverse cant of the inferior chin plane, lower on the affected side.	Chin moves to the unaffected side. No transverse cant of the inferior chin plane, which remains level.
The unilateral increase in lower face height gives rise to a sloping rima oris, the oral commissure on the affected side is displaced inferiorly but not laterally.	There is no cant to the rima oris, but the lower lip tends to be displaced horizontally to the unaffected side.
In severe cases the unilateral skeletal changes result in a typical 'corkscrew-like' rotation of the lower face.	No rotation of lower face, only a horizontal deviation of the chin and lower lip to the unaffected side.

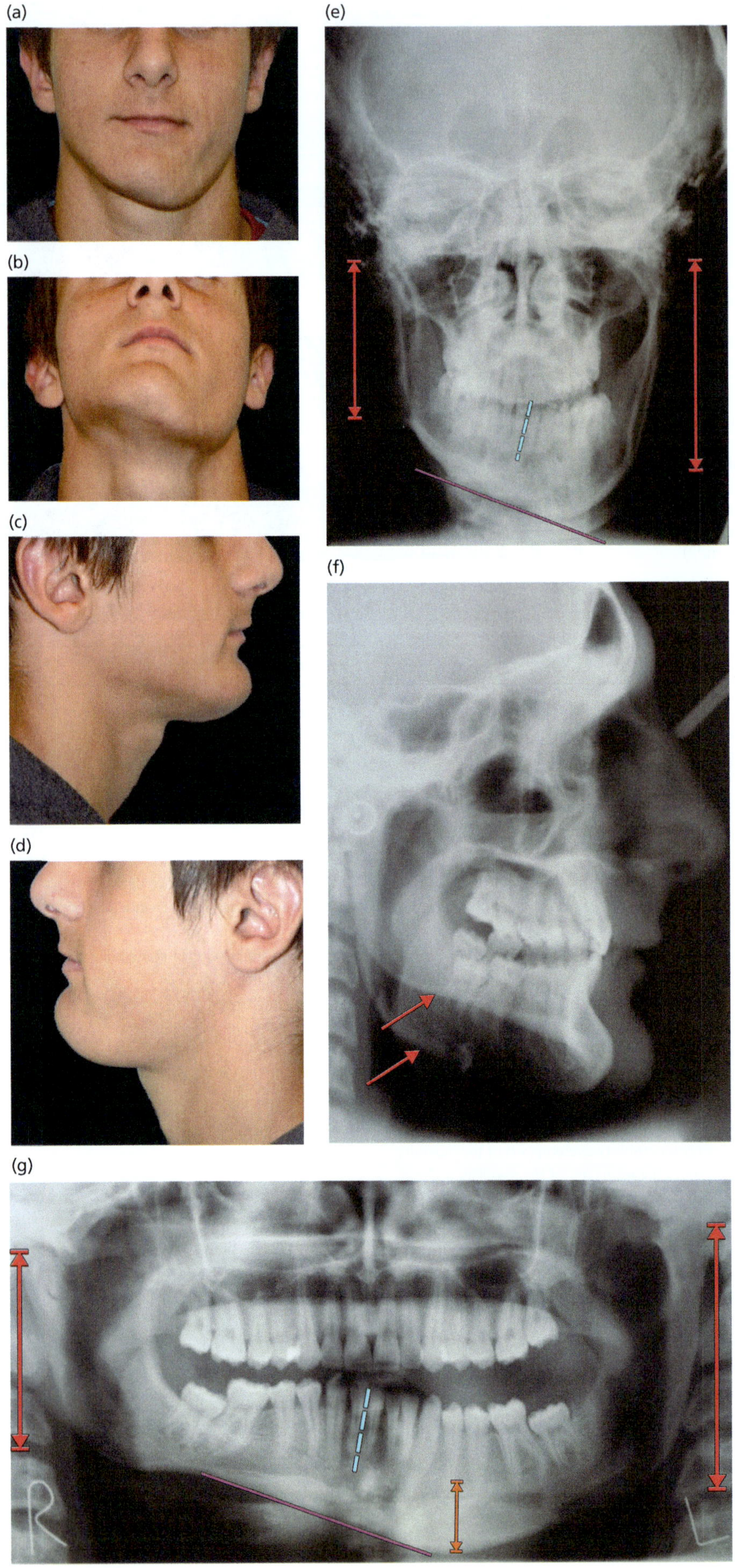

Fig. 34-6 Left-sided hemimandibular hyperplasia.

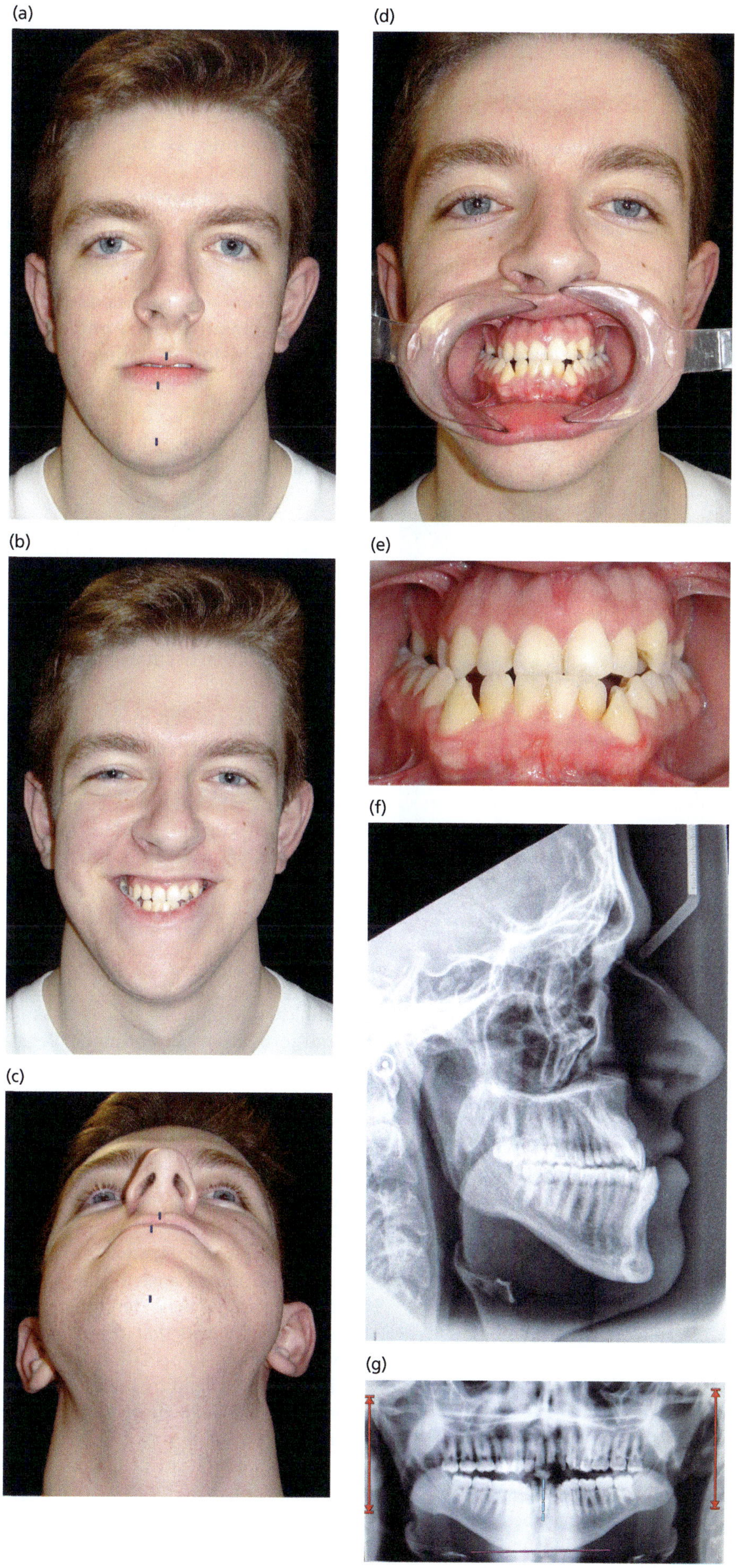

Fig. 34-7 Left-sided hemimandibular elongation.

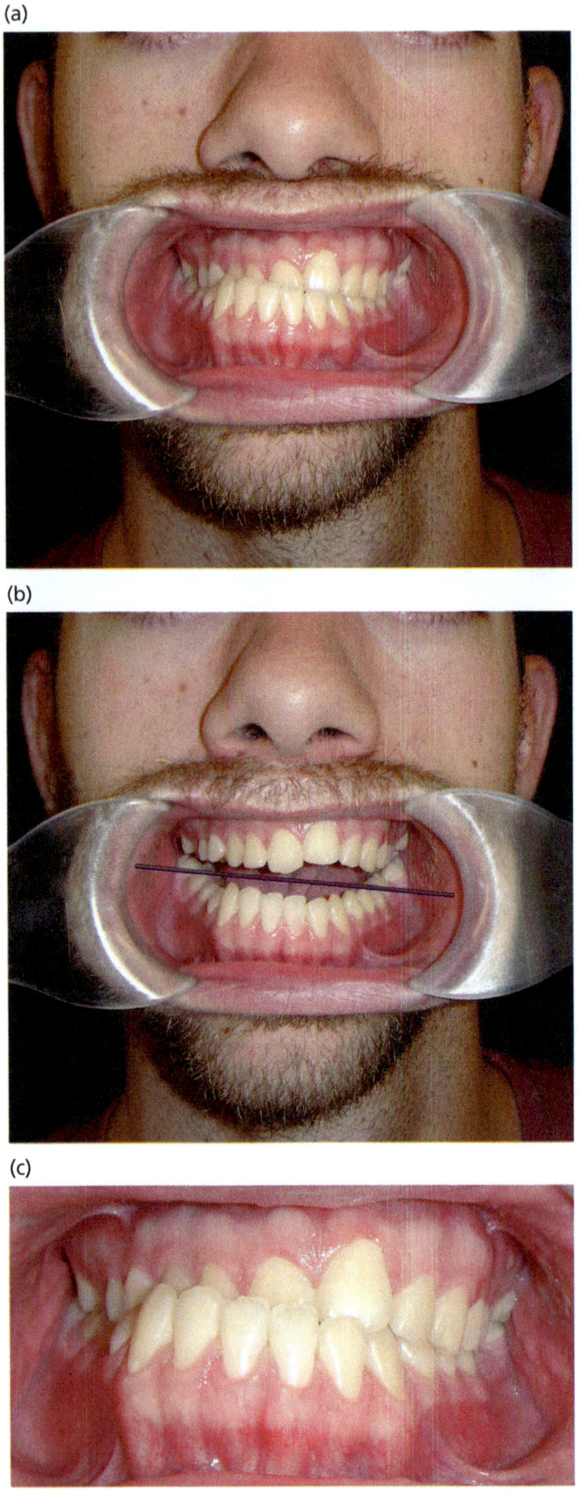

Fig. 34-8 The mandibular occlusal plane is oriented downward on the affected (left) side.

requires additional questions, specifically pertaining to the following:

- **At what age was the asymmetry first noticed (i.e. approximate age of onset)?**
  The patient's parents/family may be able to help, and the patient may need to find and check their own photographs at different ages, which may also be useful for the clinician to assess. If recently noticed, the asymmetry may well be progressing, in which case further investigation is required.
- **Is the asymmetry progressing, or has it been stable for some time?**
- **If progressing, is the patient still growing in stature?**
  Developmental jaw growth anomalies tend to stop progressing when general growth in height diminishes to negligible levels. If there is any doubt, serial cephalometric radiographs may be required after a suitable intervening time period of perhaps one year.
- **Is there a family history of facial asymmetry?**
- **Is there a history of trauma to the face or jaws?**

When evaluating the craniofacial structures for asymmetry, the purpose of the clinical examination is threefold:[16]

- **Qualitative analysis** (visual, anthroposcopic) – Identifying the specific location(s) of the facial asymmetry (skeletal and/or soft tissue).
- **Quantitative analysis** (anthropometric and cephalometric) – Objectively quantifying the degree of facial asymmetry.

Having undertaken a thorough clinical examination, the third step is:

- **Craniofacial growth assessment** – To determine, as far as possible, the location(s), magnitude and direction of any further growth of the craniofacial complex.

Note:

Clinical photographs are useful as a diagnostic aid, and form an important medicolegal record. However, although they permit further facial analyses to be undertaken, *clinical photographs are not a substitute for comprehensive clinical evaluation.*[16]

The clinical evaluation should begin with the **frontal facial examination,** and go on to assess the face from different viewpoints and using various diagnostic records. Comprehensive diagnosis of craniofacial asymmetries has been described elsewhere (see *Facial Aesthetics: Concepts and Clinical Diagnosis*),[16] but the most pertinent information related to jaw asymmetries is summarized in Table 34-4. The patient should be in **natural head position** (NHP), though the clinician may need to make minor manual adjustments to the patient's head position, as patients may have developed a *compensatory head posture* to minimize the aesthetic impact of their facial asymmetry, often tilting their heads to the right or the left, around the sagittal axis.[16]

Table 34-4 Systematic facial evaluation for bilateral symmetry of the maxilla, mandible and related structures

Clinical evaluation	

Frontal view	• Visually assess the approximate vertical distance of bilateral facial structures from a superior true horizontal line (Figure 34-9).
	• Visually assess the approximate horizontal distance of bilateral facial structures from the facial midline.
	• Mark midfacial structures with a skin pencil – Soft tissue glabella, nasion, rhinion, pronasale, labrale superius, labrale inferius and pogonion. Assess their relative positions in relation to each other and the facial midline (see Figure 5-32).
	• Assess the **relative inclination of horizontal reference lines** to each other and to the true horizontal plane (Figure 34-10):
	  ○ Interpupillary line.
	  ○ Intercommissure line.
	  ○ Maxillary occlusal plane – Assess with a wooden tongue spatula or a dental mirror handle (Figure 34-11); assess in the incisor region, and the canine, premolar and molar regions.
	  ○ Mandibular occlusal plane – Assess as for maxilla (Figure 34-12).
	  ○ Inferior chin plane.
	• Assess maxillary and mandibular occlusal plane with the transverse occlusal plane view, using an orthodontic cheek retractor (Figure 34-13) or photographic cheek retractor (Figure 34-14).
	• Assess maxillary incisor and canine exposure bilaterally in relation to the upper lip in repose and in animation (i.e. speech and smiling).
	• Assess vertical face height in midline and bilaterally in lateral aspect of chin, inferior borders of the mandible and gonial angles.
	• Is there a lateral deviation of the lower lip as well as the chin (signifying a horizontal mandibular asymmetry akin to hemimandibular elongation) (Figure 34-15), or is the lower lip aligned with the upper lip?

Profile view	Assess contour of the inferior borders of the mandible.
Submental view	• Assess the symmetry of the mandibular body and the base of the nose. • Assess the horizontal position of the lower lip in relation to the upper lip and chin (Figure 34-16).
Dynamic clinical evaluation	**Mandibular lateral displacement** Assess for a posterior crossbite (especially unilateral) – If a crossbite exists, check for a lateral displacement (functional shift) of the mandible, to ascertain whether *all or part* of the asymmetry is postural (Figure 34-17). Clinically manipulate the mandible into occlusion by placing the knuckle of your curled index finger under the patient's chin and your thumb on the mental eminence. Ask the patient to relax, and to roll the tip of their tongue to the back of their throat, then apply gentle pressure to move the mandible up and down, aiming to keep the condyles in their retruded position within the glenoid fossae. Look for an initial, premature dental contact; the patient may be better able to identify this area and point it out to you. Having established the premature contact, ask the patient to bite together and the displacement will become evident. **Asymmetrical facial animation** An asymmetrical smile where the levator muscles of one side cause greater elevation of the upper lip than the contralateral side – This may be mistaken for a transverse cant of the maxillary occlusal plane.
Maxillary dental midline	Should be aligned to the mid-philtrum of the upper lip. Assess: • Midline deviation (bodily) to the left or right in mm. • Mesiodistal angulation of incisors, and relation to maxillary occlusal plane (i.e. will the incisor angulation self-correct on correcting the jaw asymmetry?) (Figure 34-18)
Mandibular dental midline	Assess in relation to: • Maxillary dental midline • Body of the mandible • Chin proper – i.e. is the dental midline coincident with the midpoint of the chin? Assess: • Midline deviation (bodily) to the left or right. • Mesiodistal angulation of incisors, and relation to transverse occlusal plane cant (i.e. will the incisor angulation self-correct on correcting the jaw asymmetry?)
Radiographic-cephalometric evaluation	
Posteroanterior (PA) cephalometric radiograph	Assess the relative orientation of vertical reference lines drawn parallel to the midsagittal plane, through any pair of bilateral landmarks, to help identify transverse skeletal asymmetries (Figure 34-19). Horizontal reference lines may be used to assess vertical dentoskeletal asymmetries (Figure 34-20). Triangular analysis – This may be used to compare the left and right sides of the facial skeleton (Figure 34-21). *Note*: Any of these methods of analysis may also be used with 3D images, such as CT scans.
Lateral cephalometric radiograph	Assess lack of superimposition of bilateral structures, in particular significant vertical differences between two separate inferior mandibular borders may indicate evidence of mandibular asymmetry, such as hemimandibular hyperplasia (see Figure 34-6f).
Panoramic rotational tomography (OPT)	Assess the morphology and relative height of the mandibular condyle, ramus and body bilaterally (see Figure 34-6g), visually and with comparative bilateral measurements.Assess for degenerative changes to the condylar heads, such as from condylar resorption.

(continued)

Table 34-4 (*Continued*)

Three-dimensional evaluation	
Dental study models	Assess the maxillary and mandibular arch forms separately in occlusal view – One may use a transparent ruled grip oriented in the midline over the mid-palatal raphe, allowing direct observation of arch form.
	This may be useful for monitoring occlusal changes in a growing patient.
Facial soft tissue scans	May be useful for monitoring asymmetrical growth by superimposition of serial scans – This technology requires further development.
Computed tomography (CT)	Useful for more severe asymmetries, particularly panfacial/craniofacial (Figure 34-22).
	Relationship of horizontal and vertical reference planes may be compared (similar to PA cephalograph analysis), and comparison of the relative positions of trigeminal foramina.[2]
	Stereolithographic models, fabricated from CT data, may be useful in diagnosis and planning of complex surgery.

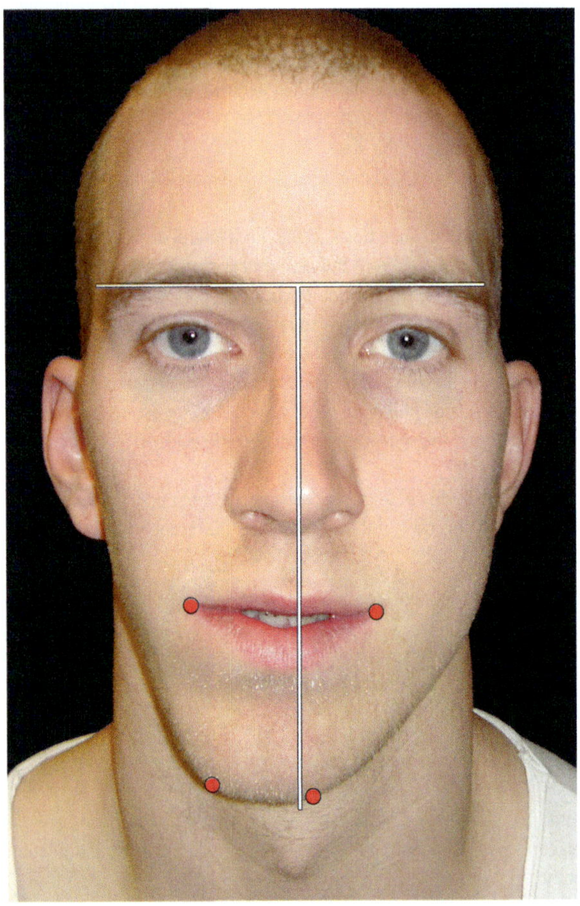

Fig. 34-9 Visually assess the approximate vertical distance of bilateral facial structures from a superior true horizontal line, and the approximate horizontal distance of bilateral facial structures from the facial midline.

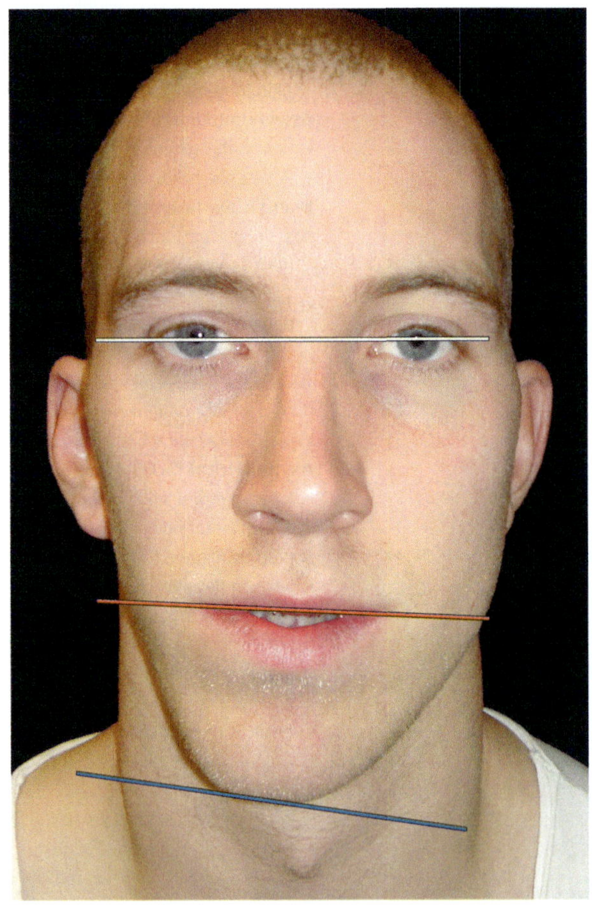

Fig. 34-10 The relative inclination of horizontal reference lines, such as the interpupillary line, intercommissure line and inferior chin plane may be compared to each other and the true horizontal plane.

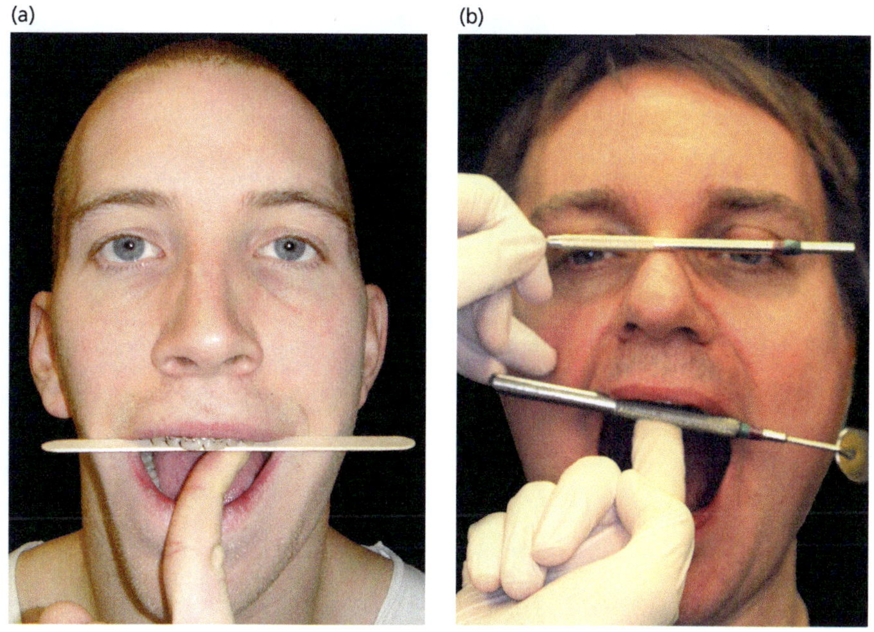

Fig. 34-11 The transverse inclination of the maxillary occlusal plane may be assessed with (a) a wooden tongue spatula or (b) a dental mirror handle.

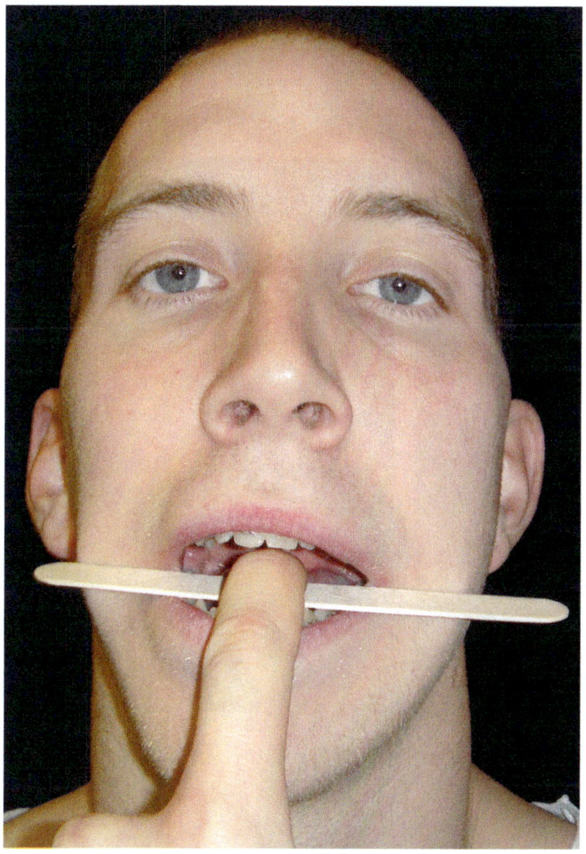

Fig. 34-12 The transverse inclination of the mandibular occlusal plane may be assessed with a wooden tongue spatula or dental mirror handle.

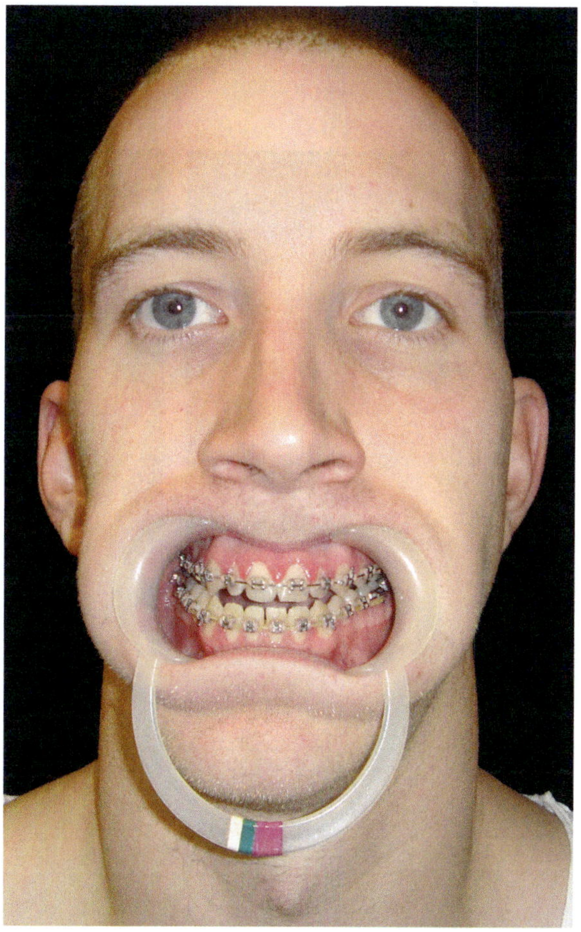

Fig. 34-13 Transverse occlusal plane view using an orthodontic cheek retractor.

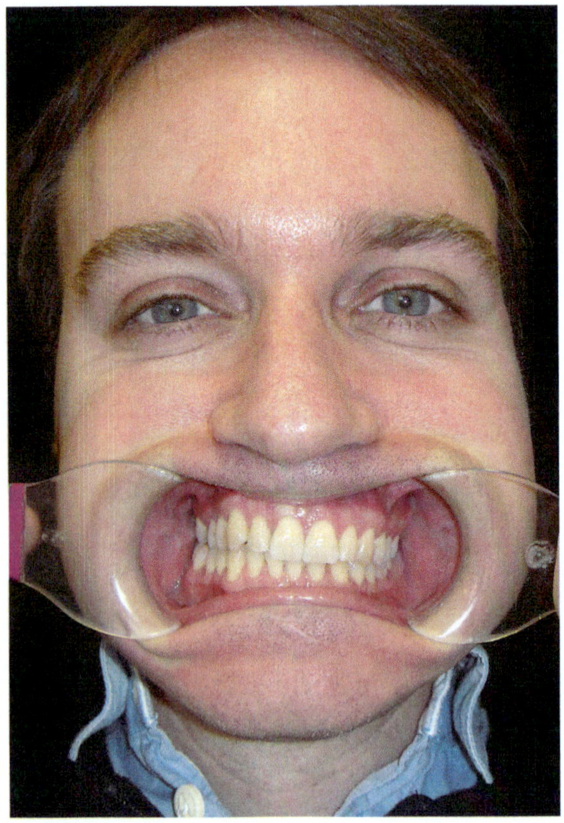

Fig. 34-14 Transverse occlusal plane view using a photographic cheek retractor.

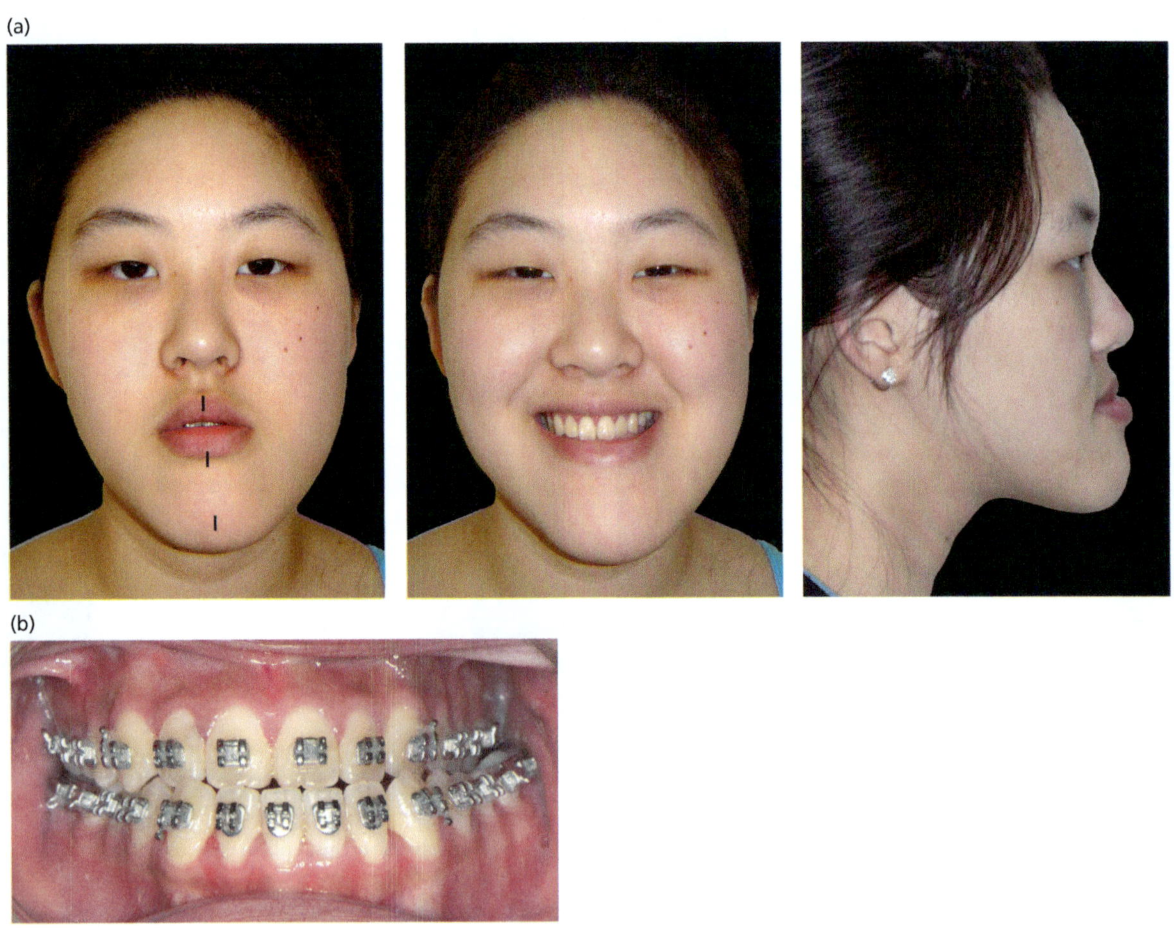

Fig. 34-15 (a) Patient with right-sided hemimandibular elongation, with her chin point and lower lip deviated to her left side. There is a severe Class III skeletal discrepancy, evident in profile view. (b) The dental arches have been orthodontically prepared, with the mandibular dental midline aligned with the chin midline.

(c)

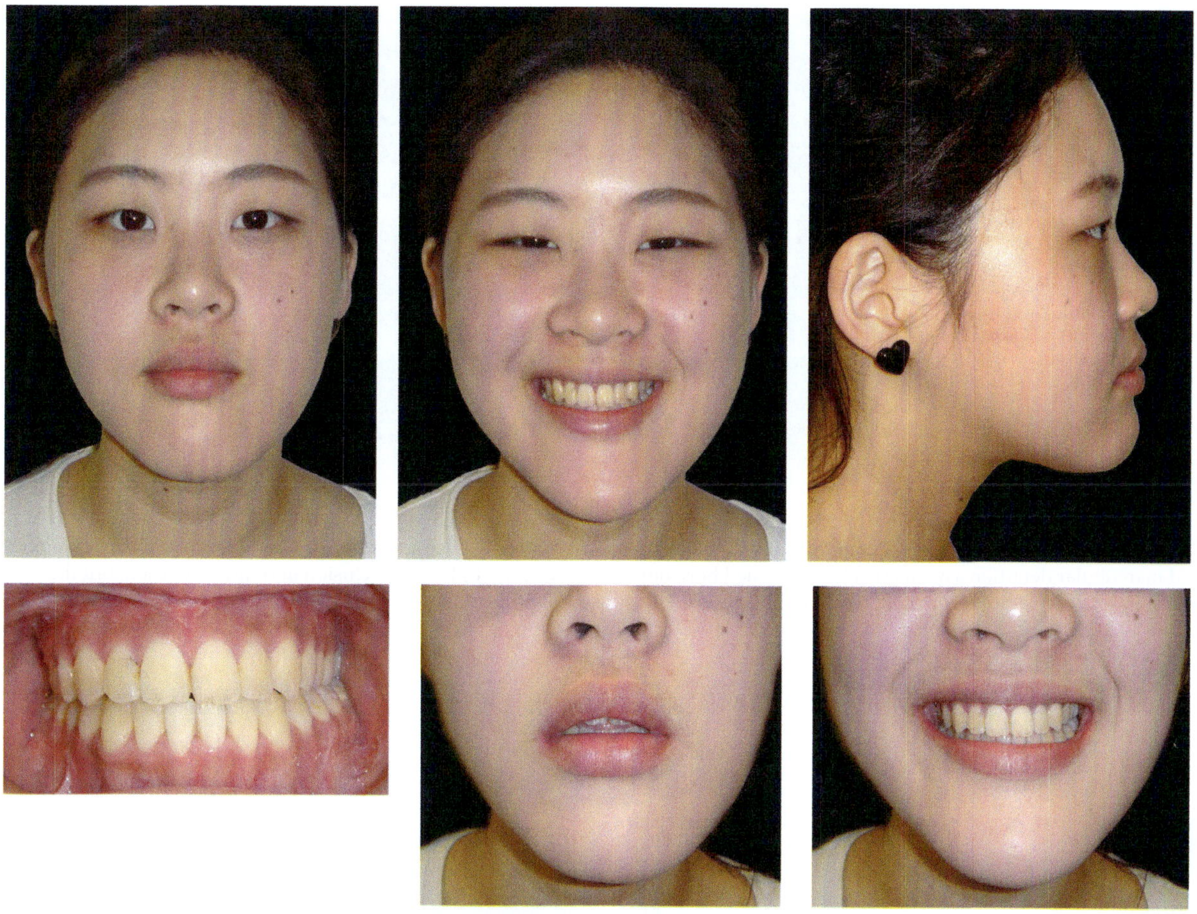

Fig. 34-15 (*Continued*) (c) Bimaxillary surgery with maxillary advancement and asymmetrical mandibular set-back has improved the symmetry of the lower lip and chin in relation to the upper lip and face.

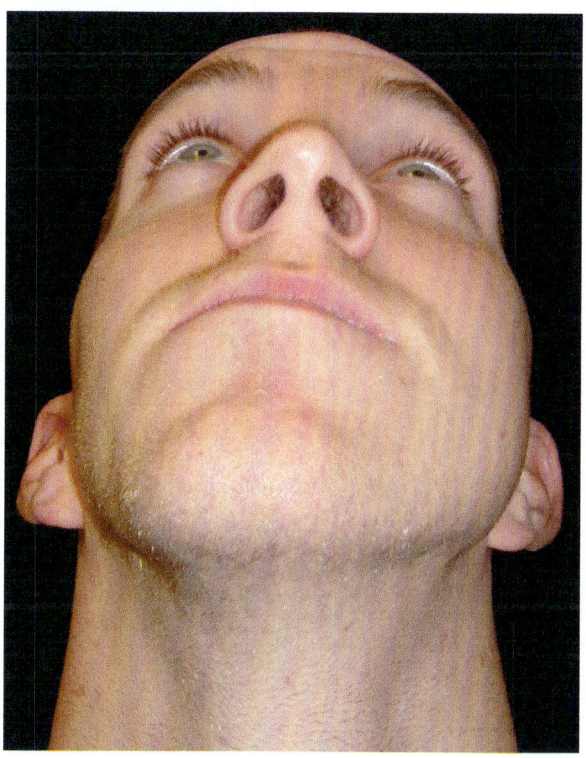

Fig. 34-16 The horizontal position of the lower lip in relation to the upper lip and chin may be assessed with the submental view.

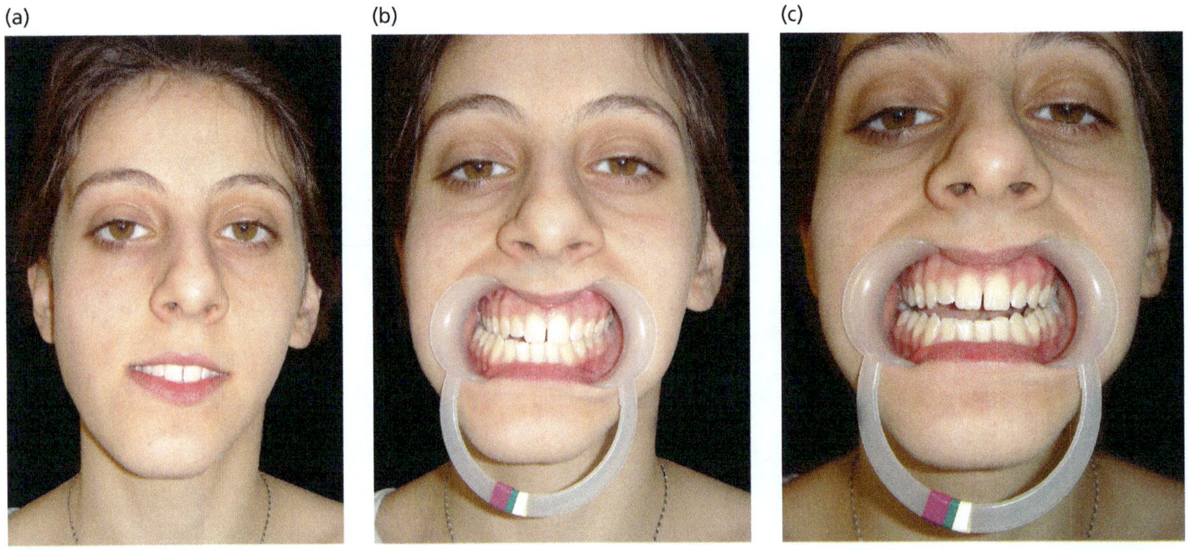

Fig. 34-17 (a) Patient with left-sided hemimandibular elongation (and right-sided hemimandibular hyperplasia), with her chin point and mandibular dentition asymmetrically positioned horizontally to her right. (b) Dental occlusion in centric occlusion, but the patient is also displaced to her right, which is evident in (c) demonstrating the undisplaced position of the mandible.

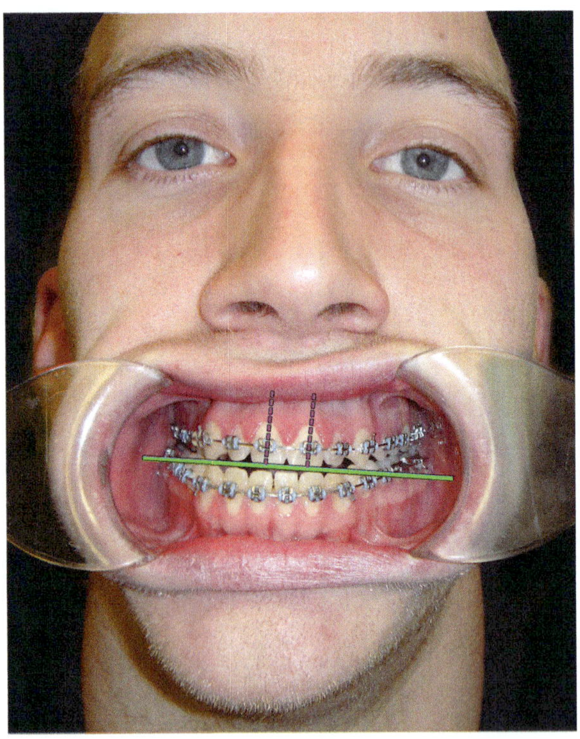

Fig. 34-18 The mesiodistal angulation of the maxillary incisors should be assessed in relation to the maxillary occlusal plane. The question is whether the incisor angulation will self-correct on correcting the jaw asymmetry or whether preoperative orthodontic preparation of the incisor angulations is required.

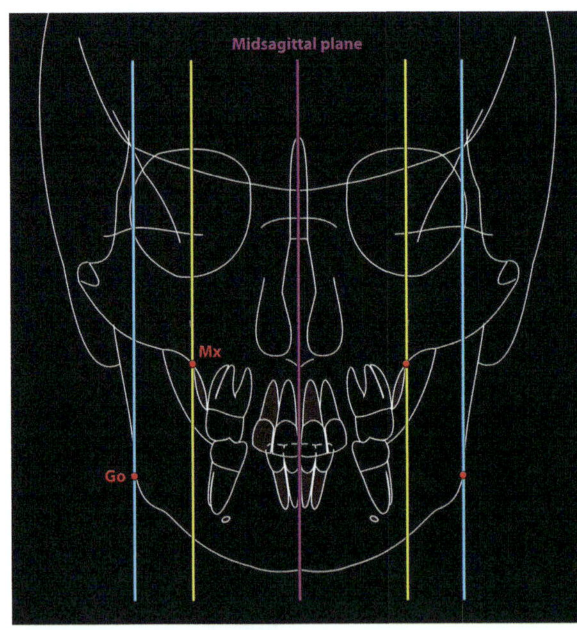

Fig. 34-19 Vertical reference lines may be drawn parallel to the midsagittal plane through any pair of bilateral landmarks to help identify transverse skeletal asymmetries. Mx, maxillare; Go, gonion. (From: Naini FB. Facial Aesthetics: Concepts and Clinical Diagnosis. Oxford: Wiley-Blackwell, 2011; used with permission.[16])

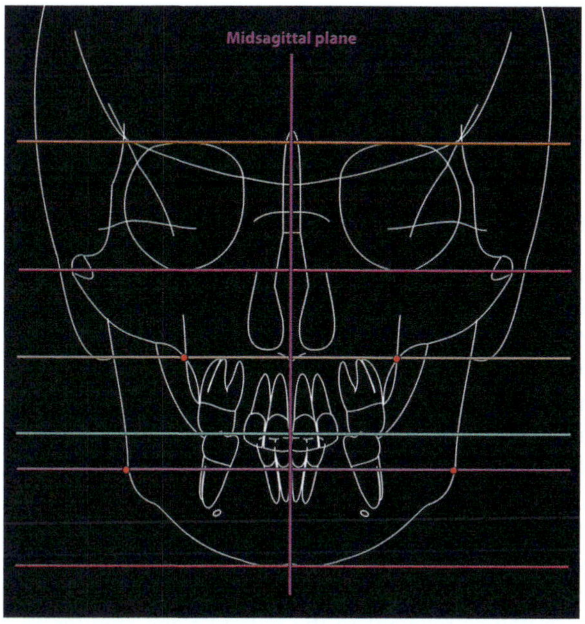

Fig. 34-20 Horizontal reference lines may be used to illustrate vertical dentoskeletal discrepancies. (From: Naini FB. Facial Aesthetics: Concepts and Clinical Diagnosis. Oxford: Wiley-Blackwell, 2011; used with permission.[16])

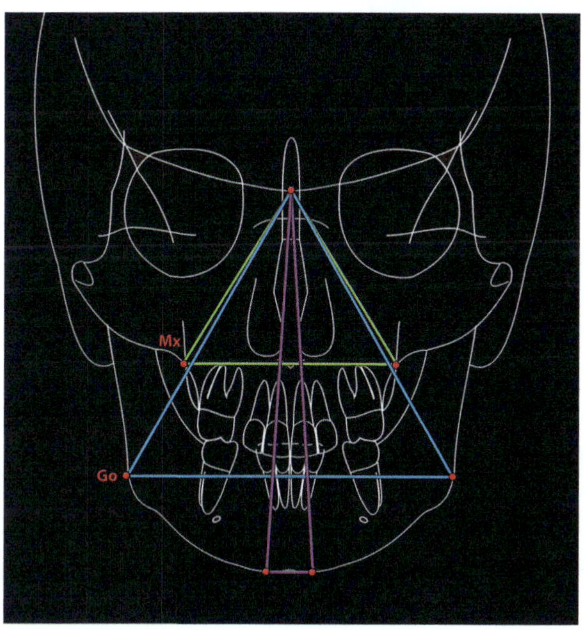

Fig. 34-21 'Triangular analysis' demonstrating the maxillary, mandibular and chin triangles. Comparison of the left and right legs of the triangles demonstrates transverse canting in relation to the cranial base. Comparison of the left and right halves of the bases of the triangles will indicate asymmetry and left-right difference in size (assuming no rotation of the patient's head around the vertical axis). (From: Naini FB. Facial Aesthetics: Concepts and Clinical Diagnosis. Oxford: Wiley-Blackwell, 2011; used with permission.[16])

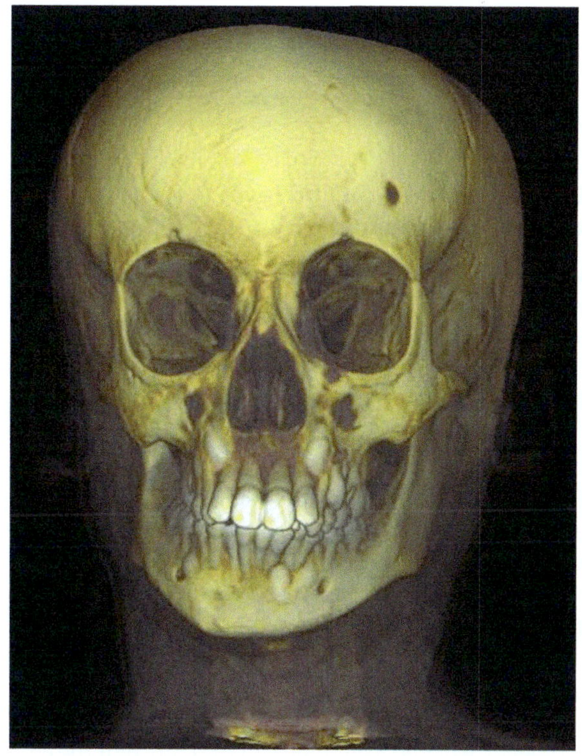

Fig. 34-22 Three-dimensional computed tomograph of a patient with hemifacial microsomia. (Courtesy of Dr Jacques Treil.)

Principles in planning the surgical correction of maxillary and mandibular asymmetry

The principles in planning the orthognathic surgical correction of maxillary and mandibular asymmetry are summarized in Table 34-5.[16]

The **management of patient expectations** has been described in Chapter 5. However, it is vitally important that patients with significant dentofacial asymmetries are made aware of the following:

- Their postoperative result will *not* be perfectly symmetrical;

Table 34-5 Principles in planning the surgical correction of jaw asymmetry

- Define the location and level of the asymmetry
- Define the type and extent of the asymmetry
- Determine which tissues are involved
- Correct transverse cants
  - Maxillary occlusal plane
  - Mandibular occlusal plane
  - Inferior chin plane
- Maintain/improve exposure of maxillary incisors
- Maintain/improve LAFH proportion
- Maintain/improve sagittal skeletal relationships
- Correct midlines
  - Maxillary dental midline
  - Mandibular dental midline
  - Chin midline
- Improve dental occlusion

LAFH, lower anterior face height.

- A degree of asymmetry is inevitable; and,
- The correction of asymmetry in one facial region may make the asymmetry of another region appear more obvious.

Define the location and level (i.e. facial thirds) of the asymmetry

With the patient in natural head position (NHP) and having assessed and adjusted the patient's head to remove any compensatory head posture, it is necessary to evaluate the facial thirds in order to assess the level (i.e. upper, middle or lower facial third) and specific location of the asymmetry (Figure 34-23). In most dentofacial deformity patients (as opposed to craniofacial deformities), the upper face will not be affected and the interpupillary line will be approximately level with the true horizontal. Midfacial asymmetries may involve the nose or zygomatic regions. Asymmetries of the maxilla are usually secondary to those of the mandible. Asymmetries of the chin are usually associated with asymmetries of the mandible, and thereby often self-correct with repositioning of the mandible. However, isolated asymmetry of the chin, or if the chin is more asymmetrical than the mandible, may require an asymmetrical repositioning genioplasty for correction. Sequential masking of the face is a useful technique in defining the location and level of facial asymmetry (see Figure 6.27a).

Define the type and extent of the asymmetry

Having assessed the level and location of the asymmetry, it is necessary to define, as far as possible, whether the asymmetry is due to unilateral *excess or deficiency* in growth, or a combination. The diagnostic determination regarding excess or deficiency depends foremost on the overall facial aesthetics and the craniofacial size in relation to the patient's standing height and stature. Quantifying the extent of the asymmetry can be aided by the patient's anthropometric and cephalometric measurements and proportional relationships being compared with normative population values relevant to the patient's age, gender and ethnicity.

The relevance of this information to treatment planning is significant. It is important to bear in mind that skeletal expansion has more predictable soft

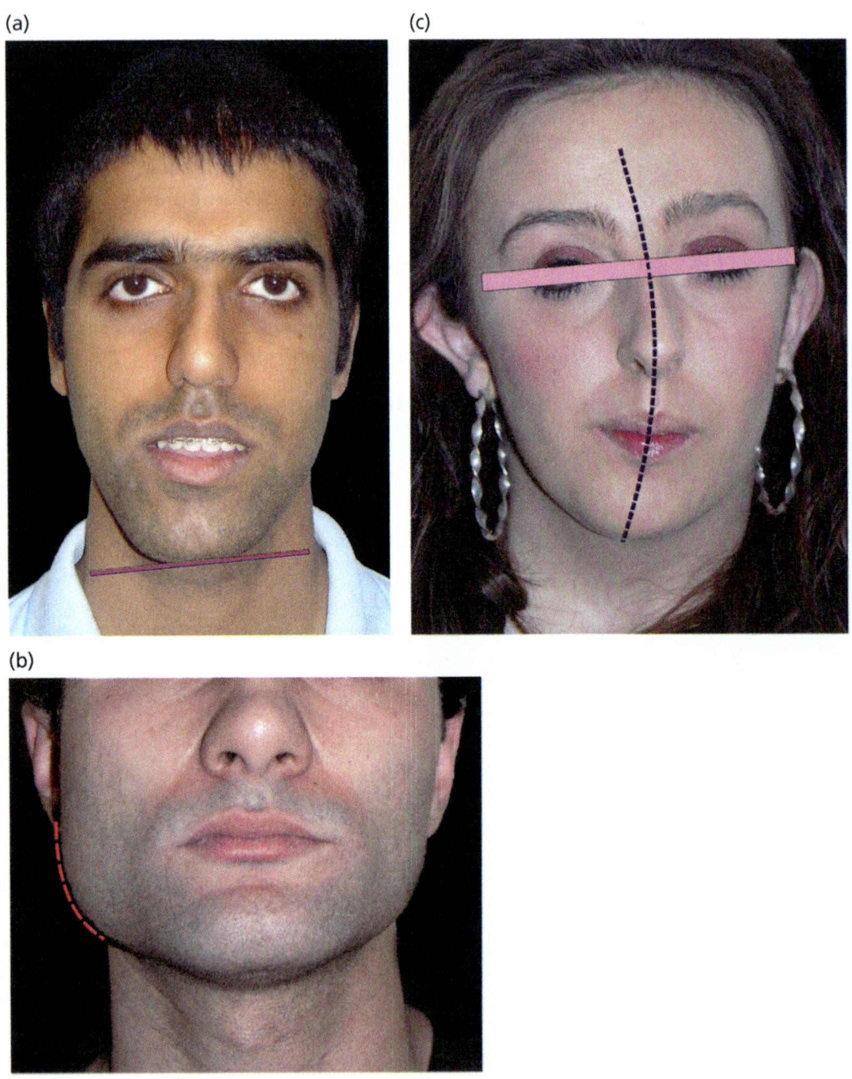

Fig. 34-23 Defining the level and location of facial asymmetries. (a) Asymmetry of the mandible and chin, with transverse canting of the inferior chin plane. (b) Asymmetry of the gonial angle region, which demonstrates greater lateral prominence on the patient's right side. (c) Panfacial asymmetry, including vertical orbital dystopia. In essence, the higher the level of the facial asymmetry, the more difficult it is to improve with surgery.

tissue results compared with skeletal reduction. Therefore, in improving facial symmetry it may be better to err on the side of skeletal expansion and soft tissue augmentation on the relatively deficient side. Alternatively, if the larger side is excessively increased in size, a decision may be made to partly reduce that side, and partly augment the contralateral side.

Determine which tissues are involved

It is important to determine whether a facial asymmetry is predominantly due to the underlying skeletal structures (e.g. skeletal mandibular asymmetry), the soft tissues (e.g. hemifacial atrophy) or both. In this way, it is possible to determine how much of the correction requires dentoskeletal repositioning or rigid consistency materials for soft tissue augmentation, and how much requires softer materials for soft tissue augmentation, such as fat grafting (see Chapter 51).

The next four sections, i.e. assessing and planning the correction of transverse cants, maintaining or improving the exposure of the maxillary incisors, the vertical proportions of the lower face, and the sagittal skeletal relationships, are not evaluated independently, but rather *need to be considered simultaneously*. Based on this, the following decisions may be made:

- Do one or both jaws need to be repositioned?
- What type of jaw movement (direction and magnitude) is required in relation to the three planes of space and the three axes of rotation?
- Which surgical procedure(s) is required to achieve the desired results?

Correct transverse cants

Maxillary occlusal plane

Perhaps the most significant decision is whether a surgical correction of a transverse maxillary occlusal plane cant is required. If there is a significant cant, the second decision is whether correction will require superior repositioning on the vertically lower side, setdown on the contralateral side, or a combination of both. This decision is made primarily based *on the aesthetic parameter of the maxillary incisor and canine exposure in relation to the upper lip at rest (and in animation), bearing in mind the lower anterior face height proportion and the implications for surgical stability*.

If the incisor and canine exposure is reduced, unilateral setdown of the maxilla is the treatment of choice. However, the requirement for a bone graft and the stretching of the musculofascial tissues on this side will be concerns for surgical stability. Additionally, if concomitant advancement or set-back of the maxilla is required to improve the sagittal skeletal relationship, the change in incisor exposure resulting from this must also be taken into account.

Mandibular occlusal plane

The maxillary occlusal plane is usually canted as a secondary response to the asymmetry of the mandible. As such, the mandibular occlusal plane is usually of a similar extent and the required rotation of the bimaxillary complex from the frontal view will correct the transverse cants of both occlusal planes.

Inferior chin plane

If the asymmetry of the chin is positional and secondary to the asymmetry of the mandible, then the inferior chin plane will also correct with the repositioning of the mandible. However, if there is an additional asymmetry of the chin, a corrective genioplasty will be required.

Other bilateral structures that may present with transverse canting are the inferior borders of the mandible and the gonial angles. These also need to be evaluated, but may require additional surgical procedures, such as augmentation or skeletal reduction, for correction.

Maintain/improve exposure of maxillary incisors

As with every aspect of orthognathic treatment planning previously discussed (see Chapter 6), the relationship of the maxillary incisors to the upper lip forms the foundation stone of treatment planning. Correction of the maxillary occlusal plane, lower face height and sagittal repositioning of the maxilla all revolve around this foundation.

Maintain/improve lower anterior face height (LAFH) proportion

This is relevant in terms of the decision to impact or setdown the lateral aspects of the maxilla when planning the correction of the maxillary occlusal plane.

Maintain/improve sagittal skeletal relationships (maxilla, mandible and chin)

The sagittal prominence of the maxilla, mandible and chin is planned as previously described (see Chapters 5 and 6). It is important to bear in mind the effect of advancement or set-back of the maxilla in relation to the maxillary incisor exposure, as discussed above.

Correct midlines (to facial midline)

The maxillary and mandibular dental midlines and the midpoint of the chin should be coincident with the facial midline. If the dental midlines are not coincident with each other or the facial midline, it is important to determine the extent of deviation from the facial midline, the angulation of the incisors, and the relationship to the underlying jaw deformity. Mesiodistal incisor angulations usually occur as a result of dental compensation for the underlying skeletal asymmetry. The incisor angulation should be corrected to the respective skeletal base with preparatory orthodontics, such that the angulation self-corrects with surgical repositioning of the jaws.

Maxillary dental midline

Maxillary dental midline deviations are usually a result of a dentoalveolar anomaly, such as crowding. Therefore, correction may well require orthodontic correction. However, space is required to correct a midline deviation with tooth movement. If dental extractions are not required for any other reason, it is possible to plan for surgical correction of maxillary midline deviations of up to 3–4 mm with rotation of the maxilla around the vertical axis. Greater rotations of the maxilla are not advisable, as they may result in problems with the posterior dental occlusion.

Mandibular dental midline

The mandibular dental midline should be aligned to the body of the mandible, such that repositioning of the mandible will correct the dental midline. This should also be made coincident with the midpoint of the chin, so long as the chin is symmetrical to the mandibular body.

Chin midline

The chin midline should be coincident with the mandibular body midline and the mandibular dental midline. Any isolated asymmetry of the chin may be corrected with asymmetrical repositioning genioplasty.

Improve dental occlusion

Improvement of the dental occlusion should be an integral part of the treatment plan. Asymmetry correction usually involves repositioning of the jaws in all three planes of space, and the effect on the proposed dental occlusion should be borne in mind.

Orthodontic preparation

Preparatory orthodontics has been described in detail (see Chapter 12). However, there are a number of specific points to consider in preparation for surgical correction of jaw asymmetries.

The primary objective of preparatory orthodontics in an asymmetry patient is to remove the dental compensations and *to make the dental-occlusal asymmetry match the skeletal asymmetry*, which will allow correction of the dental occlusion with the skeletal repositioning. Judging the arch width of the opposing jaws for arch coordination is best accomplished by hand articulating the dental study models, which will demonstrate the requirement for arch expansion or contraction. Preparing the dental midlines based on the type of surgery planned, and preparing incisor angulations in preparation for occlusal plane rotation around the sagittal axis have been described above. If maxillary surgery is not required, maxillary dental midline deviation correction may well require dental extractions to create space. This usually involves extraction of the first premolar on the side to which the dental midline is to be moved. However, all things being equal, it is better to avoid extractions in the maxillary arch only, as there is a tendency to narrowing of the arch width, making arch coordination more difficult. This is particularly true in Class III asymmetrical patients, where the maxilla may be rather small relative to the mandible.

In the asymmetrical patient, arch coordination may necessitate unilateral arch expansion and/or contralateral arch contraction of the maxilla. This may be achieved using coordinated rectangular stainless steel archwires, and the use of cross-elastics may also be useful.

Otherwise, the objectives of preoperative orthodontics are essentially as described in Chapter 12.

Preoperative model surgery

Patients with jaw asymmetries present a unique set of challenges for model surgery, and special considerations are required. *The most important principle to follow is that the direction and magnitude of the surgical movements must be decided clinically*. No attempt should be made to make alterations or adjustments when just viewing the articulator-mounted dental models. If there is a vertical discrepancy in the position of the external auditory canals, the facebow recording should avoid the ear canals, or alternatively use one canal, maintaining the facebow in relation to the true horizontal plane.

Surgical technique

The Le Fort I osteotomy and the mandibular sagittal split osteotomy have been described in Chapters 22 and 24 respectively, and osseous genioplasty has been described in Chapter 33. However, there are a number of technical modifications and nuances required in the correction of maxillary and mandibular asymmetry. Depending on the complexity of the presenting asymmetry, surgical techniques need to be individualized and may involve variations in standard osteotomies, skeletal recontouring and soft tissue augmentation or reduction (see Chapter 51).

In the first instance, the Le Fort I osteotomy allows the maxillary occlusal plane to be levelled, and the maxilla to be repositioned in relation to the three planes of space as planned. In levelling a transverse maxillary occlusal plane cant the decision regarding how much to impact on one side and/or setdown on the contralateral side, or a combination of the two, depends on the degree of maxillary incisor/canine exposure and the lower anterior face height, i.e. aesthetics vs. stability (see planning section above).

Mandibular repositioning follows, usually with a bilateral sagittal split osteotomy (BSSO). Reyneke has emphasized the importance to the surgeon and their team of being constantly 'condyle aware' during repositioning of the mandible following a BSSO.[17] Significant mandibular advancement or set-back, particularly with a rotational element of the distal segment (bearing the teeth and alveolar process) to correct a mandibular asymmetry may lead to lateral condylar torque/rotation and/or displacement within the glenoid fossa when the proximal segment is rigidly fixated to the distal segment (Figure 34-24). This effect is exacerbated with greater degrees of rotation and in an anatomically V-shaped mandible. Tucker and Thomas[18] have described special precautions required to avoid this problem:

1. Recontouring of the most posterior aspect of the distal segment, allowing close adaptation of the proximal segment without the fulcrum effect that would torque/rotate the condyle (Figure 34-25a). A conventional lag screw or a position screw may be used for fixation.
2. Use of a piece of bone as a wedge or shim to maintain any anterior space in the osteotomy site and preventing condylar displacement as a conventional lag screw is tightened (Figure 34-25b).
3. Use of position screws to engage the outer and inner cortices whilst maintaining the bony distance between the osteotomized segments, thereby preventing the fulcrum effect and lateral condylar torque/rotation (Figure 34-25c).

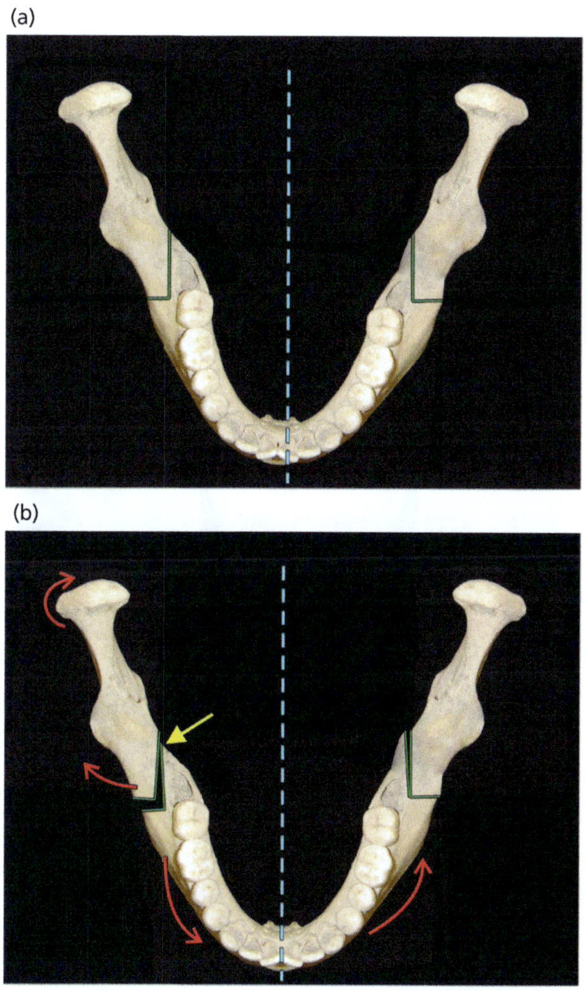

Fig. 34-24 (a) Bilateral sagittal split osteotomy (BSSO) in an asymmetrical mandible (superior view). (b) Unilateral advancement and rotation of the distal segment (bearing the teeth) to the contralateral side, in order to correct the asymmetry, may result in the posterior aspect of the distal segment engaging the medial aspect of the proximal (condyle bearing) segment (shown with the yellow arrow), thereby resulting in lateral displacement of the proximal segment and rotation/torquing of the condyle. An attempt to place rigid fixation in such a situation, squeezing the two segments together, will lead to problems, usually of an asymmetry becoming evident when the patient's muscular function returns to normal following the general anaesthesia.

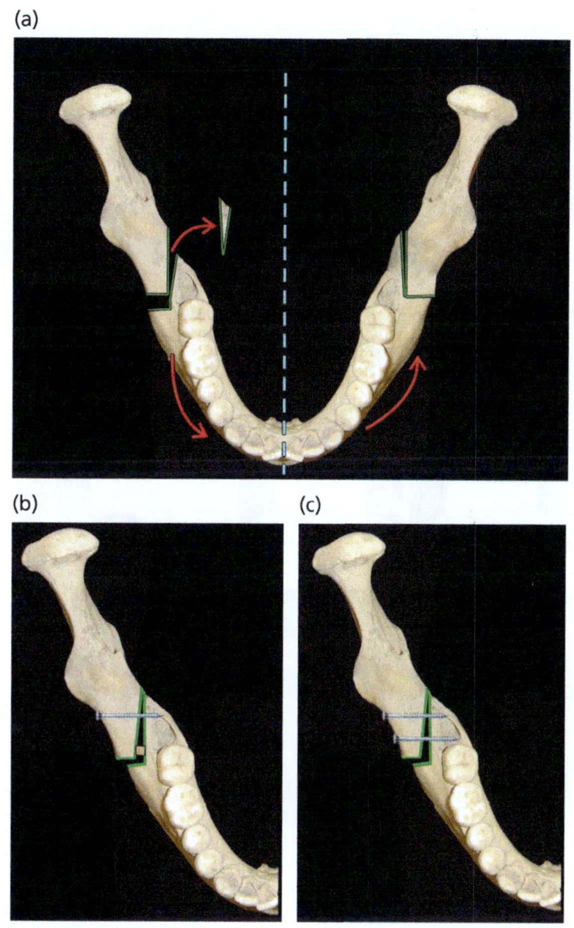

Fig. 34-25 There are three methods to avoid the problem described in Figure 34-24: (a) Recontouring of the posterior aspect of the distal segment by removing bone, as shown, prior to rigid fixation. This permits passive adaptation of the distal and proximal segments without lateral condylar torque/rotation or displacement of the condyle within the glenoid fossa. (b) Use of a piece of bone as a wedge or shim to maintain any anterior space in the osteotomy site and prevent condylar displacement as a conventional lag screw is tightened. (c) Placement of a position screw in the anterior part of the proximal segment to maintain the interbony distance. (After Tucker and Thomas.[18]).

Asymmetrical genioplasty (see Figure 2-69d) and skeletal/soft tissue augmentation (see Chapter 51) or reduction may need to be carried out as secondary procedures.

Postoperative orthodontics

The potential for slight variation in the actual postoperative dental occlusal position compared with the planned position in asymmetry cases is greater than with orthognathic surgery in more straightforward sagittal and vertical discrepancies. As such, the postoperative orthodontics may need to compensate the dentition for an essentially minor skeletal malocclusion. Asymmetrical use of intermaxillary elastics may be required in some patients if the dental occlusion and midlines are not quite coincident, but was planned to be, i.e. Class II elastic on one side and Class III on the contralateral side (see Figure 12-63k). An anterior cross elastic may also be required, which should usually only be worn at night. The elastic force should be kept light, in order to avoid unwanted vertical extrusion of teeth and potential transverse rotation of the occlusal plane. Small posterior or lateral open bites may also be present, which will require light vertical elastics on flexible archwires, allowing dental extrusion.

Case Examples

Case example 1 (Figure 34-26)

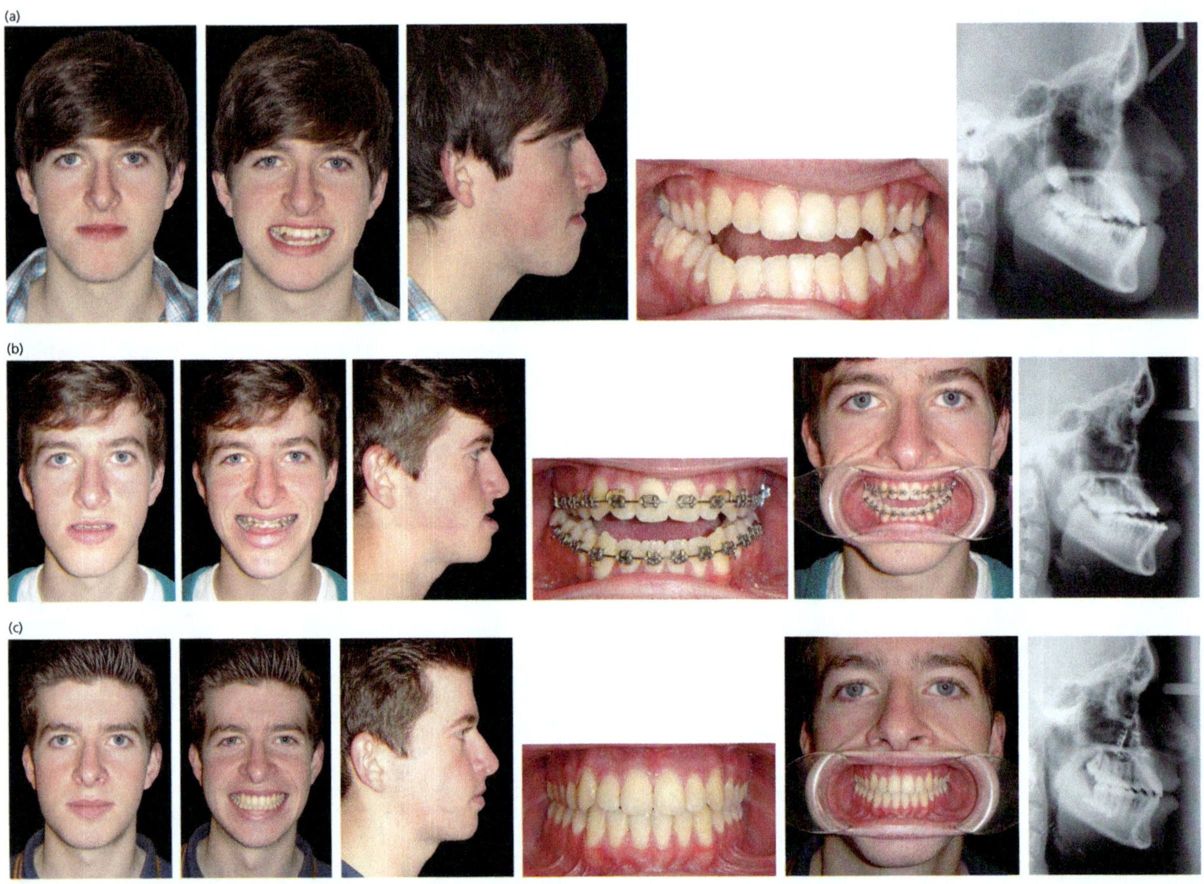

Fig. 34-26 (a) Patient with a severe Class III skeletal discrepancy (due to maxillary retrognathism and mandibular prognathism) and anterior open bite, with left-sided hemimandibular elongation, and his chin point and mandibular dental midline to his right. (b) Preoperative views. The patient was planned for a maxillary posterior differential impaction and advancement, and forward mandibular autorotation and asymmetrical mandibular set-back. (c) End of treatment views.

Case example 2 (Figure 34-27)

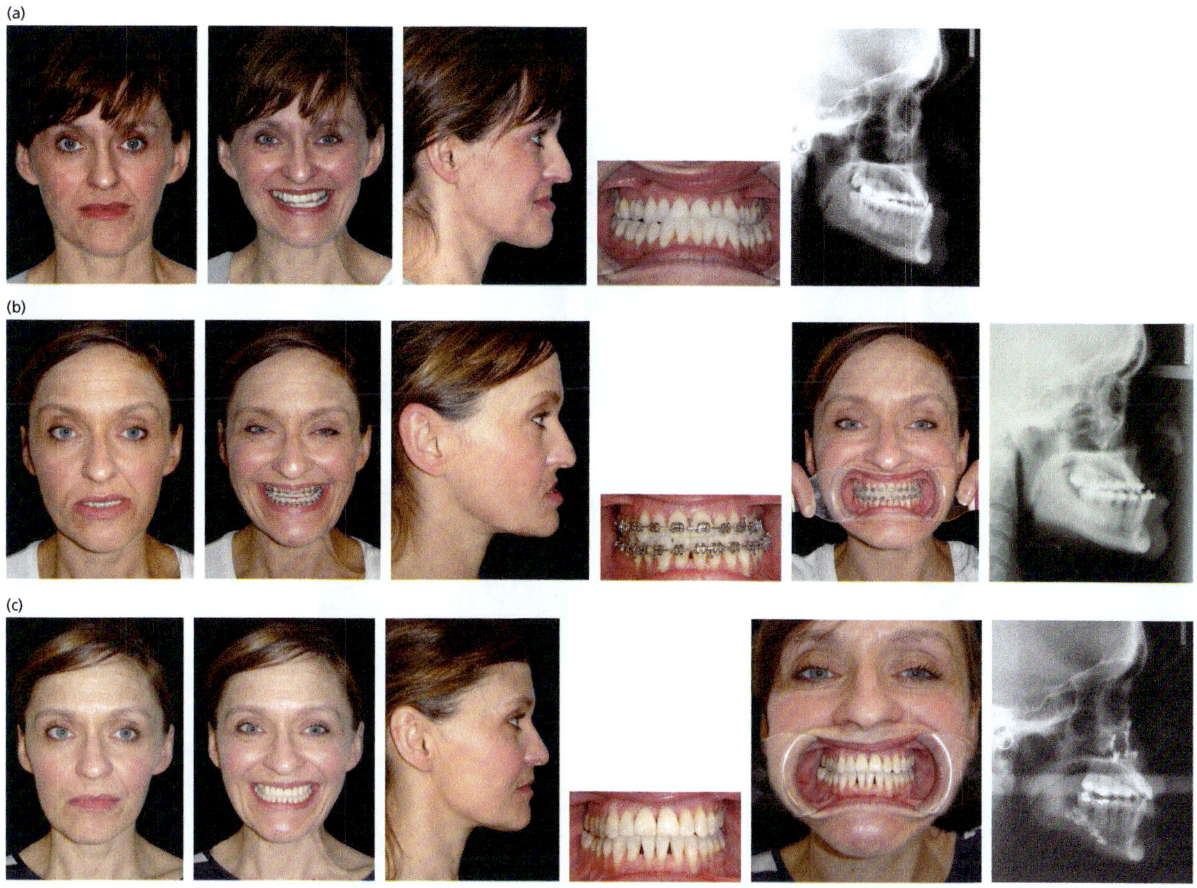

Fig. 34-27 (a) Patient with a severe Class III skeletal discrepancy (due to maxillary retrognathism and mandibular prognathism), with right-sided hemimandibular elongation, and her chin point and mandibular dental midline to her left. (b) Preoperative views. The patient was planned for maxillary advancement (2/3rds) and asymmetrical mandibular set-back (1/3rd). (c) End of treatment views.

Case example 3 (Figure 34-28)

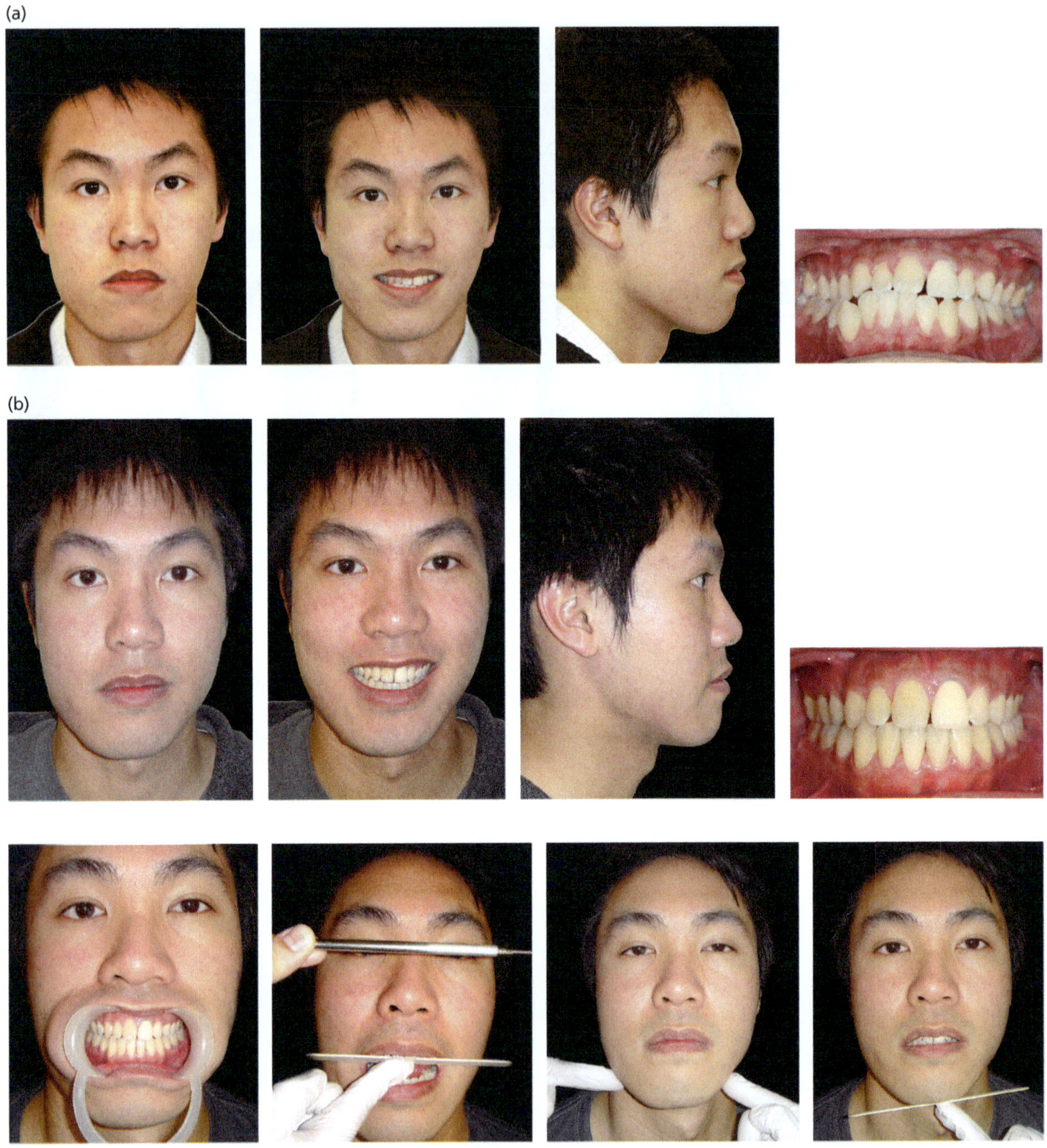

Fig. 34-28 (a) Pretreatment views of a patient with right-sided hemimandibular hyperplasia (HH) and left-sided hemimandibular elongation (HE). It is important to bear in mind that HH and HE may affect contralateral sides of the mandible. (b) Bimaxillary surgery was undertaken and the midpoint of the chin is symmetrical with the facial midline and the occlusal planes are level. However, the patient's right mandibular inferior border is still lower in position than his left side, and the inferior chin plane is transversely canted. The chin asymmetry would require an isolated genioplasty, which was planned as a potential secondary procedure, which the patient did not desire.

Case example 4 (Figure 34-29)

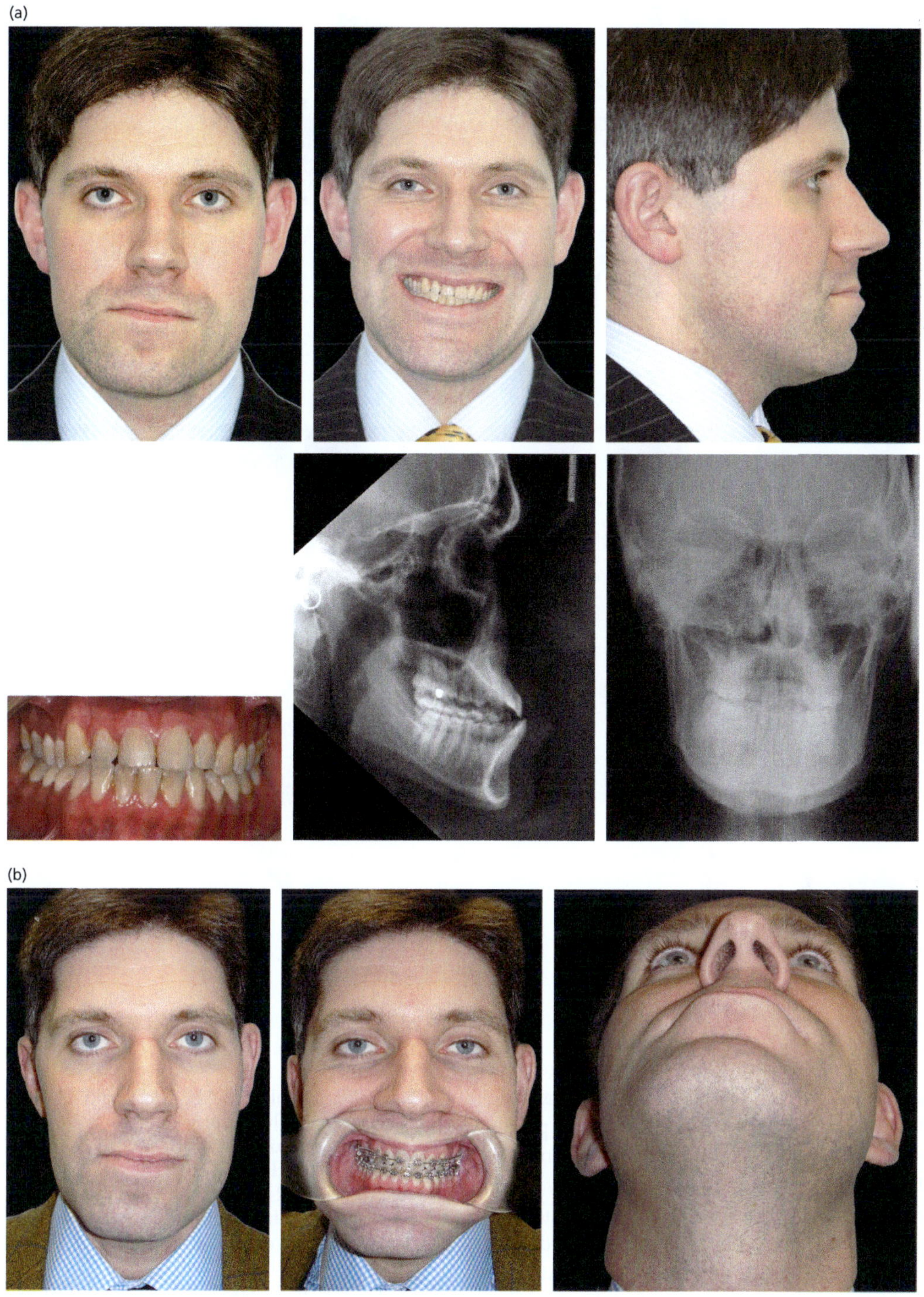

Fig. 34-29 (a) Patient with combined left-sided hemimandibular hyperplasia and elongation. The ramus height was increased on his left side, and there was a maxillary occlusal plane cant, lower on his left side (signs of hemimandibular hyperplasia). The mandibular body length was increased on his left side, and the chin point and mandibular dental midline were off to his right (signs of hemimandibular elongation). There was a mild Class III skeletal discrepancy. (b) Preoperative views. The maxillary and mandibular occlusal plane cants were maintained. The patient was planned for correction of the maxillary occlusal plane cant with impaction on his left side and setdown on his right to level the occlusal plane. The maxilla was advanced slightly. The mandible was asymmetrically set-back (with a bilateral sagittal split osteotomy), correcting the mandibular occlusal plane cant and chin point by rotation of the distal segment (tooth-bearing portion of the mandible) around both the sagittal axis and the vertical axis. (c) End of treatment views.

(c)

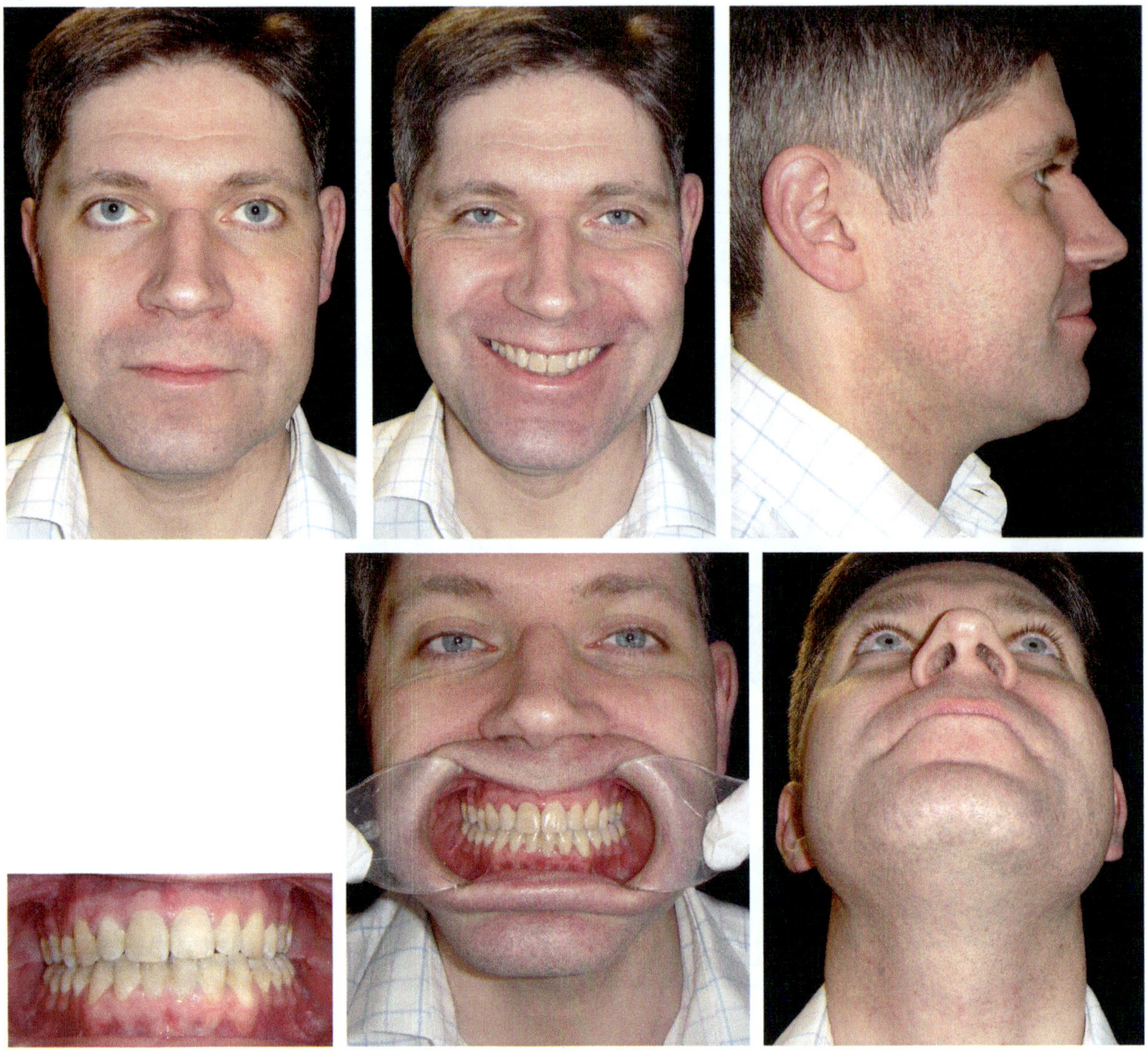

Fig. 34-29 (*Continued*)

Conclusion

The diagnosis, planning and surgical management of jaw asymmetries is among the most challenging aspects of orthognathic surgery. Two important points should be borne in mind. Firstly, surgical techniques do not allow surgeons to produce a perfectly symmetrical facial result. Therefore, surgical treatment of asymmetry should focus on improving the condition, not correcting it. Secondly, the effect of the surgical movement of the hard tissue on the facial soft tissue contour is currently the most unpredictable area of this type of surgery. For this reason, the orthognathic surgeon should also have a thorough understanding and familiarity with adjunctive surgical techniques, such as soft tissue augmentation and grafting (see Chapter 51).

References

1 Vitruvius. The Ten Books on Architecture (c. 25 BC). Trans. Morgan MH. Mineola, NY: Dover Publications, 1960.

2 Naini FB. Facial Symmetry and Asymmetry. In: Naini FB. Facial Aesthetics: Concepts and Clinical Diagnosis. Oxford: Wiley-Blackwell, 2011.

3 Naini FB, Donaldson AN, McDonald F, Cobourne MT. Assessing the influence of asymmetry affecting the mandible and chin point on perceived attractiveness in the orthognathic patient, clinician, and layperson. J Oral Maxillofac Surg. 2012;70:192–206.

4 Shackelford TK, Larsen RJ. Facial asymmetry as an indicator of psychological, emotional, and physiological distress. J Personal Soc Psychol. 1997;72:456–66.

5 Cohen MM Jr. Perspectives on craniofacial asymmetry 1. The biology of asymmetry. Internat J Oral Maxillofac Surg. 1995;24:2–7.

6 Cohen MM Jr. Perspectives on craniofacial asymmetry 3. Common and/or well-known causes of asymmetry. Internat J Oral Maxillofac Surg. 1995;24:127–33.

7 Rushton MA. Growth at the mandibular condyle in relation to some deformities. Br Dent J. 1944;76:57–68.

8 Waldron CW, Peterson RG, Waldron CA. Surgical treatment of mandibular prognathism. J Oral Surg (Chic). 1946;4:61–88.

9 Cernea P. Les déviations mandibulaires d'origine epiphysaire. Rev Stomatol. 1948;49:388–413.

10 Gottlieb OP. Hyperplasia of the mandibular condyle. J Oral Surg. 1951;9:118–35.

11 Hinds EC, Reid LC, Burch RJ. Classification and management of mandibular asymmetry. Am J Surg. 1960;100:825–34.
12 Rowe NL. Aetiology, clinical features and treatment of mandibular deformity. Brit Dent J. 1960;108:41–64.
13 Bruce RA, Hayward JR. Condylar hyperplasia and mandibular asymmetry. J Oral Surg. 1968;26:281–90.
14 Obwegeser HL, Makek MS. Hemimandibular hyperplasia–hemimandibular elongation. J Maxillofac Surg. 1986;14:183–208.
15 Naini FB. Regional Aesthetic Analysis: The Mandible. In: Naini FB. Facial Aesthetics: Concepts and Clinical Diagnosis. Oxford: Wiley-Blackwell, 2011.
16 Naini FB. Facial Aesthetics: Concepts and Clinical Diagnosis. Oxford: Wiley-Blackwell, 2011.
17 Reyneke JP. Essentials of Orthognathic Surgery (2nd Ed.). Hanover Park, IL: Quintessence Publishing, 2010.
18 Tucker MR, Thomas PM. Rigid fixation for orthognathic surgery: Current perspectives and controversies. In: Melsen B. (Ed.) Current Controversies in Orthodontics. Chicago, IL: Quintessence Publishing, 1991.

Chapter 35

Temporomandibular Joint Replacement Surgery in the Orthognathic Patient

N. Shaun Matthews, Jonas Osher and Martyn T. Cobourne

Introduction

It is important to be able to diagnose and treat temporomandibular joint (TMJ) pathology as an orthognathic surgeon. The TMJs form the foundation for any orthognathic procedure and it is important that they are stable and healthy in order to ensure satisfactory orthognathic outcome. Pathological TMJs will prevent good function, aesthetics and stability. TMJ replacement can be considered during orthognathic surgery when this type of surgical intervention alone is unable to correct the dentofacial deformity, if the stability of orthognathic surgery is in doubt due to on-going TMJ pathology, or if the symptoms of TMJ dysfunction are severe enough. Therefore, when the pathological condition dictates that the TMJs have become unsalvageable, one should always consider replacement of the joint.

History of TMJ reconstruction

TMJ reconstructive surgery has a long history, beginning in the middle of the 19th century with the use of alloplastic grafts and progressing toward autogenous grafts in the early 20th century.

Alloplastic grafts

TMJ reconstruction dates back as far as 1840 when Carnochan, a New York surgeon, placed the first prosthetic material (wood) between the joint surfaces in a patient with TMJ ankylosis. Thereafter, in the 1930s and 1940s, different surgeons used various materials as inter-positional grafts after removing the osteotomized condyles. In the 1960s, the first implant was used by Robinson for the correction of ankylosis; this consisted of a stainless steel glenoid fossa

Orthognathic Surgery: Principles, Planning and Practice. Edited by Farhad B. Naini and Daljit S. Gill.

component secured to the zygomatic arch. In the mid-1960s, Christensen developed implants for first the glenoid fossa and then the condyle in 1973, to form the first total joint replacement. In the past 30 years, many prosthetic systems have been developed, generally with poor clinical results. Currently, there are just three devices in use that have been approved and licensed. These are TMJ Implants (Christensen), TMJ Concepts, and the Biomet-Lorenz. The Christensen system was originally made from acrylic on cobalt-chrome; it was then modified to cobalt-chrome only. This 'metal-on-metal' design had superior wear properties but 10% of patients developed a foreign body reaction due to metal allergy and the high friction resulted in implant loosening. The TMJ Concepts and Biomet-Lorenz systems are more recent innovations, which use a 'metal-on-plastic' design. The fossa component is made from Ultra-High Molecular Weight PolyEthylene (UHMWPE), which is the gold standard in total hip replacements. This material has a much lower coefficient of friction and higher wear resistance. The condylar component is made from a cobalt-chrome-molybdenum alloy (or titanium if patients have an allergy to cobalt-chromium alloy).[1,2]

Autogenous grafts

Metatarsal bone was used for the first condylar reconstruction in 1909. Then in 1920, the first costochondral graft was used. In 1956, Sarat used costochondral junction grafts from actively growing samples. It was this growth potential and the capacity for remodelling that made these grafts especially beneficial in children. Another autogenous tissue of interest has been the use of sternoclavicular grafts. These were initially harvested with a pedicle flap of sternocleidomastoid muscle; however, in the early 1990s, Wolford reported the use of free partial thickness sternoclavicular grafts to reconstruct the TMJ.

Autogenous or alloplastic?

The most widely accepted autogenous technique is the costochondral graft. The advantages of this graft are its biological compatibility and its growth potential, which make it the ideal choice where further growth is anticipated. Disadvantages are the risk of fracture, donor site morbidity (which may include pneumothorax, pain, scar) and the need for rigid inter-maxillary fixation during the recovery period, which prevents early function and physiotherapy. There is also a variable biological behaviour of the graft that can cause problems, including overgrowth, resorption and particularly, recurrent ankylosis.

Alloplastic materials allow closer reproduction of the normal anatomy of the joint, avoidance of donor site morbidity, reduced surgery time and immediate function and physiotherapy. The disadvantages include financial cost, potential material wear, long-term stability and especially with regards to children, the implants will not follow growth. From orthopaedic data of total joint replacements, patients are advised that the implants may fail after 10–15 years.

Comparative studies have shown that both autogenous and alloplastic reconstructions give patients significant improvements in symptoms. However, there is a more favourable outcome and fewer long-term complications in those treated by alloplastic reconstruction. Therefore, alloplastic reconstruction is preferred in most situations. Importantly, the growth potential of the costochondral graft make it the treatment of choice for TMJ reconstruction in children.[3,4]

Guidelines for TMJ replacement

The guidelines for total alloplastic joint replacement are more stringent than those for an orthopaedic total joint replacement. They have been outlined in the United Kingdom by the National Institute for Health and Clinical Excellence (NICE) and British Association of Oral and Maxillofacial Surgeons in 2008[5] and are summarized in Table 35-1.

Surgical planning for TMJ reconstruction

TMJ reconstruction can be carried out in a number of different ways. In the past, reconstructions were carried out in two stages, with condylar resection and spacer insertion, followed by secondary reconstruction some time later. Currently, single stage procedures are being performed more frequently, which not only save time and cost but also reduce the risks and morbidity of multiple surgeries.

Conventional surgical planning has involved rapid prototyping, which is used to fabricate stereolithographic models from computerized tomographic (CT) scans. These models are used to carry out model surgery, prior to implants being fabricated on the models, or stock implants chosen to closely fit

Table 35-1 Indications and contraindications for total alloplastic TMJ joint replacement

Indications:
- Dietary score of <5/10 (liquid scores 0, full diet scores 10);
- Restricted mouth opening (<35 mm);
- Occlusal collapse (anterior open bite or retrusion);
- Excessive condylar resorption and loss of height of the vertical ramus;
- Pain score >5 out of 10 on visual analogue scale (combined with any of the others); and
- Other quality of life issues

Contraindications:
- Local infective process;
- Severe immunocompromise; and
- Severe coexistent diseases (American Society of Anesthesiologists Grade III)

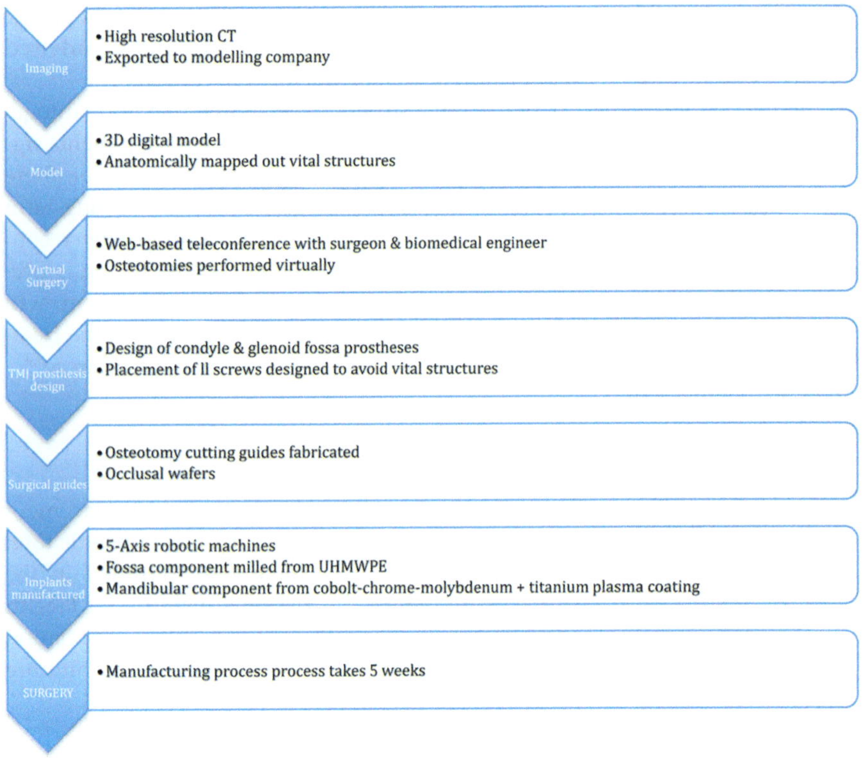

Fig. 35-1 Timeline of the TMJ replacement surgery virtual planning and manufacturing process.

them. However, this manual model surgery is work-intensive and time-consuming.

The technique that the authors favour is virtual surgical planning (Figure 35-1). By using computer-aided design (CAD) and computer-aided manufacturing (CAM) techniques, surgeons can perform virtual osteotomies and move bony segments to the required position, as performed in the operating theatre. The whole TMJ replacement procedure, as well as the orthognathic osteotomies can be planned on the same virtual model concurrently.

Virtual planning

Imaging of the facial bones is carried out with a high-resolution contrast-enhanced CT scan (with thin slices of 1.25 mm or less). The CT data in DICOM (Digital Imaging and Communications in Medicine) is then exported to the modelling company for processing and creation of 3D digital models, which includes anatomically mapped out inferior dental neurovascular bundles and maxillary arteries. The models are at 1:1 scale, therefore representing true patient anatomy. Virtual surgery is then performed using virtual surgical planning software. Virtual osteotomies including condylectomy and maxillary or mandibular osteotomies are performed and trialled until the optimal outcome has been achieved. The virtual surgery is performed during a web-based teleconference between the surgeon and the biomedical engineer from the modelling company. The 3D computer model allows the surgeon and orthodontist to conceptualize the anatomy, surgical movements, implant position and final outcome and recognize any potential problems or complications. The position of vital structures and important anatomy is visualized and the depth of osteotomy cuts and screw length can be safely designed to avoid inadvertent damage to the contents of the middle cranial fossa, maxillary artery, inferior dental nerve and the roots of the teeth. The surgical plan can be easily altered on the computer to choose the most appropriate plan (Figure 35-2).

Once the virtual surgery has been performed, the biomedical engineers at the implant company design the TMJ prostheses. The implants are designed according to the patient-specific model. The fossa component is made from UHMWPE with a minimum thickness of 3 mm. It is designed to fit the bony anatomy of the skull base perfectly with a flange onto the zygomatic arch and a minimum of four screw holes for attachment. The mandibular condyle prosthesis is then designed also fitting onto the buccal surface of the ramus anatomically, with a minimum of five screw holes for fixation. The positions of all the screw holes are designed to be away from any vital structure and are re-sited in the most solid bone available. Depth measurements are provided for each screw hole ensuring bicortical fixation.

Once the design process has been verified, the manufacturing of the implants and surgical guides (osteotomy cutting guides and occlusal wafers) begins. Using 5-Axis robotic machines, raw materials are cut to the precise size and length. By employing computerised numeric control programming, the 5-Axis robotic machine mills the patient specific contour of the fossa component from a block of UHMWPE, and the mandibular component from a block of cobalt-chrome-molybdenum alloy. Once each

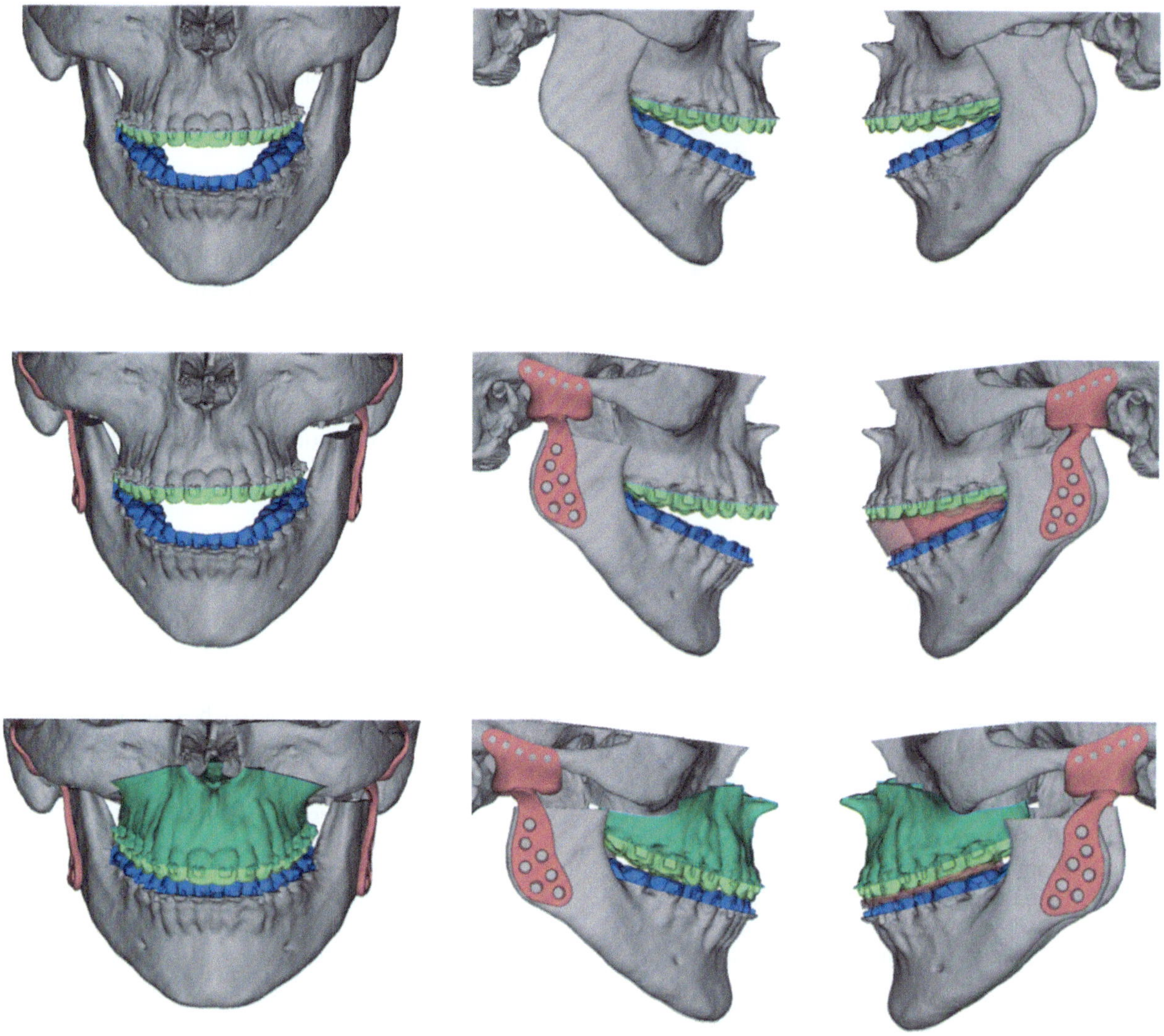

Fig. 35-2 Three-dimensional digital models. Upper panel shows the preoperative models. Middle panel shows the TMJ prostheses in situ after the TMJ replacement surgery has been carried out virtually. Lower panel shows the final digital models after a maxillary advancement has been carried out virtually.

implant is produced, meticulous inspection of the articulating surface and anatomical compatibility is performed. The medial surface of the mandibular component is finally coated with a titanium plasma spray to enable osseointegration with the mandible. The implants can then be sterilized, packaged and shipped to the surgeon. The whole planning process from initial CT scan to shipment of the implants typically takes 5 weeks.

Surgical procedure

Meticulous preoperative preparation of the patient is essential to prevent surgical site infection (SSI). The risk of SSI is around 1.5% and a number of precautions should be taken to help prevent it occurring. These include peri- and postoperative antibiotic prophylaxis with Clindamycin or Co-Amoxiclav, washing of the hair with a gentle shampoo the night before surgery, tying the hair back before surgery, trimming hair around the incision site with clippers, skin preparation with iodine solution and irrigation of the external auditory canals with iodine prior to occlusion with dressing material during the surgery.

1. Application of Leonard buttons, IMF screws or arch bars

Intra-oral procedures, such as application of intermaxillary fixation should be completed before skin preparation and final sterile draping (Figure 35-3). The oral cavity should also be barriered from the surgical site using adhesive dressing. Implants should be soaked in antibiotic solution prior to final placement.

2. Exposure of the condyle via a pre-auricular incision

The superficial temporal artery is ligated as part of the initial dissection down to the root of the zygoma. Adequate dissection of the soft tissue medial to the neck of the condyle is important to avoid haemorrhage from the internal maxillary artery and the

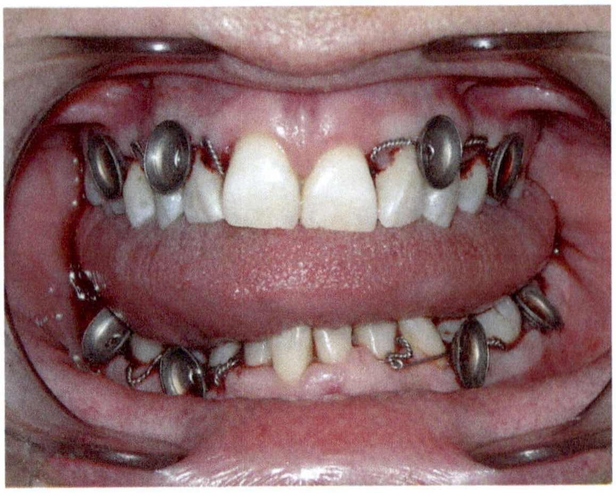

Fig. 35-3 Application of Leonard Buttons.

branches most commonly involved with haemorrhage during TMJ surgery (middle meningeal artery and deep temporal artery). This is especially important in the multiple-operated patient, where scarring and fibrosis may bring these vessels in closer proximity to the osteotomy cuts.

3. *Exposure of the mandibular ramus via a retromandibular incision*
The retromandibular incision is largely a vertical plane of dissection anterior to the sternocleidomastoid muscle. This gives greater visualization of the entire ramus for placement of the mandibular prosthesis and allows rapid access to the upper portion of the external carotid artery in case it is necessary to ligate the vessel to control haemorrhage on the medial surface of the condylar neck and superior ramus. It is important to complete the dissections for both the superior and inferior incisions before the osteotomies are performed in order to allow for optimal visualization and control of haemorrhage from branches of the external carotid artery should it occur during the procedure.

4. *Condylectomy*
The custom-made cutting guides are placed onto the ramus so they engage the posterior border and are held *in situ* with screws. The condylectomy and coronoidectomy are performed with a piezo saw.

5. *Glenoid fossa preparation*
If needed, the glenoid fossa can be prepared using a custom-made cutting guide fitted to the zygomatic arch, to remove any excess bone. All soft tissue joint material is excised. The space is then thoroughly irrigated with antibiotic (clindamycin) impregnated saline solution.

6. *Application of intermaxillary fixation*
The patient is placed into IMF using custom-made inter-positional wafers and wire loops.

7. *Trial of implant guides*
The trial prostheses are placed and secured using the corresponding screw holes and the fit is assessed. The stability and fit of the prostheses are then scrutinized.

8. *Fit of final implants*
Implants are secured using the corresponding screw holes and the fit is finally assessed before the IMF is removed and functional movement of the joint components is evaluated.

9. *Closure of wounds*
A layered wound closure is effected; no drains are placed.

Orthognathic procedures

After the surgical sites have been closed and dressed, conventional orthognathic procedures to definitively correct the jaw positions can then be carried out if necessary, through standard approaches and techniques.

TMJ pathology related to the orthognathic patient

There are a number of different disease processes that can affect the TMJ, which may warrant the consideration of specific TMJ surgery (including total joint replacement) in the orthognathic patient. All of the conditions outlined in Table 35-2 can lead to dentofacial deformities, which include condylar resorption, TMJ ankylosis or excessive condylar enlargement. They may all be associated with symptoms of TMJ dysfunction and severe pain.

Table 35-2 Pathological conditions affecting the TMJ

Causes	Examples	Deformity
Degenerative	Osteoarthritis	Condylar resorption
Systemic	Arthropathies	Condylar resorption
	• Rheumatoid	Ankylosis
	• Psoriatic	
	• SLE	
	• Juvenile	
	• Ankylosing spondylitis	
Idiopathic	Idiopathic condylar resorption	Condylar resorption
Traumatic	Condylar fractures	Ankylosis
		Condylar resorption
		Growth disturbance
Infective	Infective arthritis	Condylar resorption
	Middle ear infections	Ankylosis
Iatrogenic	Intra-articular steroid use	Condylar resorption
Neoplasia	Osteochondroma	Condylar overgrowth
	Osteosarcoma	
	Chondrosarcoma	

Condylar resorption

Condylar resorption may occur in all the systemic arthropathies, in degenerative osteoarthritis, following trauma to the condyles, after intra-articular steroid use and in idiopathic condylar resorption. It may be unilateral or bilateral, asymmetrical or symmetrical. There may be varying degrees of resorption and in severe cases, the condyle can resorb down to the sigmoid notch, causing occlusal collapse, as well as TMJ symptoms of pain and dysfunction.

Ankylosis

TMJ ankylosis is caused by bony or fibrous adhesions around the articular components of the joint resulting in loss of function and trismus. The loss of function means that patients may require a liquid-only diet. If this disease process occurs during childhood, growth will be severely disrupted on the side of the ankylosis. The resulting dentofacial asymmetry may be severe.

Condylar overgrowth

Osteochondromas are one of the most common benign tumours of bone. They represent 8–15% of all primary bone tumours. They usually develop in the metaphyses of long flat bones but rarely occur in the maxillofacial region, where they are generally associated with the coronoid process or the condyle. The deformity that develops usually includes vertical elongation of the face on the affected side with mandibular asymmetry, malocclusion with cross-bite on the contralateral side and lateral open bite on the affected side, together with possible symptoms of TMJ dysfunction.[6]

Malignant tumours of the TMJ may also present and cause significant dentofacial deformities. Osteosarcoma and chondrosarcoma of the TMJ is extremely rare. Osteosarcoma accounts for about 30% of all primary malignant bone tumours. More than half of all osteosarcomas arise in the long bones of the limbs, particularly in the knee and in the bones of the pelvis. Osteosarcoma of the jaw is a rare, aggressive malignancy constituting between 5% to 10% of all cases of skeletal osteosarcoma. Chondrosarcoma is a rare malignant tumour of cartilaginous tissue with an incidence of 5% to 12% in the head and neck region. The maxilla, nasal and paranasal sinuses are the most commonly affected regions, but chondrosarcoma of the TMJ is extremely rare.[7,8]

Surgical 'work-up'

History

A thorough history is essential to diagnose any underlying pathology. It is important to elicit any history of previous joint trauma, surgery or infection (including TMJ and middle ear infections), as well as previous orthodontic or orthognathic treatment. Any history of previous intra-articular steroid use should also be established. A medical history must be taken to include a systemic review, with particular assessment of skin lesions and musculoskeletal symptoms.

Examination

The systemic examination should include the identification of any skin lesions and other joint pathology, which may indicate an undiagnosed systemic arthropathy. General systemic examination is also mandatory to assess fitness for general anaesthetic. An orthognathic assessment for dentofacial deformity, including signs of previous trauma to the facial skeleton should also be carried out, in addition to TMJ assessment of joint pathology and signs of previous TMJ surgery.

Investigations

A number of investigations will need to be carried out prior to considering surgery:

- Blood: Systemic investigations for arthropathies should include laboratory blood tests for inflammatory markers (ESR and CRP) and rheumatoid screening (rheumatoid factor and anti-nuclear antibodies).
- Imaging: Plain films (OPT, lateral cephalograph), cross-sectional (CT or cone beam CT or MRI) and radioisotope scans (bone scans or PET CT).
- Study models.
- Stereolithographic models.

If there is an active disease process, it is important to carry out serial imaging (either plain films or bone scans) and take serial study models of the dentition. This will help to define when the disease process has ceased.

Management

The aims of any treatment of TMJ pathology should be to:

- decrease or eliminate pain
- provide a predictable, stable outcome with no further joint damage
- optimize joint function
- improve occlusion
- improve facial aesthetics.

It is important to consider the stability of any treatment regime. Many of these disorders are progressive and any definitive treatment should aim to remove the diseased components. TMJ replacement should be considered when orthognathic surgery alone is unable to correct the dentofacial deformity, if the stability of the orthognathic surgery is in doubt due to ongoing TMJ pathology, or if the symptoms of TMJ dysfunction are severe enough. Therefore, when the pathological condition is so severe that the TMJs become

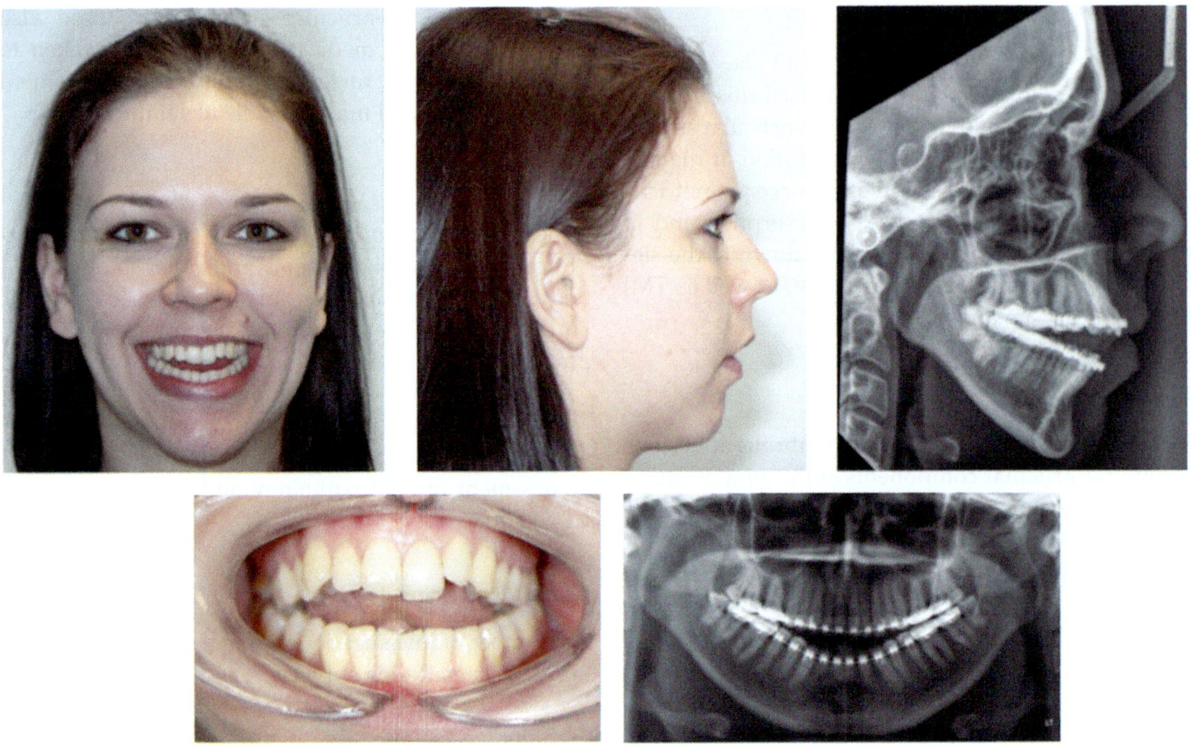

Fig. 35-4 Case 1: Preoperative extraoral and intraoral clinical photographs, panoramic and lateral cephalometric skull radiographs.

unsalvageable, one must consider replacement of the joint. TMJ replacement with concurrent orthognathic surgery can be performed as a single stage procedure.[9]

Case studies

Case 1: Idiopathic condylar resorption (ICR)

A 30-year-old female was referred from the orthodontic department of a nearby hospital where they had been unsuccessfully treating her progressive anterior open bite (AOB) with upper and lower fixed appliance therapy for 18 months. She had developed a progressive AOB and had symptoms of TMJ dysfunction. She gave no history of previous mandibular trauma, joint or middle ear infections and no history of intra-articular steroid use. The history indicated idiopathic condylar resorption.

Examination revealed a Class II division 1 malocclusion on skeletal II bases with an increased maxillary-mandibular plane angle (MMPA), decreased posterior face height and an 8 mm AOB. Serial panoramic radiographs revealed a progressive decrease in condylar size bilaterally (Figure 35-4).

Bilateral total TMJ replacements together with a Le Fort I maxillary osteotomy with posterior impaction was carried out. The surgery was uneventful and there were no complications. Details of the surgical procedure are highlighted in Figure 35-5. At 1 year follow-up, the patient had a stable Class I occlusion. Maximal inter-incisal opening was 38 mm and there were no symptoms of TMJ dysfunction (Figure 35-6).

The diagnosis and treatment of ICR is challenging. There have been many different management strategies discussed in the literature. Most do not address the disease process within the TMJs and concentrate on restoring the dental occlusion, skeletal discrepancy,

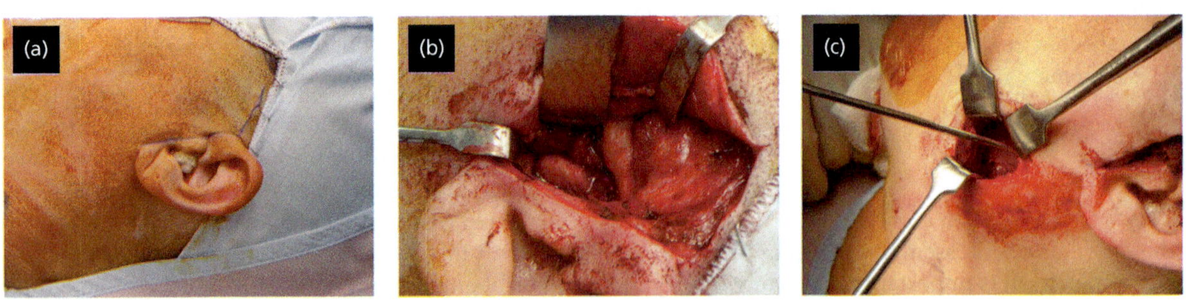

Fig. 35-5 Surgical procedure: (a) Preauricular incision marked out; (b) Exposure of the condyle via a preauricular incision; (c) Exposure of the mandibular ramus via a retromandibular incision; (d) Preauricular and retromandibular incisions in continuity; (e–g) Condylectomy; (h) Glenoid fossa preparation; (i) Trial of fossa implant guide; (j-l) Fit of final implants.

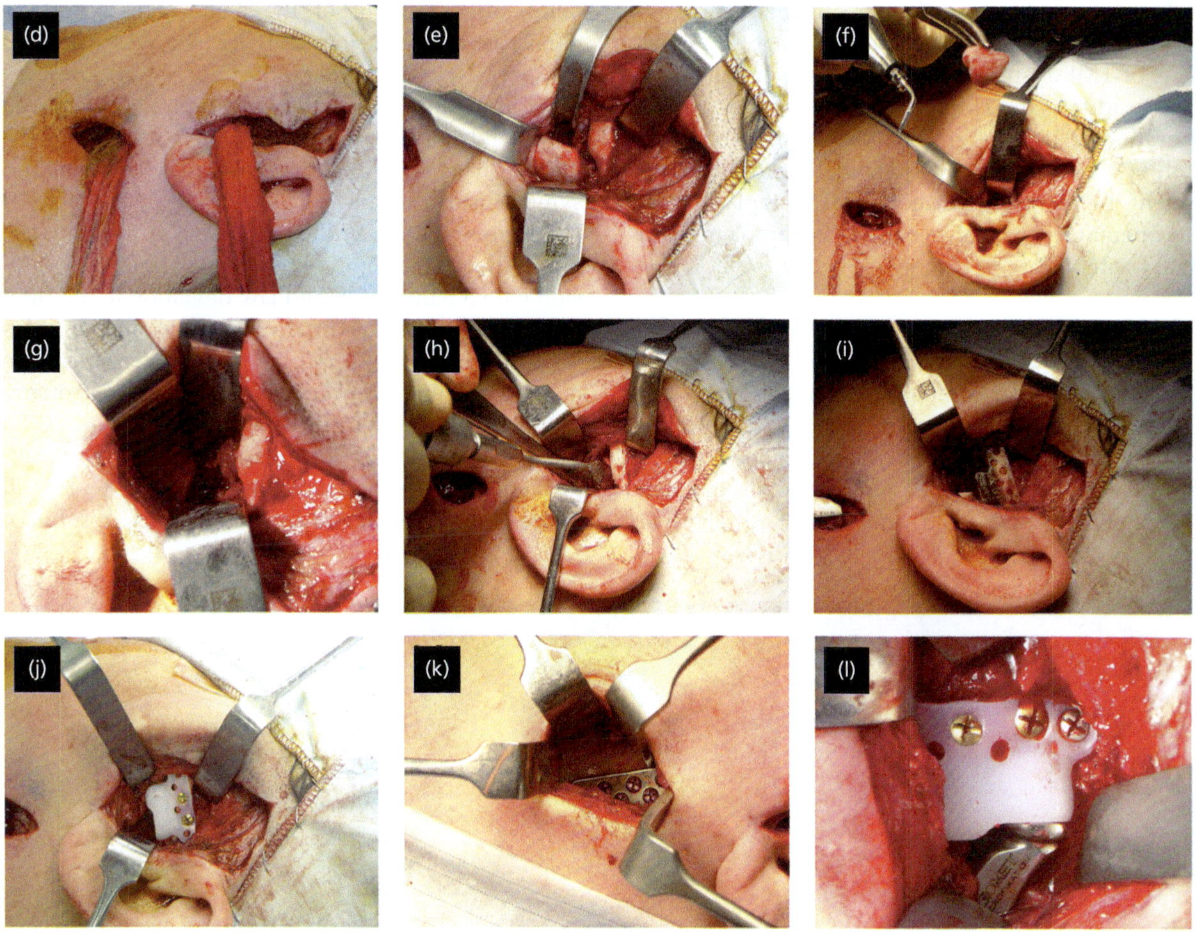

Fig. 35-5 (*Continued*).

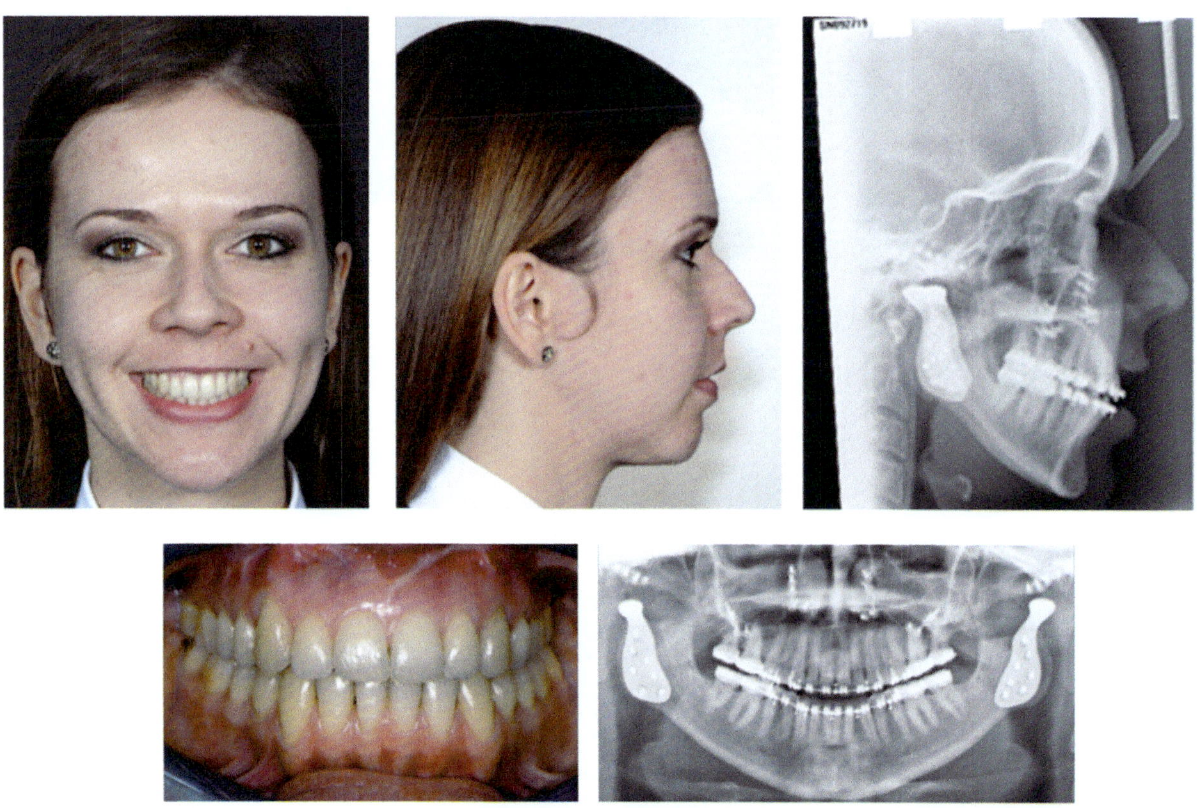

Fig. 35-6 Case 1: Postoperative extraoral and intraoral clinical photographs, panoramic and lateral cephalometric skull radiographs.

and/or facial imbalance. These treatments have a high probability of relapse and do not manage the symptoms of TMJ dysfunction. Those treatment strategies that do address the TMJs either require more than one operation or involve graft harvest from donor sites, both of which increase the potential morbidity to the patient. By using alloplastic total TMJ replacements, one operation can resolve many of the problems associated with ICR.

Case 2: Iatrogenic malocclusion

Case 2 is a 31-year-old female who presented with significant TMJ dysfunction following previous orthognathic surgery. She had undergone bilateral vertical sub-sigmoid osteotomies 10 years previously. The previous surgery had resulted in both condyles being displaced out of the glenoid fossae and a persistent malocclusion. Initially, she was managed conservatively with a flat bite splint, which provided short-term alleviation of her symptoms. However, both condyles remained out of their fossae and the patient began to experience increasing pain and symptoms of TMJ dysfunction.

On presentation, she complained of severe pain, especially on the right. She had a Class III malocclusion with a 5 mm AOB and jaw deviation to the right on opening. Her maximal interincisal opening was 32 mm (Figure 35-7). A bilateral total TMJ replacement, together with a Le Fort I maxillary osteotomy with 5 mm advancement was planned (Figure 35-8). The surgery was uneventful and there were no complications. A Class I occlusion was achieved with a full range of mandibular movement, complete resolution

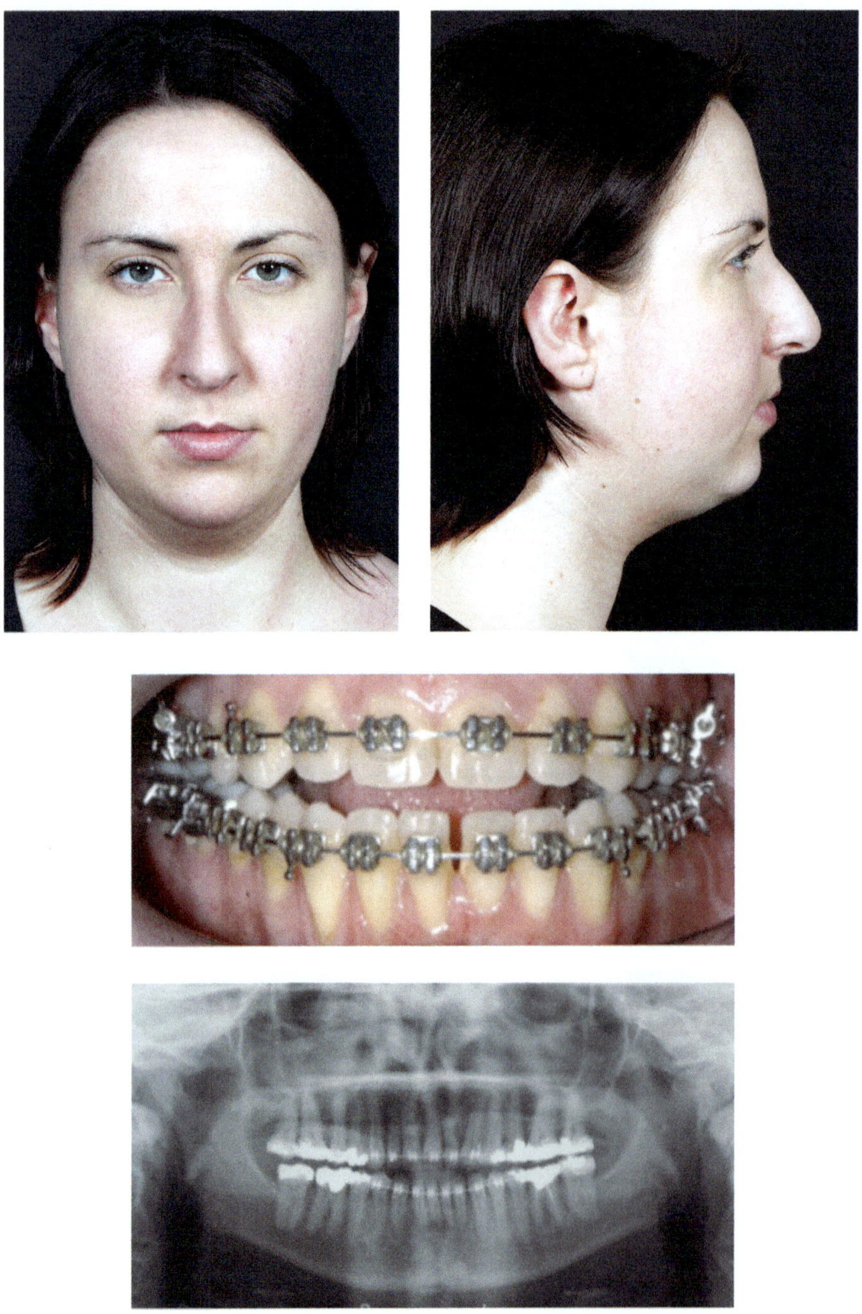

Fig. 35-7 Case 2: Preoperative extraoral and intraoral clinical photos and panoramic radiograph.

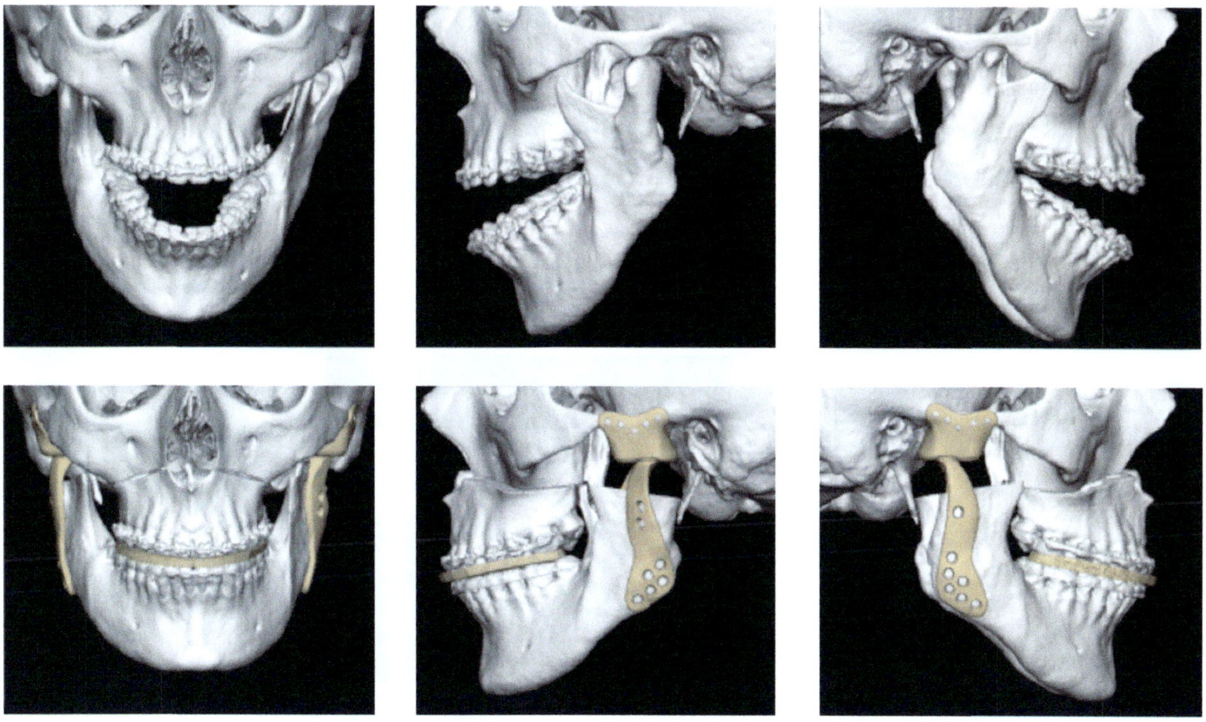

Fig. 35-8 Case 2: Upper panel shows preoperative three-dimensional digital models. Lower panels show the maxillary advancement and the position of the TMJ prostheses on the digital models.

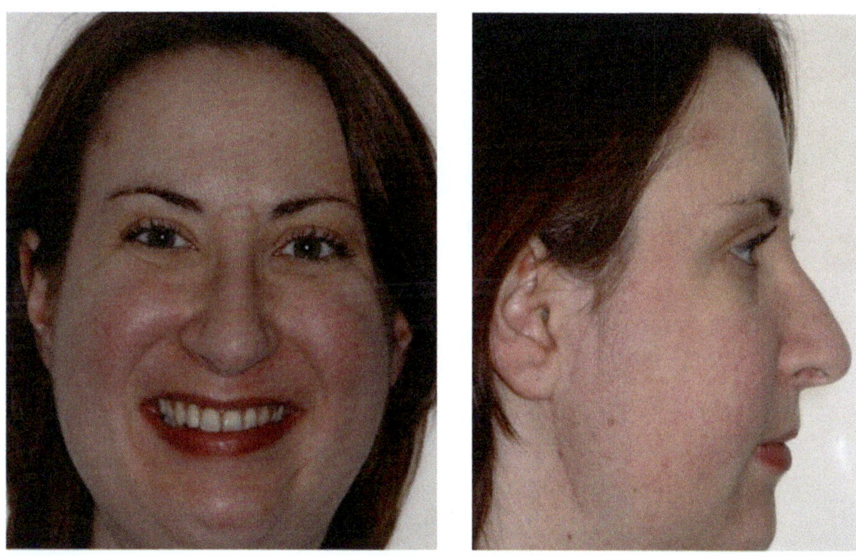

Fig. 35-9 Case 2: Postoperative extraoral clinical photographs.

of pain and good functional and aesthetic outcomes (Figure 35-9). At 2 years follow-up, these results were maintained and her long-standing pain has resolved.

Case 3: Post-traumatic facial asymmetry

Case 3 is a 36-year-old female who presented complaining of facial asymmetry and symptoms of TMJ dysfunction. She had fractured her left mandibular condyle 18 years previously following a road traffic accident and this had been treated conservatively at the time. On presentation, she had a Class I malocclusion with mandibular deviation to the left, creating a crossbite and centreline shift. Subsequent imaging of the mandible showed a marked overgrowth and deformity of the left mandibular condyle, which represented remodelling and degenerative overgrowth at the site of the previous fracture. There was a pseudo-arthrosis between the subcondylar region and a separate condylar fracture fragment that was fused to the glenoid fossa.

Following orthodontic decompensation, a left total TMJ replacement with concurrent unilateral right-sided sagittal split osteotomy and mandibular rotation to the right was planned to correct the transverse skeletal discrepancy (Figure 35-10). This was

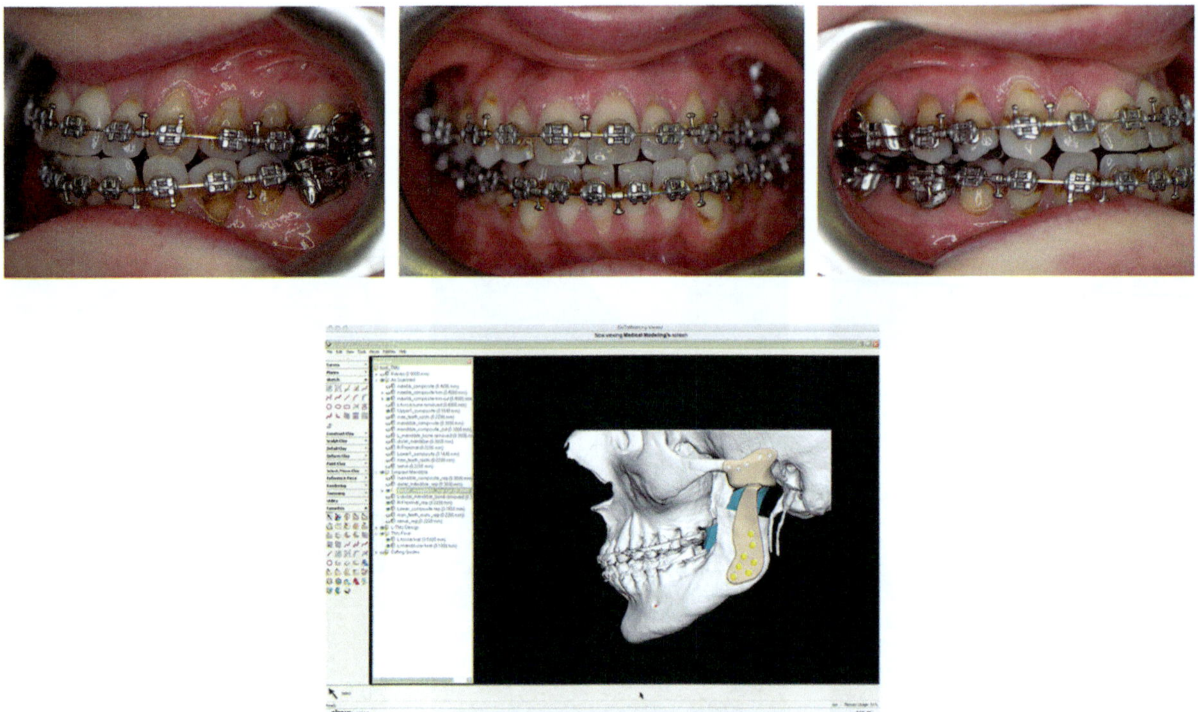

Fig. 35-10 Case 3: Preoperative intraoral clinical photographs. Virtual planning for the left TMJ prosthesis.

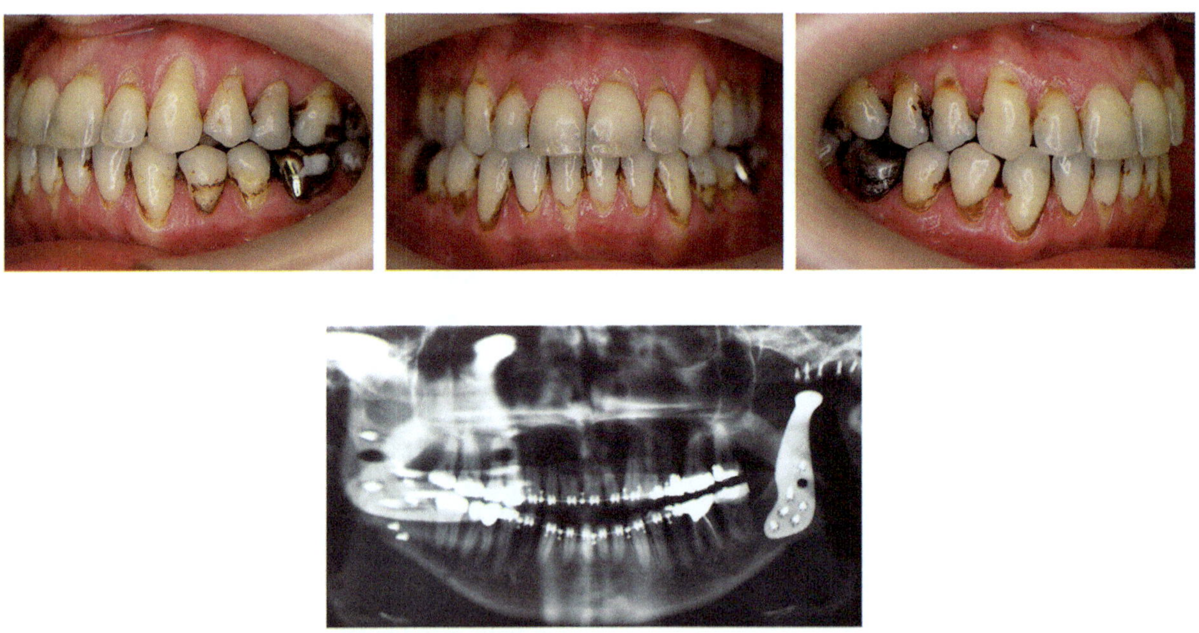

Fig. 35-11 Case 3: Postoperative intraoral clinical photographs. Panoramic radiograph showing the left TMJ prosthesis.

carried out without complication. At 2 years follow-up, the Class I occlusal relationship is stable and there are no symptoms of TMJ dysfunction (Figure 35-11).

Acknowledgements

We are grateful to Thushala Ubaya and David Young for managing the orthodontic care of Cases 1 and 2, respectively.

References

1 Driemel O, Ach T, Müller-Richter UD, et al. Historical development of alloplastic temporomandibular joint replacement before 1945. Int J Oral Maxillofac Surg. 2009;38:301–7.

2 Driemel O, Braun S, Müller-Richter UD, et al. Historical development of alloplastic temporomandibular joint replacement after 1945 and state of the art. Int J Oral Maxillofac Surg. 2009;38:909–20.

3 Saeed N, Hensher R, McLeod N, et al. Reconstruction of the temporomandibular joint autogenous compared with alloplastic. Br J Oral Maxillofac Surg. 2002;40:296–9.

4 Giannakopoulos HE, Sinn DP, Quinn PD. Biomet Microfixation Temporomandibular Joint Replacement System: a 3-year follow-up study of patients treated during 1995 to 2005. J Oral Maxillofac Surg. 2012;70:787–94.
5 Sidebottom AJ. Guidelines for the replacement of temporomandibular joints in the United Kingdom. Br J Oral Maxillofac Surg. 2008;46:146–7.
6 Morey-Mas M, Caubet-Biayna J, Iriarte-Ortabe J. Osteochondroma of the temporomandibular joint treated by means of condylectomy and immediate reconstruction with a total stock prosthesis. J Oral Maxillofac Res. 2010;1(4):e4.
7 Dos Santos D, Cavalcanti M. Osteosarcoma of the temporomandibular joint: report of 2 cases. Oral Surg Oral Med Oral Pathol Oral Radiol Endod. 2002;94:641–7.
8 Abu-Serriah M, Ahluwalia K, Shah K, et al. A novel approach to chondrosarcoma of the glenoid fossa of the temporomandibular joint: A Case Report. Oral Maxillofac Surg. 2013;71:208–13.
9 Wolford LM, Karras S, Mehra P. Concomitant temporomandibular joint and orthognathic surgery: a preliminary report. J Oral Maxillofac Surg. 2002;60:356–62.

Chapter 36

Surgically Assisted Rapid Maxillary Expansion

Nigel Taylor and Paul Johnson

Introduction

Transverse discrepancies are a common feature of malocclusion in adolescents and adults and often a feature in the commonest congenital facial anomaly, clefts of the lip and palate. The incidence of transverse maxillary deficiency is reported to be 8 to 18% of patients receiving orthodontic consultations.[1] Correction of the transverse dimension is a key factor when planning arch alignment and related correction of the vertical dimension. Inadequate assessment is common and successful management involves identification and correcting the cause of a transverse discrepancy. Most transverse discrepancies arise due to a narrow maxilla. It is possible for a normal maxilla to be associated with a wide mandible or, on occasions, a narrow maxilla and a wide mandibular arch. Widening of the maxilla is important to allow arch coordination and improve tongue space. The key question to consider when managing the transverse dimension is to select the minimal procedure required to produce consistent and stable maxillary expansion.[2] Over the years a variety of techniques have been described ranging from removable orthodontic appliances to surgical facilitated expansion and segmental osteotomies.

The first reported correction of a narrow upper arch treated by expansion was in 1860, reported by Angell (see Figure 12-33) in the Dental Cosmos published in the San Francisco Medical Press.[3] The mechanical principals described by Angell using rapid maxillary expansion (RME) to widen the arch are still used by orthodontists today in the management of children and adolescents.[4] Orthodontists use a range of removable and fixed appliances to widen the dental arch. The evidence available describing the extent of dental expansion possible varies. A Cochrane review in 1999 reported orthodontic correction of posterior crossbites in randomized controlled trials and case controlled trials between 1970 and 1997. The report identified 12 trials which satisfied the selection criteria and the review concluded that there was no evidence for the advantage of any expansion technique above any other.[5] The effects of expansion have been reviewed.[6]

Schiffman and Tuncay (2001)[7] in a meta-analysis reviewed 5000 articles between 1978 and 1999 and identified six studies for the final analysis, based on agreed inclusion criteria. The mean expansion after adjustment was 6.0 mm, falling to 2.4 mm after one year. Furthermore, they concluded that insufficient data existed to support the view that dental expansion produced any useful expansion beyond that achieved by normal growth. This conclusion is difficult to accept as orthodontists treat many cases and successfully achieve arch expansion as concluded by Petren et al.[8]

Orthognathic Surgery: Principles, Planning and Practice. Edited by Farhad B. Naini and Daljit S. Gill.

It is generally accepted that orthodontic treatment can widen the upper arch by about 5 mm with orthodontic forces alone.[9]

Corbridge et al. reported 73 cases treated with a quadhelix, which had been assessed pre-, and post-expansion with cone beam computed tomography (CBCT). Interestingly the maxillary expansion with the quad helix appliance led to an increase of palatal bone thickness and a decreased buccal bone thickness with 30% of the subjects showing little or no buccal bone on one or both sides. This finding implies that if significant expansion is achieved by dental techniques alone, future periodontal attachment could be compromised.[10] Both Goddard (1893) and Black (1893)[4] both supported the use of RME. However, RME fell out of favour in the mid-twentieth century until Korkhaus (1956)[11] re-introduced RME into the United States and Haas in the 1960s further developed the technique and appliances. Timms (1981)[12] reported 30–50% relapse with standard RME and advocated over expansion to allow for post-treatment change.

Many clinicians have recognized the limitations of expansion using RME in the mature patient. Several problems have been reported such as lack of movement of maxillary halves, tipping of anchor teeth,[13] extrusion,[14] unequal expansion, root resorption,[15,16] relapse and periodontal problems caused by teeth pushed through the buccal cortex leading to attachment loss.[17,18] Capelozza et al. (1996)[19] described moderate expansion was possible using RME in adults without surgery and Handelman et al. (2009) reported effective RME in adults with some buccal attachment loss recorded.[20] Skeletal age is an important factor in case selection[21] and may not fit with chronological age which would explain why successful RME has been reported in mature cases and where RME is unsuccessful in younger patients who may be advanced in skeletal maturity.

A main area of resistance to expansion was considered to be the mid-palatal suture. Brown in 1938 was one of the first to describe a Surgical Assisted Rapid Palatal Expansion technique (SARPE) with midpalatal splitting. Haas[22,23] described midline splitting to increase maxillary width for orthodontic reasons and believed that during RME carried out in adolescents separation of the maxillary halves occurred in a tipping fashion due to the strength of the zygomatic buttress. Issacson et al.[24] demonstrated that the facial skeletal offered increased resistance to expansion as it aged and matured. These workers concluded that the major site of resistance was not the mid palatal suture but the maxillary articulation with the zygomatic bones. Lines in 1975[25] and Bell and Epker in 1976[26] supported this view. Furthermore, Wertz[27] concluded that the main area of resistance was the zygomatic arches. Shetty et al. (1994)[28] concluded using photo-elastic studies that as the patient ages, areas of resistance become more established in both midpalatal and circum-maxillary sutures and therefore if skeletal expansion is to be achieved in an adult, release of these areas of resistance needs to be considered. Identification of the areas of resistance led to the development of various osteotomies to facilitate maxillary widening using RME appliances to apply force to the maxillary halves via the teeth. Bell (1982)[29,30] advocated releasing the osseous structures to avoid many of the complications of RME in a mature patient and described a combination of surgical and orthodontic treatment to widen the maxilla in a mature patient. The two main approaches to widen the maxilla in a mature patient are surgical expansion with segmental surgery as part of a Le Fort I osteotomy, or SARPE, sometimes described as surgically assisted rapid maxillary expansion (SARME), where the areas of resistance are relieved prior to expansion with an appliance. A series of appliances have been described from occlusal coverage splints, bands attached to teeth and more recently bone borne devices applying force directly to palatal bone. This chapter will consider the indications and rationale for surgically facilitated expansion with an evaluation of techniques and protocols for management.

Rapid maxillary expansion

During non-surgical rapid maxillary expansion, an appliance is attached to the teeth either with bands to molars and premolars or full coverage with either chrome or alternatively acrylic bonded appliances. Full coverage is considered to cause less dental tipping; however the technique has largely fallen out of favour in preference to banded appliances (Figure 36-1). A transverse directed force is applied using a jackscrew with the aim to achieve rapid expansion to open the mid-palatal suture. The aim is to achieve skeletal rather than dental expansion and minimize buccal tipping of molars. High forces have been reported between 2 and 10 kg and expansion is achieved by turning the screw 0.25 mm twice a day delivering 0.5 mm of expansion per day. The ideal period for RME is during the growth spurt or usually below 15 years of age.[6,31] A systematic review in 2005

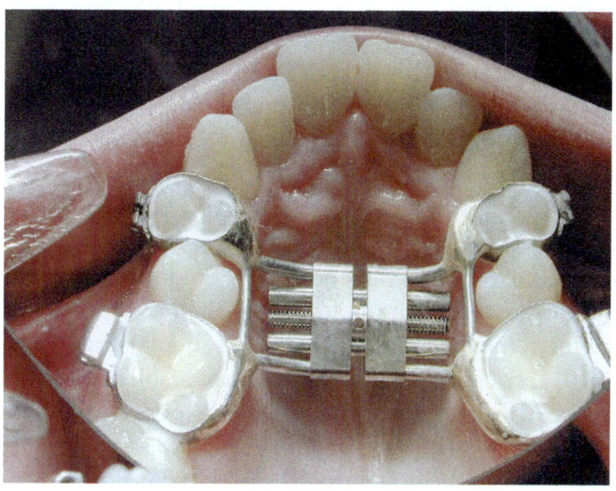

Fig. 36-1 A banded RME appliance with a hyrax screw.

by Lagravere et al.[32] confirmed optimal non-surgical expansion is achieved in pre-pubertal patients with skeletal expansion retained in the long term, representing 25% of the total expansion. Long-term stability is considered to be better in skeletally less mature individuals and questions the clinical significance of long-term maxillary expansion in skeletally mature individuals. The review confirms the need for long-term randomized clinical trials and warns that evidence was only identified from non-randomized controlled trials. There was criticism of poor controls and lack of error assessment in the studies reviewed.[32]

Proffit[33] has described a hierarchy of stability for surgical orthodontic treatment indicating that correction of the maxillary width by expansion is the least stable movement. Management of the transverse dimension is a key consideration in planning treatment. Basic principals of pre-surgical preparation involve arch coordination. Therefore if an arch is considered very narrow and non amenable to orthodontic preparation, either segmental surgery or SARPE should be considered. Moss in 1968[34] suggested that indications for rapid maxillary expansion alone or in conjunction with surgery depends on the patient's age and the condition of the mid palatal suture and not on the maxilla and mandibular relationship. Palatal closure in man has been studied from 15 to 35 years of age.[35] Haas in 1980[36] identified six indications for non-surgical rapid maxillary expansion: (1) real and relative transverse maxillary deficiency; (2) nasal stenosis; (3) Class III malocclusions; (4) the mature cleft palate patient; (5) anteroposterior maxillary deficiency; (6) selected arch length problems.

When children and adolescents present with a narrow maxillary arch and orthognathic surgery is a consideration for the future, careful assessment of arch width and coordination is important. Orthodontic arch expansion to correct the transverse discrepancy should be considered for the prepubertal patient at this early stage to reduce the need for later transverse surgery. Sokuco et al. in 2009[37] compared a sample of RME and SARPE patients treated using a bonded acrylic RME expander. They concluded that similar stability of dentoalveolar expansion was possible with both RME and SARPE which has been supported by other workers.[38] The study confirmed that expansion with RME and SARPE could be shown to have equal stability. The sample sizes were small and some would consider non-surgical expansion on some participants in the surgical sample would be more appropriate. However it is important to remember that as sutures mature the majority of orthopaedic rapid palatal expansion occurs by dental tipping and bending the alveolar bone rather than by true skeletal movement. Altug in 2006[39] and in a later study in 2010[40] concluded that the long-term stability of RME and SARPE is similar with both experiencing 50% skeletal and 30% dental relapse. It would seem reasonable to consider non-surgical rapid expansion to correct transverse discrepancies in young patients. RME has been considered a useful intervention to manage airway and rhinological problems[6,9] and, therefore, any benefits achieved by non surgical RME should be achieved with SARPE. Furthermore Magnusson et al. in 2013, in a three dimensional computed tomographic analysis of the nose, reported significant widening of the nose following SARPE.[41]

When patients have completed RME at an early age it is important to identify whether the non-surgical dental expansion achieved is sufficient or whether surgery is required to achieve additional correction of the transverse discrepancy. Clinical examination may identify buccal segments and canines already flared bucally from previous expansion indicating that significant dental compensation of an underlying transverse discrepancy already exists. Palpation of the labial sulcus above the canine is an important technique to assess the true width of the intercanine region. Assessment of skeletal width from PA radiographs can also be helpful and confirm identification of pre-existing dental compensation is important.[42] However, use of PA radiographs is not routine in many centres. Angelieri et al. (2013) described a technique to assess suture maturation using cone beam computed tomography (CBCT) rather than chronological age.[43] These findings offer an opportunity for more precise planning between a non-surgical or surgical approach and may explain why apparently successful non-surgical expansion has been reported in older patients.

Treatment planning – surgical options to widen the maxilla

SARPE can be considered as a variation of distraction osteogenesis. Codvilla described distraction osteogenesis for the shortened femur in 1905 and Ilizarov in 1990[38,44] described a group of orthopaedic patients undergoing distraction osteogenesis using gradual forces to lengthen legs following an osteotomy. Following corticotomy and a 5-day latency period, force was applied via a distractor to separate the bone segments allowing the deposition of new trabecular bone, which later mineralized. An initial callus forms but time is too short for consolidation to take place. Between day 5 and day 7 collagen fibres are formed and orientate themselves in a parallel direction to the distraction vector. Bone formation now follows the collagen fibres by intramembranous ossification, which commences, from the cortex. Later solid compact bone forms. It is important that distraction does not progress too rapidly otherwise new bone fails to form. If distraction is too slow premature consolidation occurs limiting expansion. The effect is to facilitate new bone to separate the osteotomised segments. The principles of distraction osteogenesis can be applied to the maxilla. SARPE can facilitate surgical expansion while maintaining an intact arch and can be performed early in treatment with fewer dental extractions.

Marchetti[45] compared long-term stability of SARPE and segmental Le Fort I used to expand the maxilla in adult patients. A higher relapse rate was identified in the SARPE cases, although the overall expansion achieved following each intervention was different. The average increase in intercanine and intermolar distance was 8.5 mm and 7.0 mm in the SARPE group whereas expansion in the Le Fort 1 was only 2.75 and 3.75 mm.[45] Chamberland et al. in 2011[46] described longitudinal data for short- and long-term stability with data from 38 patients enrolled in a prospective study. SARPE showed a mean relapse rate of 24% of 1.83 mm compared to expansion achieved of 7.6 mm. A mean skeletal expansion of 3.6 mm was obtained which was considered to be modest and stable with relapse in dental expansion due to lingual movement of the posterior teeth.[46]

Segmental maxillary osteotomy is a useful technique, which may be considered if three-dimensional correction in a single procedure is indicated. Reports of relapse between 30 and 40% with vascular risk to bony segments are well accepted. Marchetti et al. compared stability of SARPE and segmental Le Fort I osteotomy and described greater expansion achieved by SARPE but greater percentage relapse.[47] Kretschmer et al.[48] reported on stability of 3-piece Le Fort I osteotomy and concluded that expansion of the maxilla at its base was reasonably stable, relapsing 10% but that relapse for the dentoalveolus was 60%. It may be that stretching of the palatal gingivae causes this unfavourable change in dental expansion.[48] When more than 8 mm expansion is indicated SARPE has been considered a more stable option than segmental osteotomy to correct the transverse dimension.

SARPE provides expansion primarily in the canine region and less at the molars whereas segmental Le Fort I osteotomy produces greater intermolar expansion than in the canine region. Patients with arch length discrepancy and upper incisors in an acceptable vertical and sagittal position are good cases for SARPE. A Le Fort I osteotomy would require sectioning of the anterior segment and in effect moving the incisors. Also a V-shaped arch is more appropriate for SARPE management as the expansion will increase the intercanine width in a greater proportion. SARPE is carried out early in the orthodontic plan and is able to create space to relieve crowding as the arch widens. This may limit the need for dental extraction. Cases involving segmental osteotomy require tooth alignment before surgery to correct arch length and therefore extractions may be needed.[9]

When SARPE is included in the treatment plan the patient has two general anaesthetics if subsequent orthognathic surgery is planned whereas a Le Fort I segmental osteotomy allows all procedure under a single general anaesthetic. This must be balanced against the easier orthognathic procedure managing an intact maxilla rather than a segmented maxilla. Any extraction indicated such as removal of third molars can be carried out at the time of SARPE.

The indications for SARPE were described by Suri et al.[49] as:

1. To increase arch perimeter
2. Correction of a severe crossbite
3. Widening of the maxillary arch
4. Space creation to relieve crowding when extractions not indicated
5. Widening of the arch in patients with clefts of the palate
6. To overcome suture resistance when RME has failed.

SARPE has been shown to improve nasal breathing by increasing nasal volume.[50]

Patient selection and case assessment for SARPE

Clinical assessment, study model analysis to assess arch form and symmetry, with radiographic assessment should be used to identify the magnitude of the discrepancy. A facial appearance with paranasal flattening is often associated with a transverse width discrepancy. A V-shaped arch or arches with a high vaulted palate are also indicators of a transverse discrepancy (Figures 36-2–36-4) and narrow arches may also be associated with a mandibular displacement. Photographs, study models and vitality tests of

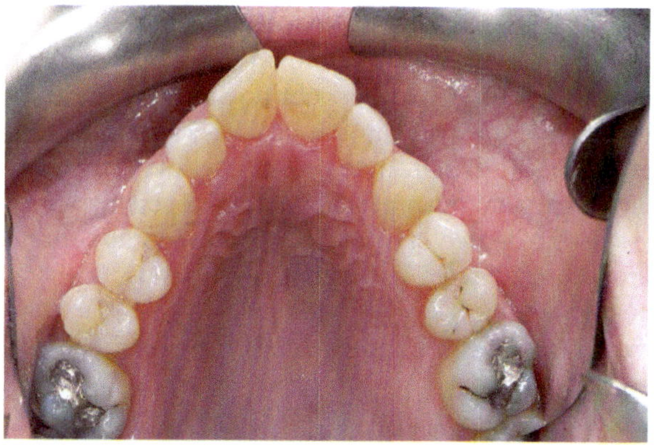

Fig. 36-2 A narrow V-shaped arch.

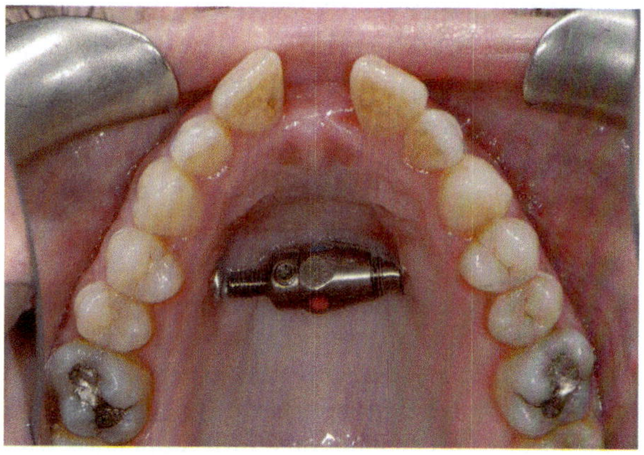

Fig. 36-3 TPD in place.

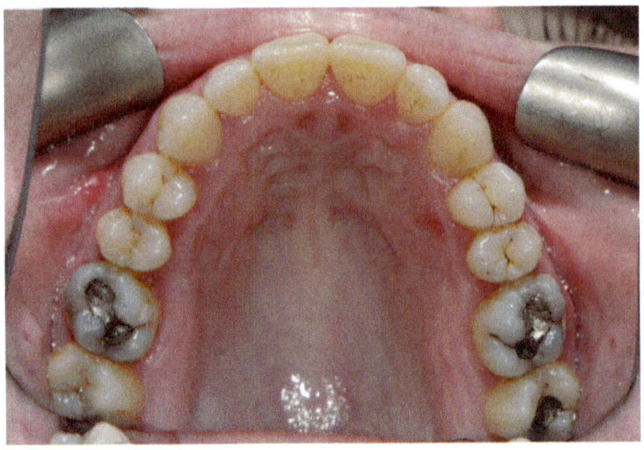

Fig. 36-4 The arch form following treatment.

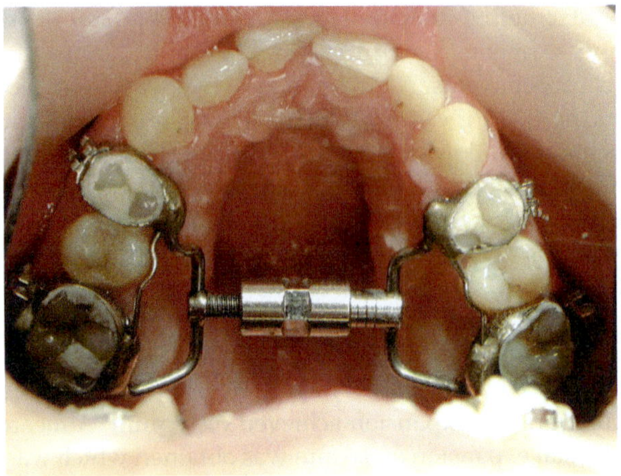

Fig. 36-5 A banded RME with a super screw.

upper incisors are important parts of the assessment process. An assessment of the periodontal attachment is essential particularly to detail buccal gingival condition. Gingiva and alveolar bone should be healthy between the roots of the central incisors. If orthognathic correction is planned it is important to complete model assessment to assess if in the corrected position a true or apparent discrepancy exists. This assessment is especially important when planning correction of skeletal Class III malocclusions. An anterior occlusal radiograph should be carried out prior to SARPE to ensure space exists between the roots of the upper incisors to allow safe surgical access. Occasionally space may need to be created between the roots using orthodontic appliances prior to surgery. The limits of the anterior occlusal view to assess the maxillary suture are well known.[51] The importance of identifying root proximity and central incisor root integrity prior to maxillary separation has been clearly demonstrated.[52] Betts et al.[42] have recommended taking a posteroanterior cephalograph to assess the degree of discrepancy between upper and lower arches from a coronal aspect using cephalometric landmarks. The landmarks are remote from the arches and this approach has not been generally accepted.

SARPE protocol

Presurgical orthodontic considerations

It is important to determine how much arch expansion is needed. Likely post-treatment change must be considered, as dental change is likely even if skeletal expansion is maintained. When the upper arch is narrow lower premolars and molars may be inclined lingually camouflaging the degree of actual discrepancy that exists. It may be helpful to decompensate lower molars prior to SARPE so as to establish more accurately assess how much upper arch expansion is actually needed. The authors favour a banded expander, which is cemented prior to surgery. The typical design is identical to a contemporary RME appliance with bands on molars and premolars. It is important to check that the screw is operational and positioned correctly. It is also important to be aware of the screw thread and turning schedule as this can vary between different screw designs (Figure 36-5).

Evaluation of surgical techniques for SARPE

There is no agreement on the on the surgical technique. A variety of techniques for each of the approaches have been described including corticotomy from the piriform rim to the maxillopterygoid junction, osteotomy of the midpalatal suture, paramedian palatal osteotomies with or without pterygoid disjunction. Release of midpalatal suture is also reported to improve mobility and to prevent deviation of the septum.

Koudstaal[53] (2005) reviewed the different surgical techniques that had been proposed. The surgical techniques vary in the degree to which the maxilla is osteotomized.[54,55] There are two main techniques which are a more conservative approach described by Glassman et al. in 1984[55] with osteotomies performed only at the lateral and anterior wall of the maxilla[12,55,56] which is less invasive, but has a greater risk of relapse, periodontal problems and unexpected fractures. Lehman et al. (1989)[57] reported stability in a case series of 56 cases using a conservative approach, however follow up ranged from 1 to 12 years. The more invasive technique with maximal mobility of the maxillary segments allows separation of the maxillary halves over greater distances with less risk of complication.[54] Anttila (2004)[58] reported 20 cases aged older than 16 years managed with a minimally invasive technique but advised more extensive osteotomies in older patients.[7] The more invasive approach facilitates more predictable and safer expansion.

The pterygoid plates are a significant site of resistance and pterygoid disjunction influences the pattern of maxillary separation. A midfacial cranial stress distribution analysis used finite element models to assess different surgical techniques and concluded that to protect the cranial base pterygoid disjunction was indicated. Pereira et al.[59] reported 70 adult patients aged 18–53 years who had completed SARPE with a subtotal Le Fort I osteotomy and pterygoid disjunction. Computerized tomography following surgical expansion showed that two-thirds of the cases did not have full palatal separation from the anterior nasal spine to the posterior nasal spine, although all cases showed full correction of the transverse maxillary discrepancy.

The authors favour a 'mini-Le Fort I' approach carried out under general anaesthesia so that the maxilla is adequately mobilized, thereby minimizing the forces on teeth necessary to expand the maxilla to allow a more predictable separation of the maxillary halves. An upper buccal sulcus incision is made from first premolar to first pre-molar and buccal bone cuts performed from piriform aperture to pterygomaxillary junction with a reciprocating saw. Pterygomaxillary disjunction and separation of the nasal septum from the maxilla is carried out using a chisel. Then a thin chisel is placed between the roots of the upper incisors the palatal split is initiated and propagated posteriorly using a wider chisel. The expansion appliance is then activated to ensure adequate mobility of the two halves of the maxilla and the mucosal incisions sutured using resorbable sutures.

General complications

SARPE is generally considered to be a low risk procedure.[9] However severe complications have been reported.[60] Ho et al.[61] reviewed records of 85 consecutive patients and reported complications in 27% of patients undergoing Le Fort I osteotomy with 14% experiencing complications specific to segmentalization such as oronasal fistulas or devitalized teeth. Increased morbidity and more lengthy surgery were also described.[61] A thorough medical history is required so that any co-morbidities or contraindications are identified prior to surgery. Following any surgical procedure bleeding and infection are possible but unusual following SARPE. The risk of intraoperative bleeding can occur following separation of the pterygoid plates. The descending palatine vessels should not be vulnerable because the lateral nasal wall remains intact and down fracturing of the maxilla is not carried out, as would be the case in Le Fort I osteotomy. Case reports of damage to the skull base, intracranial bleeding and orbital sequelae have been reported.[53] In the immediate post operative period pain during expansion and septal deviation can occur. Williams et al. (2012) reported 33% complications risk in a retrospective study of 120 patients treated with SARPE over a four-year period. Most complications were minor and resolved with local measures however 15% required additional treatment. The most common complication was asymmetrical or inadequate expansion, which was reported in 13% of the sample.[62]

Dental complications

Dental complications of SARPE when using tooth-supported appliances include those complications described for non-surgical RME.[15,16,63] Periodontal ligament compression, buccal root resorption and perforation of the buccal cortex remain as risks. As the appliance delivering expansion is attached to teeth, some tooth tipping and dental extrusion is possible but can be minimized by an overlay chrome appliance or bonded appliance. The convenience of banded appliances, which allow an easier transition to fixed appliances, has led to the use of more banded appliances in SARPE cases. Bonded acrylic appliances also have the risk that the appliance could become detached, risking loss or relapse of the expansion achieved and are not recommended for surgical expansion.

The most common dental or periodontal complication in SARPE involves the upper central incisors. Reported risks include tooth discolouration, gingival recession and periodontal bone loss which occurred in about 15% of the sample reported by Garib et al. in 2005[52] and in 2006 Garib used CT scans to assess areas of resorption on the roots of premolars and molars when these teeth contacted the buccal cortical plate.[64,65] It is also important to check the screw is functional and orientated in the correct position before cementing into position. Problems relating to the RME appliance design are rare but loosening of the appliance, stripping or locking of the screw is possible.

Postoperative management and appliance activation

1. Following surgery a latency period of three to five days is indicated. This approach is more comfortable for the patient and follows the principles of distraction osteogenesis as it allows callus development. However, it is important not to delay expansion until consolidation occurs. Expansion protocols vary from 0.25 to 1 mm per day. The authors propose expansion of 0.5 mm per day with a jackscrew equivalent to 1/4 turn (0.25 mm) morning and evening. Other screws may have different threads, however the aim should be to achieve 0.5 mm a day expansion.
2. After two to three days expansion, an anterior occlusal radiograph should be taken to assess symmetrical separation of the palatal segments (Figure 36-6). Particular note should be taken to see that the lamina dura remains intact on both central incisors. Cureton and Cuenin[52] suggest that the rate of expansion is determined by the symmetry of fracture of the alveolar bone and health of the interdental papilla and gingivae (Figure 36-7). These workers advised that the expansion schedule should be matched to the quality of split achieved as excessively rapid expansion can cause malunion or attachment loss between the

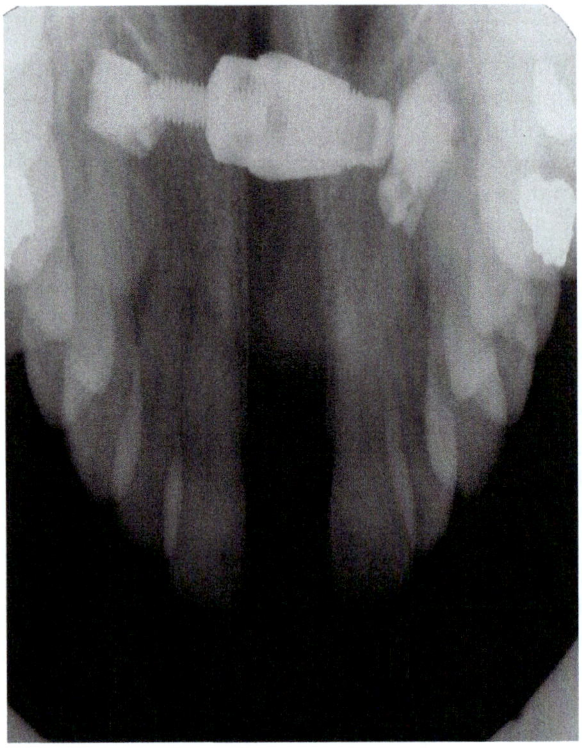

Fig. 36-6 Symmetrical separation following expansion with a TPD.

central incisors. Strategies to manage complications have been described.[52]

3. During the post-expansion phase, there is usually minimal discomfort for the patient, although tightness in the root of the nose, and posterior orbital region has been reported. Intraorally a space develops between the central incisors, as would happen with conventional non-surgical rapid maxillary expansion. This should be symmetrical. Asymmetrical expansion should invite investigation.
4. It is important to check the health and colour of the teeth at each appointment. Some tenderness and mild mobility are to be accepted however marked mobility or discolouration indicates a need for investigation with radiographs.

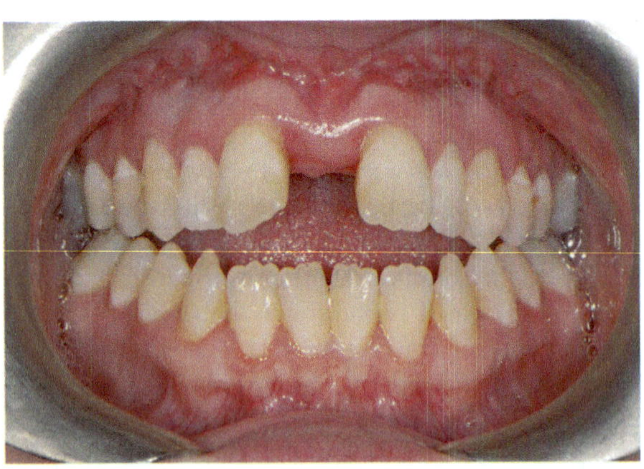

Fig. 36-7 A median diastema created following expansion. Note the healthy gingival tissue between the central incisors.

5. Immature keratinized tissue with a pinkish appearance appears between the central incisors however this should not be a grey colour, which may indicate attachment loss around the central incisors.
6. There has been significant debate as to whether over expansion should be carried out. Relapse for SARPE has been reported as 5 to 25%[38,66] with Bays and Greco[67] describing relapse less than 10% and an implication that over expansion was unnecessary. Seeberger et al. (2011)[68] reported that when using a tooth-borne distractor over expansion was indicated. When considering overcorrection in the schedule the surgical technique used to separate the sutures is very relevant and the team must be aware which sutures have been released. There are many surgical techniques and it is generally agreed that if pterygoid separation is performed, significant over-expansion is not needed whereas more conservative surgery leaves more resistance and influences the quality and pattern of expansion.
7. Various approaches to post-expansion management have been described from no retention to 12 months retention.[53,55,69,70,71] Optical density measurements from occlusal radiographs of the midpalatal suture show incomplete healing at 3 months post SARPE and the commonly held belief that consolidation in the expansion site is complete at 3 months may be premature. A transpalatal arch can replace the tooth borne rapid maxillary expander after three months post expansion, which improves patient comfort, and allow progress with orthodontic treatment.

Bone-borne appliance

Conventional SARPE applies lateral force to the maxillary skeletal halves via the teeth using an RME dental appliance. The disadvantages of using a dental appliance are well-documented.[29,70,72] If force could be applied directly to the bone and not via the teeth, the risk of periodontal membrane compression could be eliminated reducing the risk of root resorption, bone fenestration and unfavourable tipping of segments. Furthermore, a bone-borne expander could act as a retainer applying a retaining force directly to the bone while not interfering with the orthodontic treatment. Mommaerts (1999) described a bone-borne expansion attached directly to the palatal shelves using a device placed in the premolar region which he named the Trans Palatal Distractor (TPD).[66] No pterygoid maxillary separation was performed during the procedure and unequal expansion was achieved with greater expansion anteriorly than posteriorly in a 3:2 ratio.[66] Later Matteini and Mommaerts[72] investigated the influence of positioning the TPD at the level of the first molars and carrying out pterygoid disjunction to achieve parallel maxillary expansion. In a prospective study of 20 consecutive patients the change in resistance following pterygoid dysjunction and force application by placing the TPD

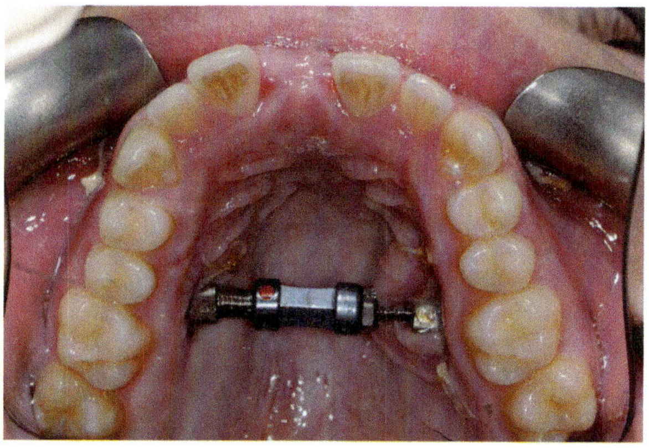

Fig. 36-8 A Martin distractor.

posteriorly delivered on average parallel expansion. Bone-borne distractors vary in designs and include the Surgitech TPD[66] (Figure 36-3), Magdenburg palatal distractor,[73] Martin Rapid Palatal Expander (Figure 36-8) (KLS Martin Group), the Rotterdam palatal distractor,[74] (KLS Martin Group), and the MDO-R device (Orthognathics, LTD, Zurich. Switzerland). The authors have treated most cases with the TPD supplied from Surgitech[R]. The pitch of the screw varies between different distractors and so it is very important to understand the manufacturer's guidelines. The TPD has three colours with the move to the next colour delivering 0.33 mm of expansion. The Rotterdam distractor is designed like a mini lifting jack and is useful in a very narrow arch. There is a progressive reduction in the distraction achieved with each progressive activation and to achieve the widening planned a complex schedule is needed.

A recent prospective randomized trial in 2009 by Koudstaal et al.[75] investigated stability, tipping and relapse of bone-borne versus tooth-borne surgical assisted cases. A comparison of 23 bone-borne and 19 tooth-borne patients showed no significant differences between the groups. Transverse expansion was comparable at canine, premolar and molar levels. Relapse was not significant and the transverse expansion was maintained. Also the maxilla was found to move slightly downwards. Segmental tipping occurred in both groups and did not influence relapse.[76] Verstraaten et al. (2010)[77] reported a systematic review of the effects of bone-borne SARPE from 10 studies and concluded that there was limited evidence to support using a bone-borne distractor. The sample sizes in this review were small and different techniques were used with significant limitations to the study designs described.

Complications

Ramieri et al. (2005)[78] examined 29 patients and difficulties reported were mainly device related. Most difficulties with bone-borne SARPE appliances relate to loosening of the distractor, mucosal inflammation and ulceration were also described. Minimal periodontal and dental damage following the midline osteotomy were reported. Neyt et al. reviewed 57 patients managed with a TPD and concluded that the expansion was achieved in all cases however loosening of the module was a major cause of patient discomfort.[79] Correct placement of the appliance is important to allow access for the spanner to turn the activation screw. Increased mobility, loss tooth vitality, tooth discolouration, gingival recession and external root resorption have been described by Koudstaal et al. (2009).[75]

Evidence for stability of expansion achieved with SARPE

In a meta-analysis reported by Vilani et al. (2012)[80] seven studies with moderate research quality were selected and five studies were finally included in the meta-analysis. Varying amounts of expansion were reported using a variety of techniques with or without pterygoid dysjunction. SARPE was found to achieve a long-term significant increase in maxillary alveolar width, intercanine width and intermolar width. Byloff and Mossaz 2004[81] reported 9 mm molar expansion and 5 mm expansion in the region of the canines with 75% of expansion retained. These workers also concluded that SARPE causes maxillary skeletal expansion by a lateral rotation of the maxillary halves with minimal translation. Koudstaal et al. (2009)[75] investigated stability and relapse in a study comparing bone-borne and tooth-borne devices and concluded that there were no significant differences between the groups. The widening achieved at dental level was found to be stable at 12 months and over correction was not considered to be required. Magnusson et al. (2009) evaluated long-term stability and concluded that SARPE is stable a mean of 6 years post-treatment with a loss of expansion most pronounced in the 3 years post-treatment.[82]

The future

Improved case assessment and monitoring using digital models, radiographs and CBCT will offer a better understanding of case selection and management. Digital assessment of models using software to assess arch size and arch form should allow simulation of expansion and should offer more predictable outcomes. The introduction of CBCT can create images that allow the clinician to carry out a true three dimensional assessment[83] allowing more precise surgical planning.[43]

There is currently no consensus on surgical technique, distractor design, protocol and relapse. Clearly the surgical approach and technique is likely to influence outcome and until large studies are reported uncertainty of decision-making will remain. SARPE is an important technique to manage the transverse dimension and improved assessment and distractor design will enhance patient acceptability and outcome.

References

1 Da Silva Filho OG, do Prado Montes LA, Torelly LF. Rapid maxillary expansion in the deciduous and mixed dentition evaluated through posteroanterior cephalometric analysis. Am J Orthod Dentofac Orthop. 1995;107:268–75.

2 Pogrel MA, Kaban LB, Vargervik K, Baumrind S. Surgically assisted rapid maxillary expansion in adults. Int J Adult Orthodon Orthognath Surg. 1992;7:37–41.

3 Angell EH. Treatment of irregularity of permanent adult teeth. Dent Cosm. 1860;1:540–54.

4 Timms DJ. The dawn of rapid maxillary expansion. Angle Orthod. 1999;69:247–50.

5 Harrison J, Ashby D. Orthodontic treatment for posterior crossbites. Cochrane Database Syst Rev. 2001;CD000979.

6 Bishara S, Staley R. Maxillary expansion: clinical implications. Am J Orthod Dentofac Orthop. 1987;91:3–14.

7 Schiffman PH, Tuncay OC. Maxillary expansion: a meta analysis. Clin Orthod Res. 2001;4:86–96.

8 Petrén S, Bjerklin K, Bondemark L. Stability of unilateral posterior crossbite correction in the mixed dentition: a randomized clinical trial with a 3-year follow-up. Am J Orthod Dentofac Orthop. 2011;139:e73–e81.

9 Silverstein K, Quinn P. Surgically-assisted rapid palatal expansion for management of transverse maxillary deficiency. J Oral Maxillofac Surg. 1997;55(7):725–7.

10 Corbridge JK, Campbell PM, Taylor R, Ceen RF, Buschang PH. Transverse dentoalveolar changes after slow maxillary expansion. Am J Orthod Dentofac Orthop. 2011;140:317–25.

11 Haas A. Palatal expansion: just the beginning of dentofacial orthopedics. Am J Orthod. 1970;57:219–55.

12 Timms DJ, Vero D. The relationship of rapid maxillary expansion to surgery with special reference to midpalatal synostosis. Br J Oral Surg. 1981;19:180–96.

13 Timms DJ. A study of basal movement with rapid maxillary expansion. Am J Orthod. 1980;77:500–7.

14 Isaacson R, Murphy T. Some Efifects Of Rapid Maxillary Expansion In Cleft Lip And Palate Patients. Angle Orthod. 1964;34:143–54.

15 Barber A, Sims M. Rapid maxillary expansion and external root resorption in man: a scanning electron microscope study. Am J Orthod. 1981;79:630–52.

16 Langford SR. Root resorption extremes resulting from clinical RME. Am J Orthod. 1982;81:371–7.

17 Pinto P, Mommaerts M. Immediate postexpansion changes following the use of the transpalatal distractor. J Oral Maxillofac Surg. 2001;59:994–1000.

18 Greenbaum KR, Zachrisson BU. The effect of palatal expansion therapy on the periodontal supporting tissues. Am J Orthod. 1982;81:12–21.

19 Capelozza Filho L, Cardoso Neto J, Da Silva Filho OG, Ursi WJ. Non-surgically assisted rapid maxillary expansion in adults. Int J Adult Orthodon Orthognath Surg. 1996;11:57–66; discussion 67–70.

20 Handelman CS, Wang L, BeGole EA, Haas A. Nonsurgical rapid maxillary expansion in adults: report on 47 cases using the Haas expander. Angle Orthod. 2000;70:129–44.

21 Melsen B. Palatal growth studied on human autopsy material. Am J Orthod. 1975;68:42–54.

22 Haas A. Rapid expansion of the maxillary dental arch and nasal cavity by opening the midpalatal suture. Angle Orthod. 1961;31:73–90.

23 Haas A. The treatment of maxillary deficiency by opening the midpalatal suture. Angle Orthod. 1965;35:200–17.

24 Zimring J, Isaacson R. Forces produced by rapid maxillary expansion: III. Forces present during retention. Angle Orthod. 1965;35:178–86.

25 Lines P. Adult rapid maxillary expansion with corticotomy. Am J Orthod. 1975;67:44–56.

26 Bell W, Epker B. Surgical-orthodontic expansion of the maxilla. Am J Orthod. 1976;70:517–28.

27 Wertz RA. Skeletal and dental changes accompanying rapid midpalatal suture opening. Am J Orthod. 1970;58:41–66.

28 Shetty V, Caridad J. Biomechanical rationale for surgical-orthodontic expansion of the adult maxilla. J Oral Maxillofac Surg. 1994;52:750–1.

29 Jacobs JD, Bell WH, Williams CE, Kennedy JW. Control of the transverse dimension with surgery and orthodontics. Am J Orthod. 1980;77:284–306.

30 Bell R. A review of maxillary expansion in relation to rate of expansion and patient's age. Am J Orthod. 1982;81:32–7.

31 Melsen B. Palatal growth studied on human autopsy material. A histologic microradiographic study. Am J Orthod. 1975;68:42–54.

32 Lagravere MO, Major PW, Flores-Mir C. Long-term skeletal changes with rapid maxillary expansion: a systematic review. Angle Orthod. 2005;75:1046–52.

33 Bailey L, Tanya J, Cevidanes LHS, Proffit WR. Stability and predictability of orthognathic surgery. Am J Orthod Dentofacial Orthop. 2004;126:273–7.

34 Moss JP. Rapid expansion of the maxillary arch. II. Indications for rapid expansion. JPO J Pr Orthod. 1968;2:215–23.

35 Persson M, Thilander B. Palatal suture closure in man from 15 to 35 years of age. Am J Orthod. 1977;72:42–52.

36 Haas A. Long-term posttreatment evaluation of rapid palatal expansion. Angle Orthod. 1980;50:189–217.

37 Sokucu O, Kosger HH, Bicakci AA, Babacan H. Stability in dental changes in RME and SARME: a 2-year follow-up. Angle Orthod. 2009;79:207–13.

38 Berger JL, Pangrazio-Kulbersh V, Borgula T, Kaczynski R. Stability of orthopedic and surgically assisted rapid palatal expansion over time. Am J Orthod Dentofac Orthop. 1998;114:638–45.

39 Altug-Ataç A T, Karasu H, Aytac D. Surgically assisted rapid maxillary expansion compared with orthopedic rapid maxillary expansion. Angle Orthod. 2006;76:353–9.

40 Kurt G, Altug-Ataç AT, Ataç MS, Karasu HA. Stability of surgically assisted rapid maxillary expansion and orthopedic maxillary expansion after 3 years' follow-up. Angle Orthod. 2010;80:425–31.

41 Magnusson A, Bjerklin K, Kim H, Nilsson P, Marcusson A. Three-dimensional computed tomographic analysis of changes to the external features of the nose after surgically assisted rapid maxillary expansion and orthodontic treatment: A prospective longitudinal study. Am J Orthod Dentofac Orthop. 2013;144:404–13.

42 Betts N, Vanarsdall R. Diagnosis and treatment of transverse maxillary deficiency. Int J Adult Orthognath Surg Orthognath Surg. 1995;10:75–96.

43 Angelieri F, Cevidanes LHS, Franchi L, Gonçalves JR, Benavides E, McNamara JA. Midpalatal suture maturation: classification method for individual assessment before rapid maxillary expansion. Am J Orthod Dentofac Orthop. 2013;144:759–69.

44 Illizarov G. Clinical application of the tension-stress effect for limb lengethening. Clin Orthop Relat Res. 1990;250:8–26.

45 Marchetti C, Pironi M, Bianchi A, Musci A. Surgically assisted rapid palatal expansion vs. segmental Le Fort I osteotomy: transverse stability over a 2-year period. J Craniomaxillofac Surg. 2009;37:74–8.

46 Chamberland S, Proffit WR. Short-term and long-term stability of surgically assisted rapid palatal expansion revisited. Am J Orthod Dentofac Orthop. American Association of Orthodontists; 2011;139:815–822.e1.

47 Marchetti C, Pironi M, Bianchi A, Musci A. Surgically assisted rapid palatal expansion vs. segmental Le Fort I osteotomy: Transverse stability over a 2-year period. J Cranio-Maxillofacial Surg. 2009;37:74–8.

48 Kretschmer WB, Baciut G, Baciut M, Zoder W, Wangerin K. Transverse stability of 3-piece Le Fort I osteotomies. J Oral Maxillofac Surg. 2011;69:861–9.
49 Suri L, Taneja P. Surgically assisted rapid palatal expansion: a literature review. Am J Orthod Dentofac Orthop. 2008;133:290–302.
50 Wriedt S, Kunkel M, Zentner A, Wahlmann U-W. Surgically assisted rapid palatal expansion an acoustic rhinometric, morphometric and sonographic investigation. J Orofac Orthop/Fortschritte der Kieferorthopädie. 2001;62:107–15.
51 Lehman JA, Haas AJ, Haas DG. Surgical orthodontic correction of transverse maxillary deficiency: a simplified approach. Plast Reconstr Surg. 1984;73:62–8.
52 Cureton S, Cuenin M. Surgically assisted rapid palatal expansion: orthodontic preparation for clinical success. Am J Orthod Dentofac Orthop. 1999;116:46–59.
53 Koudstaal M, Poort L. Surgically assisted rapid maxillary expansion (SARME): a review of the literature. Int J Oral Maxillofac Surg. 2005;34:709–14.
54 Bell WH, Epker BN. Surgical-orthodontic expansion of the maxilla. Am J Orthod. Elsevier, 1976;70:517–28.
55 Glassman AS, Nahigian SJ, Medway JM, Aronowitz HI. Conservative surgical orthodontic adult rapid palatal expansion: Sixteen cases. Am J Orthod. 1984;86:207–13.
56 Schimming R, Feller K. Surgical and orthodontic rapid palatal expansion in adults using Glassman's technique: retrospective study. Br J Oral Maxillofac Surg. 2000;38:66–9.
57 Lehman JA, Haas A. Surgical-orthodontic correction of transvers. Clin Plast Surg. 1989;16:749–55.
58 Anttila A, Finne K, Keski-Nisula K, Somppi M, Panula K, Peltomäki T. Feasibility and long-term stability of surgically assisted rapid maxillary expansion with lateral osteotomy. Eur J Orthod. 2004;31:142–9.
59 Pereira MD, Prado GPR, Abramoff MMF, Aloise AC, Masako Ferreira L. Classification of midpalatal suture opening after surgically assisted rapid maxillary expansion using computed tomography. Oral Surg Oral Med Oral Pathol Oral Radiol Endod. 2010;110:41–5.
60 Lanigan D, Mintz S. Complications of surgically assisted rapid palatal expansion: review of the literature and report of a case. J Oral Maxillofac Surg. 2002;60:104–10.
61 Ho MW, Boyle MA, Cooper JC, Dodd MD, Richardson D. Surgical complications of segmental Le Fort I osteotomy. Br J Oral Maxillofac Surg. 2011;49:562–6.
62 Williams BJD, Currimbhoy S, Silva A, O'Ryan FS. Complications following surgically assisted rapid palatal expansion: a retrospective cohort study. J Oral Maxillofac Surg 2012;70:2394–402.
63 Alpern MC, Yurosko JJ. Surgically assisted rapid palatal expansion. Am J Orthod Dentofacial Orthop. 2008;133:786.
64 Garib DG, Henriques JFC, Janson G, de Freitas MR, Fernandes AY. Periodontal effects of rapid maxillary expansion with tooth-tissue-borne and tooth-borne expanders: a computed tomography evaluation. Am J Orthod Dentofacial Orthop. 2006;129:749–58.
65 Garib D, Henriques J, Janson G. Rapid maxillary expansion-tooth tissue-borne versus tooth-borne expanders: a computed tomography evaluation of dentoskeletal effects. Angle Orthod. 2005;75:548–57.
66 Mommaerts MY. Transpalatal distraction as a method of maxillary expansion. Br J Oral Maxillofac Surg. 1999;37:268–72.
67 Bays RA, Greco JM. Surgically assisted rapid palatal expansion: an outpatient technique with long-term stability. J oral Maxillofac Surg Off J Am Assoc Oral Maxillofac Surg. 1992;50:110–113; discussion 114–115.
68 Seeberger R, Kater W, Schulte-Geers M, Davids R, Freier K, Thiele O. Changes after surgically-assisted maxillary expansion (SARME) to the dentoalveolar, palatal and nasal structures by using tooth-borne distraction devices. Br J Oral Maxillofac Surg. 2011;49:381–5.
69 Mossaz CF, Byloff FK, Richter M. Unilateral and bilateral corticotomies for correction of maxillary transverse discrepancies. Eur J Orthod. 1992;14:110–6.
70 Northway WM, Meade JB. Surgically assisted rapid maxillary expansion: a comparison of technique, response, and stability. Angle Orthod. 1997;67:309–20.
71 Kraut R. Surgically assisted rapid maxillary expansion by opening the midpalatal suture. J Oral Maxillofac Surg. 1984;42:651–5.
72 Matteini C, Mommaerts M. Posterior transpalatal distraction with pterygoid disjunction: a short-term model study. Am J Orthod Dentofac Orthop. 2001;120:498–502.
73 Gerlach K, Zahl C. Transversal palatal expansion using a palatal distractor. J Orofac Orthop. 2003;64:443–9.
74 Koudstaal M, Wal K Van der. The Rotterdam Palatal Distractor: introduction of the new bone-borne device and report of the pilot study. Int J Oral Maxillofac Surg. 2006;35:31–5.
75 Koudstaal MJ, Smeets JBJ, Kleinrensink G-J, Schulten AJM, Van Der Wal KGH. Relapse and stability of surgically assisted rapid maxillary expansion: an anatomic biomechanical study. J Oral Maxillofac Surg. 2009;67:10–4.
76 Koudstaal MJ, Wolvius EB, Schulten AJM, Hop WCJ, Van Der Wal KGH. Stability, tipping and relapse of bone-borne versus tooth-borne surgically assisted rapid maxillary expansion; a prospective randomized patient trial. Int J Oral Maxillofac Surg. 2009;38:308–15.
77 Verstraaten J, Kuijpers-Jagtman AM, Mommaerts MY, Bergé SJ, Nada RM, Schols JGJH. A systematic review of the effects of bone-borne surgical assisted rapid maxillary expansion. J Craniomaxillofacial Surg. 2010;38:166–74.
78 Ramieri G, Spada M, Austa M. Transverse maxillary distraction with a bone-anchored appliance: dento-periodontal effects and clinical and radiological results. Int J Oral Maxillofac Surg. 2005;34:357–63.
79 Neyt N, Mommaerts M. Problems, obstacles and complications with transpalatal distraction in non-congenital deformities. J Craniomaxillofac Surg. 2002;30:139–43.
80 Vilani GNL, Mattos CT, De Oliveira Ruellas AC, Maia LC. Long-term dental and skeletal changes in patients submitted to surgically assisted rapid maxillary expansion: a meta-analysis. Oral Surg Oral Med Oral Pathol Oral Radiol. 2012;114:689–97.
81 Byloff FK, Mossaz CF. Skeletal and dental changes following surgically assisted rapid palatal expansion. Eur J Orthod. 2004;26:403–9.
82 Magnusson A, Bjerklin K, Nilsson P, Marcusson A. Surgically assisted rapid maxillary expansion: long-term stability. Eur J Orthod. 2009;31:142–9.
83 Macchi A, Carrafiello G, Cacciafesta V, Norcini A. Three-dimensional digital modeling and setup. Am J Orthod Dentofac Orthop. 2006;129:605–10.

Chapter 37

Mandibular Midline Osteotomy

Dale Bloomquist and Don Joondeph

Introduction

The correction of transverse discrepancies in patients undergoing orthognathic surgery has been traditionally managed either by the orthodontist through orthopaedic maxillary arch expansion or by the surgeon with maxillary osteotomies. Young growing patients can often be treated with orthopaedic rapid maxillary expansion when the palatal suture has not yet matured and surgical intervention is not needed. However, adults with transverse problems have limited orthodontic options. Most nonsurgical attempts in the adult occur with simple dentoalveolar tipping of the teeth. This can be successful with minor expansions but is generally felt to be unstable with larger corrections. Surgery, however, offers four possible alternatives: cortical osteotomies, surgically assisted rapid palatal expansion (SARPE), maxillary Le Fort I osteotomy with two or more segments, and mandibular midline osteotomy with constriction done in conjunction with bilateral sagittal split osteotomies (BSSO). Cortical osteotomies, with or without bone grafts, are relatively new and as such long-term stability has not been well studied.[1] The use of this technique will be limited until research clearly shows a permanent benefit. Surgically assisted rapid palatal expansion has been reviewed in a number of papers with relapse being reported between 5–30%.[2,3] This large variability is likely due to the variations in both surgical technique as well as research methodology. The Le Fort I osteotomy is the most common and oldest method for surgically correcting transverse problems. However, it has been ranked as one of the most, if not the most, unstable of orthognathic surgical procedures in the North Carolina hierarchy of stability study.[4] Each of these three maxillary procedures has advantages in certain situations and surgeons generally have their preferences. It is important, however, to remember that they have in common a definite relapse potential. The last option for surgically correcting transverse discrepancies is the mandibular midline osteotomy. Not unlike all other orthognathic surgeries this procedure has a relapse potential, but a concern in discussing that potential is that all the published studies have been conducted in only one institution, the University of Washington in Seattle, USA.[5–7] This brings into question whether stability can be used as a consideration in a clinical decision of which surgical technique should be used. Therefore, although we will discuss our findings on relapse, we will also review other benefits of using this procedure.

The mandibular midline osteotomy used in conjunction with a BSSO is clearly an underused technique in orthognathic surgery. Since it was initially mentioned in the literature, almost as an afterthought,[8] it has not been discussed except in papers from Seattle. Although the reasons for this apparent oversight are unclear, the concerns brought to our attention have been: unfamiliarity with the procedure, concern over relapse, effects on the temporomandibular joint, and not addressing the skeletal problem. For that reason each of these concerns, will be reviewed in this chapter.

Orthognathic Surgery: Principles, Planning and Practice. Edited by Farhad B. Naini and Daljit S. Gill.

Literature review

Although the use of midline osteotomies for the correction of transverse skeletal problems seems recent to a number of surgeons, it was first described by Bell in 1976. Ostectomies in this region were first described even earlier, but were generally considered as techniques that had few indications. Bell only mentions the use of the midline procedure in a case report in which the mandible was set-back and widened. In his paper the midline osteotomy was considered a minor adjunct to the more major procedures of the BSSO and a genioplasty. Brusati[9] was the first to describe the value of the osteotomy and he specified the indications and limitations of the procedure. It was left to Alexander[5] to first describe application of the midline osteotomy in the era of rigid internal fixation as well as evaluate the stability of this technique. He found no statistically significant relapse and there were about an equal number of patients that had some relapse as compared to patients who had further constriction. Importantly, there was only one patient out of the 15 studied that had 2 mm of relapse. This fact is significant if this technique is going to be compared to other surgical procedures under the criteria used in North Carolina's studies of the stability of orthognathic surgeries. For the purpose of ranking stability they consider that less than 2 mm of relapse not to be significant.[10] Thus the 7% of 'potentially clinically significant' relapse seen in Alexander's study is very favourable compared with the relapse seen with segmental maxillary surgery. Pitts[6] later looked at a larger group long-term, and similarly found no clinically significant relapse. It is important to note that in neither study was there relapse into a posterior crossbite.

The potential negative effects of the midline osteotomy on the temporomandibular joint seem to be a common concern among clinicians. Both Alexander and Pitts evaluated the TMJ in their studies. Their findings were based on patient's responses to a questionnaire along with measurements of mandibular movement preoperatively and at their final examination. Alexander noted minor decrease in lateral excursions but neither authors noted any other significant change in joint signs or symptoms. Joondeph[7] compared angular and linear radiographic changes in patients who had a conventional mandibular advancement to the mandibular advancement including a mandibular midline osteotomy. Contrary to what many surgeons anticipated he found less change in condylar rotation and lateral movements in patients who had mandibular constriction along with the advancement. However, this is not surprising if one considers the mechanics of the fragment movements that occur at the sagittal split osteotomy site. Since the mandibular body is somewhat 'V' shaped the proximal fragments will tend to flare laterally as the distal segment is advanced in the correction of mandibular retrognathia. This rotation of the proximal fragment usually occurs despite the attempts by surgeons to minimize these changes. Joondeph also used a patient questionnaire to compare TMJ symptoms and found no difference between the two groups long-term.

Damage to the incisors and their supporting periodontium also has been a concern of some clinicians. Alexander and Pitts both evaluated that question without finding any evidence of damage to those tissues on either side of the osteotomy. However, as mentioned earlier, these studies were all completed at one centre. They also were operated primarily by one surgeon, which begs the question of whether the same stability and apparent lack of complications could be duplicated by other less experienced surgeons. It must be emphasized that although these studies showed significant success with midline osteotomies, the authors have had patients with relapse significant enough to result in posterior crossbite and infections that have resulted in periodontal pockets. Fortunately these complications are rare and can be minimized with a few technical suggestions that will be reviewed later.

The final areas of discussion before reviewing the technique are the criteria for choosing the midline osteotomy in conjunction with the BSSO in cases of transverse skeletal discrepancies. A major difficulty in setting clinical criteria for choosing the appropriate surgery is guidelines that are not clear as to diagnosing the cause of a transverse skeletal discrepancy. Historically, and perhaps correctly, absolute transverse problems in developmental facial-skeletal problems have been attributed to maxillary constriction. Therefore both orthodontists and surgeons have developed procedures to address that skeletal deformity. Authors who have tried to describe how the diagnosis of maxillary constriction can be made have on the most part relied on subjective clinical findings.[8,11] These findings include: narrow tapering maxillary arch form, increased curve of Wilson of the posterior maxillary teeth, deep palatal vault, 'enlarged buccal corridor', and most commonly simply a narrower arch than exists in the mandible. The one attempt at objectively describing maxillary constriction is based on PA headfilms. The use of metrics on this radiograph to evaluate maxillary width is attributed to Ricketts,[12,13] but is rarely used. The reasons for these measurements not generally being used are based on a number of factors including: relatively limited group of subjects used to the determine standards, possible variability in choosing the reference points, variability in head positioning that will influence those points, and generally the question of the relevance of the measurements advocated. Most clinicians therefore rely simply on their clinical impression of whether maxillary constriction exists. Along the same lines, a diagnosis of excessive mandibular width in most cases is simply made by clinical impression. It can be fairly said that excessive mandibular width is very rare except in cases of mandibular hyperplasia in which the mandible is larger in all three planes of space. Maxillary constriction, however, can occur without any abnormality in vertical or horizontal development.

Accepting that the diagnosis of maxillary constriction is somewhat an arbitrary call, then clinicians need to evaluate the consequences of a misdiagnosis. Vanarsdall,[11] who is an advocate of the use of a PA cephalometric radiograph, emphasizes an increased risk to the periodontium as well as the instability of the dental correction if maxillary constriction is not diagnosed. Aesthetically, clinicians are concerned about leaving the buccal corridors too wide. Most commonly, however, a mild maxillary constriction by itself has no aesthetic or functional implications. The necessity of the clinician to correctly diagnose the aetiology of a mild or possibly even moderate transverse arch discrepancy may not be biologically critical. The treatment decision in those cases then becomes more of a practical decision. The justification for the use of the mandibular midline osteotomy in conjunction with bilateral sagittal osteotomies in transverse discrepancies in most cases falls under that category of reasoning. We don't argue that the use of this osteotomy is, other than rarely, based upon a diagnosis of absolute excessive mandibular width. The most common reason for using a mandibular midline osteotomy is a situation in which there is a mild to moderate transverse problem and there is no other justification for a maxillary osteotomy,[14] (Figure 37-1). Practically, many of our corrections are for a minor, less than 5 mm as measured at the second molars, transverse discrepancy. Admittedly orthodontists can often compensate for minor transverse problems by tipping the posterior teeth. This, however, can decrease any safety factor that could prevent relapse into posterior crossbite. In cases in which the patient already has a large curve of Wilson, dental compensation may not be possible.

Techniques

The mandibular midline osteotomy is technically very simple and generally does not take more than 10–15 minutes operating time. Even with its simplicity there have been specific steps that we have found to be important in decreasing problems both intraoperatively as well as postoperatively. The orthodontic preparation like with all of orthognathic surgery is as important, if not more important, than the surgical technique in the achievement of a good result. It is not recommended that the incisors be separated, but it is important that the roots of the central incisors be parallel to each other as well as perpendicular to the incisal (occlusal) plane. This allows the surgeon to safely make a bicortical cut from the inferior border up to a point just above the root tips and into the alveolar bone. Superiorly from that point up to the attached tissue the cut should only be through the labial bone. A fine instrument such as an osteotome can then be wedged into the cut at the level of the basal bone and with some pressure the rest of the split with be completed. It has been found from the periapical radiographs that have been taken for our studies that the rest of the split generally will run up one of the periodontal ligaments. This has not resulted in any periodontal problems as has been previously mentioned.

The most important orthodontic step in preparation for a mandibular midline osteotomy is the narrowing of the mandibular archwire just before surgery. We have found in our early experience with this procedure that one of the biggest contributors to relapse was the memory inherent in a rectangular steel archwire. The surgeon can be of benefit in this preparation by informing the orthodontist of the amount of planned constriction measured at the distal of the second molars. Then within five days before surgery the wire can be constricted, at the same time surgical hooks are placed. We have tried cutting the archwire at the time of surgery but this lends to instability at the midline osteotomy, especially vertically. All oral and maxillofacial surgeons know of the importance of double plating a symphysis fracture but normally only a single plate is used for the midline osteotomy with the archwire acting as the superior 'tension' plate in the fixation. Using two plates for the fixation is possible but unnecessary and requires a larger area of bone exposure including stripping of mentalis muscle attachment. Narrowing of an archwire after surgery is generally impractical due to the limited access available in the patient's mouth for a few weeks after surgery.

The presurgical model surgery usually done by the surgeon needs to include overcorrection of the transverse correction much like is practiced with surgical expansion of the maxilla. This is done both to allow for any relapse that may occur as well to accommodate for the small amount of lingual tipping of the segments that was noted in Alexander's study. The mandibular sagittal osteotomies are completed first and the distal fragment is temporarily stabilized in the usual manner preferably with an occlusal splint and wire intermaxillary fixation. Although the teeth will not fit completely into the splint, this stabilization is very beneficial while completing the midline osteotomy. The surgical procedure itself, as previously mentioned, is simple and can be accomplished with minimal bone exposure. The bone cut is made with a sagittal saw with care being taken for the extension between the roots. It is safest to simply cut through only the buccal cortex at the alveolar bone level with the final split being made by twisting a thin instrument in the osteotomy. The teeth of the two mandibular fragments are then completely seated in the splint and secured by tightening the intermaxillary wires. A titanium non-compression 2 mm four-hole plate is then contoured with a slight overcorrection to fit across the osteotomy. It is not necessary to place the plate at the inferior border and it simply can be placed about 5 mm below the apices of the teeth. Since the exposure is minimal there is no need to resuspend the soft tissue including the mentalis muscle and the wound can be closed at the mucosa. The surgery is then completed with the fixation of the sagittal splits. External supporting dressing of the lip is not needed and the post-operative care is no different than with a standard bilateral sagittal split of the mandible.

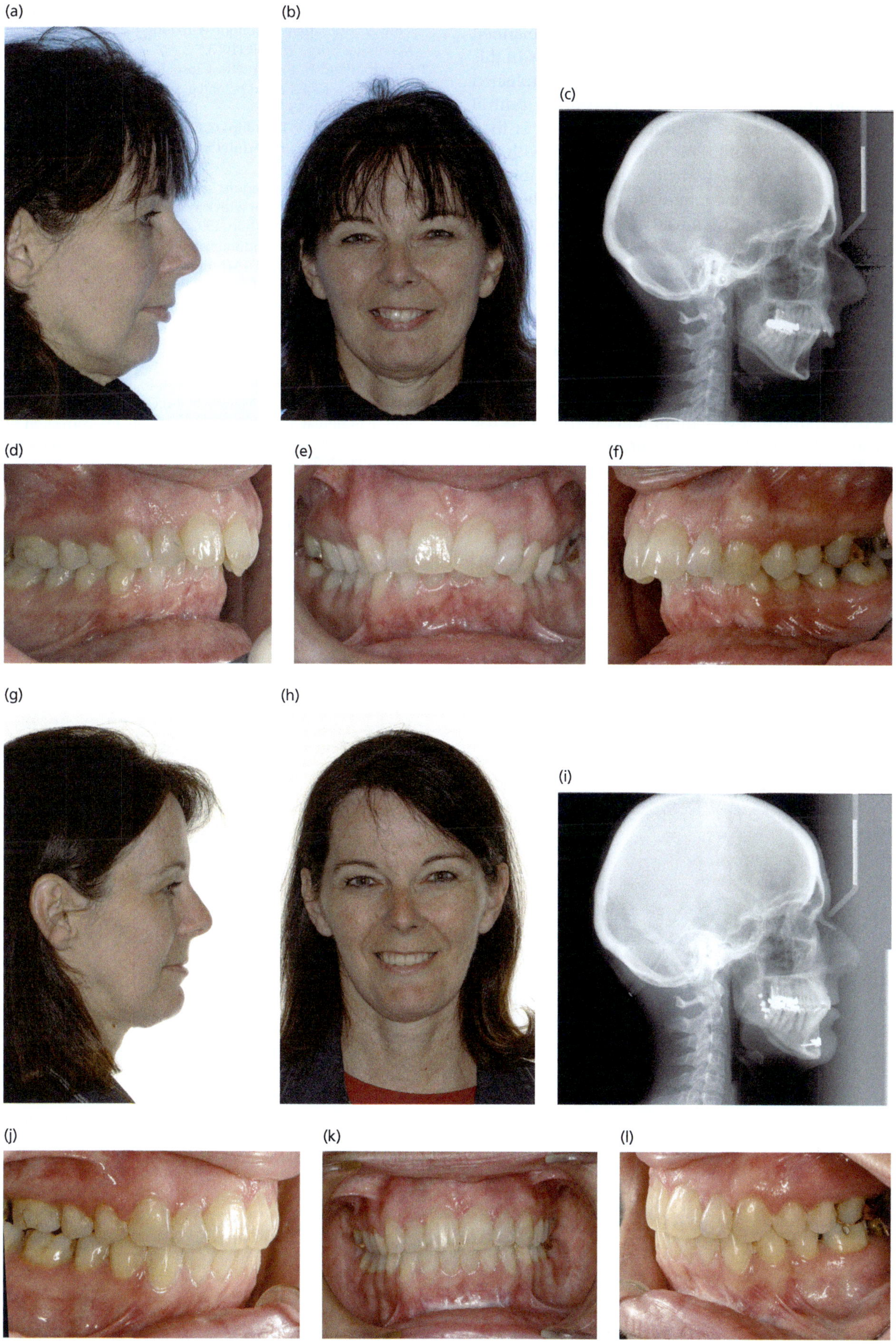

Fig. 37-1 (a–f) Pretreatment records of patient with mandibular retrognathia and narrow maxillary arch. (g–l) Final records of patient who had mild dental arch widening with orthodontics and mandibular BSSO and a midline ostetomy.

A variation of this technique can be used in cases in which a horizontal osteotomy (genioplasty) is planned to either increase or decrease chin prominence. In this situation the horizontal osteotomy is accomplished first and then the vertical cut between the central incisors can be made. The inferior fragment is then used in the fixation of the midline osteotomy with two bicortical screws placed on either side of the midline started either from the inferior fragment to the body fragments in the case of chin advancement or from the mandibular body fragments to the inferior fragment.

Conclusion

The mandibular midline osteotomy as used with a bilateral sagittal split osteotomy is a simple and extremely useful technique in orthognathic surgery. We have found that with minimum experience its use becomes standard for both the surgeon and orthodontist. Decreasing the surgical trauma associated with adding maxillary osteotomies, risks/costs, and relapse are the notable benefits of using this procedure in the correction of transverse facial skeletal deformities.

References

1 Mathews DP, Kokich VG. Accelerating tooth movement: the case against corticotomy-induced orthodontics. Am J Orthod Dentofacial Orthop. 2013;144:5–13.

2 Bays RA, Greco JM. Surgically assisted rapid palatal expansion: An outpatient technique with long-term stability. J Oral Maxillofac Surg. 1992;50:110–3.

3 Chamberland S, Proffit WR. Closer look at the stability of surgically assisted rapid palatal expansion. J Oral Maxillofac Surg. 2008;66:1895–900.

4 Proffit, W; Turvey, T; Phillips C. Orthognathic surgery: A hierarchy of stability. Int J Adult Orthodonitics Orthognath Surg. 1996;11:191–204.

5 Alexander CD, Bloomquist DS, Wallen TR. Stability of mandibular constriction with a symphyseal osteotomy. Am J Orthod Dentofacial Orthop. 1993;103:15–23.

6 Pitts A. Mandibular midline osteotomy: long term stability, periodontal status, and TMJ function (Master's thesis). University of Washington, Seattle, 1996.

7 Joondeph D. Temporomandibular effects of mandibular constriction, 1994.

8 Jacobs JD, Bell WH, Williams CE, Kennedy JW. Control of the transverse dimension with surgery and orthodontics. Am J Orthod. 1980;77:284–306.

9 Brusati, R; Sesenna, E; Mannucci, N; Gamoietti R. The midline mandibular osteotomy-ostectomy in the correction of dentofacial deformities. Int J Adult Orthodon Orthognath Surg. 1987;2:37–50.

10 Proffit, WR; Turvey, TA; Phillips C. The hierarchy of stability and predictability in orthognathic surgery with rigid fixation: an update and extension. Head Face Med. 2007;3:1–11.

11 Vanarsdall RL. Transverse dimension and long-term stability. Semin Orthod. 1999;5:171–80.

12 Ricketts RM. Cephalometric synthesis. Am J Orthod. 1960;46:647–73.

13 Ricketts RM. Perspectives in the clinical application of cephalometrics. Angle Orthod. 1981;51:115–50.

14 Bloomquist D. Mandibular narrowing: advantage in transverse problems. J Oral Maxillofac Surg. 2004;62:365–8.

Chapter 38

Segmental Surgery of the Maxilla

Jocelyn M. Shand and Andrew A. Heggie

Introduction

The indications for and role of segmental surgery in the maxilla has changed over time with the increasing sophistication of orthodontic treatment in presurgical preparation for orthognathic surgery. The first recognized report of segmental maxillary surgery was in Europe in 1921,[1] and the early procedures that followed were usually undertaken as isolated procedures. As the experience with orthognathic surgery techniques increased, together with the development of orthodontic expertise, segmental procedures where undertaken for specific occlusal or skeletal problems as part of a combined surgical/orthodontic treatment plan.

Concerns about maintaining the vascularity of the maxilla influenced the development of surgical techniques. Wassmund[2,3] described a single-stage labial (vestibular) approach for a 'set-back' osteotomy of the maxilla in the 1920s and a tunnelling approach was subsequently outlined by Axhausen.[4] Schuchardt subsequently reported on a two-stage procedure for maxillary segmental procedures where the palatal osteotomy was undertaken as the first stage, then several weeks later, the buccal approach was performed for access and subsequent mobilization.[5,6] In 1962, Wunderer described a modification of the Wassmund technique with the majority of the procedure being performed via a palatal approach.[7] This helped to improve overall access whilst maintaining a broad buccal pedicle for perfusion. Later, Obwegeser reported on his technique and experience with maxillary repositioning for the correction of small or retrodisplaced maxillae.[8] He identified the need for complete mobilisation of the segment to achieve repositioning without tissue resistance. This was followed by the landmark studies of Bell and Fonseca who reported on bone healing and revascularization of the maxilla following a total maxillary osteotomy in primates. It was found that the palatal mucosal pedicle and labio-buccal pedicle provide an adequate nutrient pedicle and that transection of the greater palatine artery had no notable effect on the circulation to the teeth, bone and soft tissues of the maxilla.[9–11] Over the following years, this became the 'work-horse' procedure for maxillary repositioning and had predictable outcomes. Subsequently, segmental procedures were undertaken as part of the Le Fort I maxillary osteotomy where it was possible to divide the maxilla into segments from the downfractured position for expansion or to manage orthodontic arch discrepancies. The procedures described used in earlier decades are now rarely undertaken but they remain available for specific indications. The posterior segmental osteotomy was introduced by Schuchardt[5,6] and a one-stage procedure was subsequently described by Kufner.[12] Specific indications for the posterior maxillary segmental procedure

Orthognathic Surgery: Principles, Planning and Practice. Edited by Farhad B. Naini and Daljit S. Gill.

were described by West and Epker such as the correction of a unilateral cross-bite or management of overeruption of a segment.[13]

In this chapter, the techniques for segmental surgery undertaken in conjunction with the Le Fort I maxillary osteotomy will be described together with an outline of the historical procedures.

Treatment planning

Among the well-established indications for undertaking segmental maxillary surgery are the management of an anterior arch length discrepancy and a narrow maxilla with posterior transverse discrepancy that can be resolved with surgical expansion. Conversely, the less commonly overexpanded maxilla can be addressed with narrowing from the midline via a segmental procedure. Malocclusions presenting with dual occlusal planes in the maxilla potentially may not be managed satisfactorily by orthodontic alignment alone due to the risk of extruding anterior teeth that would subsequently relapse. Segmental orthodontic alignment or stepped arch wires may be used to prepare for surgical levelling. Segmental surgery can facilitate space closure within the arch, address a markedly retroclined anterior segment or a prominent premaxilla that may need to be set-back by the removal of a dental unit.

Early identification of the cases potentially requiring segmental surgery will facilitate a coordinated surgical and orthodontic approach with presurgical alignment being specifically planned. In the site of a planned interdental osteotomy, the roots should ideally be either parallel or divergent to facilitate an osteotomy that will not put tooth vitality at risk nor damage root surfaces. Working study models assist in monitoring the presurgical alignment and promote an ongoing liaison between the surgeon and the orthodontist to achieve the optimal orthodontic presurgical preparation and finishing, particularly in complex segmental cases. There may also be an indication for progress imaging such as an orthopantomograph (OPT) to view the root orientation and to enable optimal orthodontic positioning prior to the presentation of the patient for the surgical phase. Studies have reported on the periodontal effects of interdental osteotomies and recommended that at least 3 mm of bone be left between the osteotomy and adjacent roots to minimise the risk.[14] The positioning of the interdental osteotomy is most commonly performed in the mid-line or between the lateral incisor/canine or first premolar regions (para-midline) depending on the management of the arch required.

There are a number of specific complications that may arise from segmental surgery. These include gingival recession, periodontal pocketing, discolouration of teeth due to pulpal haemorrhage or non-vitality. On rare occasions, there may be significant areas of ischaemia with the potential loss of teeth, alveolar bone and associated soft tissue.

Segmental surgery should be undertaken with caution in cleft lip and palate patients, particularly bilateral cases. The axial perfusion of maxillary segments may be distorted in patients who have undergone earlier procedures for closure of palatal fistulae. Segmental surgery increases the risk of complications including the serious risk of avascular necrosis in this group. In cases with transverse discrepancy, that is common in patients with a history of cleft palate, rapid maxillary expansion with a hyrax device, with or without surgically-assisted maxillary expansion procedures, should be considered prior to definitive orthognathic surgery to minimize the maxillary transverse discrepancy and reduce the requirement for segmental expansion at the time of the Le Fort I maxillary osteotomy.

Surgical technique

Segmental Le Fort I osteotomy

Following infiltration with local anaesthetic (with adrenaline) for haemostasis and postoperative pain control, access to the maxilla is achieved via a vestibular incision from first molar to first molar sites across the midline. Buccal pedicles are maintained to augment the vascularity of the maxilla. Periosteal elevators are used to deglove the anterior and lateral maxilla, up to identification and preservation of the infraorbital nerves. As the dissection moves posteriorly towards the pterygomaxillary fissures, it is tunnelled to protect the buccal mucosal pedicle. In the midline, the nasal aperture is exposed with dissection along the piriform rim and lateral nasal wall. Small periosteal elevators are used for this careful dissection of the more delicate nasal mucosa. The dissection continues to expose the anterior nasal spine and to commence separation of the nasal septum in the midline region. An osteotomy is made bilaterally at the Le Fort I level with a surgical burr or reciprocating saw from the posterior lateral maxillary region, moving anteriorly beneath the zygomatic buttress and along the thin anterior maxillary wall to the piriform apertures. Before maxillary mobilization, interdental osteotomies are undertaken in the desired areas e.g. midline, or as planned interdentally in the arch to connect to the horizontal osteotomy. A fine burr or saw begins a full thickness osteotomy superiorly and on descent towards the apices, only a mono-cortical osteotomy is made and continues inferiorly with careful reflection of the mucoperiosteum close to the interdental papillae. The separation of the posterior maxilla is undertaken by a curved osteotome either trans-tuberosity or at the pterygomaxillary junction according to operator preference. Division of the lateral wall it achieved with a straight osteotome in a posterior and inferior direction bilaterally protecting the nasal mucosa with a periosteal elevator placed submucosally on the medial side. An audible change in bone density is detected when the region of the palatine bone is reached with the osteotome. A guarded nasal

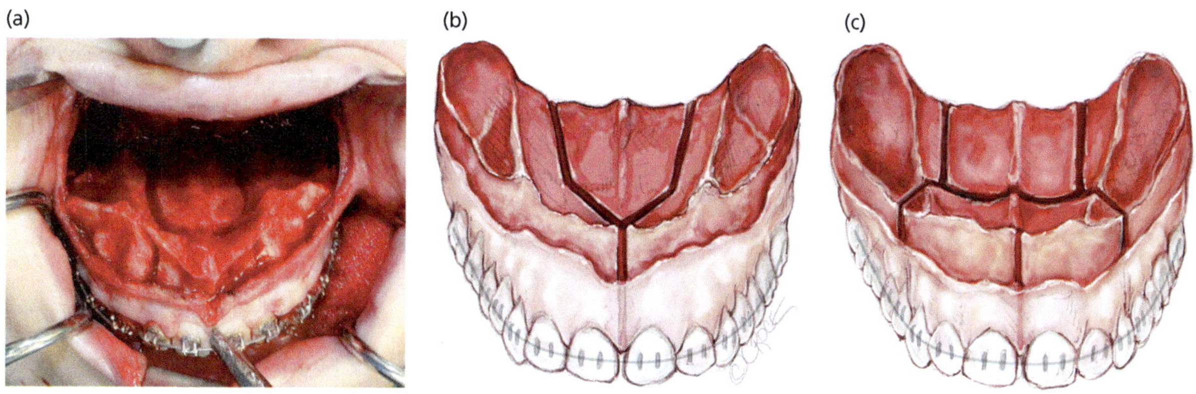

Fig. 38-1 (a) U-shaped palatal osteotomy following downfracture of the Le Fort I maxillary osteotomy. (b) Palatal osteotomy with midline osteotomy. (c) Palatal osteotomy with bilateral para-midline osteotomies.

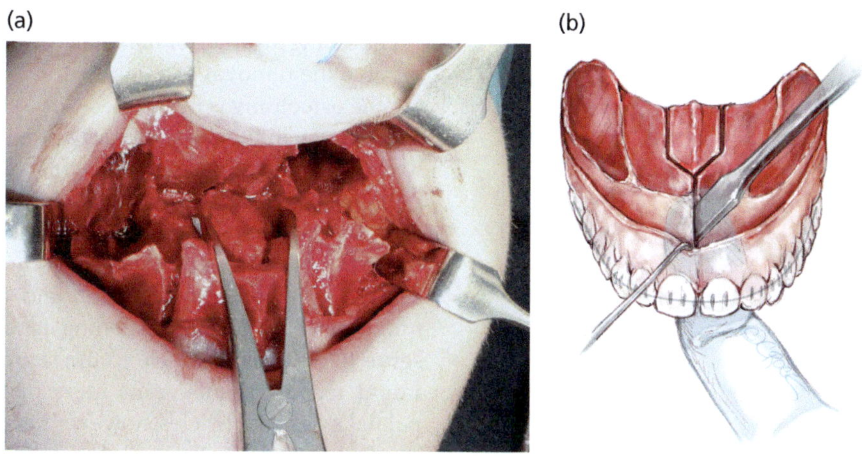

Fig. 38-2 (a) Mobilizing midline osteotomy with osteotome and finger placed on palatal mucosa. (b) Mobilizing osteotomy segments with spreader.

septal osteotome is positioned in the midline above the anterior nasal spine and advanced along the crest separating the septum along the nasal floor and maxillary crest.

The maxilla is then downfractured and mobilized using a combination of osteotomes, 'spinal' laminar spreaders or finger pressure depending on the degree of resistance encountered and the surgeon preference. The descending palatine vessels are identified bilaterally during mobilization. Bony interferences are removed in all regions with rongeurs or a 'pineapple' burr, and smoothed. A 'U-shaped' palatal osteotomy is performed in the central palate and mobilised with an osteotome. The midline or para-midline interdental osteotomy sites are then connected to the palatal osteotomy segment and fine osteotomes are used to complete the interdental osteotomy sites enabling mobilization of the dentoalveolar segments (Figure 38-1a–c). If however, a tooth or teeth are being removed for repositioning of a segment, the extraction is undertaken and bone removal with a burr is performed to allow the segment to be repositioned with space closure. Residual bony interferences in the palatal and cervical regions of the alveolar ridge require careful removal to avoid damage to the adjacent tooth roots. Segmentalization and mobilization can be challenging and must be undertaken carefully (Figure 38-2a,b).

The desired movement of the segments is achieved and a palatal splint is inserted and secured to adjacent teeth (Figure 38-3). To avoid distortion or deviation of the nasal septum, it is reduced and needed and any tears of the nasal mucosa are closed with resorbable sutures. The segments are then positioned into an occlusal wafer/surgical splint and the patient

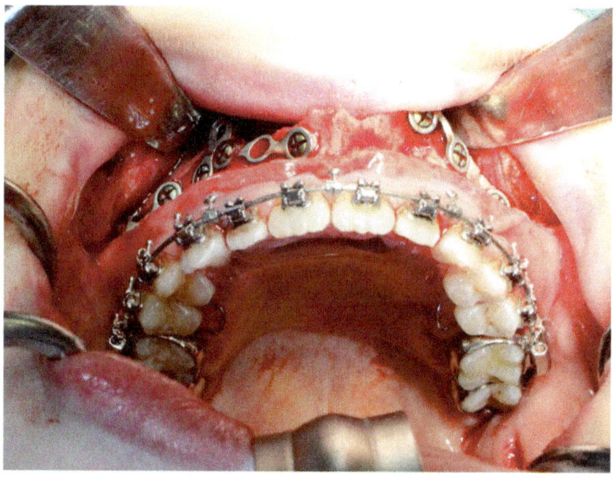

Fig. 38-3 Palatal splint wired in-situ.

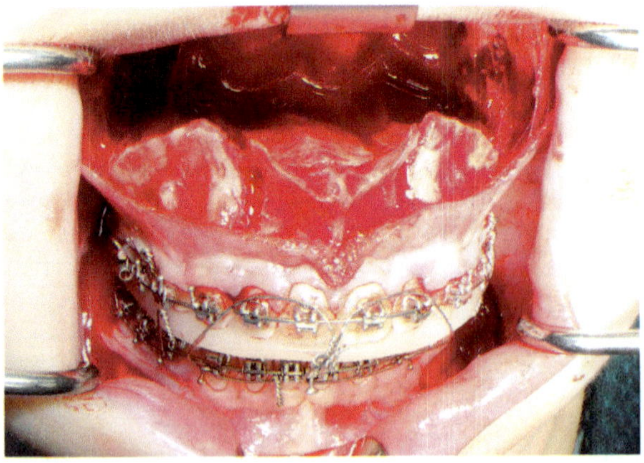

Fig. 38-4 Positioning of segments into occlusal splint and intermaxillary fixation.

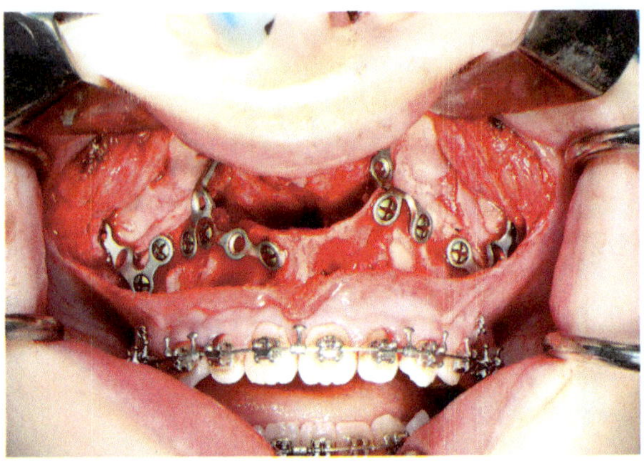

Fig. 38-5 Fixation with bone plates and screws incorporating interdental osteotomy sites.

placed into intermaxillary fixation (Figure 38-4). When the maxillomandibular complex is vertically repositioned, bony interferences are relieved before applying internal fixation with mini-plates and screws. In the placement of the bone plates, if possible, the interdental osteotomy site(s) are incorporated into the fixation (Figure 38-5). The intermaxillary fixation is released and the occlusal wafer/surgical splint is removed to check the occlusion. Palatal splints that do not cover the occlusal surfaces remain in-situ for 6-weeks post-operation before removal. Control of the nasolabial aesthetics is achieved with an alar base suture ('figure-of-8' 2/0 resorbable suture) passed through a hole made in the anterior nasal spine picking up the alar base bilaterally. The mucoperiosteal flaps are then closed starting in the midline with either a straight or V-Y closure depending on the lip dimensions with a resorbable suture such as 3/0 or 4/0 chromic gut.

Anterior maxillary segmental osteotomy

The anterior subapical or anterior maxillary segmental osteotomies are procedures that can be used for specific clinical situations such as maxillary protrusion or a markedly stepped occlusal plane.

Following an anterior maxillary osteotomy that may involve the removal of a dental unit such as a premolar, the osteotomy is performed through the extraction socket to facilitate the anterior dentoalveolar segment to be repositioned posteriorly or inferiorly. There may be bony interferences encountered secondary to the tipping movement of the dentoalveolar segments that must be removed to allow the accurate positioning of the segment. The Wassmund and Wunderer techniques used for this repositioning are designed to preserve the vascular pedicle to the segment. The Wassmund technique maintains more of the buccal and palatal mucosal pedicles, however the access provided results in a technically challenging procedure.

Wassmund technique

Following infiltration of local anaesthetic vertical mucosal incisions are made bilaterally between the canine and premolar, from the gingival margin superiorly to the nasal aperture region. Using periosteal elevators the mucoperiosteum is elevated and tunnelled until the piriform aperture is exposed and the dissection continued over the rim (Figure 38-6a). On the palatal aspect of the anterior maxilla gingival incisions are made from the incisor to second premolar region and then a palatal mucosal flap is elevated in

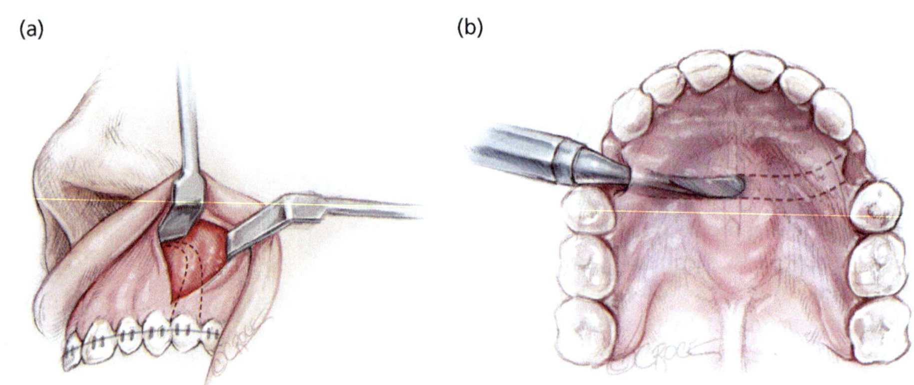

Fig. 38-6 (a) Exposure of buccal aspect of maxilla and outline of osteotomy cuts. (b) Dissection of palatal mucosal tunnel with periosteal elevator.

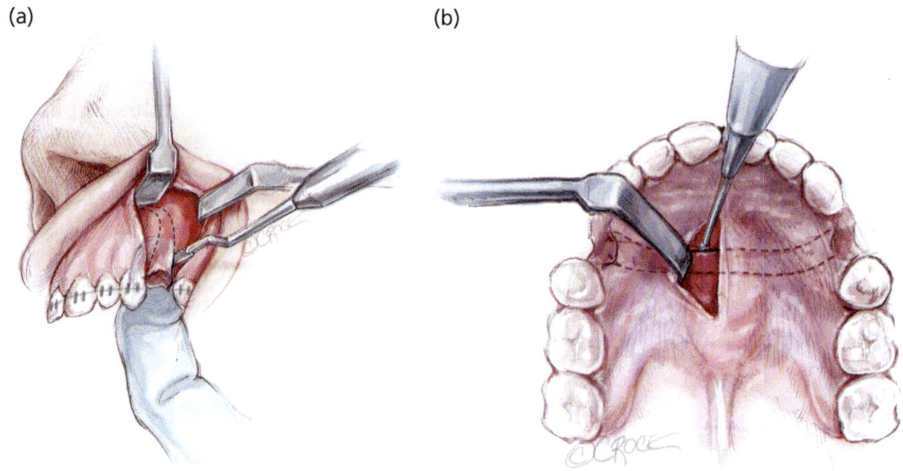

Fig. 38-7 (a) Buccal osteotomy cuts and bone removal is performed in region of extracted tooth. (b) Midline palatal incision for exposure of bone in the midline is required to complete palatal osteotomy cuts.

a tunnelling approach (Figure 38-6b). If a premolar extraction is planned, it is removed at this stage. An osteotomy is made with a burr or reciprocating saw and bone should be preserved over the surface of the adjacent teeth. The osteotomy extends from the alveolar region superiorly to the lateral aspect of the nasal sill (Figure 38-7a). The tunnelled palatal mucosal flap is retracted and a bilateral osteotomy cut is made from the mid-line to the alveolar process. This is the challenging component of the procedure as part of the osteotomy cut is not performed under direct vision. A midline palatal incision can be made for access to bone in the midline (Figure 38-7b). Osteotomes are used to complete the osteotomy and to mobilise. Palatal and labial/nasal bone removal is performed depending on the movements required to accommodate superior or posterior repositioning of the segment. In the midline a buccal mucosal incision in the region of the anterior nasal spine is undertaken to expose this area and to separate the nasal septum from the anterior maxillary segment with a guarded nasal osteotome. Once the segment or segments have been mobilized and bony interferences removed, the segments are fitted into the occlusal splint and mini-plates and screws applied for fixation above the level of the apices of the teeth.

Wunderer technique

The buccal incisions for this technique are similar to those described for the Wassmund procedure and a bone osteotomy cut is made from the nasal sill or aperture to the alveolar crest. If the extraction of a premolar is required this is performed. On the palatal aspect an anterior curved full thickness incision is made and the palatal flap is elevated posteriorly to expose the region. Using a burr or reciprocating saw an osteotomy cut is made under direct vision from one side of the alveolus to the contralateral side (Figure 38-8). Osteotomes are used to mobilize the segment

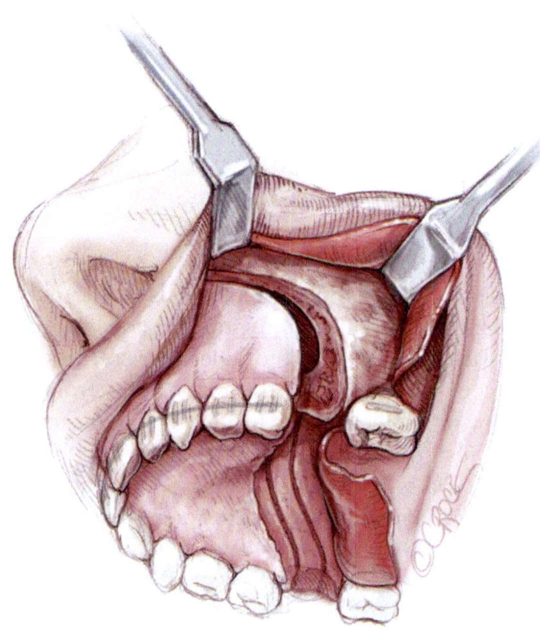

Fig. 38-8 Palatal incision with elevation of palatal flap to expose palatal bone for osteotomy and removal of segment of bone.

which can then be rotated superiorly and the nasal septum separated from the segment. Bone removal is undertaken in the required areas to facilitate the planned movement of the anterior maxillary segment. If a midline osteotomy of the anterior segment is required this is performed and then the maxillary segments placed in the surgical splint or occlusal wafer, and internal fixation placed. The intermaxillary fixation is released, the occlusion checked and the wounds closed with resorbable sutures.

Posterior maxillary segmental osteotomy

Following infiltration of local anaesthetic, a vestibular incision is made and the mucoperiosteum is reflected

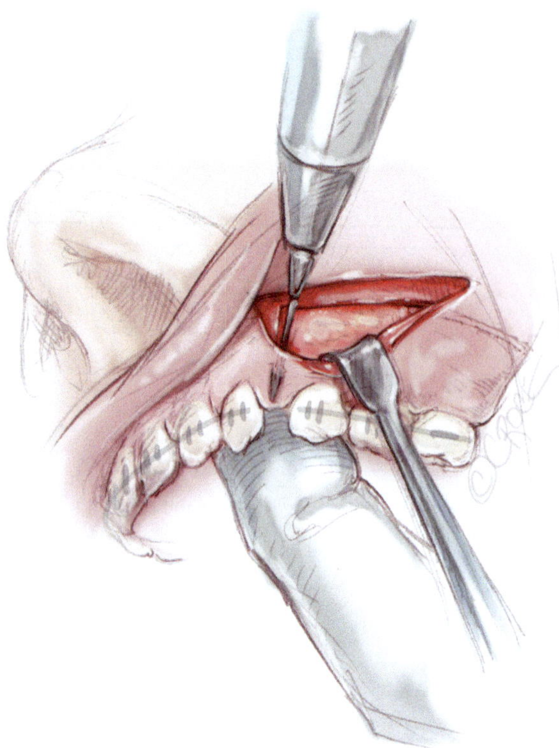

Fig. 38-9 Exposure of posterior maxillary region with vertical and horizontal buccal osteotomy cuts.

to expose the anterior and lateral walls of the maxilla, and zygomatic buttress region. A periosteal elevator is then carefully used to reflect the soft tissues inferiorly in the region of the planned interdental osteotomy or in the site of the tooth that is to be removed just prior to the extraction being undertaken. Using a burr or reciprocating saw, a horizontal osteotomy is made above the segment that is to be mobilized and the vertical osteotomy is made interdentally or through the extraction site (Figure 38-9). A curved osteotome is then used to separate the segment posteriorly through the tuberosity or pterygomaxillary regions and is also introduced via the horizontal osteotomy, to separate the hard palate. If the segment is unable to be adequately mobilized with osteotomes, a midline palatal mucosal incision may be required to expose the palatal bone to complete the division under direct vision or to perform bone removal that is required for repositioning of the posterior segment. Bone removal is performed anterior or superiorly to facilitate the planned movement and the segment is positioned into the occlusal splint/surgical wafer with intermaxillary fixation. Miniplates and screws are used to stabilize the segment, the intermaxillary fixation is then released to check the occlusion and the vestibular wound is then closed with resorbable sutures.

Case report

A 23-year-old female presented with maxillary protrusion and vertical maxillary excess with a Class II malocclusion. She had lip incompetence at rest with an acute nasolabial angle. She underwent presurgical orthodontic alignment for 11 months, and her preoperative facial and occlusal views confirm the degree of the discrepancy (Figure 38-10a–c, and Figure 38-11). She underwent a maxillary Le Fort I osteotomy with a large impaction and premaxillary set-back. The first premolars were removed bilaterally and she underwent a set-back of the segment to address the marked maxillary protrusion. A mandibular advancement and genioplasty was performed for facial balance. The postoperative images are taken at 12 months following her orthognathic surgery and debonding of her fixed appliances, with fixed lingual and palatal retainers (Figure 38-12a–c, and Figure 38-13).

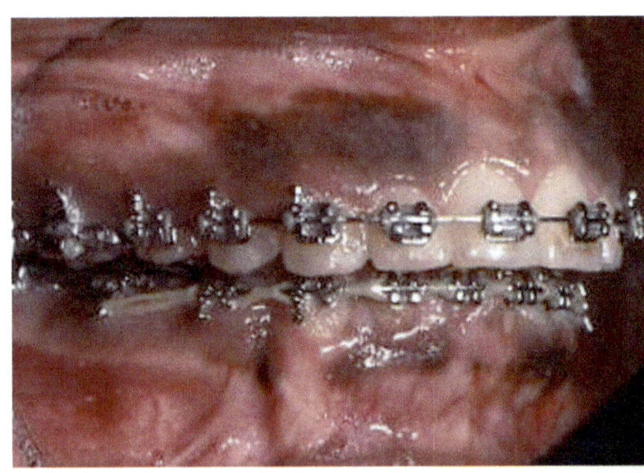

Fig. 38-11 Preoperative occlusal view.

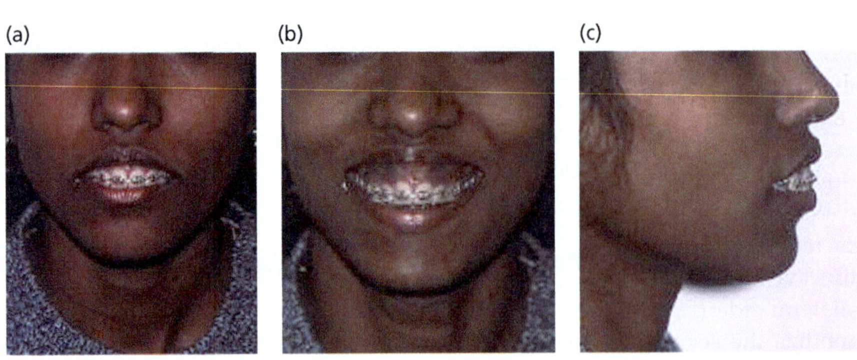

Fig. 38-10 (a) Preoperative frontal facial view at rest showing vertical maxillary excess (b) Preoperative frontal facial view on smiling. (c) Preoperative lateral facial view showing maxillary protrusion and acute nasolabial angle.

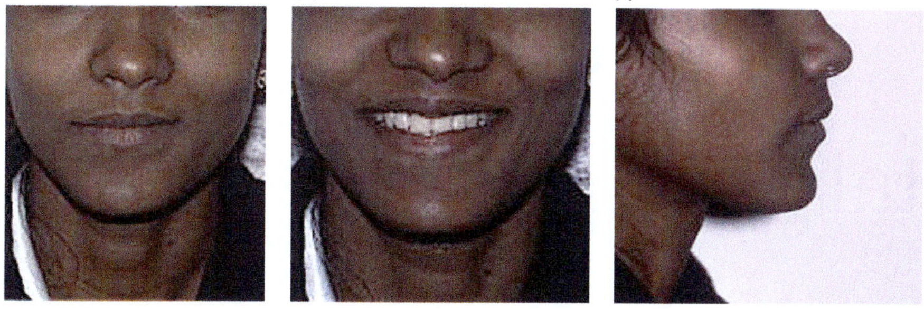

Fig. 38-12 (a) Frontal view at rest, 1-year post-surgery. (b) Frontal view on smiling, 1-year post-surgery. (c) Lateral facial view demonstrating improved facial balance with lip competence.

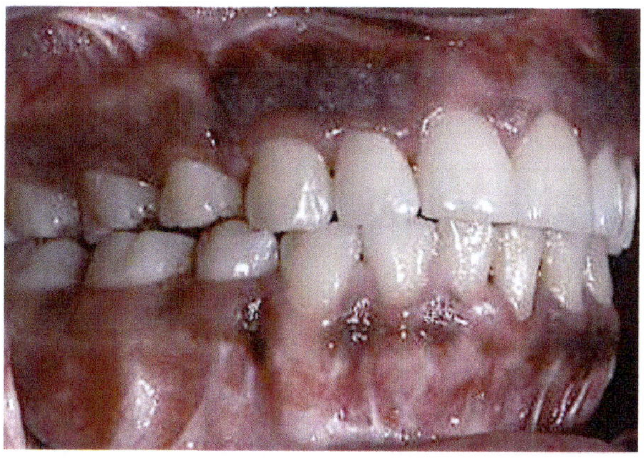

Fig. 38-13 Postoperative occlusal view following debond of orthodontic appliances.

Acknowledgment

We would like to acknowledge and thank Beth Croce, medical illustrator (© Beth Coce, Bioperspective.com).

References

1 Cohn-Stock G. Die Chirurgische-Immediatre-Julierung der Kiefer speziell die Chirurgische Behandlung der Prognathie. Vjischer Zahnheilk, Berlin. 1921;37:320.
2 Wassmund M. Frakturen und Luxationen des Gesichtsschadels. Berlin, 1927.
3 Wassmund M. From: Lehrbuch der Praktische Chiurgie des Mundes und der Kiefer 1939 Joh Ambrosius Barth, Leipzig 1926;1:277.
4 Axhausen G. Zur Bedandlung veralteter disloziert geheitter Oberkieferbruche, Dstch Zahn Mund Kieferheilk. 1937;1:334–9.
5 Schuchardt K. Chirurgie fur offense Bisses. In Bier A, Braun A, Kummel H (editors) Chirurgische Operationslehre. Leipzig: Aufl band 1954;7:2.
6 Schuchardt K. Experiences with the surgical treatment of deformities of the jaws: prognathia, micrognathia and openbite. In Wallace AG (Ed.), Second Congress of International Society of Plastic Surgeons, Livingstone, London 1959.
7 Wunderer S. Die prognathie operation mittels frontal gestiltem maxilla fragment. Osterreich Zeitschr Stomatol. 1962;59:98–102.
8 Obwegeser H. Surgical correction of small or retrodisplaced maxillae. Plast Reconstruct Surg. 1969;44:351–65.
9 Bell WH. Revascularisation and bone healing after anterior maxillary osteotomy: a study using adult rhesus monkeys. J Oral Surg. 1969;27:249–55.
10 Bell WH, Fonseca RJ, Kennedy JW, et al. Bone healing and revascularization after total maxillary osteotomy. J Oral Surg. 1975;33:253–60.
11 Bell WH. Le Forte I osteotomy for correction of maxillary deformity. J Oral Surg. 1975;33:412–26.
12 Kufner J. Experience with a modified procedure for correction of open bite. In: Walker RV (Ed.). Transactions of the Third International Congress on Oral Surgery. E & S Livingstone, London. 1970;18:18–23.
13 West RA, Epker BN. Posterior maxillary surgery: its place in the treatment of dentofacial deformities. J Oral Surg. 1972;30:562–731.
14 Dorfman H, Turvey TA. Alterations in osseous crestal height following interdental osteotomies. Oral Surg. 1979;48:120–5.

Chapter 39

Total Subapical Mandibular Osteotomy

Jonathan Sandler, Alison Murray and Peter Doyle

Introduction

In adult patients the vast majority of significant Class II division 1 malocclusions, requesting full correction, are dealt with using a combination of orthodontics and orthognathic surgery.

The most common form of mandibular surgery performed for mandibular advancement is a bilateral sagittal split osteotomy, which was first described in 1957 (see Chapters 1 and 2).[1] This operation is entirely appropriate for the vast majority of Class II division 1 malocclusions on a Class II skeletal base which almost always has some degree of mandibular retrognathia. This procedure may be combined with a Le Fort I osteotomy if there is an associated vertical discrepancy between the jaws.

A small number of patients however, whilst having a large sagittal discrepancy between the upper and lower dental arches, occasionally have a soft tissue and sometimes hard tissue pogonion which is often more or less in the correct position. If, in these cases, a mandibular advancement osteotomy is carried out using the sagittal split technique the requisite advancement of the lower dentoalveolar portion to correct the incisor overjet would result in a chin that was far too prominent producing an aesthetically unacceptable result.

Of course this chin prominence can be dealt with by performing a reduction genioplasty, but this procedure is not without its drawbacks. The exact final position of the chin is unpredictable and excessive mobility of the soft tissue chin button can sometimes be seen.

An alternative procedure, to which due consideration should be given, to fully correct these easily identifiable malocclusions, is to accept the position and shape of the mandible and advance the entire mandibular dentoalveolar process to achieve sagittal correction.

History of the technique

The total mandibular subapical osteotomy was first described in 1974 by MacIntosh (see Figure 2.27).[2] He conceded that this was an extension of previously described techniques which involved anterior mandibular osteotomies.

The initial indication for this surgical procedure suggested was infantile apertognathia,[2] i.e. an open bite from the molars forward, which develops in childhood. The second indication suggested was retreatment of previous surgical cases that have relapsed following traditional mandibular ramus osteotomy, leading to recurrence of the original malocclusion. The final indication described was condylar agenesis or hypoplasia.

The technique was described in intricate detail including an extraoral approach for the vertical osteotomies in the third molar area. A case of infantile apertognathia was illustrated showing an impressive closure of an anterior open bite. Two other

Orthognathic Surgery: Principles, Planning and Practice. Edited by Farhad B. Naini and Daljit S. Gill.

cases were described and illustrated in detail and the author admitted that he had only carried out seven cases of this procedure in total.

Treatment of a Class II division 2 case with already excessive chin development, then followed.[5] The author felt a traditional forward mandibular advancement would result in a markedly unaesthetic chin projection, as it was only really the dentition that required advancement. After 3.5 hours of surgery a dramatic occlusal and facial improvement was achieved, including a marked reduction in the previously deep labiomental fold.

From the very first reports it was noted that trauma to the inferior alveolar neurovascular bundle was a significant potential hazard and advice was given to take particular care of this anatomical area.

Another description appeared of a case involving orthodontic surgical correction of a Class II division 2 malocclusion in which a 4 mm mandibular advancement using bilateral sagittal split osteotomy was also supplemented with a 4 mm total subapical advancement, to reduce the total chin projection by 4 mm and maximize the profile improvement.[6] Possible adverse outcomes were listed by the authors as devitalisation of teeth, as well as significant nerve damage. The authors felt that the lack of evidence on the safety of the technique limits its use to cases where alternative surgical options are considered aesthetically undesirable or unpredictable.

A beautifully treated case was documented where piezosurgery and CADCAM manufactured splints enabled a total subapical osteotomy to provide the perfect solution for management of a patient with Parry–Romberg syndrome.[7] Drawbacks of the procedure were emphasized by the authors including that it was technically laborious and extremely time-consuming. Piezosurgery was thought to minimize the risks as it had been previously demonstrated that peripheral nerves exposed to direct contact with piezosurgery were not transected.

Indications for total mandibular subapical osteotomies have been described as:[8] mandibular dentoalveolar hypoplasia with good projection of the chin, vertical mandibular alveolar deficiency, lateral open bite deformity, condylar agenesis and hypoplasia, infantile open bite and correction of relapse after previous ramus osteotomies.

These authors suggested a modification of technique: to firstly carry out a sagittal split osteotomy purely to expose the nerve from lingula to within 2 cm of the mental foramen. The final 2 cm is decorticated using parallel cuts over the nerve bundle, which because of the previous sagittal split, can be directly visualized. They found this greatly simplified what can be a very time consuming, laborious technique. The ramus is then plated in its presurgical position, the actual dental advancement being performed only on the mobilized dentoalveolar segment.

The first two total subapical cases that were performed at Chesterfield Royal Hospital have been described.[9] Both were significant sagittal discrepancy Class II division 1 incisor relationships with retrognathic mandibles, but with pretreatment chin positions that would not have benefitted aesthetically from any forward movement. In both cases the 8–10 mm sagittal discrepancy was corrected by advancing the entire dentoalveolar segment. In both cases an excellent functional occlusal result complemented the greatly improved aesthetics.

Case 1

This 17-year-old female patient presented with a Class II division 1 incisal relationship on a Class II skeletal base with an overjet of 11 mm, and a full unit Class II relationship of her molars and canines (Figure 39-1a–c).

Both her upper and lower lips were 2 mm behind the E-line and her nasolabial angle was 122 degrees. Her chin was in a good position and when asked to protrude her lower jaw to simulate the effect of surgery there was significant aesthetic decline.

Her impacted but partially erupted mandibular third molar teeth were removed and preoperative orthodontics was carried out over a 16-month period. A total subapical osteotomy was carried out and her mandibular dentoalveolar fragment was advanced to fully correct the sagittal discrepancy (Figure 39-2a,b).

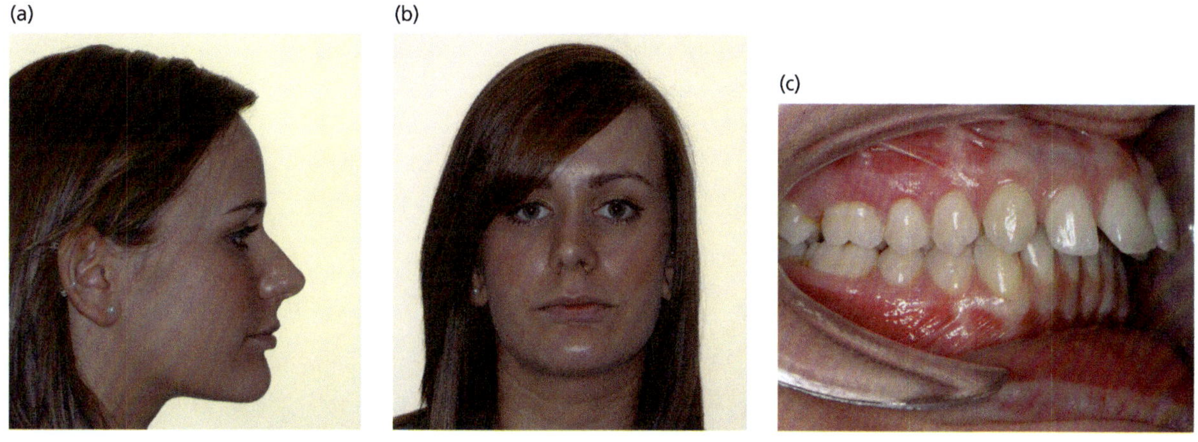

Fig. 39-1 (a–c) Pretreatment images.

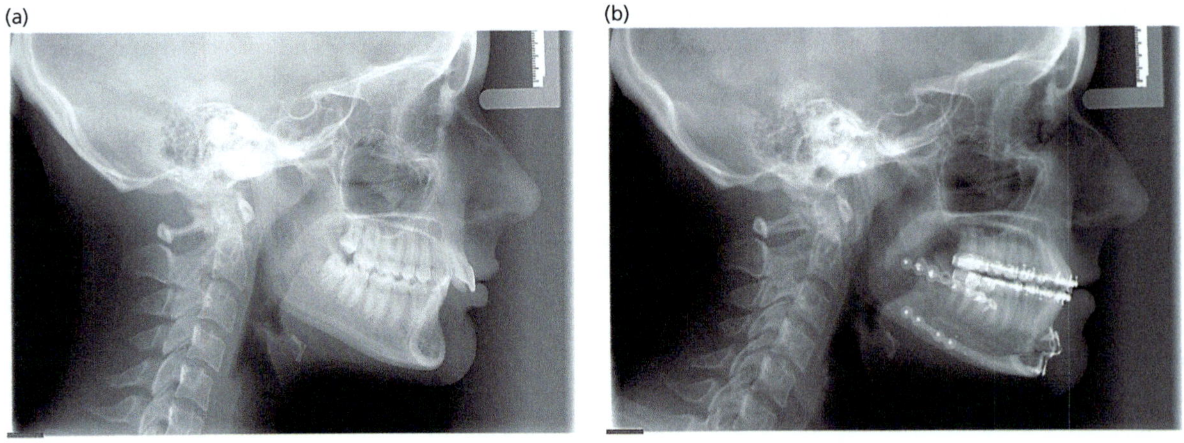

Fig. 39-2 (a) Pretreatment lateral cephalometric radiograph. (b) End of treatment lateral cephalometric radiograph.

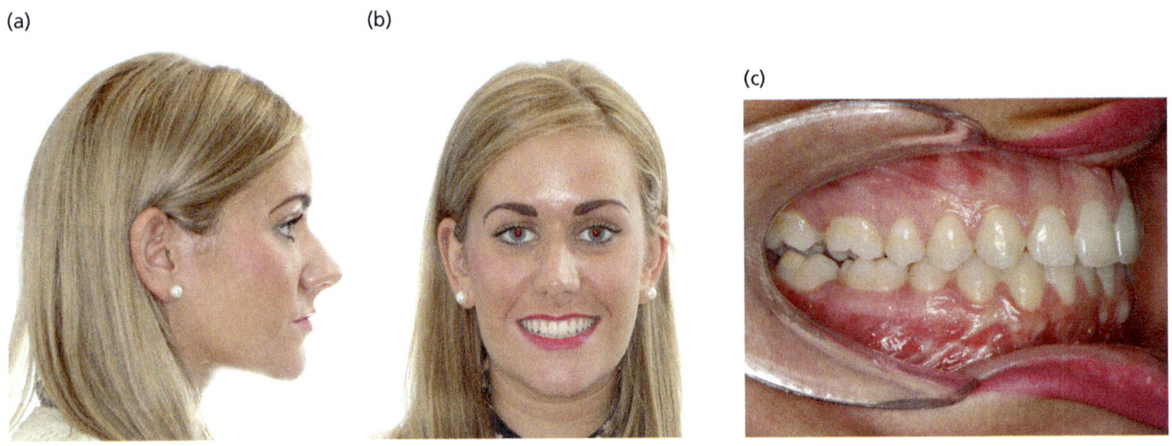

Fig. 39-3 (a–c) end of treatment images.

Postoperative orthodontics took a further 6 months. A satisfactory functional occlusion resulted and the PAR score reduced from 47 to 14 representing a 70.2% improvement. The patient was absolutely delighted with her aesthetic improvement (Figure 39-3a–c).

Case 2

This 30-year-old lady presented with a Class II division 1 incisor relationship on a Class II skeletal base with a retrognathic mandible and maxilla, a 6-degree ANB angle, and overjet of 9 mm, and a full unit Class II relationship of her molars and canines (Figure 39-4a–c). She had previously lost four premolars, but this was not followed up with a course of orthodontic treatment. Her upper lip was well behind the E-line and her nasolabial angle was already 132 degrees. Her lower incisors were already proclined at 100 degrees and she already had a prominent chin.

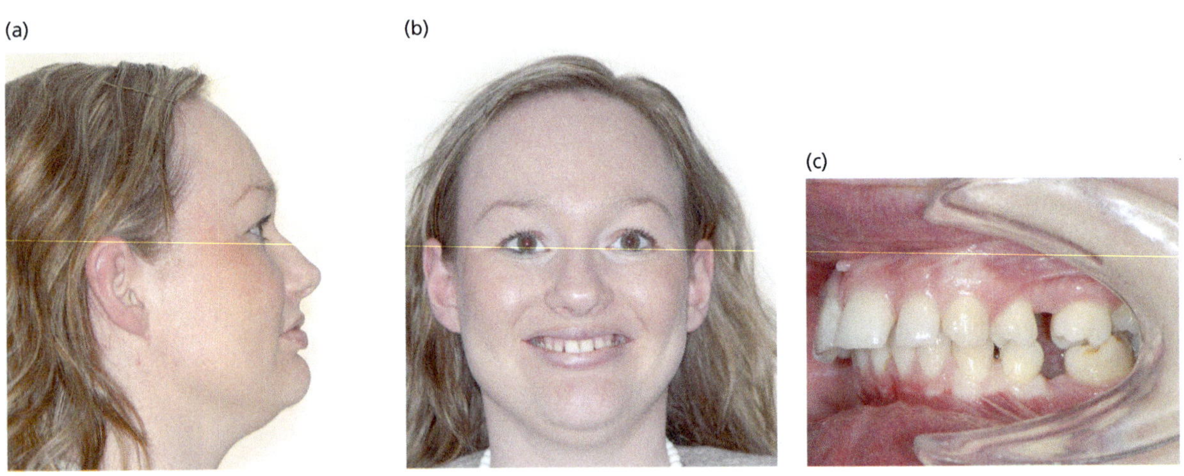

Fig. 39-4 (a–c) Pretreatment images.

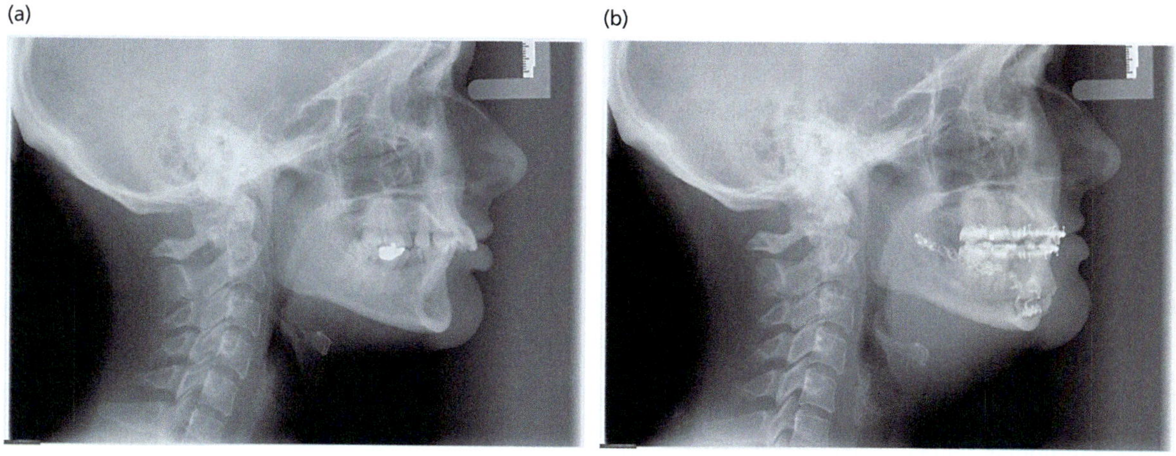

Fig. 39-5 (a) Pretreatment lateral cephalometric radiograph. (b) End of treatment lateral cephalometric radiograph.

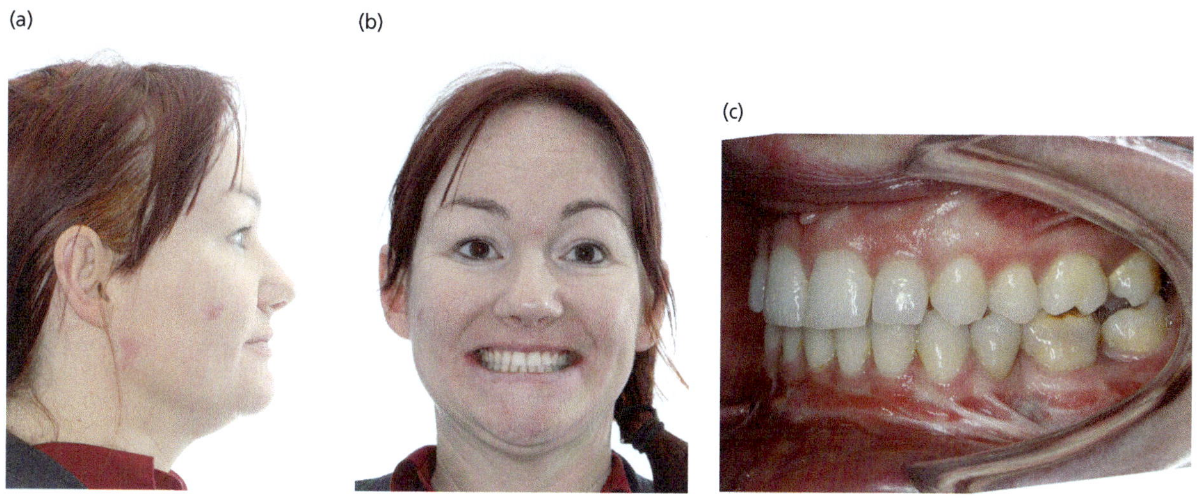

Fig. 39-6 (a–c) End of treatment images.

Retraction of the maxillary incisors was not thought to be wise, due to the already retrusive upper lip and obtuse nasolabial angle. Advancement of the mandible was also not considered advisable due to the detrimental effect on the chin protrusion. The only possibility to markedly improve aesthetics was therefore to maximize the overjet whilst achieving space closure, then to arrange a total subapical mandibular advancement osteotomy (Figure 39-5a,b).

The preoperative orthodontics took 24 months and the postoperative orthodontics a further 5 months. The objective assessment of treatment revealed a PAR score reduction from 46 to 4 which represents a 91% reduction. The patient was delighted with the achieved occlusal and aesthetic result (Figure 39-6a–c).

Discussion

From the literature we can see that the total subapical osteotomy has been successfully used in Class II division 2 cases,[5,6] and in anterior open bite cases.[2,10] We have been involved in four successfully treated Class II division 1 cases, and various other more severe craniofacial malformations have been dealt with using this technique.

All authors stress the time consuming nature of the surgery which runs the risk of nerve damage, devitalization of the teeth following interruption of their blood supply and potentially total loss of the dentoalveolar segment, although this has to date not been reported in the literature. Modifications to the surgical technique have been suggested to increase visualization of the inferior dental nerve, to ultimately reduce morbidity.

Pitched against this is the reduced morbidity during the postoperative period due to the fact that the lower border of the mandible is left intact and the muscle attachments to the mandible are largely left intact. Swelling is significantly less than with a bilateral sagittal split osteotomy, and the patients are more comfortable postoperatively and can open and close their mouths almost as normal.

Stability of the procedure was investigated in a large study involving 40 Class II division 1 patients.[11] These were divided into a group (20) having a standard bilateral sagittal split mandibular advancement and a second group (20) who had a total subapical dentoalveolar osteotomy. The same surgeon and orthodontist provided the clinical treatment for all 40 patients and the selection of the surgical procedure was based on the clinical diagnosis made by the orthodontist, which will inevitably have introduced a selection bias into the proceedings. Both of the surgical procedures yielded stable long-term results so if a profound change in the labiomental fold is one of the major aims of treatment, the authors recommend the total subapical procedure.

Conclusions

This alternative approach to correcting a severe sagittal mandibular dentoalveolar discrepancy would appear to be an excellent and stable solution for a small group of Class II cases where the chin at the start of treatment is in no way deficient. The procedure is initially technically challenging, and will take significantly longer to perform than a more conventional approach. Whilst it should certainly not be attempted by inexperienced surgeons, with practice the technique should become less arduous and time consuming. The patients will certainly benefit from the reduced discomfort and increased mobility following the surgery, and the undeniable aesthetic benefit that accompanies this approach.

References

1 Trauner R, Obwegeser H. Surgical correction of mandibular prognathism and retrognathia with consideration of genioplasty. 1. Surgical procedures to correct mandibular prognathism and reshaping of the chin. Oral Surg Oral Med Oral Pathol. 1957;10:677–89.

2 MacIntosh RB. Total mandibular alveolar osteotomy: encouraging experiences with an infrequently indicated procedure. J Maxillofac Surg. 1974;2:210–18.

3 Hofer O. Operation der prognathie und mikrogenie. Deutsche Zahn Mund Kiefer. 1942;9:121.

4 Köle H. Surgical operations on the alveolar ridge to correct occlusal deformities. Oral Surg Oral Med Oral Pathol. 1959;12:277–88.

5 Murray RB. Mandibular sagittal subapical osteotomy: A case study. Am J Orthod. 1980;77:469–85.

6 Eliadis T, Hegdvedt AK. Orthodontic-surgical correction of a Class II, division 2 malocclusion. Am J Orthod Dentofacial Orthop. 1996;110:351–7.

7 Scolozzi P, Herzog G. Total mandibular subapical osteotomy and Le Fort I osteotomy using piezosurgery and computer-aided designed and manufactured surgical splints: a favorable combination of three techniques in the management of severe mouth asymmetry in Parry–Romberg syndrome. J Oral Maxillofac Surg. 2014;72:991–9.

8 Mohammed-Ali R, Schache A, Walsh S, Sneddon K. Total mandibular subapical osteotomy: modification of the technique. Br J Oral Maxillofac Surg. 2009;47:629–30.

9 Boye T, Doyle P, McKeown F, Sandler J. Total subapical mandibular osteotomy to correct class 2 division 1 dentofacial deformity. J Cranio-Maxillofac Surg. 2012;40:238–42.

10 Pangrazio-Kulbersch V, MacIntosh RB. Total mandibular alveolar osteotomy: An alternative choice to other surgical procedures. Am J Orthod. 1985;87:319–37.

11 Pangrazio-Kulbersch V, Berger JL, Kaczynski R, Shunock M. Stability of skeletal Class II correction with two surgical techniques: the sagittal split ramus osteotomy and the total mandibular subapical alveolar osteotomy. Am J Orthod Dentofacial Orthop. 2001;120:134–43.

Chapter 40

Endoscopy in Maxillary and Mandibular Orthognathic Surgery

Katherine P. Klein, Natalie N. Tung and Maria J. Troulis

Introduction

Recognized patient-centred benefits and healthcare cost-savings have fueled the trend towards making surgical techniques as minimally invasive as possible.[1–3] Patient interest and demand for 'state of the art medical care' is reflected by the frequent popular news articles discussing 'new and improved' minimally invasive surgical techniques to replace traditionally larger procedures. Minimally invasive surgery has significant benefits, and interest in this field continues to grow.

Goals of minimally invasive surgery include less trauma to the soft and hard tissues, and therefore, faster patient recovery. With endoscopy, direct visual access, along with the capability for illumination and magnification, allows for minimal tissue dissection and an improved surgical field.[3] Decreased manipulation of soft and hard tissues minimizes the risk of extensive bleeding and swelling, and lessens postoperative morbidity for the patient, resulting in less patient pain, shorter hospital stay, and earlier return to work.[1–3]

Surgeons have increasingly used the endoscope to achieve the goals of minimally invasive surgery.[1] Modern endoscopy for use in general surgical procedures dates back to the early 1800s, and Takagi has been credited with performing the first endoscopic surgery in 1918.[4] Since this time, innovations across multiple surgical specialties (particularly gynaecology, urology and otolaryngology) have contributed to advances in both endoscopic instrumentation and its surgical application and techniques.[5] Evolving technology, increasing patient demands for minimal surgical procedures and 'state-of-the-art-medical-care,' has firmly established endoscopy as an essential tool in the armamentarium of many surgical specialists.[1–5]

Compared to other fields, the use of endoscopic techniques for exposure and reconstruction of the craniomaxillofacial skeleton is a relatively recent development.[1–3,6] Maxillofacial surgery procedures where endoscopic techniques are currently used include: the treatment of craniomaxillofacial trauma (specifically for subcondylar fracture repair,[7] and orbital floor reconstruction[8,9]), obstructive salivary gland disease,[10] orthognathic deformities,[1–3,5] maxillary sinus disorders,[5] trigeminal nerve injury,[5] facial rejuvenation and face lifts,[11] and temporomandibular joint (TMJ) disorders.[4,5]

In this chapter, endoscopic (minimally invasive surgery) orthognathic procedures are described. Additionally, principles of orthodontic tooth preparation for endoscopic orthognathic surgery, and future directions of endoscopic surgery will be discussed.

Orthognathic Surgery: Principles, Planning and Practice. Edited by Farhad B. Naini and Daljit S. Gill.

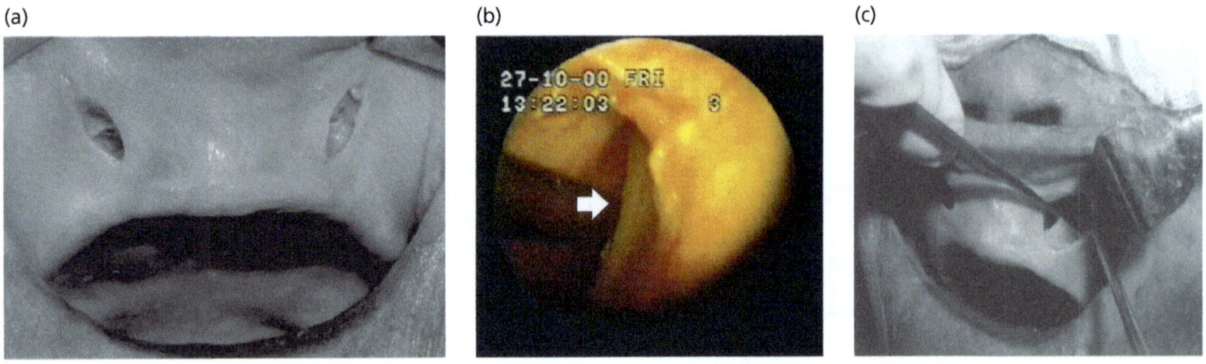

Fig. 40-1 Endoscopic-assisted Le Fort I osteotomy via limited incisions. (a) bilateral vertical incisions in the anterior region; (b) endoscopic view of lateral buttress dissection; (c) downfracture of maxilla. (Reprinted with permission from Rohner D, Yeow V, Hammer B. Endoscopically assisted Le Fort I osteotomy. J Cranio-Maxillofac Surg. 2001;29:360–65.[12])

Maxillary orthognathic surgery

For orthognathic surgery, endoscopy has been included in mandibular procedures, but few in the maxilla. In fact, few studies have described endoscopy for Le Fort I osteotomy, one of the most common orthognathic surgical procedures used to correct dentofacial deformities. The Le Fort I osteotomy is used to correct maxillary sagittal, transverse, and vertical discrepancies. This has traditionally been performed using a horizontal gingivobuccal sulcus incision with osteotomies at the lateral nasal wall, maxillary walls, and pterygomaxillary junction. Rohner et al. in 2001 described their new technique of the Le Fort I osteotomy using endoscopic techniques through limited vertical incisions[12] (Figure 40-1). Their technique was first performed successfully on six cadavers and then applied clinically to two patients. In order to preserve the labio-buccal mucosa, they used four vertical vestibular incisions, paranasally and posteriorly. They then used a Storz rigid 2.7 mm diameter, 30-degree angle endoscope to assist in direct visualization of the maxillary osteotomies as well as rigid fixation of the segments with titanium miniplates. After downfracture of the maxilla, the scope was inserted into the osteotomy gap and confirmed that the descending palatine arteries were intact. A major advantage of the endoscopic technique is the visualization of the separation of the pterygomaxillary junction, which is often done in a blind fashion.[12] Overall, this technique allowed for preservation of the descending palatine artery, decreased bleeding, and reduced postoperative oedema.[12] Comparatively, the total operative time was about 30 minutes longer than the traditional open technique.

In a separate report, Wiltfang and Kessler in 2002 similarly performed an endoscopically-assisted Le Fort I osteotomy in four human cadavers followed by application in three patients to correct maxillary transverse and sagittal discrepancies.[13] Access to the maxilla was obtained via a small, vertical vestibular incision to create a visualization port to the maxillary sinus through a bur hole. This allowed for endoscopic exposure of the maxillary sinus from within the sinus and accurate identification of landmarks. In two patients the maxilla was split sagittally for transverse maxillary expansion and, in the other patient, a buried distractor was placed to correct sagittal hypoplasia, eliminating the need for downfracture of the maxilla.

With similar rationale for minimizing bleeding, infection, and other complications, Taylor et al. in 2009 described their own endoscopically-assisted Le Fort I osteotomy using an ultrasonic scalpel in four human cadavers.[14] They utilized two small, 1-cm vertical gingivobuccal sulcus incisions to access the maxilla and carried out their osteotomies with an ultrasonic scalpel from within the maxillary sinus under direct visualization with an endoscope. This preserved the periosteal sleeve to the maxilla and therefore, its vascularity. They concluded that the advantages to the technique of endoscopically-assisted Le Fort I osteotomy using an ultrasonic scalpel include: (1) improved visualization facilitating better accuracy of the osteotomy and reducing trauma to the surrounding structures; (2) minimal disruption of the blood supply to the maxilla, including the periosteum and mucosa in addition to the named vessels; (3) decreased blood loss with the ultrasonic scalpel; and (4) reduced postoperative oedema, pain, and infection by limiting the amount of maxillary degloving via small incisions.

The other advantage of endoscopy, as noted by Pedroletti et al. in their review of endoscopic techniques in oral and maxillofacial surgery, is its use as an aid in teaching the procedure, posterior anatomy, and avoiding complications for trainees.[5] Additionally, operating theatre staff can visualize the various points of the procedure on the screen.

Mandibular orthognathic surgery

Unlike the limited use of endoscopy for maxillary procedures, its use in the mandible has been more extensive, including its use in open reduction and internal fixation of mandibular fractures as well as in mandibular orthognathic surgical procedures.[1,5,7,15]

One of the most common mandibular procedures, the sagittal split osteotomy, is often used to advance, set-back, or rotate the mandible to treat sagittal hypoplasia, mandibular prognathism, or mandibular asymmetry, respectively. Potential complications associated with this procedure include unfavorable fractures if the medial osteotomy is inadequate, leaving the inferior alveolar nerve in the proximal segment, or if the inferior border osteotomy is insufficient, resulting in a buccal plate fracture.[16,17] The horizontal medial osteotomy should be located just superior to the lingula and terminated just posterior to the lingula, carried through only the lingual cortex of the mandibular ramus. Kim and McCain in 2008 described the endoscope use in visualizing the lingula to facilitate soft tissue and inferior alveolar nerve protection as well as appropriate angulation of the medial osteotomy.[18] They further used the endoscope to verify the inferior border osteotomy to prevent an unfavourable fracture of the buccal plate.

The vertical ramus osteotomy (VRO) has traditionally been used for mandibular set-back to correct sagittal hyperplasia or prognathism. Complications of this technique include inferior alveolar nerve damage as it enters the mandible if the osteotomy is done too far anteriorly; bleeding from transection of the inferior alveolar, masseteric, or maxillary arteries; and unfavorable osteotomies if the osteotomy is placed too far posteriorly.[1–3] The use of the endoscope for improved visualization can mitigate these potential complications. The VRO can be performed via an extraoral or intraoral approach (IVRO). The IVRO offers the distinct advantage of decreased risk of inferior alveolar nerve paraesthesia, but rigid fixation is not possible, requiring the patient to be placed into maxillomandibular fixation (MMF).[3]

Robiony et al. reported in 2007 their use of an endoscope in intraoral vertical ramus osteotomy (IVRO) in conjunction with surgery.[19] After an intraoral incision is made at the level of the lower third of the anterior border of the ramus, to the area of the second molar along the external oblique ridge, a subperiosteal elevation and exposure of the lateral aspect of the mandibular ramus is completed, from the inferior border to the sigmoid notch. Then direct visualization is gained using a 45-degree Hopkins endoscope to help identify mandibular ramus landmarks and estimate the position of the mandibular foramen. The osteotomy is then completed under endoscopic visualization using the piezoelectric drill.

At our institution, the clinical results, first reported in 2001, of endoscopically-assisted extraoral vertical ramus osteotomy (EVRO) have been favourable, as published in a retrospective study by Troulis and Kaban in 2004, which included 13 patients and 23 sides.[3] In all cases, the procedure was performed via a 1.5 cm submandibular incision (Figure 40-2). The mean operating time was 37 minutes per side. The distinct advantages of the EVRO consist of: (1) mandibular set-back with rigid fixation and no MMF; (2) set-back and rigid fixation leaving in place asymptomatic third molars that are intimately involved with the inferior alveolar nerve; (3) direct visualization as the osteotomy is performed, which is beneficial in teaching institutions; and (4) less oedema compared to IVRO (from preliminary results in an animal model).[3] To date, 53 patients at our institution have been successfully treated with EVRO and rigid fixation to correct mandibular prognathism,[20] (Figure 40-3). Complication rates were very low. The hospital stay was less than 1 day for 30 of the patients and 2 days for two patients.[21]

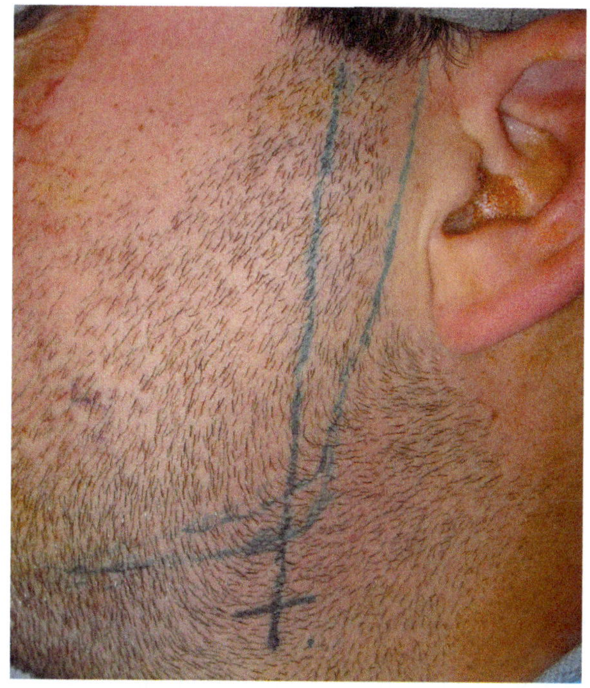

Fig. 40-2 Mandibular landmarks and 1.5-cm submandibular incision marked in malachite green.

Another use of minimally invasive surgery is in condylectomy and costochondral graft ramus-condyle unit (RCU) reconstruction for correction of condylar resorption. This condition has been reported in patients with history of trauma, rheumatoid arthritis, systemic lupus erythematosus, steroid use, and neoplasia.[22] When there is no identifiable aetiology, the condition is described as idiopathic condylar resorption, which can cause decreased posterior face height, retrognathism, and progressive anterior open bite with clockwise rotation of the mandible.[22] The traditional condylectomy and costochondral graft (CCG) RCU reconstruction consists of preauricular and submandibular incisions. With the use of an endoscope, minimally invasive access to the RCU is obtained via a 1.5 cm submandibular incision, similarly to the EVRO approach.[1,2] Specific to the condylectomy, the endoscope allows for excellent visualization of the condylar head and neck, facilitating their dissection from the adjacent soft tissues. The condylectomy is then performed from the sigmoid notch to the posterior border of the mandible. Once the CCG is harvested, the endoscope is again used to directly

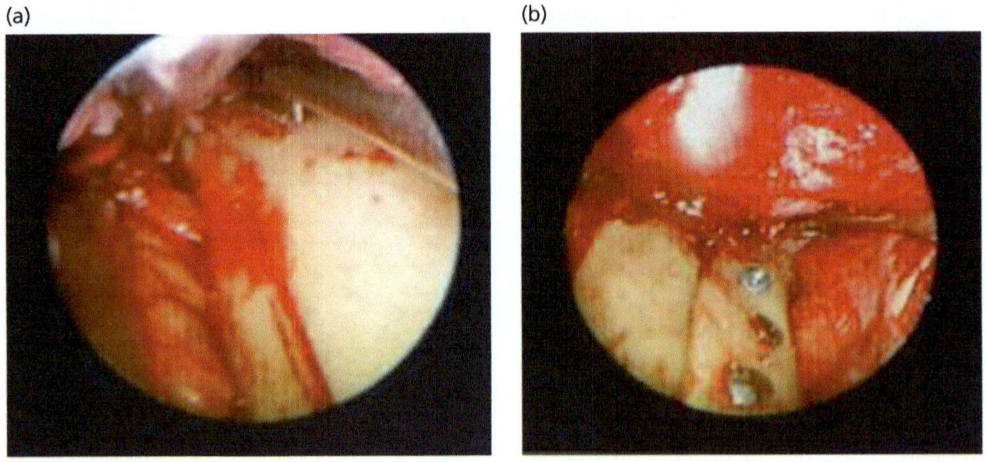

Fig. 40-3 (a) Planned osteotomy is marked using a sterile pencil. (b) Rigid fixation of the proximal and distal segments, with bony overlap seen.

visualize the articular disk and the CCG is then placed into the glenoid fossa and fixated using a titanium miniplate. The screws can be placed through the incision or via a percutaneous trocar.[1,2] In a retrospective analysis by Troulis, Williams, and Kaban in 2004, a total of 10 patients (n = 17 sides) underwent successful endoscopic condylectomy and costochondral graft RCU reconstruction.[23] All submandibular scars were aesthetically satisfactory and there were no marginal mandibular or inferior alveolar nerve injuries. Mean operating time was 52 minutes per side and the average length of stay for all patients was 2.5 days. To date, a total of 30 patients have had this procedure for treatment of idiopathic condylar resorption or degenerative joint disease, with no long-term sequelae and excellent range of motion at long-term follow-up[20] (Figures 40-4 and 40-5).

Finally, the endoscopic high condylectomy with vertical ramus osteotomy can be used to treat mandibular asymmetry associated with condylar hyperplasia, the most common acquired deformity of the condyle. Patients are usually born with a symmetrical jaw and the onset of pubertal growth then triggers the asymmetry in the mandible due to the abnormal growth centre in the condyle.[22] There are two growth patterns, vertical (with ipsilateral open bite) and rotational (with chin point deviation). The standard high condylectomy treatment for this condition involves a preauricular incision with excision of the hyperplastic condylar region, leaving the normal condylar stump in place. On the other hand, with an endoscopically-assisted high condylectomy with VRO, a small 1.5 cm submandibular incision as above is made, followed by VRO and removal of the entire proximal segment. To date, seven patients have undergone this growth-arresting procedure.[20]

Endoscopic orthognathic surgery for the orthodontist

Similar to traditional orthognathic surgical procedures, endoscopic orthognathic techniques require teeth to be coordinated in three planes of space presurgically to optimize the treatment result. The minimally invasive technique neither reduces the need for presurgical orthodontic preparation, nor necessitates more presurgical orthodontic preparation.

Orthognathic surgery cannot be executed effectively without proper presurgical tooth preparation.[24–30] When teeth are positioned in their optimal decompensated position, ideal skeletal and occlusal goals can be met during surgery. While some clinicians endorse the 'surgery first' technique (completing surgery prior to any orthodontic correction), there is little supporting research to substantiate this practice (other than in distraction osteogenesis cases; not discussed in this chapter). The three main reasons fixed appliances are placed prior to surgery include: (1) to presurgically decompensate teeth and coordinate the underlying dental and skeletal malocclusion; (2) stabilize the teeth and basal bone at the time of the surgery and during healing; (3) allow the necessary postsurgical tooth movement while retaining the surgical change.[24]

Goals of presurgical orthodontic treatment include: aligning teeth within each dental arch over the basal bone, positioning the incisors within the pre-planned anteroposterior and vertical positions, and coordinating the arches transversely to make them compatible. Successful achievement of these goals will highlight their underlying skeletal discrepancy.

Alignment of teeth over basal bone is the first step in presurgical orthodontic preparation. The principle of moving the teeth toward their proper (root determined) position in the arch remains true in both surgical and non-surgical patients.[24,25] With a standard edgewise appliance, the initial archwire should be round, undersized relative to the bracket slots and highly resilient. These wire properties minimize inadvertent root movement. Potts et al. evaluated orthognathic surgical patients to determine dental decompensation during presurgical orthodontic treatment. Their results found that only 56% of the upper incisors and 36% of the lower incisors were decompensated appropriately.[18] This finding is

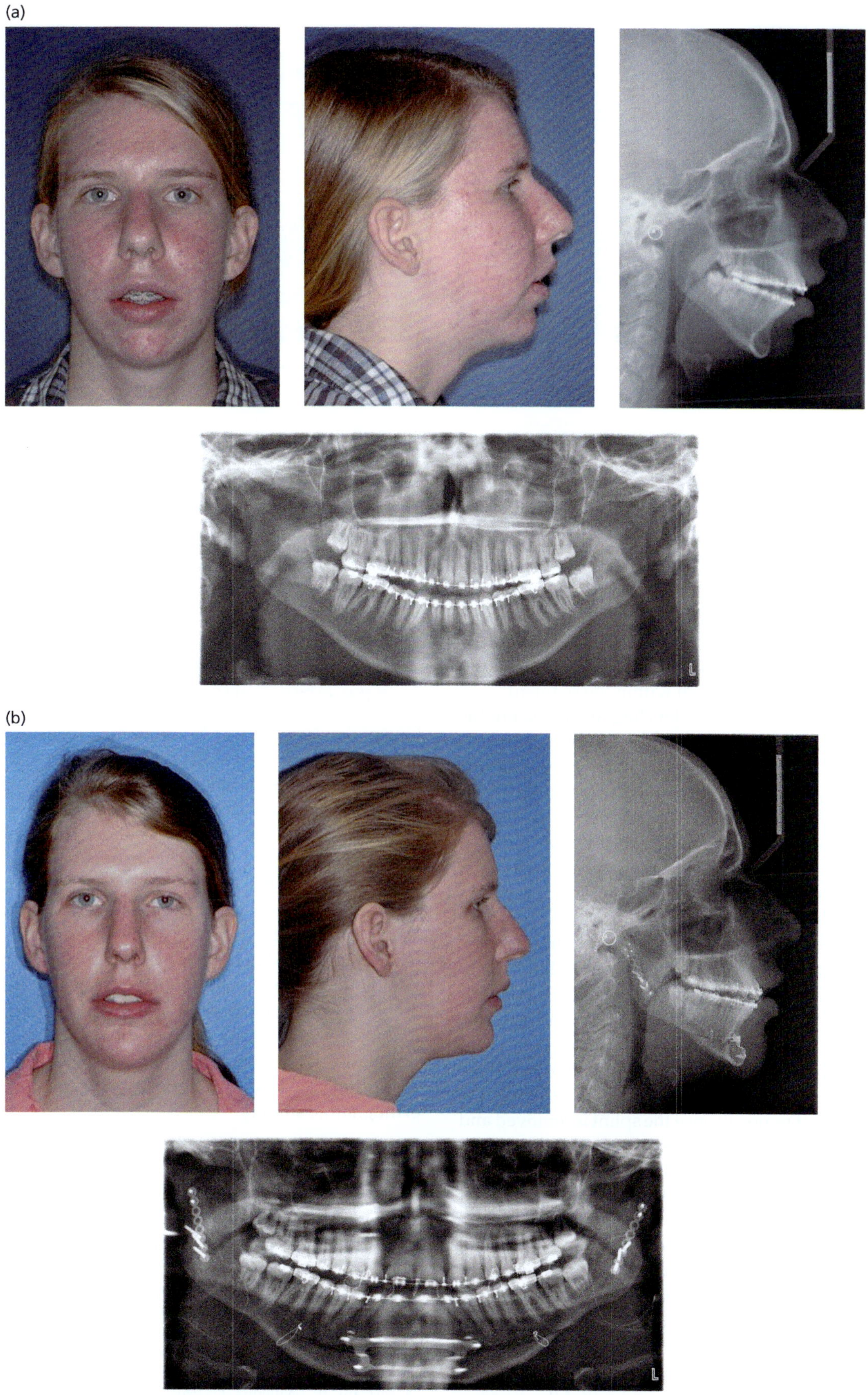

Fig. 40-4 This is a 17 year old female who initially presented with a receding chin and progressive resorption of her condyles with resulting clockwise rotation of the mandible. She was diagnosed with bilateral idiopathic condylar resorption, mandibular hypoplasia, anterior open bite, and microgenia. She underwent bilateral endoscopic condylectomies with costochondral graft for mandibular advancement and genioplasty advancement. (a) Preoperative images, lateral cephalograph and panoramic radiograph; (b) postoperative images, lateral cephalograph and panoramic radiograph.

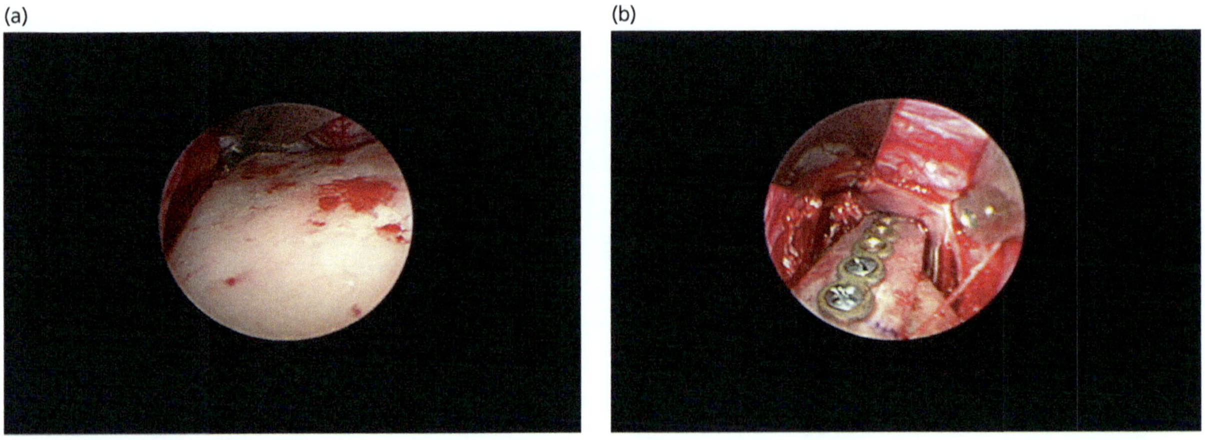

Fig. 40-5 Intraoperative endoscopic views. (a) Condylectomy; (b) Left costochondral rib graft.

particularly concerning as the relationship between surgical success and incisor decompensation has been well documented in the literature by Proffit et al., Potts et al., Burden et al. and Jang et al.[29–32]

Levelling of the maxillary arch depends on the preplanned surgical goal. If the maxilla will be moved as one piece, the maxillary teeth can be leveled as they would be in traditional non-surgical orthodontics. If segmenting the maxilla is part of the surgical plan, the teeth within each designated (intra-segment) should be aligned to the other teeth within the segment.

Presurgical mandibular leveling depends on the desired final face height. Setting the maxillary and mandibular incisors in an ideal overjet and overbite relationship can create a tripod occlusion and increase the vertical face height. After surgery, the premolars will be extruded orthodontically through a combination of archwires and elastics. This dental movement will help to maintain the increased vertical face height achieved during surgery.

The goal of post-surgical orthodontic treatment is to detail the dental occlusion. Post-surgical orthodontic treatment can begin when the surgeon is comfortable that healing has reached a stable and satisfactory point. Typically, this ranges between 3–8 weeks post-surgically. Excellent communication between the orthodontist and surgeon is needed to establish the plan for splint removal; once the splint is removed and any broken orthodontic pieces are repaired, a light and round steel wire (such as a 0.016 stainless steel archwire) can be placed. The patient will often feel that only a few teeth are touching and have a difficult time finding the best place to bite. For this reason, elastics are given immediately once the splint is removed. Elastics help to both initiate tooth movement into the ideal final occlusion, and most importantly, help to override any impulses the patient has to bite in a position that is simply 'convenient' instead of the skeletally determined condylar-based position that the surgeon worked hard to achieve.

Patients usually tire of orthodontic treatment approximately 6 months after surgery, so every effort to be efficient should be attempted. Retention for surgical patients is not particularly different than for non-surgical patients. Wearing retainers full time for the first six months, followed by 'night-time for a lifetime' is the accepted standard. The only exception for surgical patients is for those whose maxillas were segmented. To allow for maximum healing and stability, these patients should leave the transpalatal arch in place for the entire first year after surgery.

Future directions

Given the trend towards minimally invasive techniques and their appeal to patients, there needs to be greater awareness of endoscopic orthognathic surgical procedures among orthodontists. This may encourage patients who are undecided about the combined orthodontic-surgical treatment to seek care. On the other hand, for the oral and maxillofacial surgeons in training, there is a steep learning curve for endoscopic procedures and increased exposure to these techniques would help increase their use in the future among practicing oral and maxillofacial surgeons. Finally, given the limited use of endoscopy in the maxilla, mostly in cadavers and very few patients, better techniques should be developed incorporating its use to facilitate more routine endoscope use in maxillary orthognathic surgery.

References

1 Troulis MJ, Nahlieli O, Castano F, Kaban LB. Minimally invasive orthognathic surgery: endoscopic vertical ramus osteotomy. Int J Oral Maxillofac Surg. 2000;29:239–42.
2 Troulis MJ, Kaban LB. Endoscopic approach to the ramus condyle unit: clinical applications. J Oral Maxillofac Surg. 2001;59:503–9.
3 Troulis MJ, Kaban LB. Endoscopic vertical ramus osteotomy: early clinical result. J Oral Maxillofac Surg. 2004;62:824–8.
4 McCain JP, Williams L. Principles and practice of temporomandibular joint arthroscopy. St. Louis: Mosby, 1996, pp. 1–11.
5 Pedroletti F, Johnson B, McCain J. Endoscopic techniques in oral and maxillofacial surgery. Oral Maxillofacial Surg Clin N Am. 2010;22:169–82.

6 Troulis MJ, Perrott DH, Kaban LB. Endoscopic mandibular osteotomy, placement and activation of a semi-buried distractor. J Oral Maxillofac Surg. 1999;57:1110–13.
7 Troulis MJ. Endoscopic open reduction and internal rigid fixation of subcondylar fractures. J Oral Maxillofac Surg. 2004;62):1269–71.
8 Saunders CJ, Whetzel TP, Stokes RB, et al. Transantral endoscopic orbital floor reconstruction: a cadaver and clinical study. Plast Reconstr Surg. 1997;100:575–81.
9 Strong EB. Endoscopic repair of orbital blow-out fractures. Facial Plast Surg. 2004;20:223–30.
10 Nahlieli O, Shacham R, Bar T, et al. Endoscopic mechanical retrieval of sialoliths. Oral Surg Oral Med Oral Pathol Oral Radiol Endoc. 2003;95:396–402.
11 Papel ID, Lee E. The male facelift: considerations and techniques. Facial Plast Surg. 1996;12:257–63.
12 Rohner D, Yeow V, Hammer B. Endoscopically assisted Le Fort I osteotomy. J Cranio-Maxillofac Surg. 2001;29:360–65.
13 Wiltfang J, Kessler P. Endoscopically assisted Le Fort I osteotomy to correct transverse and sagittal discrepancies of the maxilla. J Oral Maxillofac Surg. 2002;60:1142–5.
14 Taylor JA, Maercks RA, Jones DC, Gordon CB. Endoscopically assisted Le Fort I osteotomy using an ultrasonic scalpel: a feasibility study in cadavers. J Oral Maxillofac Surg. 2009;67:1420–4.
15 Troulis MJ, Ramirez JL, Kaban LB. Endoscopic approach for mandibular orthognathic surgery. Facial Plast Surg Clin North Am. 2006;14:45–50.
16 Turvey TA. Intraoperative complications of sagittal osteotomy of the mandibular ramus. J Oral Maxillofac Surg. 1985;43:504–9.
17 MacIntosh RB. Experience with the sagittal osteotomy of the mandibular ramus: a 13 year review. J Oral Maxillofac Surg. 1981;8:151–65.
18 Kim K, McCain JP. Use of the endoscope in bisagittal split osteotomy. J Oral Maxillofac Surg. 2008;66:1773–5.
19 Robiony M, Polini F, Costa F, Sembronio S, Zerman N, Politi M. Endoscopically assisted intraoral vertical ramus osteotomy and piezoelectric surgery in mandibular prognathism. J Oral Maxillofac Surg. 2007;65:2119–24.
20 Troulis MJ and Kaban LB. Endoscopic Reconstruction of Ramus Condyle Unit. In: Troulis MJ (Ed.) Minimally Invasive Maxillofacial Surgery. Shelton, CT: People's Medical Publishing House, 2013;1–17.
21 Papadaki ME, Kaban LB, Troulis MJ. Endoscopic vertical ramus osteotomy: a long-term prospective study. Int J Oral Maxillofac Surg. 2014;43:305–10.
22 Kaban LB. Acquired abnormalities of the temporomandibular joint. In: Kaban LB and Troulis MJ (Eds.). Pediatric oral and maxillofacial surgery. Philadelphia, PA: Elsevier, 2004, pp. 340–75.
23 Troulis MJ, Williams WB, Kaban LB. Endoscopic mandibular condylectomy and reconstruction: early clinical results. J Oral Maxillofac Surg. 2004;62:460–65.
24 Proffit WR, White RP, Sarver DM. Contemporary treatment of Dentofacial deformity. St Louis: Mosby, 2003.
25 Proffit WR, Fields HW, Sarver DM. Contemporary orthodontics. St Louis: Mosby, 2007.
26 Potts B, Fields HW, Shanker S, Vig KWL, Beck FM. Dental and skeletal outcomes for Class II surgical-orthodontic treatment: A comparison between novice and experienced clinicians. Am J Orthod Dentofacial Orthop. 2011;139:305–15.
27 Troy BA, Shanker S, Fields HW, Vig K, Johnston W. Comparison of incisor inclination in patients with Class III malocclusion treated with orthognathic surgery or orthodontic camouflage. Am J Orthod Dentofacial Orthop. 2009;135: 146.e1–146.e9.
28 Potts B, Shanker S, Fields HW, Vig KWL, Beck FM. Dental and skeletal changes associated with Class II surgical-orthodontic treatment. Am J Orthod Dentofacial Orthop. 2009;135:566.31–566.e7.
29 Proffit WR, Phillips C, Douvartzidis N. A comparison of outcomes of orthodontic and surgical-orthodontic treatment of Class II malocclusion in adults. Am J Orthod Dentofacial Orthop. 1992;101:556–65.
30 Burden D, Johnston C, Kennedy D, Harradine N, Stevenson M. A cephalometric study of Class II malocclusion treated with mandibular surgery. Am J Orthod Dentofacial Orthop. 2007;131:7.e1–8.
31 Jang JC, Fields HW, Vig KWL, Beck FM. Controversies in timing of orthodontic treatment. Semin Orthod. 2005;11: 112–8.
32 Potts B, Shanker S, Beck FM, Vig KW. Predictors of dentoalveloar outcome of presurgical orthodontic change [abstract 128]. J Dent Res 2004; 83 (Spec Iss A).

Chapter 41

The Role of the Orthognathic Surgeon in Facial Feminization Surgery

Keith Altman

Introduction

Facial feminization surgery (FFS) is a powerful set of procedures the aim of which is to feminize the face. Most of this type of surgery is undertaken in transsexual patients who are transitioning from male to female. However, there is a small cohort of females who undergo some aspects of this type of surgery to feminize masculine aspects of their face.

The range of procedures available include, forehead reduction, orbital rim contouring, scalp advance, brow lift, rhinoplasty, cheek implants, removal of the buccal fat pads of Bichat, mandibular angle shave and taper, masseter reduction, genioplasty, lip lift and dermis graft to the upper lip and thyroid shave.

FFS was developed and popularized by Dr Douglas Ousterhout of San Francisco, California, USA, in the 1980s and 1990s. He examined several hundred dry skulls in the Atkinson skull collection at the University of San Francisco and looked at the different male and female characteristics in regard to the forehead.[1] Based on his findings he was able to develop various surgical procedures to contour the forehead in order to feminize it.

The specific procedures within facial feminization surgery of particular interest to the orthognathic surgeon include, forehead reduction, orbital rim contouring, cheek implants, rhinoplasty, mandibular angle shave and taper and genioplasty.

Male and female faces: aesthetics

It is of vital importance for the surgeon to have an appreciation of the fundamental differences between the male and female face. Feminizing the face is about converting angulated features to more rounded features. In feminizing the face it is important to appreciate that the size of the face has to be in proportion with the rest of the body.[2] The proportions of the face are important to appreciate and all orthognathic surgeons will be aware of transverse thirds and vertical fifths of the face.

Analysis of the female face demonstrates a much more heart-shaped or triangular form in which the

Orthognathic Surgery: Principles, Planning and Practice. Edited by Farhad B. Naini and Daljit S. Gill.

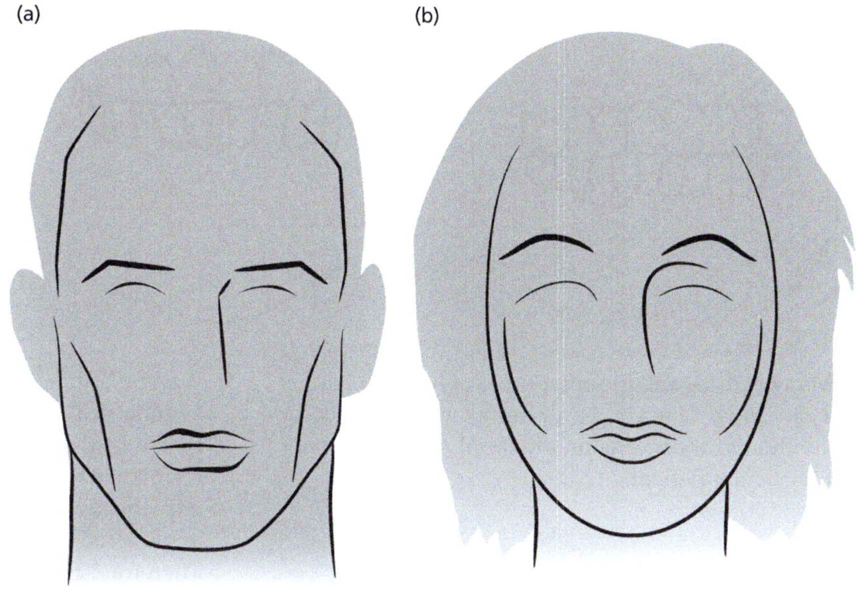

Fig. 41-1 (a and b) Line illustrations demonstrating the differences between male and female faces. Male faces are square and angulated with sharp lines and a strong jaw, while female faces are curved, round, oval and heart-shaped with smooth lines and overall are smaller. (From Altman K. Facial feminization surgery: current state of the art. Copyright © 2012 International Association of Oral and Maxillofacial Surgeons. All rights reserved. Reprinted with permission.)

base of an inverted triangle is represented by a line drawn between the maximum prominence of each cheekbone and the apex of the triangle being represented by the chin point.

The female face is softer and more rounded or oval-shaped, with soft, round, curving forms. Males faces are more square and angulated with a strong jaw and chin often in conjunction with an M-shaped hairline (Figure 41-1). The chin and lower jaw is usually longer in the male by as much as 20%,[3] and is often, but not always, more prominent in profile.

The forehead in the male may exhibit frontal bossing. This may partly be due to a large frontal sinus, but may also be due to thick supraorbital ridges. Significantly, the angle formed at the glabella between the frontal area of the forehead and nose is often acute as opposed to obtuse in the female (Figure 41-2).

Female noses tend to be smaller and shorter with narrow bridges and ala bases, often with upturning of the nasal tip giving rise to a more obtuse nasolabial angle.

Male cheeks are flat whereas female cheeks can be quite prominent as they project more anterior and are higher with some associated cheek hollowing beneath, which provides further accentuation.

The male chin is often long, square and angulated while female chins are shorter, narrower and more pointed (Figure 41-3).

The mandible in the male has a prominent angle with lipping of the bone due to the masseter muscle attachment and it is wider than in the female. The oblique ridge is thick and the masseter muscle is often bulkier.

Surgical procedures of special interest to the orthognathic surgeon

The main FFS surgical procedures of interest to the orthognathic surgeon include, forehead reduction and orbital rim contouring, rhinoplasty, cheek implants, angle shave and taper and genioplasty.

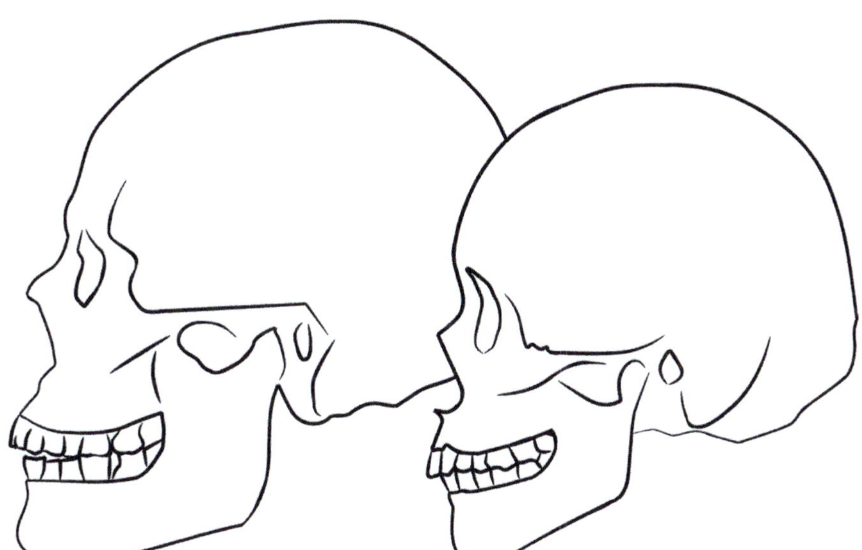

Fig. 41-2 Differences between the male and female forehead. (From Altman K. Facial feminization surgery: current state of the art. Copyright © 2012 International Association of Oral and Maxillofacial Surgeons. All rights reserved. Reprinted with permission.)

(a) (b)

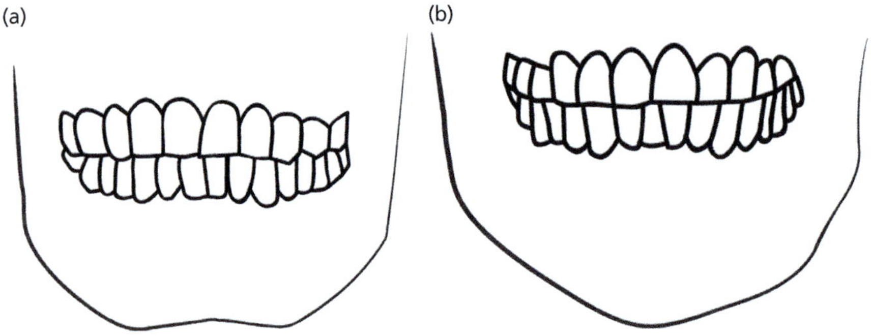

Fig. 41-3 (a and b) Differences between male and female chins. (From Altman K. Facial feminization surgery: current state of the art. Copyright © 2012 International Association of Oral and Maxillofacial Surgeons. All rights reserved. Reprinted with permission.)

Many of these and the other types of FFS procedures not described here can be undertaken all at once or individually, depending on the facial requirements of the particular patient.

Forehead reduction

Ousterhout classified forehead shape into three distinct groups:[1]

Group I

Group I has mild to moderate excessive projection of the brow and abnormal bossing. There are no frontal sinuses, or the bone anterior to the frontal sinuses is of such a thickness that its reduction will not encroach on or compromise the sinus air space.

The reduction is simply achieved with an acrylic burr in order to achieve the desired contour.

Group II

In Group II cases the brows are normal, mildly or moderately projected and there is thick bone anterior to the frontal sinuses. This bone can therefore be reduced as in Group I patients, but may become quite thin. When the bossing is reduced there may be a forehead concavity superior to the bossing, which may require filling with bone cement.

Group III

Group III cases have excessive brow fullness and the requirement for the anterior table of the frontal sinus to be set back into a more retruded position. In order to achieve this, the anterior table has to be osteotomized, reshaped and fixed with titanium mini-plate osteosynthesis.

It must be appreciated that the frontal sinus is not a symmetrical structure and one side may be larger than the other. In the glabella region the acute angle formed between the bossing of the frontal sinus and the nose must be altered to a more obtuse angle to adequately feminize this area of the face. Therefore, for Group III patients it is essential to osteotomize the inferior aspect of the anterior table of the frontal sinus precisely at the glabella and immediately above the radix area of the nose. In the author's experience, Group III cases form the majority of forehead reduction procedures undertaken.

Planning

Planning for forehead reduction is undertaken by use of computerized tomography (CT) scanning or cone-beam CT (CBCT) to measure the dimensions of the frontal sinus precisely to plan the osteotomy cuts (Figure 41-4).

In the first instance it is necessary to assess the presence or absence of a frontal sinus, its dimensions and any asymmetry as almost all frontal sinuses are asymmetric. Furthermore, frontal sinus pathology must be excluded.

The CBCT assesses the sinus in the coronal, sagittal and axial planes. The thickness of the anterior table is assessed, which in most cases is 2 to 3 mm thick away from the midline septum. The main measurements for forehead (Group) III surgery are taken from the axial and sagittal sections of the scans. The vertical height of the anterior table from the superior-most aspect to the glabella is measured as is the horizontal

(a) (b)

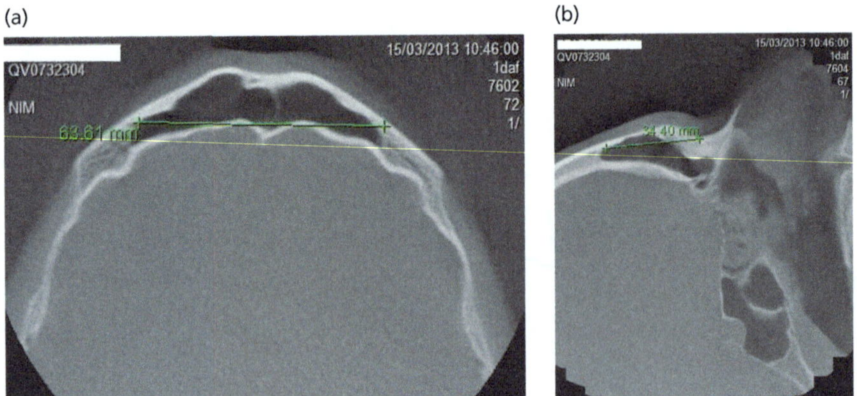

Fig. 41-4 (a and b) Cone-beam CT scans of frontal sinus demonstrating preoperative planning measurements.

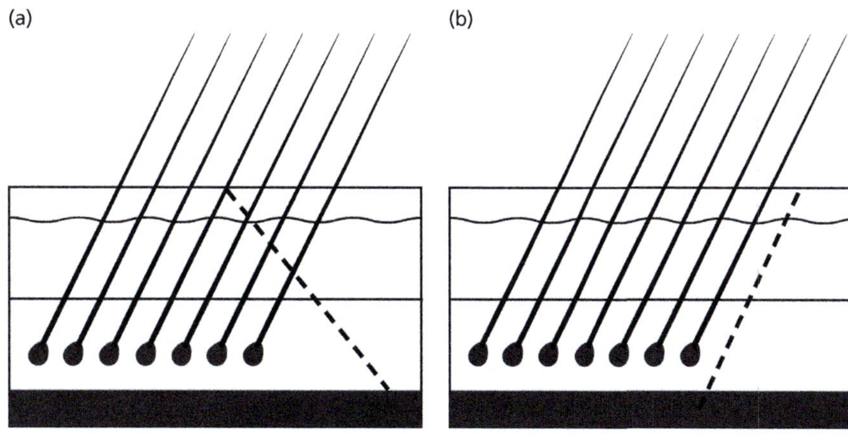

Fig. 41-5 (a) Trichophytic incision; note relationship of tangential incision to hair follicles. (b) Pre-trichial incision; note relationship of parallel incision to hair follicles. (From Altman K. Facial feminization surgery: current state of the art. Copyright © 2012 International Association of Oral and Maxillofacial Surgeons. All rights reserved. Reprinted with permission.)

maximum dimension. Both measurements are recorded as these will form the basis for the markings made at operation for the bone cuts when the anterior table is osteotomized. In addition, note must be made of the relationship of the midline of the sinus to each lateral aspect taking into account any asymmetry when planning the osteotomy cuts.

Surgical procedure

Access to the frontal area is via a coronal flap in all cases. The main decision in terms of flap design is if a scalp advance to correct the hairline is required. If it is, then a trichophytic[4,5] incision (as opposed to a pre-trichial incision) is made and run out to the temples and into the hairline above the ears (Figure 41-5). If a scalp advance is not required then a standard coronal incision further back in the scalp is used.

Standard tumescent solution is injected into the scalp and the flap raised avoiding injury to the frontal branches of the facial nerve, which is rare. The dissection proceeds in the subperiosteal plane approximately 4–5 cm superior to the glabella and the entire frontal area down to the glabella is exposed including the frontal processes of the zygomas and the superior orbital rims, dissecting 1 cm into the roof of each orbit. At this point in the dissection the supra-orbital nerves may need to be osteotomized out of their foramina in order to expose the entire superior orbital rims and additionally afford them protection.

In Group I and II cases, the bossing is reduced with the use of an acrylic trimming burr on a fast motor. In addition the frontal processes of the zygomas are also contoured if required. The addition of bone cement may be required in Group II cases. Ousterhout originally described the use of methylmethacrylate onlay implants in Group II patients,[6] though the use of bone cement has now superseded this.

Group III cases all require osteotomy of the anterior table of the frontal sinus. In terms of planning, the dimensions of the anterior table cuts are marked out on the bone from the known CT scan measurements, taking into account any asymmetry of the sinus.

The cuts are made with a Toller fissure burr or sagittal saw inclined obliquely at an angle greater than 45° to the bone surface and facing towards the sinus at all times in order to ensure correct positioning. Once the cuts are completed, a fine osteotome is used to separate the anterior table from the forehead, with great care being taken not to fracture the bone plate. Before attempting to elevate the bone plate, the osteotome must first separate the frontal sinus septum.

The sinus cavity is inspected for exposed dura at the superior aspect and the sinus lining is preserved though it is usually torn. Bony septa are trimmed and any debris is irrigated with saline.

The anterior bone plate having been adequately trimmed, is replaced with its inferior aspect placed into a retruded position in a 'tongue-and-groove' fashion, which very effectively eradicates the frontal bossing, but a precise fit is not required as steps and deficiencies cannot be appreciated on palpation of the forehead skin. On occasion, a large anterior table will need to be osteotomized transversely to prevent the superior edge protruding above the frontal bone margin.[7] The surrounding bone is further contoured.

Fixation of the bone plate is by means of titanium 1.3 mm mini-plate osteosynthesis using three X-shaped plates and short screws.

Orbital rim contouring[8] results in a larger orbital perimeter. This area of contouring is carried out at the superior and lateral area of the orbital rim. The intra-orbital periosteum is dissected approximately 1 cm into the orbital roof exposing the area of bone to be contoured. The rim is simply reduced with an acrylic burr to obtain an acceptable contour.

Forehead reduction is often carried out in conjunction with advancement of the scalp and brow lift.

During closure of the scalp the periosteum is sutured over the bone plate to ensure revascularisation. Some authors advocate periosteal preservation overlying the bone plate and carrying out the dissection in the sub-galeal plane. Preservation of the periosteum may be useful where a compression technique has been used to flatten the bone plate. Often the periosteum can also be used for suturing the bone plate rather than using mini-plate osteosynthesis.[9]

Vacuum drains are placed and their ends tunnelled under a pericranial bridge to prevent migration and being impaled by scalp clips.[10] Scalp clips are placed within the hair and 5/0 monofilament sutures are used along the trichophytic incision. It is essential that the scalp is not sutured under tension.

A head bandage is placed for 24 h and the vacuum drains removed at 48 h. After drain removal, normal hair washing may be undertaken. Sutures and clips are removed at 7–10 days.

Appropriate antibiotics are given postoperatively and patients are instructed not to blow their nose for 10 days, otherwise air may be introduced into the frontal sinus leading to surgical emphysema and possible infection.

Complications of forehead reduction include damage to the supra-orbital nerves causing anaesthesia of the forehead and scalp. These nerves however are rarely damaged making permanent forehead anaesthesia unlikely. However, due to the placement of the coronal scalp incision, all patients have scalp anaesthesia distal to and up to the vertex, which over a few months diminishes in the size of the area affected. Extremely rarely, the frontal branches of the facial nerve suffer a traction palsy resulting in frontalis weakness. Rarely frontal sinus infection may occur. In a small number of cases removal of the anterior table may lead to removal of a small portion of the posterior table resulting in dural exposure. It is unusual for the dura to be torn, but this occurrence must be looked for in all cases. If the dura is torn it may be sutured. Otherwise, Surgicel® and Tisseel® are used to seal over the area of exposed dura.

Patients commonly experience eyelid bruising and oedema along with some chemosis. The feared complication of total loss of the anterior table due to bone resorption seems to pose negligible risk.

In terms of the scalp, the main complications noted may be a thickened or stretched scar and telogen effluvium (acute hair loss).[5] The latter is more often seen in thin scalps where the blood supply may be more tenuous. Patients may report finding more hair on their hairbrush a few weeks after surgery, but spontaneous recovery may be expected after 6 months.

Rhinoplasty

The objectives of a feminizing rhinoplasty, in most cases, is to reduce any dorsal hump and to narrow the nasal bridge by in-fracture of the nasal bones. The dorsum can be left straight in the female nose, but some individuals may request more curvature to the dorsum or a retroussé nose. Skin can be excised at the nasal sills to reduce the nostril aperture. It is important to appreciate that the nose must fit the face in the sense that a small nose will not look normal on a large face however well it has been feminized. Standard techniques of rhinoplasty will not be discussed further as they are well described in standard textbooks on the subject.

Rhinoplasty is often combined with forehead reduction and both these procedures undertaken together complement each other well. If an open technique is used in conjunction with a lip lift then the columella skin flap is raised from the nasal sill to incorporate the lip lift skin excision rather than from the normal midcolumella area.

Figures 41-6 and 41-7 show two patients who had forehead III and rhinoplasty, including other procedures as part of their FFS.

The general and specific complications of rhinoplasty are also well covered in standard texts on the subject.

Cheek implants

Cheek augmentation is an important feminizing procedure. A triangle between the points of the cheeks and the chin, where the chin point forms the apex of the triangle and a line drawn between the lateral points of the cheeks forms the base of the triangle, represents the feminine appearance of the lower two-thirds of the face. This can effectively be achieved by augmenting the cheeks with implants.[11]

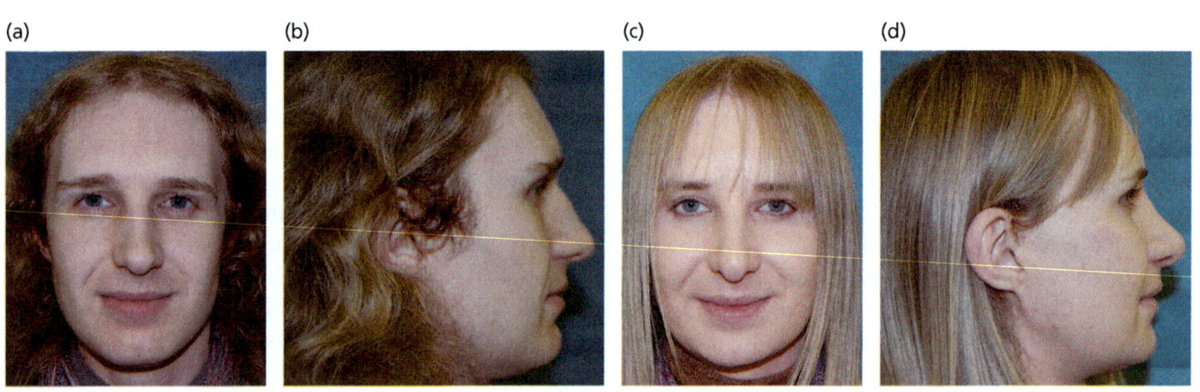

Fig. 41-6 (a and b) Preoperative frontal and profile views prior to forehead III, brow lift, rhinoplasty, cheek implants, angle shave and genioplasty. (c and d) Postoperative views at 3 months. (From Altman K. Facial feminization surgery: current state of the art.

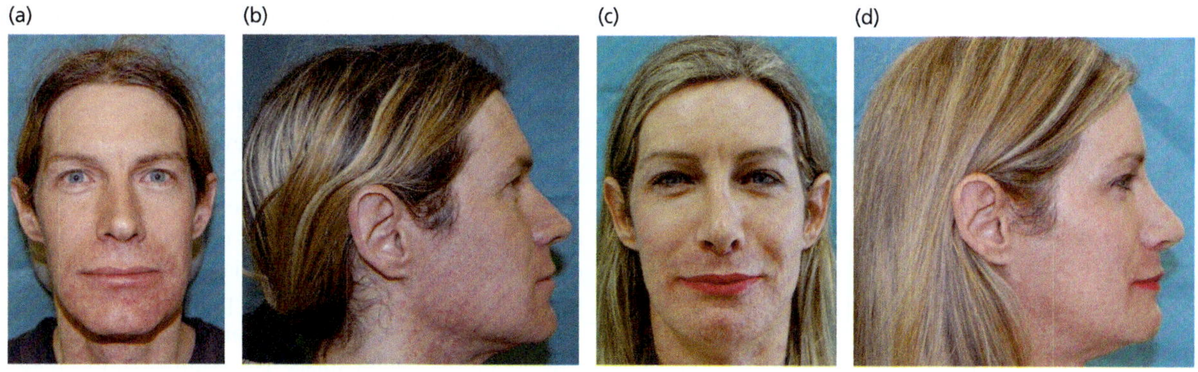

Fig. 41-7 (a and b) Preoperative frontal and profile views prior to forehead III, brow lift, rhinoplasty, cheek implants, angle shave and genioplasty. (c and d) Postoperative views at 3 months.

Medpor® (Stryker Corporation, Newnan, GA, USA) high-density polyethylene implants come in a few different malar shapes and sizes. They are easy to insert via the mouth. Silicone sizers are available to ensure the correct size is used before opening individual packs. The implants can be further carved if desired.

Surgical procedure

Following infiltration of local anaesthetic an adequately sized pocket must be dissected prior to placement and this must include dissection along the zygomatic arches to ensure the implants sit passively on the underlying bone as they are feathered in this area. Achieving symmetry of the implants can be challenging. Once the operator is satisfied with the aesthetic appearance and fit, the implants, having been immersed in suitable antibiotic solution prior to insertion, are screwed into the underlying bone with two 2.0 mm titanium screws of at least 6.0 mm length each side to prevent migration and rotation. Cheek implants also provide some degree of malar fat pad lifting.

The oral mucosa is closed with 3/0 Vicryl Rapide suture (Ethicon Inc.).

Complications of cheek implant placement include incorrect size, position and asymmetry. In thin skinned individuals caution must be exercised as cheek implants may look unsightly, however well positioned they are.

Occasionally the feathered edge of the implant overlying the zygomatic arch may appear prominent and require correction. This complication is avoided by meticulous dissection of the zygomatic arches before implant insertion. Infection is very rare and may necessitate implant removal. Finally, anaesthesia in the distribution of the infraorbital nerves, which is most often temporary, may occur.

Angle shave and taper

An angulated mandible is a very masculine feature and so in many cases of feminization surgery, the mandible needs to be contoured.

The prominent masculine feature of the mandible includes a sharp angle. It is often too square and the lipping and associated masseter bulk lead to additional width of the mandible.[12]

Planning

An orthopantomogram (OPT) is required for assessment of the mandibular angle and chin.

Width of the mandible is very much aesthetic and assessed clinically and any lipping at the angle is easily palpated for. Masseteric bulk can also be determined clinically.

An OPT is useful, in addition to clinical assessment, to assess the size of the angle and if it needs to be osteotomized or reduced. Often one side is larger than the other. The amount to be removed is predetermined from the radiograph although this can be difficult to precisely reproduce at surgery due to the difficulties with access and visualization of the operative site.

Surgical procedure

Local anaesthesia is given and the procedure performed entirely via the mouth through an incision from high on the external oblique ridge to the first molar area. The entire angle and body of the mandible is widely exposed with great care being taken to strip off the pterygomasseteric attachments completely at the lower border. It is essential to expose the entire lower border of the body, angle and ramus as this manoeuvre protects against bleeding from inadvertent muscle and vascular damage by the drill. It is entirely possible to tear the facial artery and vein during this procedure if inadequate care is not taken.

Good retraction is essential. The cortical bone is significantly reduced often exposing cancellous bone, with a high speed acrylic burr to reduce the prominence of the angle and external oblique ridge up to the mental foramen (Figure 41-8). Care must be taken not to expose tooth roots in the molar region and not to expose the inferior dental canal and as a consequence damage the inferior dental nerve.

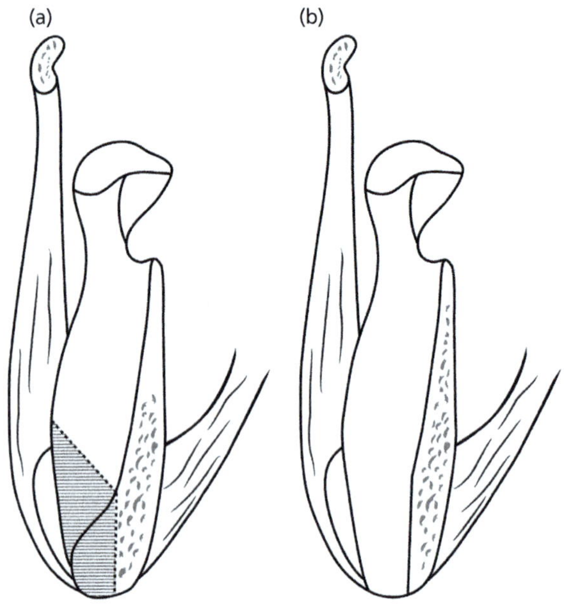

Fig. 41-8 (a and b) Angle shave by reducing the lipping at the mandibular angle and subsequent result (shading indicates area to be contoured). (From Altman K. Facial feminization surgery: current state of the art. Copyright © 2012 International Association of Oral and Maxillofacial Surgeons. All rights reserved. Reprinted with permission.)

A significant mandibular angle may require osteotomy with reciprocating and oscillating saws to give this area a more rounded and softer appearance though a smaller angle can be reduced simply with the acrylic burr[13] (Figure 41-9). This is a difficult procedure due to the limited access and visual appreciation of the cuts being made. It is very important to ensure that not too much of the angle is removed, which is unsightly.

Once the cut has been made with the saw, the osteotomy is completed with a curved osteotome. This often results in the fragment to be removed springing medially due to its retained medial pterygoid muscle attachments. The fragment is retrieved by external

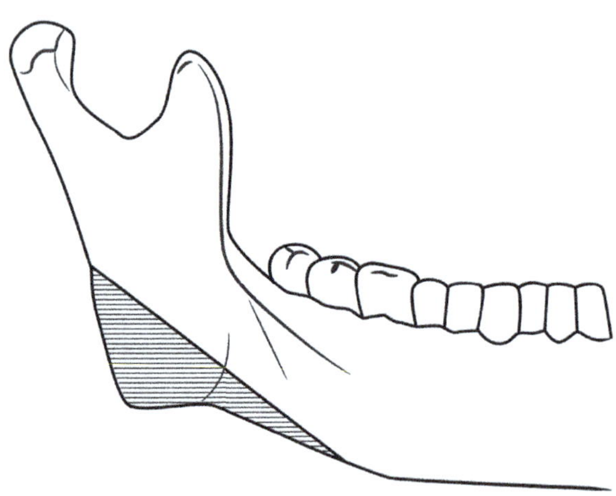

Fig. 41-9 Angle shave and osteotomy cuts to the angle of the mandible (shading). (From Altman K. Facial feminization surgery: current state of the art. Copyright © 2012 International Association of Oral and Maxillofacial Surgeons. All rights reserved. Reprinted with permission.)

digital pressure to redeliver it back to the buccal side of the mandible where it can easily be detached from the muscle and removed. Finally the lower border of the mandible is smoothed off with the drill. Further width reduction if desired can be achieved by antero-medial resection of the masseter muscle.[12,14]

Masseteric atrophy is believed likely to occur as a result of the mandible angle reduction due to the extensive muscle stripping. This effect is favourable and has been described in patients undergoing mandibular sagittal split osteotomy.[15]

Meticulous haemostasis is required and Yeates drains are placed internally without suturing and removed at 24 h. The mucosa is closed with 3/0 Vicryl Rapide sutures (Ethicon Inc.). External pressure may occasionally need to be employed in certain cases.

Post-operatively, patients may experience significant swelling, bruising and pain. The initial swelling lasts for 2–3 weeks, but full resolution may not occur for at least 6 months. Inferior dental nerve sensory disturbance may result, but this is often temporary if it occurs at all. In addition, the marginal branch of the facial nerve may suffer from temporary palsy due to the retraction used during the procedure. Wound healing can be protracted and may lead to food accumulation in the cheeks and significant scar banding.

Genioplasty

The objectives of a feminizing genioplasty are to narrow an angulated masculine chin. It is often also necessary to shorten the vertical height of the chin.[3] Chin osteotomies generally give far superior results than contouring alone, though some additional contouring is also often required.

Planning

The genioplasty is assessed clinically in terms of the requirement for midline block removal to narrow the chin point and any vertical changes required. An OPT assesses the proximity of tooth roots and any associated pathology.

Surgical procedure

Following local anaesthesia, a labial sulcus incision is made with subperiosteal dissection to expose the chin and lower border of the mandible back to the first molar area. This incision may be joined to the incisions from an angle shave. The mental nerves are identified, fully dissected and protected in order to widely expose the full lower border of the chin area. Sagittal and reciprocating saws are used to make the osteotomy cuts and vertical reduction is achieved by removal of a predetermined segment of bone depending on how much vertical height decrease is required.

Narrowing the chin is simply achieved by removal of a predetermined block of midline bone, which is osteotomized and removed. The two remaining halves

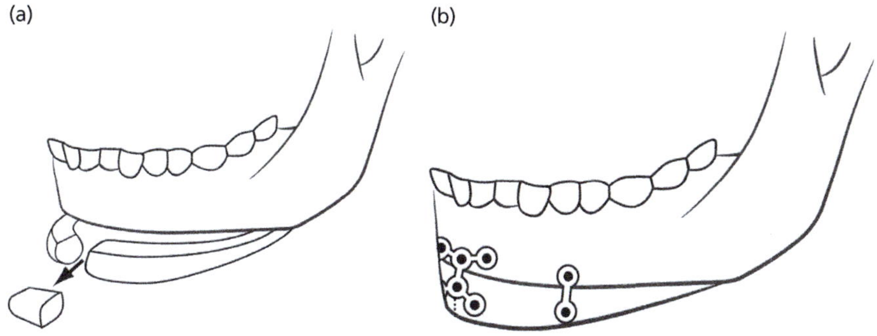

Fig. 41-10 (a and b) Chin width reduction and fixation. (From Altman K. Facial feminization surgery: current state of the art. Copyright © 2012 International Association of Oral and Maxillofacial Surgeons. All rights reserved. Reprinted with permission.)

of the chin are brought together in the midline and secured with a 1.3 mm X-shaped titanium mini-plate and two further 3-hole mini-plates placed laterally to stabilize the fragments (Figures 41-10 and 41-11). If desired the chin width posteriorly can be further narrowed by fixing the tail ends of the genioplasty fragments in a more medial position. Closure of the mentalis muscle and oral mucosa is with 3/0 Vicryl Rapide suture (Ethicon Inc.).

Complications of genioplasty include pain, swelling, bruising and sensory disturbance of the lip and chin area due to mental nerve damage.

Discussion

There is a limited role for the orthognathic surgeon in facial feminization procedures, because this area of facial surgery is so specialized and ideally surgeons involved in this surgery should be part of a multidisciplinary team.

FFS brings together a broad range of craniomaxillofacial surgical techniques whose sole objective is to convert a masculine face to a feminine one. There is no attempt to beautify or rejuvenate, though these effects may be a by-product of the feminization procedures. The main aim is for the individual to pass as a female in everyday society and to integrate as well as possible into the community.

The standards of care for transgender people is well described, though very little is written in the World Professional Association for Transgender Health (WPATH) literature with specific regard to FFS.[16]

Ousterhout was the pioneer of FFS. He carried out anthropological studies on several hundred dried skulls at the Atkinson skull collection at the University of San Francisco identifying specific features and characteristics that differentiated male from female human skulls.[1]

His findings permitted the development of surgical techniques on those areas of the face and skull that were amenable to feminization.

Most transgender females have usually lived in role for a good period of time before undergoing FFS, which is often the first surgery they have. This is important for them because they need to integrate as women in everyday society and their facial appearance is essential for them to pass. The author normally sees patients for a few consultations before surgery. Most patients are extremely knowledgeable about FFS and have researched the subject well. Some in addition have had photographs prepared from a virtual FFS website indicating what they are likely to look like following various aspects of this surgery.

All patients are photographed and detailed informed consent is taken.

Most transgender patients take various hormones, including oestrogens such as estradiol, gonadorelin analogues and anti-androgens such as cyproterone. Spironolactone is often prescribed for its testosterone suppressant properties. Hormone medication is not stopped for patients undergoing FFS, but full venous thromboembolism assessment and prophylaxis is given for the procedure.

In terms of clinical effectiveness, there are no large studies looking at this aspect of care, but the author's experience suggests that patient satisfaction overall is generally high following these procedures. Transwomen have diminished mental health-related quality of life when compared with the general

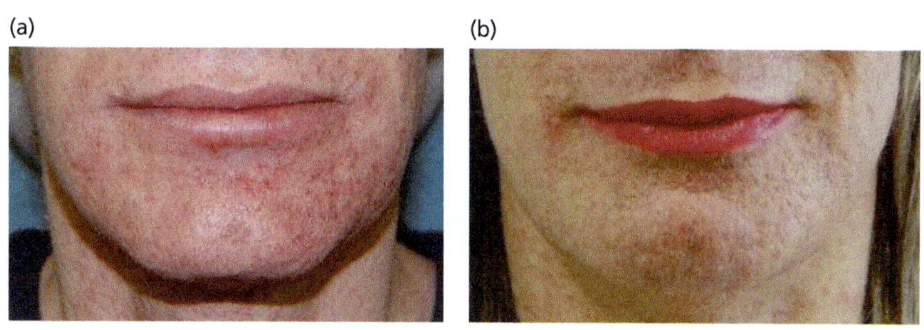

Fig. 41-11 (a) Preoperative photograph of wide and angulated chin. (b) Postoperative photograph at 3 months.

population. FFS along with gender reassignment surgery has been shown to be associated with improved mental health-related quality of life.[17]

References

1 Ousterhout DK. Feminization of the Forehead: Contour Changing to Improve Female Aesthetics. Plast Reconstr Surg. 1987;79:701–11.

2 Kolar JC. Anthropological guidelines for aesthetic craniofacial surgery. In: Aesthetic Contouring of the Craniofacial Skeleton. Ousterhout DK (Ed.) Boston/Toronto/London: Little, Brown and Company, 1991:20–21.

3 Ousterhout DK. Feminization of the chin: A review of 485 consecutive cases. In: Craniofacial Surgery (vol. 10). Salyer, K (Ed.): Bologna, Italy. Medimond International Proceedings 2003:461–3.

4 Marten TJ. Hairline lowering during foreheadoplasty. Plast Reconstr Surg. 1999;103:224–36.

5 Ramirez AL, Ende KH, Kabaker SS. Correction of the high female hairline. Arch Facial Plast Surg. 2009;11:84–90.

6 Ousterhout DK, Zlotolow IM. Aesthetic improvement of the forehead utilizing methylmethacrylate onlay implants. Aesth Plast Surg. 1990;14:281–6.

7 Komuro Y, Nishida M, Imazawa T, Koga Y, Yanai A. Combined frontal bone reshaping and forehead lift for frontal sinus hypertrophy. Aesth Plast Surg. 1999;23:361–3.

8 Flowers RS. Orbital rim contouring. In: Aesthetic Contouring of the Craniofacial Skeleton. Ousterhout DK (Ed.): Boston/Toronto/London: Little, Brown and Company 1991:243–56.

9 Rehman K-U, Johnston C, Monaghan A, Dover S. Management of the giant frontal sinus – A simple method to improve cosmesis. Br J Oral Maxillofac Surg. 2009;47:54–5.

10 Hodges S, Altman K. Simple manoeuvre to help stabilize drains when closing a coronal flap. Br J Oral Maxillofac Surg. 2009;47:162.

11 Binder WJ. Submalar augmentation: An alloplastic method for aesthetic contouring of the midface. In: Aesthetic Contouring of the Craniofacial Skeleton. Ousterhout DK (Ed.): Boston/Toronto/London: Little, Brown and Company: 1991:347–70.

12 Ousterhout DK. Feminization of the mandibular body: A review of 688 consecutive cases. In: Craniofacial Surgery (vol. 11). David DJ (Ed.): Bologna, Italy: Medimond International Proceedings 2005:135–7.

13 Chen X, Lin J, Shen J, Zhou Y, Wu X, Xu Y. Modification of square face in men. Arch Facial Plast Surg. 2011;13:244–46.

14 Lorenz HP, Schendel SA. Facial bone sculpturing. In: Maxillofacial Surgery Vol. I. Ward Booth P, Hausamen J-E, Schendel SA (Eds.). London: Churchill Livingstone: 1999:1441–56.

15 Chai G, Zhang Y, Zhu M, Xiaofei M, Zheyuan Y, Xiongzheng M, Zuoliang Q. Evaluation of dynamic morphologic changes in the masseter muscle in patients undergoing mandibular angle sagittal split osteotomy: A report of 130 cases. Arch Facial Plast Surg. 2011;13:301–4.

16 Coleman E, Bockting W, Botzer M, et al. Standards of Care for the Health of Transsexual, Transgender, and Gender-Nonconforming People, Version 7. Int J Transgend. 2011;13:165–232.

17 Ainsworth, TA, Spiegel, JH. Quality of life of individuals with and without facial feminization surgery or gender reassignment surgery. Qual Life Res. 2010;19:1019–24.

Chapter 42

Contemporary Approach to Surgical Timing in Orthognathic Surgery: The 'Surgery First' Concept

Federico Hernández-Alfaro and Raquel Guijarro-Martínez

Introduction

During the last decade, treatment concepts in orthognathic surgery have undergone a profound reassessment.[1] This re-evaluation is the natural consequence of substantial improvements in the surgical, medical, and orthodontic fields. Surgically, the combination of technical proficiency, improved rigid fixation systems, and a better understanding of bone and soft tissue healing have reduced the rate of complications, redefined surgical limits, and enabled the development of minimally invasive protocols. Medically, the routine use of hypotensive anaesthesia and subsequent reduction of bleeding and oedema have consolidated orthognathic surgery as a safe, reliable procedure that can often be performed in an outpatient context.[2] In the orthodontic field, the widespread use of skeletal anchorage systems[3–6] and the introduction of biological treatments such as interdental corticotomies[7–15] have opened a wide new range of anchorage possibilities, improved orthodontic efficiency, and reduced treatment times.[8,9,12]

In addition, the orthognathic surgery patient 'prototype' has evolved too. While the correction of a dysfunctional occlusion used to be the one and only therapeutic goal, the wish to improve facial aesthetics – in the context of a dysfunctional occlusion or not - has become the main motivation for treatment in many cases. Moreover, supported by a popular perception of surgery as safe and predictable, the number of adult patients who get involved in orthodontic or combined orthodontic–surgical therapy is increasing steadily. These patients often present with periodontal problems and job-time limitations for long treatments.[16] Some are orthodontically compensated individuals who have eventually become aesthetically concerned and opted for surgery. Others suffer sleep-disordered breathing (SDB) problems refractory to conservative therapy and cannot – or will not – undergo regular preoperative orthodontic preparation. All these new patient profiles have promoted a reconsideration of the conventional timing scheme for orthognathic surgery.[1]

Orthognathic Surgery: Principles, Planning and Practice. Edited by Farhad B. Naini and Daljit S. Gill.

Surgery first

Concept

Conventional orthognathic treatment entails a variable length of preoperative orthodontic preparation, surgery itself, and a relatively stable period of postoperative orthodontics. In particular, these phases tend to last between 15 and 24 months preoperatively[17–19] and between 7 and 12 months postoperatively.[17,19] Unfortunately, the clinician's pre-treatment estimate of duration of orthodontic treatment often tends to be too optimistic.[19] The feeling of having received inaccurate information has a negative impact on global satisfaction with treatment,[20] especially taking into account that an important percentage of patients rate the orthodontics as the worst part of their treatment due to the appliances' visibility, pain, and duration.[19,21,22] On the other hand, clinical experience has shown that routine preoperative dental alignment, arch coordination and incisor decompensation often tend to prolong treatment time with little or no clinically significant benefit for the patient.[23] In addition, preoperative axial correction of the incisors in skeletal Class III patients exacerbates a compensated anterior crossbite, thereby accentuating the prognathic profile and intensifying the patient's perception of facial disharmony.[16]

An alternative to the conventional methodology in selected cases is the so-called *surgery first* approach. This methodology proceeds with orthognathic surgery without presurgical orthodontic preparation and is followed by regular postoperative dental alignment. Although it is considered by many a revolutionary concept, the first known reference to *surgery first* dates back to 1988, when Behrman and Behrman[24] suggested that if the jaws were corrected to a proper position, the normalized surrounding soft tissues would facilitate postoperative tooth movement and reduce the length of orthodontic treatment time. They illustrated their idea by the recommendation to 'build the house and then move the furniture'. However, it was not until two decades later that the first mono-[23,25,26] and bimaxillary[16] cases managed successfully with this treatment concept were published.

During recent years, this new trend in surgical timing has been gaining popularity steadily due to several reasons:

1. The first step is the correction of the skeletal bases.[16,27] This means that the aesthetic concern, which is often the patient's chief complaint, is corrected from the beginning. Immediate aesthetic improvement and functional breathing have a positive impact in patients' compliance with postoperative orthodontics and contribute to global satisfaction with treatment notably (Figure 42-1).[1,16,28] Moreover, skeletal base correction reduces the complexity of orthodontic treatment because dental compensation is partly resolved by surgery itself, and soft tissue imbalances that may potentially interfere with certain orthodontic movements are eliminated.[26,28,29] Finally, the fact that patients can decide for themselves the surgical appointment date without the need to wait for complete arch

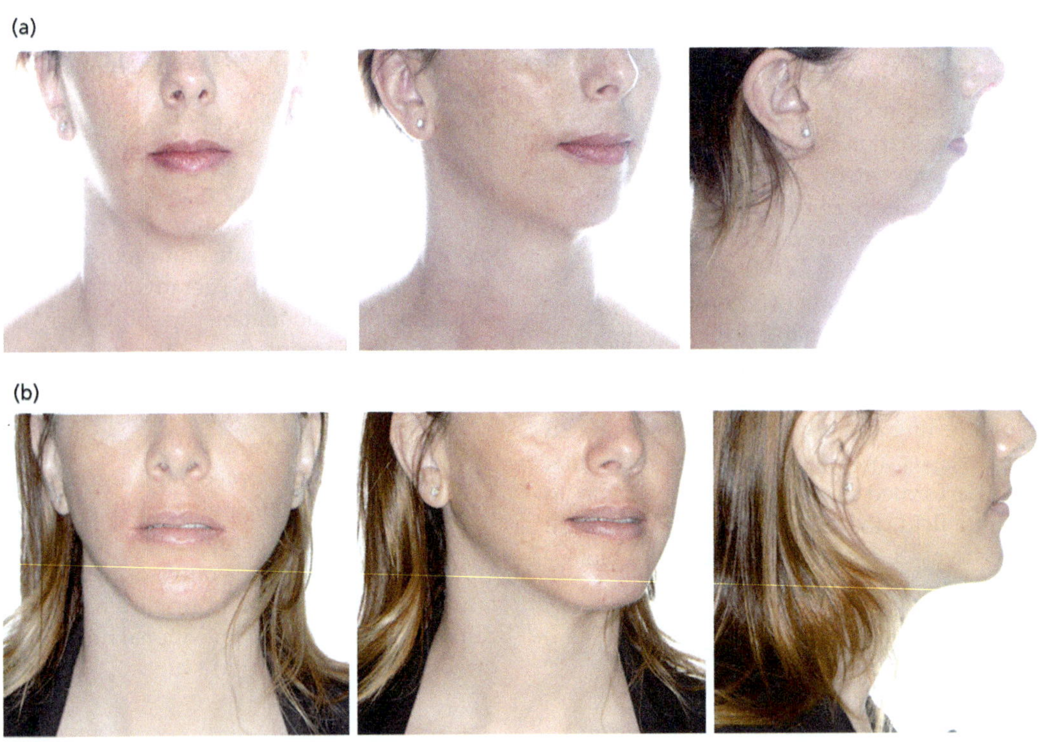

Fig. 42-1 Patient treated with a *surgery first* approach. The main motivations for treatment were aesthetic concern and sleep-disordered breathing (SDB). Preoperative (a) and one-year postoperative (b) clinical pictures after a bimaxillary procedure with anticlockwise rotation (c).

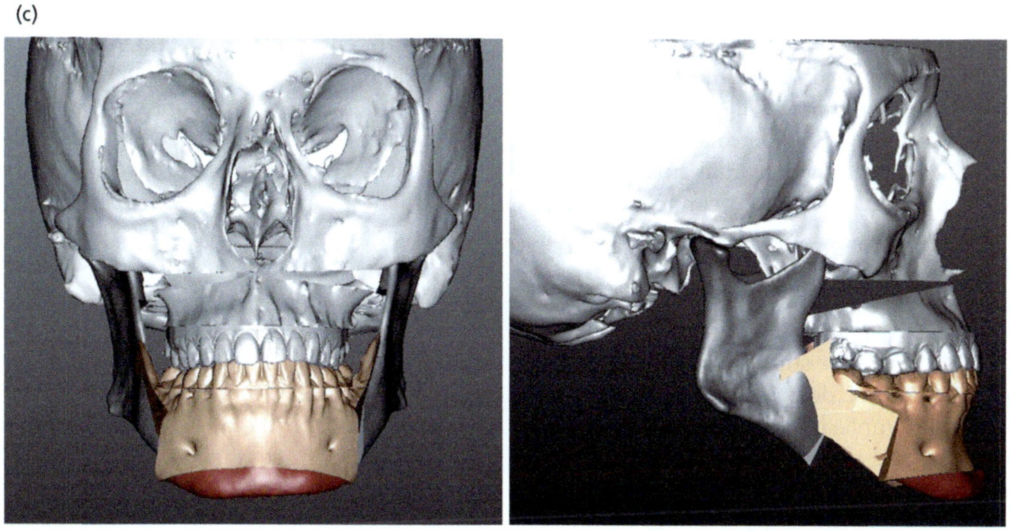

Fig. 42-1 (*Continued*).

leveling and decompensation is perceived by patients as a sign of quality.

2. Compared to the conventional approach, orthodontic treatment and hence total treatment time are significantly shortened.[1,16,23,25–28] The most numerous case series available in the scientific literature reported an average treatment time of 45 weeks.[1] Improved orthodontic efficiency is probably related to the transient demineralization of the operated bones due to the regional acceleratory phenomenon (RAP)[12–14,16,26,29,30] and to a more favourable soft tissue tone after skeletal correction.[23,28,29]
3. In the context of correct selection criteria, a *surgery first* protocol does not impair the final occlusal result or entail higher relapse rates than the traditional timing concept (Figure 42-2).[28,31,32]

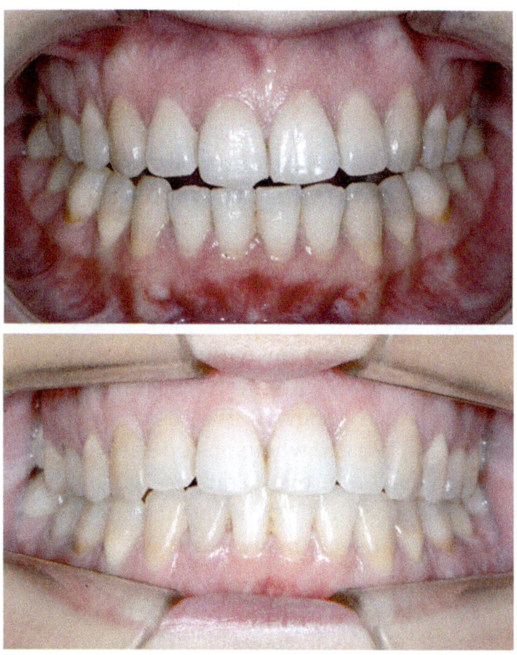

Fig. 42-2 Preoperative (top) and one-year postoperative (bottom) occlusal results of the patient shown in Figure 42-1.

Inclusion criteria

A *surgery first* approach may be considered when the following inclusion criteria are met:

1. Skeletal malocclusion requiring combined orthodontic-surgical treatment without extractions.
2. Aesthetic improvement or SDB as main motivations for treatment.
3. Orthodontic management by an officially qualified orthodontist with broad experience in orthognathic surgery.

Exclusion criteria

Whenever any of the following conditions are present, it is preferable to discard *surgery first* and opt for another timing scheme:

1. Active periodontal disease.
2. Active temporomandibular joint disease.
3. Severe crowding requiring dental extractions.
4. Severe asymmetry with three-dimensional dental compensations.
5. Transverse maxillary hypoplasia requiring previous surgically-assisted rapid palatal expansion (SARPE).
6. Class II second division with deep overbite.
7. Orthodontic management by an orthodontist with limited experience in orthognathic surgery.

Active periodontal disease and temporomandibular joint pathology are undesirable underlying conditions in any kind of orthognathic surgery procedure. However, due to the inherent characteristics of a *surgery first* methodology, in which rather demanding orthodontic movements are often required and the initial postoperative occlusion tends to be unstable, they are particularly dangerous circumstances.[28]

Criteria 3–6 refer to the underlying malocclusion. Candidates for *surgery first* must be cases with well aligned to mildly crowded anterior teeth, flat to mild curve of Spee, and normal to mildly proclined or retroclined incisors.[28,33] In addition, severe asymmetries, midline deviations, and transversal discrepancies that require a two-stage orthognathic management pose significant difficulties to the accurate anticipation of the final occlusion.[28] In these cases, a conventional timing approach continues to be the safest and most reliable option.

Finally, a conventional approach is preferable for cases managed by an orthodontist with limited experience in orthognathic surgery.[16,28] Indeed, while a *surgery first* protocol does not necessarily entail greater technical complexity from a surgical point of view, the orthodontic management can be extremely demanding. First, the patient's baseline occlusion cannot serve as a guide for the designation of treatment goals.[16] Consequently, the underlying skeletal abnormalities must be closely assessed in three dimensions in order to establish an effective treatment plan. The orthodontist must be experienced enough to foresee the extent and limitations of potential orthodontic movements accurately. Second, orthodontic treatment must start as soon as possible in order to benefit from the 'window of opportunity' provided by the RAP.[12–14,16,26,29,30] Therefore, the orthodontist must be ready to follow the patient very closely. Orthodontic appointments must be scheduled more frequently than in a conventional treatment approach. In fact, the latency period between every archwire change is approximately 2 weeks.[16,28] Third, the immediate postoperative occlusion is often unstable especially in segmented maxillae, where the end splint is left in place for 2–3 weeks. As soon as the end splint is removed, orthodontic alignment must begin. Finally, the orthodontist must be experienced in the use of temporary anchorage devices such as miniscrews and miniplates.[23,25,28] These devices play a key role in anchoring orthodontic forces such that any required vector may be used without overloading the teeth.[16] They can also help compensate surgical error or skeletal relapse.[23]

Diagnostic workup

The first step to diagnosis is a detailed interview and thorough clinical assessment of the patient by the combined surgical–orthodontic team. The patient's chief complaint, referral context, history of orthodontic treatment, underlying medical conditions, periodontal status, temporomandibular joint symptomatology, and occlusal situation must be recorded specifically.

Radiological evaluation with cone-beam computed tomography (CBCT) and dental arch anatomy registration with an intraoral digital scanner follows. Subsequently, an augmented virtual skull model with accurate representation of the bony and dental tissues is obtained by fusing the STL files of the segmented CBCT data and the intraoral scan. This method has been validated and described in detail elsewhere.[34] Although alternative methods to obtain an augmented skull representation exist,[35–45] dental anatomy registration with digital impression technology eliminates the need for dental impressions, does not require fiducial markers, reduces the number of necessary intermediate steps and hence the subsequent risk of error accumulation, and is not based on ionizing X-ray radiation.[34]

Preoperative planning

Prior to the surgeon's virtual simulation of the surgical plan, the orthodontist anticipates the necessary dental movements on the augmented skull model. This is the so-called 'three-dimensional virtual orthodontic setup'. The orthodontist must be able to foresee and predict the final – at the end of orthodontic treatment – position and axial inclination of each individual tooth accurately. This is a crucial step prior to the surgeon's skeletal base correction simulation, since the patient's current occlusion cannot serve as a guide for skeletal repositioning (Figure 42-3).

Subsequently, the planned osteotomies are simulated. An individualized treatment plan with a maxilla- or mandible-first protocol is designed, and the resulting file with the temporary intermaxillary relationship is used to obtain the intermediate splint by CAD/CAM technology. The end splint may be fabricated in a similar fashion, or it may be obtained conventionally.

Surgical protocol

With the exception of bracket bonding – normally one week before surgery – no other preoperative orthodontic preparation is required. The first soft archwire is usually placed at the first postoperative orthodontic appointment. If it is installed preoperatively, it must not be placed earlier than 24 hours before the operation in order to avoid any dental movements that could render the splints inaccurate.

Surgery itself proceeds in a standard fashion according to the surgical plan. However, some details are particularly relevant in a *surgery first* approach:

Use of temporary anchorage devices

Temporary anchorage devices play a key role in anchoring orthodontic forces such that any required vector may be used without overloading the teeth.[16] This is particularly relevant in cases managed with a *surgery first* approach, where postoperative orthodontic movements are often rather demanding, the postoperative occlusion may be unstable, and the periodontal status of many adult patients is often suboptimal.

Prior to incision, transmucosal screws (1.5 or 2.0 mm) are installed. These facilitate intermaxillary fixation during surgery and avoid excessive postoperative loading of the teeth. Four screws placed between

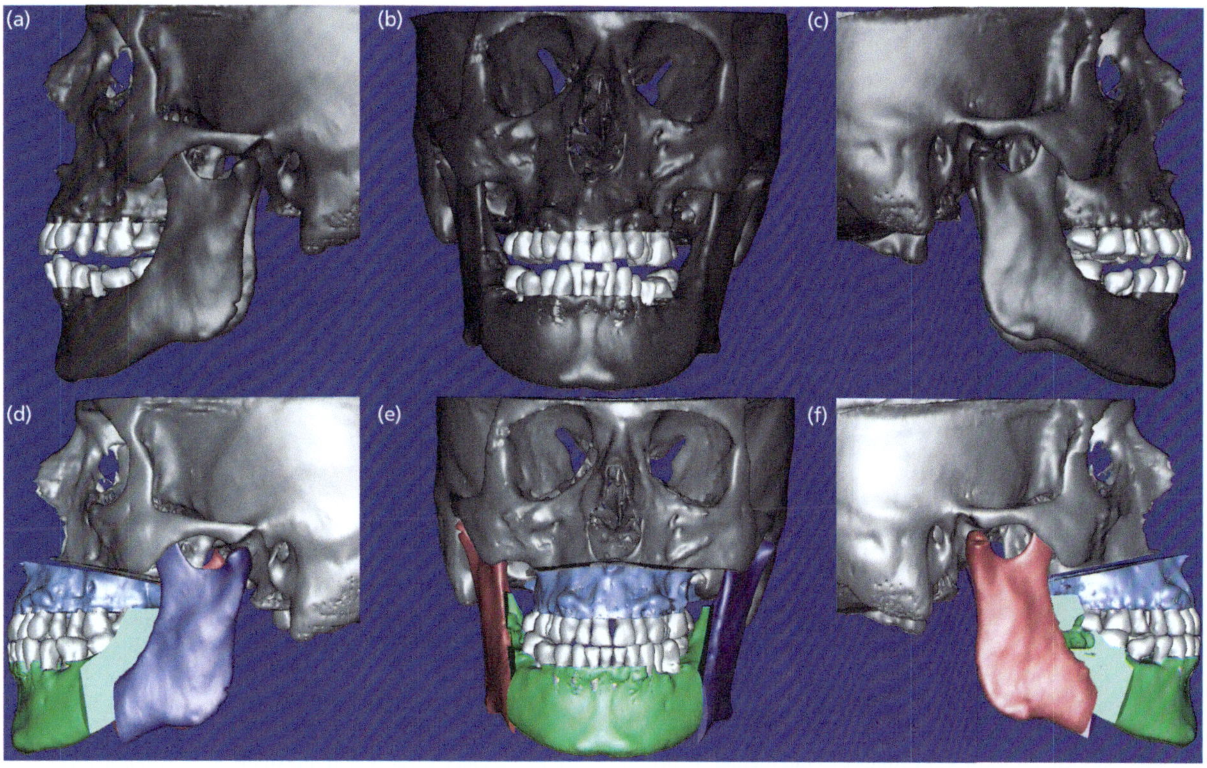

Fig. 42-3 Diagnostic workup: Baseline situation (a, b, c). Virtual orthodontic setup and simulation of surgical osteotomies (c, d, e). In this case, a bimaxillary osteotomy with maxillomandibular advancement and anticlockwise rotation of the occlusal plane with a mandible-first approach was planned.

canines and first bicuspids are enough in cases where the maxilla is not to be segmented. Whenever maxillary segmentation is planned, four additional screws are placed between the second premolars and first molars to aid in transverse and vertical control (Figure 42-4).[28] Finally, optimal control of the postoperative overbite in anterior open bite patients can be achieved by placing two interincisal screws and leaving the front maxillary segment free – in other words, not fixed with osteosynthesis plates (Figure 42-5).

Performance of interdental corticotomies

In addition to the standard maxillary and mandibular osteotomies, interdental corticotomies are executed systematically in order to accelerate postoperative orthodontic movement owing to the RAP.[8,12,30,46] Consistent with the initial phase of this phenomenon, corticotomy-facilitated orthodontics seems to entail a process of localized osteopenia in which the thin layer of bone that overlies the root prominence to be moved

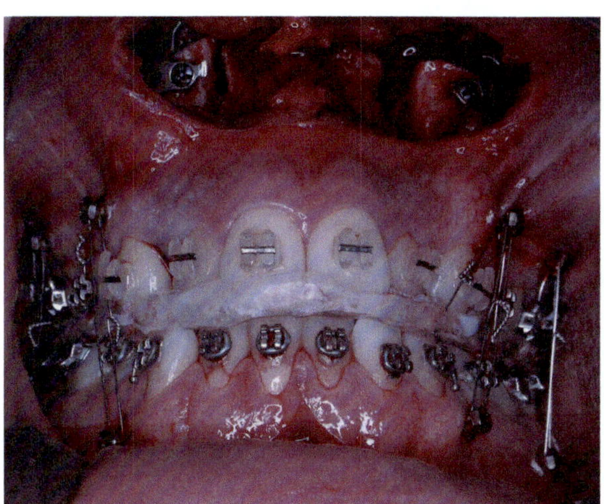

Fig. 42-4 Surgical protocol: Use of temporary anchorage devices (I). Bimaxillary surgery with maxillary segmentation. Use of eight transmucosal 2.0 mm miniscrews for intraoperative intermaxillary fixation and postoperative occlusal control.

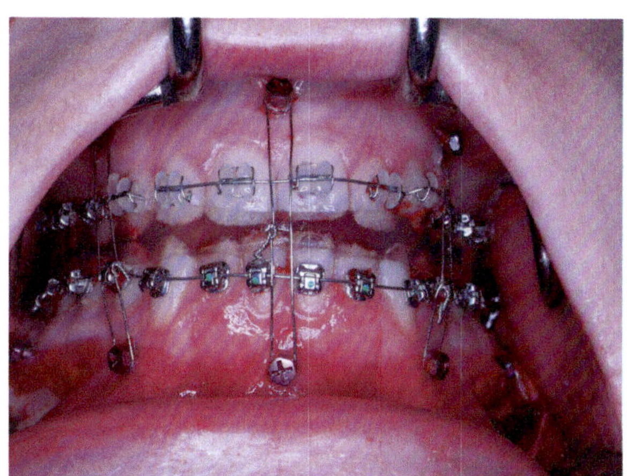

Fig. 42-5 Surgical protocol: Use of temporary anchorage devices (II). Bimaxillary surgery with maxillary segmentation in an extreme open bite case. The front segment of the maxilla was not fixed with osteosynthesis material. Two additional screws were placed between central incisors in order to facilitate postoperative overbite control.

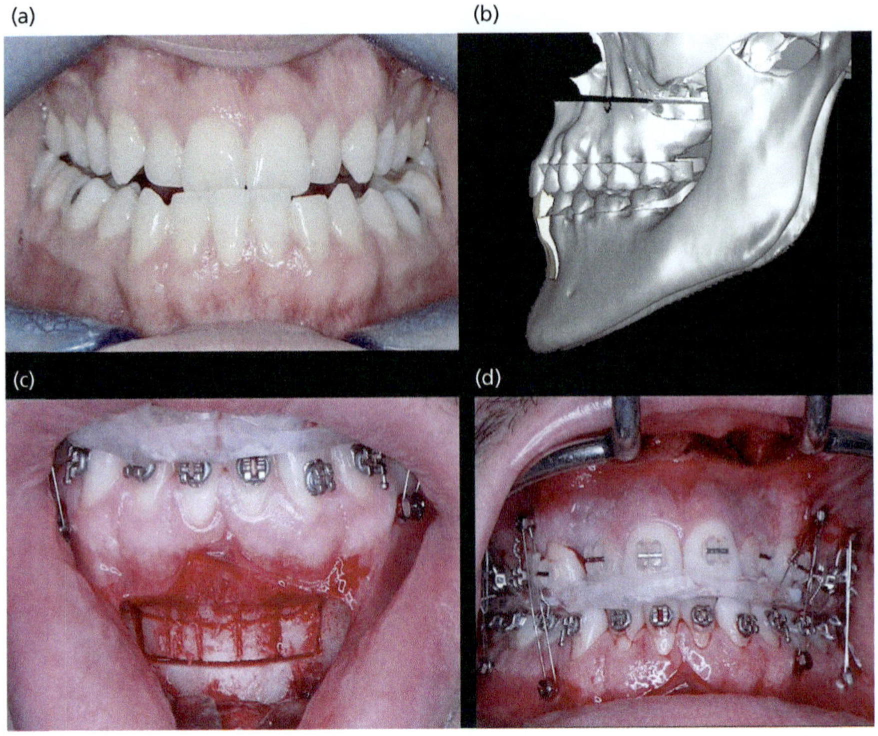

Fig. 42-6 Surgical protocol: Performance of interdental corticotomies (I). Bimaxillary surgery with maxillary segmentation and mandibular anterior segmental dentoalveolar osteotomy for axial decompensation of the anterior mandibular teeth. Preoperative occlusion (a), virtual planning of the mandibular segmental osteotomy (b) and intraoperative view (c). Interdental corticotomies were executed between the anterior mandibular teeth (c). Eight temporary screws were used for transversal and vertical stabilization (d).

demineralizes and later remineralizes at the completion of orthodontic therapy.[13,14]

Technically, these corticotomies are performed between the dental roots following the long axis of the alveolus and stopping just short of the alveolar crest. In order to minimize root damage risk, a piezoelectric saw is preferable.[8,12,15] Corticotomies are extended through the entire thickness of the buccal cortical layer and interrupted when the medullary bone is reached. In other words, the aim is not the creation of box osteotomies as in other treatment modalities,[4,47] but rather strictly to cause selective bone injury such that the biological process of the RAP is activated (Figure 42-6).

If any of the targeted teeth are not accessible through the incision required for the orthognathic procedure itself, a tunnel approach under endoscopic assistance may be used.[8] This tunnel is created subperiosteally through one to three buccal vertical incisions (5 to 10 mm) per arch (Figure 42-7). In trained hands, one single mesial incision allows access to the six anterior teeth, and one single distal incision allows access to the premolars and molars of one quadrant. This reduced access is possible thanks to the angled inserts of the piezoelectric saw and the precise control over corticotomy design and depth permitted by the endoscope.[8]

Elective bone augmentation

With the aim to maximize bone stability and accelerate bone healing, all osteotomy gaps greater than 3 mm should be grafted with bone retrieved from the orthognathic osteotomies and or artificial bone substitutes at the surgeon's preference. This is particularly important in maxillary segmentation and significant anticlockwise rotations (Figure 42-8). Similarly, selected areas with radiologically thin cortical plates or bone dehiscences detected directly or indirectly (under endoscopic assistance through a tunnel

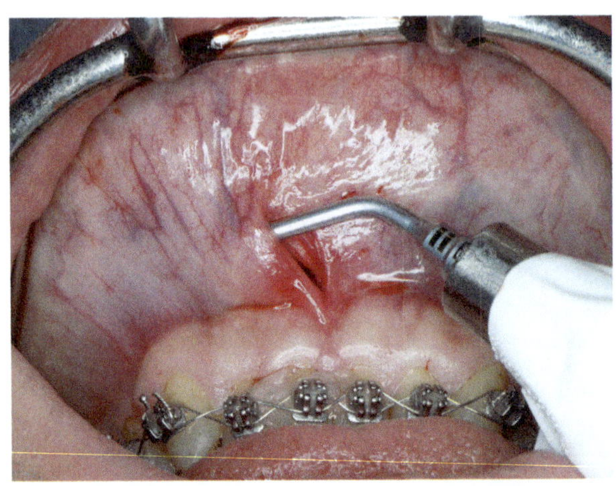

Fig. 42-7 Surgical protocol: Performance of interdental corticotomies (II). Whenever the targeted teeth are not accessible through the incisions required for the orthognathic osteotomies, an endoscopically-assisted tunnel technique may be used. Crown direction serves as an external reference, and endoscopic control permits in situ vision. In this case of mandibular setback, approach to the anterior maxillary teeth was gained through one vertical midline incision.

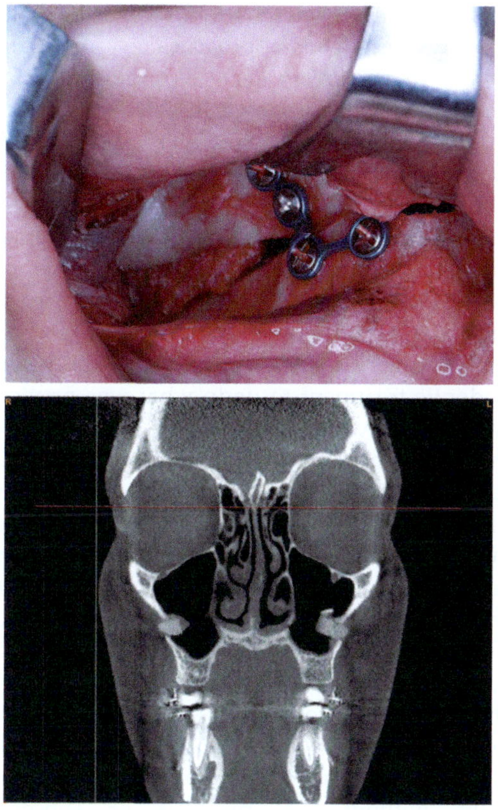

Fig. 42-8 Surgical protocol: Elective bone augmentation through an open approach. Interposition of artificial bone blocks in the posterior osteotomy gap in order to stabilize a significant anticlockwise rotation (top). Postoperative radiological view (bottom).

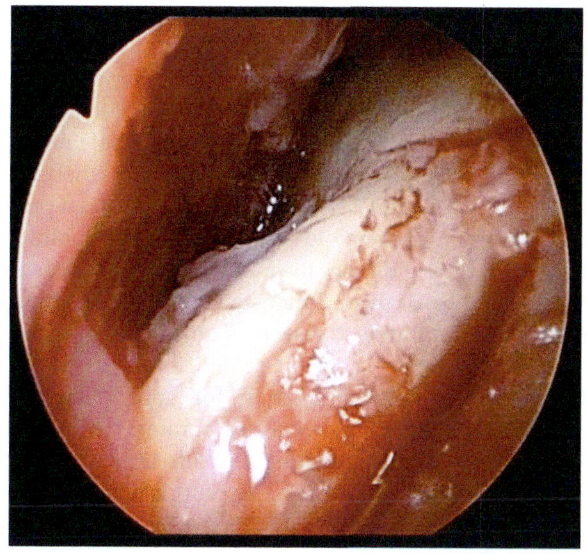

Fig. 42-9 Surgical protocol: Elective bone augmentation through an endoscopically-assisted approach. Bleeding confirms the corticotomy has reached the spongiosa. In this case, a dehiscence of the buccal cortex of the canine was detected, and primary bone augmentation was performed under endoscopic control.

approach) should be grafted prophylactically too (Figure 42-9).

Postoperative splint support

In an attempt to maximize postoperative stability, some authors propose the routine use of an occlusal splint while eating in all *surgery first* cases.[23] Nevertheless, a higher relapse rate has not been documented in comparison to cases managed with a conventional approach.[31,32] After the analysis of a long case series, Hernández-Alfaro and coworkers did not observe greater instability without the routine use of a postoperative splint; only in cases of maxillary segmentation was the end splint ligated with 0.12 mm interdental wire loops and left in place for 2 weeks.[28]

Postoperative orthodontics

In order to benefit from the RAP, orthodontic alignment should begin no later than 2 weeks after surgery. Temporary anchorage devices are especially useful during the first postoperative month, when premature loading of the orthodontic appliances could favor undesirable dental extrusions.[28]

Archwire changes are scheduled every second to third week. Therefore, a close orthodontic follow-up program is absolutely mandatory. In fact, while total treatment time is substantially shorter in comparison to a conventional timing scheme, the average number of orthodontic appointments is quite similar with both approaches.[1,28] Hernández-Alfaro et al. found mean treatment time with a conventional approach was 97.5 weeks versus 45.3 weeks with *surgery first*, but the average number of orthodontic appointments was 29 versus 21, respectively.[1]

Definition of the appropriate timing for surgery

In their retrospective analysis of all orthognathic surgery procedures performed during a three-year time period, Hernández-Alfaro and Guijarro-Martínez realized that a significant number of patients did not fall into a 'black or white' (traditional approach vs. *surgery first* approach) classification.[1] On the contrary, patients were operated on at different moments of the orthodontic treatment timeline. In an attempt to define, justify, and subsequently systematize the appropriate timing for surgical intervention, the authors described the following categories:

1. *Surgery first*
2. *Surgery early*
3. *Surgery late*
4. *Surgery last*
5. *Surgery only*
6. *Surgery never*

The *surgery late* category corresponds to the conventional approach for orthognathic surgery, that is, the traditional sequence of preoperative orthodontics, surgery, and postoperative orthodontics. Despite disadvantages such as prolonged orthodontic treatment times, aesthetic deterioration associated with dental decompensation, or the fact that the date of the intervention is strictly conditioned by the orthodontic treatment, *surgery late* continues to be the most predictable timing scheme to attain occlusal normalization. As such, it should be the method of choice in cases where the final three-dimensional dental position cannot be accurately foreseen or guaranteed, when complex dental movements are anticipated, or when the patient's main motivation for surgery is the achievement of optimal occlusal parameters.[1] Similarly, surgeons or orthodontists with limited experience in orthognathic surgery, surgically assisted orthodontics, or the use of temporary anchorage devices should select this approach.

Patients are selected for a *surgery early* approach when the inclusion criteria for *surgery first* are not completely met, or when candidates for *surgery first* need to delay surgery due to personal logistics. Regarding the first condition, it is often the case that patients with a predominantly aesthetic concern or SDB problem present with severe crowding in need for extractions, midline deviation, or complex three-dimensional dental compensations due to skeletal asymmetry. In these cases, a brief preoperative orthodontic phase takes place before surgery. As soon as most of the necessary space closure after tooth extractions has been completed and transverse compensations are resolved, surgery can proceed; complete levelling and decompensation are not necessary. Another indication for *surgery early* is patients who are candidates for *surgery first* but must postpone surgical intervention due to personal logistics (academic, professional, personal). Until an appropriate date for the surgical appointment is fixed, orthodontic treatment anticipates some dental movements before surgery. In any case, treatment planning, surgery itself and postoperative orthodontic treatment proceed with the same methodology as for *surgery first*. In other words, virtual planning includes both osteotomy simulation plus 3D orthodontic setup; intraoperatively, the regular facial osteotomies are followed by interdental corticotomies in order to further enhance the RAP, and miniscrews are placed for intraoperative intermaxillary fixation and postoperative orthodontic use; orthodontic treatment begins after two postoperative weeks and requires a high degree of technical expertise.[1]

The *surgery last* timing modality comprises patients who refused to orthognathic surgery in the past and underwent compensatory orthodontic treatment that resulted in a stable functional occlusion; at some point, however, they have become aesthetically concerned and made up their minds for surgery. In this situation, two possibilities exist: (1) The occlusion is inappropriate and requires some kind of orthodontic management. In this case, one of the previously described approaches – *surgery first, surgery early* or *surgery late* – is followed; (2) The occlusion is a stable, functional, class I occlusion. In this case, one possibility is to begin with standard decompensation and recuperate the pre-orthodontic maxillomandibular discrepancy for a *surgery late* correction. However, besides the substantial amount of time that this orthodontic retreatment implies, alveolar bone compromise and the risk for root resorption are often strong limiting factors, and many patients are very reluctant to undergo another long orthodontic treatment to undo what was previously accomplished. An alternative is the so-called *surgery last* scheme, where an occlusal plane change is introduced through clockwise or anticlockwise rotation of the maxillomandibular complex – thereby restoring facial harmony – while maintaining the preoperative occlusion. Incorrect dental inclinations from previous orthodontic compensation – in particular, the characteristic overtorqued incisors of compensated Class II and Class III patients – can be hence readjusted. No postoperative orthodontic treatment follows.[1]

A *surgery only* protocol proceeds with surgery directly, without any previous or subsequent orthodontic treatment. The difference with a *surgery last* concept is the fact that in a *surgery only* situation, the patient did not receive any orthodontic treatment in the past either. This approach is strictly limited to three specific scenarios: (1) Patients whose chief complaint is facial aesthetics and who present a stable functional occlusion as confirmed by study models; (2) Partial or total edentulous patients in whom orthodontic treatment would add little or no benefit to the final outcome, and in whom a combined prosthodontic–surgical management is foreseen; and (3) Patients with SDB – often at a stage of obstructive sleep apnoea – and a stable occlusion in whom the therapeutic goal is entirely functional (respiratory), and who cannot or will not undergo additional orthodontic treatment (Figure 42-10). As in the *surgery last* category, surgical planning requires that the preoperative occlusion be maintained. Aesthetic correction and or airway volume increase is achieved through rotational-translational movements of the maxillomandibular complex.

Finally, the *surgery never* group comprises patients with documented dentoskeletal deformities but who never undergo orthognathic surgery and are managed with orthodontics only.

Out of a total number of 362 reported orthognathic procedures, Hernández-Alfaro and Guijarro-Martínez found that the most commonly indicated approach (72%) continued to be *surgery late*, that is, the traditional timing modality.[1] For *surgery first, surgery early* and *surgery last*, the most common motivation for treatment was facial aesthetics, whereas occlusal optimization was the chief objective of patients selected

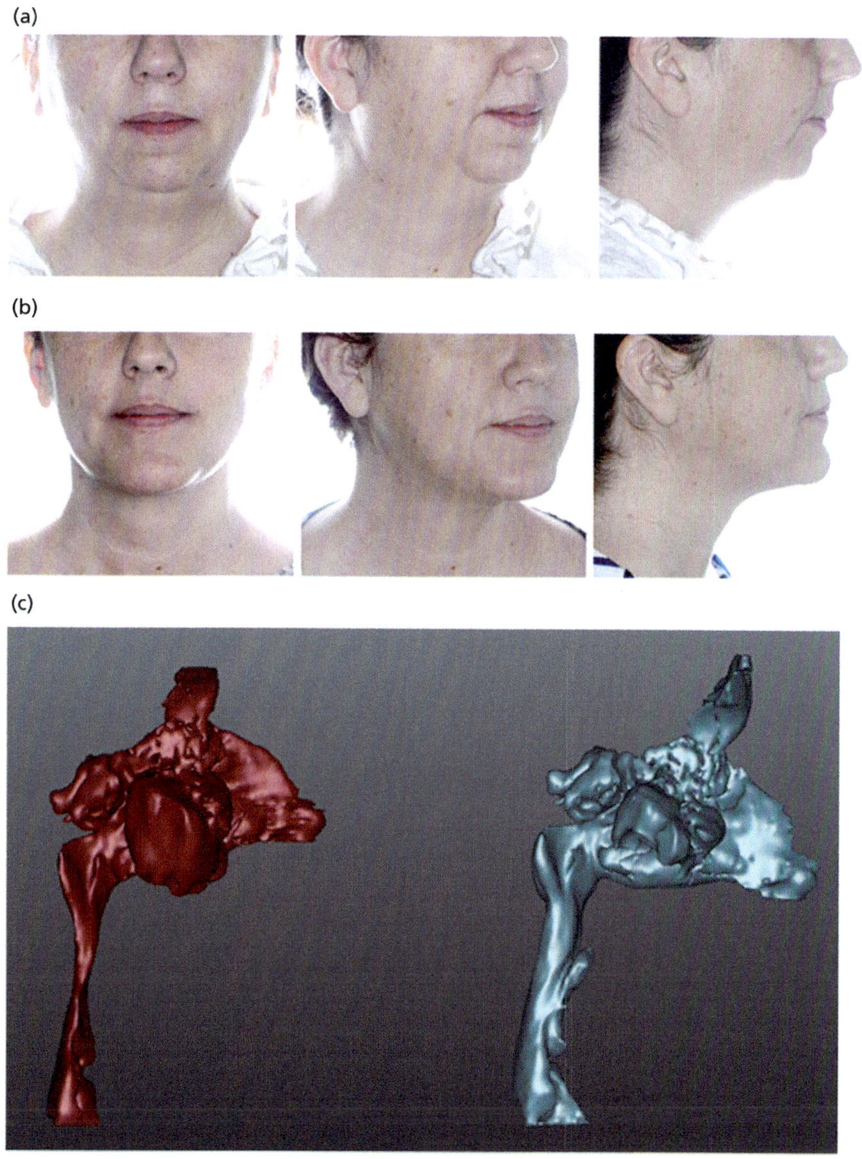

Fig. 42-10 Patient treated with a *surgery only* approach. Preoperative (a) and postoperative (b) clinical pictures. A significant volumetric increase of the airway was achieved with anticlockwise rotation and advancement of the maxillomandibular complex (c), while maintaining the preoperative occlusion.

for a *surgery late* approach. Patients who underwent a *surgery only* scheme sought functional improvement of their SDB, followed closely by aesthetic improvement. Regarding total treatment time, *surgery late* required an average of 38 and 52.2 weeks more of orthodontics than *surgery early* and *surgery first*, respectively. Nevertheless, the total number of orthodontic appointments was similar among the three timing options: 21 for *surgery first*, 28 for *surgery early*, and 29 for *surgery late*.[1]

It is important to highlight the fact that, while a high degree of orthodontic expertise is mandatory for the *surgery first* and *surgery early* timing approaches, the *surgery last* and *surgery only* modalities represent the most demanding surgical scenarios.[1] Skeletal repositioning must be accurate enough to correct the aesthetic or respiratory problem while maintaining the preoperative occlusion intact; any slight surgical inaccuracy or skeletal relapse that might cause an occlusal interference will not be compensated by subsequent orthodontics. Thus, while only expert orthodontists should manage *surgery first* and *surgery early* cases, only expert surgeons should get involved with *surgery last* and *surgery only* protocols.[1]

Figure 42-11 summarizes the characteristics of each of the above-mentioned timing modalities regarding patient motivation, treatment planning, orthodontic and surgical management, and technical particularities. Figure 42-12 displays a simple timing selection algorithm to approach selection.

The orthognathic surgeon of the 21st century should no longer conceive timing for orthognathic surgery as a constant dogma applicable to all patients and all therapeutic contexts invariably. On the contrary, contemporary management of dento-maxillofacial deformity should be based on a comprehensive analysis of various patient-, orthodontist-, and surgeon-specific variables. The ultimate goal should be the achievement of the best possible clinical outcome (in terms of facial aesthetics, occlusion, and airway) while minimizing patient morbidity and economical costs.

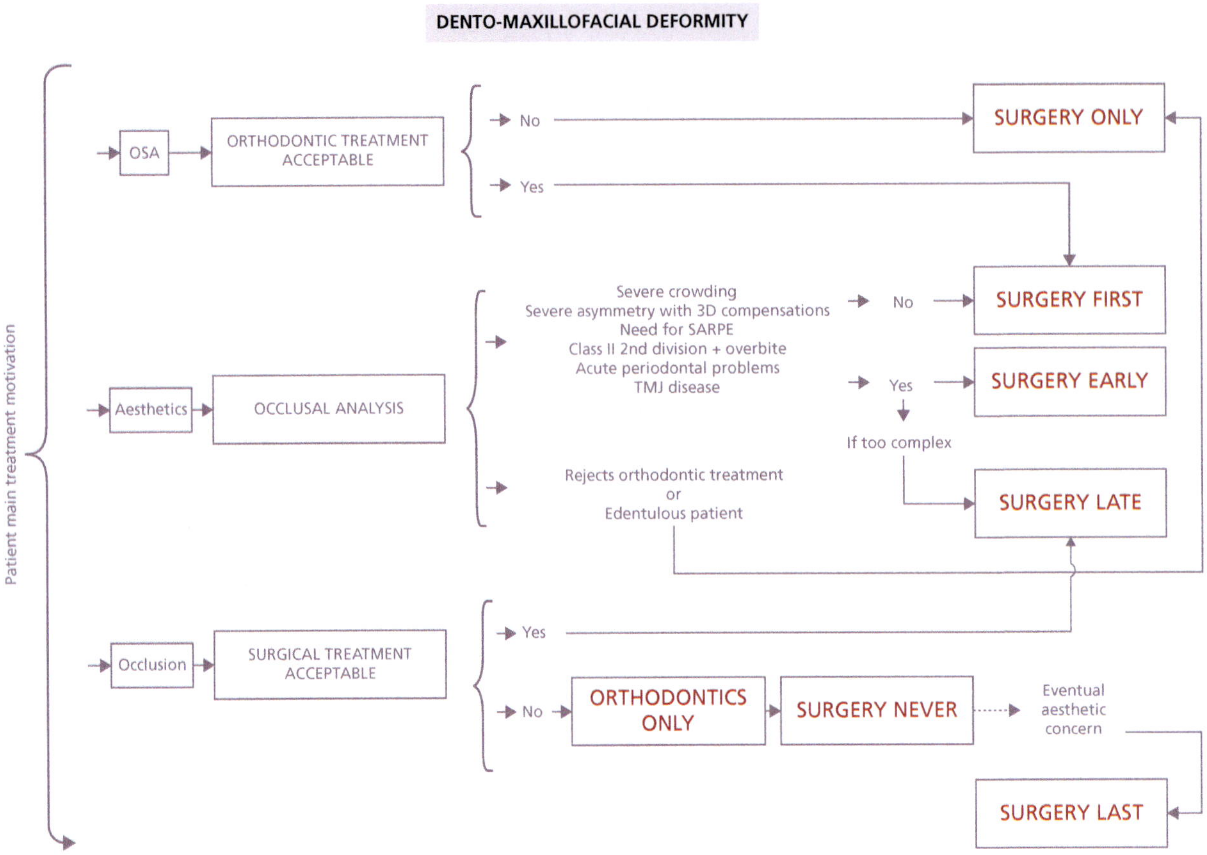

Modified from: Herninder Alfaro F, Guijarro-Martiner R. On a definition of the appropriate timing for surgical intervention in orthognathic surgery. Int J Oral Maxillolac Surg 2014; 43[7]:846-55.

Fig. 42-11 Summary of the characteristics of each of the surgical timing modalities regarding patient motivation, treatment planning, orthodontic and surgical management, and technical particularities.

OSA: Obstructive sleep apnoea
3D: Three dimensional
TAD: Temporary anchoring devices
RAP: Regional acceleratory phenomenon
NA: Not applicable

	Surgery first	Surgery early	Surgery late	Surgery last	Surgery only	Surgery never
Aesthetic motivation	•••	•••	••	•••	•••	—
Occlusal motivation	•	••	•••	—	—	•••
Respiratory motivation [OSA]	•••	•••	—	•••	•••	—
3D virtual orthodontic setup	•••	•••	•	—	—	•
Patient decides timing	•••	••	•	•••	•••	NA
Preoperative orthodontics	—	•	••	•••	—	NA
Use of TAD (miniscrews)	•••	•••	—	•••	•••	•
Corticotomies to increase the RAP	•••	•••	—	—	—	•
Orthodontic complexity	•••	•••	•	NA	NA	•••
Surgical complexity	••	••	•	•••	•••	NA

Modified from: Herninder Alfaro F, Guijarro-Martiner R. On a definition of the appropriate timing for surgical intervention in orthognathic surgery. Int J Oral Maxillolac Surg 2014; 43[7]:846-55.

Fig. 42-12 Timing selection algorithm according to patient-specific variables.

References

1 Hernandez-Alfaro F, Guijarro-Martinez R. On a definition of the appropriate timing for surgical intervention in orthognathic surgery. Int J Oral Maxillofac Surg. 2014;43:846–55.

2 Cangemi CF, Jr. Administration of general anesthesia for outpatient orthognathic surgical procedures. J Oral Maxillofac Surg. 2011;69:798–807.

3 Yao CC, Lai EH, Chang JZ, Chen I, Chen YJ. Comparison of treatment outcomes between skeletal anchorage and extraoral anchorage in adults with maxillary dentoalveolar protrusion. Am J Orthod Dentofacial Orthop. 2008;134:615–24.

4 Chung KR, Kim SH, Lee BS. Speedy surgical-orthodontic treatment with temporary anchorage devices as an alternative to orthognathic surgery. Am J Orthod Dentofacial Orthop. 2009;135:787–98.

5 Mimura H. Treatment of severe bimaxillary protrusion with miniscrew anchorage: treatment and complications. Aust Orthod J. 2008;24:156–63.

6 Upadhyay M, Yadav S, Nanda R. Vertical-dimension control during en-masse retraction with mini-implant anchorage. Am J Orthod Dentofacial Orthop. 2010;138:96–108.

7 Baloul SS, Gerstenfeld LC, Morgan EF, Carvalho RS, Van Dyke TE, Kantarci A. Mechanism of action and morphologic changes in the alveolar bone in response to selective alveolar decortication-facilitated tooth movement. Am J Orthod Dentofacial Orthop. 2011;139(4 Suppl):S83–101.

8 Hernández-Alfaro F, Guijarro-Martínez R. Endoscopically assisted tunnel approach for minimally invasive corticotomies: a preliminary report. J Periodontol. 2012;83:574–80.

9 Iino S, Sakoda S, Ito G, Nishimori T, Ikeda T, Miyawaki S. Acceleration of orthodontic tooth movement by alveolar corticotomy in the dog. Am J Orthod Dentofacial Orthop. 2007;131:448 e1–8.

10 Kim SH, Kim I, Jeong DM, Chung KR, Zadeh H. Corticotomy-assisted decompensation for augmentation of the mandibular anterior ridge. Am J Orthod Dentofacial Orthop. 2011;140:720–31.

11 Sebaoun JD, Kantarci A, Turner JW, Carvalho RS, Van Dyke TE, Ferguson DJ. Modeling of trabecular bone and lamina dura following selective alveolar decortication in rats. J Periodontol. 2008;79:1679–88.

12 Strippoli J, Aknin JJ. Accelerated tooth movement by alveolar corticotomy or piezocision. Orthod Fr. 2012;83:155–64.

13 Wilcko MT, Wilcko WM, Pulver JJ, Bissada NF, Bouquot JE. Accelerated osteogenic orthodontics technique: a 1-stage surgically facilitated rapid orthodontic technique with alveolar augmentation. J Oral Maxillofac Surg. 2009;67:2149–59.

14 Wilcko WM, Wilcko T, Bouquot JE, Ferguson DJ. Rapid orthodontics with alveolar reshaping: two case reports of decrowding. Int J Periodontics Restorative Dent. 2001;21:9–19.

15 Dibart S, Sebaoun JD, Surmenian J. Piezocision: a minimally invasive, periodontally accelerated orthodontic tooth movement procedure. Compend Contin Educ Dent. 2009;30:342–4, 6, 8–50.

16 Hernández-Alfaro F, Guijarro-Martínez R, Molina-Coral A, Badia-Escriche C. "Surgery first" in bimaxillary orthognathic surgery. J Oral Maxillofac Surg. 2011;69:e201–7.

17 Diaz PM, Garcia RG, Gias LN, Aguirre-Jaime A, Perez JS, de la Plata MM, et al. Time used for orthodontic surgical treatment of dentofacial deformities in white patients. J Oral Maxillofac Surg. 2010;68:88–92.

18 Dowling PA, Espeland L, Krogstad O, Stenvik A, Kelly A. Duration of orthodontic treatment involving orthognathic surgery. Int J Adult Orthodon Orthognath Surg. 1999;14:146–52.

19 Luther F, Morris DO, Hart C. Orthodontic preparation for orthognathic surgery: how long does it take and why? A retrospective study. Br J Oral Maxillofac Surg. 2003;41:401–6.

20 Cunningham SJ, Hunt NP, Feinmann C. Perceptions of outcome following orthognathic surgery. Br J Oral Maxillofac Surg. 1996;34:210–3.

21 Flanary CM, Alexander JM. Patient responses to the orthognathic surgical experience: factors leading to dissatisfaction. J Oral Maxillofac Surg. 1983;41:770–4.

22 Nurminen L, Pietila T, Vinkka-Puhakka H. Motivation for and satisfaction with orthodontic–surgical treatment: a retrospective study of 28 patients. Eur J Orthod. 1999;21:79–87.

23 Nagasaka H, Sugawara J, Kawamura H, Nanda R. 'Surgery first' skeletal Class III correction using the Skeletal Anchorage System. J Clin Orthod. 2009;43:97–105.

24 Behrman SJ, Behrman DA. Oral surgeons' considerations in surgical orthodontic treatment. Dent Clin North Am. 1988;32:481–507.

25 Sugawara J, Aymach Z, Nagasaka DH, Kawamura H, Nanda R. 'Surgery first' orthognathics to correct a skeletal class II malocclusion with an impinging bite. J Clin Orthod. 2010;44:429–38.

26 Villegas C, Uribe F, Sugawara J, Nanda R. Expedited correction of significant dentofacial asymmetry using a 'surgery first' approach. J Clin Orthod. 2010;44:97–103.

27 Villegas C, Janakiraman N, Uribe F, Nanda R. Rotation of the maxillomandibular complex to enhance esthetics using a 'surgery first' approach. J Clin Orthod. 2012;46:85–91.

28 Hernández Alfaro F, Guijarro-Martínez R, Peiró-Guijarro MA. Surgery First in Orthognathic Surgery: What have we learned? A Comprehensive Workflow based on 45 Consecutive Cases. J Oral Maxillofac Surg. 2014;72:376–90.

29 Liou EJ, Chen PH, Wang YC, Yu CC, Huang CS, Chen YR. Surgery-first accelerated orthognathic surgery: postoperative rapid orthodontic tooth movement. J Oral Maxillofac Surg. 2011;69:781–5.

30 Sebaoun JD, Ferguson DJ, Wilcko MT, Wilcko WM. Alveolar osteotomy and rapid orthodontic treatments. Orthod Fr. 2007;78:217–25.

31 Ko EW, Hsu SS, Hsieh HY, Wang YC, Huang CS, Chen YR. Comparison of progressive cephalometric changes and postsurgical stability of skeletal Class III correction with and without presurgical orthodontic treatment. J Oral Maxillofac Surg. 2011;69:1469–77.

32 Wang YC, Ko EW, Huang CS, Chen YR, Takano-Yamamoto T. Comparison of transverse dimensional changes in surgical skeletal Class III patients with and without presurgical orthodontics. J Oral Maxillofac Surg. 2010;68:1807–12.

33 Liou EJ, Chen PH, Wang YC, Yu CC, Huang CS, Chen YR. Surgery-first accelerated orthognathic surgery: orthodontic guidelines and setup for model surgery. J Oral Maxillofac Surg. 2011;69:771–80.

34 Hernández Alfaro F, Guijarro-Martínez R. New protocol for three-dimensional surgical planning and CAD/CAM splint generation in orthognathic surgery: an in vitro and in vivo study. Int J Oral Maxillofac Surg. 2013;42:1547–56.

35 Swennen GR, Mollemans W, De Clercq C, Abeloos J, Lamoral P, Lippens F, et al. A cone-beam computed tomography triple scan procedure to obtain a three-dimensional augmented virtual skull model appropriate for orthognathic surgery planning. J Craniofac Surg. 2009;20:297–307.

36 Gateno J, Xia J, Teichgraeber JF, Rosen A. A new technique for the creation of a computerized composite skull model. J Oral Maxillofac Surg. 2003;61:222–7.

37 Nkenke E, Zachow S, Benz M, Maier T, Veit K, Kramer M, et al. Fusion of computed tomography data and optical 3D images of the dentition for streak artefact correction in the simulation of orthognathic surgery. Dentomaxillofac Radiol. 2004;33:226–32.

38 Plooij JM, Maal TJ, Haers P, Borstlap WA, Kuijpers-Jagtman AM, Berge SJ. Digital three-dimensional image fusion processes for planning and evaluating orthodontics and

orthognathic surgery. A systematic review. Int J Oral Maxillofac Surg. 2011;40:341–52.
39 Swennen GR, Barth EL, Eulzer C, Schutyser F. The use of a new 3D splint and double CT scan procedure to obtain an accurate anatomic virtual augmented model of the skull. Int J Oral Maxillofac Surg. 2007;36:146–52.
40 Swennen GR, Mollemans W, Schutyser F. Three-dimensional treatment planning of orthognathic surgery in the era of virtual imaging. J Oral Maxillofac Surg. 2009;67:2080–92.
41 Swennen GR, Mommaerts MY, Abeloos J, De Clercq C, Lamoral P, Neyt N, et al. The use of a wax bite wafer and a double computed tomography scan procedure to obtain a three-dimensional augmented virtual skull model. J Craniofac Surg. 2007;18:533–9.
42 Swennen GR, Mommaerts MY, Abeloos J, De Clercq C, Lamoral P, Neyt N, et al. A cone-beam CT based technique to augment the 3D virtual skull model with a detailed dental surface. Int J Oral Maxillofac Surg. 2009;38:48–57.
43 Swennen GR, Schutyser F. Three-dimensional virtual approach to diagnosis and treatment planning of maxillofacial deformity. In: Bell WH, Guerrero CA (Eds). Distraction osteogenesis of the facial skeleton. Hamilton: BC Decker, 2007, pp. 55–80.
44 Xia J, Samman N, Yeung RW, Shen SG, Wang D, Ip HH, et al. Three-dimensional virtual reality surgical planning and simulation workbench for orthognathic surgery. Int J Adult Orthodon Orthognath Surg. 2000;15:265–82.
45 Xia JJ, Gateno J, Teichgraeber JF. New clinical protocol to evaluate craniomaxillofacial deformity and plan surgical correction. J Oral Maxillofac Surg. 2009;67:2093–106.
46 Frost HM. The biology of fracture healing. An overview for clinicians. Part I. Clin Orthop Relat Res. 1989;248:283–93.
47 Chung KR, Mitsugi M, Lee BS, Kanno T, Lee W, Kim SH. Speedy surgical orthodontic treatment with skeletal anchorage in adults – sagittal correction and open bite correction. J Oral Maxillofac Surg. 2009;67:2130–48.

Chapter 43

Neurosurgical Access Surgery: The Role of the Orthognathic Surgeon

Helen Witherow, Daniel Archer and Simon Stapleton

Introduction

The aim of this chapter is to provide an overview of the main facial osteotomies used to access the skull base. Skull base surgery is a highly specialized multidisciplinary approach that aims to treat a variety of rare benign and malignant lesions involving the base of the skull. The pathology may arise within the skull or brain, metastasize from other regions of the body, or spread directly from the parapharyngeal regions, the nose, sinuses, pharynx or orbits.

Principles and approaches to treating patients with skull base lesions differ from similar pathologies in other areas. The proximity in the brain and skull base to so many vital structures makes traditional en bloc resection of malignant tumours impossible because of unacceptable morbidity,[1] whereas so-called benign pathology can be fatal in the brain and skull base because of the consequences of pressure on these vital structures.

A large number of techniques have evolved using the expertise from a variety of specialties to minimize morbidity, and to preserve function with minimal scarring and deformity. Advances in endoscopic surgery, the operating microscope, intraoperative computer assisted navigation systems, interventional radiology, radiotherapy advances such as intensity modulated radiotherapy, and proton beam treatment have all resulted in fewer open craniofacial access procedures.

The endoscopic approach developed and promoted by the otolaryngological surgeon Carl H. Snyderman in Pittsburg,[2] has advanced skull base surgery significantly, reducing the morbidity frequently associated with many open techniques. Endoscopic approaches are now the main method for treating many lesions within the central areas, such as pituitary tumours. The endoscope is essential for gathering initial diagnostic information and the main method of

Orthognathic Surgery: Principles, Planning and Practice. Edited by Farhad B. Naini and Daljit S. Gill.

treating cerebrospinal fluid (CSF) leaks from the anterior cranial fossa. However, there are times when open resections are still necessary. An endoscopic technique is not appropriate for midline access when tumours invade facial soft tissue or are very vascular. Relative contraindications to endoscopic resection include extension into the orbital apex, or laterally into the infratemporal fossa or lateral pterygomaxillary space.

Choice of the appropriate technique depends on the pathology and the anatomical locations. Having the option to convert to an open approach if necessary is important.

Transfacial access to the skull base and cervical spine involves osteotomies of the mandible, the maxilla and the zygomatic bone, and careful reconstruction and suspension of the soft tissues. A number of techniques used in orthognathic surgery, aesthetic surgery, facial deformity and trauma surgery have been beneficial in developing access to the skull base. The maxillofacial surgeon is in an ideal position to work with the neurosurgeon to provide these access osteotomies.

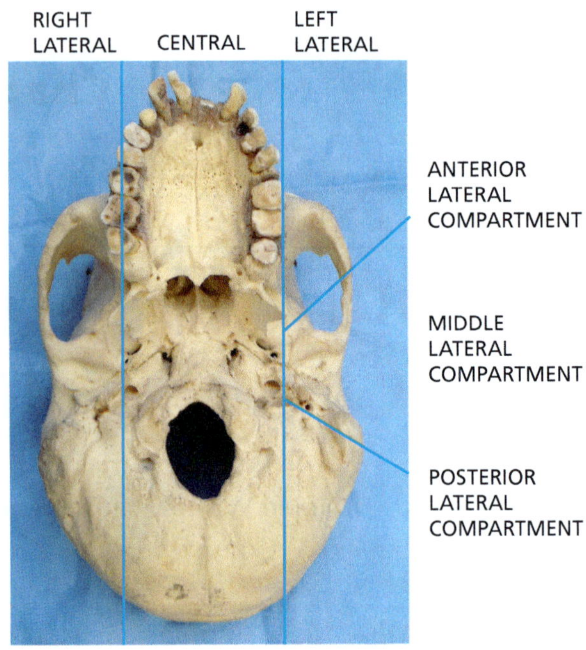

Fig. 43-1 Image showing the three regions for access, central right and left lateral. The lateral compartment is further divided into anterior, middle and posterior.

History of skull base surgery

The fact that such a variety of techniques have been described not only illustrates the difficulty in achieving optimal exposure but also reflects the expertise of interested surgeons within different specialties. In the mid-1980s it was recognized that a collaborative multidisciplinary approach was essential to further develop the specialty. On the 28 May 1992 The British Skull Base Society (BSBS) had its inaugural meeting at The Royal Marsden Hospital in London. It included a multidisciplinary group of clinicians working in the field of skull base surgery, including maxillofacial surgeons, otolaryngologists, and neurosurgeons. The founder members included David Uttley, Richard 'Dick' Haskell, Daniel Archer, Anne Moore, Iain Hutchinson and Tony Bell. The aims of the BSBS were to raise the standards of clinical care in the field of skull base medicine by supporting the coordination of multidisciplinary skull base services in the UK, promoting evidence-based clinical care and encouraging education, training and research.

The European and International meetings were started soon after and had the same objective, i.e. improving patient care by encouraging a collaborative, multidisciplinary approach.

Anatomy of the skull base

The skull base is an anatomically complex area and a comprehensive understanding of the anatomy from different aspects is essential to avoid unacceptable morbidity/mortality and optimize patient care.

Selection of the appropriate technique requires both knowledge of the pathology and the anatomical location.

The skull base

The skull base is divided anatomically into the anterior, middle and posterior skull bases. For access, however, it is divided into a central compartment and a right lateral and left lateral areas separated by the internal carotid as it crosses the temporal bone (Figure 43-1).

Anterior skull base

The anterior skull base contains the frontal lobes and the olfactory bulb. The anterior skull base extends from the posterior wall of the frontal bone, including the posterior wall of the frontal bone, to the anterior clinoid process and the planum sphenoidale, which forms the roof of the sphenoid sinus. The lateral walls are formed by the frontal bone; the floor is mainly formed by the orbital part of the frontal bone, with the ethmoids forming the central part of the floor. The frontal sinus is absent at birth but fairly well developed at age 8 and completed by puberty. It is an important structure as once the posterior wall is breached it poses a potential infection risk. If transected by trauma or by surgery it will need to be 'made safe' by cranialization (removing the posterior wall to allow the brain to expand into the area), removal of all sinus mucosa, and obliteration of the frontonasal ducts.

The cribriform plate lies in the centre and through it pass the olfactory tracts. The roof of the ethmoids, fovea ethmoidalis, is very thin medially and thicker laterally. This is important during transethmoidal approaches to the skull base.

The falx cerebri is attached to the crista galli and the foramen caecum, which communicates drainage from the nose to the superior sagittal sinus, lies anterior to the crista galli.

The optic chiasm lies posteriorly in the midline. The anterior clinoid process forms the roof of the optic canal and is an important landmark for the optic nerve and the supracavernous internal carotid artery.

The anterior skull base communicates inferiorly with the orbits and the paranasal sinuses and can be a route of spread of infection and malignancy.

A number of important structures traverse the posterior aspect of the orbit. The superior orbital fissure transmits the oculomotor, trochlear, abducens, and ophthalmic nerves as well as ophthalmic veins. Medial to this is the optic nerve and the ophthalmic artery. The posterior ethmoidal foramina transmitting the posterior ethmoidal artery is a helpful landmark on the medial wall of the orbit, lying approximately 5 mm anterior to the optic nerve.

Whilst only veins travel through the inferior orbital fissure, the maxillary division of the trigeminal nerve travels through the posterior part. The infraorbital fissure also communicates with the infratemporal fossa.

Middle cranial fossa

The important structures in the middle cranial fossa include the temporal lobe, the pituitary gland, the trigeminal ganglion, the intracranial part of the internal carotid artery, the cavernous sinus (and its contents), and the greater superficial petrosal nerve.

The anterior border of the middle cranial cavity is formed by the greater wing of the sphenoid and above it the lesser wing. The posterior wall is the clivus which is made up of the occipital bone and the sphenoid.

The clivus extends from the foramen magnum to the sphenoid sinus and it represents a surgically safe unit between the carotid artery, rostral and caudal.

The lateral wall of the middle cranial fossa is made up of the sphenoid bone. The anterior part of the floor is made up of the greater wing of the sphenoid and the posterior part, the petrous temporal bone. The central part of the middle cranial fossa formed by the body of the sphenoid makes up the sella turcica. The sella turcica is made up of three parts: anteriorly the tuberculum sellae, posteriorly is the pituitary fossa and behind that the dorsum sellae. The internal carotid artery crosses the petrous apex through the cavernous sinus lying in the sigmoid groove.

The floor and the lateral wall of the middle cranial fossa are grooved by the middle meningeal artery. At a point where four bones fuse (frontal bone, the greater wing of the sphenoid, the squamous temporal bone and the parietal bone) the pterion is formed. This bone is thin and if fractured can lead to injury to the middle meningeal artery. Anterior to the pterion a bur hole is made for the temporal craniotomy which exposes the Sylvian fissure allowing access to the middle cranial fossa.

Posteriorly a longitudinal groove runs in the petrous ridge of the temporal bone. It represents the petrosal sinus. The trigeminal ganglion lies in Meckel's cave at the most anterior and medial part of the sinus. This lies just above the point at which the internal carotid enters the cavernous sinus.

Posteriorly and laterally lies the arcuate eminence demonstrating the superior extent of the semicircular canal. It is an important landmark during the middle cranial fossa approach for finding the internal auditory canal. Lateral to the arcuate eminence the tegmen tympani and tegmen mastoideum cover the middle ear. The tegmen is very thin and separates the dura from the middle ear and the mastoid cavity.

Anterior to the middle cranial fossa lies the posterolateral wall of the maxillary sinus and laterally lies the infratemporal fossa.

Anatomy of the infratemporal fossa

The posterior wall of the maxillary sinus forms the anterior border, the inferior border is the parapharyngeal space, the lateral border the mandible, the medial border the lateral pterygoid plate, the roof the greater wing of the sphenoid and the posterior wall the styloid, the carotid sheath and the condyle. The muscles within the infratemporal fossa include the temporalis, and the medial and lateral pterygoid. The blood supply to these muscles comes from the maxillary artery, which should be preserved if at all possible. The deep lobe of the parotid gland also lies within the infratemporal fossa.

At the most anterior part of the pterygoid plate lies the pterygomaxillary fissure. The maxillary artery lies high up in the fissure (at least 1.5 cm above the inferior edge of the pterygoid plate). The maxillary division of the trigeminal nerve enters through the foramen rotundum. An important landmark of the foramen rotundum is the root of the lateral pterygoid plate. The foramen ovale lies immediately posterior, and further posteriorly the foramen spinosum.

The internal carotid artery ascends vertically and medial to the sphenoid spine and enters the middle cranial fossa.

Medially to the middle cranial fossa lies the sphenoid sinus. The sphenoid sinus is a safe and useful means by which to access to the pituitary, and below its floor is the clivus. It is important not to breach the lateral wall as both the optic nerve and the internal carotid are situated there.

Posterior skull base

The bones of the posterior skull base consist mainly of the occipital bone, together with the sphenoid and the temporal bone. The central area forms the clivus in the midline.

The posterior skull base contains the midbrain, the pons, the medulla and the cerebral hemispheres. The superior sagittal sinus, transverse, sigmoid and inferior petrosal sinuses groove the floor.

The internal auditory canal transmits the VII and VIII nerves and the nervus intermedius.

The jugular foramen transmits the cranial nerves IX, X and XI. The hypoglossal nerve travels through the hypoglossal foramen that lies medial to the jugular foramen.

The following structures traverse the foramen magnum: the medulla oblongata, part of the ligament of the dens and tectorial ligament, the spinal accessory nerve, the vertebral and posterior spinal arteries.

Access to the posterior skull base lies with the neurosurgical team; however, the maxillofacial surgeon may be involved with access anterior to the brainstem via a central approach.

Pathology

It is not within the scope of this book chapter to give a comprehensive description of the pathologies treated in skull base surgery. However, the most frequent lesions still requiring access osteotomies with a maxillofacial surgeon and neurosurgeon are sphenoid wing meningiomas, chordomas, the relatively benign chondrosarcomas, granulomas, giant cell tumours, anterior skull based trauma involving the frontal sinus orbital roof and nasoethmoidal injuries, upper cervical spine pathologies, malignant tumours (primary and secondary), those invading from the paranasal sinuses, orbits and naso and oropharynx.

Acoustic neuromas are usually treated by the neurosurgeon and the otolaryngologist, as are the pituitary tumours, paragangliomas and the anterior skull base CSF leaks.

Aneurysms and other vascular malformations are usually treated by interventional radiologists with the neurosurgeon.

However, as stressed previously, optimal patient care requires the ability to convert a closed to an open technique if it becomes necessary. This can only be offered in a multidisciplinary setting with excellent communication and with access to all the necessary specialties.

Access osteotomies

The central compartment contains the sphenoid, clivus, and upper cervical spine, whilst the lateral compartment consists of part of the greater wing of the sphenoid, the inferior part of the petrous temporal bone (the infratemporal fossa) and the posterior fossa. The lateral compartments can also be separated into anterior, middle and posterior parts. The middle segment contains the internal acoustic meatus and canal for the internal carotid and the posterior segment contains the foramen magnum, the jugular foramen and the internal jugular vein. Neither the middle nor the posterior regions are accessed transfacially. The central compartment is accessed via the mouth, and the lateral compartment extraorally. A variety of osteotomies based on this approach can be used to resect more extensive tumours.

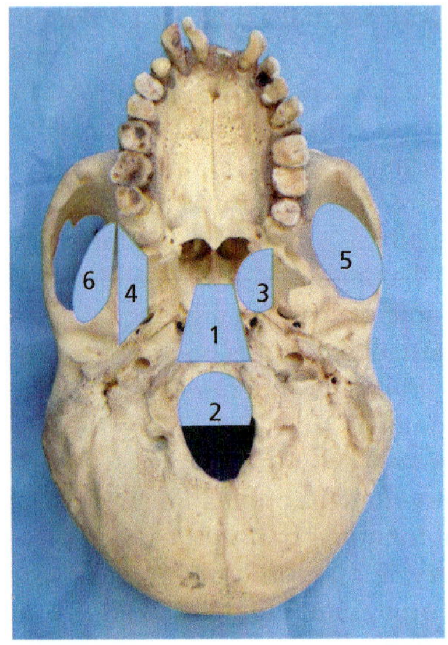

Fig. 43-2 Diagram showing the anatomical regions required to be accessed in the skull base

A number of osteotomies in the past have involved division of the hard and soft palate. These are often associated with palatal dysfunction, nasopharyngeal regurgitation and speech problems. It is possible to avoid this technique and therefore for that reason we would advise that they are not used.

For the same reason access via the facial degloving technique will not be discussed as it has significant effects on facial and nasal growth.

The regions within the skull base that require access osteotomies are shown in Figure 43-2 and the osteotomies most suitable to reach these areas are listed in Table 43-1.

Table 43-1 The most suitable open access methods to reach the following skull base regions

Clivus/sphenoid	Le Fort I, hemimaxillotomy
Upper cervical spine	Soft palate retraction ± palatal split, parasagittal mandibulotomy
Medial pterygoid retromaxillary space	Parasagittal mandibulotomy, parasagittal mandibulotomy with cervical extension, zygomaticotemporal with hemimaxillotomy
Lateral pterygoid retromaxillary space	Zygomaticotemporal, zygomaticotemporal with hemimaxillectomy, parasagittal mandibulotomy with cervical extension
Infratemporal fossa	Zygomaticotemporal (with cervical control of vessels), zygomaticotemporal with hemimaxillectomy
Middle cranial fossa	Zygomaticotemporal
Anterior cranial fossa/orbital roof/anterior cranial fossa CSF leaks/frontal sinus problems	Anterior craniotomy ± removal of superior bar

Access to the anterior cranial base is achieved by anterior craniotomy and removal of the supraorbital bar. This is discussed later.

General techniques

Coronal flap

The coronal flap is the 'workhorse' of neurosurgery and provides excellent access to the zygomatic arches, frontal and supraorbital bar, orbits and glabellar region. Two specific complications from raising the flap may occur and these are techniques specific. The first is damage to the frontal branch of the facial nerve. The frontal branch of the facial nerve supplies the frontalis muscle and is responsible for elevating the brow. In elderly patients this function is particularly important in preventing eyebrow ptosis. Severe ptosis can result in visual problems and will need to be corrected. The second complication is temporal hollowing. This is an aesthetic rather than a functional problem. The theories of why it occurs include:

1. Damage and atrophy to the temporalis muscle.
2. Atrophy of the fat pad that separates the superficial and deep layers of the deep temporal fascia.
3. Failure to adequately suspend the deep temporal fascia when it has been divided.

It is likely that all three contribute to the temporal hollowing, but the third reason, failure to correctly suspend the deep temporal fascia, is probably the most important.

Incision: There are a number of possible designs of the coronal incision (Figure 43-3). These depend on whether the patient has hair or is likely to lose it. An incision can be made posteriorly, which is useful in patients likely to go bald, but it is technically more time consuming as elevating the flap sufficient to access the nasoethmoidal region and the lateral walls of the orbit is more difficult. Tessier's manoeuvre, a vertical incision through the pericranium and galea in the region of the glabella, can help gain access to the nasoethmoidal region.

A straight incision from one preauricular region to the other following the hairline anteriorly is the most basic and offers direct access to the frontal bone.

The Stealth incision[3] is designed to help localization when closing the incision. However, the sharp points sometimes necrose. The wavy line allows good localization and also prevents the incision becoming obvious when the hair gets wet as it does not part in a straight line. It is not necessary to shave the hair. The hair can be kept out of the incision by careful platting or tying small bunches of hair with rubber bands.

Damage to the frontal branch of the facial nerve can be avoided by knowledge of the anatomy as the nerve travels across the zygomatic arch to supply frontalis. This is shown in Figure 43-4 and demonstrates where the nerve is most at risk. Pitanguy's line travels from approximately 0.5 cm below the tragus of the ear crossing the zygomatic arch to reach the frontalis muscle at a maximum of 1.5 cm above the lateral aspect of the orbit. The nerve travels in the temporoparietal fascia (superficial temporal fascia), just superficial to the superficial layer of the deep temporal fascia. The superficial and deep layers of the deep temporal fascia are fused approximately 1.5 cm above the zygomatic arch; below this they are separated by a fat pad.

The Bramley-Al-Khayat manoeuvre (Figure 43-5) is designed to preserve the frontal branch.[4]

Sharp dissection is undertaken down to the root of the zygoma close to the preauricular region. Once subperiosteal, dissection along the arch is safe within the fat pad, which lies between the superficial and deep layers of the deep temporal fascia. The incision through the superficial part of the deep temporal fascia is made at 45 degrees to the arch and is elevated to approximately 1.5 cm above the supraorbital ridge. It is important to be subperiosteally in this area as the

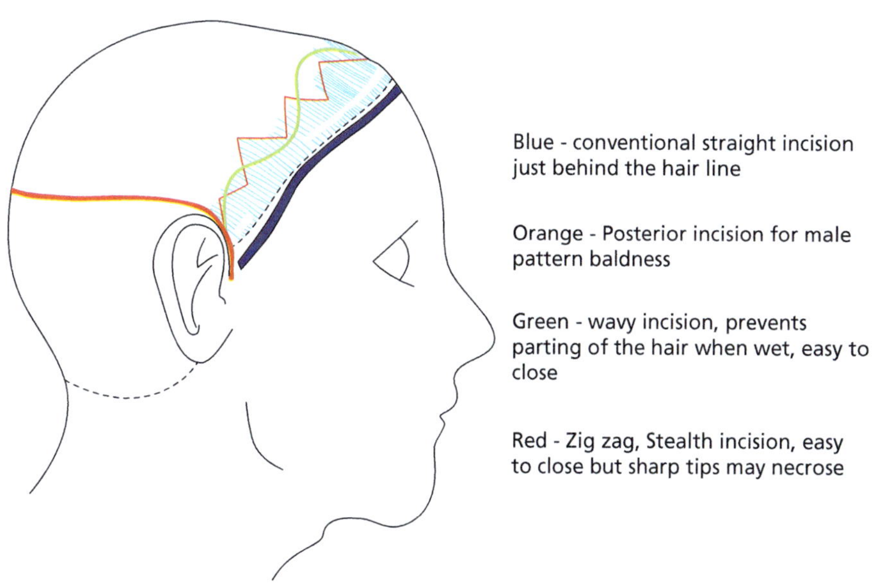

Fig. 43-3 Diagram showing some of the possible designs of the coronal incision.

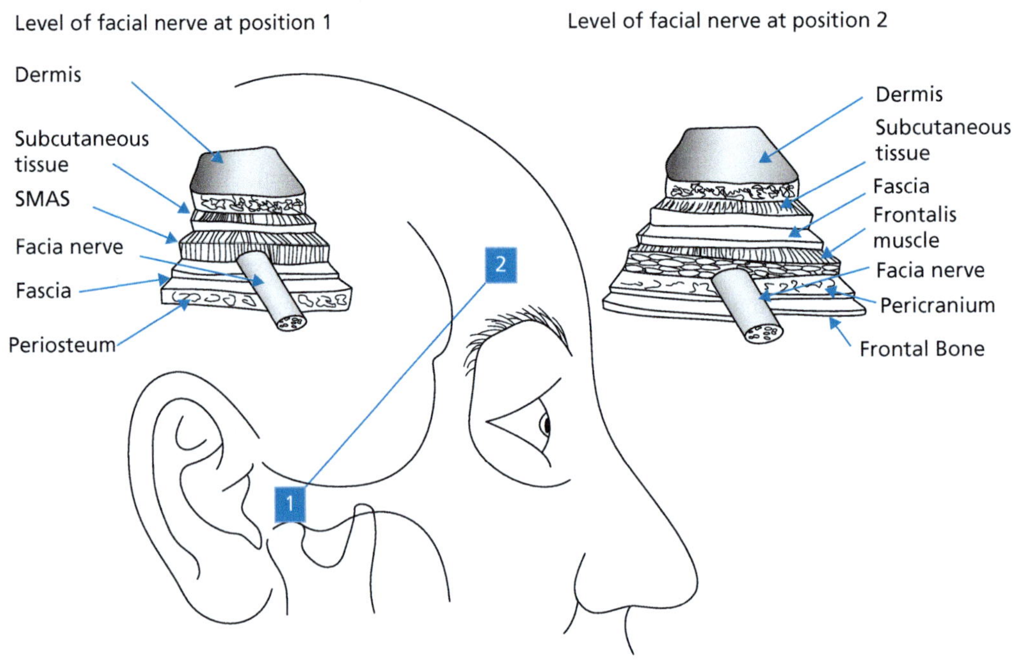

Fig. 43-4 The Pitanguy line demonstrates the position of the frontal branch of the facial nerve as it crosses the zygomatic arch, 0.3 cm in front of the tragus and 1.5cm above the supraorbital ridge, and travels cranially to supply the frontalis muscle.

frontal branch is deep to the frontalis and superficial to the pericranium. It is easy to damage the nerve again at this point by incising through the pericranium and damaging it just where it is just superficial to the pericranium The dissection proceeds subperiosteally to expose the zygomatic arch and the lateral wall of the orbit. It is essential to suspend the divided superficial part of the deep temporal fascia when closing the coronal flap as failure will cause temporal hollowing.

Calvarial bone grafts

Frequently full thickness defects in the calvarium occur when tumors are removed. The dura itself is osteogenic up until the age of 2 years and therefore defects before this age often form new bone.

In adults the defects can be replaced with allogeneic or alloplastic material. However, in young children it is preferable to use bone as their bones are still growing.

Techniques to split calvarial bone are commonly used. The easiest is to take the full thickness craniotomy and remove the inner table. This can be done with fine burs and fine saws. An alternate technique is to use the outer table of the cranium, avoiding the midline because of the possible damage to the sagittal sinus, the pterion, as the middle meningeal artery is at risk, and the sutures as the bone may fracture unpredictably in this area.

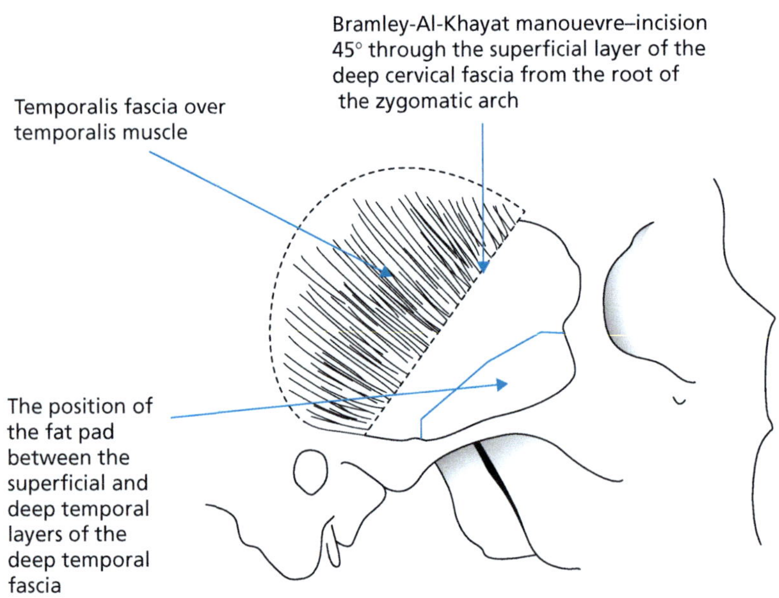

Fig. 43-5 Bramley-Al-Khayat manoeuvre to preserve the frontal branch of the facial nerve

Access to the anterior part of the anterior cranial base and treatment of the frontal sinus (removal of the frontal bandeau/frontal bar)

This technique can be used to improve access to remove tumours involving the frontal region particularly where access to the orbital roof/access to transcranial dermoids or repair of defects of the anterior part of the anterior cranial base is required. It is also necessary sometimes with trauma involving the frontal sinus.

It should be noted that the traditional view of treating frontal sinus trauma has changed over the last few years. The traditional teaching was that if the posterior wall of the frontal sinus was displaced greater than the thickness of the posterior wall then the sinus should be cranialized to 'keep the sinus safe'. This view was based on a paper published in 1990 where a predicted risk of serious life threatening complications was over 80% over a 10-year period.[5] However, large recent studies have demonstrated a more conservative approach is more appropriate.[6] Cranialization is only indicated when there is severe displacement of the posterior wall, persistent CSF leak or where there are other indications for open surgery. The complications of an anterior craniotomy and cranialization include frontal lobe retraction, anosmia and CSF leak, and should be balanced with the benefits.

Technique

Infiltration of the subcutaneous tissue with local anesthetic and adrenaline is performed. The standard coronal approach is used. An anterior based pericranial flap is raised as this may be required to repair a defect in the floor or line the frontal sinus.

The coronal flap is elevated anteriorly and the supraorbital and supratrochlear nerves either lifted out of the grooves in the supraorbital rim or elevated after small osteotomies are performed to the foramen. Dissection is continued over the orbital rim. It is important to stay in the subperiosteal plane to prevent damage to the orbital contents. Subperiosteal stripping below the trochlea on the medial aspect of the orbit roof prevents damage to the trochlea which reattaches after the coronal flap is closed. Continued dissection laterally within the orbit is possible as far as the infraorbital margin and infraorbital fissure. Care must be taken to identify and coagulate two small zygomatic vessel on the lateral wall of the orbit using bipolar diathermy.

Medially dissection should continue in a subperiosteal plane. It is often difficult to dissect over the frontonasal suture. A vertical incision through the pericranium and galea in this area can help turn down the flap (Tessier's manoeuvre) over the bridge of the nose. The bicoronal flap cannot be mobilized inferiorly any further because of the attachments of the medial canthal ligaments. Partial stripping of the anterior canthal ligament is possible; however, the posterior ligament which attached to the posterior lacrimal crest should not be removed. Care should also be taken not to damage the nasolacrimal sac lying between the anterior and posterior lacrimal crests.

An anterior craniotomy is performed, the dura elevated and the frontal lobes retracted and protected.

It is then possible to design an osteotomy to give optimal access to the roof of the orbits. The osteotomy is pre-plated to facilitate accurate repositioning. The bone is replaced as a free bone graft and rarely causes problems in terms of vascularity. It is however essential to make the frontal sinus safe if it is present. This involves cranializing the sinus, removing the posterior wall of the frontal sinus, removing the mucosa of the sinus, obliterating the frontal duct with bone, laying the pericranial flap over the frontal sinus, and allowing the brain to expand into the area. Failure to do this may lead to an unsafe sinus, and complications such as infection and mucocele development.

Access to the central compartment

The central compartment can be reached through the nose, (endoscopically), via the Le Fort I downfracture osteotomy, transorally with or without soft palate retraction and mandibular split osteotomy.[7] Splitting the maxilla and soft palate gives excellent access but in some cases unacceptable problems with swallowing.

A transoral approach by extending the head and retracting the soft palate with rubber catheters will allow access to the lower $^1/_3$ of the clivus in the midline to C1/2. One of the advantages is that it is extradural. The Le Fort I approach will enable good access to be gained to the sphenoid sinus and upper and middle clivus, but it is difficult to get to C2 easily.

The Le Fort I approach with submental intubation will enable a further 1 cm inferior displacement of the maxilla to enable access to C2 (refer to submental intubation section in Chapter 22).

Splitting the hard and soft palate should be avoided because of the possible long term morbidity/swallowing problems and nasopharyngeal incompetence. If divided, the soft palate should be divided with a lazy S-incision to one side of the uvula to reduce the risk of scarring and shortening of the soft palate, which may lead to velopharyngeal incompetence. If the maxilla is divided, the posterior pharyngeal wall can be divided from the posterior wall of the vomer to the arytenoid cartilages.

However, access to C1/2–C4 anteriorly can also be achieved by lip split and mandibulotomy division, which has fewer functional problems than splitting the maxilla vertically.

The Le Fort I osteotomy

Using this technique the superior limit of the access is to the ethmoid and sphenoid sinus, moving inferiorly the clivus and foramen magnum to the arch of the atlas. The use of the submental intubation technique (see Chapter 22 for full description) allows a little more inferior access.

The Le Fort I osteotomy is well known in orthognathic surgery, and its historical development has been described in Chapter 2. Archer described its use in treating basilar aneurysms.[9]

It has been adapted for access to the central compartment.[10–12] The standard Le Fort I osteotomy is modified by removal of the medial walls of the sinus, lateral nasal walls, turbinates and the inferior part of the nasal septum. The cleft palate/Dingman retractor was modified by Archer and provides good retraction to allow access to the central compartment.

The types of pathology that are treated include benign and malignant tumors, including meningiomas, chordomas, gliomas, craniospinal malformations, and degenerative diseases of the upper cervical spine including dislocation of the upper cervical vertebrae.

Technique

Local anaesthetic is infiltrated into the buccal mucosa. Pre-plating of the piriform aperture with adapted 2 mm plates is undertaken to ensure rapid, accurate repositioning of the maxilla. An osteotomy is performed in the traditional manner (see Chapter 22). The maxilla is downfractured, and the nasal mucosa is removed to expose the septum. The inferior turbinates need to be removed to improve access. Their blood supply enters distally and the use of the monopolar or bipolar diathermy is useful prior to their resection. The cartilaginous septum is not reduced. The inferior part of the vomerine septum is removed. The vomerine rostrum (*Latin* 'rostrum': beak) is preserved as this almost invariably is in the midline and marks the inferior extent of the sphenoid sinus. Caudal to this is the clivus.

The modified cleft palate gag is placed to produce access to the central part of the clivus and sphenoid. The superior flanges of the retractor should be positioned on the thick bone of the zygomatic buttress to prevent fracture of the maxillary bone. The inferior flanges are placed on the superior aspect of the palate. The lateral retractors abduct the cheeks. It is important not to trap the lip or tongue when the gag is opened. The posterior pharyngeal wall is incised down to bone vertically and the soft tissues elevated. Long pharyngeal retractors are placed to retract the soft tissue of the pharyngeal wall. The central region is the safe surgical area. However, the Eustachian tube openings are present superiorly either side of the midline and should be avoided. The internal carotid artery runs vertically, lateral to the Eustachian tubes.

Closure of the posterior pharyngeal wall can be technically challenging. However, the use of a J-shaped needle (W9437 4 0 Coated Vicryl suture/Ethicon) and long needle holders and a Negus suture instrument is helpful.

The maxilla is replaced with the pre-plated plates and screws and the buccal incisions closed with resorbable sutures.

The pharyngeal wound should be protected for the first 48 hours; after that a soft diet is advised for a further 4 weeks. A broad-spectrum antibiotic is given intravenously perioperatively, and orally for 5 days postoperatively.

Transmandibular approach to the central compartment

This is a useful technique that increases access centrally to the base of the clivus to the arytenoid cartilage.[7] The tongue can be divided to give slightly better access; however, this is not essential as the tongue can be displaced inferiorly through the osteotomy cut. Wide access can be achieved by using the Archer modified cleft palate gag.

Initial thought should be given as to whether a tracheostomy will be necessary. If significant floor of mouth dissection is needed and tongue division then it may be advisable. However, if access can be achieved without this, i.e. with lip split mandibulotomy and minimal floor of mouth dissection, then oral intubation alone will be adequate. The oral tube can be displaced inferiorly with the tongue to prevent it impeding access.

A number of different incisions may be used to achieve a good aesthetic result following the lip split. It is essential that the vermillion border is accurately relocated at the end of the procedure. A midline full thickness incision is made including a notch for relocation (Figure 43-6). The incision can be made straight

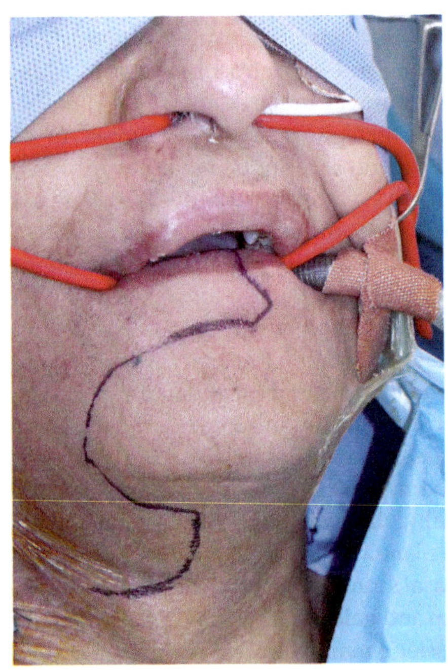

Fig. 43-6 Transmandibular approach to the central compartment. Foley catheters placed to retract the soft palate. Skin incisions are marked.

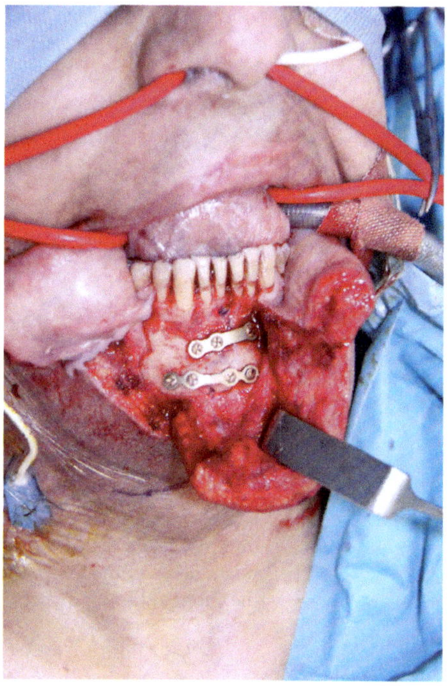

Fig. 43-7 Pre-plating of the mandible with 2mm plates and 4mm screws. The incision through the mucosa is not at the same level as the saw cut.

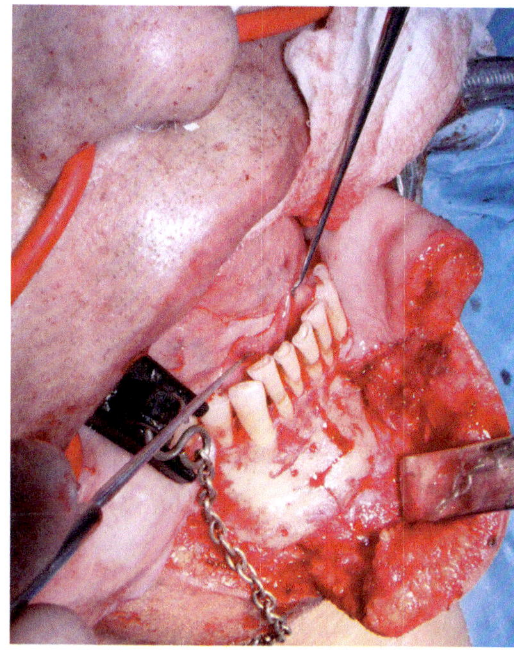

Fig. 43-8 Stepped osteotomy cut. Cuts through the bone are made with a fine saw and fine osteotome. A stepped incision improves stability. The lingual mucosa is carefully elevated prior to the bony cut.

across the chin or around it. The incision continues over the mandible to the hyoid and in an appropriate relaxation skin tension line continues laterally across the neck. The incision should be at least 2 cm below the lower border of the mandible to protect the marginal mandibular branch of the facial nerve. The platysma is divided, and the submandibular gland and muscles of the floor of the mouth exposed. If control of the major vessels of the neck inferiorly is necessary the sternomastoid muscle is retracted and the jugular, internal and external carotids are identified and loops passed round them.

An incision is made through the gingivae in a stepped manner such that the closure of the mucosa is at a different level to the bony cut. This ensures that if the wound breaks down the plates and the osteotomy line are not exposed.

The osteotomy cut is pre-plated with two miniplates to helps relocation (Figure 43-7). A step in the bone below the level of the incisor apices helps relocation and stability (Figure 43-8). Division of the bone between the incisors can be done using a fine bur through the cortex buccally and fine osteotomes between the teeth to complete the cut.

Division of the floor of the mouth can either be in the midline between the two submandibular duct orifices and if necessary continued through the tongue centrally (which is relatively avascular), or division can be extended laterally (Figure 43-9). The incision is lateral to the submandibular ducts and medial to the submandibular gland. It is important to preserve the lingual nerve that crosses the submandibular duct at the level of the first molar tooth.

The mandible can be carefully separated widely, the endotracheal tube displaced inferiorly through the mandible and carefully secured. The endotracheal tube can be wired to the inferior border of the mandible or sutured to the skin. Whichever technique is used the tube must be secured well as accidental extubation may lead to an avoidable fatality.

The Archer or other modified cleft palate gag is placed so that the tip of the epiglottis is retracted. Additional retraction of the soft palate with rubber catheters provides further access superiorly. Thus access from the base of the clivus to C3/4 can be achieved through a vertical incision in the midline through the pharyngeal muscles. The periosteum on the clivus can be elevated laterally as far as the paraclival gutters. This protects the internal carotids and associated cranial nerves.

The incisions are closed carefully. Meticulous haemostasis is essential particularly if a tracheostomy has not been performed. Closure of the floor of the mouth should be undertaken with a few interrupted sutures to allow any blood to drain. The mandible is plated with the preformed plates and the gingivae and lip sutured. Drains are placed and a nasogastric tube placed to aid postoperative feeding. This must be secured well as replacement later can be difficult and can cause damage to the repaired posterior pharyngeal wall. The posterior pharyngeal wall should be protected by gastric feeding and good oral hygiene and chlorhexidine mouth washes should be maintained.

With careful closure a satisfactory cosmetic result should be achieved.

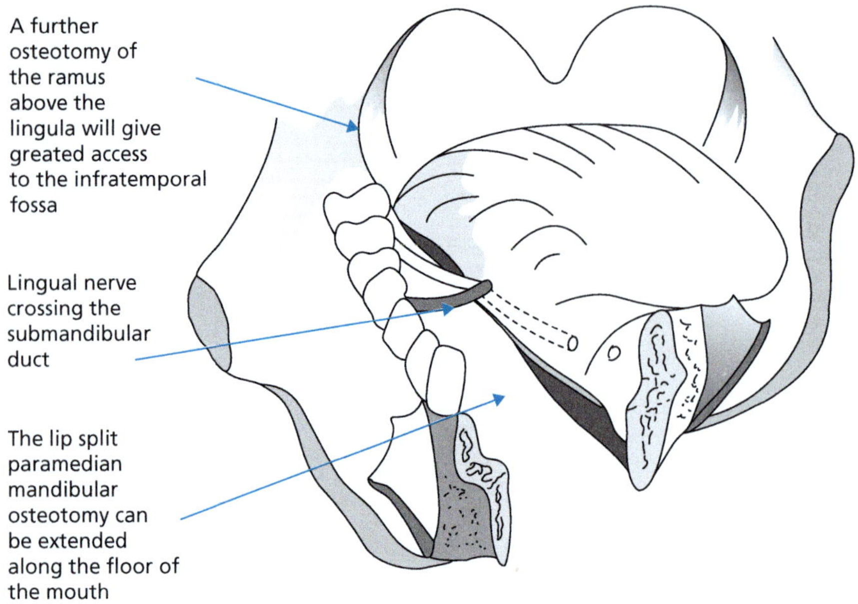

Fig. 43-9 Diagram demonstrating lateral extension of the floor of the mouth if necessary and the relationship of the lingual nerve to the submandibular ducts.

Access to the lateral compartments/ infratemporal fossa/middle cranial fossa[13]

The zygomaticotemporal approach/ frontozygomatic osteotomy (Figure 43-10)

The frontozygomatic osteotomy allows access to the sphenoid wing, lateral wall of the orbit and assists the temporal craniotomy to enter the middle cranial fossa.[14–16] An additional advantage of this osteotomy is its ability to treat proptosis; it gives excellent access to this area. Removal of the lateral wall is very effective in correcting proptosis.

A coronal flap is raised (as described above). The Bramley-Al-Kayat approach is used to protect the frontal branch of the facial nerve. The zygoma exposed from the root of the zygoma to the lateral wall of the orbit and the infraorbital rim and infraorbital fissure. Care is taken to bipolar the zygomaticofacial artery (the only branch of the internal carotid artery that appears on the face) on the lateral wall of the osteotomy.

A retractor is placed to protect the orbital contents. A 1.5 mm miniplate is used to pre-plate the frontozygomatic suture and the root of the zygoma prior to the osteotomy. The osteotomies are completed with a fine oscillating saw. The zygoma is osteotomized inferiorly where it is pedicled on the masseter muscle (Figure 43-11).

The temporalis is divided (Figure 43-12). It is useful to have a rim of temporalis superiorly to reattach the

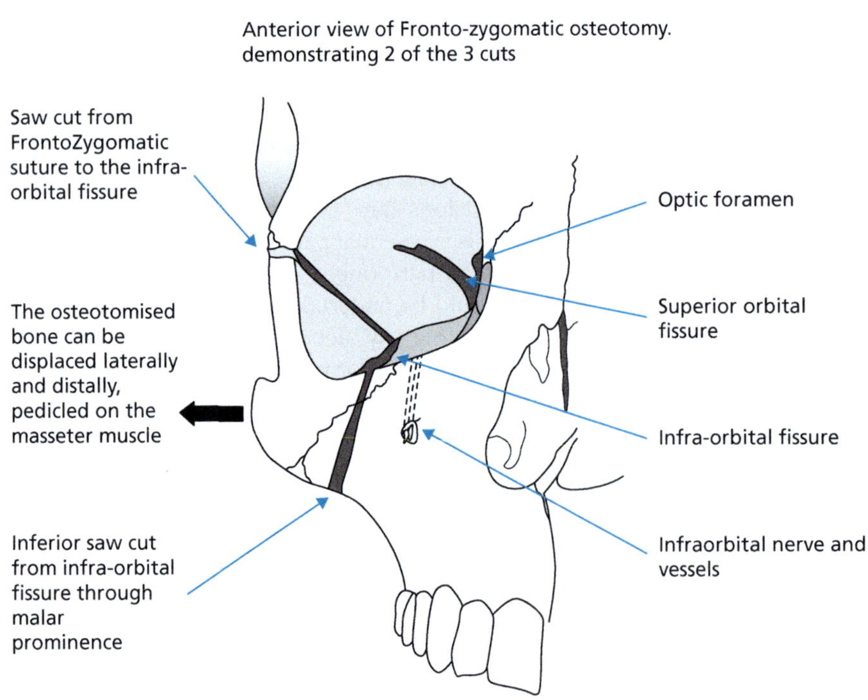

Fig. 43-10 Diagram demonstrating the osteotomy cuts for the frontozygomatic osteotomy.

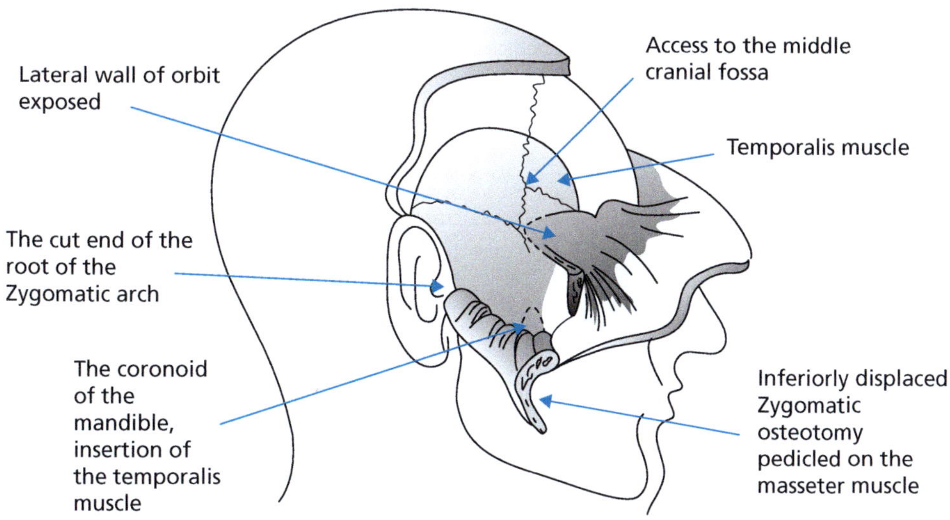

Fig. 43-11 Diagram showing the displaced zygomatic osteotomy, pedicled on the masseter muscle.

muscle and to re-suspend the divided deep temporal fascia to prevent temporal hollowing.

A temporal craniotomy is undertaken. This can be pedicled on the temporalis if necessary or can be removed as a free bone flap. Access can then be achieved to the middle cranial fossa.

Access to the retromaxillary spaces: infratemporal fossa

The retromaxillary areas (infratemporal fossa and the pterygoid space) are some of the most challenging areas to access.

Following the frontozygomatic osteotomy the temporalis obscures the infratemporal fossa. Access to the infratemporal fossa can then be achieved by elevating the temporalis muscle by dividing the coronoid process intraorally. The muscle, pedicled on the superior temporal crest is lifted superiorly to expose the infratemporal fossa (Figure 43-13).

An alternative method is to extend the coronal incision preauricularly, and mobilize the zygoma with its masseteric pedicle inferiorly. Pre-plating the mandible prior to the osteotomies is very important to prevent malocclusions postoperatively. A condylotomy can be performed, and the ramus divided above the lingula (to protect the inferior alveolar nerve). The coronoid with the ramus can then be elevated superiorly. The condylotomy prevents the condyle being dislocated, which is preferable.

One of the problems with this technique alone, however, is the safe control of the vessels, in particular the maxillary artery. It is preferable to combine the above techniques with a cervical approach to the neck vessels.

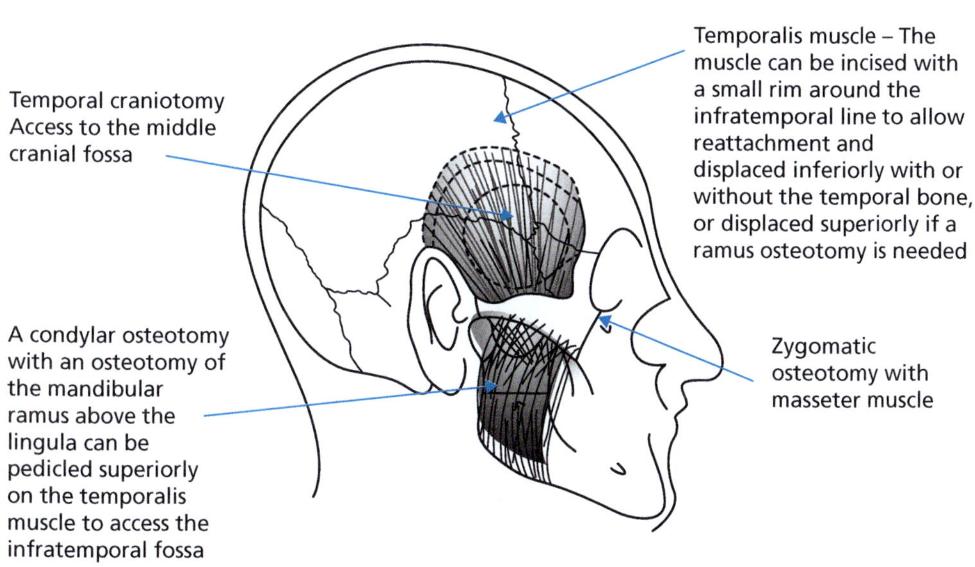

Fig. 43-12 Diagram demonstrating the different osteotomies possible to access the infratemporal fossa and the craniotomy to access the middle cranial fossa.

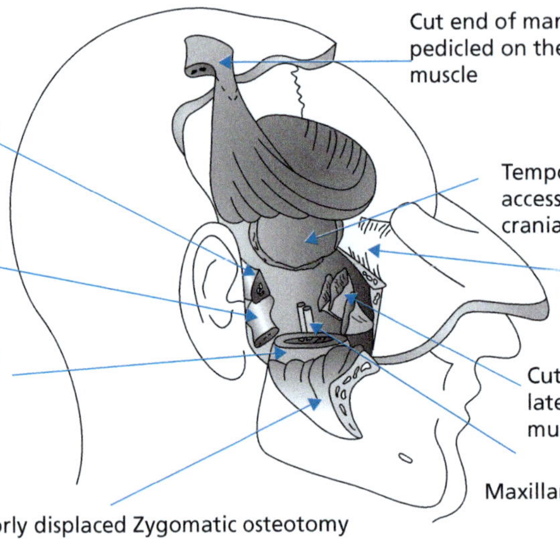

Fig. 43-13 Diagram showing the access to the middle cranial fossa, lateral orbit, and the infratemporal fossa using both the frontozygomatic osteotomy, temporal craniotomy and mandibular ramus and condylar osteotomy.

Control of the neck vessels

An incision is made in one of the neck creases approximately 2 cm below the border of the mandible (to avoid damaging the marginal mandibular branch of the facial nerve) from the mastoid to submental region. The posterior third of the incision is over the sternocleidomastoid muscle (SCM).The skin and platysma is incised and the anterior border of SCM is exposed and retracted posteriorly. The carotid sheath is identified initially by palpation. Dissection continues parallel to the carotid and the carotid artery is separated carefully from the other contents of the sheath. The internal jugular vein, ansa hypoglossi and the vagus nerve are retracted posteriorly. It is advisable to place a loop around the common carotid. The common carotid is dissected superiorly past the bifurcation of the internal and external carotid. Usually the external branch is anterior to the internal branch and is usually more superficial. Normally the internal carotid artery does not give branches off in the neck. It is important to identify at least two branches to be sure which is the external and which the internal carotid. Loops can be placed around both of these vessels to control them.

Access to the retromaxillary spaces: pterygoid space

Transoral mandibular swing technique (Figure 43.14)

The above parasagittal mandibulotomy technique is used and the incision extended along the floor of the mouth and up into the maxillary sulcus, allowing access to the maxillary antrum, pterygopalatine fossa and the infratemporal fossa. To improve access the coronoid can be divided. It can either be removed or can be replaced. It should be remembered that if it is going to be replaced it should have a wire or heavy suture placed through the bone to retrieve it.

To improve access the lip split incision should be extended into the neck. A subfascial flap is raised, the stylohyoid and digastric muscles divided and retracted superiorly with the submandibular gland, and the mylohyoid is divided parallel to the mandible. The facial artery and vein are divided and retracted superiorly. This manoeuvre protects the facial nerve.

Intraorally access to the medial aspect of the ascending ramus is achieved and an osteotomy performed above the lingula, thus preserving the inferior alveolar

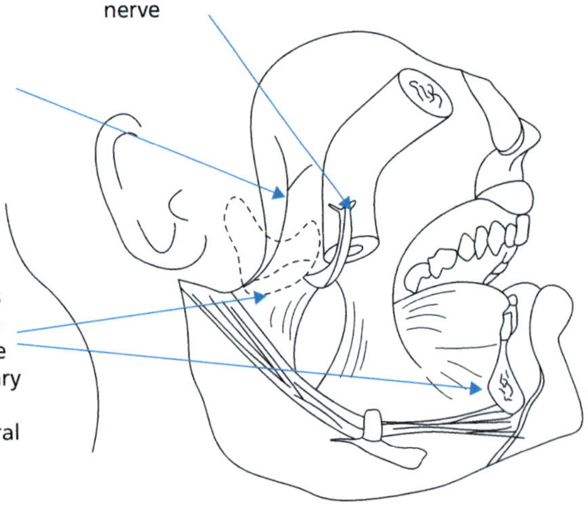

Fig. 43-14 Diagram showing how access can be increased by a further ramus osteotomy.

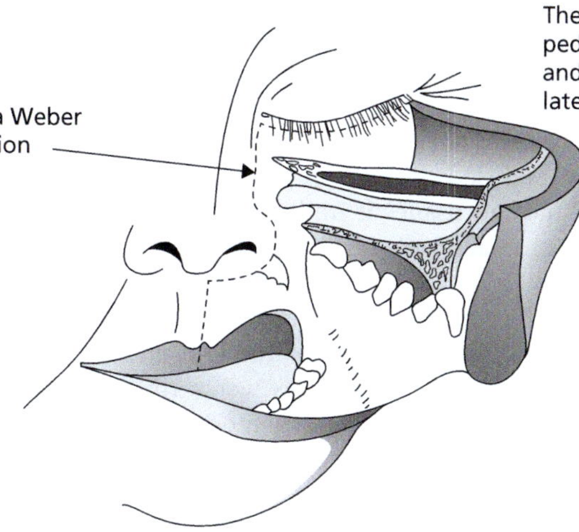

Fig. 43-15 Diagram showing the hemimaxillary osteotomy.

nerve. The mandible can then be swung upwards to expose the retromaxillary and pterygoid approach.

Careful pre-plating is necessary before the osteotomy to ensure accurate reduction and fixation preoperatively.

Hemimaxillotomy pedicled from the cheek

(See Figures 43.15 and 43.16).

This technique allows access to the central compartment, the clivus and sphenoid, the medial and lateral retromaxillary spaces and the infratemporal fossa. It involves the principle of disassembling a vascularized midface composite unit. It was popularized by Curoni and Hernández Altemir[17] and there have been a number of different modifications to this technique.

The access for this osteotomy is via a Weber–Ferguson extraoral incision. The classic Weber–Ferguson incision starts approximately 1 cm above and medial to the medial canthus, with elevation of the palatal mucosa from the tuberosity to the premolars on the opposite. It is important to maintain the viability of the palatal mucosa by preserving the greater palatine artery. It can be freed by carefully osteotomizing the artery from its bony channel. The soft tissue is dissected off the orbital floor and cheek to allow access for the osteotomies. A tunnel is also created from the anterior incision connecting with the vertical buttress incision. It is important that the cheek pedicle is maintained to ensure that the vascularity of the osteotomized bone is maintained.

A vertical incision is made along the zygomatic buttress. The soft tissue is dissected posteriorly to access the pterygomaxillary fissure when the pterygoid dysjunction occurs. The nasal mucosa is elevated and bony cuts made using a saw and fissure burr. Cuts are made between the upper incisor teeth through the cortical bone only and through the whole thickness of the hard palate. The nasal septum and vomer are separated with a septal chisel. Fine osteotomes are used to complete the bony cuts between the upper incisors. This reduces the possibility of damage to the upper incisor teeth. A high level Le Fort I cut is made from the lateral nasal wall across the infraorbital rim. The infraorbital nerve is sacrificed, dividing it with a scalpel. The cut continues laterally

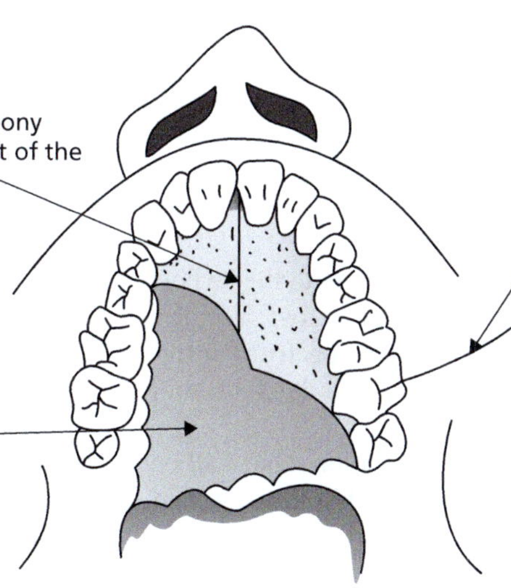

Fig. 43-16 Diagram showing palatal flap reflected as part of the hemimaxillotomy osteotomy.

across the zygomatic buttress tunnelling under the soft tissue pedicle.

The bone is pre-plated prior to the osteotomy to allow accurate repositioning of the bone. The maxilla is divided from the pterygoid plate by using a pterygoid osteotome, and the lateral nasal wall is separated with a 7 mm osteotome. The hemimaxilla is then outfractured laterally, pedicled on the soft tissue of the cheek. Closure of the soft tissues is undertaken carefully to produce a good aesthetic result. Placement of a nasogastric tube at the end of the operation is useful.

One of the complications of this operation is the permanent loss of sensation to the cheek due to division of the infraorbital nerve. This is, however, a relatively small sacrifice compared to the low morbidity and good access the technique affords.

Complications

Complications of any surgery can be divided into local or general, and early, intermediate and late. The proximity of the cranial cavity and skull base to so many vital structures means complications may result in severe morbidity, including blindness, brain damage and mortality, and therefore the decision when to treat surgically and when to manage conservatively is one of the most important and difficult.

The development of endoscopic surgery has significantly helped reduce morbidity by reducing the size of the transfacial open approaches and also by repairing CSF leaks endonasally.

The specific complications related to the transfacial osteotomies are occlusal problems, nonunion and complications secondary to damage to the frontal branch of the facial nerve, temporal hollowing and trismus.

Trismus is common after any operation that involves the temporalis muscle and usually improves over time. Active physiotherapy with mouth opening exercises is useful in patients with persistent trismus after several months.

Occlusal problems and nonunion are very rare and their problems can be prevented largely by pre-plating with miniplates, careful planning of the osteotomy and soft tissue closure. This ideally should be at a different level to the actual osteotomy so that if breakdown of the incision occurs it is not over the osteotomy or plates. Prevention of burning the bone with the saw and burr is also essential by using water irrigation, and good oral hygiene is important.

A chlorhexidine mouthwash is used with the Le Fort I osteotomy and transoral mandibular osteotomies. Two postoperative doses of broad spectrum intravenous antibiotics are given, and 5 days of oral antibiotics.

The treatment of the two complications that will be discussed further are that of temporal hollowing, and treatment of the ptotic eyebrow secondary to damage to the frontal branch of the facial nerve.

Secondary correction of complications

Temporal hollowing

The causes of this have been discussed earlier. If it occurs a number of techniques can be used to improve the appearance. Treatment strategies depend on a number of factors, whether there is also damage to the frontal branch of the facial nerve and a brow ptosis, and if there is temporal muscle underlying the hollowing of a cranioplasty. The thickness of the skin and any radiotherapy to the area is also an important consideration.

Coleman fat injection

This is a technique where autogenous fat is aspirated from usually the abdomen or the medial aspect of the thigh.[18] It is then centrifuged and the serum and oil removed and then it is injected by injecting multiple small quantities in different levels. The fat cells, which are relatively inert, gain their new blood supply from surrounding tissue. It is therefore only appropriate where there is sufficient soft tissue above the cranioplasty in which the fat can be injected.

The main advantages of this technique are that it is a closed technique and that it uses autogenous tissue. If fat is lost over time it can be repeated. However, the results are unpredictable and it does require a general anaesthetic.

Silicone implant

Custom made implants can be made either from taking a direct impression of the defect over the skin or by using 3D data from CT scans. The silicone can be made to a variety of hardnesses and can mimic muscle. Once secured with sutures or screws it is stable and rarely causes a problem. Usually a fibrous capsule forms around the implant and this makes removal very easy if necessary. The placement does, however, require an open approach. Ideally the implant should be covered with temporalis muscle.

Treatment of the ptotic brow

The main complication of the damaged frontal branch of the facial nerve is, particularly in an elderly patient, that the brow becomes ptotic and can cause problems with vision. Brow lifts can be open or closed.[19] The choice depends on a number of factors. Firstly, if a cranioplasty is present and a zygomatic osteotomy has been undertaken, the dissection is more difficult endoscopically, and fixation more problematic. If the hairline is also high an endoscopic brow lift is contraindicated as this technique will elevate the hair line.

The open approach allows direct placement of any temporal implant, makes subperiosteal dissection around the orbit easier, allows direct fixation of the suspended frontal scalp to the bone and enables excess skin to be removed. The disadvantage of this technique is that it is open and it will expose the cranioplasty. If an excessive strip of skin is removed then tension over the incision site will occur and there is a risk of wound breakdown and exposure of the cranioplasty that would necessitate its removal.

The direct brow lift is the oldest and simplest technique and there is little risk of damage to the facial nerve. It is suitable for patients with mild ptosis and thick eyebrows. However, it leaves a visible scar above the eyebrows. The mid-forehead lift involves placement of the incision line within a prominent horizontal skin crease. In patients with a frontal branch palsy this horizontal scar will mimic a skin crease and may be beneficial. The galea is shortened as much as required and the excess cutaneous tissue excised. Careful repair in layers is important. The coronal forehead lift is traditionally open but is now usually undertaken endoscopically using 3 to 5 small incisions placed in the hairline. Dissection is in the subperiosteal plane. However, lateral to the anterior temporal line the dissection should be continued below the temporoparietal fascia, on the surface of the deep temporal fascia to avoid damaging the frontal branch of the facial nerve. The supraorbital and trochlear nerves are identified and preserved. An upcutting periosteal elevator is used to divide the pericranium horizontally at a number of levels. Centrally over the glabella region the pericranium is divided and the corrugator and procerus are exposed and divided. The brow is then lifted and suspended with screws. The endoscopic approach produces less loss of hair, paraesthesia and scarring than the open coronal technique. However, it should not be used in patients with a high hairline and brow ptosis as after surgery the hairline will be higher.

A relative contraindication to the endoscopic brow lift is where previous craniotomy surgery has occurred and bony defects can make dissection more difficult. An open approach enables safer dissection. However, closure of the incision over the cranioplasty also carries the risk of wound breakdown and the subsequent need for removal of the cranioplasty. In order to reduce this risk a careful two layer closure should be undertaken and too much tension across the wound should be avoided.

References

1 Ganly I, Patel SG, Singh B, Kraus DH, Bridger PG, et al. Craniofacial resection for malignant paranasal sinus tumours: Report of an international collaborative study. Head Neck. 2005;27:575–84.

2 Snyderman CH, Carrau RL, Kassam AB, Zanation A, Prevedello D, Gargener P, Mintz A. Endoscopic skull base surgery: principles of endonasal oncological surgery. J Surg Oncol. 2008;97:658–64.

3 Munro IR, Fearon JA. The coronal incision revisited. Plast Reconstr Surg. 1994;93:185–7.

4 Al-Kayat A, Bramley P. A modified pre-auricular approach to the temporomandibular joint and malar arch. Br J Oral Surg. 1979;17:91–103.

5 Eljamel MS, Foy PM. Acute traumatic CSF fistulae: the risk of intracranial infection. Br J Neurosurg. 1990;4:381–5.

6 Choi M, Li Y, Shapiro SA, Havlik RJ, Flores RL. A 10-year review of frontal sinus fractures: clinical outcomes of conservative management of posterior table fractures. Plast Reconstr Surg. 2012;130:399–406.

7 Grime PD, Haskell R, Robertson I, Gullan R. Transfacial access for neurosurgical procedures: an extended role for the maxillofacial surgeon. I. The upper cervical spine and clivus. Int J Oral Maxillofac Surg. 1991;20:285–90.

8 Drommer RB. The History of the Le Fort I osteotomy. J Maxillofac Surg. 1986;14:119–22.

9 Archer DJ, Young S, Uttley D. Basilar aneurysms, a new transclival approach via maxillotomy. J Neurosurg. 1987;67: 54–8.

10 Uttley D, Moore A, Archer DJ. Surgical management of midline skull base tumors: a new approach. J Neurosurg. 1989;71;705–10.

11 James D, Crockard HA. Surgical access to the base of the skull and upper cervical spine by extended maxillotomy. Neurosurgery. 1991;29:411–6.

12 Roy S, Patel PK, Tomita T. The Le Fort I transmaxillary approach to skull base tumors. Clin Plast Surg. 2007;34:575–83.

13 Grime PD, Haskell R, Robertson I, Gullan R. Transfacial access for neurosurgical procedures: an extended role for the maxillofacial surgeon. II. Middle cranial fossa, infratemporal fossa and pterygoid space. Int J Oral Maxillofac Surg. 1991;20:291–5.

14 Uttley D, Archer DJ, Marsh HT. Improved actions of lesions to the central skull base by mobilization of the zygoma: experience with 54 cases. Neurosurgery. 1991;28:99–103.

15 Neil-Dwyer G, Sharr M, Haskell R, Currie D, Hosseini M. Zygomaticotemporal approach to the basis cranii and basilar artery. Neurosurgery. 1988;23:20–2.

16 Hamlyn PJ, Meredith AP, Archer DJ. A further approach to the infra-temporal fossa. J Laryngol Otol. 1986;100: 675–8.

17 Altemir HF. Transfacial access to the retromaxillary area. J. Max Fac Surg. 1986:14:165–70.

18 Pu LL, Coleman SR, Cui X, Ferguson RE Jr, Vasconez HC. Autologous fat grafts harvested and refined by the Coleman technique: a comparative study. Plast Reconstr Surg. 2008;122:932–7.

19 Withey S, Witherow H, Waterhouse N. One hundred cases of endoscopic brow lift. Br J Plast Surg. 2002;55:20–4.

Chapter 44

Obstructive Sleep Apnoea Syndrome

Ashraf Messiha, Ben Gurney and Piet Haers

Introduction

Obstructive sleep apnoea syndrome (OSAS) is a life-threatening chronic condition that can affect 5% of the population,[1] and increasingly patients are seeking help. Determining the severity of the condition through detailed assessment is crucial in deciding which therapy is most suitable for which patient.

OSAS was first identified not by a doctor, but by Charles Dickens in 1837 (Figure 44-1). In the Posthumous Papers of the Pickwick Club, Dickens describes a typical sleep apnoea sufferer, Joe, a 'fat red-faced boy who snores and who may have heart failure'.[2] The condition was subsequently referred to as Pickwickian syndrome, but obstructive sleep apnoea wasn't recognized as a clinical disorder until the 20th century.

The literature describes OSAS as a syndrome of symptoms and signs that are observed during rapid eye movement sleep. It is important to define and distinguish OSAS from the terms sleep disordered breathing (SDB) and upper airway resistance syndrome (UARS).

SDB comprises a wide spectrum of sleep-related breathing abnormalities: those related to an increase in upper airway resistance include snoring, upper airway resistance syndrome (UARS), and obstructive sleep apnoea–hypopnoea syndrome (OSAHS). Many clinicians regard SDB as a spectrum of diseases.

This concept suggests that a person who snores may be exhibiting the first manifestation of SDB and that snoring should not be viewed as normal. A patient can move gradually through the continuum, for example, with weight gain and eventual development of Pickwickian syndrome or with alcohol or sedative use, which can cause a person who simply snores to turn into a snorer with obstructive sleep apnoea (OSA).

Sleep Breathing Disorders (SBD) are a group of conditions characterized by a disruption of the normal breathing pattern when the patient is asleep.[3]

The cause of SBD (Figure 44-2) is an abnormal increase in the resistance of the airways during inspiration during the sleep. Three main factors are responsible: increase in the compliance of the walls, excess soft tissue and a reduction in their diameter.

Orthognathic Surgery: Principles, Planning and Practice. Edited by Farhad B. Naini and Daljit S. Gill.

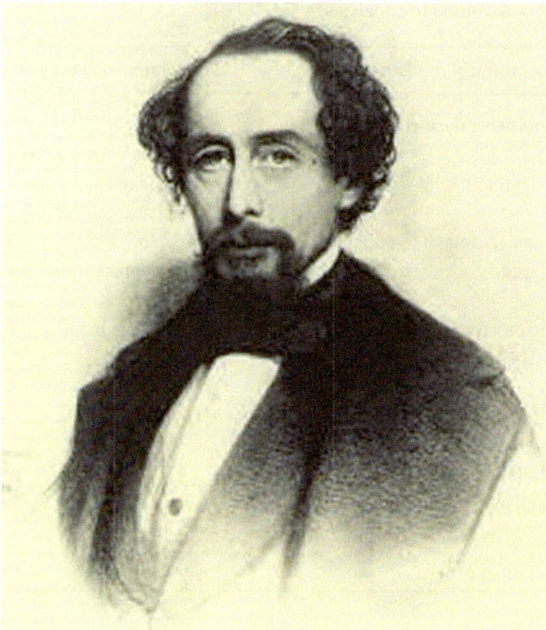

Fig. 44-1 Charles Dickens (1812–1870).

SBD can be divided as follows:

1. Simple snoring.
2. Upper Airways Resistance Syndrome (UARS).
3. Obstructive Sleep Apnoea Syndrome (OSAS).

Therefore, the clinician must recognize that this disease entity represents a continuum and that patients can continue to suffer from symptoms caused by one aspect of SBD while being treated for another aspect.

OSAS is characterized by repetitive pauses in breathing during rapid eye movement sleep, leading to apnoea despite the effort to breath. OSAS is usually associated with a drop in oxygen saturation and increased fatigue, which typically lasts 20–40 seconds and is normally accompanied by snoring witnessed by bed partners who make these individuals aware of their symptoms.

The first authors to clinically describe OSAS were Guilleminault, Tilkian and Dement in 1976.[4] UARS was described later by Guilleminault in 1992.[5] Patients with OSAS often present with unexplained excessive daytime sleepiness, restless sleep and loud snoring. Some patients have trouble concentrating or present with mood changes, irritability and anxiety.

Polysomnography (PSG) is the gold standard investigation to diagnose and classify SBD. Several parameters can be measured: heart rate, respiratory rate, noise, air passage through the nostrils, movements of the chest and abdomen, movement of the limbs, oxygen saturations, activity of the extraocular muscles, and electroencephalography (EEG).

The Respiratory Disturbance Index is the sum of the number of apnoeic and hypopnoeic episodes in one hour interval. Apnoea is defined as the complete cessation of airflow for at least 10 seconds. Hypopnoea is defined as an inspiration with a reduction of 50% or more of the tidal volume of the same patient during a normal quiet inspiration when he/she is asleep.[6]

OSAS can be classified into three stages according to the Apnoea–Hypopnoea Index (AHI) also known as Respiratory Disturbance Index (RDI):

1. Mild AHI 5–15 events/h
2. Moderate AHI 15–30 events/h
3. Severe AHI >30 events/h

Further classification systems have been described. Examination of the Nose, Oropharynx and Hypopharynx (NOH), was classified by Vicini, based on a semi-objective classification of the upper airways at flexible endoscopy (FNE) examination.[7] The scoring from 0 to 5 describes whether the region is normal or has increasing degrees of obstruction to a maximum score of 5 which describes a complete obstruction of the anatomical region.

Each patient would yield an 'obstruction grade' (e.g. N2 O1 H1 is less severe than N3 O2 H3). NOH assessment is quick, easy and informative, and the

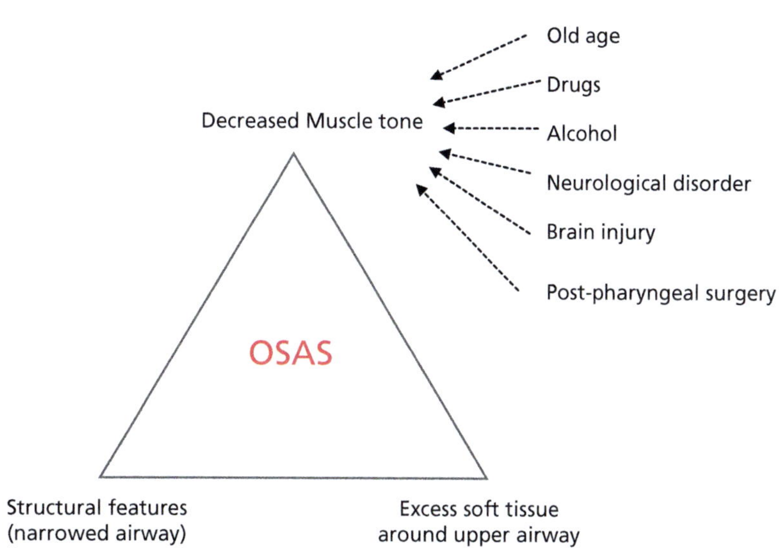

Fig. 44-2 Factors implicated in obstructive sleep apnoea.

Table 44-1 PCAV (Patient Risks, Clinical analysis, Anatomical measurements and Volumetric analysis)

Score	Patient Risk Factors	Clinical severity score	Anatomical measurements	3D Volumetric analysis
1	Middle aged male	AHI >5	Short chin neck distance <36 mm	Narrow upper nasopharyngeal air way
2	Pregnant female	ESS > 10	Chin throat angle >110	Narrow middle oropharyngeal air way
3	Post-menopausal female	SACS > 15	E-line (Pro-nasal to Pogonion) acute angle indicating retrogenia	Narrow lower laryngopharyngeal airway
4	Sedatives	Saturation drop during sleep	Increased neck circumference >38 cm	Large tongue base
5	Smoker	Class 3 or 4 Mallampati score	Retrognathic mandible	Enlarged tonsils
6	Overweight/BMI >35	NOH grade	Retrognathic maxilla	TOTAL = 5
7	Craniofacial syndrome	TOTAL = 6	Decreased transverse discrepancy	
8	Surgery upper air way		Short posterior height	
9	Hypertensive		High mandibular plane angle	
10	Type 2 diabetes		TOTAL = 9	
	TOTAL = 10			

scores correlate well with AHI values. It can be used as a screening tool before polysomnography. NOH classification takes into consideration all three levels of possible obstruction. In order to appropriately treat SBD patients, it is mandatory to pinpoint the exact level/levels of obstruction and this classification works well.

PCAV Risk Score Index

In our practice we have developed our own risk score index: **PCAV (Patient Risks, Clinical analysis, Anatomical measurements and Volumetric analysis) (Table 44-1).** This index combines several points that affect the airway, which is divided under the above four categories. The advantage of using this index is that it provides a dynamic account of a patient's risk factors, clinical examination and radiological analysis. The score is an arbitrary score of maximum severity equalling 30 points.

Patient risks

Our work up includes taking a detailed history with further assessment of the severity index. The risk factors would yield a maximum score out of 10. An example of a middle aged male, overweight, smoker and high alcohol intake would give a Patient Risk Factor score of 4/10.

Clinical analysis

This individual would then have his Apnoea–Hypopnoea Index (AHI) worked out from polysomnography, a baseline study used in diagnosing OSA.[8] Polysomnography studies characterise the pauses in breathing. To grade the severity of sleep apnoea, the AHI is reported. An AHI of less than 5 is considered normal. An AHI of 5–15 is mild; 15–30 is moderate and more than 30 events per hour characterizes severe sleep apnoea.

Apnoeic pauses are followed by a relative decrease in blood oxygen and an increase in the blood carbon dioxide. Whereas in central sleep apnoea the body's motions of breathing stop, in OSA the chest not only continues to make the movements of inhalation, but the movements typically become even more pronounced. Monitors for airflow at the nose and mouth demonstrate that efforts to breathe are not only present, but that they are often exaggerated. The chest muscles and diaphragm contract and the entire body may thrash and struggle.

An 'event' can be either an apnoea, characterized by complete cessation of airflow for at least 10 seconds, or a hypopnoea in which airflow decreases by 50% for 10 seconds or decreases by 30% if there is an associated decrease in the oxygen saturation or an arousal from sleep.[6] In patients who are at high likelihood of having OSA, a randomized controlled trial found that home oximetry (a non-invasive method of monitoring blood oxygenation) may be adequate and easier to obtain than formal polysomnography.[9]

High probability patients can be identified with an Epworth Sleepiness Scale (ESS). This scale measures daytime sleepiness by use of a very short questionnaire. This can be helpful in diagnosing sleep disorders. It was introduced in 1991 by Dr Murray Johns of Epworth Hospital in Melbourne, Australia.[10]

The questionnaire asks the subject to rate his or her probability of falling asleep on a scale of increasing probability from 0 to 3 for eight different situations that most people engage in during their daily lives, though not necessarily every day. The scores for the eight questions are added together to obtain a single number. A number in the 0–9 range is considered to be normal while a number in the 10–24 range indicates that expert medical advice should be sought. For

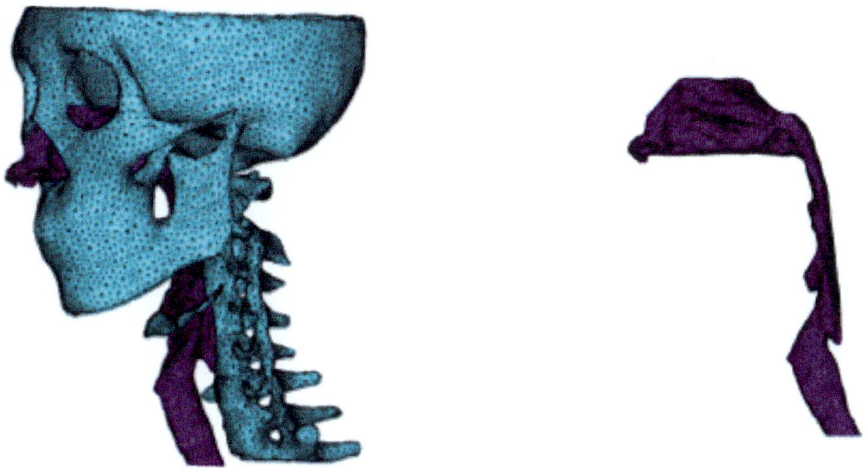

Fig. 44-3 3D representation of the narrowed airway (purple).

instance, scores of 11–15 are shown to indicate the possibility of mild to moderate sleep apnoea, whereas a score of 16 and above indicates the possibility of severe sleep apnoea or narcolepsy. Certain questions in the scale were shown to be better predictors of specific sleep disorders, though further tests may be required to provide an accurate diagnosis.[11] In addition to this, we use a further assessment, the Sleep Apnoea Clinical Score (SACS) which has been validated and has a high positive predictive value for OSAS.[12]

For the purposes of our PCAV Risk score index, the patient would score a maximum of 5 on clinical scales category if AHI is > 5, ESS > 10, SACS > 15 and a drop in oxygen saturation during sleep with a class 3 or 4 Mallampati score. Under this category the patient undergoes a flexible nasoendoscopy and an NOH grade is then given demonstrating site and severity of obstruction.

Anatomical measurements

The third category of measurement involves anatomical analysis. An important measure is neck diameter or circumference together with diagnosis of a short neck chin distance, an obtuse chin throat angle, an acute angle E line (a line drawn from the most anterior points of the nose to the chin), a retrognathic mandible, retrognathic maxilla, a decreased transverse discrepancy, short posterior height and high mandibular plane angle. The presence of all of these factors would give a maximum score of 9. This category gives an objective measure of the soft and hard tissue that surrounds the airway.

Volumetric analysis

Finally, we assess the volume deficiency, and a 3D Volumetric scan is utilized. From the scan we are able to identify the zone of narrowed airway, as well as segmentalise other anatomical areas of interest. A further maximum score of 5 here makes up the total of 30 to guide management (Table 44-1 and Figures 44-3 to 44-7).

An upper, middle or lower zone narrowing would give the severity of where the collapse is. This would guide our decision whether to carry out a maxillary advancement to improve the upper zone, mandibular advancement to improve the middle zone or an advancement genioplasty with genioglossus advancement to improve the lower zone (Figure 44-8).

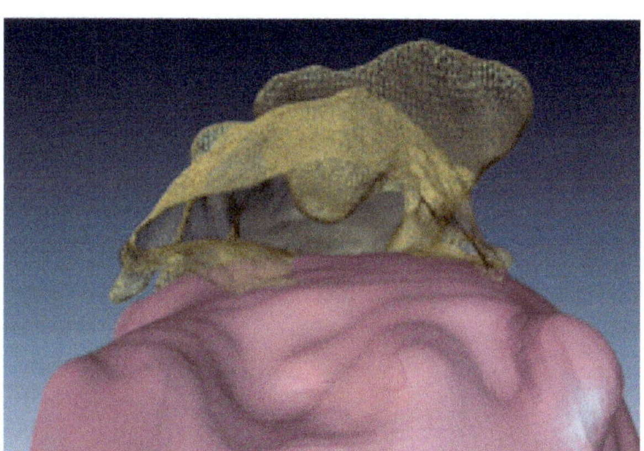

Fig. 44-4 In tra-oral view of the tongue base (pink) with soft palate and uvula above.

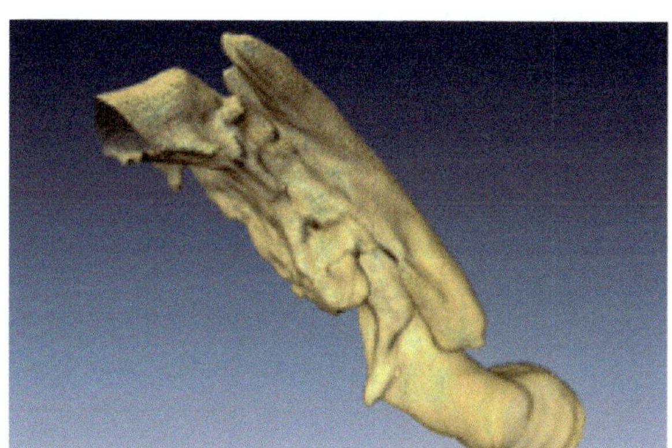

Fig. 44-5 Volumetric reproduction of the airway column from post-nasal space to larynx.

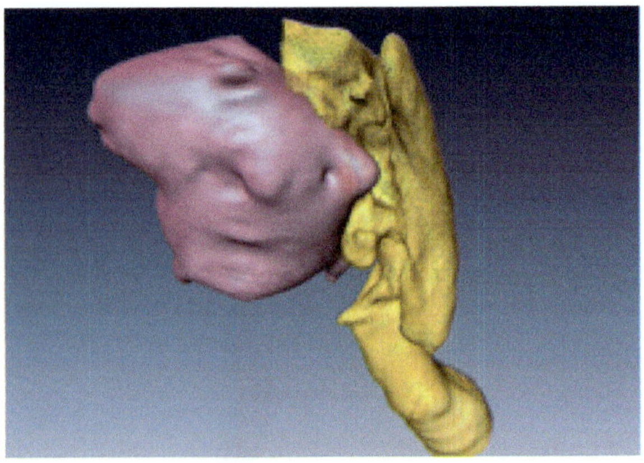

Fig. 44-6 Relationship between oral tongue volume and airway column.

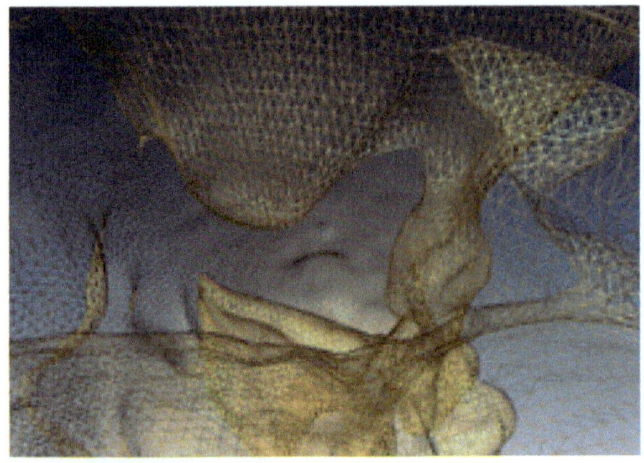

Fig. 44-7 Transoral view of soft palate (superior) and epiglottis (inferior).

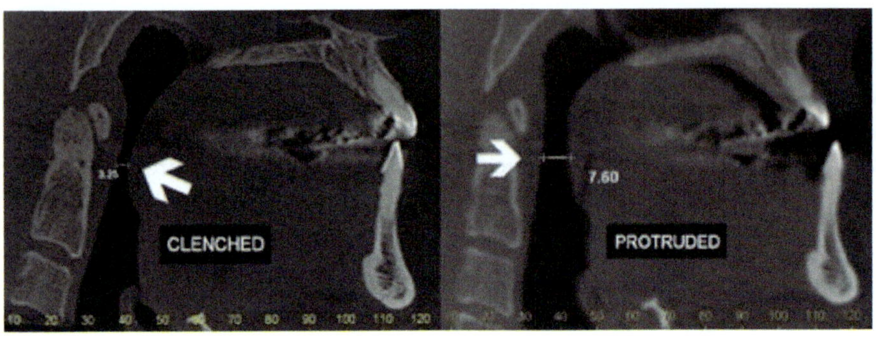

Fig. 44-8 Sagittal CT images of posterior airway space in: (a) intercuspal position and (b) mandibular protrusion.

Pathophysiology

During rapid eye movement deep sleep, the muscle tone of the throat and neck muscles relaxes and therefore the soft tissues collapse. The narrower the space in the upper airway, the more likely that obstruction is likely to occur during sleep. This may take the range of light snoring to complete collapse (Figure 44-9).

In complete collapse, the airflow is reduced to the point that oxygen concentration in the blood falls; this triggers a set of neurological arousal mechanisms. The effect of low oxygen concentration particularly affects neurons in two sensitive areas. The two areas affected by changes in oxygen concentration are the hippocampus and the right frontal cortex.

Recent research shows evidence of hippocampal atrophy in people suffering from OSAS, affecting both memory and spacial navigation.[13] Furthermore a significant portion of the OSAS cases show irreversible changes despite years of optimal CPAP treatment.[14] Therefore it is imperative that as clinicians we diagnose and treat this condition before the long lasting effects of hypoxaemia occur, potentially causing permanent neurological damage.

Treatment planning

Treatment planning is complex and successful outcomes depend on the systematic preoperative work up, choice of surgical technique and postoperative management. The initial management of OSAS starts with a thorough history and examination, evaluation of posterior airway space (normal is 11 ± 2 mm on a lateral cephalometric radiograph, but this is not taken with the patient supine), 3D cone beam CT/CT, and dental model analysis.

Wolford et al identified some clinical and radiographic characteristics that warrant documenting as part of contemporaneous recording of the severity of potential airway obstruction:[15]

1. Retruded mandible.
2. Retruded maxilla.
3. Posterior vertical maxillary deficiency.
4. Retropositioned tongue.

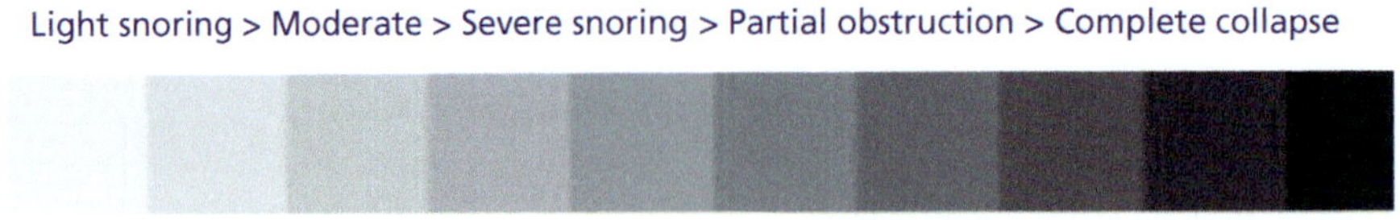

Fig. 44-9 Range of obstruction in sleep disordered breathing.

5. High occlusal plane.
6. High mandibular plane angulations.
7. Short chin-neck line and decreased PAS.
8. Nasal airway obstruction (narrow nostrils, wide columella, enlarged turbinate's, deviated septum, polyps, nasopharyngeal adenoid tissue, decreased posterior choanal height, constricted luminal valves, external nasal deformity).
9. Oropharyngeal abnormalities (elongated soft palate and uvula, medially and posteriorly positioned posterior faucal pillars, enlarged adenoids, hyperplastic tonsils, macroglossia).

Maxillomandibular advancement (MMA) involves the creation of a maxillary Le Fort I osteotomy and bilateral sagittal split mandibular osteotomy advancement. This procedure was first described with a simultaneous hyoid suspension as treatment for OSAS by Riley in 1986.[16] Holty and Guilleminault performed a meta-analysis in 2012 demonstrating a mean AHI decrease from 63.9/h to 9.5/h, $p < 0.001$, with a surgical success rate of 86% and cure rate of 43.2%. It was noted that younger age (45 years), lower preoperative weight and AHI, an increase in posterior airway space >11.6 mm, a maxillary advancement >10 mm and a mandibular advancement more than 11.3 mm improved the likelihood of success.[17] Pirklbauer et al. conducted a systematic review and analysis of data recommending a grade of A to B with regard to levels of evidence base for MMA in the treatment of OSAS.[18] On this basis, the authors have been performing bimaxillary advancements of at least 10 mm, along with advancement genioplasty, aiming for a full overlap of the symphysis menti so that the lingual plate of the distal osteotomized chin overlaps the outer buccal (facial) plate of the proximal mandible in the midline.

Preoperative work-up

The author's work-up in all cases involves:

1. OSAS arbitrary risk index score.
2. PSG work-up.
3. Radiology including: orthopantomograph, lateral cephalometric analysis, 3D spiral MRI scan of the upper airway from base of skull to bifurcation of trachea.
4. Articulated dental study models.
5. Anaesthetic evaluation.
6. Clinical photography to include: front, right and left profile, right and left 45 degrees oblique lateral, worm's eye view, lateral lower lip–chin–neck view.

For the purpose of this chapter, we will discuss surgical techniques only. As mentioned, we evaluate the level of obstruction in our work up by including a spiral 3D MRI scan of the soft tissues of the airway, from base of skull to tracheal bifurcation, traced lateral cephalometry, OPT and study models. A second appointment then is made for the patient to be seen in a multidisciplinary clinic. The participants in the clinic include the surgeon, orthodontist, sleep laboratory representative, speech and language specialists and a physician. We also prefer the presence of our regular anaesthetist to attend. We are in the process of refining who the participants of the multidisciplinary team members are. For example, we strongly believe that in order to achieve a satisfactory outcome one should look at lifestyle modification. This would involve cessation of smoking, weight reduction and reduction of alcohol intake. This important liaison is best provided by a specialist nurse with an interest in lifestyle modification.

The orthodontist role in surgical correction of the facial skeleton has been highly documented in this textbook. The authors recommend bimaxillary advancement plus advancement genioplasty with genioglossus attachments. Patients with preoperative malocclusion are evaluated for preoperative orthodontics. Due to the severity of the condition and the likely time constraints, most patients tend to undergo MMA surgery without preoperative orthodontics. The resultant malocclusion is therefore accepted in exchange for achieving the objective of having the facial skeleton in an advanced position, correcting the collapse of the upper airway posteriorly.

The orthodontist places arch wires with hooks prior to surgery or as an alternative the surgeon can place upper and lower archbars at the time of surgery. This does increase operating time and therefore the former is the preferred option.

Choice of surgical technique in treatment planning

Surgical procedures initially focused on carrying out procedures that would correct narrowing or collapse at the upper pharyngeal airway or the velopharyngeal level.

Such treatment included:

- Surgical or Laser Assisted uvuloplasty (SUPP or LAUP respectively).
- Uvulopalatopharyngoplasty (UPPP).
- Transpalatal advancement.
- Sclerotherapy injections into the soft palate.
- Radiofrequency tissue volume reduction (RFTVR) of the soft palate.
- Soft palatal pillar implantation.

Unlike a single operation to treat a condition, such as appendicectomy for appendicitis, OSAS is complex to treat and few of the earlier described surgical procedures reflected a satisfactory outcome. Dissatisfied with these techniques, clinicians started looking at lower pharyngeal airway surgery. In the first instance, soft tissue surgery to correct collapse was advocated.

Such treatment included:

- Genioglossus advancement.
- Hyoid suspension.
- Hyoid advancement.
- Tongue base reduction.

Table 44-2 A summary of higher evidence published papers on the surgical correction utilizing maxillary mandibular advancement for OSAS

Author	Year/Journal	Study type	Description	Findings
Sommer JU	2012/HNO	Metanalysis Of all OSA surgery	Medline search 310 studies, 12 RCTs	Surgical studies limited MMA favourable outcomes
Prinsell JR	2012/JOMS	Lit Review	MMA v UP3 v multilevel surgery v CPAP Outcome measure – mean % reduction AHI	AHI reduction 92.1% MMA with adjunctive procedures, 88.4% MMA alone vs 53.0% non-MMA surgery. Nasal CPAP 89.8%
Pirklbauer K	2011/JOMS	Syst Review	Pubmed literature review. 1,113 citations, 101 articles, 39 studies included.	Only 5 studies > level 2b evidence, most level 4. Recommendation for MMA Grade A to B
Randerath WJ	2011/Eur Respir J	Review (European multicentre taskforce)	Interdisciplinary European respiratory society taskforce literature review	MMA as efficient as CPAP in patients refusing conservative Rx and can be recommended as single intervention
Vicini C	2010 Am K Otolaryngol	RCT PAPvMMA Level 1b evidence	N=50	CPAP (88% AHI reduction) compared with MMA (86% AHI reduction)– no statistical difference but both effective treatments
Caples SM	2010/Sleep	Metanalysis (AASM standards of practice paper adjunct)	Systematic review and metanalysis % reduction AHI as primary efficacy outcome measure	MMA better reduction AHI (87%) than UP3 (33%), LAUP (32%) and RFA (40%)
Holty JE	2010/Sleep Med Review	Metanalysis	53 studies, 627pts	Mean AHI ↓ 63.9 to 9.5 ± 10.7 events/h post MMA 86.0% success 43.2% AHI <5 and 63% AHI<10
Pirsig W	2000/Eur Arch Otorhinolaryng	Syst Review	Study of long term results >3yrs f/u	CPAP, MMA, tracheostomy, tonsillectomy – most effective treatments of OSA

By 1983, mandibular sagittal advancement osteotomy was used for the first time in OSAS.[19] A year or two later, the same authors advocated maxillary advancement.[16] Current practice of bimaxillary advancement with modified genioplasty procedure seems to provide a satisfactory outcome in improving the posterior pharyngeal airway and in some clinical case series success rates exceed 90%.[20] Over the last 30 years, there has been increasing evidence, some of higher level, and a lot more of lower level, with the majority of papers in support of MMA as efficacious in treating OSAS, offering comparative outcomes to nasal CPAP, which still remains the gold standard of treatment. Long-term outcome data is also increasing, and this should be what is focused on when examining the evidence for this treatment (Table 44-2).

Surgical technique

MMA for OSAS follows many of the standard principles of conventional orthognathic surgery, but there are various extra factors that the surgeon must consider. To give a successful outcome, mean mandibular advances have been reported as 12 mm[21] which in orthognathic terms is considerable, and it is vital that the surgeon take all the necessary actions intraoperatively to make these movements possible and prevent the likelihood of postoperative relapse. The steps are outlined in the following section.

Perioperative

Nasal intubation, head elevation and hypotensive anaesthesia as well as intraoperative antibiotics and steroids are important anaesthetic considerations.

Maxilla

For OSAS cases, it is useful to have an external landmark reference; often a Kirschner wire or screw placed at the nasion from which to measure advances and ensure the full planned movement has been achieved. Calliper measurement from this reference point to a fixed point on the teeth such as the central incisor tip or wire of the fixed appliance allows the surgeon to more accurately position the maxilla. With OSAS, the maxillary movement is likely to be at least 5 mm, but may be more.[21] The possibility of autogenous or alloplastic bone grafting must therefore also be considered prior to the operation in terms of patient consent.

Disruption of blood supply to the maxilla after downfracture and mobilisation is very rare,[22] but due to increased advances required to treat OSAS, is probably more likely than in conventional cases. After local infiltration with lidocaine/adrenaline a high upper maxillary vestibular incision is made between the upper first molars, ensuring a broad base of non-keratinised mucosa to preserve blood supply to the alveolar segments. Periosteal stripping, exposure of inferior orbital nerves, nasal aperture, anterior nasal spine and dissection of the nasal floor mucosa is completed in usual fashion.

The osteotomy is made with a reciprocating saw from the lateral zygomatic buttress, taking care to clear the apices of the maxillary teeth superiorly. Impacted upper third molars should not influence these cuts and may require removal once the maxilla has been down fractured. The cuts are made, with care to upright the saw approaching the lateral nasal wall to avoid the likelihood of damaging the nasal endotracheal tube. A back cut is reinforced at the lateral zygomatic buttress as far posteriorly as the saw will allow. A second cut and wedge of bone is removed if the maxilla is being impacted. Pterygomaxillary dysjunction is essential to get complete posterior disassociation of the maxilla, using a curved pterygoid chisel angled medially and inferiorly at the posterior edge of the maxilla into the suture. Controlled taps aimed inferiorly can avoid propagating this split up towards the cranial base, where impingement of cranial nerves could potentially be a risk. Further use of septal and spatula osteotomes divides the nasal septum and lateral nasal wall.

Downfracture should be simple with inferior digital pressure on the anterior maxilla; Smith spreaders can be used at the nasomaxillary and zygomaticomaxillary buttresses to fully displace the maxilla.

It is critical in OSAS that the maxilla be mobilised fully, but before any further intervention, the colour of the downfractured labial gingivae should be checked. If they have turned purple, then it is safe to proceed with caution, but if they have turned white, this indicates poor vascular supply to the maxillary segment and surgery should be paused to allow this to recover before further manipulation.

It is useful to lay the patient flat at this stage and lower the bed with the surgeon positioned at the head end. Rowe's and Tessier's mobilizers can be used to dissociate all bony parts and gentle stretching of the posterior soft tissue may be required to achieve the necessary advancement. Care must be taken not to tear the palatal or buccal soft tissues, which can then propagate very quickly during this mobilisation stage: this must be checked. The descending palatine neurovascular bundle must also be examined for bleeding at this stage. It can be safely clipped or cauterised for haemostatic control, but it is obviously advantageous to preserve it. Further vasoconstrictor can be infiltrated into the pterygoid musculature if required to arrest bleeding.

At this stage the intermediate wafer and intermaxillary fixation, either with wires or running elastic power chain is applied. It is vital that all bony interferences are reduced with Rongeurs or rotary burr. The maxilla will often 'telescope' when advanced, but very careful inspection and palpation of the bony contact will alert the surgeon to where bone requires removal. The maxilla must make good bony contact with the buttresses in the new position, and vertical change checked using the external reference point, and if needed bone grafts should be considered. It is also important to remember to reduce the base of the nasal cartilaginous septum to prevent buckling or distortion if the maxilla is being impacted. Further segmentation of the maxilla may be required at this stage depending on the treatment plan.

The authors recommend four L-shaped osteosynthesis plates of at least 1.5 mm thickness to fix and stabilize the maxilla – an alternative is to use a straight plate at the nasomaxillary buttress and an L-shaped plate at the zygomaticomaxillary buttress.

Mandible

For OSAS, a bilateral sagittal split osteotomy (BSSO) offers the most consistent and versatile option for mandibular advancement, with maximal flexibility in controlling the distal tooth bearing segment and minimal disruption to the muscles of mastication. Given the significant movements, it is worth adapting the design of the osteotomies with this in mind. The buccal segment should extend further anteriorly to allow maximum overlap between the proximal and distal segments for fixation to allow advances of up to 12 mm and in some cases up to 15 mm. The constraints are in achieving a balanced aesthetic profile at the same time as advancing the maxilla.

All patients undergoing OSAS MMA surgery are consented for iliac crest bone graft. Some authors favour an anticlockwise MMA as opposed to a straight maxillomandibular advancement (S-MMA). Some feedback from our patients and a clinical observation is the unsightly fullness at the base of nose, upturned tip of nose, saddle deformity of the nasal bridge, and lack of upper lip curve. These problems are associated with large S-MMA when used to treat obstructive sleep apnoea. An anticlockwise maxillomandibular advancement (CCW-MMA) on the other hand seems to provide the balanced profile without the nasolabial problems observed with S-MMA.

Via a buccal/ramus incision with careful subperiosteal dissection of the lingula medially, osteotomy cuts are made either with a rotary instrument or an oscillating saw through the cortical bone on the medial surface of the ramus above the lingula, down the anterior ramus and then curving inferiorly through the lateral buccal cortical plate between the first and second molar teeth. The thicker cortical bone of the lower border must be adequately cut to favour the split anteriorly. The splits are then propagated, the authors favouring a controlled split technique. The surgeon must be aware of the greenstick fracture, particularly at the inferior posterior ramus, and this must be completed to allow free movement of the tooth bearing segment of bone. Once the split has been successfully completed, in OSAS patients, thorough stripping of the masseteric and medial pterygoid muscle attachments is essential. A J-stripper is used, allowing the mandible to advance and rotate anticlockwise sufficiently, perhaps even beyond the planned position to minimise the relapse potential. The condylar segment must also sit passively with no distracting muscle pull.

The final wafer and intermaxillary fixation is applied. Before fixation the proximal condylar segment must be pushed back into the glenoid fossa, although not overly so as this may predispose to postoperative condylar resorption.

The authors favour plate fixation, using an intermediate 2.0 mm adaptation osteosynthesis plate with 6 mm screws, two screws either side of the osteotomy gap. A minimum of three bicortical position screws either at the superior border or triangulated with two above and one screw beneath the nerve are an alternative option. Screws may need to be applied via a transbuccal approach to achieve right angles to the bone. Care is taken prior to committing to the fixation of the segments in making every effort to ensure that the condyles are seated well in the glenoid fossa and to avoid distracting the condyles laterally, inferiorly or anteriorly. Should this happen, it would be noticeable at the end of the procedure when temporary intermaxillary fixation elastics are removed as the mandible swings to one side (The midline would swing towards the ipsilateral side of a condyle that is distracted laterally).

Chin

Relaxation of the tongue musculature can contribute to lower airway obstruction in sleep apnoea.[23] The genioglossus and geniohyoid muscles attach to the genial tubercle and inferior mental spine on the inner mandibular symphyseal cortices. Genioglossus block/window advancement has been proposed for OSAS with moderate success as a single procedure,[24] but its success may be affected by limited lateral extension of the bony cut.[25] A genioplasty or inferior mandibular osteotomy can complement MMA in terms of additional advancement of both genioglossus and geniohyoid, a degree of hyoid suspension, whilst also providing an option to maximize the movements without compromising aesthetics. Additionally, this is a simple adjunctive procedure to maximize results without increasing morbidity.

The authors favour a horizontal sliding genioplasty ensuring that the muscle attachments are preserved posteriorly with maximum horizontal attachment. Access is via a lower vestibular incision between the lower canines, which can be stepped through a more labial positioned mucosal incision to ensure a broader base over the apices of the lower teeth. A definite horizontal division of the mentalis leaving a good cuff superiorly to re-approximate is essential. Care must be taken to identify, protect and preserve the mental nerves, with the knowledge that the nerves swerve forward and inferiorly within the canal before exiting the foramina. The midline is marked above and below the planned osteotomy line with a groove to help orientation. The cut is made with a rotary instrument or oscillating saw as described above. The chin segment is then advanced and fixed using a pre-bent right angled genioplasty plate – the authors favour an osteosynthesis 2.0 mm thickness titanium plate for this. An alternative is to use bicortical, long 2.0 mm diameter screws, normally three in number. The authors believe that the placement of screws is technique sensitive and very little forgiveness in getting an accurate placement to engage the overlapping cortices.

Closure

Special consideration should be made toward the upper lip: V-Y or double V-Y advancement to lengthen the lip if necessary and consideration should be made whether to perform a cinch suture to avoid flaring of the alar base in large maxillary advances. A resorbable 3/0 suture is preferred and can be running or continuous. When closing the genioplasty incision, a layered closure of mentalis muscle, followed by hermetic sealed closure of the mucosa is vital to avoid wound breakdown and prevent chin ptosis.

Postoperative

The patient should be closely observed on a high dependency unit with one to one nursing for at least 12 hours postoperatively. Head elevation, ice packs or cooling systems should be used, in addition to the prescription of postoperative steroids to minimize swelling and bruising. In thin bone we recommend strong elastic IMF to prevent an open bite developing.

New developments

Although the authors do not routinely use, many surgeons are now favouring piezosurgery for osteotomy cuts. This technique can be time consuming, but there are potential benefits of a more controlled cut with preservation of the soft tissues, nerves, periodontal ligaments etc.

Case report

A 55-year-old gentleman presented with general fatigue, daytime sleepiness and snoring. His Body Mass Index (BMI) was 28.3, and he was otherwise fit and well. A sleep study revealed mild obstructive sleep apnoea with an Apnoea–Hypopnoea Index (AHI) of 9 and hourly oxygen desaturation of 7.3/h. His Epworth sleepiness score (ESS) was 14. Clinical examination showed a class 2 division 1 skeletal profile and overjet of 4 mm. There was mandibular retrognathia and an obtuse submental-cervical angle (Figures 44-8 and 44-9). There was no facial asymmetry. He was given a trial of a mandibular advancement device, which reduced his snoring and gave him some degree of improvement, but he could not tolerate long-term nocturnal use of the device and sought a surgical opinion.

Pre-surgical orthodontics involved decompensation and alignment, plus extraction of lower premolar teeth

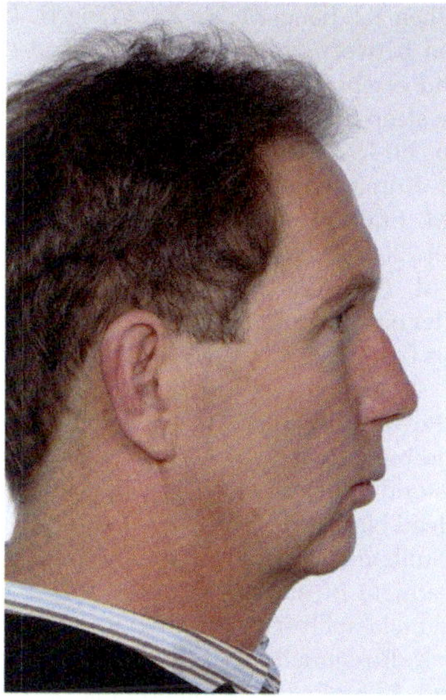

Fig. 44-8 Preoperative profile view.

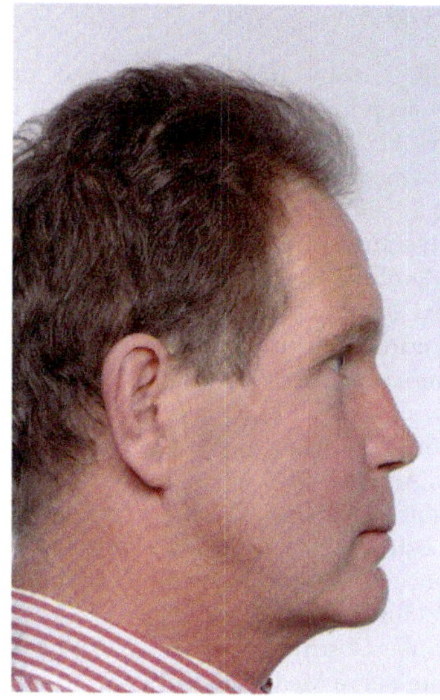

Fig. 44-10 Postoperative profile view.

to maximize the preoperative overjet. The patient underwent maxillomandibular advancement and horizontal sliding genioplasty (Figures 44-10 and 44-11). The mandibular advancement was 11 mm and the maxilla was advanced 7 mm. 2.0 mm plates were used to fix the mandible, 1.5 mm plates to fix the maxilla and 18 mm positional bicortical screws were used to fix the chin. Intraoperative intermaxillary fixation was achieved with upper and lower archbars.

The postoperative recovery was uneventful and the patient was delighted with the results, from both a functional point of view and aesthetically. His symptoms subjectively improved and he felt more rested during the day. At six months postoperatively, the ESS was reduced to 2. The sleep study was repeated and AHI had fallen to 3.1 (65.5% reduction and effective cure) and the hourly oxygen desaturations to 4/h. The posterior airway space had increased from 3.1 mm to 10.51 mm. There was no surgical relapse. A patient recorded outcome questionnaire was completed in which the patient showed high satisfaction with the procedure and would recommend to others.

Conclusions

MMA represents a clearly effective treatment for OSAS, but must be reserved for appropriate patients. It must be remembered that this option represents major surgery, and should not be undertaken lightly, or without adequate preparation. This chapter has highlighted how structured the OSAS assessment should be, and it is mandatory that a multidisciplinary approach be adopted preoperatively. If this is completed with care and attention, then the outcome of this surgical treatment for what is a debilitating medical condition can be excellent.

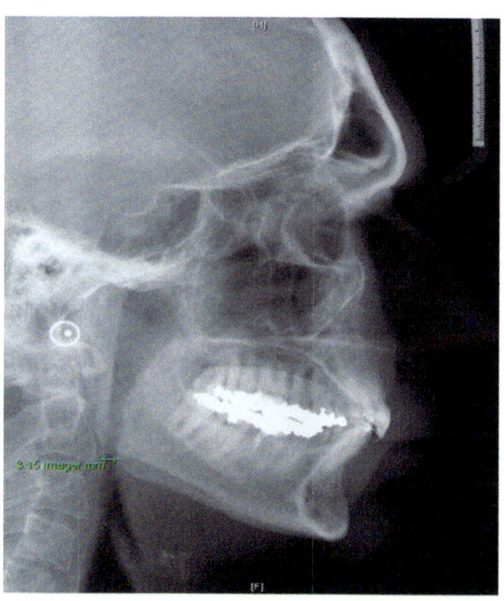

Fig. 44-9 Lateral cephalometric radiograph showed a posterior airway space of 3.15 mm.

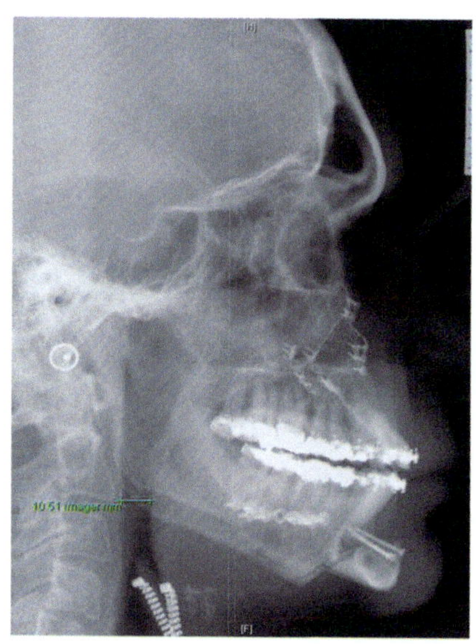

Fig. 44-11 Postoperative lateral cephalometric radiograph.

References

1 Stradling JR, Crosby JH. Predictors and prevalence of obstructive sleep apnoea and snoring in 1001 middle aged men. Thorax. 1991;45:85–90.

2 Dickens C. The Posthumous Papers of the Pickwick Club, Containing a Faithful Record of the Perambulations, Perils, Travels, Adventures and Sporting Transactions of the Corresponding Members. Chapman and Hall Publishing, 1837.

3 Sleep-related breathing disorders in adults: recommendations for syndrome definition and measurement techniques in clinical research. The Report of an American Academy of Sleep Medicine Task Force. Sleep. 1999;22:667–89.

4 Guilleminault C, Tilkian A, Dement WC. The sleep apnea syndromes. Ann Rev Med. 1976;27:465–84.

5 Guilleminault C, Stoohs R, Clerk A, Simmons J, Labanowski M. From obstructive sleep apnea syndrome to upper airway resistance syndrome: consistency of daytime sleepiness. Sleep. 1992;15(6 Suppl):S13–6.

6 De Backer W. Obstructive sleep apnea/hypopnoea syndrome. Panminerva Med. 2013;55:191–5.

7 Vicini C, De Vito A, Benazzo M, Frassineti S, Campanini A, Frasconi P, Mira E. The nose oropharynx hypopharynx and larynx (NOHL) classification: a new system of diagnostic standardized examination for OSAHS patients. Eur Arch Otorhinolaryngol. 2012;269:1297–300.

8 Epstein LJ, Kristo D, Strollo PJ Jr. Adult Obstructive Sleep Apnea Task Force of the American Academy of Sleep Medicine. Clinical guideline for the evaluation, management, and long-term care of obstructive sleep apnea in adults. J Clin Sleep Med. 2009;5:263–76.

9 Antic NA, Buchan C, Esterman A, Hensley M, Naughton MT, Rowland S, Williamson B, Windler S, Eckermann S, McEvoy RD. A randomized controlled trial of nurse-led care for symptomatic moderate-severe obstructive sleep apnea. Am J Respir Crit Care Med. 2009;179:501–8.

10 Johns MW. A new method for measuring daytime sleepiness: the Epworth sleepiness scale. Sleep. 1991;14:540–5.

11 Olaithe M, Skinner TC, Clarke J, Eastwood P, Bucks RS. Can we get more from the Epworth Sleepiness Scale (ESS) than just a single score? A confirmatory factor analysis of the ESS. Sleep Breath. 2013;17:763–9.

12 Gay PC. The value of assessing risk of obstructive sleep apnea in surgical patients: it only takes one. J Clin Sleep Med. 2010;6:473–4.

13 Peng W, Chen R2, Jiang Z1, Xu X1, Wang J1, Li J1, Liu C1. [Correlation between cognitive function and hippocampal atrophy and cerebral white matter lesions in patients with obstructive sleep apnea hypopnea syndrome]. Zhonghua Yi Xue Za Zhi. 2014;94:724–8.

14 Macey PM, Kumar R, Woo MA, Valladares EM, Yan-Go FL, Harper RM. Brain structural changes in obstructive sleep apnea. Sleep. 2008;31:967–77.

15 Wolford LM, Perez D, Stevao E, Perez E. Airway space changes after nasopharyngeal adenoidectomy in conjunction with Le Fort I osteotomy. J Oral Maxillofac Surg. 2012;70:665–71.

16 Riley RW, Powell NB, Guilleminault C, Nino-Murcia G. Maxillary, mandibular, and hyoid advancement: an alternative to tracheostomy in obstructive sleep apnea syndrome. Otolaryngol Head Neck Surg. 1986;94:584–8.

17 Holty JE, Guilleminault C. Maxillomandibular advancement for the treatment of obstructive sleep apnea: a systematic review and meta-analysis. Sleep Med Rev. 2010;14:287–97.

18 Pirklbauer K, Russmueller G, Stiebellehner L, Nell C, Sinko K, Millesi G, Klug C. Maxillomandibular advancement for treatment of obstructive sleep apnea syndrome: a systematic review. J Oral Maxillofac Surg. 2011;69:e165–76.

19 Powell N, Guilleminault C, Riley R, Smith L. Mandibular advancement and obstructive sleep apnea syndrome. Bull Eur Physiopathol Respir. 1983;19:607–10.

20 Prinsell JR. Primary and secondary telegnathic maxillomandibular advancement, with or without adjunctive procedures, for obstructive sleep apnea in adults: a literature review and treatment recommendations. J Oral Maxillofac Surg. 2012;70:1659–77.

21 Mehra P, Wolford LM. Surgical management of obstructive sleep apnea. Proc (Bayl Univ Med Cent). 2000;13:338–42.

22 Lanigan DT, Hey JH, West RA, et al. Aseptic necrosis following maxillary osteotomies: Report of 36 cases. J Oral Maxillofac Surg. 1990;48:142.

23 Gold AR, Marcus CL, Dipalo F, Gold MS. Upper airway collapsibility during sleep in upper airway resistance syndrome. Chest. 2002;121:1531–40.

24 Riley RW, Guilleminault C, Powell NB, Derman S. Mandibular osteotomy and hyoid bone advancement for obstructive sleep apnea: a case report. Sleep. 1984;7:79–82.

25 Li KK, Riley RW, Powell NB, Troell RJ. Obstructive sleep apnea surgery: genioglossus advancement revisited. J Oral Maxillofac Surg. 2001;59:1181–4; discussion 1185.

Chapter 45

Mandibular Intraoral Distraction Osteogenesis

Cesar A. Guerrero, Gisela I. Contasti-Bocco and Aura Marina Rodriguez

Introduction and history

Patients with severe mandibular deficiency have been treated previously with surgery alone or orthodontics combined with dental extractions.[1–5] Patients who underwent major surgical movements often showed limited results, severe relapse, condyliasis, temporomandibular arthrosis, postoperative sleep apnoea and failures. The experienced surgeon knows the limitations of orthognathic surgery in several clinical situations, especially in large movements and particularly in those with syndromic mandibles.

Another limiting issue is correcting deficiencies in the transverse dimension. The orthodontist usually tries to increase the intercanine distance with different mechanical methods, confronting either relapse or severe periodontal problems secondary to moving the teeth outside the alveolar bone, leading to gingival recession.[5] Extraoral distraction osteogenesis has been widely used to treat major mandibular deficiencies, with the ensuing problems of facial scars and social inconveniences.[6] However, modern technologies in intraoral distraction osteogenesis have evolved to offer a friendly and comfortable surgical technique.[7–13] The obstetrician, paediatrician and paediatric dentist are the first to evaluate patients with severe three-dimensional mandibular deficiencies, severe Class II malocclusion and anterior teeth crowding, either with or without asymmetry; they should be able to provide information to guide the patients according to state of the art technology.

Indications

This technology is indicated for patients presenting with severe mandibular deficiency (over 10 mm), temporomandibular arthritis, sleep apnoea, previous failures in advancing the mandible and inadequate anatomy (syndromic mandibles).[14,15]

Contraindications

Intraoral distraction osteogenesis biology is based on sound surgical principles that depend on vascularity and bone quantity and quality. It should not be applied after radiotherapy or conditions involving very poor bone, also this technology requires patient and family collaboration.[14,15]

Mandibular widening

(See Figures 45-1 and 45-2.)

Orthognathic Surgery: Principles, Planning and Practice. Edited by Farhad B. Naini and Daljit S. Gill.

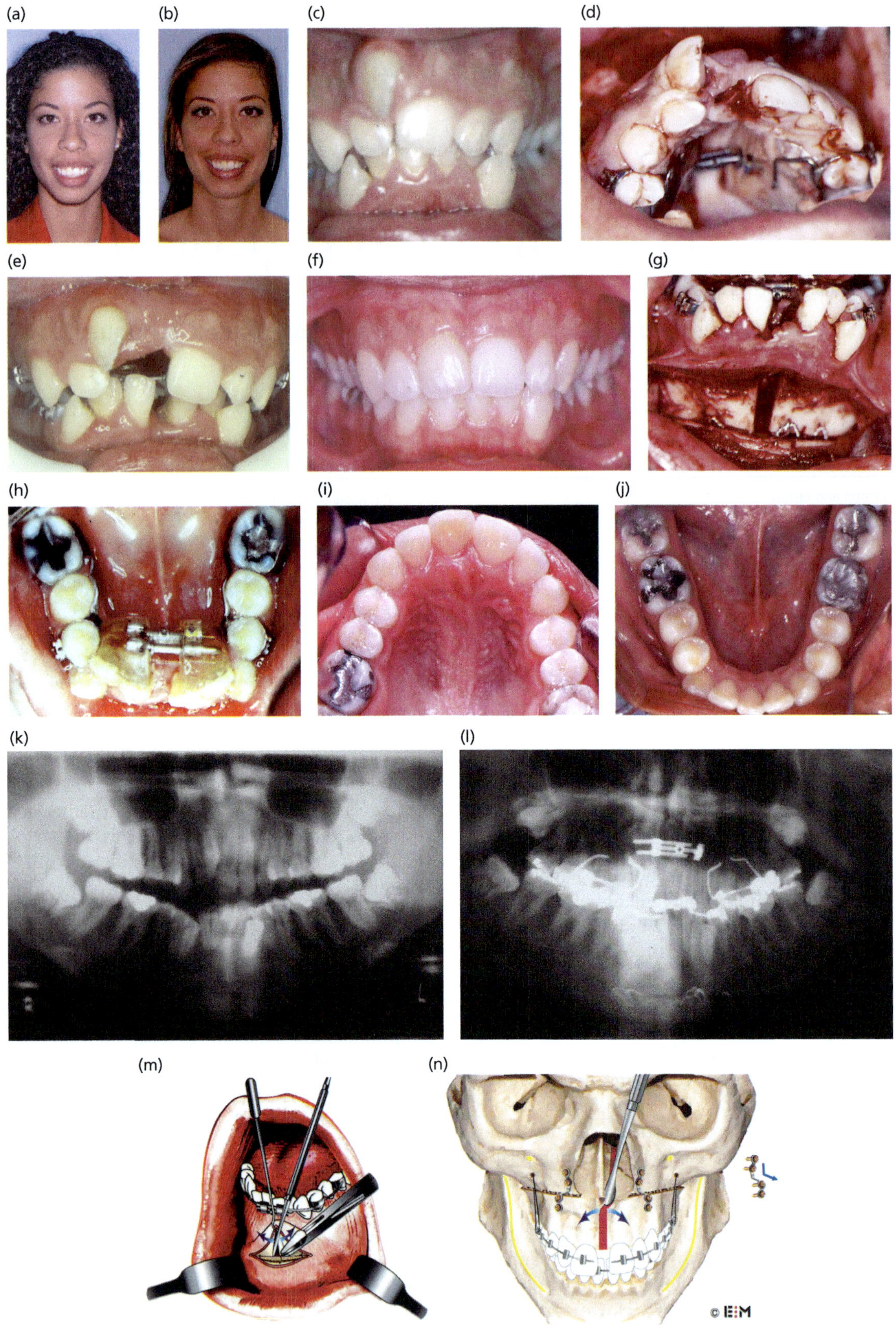

Fig. 45-1 Transverse maxillomandibular deficiency in a 15-year-old female patient, treated with Le Fort I and midline osteotomies for transverse maxillary expansion (n), mandibular widening and genioplasty (m). A periosteal elevator is kept in between the two halves of the mandible so that an acute widening at the basal bone is achieved while the wires are tightened. Preoperative (a) and postoperative (b) frontal facial views are shown. A space was needed for the right upper central incisor, and the maxillary progressive expansion forced the need for simultaneous mandibular widening (c, d). Intraoperative view (d, g) and during activation (e, h). Post-treatment dental photographs show adequate occlusion, all teeth in position, with molar and canine Class I, a lower central incisor was removed secondary to Bolton's discrepancy (f, i, j). Preoperative panoramic radiographs (k) and after distraction protocol (l). The total orthodontic-surgical treatment was 16 months. These are 2.5-year follow-up photographs.

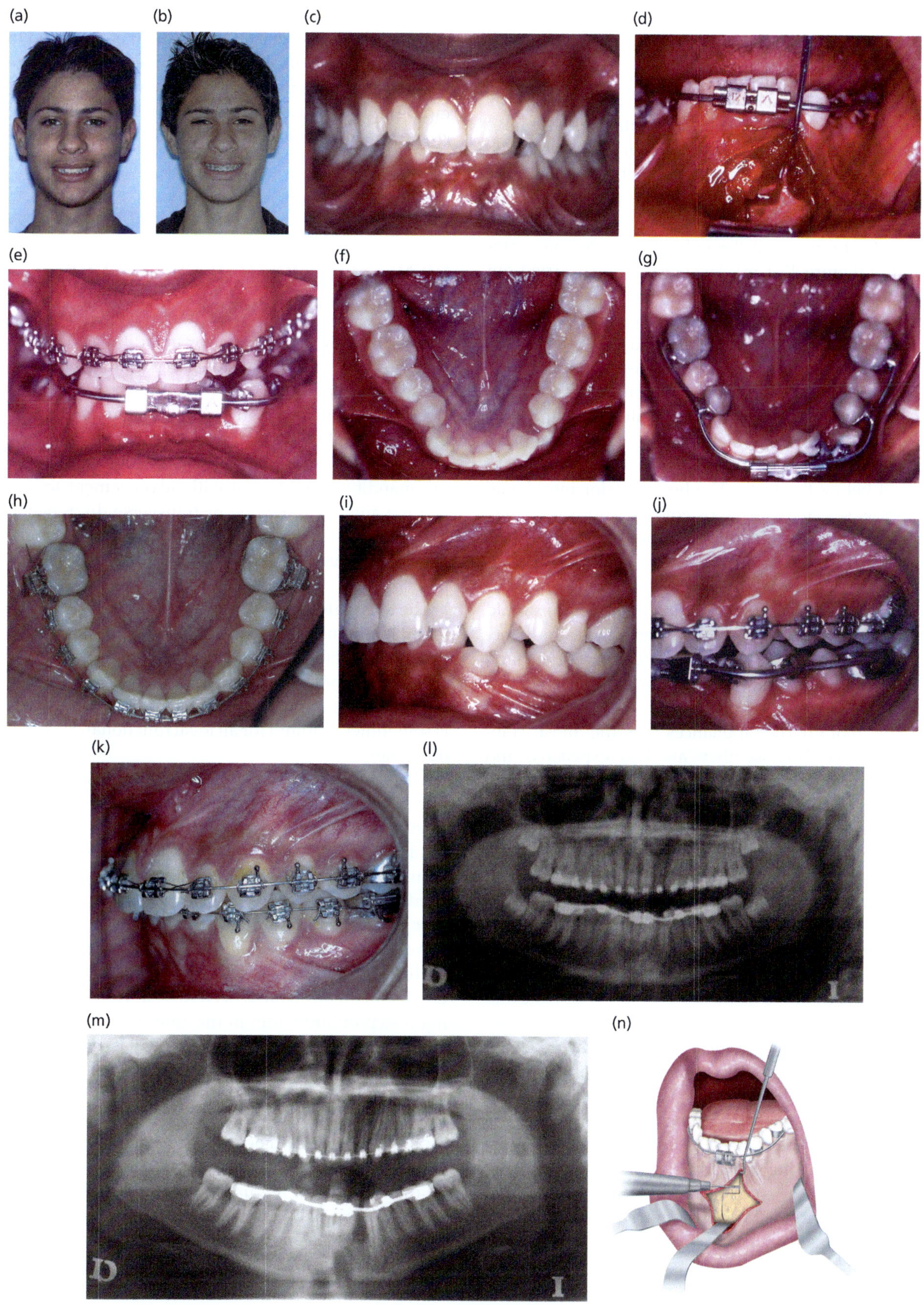

Fig. 45-2 A 15-year-old male patient with transverse mandibular deficiency, inferior left canine without space in the arch. Preoperative (a) and postoperative (b) frontal facial views; and intraoral views: frontal (c, e); occlusal (f, g, h); and buccal (i, j, k). Intraoperative view: tooth borne distractor in position (d) and symphyseal osteotomy was performed away from the midline because of lack of space between the central incisors. When the technique does not involve genioplasty, the osteotomy needs to be finished in the midline to avoid symphyseal asymmetries (d, n). Panoramic radiograph views: preoperative (l); and after distraction protocol (m); the distractor was removed 3 months after surgery.

Surgical technique

The incision is made 4 to 6 mm labial to the depth of the mandibular vestibule through the orbicularis muscle. After the muscle is transected, the dissection is directed obliquely through the mentalis muscle until contact is made with the mandibular symphysis. The periosteum is responsible for the distraction chamber healing and must be carefully reflected inferiorly to the lower border of the mandible, placing a small channel retractor to protect it throughout the osteotomy procedure (Figure 45-1 m). The osteotomy is carried out from the inferior border up to the apices with a reciprocating saw. The soft tissue between the mandibular central incisors is carefully reflected superiorly to the alveolar crest and a skin hook is used to retract and protect the soft tissues while the interdental osteotomy is completed (Figure 45-2 d,n). Initially, with a 701 burr mounted in a straight handpiece, just the outer cortex and the sectioning is finalized with a straight chisel below the teeth. The best anterior interdental space is selected for the osteotomy, and a step may be necessary to start in the symphyseal midline and finish between the lateral and canine to avoid post-surgical chin asymmetry (Figure 45-2 n). Also, those patients needing major widening (over 8 mm) should have the genioplasty osteotomy performed simultaneously, in order not to widen the lower part of the face, which is an undesirable feature, particularly in women (Figure 45-1 g).[16–18]

The tooth-borne appliances are the most commonly used because they are less expensive and save time during surgery (Figure 45-2 e,g,j). If a bone-borne device is to be used, it must be fixed before the osteotomy is completed. The upper arms of the pre-bent bone-borne appliance are wired with a 0.024-inch gauge wire to the anchorage teeth, and a 2 mm transmucosal bicortical screw is used on each side to fixate the lower arms. Acrylic is placed over the wires around the teeth to provide more rigidity. The widening obtained is similar with any distractor, but the tooth-borne distractor is easier to activate and remove.[11,15]

Most patients require an advancement genioplasty with vertical augmentation to ideally treat the three-dimensional deformity. This can be done simultaneously, by acutely widening the mandibular basal bone with an instrument, fixating the chin segment and releasing the instrument from the osteotomy site.

At this point, a 0.026-inch gauge wire could be used to tie each central incisor to the consecutive lateral incisor or canine to prevent the teeth from 'walking' into the distraction site secondary to transseptal fibres stretching during the activation period. Once the osteotomy and 2 mm activation have been performed, periosteum, muscles, and mucosa wound layers are meticulously closed using a 3-0 chromic suture. The activation is initiated 7 days later, with a rate of 1 mm a day and a rhythm of once a day; once the desired widening is obtained, acrylic is placed on the activation screw to stabilize it and the patient is advanced to a soft diet. The consolidation or mineralization stage is usually 60 days for every centimetre of distraction; radiographs are used for confirmation and then one may proceed to remove the distraction device and permit orthodontic mechanics.[15,17,18]

Bilateral mandibular lengthening

Posterior body osteotomy

This osteotomy is designed for mandibular deficiencies that present with an ideal occlusal plane. Even though most patients with a severe Class II show a steep curve of Spee with crowding, this secondary problem should be addressed either by orthodontics, inferior-repositioning subapical osteotomy or combining mandibular widening with advancement to correct the anterior crowding or transverse discrepancy. The treatment objective is to obtain an ideal canine and molar Class I occlusion relation with a flat occlusal plane.[19,20]

The adequate positioning of the distractor is fundamental to achieve the correct distraction vector, and different variables are taken into consideration for adequate planning and fixation. Obviously, the possibility of changing the distraction vector after surgery is sometimes required for an ideal functional–aesthetic outcome.

The orthodontist and surgeon should plan the positioning of the distraction appliance based on photographs, radiographs, dental models mounted on an articulator, and clinical examination, sometimes requiring a three-dimensional model. The distractors need to be parallel to the occlusal plane to avoid developing a posterior or anterior open bite.[15]

Additionally, as the mandible is transversely wider in the posterior and narrower in the anterior portion, the distractor appliances need to be adjusted by creating a step of 5 to 8 mm in the anterior fixation arms, allowing the distractor's screw to be placed parallel to the axis of distraction to compensate for this important variation in mandibular width. If this is underestimated, the reciprocal forces exerted to the mandible by the appliance will advance the mandible, moving the proximal segment not only posteriorly (this could be overcome with the use of heavy Class II elastics) but also laterally and exerting very detrimental forces to the TMJs, causing pain, dysfunction, and damage to the joints; also lateral torquing force against the condyle, loosening the screws and bending the appliance.[20,21]

Mandibular advancement needs to be planned transporting the anterior segment anteriorly into an ideal Class I occlusion and eliminating the posterior reciprocal forces with heavy Class II elastics (8–12 ounces per side for three months).[15,20,21]

Surgical procedure

A 2.5 cm full-thickness incision is made over the external oblique line, extending inferiorly over the alveolar ridge to the position of the first molar. A subperiosteal tunnelling dissection is performed to expose the alveolar ridge and the buccal cortex down to the inferior border of the mandible between the second and third molars, where a small channel retractor is placed to protect the soft tissues during the osteotomy. The periosteum, muscles, and soft tissues are minimally detached, maintaining the best blood supply possible to the area. A reciprocating saw is used to section the inferior border of the mandible bicortically at a 45° angle to increase the bony surfaces, up to around 3 mm away from the inferior alveolar nerve, continuing on the lateral mandibular cortex superiorly. A periosteal elevator is placed between the lingual soft tissues and the mandible to guard against lingual nerve injuries while the alveolar area is sectioned bicortically from the top toward the inferior alveolar nerve area 3 or 4 mm away, with the saw upside down and at a 45° angle, abundant irrigation is used throughout the osteotomy to avoid bone overheating. At this point, the uncut bone is just 6 mm around the mandibular nerve, the flaps are sutured and the distraction appliance is fixed with transmucosal bicortical screws above and underneath the nerve, an interdental wire could be used not to place interdental screws; a small incision is left open to apply a torque movement with a chisel to complete the mandibular osteotomy, a single mattress suture is placed to close the remnant of the flap; this manoeuvre ensures primary closure over the osteotomy, eliminating distraction chamber contamination and offering periosteum integrity. When both sides are to be operated, final sectioning of the ramus is deferred until the osteotomy of the opposite side is completed. A sagittal split osteotomy could also be used obtaining a broader bone surface if adequate bone width is present; this approach is beneficial in terms of avoiding pulling the mandibular nerve, especially in large advancements where the nerve is elongated 20 to 30% of its length causing paraesthesia.[15,19–21]

Parasymphyseal osteotomy

(See Figure 45-3)

This is indicated in patients with inadequate anatomy at the mandibular angle area, usually presenting with a severe anterior open bite and severe crowding, or those clinical situations requiring major movements that may jeopardize the mandibular nerve secondary to severe stretching (Figure 45-3 h,k,n). This mandibular area possesses the best bone stock with over 3 cm of height and one cm of basal bone width. It is an interdental osteotomy, which may require presurgical orthodontics to create an interdental space (Figure 45-3 h). The distraction gap would be utilized to align and level the occlusion post-surgically, or dental implants could be inserted. This technique is ideal for major movements since it is anterior to the mental nerve, and the mandibular nerve is not stretched or damaged (Figure 45-3 c,d).[15,19–21]

Surgical procedure

A 3 cm incision is made 4 to 6 mm inferior to the attached gingiva, well above the mental nerve; a subperiosteum dissection is carried out, exposing the mental nerve and inferior border of the mandible to allocate a channel retractor. The osteotomy is executed from the inferior border to the level of the dental roots, under abundant irrigation to avoid bone overheating, then a 701 burr mounted in a straight hand piece is used to complete the outer cortex bone section between the teeth and a straight chisel is utilized to complete the osteotomy. The distractor is fixed with inferior bicortical screws and interdental wires are used around the teeth and acrylic applied on top to increase rigidity and to avoid roots damaged with heat and screw placement (Figure 45-3 e,f,g).[15,19–21]

Ideally, the wound is closed before the distractor is fixed to have a close distraction chamber without food and saliva contamination.

The distraction protocol is similar, however, as the distraction chamber enlarges, the open bite increases; this is planned in the planning and prediction phases. The patient requires a major advancement at the mandibular base and a few millimeters between the teeth; once most of the activation is completed, the patient is taken to the operating theatre to change the mandibular vector, by eliminating the wires and acrylic from the antero-superior distractor arm; just keeping a single infero-anterior bicortical screw, bilaterally, the mandible rotates anticlockwise, closing the open bite. It is important to have some extra millimeters left in the distractor rod to accommodate the midline and do some final adjustments to the occlusion (Figure 45-3 i,j).[15,19–21]

Children in the primary dentition requiring mandibular lengthening need Erich arch bars during surgery for Class II elastics placement through the activation and consolidation phases and post-surgical occlusion control. The clinician needs to monitor the range of opening and avoid mandibular deviation during function; physiotherapy is mandatory to obtain at least 40 mm opening in a vertical straight fashion.[15,19–21]

The distractors are rigidly fixated with bicortical screws, avoiding teeth and the alveolar nerve; when a bicortical screw cannot be placed without damaging a dental structure, a 0.024-inch gauge wire may be used to fixate the distractor.

A transcutaneous trocar could be used to place the distractor's posterior screws, especially in small children, patients with small oral commissures, or

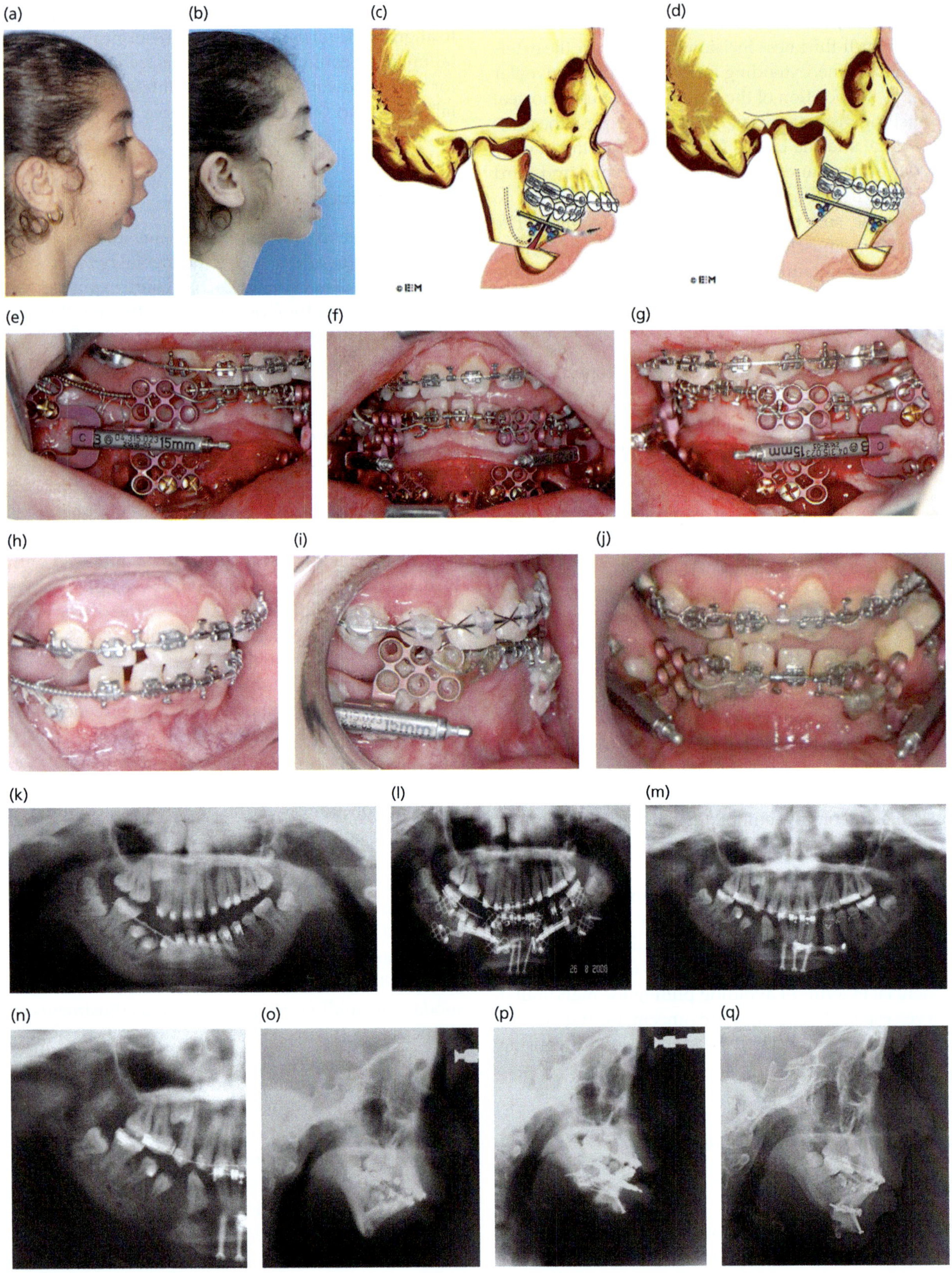

Fig. 45-3 A 15-year-old female patient with severe mandibular deficiency; bilateral mandibular lengthening was performed by parasymphyseal osteotomy because of the inadequate anatomy at the mandibular angle. Profile facial views are shown before and after 2 years of treatment (a, b). Diagram shows parasymphyseal osteotomy design anterior to the mental nerve (c) to avoid mental nerve stretch or damage, and after 15 mm of full distraction (d). Intraoperative views (e, f, g). Distractor appliance positioning and genioplasty were performed simultaneously. Intraoral views: preoperative (h); during activation period (i); acrylic is positioned at the distractor after final activation (j). Panoramic radiographs: Preoperative (k); after activation period (l); the distractors were removed 6 months after surgery (m). Adequate bone consolidation (n). Cephalometric radiographs: preoperative (o) during consolidation period (p); after 2 years of follow-up (q).

where the vertical osteotomy is located too far posterior.[15,19–21]

Distraction protocol

After surgery, a 7-day latency period is awaited for collagen type I fibres to develop, primary soft tissue to heal, and initial surgical oedema to reduce. Activation follows at a rate of 1 mm and a rhythm of once a day until the desired distraction is completed; while the patient is activating the distractors, close monitoring should take place to avoid midline deviations owing to inadequate anticlockwise or uneven activation of the distraction devices. If needed, asymmetrical activation should be done to correct a midline discrepancy.[15,19]

An important issue is the temporomandibular joint (TMJ). The presurgical orthodontic phase should include rectangular surgical orthodontic arches with welded vertical pins to apply Class II elastics, for 3 months after surgery awaiting muscles enlargement and adaptation.

After total activation is accomplished, acrylic is placed over the distractor rod for stabilization purposes and the appliances are used throughout the consolidation period as a fixation system. Radiographs are taken to verify the distraction chamber ossification, for appliance removal.

A liquid diet, including high-protein supplements, is recommended during the activation period, followed by a soft diet once the distractor is stabilized with acrylic until consolidation is achieved, between 2 and 12 months depending on the magnitude of the movement.[15,19,21]

Unilateral mandibular lengthening

(Figures 45-4 and 45-5)

Patients with unilateral craniofacial microsomia, unilateral Treacher Collins syndrome or other forms of unilateral micromandibulism may present with minimal bone stock in the post molar and angle regions, compromising the possibility of performing either traditional surgery or distraction osteogenesis. These patients frequently present requiring major movements. In these clinical cases, it is advisable to plan the surgery along the body of the mandible between the premolars, anterior to the mental nerve because of bone stock and to avoid lower lip paraesthesia. Some patients may benefit from simultaneous vertical ramus and horizontal body lengthening (Figures 45-4 and 45-5).[22,23]

Ramus lengthening procedure

When increasing mandibular ramus height the temporomandibular joint function is fundamental. The reciprocal forces exerted towards the glenoid fossa secondary to stretching the pterygomasseteric sling will maintain a continuous pressure provoking disc displacement, condylar resorption and TMJ arthrosis. This is similar to lengthening of the femur, where the orthopedic surgeon places two rings in the femur with expansible screws and another ring across the tibia and fibula, with maintenance bars, in order to avoid detrimental forces into the knee crushing the cartilages and producing arthrosis.[22–24]

There are three different scenarios in lengthening the mandibular ramus: a unilateral mandibular deficiency with a functional condyle, a unilateral

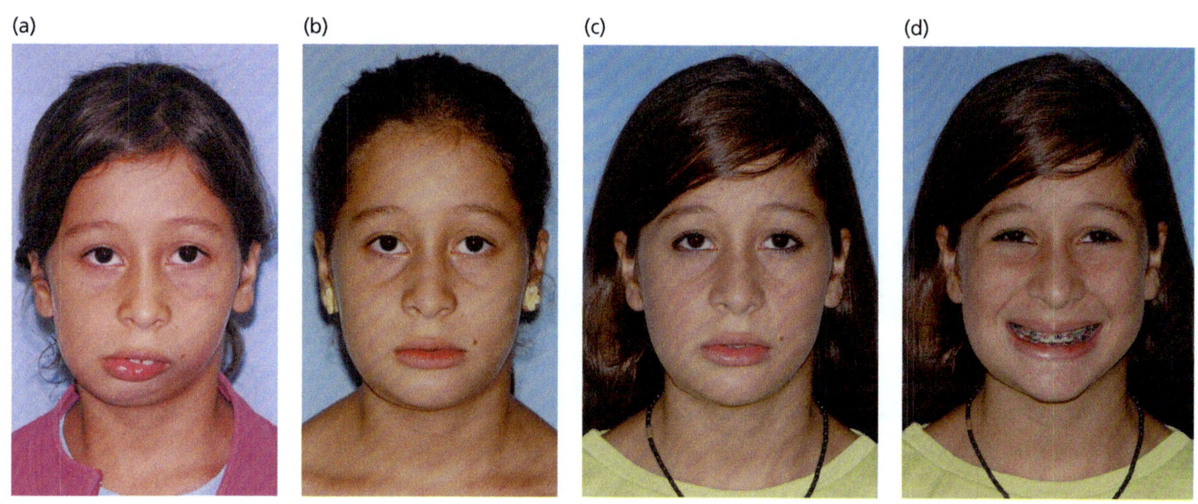

Fig. 45-4 A 10-year-old child seen long after a subcondylar fracture, with severe mandibular deficiency and mandibular hypomobility (5 mm). She was treated by unilateral mandibular ramus and body lengthening. Arch bars were used to control the occlusion and guide the physiotherapy. Before and after 3 years of treatment frontal and profile facial views are shown (a, b, c, d, e, f, g). Intraoral views: Orthodontics was continued after the archbars were removed and microscrews used to close the distraction chamber by advancing the right mandibular molars into an ideal Class I (i, j, k, l, m, n). Distractor removed and arthroplasty performed after consolidation period. Panoramic radiographs: preoperative (o), one week after surgery (p), after activation protocol (consolidation period) (q) and during remodelling period (r). Cephalometric radiographs: preoperative (s) and during consolidation period (t).

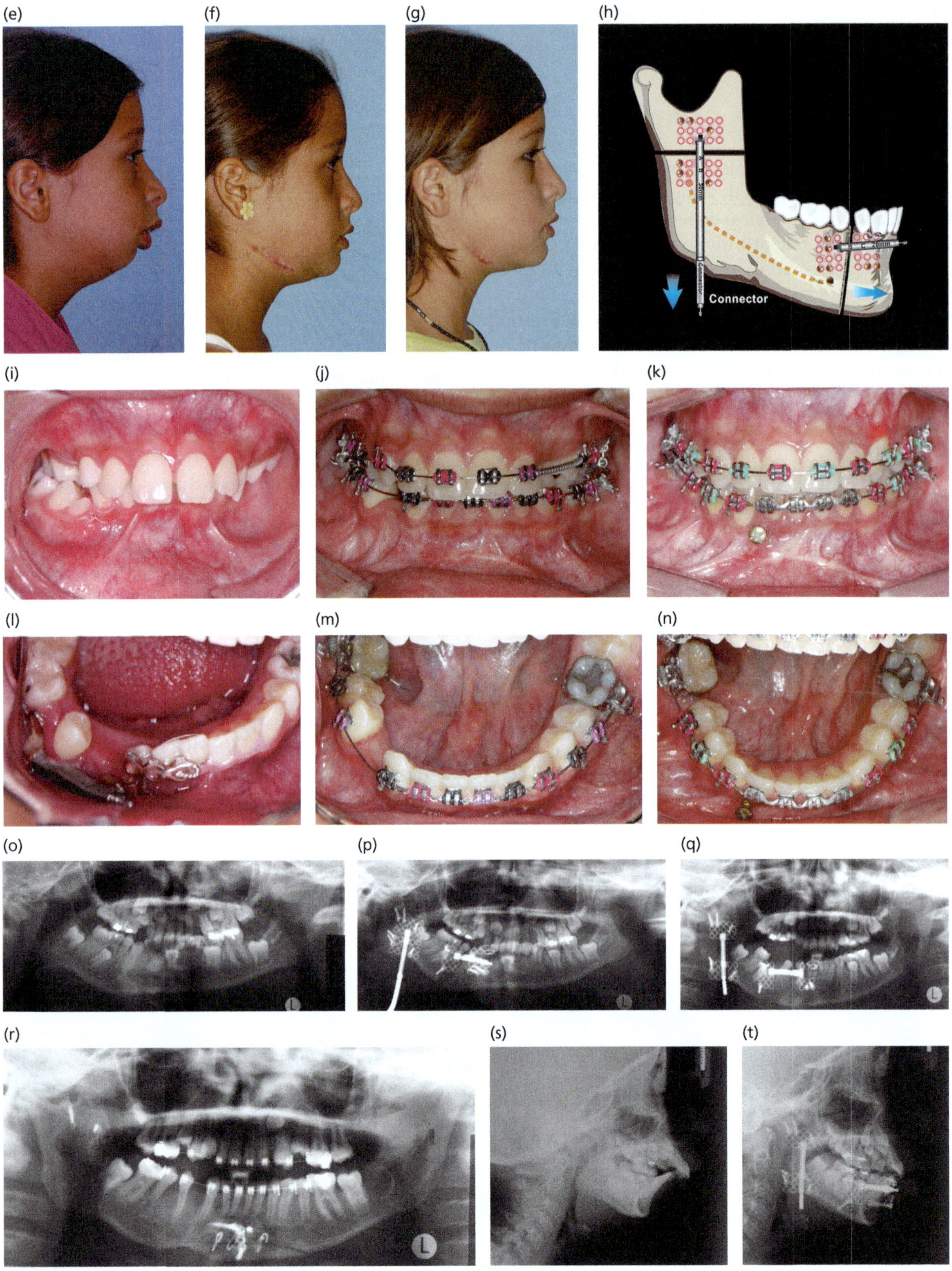

Fig. 45-4 (*Continued*).

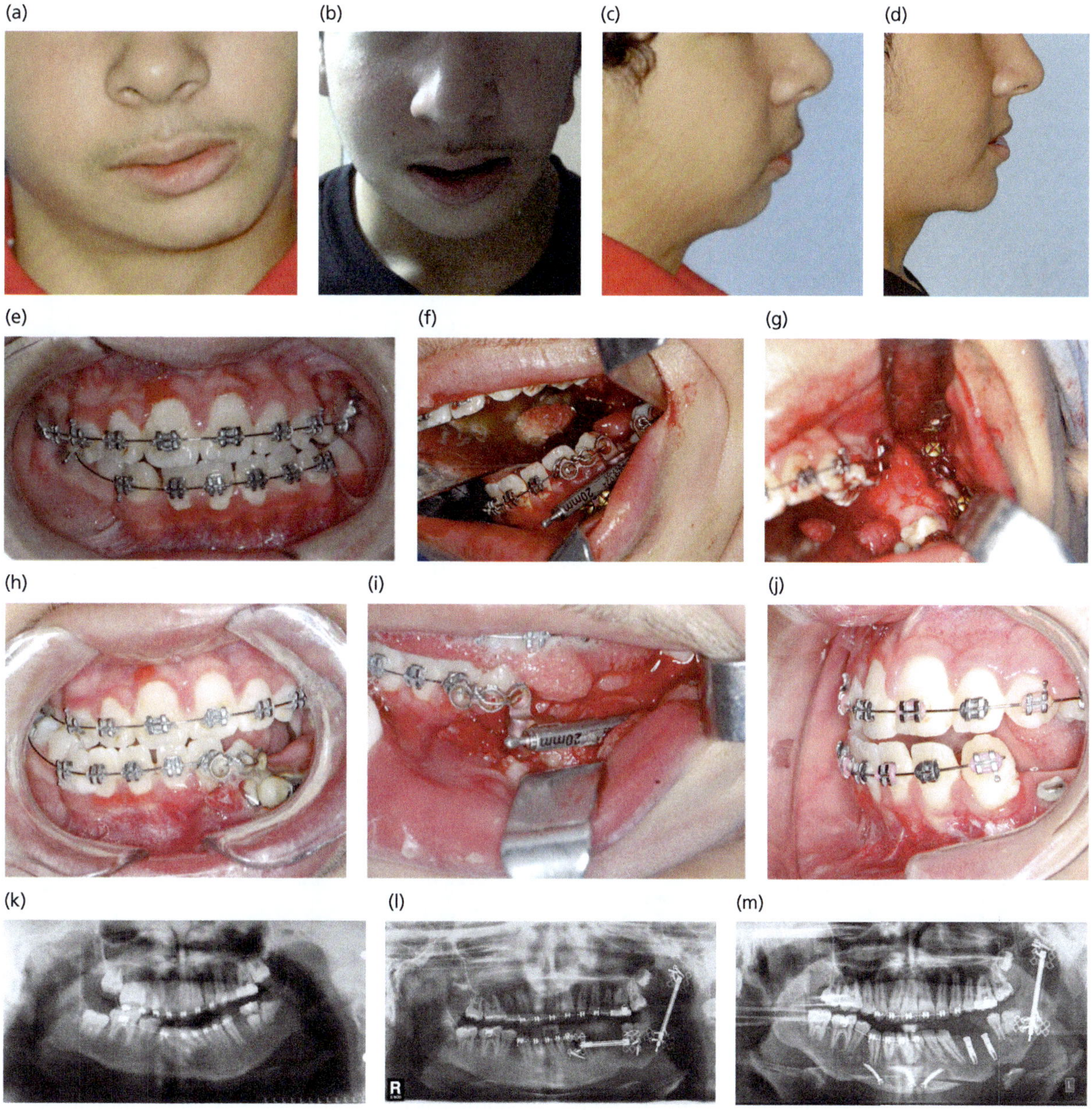

Fig. 45-5 A 13-year-old male patient with unilateral craniofacial microsomia, Pruzansky 3, treated by intraoral ramus and body intraoral distraction osteogenesis to lengthen the mandible a total of 50 mm (30 + 20 mm). Before and after 2 years of treatment frontal and profile facial views are shown (a, b, c, d). Dental views are shown: Preoperative (e) and postoperative (j). Intraoperative views (f, g): The surgery was performed completely intraorally with the exception of a 2 mm inframandibular incision to place the activation connector for the vertical device. The ramus osteotomy was done just leaving 10 mm to be transported, and the body osteotomy between the premolars avoiding the mandibular nerve before and after exiting the mandible. The appliances were activated to full length (h); the connectors were disengaged after and were left in place for 18 months (i). Once the appliances were removed, dental implants were inserted; the mental nerve was localized posterior to the body osteotomy and distraction chamber (m, p). The patient is continuing his treatment for ear reconstruction and a free fat graft is scheduled at the end of treatment. His bony structure has been meticulously augmented and ideal occlusion will be obtained after the orthodontics mechanics is finalized. Cephalometric radiographs are shown (n, o, p, q, r, s).

mandibular deficiency with a gap between the malformed condyle and the glenoid fossa, and temporomandibular joint ankylosis. Each group should be treated differently to obtain a symmetrical mandibular frame and a functional temporomandibular joint; based on function, aesthetics and stability over time. These are very complicated patients and many of them will present after numerous surgical failures; the clinician must perform all the surgical procedures in one stage, if possible, or perform as many as indicated in every surgical stage (Figures 45-4 and 45-5).[23,24]

1. Ramus procedure with a functional condyle

A 3 cm incision is made in the lateral retromolar area, to allow wide periosteal elevation of the lateral mandibular ramus, up to the coronoid process. A horizontal osteotomy is performed above the

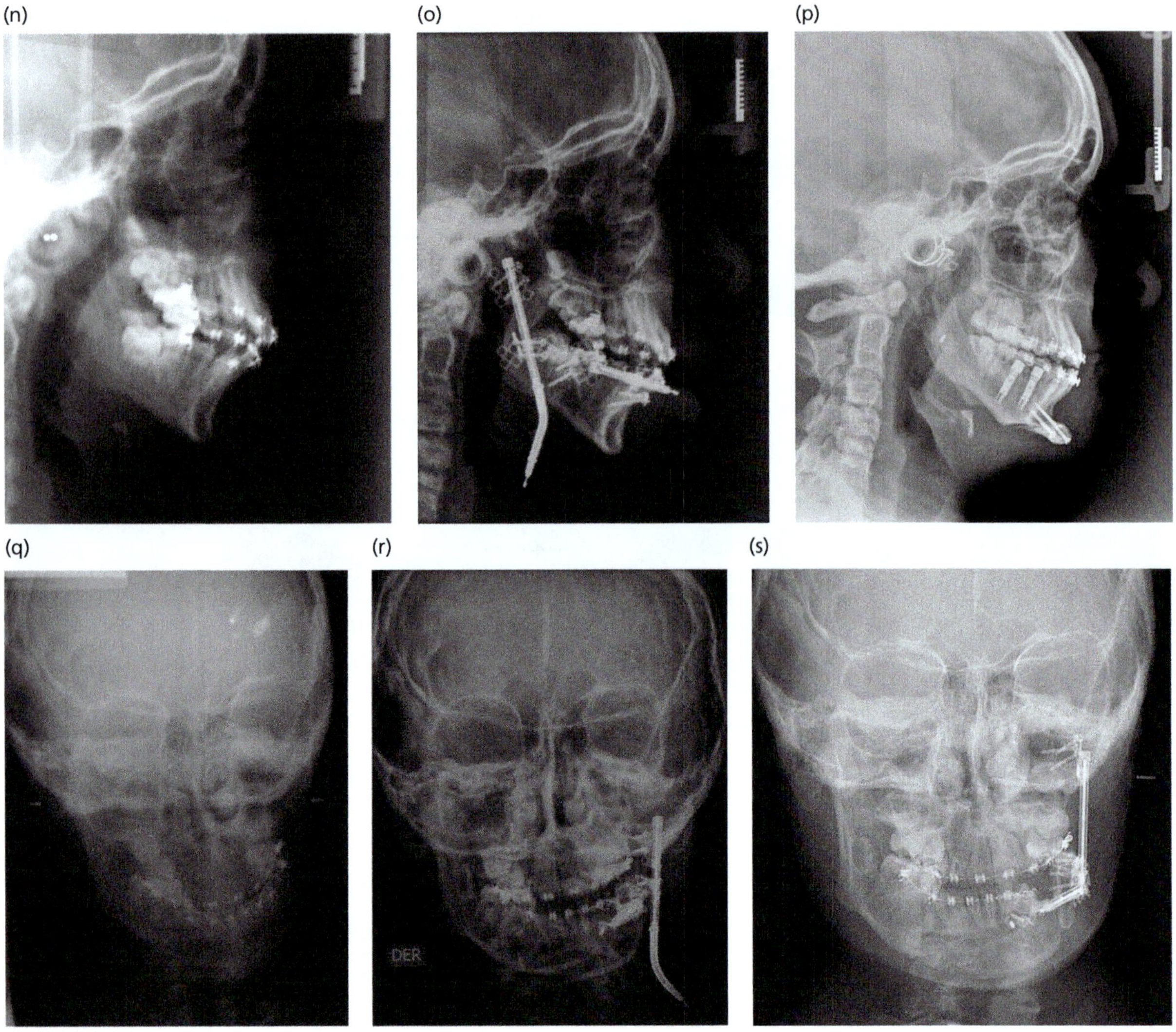

Fig. 45-5 (*Continued*).

antilingula, to ensure no damage to the mandibular nerve and vessels. Before completing the cut, rigid fixation is placed from the body of the zygoma to the upper mandibular ramus segment to stabilize the cranium to the upper mandibular ramus segment; a horizontal incision in the maxillary molar area, followed by exposing the zygoma allow insertion of at least three screws in the body, and the remaining plate is inserted through the soft tissue into the lateral mandibular area; another three screws are inserted in the coronoid area.

The mandibular osteotomy is completed after fixing the distractor into both mandibular segments; a connector emerges extraorally through a 2 mm incision. The connector will allow activation and should be removed once the clinician has completed the objectives. The distraction appliance remains in place until adequate consolidation has occurred, which may be observed radiographically. Under intravenous sedation or general anaesthesia, the distractor is removed intraorally, and the rigid fixation plate is disconnected through the retromolar incision and the maxillary incision to get to the body of the zygoma.

An alternative to the internal fixation zygoma to the mandible is David Matthew's extraoral appliance.[22,23]

2. Ramus lengthening in TMJ ankylosis (Figure 45-4)

Historically, long-term ankylosis in children leads to severe mandibular growth arrest and sleep apnoea. Most surgical procedures were wrongly planned to release the ankylosis first and in a secondary surgical stage improve the mandibular shape and size, frequently ending in re-ankylosis.[23]

The TMJ ankylosis patient (Figure 45-4 o) will require two surgical stages and long-term physiotherapy to rehabilitate the joint. The first stage would include enlargement of the mandibular frame, by lengthening the mandibular ramus and body, and a significant genioplasty. These three procedures increase the mandibular frame and lengthen the perimandibular muscles. The distractors are left in place until complete consolidation; there is no relapse because the muscles and bone have matured in a new position for over 6 months (Figure 45-4 h,p,q). On the second surgical stage, through the same Risdon approach the distraction appliance is removed, TMJ arthroplasty is performed, continuing with either a maxillary Le Fort I or partial maxillary osteotomy to close the lateral open bite and to eliminate the maxillary cant, if necessary (in younger children orthodontics may be sufficient) and secondary genioplasty to obtain ideal anterior symmetry (Figure 45-4 f,g,r).

The secondary genioplasty is needed to reduce the muscular force against the newly performed arthroplasty and to avoid ankylosis recurrence; increasing the mandibular frame in the first surgical stage creates a stable muscular environment and allows the second stage osteotomy's stability.

There may be a need for lateral ramus augmentation on the affected side. This is done a year after facial muscle healing and stability, when the physiotherapy has been completed and orthodontic appliances removed. A preformed mandibular angle prosthesis is indicated.[23]

Surgical procedure

A 3 cm skin incision is made utilizing the submandibular Risdon approach, through the skin, platysma muscle and periosteum. The mandibular angle and the ramus are exposed completely, the ankylosis area is identified, and a horizontal osteotomy is performed using a reciprocating saw protecting the anterior and posterior soft tissues with channel retractors, above the antilingula, avoiding the mandibular bundle medially. Once the segment is mobilized, the prebent, pre-shaped distraction appliance and measured screws from the 3-D model are installed, carefully checking the distraction vector, similar to the unaffected side (Figure 45-4 h).

The internal distractor is provided with a connector to be exposed extraorally at the submandibular incision site. The area is copiously irrigated and the wound is closed in layers. The appliance is activated intraoperatively 2 or 3 mm to avoid premature consolidation. This is probably the best distraction osteogenesis environment, with a close chamber and good blood supply with a wide bone contact, especially because the osteotomy is performed in a diagonal fashion (15 to 25 degree angle), secondary to the inclination working from below through the Risdon incision. Seven days after surgery the activation starts at 1 mm per day, until the desired distraction is obtained. At that point new radiographs are taken to measure in detail the facial skeleton, and then the patient is scheduled for connector removal (Figure 45-4 q); the connector is removed by twisting the screwdriver in the other direction (if the connector head has a double system, internal for the activation and external for removal) and it is released from the distractor or is cut off under the skin. Steristrips are placed over the small wound and on the second surgical stage the scar should be removed and cosmetic new closure performed. The patient resumes regular activities wearing the internal distractor, without any limitations.[23]

Once adequate consolidation is observed on the radiographs, usually 8 to 12 months after the first surgical stage, the patient undergoes surgery to have the distraction devices removed, TMJ arthroplasty and leveling Le Fort I osteotomy (Figure 45-4 r).[22,23]

3. Condylar bone transport to lengthen the ramus and close the gap (Figure 45-5)

After careful evaluation of the patient's records and 3-D models are made, the distractors are cut to length, bent and adapted to the clinical situation. The distractors are fixed to the model and acrylic section to simulate the actual surgery. The screws' length and positioning are selected and should be ready in exact order for the surgical intervention. This is a time saving manoeuver that needs to be done carefully and meticulously, to permit the desired surgical outcome.

A 3 cm incision is made at the lateral mandibular area, allowing exposure of the lateral mandibular angle and bone stomp. The medial and posterior soft tissues are left intact to ensure vascularization; this is a pedicle segment to be transported, not a free graft. The osteotomy is performed with a reciprocating saw under abundant irrigation, with a 15 to 20 degree angulation to increase bone surface. Before completion of the osteotomy, a 2 mm incision is made at the mandibular angle skin, to insert inside out, the distraction's connector and localize the selected distractor, which is fixed with three screws (tripod concept) on either side of the osteotomy; then the section is completed (Figure 45-5 a,b,o).

A second distractor is usually placed in the body of the mandible for horizontal lengthening. This second distractor is placed after the ramus surgery is concluded (Figure 45-5 i,l,o,r).[22–24]

Postoperative considerations

The distractors should be removed after proper ossification has occurred, confirmed by a radiographic evaluation, and considering the different variables involved in the healing process, such as the age of the patient, amount of movement, quality and quantity of bone, infection, inadequate stability during consolidation, poor patient selection, and some systemic diseases.

If the clinician removes the appliances before adequate bone ossification, the perimandibular muscles will force the segments away from the planned repositioning, with the consequent development of an open bite, anterior mandibular ramus rotation (proximal fragment anticlockwise rotation), disappearance of the mandibular angle projection, and TMJ pain and dysfunction. The use of maxillomandibular elastics to close the open bite is not indicated because they will extrude the maxillary incisors, the anterior open bite will relapse and prolong the post-surgical orthodontics, and the final occlusion will be unstable, heading for relapse and TMJ dysfunction symptoms.

Once the proper stabilization period has elapsed, usually 60 days for every centimetre of lengthening, the distractor is removed.[15,21]

Intraoral distraction osteogenesis allows mandibular lengthening with meticulous occlusal finishing, in a predictable and stable manner; maintaining the TMJs intact and conserving their preoperative anatomical characteristics. The surgical technique permits progressive augmentation of the hard and soft tissues, into an ideal dental occlusion. The orthodontist needs to prepare the dentition presurgically into an ideal arch situation and stabilize the tooth positions with heavy rectangular archwires to allow the use of heavy intermaxillary elastics during the early post-surgical period, but allowing complete joint unloading during the activation and consolidation phases.

References

1 Obwegeser H, Trauner R. Zur Operationstechnik bei der Progenie und anderen Unterkieferanomalien. Dtsch Zahn Mund Kieferheilkd.1955;23:1–2.
2 Bell W, Epker B. Surgical–orthodontic expansion of the maxilla. Am J Orthod. 1976;70:517–28.
3 Epker B. Distraction osteogenesis for mandibular widening. Atlas Oral Maxillofac Surg Clin North Am. 1999;7:29–39.
4 Schendel S, Wolford L, Epker B. Mandibular deficiency syndrome III. Surgical advancement of the deficient mandible in growing children: treatment results in twelve patients. Oral Surg Oral Med Oral Pathol. 1978;45:364–77.
5 Little R, Wallen T, Riedel R. Stability and relapse of mandibular anterior alignment – first premolar extraction cases treated by traditional edgewise orthodontics. Am J Orthod. 1981;80:349–65.
6 Little R, Riedel R, Artun J. An evaluation of changes in mandibular anterior alignment from 10 to 20 years post-retention. Am J Orthod Dentofac Orthop. 1988;93:423–8.
7 McCarthy J, Schreiber J, Karp N, et al. Lengthening the human mandible by gradual distraction. Plast Reconstr Surg. 1992; 89:1–8.
8 Diner P, Kollar E, Martinez H, Vazquez M. Intraoral distraction for mandibular lengthening – a technical innovation. J Craniomaxillofac Surg. 1996;24:92–5.
9 Wangerin K, Gropp H. Die intraorale Distraktionsosteotomie des mikrogenen Unterkiefers zur Beseitigung der Atemwegsobstruktion. Dtsch Z Mund Kiefer Gesichtschir. 1994; 18:236.
10 Chin M, Toth B. Distraction osteogenesis in maxillofacial surgery using internal devices: review of five cases. J Oral Maxillofac Surg. 1996;54:45–4.
11 Guerrero C. Rapid mandibular expansion. Rev Venez Ortod. 1990;48:1–2.
12 Triaca A, Minoretti R, Dimai W, et al. Multiaxis intraoral distraction of the mandible. In: Samchukov ML, Cope JB, Cheraskin AM (Eds). Craniofacial distraction osteogenesis. St. Louis Mosby, 2001:323–33.
13 Razdolsky Y, Dessner S, El-Bialy T. Correction of alveolar ridge deficiency using the ROD-5 distraction device: a case report. In: Samchukov ML, Cope JB, Cherkashin AM (Eds). Craniofacial distraction osteogenesis. St. Louis (MO): Mosby, 2001:454–58.
14 Guerrero C, Bell W, Dominguez E. Intraoral distraction osteogenesis versus sagittal split osteotomy to lengthen the mandible. In: Arnaud E, Diner PA (Eds). 4th International Congress of Maxillofacial and Craniofacial Distraction, Paris, France, July 2–5. Bologna: Monduzzi Editore, 2003: 133–8.
15 Guerrero C, Figueroa F, Bell W, Olmos Y, Rojas A, Gonzalez M. Surgical orthodontics in mandibular lengthening. In: Bell W, Guerrero C. Distraction osteogenesis of the facial skeleton. Hamilton: BC Decker, 2007:501–19.
16 Guerrero C, Bell W, Contasti G, Rodriguez A. Mandibular widening by intraoral distraction osteogenesis. Br J Oral Maxillofac Surg. 1997;35:383–92.
17 Guerrero C, Contasti G. Transverse mandibular deficiency. In: Bell WH (Ed.) Modern practice in orthognathic and reconstructive surgery. Philadelphia (PA): W.B. Saunders, 1992:2383–97.
18 Contasti G, Rodriguez A and Guerrero C. Orthodontic mandibular widening by distraction osteogenesis. Orthod Cyber J. 1998;12.
19 Gonzalez M, Bell W, Guerrero C, Buschang PH, Samchukov ML. Positional changes and stability of bone segments during simultaneous bilateral mandibular lengthening and widening by distraction osteogenesis. Br J Oral Maxillofac Surg. 2001;39:169–78.
20 Guerrero C, Bell W, Gonzalez M. Mandibular remodeling: the fifth stage in distraction osteogenesis healing. In: Arnaud E, Diner PA (Eds). 3rd International Congress on Facial Distraction Processes, Paris, France. Bologna: Monduzzi Editore, 2001: 267–73.
21 Guerrero C, Rivera H, Mujica E, Henriquez M, Gonzalez M. Principles of distraction osteogenesis. In: Bagheri S, Bell B, Khan H. Current therapy in oral and maxilofacial surgery. St Louis: Elsevier, 2012:101–11.
22 Gonzalez M, Guerrero CA, Figueroa F. Predictable mandibular ramus lengthening in TMJ ankylosis. In: Arnaud E, Diner PA (Eds). Proceedings of the 4th International Congress of Maxillofacial and Craniofacial Distraction; 2003 July 2; Paris, France. Bologna, Italy: Monduzzi Editore, 2003:169–74.
23 Gonzalez M, Egbert M, Guerrero C, Van Sickels J. Vertical and horizontal mandibular lengthening of the ramus and body. Atlas Oral Maxillofac Surg Clin North Am. 2008;16:215–36.
24 Stucki-McCormick SU. Reconstruction of the mandibular condyle using transport distraction osteogenesis. J Craniofac Surg. 1997;8:48–52.

Chapter 46

Maxillary Intraoral Distraction Osteogenesis

Cesar A. Guerrero

Introduction and history

Three-dimensional (3-D) maxillary deficiency may present in a variety of craniofacial syndromes, clefts and certain idiopathic clinical situations. The deficiency may be present at different maxillary levels and needs to be treated accordingly, i.e. Le Fort I level (either low or high), Quadrangular Le Fort I, Le Fort II, Modified Le Fort III, or Le Fort III. The issue of frontofacial deficiency is not included in this section; this chapter only covers intraoral devices.

Traditional surgery has some limitations in terms of the amount of movement possible, the need for iliac crest bone grafts, stability and quality of bone. Additionally, the soft tissues may be a limitation, especially clefts and scar tissue from multiple surgeries. Having intraoral distraction osteogenesis is an alternative surgical modality that can provide better stability, easier surgery based on performing the osteotomies and fixing the appliances, reduces the need for bone grafts and reducing costs due to earlier discharge from the hospital and the ability for the patient to resume activities within a week. Through the years, two different approaches have been described to perform distraction osteogenesis in the craniofacial region. There are extraoral distractors, with a semicircular metal structure fixed to the skull with multiple screws, with a vertical bar connected to facial plates by wires and coils to exert the anteroposterior force required to advance the midface.[1–5] There have been modifications and improvements to ensure skull stability, vector control, attachment methods and connectors by different companies on the market. The common problems are: social inconvenience, facial scars, and more importantly, all patients have the distractors removed before completing the distraction consolidation phase (in large movements this would require up to a year of treatment time) and consequently the stability is jeopardized.[2–5]

The internal maxillary distractors are based on a solid body with a barrel to be activated between anterior and posterior plates for bony fixation. Different designs have been published to improve bone anchorage, easier activation, vector control and to facilitate removal. Understanding the biology and biomechanics are fundamental to predictably correct facial anomalies. The distraction protocol is based on amount of movement, age of the patient, quality and quantity of bone; minor or standard deformities are corrected with traditional surgery.[6–12] Obviously to ideally correct facial and occlusal discrepancies, orthodontics needs to be involved; the surgery needs to be planned, with 3-D models to perform the model surgery. The distractors are pre-bent, pre-shaped and activated to full movement and the vector is planned to the objective movement required. Once the appliances are activated and perfect occlusion is obtained on the model, the actual surgery is performed with

Orthognathic Surgery: Principles, Planning and Practice. Edited by Farhad B. Naini and Daljit S. Gill.

proper vectors, size of the distractors (15, 20, 25 mm, etc.) and the screw lengths are measured and will be ready for surgery. All this work is done before the surgical intervention, and needs to be supervised by the group expert and discussed with the orthodontist. The surgeon must know that the final positioning of the midface needs to be occlusally stable and have to be maintained until bone rigidity occurs, after the distraction's consolidation phase, which may take from 3 to 12 months, according to the variables of amount of movement, age of the patient, quantity and quality of bone.[12,13] The distractor appliances are user-friendly and comfortable to remain in place for a long time, and the patient may resume many regular activities only a few days after surgery.[12–14]

Some patients will show divergences from the treatment plan, even though the appliances were prepared to obtain the best occlusion possible. The clinician needs to install a secondary method to make postoperative changes in the vector, such as circumferential vertical anterior suspension wires, or change the position of the anterior plate by changing the screws under intravenous sedation, but under no circumstances should the distraction appliances be removed, expecting the guiding elastics to improve or maintain the occlusion. The collagen fibres within the distraction chamber are under tension awaiting mineralization in the consolidation stage, and if the appliance rigidity collapses or it is removed, the fibres contract, the segments become unstable and complete relapse occurs.[10,13,16]

Chin, Guerrero, Salyer, Wangerin, and Kessler were pioneers in developing internal devices or utilizing existing mandibular technology to advance the maxilla at different levels following the correct indications for distraction osteogenesis.[17–23]

Indications

This technology is indicated for patients presenting with severe maxillary deficiency (over 10 mm), sleep apnoea, previous failures in advancing the maxilla, inadequate anatomy to perform traditional surgery and syndromic deficiency situations.

Contraindications

Intraoral distraction osteogenesis biology is based on sound surgical principles that depend on vascularity and bone quality; it should not be applied after radiotherapy or conditions involving extremely poor bone quantity or quality, and also requires patient and family collaboration.

Maxillary Le Fort I level advancement

(See Figure 46-1)

Surgical technique

The intraoral devices are ideal means to treat maxillary deficiencies in a two- or three-dimensional manner. In specific situations where there is lack of hard and soft tissues, different distraction osteogenesis techniques can be combined to solve deficiencies secondary to trauma or syndromes. This surgical approach eliminates the need for bone grafts or extraoral devices. Selecting the adequate surgical timing and surgical technique avoids permanent surgical damage to the teeth, nerves, and lacrimal ducts.[12–15]

Either arch bars in children or full orthodontics in the mixed or adult dentition are used to control the occlusion postoperatively. Once the dental objectives are met in the presurgical phase, rectangular orthodontic archwires with welded vertical pins are used to apply elastics after surgery.

3-D models may be used for planning, distraction device selection and pre-adaptation; also an acrylic interdental splint may be fabricated to be used after the maxillary downfracture and intermaxillary fixation; the splint would maintain the positioning while the distraction devices are securely fixed. The clinician needs to ensure the maxilla's total mobilization at surgery, as exerting too much pressure within the distractors and fixation screws to advance it may be detrimental for the device, may disengage bone screws, create asymmetrical movements and may create instability.[15,24]

Under general nasotracheal intubation and controlled hypotensive anaesthesia, and after local anaesthetic is infiltrated, an incision from premolar to premolar is made through the mucosa, muscles and periosteum; the tissues are superiorly elevated with two Molt no. 9 elevators anterior and posterior to the infraorbital nerve and posteriorly up to the pterygomaxillary junction through a tunnel, maintaining the lateral blood supply as much as possible. Calipers are used to measure the canine and first molar lengths and the osteotomy is performed 5 mm above (Figure 46-1 e). According to the individual clinical features the osteotomy design may vary. Careful medial dissection is made and a periosteal elevator is placed between the detached nasal mucosa and piriform rim. Reference lines are drawn in the maxillary lateral wall anteriorly and posteriorly, bilaterally. All soft tissues are meticulously reflected and separated to complete the osteotomy without tearing them. The Langenbeck–Obwegeser retractors are placed anterior and posterior to the infraorbital nerves. Through the lateral wall osteotomy line a spatula osteotome is used to wick the maxillary sinus medial wall, to avoid irregular fractures up to the orbit. A second incision is made in the tuberosity area to place a curved chisel to section the tuberosity into the palatine bone; working through tunnels permits maintenance of the best blood supply, reduces oedema and improves bone healing.[12–15]

The maxilla is downfractured and released from the posterior maxillary union using a rough periosteal elevator; the nasal airway is approached and treated if necessary (septum, turbinates, deviations, cysts removal, etc.). The nasal mucosa is closed and attention to placing the distractors is focused. The

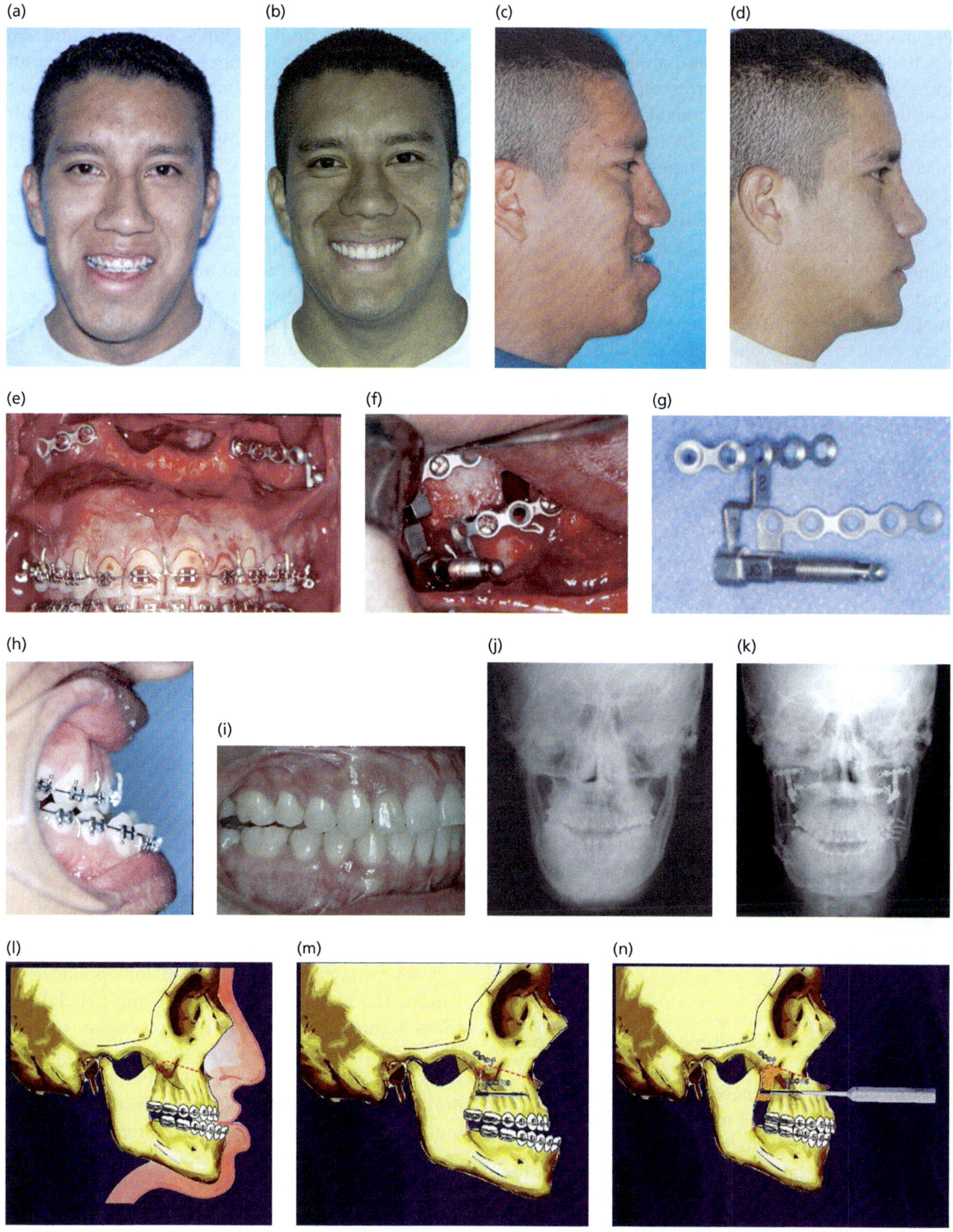

Fig. 46-1 A severe maxillary hypoplasia in a 23-year-old male patient; a maxillary advancement by a high Le Fort I osteotomy distraction osteogenesis and genioplasty were performed. Frontal and profile views were obtained preoperatively and after 10 years of follow-up (a, b, c, d). The diagram demonstrates the preoperative profile, high Le Fort I osteotomy design, and during the activation period (l, m, n). Intraoperative views: Maxillary distractor appliance (e, f); the distractors are with fixed parallelism, following the mandibular occlusal plane in order to avoid an open bite. Preoperative (j) and postoperative (k) cephalometric radiographs. Preoperative dental view (h) and final changes after 10 years (i).

positioning of the distractors is sensitive; there are two ways to approach this situation: either the distractors are placed into position before the down-fracture manoeuvre, placing the screws to serve as a guide once the maxilla has been freed, and not tighten the screws to avoid loosening during final fixation, or the distractors are fixed after the maxillary mobilization, and having references lines to avoid malpositioning (Figure 46-1 f,g). In either situation the surgeon must have a 3-D model to pre-shape, pre-bend and adapt the distractor, measure the moving distance and create the right vector of movement. The distractor is fixed with three or four screws in every plate, the upper and the lower to ensure stability; the activation rods must be as parallel as possible (Figure 46-1 k,m). The distractors offer an excellent and secure way to advance the maxilla; in large movements, minimal discrepancies in the vertical plane may create either an anterior or posterior open bite, and the solution for many surgeons is to remove the distractor and place rigid fixation plates and screws, with the inconvenience of a second major surgery, and instability of the distraction chamber collapsing, secondary to contraction of the immature callus formation.[16] An alternative solution is to create a secondary mechanism to control the distraction vector. The surgeon needs to place a 0.024″ gauge wire from the nasal bone to the anterior maxilla, using a long bur to go transcutaneous at the nasal bone region and go through from right to left; the wire is passed through the hole and using an Obwegeser passing owl needle from the anterior maxilla on the right side emerging through the skin hole and repeating the manoeuvre on the left side, the wires emerge in the anterior maxilla and embraces the maxilla; this wire is loosely placed at the time of surgery, but can be tightened or released in the event of open bite development, either anterior or posterior.[24] The soft tissues are carefully closed by advancing the facial musculature anteriorly, a V-Y lip closure is used after an adequate nasal cinch has been tightened.[25] The distractor is removed under IV sedation in the clinic, once there is radiographic evidence of mineralization, by small lateral maxillary incisions and screw retrieval. The supero-posterior plate can be cut and left in place, and resorbable sutures are utilized to close the wounds.[13]

Maxillary Le Fort I level advancement in clefts

(See Figure 46-2)

Most cleft patients after multiple surgeries will have a severe lack of 3-D maxillary growth. The clinicians confronting the problem need to elaborate a surgical-orthodontic plan including maxillary widening, vertical and anteroposterior (A-P) movements.

The single most important aspect is to convert the two or three piece maxilla, either unilateral or bilateral clefts, into a single unit; once that is completed the only remaining task is to place the maxilla in the best possible occlusion and to complete the post-surgical orthodontics; understanding the roll, yaw and pitch is fundamental to properly reposition the maxilla (see Chapters 5 and 6). The transverse correction needs to be addressed by surgical maxillary widening in a previous surgical stage, which is indicated for more than 4 mm of widening or immediate minor widening with the maxillary vertical and A-P repositioning.[24,26–30]

Surgical technique

After diagnosis and treatment planning, including 3-D models, the distraction appliances are pre-shaped, pre-bent and pre-adapted; also a palatal splint is fabricated with multiple holes for interdental wires and internal metal frame to avoid intraoperative splint fractures.[24] The splint is made from the model surgery, and will include minor maxillary widening. The patient undergoes surgery, basically utilizing the same technique; the only difference is the need to created three flaps, nasal, palatine layer and buccal layer; for alveolar bone grafts simultaneous with the maxillary repositioning. The bilateral cleft patients would need the soft tissue management on the right and left sides equally, but no incision is made on the premaxilla buccal area, which has the only vascular supply; the nasal septum can be fractured or partially resected behind the premaxilla, while maintaining the premaxillary buccal blood supply (Figure 46-2 e,f,g).

Once the two or three maxillary segments are down-fractured and the three-dimensional alveolar graft sites have been prepared (Figure 46-2 h), the palatine and nasal layers are closed in a water-tight manner; the maxillary pieces are carefully positioned into the acrylic splint with interdental wires, a 2 mm thick long titanium plate is placed above the teeth level and fixated with 6 to 8 mm long microscrews to create bone rigidity (Figure 46-2 q,r). The orthodontic rectangular archwire, rigid fixation plate and acrylic splint offer stable maxillary rigidity, creating a single-piece maxillary unit, to be fixed to the upper midface with the maxillary distractors and anterior suspension 0.024″ wire around the nasal bones and anterior maxilla.[24] Bone grafts are placed into the alveolar clefts and careful and meticulous soft tissue closure is obtained (Figure 46-2h). Exposed dental roots next to the cleft may be an indication for tooth removal in order to avoid bone graft contamination and loss; the periodontal ligament is a route for bacteria to infiltrate into the closed alveolar bone graft area.[13,24]

A seven-day period is awaited for appliance activation. The maxilla is advanced 1 mm per day, until Class I canine and molar relationship is obtained. There is no need for overcorrection. The clinician must wait for complete mineralization before the distraction devices are removed. Once the ideal positioning is obtained, the midlines are carefully monitored and more activation on one side may be necessary to localize the perfect positioning. If an anterior or posterior open bite develops, the anterior vertical suspension wire is adjusted to control the final vertical positioning.

Modified Le Fort III midface advancement

After surgical planning using the 3-D model, the distraction appliances are pre-shaped, pre-bent and pre-adapted; the patient is taken to surgery and under nasotracheal intubation and controlled hypotensive anaesthesia the surgical procedure is performed. The distraction osteogenesis healing process is based on three areas for bone mineralization; splitting the zygomatic bone in halves offers the best bone stock for

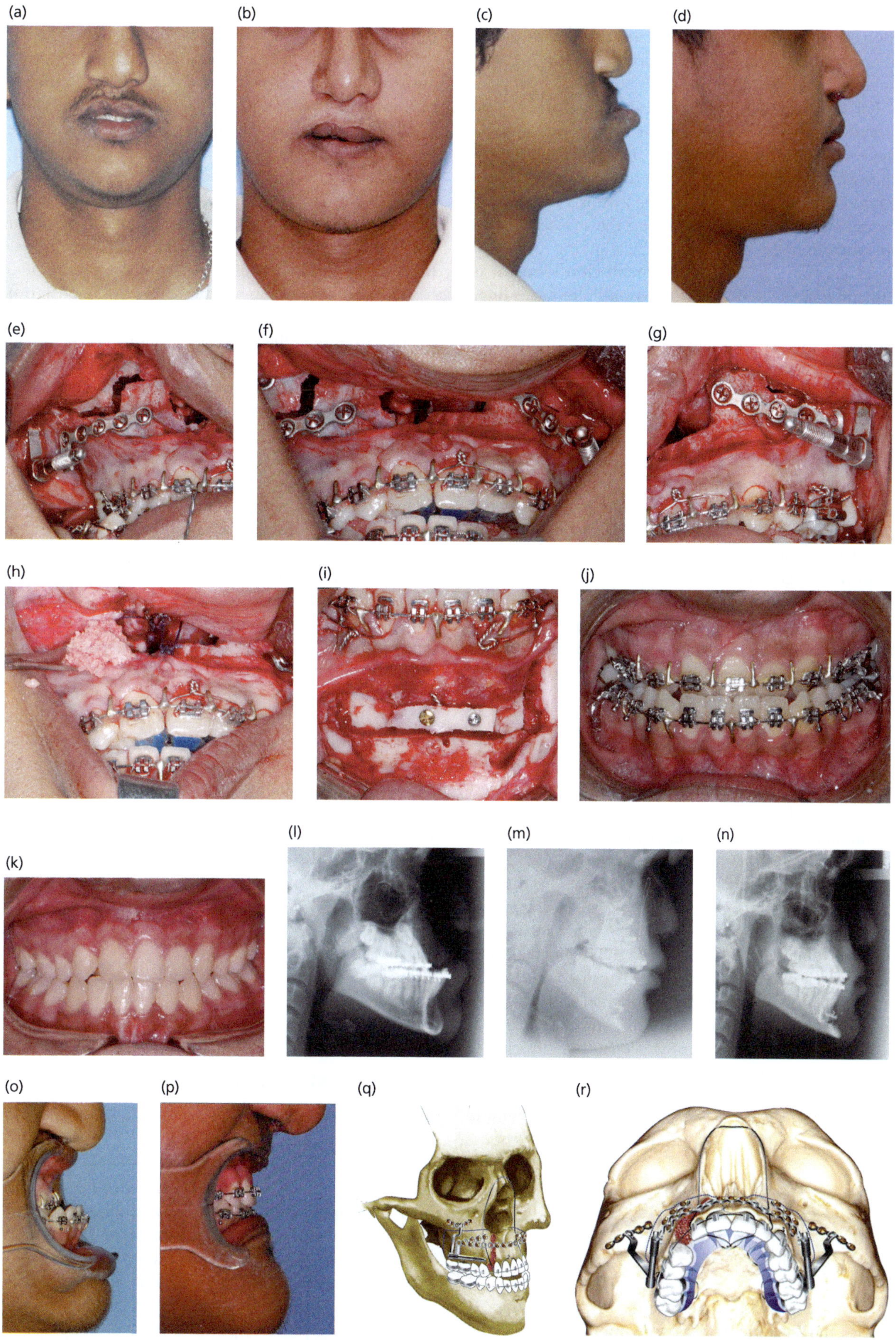

Fig. 46-2 A severe maxillary hypoplasia in a 15-year-old unilateral cleft lip and palate patient. A maxillary advancement by a high Le Fort I osteotomy distraction osteogenesis and subapical osteotomy were performed. Facial and dental photographs are shown illustrating the changes, and a diagram showing simultaneous autologous alveolar bone grafting with the maxillary advancement, intraoral distractors and vertical vector control with circumferential nasomaxillary wiring. A palatal splint was used, together with orthodontic arch and transverse rigid fixation to transform a two-piece maxilla into one single solid unit, to be advanced with intraoral distractors. Final changes after 4 years are shown; the total orthodontic treatment time was 14 months.

future mineralization, the pterygomaxillary area and the piriform rims. Osteotomies are performed under abundant irrigation to avoid bone overheating and delayed healing.[24,26–30]

For the modified Le Fort III osteotomy, an incision is made buccally from the right second premolar to the second premolar tooth on the left. The soft tissues are elevated exposing the anterior maxilla and behind the infraorbital nerve the zygoma is exposed. Dean scissors are used to section the masseter muscle junction to the zygomatic arch, allowing rapid and wide zygoma exposure and a small chin retractor is utilized to protect the soft tissues, and references lines are drawn over the body of the zygoma. The reciprocating saw sections the body of the zygoma vertically as close to the frontozygomatic apophyses as possible. An additional transconjunctival incision is used to approach the infraorbital rim; an eye globe protector is inserted, over abundant lubricant. The osteotomy divides the malar process in halves, carried out medially and above the infraorbital nerve, the orbital floor is sectioned behind the infraorbital rim, continuing underneath and obliquely anterior to avoid the nasolacrimal duct from reaching the piriform rim, the osteotomy is completed intraorally sectioning the pirifrom rim, and posteriorly, the pterygomaxillary suture is separated with a curved chisel or through the tuberosity area. The septum is sectioned with a ball osteotome from anterior to posterior, after reflecting the nasal floor mucosa.[26–30]

Two wide-curved osteotomes are placed behind the maxillary tuberosities to displace the zygoma–maxillary complex, which is slowly and progressively separated; if there is resistance, the osteotomies need to be revised, avoiding unilateral strong pull and a secondary zygoma fracture. If that happens, double 2 mm thick multiple hole plates need to be placed to ensure bone repositioning and stability. The distractor's posterior plate is fixed to the posterior zygoma, bending the plate with anchor shape, and the anterior plate to the anterior zygoma and maxillary wall. For those cases where the appliance is buried under the mucosa, a flexible connector is attached to the distractor activation head for activation, eliminating facial scars; the connector is removed once the clinician is happy with the maxillary position; ideally the connector is released by twisting the connector with the activation key in a clockwise fashion, and the connector is disengaged and pulled without any incision.[26–30]

Subcranial Le Fort III midface advancement

(See Figure 46-3)

A 3 cm long incision at the first to third molars is made; the zygoma is exposed, after sectioning the masseter muscle fibres into the zygomatic arch. A small channel retractor is used to protect the soft tissues and with a reciprocating saw the osteotomy is started at the most lateral aspect to the orbit, splitting the zygoma in two halves and continuing inferior to the pterygomaxillary junction; references lines are drawn over the body of the zygoma. The same procedure is performed on the opposite side. Then, a transconjunctival approach is utilized to section the floor of the orbit, an eye globe protector is inserted, abundant lubricant, and the osteotomy is just posterior to the rim and anterior to the lacrimal bone (Figure 46-3 e). Continuing with a 3 mm sub-glabellar incision to the supero-inferior section, the nasal bones form the frontal and the nasal septum (Figure 46-3 h). The only remaining solid junction is the posterior maxilla, and a curved osteotome is applied bilaterally to fracture either the tuberosity or pterygomaxillary junction. A careful and progressive pressure is exerted anterior and inferior to mobilize the facial structures. If there is resistance, the osteotomies need to be revised. Rowe disimpaction forceps with gauze are placed over the palate to avoid soft tissue damage, or bilateral Carroll–Girard screws combined with a straight chisel at the frontonasal osteotomy line are used to mobilize the midface (Figure 46-3 h). A 10 mm long screw is fixed in the thickest part of the frontal bone, to be used as anchorage for a suspension wire around the anterior maxilla; an Obwegeser passing owl is used from the anterior maxilla into the sub-glabellar incision, and a 0.024″ gauge suspension wire is embraced for vector control postoperatively.[13,30]

Once the bony segment is freed, bilateral internal maxillary distractors are placed over the zygoma, anterior and posterior to the line of fracture. The distraction appliance was adapted in the 3-D model to be exposed in the oral cavity, at the molar level, to facilitate activation. The wounds are closed in a standard fashion (Figure 46-3f,k).

Distraction protocol

There is a latency period of 7 days, followed by activation of 1 mm a day, until distraction is completed; a consolidation period of 60 to 90 days per each centimetre distracted is indicated. One distractor may be activated more than the other to obtain symmetry and adequate midline positioning.

Postoperative considerations

The patient resumes regular activities a few days after surgery. The activation should be done in the morning before going to school or work, and a liquid diet is indicated for the activation period. Once the midface is in the proper position, adjusted with the suspension wire or re-positioned under intravenous sedation in the clinic, the patient's diet can move on to soft food. A blender is useful; anything the patient may want or the family is having, should be previously passed through the triturating process, put in a glass or soup spoon and given to the patient.

After total activation is accomplished and the consolidation period elapses, radiographs are taken

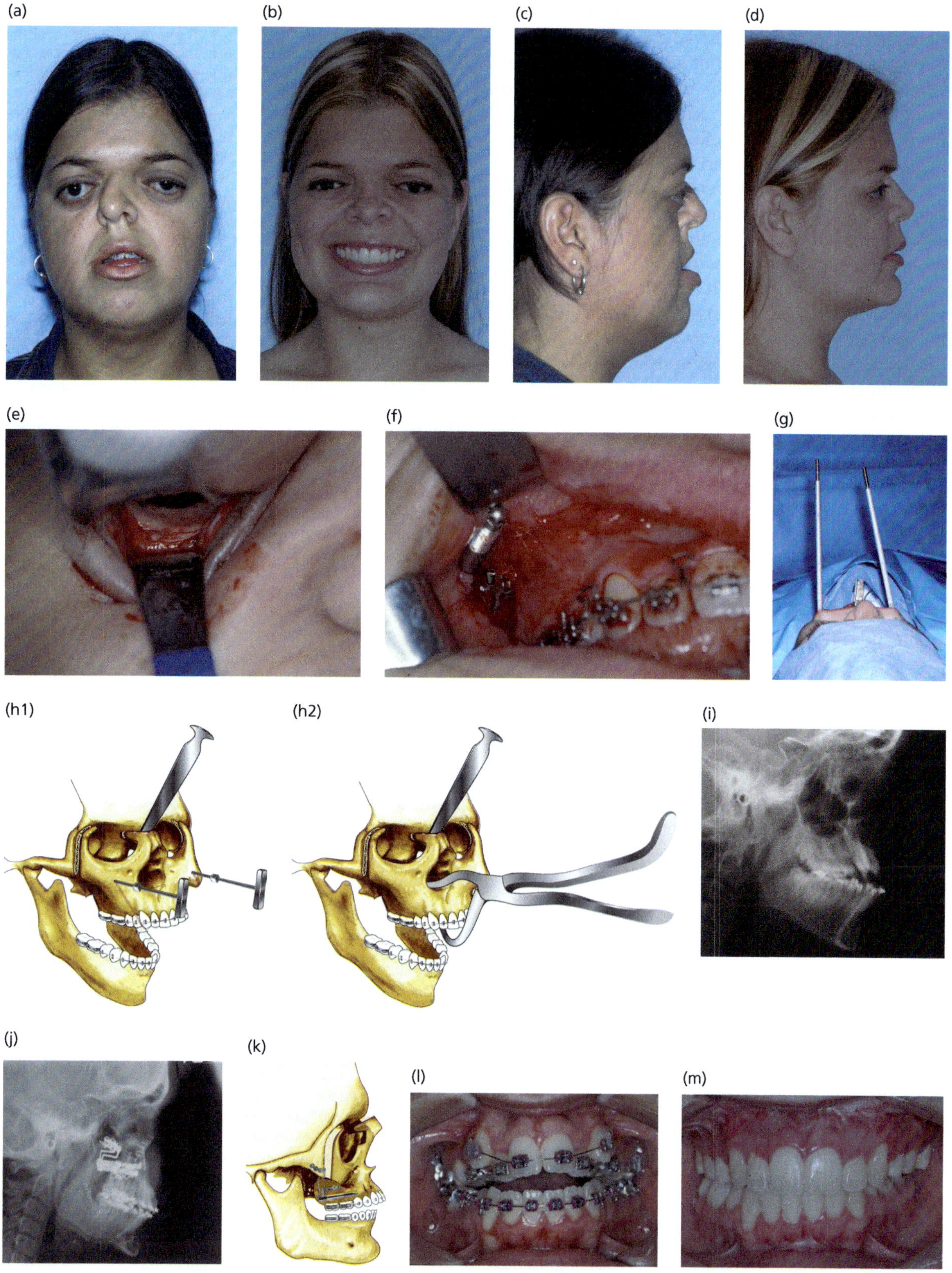

Fig. 46-3 A 16-year-old female patient with Crouzon syndrome underwent a subcranial Le Fort III maxillary advancement and genioplasty. At the second stage, the distractors were removed, and a rhinoplasty and maxillary widening were performed. Frontal and profile views were obtained preoperatively and after treatment (a, b, c, d). Intraoral and transconjunctival approaches were made with rods emerging intraorally to check positioning (e, f, g, h). This diagram shows the mineralization sites (k). Preoperative and postoperative lateral cephalometric radiographs (i, j). (l, m) Dental changes after 10 years.

to verify the distraction chamber ossification; once adequate radiopacity is observed the patient is taken to the operating theatre and under intravenous sedation the appliance's anterior plates are disengaged by removing the multiple screws and mobility is checked; the decision is made to continue removing the posterior plates and anterior suspension wire.

The distractors should be removed after proper ossification has occurred, confirmed by radiographic evaluation, considering the different variables involved in the healing process, such as the age of the patient, amount of movement, quality and quantity of bone, infection, inadequate stability during consolidation, poor patient selection, and some systemic diseases.

Intraoral distraction osteogenesis allows maxillary advancement with meticulous occlusal finishing, in a predictable and stable manner. The surgical technique permits progressive augmentation of the hard and soft tissues, into an ideal dental occlusion. It is required that the orthodontist has prepared the dentition presurgically into an ideal arch situation and fixated the dental positioning with heavy rectangular archwires to allow the use of intermaxillary heavy elastics during the early post-surgical period, but allowing complete joint unloading during the activation and consolidation phases.

References

1 Ilizarov G. The tension-stress effect on the genesis and growth of tissues. In: Ilizarov G (Ed.) Transosseous osteosynthesis. Germany: Springer-Verlag, 1992;137–255.

2 Polley J, Figueroa A. Maxillary distraction osteogenesis with rigid external distraction. Atlas Oral Maxillofac Surg Clin North Am. 1999;7:15–28.

3 Figueroa A, Polley J. Management of the severe cleft and syndromic midface hypoplasia. Orthod Craniofac Res. 2007;3:167–79.

4 Figueroa A, Polley J: Introduction of a new removable adjustable intraoral maxillary distraction system for correction of maxillary hypoplasia. J Craniofac Surg. 2009;1776–86.

5 Ching E, Figueroa A, Polley J. Soft tissue profile changes after maxillary advancemen twith distraction osteogenesis by use of rigid external distraction device: a 1-year follow-up. J Oral Maxillofac Surg. 2000;58:959–69.

6 Ilizarov G. The principles of the Ilizarov methods. Bull Hosp Joint Dis Orthop Inst. 1988;48:1.

7 Ilizarov G. The tension-stress effect on the genesis and growth of tissues: Part I. The influence of stability on fixation and soft tissue preservation. Clin Orthop. 1989;238:249–81.

8 Ilizarov G. The tension-stress effect on the genesis and growth of tissues: Part II. The influence of the rate and frequency of distraction. Clin Orthop. 1989;239:263–85.

9 Samchukov M, Cherkashin A, Makarov M, et al. Muscle adaptation during single and double level tibial lengthening. In: Stein H, Suk S, Leung P, et al. (Eds). SIROT 99 International Research Society of Orthopaedic Surgery and Traumatology, Sydney, Australia, April 16–19, 1999. Tel Aviv: Freund Publishing House, 1999:460–5.

10 Samchukov M, Cope J, Cherkashin A. Craniofacial distraction osteogenesis. St Louis, CV Mosby, 2001.

11 Bell W, Gonzalez M, Samchukov M, Guerrero C. Intraoral widening and lengthening the mandible by distraction osteogenesis and histogenesis. J Oral Maxillofac Surg. 1999;57:548–62.

12 Guerrero C, Bell W, Meza L. Intraoral distraction osteogenesis. Maxillary and mandibular lengthening. Atlas Oral Maxillofac Surg Clin North Am. 1999;7:111–51.

13 Guerrero C, Gonzalez M, Dominguez E. Bone transport by distraction osteogenesis for maxillomandibular reconstruction. In: Bell W, Guerrero C. Distraction osteogenesis of the facial skeleton. Hamilton: BC Decker, 2007:501–19.

14 Guerrero C, Bell W. Intraoral distraction. In: McCarthy JG (Ed.) Distraction of the craniofacial skeleton. New York (NY): Springer-Verlag, 1999:219–48.

15 Guerrero C, Bell W, Gonzalez M, Meza L. Intraoral distraction osteogenesis. In: Fonseca RJ (Ed.) Oral and maxilofacial surgery. Philadelphia (PA): W.B. Saunders, 2000:343–402.

16 Guerrero C, Rivera H, Mujica E, Henriquez M, Gonzalez M. Principles of distraction osteogenesis. In: Bagheri S, Bell B, Khan H. Current therapy in oral and maxilofacial surgery. St Louis: Elsevier, 2012:101–11.

17 Chin M, Toth B. Le Fort III advancement with gradual distraction using internal devices. Plast Reconstr Surg. 1997;100:819–30.

18 Guerrero C. Rapid mandibular expansion. Rev Venez Ortod. 1990;48:1–2.

19 Wangerin K, Gropp H. Die intraorale Distraktionsosteotomie des mikrogenen Unterkiefers zur Beseitigung der Atemwegsobstruktion. Dtsch Z Mund Kiefer Gesichtschir. 1994;18:236.

20 Shokirov S, Wangerin K. Transantral distraction device in correction of severe maxillary deformity in cleft patients. Stomatologija. 2011;13:25–32.

21 Kessler P, Wiltfang J, Schultze-Mosgau S, Hirschfelder U, Neukam FW. Distraction osteogenesis of the maxilla and midface using a subcutaneous device: report of four cases. Br J Oral Maxillofac Surg. 2001;39:13–21.

22 Cheung LK, Lo J. Distraction of Le Fort II osteotomy by intraoral distractor: a case report. J Oral Maxillofac Surg. 2006;64:856–60.

23 Gonzalez M, Guerrero C, Ding M. Distraction osteogenesis. In: Bagheri S, Bell B, Khan H. Current therapy in oral and maxillofacial surgery. St Louis: Elsevier, 2012:658–70.

24 Schendel S, Delaire J. Facial muscles: Form, function and reconstruction in dentofacial deformities. In Bell W, Proffit W, White R (Eds). Surgical Correction in Dentofacial Deformities. Philadelphia, WB Saunders, 1980:259–80.

25 Guerrero C. Intraoral bone transport in clefting. Oral Maxillofac Surg Clin North Am. 2002;14:509–23.

26 Guerrero C. Intraoral distraction osteogenesis. In: Selected readings in oral and maxillofacial surgery. Vol 10. Dallas: University of Texas Southwestern Medical Center at Dallas, 2002:1–30.

27 Guerrero C, Bell W, Gonzalez M, Meza L. Intraoral distraction osteogenesis. In: Fonseca RJ (Ed.) Oral and maxillofacial surgery. Vol 2. Philadelphia (PA): W.B. Saunders, 2000:359–402.

28 Cohen S, Burstein F, Stewart M, Rathburn M. Maxillary-midface distraction in children with cleft lip and palate: a preliminary report. Plast Reconstr Surg. 1997; 99:1421-28.

29 Guerrero C, Bell W, Gonzalez M, Rojas A. Maxillary advancement combined with posterior palate reposition via distraction osteogenesis: a case report. In: Samchukov ML, Cope JB, Cherkashin AM (Eds). Craniofacial distraction osteogenesis. St. Louis (MO); Mosby, 2001:531–4.

30 Guerrero C. Maxillary intraoral distraction osteogenesis. In: Arnaud E, Diner PA (Eds). Proceedings of the 3rd International Congress on Facial Distraction Processes; 2001 June 14–16; Paris, France. Bologna, Italy: Monduzzi Editore, 2001:381–87.

Section 2: Adjunctive Surgery

Chapter 47

Introduction: Adjunctive Surgery

Foad Nahai

The last decade or two have witnessed significant progress in our understanding of how the face changes with age. Establishing that volume loss, bony and soft tissue, plays a pivotal role challenged the previous widely held concept that aging of the face was a combination of descent of tissues and skin changes. Whilst there is agreement that actinic changes and loss of skin elasticity contribute to facial aging, there is debate as to which plays a greater role, deflation or descent. In reality all three play a role and the role each plays will vary from individual to individual. Not all faces age in the same way, nor should all faces be rejuvenated in identical fashion. Not all aging faces need or should undergo surgery, nor are all faces candidates for non-surgical rejuvenation.

Appropriate evaluation of the aging changes assessing deflation, descent and skin quality should guide which rejuvenation procedures are chosen: surgical, non-surgical or a combination of both. The evaluation should also include the underlying bony skeleton, which contributes significantly to facial appearance. Will soft tissue rearrangement and volume restoration be sufficient, or should the skeleton be altered or augmented? There is a limit as to how much soft tissue augmentation can improve underlying bone deficits.

In parallel with the clearer understanding of facial aging, the development of injectables has led to a paradigm shift in our approach to facial rejuvenation. Toxins and fillers have rapidly become the most popular non-surgical cosmetic procedures. According to the Cosmetic Surgery National Data Bank Statistics published in Aesthetic Surgery Journal,[1] non-surgical cosmetic procedures outnumber surgical procedures by a factor of eight. Injectables offer a relatively safe and efficacious option for those with early facial aging, and a reasonable alternative for surgical candidates who wish to delay surgery. The fillers are not limited only to soft tissue restoration but also bony enhancement.

The role of volume replacement in facial rejuvenation is the most significant and disruptive change in our approach to facial rejuvenation. Volume restoration is even more important than the description of the superficial muscular aponeurotic system (SMAS) in the mid-1970s.[2] The description of the SMAS was followed by a clearer understanding of its anatomical relations and its role in facial rejuvenation. Many modifications were and continue to be described, each claiming advantages over the other. Compared to the SMAS, the role of volume is still in its infancy with many questions yet unanswered. All agree that it is an integral part of facial rejuvenation, be it surgical or non-surgical. Whilst with fillers the questions centre around which filler and which plane, there are more questions surrounding autologous fat grafting. Questions remain and debate continues as to which donor site is best, how best to harvest and prepare the fat and how much and where to inject the fat. Should the fat be injected before or after the surgical procedure? The most relevant question is how much of the fat will survive and how can we predict that. For most it is a question of guesswork as to how much we should over inject. No such guesswork with fillers. Although tremendous advances have been made in our understanding of fat and fat grafting we still have a way to go until it is consistently predictable in all hands. The commercialization of fat grafting, claims made concerning stem cells, none of which is based on scientific evidence should raise ethical issues and be a concern to all.[3,4]

Despite the many unanswered questions on fat grafting mentioned above, grafting fat has become an integral part of facial rejuvenation either as an isolated procedure or an adjunct to surgical facelifts. Where the fat is injected, cheeks, temples, eyelids, lips, perioral or periorbital, will vary with the aging changes of each individual patient. In contrast

Orthognathic Surgery: Principles, Planning and Practice. Edited by Farhad B. Naini and Daljit S. Gill.

rejuvenation, or more appropriately put, recontouring of the neck in the majority of patients entails reduction of volume. Superficial fat is removed through liposuction or direct excision. Subplatysmal fat and rarely digastric muscle and partial submandibular gland excision may be necessary to appropriately recontour the neck and jaw line. On rare occasions in extremely thin individuals or secondary neck procedures, fat grafting may be needed.

The volume loss associated with facial aging is not limited to the soft tissues and involves the bony skeleton. The bony skeleton is the foundation of facial appearance and any change in that skeleton will alter facial size and overall appearance. Some of the most dramatic enhancements to facial appearance result from skeletal manipulations, be it bony advancements, recession or augmentation. With all of our current excitement over volume replacement, we should recognize the role of facial implants in facial reshaping and rejuvenation as the forerunners of soft tissue volume restoration. I am often asked by patients who are candidates for orthognathic surgery whether they should have their facelift first or the orthognathic procedure. Without question the answer is that they should undergo the orthognathic and any other bony procedures first. These procedures will dramatically alter facial appearance and with it my approach to their rejuvenation. *Establish a sound bony foundation first then approach the soft tissues.*

Facial rejuvenation extends from the bone to skin surface. In addition to volume restoration, rearrangement of soft tissues and redraping or excision of excess skin, some patients require skin resurfacing to complete the rejuvenation. Peels and laser resurfacing have a role as isolated procedures to treat actinic changes and rhytids and also as an adjunct in combination with surgical procedures.

Alteration of facial appearance including facial rejuvenation may involve the underlying skeleton, volume restoration, rearrangement of soft tissues, excision of excess and inelastic skin and resurfacing of the skin. Rejuvenative procedures should be based on evaluation of these changes.

References

1 Cosmetic Surgery National Data Bank: Statistics 2013. Aesthet Surg J. 2014;34(1 suppl):1S–22S.

2 Mitz. V, Peyronie, M. The superficial musculo-aponeurotic system (SMAS) in the parotid and cheek area. Plast. Reconstr. Surg. 1976;58:80–8.

3 Nayar HS, Caplan AL, Eaves FF, Rubin JP. The ethics of stem cell-based aesthetic surgery: attitudes and perceptions of the plastic surgery community. Aesthet Surg J. 2014;34:926–31.

4 Atiyeh BS, Ibrahim AE, Saad DA. Stem cell facelift: between reality and fiction. Aesthet Surg J. 2013;33:334–38.

Chapter 48

Rhinoplasty and Nasal Changes In Relation to Orthognathic Surgery

Mehmet Manisali and Leila Khamashta-Ledezma

Introduction

Facial appearance changes following orthognathic surgery can be dramatic. Change in facial appearance is also often significant after a rhinoplasty. Clearly, when indicated, both procedures can be performed for the same patient in a sequential manner, with potentially phenomenal results (Figure 48-1).

However, the relationship between the two procedures is more complex than it may appear at first sight. Firstly, there are some illusory changes; when the chin point is advanced the relative prominence of the nose appears altered, and conversely hump removal is followed by a perceptual change in the chin position in the profile view (Figure 48-2).

Secondly, certain manoeuvres in a rhinoplasty have the ability to change the observed relative relationship between the maxilla and the mandible. This is observed in the management of the **tension nose** when the anterior nasal spine is reduced and when techniques are used to alter the relationship between the caudal edge of the septum and the medial crura. The resultant reduction in the nasolabial angle converts a Class II skeletal profile to a Class I with no real change in the maxillary mandibular position (Figure 48-3). Thirdly, and most importantly, there are some real changes in the nasal appearance and function following the change in the maxillary position after orthognathic surgery. Some of these could be beneficial and should be allowed to happen for a more refined aesthetic result. A small increase in the inter-alar distance in advancement of hypoplastic maxillae is a good example. On the other hand anticipated negative features should either be eliminated at the planning stage or corrected by considering ancillary procedures, such as reduction of the anterior nasal spine, at the time of

Orthognathic Surgery: Principles, Planning and Practice. Edited by Farhad B. Naini and Daljit S. Gill.

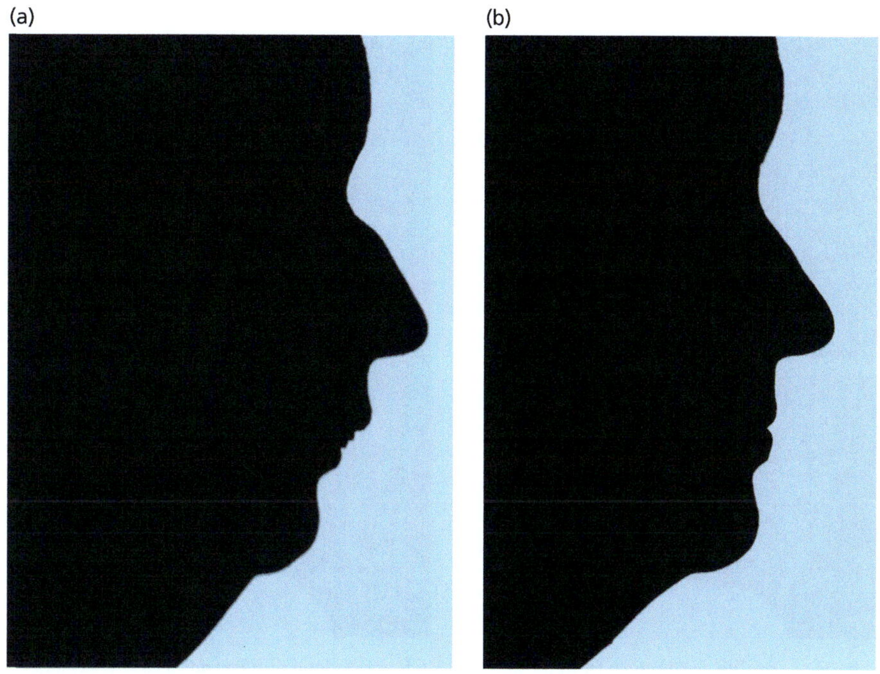

Fig. 48-1 Example of a patient who underwent combined orthodontic and orthognathic management followed by a rhinoplasty. (a) Pretreatment. (b) End of treatment.

the operation. Indeed, secondary procedures may be necessary to correct unwanted changes at a later date.

Nasal analysis

The key to a successful outcome in aesthetic rhinoplasty is a thorough analysis of the deformity. Making this diagnostic step a methodical one yields maximum information and repetition breeds thoroughness and accuracy.

The first feature to be noted is the skin quality. Thick and sebaceous nasal skin will be a significant barrier to demonstrate changes applied to the underlying osseocartilaginous framework. On the other hand, thin, translucent skin will readily show imperfections and irregularities.

Almost simultaneous to recording the skin quality, a mental note of the most characteristic feature of the nose should be made. An example of this first impression could be a 'prominent hump', 'a droopy tip' or

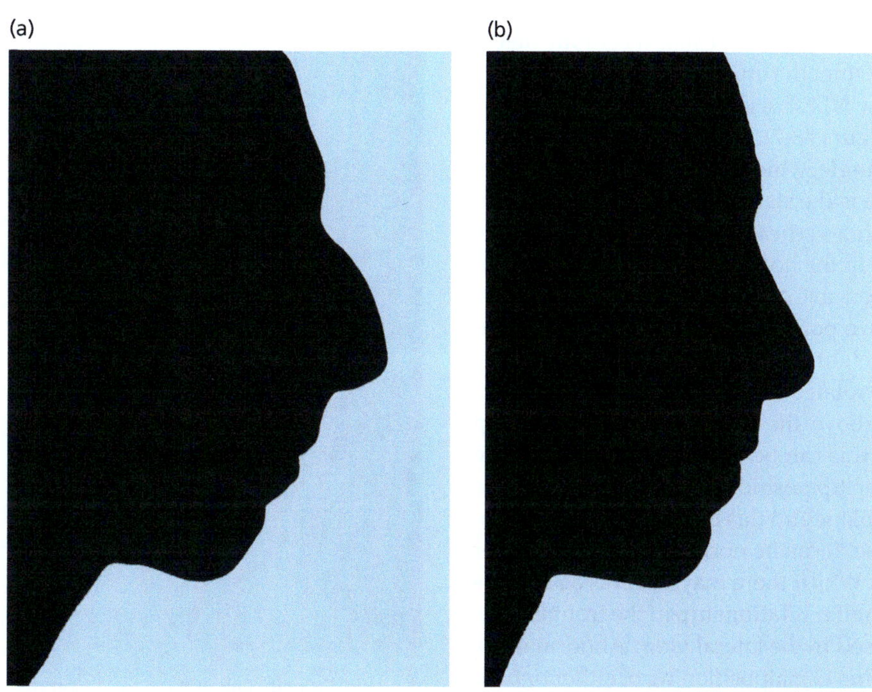

Fig. 48-2 Illusional change in the perception of the position of the chin in profile view following nasal hump removal. (a) Preoperative profile. (b) Postoperative profile.

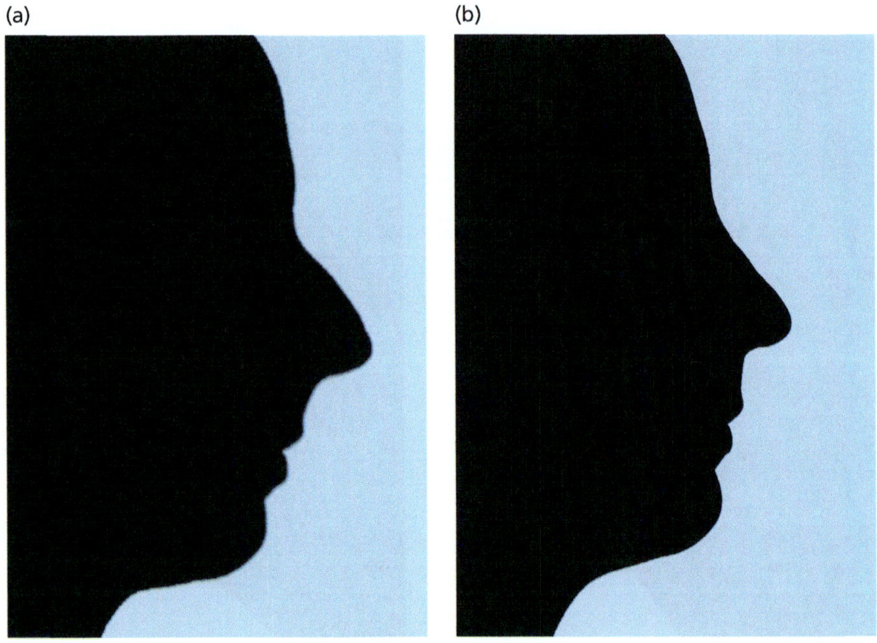

Fig. 48-3 Illusional change in profile appearance from a Class II to a Class I skeletal appearance as a consequence of a reduction in the nasolabial angle following anterior nasal spine reduction and techniques for managing the relationship between the caudal edge of the septum and the medial crura. (a) Preoperative profile. (b) Postoperative profile.

'crooked nose'. This is called the **primary descriptor** and it should be revised at the end of the assessment.

The nose should be assessed clinically and photographically from the frontal, lateral, basal and oblique views. The frontal view gives the best opportunity to assess straightness, the width in the upper, middle and lower thirds, as well as the characteristics of the tip (e.g. bulbosity) (Figure 48-4). The 'gull in flight' appearance of the nose from the frontal view gives an indication to the degree of rotation of the tip of the nose (Figure 48-5). This is also the view where a gentle curve of the brow to tip aesthetic line is observed. An underlying deformity may cause a contour defect in this otherwise smooth running line (Figure 48-6).

The lateral view is best assessed in a superior to inferior sequence (Figure 48-7). A note should be made of the **frontonasal angle**, which could be acute or obtuse. **The radix**, which is the starting point of the nose, can be high or low in a vertical orientation and it can be deep or shallow in the horizontal plane. The dorsum can be straight, concave or convex. The **nasal length** is determined by two points: the radix and the tip defining point. The height of the radix and the degree by which the tip is rotated will define the nasal length. The low point above the tip is called the **supratip depression** and this can be observed as a feminising characteristic. The tip position is also assessed in relation to the facial plane and this is referred to as the projection of the nose. It can be normal, over-projected or under-projected. Whilst there may be hints as regards to the **alar-columellar relationship** in the frontal view, this is best assessed in the lateral view. Abnormalities can be detected due to malpositioning of either or both of these two components. The nasolabial angle can be obtuse or acute and can be susceptible to changes in rhinoplasty, maxillary osteotomy procedures and maxillary incisor inclination changes in orthodontic treatment. The basal view allows the assessment of the **triangularity of the nose** (Figure 48-8). The columellar lobule ratio, which is normally two to one, can also be assessed in this view. The tip characteristics observed

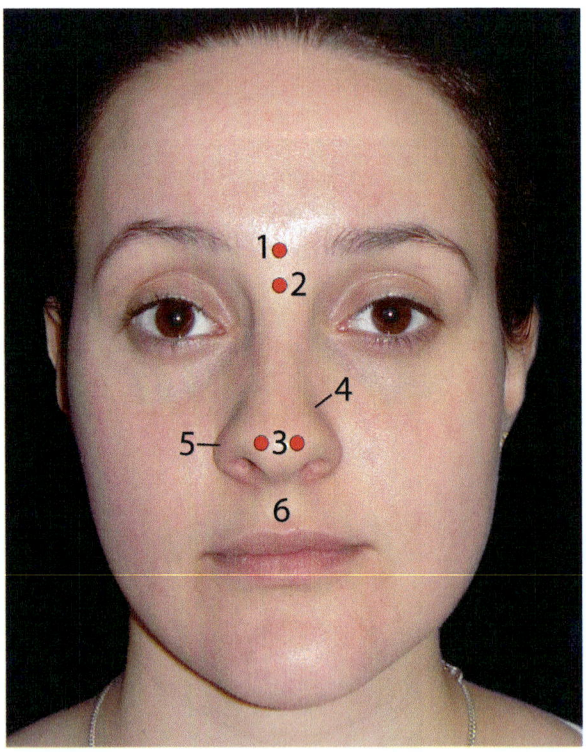

Fig. 48-4 Frontal view of the nose. 1, soft tissue glabella; 2, soft tissue nasion; 3, tip-defining points; 4, supraalar crease; 5, alar sidewall; 6, philtrum.

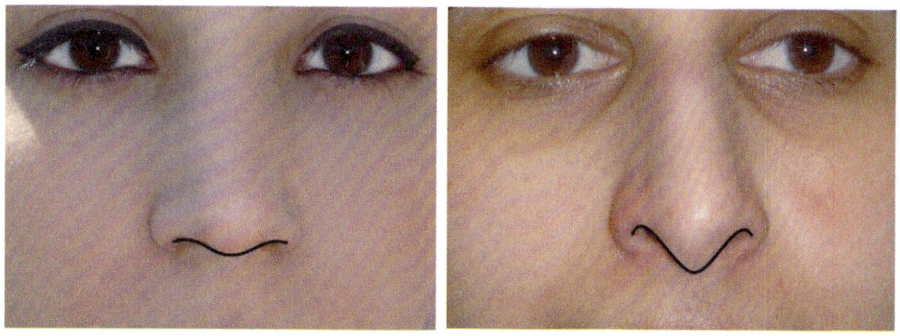

Fig. 48-5 Frontal view showing the 'gull in flight' appearance. The columella is observed to hang just inferior to the inferior alar rims, giving the infratip lobule and alae a *gentle* 'gull in flight' appearance on *frontal view*. Excessive exposure of the columella on frontal view may indicate inferior protrusion of the columella. (From: Naini FB. Facial Aesthetics: Concepts and Clinical Diagnosis. Oxford: Wiley-Blackwell, 2011[6]; used with permission.)

in the frontal view, such as tip bifidity, can also be confirmed and better characterised from the basal view. Base width and symmetry can be assessed. Caudal septum deflection can be noted if present. The oblique views often confirm the observations gathered thus far in the assessment. It is also useful in unmasking minor asymmetries.

Basic steps in rhinoplasty

This section is written for the readers not familiar with the procedure of rhinoplasty. The relevance to orthognathic surgery is better appreciated if basic steps are understood. Once the analysis of the nose is completed, a list of objectives to be achieved in surgery can be drawn up. Then, techniques that will allow the fulfilment of these objectives are selected. Generally the aims of these techniques are to reduce, augment or alter the position of the bone, the cartilage or soft tissues. For example, if one of the objectives of the procedure is to reduce a prominent hump this would require resection of the nasal bones (the osseous component of the hump) as well as reduction of the dorsal septal cartilage and resection of the upper lateral cartilages (the cartilaginous component of the hump) (Figure 48-9). By contrast, if the aim is to augment the dorsal profile then septal, auricular or costal cartilages can be used to achieve this.

Altering the position and shape of the framework is also common practice. Osteotomies are used to narrow the open roof deformity following a hump reduction. In cases where the tip form is to be changed, sutures

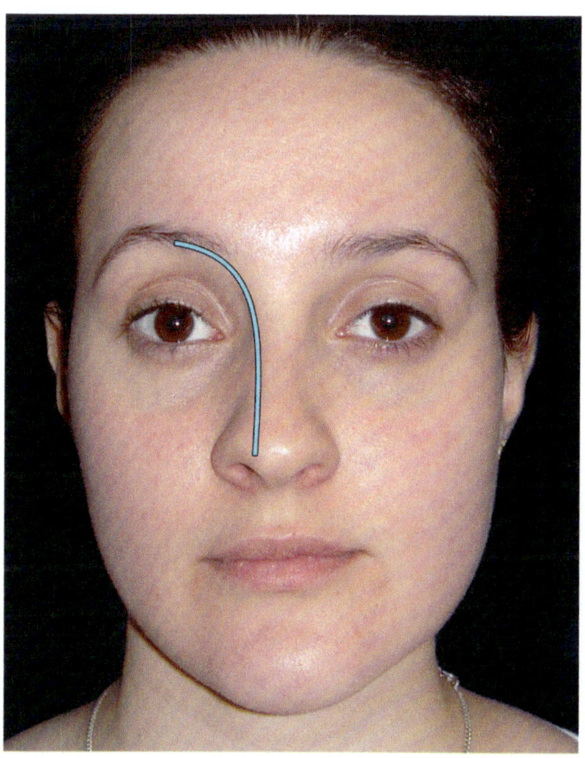

Fig. 48-6 Brow to tip aesthetic line.

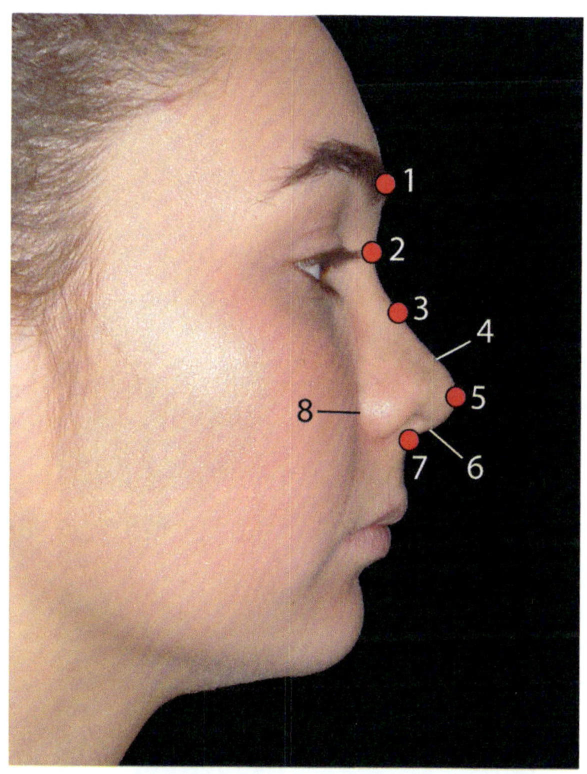

Fig. 48-7 Lateral view of the nose. 1, soft tissue glabella; 2, soft tissue nasion; 3, rhinion (osseocartilaginous junction); 4, supratip depression; 5, pronasale; 6, columella; 7, subnasale; 8, alar-facial groove/junction.

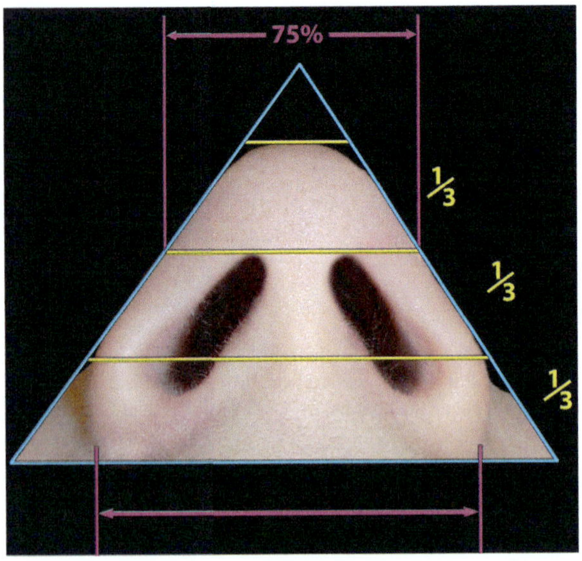

Fig. 48-8 Basal view, showing the triangularity of the nose. (From: Naini FB. Facial Aesthetics: Concepts and Clinical Diagnosis. Oxford: Wiley-Blackwell, 2011[6]; used with permission).

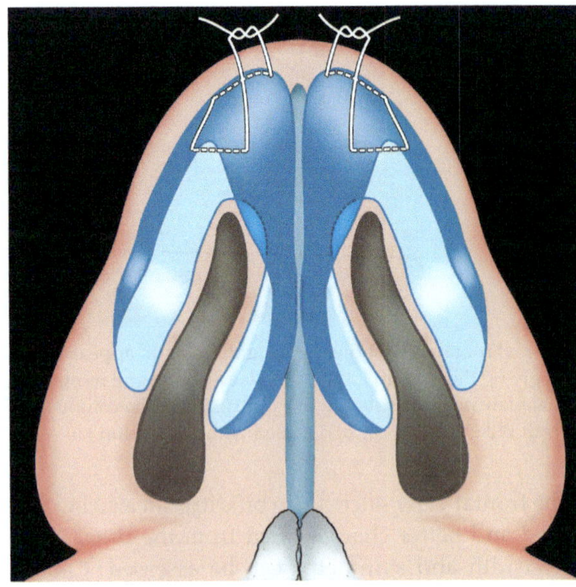

Fig. 48-10 Diagram showing a single dome suture. (Modified from: Naini FB. Facial Aesthetics: Concepts and Clinical Diagnosis. Oxford: Wiley-Blackwell, 2011[6]; used with permission).

can be used to alter the shape of the lower lateral cartilages (e.g. a single dome suture) (Figure 48-10).

Having compiled a list of techniques to be employed (subject to alteration during the procedure), the next stage is to decide on incisions and the approach required allowing the application of chosen techniques. In general, the **open tip approach** utilizing transcolumellar and marginal incisions allows generous access to carry out reduction and augmentation techniques in a symmetrical and accurate fashion (Figure 48-11). The alternative method is the **endonasal approach**, which utilizes inter-cartilaginous and transfixion incisions (Figure 48-12). If a marginal incision accompanies the inter-cartilaginous incision then the lower lateral cartilage can be delivered externally, allowing for resection and suturing techniques to be

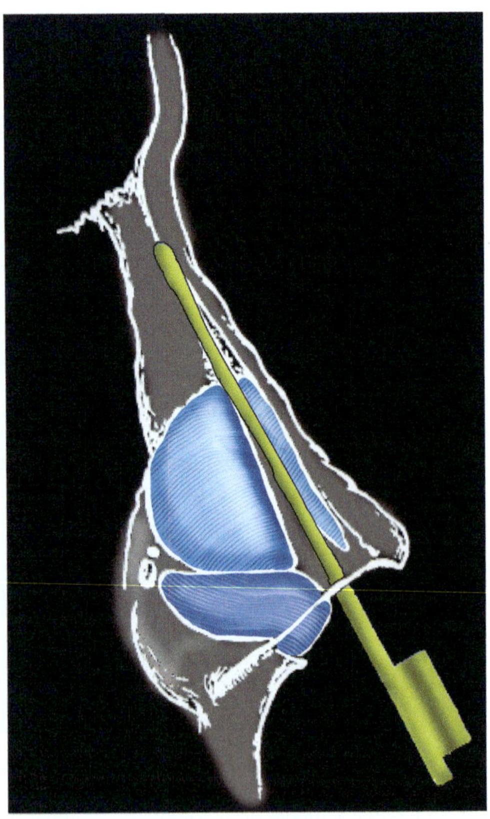

Fig. 48-9 Diagram showing nasal dorsal hump reduction.

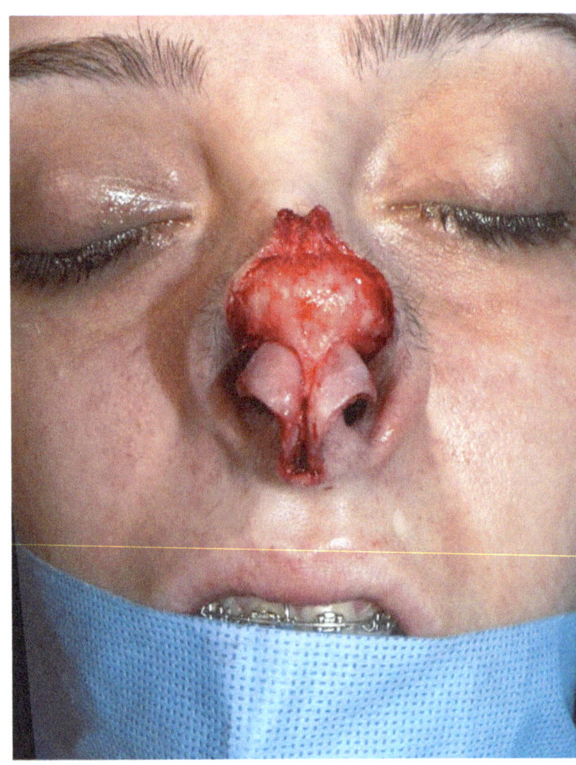

Fig. 48-11 The open tip approach.

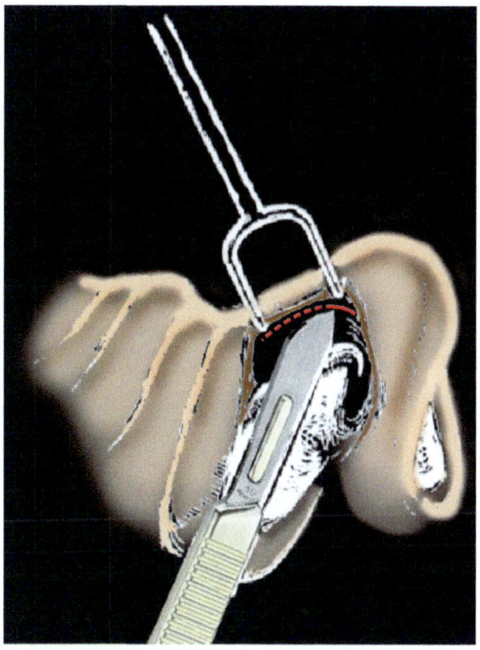

Fig. 48-12 Diagram showing the endonasal approach.

applied. This approach is called the **delivery approach** (Figure 48-13).

Nasal function following maxillary osteotomies

When performing maxillary osteotomies the anatomy and volume of the nasal cavity are altered; as a result nasal airway resistance also changes. After impaction and/or advancement of the maxilla a decrease in the nasal airway resistance may be observed.[1] This change is likely to be due to widening of the naris (external nasal valve) and opening of the internal valve. Turvey et al. reported a decrease in the nasal airway resistance in 38 of 52 patients after maxillary expansion.[2] Seventeen of the 19 patients with high preoperative nasal resistance showed a dramatic reduction to normal values postoperatively. Other studies have also shown that patients with high initial values for airway resistance had the greatest benefit.[3] A decrease in nasal resistance has been reported also after maxillary expansion; either with preoperative rapid maxillary expansion, surgically assisted rapid maxillary expansion or a transverse increase at the time of the Le Fort I osteotomy.

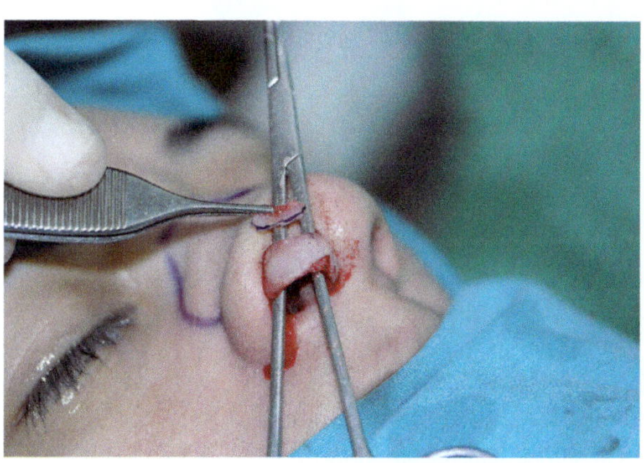

Fig. 48-13 A cephalic trim via the delivery approach.

Aesthetic changes in the nose following orthognathic surgery

Nasal appearance can improve or deteriorate following maxillary osteotomies. Careful assessment of the nose preoperatively and formulation of a treatment plan according to these findings will determine a successful outcome. Very often in skeletal Class III cases, part of the deformity is maxillary hypoplasia and poor support to the alar bases resulting in a narrowed **inter-alar distance** (Figure 48-14). Therefore, in these types of cases a mild widening of the nasal alar base width is welcomed. On the other hand, if the inter-alar distance is already wide, as is very often the case in patients of African-Caribbean ethnicity, avoidance of a further increase is of paramount importance. Different strategies in planning are the key to success in ethnic cases.

Changes following maxillary osteotomies are most frequently observed in the alar region. However, other changes also take place depending on the direction and the magnitude of the maxillary move. Rotation of the tip, exaggeration of the supratip break and softening of the dorsal hump may follow maxillary advancements.[4] Superior repositioning (impaction) of the maxilla widens the nose, particularly if it is coupled with advancement.[4] During impactions it is important to trim the cartilage of the septum appropriately to prevent its lateral deflection. If, on the other hand, this is done overzealously in front of the anterior nasal spine, in the postoperative period when scarring is taking place, columellar retraction may occur. Excessive reduction of the anterior nasal spine itself can also cause the same deformity. Whilst a minor degree of reduction of the nasolabial angle may also follow advancement of the maxilla, much less frequently performed push back is very potent in widening the nasolabial angle.[4]

Alar region

Widening of the alar base following orthognathic surgery is the most consistently reported change in the literature. Almost all of the osteotomies, independent of the direction and the magnitude of the move, result in a widening of the alar base. The most likely explanation for this is the elevation of the periosteum off the anterior surface of the maxilla, together with the muscles and ligaments stabilizing the alar region.[5] However, the most powerful association is with the advancement and impaction of the maxilla. Occasionally, moves that result in an increase in inter-alar distance may unmask pre-existing asymmetries that may require correction with secondary surgery (Figure 48-15).

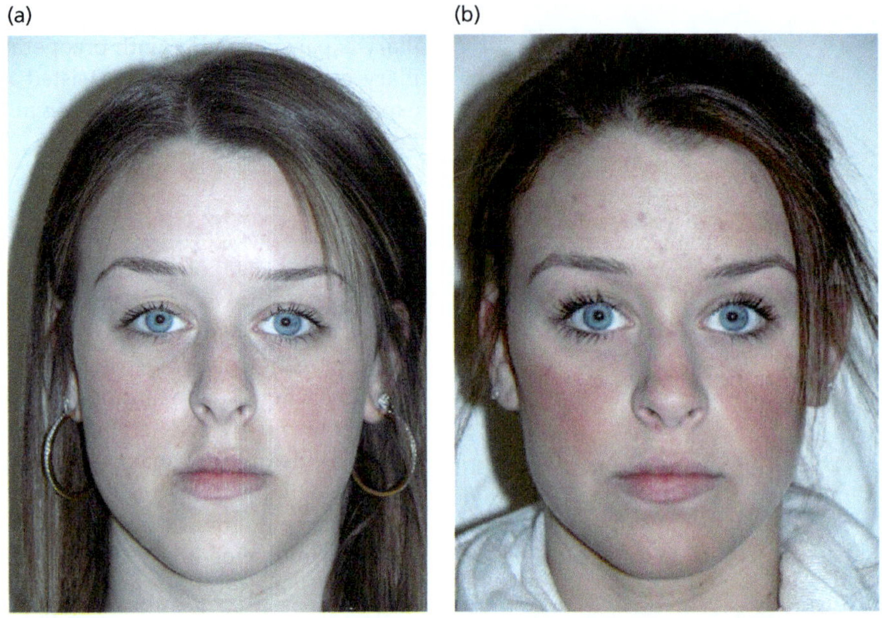

Fig. 48-14 Photographs of a patient with a Class III malocclusion and maxillary retrognathia and associated poor support to the alar base and narrowed interalar distance. The latter improved following orthognathic surgery as a result of the expected increase in interalar distance with the maxillary advancement. (a) Preoperative view. (b) Postoperative view.

Nasal tip and supratip region

Nasal tip support is provided by various components of the nasal anatomy. The nasal septum, strength of the lower lateral cartilages, attachment of the medial crura foot plates to the septum, attachment of the upper lateral cartilages to the lower lateral cartilages, and the anterior nasal spine all contribute to the tip support. Therefore, it is reasonable to assume that the dissection in this area, modification of the septal cartilage, reduction of the anterior nasal spine, and movement of the maxilla may all have an influence on the tip position. However, this association is not consistent. Probably, the most consistent association is the projection and rotation of the nasal tip with maxillary advancement (Figure 48-16). In under-projected, rotated short noses, this may result in excessive nostril show (Figure 48-17). Superior repositioning also causes elevation of the nasal tip. With inferior repositioning of the maxilla there is a loss of tip support. Equally, with the rarely performed posterior repositioning of the maxilla there is a similar trend. Changes in the supratip area follow the same pattern and is

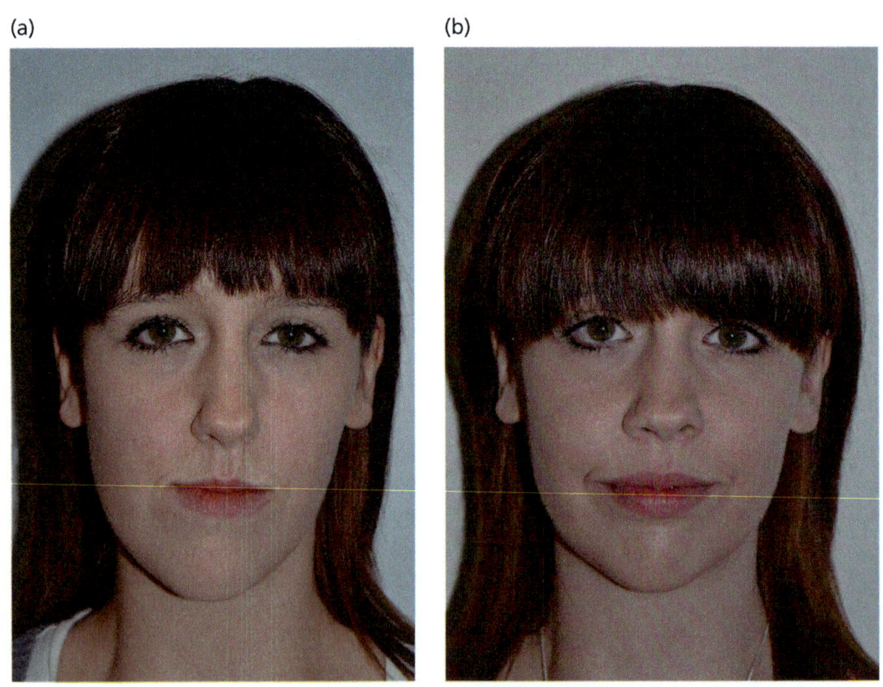

Fig. 48-15 Post-orthognathic surgery unmasking of pre-existing alar asymmetries, which were corrected with a secondary procedure. (a) Preorthognathic surgery. (b) Post-orthognathic surgery.

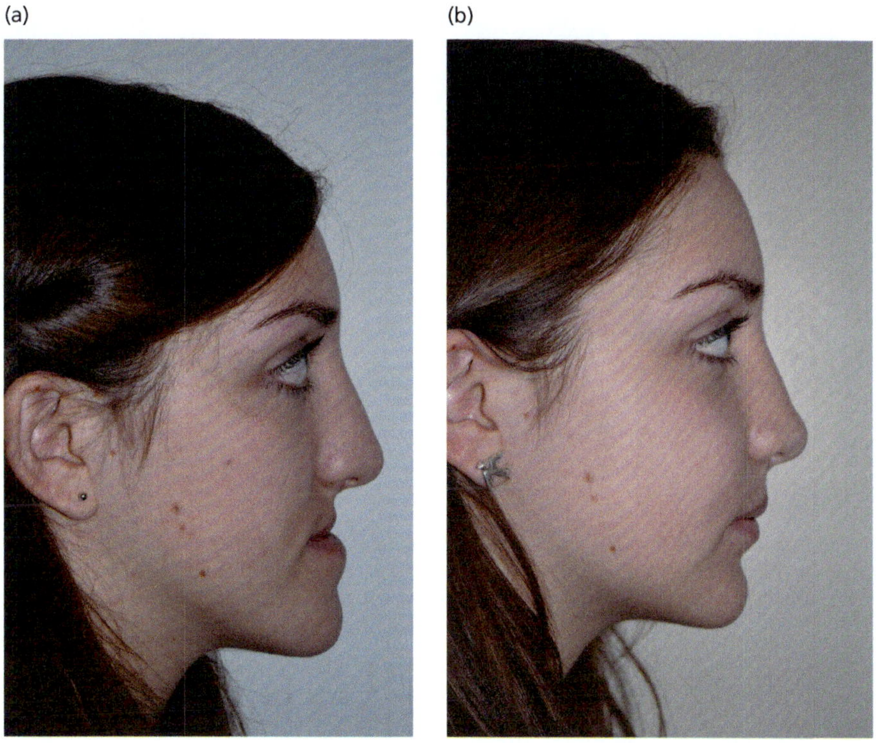

Fig. 48-16 Photographs showing increased projection and rotation of the nasal tip with a maxillary advancement procedure. (a) Preoperative profile. (b) Postoperative profile.

most noticeable by accentuation of the supratip break in advancement and impaction of the maxilla.

Nasolabial angle

In maxillary surgery a further change that takes place is in the nasolabial relationship and angle. However, in predicting the change in this angle it is helpful to consider it as being composed of two components; hence, the overall alteration will depend on the changes in the columella angle (i.e. upturning of the nasal tip) and the change in the inclination of the upper lip,[6] (Figure 48-18a). For instance, in maxillary advancement procedures the upper lip would be advanced leading to a reduction in the nasolabial angle, due to a reduction in its lower component. However, if there is considerable upturning of the nasal tip and thereby an increase in the upper component of the angle, there may be a resultant overall increase in the nasolabial angle. There tends to be a decrease in the nasolabial angle following maxillary impaction, which can also be coupled with deepening and accentuation of the nasolabial groove. On the other hand, inferior and posterior repositioning of the maxilla causes an increase in the nasolabial angle (Figure 48-18b). This could be very significant if the maxilla is set back considerably.

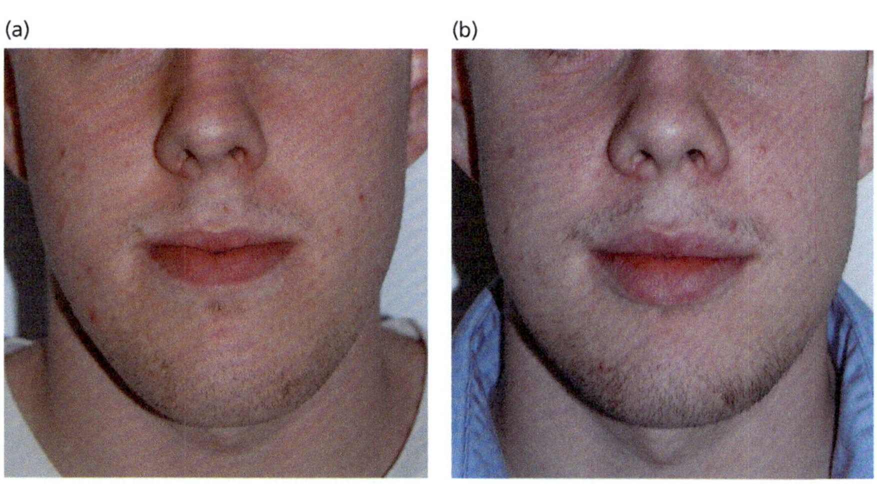

Fig. 48-17 Photographs showing excessive nostril show caused by a maxillary advancement procedure. (a) Preoperative view. (b) Postoperative view.

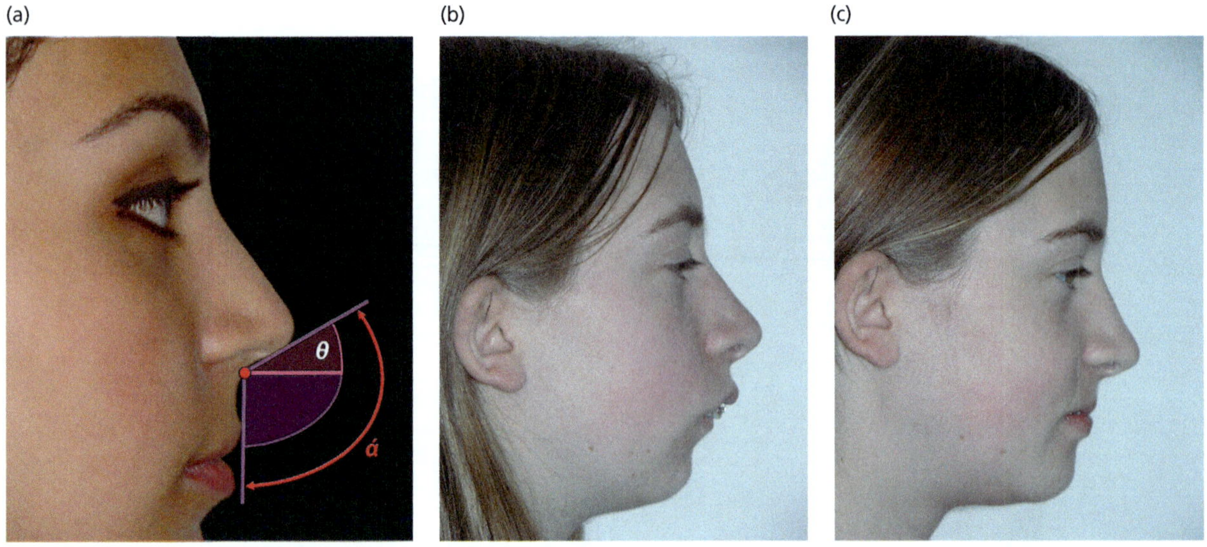

Fig. 48-18 (a) Division of nasolabial angle into upper and lower components. (From: Naini FB. Facial Aesthetics: Concepts and Clinical Diagnosis. Oxford: Wiley-Blackwell, 2011[6]; used with permission). (b) Preoperative profile, and (c) Postoperative profile showing increase in the nasolabial angle (particularly the lower component, i.e. the upper lip inclination) following a posterior set-back of the maxilla.

Nasal dorsum

Maxillary Le Fort I osteotomy has minimal direct effects on the nasal dorsum. These changes are often perceptual and relate to the tip position. Nasal tip droop often accentuates a prominent nasal dorsum. When the tip projects and rotates upwards, the hump becomes less visible. Conversely when the dorsal nasal profile is low, advancement of the maxilla may result in further flattening of the dorsum.

Columella

A retracted columella may be iatrogenic, from excessive resection of the anterior nasal spine and the caudal septum anterior to the spine. On the other hand, alar-columellar discrepancy may be due to maxillary impaction, where the alae move superiorly, leaving the columella in a relatively 'hanging' position.

Nasal septum

Small slit-like perforations in the inferior aspect of the cartilaginous septum, at the junction of the maxillary crest, are occasionally observed in the rhinoplasty of patients who have previously had maxillary osteotomies. These are often asymptomatic and probably not infrequent. However, the most common septal problem is the inadequately trimmed nasal septum in maxillary impaction cases. The lateral deflection that ensues may obstruct the nasal airway, as well as causing asymmetrical deviation of the nose (Figure 48-19).

In summary, a plethora of nasal changes may follow maxillary surgery depending on the direction and magnitude of the move. Some of these are due to postoperative oedema and will settle. Although patterns of change affecting the regions are established, their manifestations are variable, as is the compliance of the tissues. Preoperative assessment of the nose is an important part of orthognathic planning. The key to success is anticipation of changes and allowing the minor positive changes to take place, and avoiding unwanted changes that may be resistant to correction. Avoiding moves of large magnitude is of cardinal importance. Also important is taking into account ethnic features that may require different strategies.

Intraoperative procedures to manage nasal changes with orthognathic surgery

Alar base cinch suture

Alar base cinch sutures were originally described by Millard (1980) for cleft patients. Thereafter, Collins and Epker (1982) introduced these into the orthognathic

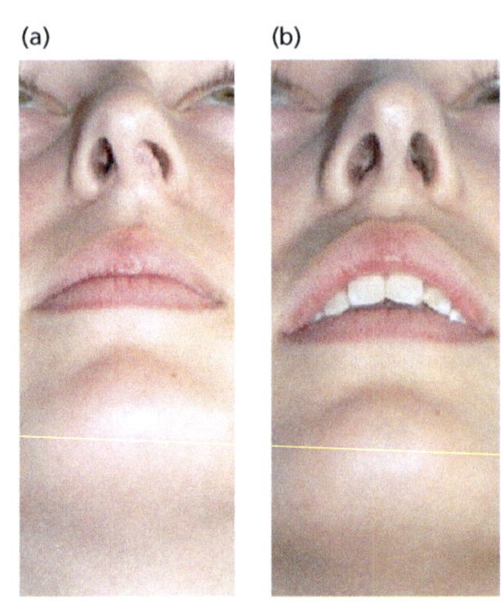

Fig. 48-19 (a) Photograph showing an example of post-orthognathic nasal septum deflection caused by insufficient trimming of the septum during a maxillary impaction, and (b) its management with a secondary procedure.

field as a technique for minimising alar base widening with maxillary surgery.[7] It was postulated that the elevation without re-approximation of the perioral and perinasal musculature was the reason for increased nasal width following Le Fort I type osteotomies.[5] Other reasons offered for this widening include release of periosteum and muscle attachments adjacent to the nose, and oedema and spatial change of the supportive bone to the nasal base superiorly or anteriorly.[8] When assessing the literature involving the use of cinch sutures it is important to identify what type of cinch suture was undertaken as a number of modifications have been introduced and reported since it was first described, as well as the type of suture material used, i.e. resorbable,[9] or non-resorbable.[7] In the classical cinch suture a 3/0 non-absorbable suture is passed through the intra-oral incision, anchoring fibro-areolar tissue under both alae and the transverse nasalis muscle. The two free ends are then pulled and the tension adjusted to achieve the desired width of the alar base before tying the knot. This suture runs in front of the anterior nasal spine. In the view of some authorities, this controlled reorientation of the perinasal muscles is thought to provide a more predictable and stable result than their random reinsertion.[10]

The placement of this suture during orthognathic surgery has been criticised by some authors as the technique was deemed inaccurate,[11] especially with the endotracheal tube in place, unpredictable and leading to other possible effects such as upper lip 'lengthening', which may not be desirable. The naso-endotracheal tube may distort the nostrils, which may make intraoperative assessment of alar width and tightening by the cinch suture difficult and inaccurate. Some surgeons have opted to address this by undertaking orthognathic surgery under submental intubation (see Chapter 22),[12] whilst others have described the replacement of the naso-endotracheal tube with an oral endotracheal tube following stabilization of the maxilla and mandible.[13]

There is controversy as to the effectiveness of alar base cinch sutures on minimizing alar flare and alar base widening; some in support,[9,13,14] whilst others stating no significant effect is provided.[15] A prospective randomized controlled trial of 28 patients (14 with and 14 without cinch suture) who had 3D surface laser scans preoperatively, 1 and 6 months postoperatively, found it provides a small and clinically insignificant decrease in alar width widening (0.5 mm) and concluded it was of 'little benefit'.[15] The authors of the study admit the results are to be viewed with caution due to the small sample size as well as the sole use of descriptive statistics. Potential inaccuracies of the scanning system should also be borne in mind. On the other hand, in a retrospective study where 38 patients received cinch sutures and 17 acted as a control, alar widening was statistically significantly reduced ($P = 0.04$) with the cinch suture compared to the control group; 1.6 mm and 2.3 mm respectively at a minimum of six months postoperatively.[9]

One of the major criticisms of the use of the cinch suture is unwanted nasal tip rotation, thought to occur due to the ventral pressure of the maxillary bone on the lateral crurae.[16] This effect, together with an increased nasolabial angle, with the use of cinch sutures has been identified in individual studies,[13] as well as in a recent systematic review of the literature in this subject.[17] Muradin and Rosenberg (2000) suggested it was the anterior positioning of the cinch suture relative to the anterior nasal spine, which may lead to nasal tip elevation as a result of antero-cranial rotation of the lateral crurae.[18] Therefore, they suggested a modified alar cinch closure, using a 2-0 Vicryl suture which passes through the nasal septum 10 mm posterior to the nasal spine to limit this effect. They combined this with a muco-musculo-periosteal V-Y closure with 3-0 Vicryl to produce a 15 mm tail on the Y, terming this the mACVY closure.[18] The mACVY technique ($n = 31$) was compared to simple closing sutures ($n = 25$) on patients who underwent Le Fort I maxillary impaction ± advancement and mandibular set-back ($n = 13$) or advancement ($n = 43$). On lateral cephalometric radiographs taken 18 months postoperatively, there was no significant difference found for vertical changes of nasal tip between the groups, but a statistically significant increase in nasal tip projection horizontally measured by the Sella–Nasion–Pronasale angle (2° versus 0.6°) was noted on the mACVY group. Therefore, the authors concluded that their mACVY modification does not cause excessive upward rotation of the nasal tip.[19] Interestingly, the horizontal and vertical changes of labrale superius were significantly greater for mACVY versus the simple closure group, producing increased soft to hard tissue ratios of upper lip movement in mACVY cases. This trend was also found in a recent systematic review of studies when a comparison was made between studies involving patients with simple continuous closures with those who received cinch, V-Y or both procedures.[17] This in turn could affect the horizontal position of the upper lip and the nasolabial angle change.

The other criticism of this technique is its long-term stability. Generally, it is accepted that postoperative oedema can take up to six months if not longer to settle,[20] hence ideally studies investigating the stability of these sutures should follow-up patients for one year or more. Shoji et al. (2012) found with their cinch sutures they were able to maintain the preoperative alar base width and one year postoperatively there was no clinically significant increase in this measurement.[13] Another study examined 36 patients prospectively, who received maxillary advancement, impaction or both as part of their skeletal II or III correction with a submental intubation technique, allowing for intraoperative nasal measurements.[14] All patients received a classical alar base cinch suture as well as a V-Y closure and clinical measurements were taken preoperatively, intraoperatively and at three, six and 12 months follow-up. Alar base and inter-alar width increased by a mean of 3 mm and 3.6 mm respectively following the osteotomy, the cinch sutures (classical cinch with 3/0 nylon) where then placed adjusting the tension to achieve the best aesthetic results leading to a reduction of these measurements by 53% (1.6 mm) and 58% (2.1 mm) intraoperatively. Though complete records were not available for all stages of the study, all were included for their one year measurement, where an increase of 1.7 mm (SD 1.0) and 2.3 mm (SD 1.6) were found in the alar base and inter-alar width measurements and judged by the authors to be of no clinical significance, suggesting good medium term stability.[14] There was no statistical analysis included and the clinical significance of the reported widening could be dependent on the clinical scenario.

Although it has not been reported or investigated, it may be that the material (resorbable or non-resorbable) used for the cinch suture could have a bearing on the stability of the procedure. The classical suture was described to be used with non-resorbable sutures; however, some surgeons prefer to use resorbable with the theory that they will hold the tissues together long enough for the reattachment to occur. Others believe this would not necessarily occur.

Some modifications to the classical cinch suture to address this have been described and in general are based on the principle of ensuring an increased grasp of the alar tissues. One of these, involved using a 0 monofilament suture with a thick needle, which was inserted from the intraoral incision to the skin exiting at the alar-facial junction and reinserting it through the same puncture site and changing its direction before exiting intraorally in order to grasp the alar base tissues.[21] This research group conducted a randomized double-blind controlled trial on 35 patients who underwent maxillary impaction ± advancement. The extraoral modified cinch suture proved to be statistically significantly ($P < 0.05$) more effective in maintaining preoperative alar and alar base width compared to the classic intraoral cinch suture at 5 months follow-up.[21] The mean alar base widening recorded on submental oblique digital photographs was 1.38 mm and 2.5 mm in the extraoral and classical cinch suture groups respectively. A further modification with a similar aim was described by Rauso et al. (2010), where to anchor more tissue a percutaneous straight needle was inserted extraorally and partly retracted without leaving the skin to then be reinserted into the oral cavity in a medial direction, taking with it the needleless suture.[22] In a prospective study of 40 patients undergoing a bimaxillary procedure by the same surgeon, the patients were randomly allocated to the latter modified cinch suture or a classical group.[22] The modified suture technique prevented nasal widening in 14 out of 20 patients versus 3 out of 20 in the classic cinch group, based on clinical measurements taken six months postoperatively compared to pre-treatment.[22] Since there was no sample size calculation, no statistical testing of the results, and stability was measured at six months only, the latter cannot be taken as conclusive.

Finally, a prospective randomized trial assessed the effectiveness of the classical cinch suture ($n = 31$) compared to their modified transseptal cinch, which was placed through the septum 10 mm posterior to the anterior nasal spine ($n = 31$).[23] The researchers found a statistically significant difference between the two groups ($P < 0.001$); whereby there was an increase in the mean alar base width of 2.66 mm (0.8 SD) in the classic cinch group compared to 0.145 mm (2.05 SD) in the modified cinch group six months postoperatively. The variation found in their modified group was large. In addition, without a control group (no cinch suture) it is difficult to determine the reduction in widening provided by the cinch sutures.

A systematic review comparing the classical cinch suture to the modifications described above (transseptal and re-insertion) found the modified versions were more effective at maintaining the preoperative alar and alar base width.[24]

Pyriform guttering

This is an optional manoeuvre during the Le Fort I osteotomy whereby bone is removed from the pyriform rim to minimize the anterior or superior displacement of alar and peri-alar soft tissues (see Chapter 22). Literature assessing the effect of this manoeuvre on nasal soft tissues is lacking.

ANS recontouring/subspinal osteotomy

Reduction of the anterior nasal spine (ANS) can be undertaken when advancing the maxilla in order to control nasal tip rotation, as advancement of the maxilla often leads to nasal tip upturning. There is little evidence in the literature regarding the effectiveness of this procedure, though it is commonly undertaken clinically. The paucity of the literature may be due to the difficulty in quantification of the amount and site of bone removal. In addition, measurement of changes on lateral cephalometric radiographs can be difficult due to the local disruption to the anatomy at the site. Nevertheless, it has been reported to lead to a reduced ratio of response of the anterior nasal tip to movement at A-point from 0.33:1 to 0.25:1.[25]

Another technique suggested for limiting changes to the nasal soft tissues is a subspinal osteotomy. The technique was described as a modification to the classical Le Fort I osteotomy for patients undergoing maxillary advancement and/or impaction with the intention of limiting nasal tip rotation.[26,27] The theory behind the technique is that preservation of the natural muscular insertions of the, transverse nasalis and depressor septi muscles can be achieved if the anterior portion of the usual circumvestibular incision is undertaken in a V-shaped full thickness manner and the rest of the osteotomy undertaken as usual except without detaching the anterior osteo-musculo-mucosal flap from the nasal septum.[26] The authors conducted a small study to test their modification on 10 selected patients who received this procedure for maxillary advancement and impaction and compared them to 10 selected patients who had a standard Le Fort I osteotomy with ANS recontouring and cinch sutures. The clinical, radiographic and photographic outcome was assessed at an average follow up of 12 months. In their view, this technique helped reduce alar base widening and tip rotation, however, this was a selected small sample with no analysis of surgical movement differences between the groups, no analysis of the results and no statistical tests. Another study, comparing the subspinal osteotomy to a conventional Le Fort I type osteotomy found there was no difference in nasal tip elevation and projection between the two groups.[16] The latter, was a retrospective study in which the lateral cephalometric radiographs of patients preoperatively and 6 months postoperatively were compared for two matched groups of 23 patients who received a conventional Le Fort I osteotomy for maxillary advancement and impaction with ANS recontouring, alar base cinch suture and V-Y closure, and the other group underwent subspinal osteotomy. The matching between groups was based on a sagittal and vertical movement within 1 mm for both directions and the choice of osteotomy was reported to be random within that period. Matching based on the amount and direction of skeletal movement allows for a more true comparison of the effect of the techniques used, reducing bias. On the other hand, a cinch suture was used in these cases, which as discussed above could also be a variable leading to effects on the nasal tip changes.

V-Y closure

The adjunctive surgical technique thought to have the greatest impact on the upper lip height and more researched with regards to this effect on the lip is the V-Y closure. This was described by Schendel and Williamson as a technique to help minimize the upper lip shortening and thinning noted with Le Fort I type osteotomies.[5] Instead of a continuous simple closure of the vestibular incision from first permanent molar to first permanent molar, there is medial advancement of the superior aspect of the vestibular incision to produce the 'Y' appearance. It is thought to help re-approximate the nasolabial musculature, reducing the tendency for thinning and shortening of the upper lip.

The results of the available literature are controversial. A retrospective study comparing ten patients with a V-Y closure and eight with simple continuous closure found no statistically significant difference in upper lip height changes.[28] However, other studies with larger sample sizes and/or executed in a prospective manner have attained different results. McCollum et al. conducted a retrospective study involving assessment of the lateral cephalometric radiographs of 26 patients who received bimaxillary surgery, 11 of whom received V-Y closures.[29] In this study, the V-Y closure allowed the upper lip to roll out by allowing stomion superius to advance by approximately 25% more than when no V-Y closure was used and reduced lip shortening by a factor approaching 2 (Stms:UIT decreased from 0.26:1 to 0.12:1). This effect seemed also to be reflected in the results of the prospective study where the sample with a mACVY had an increase in the upper lip vermillion exposure compared to the group with simple continuous closure.[19] Furthermore, in the randomized prospective trial by Peled et al. a statistically significant increase in height of the upper lip with an alar cinch suture and V-Y closure (1.10 mm ± 0.34) was found, which reflects a 23% increase compared to the shortening experienced by the simple closure group with a cinch suture (–0.79 mm ± 0.45).[30] Hence a trend towards V-Y closure helping to minimise upper lip shortening is noted and further research with larger sample sizes executed in a prospective manner may help to confirm this further. As mentioned earlier, in the latter study the mACVY showed no significant nasal tip turning although an increased projection was found. Since this group had a combination of cinch and V-Y closures it is difficult to ascertain what effects were due to which procedure. There is therefore a lack of research comparing individual techniques to controls to ascertain their impact on the result.

To investigate the effect of a V-Y closure on upper lip thinning, linear measurements on lateral cephalometric radiographs were undertaken retrospectively.[28] At 12 months postoperatively, the upper (A-Sn) and lower (cervical margin of the maxillary incisor – Ls) parts of the upper lip experienced thinning in both groups; 0.87 mm and 0.5 mm thinning in the upper part for the simple continuous ($n = 10$) and V-Y ($n = 8$) closure groups respectively, and 1.9mm and 1.7 mm thinning in the lower part respectively.[28] No statistically significant differences were noted between the groups, though they highlighted a trend towards better lip height stability and decreased thinning with V-Y closures. Whereas, statistical significance ($P < 0.05$) was achieved in the investigation executed by Peled et al.,[30] described above, where the simple closure group experienced thinning of the inferior (labial aspect of maxillary incisor – labrale superius) part of the upper lip by 1.94 mm (SE ± 0.24 mm) versus 1.14 mm (SE ± 0.31 mm) in the V-Y group.

Septal trimming and septal fixation with suture

Instead of or in addition to nasal spine recontouring, septal trimming can be undertaken to allow for its adaptation to the new anatomical position of the maxilla without it being bent and deviated if lacking space. Additionally, surgeons might use a suture to fix the septum to the surrounding anatomy in the desired position. The fixation of the septum to the anterior nasal spine could be an important stabilization manoeuvre, but one should be careful as the orthognathic surgical procedure aims to change the position of the maxilla and in doing so the anatomical landmarks generally used may have changed in position and no longer be relevant to the position aimed for the septum.

Secondary nasal procedures following orthognathic surgery

Facial assessment and analysis carried out at the outset of the orthognathic planning should make specific reference to the nose. If the patient is keen to pursue nasal surgery in the future then it is important to advise on the sequencing of procedures. Generally, nasal surgery should follow orthognathic surgery. Firstly, as discussed in the previous section, despite careful planning, there may be distortion of the nose following orthognathic surgery. Correction of these together with achievement of other objectives, based on the assessment can safely be carried out once the postoperative oedema has settled. If possible, it would be advisable to wait for a year. Secondly, finely tuned and executed nasal surgery is likely to be altered following orthognathic surgery. Therefore, it is highly desirable to delay nasal surgery to follow orthognathic surgery when sequencing overall treatment.

The concept of carrying out rhinoplasty and maxillary osteotomy at the same time is highly contentious. Whilst some authors advocate this approach,[31] if excellence is pursued, it should be avoided. Firstly, as the nose will change during the maxillary osteotomy, preoperative observations are not going to hold true making a finely tuned rhinoplasty plan impossible. If rhinoplasty is going to be carried out as a secondary procedure, enough time should elapse for oedema free analysis, and a treatment plan to be formulated offering surgery at a stable point, giving the very best chance for a successful outcome. Rhinoplasty plans are often very comprehensive, and the temptation of to meet only a few objectives at the same time should be avoided. Secondly, each procedure may take several hours, making the whole operation unreasonably long. Thirdly, anaesthetic considerations, such as change of nasal tube to oral, or a submental intubation to be carried out at the outset, may become a necessity. Combined procedures of rhinoplasty and orthognathic surgery are therefore rarely recommended.

Alar soft tissue techniques

If the distortion in the alar base is beyond the aesthetic balance and natural appearance following orthognathic surgery, alar base surgery may be considered. Ideally, the most lateral aspect of the ala should fall within a perpendicular line dropped from the medial aspect of the medial canthus. This situation is not always attainable, due to variations in facial morphology, but can be used as a guideline in assessing the need for alar base narrowing. Furthermore, referencing within the nose, i.e. nasal tip width to the alar base width ratio, is also important. Broader nasal tips can be accommodated in a wide alar base. The width of the infratip lobule should be approximately 75% of the nasal width.

As Sheen described, there are two surfaces to the ala that affect to a varying degree the width and contour of the alar base.[32] These are the cutaneous and vestibular surfaces. If these two surfaces are considered independently, maintaining or narrowing the width of the alar base, and maintaining or narrowing the nostril size can be well controlled separately.

Prior to choosing a procedure to alter the alar base the following areas should be assessed:

1. Inter-alar width and the amount of nasal sill available.
2. The presence or absence of alar flaring.
3. Nostril shape.
4. Thickness of the alar rim.

Alar base reduction is best performed in the nasal sill. The excision then can be extended at the alar facial groove to deal with the flare component. Excision may be limited to the alar facial groove if the problem is primarily one of flaring. Extension of incisions to the internal vestibular surface depends on the desire to change the shape of the naris. If the alar rim is thick a further wedge excision of the rim may be carried out to narrow it (Figure 48-20).

Septoplasty

Septoplasty for the buckled septum following maxillary impaction may be necessary to improve the nasal airway and to deal with the resultant asymmetry.

Columellar retraction

Columellar retraction resulting from overzealous removal of caudal septum and anterior nasal spine can be corrected using septal extension grafts and plumping grafts. Long-term stability is better with a septal extension graft but patients may complain of stiffness of the nose.

Dorsal augmentation

Following maxillary advancement, in cases where there is already a saddle deformity, improvement in dorsal profile can be best achieved by using diced cartilage wrapped in temporalis fascia. This gives a stable result allowing the dorsum to blend well with the neighbouring areas.

Concluding remarks

The orthognathic surgeon should include nasal aesthetic and functional analysis as part of the diagnostic process and treatment planning for orthognathic surgery. Patients should be warned comprehensively about nasal changes that may follow orthognathic

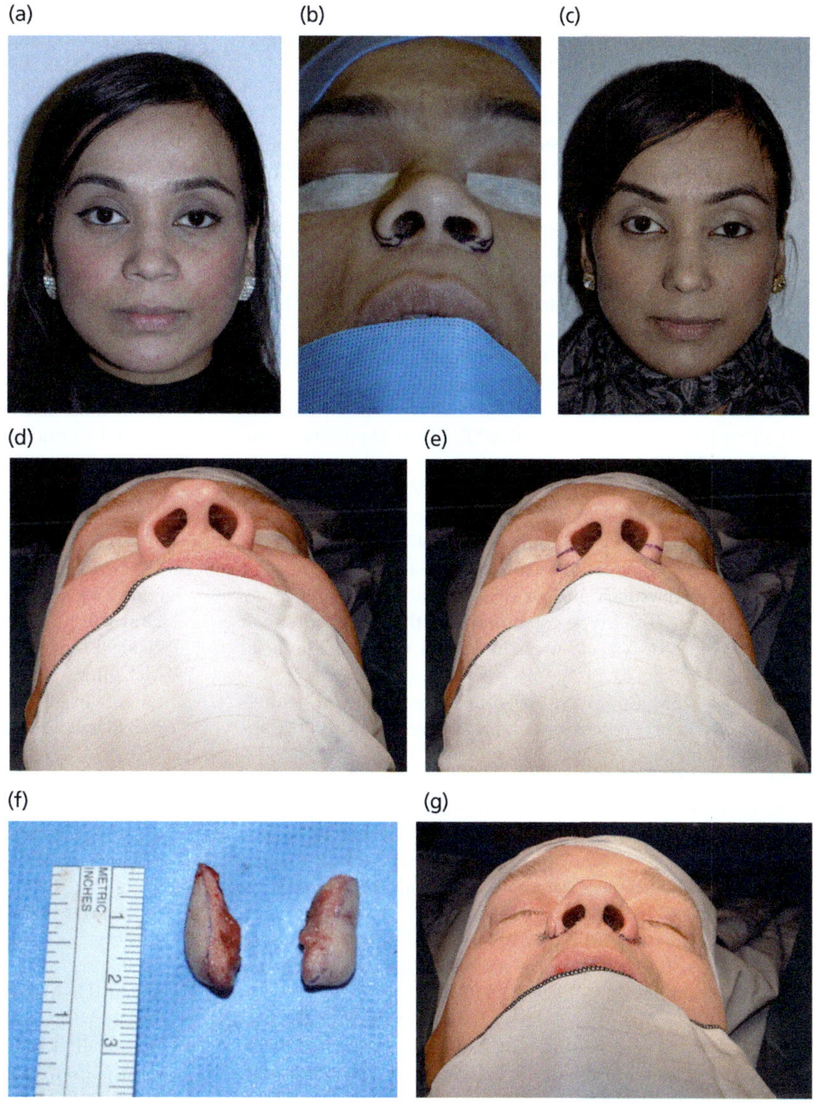

Fig. 48-20 Photographs showing two clinical examples of patients who underwent alar wedge excision. (a-c) Preoperative, intraoperative and postoperative stages shown. (d-g) Preoperative, intraoperative and post wedge resection.

surgery and associated strategies for management. Sequencing of treatment should be undertaken in such a way that nasal refinement follows other orthognathic procedures. Avoidance of excessive maxillary moves is key to minimizing unwanted effects on nasal aesthetics. On the other hand, it is an art to allow some changes to occur such as a moderate increase in interalar distance to achieve harmony. When it is felt that boundaries of harmony are breached ancillary procedures during orthognathic surgery could be considered. However, it is important to understand the limits of such manoeuvres and the surgeon should be prepared to deal with some of the adverse effects with secondary procedures. To be able to carry out a comprehensive septo-rhinoplasty either planed at the outset as needed or introduced later based on post-orthognathic surgical assessment, provides a powerful tool for the facial surgeon. Whilst there may be attraction to carrying out a rhinoplasty concurrently with a bimaxillary osteotomy, both in terms of inaccuracy of planning as well as inability to achieve a high quality technical result this temptation should be avoided. Far superior results in facial harmony can be achieved if these procedures are undertaken sequentially.

References

1 Guenthner TA, Sather AH, Kern EB. The effect of Le Fort I maxillary impaction on nasal airway resistance. Am J Orthodont. 1984;85:308.
2 Turvey TA, Hall DJ, Warren DW. Alterations in nasal airway resistance following superior repositioning of the maxilla. Am J Orthodont. 1984;85:109.
3 Williams BJD, Isom A, Jilho JRL, O'Ryan F. Nasal Airway Function after maxillary surgery: A prospective cohort study using the nasal obstruction symptom evaluation scale. American Association of Oral and Maxillofacial Surgeons. J Oral Maxillofac Surg. 2013;71:343–50.
4 Mitchell C, Oeltjen J, Panthaki Z, Thaller SR. Nasolabial Aesthetics. J Craniofac Surg. 2007;18:756–65.
5 Schendel SA, Williamson LW. Muscle reorientation following superior repositioning of the maxilla. J Oral Maxillofac Surg. 1983;41:235–40.
6 Naini FB. Regional analysis: The nose. In: Naini FB. Facial Aesthetics: Concepts and Clinical Diagnosis. Oxford: Wiley-Blackwell, 2011.
7 Collins PC, Epker BN. The alar base cinch: a technique for prevention of alar base flaring secondary to maxillary surgery. Oral Surg Oral Med Oral Pathol. 1982;53:549–53.
8 Wolford LM. Lip-nasal aesthetics following Le Fort I osteotomy-discussion. Plast Reconstruct Surg. 1988;81:180–2.
9 Westermark AH, Bystedt H, von Konow L, Sällström KO. Nasolabial morphologies after Le Fort I osteotomy. Internat J Oral Maxillofac Surg. 1991;20:25–30.

10 Carlotti AEJr, Aschaffenburg PH, Schendel SA. Facial changes associated with surgical advancement of the lip and maxilla. J Oral Maxillofac Surg. 1986;44:593–6.
11 Rosen HM. Lip-nasal aesthetics following Le Fort I osteotomy. Plast Reconstruct Surg. 1988;81:171–82.
12 Chandu A, Witherow H, Stewart A. Submental intubation in orthognathic surgery: initial experience. Br J Oral Maxillofac Surg. 2008;46: 561–3.
13 Shoji T, Muto T, Takahashi M, Akizudi K, Tsuchida Y. The stability of an alar cinch suture after Le Fort I and mandibular osteotomies in Japanese patients with Class III malocclusions. Br J Oral Maxillofac Surg. 2012;50: 361–4.
14 Stewart A, Edler RJ. Efficacy and stability of the alar base cinch suture. B J Oral Maxillofac Surg. 2011;49:623–6.
15 Howley C, Ali N, Lee R, Cox S. Use of alar base cinch suture in Le Fort I osteotomy: is it effective? Br J Oral Maxillofac Surg. 2011;49:127–30.
16 Mommaerts MY, Lippens F, Abeloos JVS, Neyt LF. Nasal profile changes after maxillary impaction and advancement surgery. J Oral Maxillofac Surg. 2000;58:470–5.
17 Khamashta-Ledezma L, Naini FB. Systematic review of changes in maxillary incisor exposure and upper lip position with Le Fort I type osteotomies with or without cinch sutures and/or VY closures. Internat J Oral Maxillofacial Surg. 2014;43:46–61.
18 Muradin MSM, Rosenberg A. Controlling nasolabial aesthetics after Le Fort I osteotomies: A retrospective study. J Craniomaxillofac Surg. 2000;28:209.
19 Muradin MSM, Seubring K, Stoelinga PJW, Bilt A, Koole R, Rosenberg AJWP. A prospective study on the effect of modified alar cinch sutures and V-Y closure versus simple closing sutures on nasolabial changes after Le Fort I intrusion and advancement osteotomies. J Oral Maxillofac Surg. 2011;69:870–6.
20 Stella JP, Streater MR, Epker BN, Sinn DP. Predictability of upper lip soft tissue changes with maxillary advancement. J Oral Maxillofac Surg. 1989;47:697–703.
21 Ritto FG, Medeiros PJ, Moraes M, Passeado DBR. Comparative analysis of two different alar base sutures after Le Fort I osteotomy: randomised double-blind controlled trial. Oral Surg Oral Med Oral Pathol Oral Radiol Endodont. 2011;111:181–9.
22 Rauso R, Tartaro G, Tozzi U, Colella G, Santagata M. Nasolabial changes after maxillary advancement. J Craniofac Surg. 2011;22:809–12.
23 Nirvikalpa N, Narayanan V, Wahab A, Ramadorai A. Comparison between the classical and a modified trans-septal technique of ala cinching for Le Fort I osteotomies: a prospective randomized controlled trial. Internat J Oral Maxillofac Surg. 2013;42:49–54.
24 Liu X, Zhu S, Hu J. Modified versus classic alar base sutures after Le Fort I osteotomy: a systematic review. Oral Surg Oral Med Oral Pathol Oral Radiol. 2014;117:37–44.
25 Freihofer HPJr. Changes in nasal profile after maxillary advancement in cleft and non-cleft patients. J Maxillofac Surg. 1977;5:20–27.
26 Becelli R, De Ponte FS, Fadda MT, Govoni F, Iannetti G. Subnasal modified Le Fort I for nasolabial aesthetics improvement. J Craniofac Surg. 1996;7:399–402.
27 Mommaerts MY, Abeloos JV, De Clercq CA, Neyt LF. The effect of the subspinal Le Fort I-type osteotomy on interalar rim width. Int J Adult Orthodon Orthognath Surg. 1997;12:95–100.
28 Talebzadeh N, Pogrel MA. Upper lip length after V-Y versus continuous closure for Le Fort I level maxillary osteotomy. Oral Surg Oral Med Oral Pathol Oral Radiol Endodont. 2000;90:144–6.
29 McCollum AGH, Dancaster JT, Evans WG, Becker PJ. Sagittal soft tissue changes related to the surgical corrections of maxillary deficient class III malocclusions. Semin Orthodont. 2009;15:172–84.
30 Peled M, Ardekian L, Krausz AA, Aizenbud D. Comparing the effects of V-Y advancement versus simple closure on upper lip aesthetics after Le Fort I advancement. J Oral Maxillofac Surg. 2004;62:315–9.
31 Seah TE, Bellis H, Ilankovan V. Orthognathic patients with nasal deformities: case for simultaneous orthognathic surgery and rhinoplasty. J Oral Maxillofac Surg. 2012;50: 55–9.
32 Sheen JH. Alar Resection and Grafting: Dallas Rhinoplasty. 2nd edn. St Louis, MO: Quality Medical Publishing, 2007.
33 Warner JP, Chauhan N, Adamson PA. Alar soft-tissue techniques in rhinoplasty: algorithmic approach, quantifiable guidelines, and scar outcomes from a single surgeon experience. Arch Facial Plast Surg. 2010;12:149–58.

Chapter 49

Deep Plane Facelift

Farhad Ardeshirpour, Craig S. Murakami and Wayne F. Larrabee

Anatomy

As the face ages, its layers (skin, fat, muscle, bone) undergo changes that result in a deflated or droopy appearance. The skin becomes thin and wrinkled from a decrease in collagen production and loss of elasticity. The effects of gravity and increased laxity in the supporting ligaments between bone and skin (i.e. zygomaticus-cutaneous ligament, mandibular-cutaneous ligaments, etc.) contribute to soft tissue descent.[1] The malar fat pad, sub-orbicularis oculi fat, jowls, and submental fat appear to descend and the melolabial folds appear to deepen. The atrophy of fat pads (i.e. buccal) and skeletal absorption (i.e. orbits, mandible, maxilla) also contribute to the loss of volume by creating space for the soft tissues to descend or retract. The thinning skin and soft tissue descent create mounds and depressions which cast shadows that create a sunken, drooping, and tired appearance.

The superficial musculo-aponeurotic system (SMAS) is an important layer of facial soft tissue support. From a surgical perspective, it is the superior fibromuscular extension of the platysma (Figure 49-1). Above the zygomatic arch the SMAS plane extends superiorly as the temporoparietal fascia although embryonically these plane may differ. It is subject of debate whether the sub-SMAS fascial layers are contiguous or separate as they condense down onto the zygotmatic arch.[2] The SMAS is thickest over the parotid and thins out medial to the zygomatic major muscle.[3] Failure of the SMAS to support the lower face and neck produces jowls and visible anterior platysma bands. The majority of blood supply to facelift flaps comes from the facial artery, with contribution from the transverse facial artery, superficial temporal, and post-auricular arteries. In theory, deep plane facelifts have less risk of skin flap necrosis because of limited subcutaneous dissection and elevation of a thick SMAS and skin complex.

The greater auricular nerve (GAN) provides sensation around the ear and is the most commonly injured nerve in facelift surgery. The course of the GAN can be predicted using palpable anatomical landmarks. A line drawn between the mastoid process and the angle of the mandible, followed by second perpendicular line that bisect the first line, will outline its course.[4]

Orthognathic Surgery: Principles, Planning and Practice. Edited by Farhad B. Naini and Daljit S. Gill.

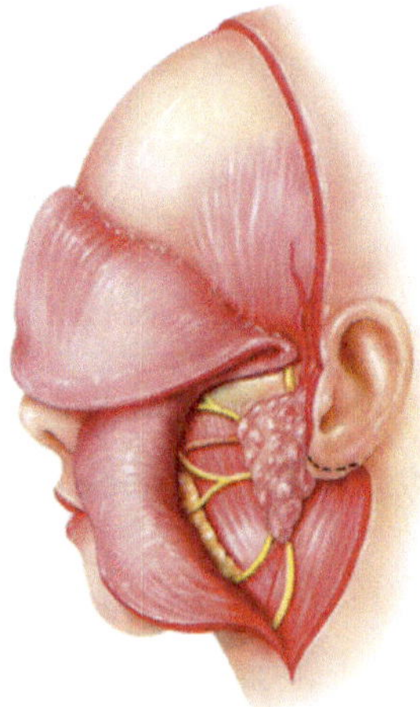

Fig. 49-1 The SMAS has been reflected showing its continuity with the temporoparietal fascia, and platysma. The facial nerve can be seen in relation to the masseter, the parotid duct, and buccal fat. (Illustration reprinted from Azizzadeh et al.[5] with permission from Saunders, Philadelphia, PA, USA.)

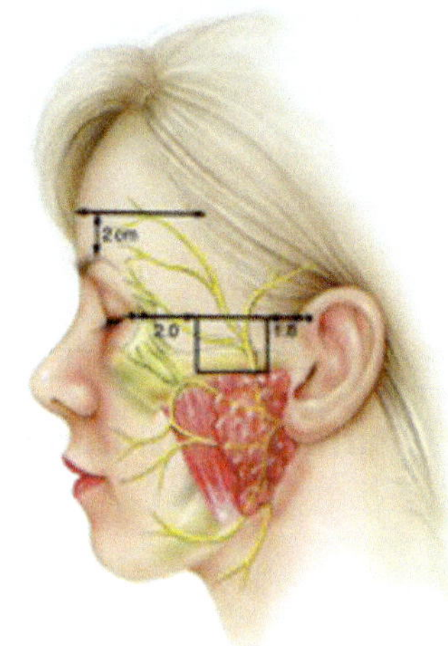

Fig. 49-2 Landmarks for identification of the frontal branches of the facial nerve. (Illustration reprinted from Azizzadeh et al.[5] with permission from Saunders, Philadelphia, PA, USA.)

The spinal accessory motor nerve (SAN), is 1 cm inferior to the GAN along the anterior border of the sternocleidomastoid muscle (SCM) and 1 cm superior to GAN along the posterior border of SCM.[4] The SAN has been described as being approximately 6.5 cm inferior to the external auditory canal. Anterior to the SCM, the SAN should not be encountered because of limited sub-platysma dissection below the angle of the mandible. However, in thin individuals the SAN can be seen in the posterior neck triangle, so it is important to keep the posterior neck dissection within the subcutaneous layer.

The facial nerve lies in the parenchyma of the parotid gland and the exits the gland remaining deep to the thin parotid-masseteric fascia. Its location in this fascial plane allows for the SMAS to be elevated without injuring the nerve. During a deep plane facelift, branches of the facial nerve can be seen beneath the thin fascia overlying the masseter muscle. It is of utmost importance not to violate this fascia, which could lead the nerve injury. The masseteric cutaneous ligaments run in a deep to superficial fashion, which is different from the facial nerve fibres that run parallel with contour of the face. Knowledge of this orientation allows the surgeon to dissect through the ligaments while preserving the nerves.

There are usually three to four branches of the frontal nerve that cross the zygomatic arch. The most posterior branch may lie 1.8 cm anterior to the external auditory canal and most anterior branch lies about 2 cm posterior to the bony lateral orbital rim (Figure 49-2). The frontal branches of the nerve remain in the temporoparietal fascia, which condenses over the periosteum of the zygomatic arch. The marginal mandibular branch is located deep to the platysma until approximately 2 cm lateral to the corner of the mouth where it becomes more superficial under the perioral musculature.[2,5]

Preoperative evaluation

Assessment

The surgeon must assess the patient's ability to endure aesthetic surgery both physically and psychologically. Any concerns about anxiety, depression, and body dysmorphic disorder should postpone the surgery until a specialist has performed proper psychological evaluation. The patient should be asked about what specifically concerns them about their facial appearance. The surgeon should listen to the goals and expectations of the patient to make sure that they are attainable before committing to the operation. Photographs from a patient's younger years may help set realistic goals about surgical outcomes. For example, many aging face patients do not like the appearance of their deep melolabial folds, but photographs may show that they had deep folds in their youth.

In the authors' experience, it is difficult to achieve significant and lasting improvement of the melolabial folds with facelift surgery alone. Even with a high SMAS incision above the zygomatic arch and superior vector suspension, the melolabial folds do not usually correct. Superior traction along the SMAS in a facelift or midface lift may actually accentuate the nasolabial folds.[3] Furthermore, subcutaneous dissection anteriomedially to melolabial folds does not create a long-lasting look. In our practice midface lifts have diminished, due to long-term postoperative oedema, chemosis, and failure to address the patient's concerns. We have been using autologous fat grafting and synthetic fillers with great success in augmenting the melolabial folds and have combined it with lower blepharoplasty to address midface concerns.

Skin must be assessed for sun damage (i.e. Glogau Scale), Fitzpatrick skin type, and cutaneous lesions. Patients who have had sun damage or exposure to tobacco may have thickened and discoloured facial skin. A facelift alone will not address sun damaged skin or deep perioral/periorbital rhytids which may require skin resurfacing (i.e. laser, chemical peel, dermabrasion). The patient's body habitus must be evaluated and questions must be ascertained about changes in weight. Submentoplasty and cervical liposuction may be necessary if the patient has excess subcutaneous fat. A history and physical must be taken about pre-existing hair loss, scarring, or keloids.

During facial analysis the surgeon should look for facial asymmetries and discuss them with the patients. Elderly patients with significant bone loss or patients with hypoplastic malar bones or chins may require alloplastic implants for better augmentation.[6]

Counselling and consent

Obtaining a detailed medical history and physical examination is critical to selecting appropriate facelift candidates and informing them of what to expect in all stages of the postoperative period. Patients, and their friends/family caring for them, should be made aware of postoperative oedema, ecchymosis, chemosis, signs of haematoma/infection, etc. Pain is generally not problematic after a facelift, and most patients do well with acetaminophen and a couple days worth of narcotic medications, if needed. Obtaining and reviewing a thorough medical history will reduce and prevent potential complications (see Complications section) such bleeding and poor wound healing (diabetes mellitus, tobacco use, alcohol intake, hypertension, previous radiation). Anticoagulants (aspirin, ibuprofen, vitamin E, etc.) should be discontinued for one week before and after surgery. Obtaining medical clearance from an internist or the patient's primary care provider is invaluable. Any concerns about the patient's history should be discussed with the anesthesiologist before the surgery.[5]

Informed consent should be a two-way conversation between the patient and surgeon in which the risks and benefits are clearly understood by the patient. Poor communication between the surgeon and patient can lead to anger, frustration, and litigation. Since cosmetic surgery is optional, the surgeon should decline to proceed with surgery if there are any significant reservations by the patient or surgeon. It is helpful for the patient to have a friend or family member present at the time of consent so that information is not overlooked and that all questions are answered. The patient can be provided with photographic examples of realistic expectations by the surgeon.[7] The surgeon should use examples of patients with similar features. Incision placement should be reviewed with the patients so that there are no surprises.

Photography

Standard pre- and postoperative photographs should be taken before and after facelift surgery. Preoperative photographs can be used to review features of the face that the patient may not appreciate on a daily basis, such as asymmetries, atypical hairlines, and skin irregularities. Often in the postoperative period, patients forget or have a misconception about how they appeared prior to surgery, and preoperative photographs are useful in reminding of their previous areas of concern. Standard photographic views for facelift patients include the frontal view (smiling and repose), bilateral obliques, and bilateral lateral views (in Frankfort horizontal plane and neck in flexion). Hair, jewellery, and clothing should not obstruct the view and the entire neck should be included.

Surgical technique

Anaesthesia and positioning

In our practices, facelifts are typically performed under general anesthesia; however the procedure may also be performed under conscious sedation with local anaesthetic. The patient is positioned in the supine position. After induction and administration of IV antibiotics (Cephalexin or Clindamycin), 1% lidocaine with 1:100,000 epinephrine is injected along the intended submental and peri-auricular incision lines with a 27-gauge needle. Then, a mixture of 0.5% lidocaine with 1:200,000 epinephrine is infiltrated broadly along the face and neck in the subcutaneous plane with a 22-gauge spinal needle. Ophthalmic ointment is applied to the eyes which are then taped shut with Tegaderm tape. The face and neck are prepped with Betadine and the patient is draped. The authors CSM suture the endotracheal tube to the anterior incisor to prevent extubation during manipulation of the head and neck.

Submentoplasty

An incision is made through the skin and subcutaneous fat in either the submental crease or slightly posterior to it (Figure 49-3). This positioning ensures that the scar will be hidden under the mandible. Blunt dissection is performed with scissors or alternatively with a 23 mm liposuction cannula in a subcutaneous plane. (Note: make sure that cannula opening faces away from the skin.) A stout pair of Mayo, Tressler–Dean, or Castenare scissors are used for direct dissection in the subcutaneous plane of the neck. If there is excess fat in the midline, it is excised under direct visualization (Figure 49-4). The anterior edges of the platysma are plicated with 4-0 polydiaxone or polypropylene sutures in an interrupted fashion (Figure 49-5).

Skin incisions

If the patient has a high hairline (above the root of the helix), an incision is made along the anterior margin of the temporal hair tuft in order to prevent further elevation of the temporal hairline (Figure 49-6).

(a) (b)

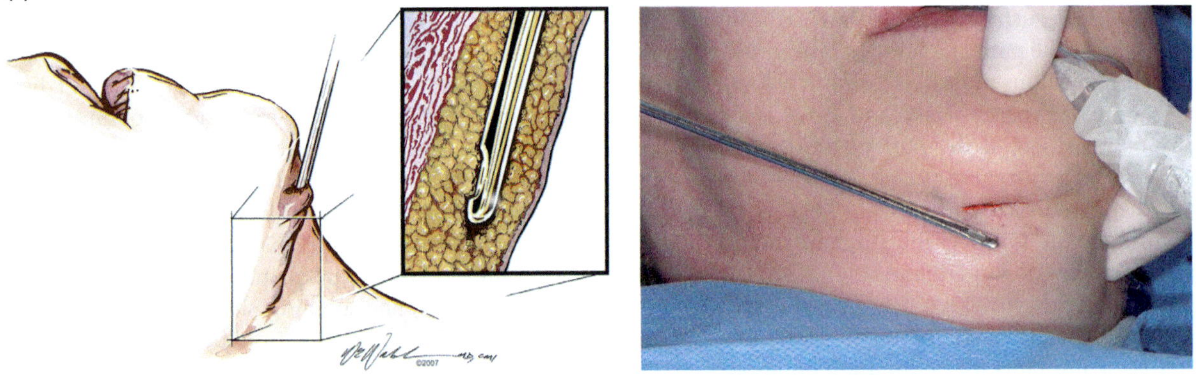

Fig. 49-3 Subcutaneous tunnels are made through the submental incision. The cannula opening should always face the platysma. (Illustration and photo are reprinted from Larrabee et al.[8] with permission form People's Medical Publishing House, Shelton, CT, USA.)

If the patient has a low hairline, an incision is made vertically in a coronal plane for 3 cm and curved slightly anteriorly. The incision is made with a 15-blade scalpel. Along the hairline, the scalpel is bevelled through the hair shafts in a trichophytic fashion that allows for growth of hair through the final scar. This helps to camouflage scars along the temporal hairline. Incisions within the temporal hair are made parallel to the hair shafts in order to avoid injury to follicles. The incision above the root of the helix is made within a pre-existing rhytid, but then transitions post-tragally just below the helical root. (Note: in men, a pre-tragal incision may be considered to avoid hair-bearing skin from being placed in the ear canal.) The incision curves around the lobule and then onto the conchal bowl. Post-auricularly the incision ascends along the conchal bowl to usually at the level of the concha cymba. At this height, it is less visible as it crosses the non-hairbearing post-auricular skin. The incision continues straight posteriorly for 1 to 2 cm into the hair before curving inferiorly for a few centimetres within the hair-bearing scalp overlying the mastoid.

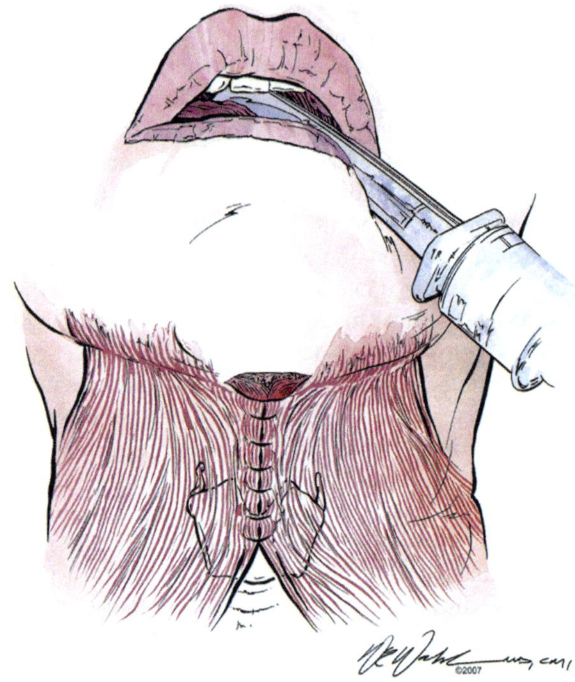

Fig. 49-5 Plication of the anterior edges of the platysma. (Illustration is courtesy of People's Medical Publishing House, Shelton, CT, USA.[8])

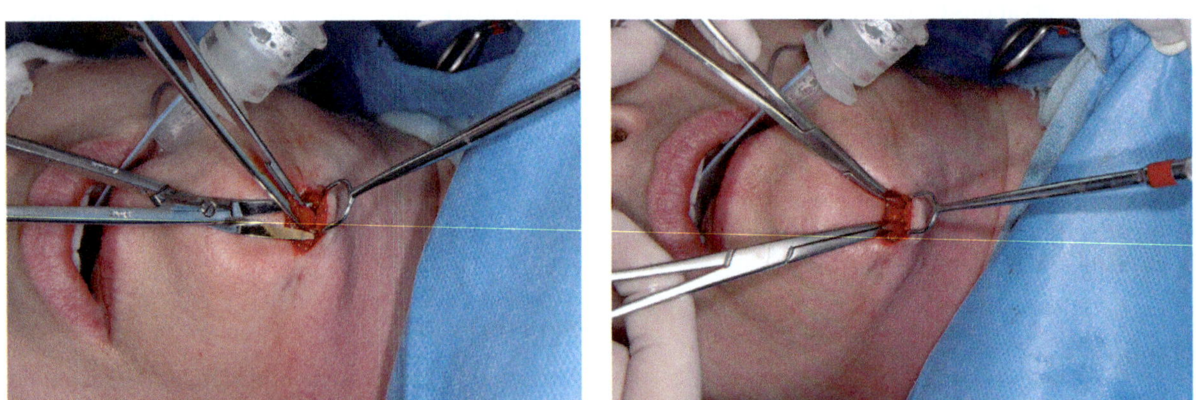

Fig. 49-4 (left) Midline fat excision through submental incision. (right) Identification of the anterior edges of the platysma muscle. (Photos are reprinted from Larrabee et al.[8] with permission form People's Medical Publishing House, Shelton, CT, USA.)

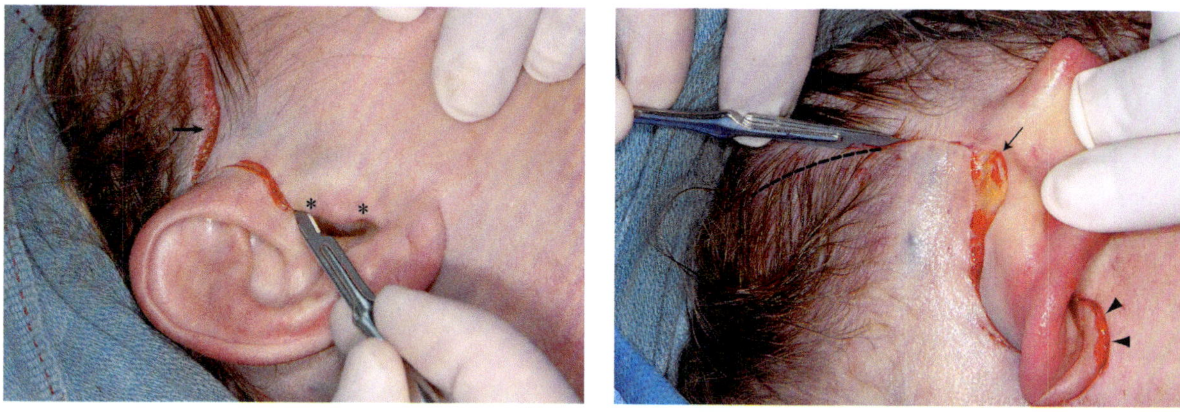

Fig. 49-6 (left) Pre-auricular incision. Asterisks mark where right angles should be made at the surperior and inferior borders of tragus when making a post-tragal incision. (right) Post-auricular incision. (Photos are courtesy of People's Medical Publishing House, Shelton, CT, USA.[8])

Skin flap elevation

Scissors and Adson Brown forceps are used to elevate the post-auricular and upper neck skin flap. The assistant should provide counter-traction on the skin during skin flap elevation to facilitate dissection. Overhead lights are aimed on to the flap to create trans-cutaneous illumination (Figure 49-7). The sub-lobule and neck skin flaps are elevated at a subcutaneous level with the scissors and skin hooks to the midlevel of the neck. The anterior limit of pre-auricular subcutaneous dissection is a line from malar eminence to the angle of the mandible. Subcutaneous dissection along the lower face extends from a line draw between the tragus and the menton. Skin flap elevation allows transection of the masseteric-cutaneous and zygomatic cutaneous retaining ligaments. Below the mandible the subcutaneous dissection connects with the previous subcutaneous submental dissection. At the level of the mandible the mandibular cutaneous ligaments are dissected. Care must be taken to stay superficial to the platysma to prevent injury to the marginal mandibular branch of the facial nerve.

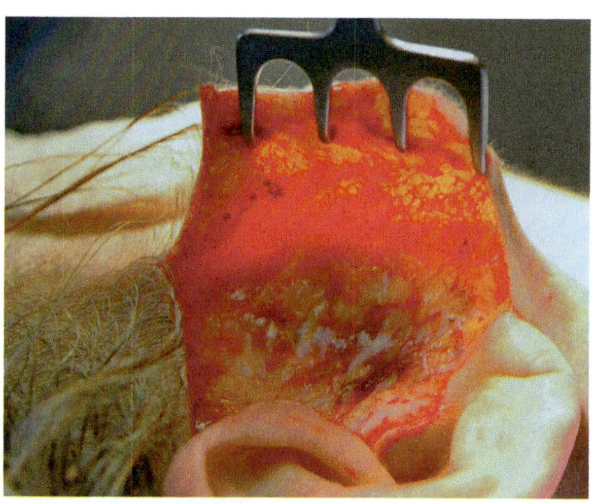

Fig. 49-7 Skin flap elevation with the assistance of trans-illumination. (Photos are courtesy of People's Medical Publishing House, Shelton, CT, USA.[8])

Superficial musculo-aponeurotic system (SMAS) flap

The inferior-lateral aspect of the malar eminence is palpated (represents the origin of the zygomatic major muscle) and then a line is marked from this point to a point 2 cm below the lobule which overlies the posterior margin of the platysma. A 15-blade scalpel is used to incise the SMAS and then a sub-SMAS flap is elevated with scissor dissection assisted with a lighted-retractor (Figure 49-8). The thin parotid-masseteric fascia should be preserved to avoid exposure of the parotid gland. Branches of the facial nerve can be seen through the fascia overlying the masseter muscle, thus the masseter muscle fibres themselves should never be dissected since this muscle lies beneath the level of the facial nerve. The majority of the sub-SMAS dissection is performed by spreading horizontally with scissor dissection, which creates multiple tunnels. The tunnels are then connected with careful transection of intervening fibres. Anterior to the parotid gland a spoon-billed elevator facilitates a safe

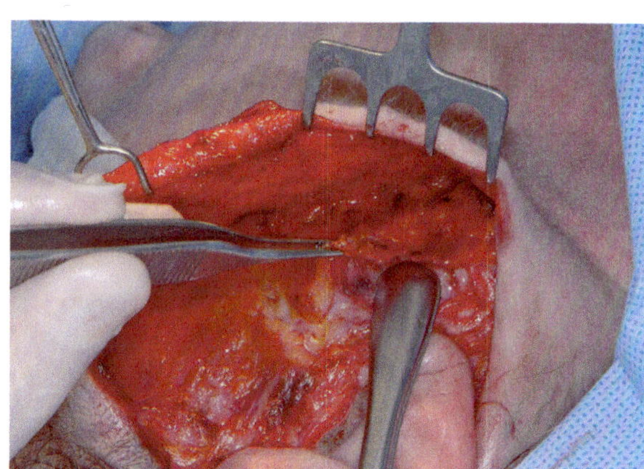

Fig. 49-8 SMAS Dissection. (Photos are courtesy of People's Medical Publishing House, Shelton, CT, USA.[8])

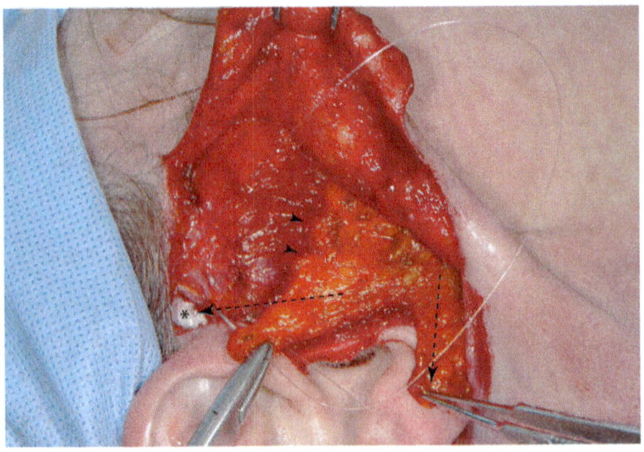

Fig. 49-9 Vectors of SMAS closure. Photo shows transposition of excess pre-auricular SMAS post-auricularly. (Photo is courtesy of People's Medical Publishing House, Shelton, CT, USA.[8])

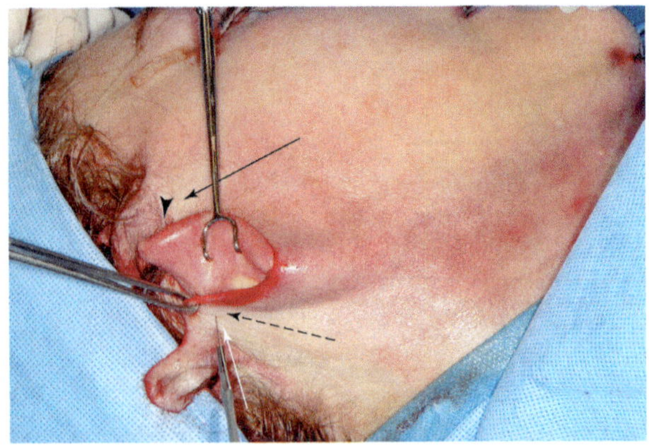

Fig. 49-10 Vectors for skin closure. (Photo is courtesy of People's Medical Publishing House, Shelton, CT, USA.[8])

dissection (Figure 49-8). The SMAS is elevated anteriorly until the zygomaticus major muscle is identified superiorly. Dissection is continued anteriorly releasing the SMAS from the zygomatic major. Inferiorly, sub-SMAS dissection continues anteriorly to the mandibular notch (where facial artery passes). It is critical to perform meticulous haemostasis with the bipolar to avoid facial nerve injury. The assistant should be examining the face for muscle twitches, which indicates a branch of the nerve is nearby.

SMAS draping

The SMAS is draped and then secured with a 3-0 polydioxanone suture to un-dissected, pre-auricular SMAS or the deep temporal fascia. The pre-auricular SMAS flap is draped in a more vertical, rather than posterior, vector (Figure 49-9). If there is excess SMAS it may be trimmed or incised to create a flap that can be transposed post-auricularly. Absorbable, barbed 4-0 V-Loc 90 (Covidien, Mansfield, MA) sutures are placed in a running fashion to further secure the flap and smooth out irregularities.

Skin redraping

Meticulous haemostasis must be achieved prior to closing the skin. The redraping process begins with cleaning off the skin with a moist sponge to ensure visualization of the surface and detection of irregularities. Allis clamps are used to grasp the edge of the skin flap and drape the pre-auricular temporal areas (Figure 49-10). The vector of the anterior flap is from the tragus to the Darwinian tubercle of the ear and the posterior flap is more vertical. Great care is taken to redrape and align the post-auricular hairline. None of the skin flaps should be under tension. At this point the skin flap, secured both pre-auricularly and post-auricularly, covers the lobule. Scissors are used to make a conservative incision along the antero-inferior direction through the skin flap overlying the lobule. Next, excess peri-auricular skin is conservatively trimmed (Figure 49-11).

Skin closure

Before the skin is closed, the contralateral face is injected with local anaesthetic to achieve haemostasis.

A few deep interrupted 5-0 polydiaxone sutures are placed to take the tension of the skin closure.

(a) (b)

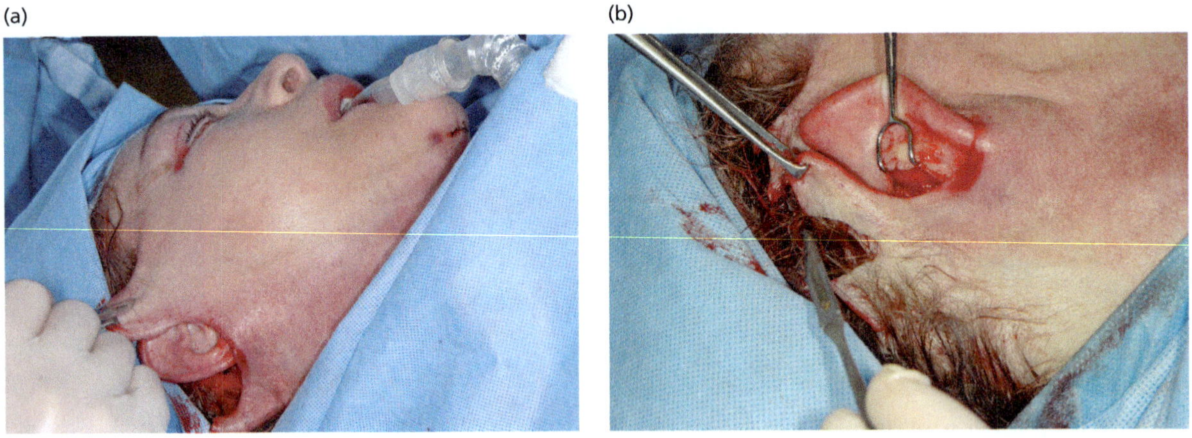

Fig. 49-11 Pre and Post-auricular skin trimming and redraping. (Photos are courtesy of People's Medical Publishing House, Shelton, CT, USA.[8])

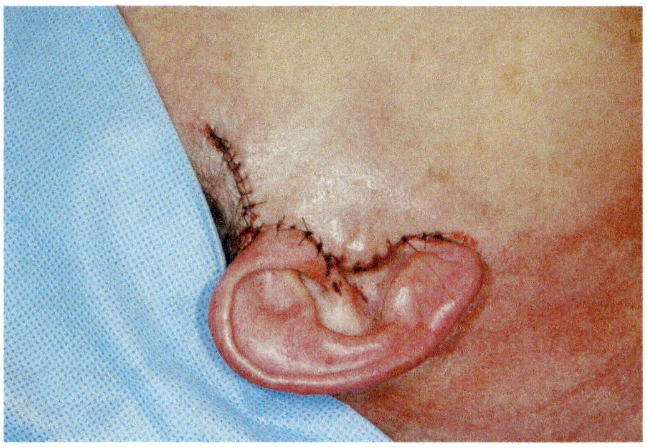

Fig. 49-12 Skin closure. (Photo is courtesy of People's Medical Publishing House, Shelton, CT, USA.[8])

A similar suture is placed along the anterior tragus to recreate the pre-tragal dimple. The temporal incision is closed with a 5-0 nylon suture in a running locking fashion and the pre-auricular incision is closed with 5-0 nylon simple interrupted sutures (Figure 49-12). The post-tragal incision is closed with 5-0 Fast Absorbing Gut simple interrupted sutures. The occipital hair-bearing incision is closed with staples and the post-auricular incision is closed with running 5-0 Vicryl Rapide sutures. The running stitch has three starting and ending points with gaps between them to allow drainage.

After the contralateral side facelift and closure are completed, the submental incision is closed with simple interrupted 5-0 nylon sutures.

Dressing

The face and hair are cleaned after smoothing out the skin and draining any excess blood via post-auricular incision gaps. Mupirocin ointment is applied to all incision lines and a dressing draped along the neck and face. A jaw-bra or Coban is used to compress the dressing, making sure there is even pressure over the face. It is important to include the post-auricular area which is the most common site for haematoma formation.

Postoperative care

The patient returns to clinic the day after surgery for evaluation and dressing change. Afterwards, they return one week later for suture removal, or earlier, if there are any concerns. Someone must escort the patient and observe them the night after surgery. Patients and their family or friends should be taught how to clean incision lines and apply ointment. Generally, the jaw-bra is not worn after the third postoperative day unless the patient chooses to do so for comfort. Patients may shower after the first dressing change, but must be careful not scrub directly over incisions and to only pat their face dry.[8]

Complications

Haematoma

Haematoma is the most common complication of facelift surgery, which occurs between 1 to 10% of patients, depending on the literature referenced.[10] Hypertension, strenuous activity, male gender, and anticoagulant medication predisposes patients to postoperative haematoma formation. Haematomas usually present in the first 24 hours, but can occur up to 2 weeks postoperatively. Patients may present with facial oedema, ecchymosis, pain, and difficulty speaking. Larger haematomas may directly compress the trachea, therefore immediate neck decompression is critical and should not be delayed. The patient may require securement of the airway via intubation. These patients should be taken to the operating room for surgical exploration, haemostasis, and drain placement. (Note: hash marks across the incision prior to suture removal will help in closure of the incision post-evacuation.) In cases of small haematomas, the surgeon can attempt manual decompression after limited suture removal or needle aspiration. Needle aspiration is typically unsuccessful until the haematoma liquefies. Needle aspiration is more successful for treatment of seromas. Patients should be seen daily after haematoma evacuation to evaluate for recurrence. Patients who developed haematomas will generally still have a good aesthetic result if they are properly managed, but will have a longer recovery due to prolonged oedema and ecchymosis.

Scarring/flap necrosis

Fibrosis or hypertrophy may be noticed along the incision, typically a few months after surgery. Scarring can be treatment with steroid injections, massage and sun precautions. It may require excision if there is no improvement after 6 months and they are not felt to be predisposed to keloid formation. Skin flap necrosis is rare due to the excellent blood supply in the head and neck region. Care should be taken when raising subcutaneous flaps to avoid buttonholes or excessive thinning of the flap, especially in patients at risk of poor wound healing (e.g. diabetics, smokers, etc). The most common area for skin flap loss is in the post-auricular region. If this occurs and the area is small, the patient should be reassured that the areas of loss usually heals well over time. Ointment should be applied frequently to these areas to keep them moist. After the area of necrosis has appeared, this area should conservatively debrided.

Alopecia

Hair loss after a facelift can cause emotional distress. Hair loss can result from direct trauma to hair follicles with cautery or scissors or from excessive tension. Hair regrowth typically returns 6 to 12 months after surgery. If the hair fails to grow, microfollicular hair grafts may be considered.[7]

Facial nerve injury

It is not uncommon to notice mild temporary weakness immediately after surgery due to the local anaesthetics. The most common permanently injured motor nerves are the frontal and marginal mandibular nerves. Although there are no data, the buccal branch is most likely the most common injured nerve, but it does not produce symptoms because of its multiple redundant branches. If more than 50% of the nerve's diameter is transected, the epineurium should be re-anastamosed with 2 to 3 simple interrupted 8-0 nylon sutures.

Loss of sensation

The most commonly injured nerve is the greater auricular nerve. The nerve should be re-anastamosed with 2 to 3 simple interrupted 8-0 nylon sutures through the epineurium. It is common for patients to experience temporary facial sensation loss around the incision, which generally improves in 1–6 months. The return of sensation usually occurs gradually in an anterior to posterior fashion. Patients should be warned not to apply hot objects (i.e. heat pads) to their face because they may they may not sense the thermal damage which is taking place to the skin.

Parotid injury

A postoperative sialocoele or fistula after facelift is rare which should not occur if the sub-SMAS dissection did not violate the parotid-masseteric fascia. If injury to the gland does occur intraoperatively, the surgeon must cover all areas of exposed parotid gland with the SMAS flap. Postoperative sialocoeles are successfully managed conservatively with aspiration and pressure dressings. Intra-parotid botulinum toxin type A injections or anticholinergic medications (i.e. glycopyrolate) can be considered in recalcitrant cases. The patient may require surgery to explore the fistula/sialocoele and excise it.[10]

Infection

The incidence of perioperative infection following facelift surgery is less than 1%, likely from the rich vascular supply of the face and neck. Risks of infections are increased in patients at higher risk for poor wound healing (smokers, diabetics, immune-compromised). Un-evacuated haematomas also increase the risk of infection. Patients must be taught about the signs and symptoms including pain, swelling, tenderness, fever, and erythema. Perioperative antibiotics often prevent infection, but once it is identified antibiotics should resume. Any infected tissue should be cultured and conservatively debrided. Abscesses should be managed with incision and drainage and systemic antibiotics should be considered. Infectious disease consultant may be helpful if there is progressive infection.[7]

Submental deformities

Cobra deformity is a complication of over-aggressive liposuction or direct lipectomy in the submentum. It may also result from inadequate plication of the anterior edges of the platysma muscle. Lateral standing cone deformities may occur if the submental incision was improperly position or designed or when too much submental skin is excised. The deformities may be revised surgically but care should be taken to chase the cone too far laterally, which will leave scar.[11]

Ear deformity

Ear lobe deformities (pixie ear) can be result from a poor incision placement, malpositioning of the lobule during closure, or tension on the skin closure. Correction may require V to Y advancement flaps with placement of the tension on the deeper tissue layers rather than the skin.[12]

References

1 Alghoul M, Codner MA. Retaining ligaments of the face: review of anatomy and clinical applications. Aesthetic Surg J. 2013;33:769–82.
2 Owsley JQ, Agarwal CA. Safely navigating around the facial nerve in three dimensions. Clin Plast Surg. 2008;35:469–77.
3 Gassner HG, Rafii A, Young A, Murakami C, Moe KS, Larrabee WF Jr. Surgical anatomy of the face: implications for modern face-lift techniques. Arch Facial Plast Surg. 2008;10:9–19.
4 Baring DEC, Johnston A, O'Reilly BF. Identification of the accessory nerve by its relationship to the great auricular nerve. J Laryngol Otol. 2007;121:892–4.
5 Honrado CP, Bradley DT, Larrabee WF Jr. Facial Embryology and Anatomy. In: Azizzadeh B, Murphy MR, Johnson CM (Eds). Master techniques in facial rejuvenation. Philadelphia, PA: Saunders/Elsevier, 2007:17–32.
6 Shaw RB Jr, Katzel EB, Koltz PF, et al. Aging of the facial skeleton: aesthetic implications and rejuvenation strategies. Plast Reconstr Surg. 2011;127:374–83.
7 Sykes JM, Kim J-E, Papel ID. In: Capone RB, Sykes JM (Eds). Complications in Facial Plastic Surgery Prevention and Management. New York: Thieme, 2012.
8 Larrabee WF, Gassner HG, Walsh WE. Face Lift. In: Larrabee WF, Gassner HG, Walsh WE (Eds).Art and Craft of Facial Rejuvenation Surgery. PMPH-USA, 2013:1–15.
9 Larrabee WF, Gassner HG, Walsh WE. Art and Craft of Facial Rejuvenation Surgery. PMPH-USA, 2013.
10 Baker SR. Rhytidectomy. In: Flint PW, Haughey BH, Niparko JK, et al. (Eds). Cummings Otolaryngology – Head and Neck Surgery. Elsevier Health Sciences, 2010:405–27.
11 Perkins S, Dayan S. Rhytidectomy. In: Papel ID (Ed.) Facial Plastic and Reconstructive Surgery. Thieme, 2011:153–70.
12 Murakami C, Ambro BT. Rejuvenation of the Lower Face and Neck. In: Snow JB, Wackym PA, Ballenger JJ (Eds). Ballenger's Otorhinolaryngology: Head and Neck Surgery. PMPH-USA, 2009:749–57.
13 DeFatta RJ, Williams EF 3rd. Evolution of midface rejuvenation. Arch Facial Plast Surg. 2009;11:6–12.

Chapter 50

Soft Tissue Resuspension

Alistair R.M. Cobb and Jonathan A. Britto

Introduction

The resuspension of the craniofacial soft tissue envelope may be used to help reduce the ptosis of the soft tissues that may result following the subperiosteal surgical degloving used to access the facial skeleton. This may be required after orthognathic surgery, trauma, reconstructive, aesthetic, oculoplastic or craniofacial surgical procedures.

Surgical fixation following midfacial procedures using devices such as the Endotine hook have proved very useful for some surgeons.[1] The use of a hypodermic needle as a transport shuttle for suture insertion is an alternative technique and obviates the need for alloplastic fixation and its attendant potential morbidity. The technique is a reasonably straight forward procedure and offers a more bespoke and accurate repositioning of the facial soft tissues. Facial shape and volume can also be modified by surgical adjustment of the position and depth of soft tissue fixation, and the extent of midface degloving from the maxilla. The technique is useful in the closing stages of midface and craniofacial surgery, after skeletal fixation has been achieved (when required) and the soft tissue envelope has been liberated subperiosteally.

Surgical technique

A 16/18 gauge hypodermic needle is passed transcutaneously through a selected point in the midface to the subperiosteal plane which has been exposed by any or a combination of transblepharoplasty, transconjunctival, temporal, coronal, and upper sublabial approaches. Typically, in a patient undergoing a Le Fort I level procedure, the vector for resuspension required will be superolateral pull – so a temporal approach will be used. The point of entry of the needle, which functions as a transport shuttle for the suture, acts together with the extent of the subperiosteal degloving to determine the volumetric shape change of the face when lifted.

The points of transcutaneous needle entry may initially be determined in a strict manner; however, with experience a more bespoke approach may be adopted to achieve the optimum vectors of pull for the individual. Care must be taken not to trap the direct course of the infraorbital nerve, extrinsic lip elevator muscles or zygomaticus major. Initial landmarks for the entry points of the hypodermic needle are described as follows. There are two points on each side: (1) the bisecting point of a line dropped vertically from the lateral canthus and a horizontal line from the superior aspect of the nasal alar crease; and (2) the bisection of a mid-pupillary vertical line in neutral gaze to a horizontal line at the level of the inferior aspect of the alar base (Figure 50-1). However, these points are modified according to the clinical indication and desired vector of movement. Where bilateral surgery is undertaken, symmetry of technique is important to the symmetry of the final result. The 'target' fat pads of the face for volume resuspension are the malar fat and the suborbicularis oculi fat pad (SOOF).

The needle 'transport shuttle' passes transcutaneously (Figure 50-2) to subperiosteally and receives the reverse unmounted end of a colourless 3/0 PDS® (polydioxanone) suture (Figure 50-3), which is passed out to the barrel of the needle. This is then withdrawn to just short of the dermis and passed back to the

Orthognathic Surgery: Principles, Planning and Practice. Edited by Farhad B. Naini and Daljit S. Gill.

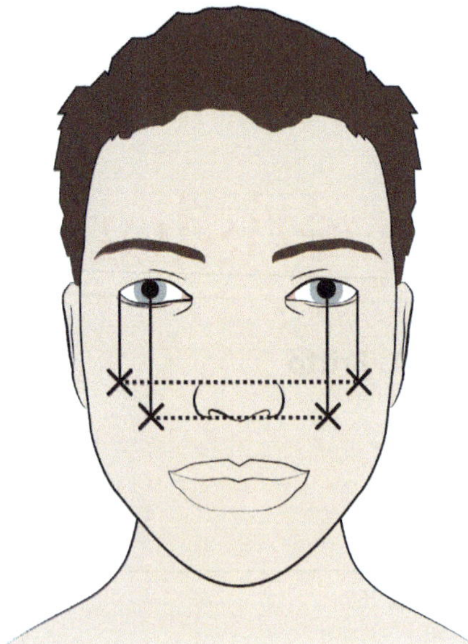

Fig. 50-1 Anatomical landmarks.

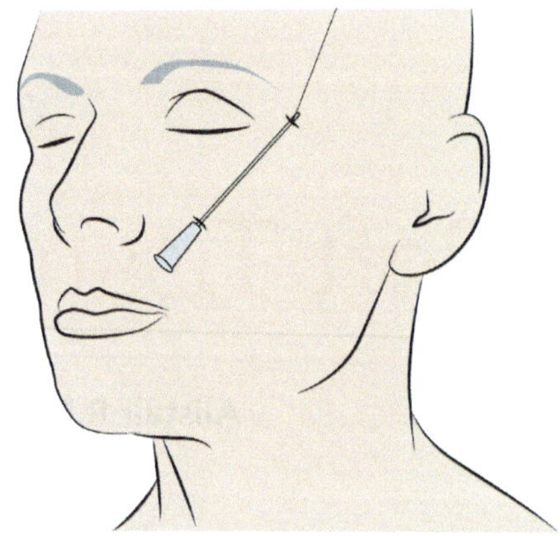

Fig. 50-3 The suture is fed into the hypodermic needle lumen and advanced until sufficiently through the other end of the hypodermic needle to allow it to be held securely.

subperiosteal plane with a different trajectory (Figures 50-4 and 50-5). The act of pulling the PDS® suture loop back into the subperiosteal plane results in a 'bite' of the soft tissue, which can be elevated on the suture for vertical fixation (Figure 50-6). The more superficial the 'bite', the greater is the likelihood of skin dimpling. It is important to avoid entering the dermis as a soft tissue dimple will result when the suture is tied. However, if the path of the suture lies too deep, then

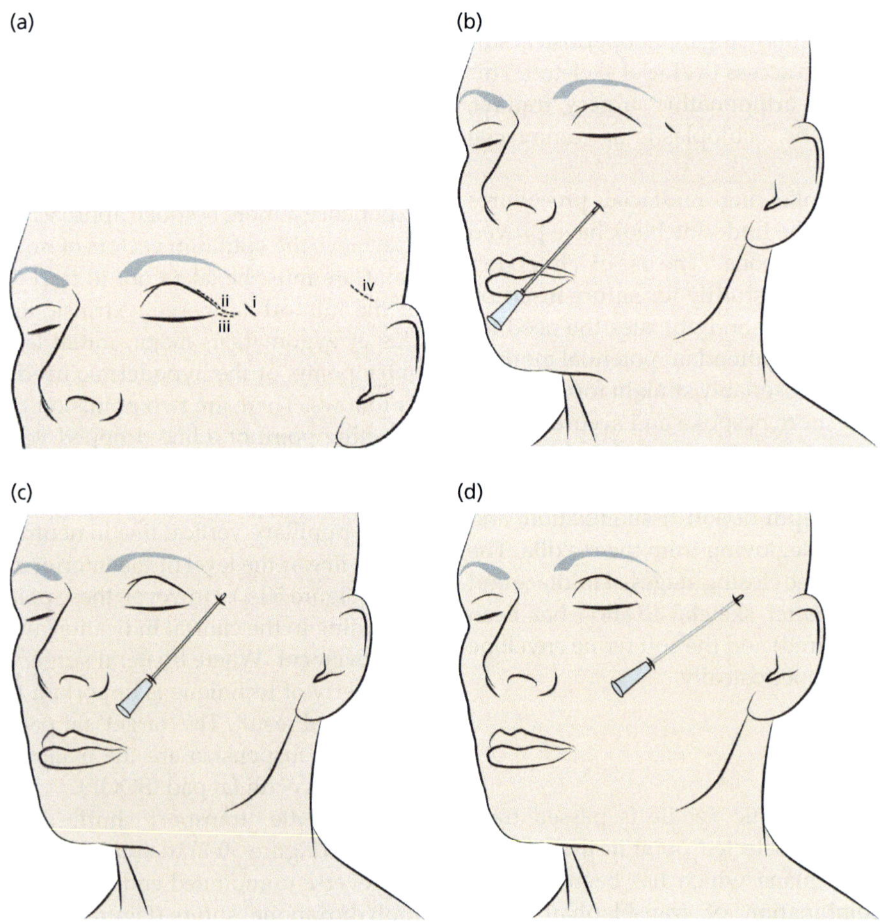

Fig. 50-2 (a)Potential fixation sites (i) lateral upper blepharoplasty incision (ii) lateral canthal incision (iii) to access the fronto-zygomatic perisoteum, or an incision in the temporal hair bearing skin (iv), the target tissue to anchor the suture to being the superficial lamina of the deep temporal fascia. (b) The needle is inserted at each of the four anatomically landmarked points in turn. Each time, the hypodermic needle is advanced superficially, subdermally. (c) Where the suture finally emerges, a small incision is made in the skin through which the hypodermic needle is passed to permit tying to the underlying anchoring tissue. (d) The temporal hair bearing skin exit point being used.

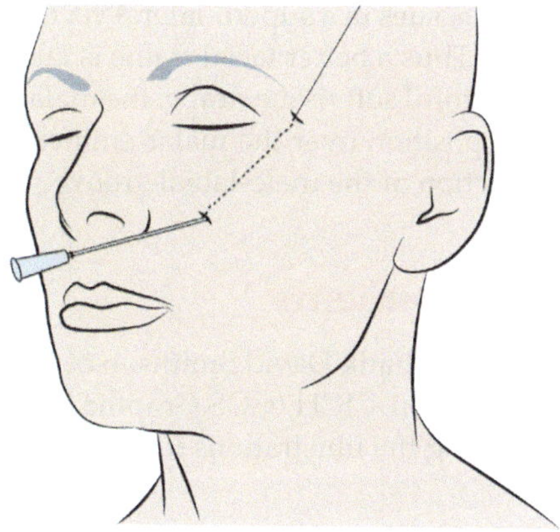

Fig. 50-4 Then the needle is withdrawn to a position below the cutis (to avoid skin puckering) before changing the orientation of the hypodermic needle to a deeper inclination; the tissue captured is usually the SOOF and/or the malar fat.

not enough volume of tissue will be captured in the 'bite' and the resuspension will not be as effective. The trajectory and volume of the soft tissue 'bite' matter greatly to the shape and elevation of the soft tissue envelope and this is particularly important in bilateral surgery. Similarly the extent of midfacial degloving and soft tissue release matters to the shape, elevation and symmetry of the result. Volume augmentation of the face results from the elevation and repositioning of the malar fat and SOOF. The suture will only hold the resuspension until it dissolves and the long-term result depends upon the re-adhesion of the midface to bone in a subperiosteal plane.

The technique of fixation of the PDS® suture depends upon the indications for use and the degree of access that has been achieved for the overall surgical procedure. Where there is wide craniofacial access via a coronal approach, the PDS® suture may be passed through a drill hole in the fronto-zygomatic process or any desired proximal fixation point; whereas for trans-blepharoplasty aesthetic surgery a proximal fixation 'bite' may be taken in the SOOF or arcus periosteum,

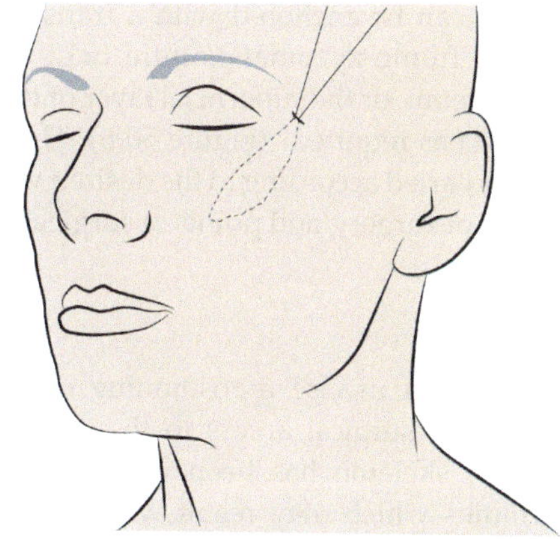

Fig. 50-5 The hypodermic needle is advanced to pick up the deeper soft tissues and then up to re-emerge from the temporal incision where the suture can be recovered and the hypodermic needle removed. The suture is then tightened to effect the appropriate degree of mid face lift, moving the tissues in a posterosuperior vector over the malar region. The suture may then be tied to the underlying fascia.

exposed via a subciliary transpalpebral approach. It is worth noting here that the lateral SOOF may be elevated subperiosteally and fixed more proximally for some indications, or may itself be the point of proximal fixation of a more distal soft tissue 'bite' in the nasolabial fold, for example to increase malar eminence. Furthermore, in a Le Fort I type osteotomy, where the wide access is via the maxillary vestibular incision (upper labio-buccal sulcus approach), the proximal fixation can be achieved via a small incision in the lower temporal hair bearing skin or at the lateral canthal creases, to allow passage of the needle and access to the underlying tissues for transosseous or deep soft tissue fixation (Figure 50-3).

Often only a single suture fixation will be required on each side, up to a total of four (two each side). All four sutures are placed in this way, following which the four vectors of pull can be checked and the tension adjusted relative to each other, to ensure the correct overall movements are achieved.

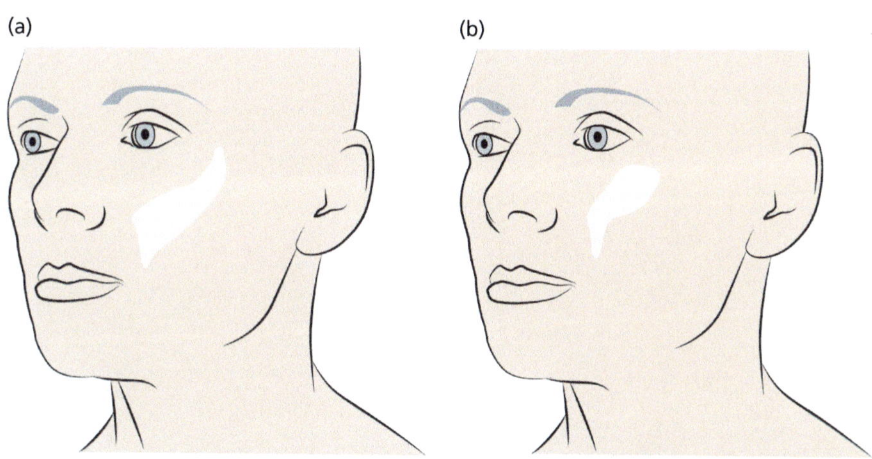

Fig. 50-6 In aesthetic applications the facial soft tissue volume lift enhances the malar definition which can be seen in a change in the pattern of the light reflected on the malar skin and an improved lid cheek harmony, blending the interface between the two. In this case a blepharoplasty incision approach has been utilized. (a) Before procedure; (b) after procedure.

The sutures can be anchored with a trans-osseous drill hole in the fronto-zygomatic suture, or by taking a 'bite' of periosteum, or the superficial layer of the deep temporal fascia as required[2] (Figure 50-6). The proximal fixation is varied according to the desired vector of lift, the nature of surgery, and points of surgical access.

Discussion

The importance of precise repositioning of the soft tissues following surgical access to the upper craniomaxillofacial skeleton has been well-described.[3–5] The deformities which may result when this is not undertaken include midface ptosis, soft tissue hollowing, malar arch protrusion, malar eminence underprojection, lower eyelid malposition or increased melolabial creasing.[3]

Surgical degloving of the tissues in the subperiosteal plane to access the facial bones liberates the tissues, which will descend down the facial skeleton unless resuspended. Initially the focus of the approach was to re-establish the premorbid position of the tissues. However, with greater understanding of the effects that can be achieved, the indications have expanded to include more aesthetic changes achievable by improving the initial facial form. Following orthognathic procedures at the le Fort I level to improve the midfacial projection, one may now consider repositioning the midfacial soft tissues in a supero-lateral vector, akin to a midface lift. Thus a better facial frame is augmented by a more youthful soft tissue drape: the malar fat pad restored in a position over the malar eminence and a marked reduction of the melo-labial groove.

Acknowledgements

We would like to thank David Smithson of UCL AISC Medical Illustration – ICH/GOS Graphic Design Studio for providing the illustrations used in this paper.

References

1 Accioli de Vasconcellos JJ, Britto JA, Henin D, Vacher C. The fascial planes of the temple and face: an en-bloc anatomical study and a plea for consistency. Br J Plast Surg. 2003;56:623–9.
2 Frodel JL Jr, Rudderman R. Facial soft tissue resuspension following upper facial skeletal reconstruction. J Craniomaxillofac Trauma. 1996;2:24–30.
3 Phillips JH, Gruss JS, Wells MD, Chollet A. Periosteal suspension of the lower eyelid and cheek following subciliary exposure of facial fractures. Plast Reconstr Surg. 1991;88:145.
4 Saltz R. Endoscopic temporal-incision only midface lift is enhanced by Endotine technique. Aesthetic Surg J. 2005;25:80–83.
5 Yaremchuk MJ, Kim WK. Soft-tissue alterations associated with acute, extended open reduction and internal fixation of orbital fractures. J Craniofac Surg. 1992;3:134.

Chapter 51

Soft Tissue Augmentation and Fat Grafting

Mehmet Manisali and Rahul Jayaram

Introduction

The objective of planning orthognathic surgery is to alter the facial bony foundation to achieve an aesthetic and functional dental and skeletal relationship. Contours, at times, are not transferred through the overlying soft tissue envelope. There is hence a need to explore techniques that independently control the volume and shape of the facial soft tissues.

There are four broad areas where facial soft tissue augmentation can be considered.

1. When soft tissue is lacking as part of the underlying pathology (e.g. Parry–Romberg syndrome).
2. Irregularities of overlying soft tissue contour following orthognathic surgery (e.g. mandibular lower border irregularities).
3. Camouflage of an essentially bony abnormality.
4. Comprehensive management of soft tissue changes associated with aging in the orthognathic patient.

The workhorse of facial soft tissue augmentation is autologous fat grafting and there are many variations to the theme. Other techniques may play a minor role. Dermis fat graft historically precedes micro fat grafting techniques, and has fallen out of favour due to scars at donor and recipient sites, as well as dimensional instability. Fascia harvested from temporalis muscle for example, is by contrast dimensionally stable, but available only in small quantities and therefore only suitable for augmentation of small areas, such as the nose and the lip. Synthetic injectable fillers have been used widely, but problems such as tissue reaction have been common. Onlay synthetic implants made of silicone and polyetheretherketone (PEEK) applied onto the underlying bony skeletal surface also indirectly bulk out the soft tissues. These can be used solely or in combination with fat grafting and orthognathic surgery where appropriate (Figures 51-1 and 51-2). Finally, use of vascularized free tissue transfer techniques have a role in the reconstruction of areas of major soft tissue deficiency.

Fat grafting

Autologous fat in many ways represents an ideal soft tissue filler: it is biocompatible, non-teratogenic and non-carcinogenic. This is inexpensive, readily available in sufficient quantities and easily acquired and repeated when needed. Although generally durable, the long-term results can be variable and at times unpredictable. Fat grafting has become increasingly popular in aesthetic and reconstructive surgery both as a primary procedure and as an adjunct.

Neuber in 1893 was the first to transplant fat from the arm to the face.[1] Two years later Czerny

Orthognathic Surgery: Principles, Planning and Practice. Edited by Farhad B. Naini and Daljit S. Gill.

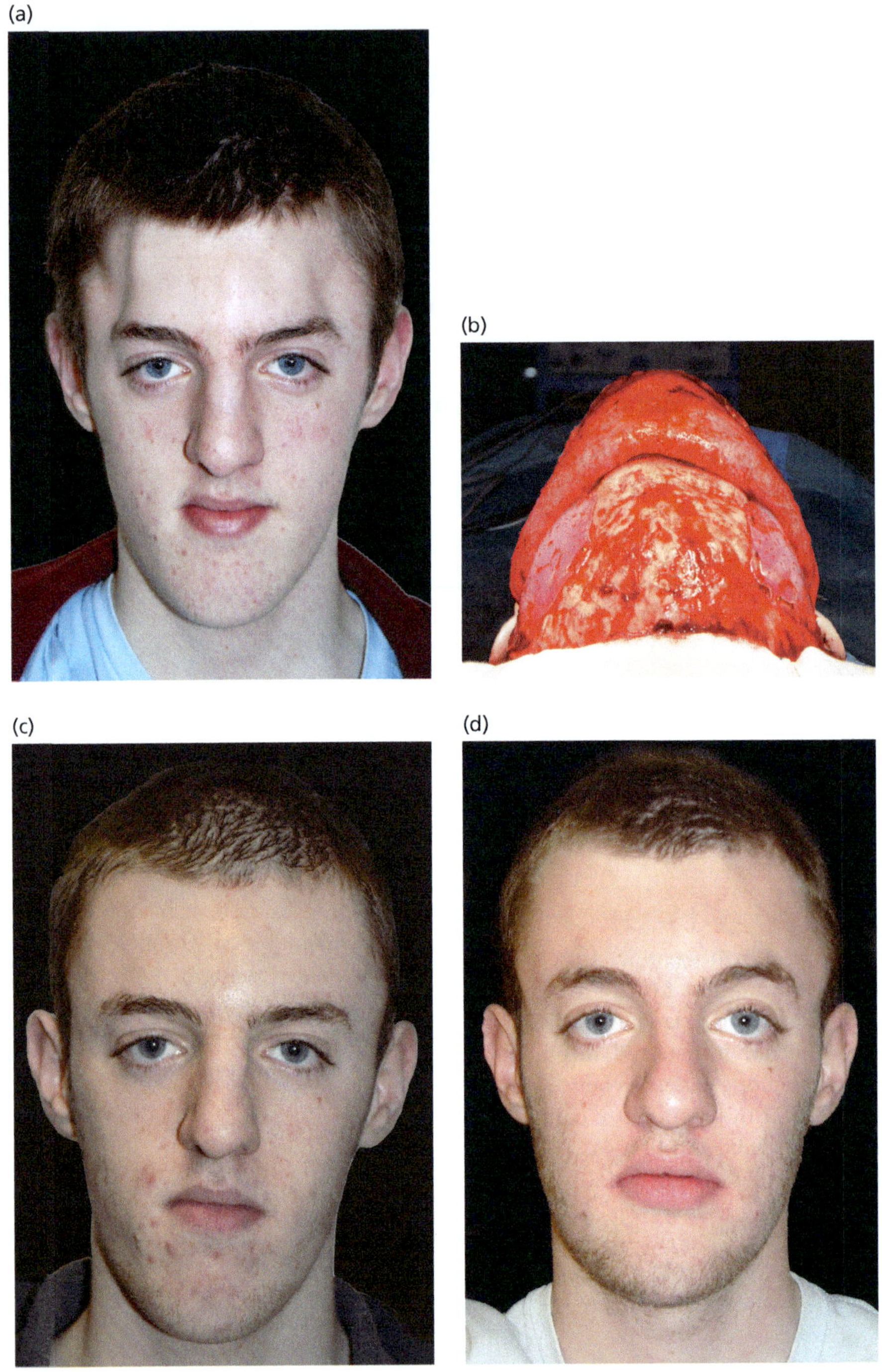

Fig. 51-1 Craniofacial abnormality in a previously treated case of trigonocephaly. Temple hollowing is noted as well as an increased face height (a). Temple hollowing treated with custom made silicone implants (b, c). Patient subsequently underwent bimaxillary osteotomy to correct the increased facial height, and rhinoplasty (d).

transplanted a lipoma from the back to a breast for augmentation.[2] In 1912 Eugene Hollander from Berlin, published two cases of lipo-atrophy treated with the infiltration of fat.[3] In 1926 Charles Conrad Miller, wrote about 36 cases of cicatricial contractures on the face and neck treated with fat injections, and reported moderate shrinkage of the fat.[4] Interestingly this technique never became widely used. This technique was re-visited in the 1980s with the increasing popularity of liposuction and Illouz's early publications described great results.[5] However, the popularity of the technique vastly increased after Coleman's publication in 1994 and maintains the pole position amongst soft tissue augmentation techniques today.[6] His technique combines the harvesting of fat with centrifuge separation prior to placement for more stable results.[7]

Biology of fat grafting

Fat develops during the fourth month in utero. Adipocytes have thin and fragile cell membranes with varying amounts of lipid. These cells are contained in a matrix of connective tissue composed of collagen and

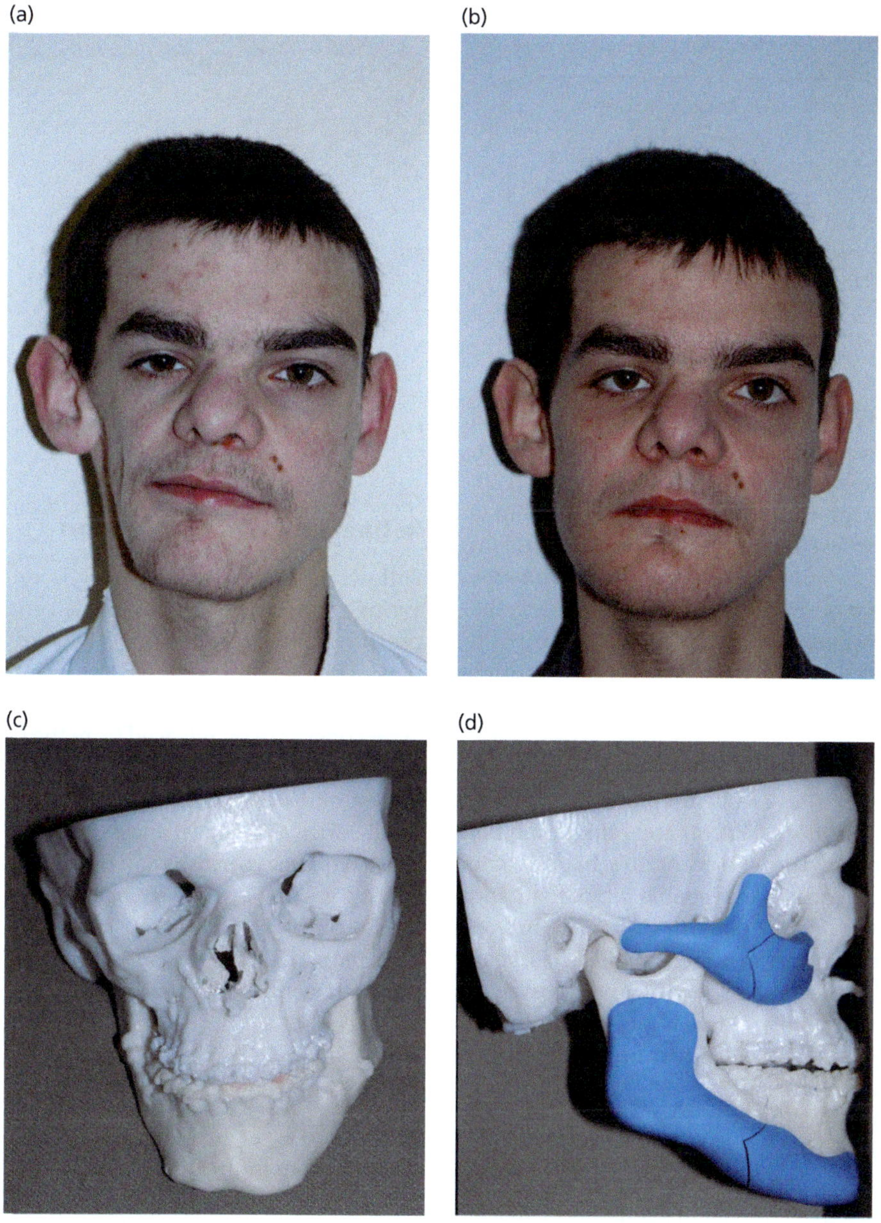

Fig. 51-2 Combination of orthognathic surgery, custom-made onlay implants and fat grafting, in correction of complex skeletal and soft tissue deformity in hemifacial atrophy.

elastic fibres, stromal cells and neurovascular structures. Each unilocular conglomeration of fat cells has its own small vascular pedicle and is supported and surrounded by the connective tissue matrix.[8] This stromal vascular fraction of the fat tissue also has adipose derived stem cells (ADSC), endothelial cells, smooth muscle cells and associated progenitor cell lines and other multipotent stem cells. Zuk et al. were the first to clearly describe the presence of stem cells in fat grafts.[9] These ADSCs have the ability to differentiate into ectodermal, mesodermal and endodermal cell lines. Early research indicates the possible role of these undifferentiated cells to induce angiogenesis, reduce fibrosis, promote wound healing and contribute to the therapeutic potential of the fat graft.[10]

Adipose derived stem cells may also be responsible for other benefits observed with fat injection. Coleman reported that fat grafted under depressed scars, not only relieved the depression, but also seemed to soften or completely eliminate the scars, making it look like normal skin. Fat grafting is also reported for the treatment of radiation damage, damaged vocal cords and even the regrowth of calvarial bone.[10] Sultan et al. have shown the attenuation of inflammation and slowing of fibrosis associated with radiodermatitis in a murine model.[11]

Preadipocytes, compared to mature fat cells are more resilient and have lower oxygen and nutritional demands once grafted.[12,13] The only survivors of fat transplantation might be preadipocytes and adipose-derived stem cells. The relative proportions of mature fat cells, preadipocytes and adipose derived stem cells and the variable survival of preadipocytes and ADSCs between individuals may be some of the reasons for the observed differences in survival of fat grafts.[10]

Table 51-1 Equipment (Coleman technique)

1.	No. 15 and No. 11 blade surgical scalpels
2.	Lamis infiltration cannula
3.	Harvesting and infiltration cannula
4.	Centrifuge
5.	10 mL and 1ml Luer–Lok syringes
6.	Local anaesthetic

Surgical technique

The Coleman technique of structural fat grafting has generally remained unchanged since its introduction and has stood the test of time (Tables 51-1 and 51-2). The procedure involves gentle harvesting to minimize damage of the harvest. Refinement of the harvested fat with centrifugation removes non-viable components. Careful placement of small aliquots of fat increase the surface area and available vascular supply to the fat grafts.[6,7,14]

Harvesting

A variety of harvest sites can be used and include the abdomen, flanks, buttocks, sacral area, thigh, medial knee and the neck. The choice of the harvest site depends on the adequacy of available fat, patient and surgeon preference. No conclusive difference in viability of fat harvested form different sites has been demonstrated. Rohrich et al. showed no difference in the adipose tissue viability at five hours after harvest, from various body donor sites including abdomen, flank, thigh, and medial knee.[15]

The authors most commonly harvest fat from the abdomen and medial thighs. A thorough skin preparation of both the donor and recipient sites is carried out with an iodine based or equivalent agent. Local anaesthetic or tumescent solution is injected with a blunt Lamis infiltrator in all four quadrants of the anterior abdominal wall, through a 3 mm stab incision in the inferior aspect of the umbilicus. Through this a harvesting cannula attached to a 10 mL Luer–Lok syringe is introduced (Figure 51-3). The plunger on the syringe is pulled back to create a gentle negative pressure and the harvesting cannula is moved in the deep layer of subcutaneous adipose tissue in a tunnelling and reaming fashion. When filled with fat the syringe is disconnected from the cannula and capped with a Luer–Lok plug. This process is repeated until adequate fat has been harvested.

Table 51-2 Steps in fat grafting

1.	Patient preparation and anaesthesia
2.	Fat harvest
3.	Refinement and preparation
4.	Fat placement
5.	Postoperative care

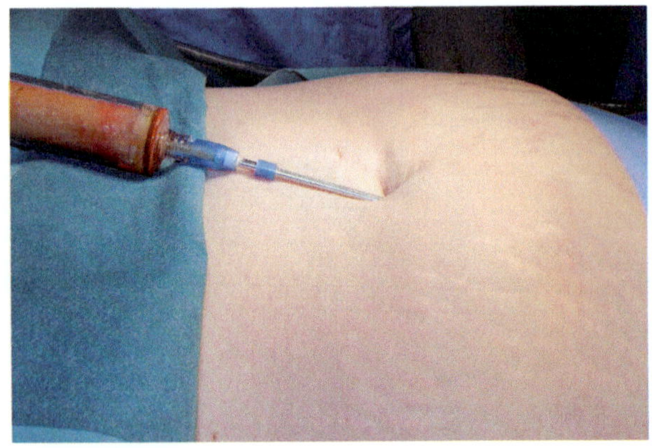

Fig. 51-3 Fat harvest from the anterior abdominal wall.

Refinement and preparation

Following harvest the plunger is removed, and the syringes are placed into a sterile centrifuge tray. The centrifugation is carried out at 3000 rpm for three minutes. This separates the aspirate into three component layers according to their density. The supernatant layer consists of oil released from the ruptured fat cells. The middle portion consists of viable fat parcels. The lowest and densest layer is blood and aqueous elements, such as the local anaesthetic and tissue fluid. At the end of the centrifugation process the oil is decanted off and wicked away with absorbent neuro pads. The Luer–Lok plug is removed to release the denser liquid layer. The plunger is replaced and the refined fat is transferred into 1 mL syringes ready for placement (Figure 51-4).

Placement

The Coleman infiltration cannulas are smaller and are available in different length, diameter and tip characterization. The tips can be blunt, semi-blunt or sharp (V-shaped dissector). A 17-gauge cannula is the most useful for fat placement in the face. The use of blunt cannulas allow placement of the fat parcels in a more

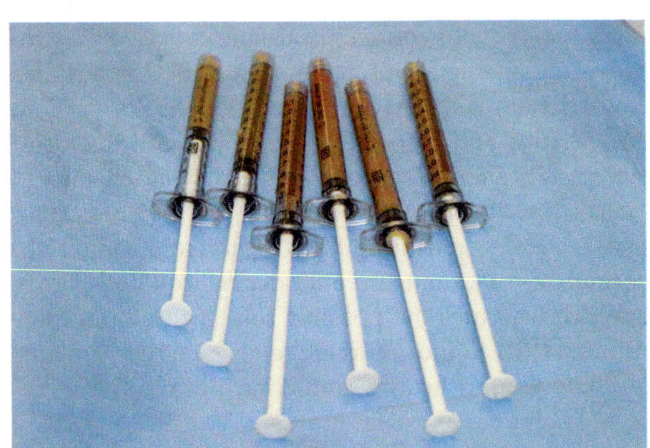

Fig. 51-4 Prepared refined and transferred to 1 ml Luer–Lok syringes, ready for placement.

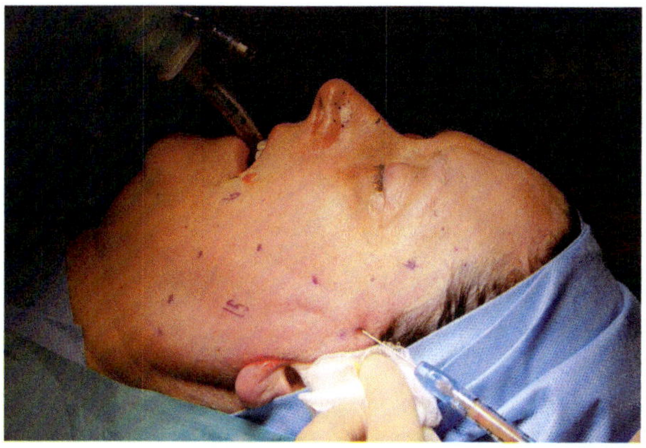

Fig. 51-5 Fat placement: Areas marked and fat transferred through small stab incisions. Attention should be given to place small aliquots of fat in multiple serial passes.

stable, less traumatic way. However, semi-blunt cannulas give more control for placement in the subdermal plane and a higher penetrating ability. Sharp cannulas are useful to release adhesions and scars. A 2 mm incision is made and the infiltration cannula is introduced. Fat is placed gently as the cannula is withdrawn, depositing a row of fat cell packets as the cannula retreats (Figure 51-5). This procedure is undertaken with small increments not exceeding the placement of one tenth of a 1 mL syringe. The structure and contour should be incrementally built up with small aliquots of fat in layers instead of inserting a large quantity and then attempting to mould the tissues. This massaging action risks displacing the fat or to necrosis of fat leading to irregular contours. The stab incisions at the donor and recipient sites are closed with interrupted nylon sutures.

Postoperative care

Cold therapy with ice packs and cooling face packs is recommended for the first 24 to 48 hours postoperatively and sutures are removed at 5–7 days. Once placed the volume of the fat content seems to stabilize at three to four months, but there may be a reduction in volume for even up to one year after the procedure (Figures 51-6). Patients should hence be counselled about the need for secondary and 'touch-up' procedures for volume restoration or subtle refinement.

Complications

The common sequelae of fat grafting are swelling, bruising and discomfort. Aesthetic problems with surface and contour irregularities are related to under or over correction of the defect, fat migration, recipient tissue characteristics, technique employed and the inherent dimensional instability of the grafted fat. Furthermore, an overgrowth of fat grafts with or without weight gain has also been reported. Infection associated with fat grafting is rare; nevertheless when this occurs, it has the potential for fat resorption and associated contour loss. Strict sterile techniques should be adopted at all times. Cannula related injuries to the nerves, muscles, glands and blood vessels are also rare, often transient and are reduced with the use of blunt cannulas and gentle tissue handling. A single case of an acute fatal stroke immediately following autologous fat injection into the glabellar region has been reported.[16] Sporadic reports in the literature exist of fat emboli to the cerebral and retinal vessels causing stroke symptoms and blindness.[17–21]

Discussion

Fat grafting, whilst universally a successful tool, the variations in harvest technique, fat refinement and placement methods causes difficulty in the interpretation of studies and guidance for best practice.

The survival rate of grafted fat has been reported by various authors from 40 to 90%.[22,23] Coleman sites studies demonstrating that fat harvest using a blunt cannula refined by centrifugation has a greater than 90% survival rate.[23] However, centrifugation is not the only purification method and success has also been reported with gravity separation, filtered and washed and simultaneous washing with filtration in a closed system. Botti et al., in a clinical study, compared filtered and washed fat with centrifuged fat in 25 patients, with injecting hemifaces in these patients with fat processed by the two methods. At 12 months, the comparable subjective and objective results were noted.[24]

Zhu et al. carried out an in vitro study to compare gravity separation, centrifugation and washing with filtration in a closed system. They concluded that graft tissue prepared by washing with filtration in a closed system produces grafts of a higher viability and lower contaminants.[25] Smith et al. found no significant differences in fat cell viability as assessed by fat cell weight, by comparing techniques of fat preparation with six different combinations of centrifugation and or washing with ringers lactate solution or normal saline harvested from three patients.[26]

Rohrich et al. found no differences in cell viability in fat removed from abdomen, flank, thigh and medial knee.[15] However, Padoin et al. reported that fat harvested from the lower abdomen had more adipose stem cell levels compared with anatomical sites.[27]

A prospective study by Pu et al. compared the Coleman versus conventional liposuction on the same patient. Higher viable adipocytes and glyceraldehyde-3-phosphate dehydrogenase enzyme activity levels were found in the Coleman method.[28] The current evidence does not support one harvesting method over the other; however techniques with low-pressure aspiration and larger bore cannulas appear to increase adipocyte activity.[22] In a recent critical appraisal of the literature on the subject, Ross et al. reviewed 103 articles on the various aspects associated with this technique. They concluded that despite a significant

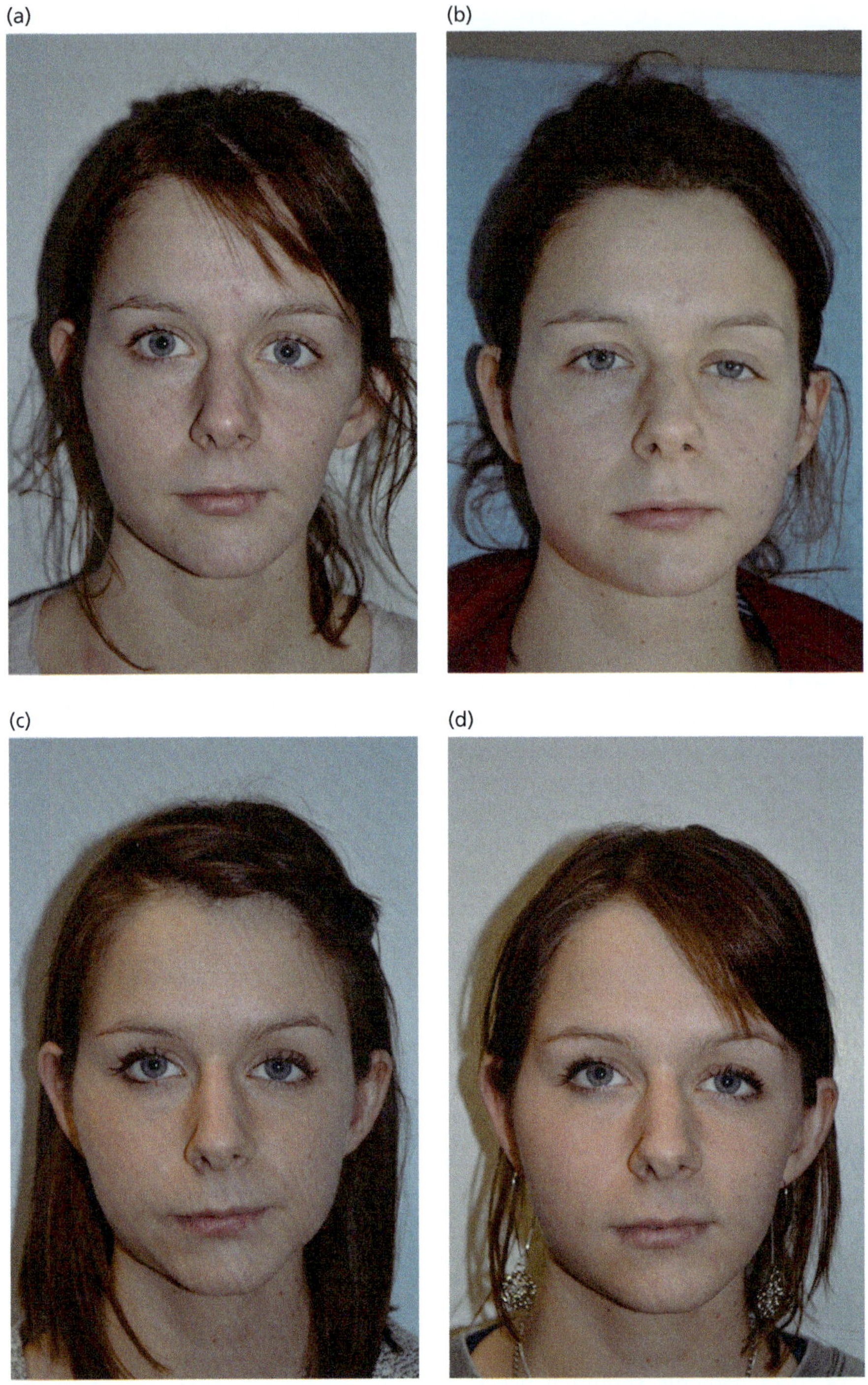

Fig. 51-6 Facial asymmetry (a) secondary to radiotherapy given to treat rhabdomyosarcoma of left temporalis at the age of 4. This deformity was treated with micro fat grafting post hyberbaric oxygen therapy. Sequential results at day 1 post-op (b), three months (c) and 6 months (d).

research effort, there was a lack of consensus on the optimum technique.[29]

Conclusions

The concept of fat grafting has existed for almost a century, but its use has exponentially increased in the last 20 years in aesthetic and reconstructive surgery. It can fill large and small defects of the face, augment facial structures, rejuvenate an aging face and act as an adjunct to orthognathic surgery to achieve a balanced and pleasing aesthetic result. As has been alluded to previously it is more than just a biofiller, but this living free graft has shown its capacity to rejuvenate and repair tissues. The use of other techniques such as dermis fat grafts, onlay implants, free tissue transfer in isolation or in combination with structural fat grafting and orthognathic surgery, have a relevant place in the current practice of facial deformity management.

The future development of fat grafting as a biological treatment modality lies in incorporating knowledge gained from further research and producing randomized controlled prospective multicentre trials to standardize techniques and improve clinical outcomes.

References

1 Neuber F. Fettransplantation. Bericht uber die Verhandlungen der Dt Ges f Chir Zbl Chir. 1893;22:66.
2 Czerny V. Plastischer Erzats de Brustdruse durch ein Lipom. Zentral Chir. 1895;22–66.
3 Holländer E. Die kosmetsche Chirurgie (S.669–712, 56 Abb.) In: Joseph M (Ed.) Handbuch der kosmetik. Leipzig: Verlag van Veit; 1912:690–1.
4 Miller CC. Cannula implants and review of implantation techniques in esthetic surgery. Chicago: The Oak Press, 1926.
5 Illouz YG. The fat cell 'graft': a new technique to fill depressions [letter]. Plast Reconstr Surg. 1986;78:122–3.
6 Coleman SR. The technique of periorbital lipoinfiltration. Oper Tech Plast Reconstr Surg. 1994;1:120–6.
7 Coleman SR. Structural fat grafting, 1st edn. St Louis, MO Quality Medical, 2004.
8 Markman B. Anatomy and physiology of adipose tissue. Clin Plast Surg. 1989;16:235–44.
9 Zuk PA, Zhu M, Mizuno H, et al. Multilineage cells from human adipose tissue: implications for cell-based therapies. Tissue Eng. 2001;7:211–28.
10 Coleman SR. Structural fat grafting: more than a permanent filler. Plast Reconstr Surg. 2006;118:108S.
11 Sultan SM, Stern CS, Allen RJ, et al. human fat grafting alleviates radiation skin damage in a murine model. Plast Reconstr Surg. 2011;128:363–72.
12 Von Heimburg D, Hemmrich K, Haydarlioglu S, et al. Comparison of viable cell yield from excised versus aspirated adipose tissue. Cells Tissues Organs. 2004;178:87.
13 Wolter TP, Von Heimburg D, Stoffels I, et al. Cryopreservation of mature human adipocytes: In vitro measurement of viability. Ann Plast Surg. 2005;55:408.
14 Coleman SR. Structural fat grafts: the ideal filler? Clin Plast Surg. 2001;28:111–9.
15 Rohrich RJ, Sorokin ES and Brown SA. In search of improved fat transfer viability: A quantitative analysis of the role of centrifugation and harvest site. Plast Reconstr Surg. 2004;113:391.
16 Yoon SS, Chang DI, Chung KC. Acute fatal stroke immediately following autologous fat injection into the face. Neurology. 2003;61:1151–2.
17 Teimourian B. Blindness following fat injections. Plast Reconstr Surg. 1988;82:361.
18 Thaunat O, Thaler F, Loirat P, Decroix JP, Boulin A. Cerebral fat embolism induced by facial fat injection. Plast Reconstr Surg. 2004;113:2235–6.
19 Egido JA, Arroyo R, Marcos A, Jimeénez-Alfaro J. Middle cerebral artery embolism and unilateral visual loss after autologous fat injection into the glabellar area. Stroke. 1993;23:615–6.
20 Feinendegen DL, Baumgartner RW, Vuadens P, Schroth G, Mattle HP, Regli F, Tschopp H. Autologous fat injection for soft tissue augmentation in the face: a safe procedure? Aesthetic Plast Surg. 1998;22:163–7.
21 Dreizen NG, Framm L. Sudden unilateral visual loss after autologous fat injection into the glabellar area. Am J Ophthalmol. 1989;107:85–7.
22 Gir P, Brown SA, Oni G, Kashefi, Mojalla A, Rohrich RJ. Fat grafting: Evidence based review on autologous fat harvesting, processing, reinjection and storage. Plast Reconstr Surg. 2012;130:249–58.
23 Coleman SR. Long-term survival of fat transplants: controlled demonstrations. Aesth Plast Surg. 1995;19: 421–5.
24 Botti G, Pascali M, Botti C, Bodog F, Cervelli V. A clinical trial in facial fat grafting: Filtered and washed versus centrifuged fat. Plast Reconstr Surg. 2011;127:2464–73.
25 Zhu M, Cohen SR, Hicok KC, Sanahan RK, Strem BM, Yu JC, Arm DM, Fraser JK. Comparison of three different preparation methods: Gravity separation, centrifugation, and simultaneous washing with filtration in a closed system. Plast Reconstr Surg. 2013;131:873–80.
26 Smith P, Adams WP Jr, Lipschitz AH, et al. Autologous human fat grafting: Effect of harvesting and preparation techniques on adipocyte graft survival. Plast Reconstr Surg. 2006;117:1836–44.
27 Padoin AV, Braga-Silva J, Martins P, et al. Sources of processed lipoaspirate cells: Influence of donor site on cell concentration. Plast Reconstr Surg. 2008;122:614–8.
28 Pu LL, Coleman SR, Cui X, Ferguson RE Jr, Vasconez HC. Autologous fat grafts harvested and refined by the Coleman technique: A comparative study. Plast Reconstr Surg. 2008;122:932–7.
29 Ross RJ, Shayan R, Mutimer KL, Ashton MW. Autologous fat grafting: Current state of the art and critical review. Ann Plast Surg. 2014;73:352–7.

Chapter 52

Aesthetic Surgery of the Submental-Cervical Region

Tirbod Fattahi

Introduction

There is very little doubt that orthognathic surgery of the upper and lower jaws can have a significant impact on the aesthetics of the nose, lower face and neck. Foundational surgery (skeletal surgery) is perhaps the best type of aesthetic surgery. Spatial movement of the maxilla and mandible induce inherent soft tissue changes that if planned appropriately, will enhance the final outcome of surgery. There are times, however, that no matter how much bony movement has occurred, there is room for further soft tissue enhancement. This is particularly true in the submental and cervical region as it relates to mandibular or chin surgery.[1] This chapter describes the pertinent anatomy, and aging process, along with surgical options and benefits of various procedures in the aesthetic improvement of the submental and cervical areas.

Anatomy

The submental and cervical areas encompass a specific portion of the lower face and neck. Specifically, the area most influenced by aesthetic surgery includes the central portion of the neck encompassed by the right and left sternocleidomastoid muscles laterally, submental skin anteriorly, thyroid cartilage inferiorly, and the platysma muscle on the deep surface. Supra- and subplatysmal fat, as well as the right and left platysma muscles are found within this space. Each component of this region will be described since various surgical procedures are available to address specific areas.

Submental fat

Fat accumulation, also known as lipomatosis, is dependent on various factors such as sex and body habitus. In the anterior neck, fatty deposition is typically found in two general regions: supra- or subplatysmal areas. Supraplatysmal fat is the superficial fat located just above (superficial) to the platysma muscle. Subplatysmal fat, on the other hand, is considered a deep fat and is located deep to the platysma and just superficial to the anterior bellies of the digastric muscles. Liposuction of the submental region involves removal of the supraplatysmal fat; there are very few indications for removal of subplatysmal fat. While there is some variability in the exact volume of fat in the anterior neck, it is generally no more than 10–15 cc, based on clinical findings at the time of liposuction. Anatomical boundaries of this fat pad have been well described by various authors.[2,3]

Orthognathic Surgery: Principles, Planning and Practice. Edited by Farhad B. Naini and Daljit S. Gill.

Platysma muscle

Platysma muscles are two flat and broad sheets of muscle which originate from the deltoid and pectoralis muscles fascia, travelling over the clavicle and inserting on the lower face, eventually forming the superficial musculoaponeurotic system (SMAS) of the face. The superficial cervical fascia covers the superficial aspect of the muscle while the superficial layer of deep cervical fascia (investing fascia) covers the deep aspect of the muscle. The exact anatomy of the platysma has been extensively studied.[4–8] An important consideration, as described by de Castro, is the anatomy of the central area of the neck where the right and left platysma muscles near each other.[6,7] Most patients will have some decussation (cross-over) of the right and left platysma in the central neck. Some patients have no decussation; this leads to the formation of an aponeurosis between the medial edges of the right and left muscles. Irrespective of decussation or lack thereof, submental fat provides a covering over this area.

Submental and cervical skin

Tone and laxity of the submental and cervical skin, similar to all other areas of the body, is directly related to the patient's age. As the aging process continues, collagen and elastin fiber concentration is diminished in the papillary and reticular dermis. This leads to laxity of the overlying skin. This fact is compounded if one has submental lipomatosis and platysmal redundancy or banding.

Position of mandible and chin

While a formal discussion as well as indication for mandibular skeletal surgery is done elsewhere in this book, it is critical to assess the anterior–posterior position of the mandible. Clearly, a 'weak' jaw will not support the overlying soft tissue drape. Furthermore, a deficient chin will have a similar impact on the appearance of the lower face. Aesthetic components of the ideal neck have been well described.[9,10] Indications for chin augmentation, either through an osteoplastic procedure or via an alloplast, are discussed later in this chapter.

Aging process

Irrespective of the body part, the aging process is multi-factorial encompassing both intrinsic (familial, congenital) as well as extrinsic (environmental, smoking, body habitus) factors. Multiple other specific elements contribute to the classical description of the aging process of the lower face, submental and cervical areas such as lack of proper foundational skeletal support (i.e., microgenia), fat deflation, and dermal/fascial/muscular descent of the facial and neck musculature. Other components unique to the anterior neck is the accumulation of fat in the submental region as well as redundancy or banding of the platysma muscle as contributing factors towards the aging process.

Surgical options and evaluation

Appropriate surgical options are predicated on appropriate preoperative evaluation and correct diagnosis. In the submental or cervical area, there are several surgical options:

- Mandibular surgery (osteotomy) – discussed in Chapters 24 and 25.
- Liposuction.
- Platysmaplasty.
- Chin surgery.

When evaluating a patient for lower face and neck rejuvenation, several factors must be taken into consideration such as skin tone, laxity and specific contributing factors to a full neck. Age of the patient will clearly have an impact on tone and laxity of the anterior neck since younger patients tend to have a 'tighter' and more elastic tone to their skin. Fullness in the anterior neck must also be discerned carefully. This fullness (obtuse cervicomental angle) can be due to underlying fat in the submental area (lipomatosis), the anatomy of the right and left platysma muscles, or both, along with other factors such as the position of the chin and hyoid bone (Figure 52-1).

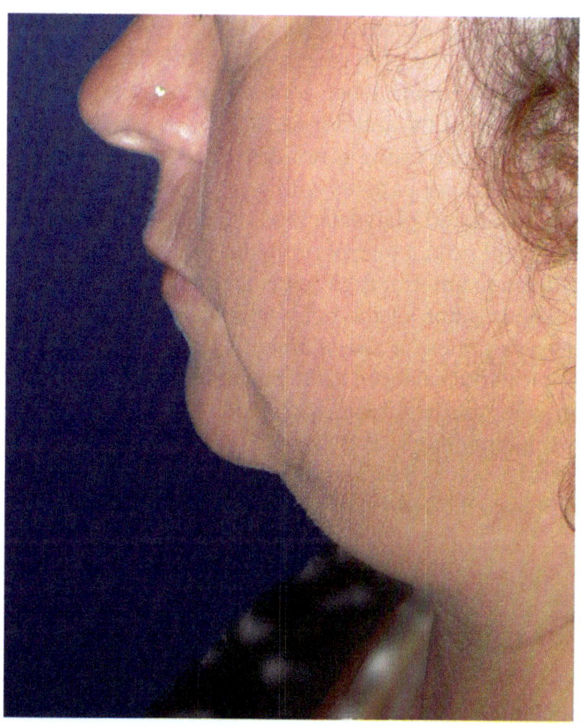

Fig. 52-1 Aging and fullness of the anterior neck. Note obtuse cervicomental angle, lack of chin projection and jowling.

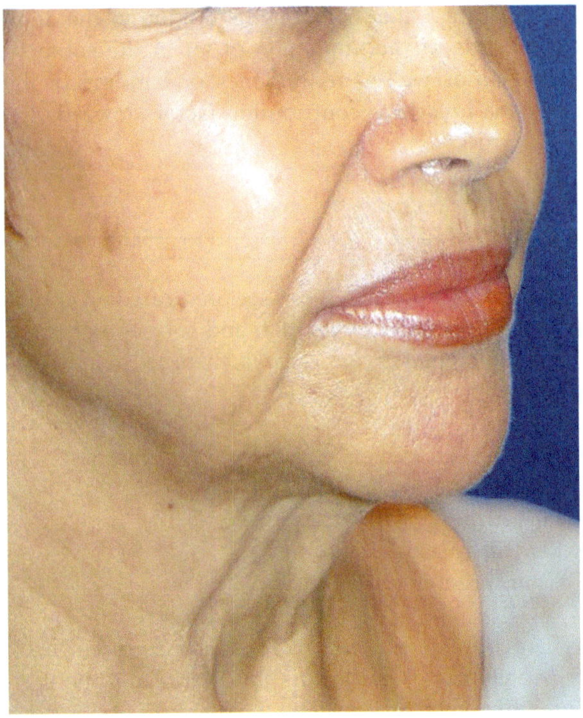

Fig. 52-2 Platysmal banding clearing visible.

The anatomy of the platysma muscles will also play a role in the appearance of the anterior neck. As previously mentioned, patients with cross-over (decussation) of the right and left platysma muscles will exhibit platysmal redundancy (fullness) in the central portion of the upper neck whereas those without decussation will have platysmal banding (visible medial edges of the right and left muscles and overlying fascia) (Figure 52-2). Both conditions may become exaggerated by contracting the platysma muscle. The superficial cervical fat may actually camouflage the underlying anatomy of the platysma muscles; this is an important consideration when contemplating isolated liposuctioning of the anterior neck.

Formal face lifting is not discussed in this chapter; however, older patients with moderate laxity of lower facial skin and platysma, jowling, and ill-defined jaw lines will need a formal cervicofacial rhytidectomy *in addition* to anterior neck rejuvenation.

The position of the bony chin also plays a role in the evaluation of the submental and cervical areas. A properly balanced chin position can enhance the anatomy of the labiomental crease as well as the cervicomental angle. It is imperative to recall that other factors such as the position of the hyoid bone can also influence the cervicomental angle.

Surgical procedures

Submental liposuction

There is no question that there exists a role, albeit small, for isolated submental liposuction. Removal of the supraplatysmal fatty deposits can enhance the appearance of the submental area. However, this should only be reserved for younger patients with no evidence of platysmal pathology (redundancy or banding) who have a good skin tone. As mentioned before, removal of fatty deposits in the submental area can at times expose the underlying platysmal issues, which if left untreated, can lead to an unhappy patient.

Submental liposuction can be done through an open approach or via a closed technique. Typically, about 10–15 cc of fat are removed. There is no skin excision; the submental and cervical skin will redrape over time. In the author's practice, isolated liposuction is only performed in the young patient who has submental lipomatosis without platysmal redundancy.[11]

Cervicoplasty

Considered the most comprehensive rejuvenative procedure for the anterior neck, cervicoplasty includes an open liposuction and a platysmaplasty.[1,8,10–18] This procedure addresses both the fat and the platysma muscles simultaneously. Cervicoplasty begins with an incision just posterior to the submental crease. A skin flap with 4–5 mm of subdermal fat is then elevated between the SCM muscles and the inferior border of the mandible, after which an open liposuction is performed until the underlying platysma muscle is well-visualized. Next, the superior edge of the platysma is elevated off the anterior mandible and a sub-muscular dissection is performed in the central compartment of the neck extending beyond the inferior extent of the platysmal bands or redundancy. The central portion of the right and left platysma is then sharply excised in a diamond shape pattern, thus creating two free edges of muscle (medial edges of right and left platysma). The free edges of the muscles are then imbricated similar to the corset platysmaplasty described by Feldman.[18] No skin excision is necessary since skin contracture will occur over the following several weeks. A pressure dressing is applied and worn for a few days. Patients are typically seen in 24 hours to rule out any haematoma or seroma formation.

Genioplasty

Altering the position of the chin can have an impressive effect on lower face aesthetics. There are numerous well established guidelines that describe the 'ideal' position of the soft tissue and bony chin. It is a well-known fact that for every 1.0 mm of bony movement of the chin (or mandible) in the anterior vector, the soft tissue of the chin will move approximately 0.8 mm. This ratio can guide clinicians as to the final position of the mandible following mandibular advancement surgery. There are many instances where further chin augmentation is necessary beyond what is accomplished by the mandibular advancement. Options for such augmentation include osseous genioplasty (sliding horizontal body osteotomy) and alloplastic augmentation using various synthetic implants. What is perhaps missing or overlooked is

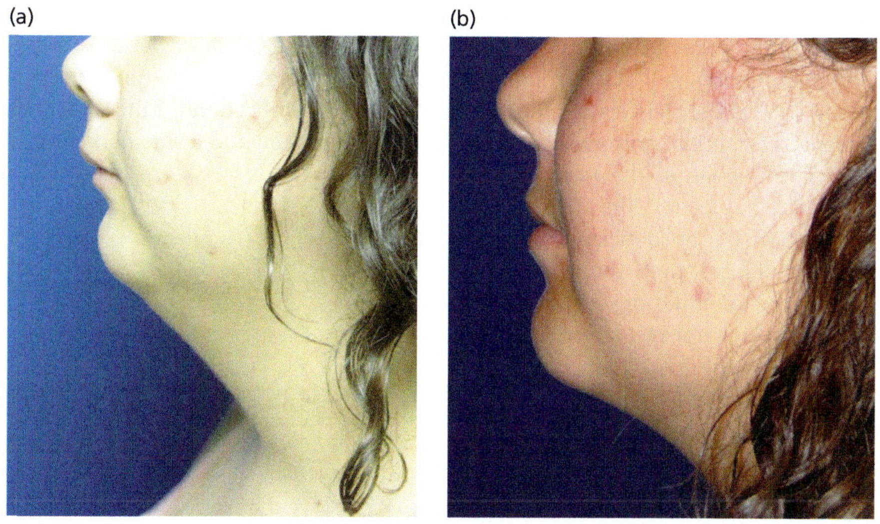

Fig. 52-3 Pre- and postoperative photographs following mandibular advancement surgery and cervicoplasty.

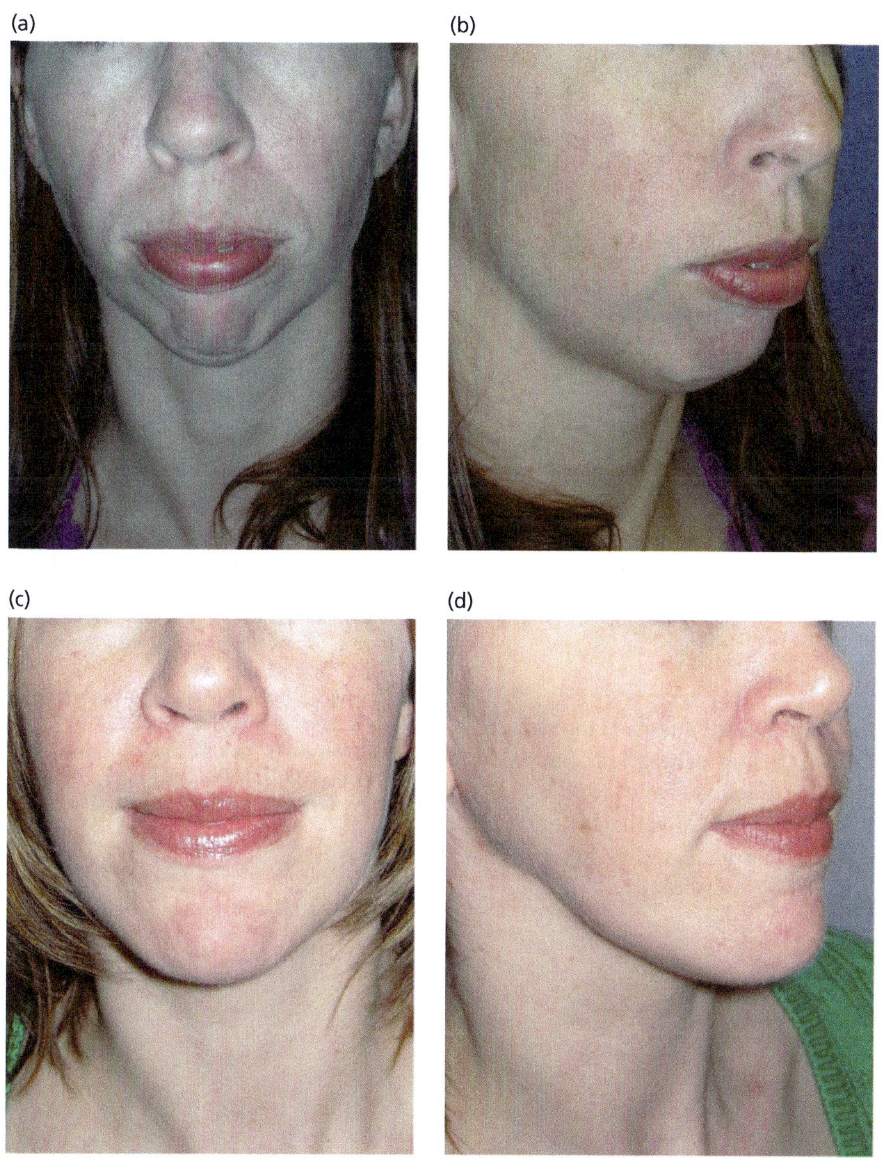

Fig. 52-4 Preoperative (a & b) and postoperative (c & d) photographs following mandibular advancement surgery and placement of extended silicone chin implants.

not just the anterior–posterior position of the chin, but also its lateral position. Many patients with a deficient chin (retrogenia or microgenia) will have a lateral deficiency of the chin. Lateral deficiencies are located just behind the mental foramina and mandibular retaining ligaments. These areas of the lateral chin are known as the 'pre-jowl sulcus'.[19] *Pre-jowl* relates to the anatomical position of the deficiency which is always anterior to or before ('pre') the formation of jowls. Augmentation of the anterior chin without addressing the lateral aspect is not ideal. Special consideration must be given to differentiation of a chin that is deficient in the anterior–posterior vector only, versus one that is deficient laterally along the pre-jowl sulcus.

In the author's practice, osteoplastic genioplasty is only performed in cases of chin asymmetry, vertical height reduction, or a set-back. All advancement surgery of the chin is performed via alloplastic augmentation using silastic (solid silicone) implants that are placed subperiosteally and secured to the bone. Various designs of these implants will allow augmentation of the entire body of the chin (A-P as well as lateral).

Discussion

Aesthetic surgery of the submental and cervical areas can be done at the time of orthognathic surgery or can be used to camouflage an underlying deformity (Figures 52-3 and 52-4). Patient with a Class II malocclusion and poor cervicomental angle can certainly benefit from a mandibular osteotomy and a simultaneous cervicoplasty.

Alternatively, a patient who has already undergone orthodontic care with a Class I occlusion, but suffers from a deficient chin, can simply undergo an alloplastic augmentation of the chin with minimal recovery time.

Conclusion

No one can argue the soft tissue benefits of moving the maxilla and mandible during orthognathic surgery. These well established guidelines have stood the test of time. However, it is critical to know that other surgical options are available in order to address the chin, as well as the fat and platysma muscles in the submental and cervical areas. Knowledge of such procedures and their incorporation at the time of orthognathic surgery can significantly enhance the final outcome, leading to a happy patient and a satisfied clinician.

References

1 Fattahi T. Aesthetic surgery to augment orthognathic surgery. Oral Maxillofac Surg Clin North Am. 2007;19:435–7.
2 Rohrich RJ, Pessa JE. The anatomy and clinical implications of perioral submuscular fat. Plast Reconstr Surg. 2009;124:266–71.
3 Ramirez OM. Advanced considerations determining procedure selection in cervicoplasty; part one: anatomy and aesthetics. Part one: anatomy and aesthetics. Clin Plast Surg. 2008;35:679–90.
4 Vistnes LM, Souther SG. The platysma muscle: anatomic considerations for aesthetic surgery of the anterior neck. Clin Plast Surg. 1983;10:441–8.
5 De Castro CC. The changing role of platysma in face lifting. Plast Reconstr Surg. 2000;105:764–75.
6 De Castro CC. Anatomy of the neck and procedure selection. Clin Plast Surg. 2008;35:625–42.
7 De Castro CC. The anatomy of the platysma muscle. Plast Reconstr Surg. 1980;66:680–3.
8 Evans TW, Stepanyan M. Isolated cervicoplasty. Am J Cosmetic Surg. 2002;19:91–113.
9 Ellenbogen R, Karlin JV. Visual criteria for success in restoring the youthful neck. Plast Reconstr Surg. 1980;66:826–37.
10 Rohrich RJ, Rios JL, Smith PD, Gutowski KA. Neck rejuvenation revisited. Plast Reconstr Surg. 2006;118:1251–63.
11 Fattahi T. Submental liposuction versus formal cervicoplasty: which one to choose? J Oral Maxillofac Surg. 2012;70:2854–8.
12 Fattahi T. Management of isolated neck deformities. Atlas Oral Maxillofac Surg Clin N Am. 2004;12:261–70.
13 Ramirez OM. Advanced considerations determining procedure selection in cervicoplasty. Part two: surgery. Clin Plast Surg. 2008;35:691–709.
14 Ramirez OM, Robertson KM. Comprehensive approach to rejuvenation of the neck. Facial Plast Surg. 2001;17:129–40.
15 Patel BC. Aesthetic surgery of the aging neck: options and techniques. Orbit. 2006;25:327–56.
16 Barton FE. Aesthetic surgery of the face and neck. Aesthetic Surg J. 2009;29:449–63.
17 Guerrerosantos J. Managing platysma bands in the aging neck. Aesthet Surg J. 2008;28:211–6.
18 Feldman JJ: Neck Lift. St. Louis, MO: Quality Medical Publishing, 2006, pp.307–361.
19 Fattahi T. The prejowl sulcus: an important consideration in lower face rejuvenation. J Oral Maxillofac Surg. 2008;66: 355–8.

Chapter 53

Surgical Options for Aesthetic Enhancement of the Lips and Perioral Region

Joe Niamtu

Introduction

The lips have been described as the only exposed sexual organ in the body and very few body parts have received as much attention over the millennia as have the lips. Voluptuous lips will never go out of style as they play such an important part in speaking, eating, communication, courtship, and persona. It does not take long to conjure up a list of female and male patients that are defined by their lips.

Cosmetic lip treatments have increased exponentially over the past 20 years as bovine collagen fillers with all their limitations have been replaced by an endless list of safe and effective injectable fillers to augment and rejuvenate the lips and perioral region.[1–6]

Although fillers are a very powerful treatment modality, they cannot serve all aesthetic lip problems encountered through heredity, development and aging. To be well versed in the aesthetic treatment of the lips, one must have surgical lip procedures in his or her armamentarium. The remainder of this chapter will deal with the surgical treatment of various diagnostic and functional conundrums concerning the lips and related structures.

Patient assessment and communication – not everyone needs bigger lips

If you ask the average practitioner what is their most common treatment to the lips, inevitably it would be augmentation. Many clinicians do not realize the worldwide popularity of lip reduction. Although I have performed lip reduction procedures for over 20 years, I was mostly targeting patients in my hometown and performed a handful of procedures. Like many surgeons, the Internet has served to provide a worldwide forum to showcase surgical offerings and talents. Due to this, I get an average of three requests per week from around the world to consult for surgical lip reduction. Obviously these requests are mainly from ethnic populations, mainly African-American. Eastern Asian patients also request this procedure and I have performed it on multiple nationalities including Caucasian patients. In any event, it is a much more popular procedure than I ever realized.

While many of these patients have larger than normal lips, even for their ethnicity, a number of these patients merely want a subtle reduction to approach a

Orthognathic Surgery: Principles, Planning and Practice. Edited by Farhad B. Naini and Daljit S. Gill.

more 'global' beauty. The majority of patients presenting for lip reduction have lips that show an increased amount of 'pink' mucosa and also frequently protrude and droop (in the case of the lower lip) more than the general population for their ethnicity.

Before reducing anyone's lips, it is important to access the biopsychosocial reasons for wanting to look different. Like any cosmetic procedure, it is important to rule out body dysmorphic disorder and ascertain why the patient wants smaller lips. Although I don't generally like it when a cosmetic patient presents with pictures of how he or she would like to look, with lip reduction it is a positive. I say this because some patients simply have totally unrealistic expectations of what the surgery can do. As it has been said many times, 'it is a scalpel, not a magic wand'.

Lip reduction is one of the few cosmetic procedures where a patient can 'functionally' show the surgeon a desired result. Any patient with overly large lips can voluntarily retract the lips toward the teeth and effectively mimic a reduction result. Not only is this a useful manoeuvre to determine if the patient has realistic expectations, but it also can provide useful diagnostic and treatment predictions.

When patients first present for lip reduction consultation numerous parameters are evaluated including the position of the teeth, the amount of tooth and gingival show in repose and full smile, the height of the teeth and the chin position.

Reducing the lips by removing excess tissue can cause the lip to be shorter and to 'roll back' toward the teeth. These are usually positive attributes, but if a patient already shows excessive incisor height or gingival excess, this will be amplified after reduction. If a patient is 'toothy' in repose and full smile, shortening the lip can be aesthetically disastrous by exposing excessive enamel or gingiva.

Another caveat is that many African-American patients have a bimaxillary protrusion of their dental and skeletal relationships coupled with a recessive chin. The larger lip combined with protrusive alveolar and incisor position is accentuated by microgenia as there is even less support for the lip posture.

Mucosal reduction cheiloplasty procedure

Many procedures have been described over the years for lip reduction.[7–24] Although this procedure can be performed with local anaesthesia, I always sedate the patient as I think it provides increased control and precision for the surgeon and is less stressful for the patient. Patients are provided with prescriptions for antibiotics (cephalosporin 500 mg four times a day), a steroid for mitigation of postoperative swelling (prednisone 60 mg per day for five days) and an appropriate analgesic. Pain is generally significant after this procedure, but oedema can be impressive in some patients and they need to be forewarned. Additionally, an anti-sialagogue such as atropine may be given immediately preoperatively to reduce salivary flow.

The first step is to dry the lips and wipe them with an alcohol pad to better retain the marking ink. Like many cosmetic surgery procedures, the surgical markings are an important part of the procedure and to maintain accuracy, the markings must not rub off before the procedure begins. The key to marking the patient is to determine how much tissue is removed. This is generally performed by handing the patient a mirror and asking them to retract their lips (pulling the lips back toward the teeth) to a position that they desire for the final result. The average patient is well aware of this position in the same manner that patients with microgenia can protrude their jaw to a more aesthetic position. Although most cases involve bilateral lip treatment, some patients present for single lip reduction.

To begin marking, the patient is asked to relax their lips and a surgical marker is used to make a dot where the lips meet (Figure 53-1a). Next, the patient is asked to retract the lips to the desired position of reduction and a surgical marker is used to make a line or dot in the retracted position (Figure 53-1b). The two marks serve to estimate the distance between the actual lip position and the desired lip position, which in this case is 7.5 mm (Figure 53-2a). The lip mucosa is very pliable and a 1:1 ratio of excision and retraction does not exist, therefore an increased amount of tissue must be removed to achieve the desired clinical result. Generally a 1.5× to 2× amount of mucosa is removed and

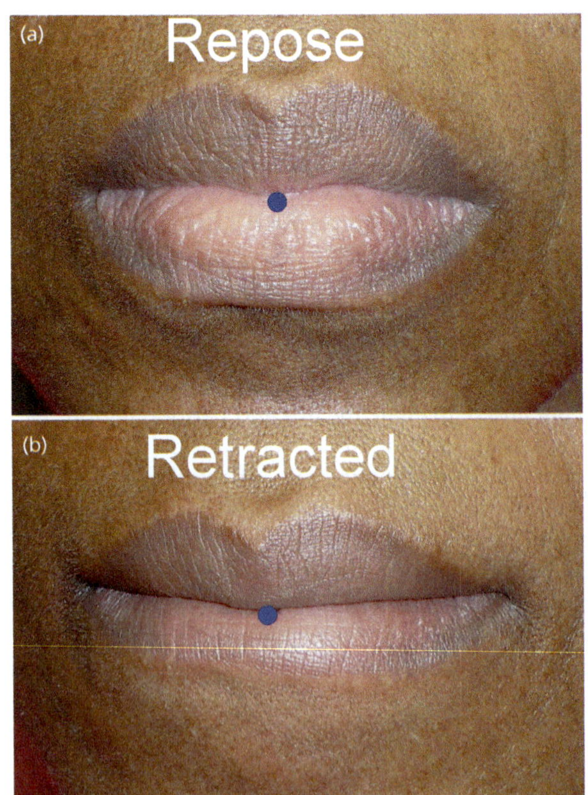

Fig. 53-1 A surgical marking is made at the lip junction in repose (a). The patient is then asked to retract the lip to the desired position and an anterior mark is made (b).

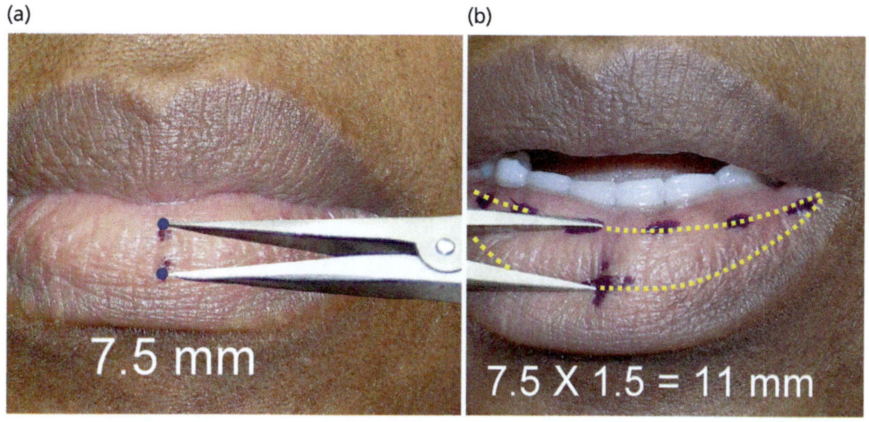

Fig. 53-2 The difference between the two markings is 7.5 mm (a) and factoring this by one and a half times equals an 11.5 mm excision. It is important that the anterior extent of the incision is not anterior to the wet/dry line or it will be visible.

novice surgeons should err on the conservative side. If the surgeon desires a 7.5 mm reduction of tissue to reduce the lip posture, an 11.5 mm ellipse of tissue is removed (Figure 53-2b). The measurement is performed for each lip and in this case the 11.5 mm excision is marked with the anterior margin at or close to the wet/dry line and the posterior margin extending inside the mouth on the mucosal lip surface. It is imperative to position the anterior margin so that it will be hidden in repose and the majority of the mucosa excision is taken from behind this margin. This is why the incision is made at or just posterior to the wet/dry line. Also, the elliptical markings need to join at an acute angle at the commissure to avoid a dog ear deformity (Figure 53-3).

After the markings are made, gauze is held in the mouth to absorb saliva and keep the markings dry and prevent their being rubbed off. Each lip is then infiltrated with several mL of 2% lidocaine with 1:100,000 epinephrine.

Although a scalpel can be used, haemostatic incisional modalities such as CO_2 laser or radiowave surgery make the procedure virtually bloodless (Figure 53-4). Less bleeding means more accurate surgery, less swelling, less bruising and less postoperative discomfort.

After this incision is outlined, one edge is grasped with a clamp and submucosal dissection begins until the entire ellipse is removed. At this point the submucosal anatomy is visible and consists of minor salivary glands, fat and muscle (Figure 53-5). For minor corrections, only a mucosal strip excision is necessary but for larger or more complex reductions, deep tissue is removed as well. This includes portions of the orbicularis oris muscle and is performed by removing a wedge through the muscle (Figure 53-6).

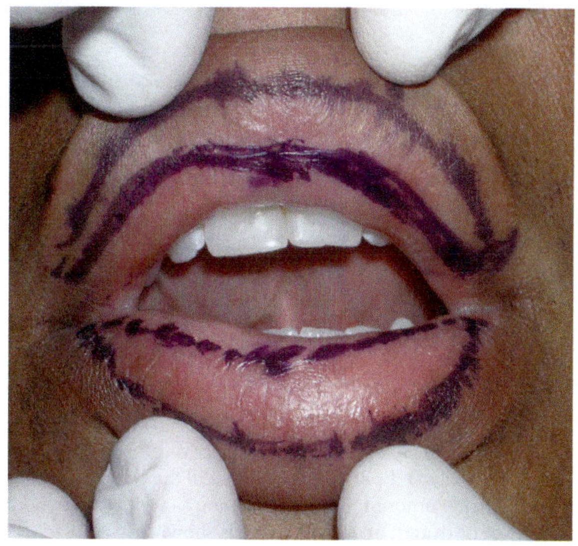

Fig. 53-3 This image shows a typical incision marking from the wet/dry line posterior and tapering at the oral commissures.

After all excess tissue is removed, haemostasis is reevaluated and controlled with fine tooth bipolar forceps. The suturing process begins with 'key sutures' utilizing 4-0 gut suture beginning in the midline and equally spacing across each lip (Figure 53-7a). At this point the final closure is performed using 5-0 silk suture or 5-0 Vicryl (poly lactic acid) suture (Figure 53-7b).

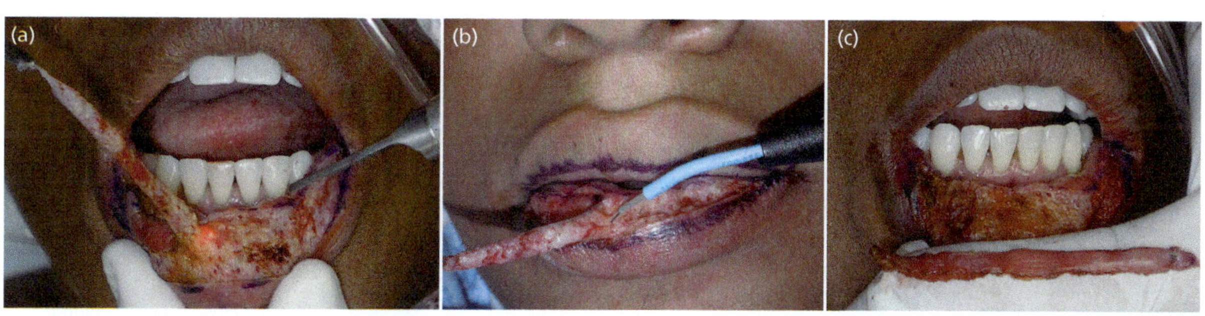

Fig. 53-4 Bloodless incision modalities such as CO_2 laser (a) or radiowave surgery (b) maintain a dry surgical field, increase operator precision and lessen the postoperative recovery. The excised tissue is shown in (c).

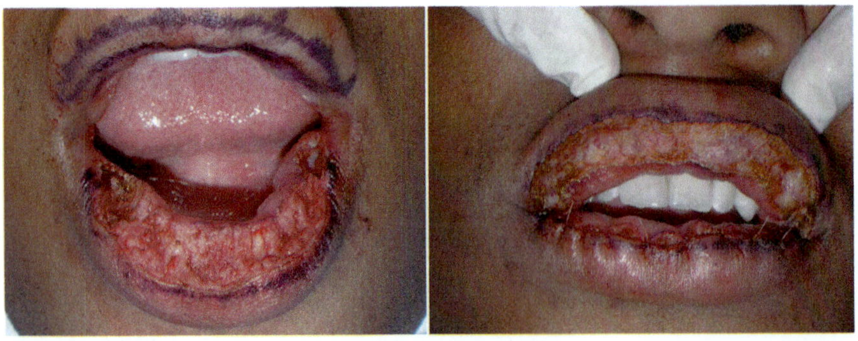

Fig. 53-5 The mucosal ellipse has been removed revealing the submucosal tissue on the lower and upper lips.

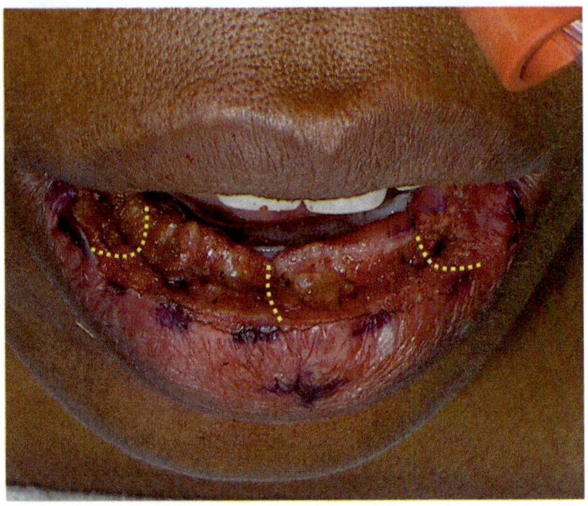

Fig. 53-6 When increased reduction is necessary, removing a wedge of muscle and parenchymal tissue in the central lip allows a greater amount of inward rotation as well as reduction. The wedge or trough of excised tissue is shown.

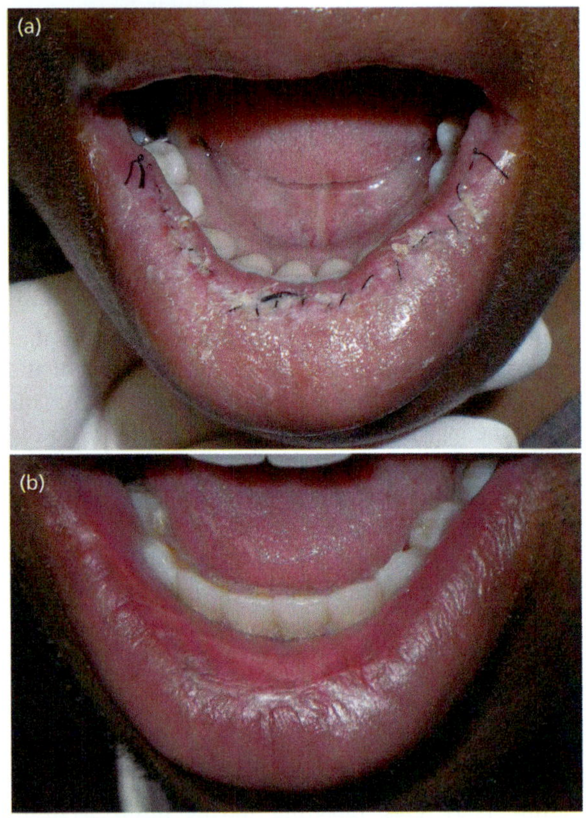

Fig. 53-8 This patient is shown one week after lower lip reduction (a) and 90 days after surgery (b).

I do not routinely use any dressing and the post-op care consists of ice for the first 48 hours and heat for several days after that. The degree of oedema is variable and some patients are fine to return to work at a week while others have significant oedema and a protracted recovery. Most patients can return to work after 7–10 days (Figure 53-8).

Complications

I have encountered very few complications from this procedure. I am always conservative in my removal and have never over-corrected a patient. I have seen several mucous retention cysts which were easily excised.

Case presentations

Figures 53.9–53.15 show before and after images of patients after mucosal lip reduction.

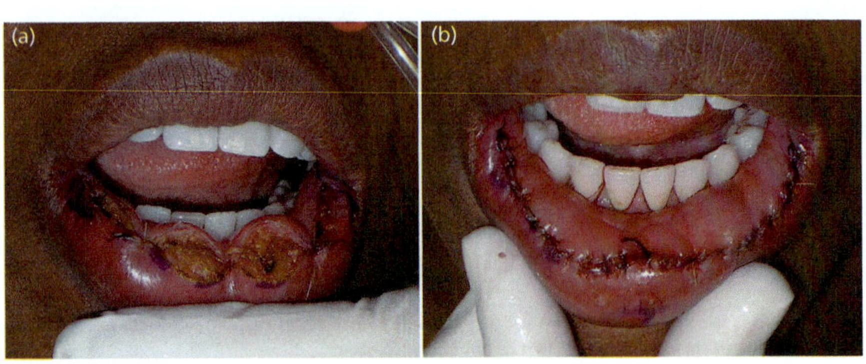

Fig. 53-7 (a) The suturing process begins with 'key sutures' utilizing 4-0 gut suture beginning in the midline and equally spacing across each lip. (b) At this point the final closure is performed using 5-0 silk suture or 5-0 Vicryl (poly lactic acid) suture.

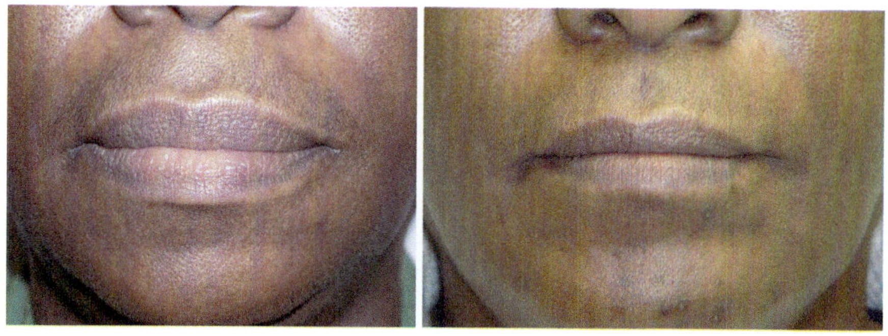

Fig. 53-9 This patient is shown before and 90 days after bilateral lip reduction.

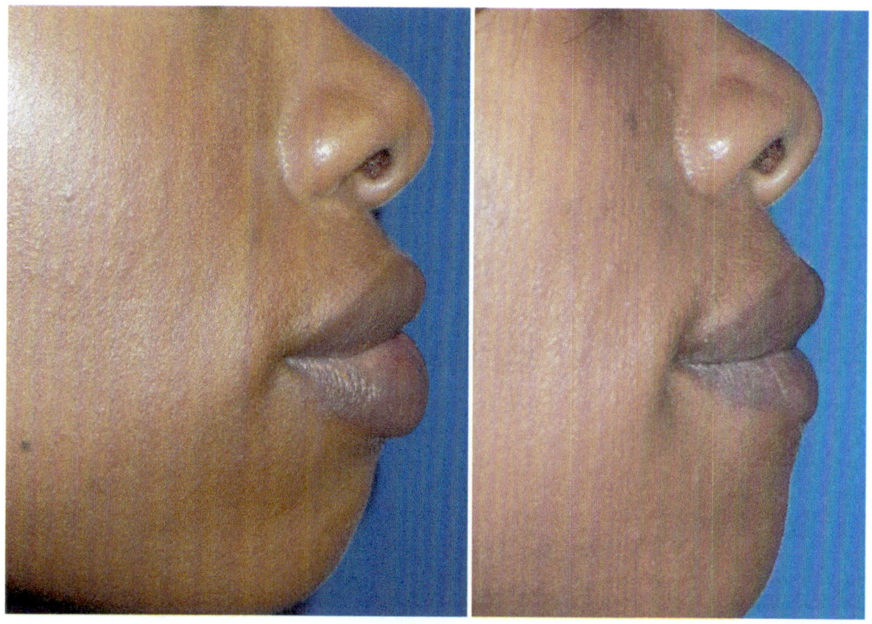

Fig. 53-10 This patient is shown before and 120 days after lower lip reduction only.

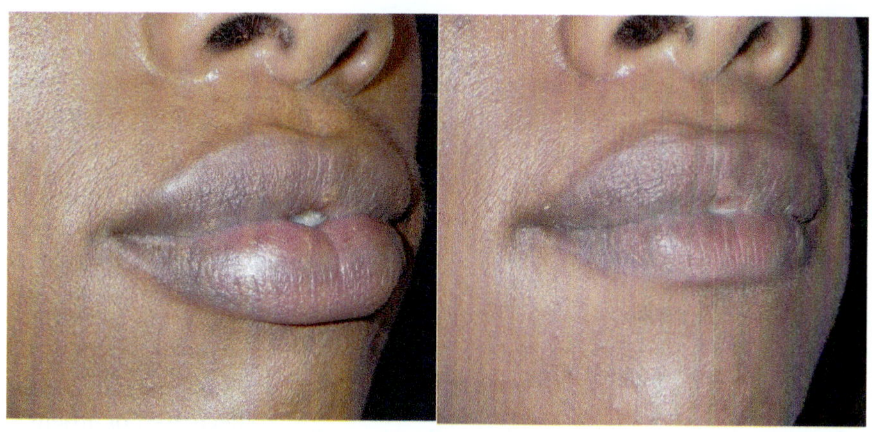

Fig. 53-11 This patient is shown before and 90 days after lower lip reduction only.

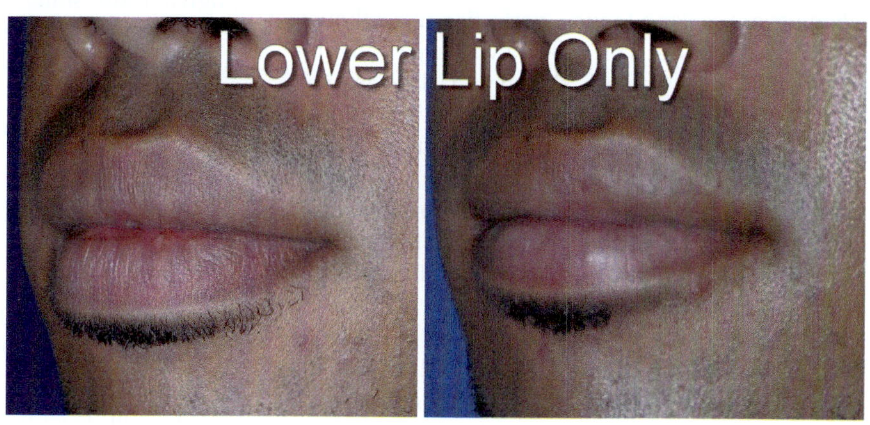

Fig. 53-12 This patient is shown before and 120 days after lower lip reduction only.

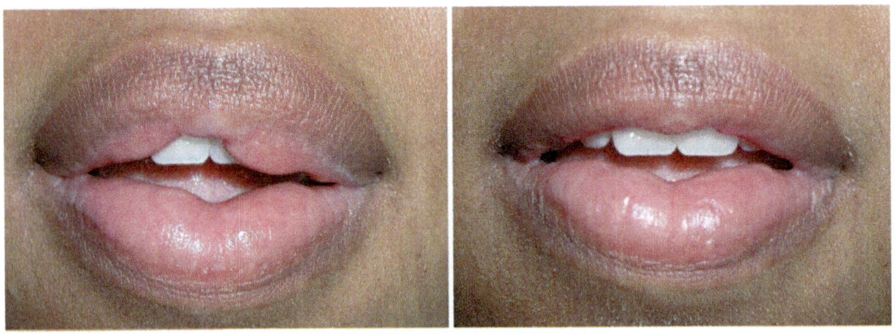

Fig. 53-13 This patient is shown before and 90 days after upper lip reduction for a 'double lip' condition which required mucosal resection only.

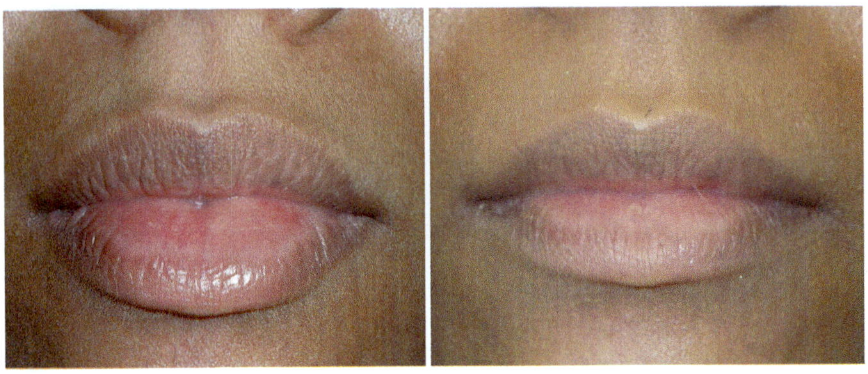

Fig. 53-14 This patient is shown before and 180 days after lower lip reduction only.

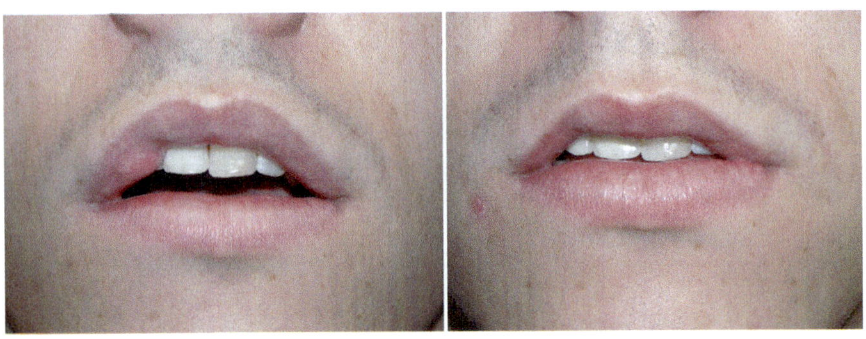

Fig. 53-15 Although less common, lip reduction is also performed on Caucasian patients.

Cutaneous lip reduction

The previous text described what could be loosely termed as 'horizontal' lip excess while the next section discusses vertical lip reduction. The aesthetics of the lips are among the most complex on the face. It is sometimes hard to pinpoint 'what is an aesthetic lip', but it is very easy to pinpoint what is not an aesthetic lip.

Youth is beauty and beauty is youth. Generally, when we are seeking to view perfection in aesthetics, we need only look at a picture of a young person. This applies to eyes, jowls, neck, skin, breasts, legs and just about everything else. The youthful lip is very curvaceous and short, when compared to the senescent lip (Figure 53-16a). As we age, the upper lip loses its youthful curvatures, becomes elongated and also loses its volume due to atrophy of hard and soft tissues. This leaves older individuals with elongated, flat and thin lips (Figure 53-16b).

Lip aesthetics are further complicated by the way they showcase the teeth and gingiva. Youthful patients with an aesthetic smile exhibit several millimetres of anterior incisal edge in repose and several millimetres of anterior gingiva when smiling (Figures 53-17 and 53-18). Patients that show too much or not enough tooth and gingiva are not aesthetic. An elongated lip measured from the subnasale to the vermillion tip is unaesthetic by virtue of excess soft tissue, but also by hiding the teeth and gingiva during animation. Patients with elongated upper lips have decreased or absent show of their upper incisors in repose and decreased or absent show of sufficient incisal edge or gingiva in full smile (Figure 53-18). This problem can be from a long lip, a vertically deficient maxilla or clinically short incisor crowns. This means that lip shortening, surgical maxillary distraction or crown lengthening can all be treatment modalities depending on the diagnosis.

For a true long lip (with normal maxillary height and crown height) surgical vertical reduction can be a definitive and aesthetic treatment as it not only shortens the lip but also 'rolls the lip out' providing more pout and vermillion show. When evaluating patients for a surgical lip lift, they must first (and obviously) possess a lengthened lip. The average length of the maxillary lip is 20 to 22 mm in young adult females

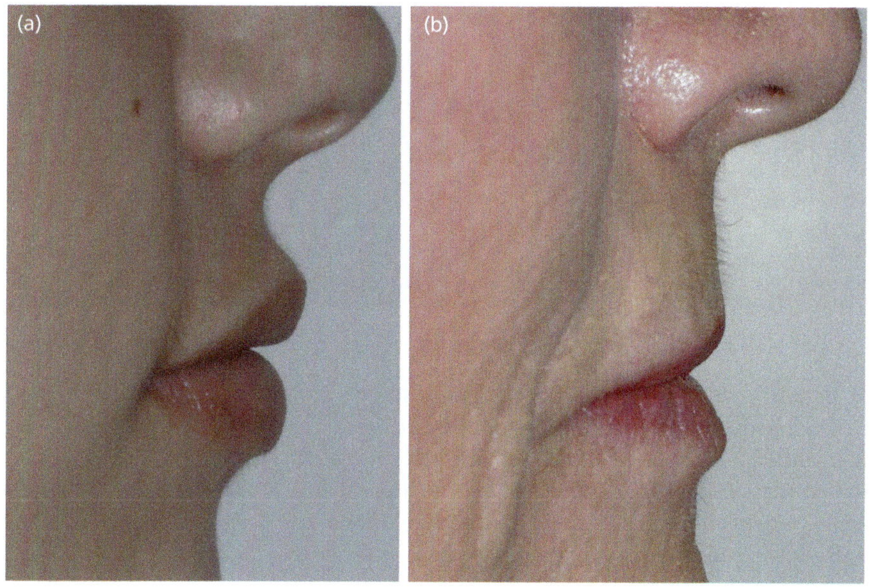

Fig. 53-16 The youthful lip (a) is shorter and with more curvature and volume when compared to the aging lip (b).

and 22 to 24 mm in young adult males.[25] The decision to use this procedure is generally based on minimal or absent incisor show in a patient with normal maxillary position and crown height. These patients will complain that they don't show any teeth in repose and little or none when smiling, giving them an edentulous appearance. By elevating the lip 6–10 mm in these patients, the smile is normalized while the lip is enhanced. One caveat when considering a surgical lip lift is the case of a patient with a long lip but excessive incisor show. This can occur with vertical maxillary excess (gummy smile) or overly long

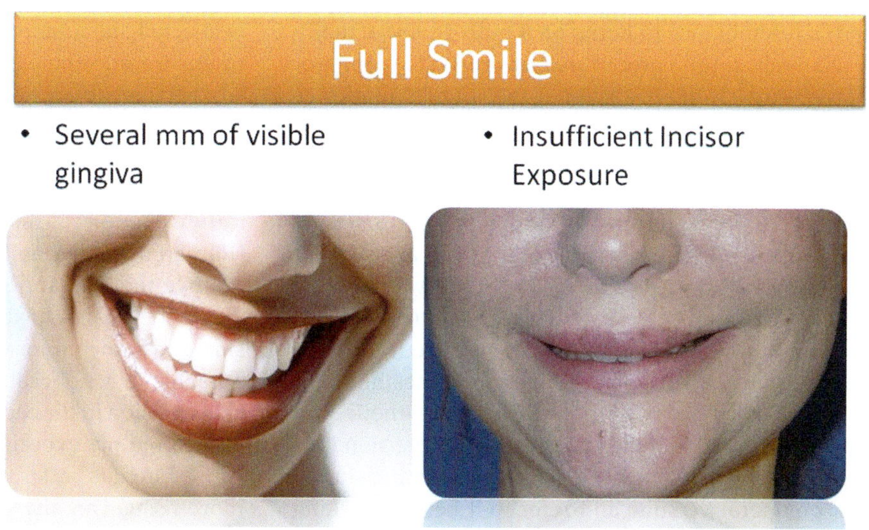

Fig. 53-17 A normal incisor and gingival relationship is shown where several millimetres of incisal edge is shown in repose and several millimetres of gingiva is shown in full smile.

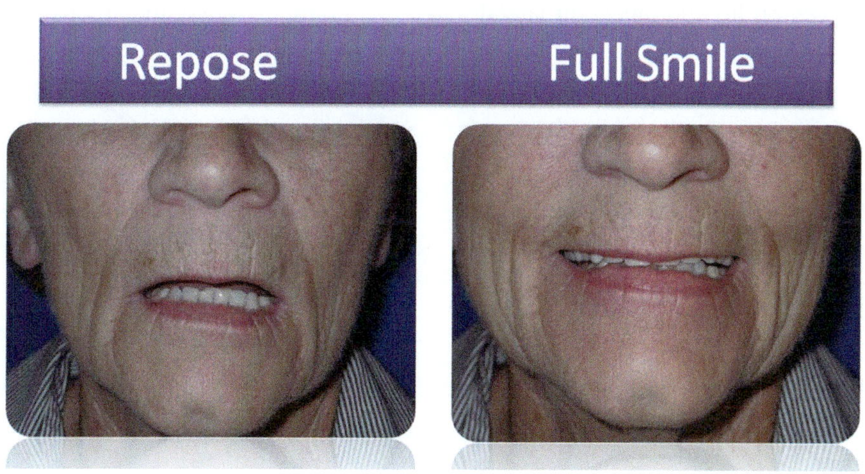

Fig. 53-18 This patient has insufficient upper incisor show in repose and no gingival show in full smile.

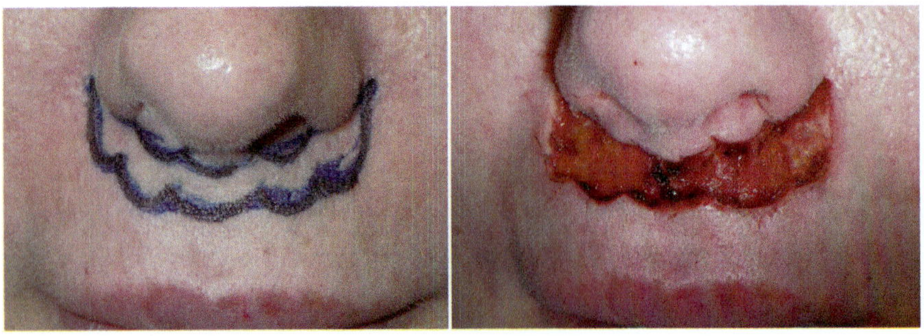

Fig. 53-19 These images show the marking and the incision for the subnasal lip lift. The incision is very precise and must include curvatures that correspond to the normal anatomy in that region.

clinical incisor crowns. Shortening the lip on this type of patient could result in a permanent aesthetic and functional disability. In most cases the procedure is not warranted in a lip shorter than 18 mm as not to create a foreshortened upper lip, but every case is different and some patients have an aesthetic lip/tooth relationship with only a centimetre of lip height. Although the scar is usually very aesthetic, the patient must understand that a visible scar will be apparent for several weeks and laser resurfacing may be necessary to improve the scar in the future.

Many articles have been published to the aesthetics and treatment of the 'gummy smile', long lip and insufficient incisor show.[25–60] The main procedure has been described in numerous ways and is known as a subnasal lip lift, but frequently called the 'bullhorn' procedure because of the excision pattern's resemblance to horns on a bull. This is actually a relatively simple procedure but similar to blepharoplasty surgery, the precision of the surgical markings is imperative for a successful procedure. I have seen this procedure performed with a simple 'smile face' incision and the result and scar are substandard. The crux of this procedure is to accurately and precisely draw the proposed excision outline. The anatomy of the nasal sill, nostrils and philtrum are very unique and delicate and can be unforgiving in terms of scarring if improperly incised. A well angulated, curvilinear incision will provide the maximum aesthetics in terms of shortening the lip as well as an aesthetic scar. I personally feel that the exactness of this incision is so critical that I keep a picture of the desired incision in my preoperative suite and refer to it before marking the patient. The incision provides most of the lifting in the central lip and tapers off laterally to a fine point at the lateral nostril. As the incision curves around the nostrils it is important to stay on the nasal sill and not in the nostril or too much below the sill or it will be more visible. When drawing the incision the surgeon should keep in mind that each transition of the upper limb is very curvilinear and the lower limb mirrors most of the upper incision and forms a fine tapered and upswept point at the terminus which is at the lateral nostril (Figure 53-19).

The patient must be marked in the upright position and before any local anaesthesia is administered. The procedure can be performed with local anesthesia, but like all cosmetic surgery procedures, I prefer intravenous sedation as a much smaller amount of local anaesthesia can be used which means less distortion of the markings and surgical site. Approximately 4 mL of 2% lidocaine with 1:100,000 adrenaline (epinephrine) is injected subcutaneously as well as deeper in the lip to ensure anesthesia and haemostasis. After the tissue becomes blanched, a number 15 scalpel blade is used to precisely outline the 'bullhorn' shape with care to follow the aforementioned guidelines. As soon as the outline is established, I prefer to use CO_2 laser, radiowave microneedle or radiowave bipolar forceps (Ellman International, Oceanview, NY) to bloodlessly remove the skin and subcutaneous tissue (Figure 53-20). If the goal is to simply shorten the lip, removing skin and some minor subcutaneous tissue will suffice. To achieve a noticeable difference, at least 6 mm of skin excision in the central lip is necessary. The average excision in my experience is 8 mm. Like any cosmetic procedure it is better to err on the conservative side as more tissue can always be excised. A skin only excision will also provide some bulk to the upper lip by rolling the lip upward and curling it back. If a greater

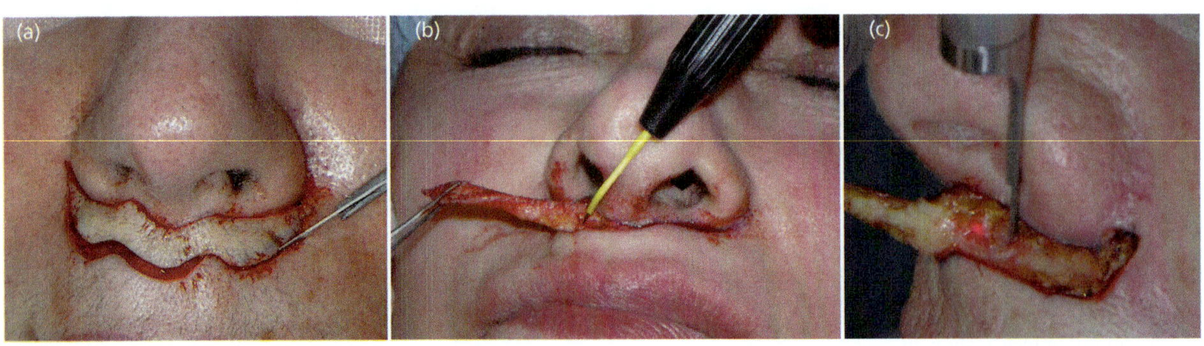

Fig. 53-20 Use of a CO_2 laser, radiowave microneedle or radiowave bipolar forceps to bloodlessly remove the skin and subcutaneous tissue.

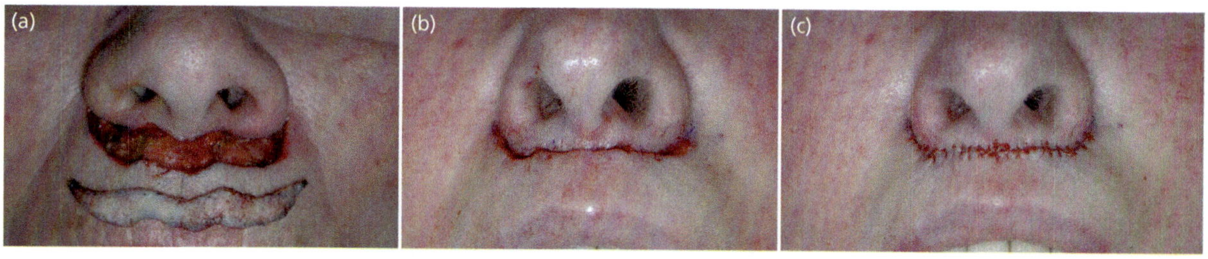

Fig. 53-21 The incision is shown before closure (a) with the subcutaneous sutures in place (b) and with the immediate final closure.

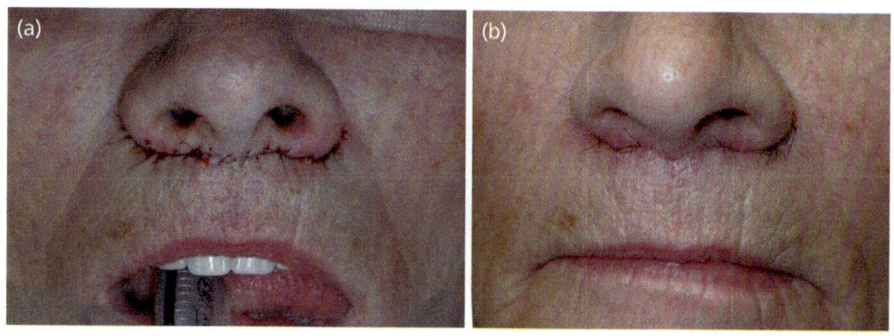

Fig. 53-22 This images show immediate closure with interrupted 6-0 nylon (a) and one week later (b).

degree of pout or 'roll up' is desired, a strip of deeper tissue, usually orbicularis oris, is also excised. The procedure is adjustable intraoperatively by paying attention to the amount of incision exposure during excision. If more incisal edge exposure is required, more skin is excised although it may not be a one to one relationship. When the desired excision is achieved, the area is rechecked for haemostasis and a 5-0 gut suture is placed subcutaneously in the midline and below each nostril. The tissue is thick in this area and easy edge approximation is achieved (Figure 53-21). Finally, interrupted or running closure is performed with a 6-0 nylon suture that remains in place for a week. Figure 53-22 shows a closure immediately and 7 days postoperatively. No dressing is necessary and patients are covered with antibiotic therapy.

The subnasal scar is usually very aesthetic, but all patients are offered CO_2 laser resurfacing, if they desire, at the six week period. Two high fluence, high density passes are made over the scar and this can greatly improve the problematic scar. Prophylactic CO_2 laser resurfacing can also be performed intraoperatively after the subcutaneous sutures but before the final closure (Figure 53-23).

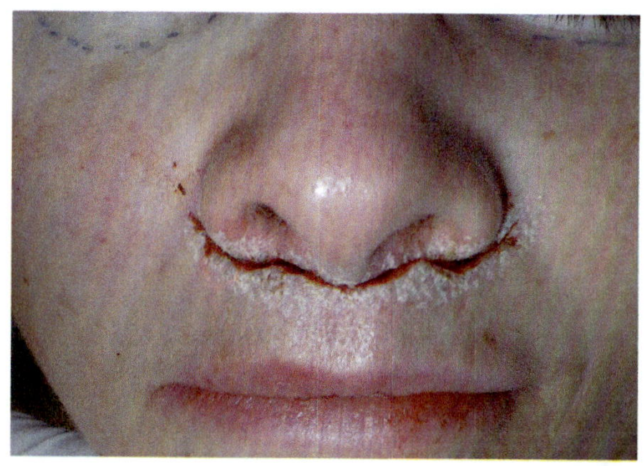

Fig. 53-23 Prophylactic CO_2 laser resurfacing can be performed at the initial surgery after the subcutaneous closure and before the final closure. This assists the wound healing and can proactively lessen scarring.

Figures 53-24 to 53-30 show before and after cases of the subnasal lip lift procedure. All pictures show improved lip/tooth aesthetics as well as improved position and volume. Many lip lift patients also desire further improvement with injectable fillers to even better showcase their new lips.

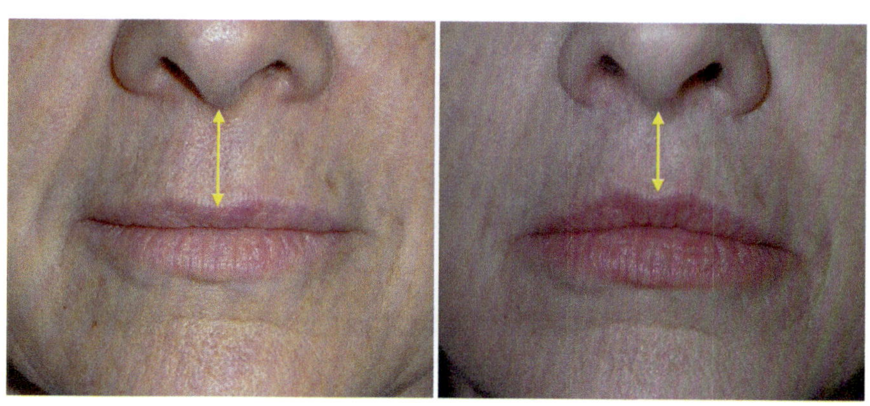

Fig. 53-24 This patient is shown before and after subnasal lip lift. The shortening of the upper lip is obvious. Note also how the 'bullhorn' pattern allows a better shaped upper lip where more lift is produce centrally and less laterally.

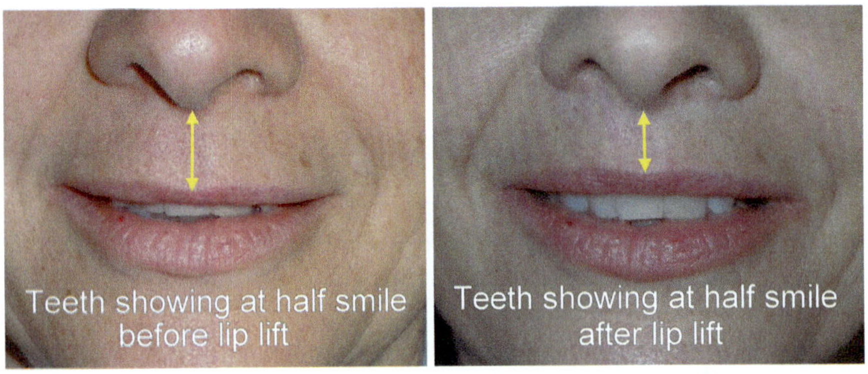

Fig. 53-25 The same patient in Figure 53-24 is shown here to illustrate the improvement in incisor show with partial smile.

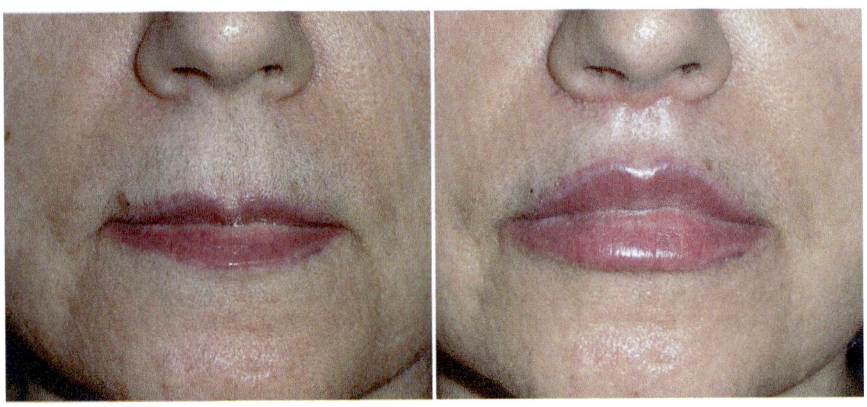

Fig. 53-26 This patient is shown before and 4 months after subnasal lip lift. Note the aesthetic scar.

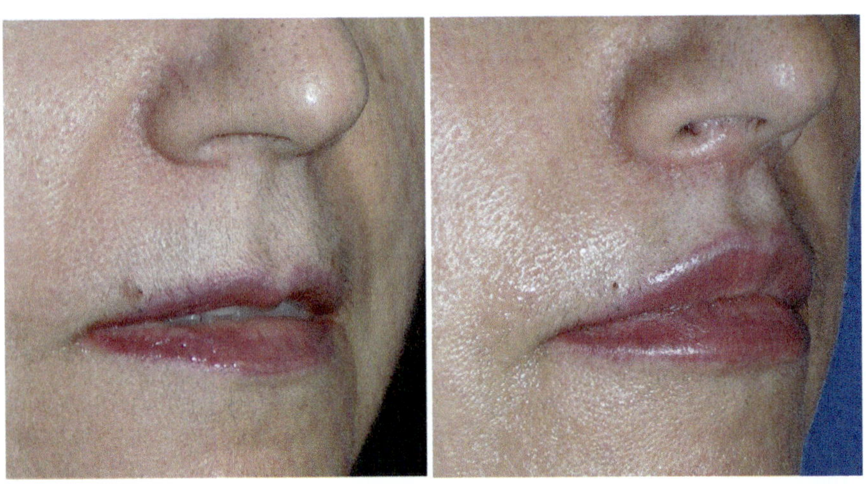

Fig. 53-27 This is another picture of the patient shown in Figure 53-26. Not only is the upper lip shortened, but the volume and 'pout' are improved from the shortening.

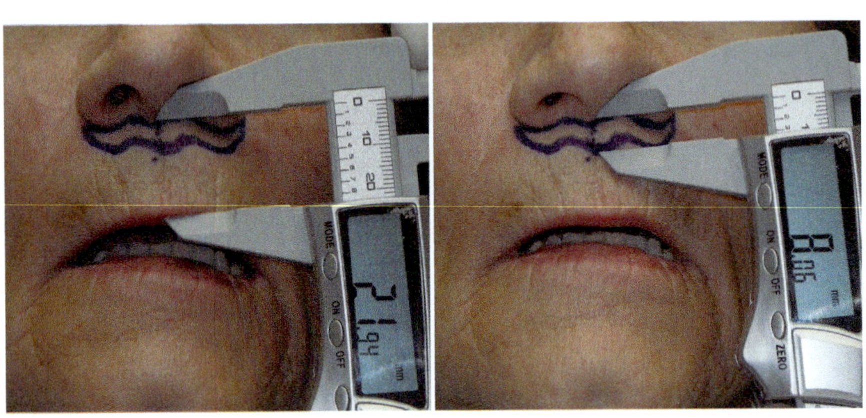

Fig. 53-28 This patient is shown preoperatively where the total lip height is 21.9 mm and the excision is 8 mm which equals a 36.5% reduction.

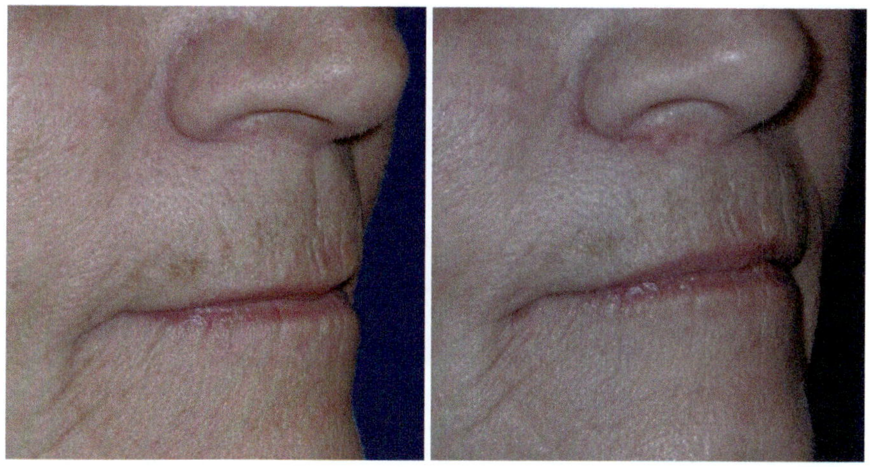

Fig. 53-29 The same patient shown in Figure 53-28 is shown before and after subnasal lip lift in the repose position.

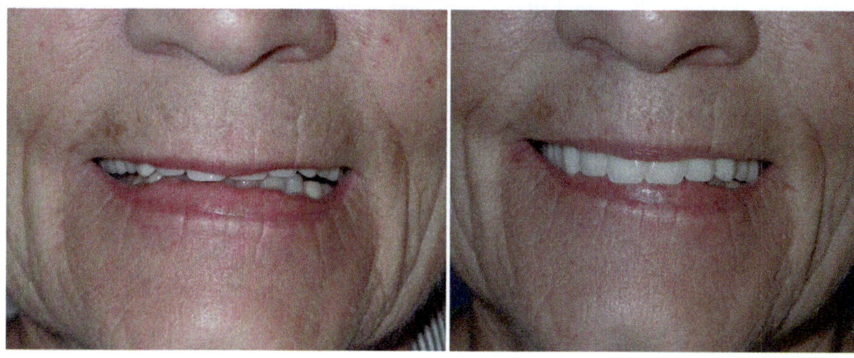

Fig. 53-30 The same patient shown in Figures 53-28 and 53-29 is shown smiling before and after subnasal lip lift. Not the increase in incisor exposure after the surgery.

Intraoral soft tissue surgery for excessive gingival display

A pleasing smile results from the harmony of the teeth, gingiva and lips but can be negatively affected by problems of any of the contributors including excessive long or short tooth crown height, short or long upper lip, maxilla or alveolus, large or small gingival band and hyper or hypoactivity of the lip elevator musculature. Singularly or a combination of these problems can lead to excessive gingival display which is generally considered to be unaesthetic by doctors and patients. In a sample of over 450 adults, aged 20 to 30 years, 7% of men and 14% of women were found to have a gummy smile.[37]

The average length of the maxillary lip is 20 to 22 mm in young adult females and 22 to 24 mm in young adult males. A congenitally short upper lip can contribute to excessive gingival display. During a full smile, the average upper lip mobility ranges from 7 to 8 mm.[37]

Hypermobility of the upper lip is caused by hyperfunction of the lip elevator muscles and can result in excessive gingival display.

Intraoral mucosal reduction is indicated for moderate reduction of excessive gingival exposure and is not indicated for extreme gingival show such as that seen with vertical maxillary excess. Class 1 gingival display is 1–4 mm, Class 2 display is 4–8 mm and Class 3 gingival display is greater than 8 mm. Mucosal reduction procedures are more appropriate for minor to moderate excess gingival display with normal maxillary length and normal lip length. With a normal length maxilla and a normal size lip, the diagnosis of lip elevator hypermobility is most relevant.

Several articles are commonly cited in relation to hypermobile lip treatment for excessive gingival display. Rubinstein and Kostianovsky[56] reports a technique that undermines the upper lip mucosa to allow further reduction and area to scar down while Humayun et al. did not undermine the upper lip mucosa.[37] In these procedures, the repositioned mucosal flap is used to reduce the excessive gingival display by shortening the vestibular (sulcular) depth (Figure 53-31).

There appears not to be any precise means of estimating the amount of mucosal reduction performed and some authors recommend excising two times the amount of the excess gingiva displayed at full smile while other reports advocate 10–20 mm of mucosa resection.[37]

The basis of these procedures consists of excising an ellipse of mucosa from several millimetres above the mucogingival junction superiorly towards the inferior part of the maxillary sulcus. Incisions can range from 10–20 mm and tapers off bilaterally into an acute angle at the second molar teeth. This taper is to prevent a dog ear deformity and gradually blend the incision where no significant vestibular reduction is required. At this point, some surgeons continue dissection to undermine the mucosa of the upper lip while others do not. After the mucosal ellipse is removed and haemostasis provided, the superior incision is advanced inferiorly

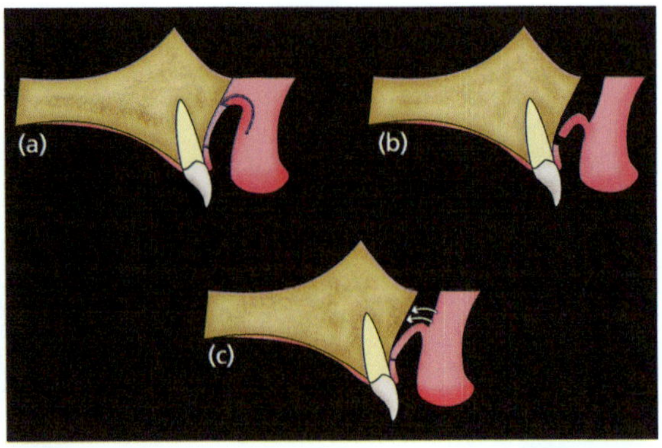

Fig. 53-31 This image shows a method of surgery to reduce upper lip mobilization when hypermobility of the upper lip is the primary aetiology of a 'gummy smile'.[56] (a) illustrates the amount of gingiva to be excised and the amount of lip to be undermined; (b) shows the wound after excision and the lip mucosa advanced and (c) shows the sutured flaps and the arrows represent the region that will scar down to the deeper tissues and assist in vestibular reduction and reduce elevation of the upper lip on smiling (from Naini FB. Facial Aesthetics: Concepts and Clinical Diagnosis. Oxford: Wiley-Blackwell, 2011; reprinted with permission).

and sutures to the mucogingival junction. Again the goal of this surgery is to shorten the depth of the maxillary vestibule to reduce the hypermobility of the lip elevators.

References

1 Niamtu J. Rejuvenation of the lip and Perioral Areas. In: Bell WH, Guerroro CA (Eds). Distraction Osteogenesis of the Facial Skeleton. BC Decker: Ontario, Canada, 2007.
2 Niamtu J. Advanta ePTFE Facial Implants in Cosmetic Facial Surgery J Oral Maxillofac Surg. 2006;64:543–9.
3 Niamtu J. Advanta facial implants. In: Minimally Invasive Cosmetic Surgery, Oral and Maxillofacial Surgery Clinics of North America 2005, 17:1, pp.29–39. Saunders: Philadelphia.
4 Niamtu J. The use of Restylane in cosmetic facial surgery. J Oral Maxillofac Surg. 2006;64:317–25.
5 Niamtu J. New lip and wrinkle fillers. In: Minimally Invasive Cosmetic Surgery. Oral and Maxillofacial Surgery Clinics of North America 2005, 17:1, pp.17–27. Saunders: Philadelphia.
6 Niamtu J. Injectable fillers. In: Niamtu J. Cosmetic Facial Surgery. Mosby Elsevier: St. Louis, 2011.
7 Niamtu J 3rd. Lip reduction surgery (reduction cheiloplasty). Facial Plast Surg Clin North Am. 2010;18:79–97.
8 Niamtu J. Lip reduction. In: Niamtu J. Cosmetic facial surgery. Mosby Elsevier: St. Louis, 2011.
9 Epker BN, Wolford LM. Reduction cheiloplasty: its role in the correction of dentofacial deformities. J Maxillofac Surg. 1977;5:134–41.
10 Dev VR, Wang P. Lip reduction. http://emedicine.medscape.com/article/1288624-overview Accessed 7.03.16.
11 Farkas LG. Anthropometry of the Head and Face in Medicine. Elsevier Science: NY, 1981.
12 Pierce HE. Cosmetic head and face surgery. In: Pierce HE (Ed.) Cosmetic Plastic Surgery in Nonwhite Patients. Grune and Stratton: New York, 1982.
13 El-Hakim M, Chauvin P. Orofacial granulomatosis presenting as persistent lip swelling: review of 6 new cases. J Oral Maxillofac Surg. 2004;62:1114–7.
14 Ali K. Ascher syndrome: a case report and review of the literature. Oral Surg Oral Med Oral Pathol. 2007;103:e26–8.
15 Fanous N, Brousseau VJ, Yoskovitch A. The 'bikini' lip reduction: an approach to oversized lips. Plast Reconstr Surg. 2008;122:23e–25e.
16 Hoffman S. A simple technique for mucosal irregularities of the lip. Plast Reconstr Surg. 1999;103:328.
17 Manstein CH. Vermilionectomy and mucosal advancement. Plast Reconstr Surg. 1997;100:1363.
18 O'Sullivan ST, O'Shaughnessy M. A simple technique for correction of mucosal irregularities of the lip. Plast Reconstr Surg. 1998;101:1146–7.
19 Cortés-Aroche S. Double lip treated with 'midmoon' incision. Report of a case. Rev Med Inst Mex Seguro Soc. 2007;45(3):277–80. [Spanish].
20 Pinto Rdos S, Marzola C. [Double lips – surgical technique]. Rev Assoc Paul Cir Dent. 1966;20:203–6. [Portuguese].
21 Kruse-Lösler B, Presser D, Metze D, Joos U. Surgical treatment of persistent macrocheilia in patients with Melkersson-Rosenthal syndrome and cheilitis granulomatosa. Arch Dermatol. 2005;141:1085–91.
22 Stucker FJ. Reduction cheiloplasty. An adjunctive procedure in the black rhinoplasty patient. Arch Otolaryngol Head Neck Surg. 1988;114:779–80.
23 Pierce HE. Cheiloplasty for redundant lips. J Natl Med Assoc. 1976;68:211–2.
24 Calnan J. Congenital double lip: record of a case with a note on the embryology. Br J Plast Surg. 1952;5:197–202.
25 Peck S, Peck L, Kataja M. The gingival smile line. Angle Orthod. 1992;62:91–100; discussion 101–102.
26 Perenack J: Treatment options to optimize display of anterior dental esthetics in the patient with the aged lip. J Oral Maxillofac Surg. 2005;63:1634–41.
27 Perenack JD, Biggerstaff T: Lip modification enhances aesthetic appearance. Atlas Oral Maxillofac Surg Clin North Am. 2006;14:51–74.
28 Holden PK, Sufyan AS, Perkins SW. Long-term analysis of surgical correction of the senile upper lip. Arch Facial Plast Surg. 2011;13:332–6.
29 Ramirez OM, Khan AS, Robertson KM. The upper lip lift using the 'bull's horn' approach. J Drugs Dermatol. 2003;2:303–6.
30 Rozner L, Isaacs GW. Lip lifting. Br J Plast Surg. 1981;34:481–4.
31 Felman G. Direct upper-lip lifting: a safe procedure. Aesthetic Plast Surg. 1993;17:291–5.
32 Penna V, Iblher N, Bannasch H, Stark GB. Proving the effectiveness of the lip lift for treatment of the aging lip: a morphometric evaluation. Plast Reconstr Surg. 2010;126:83e–4e.
33 Austin HW. The lip lift. Plast Reconstr Surg. 1986;77:990–4.
34 Guerrissi JO, Sanchez LI. An approach to the senile upper lip. Plast Reconstr Surg. 1993;92:1187.
35 Guerrissi JO. Surgical treatment of the senile upper lip. Plast Reconstr Surg. 2000;106:938–40.
36 Kamer FM. 'How I do it' – plastic surgery. Practical suggestions on facial plastic surgery. Smile surgery. Laryngoscope. 1979;89:1528–32.
37 Humayun N, Kolhatkar S, Souiyas J, Bhola M. Mucosal coronally positioned flap for the management of excessive gingival display in the presence of hypermobility of the upper lip and vertical maxillary excess: a case report. J Periodontol. 2010;81:1858–63.
38 Garber DA, Salama MA. The aesthetic smile: Diagnosis and treatment. Periodontol. 2000 1996;11:18–28.
39 Tjan AH, Miller GD, The JG. Some esthetic factors in a smile. J Prosthet Dent. 1984;51:24–8.
40 Robbins JW. Differential diagnosis and treatment of excess gingival display. Pract Periodont Aesthet Dent. 1999;11:265–72.
41 Ezquerra F, Berrazueta MJ, Ruiz-Capillas A, Arregui JS. New approach to the gummy smile. Plast Reconstr Surg. 1999;104:1143–50; discussion 1151–2.

42 Silberberg N, Goldstein M, Smidt A. Excessive gingival display – etiology, diagnosis, and treatment modalities. Quintessence Int. 2009;40:809–18.
43 Levine RA, McGuire M. The diagnosis and treatment of the gummy smile. Compend Contin Educ Dent. 1997;18:757–62, 764.
44 Polo M. Botulinum toxin type A (Botox) for the neuromuscular correction of excessive gingival display on smiling (gummy smile). Am J Orthod Dentofacial Orthop. 2008;133:195–203.
45 Niamtu J: Neurotoxins. In: Niamtu J. Cosmetic Facial Surgery. Mosby Elsevier: St. Louis, 2011.
46 Niamtu J. Botox injections for gummy smiles. Am J Orthod Dentofacial Orthop. 2008;133:782–3; author reply 783–4.
47 Niamtu J. More on Botox treatment. Am J Orthod Dentofacial Orthop. 2005;127:645–6.
48 Sucupira E, Abramovitz A. A simplified method for smile enhancement: botulinum toxin injection for gummy smile. Plast Reconstr Surg. 2012;130:726–8.
49 Mangano A, Mangano A. Current strategies in the treatment of gummy smile using botulinum toxin type A. Plast Reconstr Surg. 2012;129:1015e.
50 Gupta KK, Srivastava A, Singhal R, Srivastava S. An innovative cosmetic technique called lip repositioning. J Indian Soc Periodontol. 2010;14:266–9.
51 Marangos D. Treating the gummy smile. Dent Today. 2011;30:132, 134, 136.
52 Polo M. Myotomy of the levator labii superioris muscle and lip repositioning: a combined approach for the correction of gummy smile. Plast Reconstr Surg. 2011;127:2121–2; author reply 2123–4.
53 Mazzuco R, Hexsel D. Gummy smile and botulinum toxin: a new approach based on the gingival exposure area. J Am Acad Dermatol. 2010;63:1042–51.
54 Simon Z, Rosenblatt A, Dorfman W. Eliminating a gummy smile with surgical lip repositioning. Cosmet Dent. 2007;23:100–108.
55 Miskinyar SA. A new method for correcting a gummy smile. Plast Reconstr Surg. 1983;72:397–400.
56 Rubinstein AM, Kostianovsky AS. Cosmetic surgery for the malformation of the laugh: Original technique (in Spanish). Prensa Med Argent. 1973;60:952.
57 Rosenblatt A, Simon Z. Lip repositioning for reduction of excessive gingival display: A clinical report. Int J Periodontics Restorative Dent. 2006;26:433–7.
58 Litton C, Fournier P. Simple surgical correction of the gummy smile. Plast Reconstr Surg. 1979;63:372–3.
59 Júnior NV, Campos TV, Rodrigues JG, Martins TM, Silva CO. Treatment of excessive gingival display using a modified lip repositioning technique. Ribeiro-Int J Periodontics Restorative Dent. 2013;33:309–14.
60 Cairo F, Graziani F, Franchi L, Defraia E, Pini Prato GP. Periodontal plastic surgery to improve aesthetics in patients with altered passive eruption/gummy smile: a case series study. Int J Dent. 2012;2012:doi: 837658.

Section 3: Orthognathic Surgery in the Cleft Patient and Orthognathic Aspects of Craniofacial Surgery

Chapter 54

Introduction: Craniofacial Surgery

Jesse A. Taylor and Scott P. Bartlett

Craniofacial surgery is the art of normalizing the form and function of the bones and soft tissues of the head and neck. The birth of the specialty in modern times is Tessier's original description of moving the orbits via an intracranial approach, demonstrating its feasibility and relative safety.[1] Tessier pioneered many of the standard approaches to the orbit and began teaching these techniques to the 'second generation' surgeons – Marchac (Paris), Whitaker (Philadelphia), Ortiz-Monasterio (Mexico City), Munro (Toronto), McCarthy (New York), Jackson (Michigan), and Salyer (Dallas).[1] Each of the 'second generation' has made enormous contributions to the field, none more important than the introduction of orbito-cranial techniques in young children.[2]

As in other areas of medicine that are new, the second generation's task was both creative, i.e. the introduction of new techniques, and also normative, developing an understanding of operative indications, optimal timing of surgery, perioperative safety, and development of measurement tools. The second generation wrote an early textbook to describe techniques, *Atlas of Craniomaxillofacial Surgery*,[3] and they defined complications in various transcranial operations.[4] The second generation began the process of working through these complex topics, and have handed off the baton to subsequent generations of craniofacial surgeons whose task will be to continue the evolutionary process.

Current trends in craniofacial surgery include minimization of operative blood loss, improved perioperative safety profile, earlier return to school/work, and minimizing surgery's footprint via minimally invasive techniques. The 1990s brought about the advent of craniofacial distraction osteogenesis, allowing for larger movements and improved adaptation of soft tissues. McCarthy is credited with the first mandibular distraction,[5] and the technique has now been applied to all areas of the craniofacial skeleton. Multiple authors have recently demonstrated that cranial vault distraction, and specifically posterior cranial vault distraction, leads to greater volumetric increases, lower perioperative morbidity, improved bony stability, and potentially improved growth characteristics in treating syndromic craniosynostosis.[6,7]

Technological advances in imaging have been behind the scenes of every major surgical advancement, allowing better visualization of pre-, intra-, and postoperative phenotypic changes. Imaging modalities have also found their way into the operating room, where CT-guided operative osteotomies, as well as computer-aided design and modelling, or 'CAD/CAM', allow the surgeon to pre-plan osteotomies, develop preoperatively a 'cutting guide' and 'placement guide', and create stereolithographic models for planning, pre-bending of fixation plates, and creation of intra-operative splints in orthognathic surgery.[8] The next phase in the CAD/CAM revolution must be a clear demonstration, based on real data, that it is cost-effective and truly beneficial. In the craniofacial literature, it has led to shorter operative times, increased accuracy of osteotomies, and increased accuracy of fixation; there have been several retrospective looks at cost-benefit analyses as well, but the appropriate indications for CAD/CAM surgery are still being defined.[9]

The future of craniofacial surgery, at least in the near-term, will be shaped by the introduction and proliferation of new modalities. As prenatal diagnosis of congenital deformity, either through intra-uterine imaging with MRI or ultrasound, becomes standard-of-care, there may be an increase in fetal terminations and a decrease in the number of complex congenital craniofacial cases.[10] Prenatal diagnostic modalities may also open the door for intervening prenatally with some form of fetal surgery. Tissue engineering,

Orthognathic Surgery: Principles, Planning and Practice. Edited by Farhad B. Naini and Daljit S. Gill.

or the ability to create complex tissues ex-vivo, carry the promise of truly replacing 'like with like'. As we learn more about tissue scaffolds, growth factors, and stem cells, we may be able to apply these exciting technologies to age-old unsolved clinical problems. For instance, the largely unsolved problem of temporomandibular joint (TMJ) ankylosis which is plagued by high treatment failure rates, may benefit from the ability to replace scarred tissues with healthy, vascularized engineered joint replacements.[11] Other difficult problems whose solution may lie in tissue engineering include the Treacher Collins midfacial deficiency, soft tissue deficiency in hemifacial microsomia, and early paediatric cranioplasty.

Equally promising is the field of vascularized composite tissue allotransplantation, or as it would be applied in the head and neck, 'face transplant'. Modern immunosuppression has allowed for safe transfer of the craniofacial skeleton and overlying soft tissues in cases where conventional reconstructive techniques have fallen short.[12,13] Cost, the morbidity of long-term immunosuppression, a deficiency in donor grafts, and lack of widespread expertise have hampered the advancement of this nascent field. Many centres though, realizing the immense potential and promise of this emerging technology, have begun multidisciplinary teams to investigate its use in craniofacial surgery. It would not be difficult to imagine a future in which hundreds, or even thousands, of face transplants are done each year, especially if the 'holy grail' of immune tolerance is achieved.[14]

At its heart, craniofacial surgery seeks to normalize those structures that are at the core of our 'self-image'.[15] Our self-image develops early in life, and is likely a combination of our own view of our appearance when we look in a mirror, and the reactions of others to our appearance. A strong self-image allows for confident relationship building in an uninhibited fashion; conversely, a poor self-image secondary to post-traumatic or congenital deformity may impair one's ability to form relationships, potentially leading to isolation.[15] Perhaps the father of plastic surgery, Gaspare Tagliacozzi, said it best: 'We restore, repair, and make whole those parts which fortune has taken away, not so much that they delight the eyes but that they may buoy up the spirit and help the mind of the beset.'[16] It is this interplay between anatomy, physiology, and psychology that cannot be emphasized enough.

References

1 Oritz-Monasterio F. Notes on the history of craniofacial surgery. In: Jackson IT, Munro IR, Salyer KE, et al, eds. Atlas of Craniomaxillofacial Surgery. St. Louis: Mosby, 1982:vii–xii.

2 Whitaker LA, Schut L, Kerr LP. Early surgery for isolated craniofacial dysostosis. Improvement and possible prevention of increasing deformity. Plast Reconstr Surg. 1977;60:575–81.

3 Jackson IT, Munro IR, Salyer KE, et al. (Eds). Atlas of Craniomaxillofacial Surgery. St. Louis: Mosby, 1982.

4 Whitaker LA, Munro IR, Salyer KE, et al. Combined report of problems and complications in 793 craniofacial operations. Plast Reconstr Surg. 1979;64:198–203.

5 McCarthy JG, Schreiber J, Karp N, Thorne CH, Grayson BH. Lengthening the human mandible by gradual distraction. Plast Reconstr Surg. 1992;89:1–8.

6 Steinbacher DM, Skirpan J, Puchala J, Bartlett SP. Expansion of the posterior cranial vault using distraction osteogenesis. Plast Reconstr Surg. 2011;127:792–801.

7 Taylor JA, Derderian CA, Bartlett SP, Fiadjoe JE, Sussman EM, Stricker PA. Perioperative morbidity in posterior cranial vault expansion: distraction osteogenesis versus conventional osteotomy. Plast Reconstruct Surg. 2012;129:674e–80e.

8 Seruya M, Borsuk DE, Khalifian S, Carson BS, Dalesio NM, Dorafshar AH. Computer-aided design and manufacturing in craniosynostosis surgery. J Craniofac Surg. 2013;24: 1100–5.

9 Hanasono MM, Skoracki RJ. Computer-assisted design and rapid prototype modeling in microvascular mandible reconstruction. Laryngoscope. 2013;123:597–604.

10 Mirsky DM, Shekdar KV, Bilaniuk LT. Fetal MRI: head and neck. Magn Reson Imaging Clin N Am. 2012;20:605–18.

11 Murphy MK, MacBarb RF, Wong ME, Athanasiou KA. Temporomandibular disorders: a review of etiology, clinical management, and tissue engineering strategies. Int J Oral Maxillofac Implants. 2013;28:e393–414.

12 Dorafshar AH, Brazio PS, Mundinger GS, Mohan R, Brown EN, Rodriguez ED. Found in space: computer-assisted orthognathic alignment of a total face allograft in six degrees of freedom. J Oral Maxillofac Surg. 2014;72:1788–800.

13 Coffman KL, Siemionow MZ. Ethics of facial transplantation revisited. Curr Opin Organ Transplant. 2014;19:181–7.

14 Kumamaru KK, Sisk GC, Mitsouras D, Schultz K, Steigner ML, George E, Enterline DS, Bueno EM, Pomahac B, Rybicki FJ. Vascular communications between donor and recipient tissues after successful full face transplantation. Am J Transplant. 2014;14:711–9.

15 Masnari O, Landolt MA, Roessler J, Weingaertner SK, Neuhaus K, Meuli M, Schiestl C. Self- and parent-perceived stigmatisation in children and adolescents with congenital or acquired facial differences. J Plast Reconstr Aesthet Surg. 2012;65:1664–70.

16 Goldwyn RM. Psychological Aspects of Plastic Surgery: A Surgeon's Observations and Reflections. In: Sarwer DB, Pruzinsky T, Cash TF, Goldwyn RM, Persing JA, Whitaker LA (Eds). Psychological Aspects of Reconstructive and Cosmetic Plastic Surgery. London: Lippincott Williams and Wilkins, 2005.

Chapter 55

Developmental Disorders of the Craniofacial Complex

Martyn T. Cobourne and David P. Rice

Introduction

The human face is infinite in the individual variation that is seen, both between and within different ethnic groups. We acquire the ability to recognize different faces from an early age and the perception of facial beauty has an important influence upon human social behaviour. Within the face, the lips play an integral role in communication, social interaction and feeding; whilst the hard and soft palate are required for speech, mastication and swallowing. Acquired defects within these regions are surprisingly common and the manifestations of perturbed development can remain for a lifetime, significantly influencing the social and psychological well-being of affected individuals. Here, we will briefly review some common disorders of human craniofacial development, focusing on the clinical features and molecular basis of these varied conditions. We have used HUGO Gene Nomenclature Committee[1] assigned names for human genes and include reference numbers for syndromic conditions from the Mendelian Inheritance in Man (MIM) catalogue of human genes and disorders database.[2]

Orthognathic Surgery: Principles, Planning and Practice. Edited by Farhad B. Naini and Daljit S. Gill.

Development of the craniofacial region

The foundations of the human head are laid down within a short period of a few weeks early in embryogenesis. The skeletal elements of this region are derived primarily from cranial neural crest cells; with the musculature originating from the somites, cranial paraxial and prechordal mesoderm; skin, oral mucosa and sensory placodes from the ectoderm and glands of the neck from mesoderm and endoderm. The developmental processes that create the mature structures of the craniofacial region are dynamic, relying upon complex tissue interactions that are closely co-ordinated, both temporally and spatially.[3–5]

Growth and development of the face is strongly influenced by neural crest migration and proliferation, which directs the formation and approximation of a series of swellings or processes. Ultimately, these processes meet and fuse with each other to produce seamless regions of union and the characteristic features of a face. At the molecular level, a host of signalling molecules, transcription factors and extracellular matrix proteins control these cellular activities and underpin this complex process.[6]

Embryonic development of the face

Human facial development begins at approximately four weeks post-conception and is dominated by the appearance of five processes, which surround the early oral cavity or stomodeum. These consist of the frontonasal process and paired derivatives of the first branchial arch, the maxillary and mandibular processes. During the fourth week of development the frontonasal process rapidly enlarges as the underlying forebrain expands into bilateral cerebral hemispheres and the paired mandibular processes unite to provide continuity to the forbearer of the lower jaw and lip.

By five weeks, two further thickenings appear within the enlarged frontonasal process, the medial and lateral nasal processes, which surround paired early ectodermal thickenings or nasal placodes. These placodes give rise to highly specialized olfactory receptor cells and nerve fibre bundles, which will innervate the future nasal cavity. As the medial and lateral nasal processes enlarge, the nasal placodes sink to produce nasal pits, which begin to demarcate the nares of the future nose.

Medial growth of the maxillary processes dominates subsequent development of the face, resulting first in contact and then fusion with the lateral nasal processes to form the nasolacrimal duct, cheek and alar base of the nose. Further growth of the maxillary process towards the midline pushes the lateral nasal processes superiorly and allows fusion of the maxillary processes with the medial nasal processes inferiorly, merging them together in the midline to form the central portion of the nose, upper lip philtrum and primary palate. Thus, the upper lip is formed from the maxillary processes laterally and the medial nasal processes in the midline (Figure 55-1a–c).[7]

Embryonic development of the secondary palate

In the developing embryo, the primary palate containing the future incisor teeth contributes to the hard palate anterior to the incisive canal. The secondary palate, consisting of the hard palate posterior to the incisive canal and the soft palate, forms from the paired palatine processes derived from the maxillary process (Figure 55-1d–i). Initially, these processes descend vertically as they grow, lying adjacent to the developing tongue in the floor of the early oral cavity. However, subsequent growth and elevation of these shelves in conjunction with simultaneous inferior and forward movement of the early mandible and tongue, results in them acquiring a position above the tongue. Further growth of the palatine shelves towards the midline results first in their contact and then fusion with each other.[8] They also fuse with the nasal septum superiorly and the primary palate anteriorly; sealing and separating the oral and nasal cavities. Together, the essential structures of the human face and oral cavity have formed by eight weeks of development.

Oro-facial clefting

Clefts involving the lip with or without the palate (CLP) or isolated clefts of the palate (CP) are some of the commonest congenital anomalies to affect the craniofacial region in man. Their aetiological basis is complex and reflects a failure of the normal mechanisms involved during early embryological development of the face.[9–14] CLP and CP are distinct conditions, but they can both be broadly subdivided into syndromic and non-syndromic forms. In syndromic cases, the cleft phenotype occurs in association with deficits or structural abnormalities in other regions of the body,[11,15] whilst non-syndromic clefting occurs in isolation, unassociated with any other recognizable anomalies. CLP can range from simple notching or isolated clefting of the upper lip with or without involvement of the alveolus, to a complete unilateral or bilateral cleft of the lip, alveolus and hard/soft palate. CP can also present with a variable phenotype, ranging from a simple submucous cleft or lack of muscular continuity across the palate, to a bifid uvula or frank complete cleft involving hard and soft palates (Figure 55-2a–f).

A child born with CLP requires complex long-term treatment, depending upon the severity of the cleft, and there are often lifelong implications for affected individuals. These can extend beyond the significant functional and psychosocial effects afforded by a facial handicap. There is also increasing evidence that CLP can have a direct association with premature mortality,[16] psychiatric problems,[17] and carcinoma.[18] The

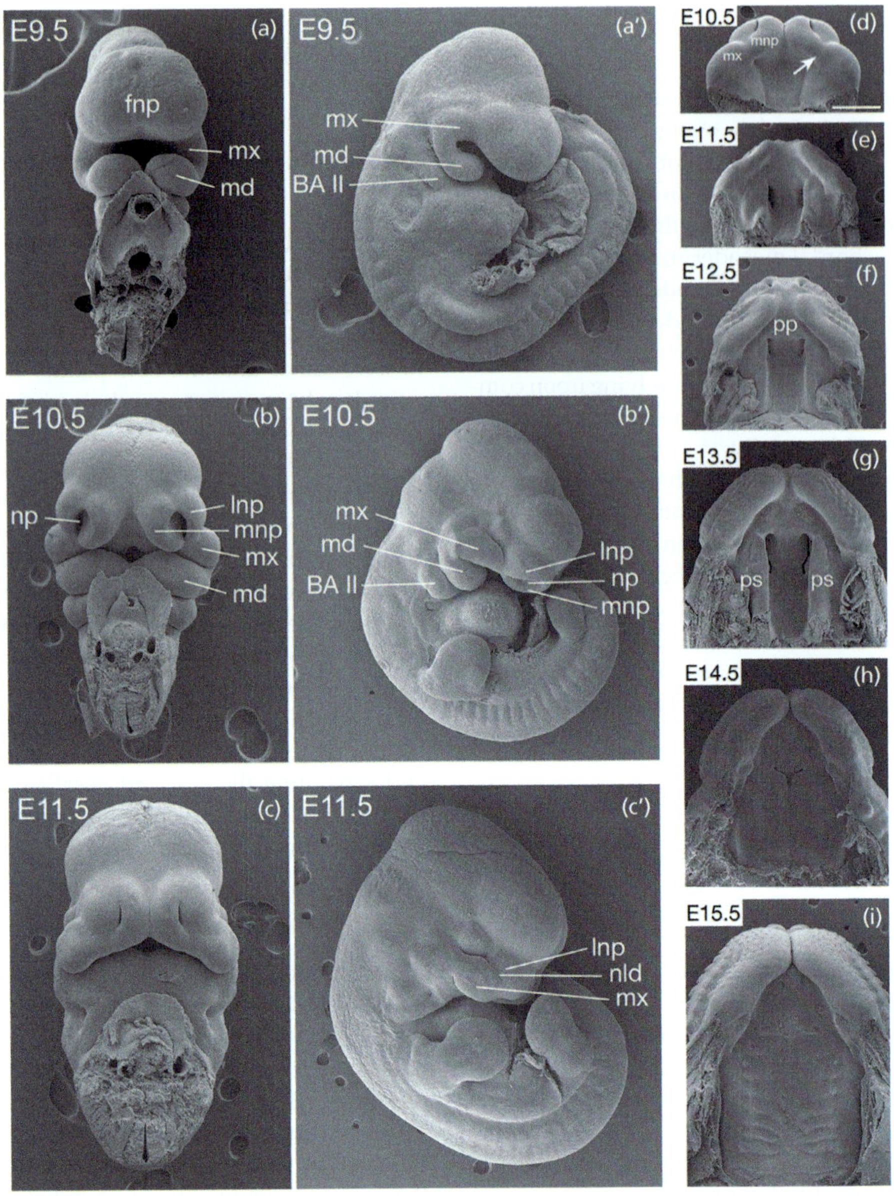

Fig. 55-1 Facial and palatal development in the mouse embryo. Facial development. (a, a′) At embryonic day (e) 9.5 the early oral cavity is surrounded by the fronto-nasal process superiorly, the paired maxillary processes laterally and the mandibular process inferiorly; (b, b′) At E10.5 the paired mesial nasal processes and lateral nasal processes have formed adjacent to the nasal pits and medial growth of the maxillary processes results in fusion with the lateral nasal process to form the outer part of the upper lip and alar of the nose; (c, c′) By E11.5, further medial growth of the maxillary processes produces fusion with the medial nasal process in the midline and their approximation to form the philtrum of the upper lip and central portion of the nose. Medial growth of the maxillary process and fusion with the medial nasal process is a key feature of facial development and is illustrated from below in d, e (the arrow delineates the point of fusion between maxillary and medial nasal process). (d–f) Development of the palate from E9.5–15.5. The primary palate is a product of the medial nasal processes. The secondary palate is derived from the palatine shelves of the maxillary processes. Medial growth of the palatine shelves results in their fusion together in the midline, in addition to fusion superiorly with the nasal septum and anteriorly with the primary palate (d–i). BAII, branchial arch II; fnp, fronto-nasal process; lnp, lateral nasal process; md, mandibular process; mnp, medial nasal process; mx, maxillary process; nld, nasolacrimal duct; np, nasal pit; pp, primary palate; ps, palatal shelf; ul, upper lip.

principles of treatment are to establish good facial appearance, good function during speech, eating and swallowing, and good hearing. If these objectives are achieved, they maximize the chances of an affected child growing up and developing normally within their social environment. The clinical management of children born with CLP is most effective when carried out by a fully integrated team, in a unit treating a high volume of patients.[19,20]

Epidemiology

In Caucasians, CLP is seen in approximately 1:700 live births, but demonstrates ethnic variation, being more common in Asians (1:500) and rarer in those of African descent (1:2500). Males are more commonly affected than females by a ratio of approximately 2:1 and in around 80% of cases, CLP is unilateral with a left-sided predominance. Around 70% of CLP cases are

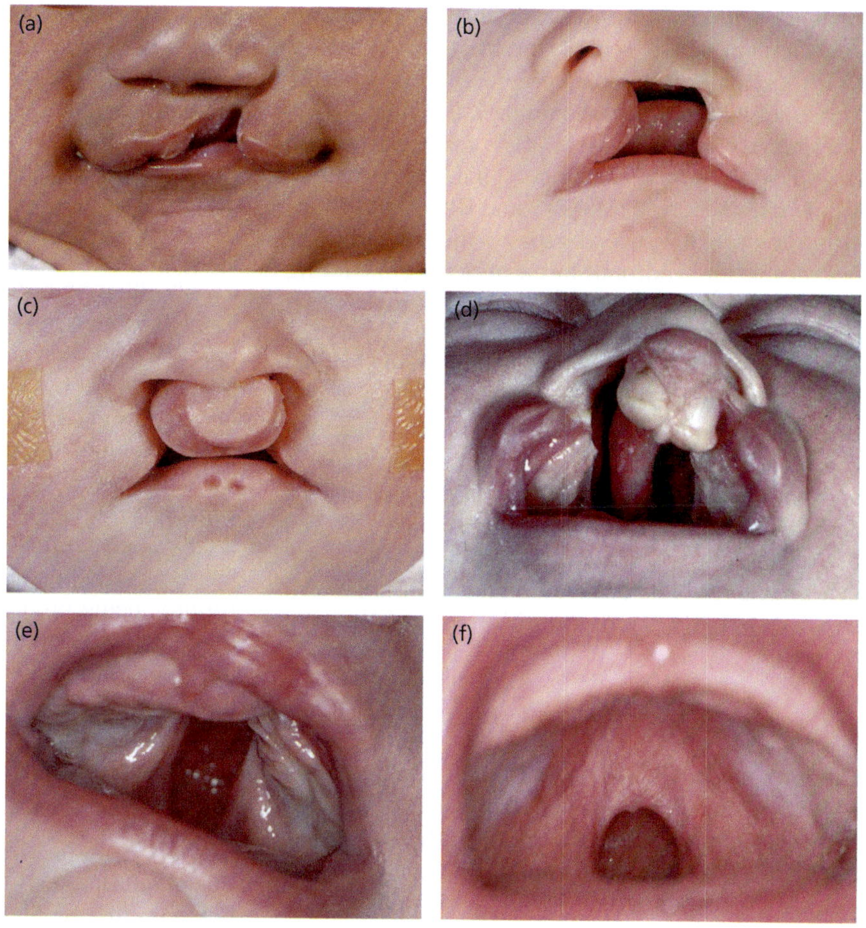

Fig. 55-2 Human facial clefting. (a) Isolated cleft lip; (b) Unilateral cleft lip and palate; (c) Bilateral cleft lip and palate in association with van der Woude syndrome (note bilateral lower lip pits); (d) Bilateral cleft lip and palate with marked displacement across the cleft; (e) Isolated cleft palate; (f) Isolated cleft of the soft palate.

non-syndromic and therefore occur in isolation, in children that are otherwise normal and healthy.

In contrast, CP is less common than CLP, seen in around 1:2000 live births and having no significant racial differences. Females are more commonly affected than males by a ratio of approximately 4:1 and only around half of cases are non-syndromic.

Molecular genetics

The identification of genes or chromosomal regions associated with syndromic forms of CLP and CP has often been achieved through linkage analysis of affected family pedigrees or direct sequencing of candidate regions suggested by an individual expression pattern or phenotype derived from an animal model. Significant progress has been made in elucidating the genetic basis of some Mendelian syndromes associated with CLP. In particular, identification of mutations in interferon regulatory factor 6 (*IRF6*) responsible for the van der Woude (#119300) and popliteal pterygum (#119500) syndromes,[21] muscle segment homeobox 1 (*MSX1*) responsible for a form of CLP or CP associated with tooth agenesis (#106600),[22] poliovirus receptor-related 1 (*PVRL1*) for CLP/ectodermal dysplasia (#225060),[23] tumor protein p63 (*TP63)* for a variety of mixed-clefting syndromes associated with ectodermal dysplasia,[24–27] and midline 1 (*MID1*) in Opitz syndrome (#300552).[28] Given that over 300 syndromes incorporate CLP as part of their phenotypic spectrum, the task of elucidating all the causal genes is a large one. Similarly, many syndromic forms of CP are also associated with single gene mutations or chromosomal rearrangements that have been discovered by similar methods of genetic analysis.

The aetiology and pathogenesis of the more common non-syndromic or isolated variants of CLP and CP are less well understood. This is a reflection of the multifactorial nature of these conditions, being the result of genetic and environmental interactions affecting development of the facial region at specific time-points during embryogenesis. A clear familial tendency does exist, the sibling risk for CLP is approximately 30 times higher in affected families than that for a normal population,[29] but there is no clearly recognizable mode of inheritance for isolated clefting.[30] It has been estimated that up to 14 different genetic loci may be involved in non-syndromic CLP,[31] either acting alone or in combination with other genes;[32,33] which means that very large and genetically pure sample sizes are required for identification.[30] Despite these difficulties, progress has been made,[13] and mutations in a number of loci have now been demonstrated, which together may account for up to a quarter of the non-syndromic clefting cases seen.[34] These loci harbour genes from many different families, which in many cases, encode proteins with established roles during embryonic development. These include Fibroblast Growth Factor (FGF) proteins and their receptors,[34] the tyrosine kinase inhibitor sprouty homolog 2 (SPRY2),[35] transcription factors such as MSX1,[36] forkhead box E1 (FOXE1), GLI family zinc finger 2 (GLI2) and muscle segment homeobox 2 (MSX2)[35] and IRF6.[37] It is interesting to note that several genes demonstrated to be responsible for syndromic forms of clefting, including *IRF6*,[37] *MSX1*,[36] and *PVRL1*,[38] have also proved to be important in the aetiology of isolated clefts.[30,39]

An increased maternal or paternal age has also been shown to contribute to isolated CLP risk,[40] and there are also known environmental causative factors, including maternal exposure to cigarette smoke,[41] and pharmacological agents such as anticonvulsants and steroids.[42] In many cases of isolated clefting, the phenotype arises from the combined effect of a genetic susceptibility and environmental insult, which is active at a particular time during the developmental process.

Holoprosencephaly

Holoprosencephaly (HPE) (#236100) is a clinically heterogeneous developmental field defect of the central nervous system (CNS), in which the embryonic forebrain fails to divide into distinct halves. It is the commonest structural anomaly of human brain development and in the most severe alobar form, the forebrain remains as a single undivided vesicle and there is cyclopia, with a single midline eye situated below a rudimentary nose or proboscis (Figure 55-3).[43] The incidence of HPE in first trimester pregnancies is around 1:250, making it one of the commonest causes of early miscarriage;[44] however, there is wide variation in severity, even amongst members of the same pedigree, which results in a live birth rate of around 1:8000.[45] The vast majority of HPE subtypes have facial anomalies, which also present with varying degrees of severity and include cyclopia, hypotelorism, premaxillary agenesis, cleft palate and solitary median maxillary central incisor (SMMCI). Moreover, microforms of HPE can also occur, presenting with normal brain anatomy but varying midline facial defects.[46]

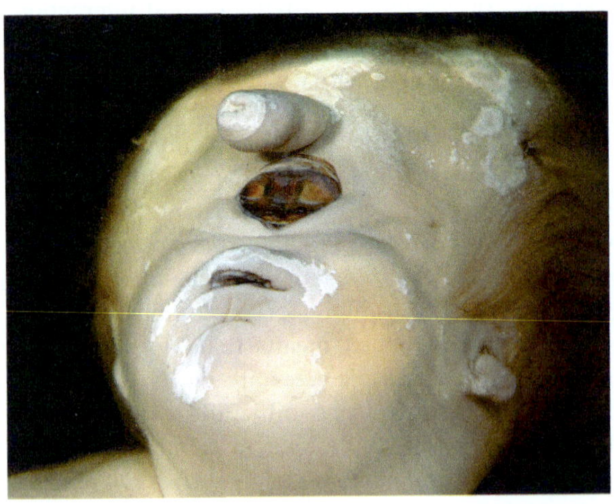

Fig. 55-3 Alobar holoprosencephaly. Alobar holoprosencephaly in a human fetus. Note the cyclopia and midline proboscis. (Courtesy of the Gordon Museum, King's College London.)

Molecular genetics

In humans, most cases of HPE are sporadic and caused by chromosomal abnormalities or syndromic disorders,[47] although both genetic and environmental factors have being implicated in the etiology of this disorder.[48] Syndromic forms of HPE are usually the most severe, with those that do survive generally having non-syndromic HPE. Currently, 14 dominant loci have been identified in association with non-syndromic HPE, encoding proteins within the Bone Morphogenetic Protein (BMP), Fibroblast Growth Factor (FGF), Nodal and Hedgehog pathways.[49,50] Amongst these, Sonic hedgehog (Shh) signalling is a major contributor, being produced in mesendoderm of the prechordal plate and required reiteratively for early forebrain subdivision and facial development. $Shh^{-/-}$ mice have alobar HPE and are cyclopic (Figure 55-4); whilst mutations in human *SHH* and other pathway members can cause both familial and sporadic HPE.[51,52]

Fetal alcohol syndrome

The manifestations of fetal exposure to maternal alcohol were first highlighted in the early 1970s,[53,54] and include both pre- and postnatal growth deficiencies, varying levels of developmental delay, mental retardation and facial anomalies, which are collectively described as the Fetal Alcohol Syndrome (FAS) (Table 55-1). The features of this condition are primarily related to the amount of alcohol ingested during pregnancy, but are also known to be influenced by other factors, including maternal age, socioeconomic status, ethnic background and underlying genetics.[55] The facial features associated with FAS include flattening of the lip philtrum, thinning of the upper lip and narrowing of the palpebral fissures. Within the CNS, FAS can induce features of HPE, including microcephaly and impaired separation of the forebrain and there is evidence from mouse models that ethanol can act as a modifier for HPE in combination with alterations in hedgehog signalling.[56]

Ectodermal dysplasia

The ectodermal dysplasias (ED) are a heterogeneous group of conditions characterised primarily by defects in the teeth, hair, nails and sweat glands.[57] Well over 100 different types of ED have been described, with hypohidrotic or anhidrotic (HED) forms occurring most frequently. Amongst these, X-linked-HED (XL-HED; #305100) is the commonest variant, with affected males having sparse, lightly pigmented hair, hypoplastic or aplastic sweat glands, nails that can be split, dystrophic or abnormally keratinized and tooth agenesis, which can affect both the primary and

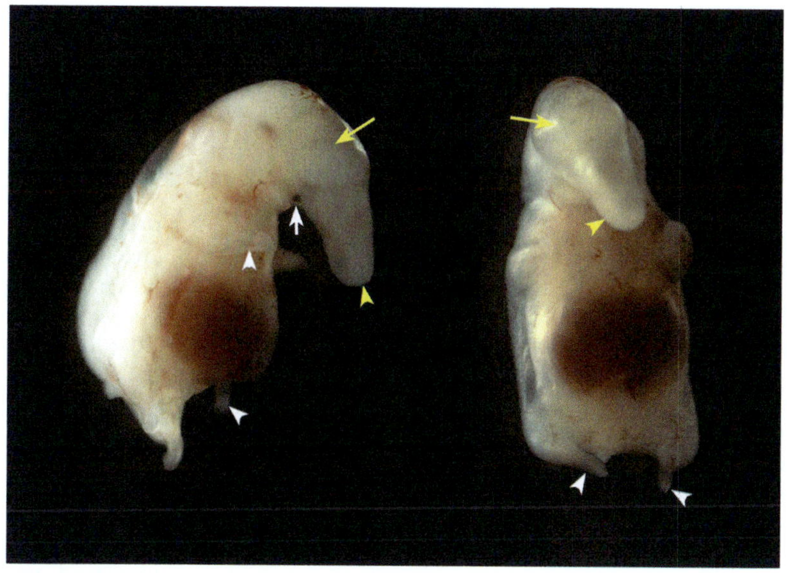

Fig. 55-4 Alobar holoprosencephaly in mice lacking sonic hedgehog function. Mice generated with targeted deletion in the sonic hedgehog gene have alobar holoprosencephaly. The forebrain is small and lacks division (yellow arrow), whilst the rudimentary face is dominated by a large midline proboscis (yellow arrowhead). There is a single eye in the midline situated below the proboscis (white arrow). Note also the absence of limb development (white arrowheads).

secondary dentitions. The teeth that do form are often small and abnormally shaped. The reduced number of functioning sweat glands means that HED subjects lack the ability to sweat correctly (hypohidrosis), which results in impaired temperature regulation that can be life-threatening. Female carriers in the heterozygous state can also be affected by XL-HED, but the clinical features are generally less severe. Autosomal recessive-HED is clinically very similar to XL-HED, with both males and females exhibiting the full spectrum of anomalies.

Molecular genetics

HED is caused by disruption to ectodysplasin A (EDA) signalling, which is a component of the large Tumour Necrosis Factor (TNF) superfamily.[58] The TNF pathway is active in organs that develop via reciprocal signalling between epithelial and mesenchymal tissues, such as sweat glands, mammary glands, hair follicles and teeth, and is essential for their development. EDA signalling occurs through binding of EDA to the TNF ectodysplasin A receptor (EDAR), which results in recruitment of an EDAR-associated death domain protein (EDARRAD).[59] EDARRAD acts as an adapter protein within the cell cytoplasm, interacting with a number of molecules, which ultimately mediate activation of transcription factor complex nuclear factor-κB [NF-κB] signalling. XL-HED is caused by mutation in *EDA*,[60,61] whilst mutation in *EDAR* and *EDARADD* can cause both AD-HED and AR-HED.[59,62]

Table 55-1 Features of fetal alcohol syndrome

Prenatal growth deficiency
Postnatal growth deficiency
Microcephaly
Developmental delay
Fine motor dysfunction
Facial dysmorphology
Short palpebral fissures
Long, smooth lip philtrum
Thin vermillion border
Maxillary hypoplasia
Cleft palate
Altered palmar creases in the hands
Cardiac defects

Adapted from Reference 55.

Pierre Robin syndrome

Pierre Robin syndrome or Robin sequence (PRS; %261800) occurs in around 1:10,000–20,000 and is characterized by mandibular micrognathia, glossoptosis (posterior positioning of the tongue) and cleft palate.[63] Micrognathia is thought to be the primary etiological factor, with a small mandible resulting in the tongue assuming a downwards and backwards position in the oropharynx and preventing closure of the palatal shelves. In addition to a large and U-shaped cleft palate, the tongue position can also cause life-threatening respiratory difficulty at birth, obstructing the epiglottis and preventing adequate inhalation of the lungs. A number of theories have attempted to explain why growth and development of the mandible is restricted during embryogenesis in PRS. These include oligohydramnios or a reduced amniotic fluid pressure compressing the chin against the sternum, a lack of mandibular movement (secondary to muscle weakness or hypotonia) or generalized growth deficiency affecting the embryo. The upper airway obstruction can present as a medical emergency at birth, requiring neonatal nasopharyngeal intubation or tracheostomy. However, once the airway is stabilized and a feeding regime put in place, infants usually thrive; with surgical repair of the cleft palate taking place during the first year of life.

Molecular genetics

It is likely that PRS may also contain a genetic component, as the features are seen in association with other syndromes, including the Stickler and 22q11 deletion syndrome (#611687). A genetic component has been further demonstrated with evidence for a potential locus at 17q24 underlying PRS.[64] Significantly, a number of translocation breakpoints have been identified in PRS upstream of the SRY (sex determining region Y)-box 9 (*SOX9*) gene, suggesting that developmental misexpression of *SOX9* may be responsible for this disorder.

Hemifacial microsomia

Hemifacial microsomia (HFM; %164210) is a relatively common congenital disorder associated with unilateral developmental defects affecting derivatives of the first and second branchial arches.[65,66] HFM occurs in around 1:5000 children and is usually sporadic, although autosomal dominant familial cases have been reported. A wide spectrum of clinical features are seen in association with HFM, but there is often marked and progressive skeletal asymmetry of the facial region, associated with unilateral aplasia or hypoplasia of the mandibular ramus and condyle. The mandible is often retrognathic and the skeletal asymmetry usually contributes to a marked canting of the occlusal plane. The facial bones are often flattened and reduced in size. The skeletal defects generally progress with facial growth. In addition to the facial skeleton, the soft tissues are also affected in HFM. In particular, the pinna of the ear is often severely malformed or absent (microtia), preauricular skin tags are common, the orbital palpebral fissures are narrowed and epibulbar dermoids are often present unilaterally. Less commonly CLP, palatal and tongue muscle hypoplasia and velopharyngeal insufficiency are also present. A related condition is Goldenhar syndrome, which incorporates vertebral anomalies and epibulbar dermoids in combination with the features of HFM.

Molecular genetics

The aetiology of HFM is not understood, but a disruption during early development of the branchial arches is consistent with the phenotype. Haemorrhage of the stapedial artery has been described as one possible mechanism,[67] and a transgenic mouse line harbouring an insertional mutation within chromosome 10 has been shown to phenocopy the syndrome; this mouse demonstrates microtia, an asymmetric bite and anomalies of the external auditory canal, middle ear and maxilla.[68]

Linkage analysis in human populations has suggested the goosecoid homeobox (*GSC*) gene as a potential candidate gene for HFM.[69] *GSC* encodes a transcription factor strongly expressed in the pharyngeal arches and mice lacking *Gsc* function have a number of craniofacial defects, including hypoplasia and a lack of coronoid and angular processes in the mandible, and defects in the maxillary, palatine and pterygoid bones.[70,71]

Treacher Collins syndrome

Treacher Collins syndrome (TCS; #154500) is a rare autosomal dominant disorder that occurs in around 1:50,000 live births.[72] The derivatives of branchial arches 1 and 2 are most commonly affected, but there can wide variation in the severity of clinical presentation. However, a characteristic facial appearance is common and frequently characterized by down-slanting palpebral fissures, hypoplasia of the zygomatic, supraorbital and mandibular regions, colobomas (areas of tissue deficiency) affecting the lower eyelids and severe malformation of the ears, including the external ear, middle ear ossicles and external auditory canal, which together often result in conductive hearing loss (Figure 55-5). In addition, cleft palate is seen in around one third of cases and there is usually a marked class II skeletal pattern with increased vertical proportions, due to mandibular deficiency and posterior mandibular growth rotation.

Molecular genetics

Treacher Collins–Franceschetti syndrome 1 (*TCOF1*) was originally identified as the gene mutated in the majority of cases of TCS.[73] *TCOF1* encodes a nucleolar phosphoprotein (Treacle), which plays a key role in ribosomal biogenesis and is essential for normal cell growth and differentiation. Mutation in RNA polymerase I and II subunits have also been identified in TCS, which further demonstrate TCS as a ribosomopathy.[74]

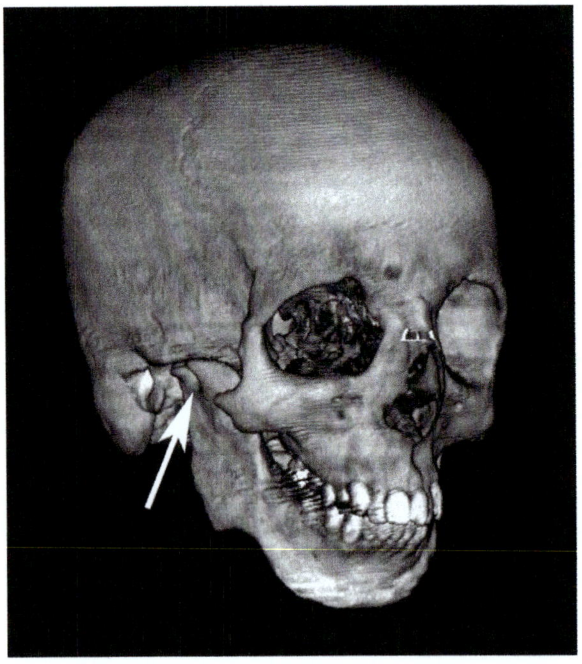

Fig. 55-5 Treacher Collins syndrome. Some of the typical features of Treacher Collins syndrome are illustrated in this CT scan, including an absent zygomatic arch (arrow) and bilateral inferolaterally slanting orbits. (Courtesy of Dr J Hukki and Dr K Hurmerinta.)

Mice lacking function of *Tcof1* have compromised production of mature ribosomes in cranial neuroepithelial and neural crest cells, which leads to reduced proliferation and increased programmed cell death associated with the early neural tube, and a reduction in neural crest cell migration into the early craniofacial region.[75] The mechanism underlying this effect appears to be increased abundance of the cell cycle regulator p53, secondary to its stabilization and prevention from degradation. Significantly, pharmacological inhibition of p53 function can rescue of the craniofacial defects associated with mice lacking Tcof1 function, albeit with some associated developmental defects.[76]

Nager syndrome

Nager syndrome (#154400) or acrofacial dysostosis 1 has similar craniofacial features to those of Treacher Collins syndrome (downslanted palpebral fissures, malar and mandibular hypoplasia, external ear abnormalities) but in addition patients with Nager syndrome also have limb defects, typically of the upper limbs (Figure 55-6). These include radial aplasia or hypoplasia and thumb aplasia or hypoplasia. Although their features are overlapping Nager syndrome is generally distinguished from the Miller syndrome spectrum by its absence of hind limb deformity.

Molecular genetics

Nager syndrome is caused by heterozygous mutations in splicing factor 3b, subunit 4 (*SF3B4*) which encodes a spliceosome-associated protein.[77] The spliceosome is part of the molecular machinery of the nucleus which removes (splices) introns from mRNA. Little is known about the role of spliceosome components and function during development but presumably abnormalities in spliceosome function will cause isoform abnormalities that affect development. Also, SF3B4 is known to inhibit BMP2 activity probably by interacting with BMP receptor 1A. BMPs are growth factors that regulate the development of facial processes, bone, cartilage and tooth. Consistent with splicing abnormalities causing Nager syndrome, another facial dysostosis mandibulofacial dysostosis with microcephaly (#610536), results from mutations in elongation factor Tu GTP binding domain containing 2 (*EFTUD2*), which encodes a spliceosomal GTPase.[78]

Miller syndrome

Miller syndrome (#263750) or postaxial acrofacial dysostosis is a rare autosomal recessive disorder which has overlapping craniofacial features to those of Treacher Collins and Nager syndromes. Patients display micrognathia, malar hypoplasia, ear defects and postaxial limb deformity.

Molecular genetics

Mutations in the dihydroorotate dehydrogenase (quinone) (*DHODH*) gene result in Miller syndrome. There is evidence that DHODH has a role in neural crest cell development and function.[79]

Craniosynostoses

Craniosynostosis is the premature fusion of intramembranous bones of the face or calvaria (skull) across obliterated sutural joints. The prevalence of craniosynostosis is 4.3 per 10,000 births, with approximately 84% of cases occurring in isolation, while approximately 16% of patients display multiple defects or are part of a syndrome.[80] Over 100 craniosynostotic syndromes have been described, many of which are inherited in a dominant fashion, such as Apert (#101200), Crouzon (#123500), Pfeiffer (#101600) and Saethre–Chotzen (#101400) syndromes. Other syndromes, such as Carpenter 1 and 2 (#201000 and #614976, respectively) and Antley–Bixler (#176943) syndromes, exhibit recessive inheritance. New mutations account for approximately 50% of patients.[81]

Craniosynostosis may be the result of a primary defect of the developing craniofacial bones and sutures or a defect secondary to another disease for example physical constraint of the fetus in the womb may limit the expansion of one or more fetal sutures

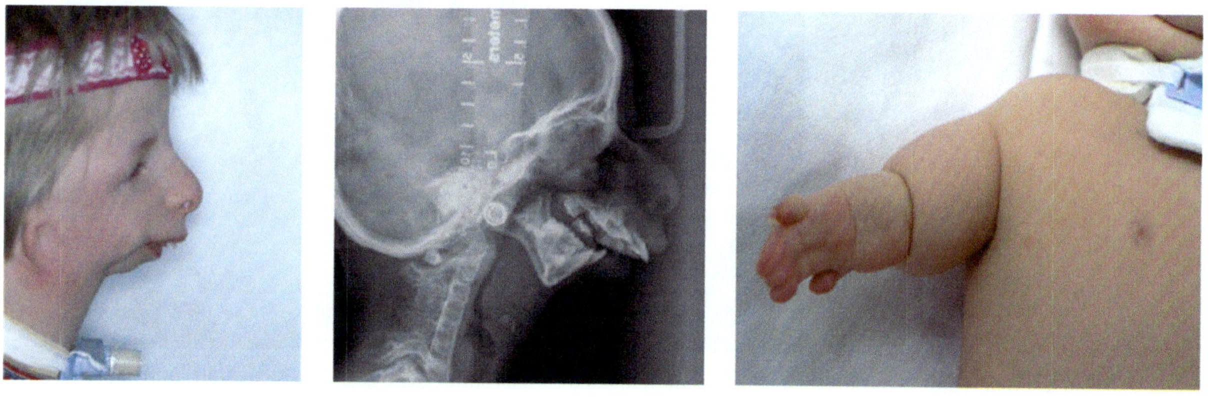

Fig. 55-6 Nager syndrome. Nager syndrome demonstrates similar craniofacial features to those of Treacher Collins syndrome (downslanted palpebral fissures, malar and mandibular hypoplasia, external ear abnormalities) but in addition, patients have limb defects, which typically affect the upper limb. (Courtesy of Dr J. Hukki and Dr K. Hurmerinta.)

and may cause craniosynostosis. Some metabolic conditions such as hyperthyroidism or rickets, and hematological disorders such as thalassaemia or sickle cell anemia are also associated with craniosynostosis.[82]

The most commonly affected suture is the sagittal suture (between the two parietal bones) followed by the coronal suture (between the frontal and parietal bones), the metopic suture (between the two frontal bones) and then the lambdoid suture (between the parietal and occipital bones). Any combination of sutures can fuse with the resulting deformity dependent on the time, location and pattern of fusing sutures. In addition to craniosynostosis, patients commonly have facial and cranial base abnormalities, which also results in abnormalities in the shape of the face and head.

Single suture synostosis

Single suture synostoses are normally classified by the anatomical suture affected and by the shape of the calvaria that results. While no growth can occur at the site of the fusion, compensatory growth can occur at other sutures, distant from the fusion site. When only the sagittal suture is affected an elongated scaphocephalic (boat-shaped) cranium will result. When the metopic suture fuses prematurely a trigonocephaly will occur with manifestations including a triangular or pointed forehead, sutural ridging, narrow bitemporal width and hypotelorism, and parietal widening. When a unilateral coronal suture fuses an anterior plagiocephalic cranium will arise with asymmetric flattening of the forehead on the affected side and a bulging of the forehead on the contralateral side due to compensatory growth of the contralateral coronal suture (Figure 55-7). Unilateral lambdoidal synostosis will result in a posterior plagiocephalic cranium (asymmetric). On the affected side, the occipitoparietal area is flattened whereas on the contralateral side there is compensatory bossing in the parietal and sometimes frontal regions. There is an ipsilateral occipitomastoid bulge and the external ear on the ipsilateral side is displaced inferiorly. This feature separates the true lambdoid synostosis from the deformational posterior plagiocephaly where the characteristics are opposite no matter how severe the deformity is. In deformational plagiocephaly, the ipsilateral ear is shifted forwards along with the flattened side and the compensatory bossing in the forehead is always on the ipsilateral side.[83]

Non-syndromic craniosynostosis

Although most non-syndromic craniosynostoses are spontaneous new mutations, approximately 2% of sagittal suture synostosis and 10% of both coronal and metopic synostoses have a family history. Genetic causes can be found in 2–5% of patients with non-syndromic craniosynostoses. These include mutations in ephrin-A4 (*EFNA4*), FGF receptors 1–3 (*FGFR1-3*), FRAS related extracellular matrix 1 (*FREM1*), insulin-like growth factor 1 receptor (*IGF1R*), leucine-rich repeat, immunoglobulin-like and transmembrane domains 3 (*LRIT3*), runt-related transcription factor 2 (*RUNX2*) and twist family bHLH transcription factor 1 (*TWIST1*) and using genome wide screening *BMP2* and Bardet–Biedl syndrome 9 (*BBS9*) have both been identified as notable candidate genes.[84,85] This low percentage compares to approximately 30% of patients with syndromic craniosynostosis suggests that in part, the genetic basis of the condition is yet to be discovered but also that the calvarial development, while clearly controlled by genetics, is influenced by epigenetic and environmental factors.

Syndromic craniosynostoses: Apert, Crouzon and Pfeiffer

Together with Crouzon syndrome, Apert syndrome occurs once in every 64,500 live births. Patients with Apert, Crouzon or Pfeiffer syndrome can all display a characteristic 'Crouzonoid-type' face with

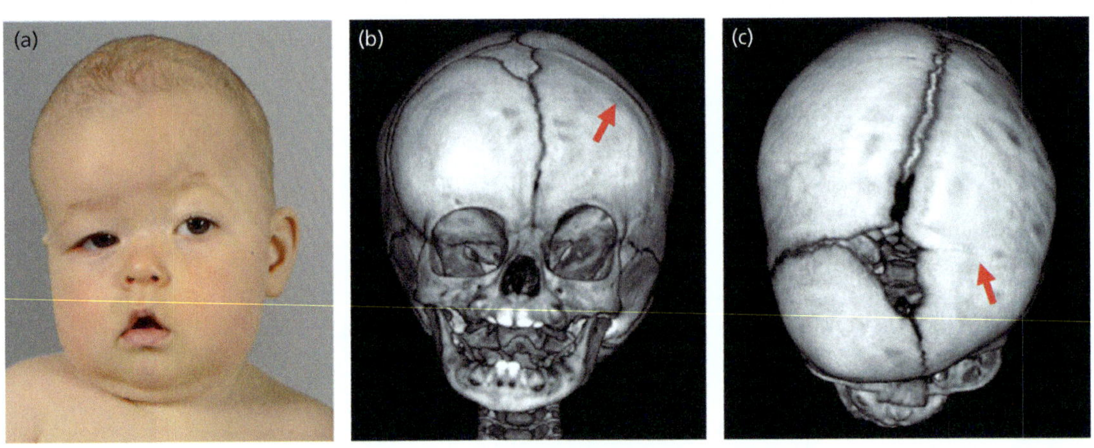

Fig. 55-7 Isolated coronal suture synostosis. Non-syndromic left-sided coronal suture synostosis in a 5-year-old child. (a) Frontal view demonstrates a resulting asymmetric deformity of the face and calvaria on the right side. CT scans of the (b) Face and (c) Calvarium show the distortion of the skull and region of synostosis (red arrows). (Courtesy of Dr J. Hukki and Dr K. Hurmerinta.)

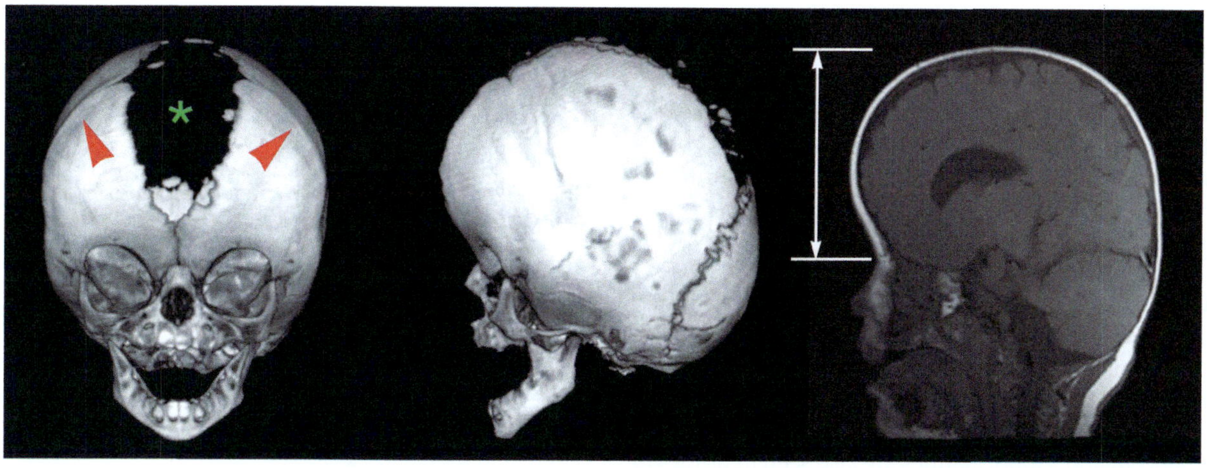

Fig. 55-8 Apert syndrome. CT scans demonstrating the typical features of Apert syndrome, which include bicoronal synostosis (red arrowheads), a wide midline defect between the frontal bones (green *) and an increase in skull height (white arrow). (Courtesy of Dr J. Hukki and Dr K. Hurmerinta.)

a short head length, increased head height, midfacial hypoplasia and ocular proptosis (Figure 55-8).

Apert syndrome is characterized by bilateral craniosynostosis of the coronal sutures, which are typically closed at birth. The metopic and sagittal sutures are usually expanded to form a wide midline defect in which ectopic bones form and coalesce. Another cardinal feature is symmetrical syndactyly of the limbs. Often the palate is cleft.[86] If the premature fusion of the cranial base synchondroses occurs it happens late in childhood. This is in contrast to the cranial base abnormalities in patients with Crouzon syndrome where very early fusion of the synchondroses is not uncommon.[87] In Crouzon syndrome, craniosynostosis usually occurs during the first year after birth. In most cases the coronal sutures are usually affected and this can be in combination with synostosis of the sagittal and/or lambdoid sutures. Patients with Crouzon syndrome have normal limbs. In addition to the craniofacial features (craniosynostosis) individuals with Pfeiffer syndrome also exhibit broad thumbs, broad great toes and syndactyly.

Molecular genetics

Heterozygous mutations in fibroblast growth factor receptor 2 (*FGFR2*), which encodes a growth factor receptor, can cause Apert, Crouzon or Pfeiffer syndromes. Rarely Pfeiffer syndrome can be caused by mutations in *FGFR1*. All three conditions are inherited in an autosomal dominant manner with most mutations arising spontaneously.[81] Together with Muenke syndrome, mutations causing Apert, Crouzon or Pfeiffer syndromes are of paternal origin and their risk of occurrence increases with increasing paternal age.[88]

Muenke syndrome

Muenke syndrome (#602849) is the most common form of syndromic craniosynostosis with an incidence of 1 in 30,000 births, accounting for approximately 5% of all cases of craniosynostosis.[89] The most common features of Muenke syndrome are either unilateral or bilateral coronal suture synostosis, tarsal and/or carpal joint fusions and deafness. Other features can include macrocephaly, midfacial hypoplasia and developmental delay. Features are of variable severity with some individuals having a very mild or even apparently no phenotype.

Molecular genetics

Muenke syndrome refers to the specific heterozygous mutation in *FGFR3* resulting in a Pro250Arg amino acid substitution. Of note is the finding that patients with Muenke syndrome have an increased risk of re-operation compared to cases of isolated coronal craniosynostosis without the Pro250Arg *FGFR3* mutation.[90]

Saethre–Chotzen syndrome

The characteristic features of Saethre–Chotzen syndrome (#101400) include craniosynostosis, although not obligatory for the syndrome, drooping eyelids (ptosis), a high forehead with a low frontal hairline and deviation of the nasal septum. External ear abnormalities are common, being low set, small and having a prominent crus of the anti-helix. Short digits (brachydactyly) and mild soft tissue syndactyly are also frequent features. There is phenotypic overlap with Muenke syndrome.[91]

Molecular genetics

Saethre–Chotzen syndrome is an autosomal dominant condition caused by mutations in the transcription factor *TWIST1* and possibly by a mutation in *FGFR2*. As an individual with Saethre–Chotzen features has been found with an *FGFR2* mutation.[92] Heterozygotic loss of *Twist1* in mice results in late onset coronal suture synostosis with associated facial distortion.[93] Twist1 negatively regulates Runx2, a transcription factor critical for osteoblast differentiation and loss of Twist1 function in the calvarial mesenchyme permits abnormal Runx2 function and bony fusion across sutures.[94]

Craniofrontonasal syndrome

Craniofrontonasal syndrome (#304110) is identified as a subgroup of frontonasal dysplasia with females exhibiting frontonasal dysplasia, craniofacial asymmetry, coronal suture craniosynostosis, hypertelorism, a broad and/or bifid nasal tip, an anterior open bite malocclusion. Abnormalities are also seen in tissues of ectodermal origin including longitudinal grooving in the finger and toe nails and thick wiry hair. Males are less severely affected, usually exhibiting only hypertelorism.[91]

Molecular genetics

Craniofrontonasal syndrome is an X-linked condition in which females are more often affected, and also exhibit a more severe phenotype. It is caused by heterozygous mutations in ephrin-B1 (*EFNB1*), which encodes a membrane protein that functions as a ligand of Eph-related receptor tyrosine kinases.[95]

With regard to the pathogenesis of craniofrontonasal syndrome, Eph-Ephrin signalling has roles in mediating osteoblast and osteoclast function, possibly in response to mechanical loading and also in embryonic boundary formation. Of note may be the maintenance of the boundary between cranial neural crest and mesodermal cells at the coronal suture and the segregation of these two cell populations.

Carpenter syndrome 1 and 2

Typical features of Carpenter syndrome are craniosynostosis and preaxial polysyndactyly of the feet, although the polysyndactyly is not an obligatory feature. Carpenter syndrome patients have craniosynostosis, usually affecting the coronal, sagittal and lambdoid sutures, with the coronal sutures being the last to fuse. The head shape is variable but may be cloverleaf-shaped and may be asymmetric. There is often accompanying midface hypoplasia, heart defects, growth retardation, mental deficiency and obesity.

Molecular genetics

Unlike most craniosynostosis syndromes which are autosomal dominant, Carpenter syndrome is autosomal recessive and caused by homozygous mutations in RAB23, member RAS oncogene family (*RAB23*) (Carpenter syndrome 1) or multiple EGF-like-domains 8 (*MEGF8*) (Carpenter syndrome 2). *RAB23* encodes a small GTPase and has been proposed to be a negative regulator of Hedgehog signalling.[96,97]

Greig cephalopolysyndactyly syndrome

The characteristic features of Greig cephalopolysyndactyly syndrome (#175700) are macrocephaly, scaphocephaly, postaxial polysyndactyly in the hands and preaxial polydactyly in the feet. Craniosynostosis is a rare finding.[91]

Molecular genetics

Heterozygous mutations in GLI family zinc finger 3 (*GLI3*) cause Greig cephalopolysyndactyly syndrome and these result in a loss of protein function. Although craniosynostsosis in patients is a rare feature, lambdoid suture synostosis occurs in 100% of *Gli3* null allele mice. *Gli3* encodes a transcription factor which, like Rab23, has been shown to be a negative regulator of the Hedgehog signalling pathway.[98,99]

Chromosomal abnormalities causing craniosynostosis

Chromosomal abnormalities make up approximately 15% of all cases of craniosynostosis and vary in the phenotype, with single to multiple sutures being affected. Many different abnormalities have been documented including deletions, duplications and trisomies and these can affect many different chromosomes. Some of these regions affected map known causal single genes of craniosynostosis such as *TWIST1*. Interestingly, when compared to single genetic causes of craniosynostosis, patients with chromosomal abnormalities resulting in craniosynostosis have a much lower re-operation rate (17% compared to 58%).[100–102]

Mouse models of craniosynostosis

Several mouse models of craniosynostosis have been developed which mimic the human condition. Using these models it has been possible to correct abnormal biomolecular signalling within sutures by altering osteogenic fate of the sutural mesenchyme and thereby preventing suture fusion.[103] These experiments confirm the postulated molecular pathology of the condition and point the way towards potential future therapeutics.

Frontonasal dysplasias 1–3

Frontonasal dysplasias 1–3 (#136760, #613451 and #613456, respectively) are a group of disorders with variable phenotype.[104] Features can include hypertelorism, median orofacial clefting, anterior cranium bifidum occultum, a V-shaped frontal hairline, nasal abnormalities which include broadening of the nasal root, lack of formation of the nasal tip, short nasal ridge, splayed nasal bones with bifid nasal tip and clefting of the alae nasi (Figure 55-9).

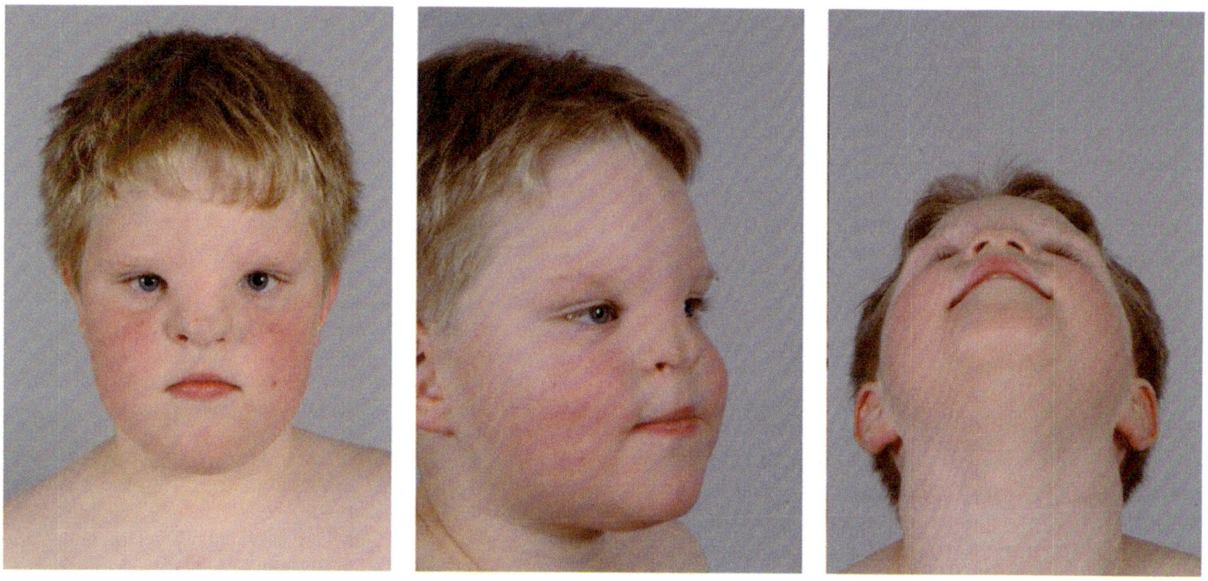

Fig. 55-9 Frontonasal dysplasia. Characteristic features of frontonasal dysplasia include hypertelorism, broadening of the nasal root, short nasal ridge and a bifid nasal tip. (Courtesy of Dr J Hukki and Dr K Hurmerinta.)

In addition, frontonasal dysplasia 1 (frontorhiny) can also exhibit other feature including widely separated slit-like nares, long philtrum with prominent bilateral swellings, and midline upper lip/alveolus notching.[105] Frontonasal dysplasia 2 is characterized by a hypertelorism, nasal deformity, cryptorchidism, agenesis of the corpus callosum, craniosynostosis, alopecia, and mental retardation.[106] Frontonasal dysplasia 3 is described as frontonasal dysplasia with severe facial clefting and microphthalmia.[107]

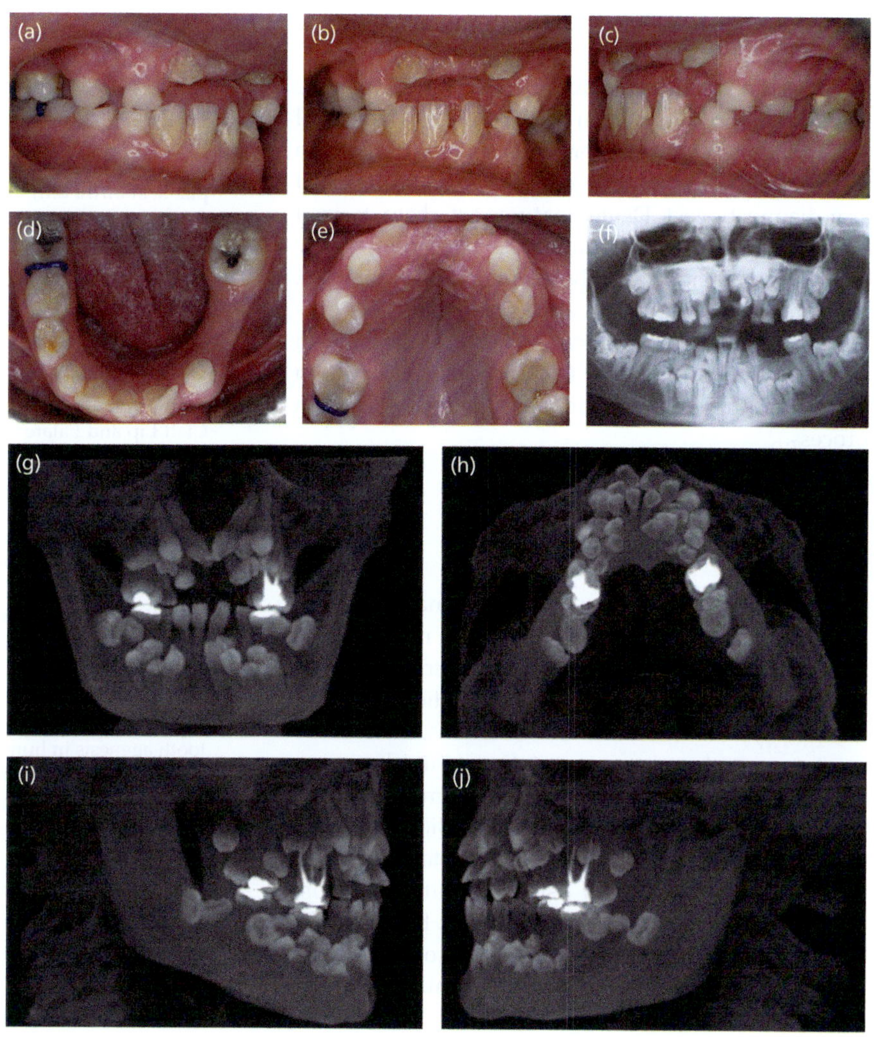

Fig. 55-10 Cleidocranial dysplasia. Cleidocranial dysplasia in an 18-year-old girl. (a–e) Intra-oral photographs demonstrating retention of the primary dentition and failure of eruption associated with the successional dentition; (f) Panoramic radiograph demonstrating multiple supernumerary teeth in all four quadrants; (g–j) CB CT imaging of the jaws.

Molecular genetics

Frontonasal dysplasia 1, 2 and 3 are caused by mutations in the ALX homeobox genes ALX3, ALX4 and ALX1, respectively. *Alx1*, *Alx3*, and Alx4 are putative transcription factors that are expressed in the embryonic facial mesenchyme and *Alx3*/*Alx4* double null mutant mice exhibit severe midfacial malformations, including orofacial clefting.[108]

Cleidocranial dysplasia

The clinical features of cleidocranial dysplasia (#119600) include widened skull sutures and fontanels, supernumerary teeth and delayed tooth eruption (Figure 55-10), clavicle bone abnormalities and short stature. Patients have a characteristic bulging of the frontal and parietal regions and consequently appear to have a small face. Skeletal development in general is affected and although patients are short, the skeletal abnormalities are most obvious in areas formed by intramembranous ossification: the calvaria, face and lateral end of the clavicles. Calvarial bone development is delayed and the sutures are wide. This is especially noticeable in the metopic and sagittal sutures and the anterior fontanel, where there may be a groove over the metopic suture. In the widened sutures, ectopic Wormian bones form and this is particularly common in the lambdoid suture. The clavicles can be missing but are more often hypoplastic in the lateral acromial third. These abnormalities allow patients to approximate shoulders together, which can be used as a diagnostic test. Dental features are characterized by the presence of supernumerary teeth, which may be numerous and generally supplemental in nature. Removal of the extra teeth and/or the preceding primary teeth does not encourage tooth eruption, which suggests that in addition to abnormalities in tooth formation, there are primary defects in the eruption process.[91]

Molecular genetics

Cleidocranial dysplasia has an autosomal dominant pattern of inheritance and is caused by mutations in the gene encoding the runt-related transcription factor 2 (*RUNX2*). Cleidocranial dysplasia patients present with many different mutations in *RUNX2*, which are most commonly missense mutations, but also occur as nonsense, splicing and frameshift mutations, as well as intragenic deletions and duplications.[109,110] Most mutations result in a loss of protein function. RUNX2 is an activator of osteoblast differentiation, which regulates most osteoblastic genes. In mice a 55–70% reduction of Runx2 mRNA and protein is sufficient to produce skeletal defects that mimics human cleidocranial dysplasia.[111]

References

1 HUGO gene Nomenclature Committee. wwwgenename sorg.
2 Online Mendelian Inheritance in Man (OMIM). wwwomi morg.
3 Chai Y, Maxson RE, Jr. Recent advances in craniofacial morphogenesis. Dev Dyn. 2006;235:2353–75.
4 Cobourne MT, Sharpe PT. Tooth and jaw: molecular mechanisms of patterning in the first branchial arch. Arch Oral Biol. 2003;48:1–14.
5 Wilkie AO, Morriss-Kay GM. Genetics of craniofacial development and malformation. Nat Rev Genet. 2001;2:458–68.
6 Francis-West PH, Robson L, Evans DJ. Craniofacial development: the tissue and molecular interactions that control development of the head. Adv Anat Embryol Cell Biol. 2003;169:III–VI, 1–138.
7 Jiang R, Bush JO, Lidral AC. Development of the upper lip: Morphogenetic and molecular mechanisms. Dev Dyn. 2006;235:1152–66.
8 Ferguson MW. Palate development. Development (Cambridge, England). 1988;103 Suppl:41–60.
9 Cobourne MT. The complex genetics of cleft lip and palate. Eur J Orthod. 2004;26:7–16.
10 Murray JC, Schutte BC. Cleft palate: players, pathways, and pursuits. J Clin Invest. 2004;113:1676–8.
11 Schutte BC, Murray JC. The many faces and factors of orofacial clefts. Hum Mol Genet. 1999;8:1853–9.
12 Stanier P, Moore GE. Genetics of cleft lip and palate: syndromic genes contribute to the incidence of non-syndromic clefts. Hum Mol Genet. 2004;13 Spec No 1:R73–81.
13 Vieira AR. Unraveling Human Cleft Lip and Palate Research. J Dent Res. 2008;87:119–25.
14 Dixon MJ, Marazita ML, Beaty TH, Murray JC. Cleft lip and palate: understanding genetic and environmental influences. Nat Rev Genet. 2011;12:167–78.
15 Jones MC. Etiology of facial clefts: prospective evaluation of 428 patients. Cleft Palate J. 1988;25:16–20.
16 Christensen K, Juel K, Herskind AM, Murray JC. Long term follow up study of survival associated with cleft lip and palate at birth. BMJ (Clin Res Ed.) 2004;328:1405.
17 Christensen K, Mortensen PB. Facial clefting and psychiatric diseases: a follow-up of the Danish 1936–1987 Facial Cleft cohort. Cleft Palate Craniofac J. 2002;39:392–6.
18 Bille C, Winther JF, Bautz A, Murray JC, Olsen J, Christensen K. Cancer risk in persons with oral cleft – a population-based study of 8,093 cases. Am J Epidemiol. 2005;161:1047–55.
19 Sandy J, Williams A, Mildinhall S, Murphy T, Bearn D, Shaw B, et al. The Clinical Standards Advisory Group (CSAG) Cleft Lip and Palate Study. Br J Orthod. 1998;25:21–30.
20 Shaw WC, Dahl E, Asher-McDade C, Brattstrom V, Mars M, McWilliam J, et al. A six-center international study of treatment outcome in patients with clefts of the lip and palate: Part 5. General discussion and conclusions. Cleft Palate Craniofac J. 1992;29:413–8.
21 Kondo S, Schutte BC, Richardson RJ, Bjork BC, Knight AS, Watanabe Y, et al. Mutations in IRF6 cause Van der Woude and popliteal pterygium syndromes. Nat Genet. 2002;32:285–89.
22 van den Boogaard MJ, Dorland M, Beemer FA, van Amstel HK. MSX1 mutation is associated with orofacial clefting and tooth agenesis in humans. Nat Genet. 2000;24:342–43.
23 Suzuki K, Hu D, Bustos T, Zlotogora J, Richieri-Costa A, Helms JA, et al. Mutations of PVRL1, encoding a cell–cell adhesion molecule/herpesvirus receptor, in cleft lip/palate-ectodermal dysplasia. Nat Genet. 2000;25:427–30.
24 Celli J, Duijf P, Hamel BC, Bamshad M, Kramer B, Smits AP, et al. Heterozygous germline mutations in the p53 homolog p63 are the cause of EEC syndrome. Cell. 1999;99: 143–53.
25 Ianakiev P, Kilpatrick MW, Toudjarska I, Basel D, Beighton P, Tsipouras P. Split-hand/split-foot malformation is caused

by mutations in the p63 gene on 3q27. Am J Hum Genet. 2000;67:59–66.
26 McGrath JA, Duijf PH, Doetsch V, Irvine AD, de Waal R, Vanmolkot KR, et al. Hay–Wells syndrome is caused by heterozygous missense mutations in the SAM domain of p63. Hum Mol Genet. 2001;10:221–9.
27 van Bokhoven H, Hamel BC, Bamshad M, Sangiorgi E, Gurrieri F, Duijf PH, et al. p63 Gene mutations in EEC syndrome, limb–mammary syndrome, and isolated split hand–split foot malformation suggest a genotype–phenotype correlation. Am J Hum Genet. 2001;69:481–92.
28 Quaderi NA, Schweiger S, Gaudenz K, Franco B, Rugarli EI, Berger W, et al. Opitz G/BBB syndrome, a defect of midline development, is due to mutations in a new RING finger gene on Xp22. Nat Genet. 1997;17:285–91.
29 Mitchell LE, Risch N. Mode of inheritance of nonsyndromic cleft lip with or without cleft palate: a reanalysis. Am J Hum Genet. 1992;51:323–32.
30 Lidral AC, Murray JC. Genetic approaches to identify disease genes for birth defects with cleft lip/palate as a model. Birth Defects Res A Clin Mol Teratol. 2004;70:893–901.
31 Schliekelman P, Slatkin M. Multiplex relative risk and estimation of the number of loci underlying an inherited disease. Am J Hum Genet. 2002;71:1369–85.
32 Jugessur A, Lie RT, Wilcox AJ, Murray JC, Taylor JA, Saugstad OD, et al. Variants of developmental genes (TGFA, TGFB3, and MSX1) and their associations with orofacial clefts: a case–parent triad analysis. Genet Epidemiol. 2003;24:230–9.
33 Vieira AR, Orioli IM, Castilla EE, Cooper ME, Marazita ML, Murray JC. MSX1 and TGFB3 contribute to clefting in South America. J Dent Res. 2003;82:289–92.
34 Riley BM, Mansilla MA, Ma J, Daack-Hirsch S, Maher BS, Raffensperger LM, et al. Impaired FGF signaling contributes to cleft lip and palate. Proc Natl Acad Sci USA. 2007;104:4512–7.
35 Vieira AR, Avila JR, Daack–Hirsch S, Dragan E, Felix TM, Rahimov F, et al. Medical sequencing of candidate genes for nonsyndromic cleft lip and palate. PLoS Genet. 2005;1:e64.
36 Jezewski PA, Vieira AR, Nishimura C, Ludwig B, Johnson M, O'Brien SE, et al. Complete sequencing shows a role for MSX1 in non-syndromic cleft lip and palate. J Med Genet. 2003;40:399–407.
37 Zucchero TM, Cooper ME, Maher BS, Daack-Hirsch S, Nepomuceno B, Ribeiro L, et al. Interferon regulatory factor 6 (IRF6) gene variants and the risk of isolated cleft lip or palate. N Engl J Med. 2004;351:769–80.
38 Sozen MA, Suzuki K, Tolarova MM, Bustos T, Fernandez Iglesias JE, Spritz RA. Mutation of PVRL1 is associated with sporadic, non-syndromic cleft lip/palate in northern Venezuela. Nat Genet. 2001;29:141–2.
39 Jugessur A, Murray JC. Orofacial clefting: recent insights into a complex trait. Curr Opin Genet Dev. 2005;15: 270–8.
40 Bille C, Skytthe A, Vach W, Knudsen LB, Andersen AM, Murray JC, et al. Parent's age and the risk of oral clefts. Epidemiology (Cambridge, Mass). 2005;16:311–6.
41 Shi M, Christensen K, Weinberg CR, Romitti P, Bathum L, Lozada A, et al. Orofacial cleft risk is increased with maternal smoking and specific detoxification–gene variants. Am J Hum Genet. 2007;80:76–90.
42 Webster WS, Howe AM, Abela D, Oakes DJ. The relationship between cleft lip, maxillary hypoplasia, hypoxia and phenytoin. Curr Pharmaceut Design. 2006;12:1431–8.
43 Cohen MM, Jr. Holoprosencephaly: clinical, anatomic, and molecular dimensions. Birth Defects Res A Clin Mol Teratol. 2006;76:658–73.
44 Leoncini E, Baranello G, Orioli IM, Anneren G, Bakker M, Bianchi F, et al. Frequency of holoprosencephaly in the International Clearinghouse Birth Defects Surveillance Systems: searching for population variations. Birth Defects Res A Clin Mol Teratol. 2008;82:585–91.
45 Nanni L, Ming JE, Bocian M, Steinhaus K, Bianchi DW, Die-Smulders C, et al. The mutational spectrum of the sonic hedgehog gene in holoprosencephaly: SHH mutations cause a significant proportion of autosomal dominant holoprosencephaly. Hum Mol Genet. 1999;8:2479–88.
46 Garavelli L, Zanacca C, Caselli G, Banchini G, Dubourg C, David V, et al. Solitary median maxillary central incisor syndrome: clinical case with a novel mutation of sonic hedgehog. Am J Med Genet A. 2004;127:93–5.
47 Kauvar EF, Muenke M. Holoprosencephaly: recommendations for diagnosis and management. Curr Opin Pediatr. 2010;22:687–95.
48 Geng X, Oliver G. Pathogenesis of holoprosencephaly. J Clin Invest. 2009;119:1403–13.
49 Bae GU, Domene S, Roessler E, Schachter K, Kang JS, Muenke M, et al. Mutations in CDON, encoding a hedgehog receptor, result in holoprosencephaly and defective interactions with other hedgehog receptors. Am J Hum Genet. 2011;89:231–40.
50 Roessler E, Muenke M. The molecular genetics of holoprosencephaly. Am J Med Genet C Semin Med Genet. 2010;154C:52–61.
51 Chiang C, Litingtung Y, Lee E, Young KE, Corden JL, Westphal H, et al. Cyclopia and defective axial patterning in mice lacking Sonic hedgehog gene function. Nature. 1996;383:407–13.
52 Roessler E, Belloni E, Gaudenz K, Jay P, Berta P, Scherer SW, et al. Mutations in the human Sonic Hedgehog gene cause holoprosencephaly. Nat Genet. 1996;14:357–60.
53 Jones KL, Smith DW. Recognition of the fetal alcohol syndrome in early infancy. Lancet. 1973;302:999–1001.
54 Jones KL, Smith DW, Ulleland CN, Streissguth P. Pattern of malformation in offspring of chronic alcoholic mothers. Lancet. 1973;1:1267–71.
55 Jones KL. The effects of alcohol on fetal development. Birth Defects Res Part C, Embryo Today: Rev. 2011;93:3–11.
56 Hong M, Krauss RS. Cdon mutation and fetal ethanol exposure synergize to produce midline signaling defects and holoprosencephaly spectrum disorders in mice. PLoS Genet. 2012;8:e1002999.
57 Visinoni AF, Lisboa-Costa T, Pagnan NA, Chautard-Freire-Maia EA. Ectodermal dysplasias: clinical and molecular review. Am J Med Genet A. 2009;149A:1980–2002.
58 Mikkola ML. Molecular aspects of hypohidrotic ectodermal dysplasia. Am J Med Genet A. 2009;149A:2031–6.
59 Headon DJ, Emmal SA, Ferguson BM, Tucker AS, Justice MJ, Sharpe PT, et al. Gene defect in ectodermal dysplasia implicates a death domain adapter in development. Nature. 2001;414:913–6.
60 Kere J, Srivastava AK, Montonen O, Zonana J, Thomas N, Ferguson B, et al. X-linked anhidrotic (hypohidrotic) ectodermal dysplasia is caused by mutation in a novel transmembrane protein. Nat Genet. 1996;13:409–16.
61 Srivastava AK, Pispa J, Hartung AJ, Du Y, Ezer S, Jenks T, et al. The Tabby phenotype is caused by mutation in a mouse homologue of the EDA gene that reveals novel mouse and human exons and encodes a protein (ectodysplasin-A) with collagenous domains. Proc Natl Acad Sci USA. 1997;94:13069–74.
62 Monreal AW, Ferguson BM, Headon DJ, Street SL, Overbeek PA, Zonana J. Mutations in the human homologue of mouse dl cause autosomal recessive and dominant hypohidrotic ectodermal dysplasia. Nat Genet. 1999;22:366–9.
63 Tan TY, Kilpatrick N, Farlie PG. Developmental and genetic perspectives on Pierre Robin sequence. Am J Med Genet C Semin Med Genet. 2013;163:295–305.
64 Benko S, Fantes JA, Amiel J, Kleinjan DJ, Thomas S, Ramsay J, et al. Highly conserved non-coding elements on either side of SOX9 associated with Pierre Robin sequence. Nat Genet. 2009;41:359–64.
65 Birgfeld CB, Heike C. Craniofacial microsomia. Semin Plast Surg. 2012;26:91–104.

66 Heike CL, Hing AV, Aspinall CA, Bartlett SP, Birgfeld CB, Drake AF, et al. Clinical care in craniofacial microsomia: a review of current management recommendations and opportunities to advance research. Am J Med Genet C Semin Med Genet. 2013;163:271–82.
67 Poswillo D. The pathogenesis of the first and second branchial arch syndrome. Oral Surg Oral Med Oral Pathol. 1973;35:302–28.
68 Cousley R, Naora H, Yokoyama M, Kimura M, Otani H. Validity of the Hfm transgenic mouse as a model for hemifacial microsomia. Cleft Palate Craniofac J. 2002;39: 81–92.
69 Kelberman D, Tyson J, Chandler DC, McInerney AM, Slee J, Albert D, et al. Hemifacial microsomia: progress in understanding the genetic basis of a complex malformation syndrome. Hum Genet. 2001;109:638–45.
70 Rivera-Perez JA, Mallo M, Gendron-Maguire M, Gridley T, Behringer RR. Goosecoid is not an essential component of the mouse gastrula organizer but is required for craniofacial and rib development. Development. 1995;121:3005–12.
71 Yamada G, Mansouri A, Torres M, Stuart ET, Blum M, Schultz M, et al. Targeted mutation of the murine goosecoid gene results in craniofacial defects and neonatal death. Development. 1995;121:2917–22.
72 Trainor PA, Dixon J, Dixon MJ. Treacher Collins syndrome: etiology, pathogenesis and prevention. Eur J Hum Genet. 2009;17:275–83.
73 Group TTCSC. Positional cloning of a gene involved in the pathogenesis of Treacher Collins syndrome. The Treacher Collins Syndrome Collaborative Group. Nat Genet. 1996;12:130–6.
74 Dauwerse JG, Dixon J, Seland S, Ruivenkamp CA, van Haeringen A, Hoefsloot LH, et al. Mutations in genes encoding subunits of RNA polymerases I and III cause Treacher Collins syndrome. Nat Genet. 2011;43:20–2.
75 Dixon J, Jones NC, Sandell LL, Jayasinghe SM, Crane J, Rey JP, et al. Tcof1/Treacle is required for neural crest cell formation and proliferation deficiencies that cause craniofacial abnormalities. Proc Natl Acad Sci USA. 2006;103: 13403–8.
76 Jones NC, Lynn ML, Gaudenz K, Sakai D, Aoto K, Rey JP, et al. Prevention of the neurocristopathy Treacher Collins syndrome through inhibition of p53 function. Nat Med. 2008;14:125–33.
77 Bernier FP, Caluseriu O, Ng S, Schwartzentruber J, Buckingham KJ, Innes AM, et al. Haploinsufficiency of SF3B4, a component of the pre-mRNA spliceosomal complex, causes Nager syndrome. Am J Hum Genet. 2012;90:925–33.
78 Trainor PA, Andrews BT. Facial dysostoses: Etiology, pathogenesis and management. Am J Med Genet C Semin Med Genet. 2013;163:283–94.
79 Ng SB, Buckingham KJ, Lee C, Bigham AW, Tabor HK, Dent KM, et al. Exome sequencing identifies the cause of a mendelian disorder. Nat Genet. 2010;42:30–5.
80 Boulet SL, Rasmussen SA, Honein MA. A population-based study of craniosynostosis in metropolitan Atlanta, 1989–2003. Am J Med Genet A. 2008;146A:984–91.
81 Johnson D, Wilkie AO. Craniosynostosis. Eur J Hum Genet. 2011;19:369–76.
82 Rice DP. Clinical features of syndromic craniosynostosis. Front Oral Biol. 2008;12:91–106.
83 Hukki J, Saarinen P, Kangasniemi M. Single suture craniosynostosis: diagnosis and imaging. Front Oral Biol. 2008;12:79–90.
84 Lattanzi W, Bukvic N, Barba M, Tamburrini G, Bernardini C, Michetti F, et al. Genetic basis of single-suture synostoses: genes, chromosomes and clinical implications. Childs Nerv Syst. 2012;28:1301–10.
85 Justice CM, Yagnik G, Kim Y, Peter I, Jabs EW, Erazo M, et al. A genome-wide association study identifies susceptibility loci for nonsyndromic sagittal craniosynostosis near BMP2 and within BBS9. Nat Genet. 2012;44:1360–4.
86 Cohen MM, Jr., Kreiborg S. Suture formation, premature sutural fusion, and suture default zones in Apert syndrome. Am J Med Genet. 1996;62:339–44.
87 Kreiborg S, Marsh JL, Cohen MM, Jr., Liversage M, Pedersen H, Skovby F, et al. Comparative three-dimensional analysis of CT-scans of the calvaria and cranial base in Apert and Crouzon syndromes. J Craniomaxillofac Surg. 1993;21: 181–8.
88 Goriely A, Wilkie AO. Paternal age effect mutations and selfish spermatogonial selection: causes and consequences for human disease. Am J Hum Genet. 2012;90:175–200.
89 Agochukwu NB, Solomon BD, Muenke M. Impact of genetics on the diagnosis and clinical management of syndromic craniosynostoses. Childs Nerv Syst. 2012;28:1447–63.
90 Thomas GP, Wilkie AO, Richards PG, Wall SA. FGFR3 P250R mutation increases the risk of reoperation in apparent 'nonsyndromic' coronal craniosynostosis. J Craniofac Surg. 2005;16:347–52; discussion 353–4.
91 Gorlin R, Cohen JM, Hennekam R. Syndromes of the head and neck, 4th edn. Oxford: Oxford University Press, 2001.
92 el Ghouzzi V, Le Merrer M, Perrin-Schmitt F, Lajeunie E, Benit P, Renier D, et al. Mutations of the TWIST gene in the Saethre–Chotzen syndrome. Nat Genet. 1997;15:42–6.
93 Carver EA, Oram KF, Gridley T. Craniosynostosis in Twist heterozygous mice: a model for Saethre–Chotzen syndrome. Anat Rec. 2002;268:90–2.
94 Bialek P, Kern B, Yang X, Schrock M, Sosic D, Hong N, et al. A twist code determines the onset of osteoblast differentiation. Dev Cell. 2004;6:423–35.
95 Twigg SR, Kan R, Babbs C, Bochukova EG, Robertson SP, Wall SA, et al. Mutations of ephrin-B1 (EFNB1), a marker of tissue boundary formation, cause craniofrontonasal syndrome. Proc Nat Acad Sci USA. 2004;101:8652–7.
96 Eggenschwiler JT, Espinoza E, Anderson KV. Rab23 is an essential negative regulator of the mouse Sonic hedgehog signalling pathway. Nature. 2001;412:194–8.
97 Jenkins D, Seelow D, Jehee FS, Perlyn CA, Alonso LG, Bueno DF, et al. RAB23 mutations in Carpenter syndrome imply an unexpected role for hedgehog signaling in cranial-suture development and obesity. Am J Hum Genet. 2007;80: 1162–70.
98 Vortkamp A, Gessler M, Grzeschik KH. GLI3 zinc-finger gene interrupted by translocations in Greig syndrome families. Nature. 1991;352:539–40.
99 Rice DP, Connor EC, Veltmaat JM, Lana-Elola E, Veistinen L, Tanimoto Y, et al. Gli3Xt-J/Xt-J mice exhibit lambdoid suture craniosynostosis which results from altered osteoprogenitor proliferation and differentiation. Hum Mol Genet. 2010;19:3457–67.
100 Wilkie AO, Byren JC, Hurst JA, Jayamohan J, Johnson D, Knight SJ, et al. Prevalence and complications of single-gene and chromosomal disorders in craniosynostosis. Pediatrics. 2010;126:e391–400.
101 Passos-Bueno MR, Serti Eacute AE, Jehee FS, Fanganiello R, Yeh E. Genetics of craniosynostosis: genes, syndromes, mutations and genotype–phenotype correlations. Front Oral Biol. 2008;12:107–43.
102 Jehee FS, Krepischi-Santos AC, Rocha KM, Cavalcanti DP, Kim CA, Bertola DR, et al. High frequency of submicroscopic chromosomal imbalances in patients with syndromic craniosynostosis detected by a combined approach of microsatellite segregation analysis, multiplex ligation-dependent probe amplification and array-based comparative genome hybridisation. J Med Genet. 2008;45:447–50.
103 Eswarakumar VP, Ozcan F, Lew ED, Bae JH, Tome F, Booth CJ, et al. Attenuation of signaling pathways stimulated by pathologically activated FGF-receptor 2 mutants prevents craniosynostosis. Proc Nat Acad Sci USA. 2006;103:18603–8.
104 Sedano HO, Cohen MM, Jr., Jirasek J, Gorlin RJ. Frontonasal dysplasia. J Pediatr. 1970;76:906–13.
105 Twigg SR, Versnel SL, Nurnberg G, Lees MM, Bhat M, Hammond P, et al. Frontorhiny, a distinctive presentation of

frontonasal dysplasia caused by recessive mutations in the ALX3 homeobox gene. Am J Hum Genet. 2009;84:698–705.
106 Kayserili H, Uz E, Niessen C, Vargel I, Alanay Y, Tuncbilek G, et al. ALX4 dysfunction disrupts craniofacial and epidermal development. Hum Mol Genet. 2009;18:4357–66.
107 Uz E, Alanay Y, Aktas D, Vargel I, Gucer S, Tuncbilek G, et al. Disruption of ALX1 causes extreme microphthalmia and severe facial clefting: expanding the spectrum of autosomal-recessive ALX-related frontonasal dysplasia. Am J Hum Genet. 2010;86:789–96.
108 Beverdam A, Brouwer A, Reijnen M, Korving J, Meijlink F. Severe nasal clefting and abnormal embryonic apoptosis in Alx3/Alx4 double mutant mice. Development. 2001;128:3975–86.
109 Ott CE, Leschik G, Trotier F, Brueton L, Brunner HG, Brussel W, et al. Deletions of the RUNX2 gene are present in about 10% of individuals with cleidocranial dysplasia. Hum Mutat. 2010;31:E1587–93.
110 Cohen MM, Jr. Biology of RUNX2 and cleidocranial dysplasia. J Craniofac Surg. 2013;24:130–3.
111 Lou Y, Javed A, Hussain S, Colby J, Frederick D, Pratap J, et al. A Runx2 threshold for the cleidocranial dysplasia phenotype. Hum Mol Genet. 2009;18:556–68.

Chapter 56

Orthognathic Surgery in the Patient with Cleft Lip and Palate

Alexander C. Cash and Alistair R.M. Cobb

Introduction

Orthognathic surgery is a well-recognized part of the clinical armamentarium utilized widely to address maxillomandibular disproportion. Planning this interdisciplinary care for the patient with an orofacial cleft will involve a large number of clinicians from many different specialities. Treatment may be lengthy, onerous and burdensome on both the patient and the team, but excellent functional, aesthetic, stable outcomes are now the norm.

Patients with any form of cleft lip and palate exhibit a myriad of different facial forms and features. These phenotypes will be expressed not only as a result of the family identity inherited from the genetic parents but also as a result of the interactions between pre-programmed facial growth and the treatment interventions that the patient may have experienced throughout their early life to address the age relevant concerns that arise as a result of their facial cleft.

We are well aware that some of our treatment interventions may restrict 'average' facial growth.[1] Perhaps, in the fullness of time, modern treatment techniques and protocols will be shown to be less restrictive to growth, but the benefits of these interventions in the patient's early years will often rightly be prioritized over the possible later effects on facial

Orthognathic Surgery: Principles, Planning and Practice. Edited by Farhad B. Naini and Daljit S. Gill.

(a) (b)

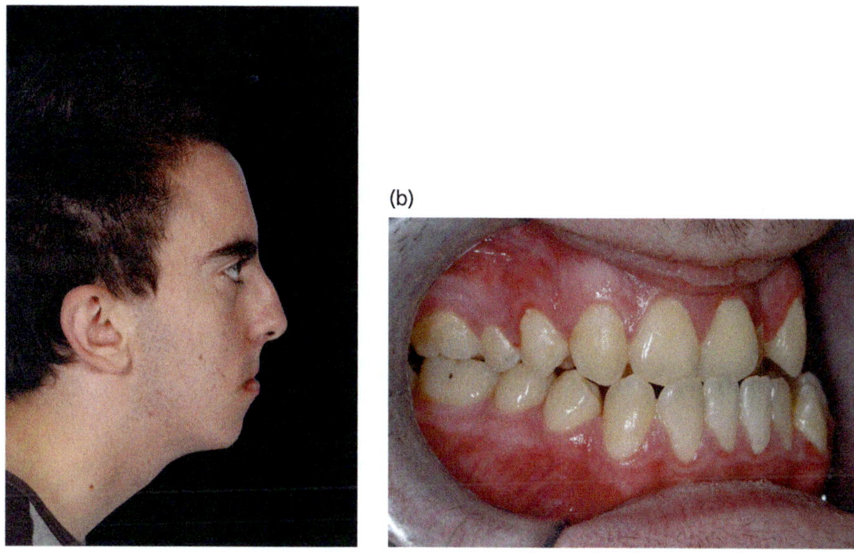

Fig. 56-1 Patient with repaired cleft palate with Pierre Robin Sequence. The patient presents with the paradox of a retrusive facial profile with Class II skeletal base elements but the presence of a Class III dental malocclusion.

harmony. These negative effects are often difficult to quantify for an individual patient because they are so varied and multifactorial; they muddy the waters of facial growth to the extent that it will take much longitudinal research to determine the precise contribution of each intervention to maxillary growth restriction.

Of course, many definitive orthognathic treatment interventions are aimed at improving the retropositioned cleft maxilla and it is suggested that 3–70% of the cleft population may benefit from this type of treatment.[2–4] However, it would be wrong to expect that all cleft faces will demonstrate a Class III facial balance. Certainly, in our clinical practice, many do, but other orofacial clefting conditions such as Pierre Robin sequence may also produce micrognathia and with that comes a Class II retrusive facial balance (Figure 56-1a,b).

It should be recognized that improving maxillomandibular relations will rely on high quality primary care and will subsequently facilitate further late corrective surgeries such as lip/nose revision. These surgeries are often more successful if the bony facial foundations are 'normalized' prior to their completion. Orthognathic jaw surgery may also produce iatrogenic concerns that may necessitate later supplemental corrective surgery. Velopharyngeal incompetence is a major risk to the speech of a cleft patient undergoing a maxillary advancement and so the consenting process must fully inform the patient of all the major risks and benefits of their care plan prior to commencing their treatment.

Prevalence

UK cleft teams aspire to an osteotomy rate similar to that of the Goteborg team where only 3% of patients require orthognathic surgery to help correct Class III malocclusion. The Swedish team produced results with no GOSLON group fives (significant Class III malocclusions) when employing a delayed hard palate closure protocol.[2]

Following a retrospective study evaluating lateral skull radiographs of cleft lip and palate (CLP) patients in Canada, it was found that 48% of their unilateral CLP patient population were considered to be likely to benefit from orthognathic surgery while the number of bilateral CLP patients was higher at 65%.[3] These findings, although worse in terms of maxillary growth than the Swedish teams' results, were better than those published in the seminal study that lead to the reconfiguration and centralization of cleft services in the UK. Prior to centralization, 39% of five-year-old UK children had a poor or very poor dental arch relationship and 70% of 12-year-olds had a Class III skeletal base relationship with midface retrusion. Less than 30% of those patients were judged by a panel of experts to have 'good facial appearance'.[4]

It is hoped that prospectively auditing the outcomes of the now centralized UK services over the coming decade will show that the patients of the new services, now over 10 years old, will have a lesser incidence of Class III and, into later teenage life, a lesser need for orthognathic surgery than prior to the UK cleft reorganization. It is universally hoped by teams and patients alike, that we do see these improvements in outcomes for patients born with cleft lip and palate.

Treatment planning

General factors

In much of the UK, cleft patients requiring more information about orthognathic treatment are likely to be invited to a multidisciplinary team clinic at around 15–16 years old. This may coincide with a cleft audit/outcome clinic but this is usually the earliest time at which orthognathic treatment may be discussed in some detail. General orthognathic and cleft associated risks and benefits are highlighted and patient information given to support the discussion on treatment in general.

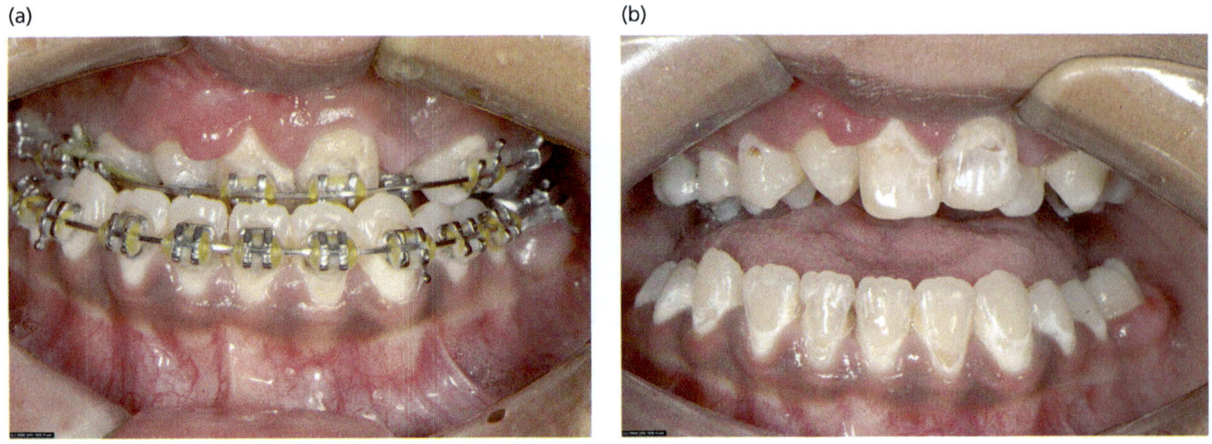

Fig. 56-2 Cleft patient's dental health needs to have been secured prior to starting orthodontic/orthognathic care. In these images orthodontic preparation for orthognathic surgery was abandoned due to poor compliance with basic oral hygiene and dietary advice.

If it is thought that general somatic growth is beginning to tail off to the extent that treatment could be commenced shortly and if the patient is keen to find out more about a specific plan for them, they are worked up through a number of direct and allied cleft team clinicians (Box 56.1). Orthognathic care for the patient with an orofacial cleft is delivered by a truly multidisciplinary team offering interdisciplinary care.

Box 56-1 Cleft and allied team clinicians for orthognathic planning and treatment

- Medical specialists
- Cleft restorative dentist
- Periodontist
- Cleft orthodontist
- Cleft psychologist
- Cleft speech and language therapist
- Cleft surgeon/orthognathic
- Cleft surgeon/speech
- Sleep physician/respiratory medics
- Orthodontic/maxillofacial technologist

Medical input

Patients with cleft lip and palate often have coexisting medical conditions, often as part of an inherited syndrome, many of which produce congenital effects on the structure of the heart. Incidence varies; European cohort statistics suggest 29% of patients have associated conditions[5] but a US cohort[6] reports rates as high as 71%. Most agree that patients with isolated cleft palate appear to have a higher prevalence of associated anomalies.[7] Appropriate medical specialists need to be involved when planning orthognathic care and strategies adopted to optimize patients for care should be employed where needed. It is obvious to say that when co-existing medical conditions exist and produce significant risk to general health, elective orthognathic surgery may be contraindicated.

Dental input and orthodontic retention

Clearly the dental team including the family dentist and the specialist team will need to ensure that the patient is dentally/periodontally fit for combined orthognathic treatment (Figure 56-2a,b). Simple restorations need to be completed, previous treatments need to have been checked as sound and oral hygiene needs to be proven to be of a consistently high standard. The periodontal status of the teeth needs assessment and particular attention paid to the teeth adjacent to sites of an alveolar cleft (Figures 56-3 and 56-4).

It is not unusual to find unattached, non-keratinized mucosa in places where one would expect to find attached, keratinized mucosa. Previous treatments, often completed in challenging clinical circumstances, may position tissues in unusual surroundings and this can produce both oral hygiene, periodontal/restorative and aesthetic complications (Figure 56-5a,b). Where such flaps overlie the alveolus in the developing dentition, normal eruption processes may be delayed and teeth may remain unerupted.

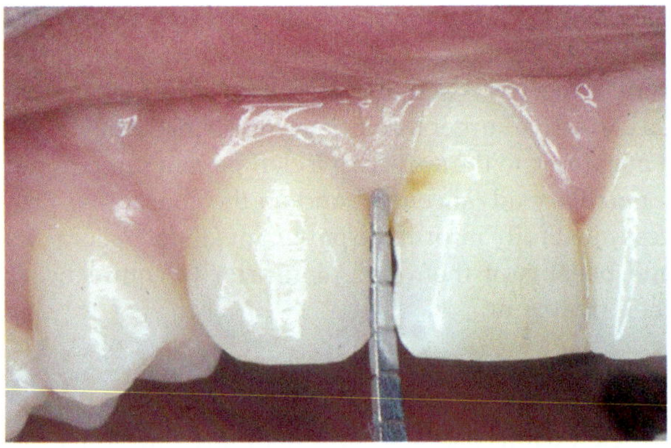

Fig. 56-3 A patient with a repaired right alveolar cleft, the patient having had an alveolar bone graft that appears successful with healthy looking supporting periodontal tissues. There is, however, a distal cavity in the upper right central incisor with some mild enamel hypomineralization and the lateral incisor is missing. Previous orthodontic treatment has nicely closed the lateral incisor space.

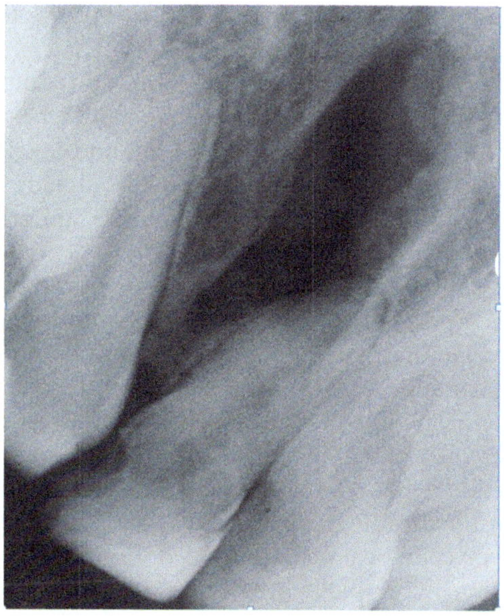

Fig. 56-4 Periapical radiographic imaging reveals that all is not well within the previously grafted alveolus and pre-orthognathic discussions must be had to determine whether or not the alveolar bone graft should be updated. Dental caries must also be addressed.

Temporomandibular joints need to be free of dysfunction, to be sound and symptom free. Often, before the orthognathic pathway opens up, patients potentially may have experienced several courses of orthodontic treatment already and there will often be evidence of enamel demineralization. This needs to be noted, monitored and used to demonstrate risks to the patient. Likewise, there may be history of previous restorative care; old restorations and tooth build-ups may require updating; hypomineralized teeth, often adjacent to an alveolar cleft, may require topical fluoride and other specialist dental treatments; and to keep on top of all this, regular liaison and maintenance with the patient's local dental team and the hygienist will also be of great benefit.

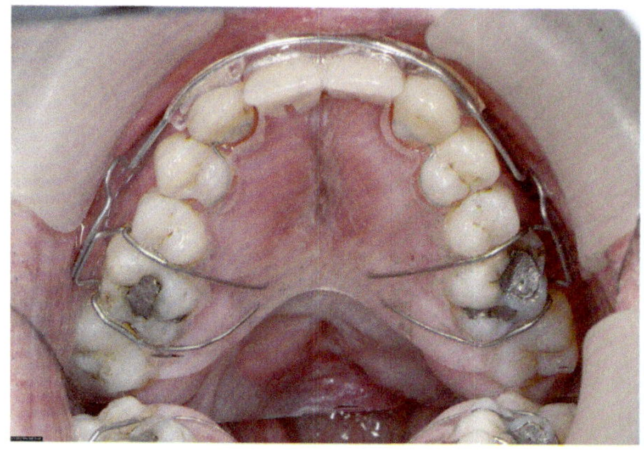

Fig. 56-6 Palatally bonded fixed retainers between both canines and first premolar teeth maintain the positions of the maxillary canine teeth in conjunction with a removable retainer carrying prosthetic upper central incisors.

Post-orthodontic treatment retention is deliberately discussed in this section – in advance of the treatment section. For the patient with a cleft lip and palate, retention is such a crucial component of treatment that this should be considered, planned and highlighted to the patient at the outset of planning the overall orthognathic care package. It has ever been so that treatment planning that involves orthodontics, should start at the end and work back towards the beginning.

In conjunction with the orthodontist, the dental specialists will consider retention, long-term restorative maintenance as well as the restoration of missing dental units. Planning retention timing, style, duration and its interaction with any restorative component is of paramount importance and should be planned in an interdisciplinary fashion. Missing units should, where possible, be restored prosthetically either by attaching teeth to the orthodontic appliance (Figure 56-6) or by making them completely removable during active orthodontic treatment. These prosthetic teeth should be replicated on removable retainers once the fixed appliances are removed. Consideration must be given

(a) (b)

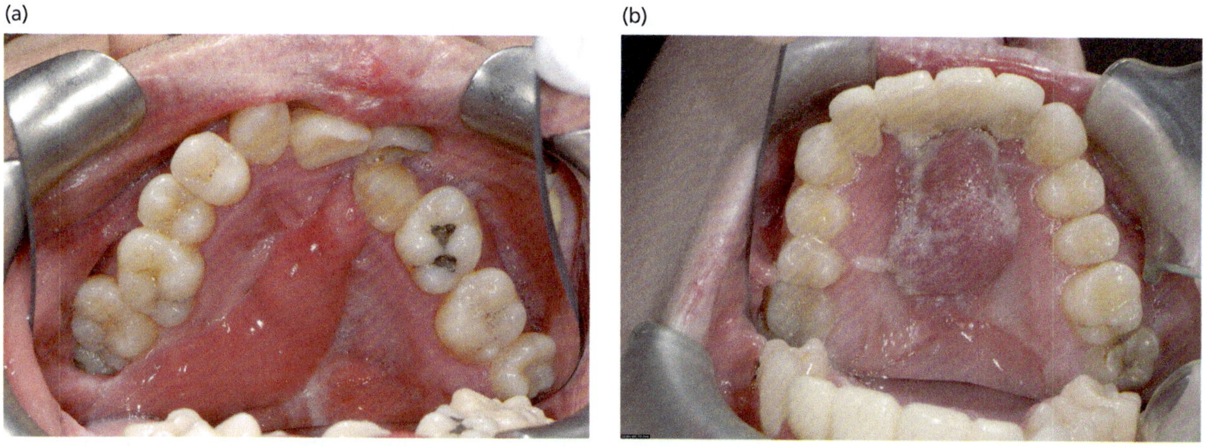

Fig. 56-5 (a) Non-keratinized, unattached mucosa, brought from a buccal flap to close a palatal fistula, lies adjacent to the palatal aspect of the upper right canine and the pedicle crosses over the occlusal surfaces of the terminal molars in the upper left quadrant. This pedicle root needs to be protected in the immediate postoperative phase as it can be traumatized by the occlusion. Once the flap has established, oral hygiene can be difficult around the flap margins. (b) Keratinized mucosa, brought from a tongue flap to close a palatal fistula, lies beneath a fixed anterior bridge in a patient with consistently poor oral hygiene.

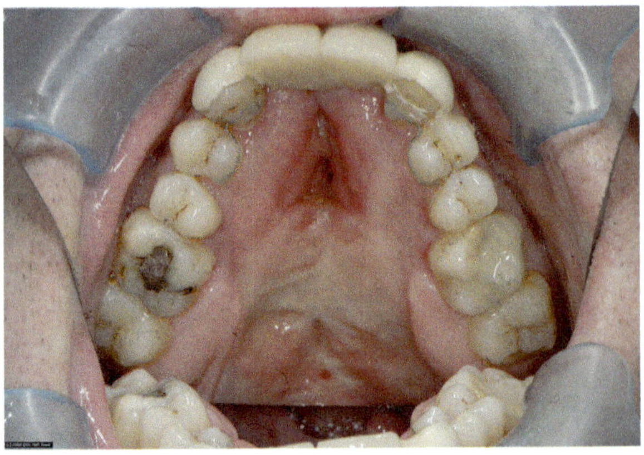

Fig. 56-7 Following provision of labially bonded cast porcelain bridge, palatal bonded retainers remain available for maintenance and upkeep of post orthodontic and restorative treatment result. Building the incisors anteriorly can also help to advance and support the upper lip, reducing a Class III profile.

to using fixed/bonded retainers to maintain tooth positions adjacent to sites where teeth are missing and where teeth were particularly rotated prior to treatment (Figure 56-7). This will often be the incisor teeth, especially those adjacent to the cleft.

Any definitive restorations need be placed, once a period of settling has been achieved. If there is a need to restore across an alveolar cleft, then a suitable period of time should be left to allow postoperative and post-orthodontic tissue maturation. There is nothing more frustrating for clinical teams *and* their patients than having to remove fixed retention devices and fixed restorations soon after their placement when things aren't allowed a suitable settling period. For example, a fistula may become symptomatic beneath a fixed bridge and may require further surgical closure. To permit complete surgical access to the cleft anatomy, the fixed retention device and/or fixed restorations will need to be removed to enable the repeated surgical closure of the fistula.

Retention, especially for those who have had alveolar clefts, is without doubt a life-long commitment and should be designed to maintain post treatment arch width. Any maxillary restriction in the transverse plane post-treatment may well have consequences for the posterior occlusion but there will likely also be effects on the incisor relationship both in an anteroposterior and vertical dimension.

Records

There is no substitute for directly planning with the patient present but clinical records are an adjunct of significant importance also forming part of the patient's legal medical record. The orthodontist will take digital records where possible and will often engage the technical team too. The digital record should include articulated study casts, two- and three-dimensional photography as well as appropriate radiography. Radiographs will usually include a lateral skull cephalometric radiograph, a dental panoramic view and, where appropriate, a cleft centred occlusal to reassess previous bone graft outcome. Dental and bone graft assessments should be made from the panoramic and occlusal films and consideration given to the loss of third molars. As already mentioned, repeat bone grafting should be undertaken where deemed to be inadequate.

The lateral skull film should allow a tracing and the incorporation of this radiograph into a digital facial planning software program from one of the many commercial providers. These produce a computer morphed prediction, which will give the patient further understanding of the aims of treatment and an indication as to possible outcome. Occasionally, three-dimensional radiography may be required. Conventional or cone beam computerized tomography may help image complex cases where two-dimensional films fail to be fully diagnostic and facilitate three dimensional software planning.

From three-dimensional radiological data, clinicians may request the production of a three-dimensional stereolithic model. This may enable a full understanding of the complexities of a three dimensional clinical problem and will also help with the production of the correct vectors when planning osteogenic distraction. Techniques are also available where the digital record can be used to directly produce the intraoperative surgical wafers for orthognathic surgery. Onlay grafting implant materials may be produced, often milled from a solid block, to accurately fit directly over the surface of an asymmetrical bone within the facial skeleton.

Timing

As for non-cleft patients, the timing for orthognathic surgery can be assessed in many different ways. Serial radiographs should be avoided to reduce the patients' radiation exposure. Clinicians may use hand wrist radiography, plot standing heights on growth charts, take serial study models or clinical photos and the orthodontist is well placed to interpret their favoured growth related record.

The premise remains true that the surgical start should be delayed in Class III, vertical growing and asymmetrical patients as they often grow longer and later than patients with opposite facial form. These short faced, often Class II patients, may start their orthognathic care earlier in their teenage years, as it is unlikely that late growth will negatively affect the outcome.

Factors in planning orthognathic care

The diagnosis and treatment planning for patients undergoing orthognathic surgery have been covered in Chapters 5 and 6. However, there are specific cleft related components to orthognathic planning that bear consideration and are discussed below (Box 56.2).

Box 56-2 Tips for cleft orthognathic surgery

- Have a back-up plan if maxillary advancement is not fully possible.
- Have an additional inter-occlusal wafer made to this prescription.
- Maximize the mobilization of the maxilla prior to fixation.
- Minimize mucosal incisions to protect as wide a vascular pedicle as possible.
- Consider distraction if full advancement cannot be achieved in one go.
- Consider the need for pre-orthognathic top up alveolar bone grafting.
- Allow longer operating time compared to non-cleft orthognathic surgery.

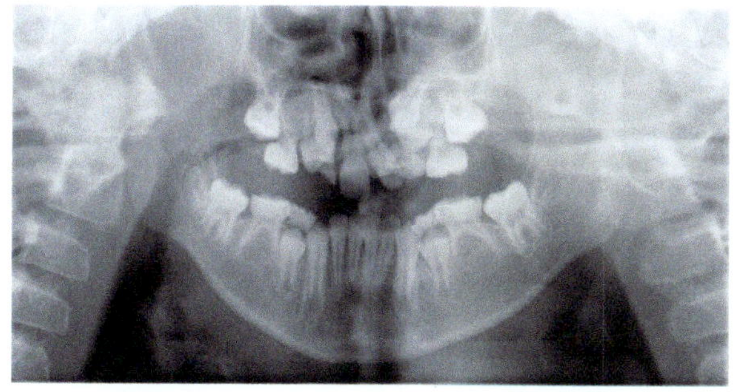

Fig. 56-8 Dental panoramic tomograph demonstrating a shortened maxillary dental arch missing both maxillary lateral incisors, upper right and both lower second premolars; with palatally impacted upper left premolars and missing maxillary second molars. The permanent upper first molars are also stacked – impacted under the distal surfaces of the second deciduous molars. This is a particularly strong sign of a small maxilla.

Surgical input (adjunctive)

Where the pre-orthognathic records reveal sub-optimal outcomes from earlier treatments, then repeat surgery may be required to facilitate the orthodontic/orthognathic care. Remedial surgery will need to be completed in advance of the orthognathic care but this may also offer an opportunity to carry out orthodontic or third molar extractions or, for example, permitting the repair of fistulae concurrently and prior to the orthognathic preparation.

Bone grafts to the maxillary alveolus cleft may require topping up – it is not an uncommon surgical experience for the unilateral cleft maxilla to separate into two parts during the surgical osteotomy in the operating theatre. Only the maxillary alveolus is repaired during bone graft surgery and, with no bony hard palate to support and strengthen the maxilla, the upper jaw is more delicate than usual in the patient with complete bony clefting.

Dental/periodontal health and tooth quality factors

Cleft lip and palate patients may well have experienced several different phases of clinical orthodontic care all with differing and varied objectives across their pre-orthognathic years. As a result of the burden of their earlier care and with an accumulation of 'dental/orthodontic load' over time, often a patient with cleft lip and palate will have a potentially compromised dentition – perhaps more heavily restored than their non-cleft peer group.

Where and when oral hygiene was less than ideal, there may be patches of decalcification affecting the dentition. This should have been treated with high dose topical fluoride and other specialist dental treatments and should be demonstrated to the patient, using its presence to motivate the patient to maintain a consistently high level of oral hygiene throughout their subsequent orthognathic orthodontics.

Teeth adjacent to the cleft are often diminutive and hypomineralized with discoloured and hypoplastic enamel as well. Care should be taken when this has been treated with composite veneers both because orthodontic bracket bonding may be compromised, but also because orthodontic bracket debonding may damage existing restorations and the patient should be made aware of this potential risk in advance. Often there may be a plan to replace/update these restorations at the end of treatment and liaison with the restoring dentist about the positioning and the timing of the placement of bonded retainers is important.

There is repeated, consistent evidence that patients with cleft lip and palate have a higher incidence of dental anomalies than the non-cleft population. Most report that over 95% of patients have at least one dental anomaly. There is an increased rate of missing teeth adjacent to the cleft site as well as an increased rate of impacted premolars[8] (Figure 56-8).

These features are very relevant to the presentation and preparation of the cleft patient for the provision of orthognathic surgery as there are consistently fewer maxillary teeth to work with. This maxillary dentoalveolar disproportion often hinders the orthodontic preparation especially when considering decompensation, co-ordination and centreline correction. Conversely, however, a lesser number of maxillary teeth may be related to a higher incidence of Class III malocclusion and this should encourage teams, correctly, to really concentrate the orthognathic treatment planning on maxillary advancement surgery. Mandibular set-back in the cleft lip and palate patient often produces very poor facial outcomes albeit with satisfactory occlusion.

It is often a challenge to bring the maxillary incisors to a reasonable position on their skeletal base when there are fewer teeth available to bond with a fixed orthodontic appliance. It is often difficult to fully express bracket prescription even when using maximum dimension archwires and to my mind, cleft orthodontics is another indication for using high

(a)

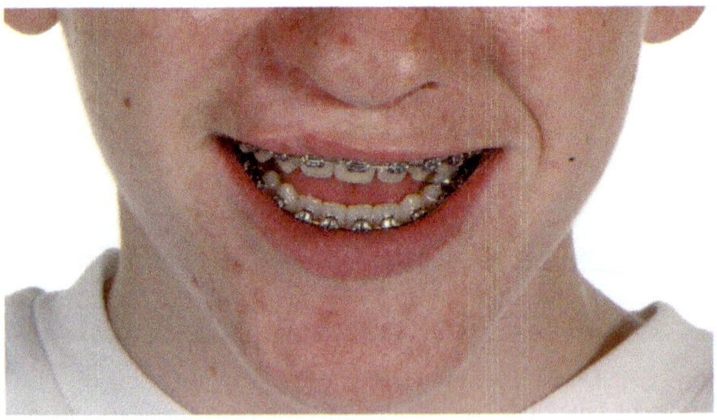

(b)

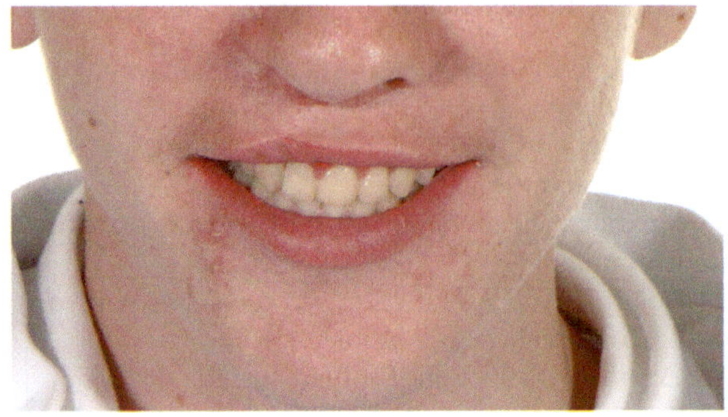

Fig. 56-9 (a & b) Images prior to bimaxillary orthognathic surgery to correct a Class III malocclusion with reduced upper incisor show and anterior openbite in a patient with a right unilateral cleft lip and palate. The missing maxillary right lateral incisor causes slight centre line discrepancy in the post bimaxillary osteotomy occlusion (b).

value bracket prescription systems. The cleft maxillary arch often has premolars missing/impacted and excluded and there is a danger that these shortened dental arches will produce upper incisor teeth that will finish retroclined and under torqued.

Missing maxillary lateral incisors brings the conundrum of whether or not to arrange the extraction of the contralateral tooth for symmetry and centreline correction (Figure 56-9a,b) at the further risk of reducing the ability to appropriately torque the upper incisors. However, failure to correct maxillary centrelines during the orthodontic preparation prior to orthognathic surgery, risks inviting surgical correction of the maxillary midline by rotating the maxilla in the horizontal plane. This will invariably introduce yaw discrepancy and these mismatches of the radial relationship of the arch width will produce one buccal segment in cross bite, the other in scissor bite. These are supremely challenging indeed to fully correct postoperatively and can give rise to significant functional occlusal disharmony.

Orthodontic factors

Anteroposterior

The majority of cleft patients undergoing orthognathic care have Class III malocclusions. Those with significant overbite and relatively minimal reverse overjet will often offer a challenge to the orthodontic team in the early stages of their care. Without the wholly compliant use of significant bite opening devices, these patients will often repeatedly fracture their brackets off the upper incisor and canine teeth where arch width and radial relations are complex (Figure 56-10). To overcome this problem, clinicians may favour starting the orthodontic treatment in the lower arch first, proclining the incisors and moving them away from the upper incisors. The uppers can then be bonded later and the arches prepared for surgery.

Vertical

Typically the patient with a complete unilateral bony cleft will have reduced incisor display and as such orthognathic planning should incorporate some increase in the exposure of the upper incisors. In some, more severe cases, this may require additional bone grafting at the time of the maxillary osteotomy to improve stability, but in other more moderate cases, angled Le Fort I maxillary bony cuts may slide the incisors down and forward, out from beneath the upper lip, as the maxilla is translated in the same direction along the bony incisions.

In the patient with a complete bilateral bony cleft there is often increased incisor display. It is a crucial part of the planning process to assess where the discrepancy lies. One must assess if the upper lip is short or whether there is true maxillary vertical excess. Typically in the bilateral cleft patient the lip is short and if maxillary impaction alone is planned as the method of reducing the incisor display, the likelihood is that the upper third of the lower anterior face height will be overly reduced producing poor facial balance and disrupting vertical facial harmony (Figure 56-11a–d).

Pre-maxillary osteotomy is a technique described for the vertical reduction of the anterior section of the

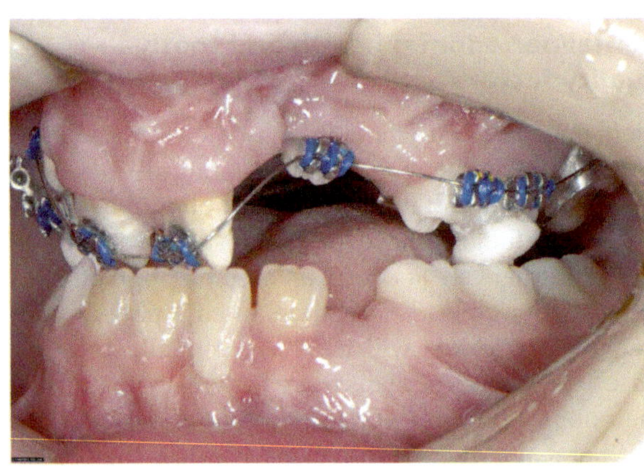

Fig. 56-10 Class III incisors with cleft centred open bite and teeth erupting high in cleft site. To enable the provision of an upper fixed appliance, a large amount of bite opening has been achieved with the addition of large volumes cement temporarily placed on the posterior teeth. This approach will enable upper arch treatment where the lower incisors consistently risk the debonding of the upper arch fixed appliance brackets.

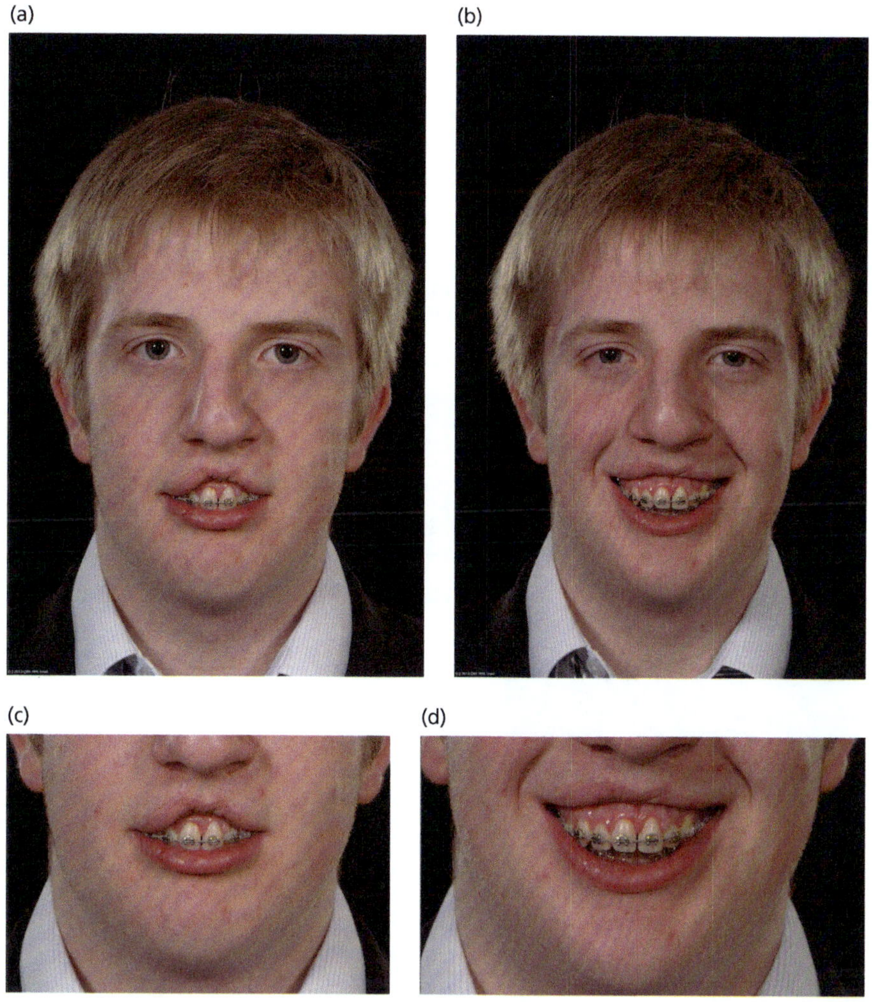

Fig. 56-11 (a, b, c, d) Increased maxillary incisor display as a result both of a short upper lip and true vertical maxillary excess in a patient with a bilateral cleft lip and palate. Surgical planning must take into account whether post orthognathic lip surgery is also planned and in a case such as this, an Abbe flap may add volume and length to the upper lip. Clearly it is crucial to assess how the incisor show will be affected both by the amount of impaction of the maxilla and by the amount of upper lip lengthening both at repose and on smiling.

maxilla that carries the upper incisor teeth. Usually employed during the growing years, it is employed as a surgical technique designed to osteotomize and intrude incisor teeth borne by the anterior maxilla. But it carries risks and may reduce growth and adds to the bony surgical burden of care. An alternative however may employ the prudent use of fixed orthodontic treatment employing Class II mechanics with incisor intrusion and perhaps coupled with lip revision surgery or sulcoplasty (Figure 56-12a–d).

Where an alveolar cleft exists, the patient will often present with a cleft centred anterior open bite. This may position the teeth adjacent to the cleft at a significantly superior position to the remaining teeth in the arch. These teeth are often levelled by orthodontic means with gentle extrusion (Figure 56-10). Despite the most gentle and prudent of mechanics, levelling teeth high up in the alveolus may produce increased relapse potential. This is yet another reason that the cleft lip and palate patient should have their post orthodontic treatment outcomes maintained into the long term with fixed bonded and removable retainers.

Horizontal

Although the maxillary arch prior to bone grafting may anteriorly be narrow with the lesser segment having collapsed towards the midline, the post bone grafting maxillary arch may be broad, with wide intermolar width. It often remains shallow, with little anteroposterior depth. Optimizing the arch co-ordination is one of the crucial aspects of pre-orthognathic surgical orthodontic preparation and in the authors experience, this is usually simply achieved with orthodontic archwires. The need for auxiliary orthodontic expansion devices is very unusual in preparatory orthodontics for orthognathic jaw surgery for the patient with orofacial clefting.

On the rare occasions where expansion is required in the patient with a repaired complete bony cleft, the maxillary arch responds readily to widening forces. Although there is bone within the alveolus, there is no bone across the bony hard palate and as such, there is little resistance from the cleft maxilla to the forces from the archwires and, as a result, maxillary arch width expansion is readily achieved.

Facial features

Typical facial features of the patient with cleft lip and palate presenting for orthognathic surgery are of a hypoplastic midface. There is a lack of midface contour with a concave rather than convex projection and a Class III facial relationship. A retruded inferior

(a) (b) (c) (d)

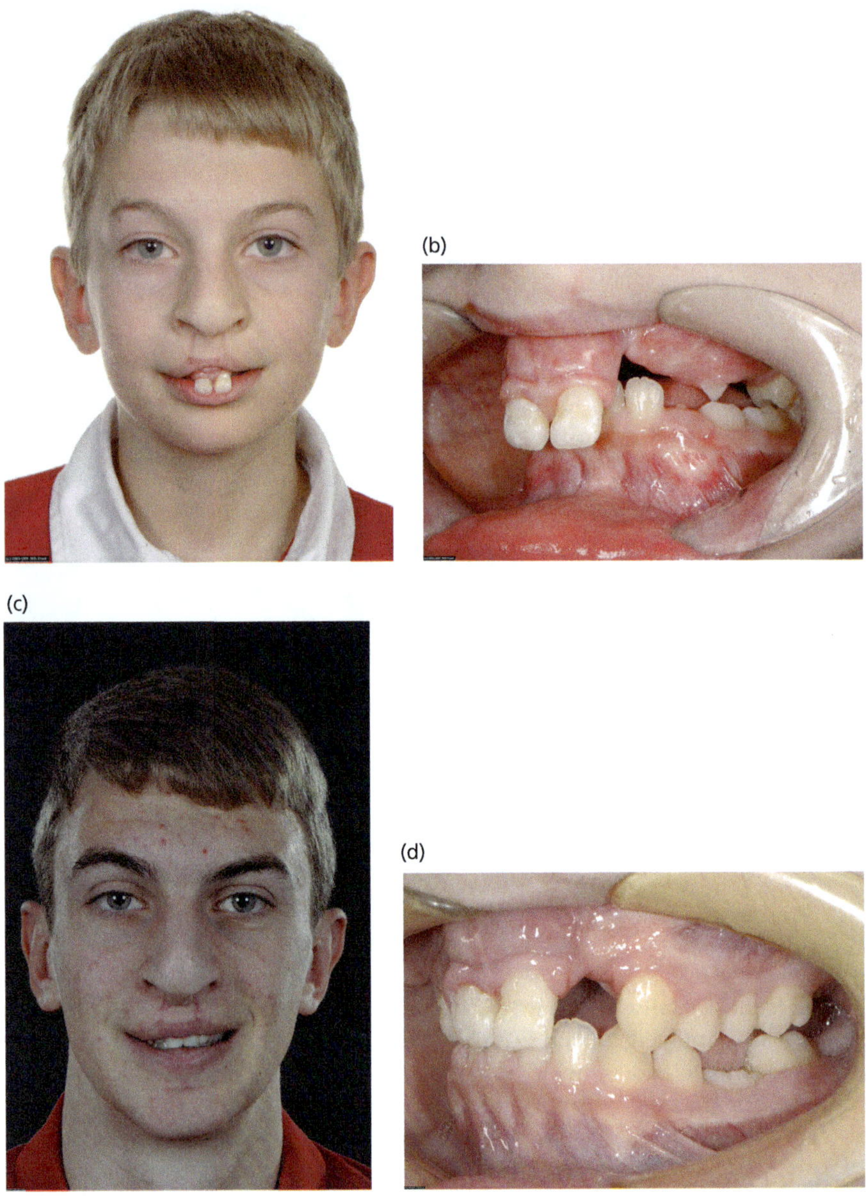

Fig. 56-12 (a, b, c, d) Severe and extreme over eruption of maxillary incisors in a patient with a bilateral cleft lip and palate. This can follow as a result of significant lip incompetence and can lead to a significant deep and traumatic overbite. In this case, intrusion and occlusal levelling has been achieved by orthodontic mechanics alone avoiding the need for premaxillary osteotomy. Later treatment involved an Abbe flap to balance the prolabium and increase upper lip volume.

orbital rim position provides poor lower eyelid support and apparent exorbitism. Paranasal flattening and posteriorized upper incisor position contribute to poor nasal tip position and upper lip support. Associated with the repaired unilateral cleft lip and alveolus there may be asymmetry of both bony and soft tissues around the nasal alar and piriform fossa.

Traditionally, Le Fort I maxillary advancement would correct the underlying AP discrepancy, normalizing the dental occlusion. If adequate advancement was not possible then commonly a '2/3 : 1/3' plan was used where the maxilla was brought forward 2 units and the mandible set-back 1 unit relatively in a bimaxillary procedure. This may still have merit as a fallback position when there is difficulty fully correcting the retropositioned maxilla. However, improved techniques of primary palatal closure and maxillary mobilization at the time of osteotomy may improve anterior repositioning of the jaw. Distraction osteogenesis therapy can be used in resistant cases to further advance the maxilla nearer to an ideal position not possible at the initial osteotomy procedure. This has become more important with more appreciation of ideal facial aesthetic outcomes of orthognathic surgery. Facial aesthetic and functional outcomes are important – sometimes requiring compromise on dental position in favour of facial form. A convex rather than concave facial form is aimed for.

Soft tissue approaches to the maxilla[9]

The vascular supply to the cleft maxilla may be compromised. The endosseous supply will be interrupted by an alveolar cleft and alveolar bone grafting may not adequately restore this. The overlying periosteum may be scarred. Therefore the typical sub-labial vestibular incision used in a non-cleft osteotomy case may be better made higher in the sulcus in cleft cases, preserving blood supply with a wider pedicle.

(a) (b)

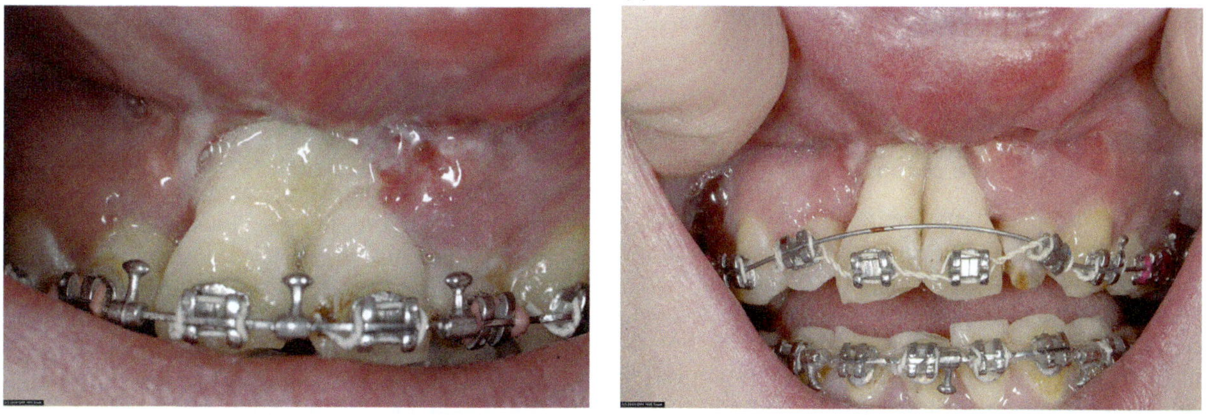

Fig. 56-13 (a) Devitalized maxillary central incisors post bimaxillary osteotomy in a patient with a bilateral cleft lip and palate. The tissues became grey and ischaemic in the weeks following the surgery and this image is from four weeks post bimaxillary osteotomy. (b) These teeth were subsequently lost and restored with a denture and subsequently a fixed bridge. An implant solution would only be possible following a block bone graft, and in a patient who is clearly unable to manage their diet/hygiene for the benefit of their dental health and is therefore not motivated with such a poor restorative status, their suitability and compliance for expensive and complex treatment should be robustly questioned.

Similarly the posterior limit of the incision should be carefully considered.

In bilateral cases, a tunnelling approach may be employed via a small midline vertical incision and a small vertical buccal incision on each side, further ensuring adequate blood supply preservation – in this case to the premaxillary segment (Figure 56-13). Where vascular compromise is thought to be a particularly risk in bilateral cleft cases, a transpalatal approach can be used for premaxillary segmental osteotomy or for segmental procedures.

Maxillary surgery

Alveolar bone grafting has largely removed the need for segmental maxillary procedures previously employed for cleft maxillary advancement. Techniques such as horseshoe and paramedian osteotomies are rarely indicated and we find that Le Fort I level advancements are usually employed – with segmental modification on occasions. This also facilitates easier access to close residual nasal floor and hard palatal fistula.[10]

Segmental advancement of the lesser segment of an ungrafted maxilla can be used to close a wide alveolar cleft. When indicated, such surgery may be performed via a small vertical incision at the anterior aspect of the lesser segment to preserve blood supply. Either a reciprocating saw or fissure burr can be used to make the subapical bone cuts, completed with an osteotome. Some clinicians still prefer to use cast cap splints with a locking slide, which obviates the need for internal fixation. Internal miniplate fixation can be used but will require further stripping of periosteum and thus potential vascular supply compromise.

With the advent of porous high-density polyethylene (PHDPE), Medpor™, malar prosthetic implants, osteotomies including the zygomatic eminences to restore malar projection are now rarely utilized. Instead a Le Fort I level advancement, with prosthetic implants, is undertaken. Hypoplastic flattening of the piriform fossa bilaterally may be addressed by higher than usual bone cuts – a so-called 'high Le Fort I' (or 'Le Fort I $\frac{1}{2}$'). More rarely, piriform fossa PHDPE implants may be used. Clockwise rotation of the midface will produce relatively more malar projection than the occlusal plane, which can be used to advantage. This will require a bilateral mandibular sagittal split procedure. However in severe cases, Le Fort II, Le Fort III or compound osteotomies (e.g. Le Fort II plus Le Fort I levels) may be employed – in which case distraction osteogenesis may be required.

Mobilization of the maxilla may be difficult because of scar tissue formation throughout the hard palate cleft, which may not be ossified. Downfracture of the maxilla may result in reopening the hard palate cleft and the patient should be warned about this prior to surgery. This palatal scarring may limit advancement and be a factor in relapse after surgery. Good mobilization is essential before positioning the maxillary segment in the wafer. Some surgeons prefer to have a second option prepared with less maxillary movement and compensatory retro-positioning of the mandible. These factors all additively contribute to a longer operative time for cleft orthognathic surgery than for non-cleft procedures.

Another option is to use a distraction device to slowly advance the maxilla in the few weeks following surgery. A second procedure may be then necessary to finally position the maxillary segment and secure with miniplate fixation. In clefts involving the hard palate it may be good practice to include wire loops onto the final interocclusal wafer so that this may be fixed onto the orthodontic archwire and left in situ postoperatively to further support the lesser segment. At the end of surgery, or the following morning, the archwire can be replaced with a heavy gauge wire. Where larger lesser segment maxillary procedures are used, some teams will still resort to the safety of traditional cast cap splints.

Segmental surgery

Maxillary horseshoe osteotomy

The horseshoe maxillary osteotomy[11–14] is an orthognathic segmental procedure moving the complete maxillary alveolus but leaving the remaining hard palate in place. It may be undertaken as an isolated segmental procedure or in conjunction with a Le Fort maxillary osteotomy. It may be difficult to apply to cleft patients since their bony palates are not intact. However, the advantage for this patient group is that the soft palate is not advanced and thus speech deterioration is avoided, and fibrous scar tissue in the hard palate may have less effect on dentoalveolar advancement. There is, though, the change of causing an anterior palate fistula.

The isolated procedure is carried out though a buccal approach. The buccal bone cuts may be made with right-angled oscillating or reciprocating saw blades, or fissure burr. The palatal bone cuts are made with a fissure burr through the access conferred by the buccal cuts. A finger placed on the palatal mucosa can be used to judge the palatal cuts but great care must be taken if palatal mucosal perforation or damage to tooth roots – particularly posterior teeth – is to be avoided.

This technique is not currently widely used in cleft surgery. However, it may have a revitalized role in distraction orthognathic surgery for people at high risk of speech deterioration following cleft orthognathic surgery. Distraction also has the advantage that slow traction on the soft tissue may facilitate their maximum advancement.

Distraction osteogenesis

After Ilizarov's first description of the process,[15] it was McCarthy who first undertook distraction osteogenesis of the facial skeleton.[16] It is a technique ideally suited to the difficult cleft cases where relatively large maxillary advancements are required but which are hampered by restrictive fibrous scar tissue in the palate and by poor vascular supply. The process involves making osteotomy cuts and then waiting 5 days for a cartilaginous callus to form (the latency period). This can then be deformed plastically, stretching out the callus at 0.5 mm twice a day by activating the distraction device to achieve advancement of the osteotomized segment (the active phase). When the desired advancement is achieved the process is stopped and a consolidation period of up to three months is observed in which the cartilaginous callus calcifies and 'new bone' has thus been created. Soft tissues are less restrictive in this form of treatment as they are liable to slowly give up their resistance compared to more immediate osteotomy surgery movements and so greater movements of the bony segment can be achieved albeit over a longer period of time.

Choice of distractor type

Distraction devices can be internally or externally placed. The rigid external distractor (RED frame) is an evolution from traditional maxillofacial halo frames. It is fixed to the temporoparietal cranium with transcutaneous screws on each side and holds a vertical bar in front of the face. Bony or dentally retained fixation of the osteotomized maxilla is anchored with wires to this vertical pin via screw thread inserting into a fixed horizontal bar on the inferior aspect of the vertical bar. These screw threads can then be turned twice daily to draw the wires and thus maxilla forward. The advantage of the external distractor is that the vector of movement can be changed mid-treatment and the device itself does not impair the distraction process so potentially more freedom of treatment is permitted. However, the obvious disadvantage is the sometime painful transcutaneous fixation and bulk of the device, which can make sleep and physical activities difficult and is very socially obvious. In cases of two level maxillary osteotomy cuts, both segments can be distracted simultaneously.

The internal distractor is placed on the bone surface and the screw thread either runs through the maxillary antrum or under the buccal mucosa. One device is required each side and must lie as parallel as possible to the axis of movement otherwise converging vectors will prevent further distraction. Vectors of movement need to be more accurately discerned before fixation of the device and are more difficult to change once the device has been placed.

Either device is left in situ until the consolidation period is completed unless internal miniplate fixation is substituted.

Le Fort I distraction

Distraction osteogenesis may be used with Le Fort I maxillary osteotomy in cases with severe maxillary deficiency. Typically advancements over 10 mm would be considered – especially given the relative difficulty of mobilizing cleft maxillas and their tendency to relapse. There is evidence that there may be less relapse of the anteriorly repositioned maxilla by distraction than by osteotomy and immediate fixation.[17]

The use of a distraction device may be helpful in cases where adequate mobilization cannot be achieved during surgery. Thus the patient must be adequately prepared for this possibility in the clinical discussions about surgery options. The slow traction on soft tissues allows greater movement.

There is evidence that distraction osteogenesis may result in lower incidence of velopharyngeal insufficiency in the cleft maxilla[18,19] (Figure 56-14).

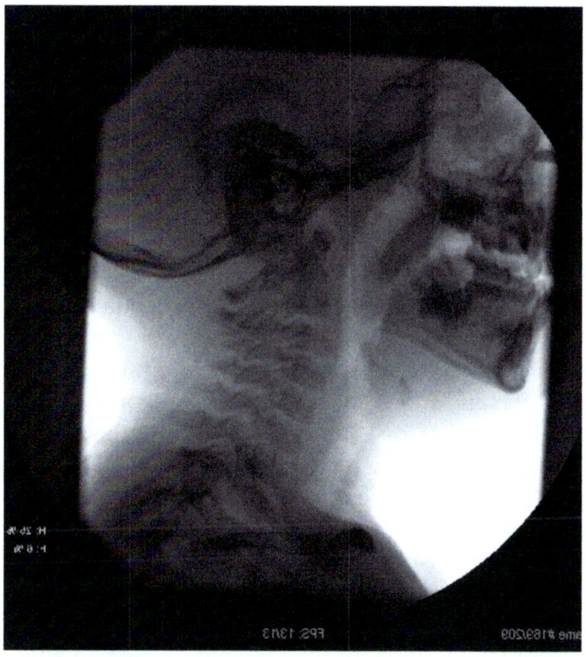

Fig. 56-14 A still frame from a lateral video X-ray of a patient having velo-pharyngeal investigations to assess palate function as the patient has cleft related nasal sounding speech with air escaping past the incompetent palate. The image demonstrates a large retropharyngeal space and a ptotic soft palate, unable to reach the posterior pharyngeal wall. Maxillary advancement is most likely to produce or further worsen VPI.

Occasionally interceptive distraction osteogenesis may be employed before facial skeletal maturity to advance a very hypoplastic maxilla. Severe lack of growth of the upper jaw leads to dental and facial problems with related functional and psychological difficulties. Interceptive distraction osteogenesis aims to bring the upper jaw forward as soon as the canines are erupted (12–14 years). A definitive procedure can be undertaken when older.

Transport distraction

Particularly wide alveolar clefts may not be amenable to the standard alveolar bone grafting technique. There is a greater volume of harvested bone required and soft tissue closure can be too difficult to effect.

First described in 2000,[20] alveolar transport distraction is an innovative method to overcome these difficulties. The procedure moves a portion of the maxillary alveolus at the lateral margin of the cleft across the cleft toward the medial aspect. Bone cuts are made horizontally apical to the tooth posterior to the cleft, and interdentally between this and the adjacent tooth. The soft tissues are left intact as far as possible using minimal incisions and tunnelling techniques. A bone saw is used to make the horizontal cut. A fissure burr is used to start the vertical interdental cut which is then completed with a fine osteotome. The distraction device may be bone or tooth borne.[21] The latency period of 3 to 5 days is observed before the device is activated twice daily to affect 0.5 mm of movement a day. The technique not only creates new alveolar bone across the cleft, but also brings with it soft tissue coverage. Once the distracted segment meets the other side of the cleft a 'docking phenomenon' is experienced – the abutting soft tissues must be removed from the cleft and closed on palatal and labial surfaces. The distractor must then be left in place for three months, or alternatively miniplate fixation may be used until consolidation of the regenerate bone has occurred. Orthodontic treatment can then be completed, the distracted tooth restored and an osseointegrated implant placed to the neo-alveolar bone for restoration.

Early mandibular distraction in Pierre Robin sequence for compromised airway

Pierre Robin sequence describes the presence of a small mandible with resultant retrogenia causing glossoptosis and thus cleft palate (because of prevention of palatal shelves fusion) and upper airway obstruction. Airway support may be required and simple measures such as nasopharyngeal airways insertion are usually sufficient. In more marked cases, however, tracheostomy, lip-tongue adhesion or mandibular advancement by distraction osteogenesis may be required. Such cases are managed by a multidisciplinary team including members of the cleft team and paediatric respiratory physician, intensivist and anaesthetic teams usually coordinated by either a neonatologist or paediatrician.

When indicated, mandibular advancement distraction osteogenesis may be undertaken in very young children using external or internal distraction devices.[22] Multivector external devices were previously popular, but it is our practice to use an univector internal device to the angle of the mandible on each side. Clinical practice has moved from external devices to semi-buried in most cases, which have fewer complications and leave less scarring.[23] The child is laid supine under oral endotracheal anaesthesia. After skin preparation and local anaesthetic injection to the overlying soft tissues, an incision is made approximately two fingerbreadths inferior to the inferior border of the mandible in the upper neck. Any higher and damage to the marginal mandibular branch of the facial nerve is possible. A soft tissue flap is raised in a plane deep to platysma. This is continued up to the inferior border of the mandible, at its angle to the ramus. Having defined the mandibular angle, a line is marked at 45 degrees back from the retromolar fossa to the angle. This is varied according to the vector of distraction required: the best combination of inferior and anterior movement.

The internal distractor is then placed on the bone and screwed lightly in place and the line position amended to ensure that the distractor sits on a suitable area of bone. The activation arm can be passed out through the mouth in the buccal sulcus in an older patient, or transcutaneously forward submentally, or posteriorly to emerge just below the ear lobule in younger patients. The distraction device is then removed but the screw holes will have ensured its correct re-positioning after the osteotomy has been completed.

Particularly in the infantile mandible, the bone is very thin and damage to the inferior alveolar nerve it contains is a risk. This is avoided by carefully marking the approximate position of the nerve as judged from CT imaging. A malleable retractor is placed deep to the bone and a fissure burr used to make cuts from the retromolar fossa from above and the mandibular angle from below, along the marked line. These are then connected superficially and a fine osteotome used to connect the cuts thus completing the osteotomy around the nerve without damaging it.

The distraction device is then placed and the procedure repeated on the contralateral side.

The devices are then gently wound out a short distance to check unimpaired function and then wound back into place. A 5-day period of new cartilage callous formation is called the latency period. The distraction period can then start – the device on each side is opened with an activation key by 0.5 mm (usually one full rotation) in the morning and evening until the desired length is required – usually 20–25 mm. Then the devices are left in situ for the consolidation phase of about 8–12 weeks during which the new bone calcifies and becomes stronger. The devices can then be removed via the original incision line. Increases in airway cross-sectional area of over 200% can be achieved.[24]

The process of mandibular distraction may need to be repeated during growth.

Management of hard palate fistulas at the time of cleft orthognathic surgery

When the maxilla is downfractured, the access to the nasal floor mucosa can afford the best opportunity for the closure of hard palate fistulas.[25] This can be achieved in two layers (oral and nasal) and, if required, with the insertion of a resorbable separating poly dioxone (PDS) sheet or a resorbable collagen membrane e.g. Biogide™. This is typically undertaken by making circumferential incisions around the fistula in the oral layer and rotating this cuff into the defect and suturing to achieve primary closure of the nasal layer. The oral layer can then be closed either by medially transposed bipedicled (von Langenbeck) flaps, or local rotational flaps – typically pedicled posteriorly permitting vascular supply from the greater palatine artery territory.

The creation of a hard palate fistula is also a complication of cleft orthognathic surgery, at the time of downfracture of the maxilla because of fibrous scar tissue attachments, or as a secondary avascular necrosis. The cleft orthognathic surgeon must thus be proficient in palatal fistula repair.

Adjunctive surgery to improve facial contouring following orthognathic procedures

Free fat grafting to the face

Ipsilateral to the repaired lip cleft there may be a degree of hemifacial soft tissue deficiency compared to the non-cleft side. There may also be poorer hard tissue support causing an apparent soft tissue deficit, which remain uncorrected despite adequate alveolar bone grafting and maxillary advancement orthognathic surgery on this side. Facial fat grafting to the peri-alar and supero-lateral (non-vermillion) aspect of the lip in cleft cases may help address this deficit. The procedure may be undertaken sequentially – fat grafting can be done at each sequential operation for other reasons over many years in severe cases, or as an adjunctive finishing procedure after other cleft related treatments have been completed.

Fat may be harvested from the abdomen, inner, anterior or lateral thigh, or over the hips. Coleman advocates the separation of the fat particles from the liquid fat and blood by centrifugation.[26] However many clinicians feel that this is not necessary and use gravity alone to separate the fat.[27] Either way, the fat is then injected into the soft tissues in multiple passes of very small amount at different angles to create a layering effect building up the deficient area. Whilst a portion of the grafted fat will resorb, the procedure can be repeated on other occasions until the desired facial contour has been produced (see Chapter 51).

Cleft rhinoplasty

Cleft associated nasal and septal differences can be complex and particularly marked in combined unilateral cleft lip and palate. Bilateral cleft lip and palate brings its own complexities but is usually a symmetrical deformity more taxing in the nasal tip and columellar restoration.

Following treatment for unilateral CLP, the septum is often very deviated. There is deviation to the non-cleft side anteriorly and the body of the septum lies diagonally across the nasal midline, causing a variable degree of obstruction of the cleft side posteriorly. There may be inferior turbinate enlargement further obstructing airflow. The cleft side alar base may be posteriorly positioned and the nasal sill and anterior nares widened, or conversely narrowed. There is very typically a slumping of the lower lateral nasal cartilage on the cleft side and a deviated asymmetrical nasal tip with underlying cartilages separation.

Maxillary advancement will usually improve the tip position, but this may be more difficult to predict in cleft cases because of the difficulty in completely achieving the desired advancement as discussed above. The greater degree of relapse in cleft osteotomy will also affect this. Septal cartilage removal may be required for obstruction alleviation but also for tip cartilage grafting. Thus cleft rhinoplasty is an integral and relatively common procedure after orthognathic surgery but usually left for at least 12 months to allow full evaluation of the stable position of the nasal tip relative to the nasal dorsum.

Cleft lip revisions and augmentation

The repaired cleft lip may be inadequately supported skeletally and dentally where the maxilla is retropositioned. After maxillary advancement, the lip support will be improved, but will then highlight any residual underlying lip volume deficiency. Closing the vestibular incision made for the maxillary orthognathic procedure in a V to Y fashion can recruit tissue in from laterally to augment the median tubercle area, but this may not be sufficient. Conventional hyaluronic acid fillers such as Restylane™ can provide improvement in such cases, but the effects are not permanent and may need repeating every year.

Alternatively augmentation may be achieved using fat or periosteum of the iliac or cranial tissues, or free fat transfer.

Better maxillary support to the lip following orthognathic surgery will also highlight any inadequacies of the cleft lip repair. Lip revision may be necessary, whether small changes in vermillion alignment or scar revision, or the need for full thickness re-repairing of the original cleft lip. Following puberty, the childhood tendency for better scar healing will have been lost and patients wishing to undergo this procedure should be cautioned about the higher chance of a thickened scar.

Facial implants

PHDPE has a high success rate for use as facial prosthetic implants. Malar implants are the most common use, then piriform fossa and chin implants. However the forwarding sliding genioplasty procedure is so straightforward and of low complication rate that chin implants are rarely required. Facial implants can be placed at the time of orthognathic surgery or at later soft tissue finishing procedures. More unusually they can be placed prior to orthognathic surgery to improve facial appearance in individuals who are struggling psychologically but who have not completed facial growth and are not ready for orthognathic surgery.

Retention and outcomes

Dental/orthodontic retention, as discussed earlier is permanent and lifelong but the cleft team may also need to provide retention to maintain the position of the maxilla in the early days and weeks post maxillary advancement osteotomy and also after maxillary distraction osteogenesis. The use of a facemask to provide additional anterior and inferior maxillary traction, over and above that provided by intraoral elastics is occasionally required. Often, it is prudent to plan this in those patients for whom previous pharyngoplasty surgery has been carried out as this velopharyngeal surgery and its incumbent scarring may produce a retraction force on the maxilla dragging the upper jaw back towards its preoperative position.

Normally, however, orthognathic surgical results may be maintained and enhanced with simple inter maxillary orthodontic elastics and weekly review in the postoperative month. The orthodontist should take a lead on this phase of treatment, altering the elastic traction to settle the occlusion in the postoperative weeks and months.

There are many different methods of assessing clinical outcome for cleft lip and palate patients who have undergone orthognathic care. Patient related outcome measures (PROMS) such as questionnaires and satisfaction scoring as well as some of the psychological testing methods and quality of life assessments are helpful to gauge patient wellbeing. No one measure is perfect and indeed the number of measures available both from the clinical and patient centred aspects of research indicate that this is an inexact science.

Clinical measures may look at dental occlusion perhaps utilising the peer assessment (PAR) rating. 2D and 3D cephalometrics may enable teams to see if they achieved the treatment objectives as initially planned and teams may also assess facial balance/facial harmony. Digital 3D stereophotogrammetry may offer a visual assessment of how the various parts of the facial surface alter as a result of the movement of the bony skeleton (Figure 56-15).

All may contribute towards the understanding of orthognathic outcomes and also aid the patient to actually see their problems, risks and benefits. Teams may build a library of treated patient records to

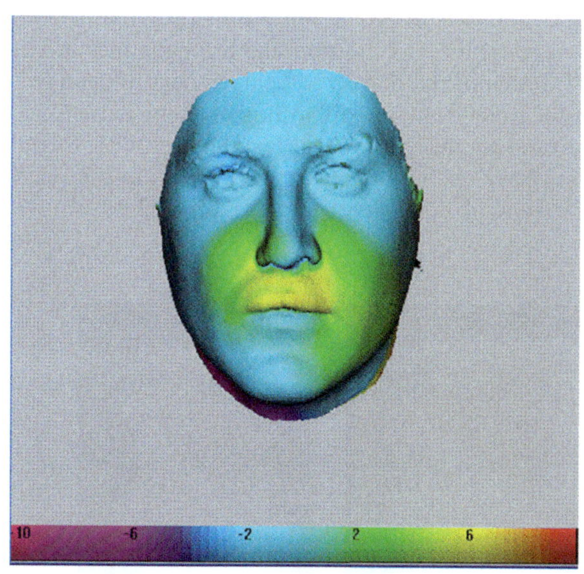

Fig. 56-15 Stereophotogrametric images illustrating facial changes as a result of Le Fort I osteotomy in a patient with cleft lip and palate. The green shades indicate maxillary advancement has increased paranasal prominence and lifted the nasal tip by in the region of 2–4 mm. The upper lip has been advanced by 6–7.5 mm.

illustrate the finer points both from a teaching perspective but also to guide patients through medical jargon with clinical images.

Psychological input

Patients should also have the opportunity to be assessed by a psychologist both to enable the patient to prioritize their concerns and to help them order those concerns into a problem/wish list. The cleft clinical psychologist will also help the patient to understand the adjustments that may need to be made as a result of a change in their facial/dental appearance on completion of the orthognathic care.[28] Patients with unrealistic concerns may be identified during this process and, although complex to treat, it is important to diagnose patients with body dysmorphic disorder prior to starting any treatment as, when treating patients with this condition, expectations of outcome may not be fully met (see Chapter 9).

Speech and language input

From a speech and language perspective, a full video recorded speech assessment will be complimented by velopharyngeal investigations with lateral video fluoroscopy (see Figure 56-14). This can be very accurate in determining patients at risk of velopharyngeal insufficiency (VPI), a hypernasal sounding speech deterioration, as a result of maxillary advancement.[29] Nasendoscopy may augment speech assessment.[30] In such cases appropriate remedial treatment should be discussed. Although prediction of post-orthognathic surgical VPI is an inexact science[31] cleft speech surgeons may be able to advise patients on which type of remedial speech surgery may be most appropriate for them prior to the orthognathic care and outline the risks and benefits going on to providing that speech surgery some months after the orthognathic care. It has been noted that short soft palates measured on pre-orthognathic lateral skull radiographs are more likely to produce velopharyngeal insufficiency.[32] However, maxillary advancement may help the Class III cleft patient with anterior articulatory difficulties.[33]

Previous speech surgery that has involved a pharyngoplasty may compromise the amount of maxillary advancement that is possible. In these cases, the soft palate, or parts of it, has been deliberately and directly tethered to the posterior pharyngeal wall to reduce VPI. This may inadvertently restrict the surgeon's ability to advance the maxilla the full distance required. Here, a difficult decision needs to be made. Does one opt for an orthognathic compromise possibly involving mandibular retro-positioning to compensate for the inability to advance the maxilla the full distance? Alternatively, and not without complication, the pharyngoplasty may be taken down prior to the orthognathic surgery and subsequently post orthognathic surgery, adjunctive speech surgery may follow or distraction osteogenesis may be considered. However, maximum effort should be exerted to achieve optimum facial balance as any compromise that involves accepting a retro-positioned maxilla will also achieve acceptance of a retro-positioned mandible. This compromise may also increase the likelihood of sleep disordered breathing or sleep apnoea, a condition with significant medical risk.

Patient input

The patient themselves must also manage their own commitments to enable the clinical team to deliver a good outcome (Figure 56-16a–d). Although teams will try to reduce the burden of care as much as is reasonably possible by having joint appointments or appointments with different specialist team members on the same day, the patient needs to be able to give their time to the process and keep to the appointment schedule as closely as possible. This may be challenging and complex as often these patients are seeking their care within their final stages of their school education with exams and other commitments to balance with their clinical treatment.

From a clinical perspective, maintaining and securing a scrupulous level of dental / oral health is a prerequisite of any complex care. If elastics are to be worn as a part of the orthodontic treatment then the

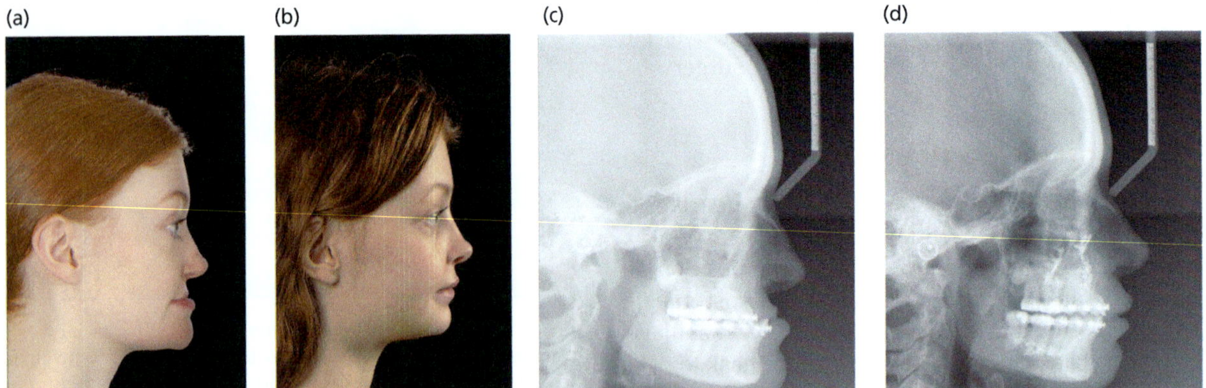

Fig. 56-16 (a & b) Patient requiring a bimaxillary osteotomy with a large maxillary movement and smaller mandibular movement. (c & d) Cephalometric changes and rigid fixation with titanium miniplates.

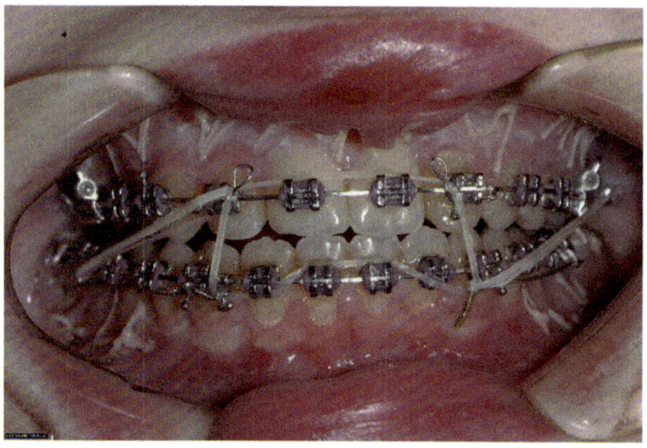

Fig. 56-17 Post-orthognathic surgery orthodontic occlusal seating elastics to guide the patient into the new occlusion and to settle the maxillae into position.

patient must be able to commit to that aspect of their care as well. Certainly elastics will need to be worn as directed in the postoperative phase to settle the occlusion (Figure 56-17). A good outcome will only be achieved where the patient is willing and able to accept all aspects of the overall plan and their clinical team has taken them through the lengthy process of preparing them for treatment giving them as much information as is possible. The psychologist may be able to support the patient where possible and teams may also facilitate prospective patients meeting former patients where appropriate.

Delivering complex interdisciplinary care involves a whole team approach and one must consider that the patient is an active member of that team. A passive patient is not conducive to clinical excellence and all patients should be encouraged to question, research and challenge the clinicians at every available opportunity – after all it is *their* treatment. Patient satisfaction remains one of several important outcome measures available to clinicians to assess overall treatment outcome. A fully engaged patient will understand the risks and therefore can enjoy the benefits of treatment.

Acknowledgements

ACC would like to remember Mr Raymond Edler, my consultant colleague. Ray was an invaluable sage and support in the early part of my career. My patients, my team and I deeply miss his wisdom. ARMC would like to acknowledge the teaching and clinical practice of Peter Ayliffe, Piet Haers and Tim Lloyd, some of whose ideas and thoughts are inevitably represented in this text.

References

1 Mars M, Houston WJ. A preliminary study of facial growth and morphology in unoperated male unilateral cleft lip and palate subjects over 13 years of age. Cleft Palate J. 1990;27:7–10.

2 Lilja J, Mars M, Elander A, Enocson L, Hagberg C, Worrell E, Batra P, Friede H. Analysis of dental arch relationships in Swedish unilateral cleft lip and palate subjects: 20-year longitudinal consecutive series treated with delayed hard palate closure. Cleft Palate Craniofac J. 2006;43:606–11.

3 Daskalogiannakis J, Mehta M. The need for orthognathic surgery in patients with repaired complete unilateral and complete bilateral cleft lip and palate. Cleft Palate Craniofac J. 2009;5:498–502.

4 Williams AC, Bearn D, Mildinhall S, Murphy T, Sell D, Shaw WC, Murray JJ, Sandy JR. Cleft Lip and Palate Care in the United Kingdom – The Clinical Standards Advisory Group (CSAG) Study. Part 2: Dentofacial Outcomes and Patient Satisfaction. Cleft Palate Craniofac J. 2001;38:24–9.

5 Calzolari E, Pierini A, Astolfi G, Bianchi F, Neville AJ, Rivieri F. Associated anomalies in multi-malformed infants with cleft lip and palate: An epidemiologic study of nearly 6 million births in 23 EUROCAT registries. Am J Med Genet A. 2007;143:528–37.

6 Shaw GM, Carmichael SL, Yang W, Harris JA, Lammer EJ. Congenital malformations in births with orofacial clefts among 3.6 million California births, 1983–1997. Am J Med Genet A. 2004;3:250–6.

7 Rittler M, Cosentino V, López-Camelo JS, Murray JC, Wehby G, Castilla EE. Associated anomalies among infants with oral clefts at birth and during a 1-year follow-up. Am J Med Genet A. 2011;7:1588–96.

8 Akcam MO, Evirgen S, Uslu O, Memikoğlu UT. Dental anomalies in individuals with cleft lip and/or palate. Eur J Orthod. 2010;32:207–13.

9 Ayliffe PR. Secondary Cleft lip and palate deformities. In: Harris M and Hunt N (Eds). Fundamentals of Orthognathic surgery (second edition). London: Imperial College Press, 2008.

10 Posnick JC, Ricalde P. Cleft-orthognathic surgery. Clin Plast Surg. 2004;31:315–30.

11 Hall H D, Reddy SC Jr. Treatment of maxillary alveolar hyperplasia by total maxillary osteotomy. J Oral Surg. 1975;33:180–8.

12 Wolford LM, Epker BN. The combined anterior and posterior maxillary osteotomy: a new technique. J Oral Surg. 1975;33:842–51.

13 West RA, McNeill RW. Maxillary alveolar hyperplasia, diagnosis and treatment planning. J Maxillofac Surg. 1975;3:239–50.

14 Bell WH, McBride KL. Correction of the long face syndrome by Le Fort I results. A report on some new technical modifications and treatment results. Oral Surg Oral Med Oral Pathol. 1977;44:493–520.

15 Ilizarov GA. The principles of the Ilizarov method. Bull Hosp Jt Dis Orthop Inst. 1988;48:1–11.

16 McCarthy JG, Schreiber J, Karp N, Thorne CH, Grayson BH. Lengthening the human mandible by gradual distraction. Plast Reconstr Surg. 1992;89:1–8.

17 Figueroa AA, Polley JW, Friede H, Ko EW. Long-term skeletal stability after maxillary advancement with distraction osteogenesis using a rigid external distraction device in cleft maxillary deformities. Plast Reconstr Surg. 2004;114:1382–92.

18 Kumar A, Gabbay JS, Nikjoo R, Heller JB, O'Hara CM, Sisodia M, Garri JI, Wilson LS, Kawamoto HK Jr, Bradley JP. Improved outcomes in cleft patients with severe maxillary deficiency after Le Fort I internal distraction. Plast Reconstr Surg. 2006;117:1499–509.

19 Scolozzi P. Distraction osteogenesis in the management of severe maxillary hypoplasia in cleft lip and palate patients. J Craniofac Surg. 2008;19:1199–214.

20 Liou EJ, Chen PK, Huang CS, Chen YR. Interdental distraction osteogenesis and rapid orthodontic tooth movement: a novel approach to approximate a wide alveolar cleft or bony defect. Plast Reconstr Surg. 2000;105:1262–72.

21 Dolanmaz D, Karaman AI, Durmus E, Malkoc S. Management of alveolar clefts using dento-osseous transport distraction osteogenesis. Angle Orthod. 2003;73:723–9.

22 Kelly N. Evans, Kathleen C. Sie, Richard A. Hopper, Robin P. Glass, Anne V. Hing and Michael L. Cunningham. Robin sequence: from diagnosis to development of an effective management plan. Pediatrics. 2011;127:936–48.
23 Davidson EH, Brown D, Shetye PR, Greig AV, Grayson BH, Warren SM, McCarthy JG. The evolution of mandibular distraction: device selection. Plast Reconstr Surg. 2010;126:2061–70.
24 Looby JF1, Schendel SA, Lorenz HP, Hopkins EM, Aizenbud D. Airway analysis: with bilateral distraction of the infant mandible. J Craniofac Surg. 2009;20:1341–6.
25 Posnick JC, Tompson B. Cleft-orthognathic surgery: complications and long-term results. Plast Reconstr Surg. 1995;96:255–66.
26 Coleman SR. Facial augmentation with structural fat grafting. Clin Plast Surg. 2006;33:567–77.
27 Fisher C, Grahovac TL, Schafer ME, Shippert RD, Marra KG, Rubin JP. Comparison of harvest and processing techniques for fat grafting and adipose stem cell isolation. Plast Reconstr Surg. 2013;132:351–61.
28 Cadogan J, Bennun I. Face value: an exploration of the psychological impact of orthognathic surgery. Br J Oral Maxillofac Surg. 2011;5:376–80.
29 Phillips JH, Nish I, Daskalogiannakis J. Orthognathic surgery in cleft patients. Plast Reconstr Surg. 2012;129:535e–548e.
30 Phillips JH, Klaiman P, Delorey R, MacDonald DB. Predictors of velopharyngeal insufficiency in cleft palate orthognathic surgery. Plast Reconstr Surg. 2005;115:681–6.
31 Chua HD, Whitehill TL, Samman N, Cheung LK. Maxillary distraction versus orthognathic surgery in cleft lip and palate patients: effects on speech and velopharyngeal function. Int J Oral Maxillofac Surg. 2010;7:633–40.
32 McComb RW, Marrinan EM, Nuss RC, Labrie RA, Mulliken JB, Padwa BL. Predictors of velopharyngeal insufficiency after Le Fort I maxillary advancement in patients with cleft palate. Oral Maxillofac Surg. 2011;69:2226–32.
33 Janulewicz J, Costello BJ, Buckley MJ, Ford MD, Close J, Gassner R. The effects of Le Fort I osteotomies on velopharyngeal and speech functions in cleft patients. J Oral Maxillofac Surg. 2004;3:308–14.

Chapter 57

Craniofacial Asymmetry: Causes and Management

Pravin K. Patel, Ronald Jacobson and Linping Zhao

'You boil it in sawdust: you salt it in glue:
You condense it with locusts and tape:
Still keeping one principal object in view –
To preserve its symmetrical shape.'

Lewis Carroll

Introduction

The face has a remarkable degree of symmetry. It is even more remarkable that the symmetry is maintained through the complex choreography of its embryological development. What begins as a simple spherical object, divides, folds and undergoes a multitude of transformations, and always maintaining symmetry.[1] Asymmetry should be the norm; and that it is not, is remarkable.

Symmetry is fundamental. It is a fundamental characteristic of nature: from snowflakes to flowers to the human face. While the multitude of facial variations defined by the size, shape and relationship of the dental, skeletal and soft tissue facial structures are important in providing each individual with his or her own identity, all faces possess a certain degree of symmetry. While no face has true mirror-image symmetry, there is a deviation from symmetry that catches the eye, and the distorted face becomes deformed (Figure 57-1).[2–4] The point at which 'normal' asymmetry becomes 'abnormal' is not easily defined and is often determined by the clinician's sense of balance and the patient's perception of the imbalance.[5]

Our focus will not be on those cases that define the subtle transition point,[6,7] but more on those cases in which there is gross deviation from the norm. There are a multitude of conditions that can cause craniofacial asymmetry, to each of which can be devoted an individual chapter or even a textbook. This chapter will provide a broad overview to conditions, while uncommon, the clinician should be aware of, and the general principles that would guide surgical management with supportive orthodontic treatment.

Causes and classification of craniofacial asymmetry

Craniofacial asymmetries can be classified based on aetiology and on the anatomical structures involved.[8–12] While the causes of facial asymmetry are numerous, they are best divided into three categories: congenital, developmental and acquired (Table 57-1). The asymmetrical birth defects that arise from in utero development represent a wide spectrum of conditions that arise from abnormal embryogenesis resulting in anatomical deformities, malformations and disruptions. These include conditions such as the unilateral cranial synostosis, atypical facial clefts

Orthognathic Surgery: Principles, Planning and Practice. Edited by Farhad B. Naini and Daljit S. Gill.

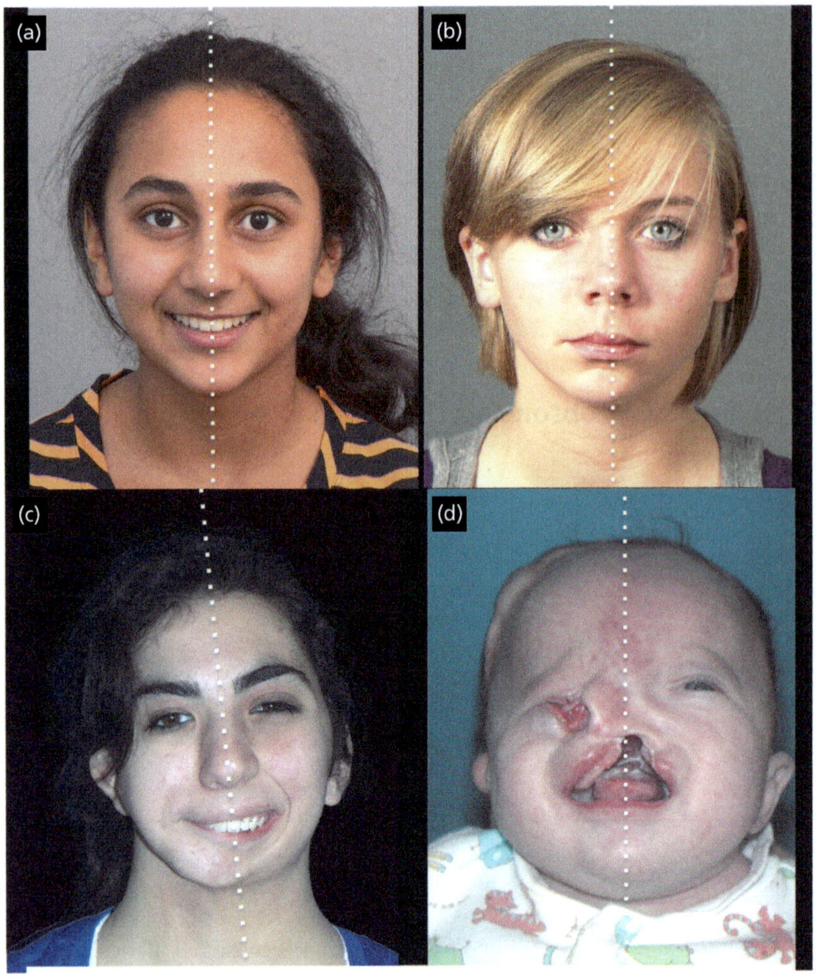

Fig. 57-1 Facial symmetry affected by craniofacial anomalies. (a) Unaffected. (b) Right hemifacial microsomia. (c) Goldenhar syndrome. (d) Atypical craniofacial cleft.

and craniofacial microsomia among others. These conditions perhaps represent not only the most severe forms clinically seen but also the most challenging in restoring the symmetry, as many involve not only the facial structures but also the orbit, skull base and cranial vault. The developmental asymmetries become evident later in childhood and adolescence, at a time when many are brought to the attention of the orthodontist primarily because of the occlusal asymmetry. Perhaps the most common cause of the asymmetry in this group occurs because of a differential in condylar activity between the two sides in conditions of unilateral condylar hyperactivity. The acquired asymmetrical deformities include facial trauma, surgical resections and pathological lesions. While the management of the acquired traumatic asymmetries is in most instances straightforward, those that arise from pathological conditions are profoundly more challenging. The pathology can significantly distort the facial soft tissue and the underlying skeletal frame work.

Table 57-1 Causes of craniofacial asymmetry

Congenital	Developmental	Acquired
Craniosynostosis Unilateral coronal Unilateral lambdoid	Condylar hyperactivity	Facial trauma
Deformational Plagiocephaly Muscular torticollis Facial clefts Craniofacial microsomia	Idiopathic causes	Parry–Romberg disease Fibrous dysplasia Skeletal tumours Soft tissue tumours

Kawamoto, in discussing causes of the idiopathic laterally deviated mandible, proposed a classification scheme that is relevant to the clinician.[13] The causes can be divided into those that are based on skull base asymmetry affecting the spatial position of the glenoid fossa and consequently the mandible, and those that are intrinsic to the condyle. In the former are conditions that affect primarily the skull base such as unilateral craniosynostosis, deformational plagiocephaly and muscular torticollis. In the latter are conditions that are intrinsic to the mandible and include condylar anomalies of hyperactivity, hypoactivity, fractures and craniofacial microsomia.

Congenital causes of asymmetry

Craniosynostosis

Craniosynostosis is the pathological premature fusion of one or more sutures in the cranial vault.[14] When a suture fuses prematurely, the normally expanding skull driven by the growing brain beneath it is restricted in the plane perpendicular to the fused suture. With the remaining skull sutures patent, compensatory expansion and growth of the brain occurs resulting in distinct patterns of the cranial vault that are readily recognizable by the clinician. The incidence of non-syndromic craniosynostoses is between 0.4 and 1/per 1000 live births, with the syndromic conditions, of which the most common are the Crouzon, Apert, Pfeiffer and Saethre–Chotzen with a genetic basis much less in frequency.

Of the various cranial vault sutures that can prematurely fuse, unilateral coronal synostosis and unilateral lambdoid synostosis are relevant to this chapter as they can result in asymmetry that not only involves the cranial vault but also the asymmetry that is propagated subcranial via the skull base and subsequent facial development.

Unilateral coronal synostosis

The premature fusion of the coronal suture with extension to involve the frontosphenoidal suture of the cranial base affects the normal development of the orbital-frontal-parietal region on the involved side (Figure 57-2). The growth of the anterior cranial vault is restricted resulting in a flattened appearance to the forehead. The lesser sphenoid wing is more vertical and the greater sphenoid wing is retracted medial resulting in altering the lateral orbital wall angle. The affected cranial base deformity of the sphenoid results in effacement of the temporal fossa, which, combined with shortening of the lateral wall of the orbit, produces proptosis of the globe. There is widening of the ipsilateral palpebral fissure, superior and posterior displacement of the ipsilateral orbital rim and corresponding eyebrow, and deviation of the nasal dorsum from the affected side toward the contralateral side. This lack of descent of the greater wing of the sphenoid results in the appearance of a 'harlequin' orbit deformity and is pathognomonic for unilateral coronal synostosis. With continued expansion of the brain, compensatory overgrowth occurs asymmetrically at the open sutures that border the now fused single frontoparietal bone plate. This accounts for the prominence in the ipsilateral squamous portion of the temporal bone, the contralateral frontal and parietal bones, and, to a lesser degree, the occipital bones.[15–17]

The asymmetry of the cranial vault affects the subsequent facial skeletal development. There is deviation of the nasal bone and septum with the nasal root 'pulled' ipsilateral. A subcranial view shows that there is displacement of the glenoid fossa with foreshortening of the zygomatic arch length on the affected side. Thus there is a corresponding displacement of

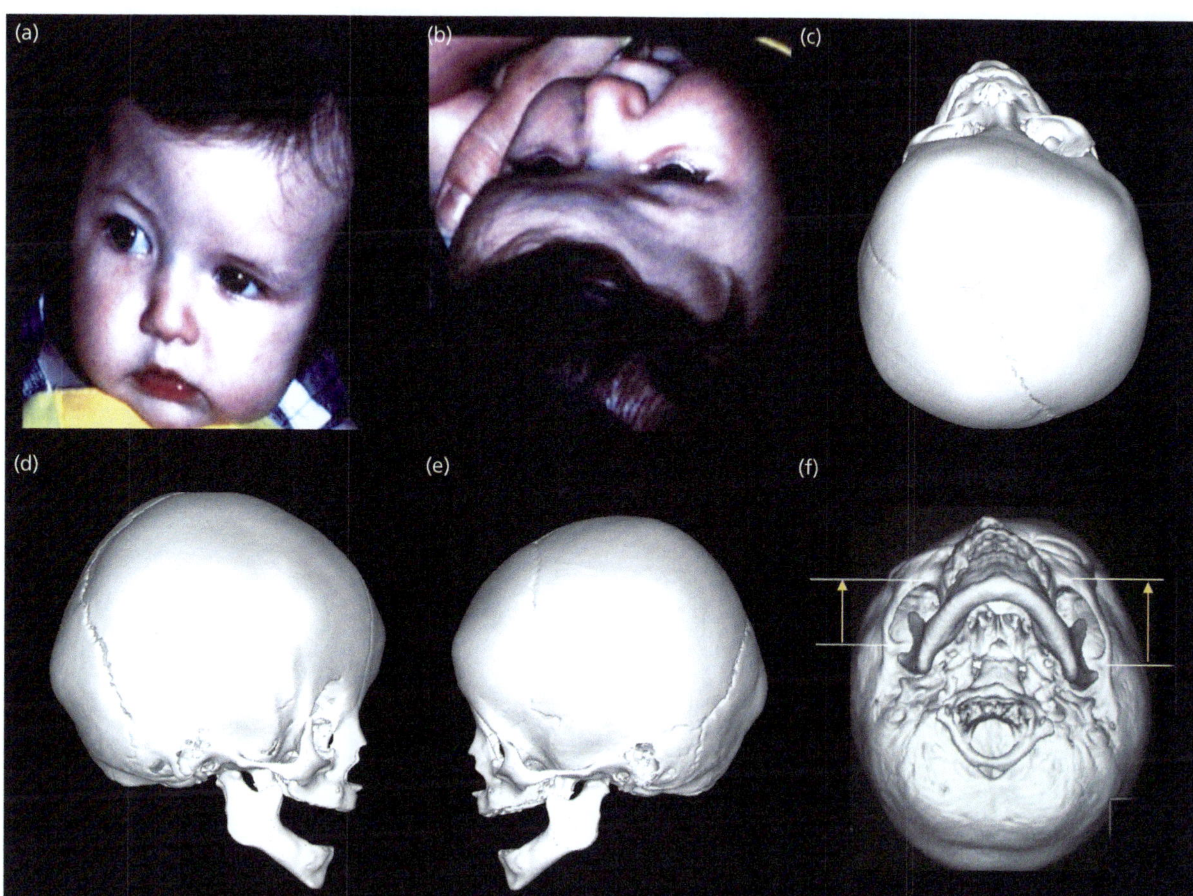

Fig. 57-2 Patient with right unilateral coronal synostosis. (a) Recessed right frontal bone and supraorbital rim with increased palpebral width. Left frontal bone prominence. (b) Vertex view of the deformity. (c) Fused right coronal suture on CT. (d) Fused right coronal suture. (e) Patent left coronal suture. (d) Asymmetry in the zygomatic arch and body. Asymmetry of the glenoid fossa, condyle and mandible.

the zygoma, with the malar eminence positioned more anterior on the affected side. With the asymmetry of the spatial relationship of the glenoid fossa, there is the corresponding asymmetry of the mandible. The chin point deviates to the contralateral side. Thus the unilateral coronal synostosis results in a rotational asymmetry in the transverse plane (yaw) of the developing facial skeleton.[18–21]

Unilateral lambdoid synostosis

Lambdoid synostosis is uncommon when compared to the other patterns of single suture synostosis. When compared to all forms of synostosis it accounts for only 3% and 0.01 per 1000 live births. Fusion of the lambdoid suture affects the posterior parietal occipital bone plate resulting in flattening of the involved region (Figure 57-3). There is typically a bony ridge that extends to involve the mastoid bone, resulting in a visible prominence of the mastoid, pathognomonic of the condition. When viewed from the posterior vantage point, the head has a distinctive appearance with inferior displacement of the occipital mastoid region and along with it the inferior displacement of the ear. With restriction in the growth on the affected side, there is compensatory growth of the contralateral parietal plate resulting in an increased posterior superior width that is visibly noticeable from the frontal view. In addition there may be a compensatory increased frontal prominence on the contralateral side. Viewed from the vertex the skull has a tendency toward a trapezoidal shape. At the cranial base level, there is an acute petrous ridge angle, deviation of the midline of the posterior cranial fossa along with the foramen magnum toward the affected side and enlargement of the contralateral middle fossa. With twisting of the skull base, there is a rotational asymmetry of the midface with prominence of the malar eminence on the unaffected side. The mandible itself appears to remain unaffected, but rotated positionally.[22–25]

Positional plagiocephaly and congenital muscular torticollis

Plagiocephaly is purely a descriptive term derived from Greek plagios (oblique) and kephale (head) and requires a qualifier as its causes are varied from unilateral forms of craniosynostosis discussed in the previous section to the non-synostotic secondary causes of asymmetry.[26] Deformational, non-synostotic forms of cranial vault deformities are the most common forms of the asymmetrical cranial vault that are clinically encountered. The pathology of such deformities arise from secondary causes (intra-uterine, postnatal

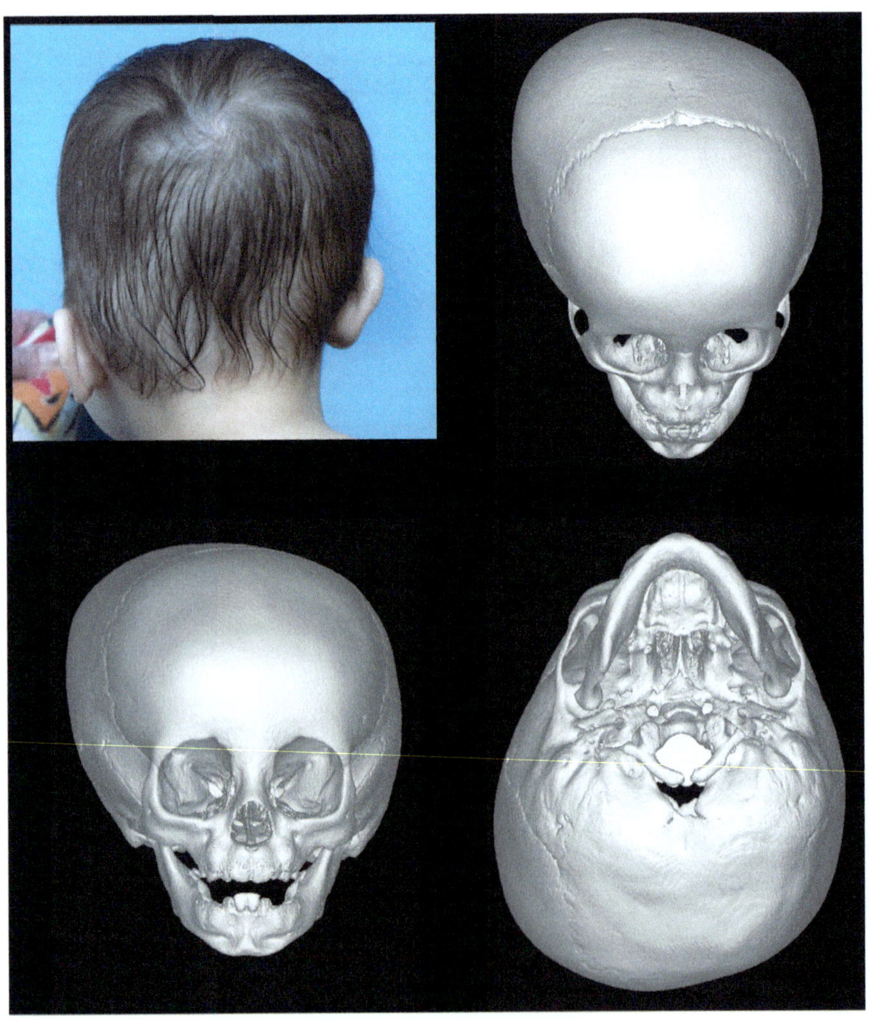

Fig. 57-3 Patient with left lambdoid suture synostosis resulting in posterior cranial vault and corresponding skull base asymmetry.

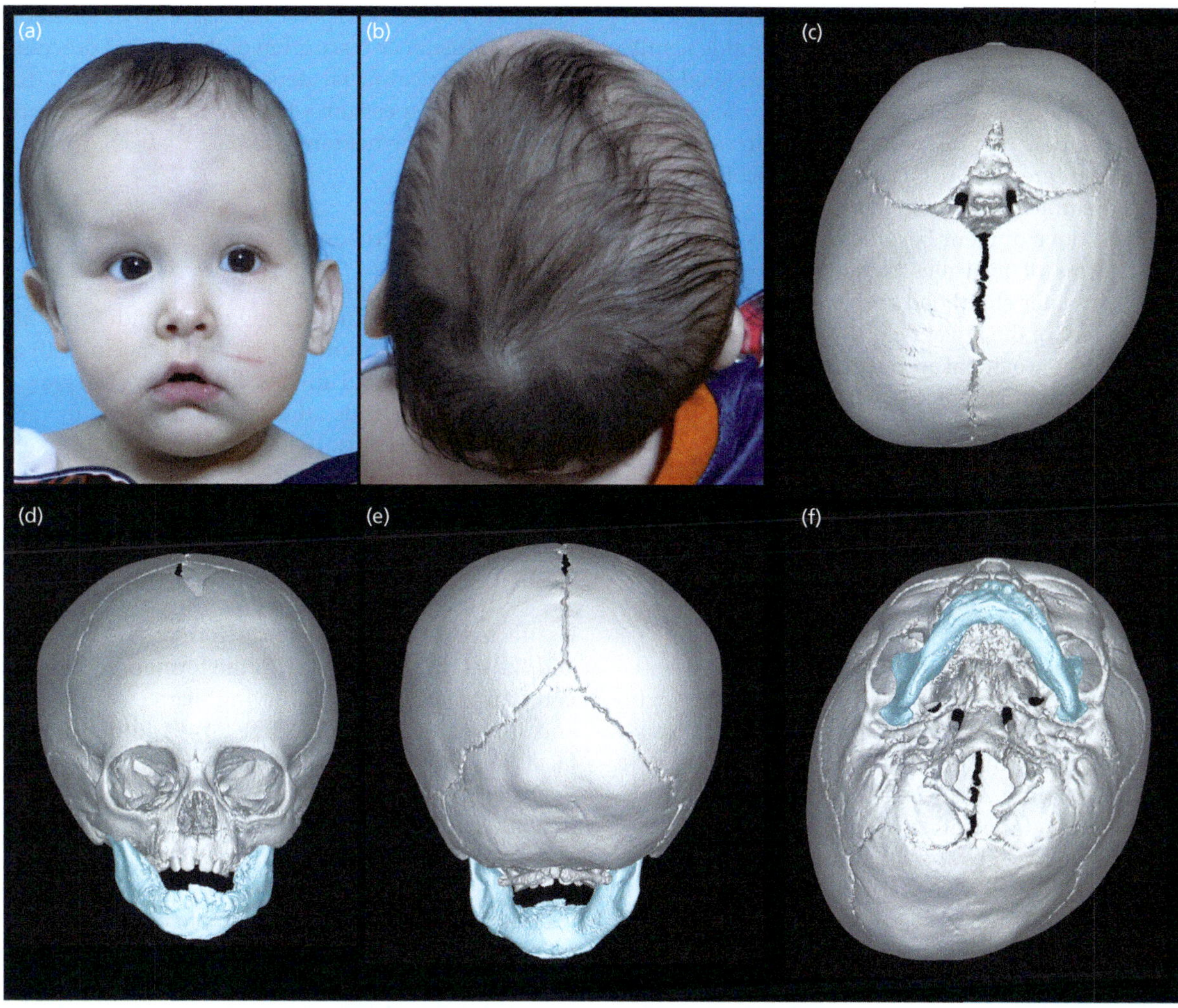

Fig. 57-4 Non-synostotic positional skull asymmetry. (a) Right frontal prominence. (b) Right occipital flattening. (c) Cranial vault asymmetry with patent coronal sutures. (d) Frontal view with symmetrical orbital rims. (e) Posterior view with patent lambdoid sutures. (f) Cranial base asymmetry.

positioning, muscular torticollis) that involve external compressive forces on the malleable neonatal and infant skull (Figure 57-4).

In gestational plagiocephaly, the normal symmetrical growth of the craniofacial region is restricted by intrauterine constraint. Early descent of the head into the true pelvis results in asymmetrical growth because of the geometry of the pelvis. The majority of the newborns with anterior plagiocephaly present with left frontal flattening in agreement with the observed 85% of vertex presentation in the left occipital anterior position. Other causes of intrauterine constraints include multiparity and maternal uterine malformations.

In 1992, the American Academy of Pediatricians recommended that infants be placed on their back or sides to reduce the risk of sudden infant death syndrome.[27] With this campaign, a sharp rise in the number of misshapen heads arose with primary posterior plagiocephaly that posed a dilemma for distinguishing the synostotic occipital deformity (lambdoid synostosis) requiring surgery from the vast majority of non-synostotic secondary positional deformities not requiring surgical intervention. Up until then children who presented with cranial vault deformity had a high index of suspicion requiring surgical consultation. The asymmetrical positional cranial vault deformity occurs by the child's preference to be supine on either the left or right occiput that quickly becomes ingrained within the first few weeks of life. With the numbers of hours that the newborn sleeps, constant and repetitive pressure results in asymmetrical 'flattening' of the involved occiput. Secondary deformational forces occur with anterior displacement of the parietal plate and the frontal bone plate on the involved side. Viewed from the vertex, the symmetry of the cranial vault appears shifted as a parallelogram. The secondary deformation that occurs at the cranial base and glenoid fossa affects the mandible with a rotational deviation toward the contralateral side.[28]

Congenital muscular torticollis, with an incidence between 0.3 to 1.3% of live births, can also be an external cause of a cranial vault plagiocephaly and facial asymmetry. Aetiologically it is attributed to intrauterine or trauma at the time of delivery resulting in a dysfunctional sternocleidomastoid muscle. With a tight, foreshortened sternocleidomastoid muscle, the cervical range of motion of the head is restricted resulting in a rotational asymmetry in the coronal (roll) and transverse plane (yaw). With this restriction, there is a preference for the child to sleep on one side resulting in a deformational positional skull and skull base deformity. The concordance of muscular torticollis and plagiocephaly is one in every 300 live births. With a significant degree and persistence of torticollis refractory to treatment, the secondary effect on the cranial vault development becomes obvious. However, milder forms of torticollis frequently go unnoticed; and only in later childhood and adolescence with the development of the lower face, the resulting asymmetry may become evident and search for the asymmetry by the orthodontist may lead to the patient's family recalling a history of torticollis. The occlusal pattern is typically Class II on the affected side and Class III on the contralateral side with a mandibular shift from the ipsilateral to contralateral.[29–31]

Facial clefts

Facial asymmetries of the typical unilateral facial clefts and the atypical craniofacial clefts are self-evident.[32] In the typical unilateral cleft lip and palate, the anatomical structures are distorted by the embryological disruption in failure of fusion between the maxillary prominence and medial nasal processes and between the palatine processes and the nasal septum that contribute to the palatal cleft. The premaxilla typically is rotated outwardly and projects anterior in relation to a relatively retropositioned lateral maxillary alveolar element. The nasal structures of the alar base, nasal sill, vomer and septum are distorted significantly. The lower lateral cartilage on the cleft side is positioned inferiorly, with an obtuse angle as it flattens across the cleft. The alar base is rotated laterally, inferiorly and posteriorly. The developing nasal septum pulls the premaxilla away from the cleft, and the septum and the nasal spine are deflected toward the non-cleft side. The cleft continues through the maxillary alveolus and palatal shelf, extending to the palatal bone and soft palate. In the atypical craniofacial clefts, the fault lines follow the classic patterns described by Tessier as failure of fusion or disruption of the normal processes of embryological facial development (Figure 57-1d). The resulting spectrum of the anatomical structures involved is overwhelmingly broad.[33]

Craniofacial microsomia

After cleft lip and palate, craniofacial microsomia is the second most common congenital condition of the head and neck encountered by the clinician with an incidence as high as 1 in 3500 live births. The craniofacial condition affects all three tissue planes to varying degrees of severity. It affects the underlying skeleton – mandible, maxilla, zygoma, orbit and cranium – resulting in an asymmetry in all three planes. Within its wide spectrum, the vertebrae may be involved. The overlying facial musculature and subcutaneous tissue is deficient and along with it the skin envelope is affected. The embryological formation of the ear and the lateral commissure in the formation of the lip is disrupted resulting in varying degrees of microtia and macrostomia (lateral cleft lip). Additionally the facial nerve and its branches are affected to varying degrees. In addition to craniofacial anomalies, there may be associated oculopalpebral anomalies (clefting and epibulbar dermoid), cardiac and central nervous system defects.[34,35]

Because of its wide range of phenotypic presentation (Figure 57-5), the condition has been known through a variety of nomenclature. These have included first and second branchial syndrome, lateral facial dysplasia, otomandibular dysostosis, oculoauriculovertebral dysplasia (Goldenhar syndrome), and within the Tessier clefting classification, a number 7 cleft. In the vast majority of cases, the condition is unilateral hence the term hemifacial microsomia, as it is more commonly known. However, in 10–15% of the cases there is bilateral involvement (bilateral hemifacial microsomia); and when present in the bilateral form, the two halves of the face are

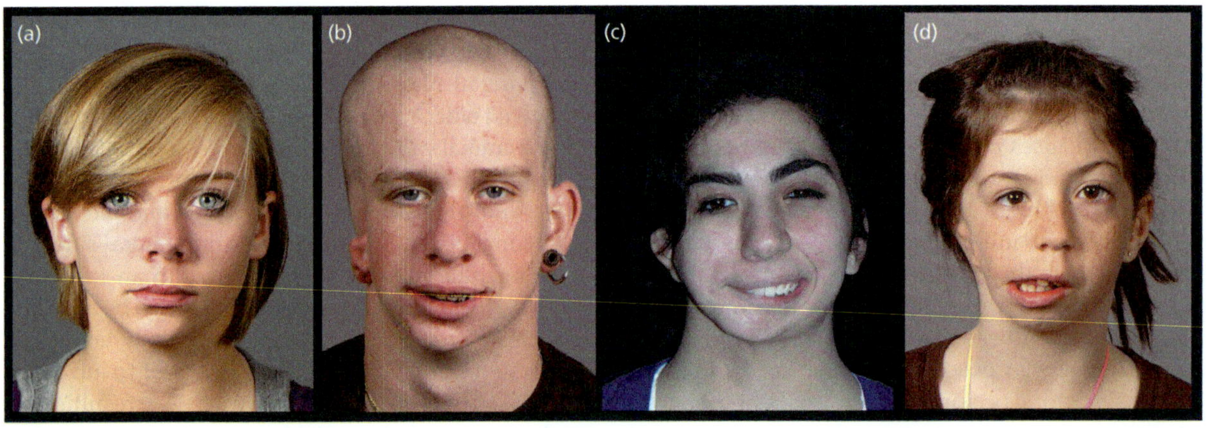

Fig. 57-5 The variability in the phenotypic expression of craniofacial microsomia. (a) Right mandibular hypoplasia (Type1 Pruzansky). (b) Right mandibular and maxillary deformity. Right microtia (Type IIA Pruzansky). (c) Right mandibular and maxillary deficiency, Right microtia. Right marginal nerve palsy, cervical scoliosis (Type IIB Pruzansky). (d) Right mandibular and maxillary deficiency. Right orbital dystopia. Right microtia. Right macrostomia. (Type III Pruzansky).

differentially involved and the face is asymmetrically affected. Thus the term craniofacial microsomia is more appropriate and the two subtypes are distinguished as unilateral craniofacial microsomia and bilateral craniofacial microsomia. Additionally the term craniofacial microsomia allows the wide spectrum of presentation and is more inclusive of a term. The nosology of the condition can then be further parsed depending on the context of the discussion. Correspondingly multiple classification schemes exist, each emphasizing an aspect of the range of deformity and the extent of involvement of any component of the deformity.[34,35]

While the overwhelming cases are sporadic in occurrence, there are rare familial cases that exhibit autosomal dominant inheritance in 2–3% of the cases. Whether these extremely rare cases with genetic basis should properly be classified within the overwhelming sporadic cases is debated. Multiple aetiologies have been proposed to account for sporadic occurrence; and among them, the most widely accepted is vascular insult to the stapedial artery. The stapedial artery is only temporarily present in the embryological development of the first and second branchial arches that is replaced by the eventual external carotid artery system. Thus a vascular insult to the stapedial artery can account for the broad range of disruption to the development of the craniofacial structures. Murine and mammalian models in which the stapedial artery is disrupted have been shown to remarkably reproduce the spectrum of pathology depending on the timing of the insult and the extent of the haemorrhage and haematoma formation.[34,35]

Even though the extent of the deformity may include the entire hemi-craniofacial skeleton, the mandibular deformity is considered the cornerstone (Figure 57-6). Asymmetrical mandibular growth and development presents in the vast majority as the initial presentation for clinical assessment and management. The mandible plays a pivotal role in progressive distortion of the facial skeleton on the affected side with secondary compensation on the contralateral side. The natural history is that the deviation toward the affected side progresses with time until the end-stage deformity is established at skeletal maturity. The normal downward vertical growth of the maxilla is restricted by the hypoplastic mandible resulting in multiplanar deficiency of the hemi-maxilla and obliquity of the occlusal plane ((coronal-roll, transverse-yaw and sagittal-pitch). The zygomatic arch with the glenoid fossa may range from fully present to rudimentary to complete absence. The zygomatic-orbital complex may also be affected in up to 15% with varying degrees of inferior, medial and rotational displacement of the orbit to degrees of microphthalmia. In the more extensive cases the temporal bone and ipsilateral frontal bone are involved. In addition,

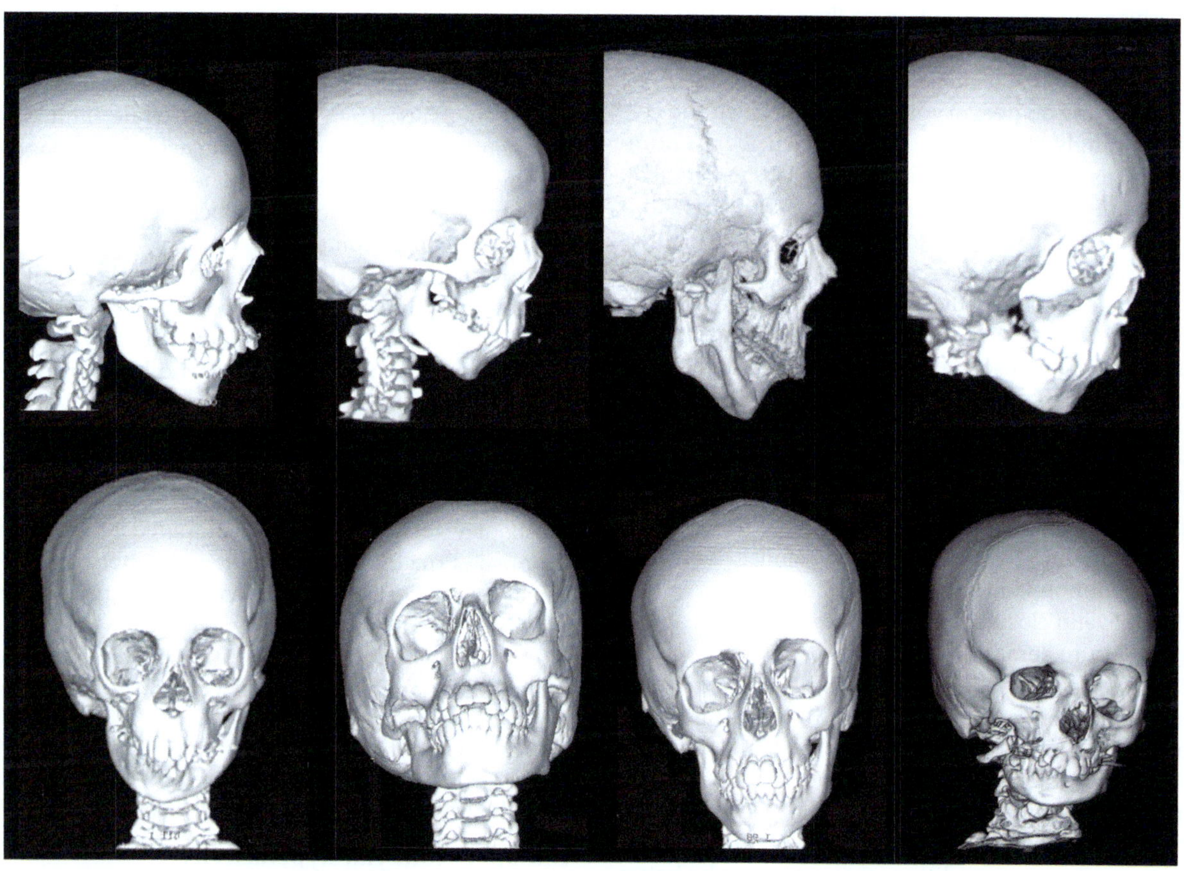

Fig. 57-6 The variability in the skeletal deformity of craniofacial microsomia is illustrated in a series of CT scans. Common to all of the cases is the mandibular deformity with various components affects. With increasing severity the maxilla, zygoma, orbit and cranial vault are affected as part of the broad spectrum.

malformations of the cervical vertebrae are not uncommon and include the presence of hemivertebrae and fused vertebrae. In the cases of craniofacial microsomia where there is involvement of the orbit, cranium and vertebrae, the clinician needs to not solely focus on the mandibular asymmetry, but understand that any intervention must be within the context of entire spectrum of involvement. Correction of the mandibular–maxillary relationship does not necessarily correct the upper midfacial involvement, and the symmetry with respect to the absolute reference plane must be clearly understood.

Associated with the hypoplastic skeletal components, the muscles of mastication are variably involved to the extent that the origins and insertions are affected. The temporalis muscle would normally insert onto the coronoid process, the lateral pterygoid muscle insert into the condyle and the medial pterygoid insert into the mandibular angle. However, when the skeletal components of the mandible are diminutive or absent then the corresponding muscles are affected. When the zygomatic arch is not present, the origin of the masseter is affected, and in such cases the temporalis and masseter muscle may become confluent. Functionally the chin deviates to the affected side both with opening and closing. Thus symmetry achieved with skeletal reconstruction, including a construction of a pseudo-TMJ, is only a static symmetry and cannot restore normal symmetrical oromotor function. There is always lateral gnathism with the exception of the mildest forms of craniofacial microsomia.

The skin and subcutaneous tissue are also involved with varying degrees of volumetric deficiency and correspondingly skin surface area deficiency. In a number of cases the parotid gland may also be deficient. Intraorally the hemi-palate may be involved with a hypoplastic levator palatini. While ear abnormalities (microtia) and lateral cleft of the lip (macrostomia) can occur independent of the skeletal component, involvement of these structures are considered part of the craniofacial microsomia spectrum because of their frequent association to the underlying skeletal pathology.

The various branches of the facial nerve can be involved, and each to varying degrees. Most commonly involved is the marginal mandibular nerve resulting in lower lip asymmetry that is distinctly more noticeable when the patient smiles. The next most common is involvement of the facial nerve that affects eyelid closure that may place the patient at risk for exposure keratitis.

In as many as 55% of the patients there is extra-cranial involvement, 13% with one extra-cranial anomaly, and in 42% anomalies that affect multiple organ systems (skeletal, cardiac, central nervous system, pulmonary and renal). The spectrum that exists is incredibly more complex and likely represents overlapping conditions that remain to be better elucidated.[36]

Of the various skeletal classification schemes, the Pruzansky classification, and its later modification by Mulliken and Kaban (Table 57-2), of the mandibular involvement provides the most workable scheme for treatment management.[37,38] In Pruzansky I, all the anatomical elements of the mandible are present, but of diminutive size volumetrically compared to the unaffected side. In Pruzansky III, there is complete absence of formation of the ascending ramus, the coronoid process, the condyle and the corresponding glenoid fossa. The mandible tapers at what would be the angle in the normal mandible. Between these two extremes, all remaining hypoplastic mandible elements (ramus, condyle and coronoid process) are classified as Pruzansky II. The later modification by Mulliken and Kaban further subdivided Pruzansky II into subtype IIA in which the glenoid fossa–condyle relation was spatially maintained at the cranial base compared to the contralateral temporomandibular joint position. However, in subtype IIB the mandible, and the corresponding glenoid fossa if present, is displaced medially. The classification, while limited to the mandible, serves the clinician well in managing the lower skeletal asymmetry. The scheme proposed by Munro and Lauritzen addresses the midfacial and orbital skeletal asymmetry.[39]

Table 57-2 Kaban-Pruzansky mandibular deformity classification in craniofacial microsomia

I	Mandible, body, ramus, condyle, coronoid are present but diminutive.
IIA	Ramus is present but hypoplastic and in an anatomically acceptable relationship to the glenoid foss.
IIB	Ramus is present but hypoplastic and is medially displaced.
III	Ramus: absent or minimally present.

Kaban's modification of the Pruzansky classification system (Kaban LB, Moses MH, Mulliken JB. Surgical correction of hemifacial microsomia in the growing child. Plast Reconstr Surg. 1988;82:9–19.)

More inclusive is the OMENS-Plus classification that evolved from a series of proposed classification schemes by David, Mulliken and Horgan.[40–42] The acronym stands for orbit, mandible, ear, nerve and soft tissue with each variable assigned a severity index (Table 57-3). The plus indicates the extracranial involvement. The more recent pictorial classification of OMENS by Birgfeld et al. provides an excellent visual tool.[43] When compared to the more simplistic Pruzansky classification, the more comprehensive classifications are not as clinically practical in guiding the treatment planning. However, they have the benefit of ensuring that all the components of the anomaly are assessed and objectively noted for management.

Developmental causes of asymmetry

Unilateral condylar hyperactivity

Idiopathic overgrowth of the mandibular condyle is unilateral, presents itself during pubertal growth as a developing mandibular asymmetry and is self-limited

Table 57-3 OMENS classification system of craniofacial microsomia

Orbit	
O0	Normal orbit: size and position
O1	Abnormal orbit: size
O2	Abnormal orbit: position
O3	Abnormal orbit: size and position
Mandible	
M0	Normal mandible
M1	Mandible, body, ramus, condyle, coronoid are present but diminutive
M2A	Ramus is present but hypoplastic and in an anatomically acceptable relationship to the glenoid fossa
M2B	Ramus is present but hypoplastic and is medially displaced
M3	Ramus: absent or minimally present.
Ear	
E0	Normal ear
E1	Ear: all structures present, but hypoplastic
E2	Absent external auditory canal with hypoplastic concha
E3	Absent auricle, malpositioned lobule remnant
Facial nerve	
N0	Normal facial nerve function
N1	Upper facial nerve involvement
N2	Lower facial nerve involvement
N3	Upper and lower facial nerve involvement
Soft tissue	
S0	Normal soft tissue and muscle
S1	Minimal soft tissue and muscle deficiency
S2	Moderate soft tissue and muscle deficiency
S3	Severe soft tissue and muscle deficiency

More inclusive classification of craniofacial microsomia. (Vento RA, LaBrie RA, Mulliken JB. Cleft Palate-Craniofac J. 1991;28:68–76.)

by adulthood. It is not evident at birth. The asymmetry becomes increasingly more noticeable in later childhood through adolescence, when many parents begin to seek treatment for their affected children. Often it is useful to ask the parents to bring the annual school photographs to review the progression of the asymmetry and the diagnosis becomes clear.

While the underlying aetiology remains unclear and may be multi-varied, the final outcome is a misregulation in growth that occurs within the cartilaginous region of the condylar head. During this active period, technetium-99 scintigraphy can confirm the condylar hyperactivity when compared to the contralateral unaffected condyle. However, while the nuclear scan does not shed insight into the aetiology once growth is completed (i.e. at the time of end-stage mandibular asymmetry), its value to the clinician is in confirming the timing of surgical intervention if there is any reservation with serial confirmation of radiographs.[44]

The terminology of unilateral condylar hyperplasia has been used by many authors; however, the term unilateral condylar hyperactivity suggested by Obwegeser is more appropriate as it more accurately encompasses the various clinical presentations seen (Figure 57-7).[44] Obwegeser and Malek provided a simple classification scheme that delineates the three clinical variations (Table 57-4).[45] In Type I (hemimandibular hyperplasia) the anatomical components of the mandible are volumetrically enlarged: the condyle, the condylar neck, the ramus and mandible on the affected aside. Clinically, the mandible on the affected side is inferiorly displaced with an increased distance between the tooth apices and the canal. The chin is not translocated to the contralateral side but remains centred. There is either a posterior open bite or the bite is closed by maxillary inclination. There is no crossbite, but there is a rotational asymmetry (yaw). In Type II (hemimandibular elongation), there is elongation without increase in volumetric mass of the various components of the mandible in the vertical and/or the horizontal planes. Characteristically, the dental midline and chin are deviated to the contralateral side with a resulting crossbite and in infraocclusion on the affected side. In Type II, a hyperplastic condyle does not occur and the term condylar hyperplasia would not be appropriate to this group of hemimandibular asymmetries. In Type III (hemimandibular hyperplasia and elongation), the resulting mandibular asymmetry is of a combination or a hybrid form of Type I and Type II. The hybrid form results in vertical elongation of the affected mandibular border along with displacement of the chin to the contralateral side.

Acquired causes of asymmetry

Traumatic

Perhaps the most common cause of dentofacial skeletal asymmetry is trauma.[13,46,47] The asymmetry can affect any component depending on the original fracture pattern, from isolated fractures to pan-facial fractures. In the upper midface, post-traumatic nasal asymmetries and residual malar asymmetries are common. In the lower face, traumatic injuries to the mandible of which nearly 25% involve the condyle are among the more common causes of facial asymmetry in children and young adults. Complications from either untreated or unsatisfactory treated outcome include skeletal facial asymmetry, occlusal crossbite, lateral gnathism, various degrees of restricted motion to complete ankylosis and osteoarthritis. For many, the early trauma goes unnoticed by the family and medical attention is not sought; and when medical attention is sought, the condylar injury is undiagnosed at the time of the assessment. The haemarthrosis that occurs with condylar compression injuries is often difficult to diagnose and becomes evident with restriction and ankylosis as functional asymmetry progresses. With condylar neck fractures medial displacement by the lateral pterygoid muscle occurs, affecting the TMJ kinematics and the posterior mandibular height on the affected site. The condylar head remodelling adapts to maintain TMJ function. The extent to which subsequent facial development can remain symmetric within an acceptable tolerance depends on the timing of the insult in the growth and development of the child and the extent of the injury.

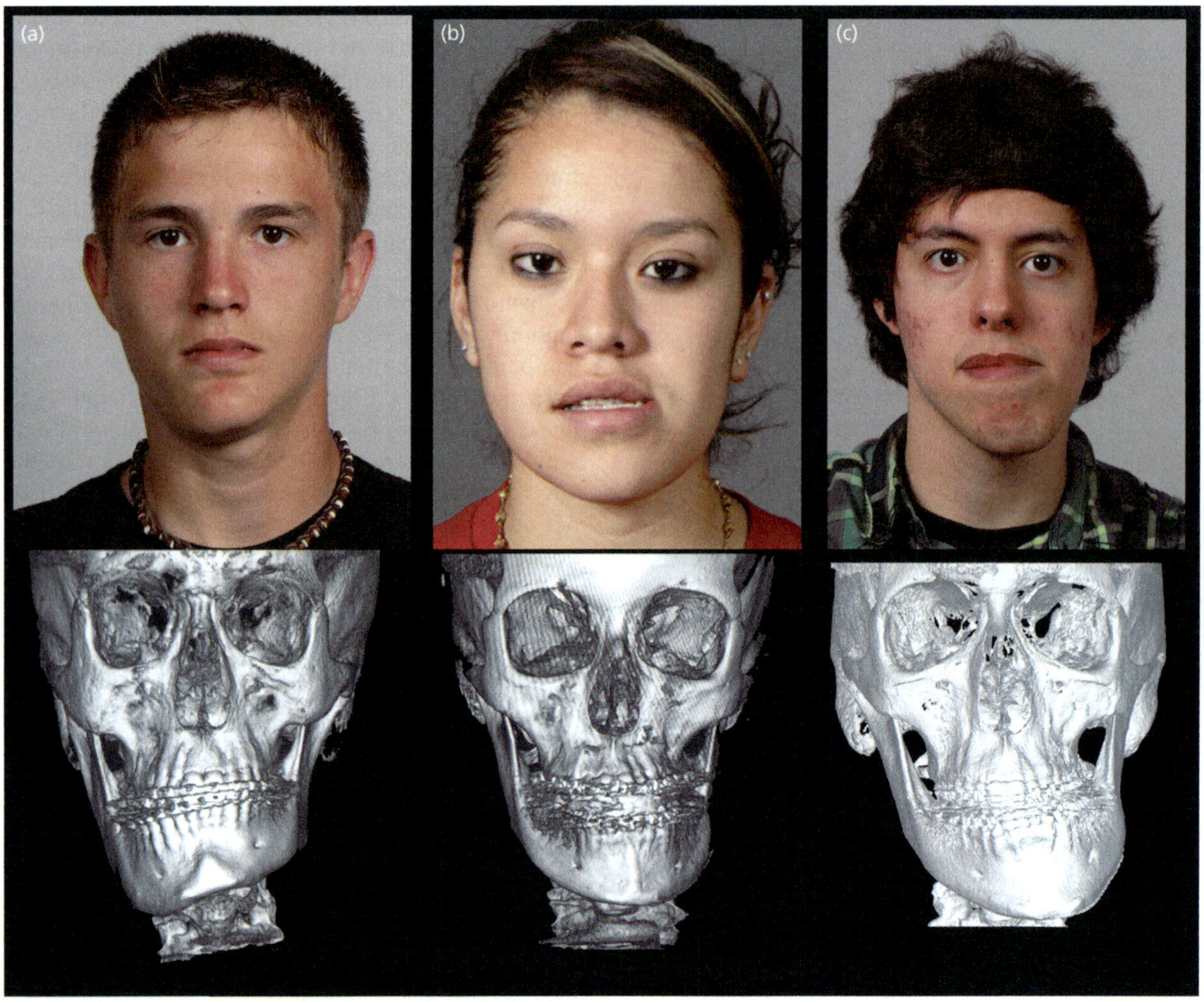

Fig. 57-7 Classification of condylar hyperactivity after Obwegeser. (a) Type I hemimandibular hyperplasia. (b) Type II hemimandibular elongation. (c) Type III hybrid form of hemimandibular elongation and hyperplasia.

Parry–Romberg disease

Of the facial asymmetries, those affected by Parry–Romberg condition are characterized by a striking 'sunken' appearance to the affected side of the face (Figure 57-8a). There is a sharp demarcation from the normal hemiface. Frequently there is a characteristic soft tissue crease in the forehead, a coup de sabre, that is a characteristic hallmark of the disease. The disease is progressive in nature with atrophy of the skin, the subcutaneous tissue, muscle and the dento-osseous framework in its severest forms. Intraoral findings of the atrophic process may involve the alveolar process, the palate and tongue on the affected side. In nearly 35 to 40% of the patients, the orbital region and eyelid adnexal structures are involved resulting in enophthalmos with the loss of the peri-orbital fat, eyelid atrophy with ptosis, loss of eyelashes and eyebrow hair. Visual acuity may be affected with involvement of the retina and optic nerve.[13,48]

The disease is of unknown aetiology. It begins insidiously in childhood to mid-adolescence with relentless progression until it stabilizes typically in adulthood. The active phase of the disease process has a broad range of variability extending from 2 years to up to over a decade. Any orthodontic-skeletal and soft tissue reconstruction must take into account this variability in the length of the active phase. While there is little correlation between the severity of the soft tissue involvement and the age of onset, the effect on the dento-skeletal involvement does correlate with the age. In an overwhelming 85% of patients with osseous involvement, the disease had started before the age of 9. With skeletal involvement of the maxilla and the mandible, the dental arch alignments are affected and there is typically a lateral open bite on the affected side.

Table 57-4 Obwegeser and Makek classification of condylar hyperactivity

Type 1	Hemimandibular hyperplasia (HH)	Condylar hyperplasia
Type 2	Hemimandibular elongation (HE)	Not condylar hyperplasia
Type 3	Hybrid HH+HE	Condylar hyperplasia

Obwegeser HL, Makek MS. Hemimandibular hyperplasia-hemimandibular elongation. J Maxillofacial Surg. 1986;14:183–208.

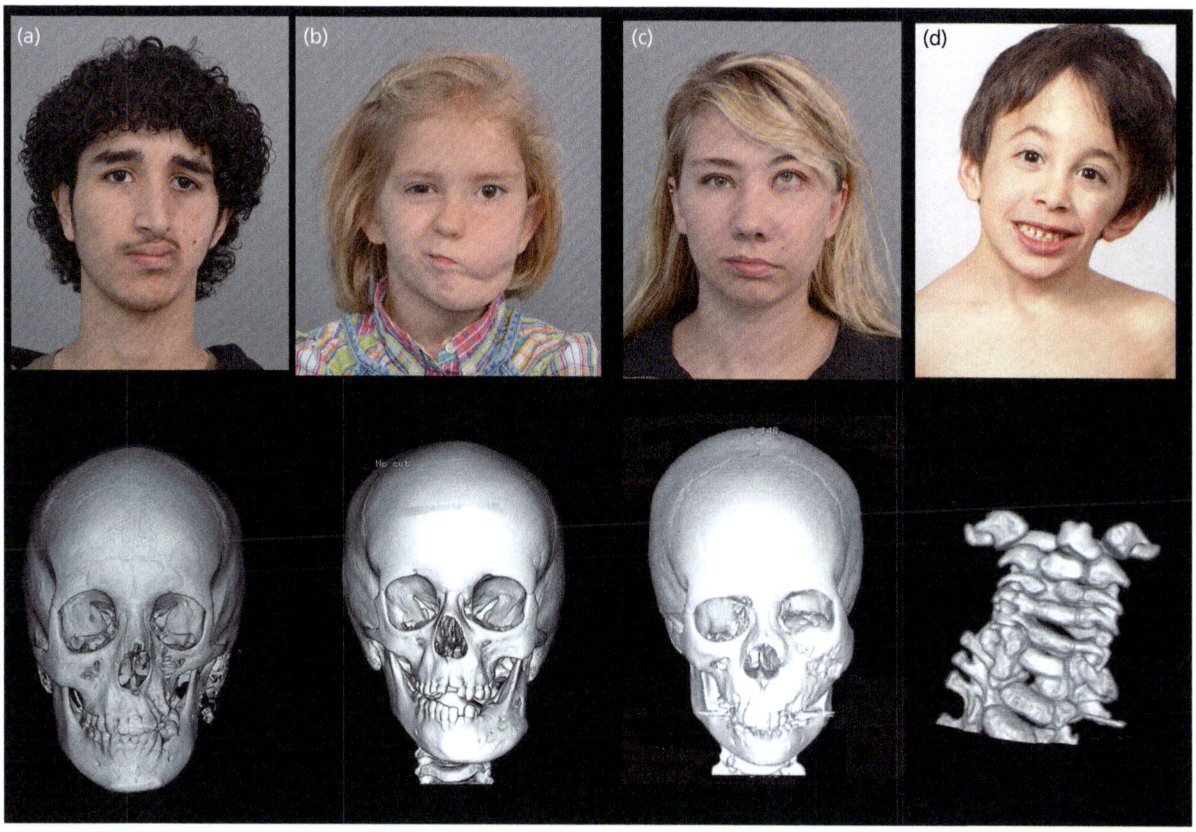

Fig. 57-8 Various aetiological causes of craniofacial asymmetry. (a) Parry–Romberg disease. (b) Hemangioendothelioma tumour. (c) Fibrous dysplasia. (d) Cervical scoliosis with hemivertebrae fusion.

Fibrous dysplasia

Among the intrinsic skeletal causes of facial asymmetry is fibrous dysplasia (Figure 57-8c), a progressive benign osseous lesion in which there is gradual expansion of the involved bone beyond its bony margin as it is replaced by fibrous tissue and haphazardly woven bone. The condition affects a single skeletal region (monostotic) in the majority of the cases (70–80%) and multiple distinctly separate bony regions (polyostotic) involving the craniofacial region, proximal femur and ribs in the remaining 20–30% of the cases. Of the patients with polyostotic disease, 3–5% have in addition precocious puberty and skin pigmentation (cafe-au-lait) known as McCune–Albright syndrome. The craniofacial involvement occurs in 25% of the monostotic forms and in 50% of the polyostotic cases. Of the craniofacial region, the maxilla, zygoma and orbital regions are more commonly involved. With the maxillary involvement involving the alveolus, dental arch and occlusal plane asymmetry occurs. With peri-orbital involvement, the orbit becomes dysmorphic with vertical orbital dystopia and exorbitism. The optic nerve can be at risk with expansile extension into the sphenoid. However, many are at first asymptomatic and first come to attention when minor asymmetry is noticed by family members, in photographs, or as an incidental finding in routine dental radiographs. Ninety percent of the patients with craniofacial involvement clinically present by the age of 10, and are radiographically detected as early as 3 years of age. Growth of the lesion begins to diminish after adolescence and becomes quiescent into early adulthood.[49,50]

Evaluation and assessment

Component facial analysis

Objectively assessing the patient who presents with a craniofacial asymmetry requires a systematic approach (Figure 57-9). Each of the components: skeletal, dental and soft tissue must be assessed in all three anatomical planes with respect to each other (intrinsic spatial relationship) but also importantly to an external three-dimensional space in which they are embedded. The natural head position (external reference frame) must be noted. Knowing where the head is held in three-dimensional space is critical in understanding where one begins to establish the planes of symmetry. Many patients with craniofacial asymmetry may present with a 'head tilt' because of ocular muscle imbalance, orbital dystopia, persistent muscular torticollis or C-spine abnormalities. For such patients dentofacial correction of asymmetry must begin with a discussion with the patient that the asymmetrical position of the head in 3D space is to be distinguished from the internal asymmetry of the facial components. The question must be clarified whether treatment planning is with respect to the

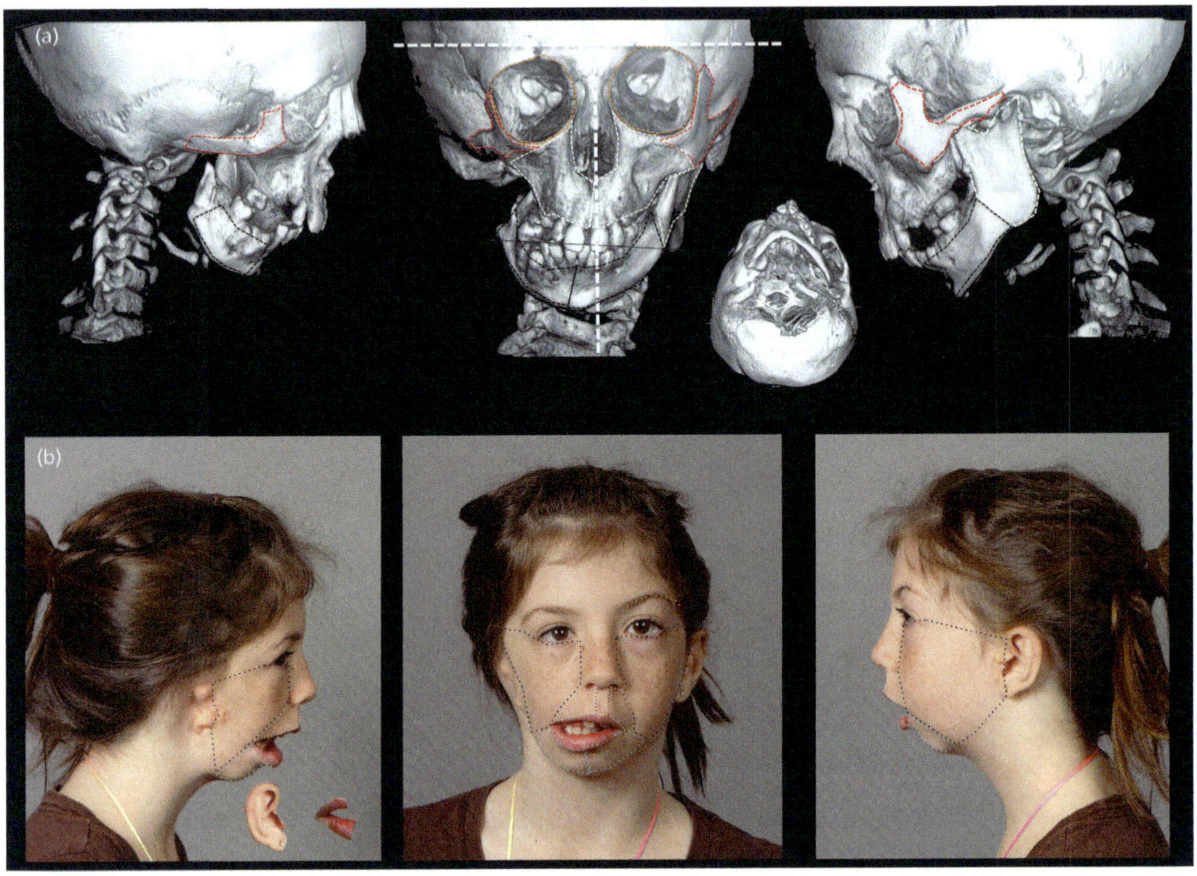

Fig. 57-9 Illustration of a component analysis of the facial asymmetry. (a) The facial skeletal is assessed regionally based on each of the skeletal elements in terms of its three-dimensional spatial relationship to the facial midline axis and to its shape to the 'mirror-image' counterpart. Osteotomies can be made and the elements repositioned. Autogenous bone grafts are used to support the gaps. Distraction can be used when there is sufficient bone; however, vascularized free flaps are used for missing elements. Alloplastic implants may be required to restore the surface topography that cannot be achieved by repositioning the bone elements alone. This particular patient will require all available surgical options. (b) The soft tissue envelope is assessed regionally and autogenous soft tissue augmentation is nearly always needed despite restoring symmetry to the skeletal framework. Additionally the auricular element and the macrostomia will need to be reconstructed.

horizon, to the level of the pupils or to an agreed upon external reference plane.

To determine the internal relationship of the facial components of symmetry, one must establish the true facial midline, 'mirror-image' plane of symmetry in which the reflection about the plane can be compared. However, in many patients with craniofacial asymmetry that involve the cranial-orbital region, defining that plane is often operationally difficult. Geometrically bisecting the inter-pupillary line is not always reliable. For example, in the atypical craniofacial clefts with resulting asymmetrically positioned orbits, the plane that bisects the inter-pupillary distance does not necessarily match that of a plane defined by the skull base (crista galli–sella). Moreover in cases of unilateral frontosphenoidal and coronal craniosynostosis, the anterior skull base itself is skewed and as a consequence needs to be referenced to the posterior skull base untouched by the pathology. However, both the anterior and posterior skull base can be skewed and any obvious plane of symmetry is difficult to clearly establish. Thus with the more severe forms of craniofacial asymmetry, the plane of symmetry is difficult to define objectively and is defined by the clinician's judgment and by what elements can be surgically altered to an acceptable appearance.

Reyneke provided a simplified asymmetry classification based on chin, mandible and maxilla to guide the orthodontic and surgical management.[51] However, once the asymmetry includes the cranio-orbital structures and extends to involve the soft tissue and facial elements, each of the components of the face must be analyzed independently in terms of (1) spatial position, and (2) shape. Any geometric object in three-dimensional space has 6 degrees of freedom to determine its spatial position: three translational (delta x, delta y, delta z) and three rotational (roll, yaw and pitch) (see Figures 5-7 to 5-9). Definition of the shape is more complex, but intuitively represented by volume and surface topography.

In any comprehensive analysis of asymmetry, the face must be anatomically broken down into its 'geometric' components: the skeletal masses, the dental arches, the soft tissue envelope and the individual facial elements. Each of these components then must be defined by its spatial position in space relative to the reflection plane or plane of symmetry, and by its individual shape relative to its counterpart.

The skeletal masses are the building blocks that structurally define the framework of the face. These include: the frontal bone, the orbital complex, the malar/zygoma, the maxilla, and the mandible. The mandible itself is a composite of the ramus, body and symphysis. Each of the maxillary and mandibular dental arches needs to be assessed independently in terms its dental midline, arch form, roll, yaw and pitch. Each is then assessed with respect to its skeletal bases: the maxillary dental arch to the maxilla and the mandibular dental arch to the mandible. Finally the inter-relationship between dental arches is assessed. The soft-tissue envelope of the skeletal framework is assessed in regional subunits,[52,53] in terms of its thickness measured from the skeletal surface (volume deficiency or excess) and surface topography to achieve the desired symmetry as the correction of the underlying framework does not necessarily correct the soft-tissue envelope. Finally the individual facial elements such as the ears, ocular adnexa, nose and lips that ultimately define the face must also be assessed in terms of both the spatial position and the individual shape.

Thus when a patient presents with asymmetry, regardless of its aetiology, every component must be carefully assessed. Only then can a systematic multistage reconstructive blueprint be developed.

Three-dimensional data acquisition and manipulation

Traditionally surgical planning for maxillofacial surgery was based on clinical examination, two-dimensional photographs, lateral and frontal cephalometric radiographs, and facebow mounting of dental casts. While this well-established approach for half-a-century provided reliable results in many patients, the outcomes were inconsistent for the patients who presented with complex facial asymmetries. The 2D analysis in the orthogonal planes was difficult to integrate in the surgical planning with any degree of confidence. While the facebow transfer provided guidance, many of the patients with significant facial asymmetries have displaced orbits and auricular asymmetry. With each step of the two-dimensional planning of a three-dimensional problem – from cephalometric analysis to dental model surgery– the errors accumulated and were incorporated into the occlusal splint fabrication.[54] Thus the surgeon found himself or herself in the operating room with an undesired clinical outcome. Inaccurate surgical planning led to inaccurate surgery. Surgical planning at best was a guide in such cases, and the final judgment of the planning was based on intraoperative assessment that required considerable judgment and experience. Thus the conventional 2D surgical planning was limited for all but the simplest cases in which there was an acceptable degree of symmetry in the frontal plane, and the surgeon had only to solve the patient's problem in the sagittal plane. Accurate presurgical planning was a challenge for all but the simplest of cases.

Thus surgical planning of patients with complex craniofacial abnormalities as described in this chapter was largely based on the surgeon's experience and abilities to achieve the desired outcome. It is only within recent years that accurate surgical planning came within the reach of the surgeon and the orthodontist with our ability to capture the 3D surface facial skeletal anatomy with the lower radiation dosage cone beam CT scan, 3D optical and laser surface image capture of the colour and texture of the facial appearance and software that allowed manipulation of that data.

The anatomical landmarks can now be more accurately located without the averaging of a 3D projection on to a 2D cephalometric radiograph. Cephalometric analysis no longer needed to be confined to the mid-sagittal plane. Analysis can now be performed in three-dimensions to allow the surgeon and the orthodontist to visualize and address asymmetry in all three planes.

Today the software for virtual surgical planning (VSP) is capable of simulating surgical procedures with ever increasing user applicability: from the imaging research lab to routine daily clinical application.[55–57] The facial skeleton is treated as a solid 3-dimensional object in virtual space that can be digitally manipulated. Osteotomy planes can be defined and the 3D facial skeletal object can be digitally sectioned into two separate solid objects, where each can now be moved independent of the other. The software treats the CT data set as solid objects on which Boolean algebra can be performed. 3D visual objects can be added and subtracted digitally. The registration and superimposition technique makes it possible to build a composite model based upon both volumetric information from CT or CBCT scan and surface information of the dentition from laser or optical scans with greater clinical accuracy can be integrated. Surgical planning can now be done in 3-dimensional space instead of in planar projection 2-dimensional cephalometric films. The complex facial skeletal asymmetries can be addressed. Moreover the conventional the inaccuracies and the time consuming laboratory process of facebow transfer, plaster mounting of dental casts, sectioning, repositioning and remounting of the dental casts are all eliminated. The surgeon now has the ability to easily execute various surgical options to optimize outcome. Regions of interference during the skeletal movement can be assessed and detected (such as with maxillary impaction and mandibular rotation cases), the dental roots can be visualized within a skeletal framework for interdental osteotomies and the course of the inferior alveolar nerve can be visualized for mandibular osteotomies.

Principles of symmetry reconstruction

Surgical armamentarium

The surgeon must have within his or her armamentarium a large number of procedures to be able to address each of the components of facial asymmetry involved – skeletal, soft tissue and functional facial elements (Figure 57-10).

Obwegeser, Tessier, Ortiz-Monasterio and others that followed firmly established the principles involved in complete disassembly and reassembly of the craniofacial skeleton through safe transcutaneous/transoral approaches, carefully designed osteotomies and rigid skeletal fixation systems supported by bone grafts.[58] The skeletal components that the surgeon can manipulate include the cranial vault, the frontal bones, the orbits, the zygoma, the maxilla, the mandible and the chin symphysis. These procedures can be done with the conventional approach of established osteotomies, and repositioning and fixation of the bone elements to their desired position. When there is concern of skeletal stability with the amount of advancement desired (bone length) and relapsing soft tissue and muscular forces, skeletal distraction is added to the surgeon's armamentarium.[59,60] When there is insufficient bone for distraction then the alternatives for the surgeon are non-vascularized bone grafts (costochondral rib grafts, iliac bone grafts) and vascularized bone transfer (fibula, scapula, radial) through microsurgery techniques.[61] Finally repositioning of the existing bone in craniofacial asymmetry cases cannot in general restore a 'mirror-image' symmetry without the use of custom onlay alloplastic implants to restore the shape or the surface topography of the involved skeletal element.[57]

Once the skeletal form is addressed, then soft tissue asymmetry of the overlying skin envelope can be addressed through microsurgical vascularized adipofascial tissue transfer, non-vascularized dermal fat grafting and structural fat grafting. When a large volumetric amount is needed then microvascular tissue transfer provides the best solution in patients with severe deficiency.[62] The choices for the surgeon include scapula, parascapula, anterolateral thigh, and deep inferior epigastric perforator, among others. However, tailoring the augmentation to specific facial regions is difficult and many will require debulking and refinement procedures. Moreover, the appearance of the donor site needs to be carefully discussed. In many patients whose soft tissue deficiency is mild to moderate, non-vascularized dermal fat grafting is an appropriate choice. As there is nearly always some degree of volumetric resorption with non-vascularized grafts, the augmentation is overcorrected generally by 20–25% and some will require additional grafting. In recent years the introduction of serial staged structural fat grafting has revolutionized the soft tissue asymmetry management in many patients. Fat is harvested from the abdominal and flank regions, purified and then injected in small aliquots (0.1 cc) in a highly controlled manner in multiple planes, giving the surgeon a degree of precision that cannot be achieved by the other approaches. As with dermal fat grafting there is resorption and structural fat grafting is repeated until the desired symmetry is acceptable.[63–65]

Finally symmetry requires restoring the unique facial elements that include the lip, nose, ocular adnexa (eyelids and canthi) and ears. Moreover in a number of conditions the various branches of the facial nerve may be involved. Functional nerve balancing

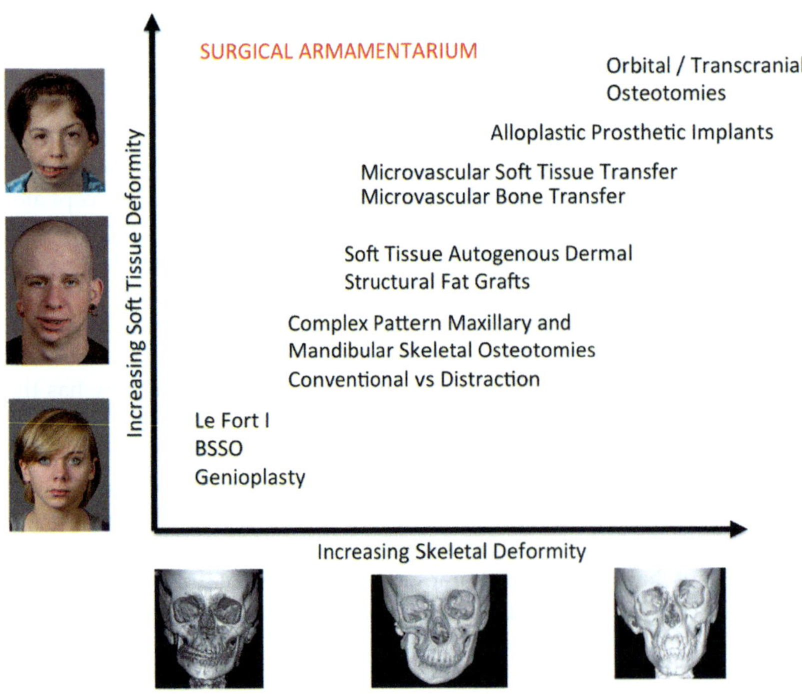

Fig. 57-10 Surgical options for skeletal and soft tissue reconstruction must be tailored to the degree of severity for each of the components. The basic principles regardless of cause of asymmetry include: (1) establish an axis of symmetry to correct roll, yaw and pitch; (2) rearrange the existing skeleton though osteotomies and repositioning each of the elements; (3) include bone grafts, skeletal distraction and microvascular bone transfer for restoration and skeletal stability; (4) refinements with custom prosthetic implants to improve surface topography; (5) soft tissue augmentation through autogenous grafts and microvascular tissue transfer; and (6) reconstruct missing elements such as the ear, eye and lips.

procedures (such as eyelid gold weight) and facial reanimation procedures may be required.

Reconstruction of each of the elements, anatomical and functional, requires a more detailed discussion that is beyond the scope of this chapter and is best found in the literature related to the specific cause of the craniofacial asymmetry. However, a number of clinical cases will elucidate the above approach.

In patients who present with an isolated malar/zygoma fracture, there are two situations each with a different aspect of asymmetry that need to be addressed. When the fracture is acute then all that needs to be corrected is its spatial position relative to its unaffected counterpart as the shape remains unaltered. However, when the malar fracture has been allowed to heal in malposition, then not only is it altered in its position in three-dimensional space by the fracture but also its shape (i.e. its volume and surface) is altered over time by asymmetrical functional loads. Thus repositioning an 'old' zygoma fracture by osteotomy cannot restore the original symmetry without also addressing the changes in the surface bony topography that have occurred over the interval of time. In either situation, the soft tissue is not involved and restoring the malar skeletal symmetry would be expected to restore the overlying soft tissue envelope.

Patients who present with skeletal asymmetry limited to the maxillofacial region can be managed with classically described osteotomies described by Obwegeser: the Le Fort I type osteotomy, the bilateral sagittal split osteotomy of the mandible and osseous genioplasty (Figure 57-11).

More complex are the patients who present with cranial–orbital asymmetry with a facial component. Reconstruction requires disassembling the anterior cranial vault and the supra-orbital rim. The orbital rim is then repositioned in all three planes to its mirror-image counterpart with the goals of restoring the palpebral shape and dimensions. The anterior cranial vault is then reconstructed to restore the symmetry of the frontal bones (Figure 57-12). The associated facial skeletal asymmetry as a result of the skull base remains uncorrected until adolescence when at the time of skeletal maturity this is typically addressed (Figure 57-13).

Perhaps of all the asymmetries, the most challenging reconstruction are patients who present with atypical craniofacial clefting pattern well described by Tessier and Kawamoto.[33] While the skeletal framework can be restored by classic procedures, the challenge is restoring the overlying fabric and the internal neural muscular facial function. Moreover, restoring the correct spatial relationship and form of the ears, the eyes, lips and nose poses in many cases a challenge that taxes the ingenuity of the surgeon. The anaplastologist and ocularist are needed when surgical limits are reached. Because of the rarity and unique nature of the clinical expression of the variety of atypical clefts, the reconstruction must be individualized in comparison

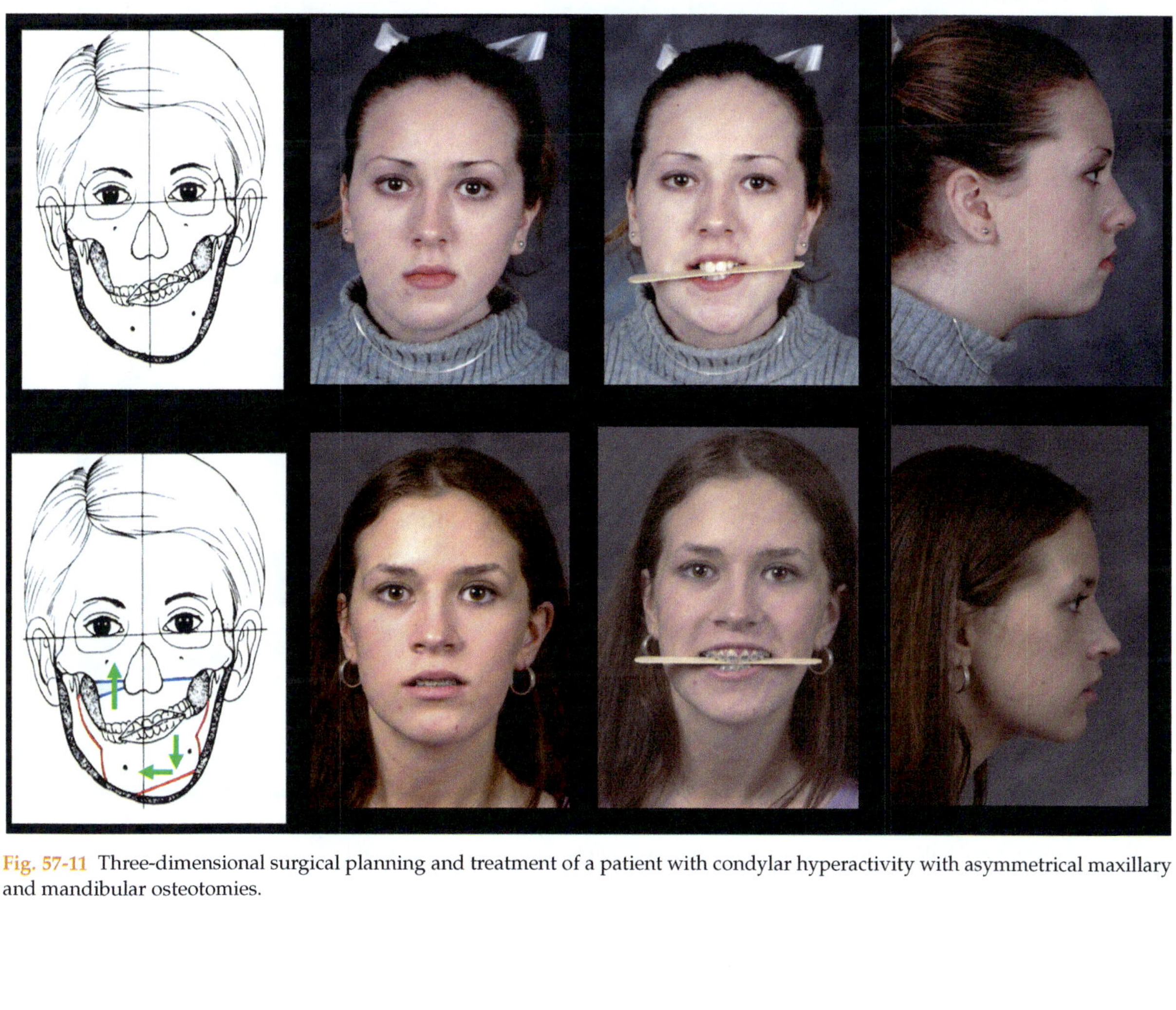

Fig. 57-11 Three-dimensional surgical planning and treatment of a patient with condylar hyperactivity with asymmetrical maxillary and mandibular osteotomies.

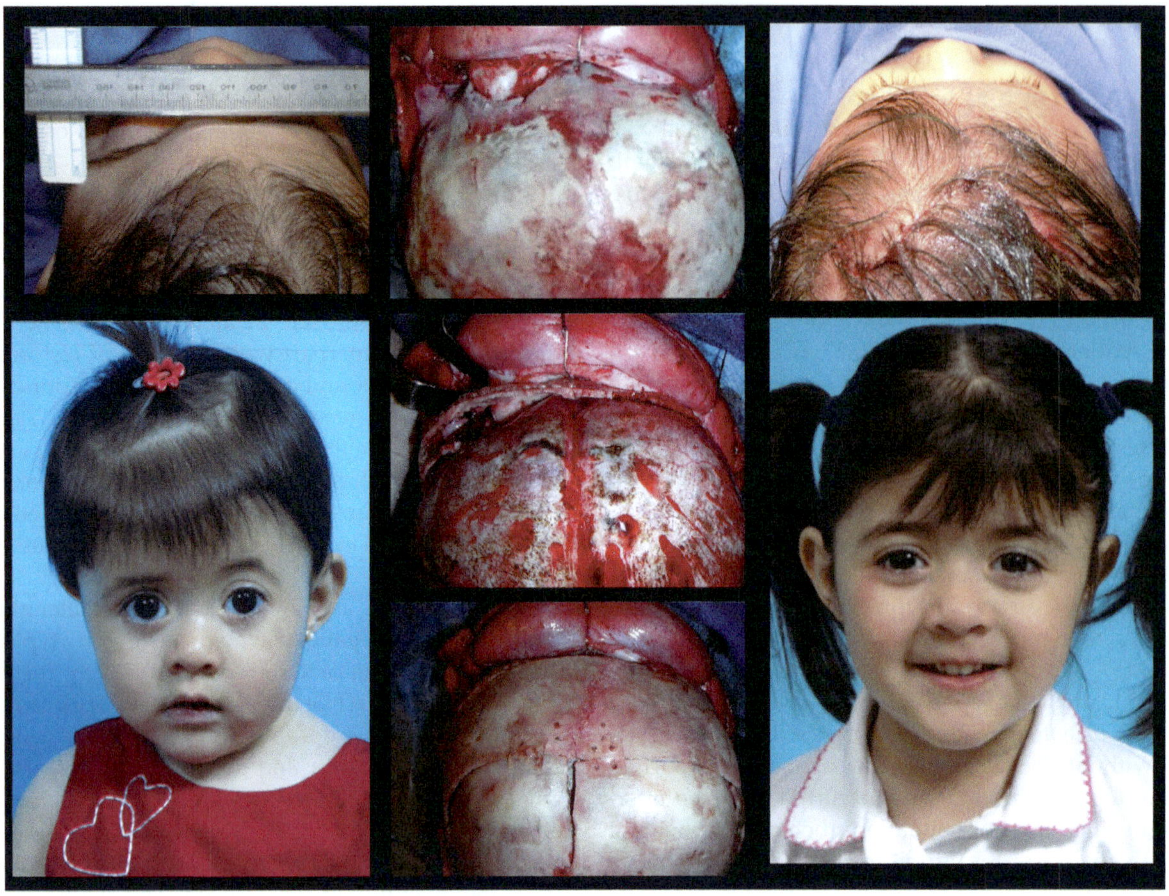

Fig. 57-12 Cranio-orbital reconstruction of a child who presents with left unilateral coronal synostosis. The anterior cranial vault (frontal and parietal bones) and the supra-orbital rim is repositioned to restore symmetry.

(a)

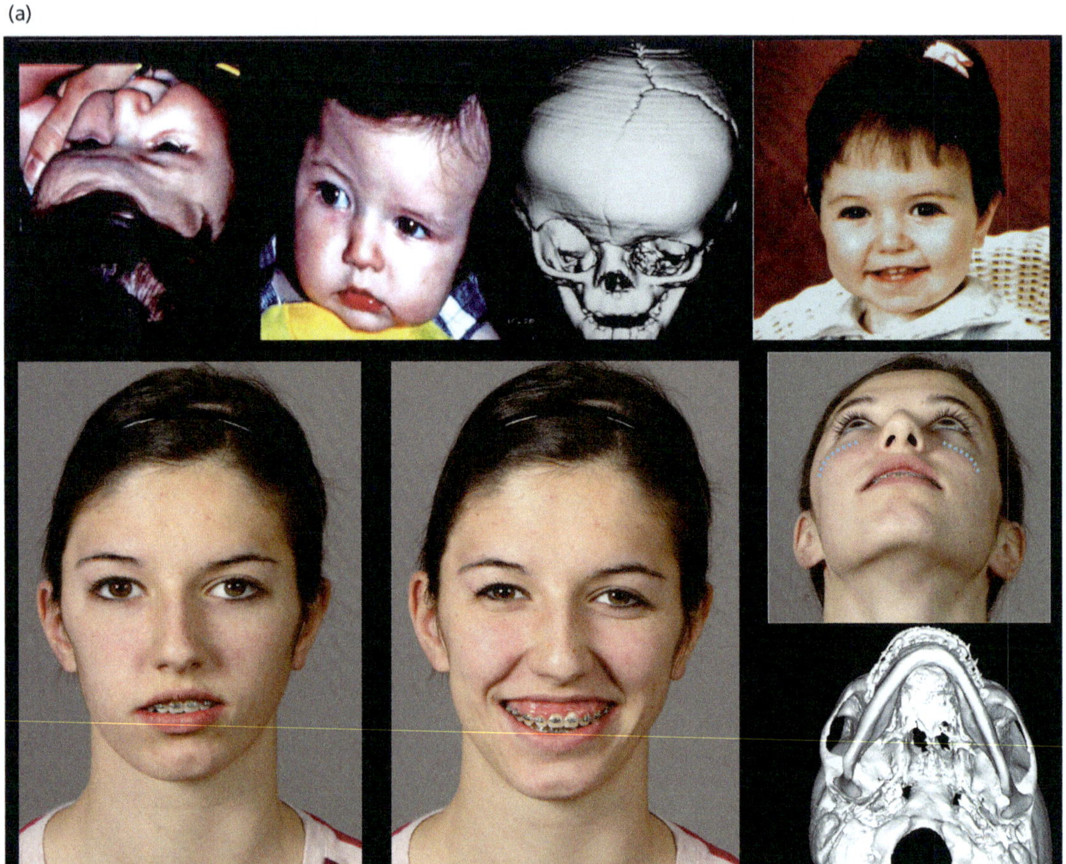

Fig. 57-13 (a) Patient 15 years after correction of the unilateral coronal synostosis illustrated in Figure 57-2. She presents with residual maxillary-mandibular asymmetry. (b) Three dimensional planning for asymmetrical Le Fort I impaction, secondary left malar osteotomy and asymmetric mandibular ramal osteotomies. (c) Outcome at approximately 6 months after surgery. Note the residual asymmetry.

(b)

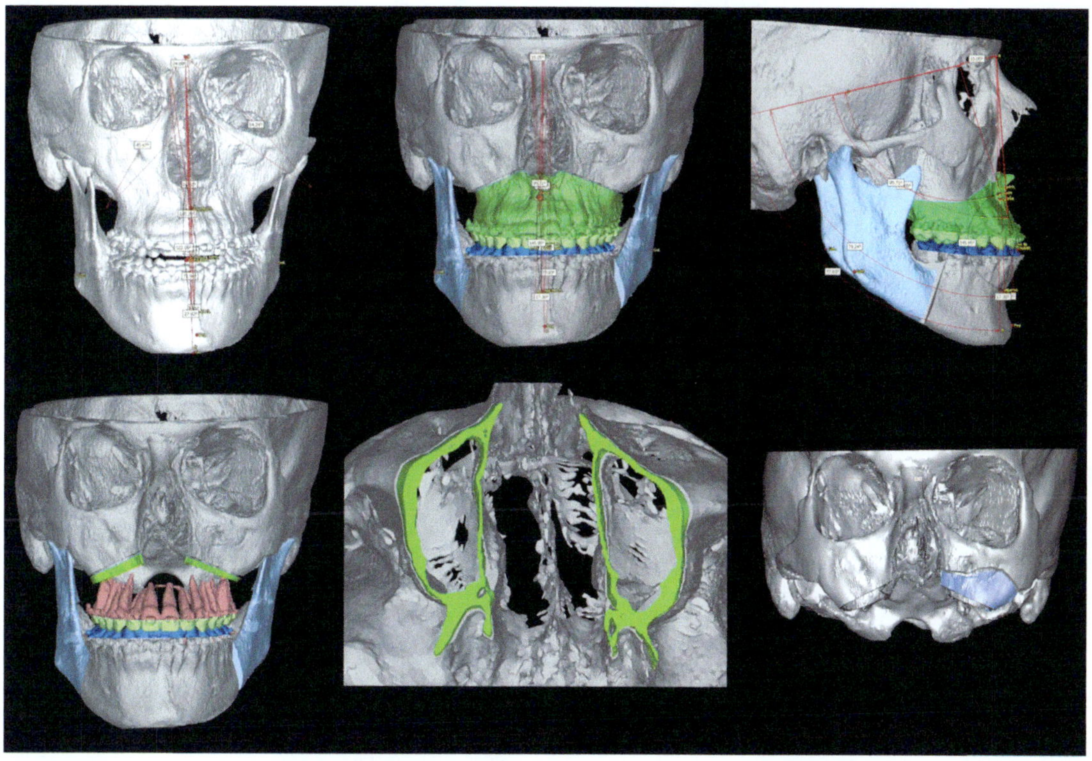

(c)

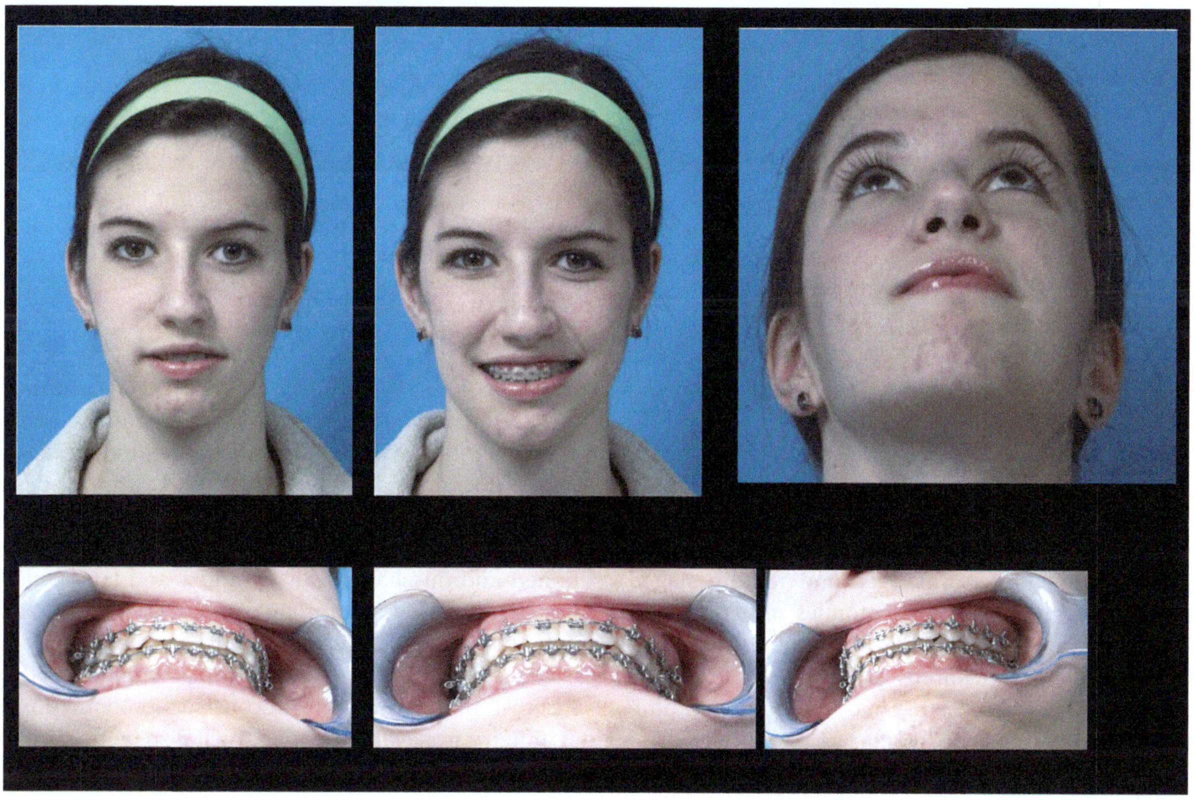

Fig. 57-13 (*Continued*).

to well-established approaches in patients with typical facial characteristics (Figure 57-14).

The adolescent facial cleft may present with midfacial deficiency. While the focus is to coordinate the dental arches with a classic Le Fort I osteotomy, it is important to assess the maxillary–malar symmetry as many will exhibit asymmetry in both the spatial relationship in three-dimensional space and in the intrinsic shape of the midfacial skeleton between the two halves. A classically designed symmetrical Le Fort I osteotomy pattern while addressing the occlusal relationship will fail to correct the maxillary–malar

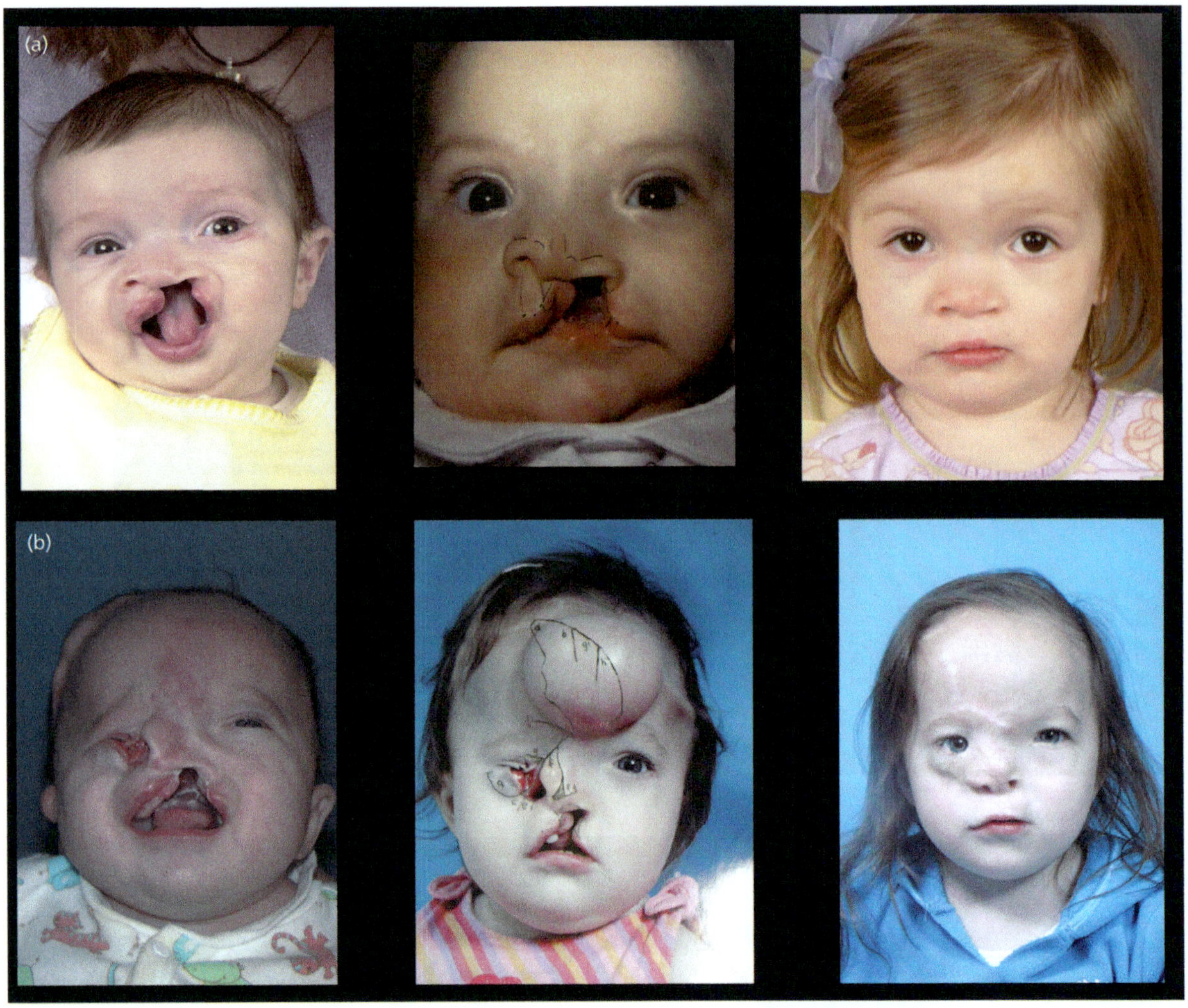

Fig. 57-14 There is a broad spectrum of asymmetric facial clefts whose reconstruction must be tailored to the extent and severity of the involved anatomical structures. (a) Typical cleft lip and palate reconstruction whose reconstruction and supportive orthodontic treatment is well established (PK Patel MD). (b) Atypical craniofacial cleft whose reconstruction remains as an unfinished surgeon's and orthodontist's task. Initial reconstruction involved tissue expansion, complex tailoring of the various skin flaps, structural bone reconstruction with rib grafts and an ocular prosthesis. (Courtesy of BS Bauer MD & PK Patel MD.)

asymmetry. Such patients are better suited with an asymmetrical Le Fort I osteotomy pattern (Figure 57-15), and when needed as a refinement, followed by onlay autogenous bone graft or alloplastic implant to match the surface contour.

In patients with craniofacial microsomia, all the facial components are involved and require staged reconstruction.[66–69] The osteotomies must be tailored to the individual deformities and not necessarily follow classic osteotomy patterns. Repositioning osteotomy and when needed maxillary and mandibular distraction are needed to correct the roll, yaw and pitch of the skeletal framework integrated with the dental arches (Figures 57-16 and 57-17). In patients with Pruzansky III mandibular deformity, patients will require costochondral rib grafts and microvascularized fibular transfer (Figure 57-18). However, skeletal repositioning alone is insufficient to achieve the desired skeletal symmetry because of the intrinsic asymmetry in the shape of the involved bony elements. Thus onlay bone grafts and alloplastic implants are needed to restore volume and surface contours (Figure 57-19). In addition to the skeletal asymmetry, these patients have a soft tissue asymmetry with deficiency that will require soft tissue augmentation with autogenous dermal grafting, fat grafting and/or vascularized microvascular free tissue transfer. Moreover, symmetry is not completed until the malpositioned and misshapen ear deformity and lateral cleft lip are addressed. Microtia reconstruction either with autogenous costocartilage graft or prosthetic implant is needed. In some there is also a lip asymmetry with a macrostomia that requires reconstruction. Functional symmetry in facial animation must also be taken into account.

Staging and timing of intervention

While the principle of skeletal reconstruction to establish the foundation first, followed by soft tissue reconstruction as a covering envelope, is a reliable guide, there are exceptions of necessity. Patients with asymmetry will present long before they reach skeletal maturity when the surgeon can address the end-stage

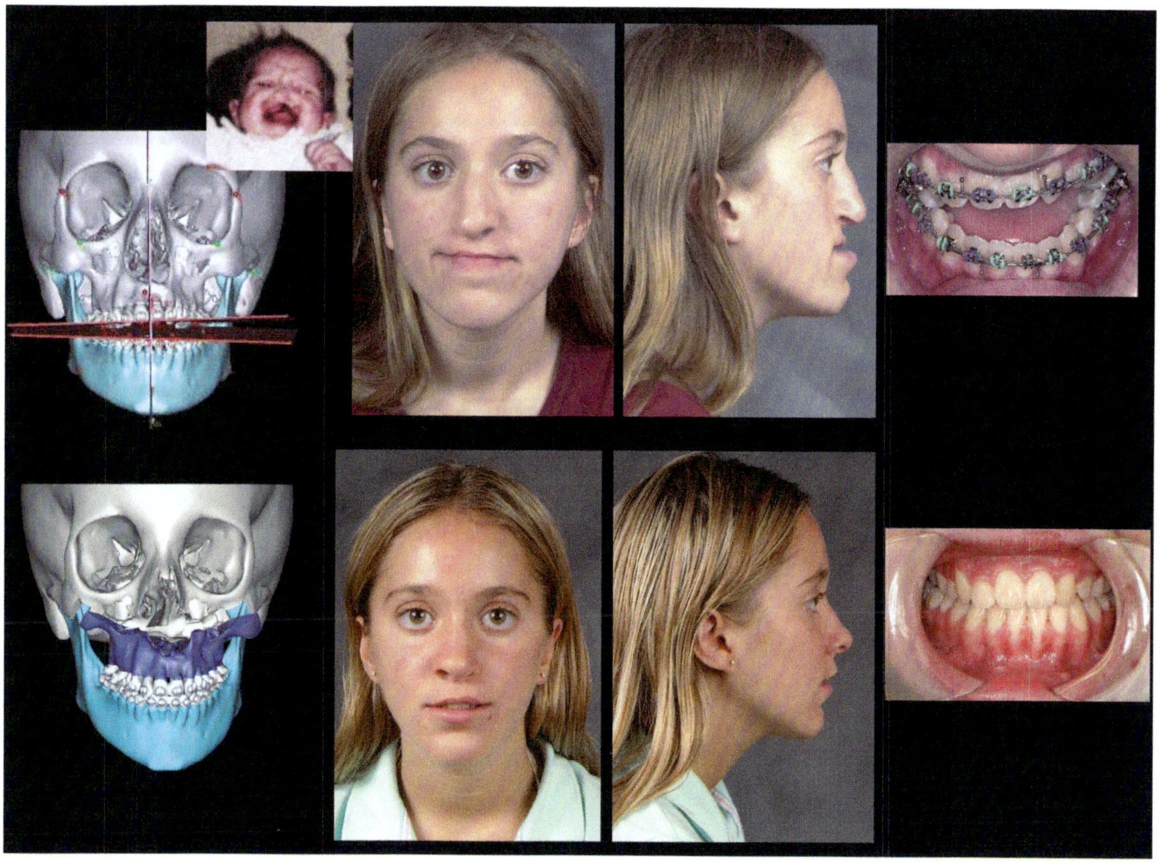

Fig. 57-15 Patient with left cleft lip and palate who required an asymmetrical Le Fort I to correct the residual facial skeletal asymmetry.

(a)

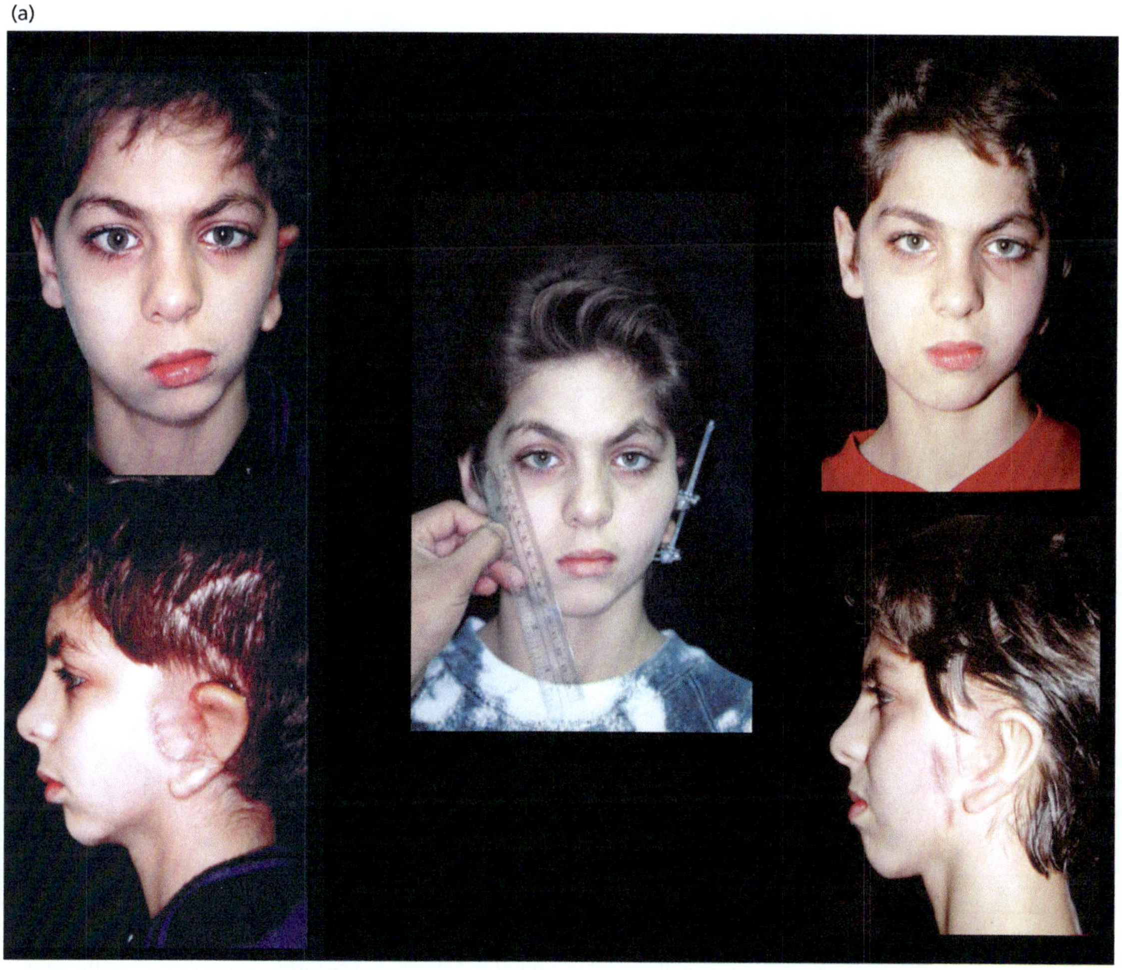

Fig. 57-16 Patient with left craniofacial microsomia. (a) Clinical outcome from left mandibular distraction. (b) Management of the occlusal open bite from the resulting left mandibular lengthening. The crossbite could have been addressed with a simultaneous palatal expansion.

(b)

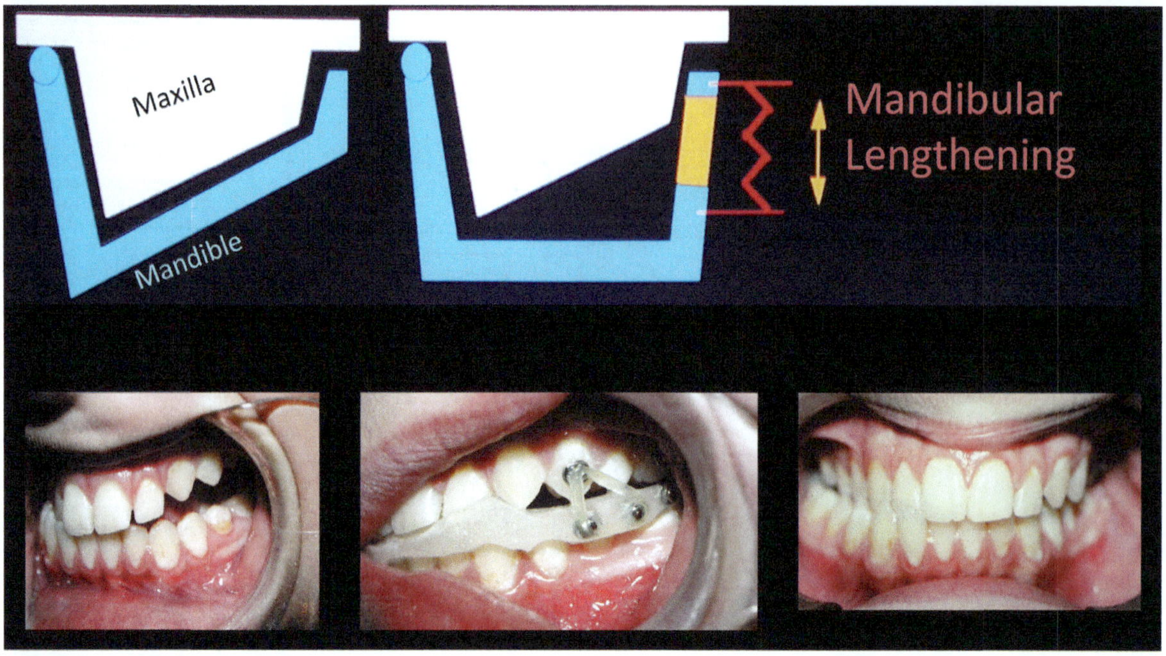

Fig. 57-16 (*Continued*).

(a)

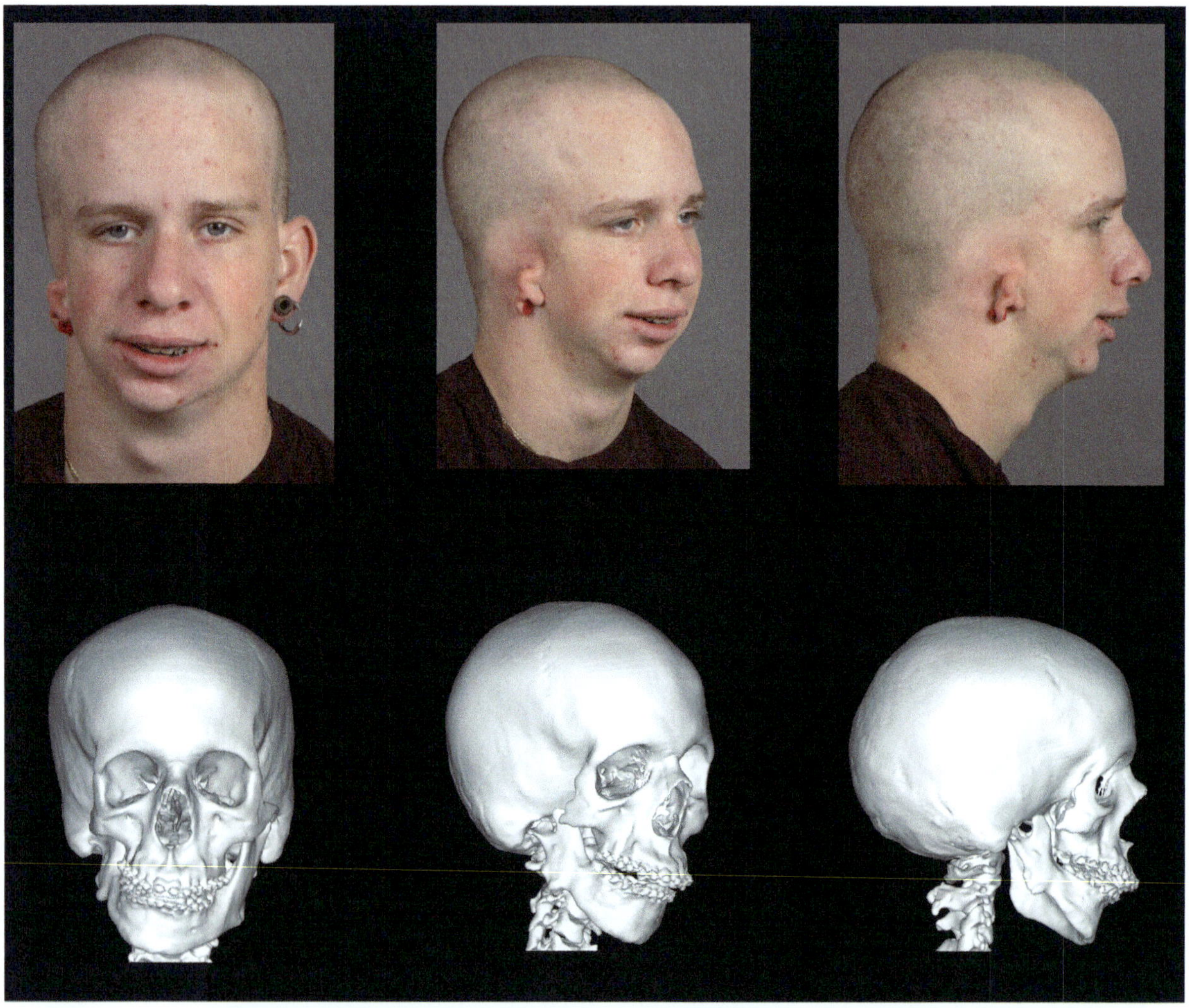

Fig. 57-17 Patient with right craniofacial microsomia. (a) Preoperative clinical images and CT scan showing the underlying skeletal anatomy. (b) Surgical simulation of simultaneous maxillary and mandibular distraction. The virtual simulation gives the surgeon an opportunity to optimize the vector of distraction with the understanding that the true kinematics of the right TMJ cannot be reproduced. (c) The outcome at 8 weeks with the internal device maintained until consolidation.

(b)

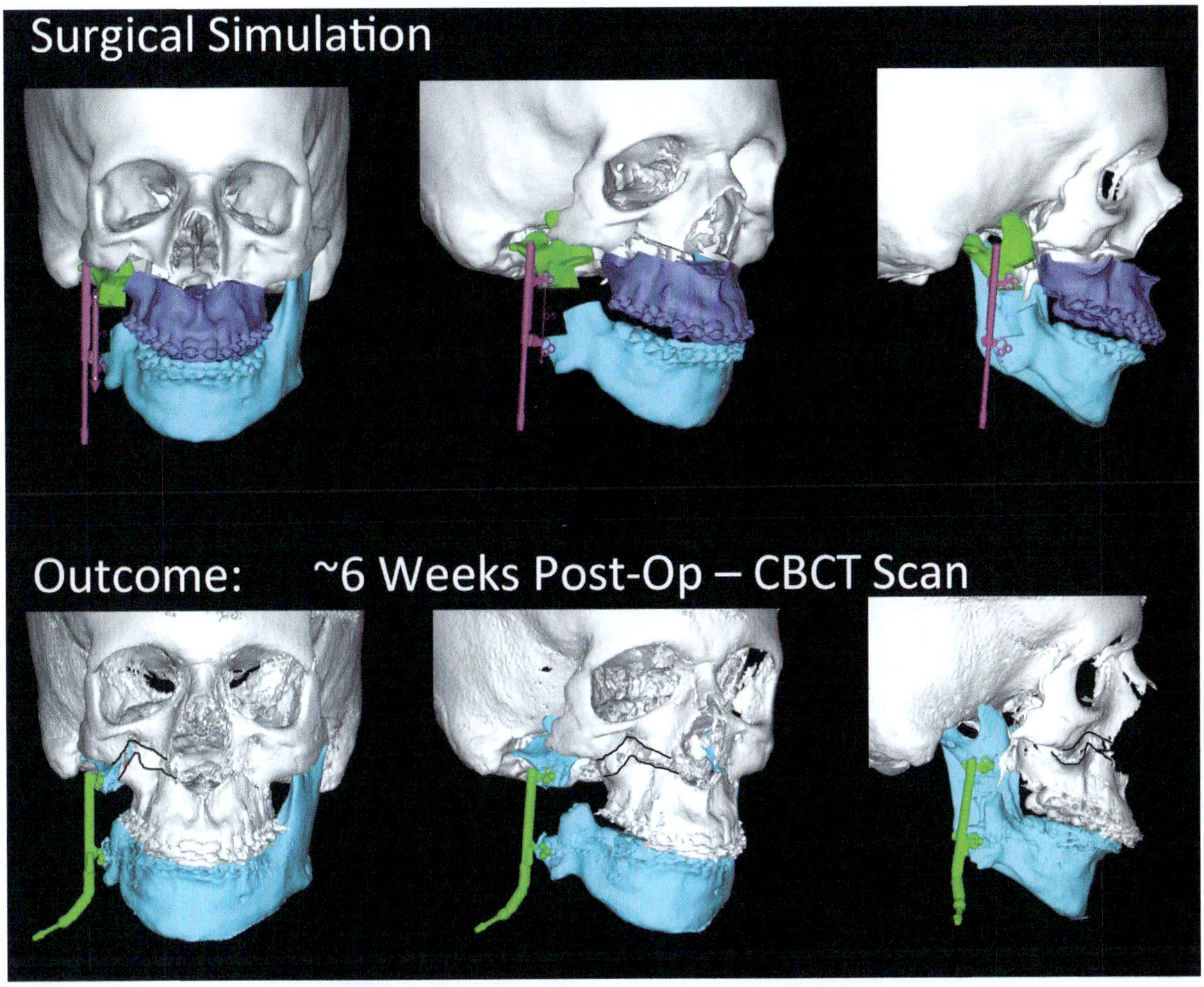

(c)

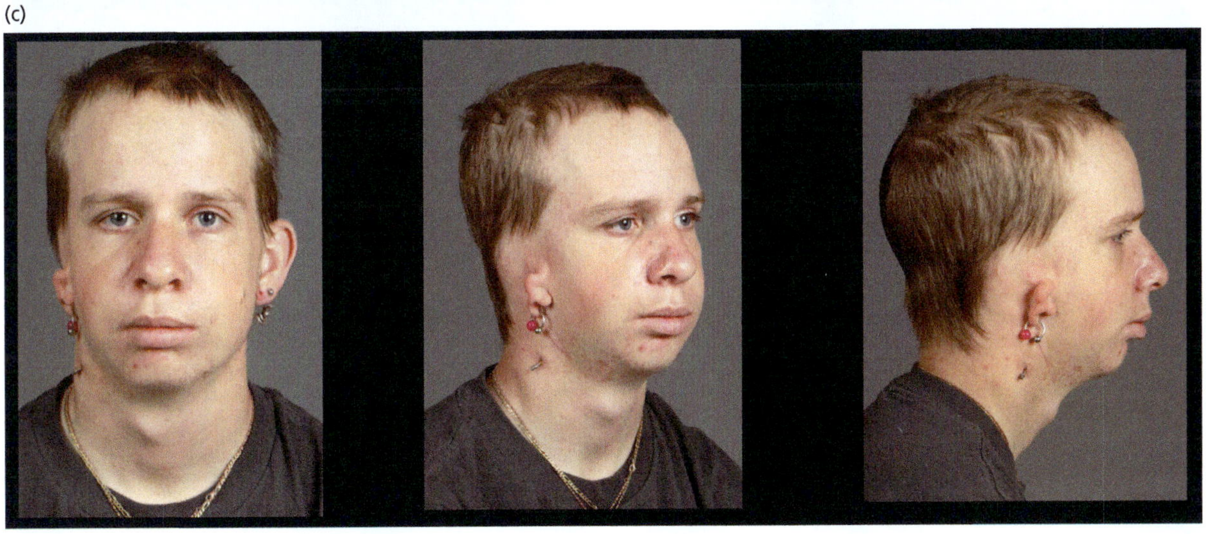

Fig. 57-17 (*Continued*).

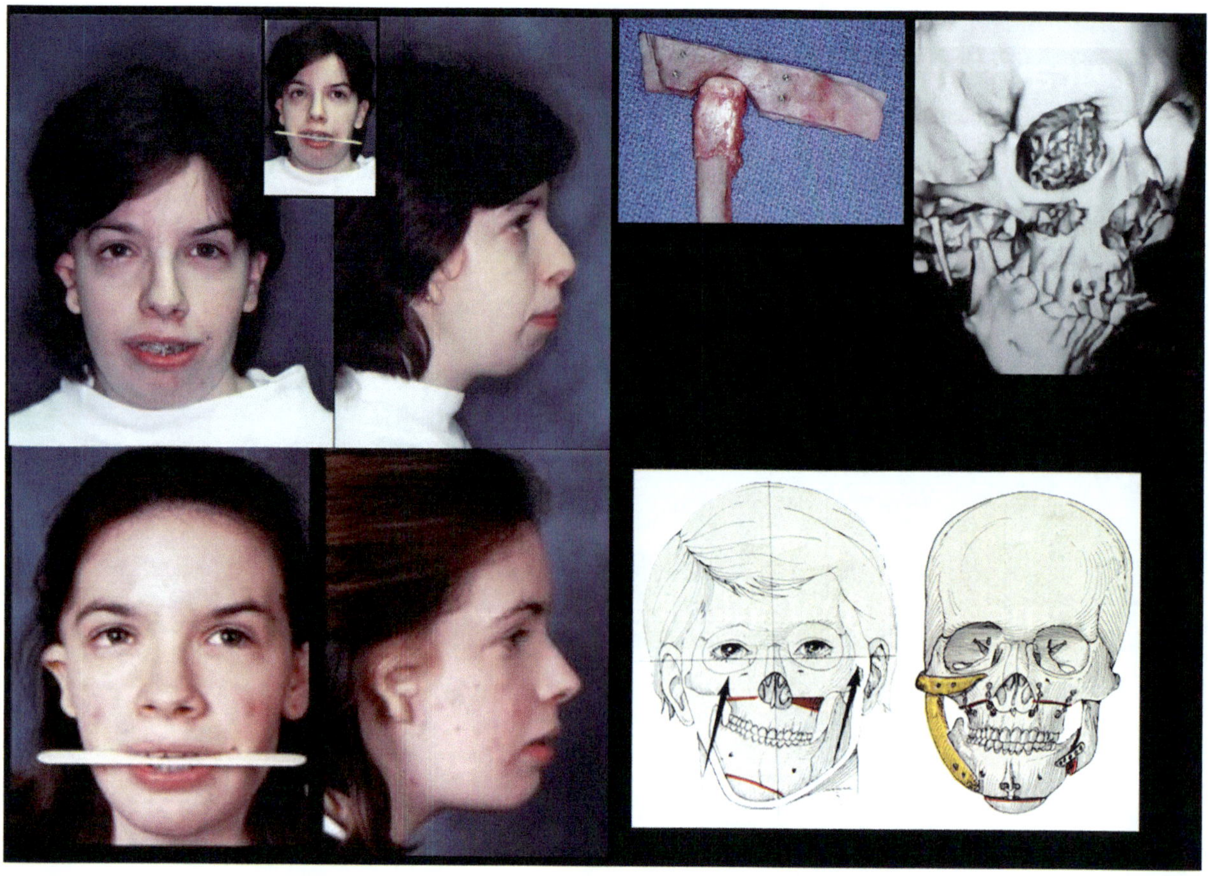

Fig. 57-18 Patient with right craniofacial microsomia who underwent asymmetrical Le Fort I, left sagittal split osteotomy of the ramus and a right rib graft and fibular reconstruction.

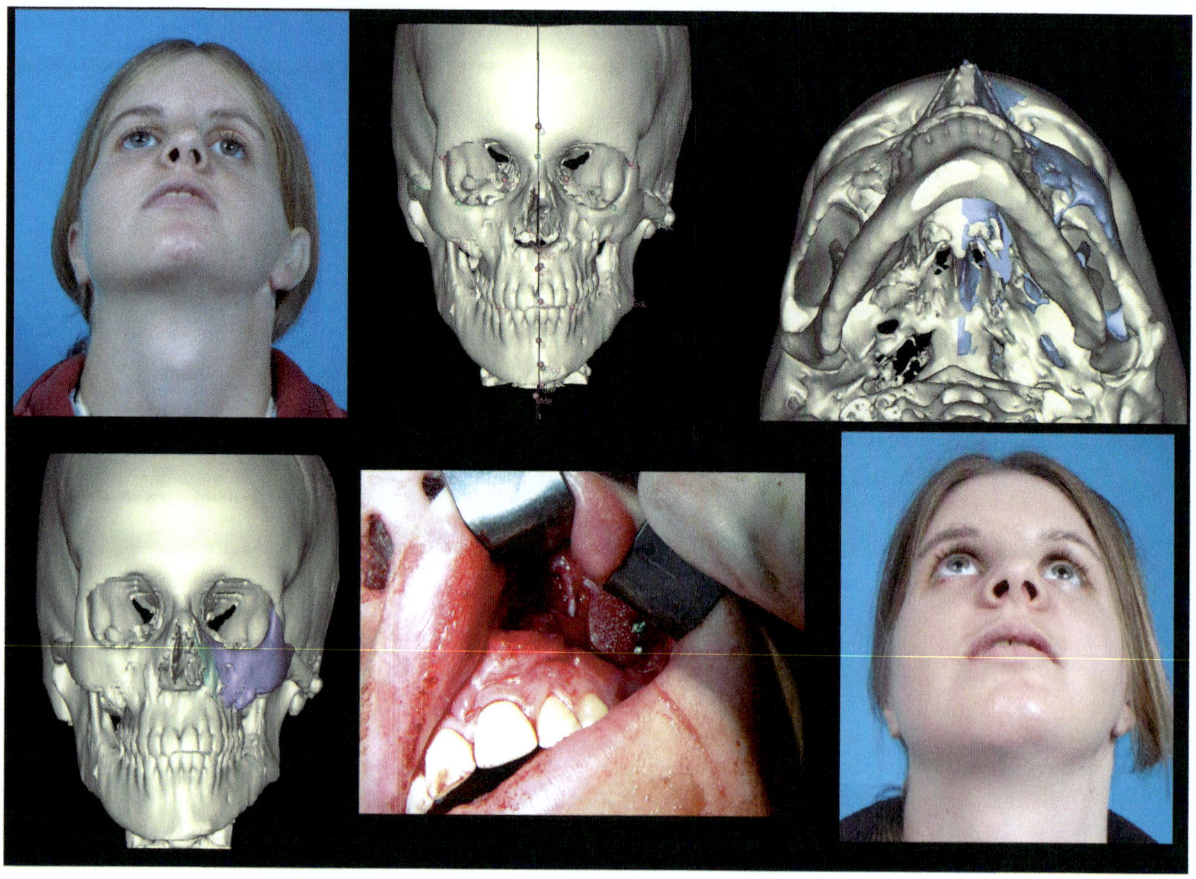

Fig. 57-19 Patient with left craniofacial microsomia after Le Fort I and BSSO. The residual zygomatic asymmetry is corrected with an alloplastic implant.

deformity. Leaving the multi-staged skeletal and soft tissue reconstruction till late in adolescence, and waiting for dentofacial maturity will for many patients have a significant detrimental impact on their education at a time when they can least afford to miss school, around the time of entrance to higher education. Moreover functional and psychosocial consequences will drive earlier intervention. Patients with significant asymmetry will benefit from earlier soft tissue augmentation procedures rather than waiting to correct the skeletal asymmetry. Most children are not as concerned about the skeletal asymmetry if the soft tissue correction can camouflage the underlying dentoskeletal asymmetry. Autogenous ear reconstruction well before skeletal surgery is of benefit not only in terms of appearance, but also for those who may need to wear corrective glasses. Appropriately positioning the ear before skeletal symmetry requires careful planning and in reality can rarely if ever be achieved even when the skeletal foundation is restored.

There is also the benefit of harnessing the patient's normal growth and development with earlier intervention. In patients with craniofacial microsomia the benefit from earlier mandibular distraction lengthening procedure includes improvement in the airway by repositioning the tongue base and lessens the secondary impact on the midfacial skeleton by removing the anatomical restriction of the mandible.[70] This is even with the understanding that patients are likely to need further mandibular lengthening later in childhood supported by orthodontic management and conventional orthognathic surgery in adolescence. There is a definite role for early interceptive orthodontics and when needed combined with surgery that can lessen the degree of asymmetry until more definite skeletal procedures can be accomplished.

Orthodontic considerations

The basic principles of surgical orthodontic management remain unchanged in the patient with skeletal maturity (end-stage deformity). The permanent dentition needs to be appropriately positioned in each of the respective basal bones, the dental arches well-coordinated to each other, and the maxillary dental midline coincident with the mandibular dental midline. It is the surgeon who must reposition the skeleton so that the dental midline can be coincident with the facial midline and correct the yaw and roll and pitch. However, with such significant asymmetry the reality is that there are frequently both skeletal and dental compromises. The surgeon is limited by the muscular and soft tissue compromises made in repositioning the jaws in a way that is functionally stable; and the orthodontist, by what the surgeon can realistically achieve. Simultaneous gradual maxillary–mandibular distraction in severe asymmetry with orthodontic guidance can overcome many, but not all, of the skeletal and soft tissue limitations.

Where orthodontic intervention can play a role is in the early and mixed dentition when intervention with functional appliances can mitigate the progressive nature of asymmetry in an actively growing and developing facial skeleton.[71–73] Various orthodontic appliances and techniques have been designed to affect the growth of the jaws by altering the functional matrix. In a child with mild to moderate hemifacial microsomia, functional appliances like the Herbst, MARA and removable Twin Block all have the similar force mechanism of holding the mandible in a protruded position to stimulate growth in the condyle and fossa. In asymmetrical growth patterns, the appliances can be adjusted to reposition the mandible downward, forward and laterally to slightly overcorrect the dental midline relation. The earlier treatment can be initiated, the less secondary maxillary growth inhibition will occur. In severe cases, where surgical intervention at an early age is indicated, the mandible is advanced on the affected side creating a large lateral open bite. The object of an orthodontic functional appliance is to then encourage the maxilla, which is vertically deficient on the affected side, to grow vertically and level the lateral occlusal cant. This does not mean eruption of teeth on that side, but downward vertical maxillary skeletal growth. Unlike surgery, this may take years and significant orthodontic guidance to accomplish the goals. In combination with surgery (mandibular distraction), the simultaneous use of a temporary skeletal anchorage device with functional appliances to hold the mandibular position, we can use an elastic force on the maxillary bone to assist the maxillary downward growth to limit treatment time. However, the stability of the long-term outcome is unpredictable and further orthodontic and surgical intervention is the norm.[74,75]

Summary

In a chapter such as this that covers the broad spectrum, the specific management of each of the specific conditions cannot be detailed. The above discussion provides principles tailored to the clinical presentation and the accompanying clinical cases and tables illustrate a number of principles.

Restoring facial symmetry is one of the most challenging of all reconstructive procedures. Its difficulty lies in the extent of the involvement that ranges from purely skeletal asymmetry, as in patients with unilateral condylar hyperactivity, to involvement of all components of the facial structures as in craniofacial microsomia. Moreover expansile bony tumours and destructive diseases such as Parry–Romberg significantly add composite tissue challenges. Restoring facial symmetry requires establishing a plane of symmetry that is increasingly difficult with the severity of involvement. While the craniofacial skeleton can be disassembled from the sphenoid and sectioned into its anatomical units, the challenge is knowing where to position each of its bony elements relative to the facial axis and then addressing the soft tissue surface and volumetric asymmetry. Today the surgeon and the orthodontist have the benefit of viewing the three-dimensional asymmetry at multiple levels with cone beam CT scans and 3D surface images, allowing more accurate visualization of the morphological deformity and planning the surgical approach.

No other patient, than the patient with facial asymmetry, will require the degree of imagination, innovation and patience on both the part of the surgeon and the orthodontist. Similarly the patients and their families face similarly difficult challenges. From birth through adolescence into adulthood, the patients and their families are faced with a multitude of clinic appointments, surgical procedures and supportive treatment adversely impacting their education, time off from work for their parents and loss of revenue. Thus it is not surprising that a number of patients and their parents become tired, frustrated and, at times, even uncooperative. It is important that they do not feel that there is no end in sight. Treatment should be planned with definite goals within a definite time frame. The orthodontist must accomplish as much as possible in a first phase of treatment, not allowing a first phase to melt unnoticed into a second phase and subsequent orthodontic phases. The patient will definitely notice, and the result may be a precipitous drop in rapport and cooperation as the patient becomes more frustrated and disheartened. Similarly, the surgeon must have definite goals and carefully determine the number and timing of the surgical interventions in the first two decades of life. Ultimately success requires not only a close working relationship between the surgeon and the orthodontist, but other members of a supportive multidisciplinary team that includes psychologists, speech and language pathologists, prosthodontists and anaplastologists, to provide the most efficient care possible within the first two decades of life.

References

1 Jehle H. Bilateral symmetry in morphogenesis of embryos. Proc Nat Acad Sci. 1970;67:156–63.

2 Rhodes G, Proffitt F, Grady J, et al. Facial symmetry and the perception of beauty. Psychon Bull Rev. 1998;5:659.

3 Wade TJ. The relationships between symmetry and attractiveness and mating relevant decisions and behavior: a review. Symmetry. 2010;2:1081–98.

4 Zaidel DW, Cohen JA. The face, beauty, and symmetry: Perceiving asymmetry in beautiful faces. Int J Neurosci. 2005;115:1165.

5 Bishara SE, Burkey PS, Kharouf JG. Dental and facial asymmetries: a review. Angle Orthod. 1994;64:89–98.

6 Haraguchi S, Iguchi Y, Takada K. Asymmetry of the face in orthodontic patients. Angle Orthod. 2008;78:421–26.

7 Naini FB, Donaldson AN, McDonald F, Cobourne MT. Assessing the influence of asymmetry affecting the mandible and chin point on perceived attractiveness in the orthognathic patient, clinician, and layperson. J Oral Maxillofac Surg. 2012;70:192–206.

8 Cohen MM Jr. Perspectives of craniofacial asymmetry. Part I. The biology of asymmetry. Int J Oral Maxillofac Surg. 1995;24:2–7.

9 Cohen MM Jr. Perspectives of craniofacial asymmetry. Part II. Asymmetric embryopathies. Int J Oral Maxillofac Surg. 1995;24:8–12.

10 Cohen MM Jr. Perspectives of craniofacial asymmetry. Part III. Common and/or well known causes of asymmetry. Int J Oral Maxillofac Surg. 1995;24:127–33.

11 Cohen MM Jr. Perspectives of craniofacial asymmetry. Part IV. Hemi-asymmetries. Int J Oral Maxillofac Surg. 1995;24:134–41.

12 Cohen MM Jr. Perspectives of craniofacial asymmetry. Part V. The craniosynostoses. Int J Oral Maxillofac Surg. 1995;24:191–4.

13 Kawamoto HK, Kim SS, Jarrahy R, Bradley JP. Differential diagnosis of the idiopathic laterally deviated mandible. Plast Reconstr Surg. 2009:124:1600–1609.

14 Knoll BI, Persing JA. Craniosynostosis. In: Bentz ML, Bauer BS, Zuker R (Ed.) Principles and Practice of Pediatric Plastic Surgery. St Louis, Missouri: Quality Medical Publishing, 2008;541–70.

15 Marsh JL, Gado MH, Vannier MW, Stevens WG. Osseous anatomy of unilateral coronal synostosis. Cleft Palate J. 1986;23:87.

16 Posnick JC. Anterior plagiocephaly: unilateral coronal synostosis and skull molding. In: Posnick JC. Craniofacial and Maxillofacial Surgery in Children and Young Adults. WB Saunders: Philadelphia, 2000;127–61.

17 Rogers GF, Mulliken JB. Involvement of the basilar coronal ring in unilateral coronal synostosis. Plast Reconstr Surg. 2005;115:1887.

18 Loomis M, Radkowski M, Pensler J. Maxillary deformation in unilateral coronal synostosis. J Craniofacial Surg. 1990;1:73–76.

19 Kane AA, Lo LJ, Vannier MW, Marsh JL. Mandibular dysmorphology in unicoronal synostosis and plagiocephaly without synostosis. Cleft Palate Craniofac J. 1996;33:418–2.

20 Kane AA, Kim YO, Eaton A, et al. Quantification of osseous facial dysmorphology in untreated unilateral coronal synostosis. Plast Reconstr Surg. 2000;106:251.

21 Becker DB, Fundakowski CE, Govier DP, Deleon VB, et al. Long-term osseous morphologic outcome of surgically treated unilateral coronal synostosis. Plast Reconstr Surg. 2006;117:929.

22 Menard RM, David DJ. Unilateral lambdoid synostosis: Morphological characteristics. J Craniofac Surg. 1989;9:240–6.

23 Posnick JC. Posterior plagiocephaly: unilateral lambdoid synostosis and skull molding. In: Posnick JC. Craniofacial and Maxillofacial Surgery in Children and Young Adults. WB Saunders: Philadelphia, 2000;131–248.

24 Ploplys EA, Hopper RA, Muzaffar AR, et al. Comparison of computed tomographic imaging measurements with clinical findings in children with unilateral lambdoid synostosis. Plast Reconstr Surg. 2009;123:300–9.

25 Smartt JM, Elliott RM, Reid RR, Bartlett SP. Analysis of differences in the cranial base and facial skeleton of patients with lambdoid synostosis and deformational plagiocephaly. Plastic Reconstr Surg. 2011;127:303–12.

26 Bruneteau RJ, Mulliken JB. Frontal plagiocephaly: synostotic, compensational, or deformational. Plast Reconstr Surg. 1992;89:21.

27 Turk A, McCarthy J, Thorne C, et al. The 'back to sleep campaign' and deformational plagiocephaly: is there cause for concern? J Craniofac Surg. 1996;7:12.

28 Mulliken JB, Van der Woude DL, Hansen M, LaBrie RA, Scott RM. Analysis of posterior plagiocephaly: Deformational versus synostotic. Plast Reconstr Surg. 1999;103:371.

29 Hollier L, Kim J, Grayson BH, McCarthy JG. Congenital muscular torticollis and the associated craniofacial changes. Plast Reconstr Surg. 2000;105:827.

30 Yu C-C, Wong F-H, Lo L-J, Chen Y-R. Craniofacial deformity in patients with uncorrected congenital muscular torticollis: an assessment from three-dimensional computer tomography imaging. Plast Reconstr Surg. 2004;113:24–33.

31 Chate RAC. Facial scoliosis from sternocleidomastoid torticollis: longterm postoperative evaluation. Br J Oral Maxillofac Surg. 2005;43:428–34.
32 Ras F, Habets LL, van Ginkel FC, Prahl-Anderson B. Three-dimensional evaluation of facial asymmetry in cleft lip and palate. Cleft Palate Craniofac J. 1994;31:116-21.
33 Patel PK, Kawamoto HK. Atypical craniofacial clefts. In: Bentz ML, Bauer BS, Zuker R (Ed.). Principles and Practice of Pediatric Plastic Surgery. St Louis, Missouri: Quality Medical Publishing, 2008;583–636.
34 McCarthy JP. Craniofacial microsomia, In: Thorne CH (Ed.) Grabb and Smith Plastic Surgery, 6th edn. Philadelphia: Lippincott Williams and Wilkins, 2007;248–55.
35 Birgfeld CB, Heike C. Craniofacial microsomia. Semin Plast Surg. 2012;26:91–104.
36 Singhal V, Hill ME. Craniofacial microsomia and craniofacial distraction. In: Bentz ML, Bauer BS, Zuker R (Ed.) Principles and Practice of Pediatric Plastic Surgery. St Louis, Missouri: Quality Medical Publishing, 2008:755–97.
37 Pruzansky S. Not all dwarfed mandibles are alike. Birth Defects. 1969;2:120–9.
38 Kaban LB, Moses MH, Mulliken JB. Surgical correction of hemifacial microsomia in the growing child. Plastic Reconstr Surg. 1988;82:9–19.
39 Lauritzen C, Munro IR, Ross RB. Classification and treatment of hemifacial microsomia. Scand J Plast Reconstr Surg. 1985;19:33–9.
40 David DJ, Cooter RD. Hemifacial microsomia: a multisystem classification. 1987;80:525–33.
41 Vento AR, La Brie RA, Mulliken JB. The OMENS classification of hemifacial microsomia. Cleft Palate Craniofac J. 1991;28:68.
42 Horgan JE, Padwa BL, LaBrie RA, et al. OMENS-Plus: analysis of craniofacial and extracranial anomalies in hemifacial microsomia. Cleft Palate Craniofac J. 1995;32:405–12.
43 Birgfeld CB, Luquetti DV, Gougoutas A, et al. A phenotypic assessment tool for craniofacial microsomia. Plast Reconstruct Surg. 2011;127:313–20.
44 Obwegeser HL. Hemimandibular hyperplasia. In: Obwegeser HL. Mandibular growth anomalies. Berlin: Springer-Verlag, 2001;145–98.
45 Obwegeser HL, Makek MS. Hemimandibular hyperplasia–hemimandibular elongation. J Maxillofac Surg. 1986;14:183–208.
46 Proffit WR, Vig KW, Turvey TA. Early fracture of the mandibular condyles: frequently an unsuspected cause of growth disturbances. Am J Orthodont. 1980;78:1–24.
47 Hovinga J, Oering B, Stegenga B. Long-term results of non-surgical management of condylar fractures in children. Int J Oral Maxillofac Surg. 1999;28:429–40.
48 Pensler JM, Murphy GF, Mulliken JB. Clinical and ultrastructural studies of Romberg's hemifacial atrophy. Plast Reconstr Surg. 1990;85:669–74.
49 Chen Y-R, Noordhoff MS. Treatment of craniomaxillofacial fibrous dysplasia: how early and how extensive. Plast Reconstruct Surg. 1990;86:835–42.
50 Gabbay JS, Yuan JT, Andrews BT, Kawamoto HK, Bradley JP. Fibrous dysplasia of the zygomaticomaxillary region: outcomes of surgical intervention. Plast Reconstruct Surg. 2013;131:1329–38.
51 Reyneke JP, Tsakiris P, Kienle F. A simple classification for surgical planning of maxillomandibular asymmetry. Br J Oral Maxillofac Surg. 1997;35:349–51.
52 Fattahi TT. An overview of facial aesthetic units. J Oral Maxillofac Surg. 2003;61:1207–11.
53 Menick FJ. Defects of the nose, lip, and cheek: rebuilding the composite defect. Plast Reconstruct Surg. 2007;120: 887–98.
54 Quevedo L, Ruiz JV, Quevedo C. Using a clinical protocol for orthognathic surgery and assessing a 3-dimensional virtual approach: current therapy. J Oral Maxillofac Surg. 2011;69:623–37.
55 Xia JJ, Gateno J, Teichgraeber JF. New clinical protocol to evaluate craniomaxillofacial deformity and plan surgical correction. J Oral Maxillofac Surg. 2009;67:2093–106.
56 Barbenel JC, Paul, PE, Khambay BS, et al. Errors in orthognathic surgery planning: the effect of inaccurate study model orientation. Internat J Oral Maxillofac Surg. 2010;39:1103–08.
57 Zhao L, Patel PK, Cohen M. Application of virtual surgical planning with computer assisted design and manufacturing technology to cranio-maxillo-facial surgery. Arch Plastic Surg. 2012;39:309–16.
58 Wolfe SA, Berkowitz S. Plastic Surgery of the Facial Skeleton. Boston, Little. Brown and Company, 1989.
59 McCarthy JG, Schreiber JS, Karp NS, et al. Lengthening of the human mandible by gradual distraction. Plastic Reconstr Surg. 1992;89:1.
60 Molina F, Ortiz-Monasterio F. Mandibular elongation and remodeling by dis- traction: a farewell to major osteotomies. Plast Reconstr Surg. 1995;96:825.
61 Guo L, Ferraro NF, Padwa BL, et al. Vascularized fibular graft for pediatric mandibular reconstruction. Plast Reconstr Surg. 2008;121:2095–105.
62 Longaker MT, Siebert JW. Microvascular free flap correction of hemifacial atrophy. Plast Reconstr Surg. 1995;96:800.
63 Coleman SR. Facial recontouring with lipostructure. Clin Plast Surg. 1997;24:347.
64 Moscona R, Ullman Y, Har-Shai Y, et al. Free-fat injection for the correction of hemifacial atrophy. Plast Reconstr Surg. 1989;84:501–7.
65 Grimaldi M, Gentile P, Labardi L, et al. Lipostructure technique in Romberg syndrome. J Craniofac Surg. 2008;19:1089–91.
66 Mulliken JB, Kaban LB. Analysis and treatment of hemifacial microsomia in childhood. Clin Plast Surg. 1987;14:91.
67 Obwegeser HL. Correction of the skeletal anomalies of otomandibular dysostosis. J Maxillofac Surg. 1974;2:73.
68 Kim S, Seo Y-J, Choi TH, Baek S-H. New approach for the surgico-orthodontic treatment of hemifacial microsomia. J Craniofac Surg. 2012;23:957–63.
69 Kaban LB. Mandibular asymmetry and the fourth dimension. J Craniofac Surg. 2009;20(suppl 1):622–31.
70 Shetye PR, Grayson BH, Mackool RJ, McCarthy JG. Long-term stability and growth following unilateral mandibular distraction in growing children with craniofacial microsomia. Plast Reconstr Surg. 2006;118:985–95.
71 Sidiropoulou S, Antoniades K, Kolokithas G. Orthopedically induced condylar growth in a patient with hemifacial microsomia. Cleft Palate Craniofac J. 2003;40: 645–50.
72 Leonardi R, Barbato E. Technical strategy mandibular asymmetry treated with a modified activator appliance. J Craniofac Surg. 2007;18:939–43.
73 Kahl-Nieke B, Fischbach R. Effect of early orthopedic intervention on hemifacial microsomia patients: an approach to a cooperative evaluation of treatment results. Am J Orthodont Dentofac Orthoped. 1998;114:538–50.
74 Meazzini MC, Mazzoleni F, Bozzetti A, Brusati R. Does functional appliance treatment truly improve stability of mandibular vertical distraction osteogenesis in hemifacial microsomia? J Cranio-Maxillofac Surg. 2008;36:384–89.
75 Işeri H, Kişnişci R, Altuğ-Atac AT. Ten-year follow-up of a patient with hemifacial microsomia treated with distraction osteogenesis and orthodontics: an implant analysis. Am J Orthodont Dentofac Orthoped. 2008;134:296–304.

Chapter 58

High Level Maxillofacial Osteotomies

Stephen Dover

Introduction

The historical development of maxillary and higher level facial osteotomies has been described in Chapter 2. The first maxillary osteotomy has been attributed to the American surgeon, David W Cheever. He is reported to have undertaken a Le Fort I downfracture as an access procedure to allow removal of a naso-pharyngeal tumour.[1] Surgery to change the position of the upper jaw was developed in Germany from 1920 onwards with Cohn-Stock, Wassmund and Wunderer, who all contributed techniques directed towards moving the pre-maxilla. Wassmund developed the Le Fort I procedure in 1927, with Axhausen using the approach to advance the maxilla with elastics in 1934. Schuchardt achieved better and more predictable advancement with pterygoid disjunction and external traction in 1942.

In that same year, the first upper midface osteotomy was performed, at the Le Fort III level, by Sir Harold Gillies (1882–1960). He was operating on a patient with Crouzon syndrome. Bone grafts were not used and relapse occurred. The procedure had to be repeated in 1949, following which, Gillies has been reported as saying this operation should 'never be done again'.[2]

It took the pioneering work of Paul Tessier (1917–2008) to develop the Le Fort III osteotomy into a reliable procedure to advance the whole of the midface at a subcranial level. It has proved to be particularly useful in the management of patients with syndromic craniosynostosis in whom prominence of the eyes (proptosis) due to under development of the orbits, and Class III skeletal jaw relationships are secondary to significant midface hypoplasia.[3] Further refinements of the Le Fort III procedure, including a trans-cranial approach, facial bi-partition to allow rotation and medialization of the orbits and facial advancement in combination with the forehead – the so called monobloc or fronto-facial procedure – followed. Fernando Ortiz-Monasterio (1923–2012) and Jacques van der Meulen (b. 1929) all contributed to this work as well as Tessier himself.

Between the Le Fort I level and Le Fort III level osteotomies, there exist a variety procedures to address various aspects of midface deformity.

The Kufner procedure describes the advancement of the maxilla together with the zygomas.[4] The nasal skeleton and soft tissues of the midface are not moved.

A variant of this is the so called 'high Le Fort I', in which the horizontal maxillary cut is made just below the infraorbital foramen rather than just above the maxillary teeth apices. In advancing the maxilla, greater support is given to the soft tissues of the cheeks, without the complexity of an osteotomy inside the orbital rim.

The Le Fort II osteotomy, analogous to the Le Fort II fracture pattern, allows for repositioning of the maxilla and the nose, leaving the zygomas in their original position. It was described by Henderson and Jackson in 1973.[5]

It is possible to combine these various approaches. For example, the Le Fort II or Le Fort III osteotomies

Orthognathic Surgery: Principles, Planning and Practice. Edited by Farhad B. Naini and Daljit S. Gill.

can be used with a Le Fort I to move the nasal skeleton or face and the maxilla differentially.

Indications for midfacial osteotomies

Osteotomies at the Le Fort I level are usually undertaken for the correction of dentofacial disproportion. This can occur without or without an obvious underlying cause. Conditions that can contribute to the need for low level procedures include cleft palate, where patients often suffer from some degree of maxillary retrusion and those with hemifacial microsomia, who can present with facial asymmetry and an occlusal cant. In contrast, most patients requiring high level mid-facial osteotomies have a recognized underlying condition, usually a craniofacial syndrome, the features of which dictate the deformity and the subsequent management.

Of the many craniofacial syndromes, the autosomal dominant and eponymous Crouzon, Pfeiffer and Apert syndromes are the most well-known. These syndromes are caused by genetic mutations in the fibroblast growth factor receptors, particularly FGFR2, which are found on chromosome 10.[6] They are characterized by premature fusion of the skull sutures, resulting in reduced calvarial volume. The brain continues to grow within a small, fused skull resulting in raised intracranial pressure in a significant number of affected children.

Apert syndrome affected patients are characterized by complex syndactyly of the hands and feet. Two genotypes are recognized, Ser252Trp and Pro253Arg, with the former having a higher incidence of cleft palate and the latter being associated with a more severe form of syndactyly.[7]

Pfeiffer syndrome affected patients often have very severe cranial fusion with a clover leaf deformity (kleeblattschadel), variable intelligence, a high arched palate and broad thumbs and first toes with a varus deformity.[8] They can be the most challenging group of patients to treat as they have multiple issues, with a predisposition to early skull fusion even after aggressive attempts at calvarial remodelling.

Fusion of the skull base sutures, particularly in the region of the pterygoid plates, (which are a part of the sphenoid bone), prevents the normal downward and forward growth of the midface. This results in the characteristic midfacial retrusion that is apparent to a varying degree in childhood. However, in this group of affected individuals it becomes more obvious towards the end of the pubertal growth spurt when mandibular growth far exceeds that of the maxilla. The maxilla effectively becomes a single structure, fused to the skull base, which has implications for surgery.

Many patients with syndromic craniosynostoses have characteristic features, midface hypoplasia being one of the most recognizable of them. The phenotype, that is, the degree of expression of the genetic condition, is very variable. It can be seen in the different degree of midface retrusion and proptosis (prominence of the eyes) present between an affected parent and their child.

The small skull and retro-positioned maxilla result in prominence of the eyes as the supra-orbital rim of the forehead and the infra-orbital rim of the midface fail to develop. The globe, which is of normal size appears to protrude from the face. Growth of the globe is largely complete by the age of 6 or 7, so affected individuals often present with proptosis early in life due to under-development of the bones that make up the orbit.[9,10]

The other significant feature is a Class III skeletal and dental relationship. This becomes more apparent during the teenage years. Normal facial growth during the pubertal growth spurt is only really apparent in the mandible as maxillary growth is retarded due to the fusion with the skull base. This discrepancy between maxillary and mandibular development results in the Class III deformity that is so typical of these conditions.

Intra-nasal anatomy is often abnormal, with narrowed airways, or obstruction by bony spurs. This can sometimes extend to choanal atresia, where the posterior aspects of one or both of the nasal passages are blocked.

Retrusion of the maxilla results in the retro-positioning of the soft palate. This can interfere with the patency of the Eustachian tube, and middle ear dysfunction is not uncommon. In Apert syndrome particularly, the hard palate is high and a cleft of the soft palate is present in about 30%.[11]

The retro-positioned maxilla can result in the soft palate being pushed against the posterior pharyngeal wall where it comes to lie vertically rather than horizontally. In occupying the space between the tongue base and the posterior pharyngeal wall, the soft palate obstructs the airway to an extent that some patients require a tracheostomy in early life. Other major reasons for a tracheostomy in this group of patients are abnormalities of the larynx, including laryngomalacia. This is a feature of some craniosynostosis syndromes where these is an abnormality of the laryngeal cartilages such that they collapse on inspiration, due to the decreased intra-tracheal pressure. This results in an obstruction of the lower airway. It is important to differentiate between upper and lower airway obstruction in these patients. Surgery that improves the upper airway, such as midface advancement, will do nothing to address obstruction at or below the level of the tongue base. These features are important when considering the anaesthetic needs of these patients.[12]

Many of the previously mentioned problems can be addressed with surgical re-positioning of the maxilla. This is usually in a forward direction in childhood and a forward and downward direction later in life, often as a differential movement of the midface, undertaken at different levels.

Bringing the orbital rims forward effectively increases orbital volume. The proptosis is addressed as the eyes appear to 'sink' into newly constructed socket. The soft palate is pulled forward with the advanced maxilla and the posterior nasal airway is improved. Splitting the maxilla in the mid-sagittal plane, as in a facial bi-partition, widens the nasal airway and can improve air entry. Intra-nasal obstruction such as from bony spurs or atresia also needs to be addressed.[13]

Advancement should bring the midface into a Class I, or even Class II skeletal and dental relationship resulting in a significant improvement in facial appearance and oral function.

In children, the emphasis is on addressing the proptosis. Consequently, the midface is advanced along the Frankfort plane – the line joining the upper border of the external auditory meatus with the inferior border of the orbital rim. This optimizes orbital volume. Where inferior movement is combined with advancement in children, enophthalmos can result.

It is the norm to over advance the maxilla in children, producing a Class II skeletal relationship with the lower jaw. In time, mandibular growth will minimize the discrepancy, even to an extent where further maxillary advancement is required. This is often undertaken at a Le Fort I level, to correct the secondary Class III dentofacial relationship that results from the inherent restriction of midfacial growth during puberty. One of the primary aims of midfacial advancement is that the tracheostomy can be removed.

Cranio-fronto-nasal dysplasia was described by Cohen in 1979.[14] It results from a mutation in the EFNB-1 gene, is X-linked and more common in females who are more significantly affected. The incidence is >1:100,000. The phenotype is variable and the presentation dictates the surgical plan. The craniofacial features include fusion of the coronal sutures, orbital hypertelorism (increased inter-ocular distance), bifid nasal tip, and dry frizzy curled hair. Treatment involves the medialization of the orbits and the widening of the narrow maxilla. This is often best approached by a facial bi-partition procedure. This is in essence a Le Fort III level osteotomy, divided in the mid-sagittal plane and with a midline wedge removed from the nasal bridge area. The two orbits can be rotated together and the palate widened.[15]

This technique also has value in the treatment of the Apert patient in whom medial rotation of the orbits corrects the downward and outward axis of rotation and lowers and widens the high arched palate.

Binder's syndrome was first described in 1939 by Noyes, but not recognized as a distinct entity until von Binder described naso-maxillary hypoplasia in 1962.[16,17] The condition is characterized by a number of features including an arhinoid face with abnormal position of the nasal bones, maxillary hypoplasia with a Class III dental and skeletal malocclusion and reduced or absent anterior nasal spine.

The management of the condition requires a re-positioning of the retruded midface and enlargement of the nose. A variety of surgical procedures have been described to address the characteristic facial features including Le Fort II advancement, Le Fort II with Le Fort I re-positioning to individualize the movements required of the nasal and maxillary components of the condition and Le Fort I alone with nasal reconstruction using cartilage and/or bone grafts.[18]

Preoperative assessment

Planning for surgery in this group of patients should be done within a specialist multidisciplinary team, including (but not restricted to), craniofacial surgeons, neurosurgeons, specialist anaesthetists, ENT and ophthalmic surgeons, geneticists, paediatric dentists, orthodontists, colleagues from speech and language, psychology, clinical nurse specialists and dedicated ward and theatre staff who understand the complexities of managing patients with these problems.

Abnormalities of the craniofacial region can have a profound impact on all of the senses. Irrespective of the age of the patient, a full assessment is essential. This should include a thorough clinical examination of the head and face, supplemented by CT and MRI scanning of the brain, face and cervical spine.

It is important to understand the anatomy of the airway, particularly in the newborn who are obligate nasal breathers.

Premature fusion of the skull sutures can result in raised intra-cranial pressure, which can be hinted at on the scans (scalloping or perforation of the calvarium, small ventricles, Chiari malformation – a hind brain hernia), and demonstrated through visual electrophysiology (visual evoked potentials), papilloedema evident on retinal examination and intra-cranial pressure monitoring.

Ophthalmic examination should also assess corneal exposure in those with prominence of the globes. The eyelids may be incompetent and in failing to close over the cornea they cannot protect or lubricate the eye.

The dentition, hearing, speech and language and general development must be assessed as well as the abilities of the parents to look after these children or affected adults to look after themselves.

In conventional orthognathic surgery, considerable weight is given to the role of cephalometric assessment in planning surgery. Whilst this does have a place in older syndromic patients, the emphasis has to be on managing the functional issues. With function comes form, and facial balance can usually be achieved once the cranial volume, airway, soft palate position and maxillary and mandibular relationship are optimized. A class I dental relationship is less important than a maxilla advanced to the point where the eyes and airway are protected and safe.

Current software planning programmes do not offer the same degree or accuracy of prediction planning for this group of patients as their anatomical landmarks are so far outside the normal reference ranges. Indeed, some of the traditional bony landmarks may not even exist on these patients. In addition, previous skull base surgery and the underlying condition itself may distort the anterior skull base to such an extent that the SN line (running for the midpoint of the sella turcica to nasion at the fronto-nasal junction), may be so abnormal as to make any assessment using SNA (where A relates to the anterior maxilla) and SNB (where B relates to the anterior mandible) meaningless.

It is important to have a photographic record of these patients as treatment may extend beyond the working life of most surgeons and it is only with time and skeletal maturity that the effect of early surgery can be assessed and critically appraised.

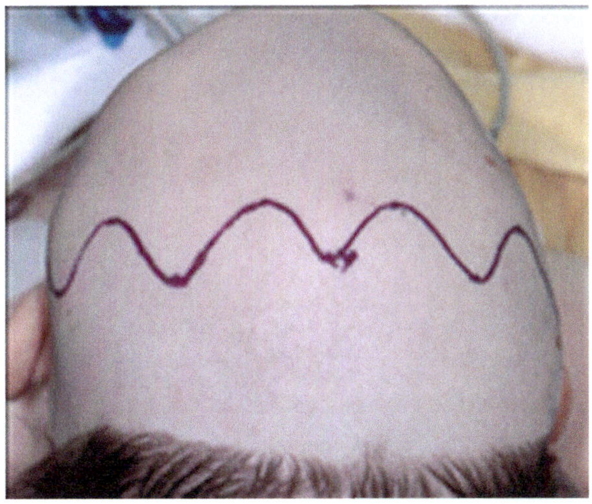

Fig. 58-1 Curved stealth incision line (in this case with a head shave).

Surgical procedures

The traditional approach to high level midface osteotomies has been to advance the midface into the correct position and stabilize it using a combination of internal fixation with plates and screws, bone grafts and intermaxillary fixation between the jaws.[19] Inevitably, the bigger the advance required, the greater the risk of relapse. Recent attempts to overcome this have seen a return to the use of traction through external frames as advocated by the early pioneers; this technique is now known as distraction osteogenesis. Distraction has probably been the most significant surgical development in craniofacial surgery, introduced over the last 20 years.

The technique was originally developed by Gavril Ilizarov (1921–1992), an orthopaedic surgeon working in isolation in Kurgan Oblast, Siberia.[20] He established the principles for successful elongation of bone and transport of segments of bone by a gradual application of traction, via an external frame, on to a surgically created fracture site in the lower limb. The technique has found application in all areas where bone 'growth' is required not least in the craniofacial region. Movements in excess of 30 mm can be achieved using either external frames, intra-oral devices or a combination of both. However, irrespective of the technique used in advancing the midface, the overall principles of the osteotomies remain essentially the same.

Most high level osteotomies are undertaken through a coronal flap combined with an intra-oral 'horseshoe' upper buccal sulcus incision. With careful dissection, the whole of the upper and midface can be safely exposed without the need for incisions through the skin of the face. On the rare occasions when a more direct approach is required to the orbital floor, the trans-conjunctival approach popularized by Tessier is recommended.

It is preferable to raise the coronal flap through a curved, wavy zigzag 'stealth' incision which heals well. In children we shave the head, in adults we shave just along the line of the proposed or previous incision (Figure 58-1).

This incision leaves a less visible scar within the hair line and is much less obvious particularly when the hair is wet. The flap is raised in the sub-galeal plane with due care being taken to safeguard the upper branches of the facial nerve where they traverse the zygomatic arch. If only the anterior skull is being accessed then the biplanar approach retains the anatomical relationship between the temporalis muscle and the overlying layers of the scalp.[21]

The coronal flap can be reflected down to expose the glabella and nasal bones in the midline and the orbital rims laterally. The supra-orbital nerves often sit within a notch in the rim. Where they traverse a canal, they can be released with an osteotome. The temporalis muscle is reflected postero-laterally if access is required to the zygoma and lateral orbital wall. Dissection over the nasion will allow the surgeon to gain access to the medial orbital walls, medial canthus, lacrimal groove and upper aspects of the anterior maxilla if the medial canthal tendon is released or if it has been avulsed as is occasionally seen in the trauma patient. Wherever possible, the medial canthal apparatus should retain its attachment to the lacrimal ridge. If it becomes detached during surgery, it is essential that the attachment is reconstructed once the osteotomies are complete and the midface advanced.

Dissection downwards and forwards over the zygoma with careful retraction of the globe allows the lateral aspects of the midface and infra-orbital rim to be exposed. A pre-auricular extension to the coronal flap (Figure 58-2) or an aesthetically more acceptable post-auricular extension allows the whole of the arch to be visualized and the upper branches of the facial nerve to be protected.

The lower aspects of the midface can be accessed through the mouth, using the standard, upper buccal sulcus approach. The incision is placed in the mobile tissue, 3 mm above the keratinized, attached mucosa allowing for easy closure of the wound at the end of the operation. Careful dissection exposes the pyriform aperture and infra-orbital rim from below, and allows the identification of the infra-orbital nerve. Lateral

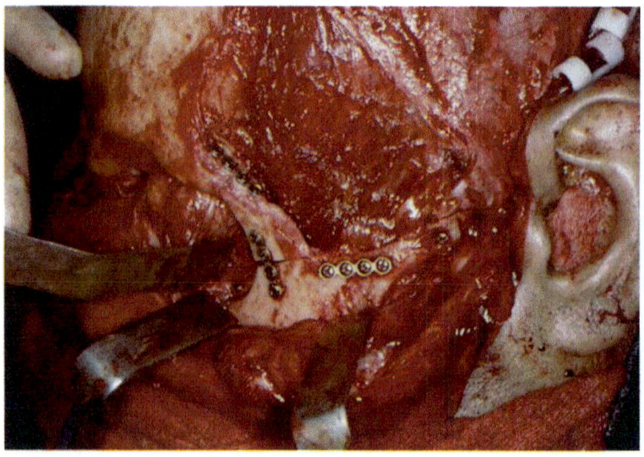

Fig. 58-2 A coronal flap, demonstrating the extensive de-gloving and exposure of the left orbit and zygoma that can be achieved through this approach.

dissection and release of the masseteric tendon using diathermy allows exposure of the inferior aspects of the zygomatic arch. It is important to stay in the subperiosteal plane so that the buccal fat pad does not prolapse into the wound and obscure vision in this area.

Posterior dissection behind the zygomatic buttress allows the surgeon to gain access to the pterygomaxillary junction. This can be fused in syndromic patients and the pterygomaxillary fissure is absent and filled with bone.

Where more exposure to the midline and nasal structures is required then a facial de-gloving procedure is recommended. The intra-oral exposure can be combined with endonasal, intercartilaginous, septal transfixation and pyriform floor incisions. The soft tissues of the nose can be dissected off the nasal cartilages and bones allowing for exposure up to the ethmoid region. In practice, this approach is usually reserved for the wide access required in ablative oncology surgery rather than in those patients requiring midfacial osteotomies.

The Le Fort III osteotomy is the most commonly undertaken procedure in patients requiring advancement of the total midface. It has evolved so that the osteotomy cuts ensure that the facial bones can be safely disengaged from the cranial base. Ideally, the midface should be separated as a single unit; this demands careful attention to the detail of the osteotomies.

Starting superiorly, the lateral orbital rim is divided using a saw at or near the zygomatico-frontal suture. The supraorbital rim also needs to be advanced, then this can be included in the osteotomy. The bony cuts are extended along the orbital floor towards the lacrimal groove using a chisel or saw. This area is often best approached via the lateral orbit wall osteotomy. The zygomatic arch is divided in an oblique sagittal plane to maximize bone overlap with facial advancement.

A transverse bone cut at the nasal bridge divides the root of the nose from the frontal bone. Care is required to avoid too deep an osteotomy so as to avoid inadvertently entering the anterior cranial fossa. This is particularly important in those syndromic patients with a foreshortened anterior skull base, in whom the floor may lie below the nasion.

Either side of the nasal bridge, the horizontal cut joins a vertical, medial orbital wall osteotomy, that is placed just anterior to the posterior lacrimal ridge. Wherever possible, it is important that the medial canthal attachment is retained and not detached from its complex insertion in the region of the anterior lacrimal crest.[22] This medial orbital wall cut joins with the orbital floor osteotomy. The above procedure is repeated on the contralateral side to achieve a symmetrical osteotomy.

In syndromic patients, the posterior maxilla is fused to the pterygoid plates of the sphenoid bone, which is a skull base structure. As such, there needs to be a formal pterygomaxillary dysjunction if the midface is to be advanced. The pterygomaxillary area can either be approached from above via the coronal flap and behind the body of the zygoma, or intra-orally. The author prefers the latter approach as it allows for separation of the maxillary tuberosity from the sphenoid bone in a more controlled manner with careful use of the osteotome medially and superiorly towards the orbital floor as required.

Once the orbital and posterior bone cuts have been completed, the nasal septum and lateral nasal walls are divided. The short maxilla means that great care is required to direct the osteotome correctly (red line) and avoid angling the midline osteotome too vertically, thereby prejudicing the base of skull and cervical spine (black line) (Figure 58-3).

The maxilla is grasped with Rowe's disimpaction forceps and the midface gently and gradually

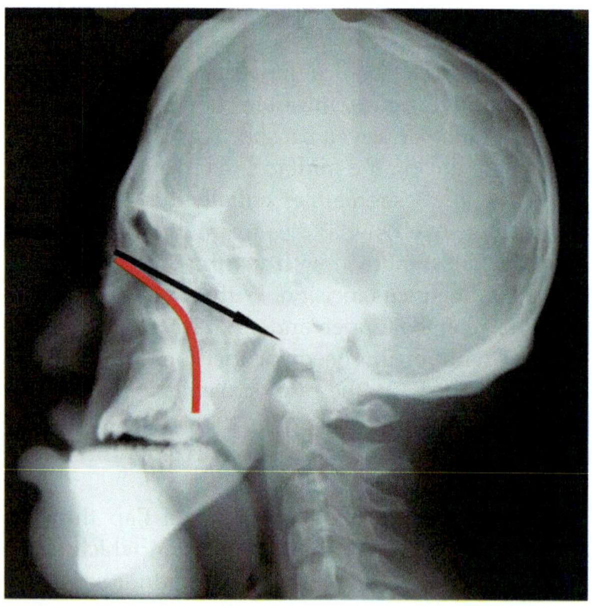

Fig. 58-3 Lateral cephalometric radiograph of a Crouzon syndrome patient demonstrating the short maxilla and the correct nasal septum division (red line) and the incorrect (black line).

downfractured off the skull base. Should facial mobilization prove difficult then the completeness of each osteotomy should be confirmed particularly in the posterior aspects of the maxilla. It is often at this anatomical site that the full midfacial downfracture fails. The temptation is to then apply lateral force to the zygoma in the hope of pushing the maxilla forwards. The zygoma then becomes detached from the central part of the midface and will need to be re-attached with plates if a successful advance is to be achieved.

It is not unusual for there to be significant bleeding from the posterior maxilla at this stage of the operation. This can be minimized with judicious use of hypotensive anaesthesia and gradual mobilization of the midface rather than an aggressive downfracture.

If a conventional procedure is undertaken then the face is held forward with plates at the zygomatic arch, zygomatico-frontal suture and nasal bridge, in combination with intermaxillary fixation if appropriate. Bone grafting is required to contribute to stability of the advancement and minimize relapse.[23] Self-stabilizing osteotomies at the orbital rim and bone grafts in the orbital walls and zygomatic arch regions contribute to early healing. As these patients have a predisposition to form bone particularly in the skull base, grafting in the posterior maxilla is not usually required.

Where advancement is to be achieved gradually by distraction, either an internal or external device can be used. The author favours the flexibility of the external halo device and the greater advancement that can be achieved with it. The internal devices have their proponents. However, if not carefully placed, they can lead to bowing of the lateral face around the midline resulting in an unfavourable advance and failure to achieve the dentofacial and soft palate changes that are often essential in this type of surgery (Figure 58-4).[24]

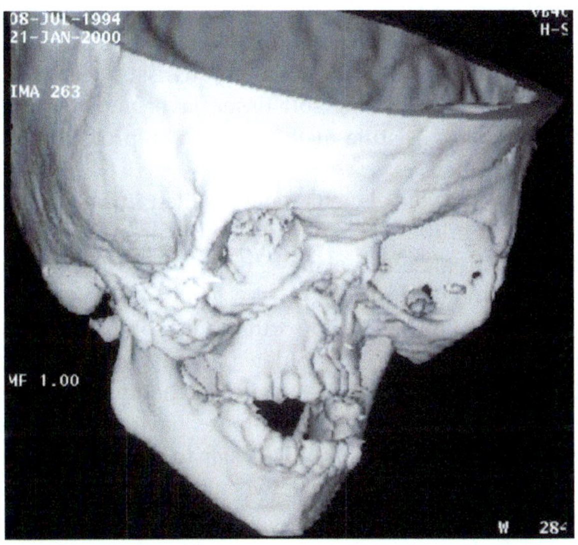

Fig. 58-4 CT scan demonstrating the bowing of the lateral face at the expense of midface advancement in an Apert syndrome patient who was treated with internal distraction rather than an external frame.

The external devices are developments of the halo frames originally used as external fixators in the treatment of midfacial fractures. The newer devices use 4–8 screws on each side, which pass through the soft tissues of the scalp and engage with the calvarium. The frame is then attached to the midface either directly using underlying plates and screws with transfacial wires, or with a per-oral bar fixed to a dental splint or with transcutaneous screws attached to customized plates. Whichever means of attachment is used, it is essential that this is robust enough to bring the midface forwards without detaching the dental or skeletal fixation from the facial skeleton.

The face is advanced at approximately 1 mm per day, starting a day or so after surgery in the very young (who heal quickly) and after 5 days in adults, once the callus has begun to form.

Once the correct advancement has been achieved, the distractors are left on for a consolidation period to allow the callus to mature. In practice, this is up to 3 months. The significant volume of bone that can be generated in these patients can be seen in Figure 58-5. The quality and quantity of this bone in the pterygomaxillary region goes some way to minimizing relapse. This is despite degrees of maxillary advancement that would be very difficult to achieve by conventional surgery.

In patients with a cleft palate who are at risk of developing velopharyngeal incompetence (VPI) due to too great a midfacial advancement, distraction allows for gradual advancement to a point where VPI is just occurring. The patient can then have a second surgical procedure where the midface is plated in the advanced position, the distractor removed and the mandible set-back to achieve a Class I occlusion and the best possible functional outcome.

In syndromic patients with a combination of small skull and small midface, the anterior skull expansion can be undertaken with midface advancement at the Le Fort III level simultaneously. This fronto-facial

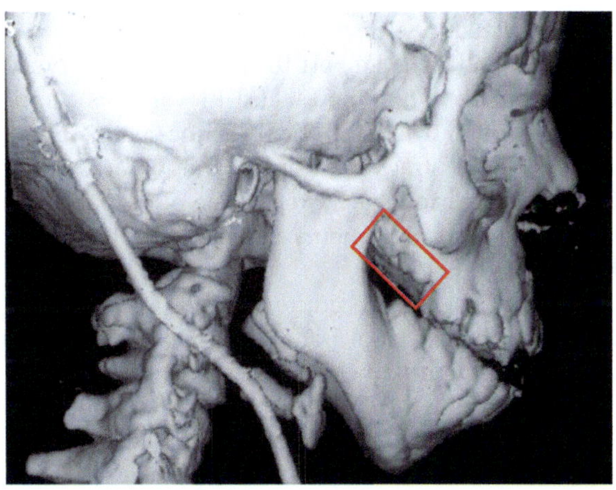

Fig. 58-5 CT scan demonstrating the volume of bone that can be created during distraction in the pterygomaxillary region.

advancement simultaneously achieves cranial vault expansion and midfacial advancement.

The procedure is usually reserved for young children with a severe phenotype of their underlying syndrome.

Occasionally, the monobloc procedure is undertaken in adults who have not had previous surgery or in whom previous surgery was unsuccessful.

The procedure of simultaneous advancement of the forehead, orbits and face was first described by Ortiz-Monasterio.[25] The major disadvantage is that the anterior skull base is divided through the cribriform plate leaving the patients at risk of meningitis via a cranio-nasal fistula. Anderl modified the technique so that the supraorbital bar and forehead were removed as one piece and the Le Fort III segment as a separate second bone fragment.[26] The cribriform plate therefore retains its integrity. With the advent of distraction, the anterior skull base may require support from a pericranial flap, but in practice, it remains intact and the leaks associated with a single surgical advancement are not the problem they once were.

A transcranial approach allows the orbital roof on each side to be exposed. In the traditional approach, the forehead remains attached to the Le Fort III midfacial segment, and both forehead and maxilla can be advanced simultaneously. Direct skeletal fixation of an external frame to the underlying bone is achieved with percutaneous wires passed through the pyriform rims and eyebrows to underlying plates, secured to the facial bones with screws. At the end of the consolidation period, the wires are withdrawn through the skin, the frame removed and the plates and screws left in situ.

Frontofacial advancement allows the face to be brought forward as a single unit. This presupposes that this will achieve the desired facial balance. In practice, differential movements are often required between the upper midface, where maximum orbital volume is normally achieved by the age of 8, and the lower tooth bearing portion of the midface where skeletal maturity and dentofacial relationship is not achieved until the late teenage years.

To overcome this discrepancy, the midface can be segmentalized in terms of simultaneous surgery with advancement at the Le Fort III level, being combined with advancement at the Le Fort I level. This can be achieved either by conventional advancement surgery alone, or by distraction. Using this approach, better facial balance can be achieved in the older patient in whom different movements are required at different levels.

Le Fort II level procedure involves a pyramidal osteotomy of the nasal bones and maxilla, with the orbital cuts running behind the medial canthal tendon and through the medial aspects of the orbital rim. The cuts then run backwards towards the pterygomaxillary fissure where dysjunction is performed. Division of the nasal septum and the lateral nasal walls allows downfracture of the nasomaxillary complex and advancement, conventionally supported by bone grafts or by distraction.

A modification of the Le Fort III procedure is the facial bipartition. It involves mobilizing the midface as for the standard procedure and then dividing it vertically in the mid-sagittal plane. This allows the two halves of the midface to be moved independent of each other. One option is to 'bookend' the midface so that the lateral part of the osteotomized section is rotated posteriorly and the central portion moves forward. This technique applies a more normal contour to individuals with flat faces such as those with Apert syndrome. Once the facial contour has been corrected, the midface can be advanced either conventionally or by distraction. The advantage of the latter approach is that by placing the distraction forces towards the centre of the unit, the advancement of the face in the new form is exaggerated. This is useful as there is a tendency for the face to relapse back to the norm and over correction is appropriate.

In those patients with cranio-fronto-nasal dysplasia, or midline facial clefts through developmental anomaly or the presence of an anterior meningocoele, there is an option with this technique of resecting the excess tissue in the midline, repairing any dural defect if a meningocoele has been resected and rotating the two halves of the midface together. In this situation it is not always necessary to advance the midface.

The procedure also has the benefit of lowering a high arched palate and levelling the occlusal plane across the Curve of Monson. Care is needed when dividing the anterior maxilla at the level of the teeth, as rotation of the dentoalveolar segment laterally creates a midline diastema. This can result in loss of periodontal support to the central incisors. The author minimizes this risk by raising a buccal muco-periosteal flap from one upper canine tooth to the other and then redraping this flap over the widened midline. In this approach it is also useful to carefully elevate the nasal mucosa from the nasal floor. The midline split should lie between the two nasal flaps either side of the septum so that any palatal soft tissue tear is at least protected by one soft tissue layer and the risk of an oronasal fistula at the end of the procedure is minimized.

Where rare facial clefts have resulted in significant facial and orbital asymmetry, then the procedures can be individualized to achieve the best possible facial balance and contour.

Whilst some degree of orthodontic preparation is ideal in many of the older patients, in practice, there is significant post-surgical orthodontic movement required as the skeletal bases have changed so much with surgery that it is easier to move the teeth once better co-ordination between the arches has been achieved.

The Kufner procedure is reserved for those patients in whom there is adequate nasal projection, but an under developed upper jaw and cheekbones.[4] Correction of this deformity can also be undertaken using a Le Fort I level maxillary advancement with alloplast malar implant onlays. This technique is simple, but there is a risk of infection where the implants are placed at the same time as the Le Fort I. This can therefore commit the patient to two operations.

The Kufner procedure advances the maxilla and the zygomas as one unit. Some surgeons prefer to limit the zygomatic component to the anterior wall of the maxilla, in effect undertaking a 'high' Le Fort I. This does not address the infra-orbital margin deficiency and may not extend laterally enough to involve the body of the zygoma where most of the deficient exists. The classical approach involves the zygomatic body with the upper limit of the osteotomy being behind the orbital rim within the orbital floor. The maxilla can be difficult to plate in place if the traditional medial cut is brought across the orbital rim into the nasal cavity. The author prefers to bring the medial cut parallel to the lateral nasal wall and across the pyriform buttress where plating the re-positioned maxilla is much simpler. The procedure can be combined with a mandibular set-back.

The midface is blessed with an excellent blood supply. A variety of osteotomies can be undertaken with little consideration for the viability of the bony segments unless a cleft is present. As such, and given the range of procedures available, treatment plans can be tailored to the individual needs of the patients. The normal values against which most orthognathic patients are planned do not easily apply to the more complex upper midface deformities described. Computer software is under development which allows complex three dimensional movements to be plotted in this group of patients whose deformities lie outside the range normally seen. Virtual planning and splint construction from scanning of the dental arches rather than impressions is already a reality. How far this will progress in the assessment and management of these patients and how they can be converted into operative procedures remains to be seen, but there will always be the need for a clinical assessment and an 'eye for the aesthetic' if these patients are to be managed in an effective way.

References

1 Cheever DW. Displacement of the upper jaw. Med Surg Rep Boston City Hosp. 1870;1:156.

2 Gillies HD, Millard DR Jr. The Principles and Art of Plastic Surgery. Boston, Little, Brown, 1955.

3 Tessier P. The definitive plastic surgical treatment of the severe facial deformities of craniofacial dysostoses. Crouzon's and Apert's diseases. Plast Reconstr Surg. 1971;48:419–42.

4 Kufner J. Four-year experience with major maxillary osteotomy for retrusion. J Oral Surg. (American Dental Association: 1965) 09/1971; 29:549–53.

5 Henderson D, Jackson IT. Nasomaxillary hypoplasia – the Le Fort II osteotomy. Br J Oral Surg. 1973;11:77–93.

6 Wilkie AOM, Slaney SF, Oldridge M, Poole MD, et al. Apert syndrome results from localized mutations of *FGFR2* and is allelic with Crouzon syndrome. Nat Genet. 1995;9: 165–72.

7 Slaney SF, Oldridge M, Hurst JA. Differential effects of FGFR2 mutations on syndactyly and cleft palate in Apert's patients. Am J Hum Genet. 1996;58:923–32.

8 Muenke M, Schell U. Fibroblast growth factor receptor mutations in human skeletal disorders. Trends Genet. 1995;11:308–13.

9 Bentley RP, Sgouros S, Natarajan K, Dover MS, Hockley AD. Normal changes in orbital volume during childhood. J Neurosurg. 2002;96:742–6.

10 Bentley RP, Sgouros S, Natarajan K, Dover MS, Hockley AD. Changes in orbital volume during childhood in cases of craniosynostosis. J Neurosurg. 2002;96:747–54.

11 Forrest CR. Hopper RA. Craniofacial syndromes and surgery. Plast Reconstr Surg. 2013;131:86e–109e.

12 Hughes C. Thomas K. Johnson D. Das S. Anaesthesia related to surgery for craniosynostosis. Paediatr Anaesthes. 2013;23:22–7.

13 Tamburrini G, Aldarelli M, Massimi L, et al. Complex craniosynostoses: a review of the prominent clinical features and the related management strategies. Childs Nerv Syst. 2012;28:1511–23.

14 Cohen MM, Jr. Craniofrontonasal dysplasia. Birth Defects Orig Art Ser. 1979;XV(5B):85–9.

15 Posnick JC. Monobloc and facial bipartition osteotomies: a step-by-step description of the surgical technique. J Craniofac Surg. 1996;7:229–50.

16 Noyes FB. Case Report. Angle Orthod. 1939;9:160–5.

17 Binder KH. Dysostosis maxillo-nasalis, ein archinencephaler Missbildungskomplex. Deutsche Zahnarztuche Zeitschift. 1962;17:438–44.

18 Posnick JC. Surgical management of Binder's syndrome: Lessons learned. Aesthetic Plast Surg. 2010;34:722–30.

19 Tiwana PS, Turvey TA. Subcranial procedures in craniofacial surgery: the Le Fort III osteotomy. Oral Maxillofac Clin North Am. 2004;16(4):493–501.

20 Ilizarov principles of deformity correction. Spiegelberg B, Parratt T, Dheerendra SK, Khan WS, Jennings R, Marsh DR. Ann Royal Coll Surg Engl. 2010;92:101–5.

21 Srinivasan D, White N, Rodrigues D, Solanki G, Dover MS, Nishikawa H. Dual plane approach for calvarial exposure. J Craniofac Surg. 2010;21:506-7.

22 Ayliffe P, Ward Booth P. Nasoethmoid fractures. In: Ward Booth P, Eppley BL, Schmelzeisen R (Eds). Maxillofacial trauma and esthetic facial reconstruction. Edinburgh: Churchill Livingstone, 2003;215–228.

23 Elsalanty ME, Genecov DG. Bone grafting in craniofacial surgery. Craniomaxillofac Trauma Reconstr. 2009;2: 125–34.

24 Chin M, Toth B. Le Fort III advancement with gradual distraction using internal devices Plast Reconstr Surg. 1997;100:819–30.

25 Ortiz-Monasterio F, del Campo AF, Carrillo A. Advancement of the orbits and the midface in one piece, combined with frontal repositioning, for the correction of Crouzon's deformities. Plast Reconstr Surg. 1978;61:507–16.

26 Anderl H, Mühlbauer W, Twerdy K, Marchac D. Frontofacial advancement with bony separation in craniofacial dysostosis. Plast Reconstr Surg. 1983;71:303–7.

27 Tessier P. Facial bipartition: A concept more than a procedure. In: Marchac D (Ed.): Craniofacial Surgery 1987; pp.217–45.

Chapter 59

Le Fort-based Maxillofacial Vascularized Transplantation

Chad R. Gordon, Harlyn K. Susarla, Edward Swanson, Seenu Susarla, Mehran Armand, Gerald Grant, Leonard B. Kaban and Michael J. Yaremchuk

Introduction

Over the past decade, the surgical community has seen the advent and advancement of maxillofacial vascularized composite allotransplantation (VCA). More than 20 maxillofacial allotransplantations have been performed, to date, with a high level of success, insofar as acceptance of tissue transfer and restoration of varying degrees of function.[1–11] The majority of transplants of the midfacial skeleton have utilized alloflap designs based on the classical patterns of skeletal disjunction described by Le Fort. The advantage of such designs, which are based on the skeletal disjunction at the Le Fort-II or Le Fort-III levels, are that the bulk of midfacial elements for orbital, nasal, zygomatic, and maxillary projection and contour are restored in the donor. The transplantation of the maxilla, along with the palate and dentition, also allows for some degree of restoration of a 'hybrid occlusion', masticatory function, and deglutition.

The purpose of this chapter is to review the historical evolution of Le Fort-based maxillofacial allotransplantation, beginning with human cadaveric studies, review some of the clinical transplants to date and ongoing translational animal investigation, and to provide the clinician with a primer on orthognathic planning for maxillofacial allotransplantation. While a surgical undertaking such as maxillofacial VCA is, by no means, an isolated endeavour, the clinician who participates as a team member would be well served to understand the basic surgical and planning principles behind maxillofacial VCA, many of which trace their origins to maxillary orthognathic surgery.

A brief review of the fracture patterns originally described by Le Fort in his seminal series demonstrates the utility of using natural fracture patterns as a basis for designing maxillofacial allotransplants.[12,13] Complex midfacial defects not amenable to standard autologous reconstruction often involve transition zones between several distinct anatomical skeletal subunits, e.g. the orbit and midface, with the corresponding soft tissue analogues (e.g. the lid–cheek junction). Reconstituting the missing structures within any given soft tissue or skeletal plane is challenging in its own right. However, recapitulating the contour and projection of several tissue layers across subunits with standard autologous technique becomes an insurmountable task, with unpredictable results.

Orthognathic Surgery: Principles, Planning and Practice. Edited by Farhad B. Naini and Daljit S. Gill.

Le Fort II-based allotransplantation

In this setting, the use of maxillofacial allotransplantation has been a major advance. Early studies utilizing Le Fort-based flaps for studying allotransplantation demonstrated the efficacy of using 'nature's foundation' for designing flaps. The Le Fort II fracture, originally described as a 'pyramidal fracture', involving fracture through the pterygoid plates, extending superiorly and obliquely along the anterior surface of the zygoma and maxilla, through the medial orbit, to the nasofrontal sutures, is an appropriate foundation to replace a central facial defect, including the nose and palate. Yazici et al. originally studied Le Fort II-based alloflaps.[14] Using magnetic resonance studies and angiography, these authors identified the critical vascular territories for a Le Fort II-based flap. They described the key vascular structures within the masticatory space and around the infratemporal fossa, consistent with the course of the internal maxillary artery.

Using this basis, several groups have demonstrated the clinical applicability of the Le Fort II-based allotransplant. Lantieri et al. utilized a Le Fort II-based flap to reconstruct a central midfacial defect (along with a chin defect) in a 27-year-old gunshot victim.[15] This was followed by a vascular Le Fort II-based maxillary transplant by Pomahac et al. in Boston, to reconstruct a central midfacial defect in a 59-year-old male who had suffered a devastating electrical injury.[16] This allotransplant included a dentate maxilla, hard palate, as well as the soft tissues of the nose and upper lip. Lantieri's group subsequently performed a second Le Fort II midfacial allotransplant this time with a concomitant mandibular transplant in a 33-year-old gunshot victim.[15] To date, all patients have achieved a functional restoration of the midfacial anatomy, with some restoration of mastication and occlusion.[6,15]

The advantages of a Le Fort II-based allotransplant, in this regard, are restoration of the anterior and central midfacial anatomy. This flap design has been successfully used in patients with high energy injuries (gunshot wounds) or injuries with significant loss of tissue and contracture of the overlying soft tissues (complex burns). A Le Fort II-based alloflap is ideally suited for central midfacial defects involving the maxillary occlusion, palate, nasal cavity and associated nasal soft tissue. More extensive defects, such as those involving the lateral orbital structures, orbital floor, or portions of the lateral midface projection, are more adequately addressed with Le Fort III-based alloflaps.

Le Fort III-based allotransplantation

Whereas the Le Fort II-based alloflap is useful for central midfacial defects involving the anterior maxilla, nose, upper lip, and hard palate, it is insufficient for more complex orbitozygomatic defects. For these defects, the use of the Le Fort III-based alloflap is more appropriate. The originally described Le Fort III fracture or 'craniofacial disjunction', includes the lateral orbital structures, orbital floor, medial orbital wall, nasal complex, as well as the dentate maxilla and hard palate. For bilateral orbitozygomatic defects with central tissue loss, this is the most appropriate method of reconstruction. The key advantages are the reconstitution of orbital volume, nasal structure, maxillary occlusion, oral cavity reconstitution via hard palate restoration, zygomatic projection, and addition of the maxillary sinuses. The numerous advantages of a Le Fort III-based design are evident in its more frequent use in experimental models as well as clinical reports.

Baccarani et al. were the first to describe the Le Fort III-based alloflap in a cadaveric model.[17] In 2006, these authors studied the efficacy of a subperiosteal harvest of an osteocutaenous flap based on skeletal disjunction at the Le Fort III level. They concluded that it was technically feasible to include a vascularized maxilla with the alloflap, based on a Le Fort III design. Further studies by Pomahac et al. demonstrated that the facial and angular blood vessels are contiguous with the maxillary vasculature via a complex micro-architecture that exists within the midfacial skeleton. Banks et al. furthered the study of the Le Fort III flap and identified the perfusion boundaries of the critical components of the flap.[18] They proposed that a single external carotid artery supplies the nasal dorsum and nasal tip, with ipsilateral perfusion of the zygomaticomaxillary complexes, and bilateral perfusion to the maxilla. These critical findings suggested that bilateral internal maxillary artery vascular pedicles were required for a Le Fort III (or Le Fort II) based maxillofacial alloflap.

The cadaveric studies on Le Fort III flaps have been validated by the clinical success of Le Fort III alloflaps for reconstruction of large, bilateral, central midfacial defects that include the orbitozygomatic regions. The first clinical example was the use of a Le Fort III based alloflap to reconstruct a complex midfacial defect in a 45-year-old female who had suffered a close-range ballistic injury.[1,2] The donor was a 44-year-old female. The composite alloflap consisted of the Le Fort III skeletal structures (bilateral zygomae, orbital floors, nasal complex, maxilla and hard palate), with the overlying soft tissue structures (nose, lower eyelids, upper lip, cheeks, oral mucosa). The flap was pedicled off of the bilateral external carotid arteries, with venous drainage from the bilateral external jugular/posterior facial veins. Bilateral parotid glands and facial nerves were also included. Several groups have since used varying designs based on the Le Fort III skeleton, with noted clinical success at restoring orbital volume, midfacial contour and projection, nasal anatomy, and maxillary occlusion and palatal integrity.

Orthognathic planning for maxillofacial allotransplantation

While there is no dearth of clinical evidence suggesting that maxillofacial allotransplantation is a suitable technique for reconstruction of complex midfacial defects, there has been minimal emphasis on the use of orthognathic surgery planning principles for planning.[19,20] In context, the initial studies have focused on the critical elements of vascular territories and pedicle design. The initial clinical efforts have been focused on technical execution and patient management through the initial transplantation with complex medical care involving immunosuppression, worries about graft rejection, and functional rehabilitation. Now that there is an adequate body of literature and clinical data verifying the initial clinical successes, the next stage in the evolution of planning for maxillofacial allotransplantation is underway. Akin to the initial planning involving well-established anatomical principles (i.e. Le Fort fracture patterns), one adjunct for the next stage of allotransplantation planning is the use of orthognathic surgical planning principles. This is of critical importance when considering the necessity for functional rehabilitation as a necessary corollary to aesthetic rehabilitation. There is a paucity of literature discussing the reconstitution of occlusion within transplant recipients. As the restoration of form is successful only insofar is function is restored, the next generation of maxillofacial allotransplants will benefit from planning based on principles in orthognathic surgery.

Such planning begins with an analysis of the donor and recipient facial forms and occlusion (Figure 59-1). While this is often a secondary consideration, given the constraints of donor availability, there is work that can be done on the recipient to not only quantify the size and shape of the defect, but also to address the functional loss in terms of skeletal profile and occlusion. Pre-injury photographs, dental models, and orthodontic records are all critical in this regard. While it is unrealistic, with a limited donor pool, to expect to identify a donor with an 'orthognathic' match to the recipient, considering the recipient defect in terms of orthognathic factors can allow teams to anticipate the need for primary bone grafts, challenges for occlusal rehabilitation, and the need for secondary surgical interventions (e.g. orthognathic surgery, soft tissue contouring, etc.).

The key components of an orthognathic evaluation for a transplant recipient include a clinical examination, photographs, radiographs, and cephalometric/dental analyses. The clinical examination should include an assessment of symmetry, facial proportions (vertical thirds and horizontal fifths), nasal/malar/periorbital contour and projection, profile (skeletal Class I, II, III), vertical and sagittal maxillary and mandibular position, as well as transverse facial form and facial shape (see Chapter 5).

Photographs in frontal repose, smiling, right and left lateral and three-quarter oblique views, as well as

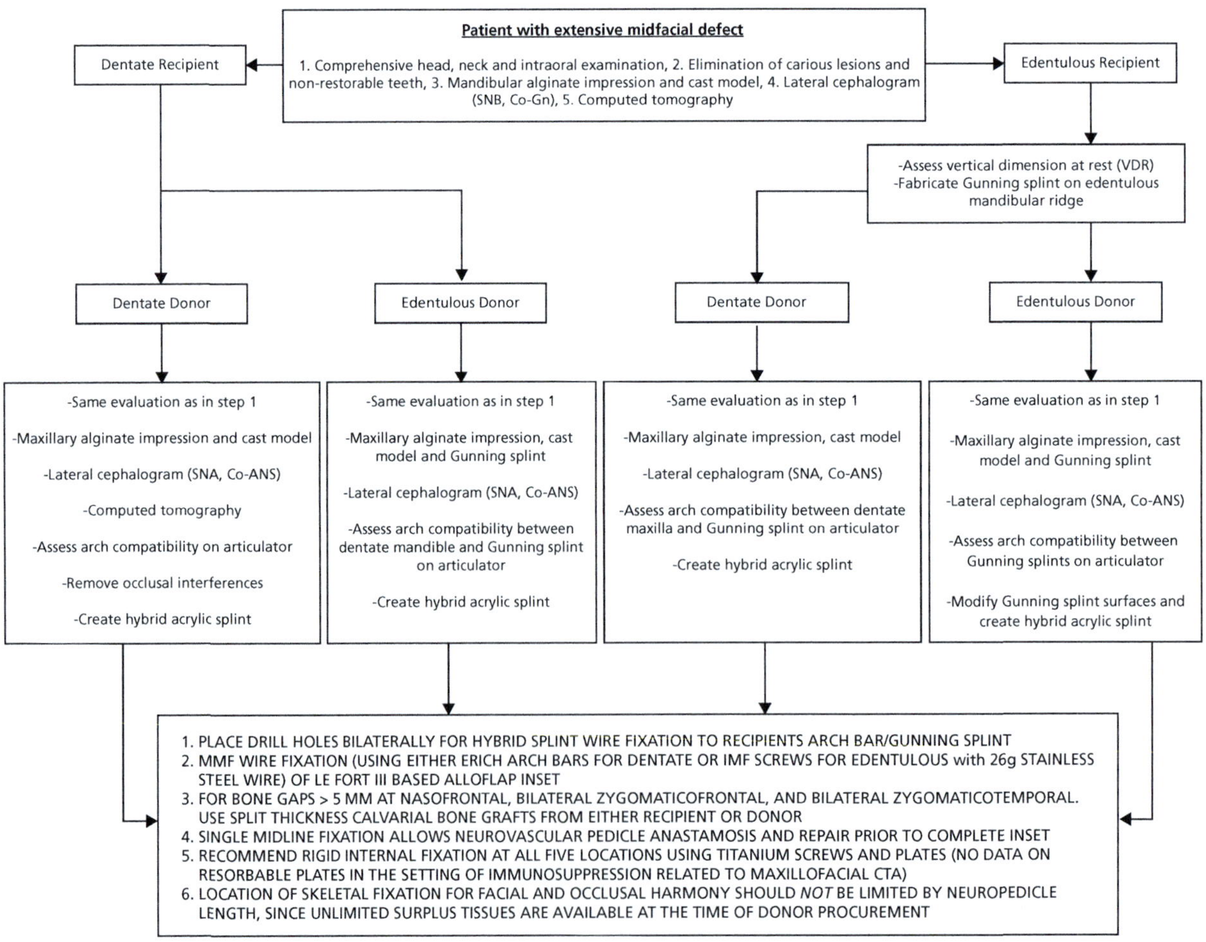

Fig. 59-1 Schematic for orthognathic planning for maxillofacial composite tissue allotransplantation (CTA). (From reference 19.)

superior (bird's eye) and inferior (worm's eye) views of the patient in their current state are a suitable starting point for planning. If available, comparable pre-injury photographs should be analyzed to identify 'what is missing', not only in terms of gross anatomical elements, but also functional components and important interfaces (e.g. nasolabial folds, lid-cheek junctions, upper lip/nasal contours, etc.).

Though plain film radiographs are a part of a standard orthognathic analysis, all patients undergoing maxillofacial VCA should have three-dimensional computed tomography scans. CAD-CAM technology is an essential tool for planning in this regard, as the missing hard and soft tissue landmarks can be replicated and an 'ideal' alloflap can be designed. The quantitative data from this ideal flap can be then used to analyze the donor alloflap, to identify areas of deficiency that can be addressed at the time of inset, or planned as secondary corrections using ancillary procedures.

Dental cast models evaluating the position of the donor maxilla to the recipient mandible are critical for assessing the magnitude of the dental discrepancy when the jaws are placed into occlusion. Size discrepancies in the sagittal and transverse planes are not critical in terms of the technical success of the transplant, as seen is the majority of clinical examples, where there are significant occlusal discrepancies. However, identifying such discrepancies prior to inset can help teams identify, preoperatively, what would constitute an acceptable intraoperative occlusion. One proposed schema describes an acceptable 'hybrid occlusion' as one, when the mandibular condyles are in centric relation, with: (1) bilateral posterior contacts; (2) overbite and overjet relationships in the range of 0–2 mm; and (3) no open bites, crossbites >4 mm, midline asymmetry, or significant occlusal prematurity wherein there are fewer than three occlusal contacts across the arch (i.e. lack of a tripod occlusion). To the extent possible, once an acceptable occlusion is identified between the donor maxilla and recipient mandible, an acrylic splint should be fashioned to assist with intraoperative positioning. This may optimize the efficiency of alloflap inset.

Orthognathic surgery principles can also be of benefit in edentulous scenarios, where one or both of the jaws in edentulous. In these instances, the use of Gunning-type splints can prevent malpositioning of the midface, which may result in mandibular overclosure, or worse, condylar dislocation. Appropriate midfacial positioning in this regard will allow for suitable anterior vertical facial height and sagittal positioning of the anterior maxillary and mandibular skeletal and soft tissue structures.

Facial identity and cross gender transplants

Prior to acceptance of facial transplantation, fear of transferred identity raised ethical concerns of proceeding with the procedure. A pilot study utilizing computer-simulated hybrid pictures of volunteer subjects demonstrated that identity is retained in recipients of midfacial transplants.[21] It is hypothesized that transplanting increasing amounts of facial skeleton results in increased transfer of donor identity. However, clinical cases of facial transplantation have not resulted in significant identity transfer, including a Le Fort III with mandible transplantation, essentially including the entire mid and lower facial skeleton.[11]

Little attention has been paid to the potential for cross-gender transplantation. The majority of facial transplant centres consider gender-mismatched donor-recipient pairs a *contraindication* to craniomaxillofacial allotransplantation. Gender specific anthropometrics and skin/hair aesthetic mismatch have led to concerns that cross-gender facial transplants will produce inferior hybrid results. However, cross-gender facial donation would increase the donor pool, decrease wait times, and potentially provide the most appropriate facial skeletal size match for recipients.

Pre-clinical investigation in swine

As with applying orthognathic surgery planning principles to facial transplantation described above, CAD-CAM presurgical planning can optimize hybrid facial skeletal matching to allow for cross-gender facial transplantations with equivalent results to gender matched pairs, as shown in both preclinical cadaveric and large animal live studies by Gordon et al.[22] Since 2011, our laboratory has chosen to establish a orthotopic large animal model employing swine due to its analogous craniomaxillofacial skeleton. As such, it allows an ideal environment for innovation, planning, and team practice. By obtaining preoperative 3D CT reconstructions for both donor and recipient, creating an optimal hybrid facial skeleton virtually, and utilizing intraoperative cutting guides to execute pre-surgical plans developed in our large animal laboratory, the surgical aspect from our standpoint has been improved. Practice and planning within a translational swine model, together with computer-enhanced technology developed by our team for navigational feedback and predictions in complex craniomaxillofacial surgery – will allow future outcomes in Le Fort-based maxillofacial transplantation to be optimized (Figure 59-2). The use of virtual surgical evaluation and planning, can result in not only the ability to quickly review different positions and techniques, but provides the information to fabricate surgical guides, interocclusal records, and custom reconstruction plates.

Planning and practice

Preoperatively, emphasis is placed on retaining proper occlusion, facial height proportions, and facial depth, allowing for acceptable aesthetic appearance upon transplantation. Not only can cross-gender facial

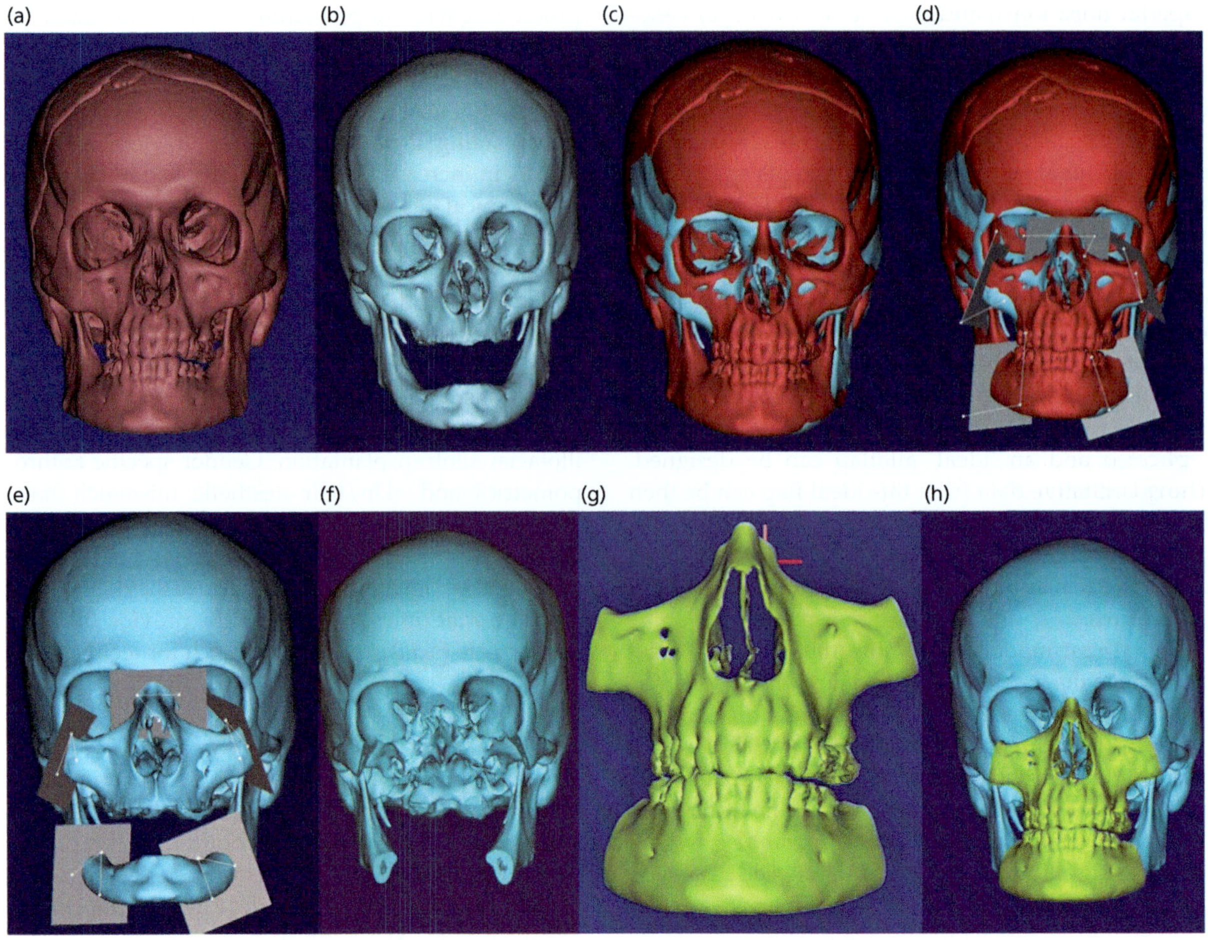

Fig. 59-2 Computer aided design and custom cutting guide fabrication for cross-gender transplantation. Preoperative virtual surgical planning utilizing donor and recipient 3D CT reconstructions (a,b) to plan optimal onlayed hybrid facial skeleton (c) and cutting guide planes (d,e) to dictate the recipient defect (f), donor midface (g), and ultimate crossgender hybrid facial skeleton (h). (From reference 22.)

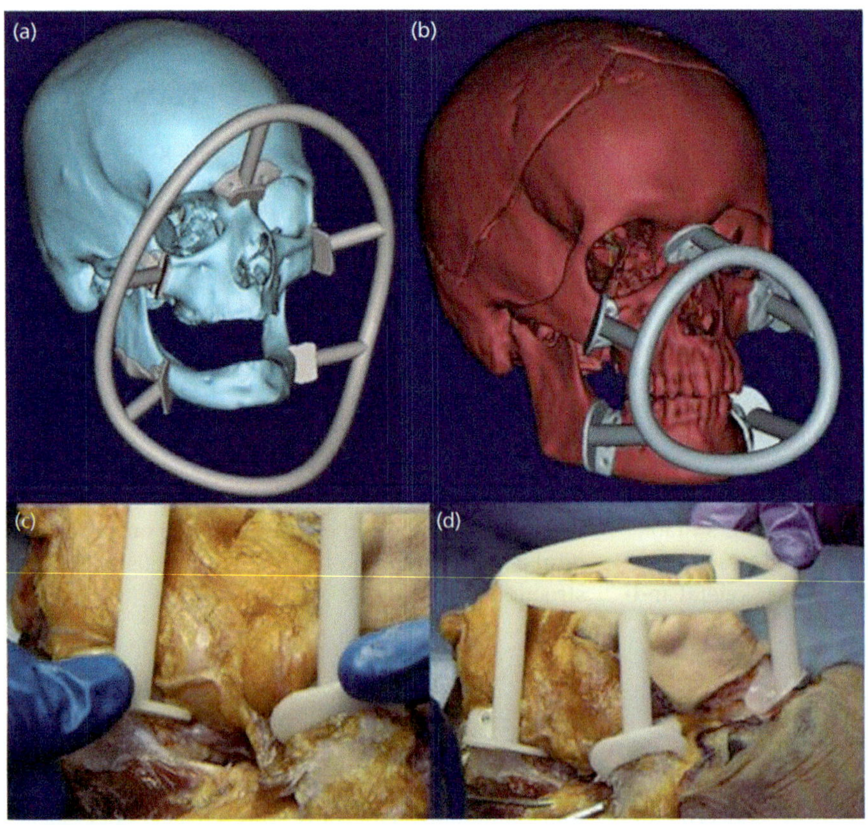

Fig. 59-3 Intraoperative cutting guides with retention of donor occlusion through intermaxillary fixation. Concentric cutting guides fabricated based on preoperative 3D CT reconstructions and determined cutting planes of the recipient and donor (a and b). Intraoperative application of custom cutting guides on donor facial skeleton, showing retained occlusion while in maxillomandibular fixation for transfer (c and d). (From reference 22.)

skeletal donation increase the donor pool, but size-matching may be improved. For example, a relatively small male recipient may be better suited by a female facial skeleton and vice-versa. Transplanting both maxilla and mandible, as shown in the cadaveric study by Gordon et al. (Figure 59-3),[22] allows for retention of donor occlusion. Concentric cutting guides, used to precisely achieve cutting planes planned preoperatively, are utilized to retain the donor maxillomandibular unit in fixation and transfer native donor occlusion. Using careful preoperative planning, desired cephalometric measurements can be achieved in the cross-gender hybrid facial skeleton. Disparities in skeletal contour due to gender specific morphology could be addressed during secondary procedures using bone graft, osteotomies, or alloplastic implants. The recipient's hormonal milieu would likely dictate the donor alloflap skin texture and hair growth pattern, as seen in transgender reassignment patients. Moreover, cross-gender facial transplantation likely poses no increased risk for identity transfer when compared to gender-matched pairs when preoperative planning is employed.

Conclusions

The use of Le Fort-based alloflaps has been the standard for maxillofacial VCA, substantiated by detailed cadaveric studies and noted clinical successes. The next step in evolution is a greater emphasis on orthognathic surgery planning principles in planning flap inset, employing custom cutting guides developed within a functional swine model, and utilizing enhanced computer-assisted technology developed specifically for Le Fort-based facial transplantation.[22] Given the scarcity of suitable donors for patients with massive central and bilateral orbitozygomatic defects, the emphasis on orthognathic planning should not be to identify an ideal donor, but rather to identify the ways in which the available donor and recipient are different, to allow for optimization of the result via ancillary techniques, either at the time of inset or as secondary interventions. Given the medical and surgical complexity of this new population of reconstructive patients, anticipation of further interventions has the potential to improve immediate and long-term functional results.

Disclosures

None of the authors have conflict of interests, commercial associations or financial disclosures to report for this book chapter.

Outside funding from various grants were used for a portion of this work. This includes grant support by the *American Society of Maxillofacial Surgery's* (2011 ASMS Basic Science Research grant), *American Association of Plastic Surgeons* (2012–14 Furnas' Academic Scholar Award), and the *Accelerated Translational Investigational Program* at Johns Hopkins (funded by the National Institute of Health).

Portions of this study were made possible by the Johns Hopkins Institute for Clinical and Translational Research (ICTR) which is funded in part by the National Center for Advancing Translational Sciences (NCATS), a component of the National Institutes of Health (NIH), and NIH Roadmap for Medical Research. Its contents are solely the responsibility of the authors and do not necessarily represent the official view of the Johns Hopkins ICTR, NCATS or NIH.

The views expressed in this chapter are those of the authors and do not necessarily reflect the official policy, position, or endorsement of the Department of the Navy, Army, Department of Defense, nor the U.S. Government.

References

1 Siemionow MZ, Papay F, Djohan R, et al. First U.S. near-total human face transplantation: a paradigm shift for massive complex injuries. Plast Reconstr Surg. 2010;125:111–122.
2 Alam DS, Papay F, Djohan R, et al. The technical and anatomical aspects of the World's first near-total human face and maxilla transplant. Arch Facial Plast Surg. 2009;11:369–77.
3 Gordon CR, Siemionow M, Papay F, et al. The world's experience with facial transplantation: what have we learned thus far? Ann Plast Surg. 2009;63:572–8.
4 Siemionow M, Ozturk C. Face transplantation: outcomes, concerns, controversies, and future directions. J Craniofac Surg. 2012;23:254–9.
5 Siemionow M, Ozturk C. An update on facial transplantation cases performed between 2005 and 2010. Plast Reconstr Surg. 2011;128:707e–20e.
6 Pomahac B, Pribaz J, Eriksson E, et al. Three patients with full facial transplantation. N Engl J Med. 2012;366:715–22.
7 Barret JP, Serracanta J, Collado JM, et al. Full face transplantation organization, development, and results – the Barcelona experience: A case report. Transplant Proc. 2011;43:3533–4.
8 Petruzzo P, Kanitakis J, Badet L, et al. Long-term follow-up in composite tissue allotransplantation: In-depth study of five (hand and face) recipients. Am J Transplant. 2011;11:808–16.
9 Petruzzo P, Testelin S, Kanitakis J, et al. First human face transplantation: 5 years outcomes. Transplantation. 2012;93:236–40.
10 Guo S, Han Y, Zhang X, et al. Human facial allotransplantation: A 2-year follow-up study. Lancet. 2008;372:631–8.
11 Dorafshar AH, Bojovic B, Christy MR, Borsuk DE, Iliff NT, Brown EN, Shaffer CK, Kelley TN, Kukuruga DL, Barth RN, Bartlett ST, Rodriguez ED. Total face, double jaw, and tongue transplantation: an evolutionary concept. Plast Reconstr Surg. 2013;131:241–51.
12 Tessier P. The classic reprint. Experimental study of fractures of the upper jaw. I and II. René Le Fort, M.D. Plast Reconstr Surg. 1972;50:497–506.
13 Tessier P. The classic reprint: experimental study of fractures of the upper jaw. 3. René Le Fort, M.D., Lille, France. Plast Reconstr Surg. 1972;50:600–7.
14 Yazici I, Cavusoglu T, Comert A, et al. Maxilla allograft for transplantation: an anatomical study. Ann Plast Surg. 2008;61:105–13.
15 Lantieri L, Hivelin M, Audard V, et al. Feasibility, reproducibility, risks and benefits of face transplantation: a prospective study of outcomes. Am J Transplant. 2011;11:367–78.
16 Pomahac B, Pribaz J, Eriksson E, et al. Restoration of facial form and function after severe disfigurement from burn

injury by a composite facial allograft. Am J Transplant. 2011;11:386–93.
17 Baccarani A, Follmar KE, Baumeister SP, Marcus JR, Erdmann D, Levin LS. Technical and anatomical considerations of face harvest in face transplantation. Ann Plast Surg. 2006;57:483–8.
18 Banks ND, Hui-Chou HG, Tripathi S, et al. An anatomical study of external carotid artery vascular territories in face and midface flaps for transplantation. Plast Reconstr Surg. 2009;123:1677–87.
19 Gordon CR, Susarla SM, Peacock ZS, et al. Le Fort-based maxillofacial transplantation: current state-of-the-art and refined technique. J Craniofacial Surg. 2012;23:81–7.
20 Gordon CR, Susarla SM, Peacock ZS, et al. Osteocutaneous maxillofacial allotransplantation: lessons learned from a novel cadaver study applying orthognathic surgery planning principles and practice. Plast Reconstr Surg. 2011;128:465–79.
21 Pomahac B, Aflaki P, Nelson C, Balas B. Evaluation of appearance transfer and persistence in central face transplantation: A computer simulation analysis. J Plast Reconstr Aesthet Surg. 2010; 63:733–8.
22 Gordon CR, Swanson EW, Susarla SM, et al. Overcoming cross-gender differences and challenges in Le Fort-based, craniomaxillofacial transplantation with enhanced computer-assisted technology. Ann Plast Surg. 2013;71: 421–8.

Section 4: Appendix

Chapter 60

Orthognathic Surgery – One Patient's Perspective

Tania Murphy

Introduction

Patient satisfaction rates following orthognathic surgery are generally high and a review of the literature suggests that 92–100% of orthognathic patients are satisfied with their result.[1] Patients frequently underestimate, however, the impact of the treatment with respect to overall life changes, general appearance and performance at work or college.[2]

The major motivation for patients undergoing orthognathic treatment is to improve their appearance – females are more likely to undergo treatment for internal psychosocial reasons, to improve their appearance and self-esteem, while males are more practical, hoping that treatment will not only improve their social life but will also prevent dental problems in the future.[3]

Research has shown, however, that patients tend to be unhappy with the amount of information received from their orthodontist and fail to recall the majority (70%) of information given to them at an orthodontic consultation after just 10 days.[4] Providing the patient with adequate information may result in increased compliance during treatment, and post-treatment satisfaction has been shown to be strongly related to feeling fully prepared for surgery. Reports show that the majority of patient complaints are related to communication rather than clinical competence or treatment outcomes.[5]

A study in 2012[6] looked at the quality and reliability of UK websites providing information on orthognathic and jaw surgery to patients. The range in the consumer information found was wide and the authors comment that clinicians must ensure they direct their patients to validated websites and that further development of websites is required.

Using the term 'orthognathic surgery' on an internet search engine generates tens of links to 'blog-spots' with patients reporting in quite graphic detail their experiences of undergoing orthognathic surgery – the highs, lows and everything else in between.

At the age of 30, I was a third-year orthodontic Specialist Registrar who decided to undergo a bimaxillary osteotomy to correct my Class III malocclusion. During this period, I too, kept a diary that recorded all the good and bad points that accompanied my 'new face'.

Prior to being an Orthodontic Registrar, I had completed a year as a Vocational Trainee dentist, spent time in General Practice and also worked for two years as Senior House Officer in Oral and Maxillofacial Surgery where I assisted on approximately one orthognathic list a week. So when I decided to undergo my bimaxillary osteotomy I thought I had probably the most informed 'Informed Consent' a patient could have!

In this chapter, I hope to give the reader an insight into the thoughts of one orthognathic patient and hopefully highlight what we fail to tell our patients but also what they fail to tell us.

Orthognathic Surgery: Principles, Planning and Practice. Edited by Farhad B. Naini and Daljit S. Gill.

My orthognathic surgical treatment

At 29, I was just about to begin my second year of orthodontic training. I was happily married, had a great social life and I feel a fairly well-adjusted individual. It was at this point, that I was asked by my Consultant Maxillofacial Surgical colleague whether I had ever considered having orthognathic surgery! I have to be honest, surgery had crossed my mind several times throughout my dental training, but for me it was the prospect of wearing fixed appliances that had prevented me from pursuing the matter further, *not* the prospect of having surgery, which I think is an important point to remember whilst reading this chapter. The more I thought about it, however, the more I thought that now probably was the right time for me.

Full orthodontic records were taken. These showed a Class III incisor relationship with a reverse overjet of 3 mm on a Class III skeletal base with an increased Frankfort–mandibular plane angle. My upper right central and lateral incisors had been previously lost due to trauma. The central incisor had been replaced with a dental implant and the upper right canine had been camouflaged to resemble the missing lateral incisor. My lower centre line was displaced to the left by 3 mm.

Radiographs helped confirm the clinical diagnosis of a moderate Class III skeletal pattern with an ANB of –6°. My upper incisors were slightly proclined at 115° and my lower incisors were retroclined at 71°. Evidence of a previous dalliance with oral surgery whilst I was a dental student was also visible, with the presence of a titanium plate following a genioplasty to correct the asymmetry of my chin point.

The orthodontic phase of my treatment progressed in a relatively straightforward manner. After just over a year of orthodontic treatment, I was fully decompensated and ready for surgery. The upper right first premolar had been rotated and intruded so that it could be camouflaged at the end of treatment to resemble an upper right canine. The radiographs confirmed the decompensation and showed that my lower third molars were removed 6 months prior to the orthognathic surgery.

I was fortunate enough to be able to spend the evening before my operation at home. On the morning of the surgery, I was quite apprehensive about what was to follow; however, in the name of consumer research I plucked up the courage and went for it!

A Le Fort I osteotomy enabled my maxilla to be brought forward 6 mm and a bilateral sagittal split osteotomy (BSSO) allowed my mandible to be set-back 3 mm, but also rotated to help correct the centre line discrepancy.

Advice on preoperative patient preparation

So what can I tell you that may make your patients better prepared?

I left hospital two days following my operation. I was totally euphoric that I was still alive and couldn't wait to get home. I was oblivious, however, to the fact that 'day 3' was to follow. Several people had warned me that this would be my worst day as it is very common for steroids to be given during surgery to reduce the postoperative swelling – this leads to patients having a 'steroid high' immediately postoperatively, but this is then followed by a 'steroid low' after two or three days. I really wasn't prepared for how low I would feel on that day and how much I would regret having put myself through surgery. I hated my new face with a passion and totally regretted putting myself through the procedure. I think it is incredibly important to pre-warn patients, parents and family that this may happen in the hope that it will help reduce the impact of this unfortunate but unavoidable phase of treatment before the patient can then start on the recovery process.

The first post-op review appointment is the appointment where you arrive still feeling very sorry for yourself, swollen, bruised and everybody tells you that you look great! I know that as a clinician, I have been guilty of using this phrase. As a patient, however, 'great' would not be the adjective that would instantly spring to mind. This look is not what you underwent hours of surgery for and you really can't see that it is ever going to improve. I think most patients at this stage are looking for reassurance that the surgery has gone well and that their face is *going* to look great. It actually took several months for me to become used to my 'new face'. I became prepared for what I was going to see when looking in mirrors but the surprise of not recognizing yourself when catching a glimpse of your reflection in windows is something that I will remember for a very long time.

I knew that with maxillary surgery there was a possibility that my nose may flare and I had therefore asked my surgeon to place a cinch stitch during the procedure. It soon became apparent, however, during the first few days following the surgery, that this was to be the least of my worries. My postoperative swelling produced a rather upturned and lopsided nose which during my initial recovery caused me to think that by correcting my Class III malocclusion I may have set myself up for a nose job! Thankfully, over the first two to three weeks the swelling around my nose subsided, as did my fears. I didn't voice these concerns at any of my appointments following the surgery and noticed that many of my patients didn't make any comment on their noses either. I now routinely reassure my patients that they will see quite dramatic improvements over the first few weeks of healing and it appears that it is only then that many of them volunteer that they were incredibly concerned regarding the change to the appearance of their nose, more so, than any of the other facial swelling.

I didn't get to see a dietician following my operation and sadly it appears the same happens to many patients. I started off on a very soft diet of soup and porridge. After about 4 days of this, the boredom of such a limited diet and the general starvation that was associated with it made me realise that I had to think of another way to feed myself. My light-bulb moment was when I suddenly realized that if what I wanted to eat could go in a food blender it could be eaten! I think this was probably the turning point in my recovery as it enabled me to continue to consume a well-balanced and healthy diet, which is obviously important with regards to healing. In the lead-in appointments to surgery, I now advise all of my patients and their carers to invest in a blender before they undergo their surgery and provide them with an accompanying leaflet with examples of food they may wish to try.

Today, all patients are warned about the possibility of numbness following surgery both immediately post-surgery and also long term. All patients should be warned that they will have some alteration of sensation immediately postoperatively. Some units provide their patients with results of audit projects that have looked at the incidence of paraesthesia of their particular surgeon. If not, the patient should be informed of regional or national statistics. What I had failed to realize is that during the first few days after the operation a swollen, numb lip can quickly ulcerate as it rubs against a fixed appliance. I awoke one morning to find a row of large ulcers on my upper lip which aligned perfectly with the brackets of the appliance. I now advise patients to wear comfort wax continually on their brace for the first two weeks of their recovery to help prevent this.

Deterioration of speech is not a common problem for patients unless they have a predisposing factor such as a repaired cleft palate or pharyngeal surgery, but it can still happen in patients where there is no obvious cause and when the movements are not particularly severe. Initially I had great problems pronouncing some sounds, especially 'sh'. However, my speech did improve quite rapidly. I feel that some patients probably don't even notice a change, however, for others it appears that it may be one more challenge for them to face when they are already feeling incredibly low.

Four months following the surgery, I had turned into the average orthognathic patient and was desperate to have my appliances removed. Unfortunately being 'in the job' doesn't necessarily prolong compliance. It seems that most orthognathic patients use up the majority of their goodwill during the surgical stage of treatment. Maybe it would be of benefit to the patients to maximize the orthodontic phase of treatment pre-op. My appliances were finally removed 8 months following my surgery.

Conclusions

So would I do it again? The short answer to this is, YES! Although, I can honestly say that initially, I really did wonder what I had done; however, I look back now and can't believe I didn't do it years ago. I love the result and wouldn't hesitate in recommending it to my patients – although hopefully with more understanding than I did before!

My top ten tips for orthognathic patients include:

1. Make sure you have some front opening shirts or blouses for immediately after your surgery – you will not feel like pulling a top over your head.
2. You will feel awful on the third day after your surgery; this is normal and after that every day should be an improvement.
3. You will be bruised and swollen after your surgery – so the face you see immediately following the surgery will not be the face you have at the end of treatment.
4. You may also have facial abrasions around your lips immediately after the surgery.
5. Nasal congestion is common after maxillary surgery – it will eventually clear.
6. Try and sleep sitting up for the first few weeks following the surgery, it helps reduce the swelling more quickly and aids with breathing if you are suffering from nasal congestion.
7. It is highly likely that you will have some numbness following the surgery – this is likely to resolve but may mean that you can't feel that the brace is rubbing your swollen lip. Therefore, use plenty of comfort wax for the first few weeks following the surgery.
8. As the nerves begin to regenerate they are likely to produce a tingling sensation in the soft tissues. If you do end up with permanent numbness – you will still be able to move your lips and will NOT look like you have had a stroke.
9. Your speech may well be different after your surgery but will return as healing occurs.
10. Be creative with food! Stock up in advance with numerous soups, porridge and pasta but also invest in a food blender; this helps provide a much more interesting, varied and balanced diet.

References

1 Flanery CM, Barnwell GM, van Sickels JE, Litterfield JH, Rugh AL. Impact of orthognathic surgery on normal and abnormal personality dimensions: a two-year follow up study of 61 patients. Am J Orthod Dentofac Orthop. 1990;98:313–22.
2 Cunningham SJ, Crean SJ, Hunt NP, Harris M. Preparation, perceptions and problems: A long-term follow-up study of orthognathic surgery. Int J Adult Orthod Orthognath Surg. 1996;11:41–7.
3 Williams AC, Shah H, Sandy JR, Travess HC. Patients' motivations for treatment and their experiences of orthodontic preparation for orthognathic surgery. J Orthod. 2005;32:191–202.
4 Ryan F, Shute J, Cedro M, Songh J, Lee E, Lee S, Lloyd TW, Robinson A, Gill D, Hunt NP, Cunningham SJ. A new style of orthognathic clinic. J Orthod. 2011;38:124–33.
5 Richards T. Chasms in communication. BMJ. 1990;301:1407–8.
6 Aldairy T, Laverick S, McIntyre GT. Orthognathic surgery: is patient information on the Internet valid? Eur J Orthod. 2012;34:466–9.

Chapter 61

Responding to Patients' Psychological and Social Needs Following Orthognathic Surgery

Henrietta Spalding

Introduction

> 'The mental effort of going through jaw surgery is equal to the physical.' 40-year-old woman receiving treatment for cancer of the jaw

In a society where good looks are increasingly prized very highly, coming to terms with a jaw that looks different from the 'norm', whether as a result of a congenital condition, acquired through trauma or disease or following surgery can be far from easy. Many patients struggle to feel good about themselves and experience psychological distress and anxiety when faced with staring, comments and awkward questions. The aim of this chapter, like the UK charity, Changing Faces, which supports and represents people with any condition that affects their appearance, is to first examine the psychological and social aspects associated with a disfiguring jaw condition; and then to explore how healthcare professionals can help their patients deal successfully with the anxiety and challenges of looking 'different'. It should be noted that the term 'disfigurement' is used as a helpful generic word to describe the visual impact of these conditions, but not to describe an individual's condition.

Living with a disfiguring jaw condition

The reality of living with a disfiguring condition is that social norms change when a person looks or sounds different.[1] The visible facial disfigurement and related functional disorders associated with conditions such as developmental facial deformities or head and neck cancer surgery predispose this patient population to unique physiological and psychosocial needs.[2] Treatments for patients with craniofacial deformities, trauma and cancer are some of the most debilitating and are often associated with chronic functional impairment. Because of its location and the effects of treatment on social interaction, patients with head and neck cancer are at particular risk of psychological concerns, particularly social anxiety and depression.[3] Research shows that 40–66% of patients with head and neck cancer meet the criteria for a

Orthognathic Surgery: Principles, Planning and Practice. Edited by Farhad B. Naini and Daljit S. Gill.

psychological diagnosis. If undetected and untreated, psychological needs are associated with reductions in quality of life, increased risk of suicide, increased length of hospital stay, more complications with treatment and increased non-compliance with treatment.

The face particularly holds both visual and functional significance, both literal and symbolic. It is how an individual is recognized, an outlet for inner feelings, thoughts and fears, enables interaction, such as eye contact, and permits a range of emotions to be displayed. In addition, it is not only a means of expression but also function, e.g. eating, seeing, speaking and enabling social interaction of all sorts. Furthermore, an individual's facial features are also inherited, and may form a link to one's family and history. Visible facial differences, and surgery that may alter facial appearance, may have effects on an individual's sense of identity.

Here are some examples of those changes:

- There is a sense of being invisible – patients are ignored, but at the same time they are highly visible – people stare.
- Strangers feel they have permission to comment and ask questions about a patient's appearance, e.g. 'What happened to you?'
- A patient may feel uncertain of what to expect from others, or what to say in response.
- Many feel they are 'on duty' all the time, and have to maintain a near constant vigilance, which can result in increased self-consciousness and considerable effort.
- Some will feel alone and isolated, and therefore cannot go out, or believe they cannot have intimate relationships.
- Others express feelings of anger, embarrassment, and a 'need to be fixed.'
- Sometimes there is a lack of communication with family and friends.

It is not therefore surprising that a patient with a different looking jaw may feel and act:

- **S:** Self-conscious, Shy
- **C:** Conspicuous, Cavalier
- **A:** Angry, Awkward
- **R:** Rejected, Retreating
- **E:** Embarrassed, Evasive
- **D:** 'Different', Defensive.

(Created by Changing Faces)

Many will feel the social pressures associated with stereotyping and myths associated with an altered appearance.

The psychosocial difficulties can be summarized as follows:[4]

- *Intra-personal*: In our appearance-focused society, any difference in appearance is a challenge to a person's self-confidence and sense of identity. Feelings of sadness, grief, guilt, anger, and depression are frequent.
- *Inter-personal*: Disfigurement poses many everyday challenges in social encounters, especially being stared at, avoided, asked curious questions, patronized, called names, and worse – ridiculed or rejected. If encounters go badly, a person can become socially anxious, withdrawn and isolated, potentially leading to depression and occasionally even suicide. Making friends and forming intimate relationships may become complicated, while getting work or promotion can be very challenging despite the fact that 'severe disfigurement' is covered by the UK's Equality Act 2010.

Case study

A young person born with Crouzon syndrome has undergone several surgical interventions to 'normalize' his appearance. He has needed to face profound life challenges:

- How can I fit in?
- How will I make friends?
- Will the teacher pick me to represent the class?
- How will I ever get a girlfriend?
- Will I be able to be a successful lawyer?

The cultural context

Prevailing assumptions about what life is like for someone with a disfigurement are deeply embedded in our culture and distort our view of the reality of disfigurement. In fact, these are myths without foundation.[5] However, the thoughts and perceptions people may have formed about what it means to live with a disfigurement, in terms of the various ways it might impact on different areas of a person's life, may influence how they themselves deal with their own emotions and beliefs when they, a member of their family, or a friend, personally experience a changed appearance.

Nine out of ten people unwittingly judge people with disfiguring conditions less favourably than those without, so that individuals with such visible facial differences, and their families, are often unfairly treated for their looks alone. The assumptions – and the subsequent behaviours – mitigate against an equal relationship.[6]

There are three significant cultural assumptions – stereotypes or misconceptions – about people with disfigurements, which tend to be reinforced by the media, film and advertising:

1. *'Good looks' are the key to success and happiness, so people with disfigurements can expect to live only second-rate lives.* As a result, this can lead to feelings of failure or being a 'write-off', and may result in the

general lowering of expectations: not only those of the person with the disfigurement, but also other people. The reality is that many people with a facial disfigurement live normal, successful lives and have fulfilling relationships and achievements.

2. *People with scars and disfigurements are 'different', not 'normal' – hence they are justifiably caricatured in film and literature as villainous or nasty.* As a result, many people may be afraid of someone with a disfigurement, or feel free to ridicule them. In reality, of course, a facially disfigured person is in no way intrinsically frightening or 'evil', and a disfigurement certainly does not influence moral character or intelligence.
3. *Reconstructive and aesthetic (or cosmetic) surgery can transform people's faces, make them perfect and make them happy, so everyone who has a disfigurement should get it 'fixed' by medical or surgical treatments.* This can lead to false expectations, not only on the part of the patient, but also by the general public. For, while surgery may help reduce the conspicuousness of a disfigurement for some and/or improve functioning, it rarely does this without leaving other scars.

Ironically, patients and their parents/families can often apply these same cultural assumptions to themselves – lacking optimism about their prospects, feeling uncomfortable with their 'less-than-good looks' and associating them with inferiority, even immorality.

Historically, beauty has been held in high regard, and advertising images endorse this. The success of the booming beauty, cosmetic surgery, and diet and fashion industries demonstrates how much people are prepared to invest in their appearance.[7]

Television and film portrayals, computer games and children's stories perpetuate the myth that heroes and heroines are handsome and beautiful. Bad people are portrayed as ugly – with scars, warts or distortions. Cinderella (and her Ugly, i.e. nasty, Sisters), the orcs in The Lord of the Rings, and Freakface in the Moshi Monsters series illustrate this well, whilst the Bond and Batman movies frequently equate scarring with evil. There are also sad images, with the Phantom of the Opera living tragically in the sewers of society. Only a few anti-archetypes are portrayed sympathetically – Shrek and Harry Potter being the shining examples.[8]

The cultural context helps to explain the many reports from people with disfigurements who say they detect 'scaredness' in those they meet. People meeting somebody with a disfigurement may feel and act:

- **S:** Sorry, Staring
- **C:** Curious, Clumsy
- **A:** Anxious, Anguish
- **R:** Recoil, Rude
- **E:** Embarrassed, Evasive
- **D:** Distressed, Dread.

(Created by Changing Faces)

How do facial deformities affect patients and their families?

The psychological effect of a disfigurement may occur at many stages throughout a patient's life and care pathway. With a congenital condition, e.g. Apert syndrome or Crouzon syndrome, it will commence right from birth through early childhood and into adulthood. The social and cognitive processes during the early years of a child's life, in relation to how their family, friends and other people around them react to their appearance, can affect their self-esteem, their sense of worth and their self-confidence (coping with other people and situations), and may result in low expectations later in life regarding relationships and work. Children with disfigurements and their parents often show signs of stress, anxiety and depression and a sense of social isolation.[9] Parents of a newborn baby with a craniofacial condition may feel and react in a variety of ways. Feelings may range between total acceptance, joy, distress, anger, guilt, grief for the 'perfect' child, or a need for surgery before attachment. In social situations, too, behaviour may range between normality, avoidance (unless the disfigurement is concealed), or being defensive.

Another important aspect is the effect having a child with a disfigurement may have on the relationship between parents or other members of the family. This, too, can range from drawing the family closer together, a breakdown of a relationship, immediate adjustment, or long-term difficulty adjusting to the situation. In addition, there will be many practical considerations for the family to manage, including treatment being miles from home, build up and preparation to discharge, threat to life and fear of recurrence, pain and loss of functions, repeated and on-going hospitalizations, looking in the mirror for the first time, and respective life stages, e.g. making friends, going to school, becoming a teenager, dating.

With an acquired jaw condition such as head and neck cancer or following violence or an accident, there is the trauma of diagnosis, followed by rapid medical investigation and treatment. However, for many patients, the effects of the disfigurement can actually be more troubling than the medical condition itself, especially after the initial immediacy of the treatment. As with children there will be many practical implications including support from loved ones, loss of income, medical concerns, survivorship, family responsibilities, return to professional activity, etc. Facial disfigurement can have a profound psychological impact, and people often have difficulties living with their appearance – emotional, social and economic, as well as those associated with surgical treatment. Self-esteem, body image and quality of life can be adversely affected.[10] The psychological and emotional effects of a changed appearance may result in social isolation and a process of bereavement for the loss of a patient's former face and identity.

A useful framework for understanding this process is the model of the five stages of loss:[11]

1. **Denial and isolation** – 'No, not me. It cannot be true'
2. **Anger** – 'Why me?'
3. **Bargaining** – 'Yes, me ... but'
4. **Depression** – 'Yes, me'
5. **Acceptance** – 'It's OK'.

However, it is important to remember that this is not a linear model – the patient can move back and forth according to what may be happening at various points in their recovery and future.

The whole family and social circle will also experience the effects of the disfigurement, in different ways. Partridge[12] highlights that they will find it hard to come to terms with the first sight of facial wounds, and even harder to accept that they are bound to leave disfiguring scars. He adds that relatives, especially spouses, partners or loved ones, will have to make some major adjustments, and some may be unable to do so. Reactions may range between commitment to help and support, feelings of sorrow, avoidance, worrying what to say and, sometimes, complete rejection.

Parents of a child who has experienced surgery or a traumatic injury resulting in disfigurement will also react in a number of ways, ranging between depression, guilt, distress and anger. Siblings, too, may become overprotective of their brother or sister, or may be ashamed of their appearance, or indeed bullied because of their brother or sister's disfigurement.

Many patients do adjust well to their disfigurements and even report positive consequences from living with a visible difference, such as personal growth, and increased empathy with others.[13] The literature also indicates that most people eventually adjust reasonably well to a disfiguring condition, though time is by no means an automatic healer. Most people, however, experience some psychosocial problems for several months, even years, as do their parents, partners and families. It is likely that if the healthcare systems fail to recognize or respond to those problems, in a timely fashion, they may lead to long-term damage.

Examples of how patients and their families might behave:

Flight

- Fear/avoidance of public places, shops, public transport, hairdressers.
- Avoiding mirrors and reflective surfaces.
- Fear of intimate relationships.
- Avoiding children and relating with own children, old friends.
- Shy, self-conscious, embarrassed.
- Clumsy, awkward.
- Retreating, evasive, defensive, shut down.

Fight

- Aggressive, irritable, snappy.
- Blaming, envious, bitter.
- Inappropriate, over-familiar.

Case study - Sandra

A 40-year-old woman developed spindle cell cancer in her jaw requiring major surgery. She was overwhelmed with questions and anxieties:

- How will I look after the operation?
- Can I face seeing myself for the first time?
- Will I be able to cope with looking different?
- What will my partner think of me – will I still be attractive to him?
- How will my child react to me?
- How will I go back to work?

The degree of emotional and social distress caused does not correlate with the extent or severity of a disfigurement. This means that treating it medically or surgically (even virtually correcting it) is no guarantee that the patient will adjust psychologically. Indeed, studies have identified perceived severity or noticeability, as opposed to objective severity, as the important factor of good or poor outcome.[14]

If a person's disfigurement is perceived by others as causing less distress because it appears to them to be less severe, this diminishes not only the disfigurement, but also the very real need to understand the extent to which that person might be experiencing their visible difference emotionally.

How to respond to patients' needs

Any patient and their family, in coming to terms with their appearance, may need to have ready access to advice, information and support which can help them develop the coping strategies necessary to living confidently. These might include emotional support, self-confidence building, self-help literature and skin camouflage services. In the early days following surgery and post discharge from hospital, a person will need to surround themselves with family and friends so that they feel cared for, loved and supported.[15] In addition, a person might need to be shielded from the social intrusion characteristic of many first encounters.[16] However, it is important to recognize that not every patient will have access to a supportive family network or group of friends. Some will rely solely on support from health and or social services or a local support group. It is therefore necessary to identify: (a) the patient's needs; (b) how the patient's social network responds to the changing needs; and (c) the family's needs, so that healthcare professionals can play their crucial part in helping their patients deal successfully with the anxiety and challenges a person faces when they look 'different'.

> **Case study**
>
> A man developed a cancerous growth requiring his parotid gland to be removed. He was informed that it would be removed and a flap created. However, he did not fully understand the impact of the surgery leaving him deaf in one ear, paralysis of one side of the face, and difficulties with speech and eating. 'My biggest gripe is the lack of information before the operation. Of course surgeons do not know the extent of surgery until the patient is opened up. However they did know beforehand about the flap and must have known the consequences…'

In orthognathic surgery, communication with patients prior to their surgery is equally important, so that both they and their families are well-prepared for the post-operative recovery period.

How healthcare professionals can support their patients adjusting to their different appearance

Changing Faces has found consistently through supporting patients and their families that the best long-term, psychosocial adjustments are achieved if patients have access to an effective package of help and support designed to promote living with confidence. The package is best delivered by a trained professional but can also be provided in a self-help format. It is essentially a cognitive-behavioural approach combining a mix of psycho-educational direction and psycho-therapeutic support, known as FACES:

- **F:** FINDING OUT – gaining realistic information about their condition and its treatment.
- **A:** ATTITUDE – developing a positive outlook and beliefs about the future.
- **C:** COPING with feelings – managing them better with help from a trained professional.
- **E:** EXCHANGING – sharing experiences with others in similar situations.
- **S:** SOCIAL SKILLS – learning the skills to handle the reactions of strangers, friends etc.

What does each element of FACES mean in practice?

Here is a brief overview with an example of how it can work with an individual patient, Sandra (case study above), who made contact with Changing Faces about the impact of surgery on her jaw following head and neck cancer, though many of the points are pertinent to patients undergoing orthognathic/reconstructive jaw surgery as well:

F: Finding out

Patients/families receiving treatment should have adequate opportunity to read about and discuss their condition prior to surgery. Uncertainty about what will happen, or when, simply increases anxiety. Both patients and relatives need reassurance, acknowledgement, and information to be empowered and cope well. Medical staff have a major role to play in empowering patients to take the right decisions – but *finding out* is not just important for that reason. One research study[17] highlighted the significance of the timing of information. It found that information needs do change and fluctuate; thus, while there was some agreement that doctors often dictate the timing of information, some people preferred not to be given a lot of information, wanting time to come to terms with their situation first. It is therefore very important that each patient should be assessed individually and regularly regarding their ability to take in information.

Another study[18] with patients who had undergone head and neck surgeries found that early involvement in self-care, managing dressings and socialization on the ward all contribute to an ethos of self-management and independence which are the precursors to effective long-term coping. Furthermore, self-care, which requires close up viewing and touching the changed areas, appears to precede reduction in anxiety.

Gaining realistic information also means that they:

- can explain things more easily to their family, friends, employers and others;
- are informed about and referred to other agencies, for example, to a skin camouflage clinic, if appropriate;
- feel more in control of their condition.

> **Case study**
>
> Sandra was given lots of information about the cancer, the surgery and the rehabilitation.
>
> > 'The staff were so supportive, giving me lots of information about the whole journey. I couldn't have been better looked after… I felt so safe.'
>
> But she was not provided with any information about the impact of the surgery on her appearance by the head and neck cancer team, or prepared for her altered appearance. She was particularly concerned how her small son was going to respond to her new look and how she was going to explain it to him and help him through it.

A: Attitude

In our appearance obsessed world, it is important for patients and their families to develop positive beliefs about their future and to debunk negative thinking about appearance issues. This can be done by attending workshops, looking at websites, reading self-help literature and/or people's personal accounts so they can:

- start to think positively about their futures;
- be encouraged to think about their strengths and interests, not just their appearance.

Case study

Post-surgery, Sandra experienced some very low times. She was supported to explore how life might become better once again. What might it look like, what did she need to do to make it happen. She started to see that her prospects in life need not be controlled by her looks.

C: Coping

Patients should have access to excellent psychotherapeutic support to help them manage their feelings.

Health professionals can help patients to manage their feelings by:

- Acknowledgement of the problem: 'It will take you a bit of time to get used to your new face,' rather than 'you are lucky to be alive.'
- Legitimizing: 'It's okay to feel upset after a car accident.'
- Normalizing: 'Many children feel distressed if they are being bullied because of a craniofacial condition.'

Case study

Sandra attended a number of one to one sessions where she could talk freely about the impact of the cancer and her change in appearance without judgement.

> 'I felt so alone, it was so scary – I needed to share what I was going through with someone so badly.'

Her concerns were normalized and she was provided with positive encouragement. A trusting relationship was established.

She now contributes to a buddying system established in her maxillofacial unit to support patients going through similar interventions.

E: Exchanging

Patients and families should be offered the chance to connect with others going through similar experiences (not all will want to) through workshops or by connecting with a relevant support group. This enables them to gain mutual support.

Case study

Sandra was directed to Macmillan Cancer support and the hospital head and neck cancer support group. She also joined Changing Faces' User Council where she meets with other patients who 'have been there'.

S: Social skills training

Patients need to learn new skills for handling others' reactions to their looks and develop effective strategies to manage social situations, for example through self-help guides, workshops covering topics such as assertiveness or intimacy. One of the factors clearly identified as predictive of good outcome is the number and variety of positive non-avoidant coping strategies employed by the individual,[19] while social competence has been found to be one of the better predictors of adjustment.[20] Another study[21] showed that a high level of social skill can serve to overcome any potentially negative effects of disfigurement on social interactions.

Several studies have suggested that social skills are central to managing the impact of disfiguring injury or disease, and most importantly, that these skills can be learned.[22] Indeed *it is behaviour rather than disfigurement that predicts successful outcome in social situations;*[23] and providing individuals with the skills to deal with difficult social interactions is likely to be empowering.[24]

Recent research has demonstrated that large numbers of individuals with visible differences experience psychosocial disturbances and have reported a need for such (psychosocial) interventions to help them cope more effectively.[25]

Changing Faces suggests that all patients should be introduced to the idea of how to answer questions about their physical appearance *before* discharge home, and for *at least two years afterwards in out-patient appointments*. The aim here is to avoid the pattern of social avoidance which follows the fear of intrusive questions, comments and staring.

Teaching the patient how to assist in dressings introduces the idea of self-management in the immediate postoperative period. This one-to-one setting within the hospital environment can also be used to discuss the importance of developing basic conventional strategies, for example, answering questions about appearance.[26] Indeed, equipped with some key sentences, nurses are in a very good position to explore and identify some of the social difficulties and concerns encountered by their patients, particularly in community settings, following hospital discharge and during routine health monitoring.[27] For example:

- 'Do you feel that your medical condition affects your appearance?'
- 'How noticeable do you feel it is to other people?'

- 'How much does this worry you?'
- 'Is there anything that you don't do as a result of your concerns about your appearance?'
- 'Are there any particular strategies that you find helpful in coping with your concerns?'
- 'What do you say if someone asks you about your appearance?'

Two models developed by Changing Faces can help:

The Reach Out Model

This model developed by Changing Faces consists of a toolkit of communication strategies to prepare for social situations so as not to be caught off-guard and to enable the individual to take the initiative:

R Reassurance – putting someone at their ease
E Energy – creating interest in what they are saying
A Assertiveness – taking the initiative
C Courage – being strong and taking control
H Humour – introducing fun or a joke
O Over there! – distracting away from the scarring
U Understanding – being aware that seeing a reconstructed jaw can be difficult
T Tenacity – try again – use a different strategy if the first does not work.

3-2-1 Go! – How to prepare a patient with a disfigurement

Three things to do if someone stares at you:

- Look back and smile.
- Look back, smile and say, 'I'm sorry, do we know one another?' if staring persists.
- Ask them not to stare.

Two things to say if someone asks you what happened:
- 'I had surgery on my face but I'd rather not talk about it.'
- 'I was born with a rare syndrome but it doesn't hurt.'

One thing to think if someone appears to turn away:
- 'It's okay, they didn't mean any harm.'

> **Case study**
>
> Sandra was encouraged to develop a number of strategies to try out in order to deal with comments or questions about her face. The ones most favoured were:
>
> - Introducing a subject, use of a distraction technique 'over there' – 'what did you do last night?', 'what meeting are you off to?' – This line allows her to take control of the conversation.
> - Assertive/confident responses – 'can we talk about something else', 'I can think of more interesting things to talk about'. These responses help to redirect the conversation.
> - Having something to say – 'I had cancer. I'm on the mend now.'

The graded approach

Changing Faces recommends that a *graded approach* be adopted to help patients increase the number and variety of coping strategies with which they feel comfortable. This approach will enable patients to feel prepared and to develop strategies during controlled exposure, for example, on visits to the patient common room, taking meals with other patients, or on accompanied trips around the hospital.

At the very beginning of this gradual process, patients may feel they are only comfortable simply nodding to another person in acknowledgement, before they feel able to perhaps smile at them or say 'hello'. Practising these strategies within the safe environment of a hospital setting will help build up their confidence for when they encounter people for the first time.

Another example of the graded approach is the way in which patients might think about what they would like to say in response to others' questions about their appearance; beginning within the hospital setting, and then after their discharge from the ward. Here are four graded ways of responding to the question: 'What happened to your face?' beginning with minimum information, and graduating to a more interactive conversation.

Minimum information and close the subject:
'I had jaw surgery, but I'd rather not talk about it at the moment.'
Answer and change the subject:
'I was born with a syndrome … Are you new to this area?'
Potentially open up the topic:
'I have Apert's and I've recently had some excellent surgery.'
Use humour to break the ice:
'At least people don't forget me!'

Helping patients to experiment and experience these graded strategies and responses in a 'safe' one-to-one setting will encourage them to decide the type of response with which they feel comfortable, and will gradually build up their self-confidence to expand their repertoire.

It should be noted, however, that, depending on mood or circumstances at any particular time, a person with a disfigurement may not always wish to respond in the same way to questions about their appearance; neither should they feel obliged to do so. An individual can respond in a firm and assertive manner in these situations, without appearing rude.

The delivery of FACES in a healthcare setting

The psychosocial aspects of disfigurements, whether developmental dentofacial/craniofacial deformities or following reconstructive jaw surgery, are frequently a priority for patients which need to be recognized.

Table 61-1 Roles of the clinical team members in promoting access to psychosocial care

Tier	People and professionals	The role they should play
1.	The whole team (clinical and non-clinical staff)	Recognition of psychological needs (including privacy and boundaries)
2.	Professionals with additional expertise such as nurses, physiotherapists, occupational therapists and social workers.	Identifying and basic screening for psychological distress in all patients, and flagging up issues to Tier 3 specialists.
3.	Trained and accredited psychosocial professionals e.g. counsellors, assistant psychologists, community psychiatric nurses, Changing Faces Practitioners.	Assessing and diagnosis of all patients/families for psychological distress; management of basic psycho-pathology.
4.	Mental health specialists such as clinical psychologists, psychotherapists and psychiatrists.	Diagnosis and treatments of psychopathology; supervision of Tier 2 and 3 staff.
5.	Psychosocial Care Co-ordinators, such as consultant clinical psychologists or psychotherapists.	Management of psychosocial rehabilitation for the whole team.

The FACES model can be adapted to a clinical setting with delivery by the whole care team ranging from non-clinical staff to psychologists, therapists and Changing Faces Practitioners, depending on the severity of patient need.

Every member of the clinical team, its leadership and management has a role to play in promoting access to psychosocial care and interventions, overseen by a trained psychologist or similar (Table 61-1) (Box 61.1).

Box 61-1 How can healthcare professionals support patients as part of their treatment learning to live with a disfiguring condition?

Assess a patient's psychosocial needs:

- Social support
- Coping mechanisms
- Self-esteem
- Anxieties
- Attitude
- Your own attitudes and terminology

Give:

- Full information and advice – especially when there are a variety of treatment options.
- Hints and tips for dealing with comments, stares, unwanted attention.

Refer:

- To other professionals for emotional support/counselling as appropriate.
- To a trained skin camouflage practitioner to teach how to self-apply specialist cover creams.
- To patient/voluntary support networks or condition specific support groups.
- For social interaction skills training.

Examples of how to respond to your patients and what to say

1. **Acknowledgement of the problem**
   There are not necessarily immediate or even right answers to a patient's distress of concerns, but it is important not to dismiss or negate the problem:

   'It must be difficult for you.'
   Your change in appearance will take time to get used to,' rather than 'you are lucky to be alive.'

2. **Legitimizing**
   Patients often need reassurance that the feelings and anxieties that they are experiencing are real and valid:

   'It's OK to feel upset when you have been given a flap.'

3. **Normalizing**
   Patients need to be reassured that their emotional response is not out of the ordinary and generally not pathological. There is the risk that if this is not addressed then the 'elephant in the room' is reinforced.

   'Many people feel distressed losing part of their tongue.'

4. **Information**
   It is helpful to patients to explain about psychological change as well as physical change – both adults and children and young people.

   'You will need to learn how to manage other people's reactions to your different looking face.'

5. **Inclusion**
   Patients and families report how helpful it is to be included in decision making and the chance to talk to other survivors.

6. **Maintaining an empathetic yet professional relationship (e.g. non-regular contact)**
   Some phrases to help 'contain' the situation, making it more manageable for both you and your patient:

   'I can hear how upset you are. I wonder if you have thought about talking your feelings through with someone?'

   'It does sound as if you've been through a rough time lately. You know, it often helps to talk it through with someone.'

Make sure you have available some resources or information with which to guide your patient.

> **Case study**
>
> A member of the Changing Faces Young People's Council born with a craniofacial syndrome: 'I think those in need could benefit from support in building up to surgery and coming to terms with the results and how to get on with life. I feel strongly that it would be a useful service.'

References

1 Bradbury ET. Psychological issues in aesthetic surgery. Aesthet Plast Surg. 1994;18:301–5.
2 Dropkin MJ, Malgady RG, Scott DW, Oberst MT, Strong EW. Scaling of disfigurement and dysfunction in postoperative head and neck patients. Head Neck Surg. 1983;6:559–70.
3 Neilson KA, Pollard AC, Boonzaier AM, Corry J, Castle DJ, Mead KR, et al. Psychological distress (depression and anxiety) in people with head and neck cancers. Med J Aust. 2010;193:48–51.
4 Changing Faces. Face equality for patients with disfiguring conditions: How health and social care professionals can support and empower, 2009.
5 Coutinho W. Facing changes: Don't let the way I Look affect the way you see me. Changing Faces, London, 2006.
6 Goode A. Public attitudes survey. Summary of COG research's survey. Findings available on (www.changingfaces.org.uk). The face equality survey is available at (www.changingfaces.org.uk/face-equality/take-the-face-equality-survey), 2008.
7 All Party Parliamentary Group on Body Image and Central YMCA. Reflections on Body Image, 2012.
8 Changing Faces. Face equality for patients with disfiguring conditions: How health and social care professionals can support and empower, 2009.
9 Bradbury E. Psychological approaches to children and adolescents with disfigurement: a review of the literature. ACPP Rev Newslett. 1993;15:1–6.
10 Rumsey N, Harcourt D. Body image and disfigurement: issues and interventions. Body Image. 2004;1:83–97.
11 Kubler-Ross E. On Death and Dying. New York: Simon & Schuster, 1997.
12 Partridge J. Changing Faces: the Challenge of Facial Disfigurement. Penguin: London, 1990.
13 Egan K. A qualitative study of the experiences of people who identify themselves as having adjusted positively to a visible difference. J Health Psychol. 2011;16:739–49.
14 Rumsey N, Clarke A, White P. Exploring the psychosocial concerns of outpatients with disfiguring conditions. J Wound Care. 2003;12:247–52.
15 Cobb S. Social support as a moderator of life stress. Psychosomat Med. 1976;38:300–14.
16 Partridge J. Professional Reintegration of Burn Patients: Dream or Reality? Belgium, 1994.
17 Picker Institute. Information for People Living with Conditions that Affect their Appearance, 2007.
18 Dropkin MJ. Anxiety, coping strategies, and coping behaviours in patients undergoing head and neck cancer surgery. Cancer Nurs. 2001;24:143–8.
19 Clarke A. 'Psychosocial aspects of facial disfigurement; problems, management and the role of a patient-led organization'. Psychol Health Med. 1999;4:129–42.
20 Kapp-Simon K, Simon D, Kristovich S. Self-perception, social skills, adjustment and inhibition in young adolescents with craniofacial anomalies. Cleft Palate-Craniofac J. 1992;29:352–6.
21 Rumsey N, Bull R, Gahagan D. A preliminary study of the potential of social skills for improving the quality of social interaction for the facially disfigured. Soc Behav. 1986;1:143–5.
22 Robinson E, Rumsey N, Partridge J. An evaluation of the impact of social interaction skills training for facially disfigured people. Br J Plast Surg. 1996;49:281–9.
23 Clarke A. Psychosocial aspects of facial disfigurement; problems, management and the role of a patient-led organisation. Psychol Health Med. 1999;4:129–42.
24 Thompson A, Kent G. Adjusting to disfigurement: processes involved in dealing with being visibly different. Clin Psychol Rev. 2002;21:663–82.
25 Bessell A, Moss TP. Evaluating the effectiveness of psychosocial interventions for individuals with visible differences: A systematic review of the empirical literature. Body Image. 2007;4:227–38.
26 Clarke A Cooper C. Psychosocial rehabilitation after disfiguring injury or disease: investigating the training needs of specialist nurses. J Adv Nurs. 2001;33:1–9.
27 Rumsey N, Clarke A, Musa M. Altered body image: the psychosocial needs of patients. Br J Commun Nurs. 2002;7:563–6.

Index

Note: page numbers in *italics* refer to figures; those in **bold** to tables.

Orthognathic Surgery: Principles, Planning and Practice. Edited by Farhad B. Naini and Daljit S. Gill.